Textbook of Audiological Medicine

Textbook of Audiological Medicine

Clinical Aspects of Hearing and Balance

Edited by

Linda M Luxon BSc(Hons) MB BS(Hons) FRCP

Professor of Audiological Medicine, University College London (Institute of Child Health), University of London; and Consultant Physician in Neuro-otology, National Hospital for Neurology and Neurosurgery, Queen Square, London, UK

Co-edited by

Joseph M Furman MD PhD

Professor, Departments of Otolaryngology, Neurology, Bioengineering and Physical Therapy
University of Pittsburg, Eye and Ear Institute Building, Pittsburg PA, USA

Alessandro Martini MD

Professor of Audiology, Chairman of Otolaryngology & Audiology Department
Ferrara University, Ferrara, Italy

Dafydd Stephens FRCP

Consultant in Audiological Medicine
Welsh Hearing Institute, University Hospital of Wales, Cardiff, Wales

MD Martin Dunitz
Taylor & Francis Group

First published in the United Kingdom in 2003
by Martin Dunitz, an imprint of Taylor & Francis Group, 11 New Fetter Lane, London EC4P 4EE

Tel.: +44 (0) 20 7583 9855
Fax.: +44 (0) 20 7842 2298
E-mail: info@dunitz.co.uk
Website: http://www.dunitz.co.uk

A CIP record for this book is available from the British Library.

ISBN 1–90186–534–7

Distributed in the USA by
Fulfilment Center
Taylor & Francis
10650 Tobben Drive
Independence, KY 41051, USA
Toll Free Tel.: +1 800 634 7064
E-mail: taylorandfrancis@thomsonlearning.com

Distributed in Canada by
Taylor & Francis
74 Rolark Drive
Scarborough, Ontario M1R 4G2, Canada
Toll Free Tel.: +1 877 226 2237
E-mail: tal_fran@istar.ca

Distributed in the rest of the world by
Thomson Publishing Services
Cheriton House
North Way
Andover, Hampshire SP10 5BE, UK
Tel.: +44 (0)1264 332424
E-mail: salesorder.tandf@thomsonpublishingservices.co.uk

Typeset in Great Britain by J&L Composition
Printed and bound in Spain by Grafos SA

Contents

Contributors

Gerhard Andersson
Department of Psychology and
Department of Audiology
Uppsala University,
Box 12 25, SE–751 42 Uppsala, Sweden

Paul Avan
Laboratory of Sensory Biophysics (EA 2667)
School of Medicine
PO Box 38
63000 Clermont-Ferrand, France

Robert W Baloh
UCLA Neurology
Reed Neurological Research Center
710 Westwood Plaza, Rm C–246A
Los Angeles
CA 90095–1769, USA

Doris-Eva Bamiou
Neuro-otology Department
National Hospital for Neurology and Neurosurgery
Queen Square
London WC1N 3BG
UK

Jane A Baran
Department of Communication Disorders
6 Arnold House
School of Public Health and Health Sciences
University of Massachusetts
715 North Pleasant Street
Amherst MA 01003-9304, USA

Marie-Louise Barrenäs
The Sahlgrenska Akademy at Göteborg University
Institute for the Health of Women and Children
Göteborg Pediatric Growth Research Center
Department of Pediatrics
The Queen Silvia Children's Hospital
SE–416 85 Göteborg
Sweden

Pierre Bonfils
ENT Department and UMR CNRS 7060
European Hospital G. Pompidou
75015 Paris, France

An Boudewyns
Department of Otorhinolaryngology and
Head and Neck Surgery
University Hospital Antwerp
Wilrijkstraat 10
2650 Wilrijk (Antwerp)
Belgium

Thomas Brandt
Neurological University Clinic
Grosshadern Clinic
Marchioninistrasse 15
81377 Munich, Germany

Jan Brokx
Department of Otorhinolaryngology and
Head and Neck Surgery
University Hospital Antwerp
Wilrijkstraat 10
2650 Wilrijk (Antwerp)
Belgium
and *University Hospital Maastricht, The Netherlands*

Adolfo M Bronstein
Department of Neuro-otology
Division of Neuroscience and Psychological Medicine
Faculty of Medicine, Imperial College
Charing Cross Hospital
Fulham Palace Road,
London W6 8RF, UK

Stephen P Cass
University of Colorado Health Sciences Center
4200 E Ninth Avenue
Denver CO 80262, USA

Jan W Casselman
Department of Medical Imaging—MRI
A.Z. ST. Jan Brugge A.V.
Brugge, Belgium

Borka Ceranic
Department of Neuro-otology
The National Hospital for Neurology & Neurosurgery
Queen Square
London WC1N 3BG, UK

Jos Claes
Department of Otorhinolaryngology and
Head and Neck Surgery
University Hospital Antwerp
Wilrijkstraat 10
2650 Wilrijk (Antwerp)
Belgium

Graeme M Clark
The Human Communication Research Centre
and Department Of Otolaryngology
384–388 Albert Street
East Melbourne
VIC 3002, Australia

Bernard Cohen
Department of Neurology, Box 1135
Mount Sinai School of Medicine
1 East 100th Street
New York NY 10029–6574, USA

Phillip D Cremer
Neurology Department
Royal Prince Alfred Hospital,
Camperdown, NSW 2050
Sydney, Australia

Ian S Curthoys
School of Psychology
University of Sydney, NSW 2006
Sydney, Australia

Rosalyn A Davies
Department of Neuro-otology
The National Hospital for Neurology & Neurosurgery
Queen Square
London WC1N 3BG, UK

Adrian C Davis
MRC Institute of Hearing Research
University Park
Nottingham NG7 2RD, UK

Frank Declau
Department of Otorhinolaryngology and
Head and Neck Surgery
University Hospital Antwerp
Wilrijkstraat 10
2650 Wilrijk (Antwerp)
Belgium

Dirk De Ridder
Department of Otorhinolaryngology and
Head and Neck Surgery
University Hospital Antwerp
Wilrijkstraat 10
2650 Wilrijk (Antwerp)
Belgium

Joanna Downton
St Thomas's Hospital
Shaw Heath
Stockport SK3 8BL, UK

Soly Erlandsson
Department of Audiology
Sahlgrenska Academy
University,
SE 405 30 Göteborg, Sweden

Edward F Evans
MacKay Institute of Communication and Neuroscience
Keele University
Keele ST5 5BG, Staffordshire UK

Andrew Faulkner
Department Phonetics and Linguistics
UCL (University College London)
Gower Street,
London WC1E 6BT, UK

Joseph M Furman
Eye and Ear Institute Building
Suite 500
203 Lothrop Street
Pittsburgh PA 15213, USA

Stuart Gatehouse
MRC Institute of Hearing Research
Royal Infirmary
16 Alexandra Parade
Glasgow G31 2ER, UK

Martin Gizzi
New Jersey Neuroscience Institute
Seton Hall University
65 James Street
Edison, NJ 08818, USA

Joseph W Hall
Division of Otolaryngology
University of North Carolina at Chapel Hill
Chapel Hill NC 27599., USA

G Michael Halmagyi
Neurology Department
Royal Prince Alfred Hospital,
Camperdown, NSW 2050
Sydney, Australia

Erwin Hamans
Department of Otorhinolaryngology and
Head and Neck Surgery
University Hospital Antwerp
Wilrijkstraat 10
2650 Wilrijk (Antwerp)
Belgium

Ronald Hinchcliffe
Institute of Laryngology and Otology
330 Grays Inn Road
London WC1X 8EE, UK

Kajsa-Mia Holgers
Tinnitus Team
Department of Audiology
Sahlgrenska University Hospital/Sahlgrenska
SE–413 45 Göteborg
Sweden

Michael J Holmes
Lycoming College
Department of Psychology
700 College Place
Campus Box 1
Williamsport, PA 17701, USA

Rolf G Jacob
Department of Psychiatry
Thomas Detre Hall of the Western Psychiatric Institute and Clinic
University of Pittsburgh
3811 O'Hara Street
Pittsburgh PA 15213, USA

Brian J Jian
University of Pittsburgh
School of Medicine
Department of Otolaryngology
Eye & Ear Institute Building
203 Lothrop Street, Room 113
Pittsburgh, PA 15213, USA

Christopher Kennard
Division of Neuroscience & Psychological Medicine
Charing Cross Campus
Faculty of Medicine
Imperial College of Science, Technology and Medicine
Fulham Palace Road, London W6 8RF
London, UK

Rose Anne Kenny
Department of Geriatric Medicine
Royal Victoria Infirmary
Newcastle upon Tyne NE1 4LP, UK

Ilan A Kerman
University of Michigan
Mental Health Research Institute
Department of Psychiatry
205 Zina Pitcher Place
Ann Arbor, MI 48109, USA

Herman Kingma
Maastricht Research Institute Brain and Behaviour
and *Department of ORL and Head and Neck Surgery*
University Hospital Maastricht
P. Debyelaan 25
6229 HX Maastricht
PO Box 5800
6202 AZ Maastricht, The Netherlands

Erwin Koekelkoren
Department of Neurosurgery
University Hospital Antwerp
Wilrijkstraat 10
2650 Wilrijk (Antwerp)
Belgium

Izumi Koizuka
Department of Otolaryngology
St Marianna University School of Medicine
Kanagawa, Japan

Mireille Lavigne-Rebillard
INSERM
University Montpellier 1
71, rue de Navacelles
34090 Montpellier, France

Harold Ludman
Neuro-otology,
National Hospital for Neurology & Neurosurgery
Queen Square
London WC1N 3BG, UK

Linda M Luxon
Audiology
Old Building
Great Ormond Street Hospital
London WC1N 3JH, UK

Brian Maki
University of Toronto
and *Sunnybrook and Women's College*
Health Sciences Centre
Centre for Studies in Aging
2075 Bayview Avenue
Toronto, Ontario
CANADA M4N 3M5

Robert Marchbanks
NIPA Unit
Mail Point 29
Medical Physics Department
Southampton General Hospital
Tremona Road
Southampton SO16 6YD, UK

Alessandro Martini
Clinical Institute ORL
Faculty of Medicine and Surgery
University of Ferrara
Corso Giovecca 203
44100 Ferrara, Italy

William E McIlroy
Department of Physical Therapy
University of Toronto
256 McCaul Street
Toronto ON M5T 1W5, Ontario, Canada

Laurence McKenna
Audiology Centre
Royal National Throat Nose and Ear Hospital
330 Grays Inn Road
London WC1X 8DA, UK

Leslie Michaels
Department of Histopathology
Royal Free and UCL Medical School
University Street
London WC1E 6JJ, UK

Claes Möller
Department of Audiology
Sahlgrenska University Hospital
41345 Göteborg, Sweden

Beth Morchower Douek
Programme of Communication Sciences and Disorders
Callier Center for Communication Disorders
University of Texas at Dallas
1966 Inwood Road
Dallas TX 75235, USA

Padma Moorjani
MRC Institute of Hearing Research
University Park
Nottingham NG7 2RD, UK

Frank E Musiek
Department of Communications Sciences
University of Connecticut
Connecticut, Storrs CT 06269, USA

Valerie Newton
Human Communication and Deafness,
Humanities Building
University of Manchester
Oxford Road
Manchester M13 9PL, UK

Cliodna OMahoney
Northern Area Health Board
Community Care Area 7
161 Richmond Road
Dublin 3, Eire

Victoria B Oxholm
Section of Otolaryngology and Audiology
Dartmouth-Hitchcock Medical Center
One Medical Center Drive
Lebanon NH 03756–0001, USA

Agnete Parving
Department of Audiology
H:S. Bispebjerg Hospital
Bispebjerg Bakke 23
2400 CPH.NV.
Denmark

Tim Petterson
Department of Geriatric Medicine
Royal Victoria Infirmary
Newcastle upon Tyne NE1 4LP, UK

Hillel Pratt
Evoked Potentials Laboratory
Behavioral Biology
Technion—Israel Institute of Technology, Israel

Silvano Prosser
Clinical Institute ORL
Faculty of Medicine and Surgery
University of Ferrara
Corso Giovecca 203
44100 Ferrara, Italy

Rémy Pujol
INSERM
University Montpellier 1
71, rue de Navacelles
34090 Montpellier, France

Ilmari Pyykkö
Tampere University Hospital
P.O. Box 2000
33521 Tampere
Finland

Ewa Raglan
Audiology Department
Old Building
Great Ormond Street Hospital
London WC1N 3JH

Andrew P Read
Department of Medical Genetics
St Mary's Hospital
Hathersage Road
Manchester M13 0JH

Ulf Rosenhall
Hörselkliniken
Karolinska sjukhuset
171 76 Stockholm, Sweden

Francesco Scaravilli
Department of Neuropathology
Institute of Neurology
The National Hospital
Queen Square
London, UK

Jukka Starck
Department of Physics
Finnish Institute of Occupational Health
Topeliuksenkatu 41
00250 Helsinki
Finland

Dafydd Stephens
Welsh Hearing Institute
University Hospital of Wales
Cardiff CF14 4XW
Wales

John Stevens
Departments of Medical Physics and Clinical Engineering
and North Trent Medical Audiology
Sheffield Teaching Hospitals, Sheffield, UK

Emily A Tobey
Advanced Hearing Research Center
Callier Center for Communication Disorders
University of Texas at Dallas
1966 Inwood Road
Dallas TX 75235, USA

Esko Toppila
Department of Physics
Finnish Institute of Occupationa Health
Topeliuksenkatu 41
00250 Helsinki
Finland

Richard S Tyler
University of Iowa Hospitals and Clinics
Department of Otolaryngology-Head & Neck Surgery
21256 PFP
200 Hawkins Drive
Iowa City, IA 52242, USA

Mats Ulfendahl
Laboratory Bldg M1—ENT
Karolinska Hospital
SE–171 76 Stockholm, Sweden

Guy Van Camp
Department of Medical Genetics
University of Antwerp
Universiteitsplein 1
2610 Antwerp, Belgium

Paul Van de Heyning
Department of Otorhinolaryngology and
Head and Neck Surgery
University Hospital Antwerp
Wilrijkstraat 10
2650 Wilrijk (Antwerp)
Belgium

Karl R White
2810 Old Main Hill
Utah State University
Logan, UT 84322, USA

Floris L Wuyts
Department of Otorhinolaryngology and
Head and Neck Surgery
University Hospital Antwerp
Wilrijkstraat 10
2650 Wilrijk (Antwerp)
Belgium

Bill Yates
University of Pittsburgh
School of Medicine
Department of Otolaryngology
Eye & Ear Institute Building
203 Lothrop Street, Room 106
Pittsburgh, PA 15213, USA

Yoshior Yazawa
Department of Otolaryngolgy and Head and Neck Surgery
Shiga Medical University, 520–2192 / Seta Tsukinowa-cho
Otsu City, Shiga, Japan

Tai-June Yoo
Molecular Sciences and Neurosciences Program
Allergy and Immunology Division
University of Tennessee,
Knoxville, 37996 TN, USA

Foreword

It is a joy for academic and personal reasons to support the publication of *Textbook of Audiological Medicine*. The contemporary avalanche of medical information is extending the boundaries in every area of medical specialization, not least in audiological medicine. Sophisticated new methods have enabled the acquisition of important basic and clinical information that provides us with the extended capacity for understanding the pathophysiology of auditory and vestibular disorders. Often, though, the diversity of sources and the time required to obtain these extensive new data limit the access of the practitioner to new treatments.

This book is a courageous attempt to define what is valuable and necessary in these areas for the diagnosis and management of a variety of audiological and vestibular disorders. *Textbook of Audiological Medicine* will fill a critical need for information about recent discoveries that can significantly improve the management of patients. Given the fragmentation in the sources of knowledge, the book should be welcomed by scientists and clinicians alike since it will contribute to a more integrated exposition of these medical problems. In addition, the material in it reinforces the need to proceed in the search of newer horizons in the alleviation of the suffering associated with inner ear disorders.

From a personal point of view and with a sense, perhaps undeserved, of personal pride for the limited but memorable interaction I had with them, first as students and now as colleagues, I wish to wholeheartedly congratulate the editors for their efforts.

Vicente Honrubia
UCLA School of Medicine
USA

Acknowledgments

My deepest thanks are due to Professor Ronald Hinchcliffe who first raised the need for a textbook in the specialty of audiological medicine and has been fundamental in providing the enthusiasm, support and guidance throughout the production of this book. My thanks are also due to Dr Ewa Raglan, my longstanding consultant colleague, who has repeatedly and unstintingly provided academic and practical support, enabling me to devote myself more fully to the editing of the textbook.

I should also like to thank in particular Professor S Dafydd G Stephens, Dr Robert W Baloh and Dr Vicente Honrubia, who unknowingly engendered my enthusiasm and interest in auditory and vestibular disorders, resulting in the motivation to undertake this task. Many others have read and advised on parts of the text, and I am most grateful to them. They include Joe Furman and Alessandro Martini, who have been excellent co-editors, bringing a balanced and different perspective in a number of areas. Finally, Abi Griffin, Senior Production Editor at Martin Dunitz Ltd, who has provided unfailing support and goodwill over the last year of production; and the final result would not have been achieved without the constant support of my secretary, Lesley Gibson.

Much of my free time has been devoted to the editing of the book, and I particularly thank my children, Rupert, Cordelia, Clementine and Christianna for their continual patience, encouragement and love.

I would finally like to dedicate my effort to my dear parents and brother for their unending support.

Linda Luxon
Editor

Preface

Audiological medicine is a relatively new specialty spanning the investigation, diagnosis and medical management of hearing and balance disorders. In some centres, communication disorders, particularly in children, are also included within the clinical framework. Medical science is expanding at an ever-increasing rate, and it becomes increasingly difficult to produce a comprehensive overview of even a single subject, let alone two quite disparate clinical disciplines, such as hearing and balance, albeit linked by similarities of anatomy and physiology and inter-related pathologically. Moreover, the practice of audiological medicine depends not only upon a clear understanding of the basic sciences relevant to auditory and vestibular function, but also upon experience and knowledge in a wide range of clinical disciplines relevant to hearing and balance disorders, including genetics, immunology, paediatrics, geriatrics, neurology, otolaryngology, ophthalmology, psychiatry and general internal medicine. Thus, far from being a narrow topic as might be assumed by those unfamiliar with the subject, audiological medicine is a specialty spanning the depth and breadth of medicine.

Hearing impairment is reported by the WHO as the commonest sensory disability worldwide, yet tragically much of the resultant disablement could be prevented by vaccination programmes in the Third World, noise prevention measures and regulation of the prescription of ototoxic drugs. Equally, balance disorders have a significant economic and social morbidity. In the UK, one in four of the population of working age reports dizziness, causing some limitation in function, and it is well recognized as the second commonest symptom preventing attendance at work. Moreover, between one third and one half of the entire population have experienced some symptoms of disequilibrium by the age of 60 years.

The growth of audiological medicine as a separate medical discipline has been prompted, in part, by necessity based on these epidemiological data and in part by other factors: the decline in middle ear surgery, associated with improved public health in the developed world; developments in pathophysiology and pharmacology, leading to the possibility of medical intervention for sensorineural hearing loss; the explosion of genetics and the possibility of gene therapy; technological developments, e.g. otoacoustic emissions leading to universal neonatal screening and the earlier identification of hearing impairment and cochlear implantation, requiring sophisticated, multidisciplinary rehabilitation programmes. In the context of vestibular diseases, the understanding of the interaction of autonomic and psychological factors in both the development and the treatment of balance disorders and the lack of good evidence to support the value of surgical intervention in the majority of balance disorders and the efficacy of vestibular rehabilitation programmes have lent support to specialist care.

Fundamental to the need for this book has been the longstanding and widespread, cursory and dismissive approach to hearing and balance disorders both by the public and the professions. Frequently, hearing impairment has been felt to require no more than the provision of a hearing aid, with little understanding of the need for thorough aetiological investigation to ensure prevention and remediation where possible and dedicated, structured rehabilitation programmes, if the devastating personal and social consequences of hearing impairment are to be avoided. In addition, dizzy patients are frequently considered as 'heart sink' problems and passed backwards and forwards between specialists, with no clear diagnosis, no rational management and a gloomy prognosis.

This volume aims to integrate the science and medicine of auditory and vestibular disorders, providing the first comprehensive *Textbook of Audiological Medicine*. This title has been written by authors from a wide range of disciplines, but each is authoritative in his/her field. The chapters have been scrutinized, modified and integrated by the editors, in order to produce a volume which, it is hoped, will be of value to the expert in the field, but which can be negotiated by the novice to provide the necessary scientific background, while emphasizing the relevant clinical aspects of each subject. There are five main sections, the first dealing with areas of common knowledge to both the auditory and vestibular systems, and then each system is considered in terms of the relevant basic sciences and clinical disorders.

Thus, the *raison d'être* for this textbook is to provide clinicians with the armamentarium necessary to improve the quality of care for these large groups of patients with personally distressing symptoms. We hope that the new and expanding band of physicians and paediatricians practising audiological medicine will find this book of value, not only during their training, but also in their professional careers, as a text to dip into for information related to all aspects of the subject. Equally we hope that the text provides a comprehensive introduction to auditory and vestibular disorders that will be of value to both doctors and scientists in many differing disciplines, who work with and for hearing and balance disordered patients.

Linda Luxon
Editor
Joseph Furman, Alessandro Martini and Dafydd Stephens
Co-Editors

Section I

Fundamentals of audiological and vestibular medicine

1 Anatomy of peripheral auditory and vestibular systems

Paul Avan, Pierre Bonfils

The temporal bone is made of three portions of different embryological origins, namely the squamous, tympanic and petrous portions. This last portion is of particular interest in this chapter, since it contains the cochleovestibular sensory organs. The petrous bone is a part of the base of the skull, made of compact bone, with a pyramidal or roughly triangular external shape. It is hollowed out by several cavities, facial and carotid canals, petrous pneumatic cells, and cochleovestibular cavities. The cochlea corresponds to the anterior part of these cavities, and it is devoted to the auditory perception of sound at frequencies ranging from 20–20 000 Hz in humans. The vestibule, situated posterior to the cochlea, responds to the effects of acceleration, either in static (gravity) or dynamic conditions (movement at varying linear or angular velocity). In this chapter, the anatomy of the cochlea and vestibule will be presented in two separate parts.

Auditory system

The peripheral auditory system consists of a complex arrangement of many different structures ensuring the conduction of acoustical vibrations from the external air to the liquids of the inner ear, and to the sensory cells, and then the transduction of sound into electrical messages. These messages are transmitted as action potentials by the auditory nerve fibres towards more central parts of the brain. The first stages of sound processing provide for impedance adaptation and pressure gain through the passive transformer system of the middle ear. Another key stage takes place in the cochlea before the occurrence of transduction processes: following the physicist Gold[1] and his theoretical suggestions, Davis[2] coined the term 'cochlear amplifier' to describe the effect resulting from the mechanical feedback of the active, electromotile outer hair cells (OHCs) on the cochlear partition. The cochlear feedback loop not only enables a high sensitivity to be obtained, but also results in an exquisite filtering of incoming stimuli. The macroscopic and microscopic (i.e. cellular, subcellular and molecular) structures involved in these complex processes have been more and more thoroughly identified, and the relationships between structure, function and physiopathology can no longer be dissociated. Thus this chapter will endeavour to emphasize the most significant functional consequences of the anatomy of the peripheral auditory system.

The description of the peripheral auditory system is classically divided into three parts, external, middle and inner ear, the first two corresponding to structures devoted to transmitting vibrations from a low-impedance gaseous medium to a high-impedance liquid one. Direct coupling between air and inner ear fluids would allow only 1/1000 of the incoming acoustical energy to be transmitted. Actually, sound transmission through a normal middle ear allows about half of this energy to reach the inner ear liquids.

External ear

The external ear consists of the pinna and external auditory meatus, up to the external border of the tympanic membrane. The human pinna is composed of cartilage. The external auditory meatus forms a canal about 25 mm deep; at its external orifice, its diameter is about 8–10 mm, decreases to 5–6 mm in the deeper portions, and enlarges again when reaching the tympanic membrane. The outer third of the canal has a cartilaginous wall, which is prolonged by a bony portion leading to the tympanic membrane. The cartilaginous portion contains numerous cerumen glands and hair follicles with a cleaning role, although an excessive accumulation may lead to a conductive hearing loss.

The role of the external ear is limited in humans, because the pinna is motionless, its muscles being largely ineffective.

However, the frequency spectrum of sounds reaching the tympanic membrane is significantly influenced by the combined transfer functions of the pinna and external ear canal. As a whole, this system presents a resonance peak of about 10–15 dB around 3 kHz. This resonance is partly responsible for the frequency-dependent sensitivity of the inner ear to noise-induced hearing loss. It also has to be taken into account when fitting a hearing aid.

The external auditory canal is S-shaped, initially running in an anterior direction, with its medial part running in a posterior direction. For otoscopy to be carried out properly, the bend of the canal has to be straightened as much as possible by gently pulling the pinna upwards and backwards. This manoeuvre allows the observer to see the part of the tympanic membrane at the bottom of the external auditory canal (Figure 1.1).

Tympanic membrane

The tympanic membrane is a translucent membrane, about 0.6 mm thick. It forms an angle of about 45° with the axis of the ear canal and its overall shape is conical, with the deepest point or umbo being attached to the tip of the manubrium of the malleus (Figure 1.1). The fibrocartilaginous peripheral ring of the tympanic membrane, inserted into the temporal bone, is roughly circular in shape (diameter 8–10 mm). The tympanic membrane is composed of three layers, namely an outer layer of keratinized epithelium prolonging that of the ear canal, an inner layer prolonging the middle ear mucosa, and a fibrous intermediate layer called the lamina propria. The lamina propria is made up of a complex arrangement of circular fibres, and radial fibres attached to the manubrium of the malleus.

The peripheral ring has a defect in its superior part, so that the tympanic membrane tends to fold at this level and extends toward the short process of the malleus (Figures 1.1 and 1.2). The part of the tympanic membrane above this limit is called the pars flaccida, whereas the largest, inferior part is called the pars tensa. The area of the pars tensa is about 30 times that of the pars flaccida in humans. The two names refer in an obvious manner to the respective stiffnesses of the membrane. The rigid lamina propria being absent in the pars flaccida, it can more easily bulge inside the tympanic cavity whenever the pressure in this cavity is not properly regulated as a result of auditory tube dysfunction (Figure 1.2). It is thought that such a mechanism is relevant to cholesteatoma generation.

Middle ear

The middle ear includes the tympanic cavity, connected to the mastoid air cells, and to the pharyngeal spaces by the auditory (Eustachian) tube. The sporadic openings of the auditory tube, either occurring spontaneously or triggered by muscular activity, e.g. due to swallowing, enable the static air pressure in the cavity to be kept close to atmospheric pressure. The tympanic cavity contains the ossicular chain (malleus, incus and stapes,

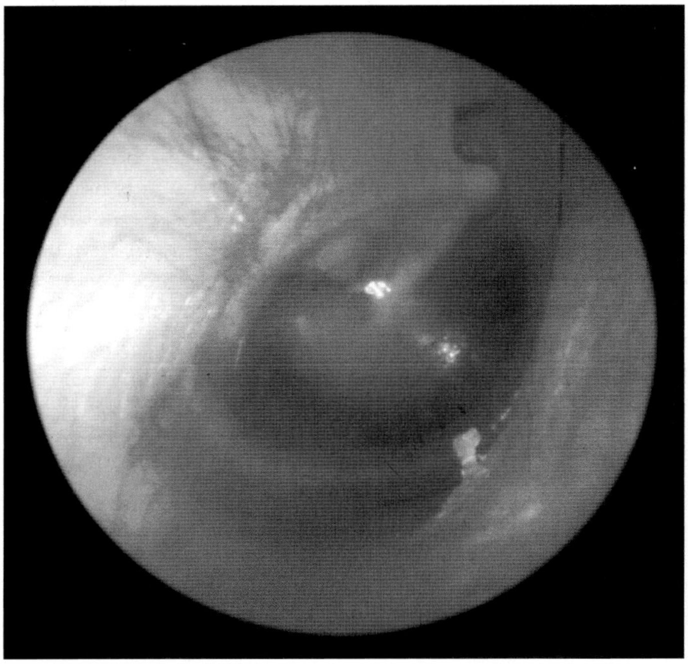

Figure 1.1 Normal tympanic membrane as seen by otoscopy. The malleus is visible through the translucent membrane. The pars flaccida corresponds to the upper part of the membrane. The bright triangle in the anteroinferior part of the tympanic membrane, starting from the umbo, is due to reflection of light on the pars tensa.

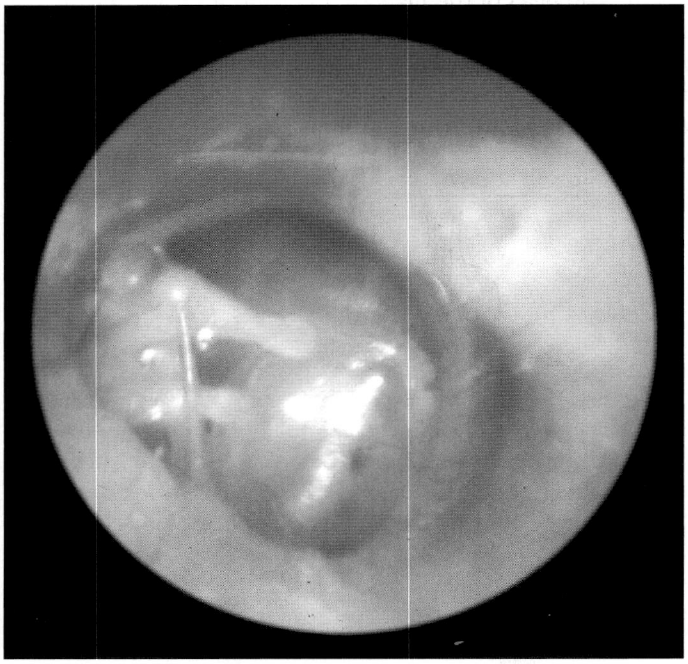

Figure 1.2 As a sequela of otitis media, the whole tympanic membrane has become retracted, so that the ossicles are moulded and clearly visible.

suspended by supporting ligaments), allowing the vibrations of the tympanic membrane to be transmitted to the inner ear fluids (Figure 1.3).

The tympanic cavity presents six faces around a central cavity in front of the tympanic membrane, the mesotympanum. This central cavity is prolonged in its superior part by the attic or epitympanum, containing the heads of two ossicles, the malleus and incus. The attic also has a close relationship with the pars flaccida of the tympanic membrane and is the usual starting place for cholesteatoma development. The floor of the tympanic cavity corresponds to the jugular bulb and the carotid artery, its anterior wall to the opening of the auditory tube, its posterior wall to the mastoid cell system, and its outer wall to the tympanic membrane. On the inner, labyrinthine wall separating the middle from the inner ear, several features can be identified, namely the promontory corresponding to the bulk of the first cochlear turn, the canals of the facial nerve and tensor tympani muscle, together with the round and oval windows. Finally, it must be borne in mind that the superior and posterior walls of the tympanic cavity have close relationships with several brain structures such as the posterior fossa and cerebellum, so that any defect in these walls due to prolonged middle ear infection can have dangerous consequences.

The three ossicles are articulated so as to make possible the transmission of sound from the tympanic membrane to the oval window. The malleus consists of a manubrium and a head. The tip of the manubrium corresponds to the umbo, and the manubrium is attached to the tympanic membrane along its length. The head of the malleus is suspended in the epitympanum by ligaments. The tensor tympani muscle is inserted on the manubrium just below the neck corresponding to the boundary between manubrium and head. The head of the malleus articulates with the incus in its posterior part. A short and a long process emerge from the body of the incus. The short process is oriented posteriorly toward the aditus ad antrum at the entrance of the mastoid air cells, while the long process is oriented downwards, then bends inwards at right angle and terminates in the lenticular process. The lenticular process articulates with the head of the stapes. The overall shape of the stapes resembles a stirrup, with two branches forming an osseous arch and a footplate inserted in the oval or vestibular window. The stapedius muscle attaches to the head of the stapes, and the annular ligament closes the footplate insertion in the oval window.

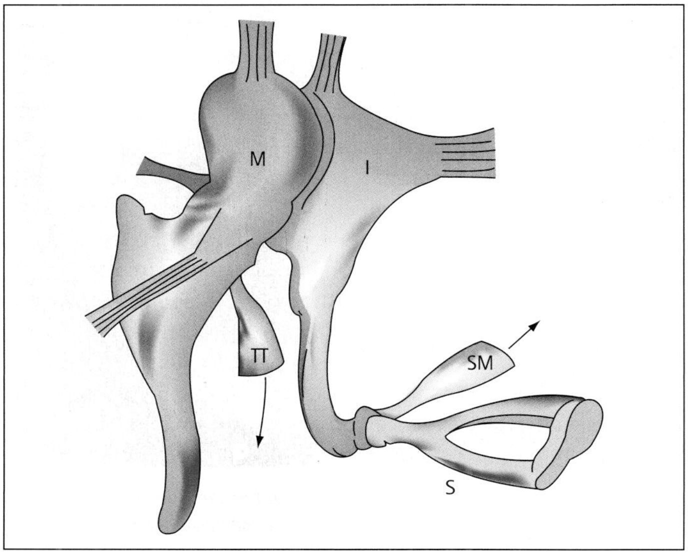

Figure 1.3 Ossicular chain (M, malleus; I, incus; S, stapes), muscles (arrow. TT, tensor tympani muscle; SM, stapedius muscle) and ligaments.

The middle ear acts as a transformer between the low-impedance air and the high-impedance fluid-filled cochlea. A simple physical model allowing for the surface ratio of the tympanic membrane to the stapes footplate, and the lever effect due to the difference in length of the manubrium of the malleus and the long process of the incus, predicts a flat pressure gain of 25–30 dB. Actually, the combined effects of the acoustical properties of the head and external and middle ear have to be taken into account to determine more accurately the input pressure level in the cochlea, from a given free-field stimulus level. The real transfer function is a little more complex than that predicted from the simple transformer model and is flat only in the mid-frequency range.[3] This issue is important, because it is thought that the external + middle ear transfer function fully accounts for the frequency range of human hearing, whereas the cochlear response would be basically frequency-independent.

Two striated muscles are located in the middle ear. The tensor tympani attaches to the malleus, and is innervated by a branch of the trigeminal nerve. The stapedius muscle attaches to the head of the stapes and is innervated by a branch of the facial nerve. In spite of their very small size, they have a surprisingly rich innervation, e.g. about 1000 nerve fibres for the stapedius.[4] The physiological role of these muscles is not fully understood. Their reflex contractions obviously lead to an increased stiffness of the ossicular chain, which tends to decrease the sound energy transmitted to the inner ear at low frequencies. In most natural situations of sound-induced contractions, only the stapedius muscle is active in humans and the resulting attenuation is only a few decibels; furthermore, its onset has a delay and it is ineffective at frequencies above 1 kHz. Vocalization seems to induce stronger contractions of both muscles. Middle ear muscle activity might contribute to some protection of the inner ear against excessive stimulation, a decrease of low-frequency masking, and an enhancement of signal-to-noise ratio for speech-like sounds.[5] Alternatively, it has been suggested quite recently that, as middle ear muscle contractions induce sharp intermittent movements of the stapes, they might thereby contribute to the long-term regulation of inner ear fluid pressure by forcing endolymph to flow to or from the endolymphatic sac.[6]

Cochlea

The cochlea is a bony tube, coiled around a central axis, the modiolus, thereby forming a spiral of two and a half turns in humans. The bony cochlea is connected to the vestibule through a wide orifice, and then leaves the vestibule to form the basal turn. The tube has a total length of about 30 mm. Its internal diameter tapers from 2 mm at the window level, to about 1 mm at the apical end. The overall size of the coiled cochlea also decreases from the basal turn (about 10 mm in diameter) to the apical one.

The cochlea is divided by the anterior membranous labyrinth into three compartments or scalae, the scala vestibuli, scala tympani and scala media (Figure 1.4). The scala media is bounded by the osseous spiral lamina projecting from the modiolus and prolonged externally by the basilar membrane, by Reissner's membrane and by the lateral wall. Its cross-section is thus approximately triangular. The basilar membrane, extending from the spiral lamina to the spiral ligament, supports the organ of Corti (Figure 1.4) containing the sensory cells. The lateral wall is lined by the spiral ligament and the heavily vascularized stria vascularis.

The scala vestibuli is above the scala media, bounded by Reissner's membrane. The oval window, closed by the stapes footplate and annular ligament, opens into the vestibule, connected to the scala vestibuli by the fenestra vestibuli. Therefore, stapes movements directly result in pressure variations in scala vestibuli.

The scala tympani is below the scala media, bounded by the basilar membrane. The round window opens into the scala tympani at the beginning of the basal turn. It is separated from the gaseous middle ear cavity by the round window membrane. On the apical side of the cochlea, since the scala media is shorter than the cochlear tube, a small opening called the helicotrema connects the scala vestibuli and tympani.

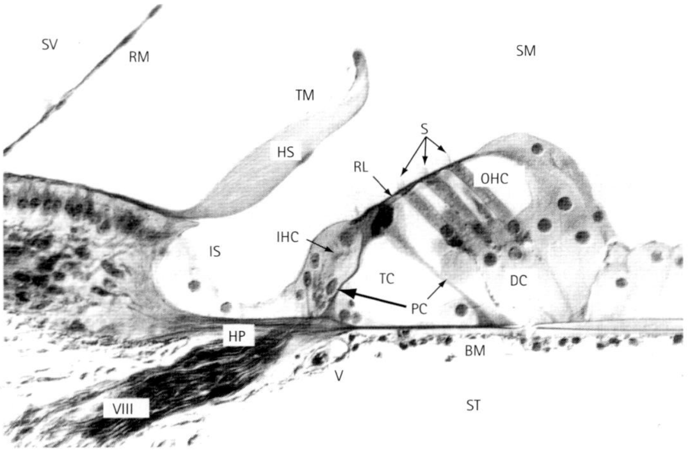

Figure 1.4 Transverse section of the organ of Corti of a guinea pig (optical microscopy). OSL, osseous spiral lamina; BM, basilar membrane; TM, tectorial membrane; HS, Hensen's stria; RM, Reissner's membrane; IS, inner sulcus; IHC, inner hair cell; OHC, outer hair cells; S, stereocilia; RL, reticular lamina; VIII, cochlear nerve fibres; TC, tunnel of Corti; PC, pillar cells; DC, Deiter's cells; ST, scala tympani; SM, scala media; SV, scala vestibuli; V, spiral vessels; HP, habenula perforata. (Courtesy of Dr Marc Lenoir, INSERM 254, Montpellier, France.)

The scala media is filled with a few microlitres of endolymph, which has a high K^+ concentration of about 150 mM, and a low Na^+ concentration (1 mM). Owing to the function of the stria vascularis, a large positive DC endocochlear potential can be measured in the cochlea: 80–90 mV. The scalae vestibuli and tympani contain perilymph, an extracellular-like fluid with a low K^+ concentration and a high Na^+ concentration (respectively about 4 and 140 mM). As these two scalae are connected through the helicotrema, there is little difference between their ionic contents. The DC resting potential in perilymph is 0 mV.

The organ of Corti, first described thoroughly by Alfonso Corti in 1851, rests on the basilar membrane and osseous spiral lamina (Figure 1.4). The basilar membrane is made up of fibres embedded in extracellular amorphous substance. Two zones are separated, the pars tecta or arcuate zone extending from the spiral lamina, and the pars pectinata or pectinate zone reaching the spiral ligament. The structure of the basilar membrane is responsible for the passive resonant properties of the cochlea, i.e. of the residual post-mortem frequency tuning first described by von Békésy. The mechanical properties of the basilar membrane, and particularly its stiffness, vary gradually from base to apex and, as a result, its resonance frequency decreases while the distance from the round window increases (with a rate of about one octave every 3 mm). This progressive decrease is mainly due to two geometrical factors: in a basoapical direction, the width of the membrane from the osseous spiral lamina to the spiral ligament increases from about 0.12 mm at the base to about 0.5 mm at the apex, while its thickness decreases by a similar amount.

The major components of the organ of Corti are the inner and outer hair cells (Figures 1.4 and 1.5), resting on the basilar membrane, surrounded by supporting cells (particularly pillar cells, Deiter's cells, Hensen cells and Claudius cells). The tops of sensory cells bathe in endolymph and are covered by a flap of gelatinous substance called the tectorial membrane. The apical parts of the inner and outer hair cells and the supporting cells form the reticular lamina (Figure 1.6). Its cell junctions are tight, and thus, the reticular lamina acts as an ionic barrier between the endolymph and the perilymph. Conversely, perilymph can diffuse through the basilar membrane. Thus a perilymph-like fluid bathes the cell bodies of sensory and support cells.

Aligned with the length of the cochlea from base to apex, one row of inner hair cells (IHCs) and about three parallel rows of OHCs can be found. Close to the apex, the rows of OHCs are less strictly aligned and supernumerary cells or additional rows are often found, especially in primates. The overall number of IHCs is around 3500 in humans, whereas about 12 000 OHCs are found. Both types of cells have apical 'stereocilia' bundles (Figures 1.6 and 1.7). Rather than being true cilia made of tubulin, the stereocilia are microvilli, made of actin filaments inserted into the cuticular plate. They vary in height, particularly those of OHCs, as a function of distance to the oval window.

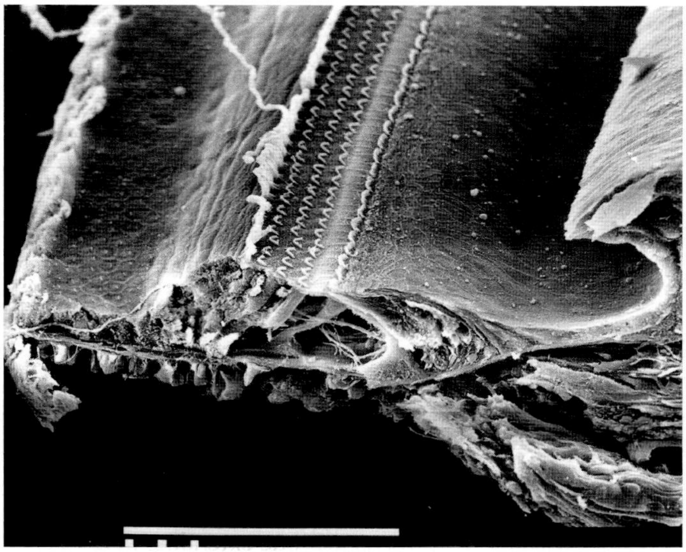

Figure 1.5 Organ of Corti of a guinea pig cochlea, seen from above with scanning electron microscopy. The tectorial membrane, attached to the top of supporting cells, has been removed, thereby uncovering the reticular lamina and the rows of outer and inner hair cells. (Courtesy of Dr Marc Lenoir, INSERM 254, Montpellier, France.)

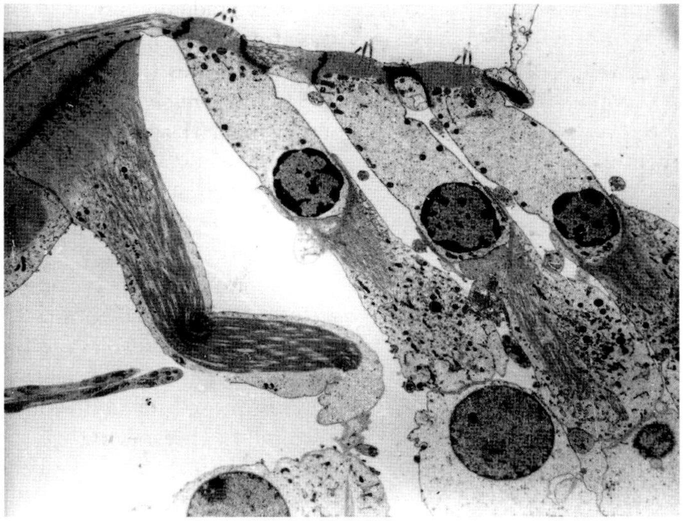

Figure 1.6 Section of the OHC region of the organ of Corti in transmission electron microscopy. Three cylindrical-shaped OHCs are visible, surrounded by Nuel spaces and supported by Deiters cells. The cuticular plate of OHCs and the apical part of supporting cells contribute to the reticular lamina. Hair-like extensions stem from the cuticular plates, forming the stereocilia bathing in the endolymph compartment. The tectorial membrane that normally tops OHC stereocilia has been retracted and elevated by the fixation process and is no longer present. On the modiolar, left side, one inner pillar cell is visible (Courtesy of Dr Marc Lenoir, INSERM 254, Montpellier, France).

Tip and lateral links connect neighbouring stereocilia. They are aligned in about four V- or W-shaped rows, with the tallest stereocilia being on the outer, lateral-wall side of the cells (Figure 1.7). In mammals, the tallest stereocilia of the OHCs are strongly embedded in the tectorial membrane, whereas the

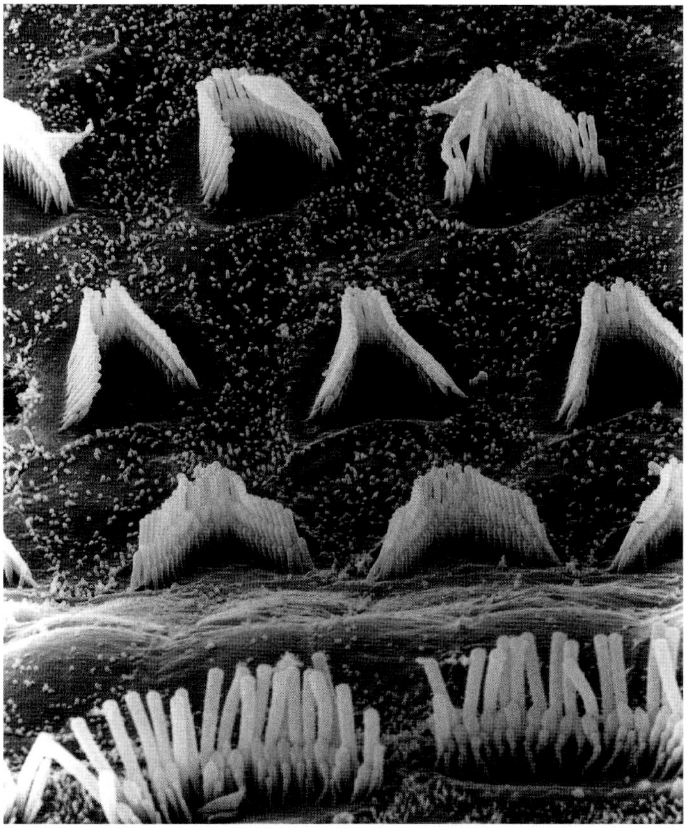

Figure 1.7 Close-up view of the stereocilia bundle of hair cells in a guinea pig cochlea (scanning electron micrograph) (modiolar side: bottom of figure). A few tip links are visible in the IHC bundles. (Courtesy of Dr Marc Lenoir, INSERM 254, Montpellier, France.)

stereocilia of IHCs do not seem to touch the tectorial membrane. Instead, their tips are very close to Hensen's stria, forming a groove along the lower surface of the tectorial membrane.

Owing to the piston-like action of the stapes footplate in the oval window, a differential pressure occurs between the scala vestibuli and the tympani. It is thought that Reissner's membrane fully transmits pressure waves from the scala vestibuli to the scala media, and thus the differential pressure is actually applied on the two sides of the basilar membrane and induces vibrations at the level of the organ of Corti. Stereocilia bundles are deflected by two different mechanisms: shearing for the OHCs due to the movement of the tectorial membrane relative to the reticular lamina, and the movements of subtectorial endolymph acting on IHC stereocilia through viscous forces. Deflection of stereocilia by sound waves alternately opens and closes ion channels, presumably at or near the tip links (Figure 1.7). These tip links are therefore believed to be of great functional importance.[7] As a result of the strong electrochemical gradient existing between endolymph (+80 mV) and intracellular space (−40 to −70 mV), K^+ ions flow into the sensory cells and induce a decrease in the membrane potential. This depolarization acts in dramatically different ways on IHCs and OHCs. IHCs release their neurotransmitter (glutamate) in the synaptic spaces and subsequently activate the afferent nerve fibres. OHCs exhibit electromotility, i.e. they respond by length and stiffness changes to changes in membrane potential, thereby contributing to shaping the mechanical excitation of IHCs. Electromotility is a unique type of mechanical response in that it does not require metabolic energy other than that needed to generate membrane potential changes. Its bandpass seems very high: in vitro, responses have been found up to more than 30 kHz. Although not yet fully delineated, its molecular origin seems to arise from specific ion-exchanging protein motors, such as prestin, identified by Dallos's team.

Another conspicuous difference between IHCs and OHCs, in line with their totally different response to depolarization, stems from the study of their innervation.[8] The spiral ganglion contains the cell bodies of afferent auditory nerve fibres. About 25 000 such fibres are found in mammals. Their dendrites come from the base of the hair cells, through small holes distributed along the osseous spiral lamina. About 95% come from IHCs and are called type I neurones. These neurones have a large diameter and are covered with a myelin sheath, enabling fast conduction of action potentials towards the first relay, in the cochlear nucleus. The pattern of innervation of IHCs is a converging one (Figure 1.8); about 10 type I fibres, or more, connect to one IHC. The remaining 5% of nerve fibres innervate OHCs. In contrast to type I fibres, they are unmyelinated. A type II fibre has to travel basally, by about 0.6 mm, before sending dendrites to about 10 OHCs, the ramifying innervation of OHCs by a single neurone is divergent (Figure 1.8). Its role is completely unknown to date. The auditory nerve also contains about 2000 efferent fibres, originating from the superior olivary complexes on both sides of the brainstem. Two neural bundles reach the cochlear area, one from the medial superior olive synapses with the base of OHCs, whereas another comes from the lateral olivary complex and projects on the afferent dendrites coming from IHCs. The medial olivocochlear neurones have large, mostly cholinergic, synapses with the OHCs, and presumably modulate their motility. The lateral olivocochlear neurones involve more complex neurotransmission. They probably regulate the function of type I afferent neurones and may also play a role when these neurones are damaged, e.g. swollen after overstimulation.[9]

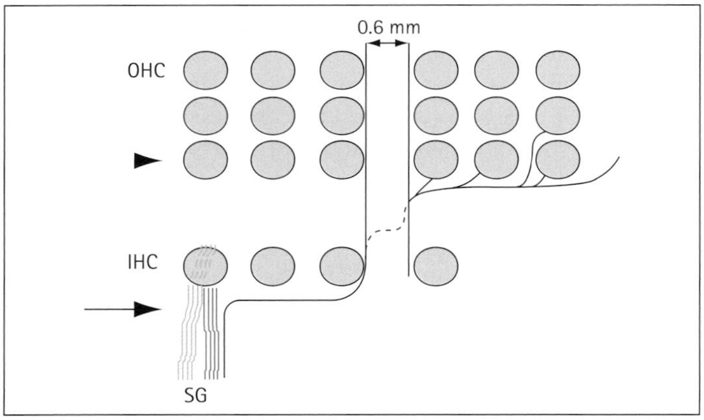

Figure 1.8 Diagram of the innervation of hair cells in the organ of Corti. The type I neurones connected to the external part of the IHCs have a larger diameter and higher spontaneous discharge rate than the fibres connected to the internal, modiolar side. Type II neurones are unmyelinated and contact OHCs. Medial olivocochlear efferents contact the basal part of the OHC (arrowhead), whereas lateral olivocochlear efferents (arrow) synapse on the dendrites of type I neurones. (SG, spiral ganglions.)

Anatomical changes due to ageing

The cochlea and the sensorineural structures it contains are morphologically fully mature at birth in humans. The performance of these structures tends to decline with ageing, and even soon after birth. Although usually very slow, this decline, sometimes referred to as presbyacusis, eventually concerns most subjects over 60 years of age. It is partly a direct consequence of ageing, although ageing alone does not necessarily result in significant audiometric losses. It is thought accordingly that 'presbyacusis' also involves external causes such as prolonged exposure to occupational or recreational noise, or other potentially damaging factors, in addition to possible genetic factors. Presbyacusis is associated with anatomical alterations, such as an atrophy of the lower basal turn, concerning a few millimetres from the basal end of the organ of Corti. Schuknecht[10] described four basic features of sensorineural changes associated with ageing, which he observed isolated or in association, namely loss in the sensory cell populations, metabolic changes in relation to atrophy of the stria vascularis, mechanical changes, perhaps due to basilar membrane stiffening and resulting in a sort of conductive cochlear hearing loss, and neuronal degeneration. The first and last types are the most commonly observed, or at least those most easily ascertained using audiological tests.

Scant detailed data are available from human temporal bones and most of them were published by a joint-study group[11] combining different microscopy techniques. While the normal number of IHCs is around 100/mm, it is found to decrease to about 30/mm after 70 years, at a distance from the basal end of about 10% of the overall cochlear length. This corresponds to a rate of decrease of IHC density of about 0.7%/year. The IHC loss is closer to 0.3% elsewhere along the cochlea. As for OHCs, they amount to about 400/mm of cochlear length, and seem to undergo a larger decrease, i.e. about 1%/year at the basal end and 0.5% elsewhere. The rate of ganglion cell loss is less than 1%/year for neurones of the lower basal part, whereas it is about 0.5%/year in the middle coil. The functional consequences of such losses are easy to predict as a predominantly high-frequency hearing loss, the boundary frequency between near-normal and pathological areas tending to get lower with age.

Vestibular anatomy

The bony labyrinth, containing the balance organs, is located posterior to the cochlea. It is made of two main compartments, the vestibule, containing the utricle and saccule, and the semicircular canals. As with the cochlea, the membranous labyrinth, filled with endolymph, is completely surrounded by the bony labyrinth. The space between osseous and membranous labyrinths is full of perilymph.

The vestibule (Figure 1.9) is just medial to the tympanic cavity, separated from it by the oval window. It is divided in two recesses containing the two otolith organs, the saccule and utricle. The saccule is a spherical vesicle resting on the floor of the vestibule. The ductus reuniens, starting from the inferior pole of the saccule, connects it to the cochlea, whereas the utriculosaccular duct leads to the utricle. The sensory organ of the saccule or macula rests on the medial face of the saccule, and its plane forms an angle of 30° with the vertical. The utricle is elliptical, and its macula is located on the anterior part of the floor. Its plane is about 30° off the horizontal plane of the head. Thus, the planes of the two otolith organs lie approximately at right angles to each other.

The semicircular canals are posterior and superior to the vestibule. They consist of three ducts called the horizontal, posterior and superior canals (Figure 1.9). Their two ends open into the vestibule, through only five orifices, because the posterior part of the superior canal meets the superior part of the posterior canal, forming the common crus prior to entering the utricular recess. Each semicircular canal forms about two-thirds of a planar torus, and the three canals are aligned so that their planes are approximately perpendicular. The horizontal canals form an angle of about 30° with the axial plane. The posterior and superior canals lie in a vertical plane, at about 45° from the sagittal plane, so that the posterior canal on one side is parallel to the superior canal on the opposite side. Each semicircular canal contains a membranous duct occupying only a quarter of its diameter. One end of each canal is dilated very near its entrance to the utricle. The sensory cells lie in this dilated portion, called the ampulla. The medial part of the ampullae present a sort of fold or ridge covered with sensory epithelium: this thickening of the basal membrane is termed the ampullary crest or crista ampullaris.

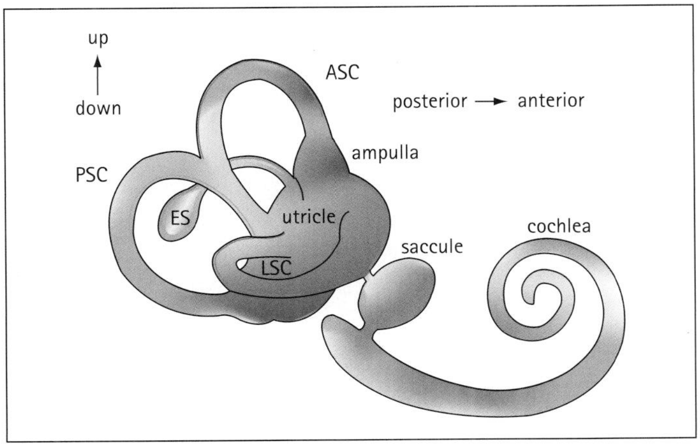

Figure 1.9 Lateral view of cochlea, vestibule and semicircular canals. ASC, anterior semicircular canal; LSC, lateral semicircular canal; PSC, posterior semicircular canal; ES, endolymphatic sac.

Although the ionic contents of vestibular perilymph and endolymph do not differ much from those of the cochlea, the endolymphatic potential is close to zero in the vestibular organs. The sensory hair cells of the vestibular system are roughly similar to those in the cochlea. They lie in the maculae and ampullae, corresponding to highly differentiated epithelial areas made of one layer of sensory cells surrounded by supporting cells. Stereocilia and a kinocilium extend from the body of the sensory cells. In contrast to the cochlea, the kinocilium of vestibular cells persists in mature cells. It is a true cilium with nine pairs of microtubules. A group of stereocilia is found on one side of the kinocilium, and, as in the cochlea, these stereocilia are made of thin extensions of the cell membrane. They are always shorter than the kinocilium, and their height decreases as the distance from it increases. The whole group of hairs is considered to be oriented as determined by the direction of the kinocilium. The kinocilium and stereocilia of all vestibular sensory cells are covered with a gelatinous flap, called the cupula in the semicircular canals. In the maculae only, this gel also contains embedded calcium carbonate crystals termed otoconia, forming the otolith membrane. The density of otoconia with respect to endolymph is about 3, so their presence results in an increase of the mass weighting the hair bundles and makes them sensitive to gravity. Deflection of hairs in the appropriate direction, i.e. from the stereocilia to the kinocilium, opens ion channels. This results in a depolarization of the cell membrane, leading to neurotranmitter release. Movement of hairs in the opposite direction is inhibitory. The structures responsible for transducing the mechanical stimulus into an electrical response of the cell membrane are probably the stereocilia, since the kinocilium can be removed without altering the responses to stimulation.

Two types of sensory cells are found in the maculae of the utricle and saccule, and in the ampullae of the semicircular canals: chalice cells (type I) and cylindrical cells (type II). They differ in morphology, innervation and location. The piriform body of type I cells (Figure 1.10) is completely surrounded by one afferent nerve calyx, giving at least 10 synaptic contacts. The columnar type II cells (Figure 1.10) are supplied at their basal end by several afferent and efferent nerve endings. Type I cells are most abundant along the striolae and on top of the cristae ampullaris, and type II cells are denser in the periphery of the sensory areas. The arrangement of sensory cells depends on the organ under consideration. In the maculae, the polarities of hair cells vary in a systematic manner. The shapes of the two maculae are different, comma-shape for the saccular macula (Figure 1.11) and more rounded for the utricular one, but both are separated into two halves by a curved boundary called the striola, corresponding either to an excess (for the utricle) or defect (for the saccule) of otoconia. All the kinocilia point away from the striola in the saccule, and towards the striola in the utricle. Unlike the macular cells, the ampullar hair cells (Figure 1.12) are all polarized in the same direction, namely towards the utricle for the horizontal canal, and away from the utricle for the other two canals.

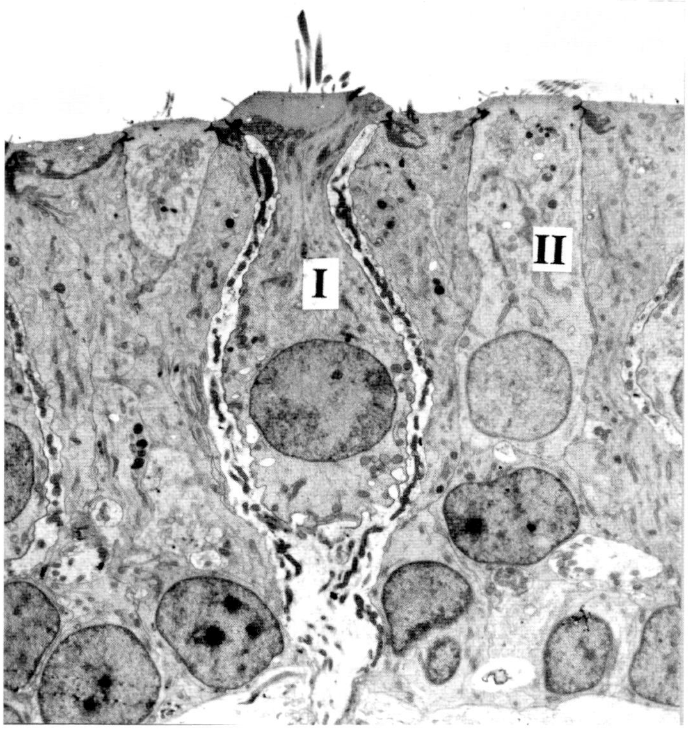

Figure 1.10 Type I and type II cells in vestibular epithelium of guinea pig (transmission electron microscopy). (Courtesy of Dr D. Demêmes, INSERM 432, Montpellier, France.)

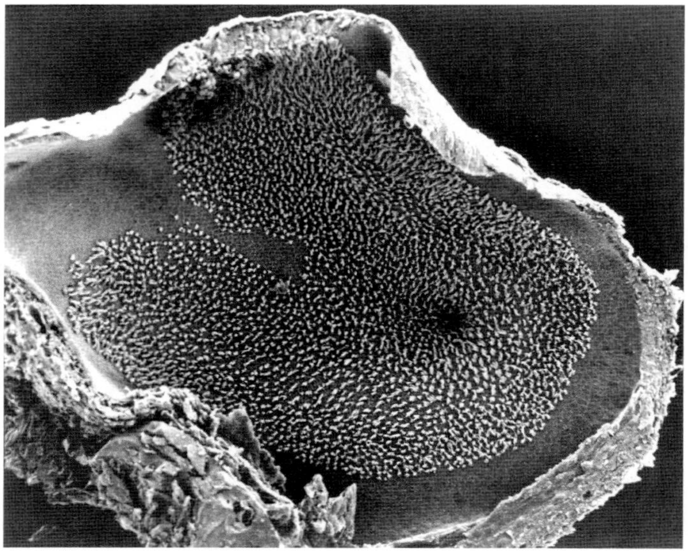

Figure 1.11 Rat saccule seen with scanning electron microscopy. (Courtesy of Dr Claude J. Dechesne, INSERM 432, Montpellier, France.)

The maculae send afferent fibres through the utricular and saccular branches of the vestibular nerve. Efferent fibres originate in the vestibular nuclear complex. They synapse not only directly on type II cells, but also on the primary afferent fibres surrounding type I cells.

Blood supply of the cochleovestibular system

The whole membranous labyrinth receives its terminal arterial supply from the labyrinthine or internal auditory artery, arising either from the anterior inferior cerebellar artery, or sometimes directly from the basilar artery. The vasculature of the bony labyrinth is completely independent. The labyrinthine artery travels within the internal auditory canal, on the surface of the neural bundles. It is divided into three branches, the anterior vestibular, vestibulocochlear and cochlear arteries. The cochlear artery enters the modiolus and ramifies into spiral arteries (see Figure 1.4), supplying most of the cochlea. The basal quarter of the cochlear duct receives its supply from the vestibulocochlear artery. The anterior vestibular artery irrigates the posterior sides of the saccule and utricle, as well as the anterior and lateral semicircular canals. The posterior vestibulocochlear branch supplies the inferior parts of the saccule and utricle, and the posterior semicircular canal.

Perilymph and endolymph connections to external spaces

The fragile sensory structures of the hearing and balance organs are bathed in liquids contained in a rigid bony structure. Sudden pressure changes or steady volume changes of perilymph or endolymph would be detrimental if the cochleovestibular cavities were not properly connected to the outside world through various channels. The cochlear aqueduct connects the termination of the scala tympani, close to the round window, to the subarachnoid space, after running

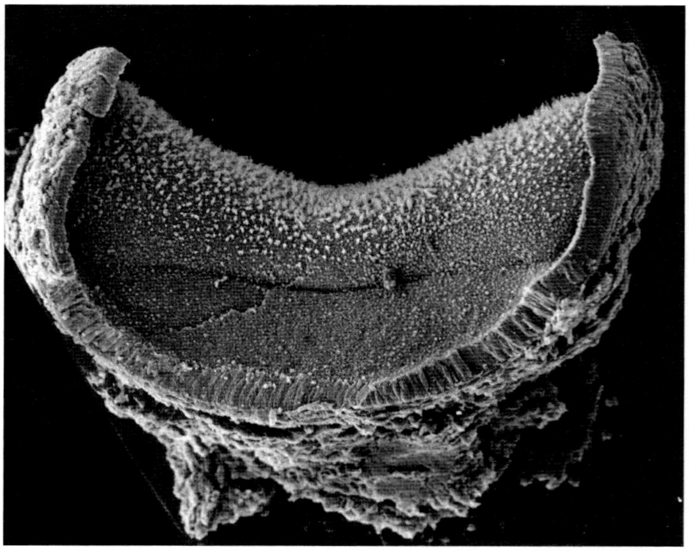

Figure 1.12 Lateral ampullary crest in a human fetus, by scanning electron microscopy. (Courtesy of Dr Claude J. Dechesne, INSERM 432, Montpellier, France.)

inferior to the internal auditory canal. Though it probably does not allow the perilymph to flow through it in general, it enables the perilymphatic pressure to equalize with that of the cerebrospinal fluid. The vestibular aqueduct also connects the vestibular perilymph to the subarachnoid spaces.

The endolymphatic duct is formed by the reunion of two small canals coming from the saccule and utricle. It first presents an enlarged intravestibular section, then tapers, penetrates the vestibular aqueduct and ends intracranially in the 10-mm-wide endolymphatic sac. The endolymphatic sac can absorb the excess endolymph together with cellular and otoconial debris. Recent data[6] suggest that the endolymph flow through the endolymphatic duct can be bidirectional in various physiological conditions, thereby contributing to buffering pressure or volume changes.

References

1. Gold T. Hearing II. The physical basis of the action of the cochlea. *Proc R Soc Lond B* 1948; **135**: 492–8.
2. Davis H. An active process in cochlear mechanics. *Hear Res* 1983; **9**: 79–90.
3. Rosowski JJ. Models of external- and middle-ear function. In: Hawkins HL, McMullen TA, Popper AN, Fay RR, eds. *Auditory Computation*. New York: Springer, 1996: 15–61.
4. Vacher SR, Guinan JJ Jr, Kobler JB. Intracellularly labeled stapedius motoneuron cell bodies in the cat are spatially organized according to their physiologic responses. *J Comp Neurol* 1989; **289**: 401–15.
5. Borg E, Counter SA, Rosler G. Theories of middle ear muscle function. In: Silman S, ed. *The Acoustic Reflex*. Orlando: Academic Press, 1984: 63–99.
6. Salt AN, DeMott JE. Longitudinal endolymph movements induced by perilymphatic injections. *Hear Res* 1998; **123**: 137–47.
7. Pickles JO, Comis SD, Osborne MP. Cross-links between stereocilia in the guinea pig organ of Corti and their possible relation to sensory transduction. *Hear Res* 1984; **49**: 103–12.
8. Spoendlin HH. Innervation pattern of the organ of Corti of the cat. *Acta Otolarygol (Stockh)* 1969; **67**: 239–54.
9. Puel JL. Chemical synaptic transmission in the cochlea. *Prog Neurobiol* 1995; **47**: 449–76.
10. Schuknecht HF. Presbyacusis. *Laryngoscope* 1955; **65**: 402.
11. Wright A, Davis A, Bredberg G et al. Hair cell distribution in the normal human cochlea. A report of a European working group. *Acta Otolaryngol Suppl* 1987; **436**: 15–24.

2 Ageing in the auditory and vestibular systems

Ulf Rosenhall

Introduction

A gradual demographic change is apparent, especially in the developed countries, resulting in a considerable increase in the number of elderly persons. The proportion of elderly people in the total population in a typical European country was about 10% fifty years ago, is about 17% today, and is expected to reach approximately 20% during the first 25 years of the new millennium. The largest relative increase is expected to occur in the group of very old persons, over 80 years of age. This group is not extremely large, but the demands on the society and on relatives in terms of health care and social care are considerable. In Sweden, the total population has grown by 25% during the last 35 years, and the increase is expected to continue during the coming decades, such that the total number of those older than 90 years will not be very large, but the relative increase is very pronounced. In these older age groups, the number of women is considerably greater than the number of men.

The ageing processes interfere with all bodily and mental functions, including the sensory systems. The influences of ageing on both the auditory and the vestibular systems are pronounced. Age-related hearing loss, previously called **presbyacusis**, is a very common type of auditory dysfunction. Age-related hearing loss is one of the three most frequently reported chronic health problems in old age, and is also the most prevalent cause of hearing loss. Quality of life depends greatly on communication with other people, and the auditory system is the most important link in communication. Presbyacusis often has a devastating effect on the social life of many elderly people.

Audiometric characteristics of age-related hearing loss

In age-related hearing loss, the pure tone audiogram shows a high frequency, symmetrical, sensorineural hearing loss in a vast majority of the cases. The configuration is either gently sloping (Figure 2.1), or steeply sloping (Figure 2.2). In one audiometric variety the pure tone loss is relatively flat over the entire frequency range (Figure 2.3). For comparison, the audiometric pattern of a typical case with noise induced hearing loss is shown in Figure 2.4. There is a marked gender effect, high-frequency

> **AUDIOMETRIC PATTERNS OF PRESBYACUSIS**
>
> - Gently or steeply sloping sensorineural high-frequency hearing loss
> - Sensorineural flat hearing loss might occur
> - Men have poorer high-frequency hearing than women
> - Women have somewhat poorer low-frequency hearing than men

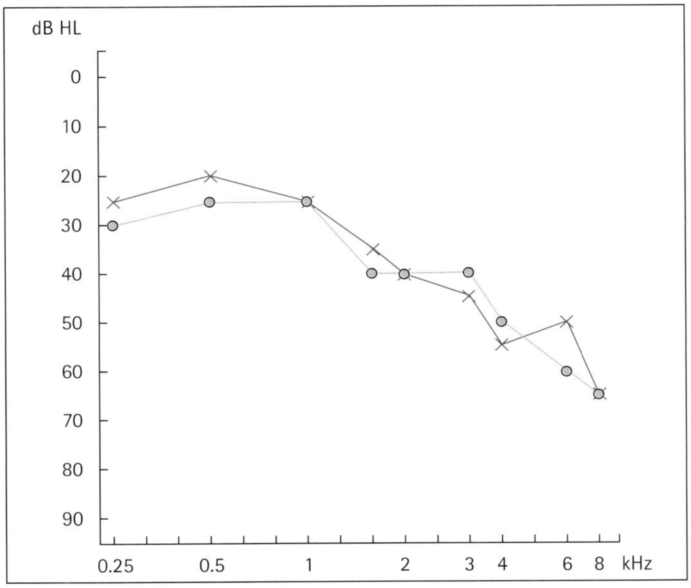

Figure 2.1 Pure tone audiogram from an 80-year-old woman. The configuration of the hearing loss gently slopes towards the high-frequency area, but hearing at the low frequencies is also impaired.

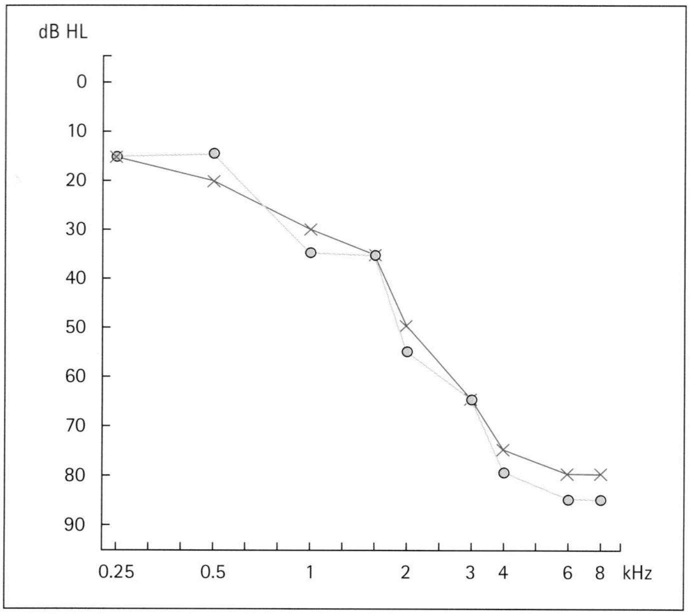

Figure 2.2 Presbyacusis pattern from a 77-year-old man. The hearing is normal in the low-frequency area. The high-frequency hearing is poor, and there is a gradual increase of the hearing impairment with increasing frequency

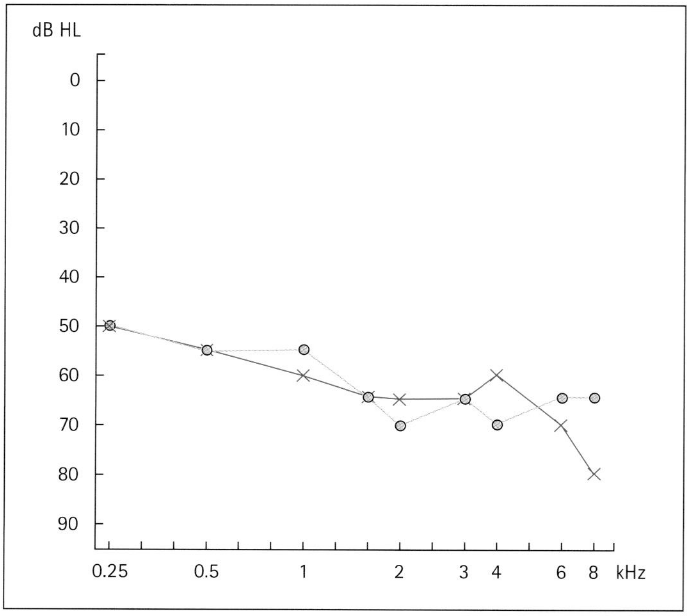

Figure 2.3 A flat audiometric pattern in an 89-year-old woman.

hearing being significantly poorer in men than in women. For the low frequencies, there is a tendency in the opposite direction, women having poorer hearing function than men in this frequency range.[1]

Speech perception in old age has been discussed over the years. In the earlier literature, it was suggested that speech discrimination of the elderly is worse than would be expected from their ability to hear pure tones. However, speech perception in quiet is often well preserved in old age. There are three basic hypotheses explaining difficulties with the understanding of speech in old age: peripheral hearing loss, central auditory dysfunction and cognitive problems.[2] Speech perception is generally fairly well preserved in the elderly, peripheral hearing loss being the single most influential factor.[3] Speech recognition in quiet, as well as in noise, is influenced by peripheral dysfunction, as in younger age groups, but there is also evidence of central auditory dysfunction in elderly subjects.[4]

Aetiology of age-related hearing loss

According to one definition, presbyacusis is the physiological change in hearing that occurs with age per se: **primary** or **pure presbyacusis.**[5] Pure presbyacusis is to some degree only a theoretical construction, probably with little relevance in a modern industrialized society. In studies of pure presbyacusis, participants with hearing loss caused by factors other than age have been excluded. In other studies, the hearing capacity of isolated populations relatively uncontaminated with possible noxious factors, typical for Western societies, has been investigated.

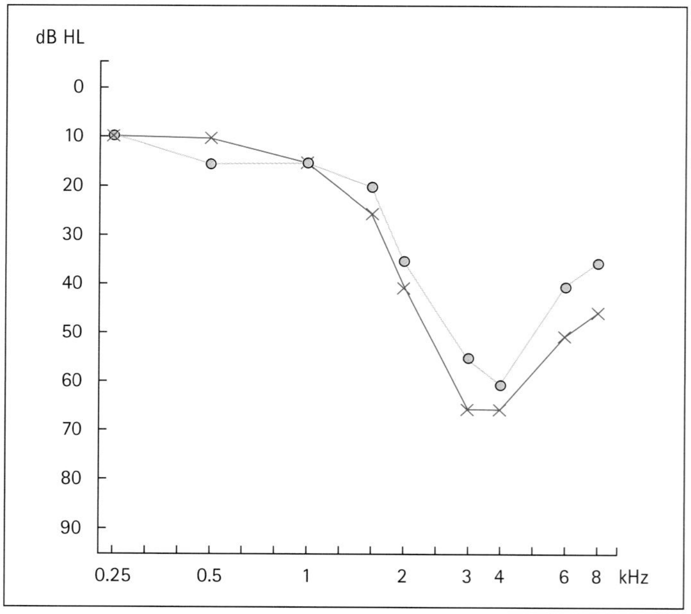

Figure 2.4 For comparison with the presbyacusis audiograms, noise-induced hearing loss affecting a 54-year-old man is shown. The audiogram sharply slopes above 1.5 kHz, and the maximal hearing loss is seen at 3–4 kHz.

Pure presbyacusis is by definition the hearing loss caused by biological, ageing processes and the term is nowadays often replaced with presbyacusis only.

Genetic mechanisms are important for the development of hearing with increasing age. Some persons have excellent hearing in advanced age, while others get presbyacusis when they are middle-aged. Genetic factors are apparent in **familial**

presbyacusis, an entity with relatively early onset of hearing loss, and affecting many members of the same family. The existence of familial presbyacusis has been verified in an epidemiological investigation.[6] Based on a temporal bone material, a mitochondrial genetic model of presbyacusis has been proposed.[7]

With the industrialization of societies throughout the world, the adverse effects of noise on hearing have become obvious. Exposure to noise is one extraneous noxious factor causing hearing loss, and increased after the industrial revolution and the migration from the country to the cities. Although the levels of environmental noise are not often directly harmful to hearing, the effects of such noise in the long term are not known. The increased exposure to vocational and non-occupational noise could result in generation effects concerning age-related hearing loss. These effects are difficult to predict, since increased exposure to occupational noise could be neutralized by a successful hearing conservation programme. The influence of noise on age-related hearing loss is not known in detail. Glorig and Nixon[8] coined the term **sociocusis**, emphasizing their opinion that age-related hearing loss, to a great extent, has extraneous causes other than occupational noise exposure. In the classical study of the hearing of the Mabaan tribe in southern Sudan, which is isolated from the noise of the industrialized society, Rosen et al[9] concluded that sociocusis is caused by wear and tear of the ear during many decades of life, with exposure to noise being the most important factor. However, the noise-free environment is only one possible explanation for the stability of hearing capacity in an isolated population, another factor could be a marked population homogeneity. In earlier investigations it has been shown that the deterioration of hearing related to ageing is reduced within the noise frequencies in noise-damaged ears. Gates and collagues reported an intriguing finding.[10] They confirmed the reduced age-related hearing deterioration within the noise frequencies (3–6 kHz region) in elderly men with noise-induced hearing loss as well as presbyacusis, but an accelerated hearing loss in frequency areas adjacent to the noise-damaged frequencies, especially 2 kHz. Their findings suggest that a noise-damaged ear does not 'age' at the same rate as an ear not exposed to noise, and that the increased loss at 2 kHz suggests that the effects of noise damage may continue even after the noise exposure.

The term **nosocusis** has been used to describe hearing loss in elderly people due to ototraumatic events other than noise.[11] Such factors include influence from ototoxic agents and environmental ototoxic insults, smoking, head trauma, and alcohol abuse.[12] Health factors, e.g. otological diseases and cardiovascular disorders, have been related to the presence of presbyacusis.[13]

Different factors related to age-related hearing loss have been studied by Stephens[14] and Lim and Stephens,[15] who studied elderly patients with hearing problems attending a rehabilitation clinic. About 17–19% of these patients were considered to have presbyacusis only. One-third had a history of vascular disease, 14–33% had chronic otitis media, 12–15% had noise-induced or traumatic hearing loss, 6–9% had familial/genetic background factors, and 3–5% had possible metabolic influence. The studies showed that hearing loss in old age often had an origin earlier in life. There was a greater risk of having vascular or biochemical abnormalities in those with hearing loss than in members of an age-matched control group.

AETIOLOGY OF AGE-RELATED HEARING LOSS

- Intrinsic factors
  - Biological ageing
  - Genetic
  - Endocrinological-metabolic
- Extrinsic factors
  - Noise exposure
  - Ototoxic agents
  - Middle ear disease
  - Trauma
  - Socio-economic
- Health factors
  - General health
  - Cardiovascular disease
  - Endocrinological disease

Histopathology of age-related hearing loss

The morphological correlate to presbyacusis has been studied in inner ears from humans as well as research animals. Two strains of mice have been used extensively for this purpose. One is the C57 strain, consisting of mice which show severe age-related changes. The other is the CBA strain, which is resistant to age-related changes of hearing function (reviewed in reference 15). The high-frequency hearing loss seen in presbyacusis is correlated with degenerative processes within the apical and basal regions of the cochlea (Figures 2.5, 2.6).

The most pronounced degeneration of the two types of cochlear hair cells is found in the basal coil.[17] The outer hair cells (OHCs) show patchy degeneration most pronounced in the apical and basal coils.[18] The degeneration of inner hair cells (IHCs), and also the nerve fibres, is predominantly confined to the basal coil. Over the age of 50 the degeneration of OHCs is more severe than the degeneration of IHCs.[18] Atrophy of the spiral ganglion and the nerves in the osseous spiral lamina is another finding.

Presbyacusis is related to dysfunction on a cellular level. Derangement of the hair bundles and formation of giant cilia are findings often seen in aged human inner ears. Lipofuscin, also called the pigment of ageing, is assumed to be the waste product of lysosomal activity. The presence of these inclusions is a sign of exhaustion of enzymatic activity leading to decreased function and cell death. Lipofuscin inclusions and other osmiophilic structures have been reported to be among the most prominent intracellular alterations in the ageing cells of the cochlea.[19]

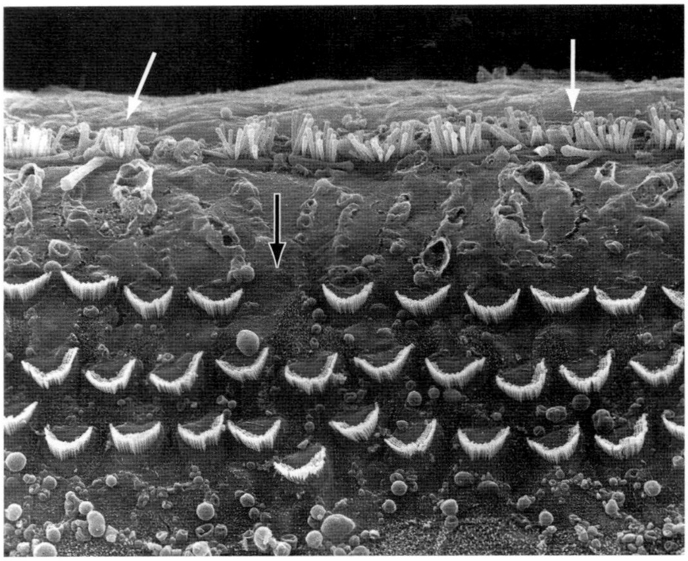

Figure 2.5 Scanning electron microscope (SEM) photomicrograph showing a short section of a human cochlea from an old individual. One outer hair cell (OHC, black arrow) is missing, indicating the presence of discrete degeneration. Some of the inner hair cells (IHC, white arrows) (in the background) have derangement of the hair bundles, and two giant cilia are present. (Courtesy of Berit Engström.)

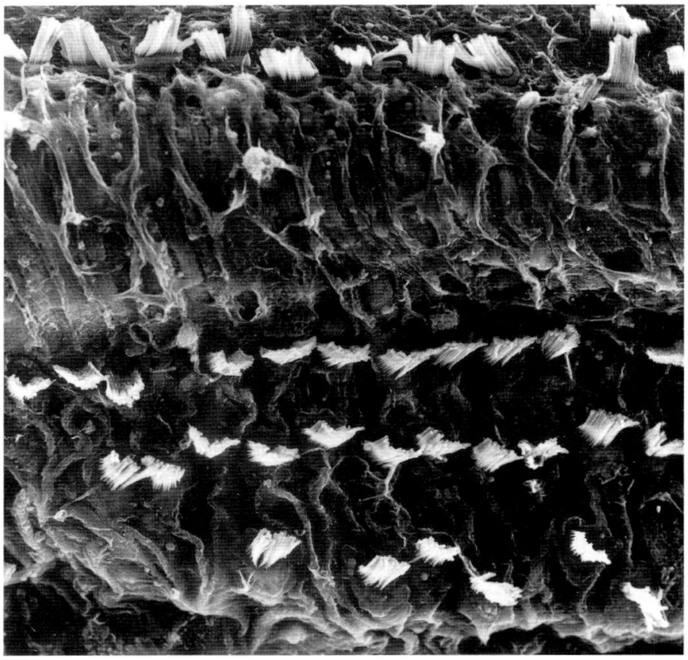

Figure 2.6 SEM photomicrograph from a human cochlea from an elderly person. Many of the OHCs are missing and the third row is disrupted, indicating age-related degeneration. Degenerative changes also affect the IHCs (upper row) with alterations of the hair bundles. (Courtesy of Berit Engström.)

Earlier histopathological studies also demonstrated degenerative changes in the central auditory nervous system. Loss of neurones has been found in the cochlear nuclei[20] and in the central auditory pathway[21] with increasing age. This concept has, however, been challenged, and presbyacusis-related histopathological alterations have been focused in the inner ear.[16]

HISTOPATHOLOGY OF AGE-RELATED HEARING LOSS

- Cochlear
  - OCH degeneration in basal and apical coil
  - IHC degeneration in basal coil
  - Alterations and derangement of hair bundles
  - Intracellular inclusions
  - Strial degeneration
- First order neurone
  - Spiral ganglion degeneration
  - Cochlear nerve degeneration
- Central auditory system degeneration

Schuknecht[22] proposed four types of presbyacusis, based on morphological findings, in some occasions correlated with audiometric measurements. He called the first type **sensory presbyacusis**, with a loss of sensory cells as well as supporting and neuronal cells, mostly in the basal coil of the cochlea. The hearing impairment in this type of presbyacusis is a high frequency loss with relatively normal speech perception. The second type, called **neural presbyacusis**, is characterized by a loss of neurones more than sensory cells. This neuronal loss is seen in the entire spiral ganglion but is more severe in the basal turn. Audiometrically, speech recognition is reduced in relation to the pure tone audiogram. The rarity of the condition[23] and the possibility that its background could be a central auditory disorder rather than a peripheral one are reasons for hesitation. Schuknecht called the third type **strial presbyacusis**. The stria vascularis shows a patchy atrophy seen in the entire cochlea but most pronounced in the middle and apical turns. The audiometric pattern is a flat hearing loss. The progression of the hearing loss is slow, and the speech recognition ability good. The fourth type, **cochlear conductive presbyacusis**, could be caused by a disturbance of the mechanics of the spiral ligament, but no morphological changes have been demonstrated, and the validity of this proposed entity has been challenged.

Correlations between hearing impairment and histopathological changes in the cochlea have been studied in humans, but the results are contradictory. One extreme is represented by Suga and Lindsay,[24] who found no correlations with the lesions in the sensory, neural or vascular elements of the cochlea and audiometry. Some degree of pathology, up to 20% hair cell loss, does not necessarily correlate with any significant hearing loss. Loss of OHCs in the apical coil can also be consistent with normal hearing. A massive loss of basal OHCs (≥50%) correlates with audiometrically verified hearing loss. Bredberg[18] found that the number of OHCs correlated rather well with the audiogram while the number of IHCs did not.

Since presbyacusis and noise induced hearing loss are closely connected, it is of interest to compare the histopathology of the two entities.[25] The most pronounced degenerations in the ageing ear are seen in the peripheral third row of the OHCs, while the most noise-susceptible sensory cells in the organ of Corti are, in decreasing order: OHCs of the first, second and third row and IHCs. The degeneration in the ageing ear is patchy and is present in all coils of the cochlea, but is most pronounced in the basal and apical regions. Two patterns of degeneration have been described in ears exposed to intense noise. One involves the lower basal turn in a sharply demarcated area and is associated with the 4-kHz dip in the audiogram. The second pattern consists of a more widespread pathology of the basal part of the cochlea and is associated with a sloping audiogram.

Epidemiology of age-related hearing loss

The extent of presbyacusis, its progress with increasing age, its distribution within different populations and calculations of rehabilitative needs can be studied using epidemiological methods. The overall state of hearing can be studied using unscreened populations. Such studies include all subjects in the study populations, even participants with hearing loss not related to ageing. The intention is to study hearing among elderly persons, regardless of the cause of any hearing impairments present. Other studies have used screened or selected populations to identify pure presbyacusis and avoid extraneous factors that could have negative influences on the hearing. Subjects with noise exposure or any kind of otological disease have been excluded from these studies.

In a cross-sectional study, the hearing of the subjects is measured in age bands during one limited period of time. In a longitudinal study, the same subjects are tested on different occasions, covering a time span of up to decades, which makes it time-consuming. The longitudinal design, in contrast to the cross-sectional design, controls different variables such as the genetic composition of the population, cultural background, level of education, and variation of noise exposure. Generation effects can be studied by comparing different cohorts of similar age on different occasions (time-lag studies). Variations between different publications could be the result of differences in selection criteria of the test populations, in study design, in generation effects, in methodology used, and in how the results are presented.

A number of epidemiological studies, covering various ages, have been published. In some reports, results from such studies have been compiled.[26] The ISO 1999[27] database A comprises age-related hearing threshold levels of otologically normal populations (highly screened regarding exposure to noise and otological diseases) from industrialized societies, and database B comprises unscreened populations.

A large-scale and very comprehensive epidemiological study with a cross-sectional design is the MRC National Study of Hearing.[28,29] The study population, living in four major cities in Great Britain, was unselected with regard to otological disorder. The prevalence of hearing impairment at ages 71–80 in the better ear was calculated. If subjects with minor hearing impairments were included, the prevalence of hearing impairment was 60%. If moderately impaired persons were included, the figure was 18%. Four per cent of the included subjects were severely impaired.

The Edinburgh study[30] was a longitudinal study with a time span of up to 17 years. The authors reported increases in hearing loss in the entire frequency range with advancing age. The deterioration rate of age-related hearing loss was more pronounced for the higher frequencies and continued steadily into the ninth decade.

In the Gerontological and Geriatric Population Study of Göteborg, Sweden, four age cohorts of elderly persons were investigated, with both longitudinal and cross-sectional designs.[31,32] From 70 to 81 years, deterioration of hearing was apparent in the entire frequency range and was about 1–2 dB/year. From 80 to 90 years of age a levelling of the deterioration was noticed, indicating a slowing down of presbyacusis. The Copenhagen male study and the Valby study[33–34] had longitudinal and cross-sectional designs, describing, among other things, gender differences. The studies also included various aspects of rehabilitation of elderly subjects. The Framingham study was conducted in Massachusetts.[23,36,37] Two age cohorts, with a time-lag of 5 years, were investigated longitudinally and cross-sectionally. Considerable differences were reported between the two cohorts, the participants of the second cohort having better hearing in old age than those of the first cohort. In the first cohort, a slowing-up of the deterioration was discernible in advanced age, but this was not seen in the second cohort. The Baltimore Longitudinal Study of Aging[38,39] was a longitudinal study. The subjects were not selected with regard to noise exposure or otological disease, but the participants predominantly had high education and socio-economic status. Changes in hearing thresholds occurred in all age groups during the follow-up period. The rate of change was faster in the speech frequencies than in the higher frequencies. The men's hearing declined faster than that of the women. Other important epidemiological contributions have been reported from Italy[40] and Finland.[41] In the Finnish study, the prevalence of hearing loss in a 55–75-year-old population was calculated. Mild hearing impairment was demonstrated in 10–30%, moderate in 4–8%, and severe in 0.2–1.1% of the participants, according to two classification systems.

The results of the cited investigations coincide reasonably well. The unscreened studies are fairly similar, but a difference of up to 10 dB or more at some octaves exists. The selected studies also coincide rather well, with some variability. The unscreened populations have 5–15-dB poorer threshold values than the screened populations, this being especially pronounced in the high frequencies.

The noise factor has been shown to be important in many studies, in which populations screened for noise exposure have been compared with populations that have not been screened. One example is the Baltimore Longitudinal study of Aging.[39] The hearing function is reported to be better in this screened study compared to the results of other investigations of unscreened populations. However, the situation is not unequivocal, since the difference between screened and unscreened populations in the MRC study from the UK is not very striking.[29]

A compilation of five epidemiological investigations of unscreened populations is presented in Figures 2.7 and 2.8 for the age groups 70–80 and 80+, respectively.[29,32,35,37,43]

The annual decline of hearing varies considerably. From ages 70–80, the mean deterioration rate is about 1 dB per year, except in the high frequencies where the decline can reach 2-3 dB/year. Two patterns can be discerned: one with a markedly greater deterioration rate in the high frequencies than in the low ones,[27,33] and another with deterioration involving the entire frequency range.[31,32,37] Hearing impairment is an especially common problem for the oldest people.[42]

Gender differences have been reported in many studies. Elderly women have generally better hearing than men of the same age. Women have better threshold values at 2–8 kHz than men, with a difference of up to 20 dB at 4 kHz.[23,26,31,32,36] The gender difference is marked in unselected cases, where the difference is 15–25 dB at 4 kHz at age 70. In the low-frequency area, there is a tendency for women to present with somewhat poorer thresholds than men. The difference between genders is as apparent at age 80 as at age 70. A complication of six epidemiological studies regarding gender differences at ages 70–80 years and 80–90 years is presented in Figure 2.9. Extrinsic ototraumatic factors, above all exposure to noise, differ between genders and are likely to be responsible for at least part of the difference.[11] However, results regarding gender differences have been somewhat contradictory. Cruickshanks et al[43] reported that the male excess of hearing loss remained statistically significant after adjusting for age, education, noise exposure, and occupation. No significant gender difference has been found in animal studies.[44] The controversy over how much noise-induced hearing loss accounts for the development of presbyacusis and for the development of presbyacusis and for the gender difference remains to be resolved.

Reported hearing disability and handicap

Pure tone audiometry gives only limited information regarding hearing disability and handicap. Listening involves many non-auditory factors, such as visual clues and mental alertness. People with an active, extrovert lifestyle place greater demands on auditory function than those with few social contacts. Other aspects of presbyacusis than measured hearing have been investigated by using instruments designed to screen hearing problems. Weinstein and Ventry[45] constructed an instrument especially designed to study the effects of presbyacusis, the Hearing Handicap Inventory for the Elderly (HHIE). This instrument has been used extensively both in the original form and in a screening version (HHIE-S). Pure tone audiometry explained less than half the variance of hearing handicap. The consequences of hearing loss are difficult to predict from the audiogram, especially if the impairment is mild, and it was

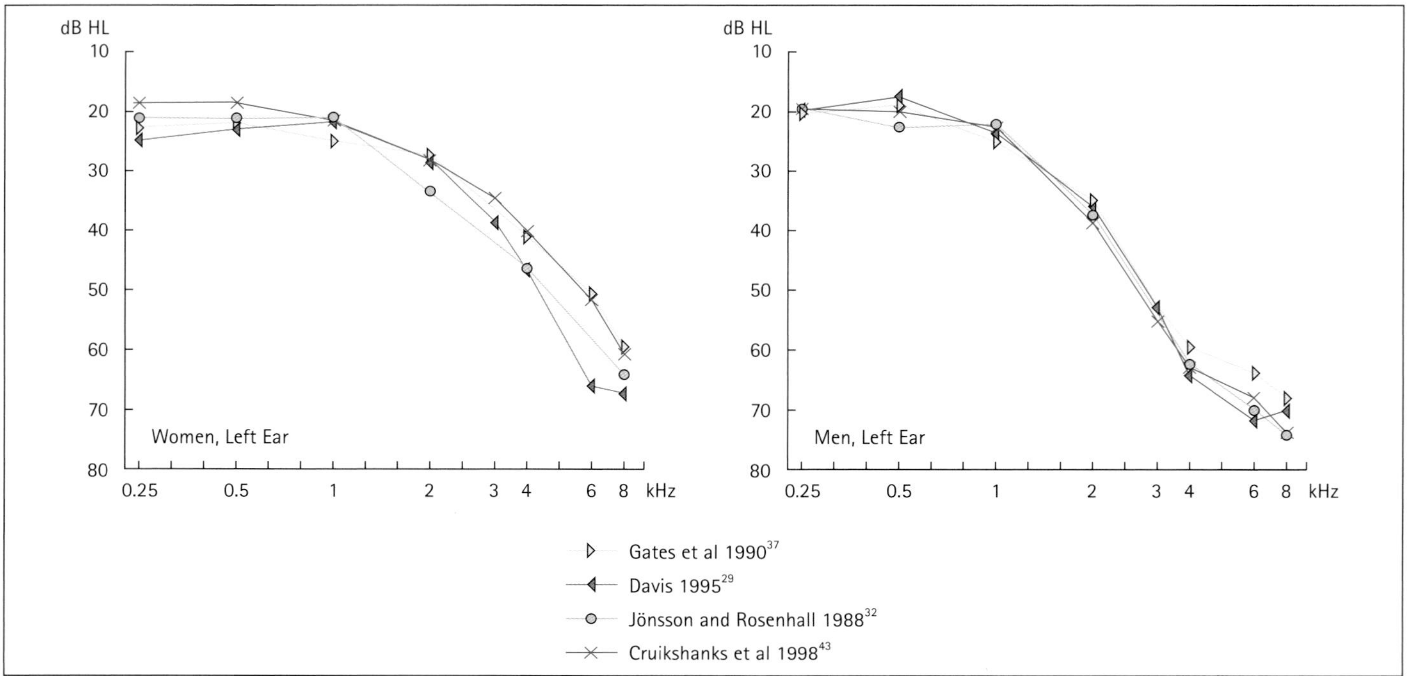

Figure 2.7. A compilation of the results of 70–80-year-old women and men, unscreened populations.[29,32,37,43] Median pure tone thresholds in dB HL at 0.25–8 kHz are presented.

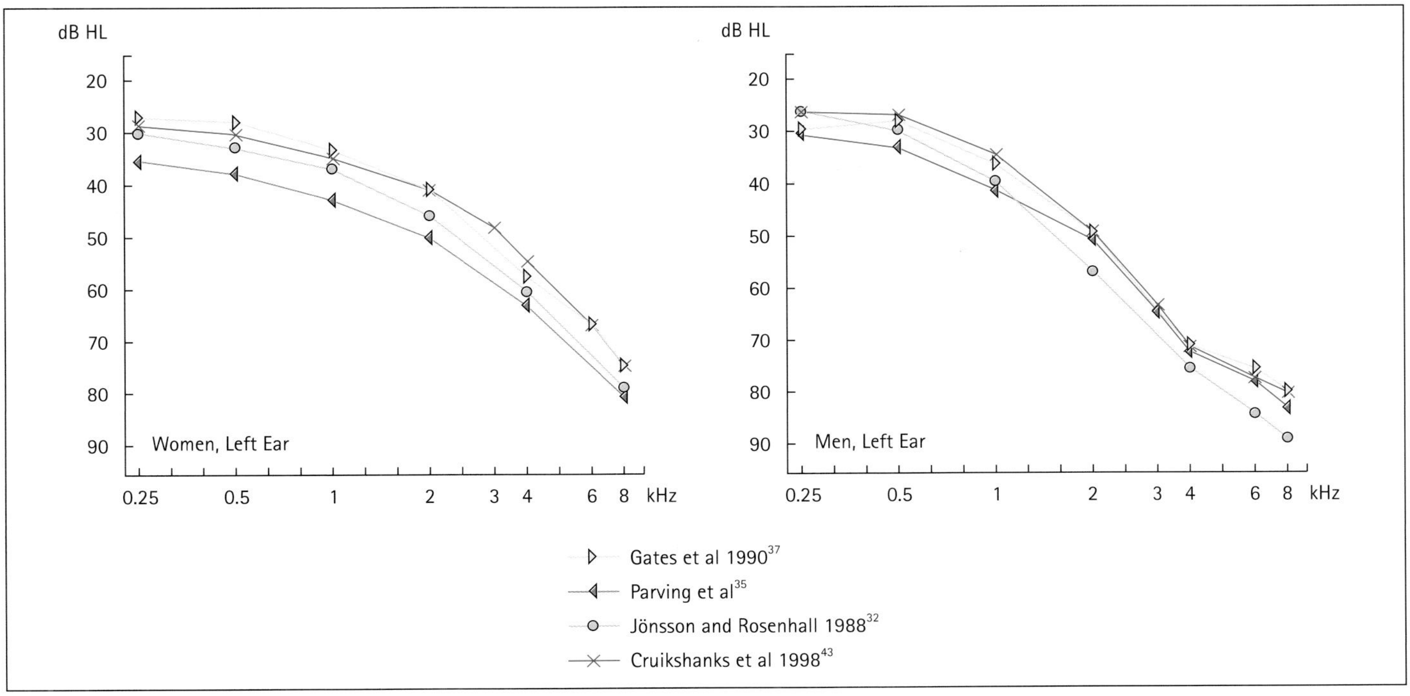

Figure 2.8. A compilation of the results of four epidemiological investigationsof 80–90-year-old persons, unscreened populations.[32,35,37,43]

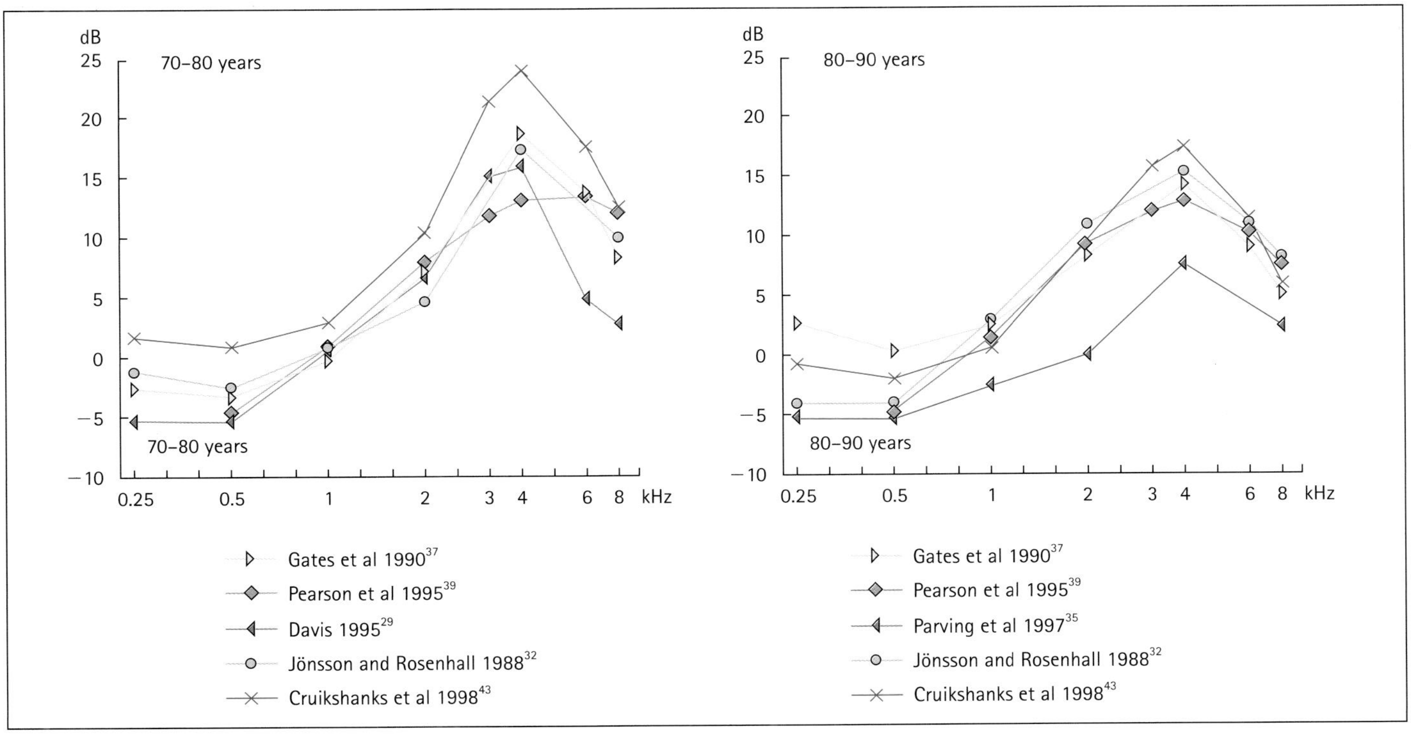

Figure 2.9. Gender differences in dB (male threshold values minus female values) for the frequencies 0.25–8 kHz. Results of six epidemiological investigations.[29,32,35,37,39,43]

suggested that self-reports would be more appropriate than measured hearing to estimate the effects of presbyacusis.[45] It has been shown that higher HHIE-S scores are related to age and measured hearing loss.[46] After adjusting for hearing loss, elderly persons tend to rate their problems as less pronounced than younger ones, especially if the hearing impairment is mild.[47–49] Jerger and Chmiel[50] reported that perceived hearing handicap emerged as a separate factor, not strongly related to either audibility, speech perception or central auditory processing.

In the MRC National Study of Hearing, the cross-sectional study of adults in Great Britain, a questionnaire was sent to a large population of adults.[28,29,51] The prevalence of persons without hearing complaints was 65%. Great difficulty in hearing in noise was reported by 44–60%, depending on the age.[51] When participants were asked about hearing difficulty in quiet, slight difficulty was reported by 14% (71–80 years) and 18% (≥80 years). Moderate difficulty was reported by 7% (71–80 years) and 10% (≥80 years). Pronounced difficulty was reported by 4% (71–80 years) and 9% (≥80 years).

In the study of Danish men with a mean age of 60 years, 64% had no complaints about their hearing capacity.[52] In the Göteborg study,[53] 1–2% of the women and about 8% of the men complained of serious hearing problems at age 70. The number of participants with subjective problems increased with age. However, at age 79, a majority of the respondents (86%) had no or only slight to moderate problems.

Aural rehabilitation in old age

Since presbyacusis is a sensorineural impairment, aural rehabilitation is the important remedy available. The basis of this rehabilitation is amplification, using hearing aids and other technical devices. Hearing aid prescription follows general principles independent of age,[54] but there are some specific comments regarding amplification in old age. Pensioners are by far the largest single recipient group of hearing aids in the developed countries. The indications for hearing aid amplification in old age can be unclear. Old persons often need extensive training to be able to appreciate a hearing aid. Since presbyacusis develops very gradually, there is a risk of development of a maladaptive coping process, dominated by avoidance of demanding communicative situations. The resulting limitations of social contacts and isolation can be avoided by a rehabilitation programme, but this is not always obvious for the hearing impaired. The 'younger' olds often have only mild hearing loss with marginal need for rehabilitation. However, when they become older and the hearing has deteriorated, many of them are debilitated by age and disease, which renders the rehabilitation difficult or even impossible. Starting a training programme relatively early pays off later on, but increases the efforts and the costs. Binaural amplification is most often superior to monaural, but for practical and economical reasons, only one hearing aid is often prescribed for elderly persons. It should, however, be noticed that pensioners also benefit from the better soundscape effects and the increased speech perception in noise obtained by binaural amplification. Assistive devices can often be recommended for the elderly. For a mildly impaired person, a simple assistive listening device might provide the necessary training up to the time when a hearing aid is needed. Signal amplifiers are examples of other unsophisticated but valuable devices.

Hearing aid fitting includes counselling in order to ensure that the device is handled properly. People with hearing impairment can be offered more extensive training programmes. Such programmes are designed very differently in different countries, e.g. as individual counselling or group training courses. The goals are to provide information about hearing impairment and the impact on activities and participation in society, to teach about hearing aids and their management, and to provide communication abilities.

HEARING REHABILITATION OF THE ELDERLY

- Hearing aid amplification
- Assistive hearing devices
- Counselling
- Training courses
- Tinnitus rehabilitation

Tinnitus

Tinnitus occurs in all age groups, and in most studies it increases, like hearing loss, with age. However, this increase with age is not as pronounced as the hearing decline caused by presbyacusis, and, according to Davis,[29] no or only little increase occurred in the total prevalence with increasing age. The total prevalence of tinnitus, both continuous and variable, has been reported as less than 20% to more than 40% in elderly people.[29,55] According to Davis,[29] no increase occurred in the total prevalence of tinnitus with increasing age. Severely annoying tinnitus was reported in 3–4%. The prevalence of tinnitus was similar between men and women in the studies cited. Tinnitus in old age is considered to have a similar aetiological background as that in younger age. A peripheral hearing loss is most often present, in old age presbyacusis, or some other type of hearing loss achieved earlier in life. A significant correlation between tinnitus and previous exposure to occupational noise has been reported by Rosenhall and Karlsson.[56]

Balance and ageing

Balance disorders are very common, and complaints of this kind increase with age.[57] Disequilibrium of ageing, sometimes called **presbybalance**, is a major problem in geriatric care. Dizziness/vertigo in the elderly often results in inactivity, and is also an important factor for fall accidents. Balance problems and falls are a common cause of morbidity and mortality in old age.[58] Prevalence figures of disequilibrium in elderly persons vary considerably. Sixt and Landahl[59] reported prevalence figures of dizziness for 75-year-olds of 30% (men), and 40% (women). Hobeika[60] found that 65% of individuals older than 60 years of age experience dizziness or loss of balance.

The equilibrium is regulated by the postural system, which gets information from three sensory systems: the vestibular, the visual and the proprioceptive. The sensory input is conveyed to different central nervous system (CNS) centres, and is integrated and stored in a memory bank. The efferent part of the postural system is mediated by the motor system to peripheral muscles for maintenance of gait and for locomotion. The vestibular apparatus consists of the semicircular system, in which cristae ampullares register angular acceleration, and the otolithic organs, which register linear acceleration, above all gravity. The vestibular input is brought via the vestibular nerve to the vestibular nuclei in the brainstem, which are in contact with different CNS centres involved in the balance system.

The morphological background of balance disorders in old age is, at least partly, similar to what has been reported in the cochlea in presbyacusis. Histopathological studies from humans and research animals have shown reductions of both vestibular hair cell populations and neurones in the vestibular nerve with age.[61,62] In the vestibular sensory epithelia, the degenerative changes are pronounced in the semicircular cristae, and, to a lesser degree, in the vestibular maculae. The vestibular hair cells show morphological changes, such as the presence of intracellular inclusions and alterations of the hair bundles.[60–62] Changes involving the otoconia have also been reported.[63] Accordingly, peripheral vestibular dysfunction is one factor responsible for disequilibrium of ageing.

MORPHOLOGICAL CHANGES IN PRESBYBALANCE

- Pronounced degeneration of cristae ampullares
- Slight to moderate degeneration of maculae
- Hair cell alterations
- Otoconial changes
- Vestibular nerve degeneration
- Degeneration of the central vestibular system

Physiological methods, measuring the peripheral vestibular function, have demonstrated declining responses with increasing age. According to Paige,[65] such age-related changes in response characteristics are similar to reported morphological deterioration of the vestibular apparatus with ageing. However, the results of peripheral vestibular tests are ambiguous: poor correlation with anatomical changes has also been reported, possibly suggesting that adaptive mechanisms in the CNS are equally important.[66]

The postural control system is very complex, and age-related changes also affect CNS functions responsible for balance regulation. One result is that central integration of postural information becomes less efficient with age.[67] The musculoskeletal system is also affected, including decreases in muscle strength and delayed motor commands, problems which result in balance impairments.[68] Numerous studies, utilizing posturographic methods, have demonstrated increased body sway in old age, especially in older subjects who complain of imbalance.[69]

AETIOLOGY OF PRESBYBALANCE

- Peripheral vestibular dysfunction
- Decline of central postural integration
- Central vestibular dysfunction
- Impaired motor control
- Overconsumption of pharmaceutical drugs

Balance problems in old age have, accordingly, a complex, often multifactorial background. One factor is the ageing process, but the resulting symptoms and signs are often vague and elusive. Peripheral vestibular disorders, e.g. BPPV (benign paroxysmal positional vertigo) and vestibular neuritis, show increasing incidence in old age. It is important to diagnose such conditions, which can be easy to treat. Central vestibular disorders must be considered, since posterior fossa stroke must be identified. In addition to decreased peripheral and central balance function in old age, ailing health and declining vision contribute to problems with the equilibrium. Overconsumption of pharmaceutical drugs is one factor that should be noted. Sedation by psychoactive drugs reduces alertness and reaction time, and increases the risk of fall accidents. Removal of unnecessary medication is therefore important. Training programmes aimed at improving the balance in old age have been devised. Postural exercises, including balance training, physical exercise, and muscular strengthening, have been demonstrated to decrease body sway and can therefore be a valuable contribution to the treatment of age-related dizziness and the prevention of fall accidents.[70]

Concluding remarks

Poor hearing and balance in old age are common problems. Age-related hearing loss is a multifactorial phenomenon and includes a variety of aetiological factors. Due to its indistinctness and the problem of defining it, age-related hearing loss can be an alternative expression. The situation is similar with presbybalance. Both conditions have often profound effects on the quality of life in old age, but in very different ways. The demands on society in terms of care are considerable. Since the number of elderly persons is increasing, the incidence of both presbyacusis and presbybalance is expected to increase in the future.

The most common audiometric configuration of age-related hearing loss is a gently sloping audiogram, above all affecting the high frequencies. Other types of auditory dysfunctions, such as noise-induced hearing loss and ototoxic hearing loss, have similar audiometric configurations. Therefore, the differentiation between presbyacusis and other lesions based on the audiogram is difficult or impossible to accomplish. Efforts to improve the auditory communication in old age are important and can be expected to result in better quality of life for elderly persons and to more efficient public expenditure. The alleviation of age-related hearing handicap includes aural rehabilitation with hearing aid fitting and training programmes. Procedures and devices especially designed for the elderly are needed. Accessibility is important. Close co-operation with general practitioners and special counsellors is important.

Hearing loss is often combined with other handicaps, such as dementia, immobility and poor vision. The synergistic effects of multiple handicaps can be pronounced. It has been reported in some studies that elderly persons in institutions have poorer hearing than those who live at home. Is this a result of ailing health, or the probability that the elderly with hearing loss develop pseudodementia, or both?

Balance disorders in old age are very often severely debilitating, and they too often result in inactivity and fall accidents, and represent thus a severe threat to health and life. It is problematic that diagnostic and treatment programmes are still so imperfect, and the demand for further research is obvious.

Prevention is an issue which is both challenging and problematic. Obviously, for hearing, the most important prevention involves noise reduction. Prevention must start early in life and not shortly before retirement. It is, however, not an easy task to change attitudes early in life for a gain decades later. Is it possible to convince young people in their twenties to avoid exposure to excessive sound, which they may not even regard as noise? Are there other preventive measures that can be of importance in the future? Diet, food additives, reduction of cardiovascular disease, and changes of life style, e.g. smoking, are possible factors. We know very little about this, and more research is needed. The possible benefits are, however, great, both in personal and economic terms.

References

1. Jerger J, Chmiel R, Stach B, Spretnjak M. Gender affects audiometric shape in presbycusis. *J Am Acad Audiol* 1993; **4**: 42–9.
2. Humes LE. Speech understanding in the elderly. *J Am Acad Audiol* 1996; **7**: 161–7.
3. Humes LE, Watson BU, Christensen LA, Cokely CG, Halling DC, Lee L. Factors associated with individual differences in clinical measures of speech recognition among the elderly. *J Speech Hear Res* 1994; **37**: 465–74.
4. Frisina DR, Frisina RD. Speech recognition in noise and presbyacusis; relations to possible neural mechanisms. *Hear Res* 1997; **106**: 95–104.
5. Gilad O, Glorig A. Presbyacusis: the aging ear. Part 1. *J Am Aud Soc* 1979; **4**: 195–206.
6. Gates GA, Couropmitree NN, Myers RH. Genetic association in age-related hearing thresholds. *Arch Otolaryngol Head Neck Surg* 1999; **125**: 654–9.
7. Bai U, Seidman MD, Hinojosa R, Quirk WS. Mitochondrial DNA deletions associated with aging and possible presbyacusis: a human archival temporal bone study. *Am J Otol* 1997; **18**: 449–53.
8. Glorig A, Nixon J. Distribution of hearing loss in various populations. *Ann Otol Rhinol Laryngol* 1960; **69**: 497–516.
9. Rosen S, Bergman M, Plester D, El-Mofty A, Satty M. Presbycusis study of a relatively noise-free population in the Sudan. *Ann Otol Rhinol Laryngol* 1962; **71**: 727–42.
10. Gates GA, Schmid P, Kujawa SG et al. Longitudinal threshold changes in older men with audiometric notches. *Hear Res* 2000; **141**: 220–8.
11. Kryter KD. Presbycusis, sociocusis and nosocusis. *J Acoust Soc Am* 1983; **73**: 1897–916.
12. Rosenhall U, Sixt E, Sundh V, Svanborg A. Correlations between presbyacusis and extrinsic noxious factors. *Audiology* 1993; **32**: 234–43
13. Gates GA, Cobb JL, D'Agostino RB, Wolf PA. The relation of hearing in the elderly to the presence of cardiovascular disease and cardiovascular risk factors. *Arch Otolaryngol Head Neck Surg* 1993; **119**: 156–61.
14. Stephens SDG. What is acquired hearing loss in the elderly? In: Glennerding F, ed. *Acquired Hearing Loss and Elderly People*. Stoke on Trent, Beth Johnson Foundation Publications; 1982: pp. 9–26.
15. Lim DP, Stephens SDG. Clinical investigation of hearing loss in the elderly. *Clin Otolaryngol* 1991; **16**: 288–93.
16. Willott JF. Anatomic and physiologic aging: a behavioural neuroscience perspective. *J Am Acad Audiol* 1996; **7**: 141–51.
17. Soucek S, Michaels L, Frohlich A. Pathological changes in the organ of Corti in presbycusis as revealed by microslicing and staining. *Acta Otolaryngol* 1987; Suppl 436: 93–102.
18. Bredberg G. Cellular pattern and nerve supply of the human organ of Corti. *Acta Otolaryngol* 1968; Suppl 236: 1–135.
19. Engström B, Hillerdal M, Laurell G. Selected pathological findings in the human cochlea. *Acta Otolaryngol* 1987, Suppl 436: 110–16.
20. Arnesen AR. Presbycusis loss of neurons in the human cochlear nuclei. *J Laryngol Otol* 1982; **96**: 503–11.
21. Kirikae I, Sato T, Shitara T. A study of hearing in advanced age. *Laryngoscope* 1964; **74**: 205–20.
22. Schuknecht H. *Pathology of the Ear*. Cambridge, Massachusetts: Harvard University Press, 1995.
23. Gates GA, Cooper JC. Incidence of hearing decline in the elderly. *Acta Otolaryngol* 1991; **111**: 240–8.
24. Suga F, Lindsay JR. Histopathological observations of presbycusis. *Ann Otol Rhinol Laryngol* 1976; **85**: 169–84.
25. Willott JF. *Aging and the Auditory System. Anatomy, Physiology, and Psychophysics*. San Diego: Singular Publishing Group, 1991.
26. Robinson D. Threshold of hearing as a function of age and sex for the typical unscreened population. *Br J Audiol* 1988; **22**: 5–20.
27. International Standards Organisation. *Acoustics – Determination of Occupational Noise Exposure and Estimation of Noise-induced Hearing Impairment* 2nd edition, Geneva, ISO, 1990.
28. Coles R, Davis A, Haggard M. Population study of hearing disorders in adults: preliminary communication. *J R Soc Med* 1981; **74**: 819–27.
29. Davis AC. *Hearing in Adults. The Prevalence and Distribution of Hearing Impairment and Reported Hearing Disability in the MRC Institute of Hearing Research's National Study of Hearing*. London: Whurr Publishers, 1995.

30. Keay D, Murray J. Hearing loss in the elderly: a 17-year longitudinal study. *Clin Otolaryngol* 1988; **13**: 31–5.
31. Pedersen KE, Rosenhall U, Møller MB. Changes in pure-tone thresholds in individuals aged 70–81: results from a longitudinal study. *Audiology* 1989; **28**: 194–204.
32. Jönsson R, Rosenhall U. Hearing in advanced age. A study of presbyacusis in 85-, 88- and 90-year-old people. *Audiology* 1998; **37**: 207–18.
33. Ostri B, Parving A. A longitudinal study of hearing impairment in male subjects — an 8-year follow-up. *Br J Audiol* 1991: **25**: 41–8.
34. Bech B, Christensen, Parving A. The Valby project: a survey of the hearing in the elderly >80 years of age provided with hearing aids. *Scand Audiol* 1996; **25**: 247–52.
35. Parving A, Biering-Sorensen M, Bech B, Christiansen B, Sorensen MS. Hearing in the elderly >80 years of age. Prevalence and sensitivity. *Scand Audiol* 1997: **26**; 99–106.
36. Moscicki E, Elkins E, Baum H, McNamara P. Hearing loss in the elderly: an epidemiologic study of the Framingham Heart Study Cohort. *Ear Hear* 1985; **6**: 184–90.
37. Gates GA, Cooper JC, Kannel WB, Miller N. Hearing in the elderly: the Framingham cohort, 1983–1985. Part 1. Basic audiometric test results. *Ear Hear* 1990; **11**: 247–56.
38. Brant LJ, Fozard JL. Age changes in pure-tone hearing thresholds in a longitudinal study of normal human hearing. *J Acoust Soc Am* 1990; **88**: 831–20.
39. Pearson J, Morrell CH, Gordon-Salant S et al. Gender differences in a longitudinal study of age-associated hearing loss. *J Acous Soc Am* 1995; **97**: 1196–205.
40. Quaranta A, Assennato G, Sallustio V. Epidemiology of hearing problems among adults in Italy. *Scand Audiol* 1996; Suppl. 42: 9–13.
41. Uimonen S, Maki-Torkko E, Jounio-Ervasti K, Sorri M. Hearing in 55 to 75 year old people in northern Finland — a comparison of two classifications of hearing impairment. *Acta Otolaryngol* 1997, Suppl 529: 69–70.
42. Rosenhall U, Jönsson R, Davis A, Parving A. Hearing in the 'oldest old' — a cross-sectional collaborative study from three European countries. *J Audiol Med.*
43. Cruickshanks KJ, Wiley TL, Tweed TS et al. Prevalence of hearing loss in older adults in Beaver Dam, Wisconsin. The epidemiology of hearing loss. *Am J Epidemiol* 1988; **148**: 879–86.
44. Hunter KP, Willott JF. Aging and and the auditory brainstem response in mice with severe or minimal presbycusis. *Hear Res* 1987; **30**: 207–18.
45. Weinstein BE, Ventry IM. Audiometric correlates of the Hearing Handicap Inventory for the Elderly. *J Speech Hear Disord* 1983; **48**: 379–84.
46. Wiley TL, Cruickshanks KJ, Nondahl DM, Tweed TS. Self-reported hearing handicap and audiometric measures in older adults. *J Am Audiol* 2000; **11**: 67–75.
47. Lutman ME. Hearing disability in the elderly. *Acta Otolaryngol* 1990; Suppl 476: 239–48.
48. Gatehouse S. Determinants of self-reported disability in older subjects. *Ear Hear* 1990; **11**: 578–658.
49. Chmiel R, Jerger J. Some factors affecting assessment of hearing handicap in the elderly. *J Am Acad Audiol* 1993; **4**: 249–57.
50. Jerger J, Chmiel R. Factor analytic structure of auditory impairment in elderly persons. *J Am Acad Audiol* 1997; **8**: 269–76.
51. Davis AC. The prevalence of hearing impairment and reported hearing disability among adults in Great Britain. *Int J Epidemiol* 1989; **18**: 911–17.
52. Parving A, Ostri B, Katholm J. Parbo J: On prediction of hearing disability. *Audiology* 1986; **25**: 129–35.
53. Rosenhall U, Pedersen K, Møller MB. Self-assessment of hearing problems in an elderly population. A longitudinal study. *Scand Audiol* 1987; **16**: 211–17.
54. Valente M (ed.). Hearing Aids: Standards, Options and Limitations. New York: Georg Thieme Verlag, 1996.
55. Axelsson A, Ringdahl A. Tinnitus — a study of its prevalence and characteristics. *Br J Audiol* 1989; **23**: 53–62.
56. Rosenhall U, Karlsson A-K. Tinnitus in old age. *Scand Audiol* 1991; **20**: 165–71.
57. Tibblin G, Bengtsson C, Furunes B, Lapidus L. Symptoms by age and sex. The population studies of men and women in Gothenburg, Sweden. *Scand J Prim Health Care* 1990; **8**: 9–17.
58. Luxon LM. Disturbance of balance in the elderly. *Br J Hosp Med* 1991; **45**: 22–6.
59. Sixt E, Landahl S. Postural disturbances in a 75–year-old population: I. Prevalence and functional consequences. *Age Ageing* 1987; **16**: 393–8.
60. Hobeika CP. Equilibrium and balance in the elderly. *Ear Nose Throat J* 1999; **78**: 558–62.
61. Engström H, Bergström B, Rosenhall U. The vestibular sensory epithelia. *Arch Otolaryngol* 1974; **100**: 411–18.
62. Park JC, Hubel SB, Woods AD. Morphometric analysis and fine structure of the vestibular epithelium of aged C57BL/6NNia mice. *Hear Res* 1987; **28**: 87–96.
63. Nakayama M, Helfert RH, Konrad HR, Caspary DM. Scanning electron microscopic evaluation of age-related changes in the rat vestibular epithelium. *Otolaryngol Head Neck Surg* 1994; **111**: 799–806.
64. Igarashi M, Saito R, Mizukoshi K, Alford BR. Otoconia in young and elderly persons: a temporal bone study. *Acta Otolaryngol* 1993; Suppl 504: 26–9.
65. Paige GD. Senescence of human visual–vestibular interactions. 1. Vestibulo-ocular reflex and adaptive plasticity with aging. *J Vestib Res* 1992; **2**: 133–51.
66. Peterka RJ, Black FO, Schoenhoff MB. Age-related changes in human vestibulo-ocular reflexes: sinusoidal rotation and caloric tests. *J Vestib Res* 1990; **1**: 49–59.
67. Perrin PP, Jeandel C, Perrin CA, Bene MC. Influence of visual control, conduction, and central integration on static and dynamic balance in healthy older adults. *Gerontology* 1997; **43**: 223–31.
68. Konrad HR, Girardi M, Helfert R. Balance and aging. *Laryngoscope* 1999; **109**: 1454–60.
69. Baloh RW, Spain S, Sochotch TM, Jacobson KM, Bell T. Posturography and balance problems in older people. *J Am Geriatr Soc* 1995; **43**: 638–44.
70. Hamman R, Longridge NS, Mekjavic I, Dickinson J. Effect of age and training schedules on balance improvement exercises using visual biofeedback. *J Otolaryngol* 1995; **24**: 221–9.

3 Pathology of the ear

Leslie Michaels

The ear is affected by a wide range of pathological conditions. Considerations of space require that the pathology of conditions dealt with by medical audiologists should be emphasized in this chapter at the expense of purely surgical ones.

Otitis media

Otitis media is one of the most common of all diseases, particularly in young children. The clinical forms of the acute and chronic conditions correspond to the pathological changes, but intermediate or mixed states are frequent. Perforation of the tympanic membrane may occur at any phase of otitis media, but an effusion is often present behind an intact tympanic membrane (see below). It is important that an advanced degree of otitis media may exist, but may remain undetected clinically and even be undetectable.

Microbiology

In the acute phase, *Streptococcus pneumoniae* and *Haemophilus influenzae* are the most common causative organisms. *Staphylococcus aureus* and *Streptococcus pyogenes* are also causative in a lesser number. Epidemiological studies have indicated that the respiratory viruses, influenza viruses A and B, enterovirus, rhinovirus, parainfluenza virus, adenovirus, and respiratory syncytial virus, may be agents in the early phases of the illness. In the chronic phase, Gram-negative organisms, particularly *Proteus* and *Pseudomonas*, are found, although *Staphylococcus pyogenes* and β-haemolytic streptococci are sometimes isolated from the discharging pus of chronically inflamed ears. Anaerobes may sometimes be isolated, including anaerobic Gram-positive cocci, *Bacteroides* spp., and *Clostridium* spp.

Although much less frequent than the above organisms, *Mycobacterium tuberculosis* may be the causative agent of chronic inflammation of the middle ear. In such cases, the inflammatory reaction is quite distinct, with giant cells, epithelioid cells and caseation.

General pathological changes

Not only is the acute phase of otitis media characterized by severe congestion of the mucosa of the middle ear and the tympanic membrane, but a similar change is also present in chronic otitis media (Table 3.1). The exudation of blood products may leave a deposit of fibrin in the tissues or in the tympanic and mastoid air cell cavities. A fluid or gelatinous exudate in the middle ear cavity is frequently a prominent component of the inflammatory reaction, giving rise to a specific form of the disease known as otitis media with effusion (serous otitis media or glue ear). In these cases, mucus may be secreted by newly formed glands in the middle ear mucosa and contribute to the fluid 'exudate'.

In acute inflammation, neutrophils are prevalent. It is likely that the immigration of these cells is mediated by the local production of cytokines, such as interleukin-1, interleukin-2, or tumor necrosis factor. In chronic inflammation, histiocytes, lymphocytes and plasma cells form the characteristic infiltrate. There is evidence that cytokine production is also present in the chronic phase of otitis media.

PATHOLOGICAL CHANGES IN CHRONIC OTITIS MEDIA

- Congestion of mucosa of middle ear
- Histiocytic, lymphocytic and plasma cell infiltration of mucosa
- Haemorrhage leading to cholesterol granuloma
- Necrosis leading to perforation of the tympanic membrane
- Erosion of ossicles and bony wall
- Glandular metaplasia
- Fibrosis: adhesive otitis
- Fibrosis: tympanosclerosis
- Cholesteatoma

Table 3.1 Pathological processes in chronic otitis media

Process	Cell or tissue	Pathological change
Congestion	Blood vessels	
Exudation	Plasma	Serous otitis media
	Histiocytes, lymphocytes, plasma cells	Chronic inflammation
	Red cells	Haemorrhage Cholesterol granuloma
Proliferation	Columnar epithelium	Glandular metaplasia with mucus secretion
	Squamous cell epithelium	Cholesteatoma
	Blood vessels, fibroblasts, mononuclear cells	Granulation tissue
	Fibroblasts, collagen	Adhesive otitis Tympanosclerosis
	Bone	Woven and lamellar bone formation
Necrosis	Tympanic membrane	Perforation
	Bone	Rarefying osteitis

In newborn infants, an inflammatory reaction may be the result of the contamination of the middle ear by inhaled amniotic squames. In these cases, the histiocytes reacting to the foreign material fuse to form giant cells.

Haemorrhage is a common result of the congestion of otitis media. It may lead to cholesterol granuloma (Figure 3.1).

Local tissue cells frequently react to the inflammatory process by dissolution or proliferation. Necrosis may occur, as is characteristic of perforation of the tympanic membrane or rarefying osteitis of the ossicles. Several factors may produce the necrosis. It is likely that rupture of the tympanic membrane takes place as a result of ischaemic necrosis caused by pressure at a focal point. Ossicular loss may, on the other hand, be caused by cytokine substances such as tumor necrosis factor-alpha.

At the same time as the process of necrosis, proliferative activity of middle ear tissue occurs and may represent an important part of the pathological picture. The columnar epithelium of the middle ear has, in the presence of inflammation, the remarkable property of invaginating itself to produce glands, which often develop luminal secretion (Figure 3.2). The glandular transformation (metaplasia) of the middle ear mucosa may be seen in any part of the cleft, including the mastoid ear cells. The secretion of the glands contributes to the exudate in otitis media with effusion. Fibrous tissue proliferation may also occur in combination with glandular transformation—a process which, in the advanced state, has been called 'fibrocystic sclerosis'. Squamous cell epithelium may likewise proliferate in the middle ear—a process known as cholesteatoma (see below). A specific form of reparative reaction following inflammation is the development of granulation tissue. In this process, the endothelium of blood vessels and fibroblasts are the newly formed cells. Mononuclear inflammatory cells usually accompany the latter. Fibroblasts and collagen are abundant in the terminal phase of the reparative stage. A normal degree of cellularity in the fibrous reaction is seen in adhesive otitis. A peculiar form of scar tissue production occurs in the middle ear, in which the collagen is poorly cellular and hyalinized. This condition, known as tympanosclerosis (Figure 3.3), is characterized also by deposition of calcium salts in the hyaline fibrous tissue. The bony walls of the middle ear frequently react to the inflam-

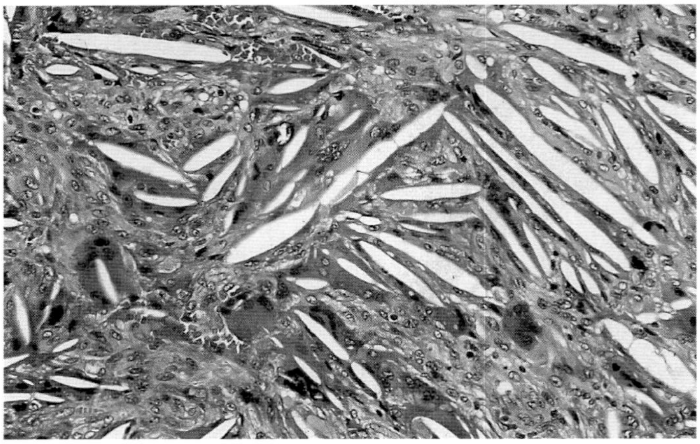

Figure 3.1 Cholesterol granuloma of the middle ear. Sheaves of elongated empty spaces are produced by crystals of cholesterol and its esters which have been dissolved in the processing of the specimen. The crystals are surrounded by foreign body giant cells.

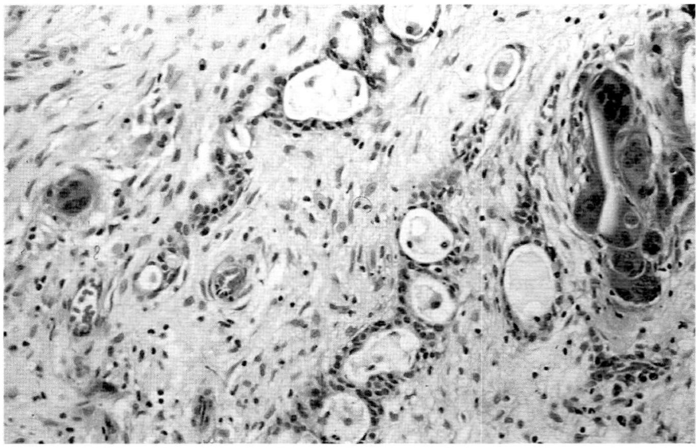

Figure 3.2 Glandular metaplasia of middle ear epithelium.

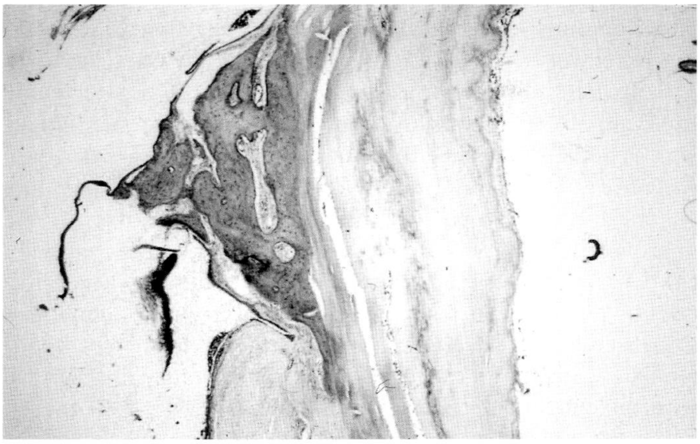

Figure 3.3 Tympanosclerosis of the middle ear. This deposit consists of collagen which is poorly cellular and hyalinized with darker areas produced by calcification. There is an area of woven bone (stained red in the original) on the left.

matory process by new formation of bone. This is woven in the early stages and lamellar later.

Cholesteatoma

Cholesteatoma is an important concomitant of many cases of chronic otitis media. It is a mass of keratin produced by a layer of stratified squamous epithelium within the middle ear cavity (Figure 3.4).

FORMS OF CHOLESTEATOMA

- Acquired—open or closed
- Congenital—open or closed

It has now become apparent that there exists a congenital or primary form of cholesteatoma, present behind an intact tympanic membrane, which is distinct from an acquired form,

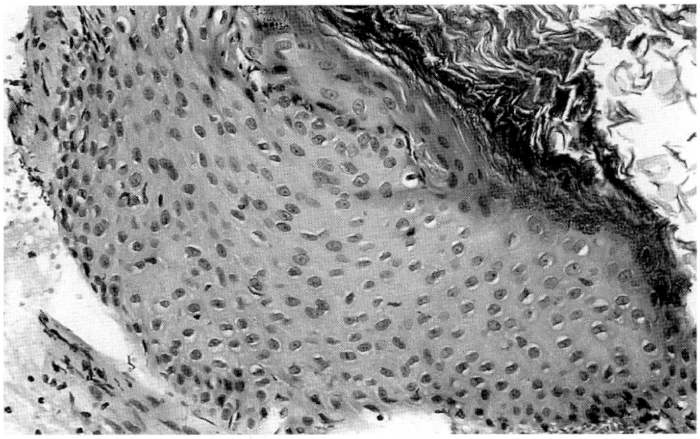

Figure 3.4 Cholesteatoma of middle ear, composed of benign stratified squamous epithelium with keratin (stained red in the original) on the surface.

in which there is a perforation of the tympanic membrane. The term congenital cholesteatoma is also applied to a squamous epithelial cyst arising at the petrous apex of the temporal bone, which causes damage by erosion of the skull. This is quite a different entity from the middle ear cholesteatoma (see below).

Both acquired and congenital cholesteatoma may take one or other of two forms: (1) a closed, keratinous cyst; or (2) an open lesion comprising multiple layers of dead keratinous squames, which is carpeted by the living epidermoid epithelium (matrix) that covers part of the middle ear surface. In most cases of acquired cholesteatoma the lesion is open. Most cases of congenital cholesteatoma, on the other hand, are described as being in the first category, presenting as a simple closed cyst.

Acquired cholesteatoma

Gross appearances

The cholesteatoma appears as a pearly grey or pale yellow cyst-like structure in the middle ear cavity. The wall of the cyst may often be seen as a thin membrane.

The cholesteatoma is usually situated in the upper posterior part of the middle ear cleft and discharges usually through a perforation of the pars flaccida of the tympanic membrane, sometimes through a perforation located at the edge of the tympanic membrane near the annulus. The cholesteatoma may extend through the aditus into the mastoid antrum and mastoid air cells. Frequently, the outline of the cholesteatomatous sac is adapted to that of normal structures such as ossicles. Chronic inflammatory changes are always present. In most cases, at least one ossicle is seriously damaged, so interrupting the continuity of the ossicular chain. The scutum, the upper part of the bony ring of the tympanic opening, is eroded in most cholesteatomas.

Microscopic appearances

Under the microscope, the pearly material of the cholesteatoma consists of dead, fully differentiated anucleate keratin squames. This is the corneal layer of the squamous cell epithelium. Sometimes, biopsy material shows only squames when the so-called capsule has not been excised. This capsule, often called the matrix, is composed of fully differentiated squamous epithelium similar to the epidermis of skin, and resting on connective tissue. As in any normal stratified epithelium, there are one to three basal layers of cells, above which is a prickle (malpighian or spinous) layer composed of five or six rows of cells with intercellular bridges. The deeper layers of the epithelium of the cholesteatoma matrix frequently show evidence of activity in the form of downgrowths into the underlying connective tissue. These often separate the cholesteatoma into lobules. A thin granular layer lies between the malpighian layer and the extensive corneal layer.

The eroded ossicles may be invested by the squamous epithelial wall of the sac. There is always, even in these circumstances, a layer of granulation tissue in contact with the bone, and it seems likely that it is the chronic inflammatory covering, not the squamous epithelium, that produces the erosion.

Pathogenesis

> **PATHOGENESIS OF ACQUIRED CHOLESTEATOMA**
>
> - Invasion of canal and tympanic membrane epidermis into the middle ear
> - Invagination of tympanic membrane as retraction pocket
> - Trauma such as blast injury or insertion of ventilation tubes into eardrum

Four concepts of the pathogenesis of acquired cholesteatoma have been put forward. It has been suggested that it may arise:

1. From invasion of canal and tympanic membrane epithelium into the middle ear.
2. From invagination of tympanic membrane in the form of a retraction pocket.
3. From metaplasia of the epithelia of the middle ear.
4. From trauma such as blast injury or insertion of ventilation tubes into the eardrum.

There is evidence to favour (1), (2) and (4), and it is likely that cholesteatoma may arise as a result of any of these three different mechanisms under different circumstances.

Congenital cholesteatoma

In contrast to acquired cholesteatoma, which has been established as a clinicopathological entity for more than a century, congenital cholesteatoma has been recognized only recently (Figure 3.5). Although not common, it is seen now with some regularity in some parts of North America, although still described as rare in other parts of the world. The mean age of presentation is 4.6 years. Many patients present with a lesion in the anterosuperior part of the middle ear. In one-quarter of patients, the cholesteatoma occupies much of the tympanic cavity. In 3% of patients, the congenital cholesteatoma is bilateral. Possible reasons for the much greater recent frequency of this entity, which was formerly considered extremely rare, are: (1) the use of the operating microscope in diagnosis; (2) the improved lighting of otoscopes by the use of the halogen bulb; (3) the screening of tympanic membranes of normal young children by paediatricians; and (4) the possibility that many cases of congenital cholesteatoma which formerly underwent 'spontaneous abortion' following acute otitis media may now survive with the cure of the otitis with antibiotics.[1]

Pathogenesis

Cell rests of epidermoid tissue have been suggested from time to time as the origin of the primary form of cholesteatoma. The discovery of a cell rest in the anterior superior part of the middle ear in 1936[2] was forgotten, but it was described again in 1986, and called the epidermoid formation (EF)[3] and confirmed in 1987[4] (Figure 3.6). It is now generally accepted that the EF is the source of congenital cholesteatoma by continuing to grow instead of disappearing, as it normally does in late development or in infancy.

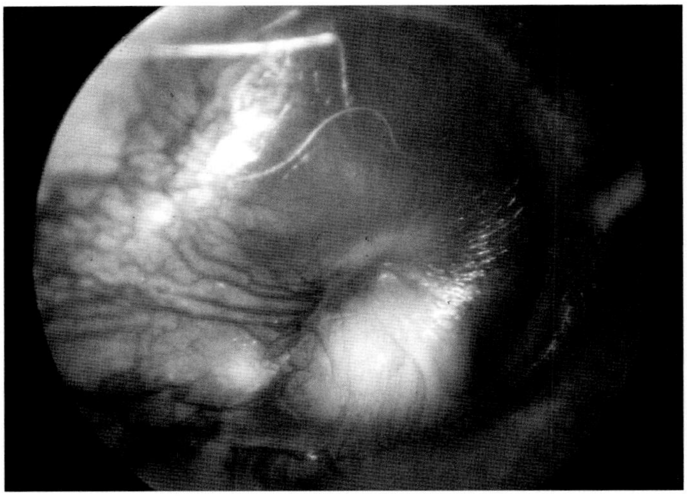

Figure 3.5 Otoscopic photograph showing tympanic membrane behind which is a congenital cholesteatoma that is situated in the anterior superior region of the middle ear.

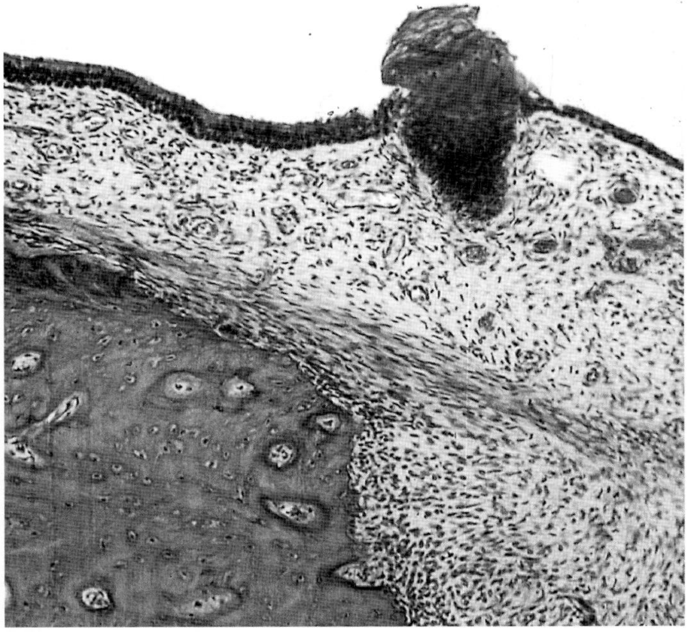

Figure 3.6 Epidermoid formation, showing a focus of stratified squamous epithelium and keratin at the junction of the columnar epithelium of the Eustachian tube (left) with that of the middle ear (right). This is found in all older fetuses and some young children.

Otitis media with effusion (OME)

Synonyms commonly in use for OME are: secretory otitis media, serous otitis media, catarrhal otitis media, tubotympanitis and glue ear. It is a very common cause of hearing loss in children characterized by an effusion behind a non-perforated eardrum in the absence of frank symptoms of acute infection. Few biopsy or temporal bone pathological studies have been described. All the features of chronic otitis may be present, including cholesterol granuloma, chronic inflammatory granulation tissue, ossicular destruction and tympanosclerosis. The most prominent feature of the histopathology in childhood OME seems to be new formation of glands in the middle ear mucosa.

OME also occurs in adults, often in association with neoplasms of the nasopharynx, probably as a result of occlusion of the distal orifice of the Eustachian tube. It is important to exclude a nasopharyngeal tumour in any adult patient presenting with OME. Histopathological examination of the middle ear mucosa in adult OME at autopsy in one study also showed such glandular metaplasia accompanying the secretion, but with more inflammatory infiltrate than in the childhood cases of OME.

Complications of otitis media

The inflammatory process may extend from the middle ear to involve adjacent structures. Inflammation of the labyrinth may occur as a result of extension of the infection through the round or oval windows. The petrous bone may become involved by spread of the inflammation through the bone marrow or air cells (see Chapter 5). Adjacent intracranial and cranial nerve structures may become inflamed by spread of the infection outside the temporal bone. Meningitis, sinus thrombophlebitis, extradural abscess or brain abscess are important possible sequelae of otitis media.

Neoplasms and similar lesions of the middle ear

The middle ear is only occasionally the site of a new growth. Because of its deep-seated position, primary malignant tumours of the middle ear do not usually manifest themselves until they are well advanced. Table 3.2 lists the developmental tumour-like anomalies and neoplasms which have been located there.

Table 3.2 Neoplasms and similar lesions of the middle ear

Developmental tumour-like anomalies
Salivary choristoma
Glial deposit
Sebaceous choristoma
Neoplasms
Primary
Adenoma
Papillary adenocarcinoma
Meningioma
Paraganglioma:
Jugular vein region origin
Tympanic cavity origin
Squamous cell carcinoma
Secondary
Metastatic neoplasms

Malformations of the middle and inner ear

Middle ear

Most of the clinically important malformations affecting the ear involve the inner ear. For convenience, a short section here describes the malformations of the middle ear. The ossicles and skeletal structure of the middle ear are formed by a complex association of the first and second branchial arches with the skull bones. The malleus is more often malformed than the stapes and incus. It may be fused with the body of the incus, or fixed to the epitympanum by bone. The incus may also be fixed to the medial wall of the epitympanum. Its long process can be short and placed in an abnormal position in the middle ear cleft. The stapes may be congenitally fixed, or the crura distorted. The stapes may show a variety of other anomalies, including complete absence. In one lesion, the anterior crus of the stapes is markedly bowed, so that the whole of it appears to be curved forwards over the promontory. Congenital dehiscence of the bony facial canal in the region of the oval window occurs frequently. Persistence of the stapedial artery and total absence of the round window are rare conditions. The whole middle ear cavity may be incompletely developed, retaining primitive mesenchyme. Anomalies of the internal and external ear are usually present in conjunction with this lesion.

Syndromes involving the middle ear

A number of congenital syndromes are seen in which middle ear lesions are combined with abnormalities elsewhere.

Treacher Collins syndrome (mandibulofacial dysostosis)

Treacher Collins syndrome is a hereditary malformation, predominantly due to abnormal development of the first branchial arch. The ossicles may be small, deformed or absent, producing mainly conductive deafness. Other anomalies of this syndrome include notching of the lower eyelids, diminished frontonasal angle, flatness of the cheeks, receding mandible, anomalies of the teeth, and deformity of the auricle. The defect is usually bilateral but may be unilateral.

Crouzon's syndrome (craniofacial dysostosis)
Crouzon's syndrome is characterized by hypertelorism, exophthalmus, optic atrophy, underdeveloped maxillae and craniosynostosis. Convulsions and dementia can also occur. Conductive deafness is due to fixation of the stapes footplate and deformed crura. The malleus and incus may also be fixed.

Hunter–Hurler syndrome (gargoylism, mucopolysaccharidosis type II)
Hunter–Hurler syndrome, an X-linked disorder, is one of the mucopolysaccharidoses, characterized by a deficiency of the lysosomal enzyme iduronate sulphatase. It produces skeletal deformity, blindness, deafness, low-set ears, mental deficiency and hepatosplenomegaly. The changes are due to the deposition of glycosaminoglycans in many tissues, particularly of the head and neck. Deafness is conductive and sensorineural. The middle ear mucosa and vestibular and spiral ganglia of the inner ear may be filled with foamy histiocytes containing one of the abnormally metabolized mucopolysaccharides in their cytoplasm ('gargoyle cells'). This material stains red by the periodic acid–Schiff reaction. An association with childhood otosclerosis has been claimed.

Klippel–Feil syndrome
Klippel–Feil syndrome consists of congenital fusion of the cervical vertebrae, causing shortening of the neck, low hair-line posteriorly and deafness. The conductive component in the deafness is due to deformed and ankylosed ossicles, and the sensorineural to a rudimentary cochlea and labyrinth.

Inner ear

Classifications

Eponymous
A classification of inner ear malformations widely used until recently was that of Ormerod[5]. Although eponymous the system was approximately based on the normal developmental processes of the inner ear. Four broad types of lesion were delineated.

> **MALFORMATION OF INNER EAR**
>
> - Morphogenetic—can be recognized by MRI and CT scan, e.g. Mondini deformity, X-linked hearing loss deformity, common cavity deformity, dilated vestibular aqueduct
> - Non-morphogenetic(>80%)—cannot be recognized by imaging methods, e.g. Scheibe's deformity

1. Michel type: complete lack of development.
2. Mondini–Alexander, more usually known as the Mondini, type: development of only a single curved tube representing the cochlea and the presence of similar immaturity of the vestibule and canals.
3. Bing-Siebenmann type: underdevelopment of the membranous labyrinth, particularly its sense organ, with a well-formed otic capsule.
4. Scheibe type: malformation restricted to organ of Corti and saccular neuroepithelium.

There are many defects not included within this classification.

A new system of malformations of the inner ear has arisen as a result of the remarkable access to inner ear structure in the living that has been provided by modern imaging techniques. The structural studies performed by meticulous use of the radiological techniques of polytomography and thin-slice high-resolution computed technology have allowed some inner ear alterations to be discerned. The availability of computerized scanning and magnetic imaging resonance scanning techniques has more recently resulted in the further description of structural anomalies. A practical approach has arisen from these now widespread facilities, whereby two broad groups of malformation are recognized[6]:

- Morphogenetic—those that can be recognized by modern imaging methods
- Non-morphogenetic—those that cannot be recognized by modern imaging methods

Extensive advances in our knowledge of malformations of the temporal bone have taken place in recent years. These have resulted not only from the use of computed tomography and magnetic nuclear resonance in the living patient, but also from the massive growth in molecular genetics that provides the blueprints for the development of most of these malformations (see below).

The classification of the morphogenetic malformations brought to light by imaging is still in a state of flux, and it must be said that knowledge is incomplete, because some of the structural changes described by imaging have not yet been confirmed or clarified by histopathological studies.

Morphogenetic malformations involve the wide range of structural abnormalities. Three of them—diminished cochlear coiling, large endolymphatic duct and sac and modiolar deficiency—have been extensively investigated by imaging methods; the observation of a 'gusher' of perilymph or a perilymphatic fistula has also been frequently found in morphogenetic malformations.

Diminished coiling of the cochlea is often detected only by the absence of the interscalar septum between the middle and apical coil, so that the upper part of the cochlea lacks a bony framework. It is associated with the classical Mondini malformation (Figure 3.7). More severe forms may be found in which the cochlea comprises a single chamber only. The severity of hearing loss in these conditions seems to reflect the severity of defective cochlear coiling.

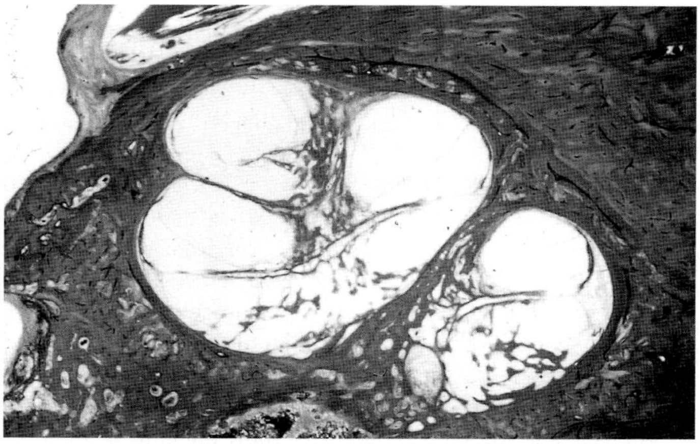

Figure 3.7 Mondini malformation of cochlea showing diminished coiling of cochlea, which normally has 2½ coils.

A dilated endolymphatic duct and sac is present in some conditions. The relationship of this change to hearing loss or vestibular symptoms is not yet understood. The classical Mondini malformation comprised both the diminution of cochlear coiling and the dilated endolymphatic duct.

Deficiency of the modiolus is an important aspect of the structural change in some malformations, because it seems to enable a direct communication between the cerebrospinal fluid (CSF)-containing subarachnoid space in the internal auditory canal and the perilymph-containing space of the scala vestibuli, which in turn communicates with the perilymph-containing space of the vestibular cavity. Thus the latter will take on the higher pressure of the CSF. When surgical entry into the vestibule from the middle ear is effected, as in the removal of an ankylosed stapes footplate or the insertion of a cochlear implant, a 'gusher' will result. This is the forcible ejection of perilymph/CSF through the opening as a result of the greater pressure of CSF in the vestibule. Another possible result of the deficiency of modiolus and the rise in perilymph pressure that this causes is the erosion of the footplate of the stapes, with the eventual production of a perilymphatic fistula from the vestibule into the middle ear through the footplate defect. Since this allows direct communication between the potentially infected middle ear space and the subarachnoid space, attacks of meningitis are likely. Treatment of this lesion to prevent further attacks of meningitis is by removal of the footplate, filling up the vestibule with muscle, and inserting a prosthesis to the incus as in otosclerosis.

Aetiology

A great deal of genetic work has been carried out to unravel the basis of malformations of the inner ear. Many of them are part of a 'disease' or 'syndrome' usually associated with other defects.

Many families of genetic non-syndromic hearing losses have also been studied and several genes located. Three recessive genes have been identified, one on chromosome 11q, one on chromosome 13q, and one on chromosome 17p. In addition, two genes causing dominant hearing impairment have been located, one on chromosome 1p and another on chromosome 5q.

The number of known genes causing hearing impairment is growing, and it is likely that many more will be unravelled in the future. The new knowledge is certain to impact on the diagnosis of disorders of hearing impairment by molecular techniques. It is probable also that this basic genetic information about hearing impairment will lead to a better understanding of the pathogenesis of malformations.

Trauma; haemorrhage; ototoxicity

Trauma

Fractures

The temporal bone is affected in the majority of fractures of the base of the skull. Although such lesions are frequent at autopsy, there has hardly been any study of fractures of the temporal bone in pathological material, and what knowledge there is has largely been derived from clinical and radiological observations.

It has been found that fractures of the petrous portion of the temporal bone fall within two anatomical groups: longitudinal and transverse. The effects on the cochlea of these two types of lesion are quite different. Longitudinal fractures arise as a result of direct blows to the temporal and parietal areas of the head. The fracture line starts in the squamous portion of the temporal bone, usually involves the external auditory canal, the tympanic membrane and one or more of the ossicles of the middle ear, and ends in the region of the foramen lacerum near the apex of the petrous temporal bone. The cochlea is spared. Transverse fractures are caused by blows to the front or back of the skull, producing a sideways tearing effect. The fracture line in these cases passes from the dural membrane on the posteromedial aspect of the petrous temporal, often through the internal auditory meatus to involve the seventh and eighth cranial nerves, and then into the cochlea in the region of the basal turn at its posterolateral side. The adjacent vestibule and round and oval windows are also frequently damaged. Thus, in the case of a longitudinal fracture, the hearing loss is usually mild or moderate and of the conductive type, which may be helped by surgery. By contrast, a transverse fracture, involving as it does both the sensory organ and the afferent nerve derived from it, produces severe sensorineural deafness in which little improvement is to be expected. A further serious side-effect of transverse fractures is the result of their establishing a communication between the meninges and the middle ear, so that there may be a leak of CSF which invariably leads to infection spreading to the meninges. This may cause death if not controlled by antibiotic therapy. Another form of fluid leakage in transverse fractures, that of perilymph, may be associated with symptoms like those of Menière's disease. The pathological changes in these cases come about from the lowering of perilymph pressure with secondary endolymphatic hydrops.

Reissner's membrane is seen to be grossly distended throughout the cochlear duct, and the saccule may be dilated.

In the temporal bone, callus does not form; the union of the two fractured portions is by fibrous tissue, not bone. This type of fracture healing seems to be general in skull fractures and may be related to the immobility of these affected bones.

Small fractures, which may or may not be united by fibrous tissue, are often found in sections of temporal bone at postmortem in cases with no history of trauma and no symptoms related to the bone damage, which is usually insignificant. These fractures are found most frequently between the vestibule or cochlea and the middle ear. Their pathogenesis is uncertain, but it is likely that they are produced at autopsy during removal of the temporal bone.

Microscopic cochlear damage in head injury

After a head injury, a sensorineural type of deafness may develop without any detectable macroscopic damage to the cochlea. The hearing loss is in the higher frequency ranges from 3000 to 8000 Hz. Experimental studies have revealed microscopic cochlear damage following direct head injury. A constant change was found to be a loss of outer hair cells in the upper basal coil region. In some animals, damage was more marked, and in a few there was a complete disappearance of internal and external hair cells in some areas. Nerve fibres and ganglion cells were correspondingly reduced in these areas.

Blast and gunshot injury

Peripheral damage to the ear, particularly rupture of the tympanic membrane, is the most striking result of explosive blast and gunshot injury; however, permanent damage to the internal ear and its hearing mechanism is also a likely sequel. The effects of blast and gunshot injury fall initially on the outer hair cells of the basal coil. When this type of trauma is particularly severe, outer hair cells in long stretches of the cochlea may be destroyed, and the supporting cells in these areas may become disrupted.

Sound-wave injury

Sound waves of high intensity damage the cochlea. Again, on pathological examination there is destruction of hair cells. The earliest changes affect isolated outer hair cells. As the intensity of the sound is increased, large groups of outer hair cells perish, and their supporting cells are lost with them. The basal coil is once more the main centre for outer hair cell loss. These findings have been obtained mainly in animal experiments, but there is a little material from human pathology replicating the same pattern of injury.

'Stimulation deafness'

The changes in the inner ear following the trauma of direct blows to the head, of explosive blasts and of high-intensity sound waves, which together produce a condition that may be designated as 'stimulation' deafness, all seem to be directed particularly to the outer hair cells of the basal coil. Inner hair cells and higher cochlear coils may be affected by greater degrees of these insults to the inner ear. Although there have been a number of studies of stimulation deafness to determine its pathogenesis, the mechanism of hair cell damage is not understood.

Haemorrhage

Haemorrhage into the cochlea may occur from trauma to the temporal bone, as a result of a blood dyscrasia, or blood may enter the cochlea or vestibule from haemorrhage into a neighbouring structure. There is experimental evidence that blood may enter the scala tympani from haemorrhage in the subarachnoid space through the cochlear aqueduct. There seems indeed to be a flow of this blood from the scala tympani of the basal coil upwards to the apex, following which it may move into the scala vestibuli.[7] Following intracranial operations or other causes of intracranial haemorrhage, such as ruptured aneurysm of the circle of Willis or intracerebral haemorrhage caused by blood dyscrasias such as thrombocytopenic purpura, blood can spread into the perilymphatic spaces of the inner ear through the cochlear aqueduct by that mechanism.

Fibrosis of the blood remaining in the cochlear or vestibular spaces after haemorrhage has been observed after surgery for vestibular schwannoma or craniotomy and following haemorrhage caused by leukaemia. The fibrosis may be seen as a fine web of fibroblasts across the cavity of the scala tympani or the perilymph space of a semicircular canal. Residua of the haemorrhage in the form of red blood cells may be seen in the fibrous web (Figure 3.8).

Haemorrhage in the inner ear in very low birthweight infants

Attention has been drawn to the possibility that haemorrhage into the cochlea around the time of birth may be a cause of deafness. The haemorrhage in these cases is probably the result of anoxia, like the frequently concomitant intracranial haemorrhage of the newborn, especially if premature. Thus haemorrhage into the inner ear is common in very low birthweight

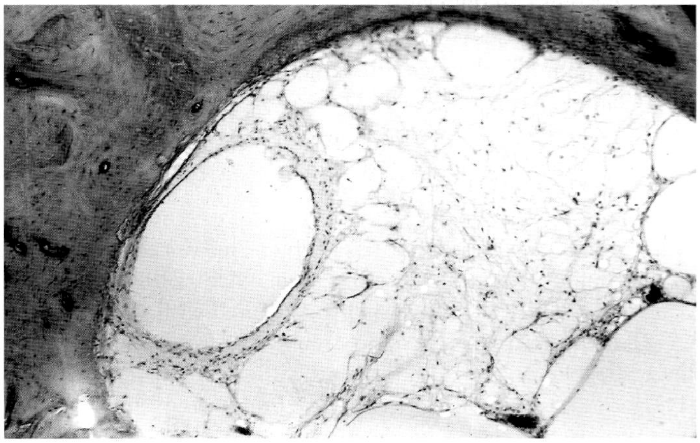

Figure 3.8 Fibrosis of the lateral semicircular canal following haemorrhage.

infants, but evidence is still lacking that this may have any connection with the sensorineural hearing loss that these infants suffer.

Sensorineural hearing loss in very low birthweight infants

Very low birthweight infants are known to be at an increased risk of sensorineural hearing loss. There have been few postmortem studies on those infants who do not survive to ascertain the possible pathological basis for the hearing loss. In cases of neonatal hyperbilirubinaemia, it is well known that the cochlear nucleus may be damaged by the toxic effect of unconjugated bilirubin. The use of anti-D prophylaxis has greatly reduced the incidence of this complication, however.

There is growing evidence of the existence of a form of hair cell damage in preterm infants characterized by inner hair cell loss unaccompanied by outer hair cell loss.[8] This would give rise to a form of hearing loss which would not be associated with loss of otoacoustical emissions, although brainstem-evoked responses would be absent. Accordingly, newborn infants affected by this condition would not be detected by those forms of screening for congenital hearing loss which rely on otoacoustical emissions only in the first instance.

Ototoxic damage to the inner ear

Ototoxic injury to the inner ear has been observed with a variety of drugs. There are five classes of substances the ototoxicity of which has been carefully investigated clinically and experimentally, because they are so frequently used in practice: (1) aminoglycoside antibiotics; (2) loop diuretics; (3) salicylates; (4) quinine; and (5) cytotoxic drugs used in the treatment of malignant disease.

> **LABYRINTHINE PATHOLOGY IN OTOTOXIC DAMAGE TO THE INNER EAR**
>
> - Aminoglycoside antibiotics—cochlear and vestibular hair cell damage
> - Loop diuretics—damage to stria vascularis followed by hair cell damage in cochlea and vestibule
> - Salicylates—unknown
> - Quinine—degeneration of the organ of Corti, particularly in the basal coil, of cochlear nerves and of stria vascularis
> - Cisplatin used in the treatment of malignant disease—degenerative changes in cochlear hair cells, maculae and cristae, and stria vascularis, and decrease in spiral ganglion cells of upper coils

Aminoglycoside antibiotics

Aminoglycoside antibiotics are in common clinical use in the treatment of a variety of infections. The following members of this group have all been found to be associated with ototoxic effects on the inner ear: streptomycin, kanamycin, gentamycin, tobramycin, viomycin and amikacin.

The aminoglycosides produce toxic effects on the renal tubules as well as the inner ear. Excretion is mainly by glomerular filtration. Disturbance of renal function may lead to impaired excretion of the drug. The raised blood levels so produced will increase the tendency for the drug to cause ototoxicity. It would seem from numerous animal studies that the ototoxicity of aminoglycosides is the result of a direct effect of the drug on the sensory cells of the cochlea and vestibule. To reach these cells, it is likely that there is passage from the bloodstream into the endolymph via the stria vascularis or spiral lamina. High levels of streptomycin in the subarachnoid space were noted during the early days of therapy for tuberculous meningitis to be particularly likely to result in ototoxicity. This suggests that there is transport of the substance to the perilymph via the cochlear aqueduct in such cases.

Clinical investigations and postmortem studies indicate that aminoglycosides do damage hair cells, particularly the outer hair cells of the basal coil of the cochlea and also those of some vestibular structures. It is also possible that the ganglion cell loss is a late manifestation of ototoxic change.

Loop diuretics

Ethacrynic acid, a loop diuretic, has been associated with ototoxicity. In laboratory animals the first sign of cochlear damage is in the stria vascularis. Later the hair cells of cochlea and vestibular structures are affected. In humans the clinical effects of ototoxicity of ethacrynic acid, like those of aminoglycosides, are both hearing loss and vestibular disturbance. Vestibular pathological changes are reported as well as cochlear hair cell damage.

Salicylates

The ototoxic effect of salicylates is well known in clinical practice, but no morphological changes have been noted in experimental animals in cochlear or vestibular structures after salicylate overdose.

Quinine

Sensorineural hearing loss of temporary duration with smaller doses, but permanent with heavier doses, is an important complication of treatment with quinine, the first and oldest drug known to cause deafness. In experimental animals, severe degeneration of the organ of Corti, particularly in the basal coil, of cochlear nerves and of the stria vascularis has been observed.

Cytotoxic drugs

Cisplatin (*cis*-platinum; *cis*-dichlorodiammineplatinum) is a cytotoxic drug which is frequently used in the treatment of advanced malignant disease. Ototoxicity is an established side-effect of the use of this drug, and the hearing of the patient is tested routinely to monitor its dosage. Degenerative changes in cochlear hair cells, severe degeneration of the maculae and cristae, degeneration of the stria vascularis and a significant decrease in spiral ganglion cells predominantly in the upper turns have been reported.

Infections of the inner ear

Infection of the inner ear may be produced by viruses, bacteria, treponemes or fungi.

Viral infections

Four viral infections which infect the labyrinth are thought to reach it by the bloodstream: cytomegalovirus infection, measles, mumps and rubella. Another infecting virus, that of herpes zoster oticus (the varicella zoster virus), enters the inner ear along the seventh and eighth cranial nerves.

Cytomegalovirus (CMV) infection

Cytomegaloviruses are DNA-containing members of the herpesvirus group. General infection is frequent, an intra-uterine source often being incriminated.

The developing human ear has been thought to be particularly susceptible to CMV infection, and the virus has been incriminated on clinical and virological grounds as the most common cause of congenital hearing loss.[9] CMV inclusion-bearing cells are present in the endolabyrinth (Figure 3.9). All cases have generalized cytomegalic inclusion disease.

CMV infection is commonly seen in patients with AIDS. Thirty-nine per cent of patients with AIDS are found to have a hearing loss of the sensorineural type. At autopsy, inclusions are found in the vestibular nerve in the internal canal, in the stria and in the saccule, utricle and lateral semicircular duct. It is likely, therefore, that the hearing loss in patients with AIDS is due to cochlear CMV infection.[10]

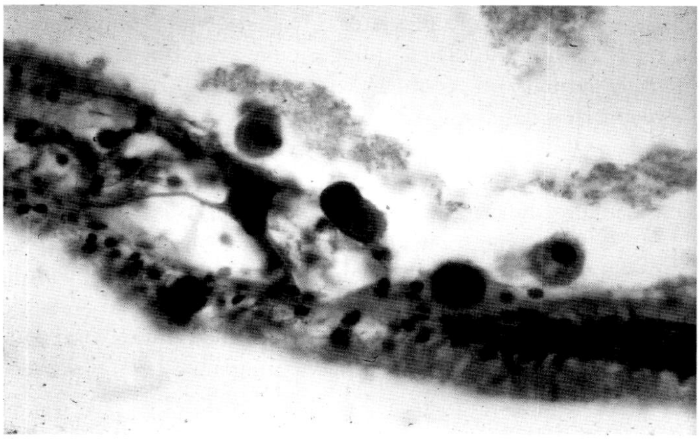

Figure 3.9 Cytomegalic inclusion disease of the cochlear region of the membranous labyrinth. Cells infected with the virus are seen with a darkly staining inclusion of the nucleus surrounded by a pale-staining halo.

Rubella

Maternal rubella is an important factor in the genesis of congenital sensorineural hearing loss. The virus is of the RNA type. There is partial collapse of Reissner's membrane, with adherence to the stria vascularis and organ of Corti. The tectorial membrane is rolled up. The stria vascularis is usually atrophic, often with cystic areas, and there may be inflammatory collections at the upper end, near the junction with Reissner's membrane and adherent to it.

Herpes zoster

In herpes zoster auris (Ramsay Hunt syndrome), the virus (the DNA herpes varicella virus) enters the inner ear along the seventh and eighth cranial nerves, presumably from nerve ganglia, where it lies dormant until a change in the immunological status of the patient. There are extensive lymphocytic infiltrates in the nerves, modiolus and skin of the external auditory meatus. Herpes varicella-zoster viral DNA has been identified, using the polymerase chain reaction, in archival celloidin-embedded temporal bone sections from two patients who clinically had Ramsay Hunt syndrome (herpes zoster oticus).[11]

Bell's palsy

A condition possibly due to viral infection in the inner ear is that of Bell's palsy, which is manifested clinically as a peripheral facial paralysis. There is pathological support for the suggestion that this condition is the result of infection with herpes simplex virus, type 1.[12] Histological findings are those of a geniculate ganglionitis. The genu region there shows constriction of the facial nerve by inflammatory tissue, which forms a sheath around it and encroaches on its interior. The adjacent bone shows foci of resorption with abundant osteoclasts. The geniculate ganglion is infiltrated by lymphocytes. The descending part of the facial nerve presents swelling and vacuolation of myelin sheaths, with some loss of axis cylinders.

Bacterial infections

Petrositis

Bacterial infections of the inner ear may involve both the petrous bone itself and the labyrinthine structures within it. Bacterial infection of the petrous bone is frequently derived by extension from middle ear infection. There are four possible routes by which infection may extend from the middle ear into the petrous bone:

1. Via air cells. Mastoid air cells frequently extend in the temporal bone as far as the apical region. It is possible, therefore, that infection to the petrous apex may extend from the middle ear by the medium of infection of air cells.
2. As direct spread of the inflammatory process by bone necrosis (osteitis).

3. By extension through the bone marrow of the petrous bone (osteomyelitis).
4. Along vessels and nerves.

In addition to inflammatory infiltration, the pathological process of petrositis comprises three main changes in the bone tissue, all of which may be seen simultaneously: (1) bone necrosis; (2) bone erosion; and (3) new bone formation. It should be noted that these three processes are frequently seen in the bony wall of the middle ear in many cases of otitis media in which extensive petrositis has not taken place. The inflammatory changes which accompany the bony ones may be 'acute', i.e. with an exudate largely of neutrophils, or 'chronic', i.e. with lymphocytes, plasma cells, histiocytes and fibroblasts forming fibrous tissue. These two forms of inflammatory infiltrate are often found in the same ear in the very variegated pathological picture of otitis media when the whole temporal bone is examined in sections.

Petrositis is of great importance, because involvement of the labyrinth, nerves, artery, veins, meninges and cerebral tissue embedded in and surrounding the petrous bone may each cause serious symptoms, and perhaps death:

- Extension to the labyrinth may lead to labyrinthitis with destruction of the organs of hearing and balance.
- Important nerves may be damaged. The facial nerve is at risk early. Involvement of the trigeminal ganglion and the sixth cranial nerve leads to 'Gradenigo's syndrome'. Extension to the jugular foramen region by the inflammatory process may cause palsy of the ninth, tenth and eleventh cranial nerves ('jugular foramen syndrome').
- The wall of the internal carotid artery may become inflamed, and this may lead to thrombosis of the vessel.
- Similarly, the lateral sinus may become thrombosed, and this and/or extension of the thrombus to the superior sagittal sinus may be associated with the somewhat arcane syndrome of otitic hydrocephalus.
- Spread of the infection to the immediately adjacent cranial structures will lead to meningitis and cerebral abscess.

It should be pointed out that patients with diabetes mellitus are especially prone to develop an extension of otitis media as outlined above. A concept of 'malignant otitis externa' has developed with regard to diabetics in whom, because of the presence of external otitis which frequently coexists with otitis media, it is postulated that the infection (usually by *Pseudomonas aeruginosa*) spreads from the ear canal to the petrous apex under the temporal bone. It is likely that spread of infection in these cases is from severe otitis media with osteomyelitis of the adjacent bone.

Labyrinthitis

Infection of the membranous labyrinth may result from otitis media or from meningitis.

> **ORIGINS OF LABYRINTHITIS**
>
> - Otitic—spread of bacteria by penetration of the oval or round window, rupture of infected air cells into the labyrinthine system, or development of a fistula between the middle ear and the labyrinth (usually in the lateral semicircular canal by cholesteatoma)
> - Meningitic—spread of bacteria from the infected meninges through both the cochlear modiolus and cochlear aqueduct

Otitic

The source of labyrinthitis is, in many instances, otitis media, as with petrositis. Infection may enter the labyrinth by penetrating the oval or the round window. An infected air cell may rupture into the labyrinthine system at some point of its complex periphery. Occasionally, damage to bone by the inflammation may produce a fistula between the middle ear and the labyrinth, usually in the lateral semicircular canal, because this is the nearest vulnerable point to the middle ear. The latter complication takes place in most cases when a cholesteatoma is present, which has the effect of stimulating the inflammatory process.

Meningitic

There is another possible source of infection of the labyrinth—the meninges—and the two ducts that join them, the cochlear aqueduct and the internal auditory meatus, may convey infection from meningitic lesions into the labyrinth. Sensorineural hearing loss is an important sequel of acute bacterial meningitis. It seems likely that the origin of the hearing loss is labyrinthitis produced by the spread of bacteria from the infected meninges through both the cochlear modiolus and cochlear aqueduct.[13] Spiral ganglion cells may be severely degenerated, suggesting that subsequent cochlear implantation may not be successful in this type of labyrinthitis.

In suppurative labyrinthitis, the perilymph spaces usually display a massive exudate of neutrophils. If the process extends to the endolymphatic spaces, there is concomitant destruction of membranous structures and irreparable damage to sensory epithelia.

Healing is at first by fibrosis, but later, osseous repair is frequent, leading to a condition of 'labyrinthitis ossificans'. In this condition, the spaces of the bony labyrinth are filled in by newly formed bone, which appears in striking contrast to the normal bone surrounding the bony labyrinth.

Syphilis

Syphilis has not been fully eradicated by penicillin treatment. Sensorineural hearing loss is common in all forms of acquired syphilis. In secondary syphilis, the pathological changes of the labyrinth seem to be part of lymphocytic meningitis. In tertiary syphilis, the pathological changes are similar to those of late congenital syphilis described below. Hearing loss is also an important feature of congenital syphilis, forming one of the constituents of Hutchinson's triad (interstitial keratitis, deformed incisor teeth and deafness). More than one-third of patients with congenital syphilis develop deafness. In infantile congenital syphilis, the labyrinthine symptoms represent an insignificant aspect of a widespread and often fatal illness.

Late congenital syphilis

The lesions of congenital syphilis assume two forms: (1) gummatous involvement of bone marrow and periosteum; and (2) diffuse periostitis. Fibrosis is a prominent component of the lesion. Also, new bone formation, both lamellar and woven, contributes to the complex appearances of the pathology of syphilitic osteitis.

There is frequently a process of hydrops identical in appearance to that seen in Menière's disease.

Mycotic infections

Fungal infections of the inner ear are rare. Cryptococcosis is a fungal infection which usually infects the meninges, but progression to the labyrinth may complicate the meningitis, particularly in cases of AIDS.

Menière's disease: hydrops and its causes

LABYRINTHINE HYDROPS

- Causes: inflammatory or neoplastic involvement of the perilymphatic spaces.
  Unknown—Ménière's disease
- Pathology
  Bulging of Reissner's membrane
  Swelling of saccule
  Rupture of Reissner's and other membranes
  Fibrosis in scala vestibuli and in vestibule
  Obstruction of endolymphatic duct by fibrosis etc. in some cases
  Changes in sensory epithelia—late

Menière's disease is an affection of both the hearing and balance organs of the inner ear, characterized by episodes of vertigo, hearing loss and tinnitus. Its pathological basis is 'hydrops' i.e. distension of the endolymphatic spaces of the labyrinth by fluid. The cause of the hydrops in Menière's disease is unknown (Figure 3.10). There are, however, other diseases of known aetiology in which hydrops may be present as a complication. The common feature of these conditions is the presence of inflammatory or neoplastic involvement of the perilymphatic spaces. Thus otitis media complicated by perilymphatic labyrinthitis, syphilitic involvement of the labyrinth, leukaemic deposits in the perilymph spaces or vestibular schwannoma may be associated with hydrops.

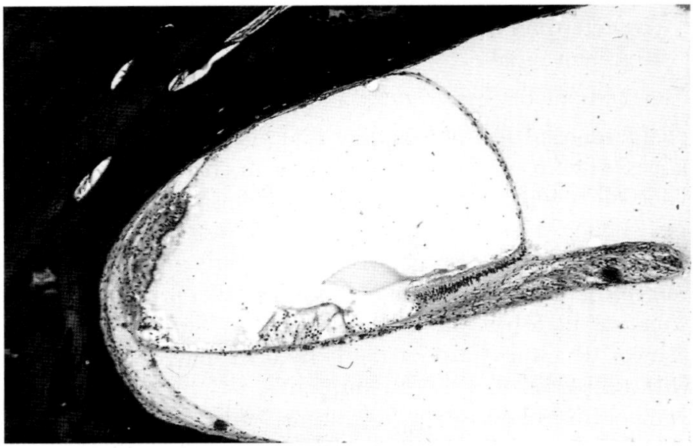

Figure 3.10 Hydrops involving the cochlea. Reissner's membrane is distended to such a degree that it reaches the top of the scala vestibuli.

Idiopathic endolymphatic hydrops may be present in patients who do not have the clinical symptoms of Menière's disease.[14,15] The patients who have Menière's symptoms seem to show a more severe degree of hydrops and a greater number of membrane ruptures than those without.

Pathological appearances

The hydrops of Menière's disease may affect one or both inner ears. In most cases, the cochlear duct and saccule are involved, but the utricle and semicircular ducts are usually not. In some cases, the cochlear duct alone is hydropic. A rare and debatable form of Menière's disease is thought to affect the vestibule, but not the cochlea. Symptoms are those of vertigo, but not hearing loss. Another rare syndrome—Lermoyez's syndrome—in which tinnitus and hearing loss precede an attack of vertigo has been associated with endolymphatic hydrops limited to the basal turn of the cochlea and the saccule.[16] In the hydropic cochlear duct, Reissner's membrane, which is elastic, shows a variable degree of bulging. In the most severe cases, the membrane reaches the top of the scala vestibuli and may be in contact with a wide area of the cochlear wall. In the apical region, it may bulge to such an extent that it fills the helicotrema. In this way, the distended scala media may even enter the scala tympani. The saccule swells up from its position on the medial wall of the vestibule and frequently touches the vestibular surface of the footplate of the stapes. The utricle may be compressed in the process. In some cases, the swollen saccule may herniate from the vestibule into the semicircular canals. Less frequently, the utricle may be distended, sometimes with small infoldings producing a scalloped appearance.

Changes in the walls of the membranous labyrinth

Changes may be seen in the thin distended membranes of the hydropic endolymphatic spaces. Ruptures may be present, particularly in Reissner's membrane, and the terminal end of the ruptured membrane may be curled up. Such ruptures have been incriminated as possible pathological bases of the fluctuations in pure tone thresholds which patients with Menière's disease may suffer. It has been suggested that the flooding of the perilymph with endolymph with its high potassium level may inhibit the bioelectric activity of the cochlea. It is likely, however, that many of these ruptures are artefactual. Fibrous tissue may be present in cases of Menière's hydrops external to the endolymphatic space in the scala vestibuli and in the vestibule deep to the footplate of the stapes. It is possible that the foci of connective tissue in these two situations are reactions to the irritation produced by repeated distension and subsidence of the adjacent cochlear duct and saccule respectively.

Changes in vestibular aqueduct and endolymphatic duct

While hydrops involving the scala media and saccule is accepted by all as a basic feature of the pathology of Menière's disease, there is no such unanimity with regard to the alterations in the endolymphatic duct and its surrounding vestibular aqueduct. There have been many descriptions of obstructive or potentially obstructive lesions of these structures associated with Menière's disease, whereby restriction of the flow of endolymph may have caused the hydrops. The most frequent of such lesions is fibrosis. In contrast to these observations, it must be pointed out that some careful studies of Menière's hydropic temporal bones have shown no changes whatever in the endolymphatic duct or vestibular aqueduct.

Changes in the sensory epithelia of the labyrinth

Alterations of the sensory cells of the organ of Corti have been described in Menière's disease, but it is still not clear whether these changes actually exist in the living patient or whether they are the result of postmortem autolysis or even the effects of acid used in decalcification of the temporal bone. The possibility that some of the changes may be artefactual has been ignored in some reports. Changes in the hair cells, particularly in the apical region, have been described and associated with low-frequency hearing loss. Atrophy of the macula of the saccule may also be found, and does not appear to be artefactual.

Relationship of symptoms to pathological changes

Image analysis of the areas in histological section of the cochlear duct (corresponding to volume in the whole structure) has been carried out in two studies and related to the hearing loss. In one study,[17] the area of the cochlear duct was significantly increased in relation to the degree of hearing loss. Losses of over 70dB showed a particularly high degree of hydropic expansion. In another study,[18] a similar relationship was found between cochlear duct size and the total average hearing loss. There was also a correlation of those dimensions with the duration of the disease: the longer the history of symptoms, the more pronounced the cochlear duct dilatation. A relationship also seemed to be present between (1) the amount of dilatation of vestibular structures, and (2) the response to caloric tests and the presence of positional nystagmus, but this was less definite than the cochlear duct–hearing loss association.

Pathology of the vestibular system

Malformations

A wide variety of malformations may affect the vestibular structures and semicircular canals (see above).

Ageing changes

Changes comparable to those in the cochlea in presbyacusis (see below) have been described for the vestibular structures. With advancing age there is degeneration of the saccular macula and, to a lesser degree, of the utricular macula. Type 1 cells are more prone to disappear than type 2 cells. These changes are accompanied by a loss of otoconia.[19] Epithelial cysts have also been seen in the sensory epithelium of the posterior and superior ampullary cristae in advanced old age. There does not appear to be a reduction of vestibular ganglion cell numbers in old age comparable to that seen in the spiral ganglion.

Trauma

Fractures may involve the vestibular system. Surgical operations may be complicated by accidental penetration of the vestibule or semicircular canals. The production of a fistula from the lateral semicircular canal, by design, into the middle ear was part of the now-abandoned operation of fenestration for otosclerosis. This procedure was replaced by stapedectomy; a fistula may occur from the vestibule into the middle ear as a complication of this operation.

Ototoxicity

Part of the damage produced by aminoglycoside antibiotics such as gentamicin may be to the sensory epithelium of the cristae and maculae.

Virus infection

In measles, rubella and cytomegalovirus infection changes have been observed in the utricle and saccule.

Bacterial infection

Bacterial infection may involve the vestibular system as part of labyrinthitis. In most bacterial infections, spread occurs from the middle ear via the oval window. A direct fistula resulting from the bone erosion of otitis media may take place, leading into the lateral semicircular canal, particularly in the presence of cholesteatoma.

Syphilis

The diffuse periostitic form of syphilis has a special tendency to involve the semicircular canals, and the lumina of the canals may be completely obliterated by bone and fibrous tissue.

Bone diseases

Paget's disease frequently involves the bony vestibule and semicircular canals to a severe degree, and as a result clinical symptoms referable to this system are likely to occur. Otosclerosis, although frequently present in relation to the bony wall of the vestibule, rarely involves the membranous structures of the vestibular system, so that vestibular symptoms are rare in this condition.

Hydrops

Hydrops of the saccule, which sometimes extends to the utricle, is the major pathological feature of Menière's disease (see above). Saccular hydrops may also be a manifestation of syphilitic and bacterial inflammation involving the labyrinth.

Atelectasis

A process of collapse of the walls of the ampullae and utricle termed 'vestibular atelectasis' has been described, but not yet confirmed.[20]

Positional vertigo

Positional vertigo is a condition in which vertigo is induced in the patient by alteration in the position of the head. Since nystagmus is used clinically as an objective test of this condition, the term 'positional nystagmus' is often preferred. It has been suggested that the deposition of a basophilically stained homogeneous deposit on the cupula of the posterior semicircular canal (the lowest region of the labyrinthine sensory epithelium) derived by gravitational descent from the otoconia of the utricle, a process known as cupulolithiasis, may explain the symptomatology of this condition.[21]

Neoplasms

The most important neoplasm of the vestibular system is schwannoma of the vestibular division of the eighth cranial nerve (acoustic neuroma; see below).

Presbyacusis

The late Harold Schuknecht and his coworkers detected morphological and audiological evidence of involvement of four regions of the cochlea in four different forms of presbyacusis. In addition, a fifth form of presbyacusis associated with hypothetically dimished qualities of the cochlear duct, and a sixth comprising a mixture of the other five, have been added.[22] Thus the six types of presbyacusis presented by Schuknecht and accepted by many as a valid summary of the pathological basis of presbyacusis, are:

- sensory, loss of organ of Corti hair cells
- neural, loss of spiral ganglion cells and nerve fibres
- strial, loss of stria vascularis cells
- cochlear conductive, diminution of conductivity of basilar membrane
- cochlear duct, alterations in the physical characteristics of the cochlear duct
- mixed, any mixture of the other five.

Pure tone audiometry has been the usual means of testing the hearing in presbyacusis. However, Soucek et al found in a study of extratympanic electrocochleograms in geriatric patients that the cochlear nerves were functioning adequately in all cases, in spite of hearing loss in all of them. These findings suggested that, contrary to the elaborate schema presented above, it was in the hair cells that the primary deficit of the hearing loss of the elderly people was to be sought.[23]

Pathological appearances

Investigations by histological section

In most investigations of the pathological basis of presbyacusis, histological sections were used. In some of these investigations, hair cells were incriminated as showing pathological changes. Statements about the appearances of these cells in histological section must be regarded with caution, however, since they are very liable to undergo postmortem autolysis. Moreover, representation of the functionally most important part of the hair

PATHOLOGY OF PRESBYACUSIS IN RELATION TO CLINICAL FEATURES

- Atrophy of the outer hair cells—moderate hearing loss across all frequencies
- Giant stereociliary degeneration of outer hair cells in middle and apical coils—a precursor of outer hair cell loss in these regions
- Complete necrosis of outer and inner hair cells in a variable length of terminal basal coil—severe high-frequency hearing loss

cells—the stereocilia—in a histological section is very small, even when adequately fixed. Clear-cut losses in the spiral ganglion cells and the nerve fibres derived from them are, however, well documented. Careful analysis of the cochlear nuclear cells in the brainstem has also shown some loss in presbyacusis. It is difficult to accept nerve cell atrophy as the basis of a universal defect, and it seems more likely that there is some more fundamental disturbance giving rise to it. Vascular thickening in the cochlea has been incriminated by some, but its importance has been difficult to assess.

Surface preparation appearances

The use of surface preparations in human cochlear autopsy material (Figures 3.11 and 3.12) has indicated two major pathological changes:[23–25]

1. atrophy of the outer hair cells
2. giant stereociliary degeneration in some of those outer hair cells which survived.

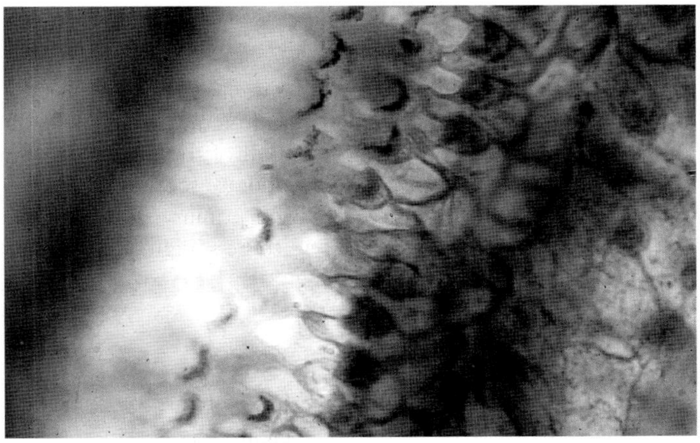

Figure 3.11 Surface preparation of outer hair cell region of the basal coil of the cochlea from patient with presbyacusis. There is a marked loss of outer hair cells. (Stained with Alcian blue–osmic acid.)

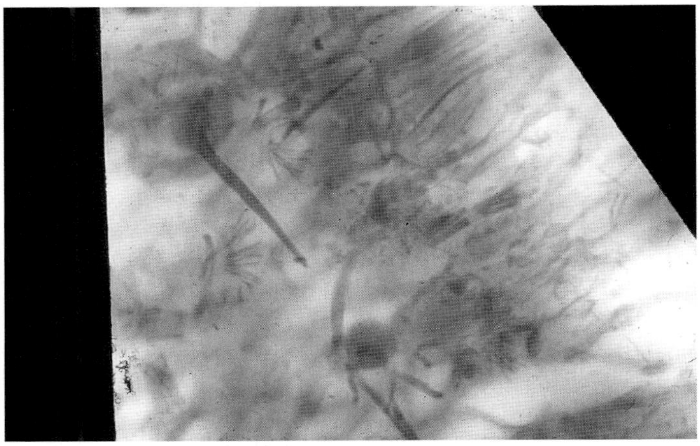

Figure 3.12 Surface preparation of outer hair cell region of the middle coil of the cochlea, showing giant stereociliary change. (Stained with Alcian blue–osmic acid.)

A severe degree of loss of outer hair cells is present in all coils of all cochleas from elderly patients. Approximate estimates of hair cell losses show that the inner hair cells sustain little loss, the first row of outer hair cells have a greater loss, the second row loss is even greater, and in the third row hair cells are very scanty or absent. In addition, there is a complete loss of all hair cells of all rows, inner and outer, at the extreme lower end of the basal coil in every elderly cochlea.

The other change is the presence of enormously lengthened and thickened stereocilia emanating from some surviving hair cells. These giant structures measure as much as 60 μm in length and are thickened due to adhesion of hairs to each other longitudinally. Giant stereocilia are found only in the outer hair cells of middle and apical coils, not in the outer hair cells of the basal coil.

Relationship of surface preparation changes to functional findings

The loss of outer hair cells throughout the cochlea may be the cause of the general hearing disability shown by Soucek et al[23] to be present at all frequencies. The exacerbation of hearing loss in the higher tones found by these and other workers using audiometry is explained by the short segment at the lower end of the basal coil with complete atrophy of both inner and outer hair cells.

Pathogenesis

It is possible that giant stereociliary degeneration is a stage in the dissolution of the outer hair cells in the apical and middle coils. In the basal coil, the stereocilia are normally different, in being shorter than in the other two coils. Perhaps giant stereociliary degeneration is an alteration that is slowly taking place throughout life, resulting eventually in presbyacusis, for it is not until the later years have been reached that hair cells will have been lost to a sufficient extent to produce significant deafness.

Molecular biology of presbyacusis

Mitochondria in the cytoplasm contain a set of genes which contribute to the phenotype of the individual. It is the mother only whose genotype is inherited. The membrane hypothesis of ageing proposes an association between reactive oxygen metabolites and the ageing process, the former leading to damage to mitochondrial DNA, resulting in cellular dysfunction and eventually death.[26] A form of mitochondrial DNA damage, that of deletion of mtDNA 4977 bp, has been discovered which accumulates in human tissues, especially those of neural and muscular type, with increasing age. Using the polymerase chain reaction on celloidin-embedded archival sections of human cochleas to determine deletion of the mtDNA 4977 bp in that structure, it has been found that 14 of 17 patients with sensorineural hearing loss, mainly associated with ageing, exhibited such deletion, while only 8 of 17 patients with normal hearing exhibited the same deletion.[27] Thus this 4977-bp mitochondrial deletion may cause presbyacusis.

Bony abnormalities

Paget's disease

Paget's disease (osteitis deformans) is a common condition affecting particularly the skull, pelvis, vertebral column and femur in people over 40 years of age. The cause is not yet certain, but the presence in many cases of paramyxovirus-like structures seen within osteoclasts has prompted the suggestion that Paget's disease may be of viral aetiology and the measles virus and canine distemper viruses have been under scrutiny as candidates. The pathological change is one of active bone formation proceeding alongside active bone destruction. The affected bones are enlarged, porous and deformed (Figure 3.13).

Microscopically, bone formation is seen in trabeculae of bone with a lining of numerous osteoblasts. A mosaic appearance is formed by the frequent successive deposition of bone, cessation of deposition resulting in thin, blue 'cement lines', followed again by resumption of deposition and its cessation, and so production of further cement lines. Bone destruction is shown by the presence of numerous, large osteoclastic giant cells with Howship's lacunae. Areas of chronic inflammatory exudate intermixed with the bone are common.

The pathology of involvement of the temporal bone by Paget's disease has been well studied. The petrous apex, the mastoid and the bony part of the Eustachian tube are most frequently affected. The periosteal part of the bony labyrinth is the first to undergo pagetoid changes. The endochondral layer is also affected in many cases, but the endosteal layer and modiolus infrequently. The internal auditory meatus may show protuberances of pagetoid tissue into its lumen. In a few cases, the stapes may be tethered by pagetoid change of its footplate. Calcification of the annulus fibrosis is cited as another cause of such fixation. Involvement of other ossicles is unusual. An alternative means of ossicular fixation may be involvement of the malleus by pagetoid tissue in the epitympanum. Fissure fractures, occurring during life, are more frequent in the temporal bone of patients with Paget's disease. The round window niche may be narrowed by the bony overgrowth. The sensorineural hearing loss which Paget's disease patients may experience is probably caused by encroachment on the membranous cochlea.

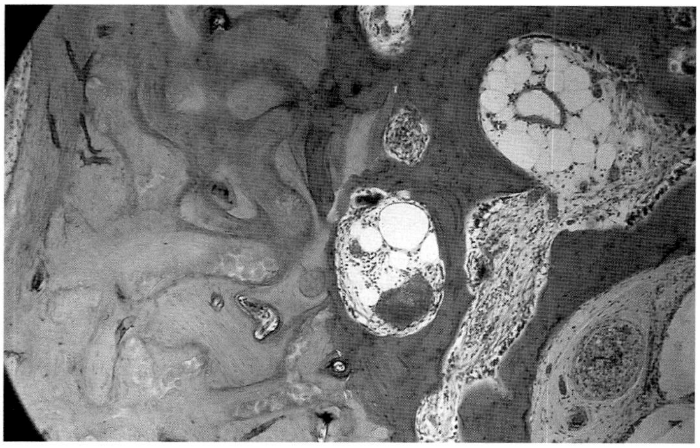

Figure 3.13 Paget's disease involving bony cochlea. The paler bone (left) is residual normal bony cochlea, containing globuli ossei. The darker bone on the right (red-staining in the original) is pagetoid bone, showing closely packed osteoid layers and prominent osteoblasts and osteoclasts.

Osteogenesis imperfecta

Osteogenesis imperfecta is a general bone disease with a triad of clinical features: multiple fractures, blue sclerae and conductive hearing loss. There is a congenital recessive form which is often rapidly fatal, and a tardive one in adults that is inherited as a mendelian dominant and is more benign. Mutations of type I collagen genes have been established as the underlying cause, leading to a general disturbance in the development of collagen; hence the thin (blue) sclerae as well as poorly formed bone tissue.

The pathology is well seen in the long bones, where resorption of cartilage in the development of bone is normal, but the bony trabeculae themselves are poorly formed. In the temporal bone, the bony labyrinth is sometimes deficient in bone. The ossicles in the tardive form are very thin and subject to fractures. The stapes footplate is also frequently fixed. The disturbance in lamellar bone formation can lead to extreme thinness, dehiscence, and non-union of the stapedial superstructure with the footplate or thickening with fixation of the footplate. The nature of the bony tissue causing fixation is problematical. It has been suggested that osteogenesis imperfecta can be associated with otosclerosis, so that the fixation is indeed otosclerotic. Otosclerosis, like osteogenesis imperfecta, may indeed be part of a general connective tissue disturbance. Indeed, some cases of clinical otosclerosis may be related to mutations within the *COL1A1* gene that are similar to those found in mild forms of osteogenesis imperfecta.

Osteopetrosis

Osteopetrosis (often known as marble bone disease) is a rare disease of bone, in which there is a failure to absorb calcified cartilage and primitive bone due to deficient activity of osteoclasts. A relatively benign form, inherited in a dominant fashion, presents in adults, and a malignant one, inherited in a recessive fashion, in infants and young children. The patients with the benign form often survive to old age and present prominent otological symptoms. The intermediate, endochondral portion of the otic capsule is swollen and appears as an exaggerated, thickened form of the normal state. Globuli ossei composed of groups of calcified cartilage cells are normally present in this region, and in osteopetrosis they are greatly increased in number and are arranged into a markedly thickened zone. The periosteal bone is normal. The organ of Corti is usually normal, but in a few cases has been said to be atrophied. The ossicles are of fetal shape and filled with unabsorbed, calcified cartilage. The canals for the seventh and eighth cranial nerves are greatly narrowed by the expanded cartilaginous and bony tissue, and these changes are probably responsible for the characteristic symptoms of facial palsy and hearing loss respectively.

Otosclerosis

Prevalence

Otosclerosis is a common focal lesion of the otic capsule, and is found principally in relation to the cochlea and footplate of the stapes. 'Histological otosclerosis' refers to a disease process without clinical symptoms or manifestations that only can be discovered by routine sectioning of the temporal bone at autopsy. 'Clinical otosclerosis' concerns the presence of otosclerosis at a site where it causes conductive hearing loss, usually by interfering with the motion of the stapes. The mean prevalence of histological otosclerosis has been estimated from temporal bone studies at 8.3%.[28] According to Guild,[29] 15% of temporal bones with histological otosclerosis demonstrate ankylosis of the stapediovestibular articulation: hence $8.3 \times 15/100 = 1.2\%$ of all temporal bones studied could, by such extrapolation, be considered as having clinical otosclerosis. The figure derived from actual clinical studies of large populations is 0.3%.[30] It is likely that the temporal bones studied by Guild and others are biased towards greater numbers of cases of otosclerosis by the fact that a large proportion of the patients had been investigated during life for otological conditions. In a study that was not so biased, consisting of unselected consecutive autopsied patients in one hospital,[28] 2.5% of 236 temporal bones showed otosclerosis, with an extrapolated figure for clinical otosclerosis of 0.37%. This correlates well with the clinically derived figure of 0.3%.[30]

Aetiology

Otosclerosis seems to have some features of a hereditary disease, but its genetics still remain incompletely elucidated. There is a histological similarity between otosclerosis and Paget's disease of bone. Because of the finding of measles-like virus particles in Paget's disease of bone osteoclasts (see above), a search for a similar connection has been made in otosclerosis. Ultrastructural and immunohistochemical evidence has indeed been found for measles virus in otosclerotic tissue. Using a method for isolation and identification of both DNA and RNA sequences in archival human temporal bone specimens with the polymerase chain reaction technique, a 115-bp sequence of the measles nucleocapsid gene has been identified in otosclerosis.[31] It thus seems likely that otosclerosis is associated with the measles virus, possibly through the intermediary of an immune reaction.

Gross appearances

Otosclerosis usually affects both ears symmetrically. The disease process is probably confined to the temporal bone. In cases with prominent otosclerotic involvement of the otic capsule, the lesion may be seen as a smooth prominence of the promontory. The stapes is sometimes fixed. The pink swelling of the otosclerotic focus may sometimes even be detected clinically through a particularly transparent tympanic membrane. In temporal bone specimens, the focus appears well demarcated and pink (Figure 3.14). Blood vessels are prominent and evenly distributed. X-rays of temporal bone specimens show the well-defined lesion as a patch of mottled translucency.

Microscopic appearances

The histological characteristic of otosclerosis is the presence of trabeculae of new bone, mostly of the woven type. This contrasts with the well-developed bone under the outer periosteum, the endochondral middle layer and the endosteal layer of the otic capsule, a sharply demarcated edge between normal otosclerotic bone being a prominent feature. The pathological

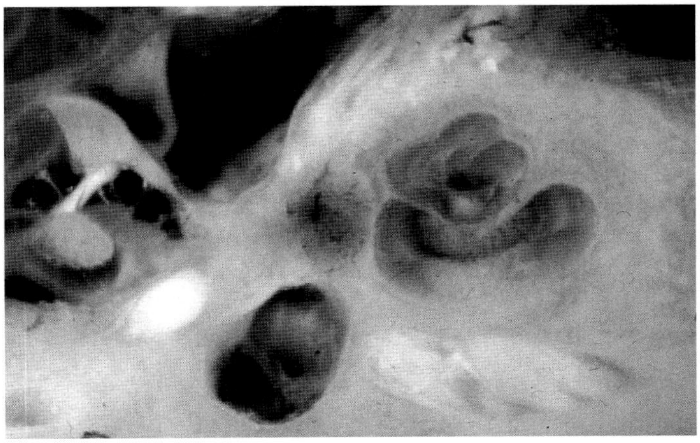

Figure 3.14 Otosclerotic focus in a slice of temporal bone showing a pink deposit between the footplate of the stapes and the cochlea.

> **PATHOLOGY AND CLINICAL RELATIONS OF OTOSCLEROSIS**
>
> - Aetiology: strong genetic aspects; measle virus relationship
> - Commences in bone anterior to footplate of stapes; then spreads
> - Gross: pinkish well-defined area in region of bone anterior to footplate
> - Microscopic: woven bone, very vascular; very cellular
> - Conductive hearing loss related to stapes footplate fixation
> - Sensorineural hearing loss related to involvement of cochlear perilymph spaces

bony tissue has a variable appearance, with areas of differing cellularity. In most places osteoblasts are very abundant within the woven bone. Osteoclasts may be present and are accompanied by evidence of bone resorption. Marrow spaces contain prominent blood vessels and connective tissue (Figure 3.15).

The commonest site for the formation of otosclerotic foci is the bone anterior to the oval window. The fissula ante fenestram, a normally appearing slit connecting middle ear with vestibule, is present in the same region, but the significance of this relationship is still not understood. Cartilaginous rests are also normal in this area and may be seen nearby. Otosclerotic foci may also be seen in the bone near the round window membrane (Figure 3.16), in the inferior part of the cochlear capsule or in the bone around the semicircular canals.

Otosclerotic involvement of the stapes footplate leading to functional fixation of the stapes may occur in two ways:

1. There may be actual participation by the stapes footplate in the formation of otosclerotic bone so that the otic capsular focus of pathological bone is continuous with the former, the annulus fibrosis being obliterated. Involvement of the oval window takes place at any point of its circumference, or indeed around most of it. The process may also occasionally be associated with similar alterations in the lower parts of the stapedial crura
2. Frequently the footplate is not affected by the otosclerotic process, but the bone surrounding it proliferates to such an extent that the oval window is distorted and narrowed. Fibrous thickening of the annulus fibrosis may be prominent. The otosclerotic focus may also encroach on the round window, narrowing it in the same fashion.

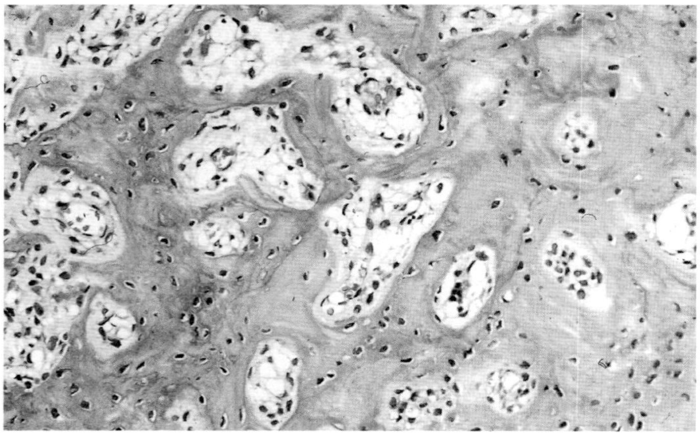

Figure 3.15 Otosclerotic bone shows an increase of cellularity of bone trabeculae and of vascularity of the marrow spaces.

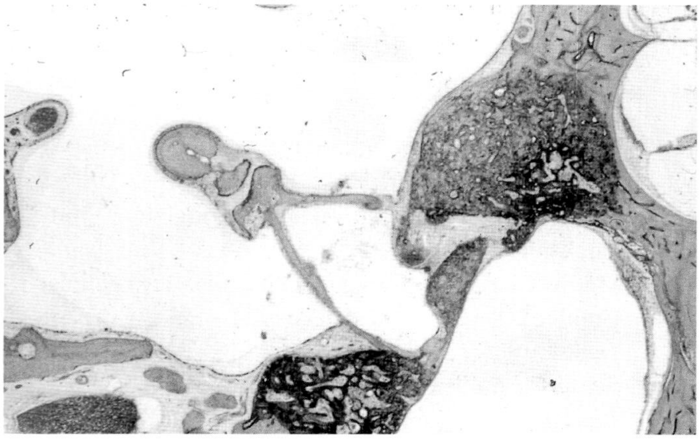

Figure 3.16 Otosclerosis involving both anterior and posterior crura of stapes.

Otosclerotic bone frequently reaches the endosteum of the cochlear capsule. In some cases, it may lead to a fibrous reaction deep to the spiral ligament. Overgrowth of otosclerotic bone may, rarely, cause distortion of the cochlear contours and even affect the modiolus and lead to spontaneous fractures of the modiolar septa.[32]

An entity of 'otospongiosis' is often referred to by radiologists, implying a more vascular and less bony lesion. In histological sections, 'otospongiotic' and 'otosclerotic' lesions are found side by side in both active and inactive lesions,[33] so that whether the lesion is 'otospongiotic' or 'otosclerotic' appears to have no relation to the activity of the condition.

Hearing loss in relation to otosclerotic foci

By far the commonest form of hearing loss in otosclerosis can be accounted for by oval window fixation, as described above, and is conductive in type. Depression of sound waves derived from air conduction also occurs following obstruction of the round window by otosclerosis. It is likely that otosclerotic involvement of the cochlea may lead to sensorineural hearing loss—'cochlear otosclerosis'.

Neoplasms of the inner ear

The cellular constituents of the inner ear, apart from bone, are, for the most part, fully differentiated non-mitotic structures—nerve cells and sensory epithelia—so that neoplasms would be expected to be of unusual occurrence in them. Primary neoplasms are indeed rare, except for vestibular schwannoma.

Internal auditory canal and cerebellopontine angle tumours

Tumours occurring in the internal auditory canal are the solitary vestibular schwannoma, and the bilateral vestibular schwannoma (neurofibromatosis 2), the latter usually accompanied in this situation by neoplasm-like masses of meningioma and neurofibroma. Primary meningiomas and lipomas are also seen in this region. Tumours of the internal auditory canal, on enlargement, extend into the cranial cavity, filling the cerebellopontine angle.

Vestibular schwannoma (acoustic neuroma)

> **PATHOLOGY OF VESTIBULAR SCHWANNOMA**
>
> - Solitary form (not familial) slowly growing. Bilateral form (neurofibromatosis 2–familial) more aggressive
> - Arises on the vestibular branch of the eighth nerve in the internal auditory canal
> - Gross: spherical tumour at first, but adopts a mushroom shape when it leaves the canal and expands in the cerebellopontine angle. The cochlear branch is stretched over the surface of the tumour. With growth, it produces a funnel-shaped canal (expanded centrally)
> - Microscopic appearances of neoplasm: Antoni A appearances—palisading of nuclei. Antoni B appearances—loose foamy cells
> - Labyrinth contains proteinaceous fluid, probably due to compression of labyrinthine veins in the canal

This neoplasm may cause characteristic symptoms of hearing loss or vertigo, or it may grow slowly for years without causing symptoms and may be first diagnosed only at postmortem, where it can be expected in about 1 in 220 consecutive adults. It is stated to arise most commonly at the glial–neurilemmal junction of the eighth nerve, which is usually within the internal auditory meatus. When seen at surgery or autopsy, however, vestibular schwannoma in most cases is found to occupy a much greater part of the nerve. Usually, it is the vestibular division of the nerve which is affected; in a few cases, the cochlear division is the source of the neoplasm. Growth takes place from the origin, both centrally onto the cerebellopontine angle, and distally along the canal. Vestibular schwannoma is usually unilateral, but may be bilateral (see below). In a large series, 129 cases were unilateral and 11 bilateral.[34]

Gross appearance

The neoplasm is of variable size and of round or oval shape. Small tumours either do not widen the canal at all or produce only a small indentation in the bone. The larger tumours often have a mushroom shape, with two components: the stalk—an elongated part in the canal; and an expanded part in the region of the cerebellopontine angle. The bone of the internal auditory canal is widened funnelwise as the neoplasm grows (see Figure 3.17). The tumour surface is smooth and lobulated. The cut surface is yellowish, often with areas of haemorrhage and cysts. The vestibular division of the eighth nerve may be identified on the surface of the tumour.

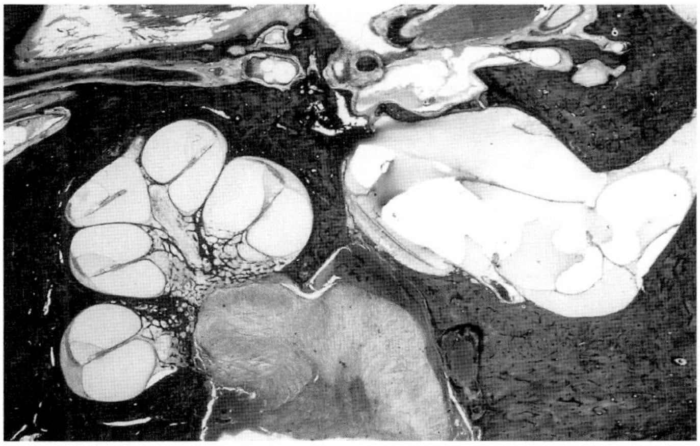

Figure 3.17 Vestibular schwannoma causing marked widening of the bone surrounding the internal auditory meatus. The tumour had been surgically excised during life, producing haemorrhage over part of the cut surface externally. Note the pale-staining eosinophilic deposit in the cochlear and vestibular cavities.

Histological findings

Vestibular schwannoma has the features of a neoplasm of schwann cells showing Antoni A and Antoni B types. Antoni A areas display spindle cells closely packed together with palisading of nuclei (Figures 3.18 and 3.19). Verocay bodies, which may be present in the Antoni A areas, are whorled formations of palisaded tumour cells resembling tactile corpuscles. The spindle cells of the tumour may lack palisading and Verocay bodies, however. The degree of cellularity of the neoplasm can be high or low. The spindle cells are frequently moderately pleomorphic, but mitotic figures are rare. The presence of pleomorphism does not denote a malignant tendency. Antoni B areas, probably a degenerated form of the Antoni A pattern, show a loose reticular pattern, sometimes with histiocytic proliferation. Thrombosis and necrosis may be present in some parts of the neoplasm. A mild degree of invasion of the modiolus or vestibule along cochlear or vestibular nerve branches may

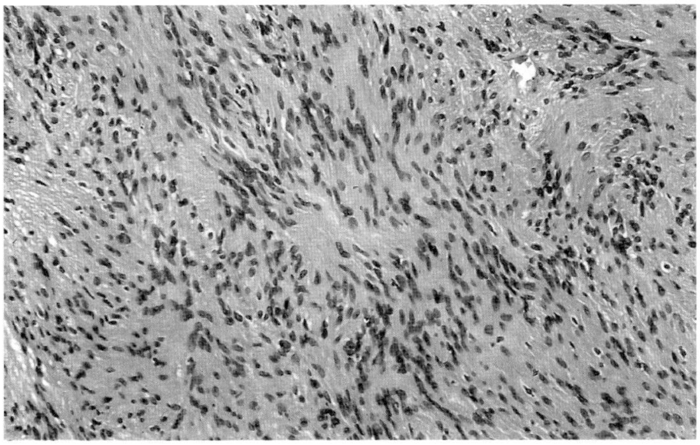

Figure 3.18 Antoni A area of vestibular schwannoma, showing palisading of nuclei.

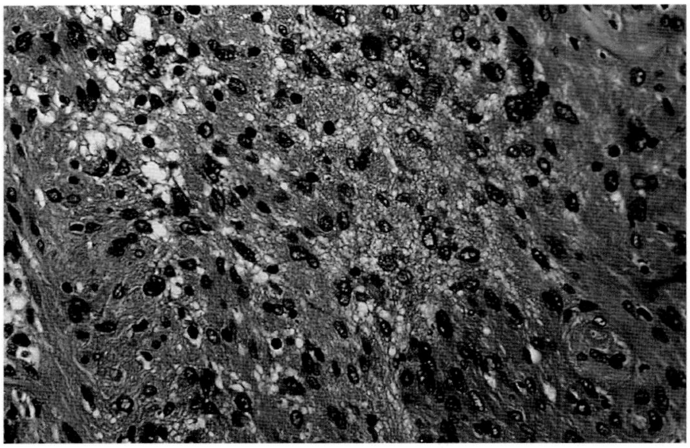

Figure 3.19 Antoni B area of vestibular schwannoma, showing a looser pattern.

be present even in solitary vestibular schwannomas. Granular or homogeneous fluid exudate is usually present in the perilymphatic spaces of the cochlea and vestibule. This may arise as a result of pressure by the neoplasm on veins draining the cochlea and vestibule in the internal auditory meatus. Hydrops of the endolymphatic system may occur, and in larger tumours there is atrophy of spiral ganglion cells and nerve fibres in the basilar membrane.[35]

Neurofibromatosis 2 (bilateral vestibular schwannoma)

Bilateral vestibular schwannoma acoustic neuroma (neurofibromatosis 2, NF2), unlike neurofibromatosis 1 (von Recklinghausen's disease), is not associated with large numbers of cutaneous neurofibromas and cafe-au-lait spots, but the temporal bone locality of the neural tumour and its bilaterality are inherited as an autosomal dominant trait. This condition has been related to a gene localized near the centre of the long arm of chromosome 22. At autopsy of cases of neurofibromatosis 2, neural neoplasms are present in both eighth nerves and other central nerves. There are often many small schwannomas and collections of cells of neurofibromatous and meningiomatous appearance growing on cranial nerves and on the meninges in the vicinity of the vestibular schwannomas and sometimes even intermixed with them. The NF2 tumours are histologically similar to the single tumours, except that the former have more Verocay bodies and more foci of high cellularity. The NF2 tumours are more invasive, however, tending to infiltrate the cochlea and vestibule more deeply.

Apex of petrous temporal bone and cerebellopontine angle tumours

A variety of neoplasms and tumour-like lesions may present at the apex of the petrous temporal bone. These include the following: jugular paraganglioma, jugular foramen schwannoma arising usually from the vagus nerve, low-grade adenocarcinoma of probable endolymphatic sac origin, and the tumour-like entities of cholesteatoma (epidermoid cyst) and cholesterol granuloma. Such lesions, on enlargement, may extend into the cerebellopontine angle.

Low-grade adenocarcinoma of probable endolymphatic sac

There is evidence of the existence of a rare epithelial neoplasm of the endolymphatic system, mainly in the endolymphatic sac. Although of benign glandular histological appearance and of slow growth, the neoplasm seems to have considerable invasive capacity, and therefore the term 'low-grade adenocarcinoma of probable endolymphatic sac origin' has been applied.[36] Some cases have presented bilateral neoplasms of the same type and some have also been associated with von Hippel–Lindau disease.[36] The course of the tumour's growth may extend over many years. Tinnitus or vertigo, similar or identical to the symptoms of Menière's disease, is present in about one-third of patients. It is presumed that early obstruction of the endolymphatic sac leads to hydrops of the endolymphatic system of the labyrinth and so to the Menière's symptoms. Imaging reveals a lytic temporal bone lesion, appearing to originate from the region between the internal auditory canal and sigmoid sinus (which is the approximate position of the endolymphatic sac). There is usually prominent extension into the posterior cranial cavity and invasion of the middle ear.

In most cases, the tumour has a papillary–glandular appearance, the papillary proliferation being lined by a single row of low cuboidal cells. The vascular nature of the papillae in some cases has given the tumour a histological resemblance to choroid plexus papilloma. In some cases, the tumour also shows areas of dilated glands containing secretion which has some resemblance to colloid and, under these circumstances, the lesion may resemble papillary adenocarcinoma of the thyroid. Such thyroid-like areas may even dominate the histological pattern. A few cases show a clear cell predominance resembling carcinoma of the kidney.

Tumour-like lesions

Cholesteatoma (epidermoid cyst)

This lesion usually presents with symptoms relating to its involvement of the seventh and eighth cranial nerves in the cerebellopontine angle. The histological appearance is similar to that of middle ear cholesteatoma. It is probably of congenital origin, but no cell rest has been discovered from which it might arise.

Cholesterol granuloma

A lesion of the petrous apex with the typical features of cholesterol granuloma as seen in the middle ear and mastoid in chronic otitis media has been revealed by MRI scan with increasing frequency. At operation it appears cystic, the contents being altered blood and cholesterol clefts with a foreign body giant cell reaction.

Microscopic examination shows non-specific granulation tissue and haemosiderin deposits in its wall. It is believed to result from an inflammatory response to an obstruction of the pneumatized air cells at the apex of the temporal bone. Haemorrhage into the air cells breaks down to hemosiderin and cholesterol, with a foreign body reaction and progressive granuloma formation. As the process develops, bone is eroded by this expansile lesion, often involving the petrous apex, the cerebellopontine angle and the middle ear.

Leukaemia

Leukaemia may involve the inner ear in several ways. The most important is haemorrhage into the membranous spaces, to which leukaemic patients are particularly prone. The haemorrhage may be into the perilymphatic spaces alone or into both perilymphatic and endolymphatic spaces. If the patient survives a massive intracochlear leukaemic haemorrhage for several months, the organ of Corti and spiral ganglion will become severely degenerated, and connective tissue and new bone will grow into the scalae. Another type of involvement may occur in chronic lymphocytic leukaemia, in the form of severe leukaemic infiltration of the perilymphatic spaces of the cochlea. The leukaemic cells are probably conveyed from the cerebrospinal fluid via the cochlear aqueduct.

References

1. Friedberg J. Congenital cholesteatoma. *Laryngoscope (suppl)* 1994; **104**: 1–24.
2. Teed, RW. Cholesteatoma verum tympani. Its relationship to the first epibranchial placode, *Arch Otolaryngol* 1936; **24:** 455–74.
3. Michaels L. An epidermoid formation in the developing middle ear; possible source of cholesteatoma. *J Otolaryngol* 1986; **15:** 169–74.
4. Wang R-G., Hawke M, Kwok P. The epidermoid formation (Michaels' structure) in the developing middle ear. *J Otolaryngol* 1987; **16:** 327–33.
5. Ormerod F. The pathology of congenital deafness. *J Laryngol Otol* 1960; **74:** 919–50.
6. Michaels L, Hellquist H. *Ear, Nose and Throat Histopathology*, 2nd edn. London: Springer, 2001.
7. Walsted A, Garbarsch C, Michaels L. Effect of craniotomy and cerebrospinal fluid loss on the inner ear. An experimental study. *Acta Otolaryngol (Stockh)* 1994; **114:** 626–31.
8. Amatuzzi MG, Northrop C, Liberman MC, Thornton A, Halpin C, Herrmann B, Pinto LE, Saenz A, Carranza A, Eavey RD. Selective inner hair cell loss in premature infants and cochlea pathology patterns from neonatal intensive care unit autopsies. *Arch Otolarygol Head Neck Surg* 2001; **127**: 629–36.
9. Hanshaw JP. School failure and deafness after 'silent' congenital cytomegalovirus infection. *N Engl J Med* 1976: **295:** 468–70.
10. Soucek S, Michaels L. The ear in the acquired immunodeficiency syndrome. II. Clinical and audiologic investigation. *Am J Otol* 1996; **17:** 35–9.
11. Wackym PA. Molecular temporal bone pathology: II. Ramsay Hunt syndrome (herpes zoster oticus). *Laryngoscope* 1997; **107:** 1165–75.
12. Burgess RC, Michaels L, Bale JF, Smith RJ. Polymerase chain reaction amplification of Herpes simplex viral DNA from the geniculate ganglion of a patient with Bell's palsy. *Ann Otol Rhinol Laryngol* 1994; **103:** 775–9.
13. Merchant SN, Gopen Q. A human temporal bone study of acute bacterial meningogenic labyrinthitis. *Am J Otol* 1996; **17:** 375–85.
14. Rauch SN, Merchant SN, Thedinger BA. Menière's syndrome and endolymphatic hydrops. Double-blind temporal bone study. *Ann Otol Rhinol Laryngol* 1989; **98:** 873–83.
15. Sperling NM, Paparella MM, Yoon TH, Zelterman D. Symptomatic versus asymptomatic endolymphatic hydrops: a histologic comparison. *Laryngoscope* 1993; **103:** 277–85.
16. Xenellis JE, Linthicum FH, Galey FR. Lermoyez's syndrome: histopathologic report of a case. *Ann Otol Rhinol Laryngol* 1990; **99:** 307–9.
17. Antoli-Candela F Jr. The histopathology of Menière's disease. *Acta Otolaryngol Suppl (Stockh)* 1976; **340:** 5–42.
18. Fraysse BG, Alonso A, House WF. Menière's disease and endolymphatic hydrops. Clinicopathological correlations. *Ann Otol Rhinol Laryngol* 1980; **8** (suppl 76): 2–22.
19. Gleeson M, Felix H. A comparative study of the effect of age on the human cochlear and vestibular neuroepithelia. *Acta Orolaryngol (Stockh) Suppl* 1987; **436:** 103–9.
20. Merchant SN, Schuknecht HF. Vestibular atelectasis. *Ann Otol Rhinol Laryngol* 1988; **97:** 565–76.
21. Schuknecht HF. Cupolithiasis. *Arch Otolaryngol* 1969; **90:** 765–78.
22. Schuknecht HF, Gacek MR. Cochlear pathology in presbycusis. *Ann Otol Rhinol Laryngol* 1993; **102:** 1–16.
23. Soucek S, Michaels L, Frohlich A. Evidence for hair cell degeneration as the primary lesion in hearing loss of the elderly. *J Otolaryngol* 1986; **15:** 175–83.
24. Bredberg G. Cellular patterns and nerve supply of the human organ of Corti. *Acta Otolaryngol Suppl (Stockh)* 1965; **236:** 1–135.
25. Johnsson LG, Hawkins JE. Sensory and neural degeneration with aging, as seen in microdissection of the human inner ear. *Ann Otol Rhinol Laryngol* 1972; **81:** 1–15.
26. Seidman MD, Bai U, Khan MJ, Quirk WS. Mitochondrial DNA deletions associated with aging and presbycusis. *Arch Otolaryngol Head Neck Surg* 1997; **123:** 1039–45.
27. Bai U, Seidman MD, Hinojosa R, Quirk WS. Mitochondrial DNA deletions associated with aging and possibly presbycusis: a human archival temporal bone study. *Am J Otol* 1997; **18:** 449–53.
28. Declau F, Van Spaendonck M, Timmermans JP, Michaels L, Liang J, Qiu JP, Van de Heyning P. Prevalence of otosclerosis in an unselected series of temporal bones.*Otol Neurotol* 2001; **22**: 596–602.
29. Guild SR. Histologic otosclerosis. *Ann Otol Rhinol Laryngol* 1944; **53:** 246–67.
30. Causse JR, Causse JB. Otospongiosis as a genetic disease. Early detection, medical management and prevention. *Am J Otol* 1984; **5:** 211–23.
31. McKenna MJ, Kristiansen AG, Haines J. Polymerase chain reaction amplification of a measles virus sequence from human temporal bone sections with active otosclerosis. *Am J Otol* 1996; **17:** 827–30.

32. Nager GT. Sensorineural deafness and otosclerosis. *Ann Otol Rhinol Laryngol* 1966; **75:** 481–511.
33. Parahy C, Linthicum FH Jr. Otosclerosis and otospongiosis: clinical and histological comparisons. Laryngoscope 1984; **94**: 508–12.
34. Erickson LS, Sorenson GD, McGavran MH. A review of 140 acoustic neurinomas (neurilemmoma). *Laryngoscope* 1965; **75:** 601–27.
35. Sidek D, Michaels L, Wright A. Changes in the inner ear in vestibular schwannoma. In: Iurato S, Veldman JE, eds. *Progress in Human Auditory and Vestibular Histopathology*. Amsterdam: Kugler Publications, 1996: 95–101.
36. Heffner DK. Low-grade adenocarcinoma of probable endolymphatic sac origin. A clinicopathologic study of 20 cases. *Cancer* 1989; **64:** 2292–302.
37. Poe DE, Tarlov EC, Thomas CB, Kveton JF. Aggressive papillary tumors of temporal bone. *Otolaryngol Head Neck Surg* 1993; **108:** 80–6.

4 Genetics of auditory and vestibular disorders

Guy Van Camp, Andrew P Read

Identifying disease genes

Unravelling the genetics of any human disorder normally follows the three stages shown in Table 4.1. As indicated, at each stage there are clinical and scientific benefits.

Defining a genetic condition

The simplest genetic conditions are Mendelian, i.e. they are caused by the segregation of mutant alleles at a single gene. Single-gene (monogenic) conditions give rise to recognizable pedigree patterns (Figure 4.1). The patterns reflect the behaviour of chromosomes during the meiotic cell divisions that produce sperm and eggs. Mitochondrial inheritance is a special case, but important in hearing loss. Mitochondria have their own small genome, mutations of which cause various clinical problems, including hearing loss. Since all of a person's mitochondria come from the egg, and none from the sperm, the inheritance pattern of mitochondrial diseases is matrilineal. All known human single-gene characters are listed in McKusick's *Online Mendelian Inheritance in Man (OMIM)*, which is freely accessible as an Internet resource at http://www3.ncbi.nlm.nih.gov/Omim. A specialized database of genetic hearing problems is maintained at http://dnalab-www.uia.ac.be/dnalab/hhh/. Given the small size of most human families, the variability of many genetic conditions and the frequent occurrence of new mutations in some conditions, patients seen in the clinic very seldom show the unambiguous pedigree patterns of Figure 4.1. Some syndromic forms of hearing loss are recognizable clinically, but for non-syndromic forms, genetic causation is usually suspected only when no other explanation seems attractive. The mode of inheritance for a particular patient is rarely more than a hypothesis.

Table 4.1 Three stages in the investigation of a genetic disease.

Stage	Benefits
1. Define a genetic condition	Allows counselling based on monogenic risks (e.g. a 50% recurrence risk for autosomal dominant disease)
2. Map the gene to a particular chromosomal location	Allows DNA diagnostics for large linked families, but not yet for small families and for individual patients
3. Identify the gene	Allows precise genetic diagnosis, also for individual patients Possibility of novel treatments

THE HEREDITARY HEARING LOSS HOMEPAGE

http://dnalab-www.uia.ac.be/dnalab/hhh

This web-site contains continuously updated tables with information for all known loci for non-syndromic hearing impairment and for many of the best-known syndromic forms. The information includes chromosomal locations, genetic markers, identified genes, reserved and withdrawn symbols, and potential mouse models. Many references for gene localizations and identifications are given, and direct links to abstracts of these publications are provided.

Recessive inheritance is suspected when an affected child has unaffected parents, especially if there is an affected sib or parental consanguinity. As discussed below, recessive hearing loss is most often prelingual and profound, while dominant loss is more often milder, of later onset and progressive.

Many conditions show some familial tendency without giving clear monogenic pedigree patterns. The reason for this can lie in the fact that more than one gene is involved. In addition, since humans give their children both their genes and their environment, conditions can run in families due to environmental factors, without being genetic. Diseases that are caused by a combination of genetic and environmental factors are called complex, and analysing such complex conditions is a major challenge, which geneticists are only beginning to address. As inherited genetic susceptibility is believed to play a part in the causation of many common diseases, including presbyacusis, otosclerosis and Menière's disease, the identification of the genetic risk factors could lead to improved diagnostics and therapy.

Mapping a disease gene to a chromosomal location

For mitochondrial and X-linked conditions, the pedigree pattern tells the geneticist where to look for the gene. For autosomal dominant and autosomal recessive diseases, the gene can be located on each of the chromosomes, except for the sex chromosomes, and the mitochondrial DNA. The gene must somehow be localized to a particular chromosome and subchromosomal region. To do this, we require families where a parent could have passed on either the disease gene or its normal version (allele) to each of several children, and where we know which allele was in fact passed on. The trick is to check each chromosome with genetic markers until one is found that segregates in exactly the same pattern as the disease. If this happens too often to be coincidence, that chromosome must carry the disease gene.

In practice, of course, it is not quite so simple.

- A parent such as individual II-1 in Figure 4.2 (the first person along in the second generation down) does not simply pass on to each child an intact copy of each chromosome as inherited from the grandparents in generation I. During meiosis, chromosomes pair up and swap segments (crossing over). On average, there are about 60 crossovers in male meiosis and about 90 in female. Thus every chromosome pair crosses over several times, more or less at random, and each chromosome transmitted to a child is a patchwork of the grandpaternal and grandmaternal chromosomes. Therefore, rather than simply checking each chromosome once for co-segregation with the disease, we need to check about 10–15 segements for an average chromosome, or 200–350 for the whole genome.
- We cannot distinguish between grandpaternal and grandmaternal segments simply by looking down the microscope.

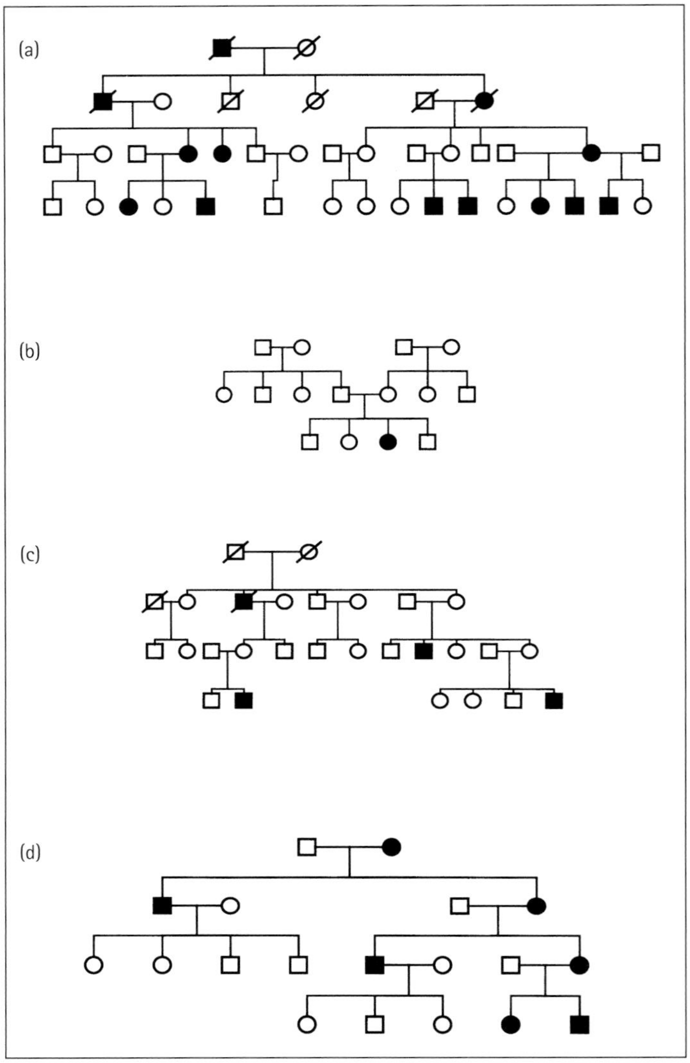

Figure 4.1 Pedigree patterns. (a) Autosomal dominant. (b) Autosomal recessive. (c) X-linked recessive. (d) Mitochondrial inheritance. Squares represent males, and circles females. Blacked-in characters are affected. Without further evidence, it would not be possible to recognize the pedigree in (b) as showing a genetically determined hearing loss.

Instead, minor non-pathogenic variants in the DNA (DNA markers) are used. Fortunately, innumerable such variants exist. The most widely used, called microsatellites, are small runs of di- or tri-nucleotide repeats, typically $(CA)_n$, in non-coding parts of the DNA where they are harmless. At a given chromosomal location, everybody will have a CA repeat, but different people will have different sizes of $(CA)_n$ run. Standard molecular biology techniques (PCR and gel electrophoresis[1] can be used to see the repeats as bands on a gel (Figure 4.2). During the last 10 years, about 10 000 such markers have been defined and placed on accurate maps covering the whole of every chromosome.

In Figure 4.2 it is easy to see that marker A segregates in a way that has no relation to the disease, but for marker B the band

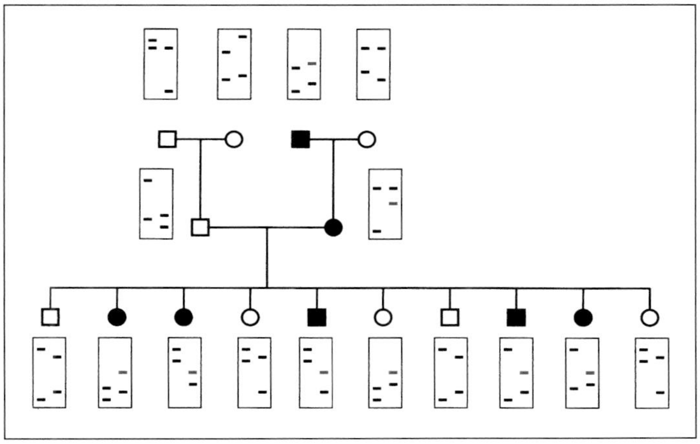

Figure 4.2 Linkage analysis. Symbols as in Figure 4.1. The pedigree shows a family with autosomal dominant hearing loss. The boxes show the bands that each person's DNA gave when tested with two microsatellite markers from different chromosomes. The two bands in the left half of each box are for marker A, from chromosome 6. Each band is inherited from one parent, but there is no relation between which band a person inherits and whether or not they inherit the disease. The two bands in the right-hand half of each box are for marker B, from chromosome 15. With one exception, anybody who inherits the disease from a parent also inherits the band marked with an arrow from that parent, and anybody who does not inherit the disease from an affected parent does not inherit the band. Thus marker B is tending to track with the disease, suggesting that the disease gene may be located on chromosome 15, near to marker A. The one exception is the sixth person in the bottom generation. This person is a recombinant (see text).

indicated with an arrow tracks with the disease perfectly in every case except for individual III-6, who inherited the band but not the disease. This particular pedigree is relatively small, and the co-segregation might be coincidental. However, if such co-segregation is seen in a big enough family (or in a big enough collection of smaller families), the result may be statistically significant. The statistic used for linkage analysis is called the lod score, and is the logarithm of the odds favouring linkage over non-linkage. Lod scores are calculated by computer. The thresholds of significance are +3.0 (significant evidence for linkage) and −2.0 (significant evidence against linkage). Individual III-6 in Figure 4.2 inherited the coloured band but not the disease. She is a recombinant. When the egg that gave rise to her was being made, a crossover must have separated the disease gene from the associated marker allele. The probability of this happening is a measure of how far apart the disease gene and the marker are. Thus the percentage recombination (measured in units called centiMorgans) is a measure of the genetic distance between two loci. If the rest of the pedigree shows sufficient evidence of linkage, each recombinant provides a means to move closer to the disease gene. Other adjacent markers, chosen on the basis of the established genetic map of markers, are tested until one is found that gives no recombinants. This then marks the best localization of the disease gene.

How closely a disease gene can be thus localized depends on the number of meioses that can be tested. Thus genetic mapping relies on unusually large families. For autosomal recessive conditions this is a big problem, because most European families consist simply of unaffected parents and one, or at most two or three, affected children. This problem was solved by going to countries where inbreeding is common, producing large extended kindreds with multiple affected sibships.

Once a disease has been mapped, it may become apparent that a supposedly unitary condition is actually a collection of different diseases (as happened with Usher syndrome). Conversely, two supposedly different conditions can map to precisely the same location, implying that they are probably caused by mutations in the same gene (as happened with the dominant *DFNA3* and recessive *DFNB1* forms of non-syndromic deafness).

Identifying the disease gene

Figure 4.3 summarizes the many possible routes to identifying a disease gene. In all cases, the strategy has two stages: define a candidate gene, and then seek mutations in that gene in affected people. Maybe if we knew enough about how hearing works, we could use that knowledge to suggest candidate genes for each disorder in the absence of the chromosomal location. For a very limited number of diseases, such an educated guess about the responsible gene has a chance of success, and this procedure is called the candidate gene approach (shortcut 1 in Figure 4.3). However, we know very little about how hearing works, and in fact one of the main reasons for researching genetic deafness is to find the genes responsible for normal hearing. Fortunately, as the Human Genome Project moves forward, a rapidly growing proportion of all human genes are already at least partially cloned, and limited information about the DNA sequence, chromosomal location and expression pattern (by tissue and by stage of development) of many genes is now available in public databases.

Thus once a gene affecting hearing has been mapped, the next step is to search the databases for genes located within the candidate region. If a gene is expressed especially in the inner ear, or if its sequence resembles the sequence of another gene known to be involved in hearing loss, that gene is a good candidate for the disease gene. This procedure is called the positional candidate approach (shortcut 2 in Figure 4.3) and was successful in identifying the *DFNA8* gene. In several families, autosomal dominant hearing impairment mapped to a rather poorly defined location on the long arm of chromosome 11. This locus was called *DFNA8* or *DFNA12* (the two later turned out to be identical). The gene for α-tectorin was known to map within this candidate region. α-Tectorin is a structural protein that is an important component of the tectorial membrane in the inner ear. This provided an obvious candidate gene, and when it was examined in affected family members, changes were identified. Animal models are also invaluable – mice in particular have almost exactly the same genes as humans, and the many mapped mouse mutants can suggest candidates for human disease. The *PAX3* and *MITF* genes that go wrong in Waardenburg syndrome types 1 and 2 respectively were

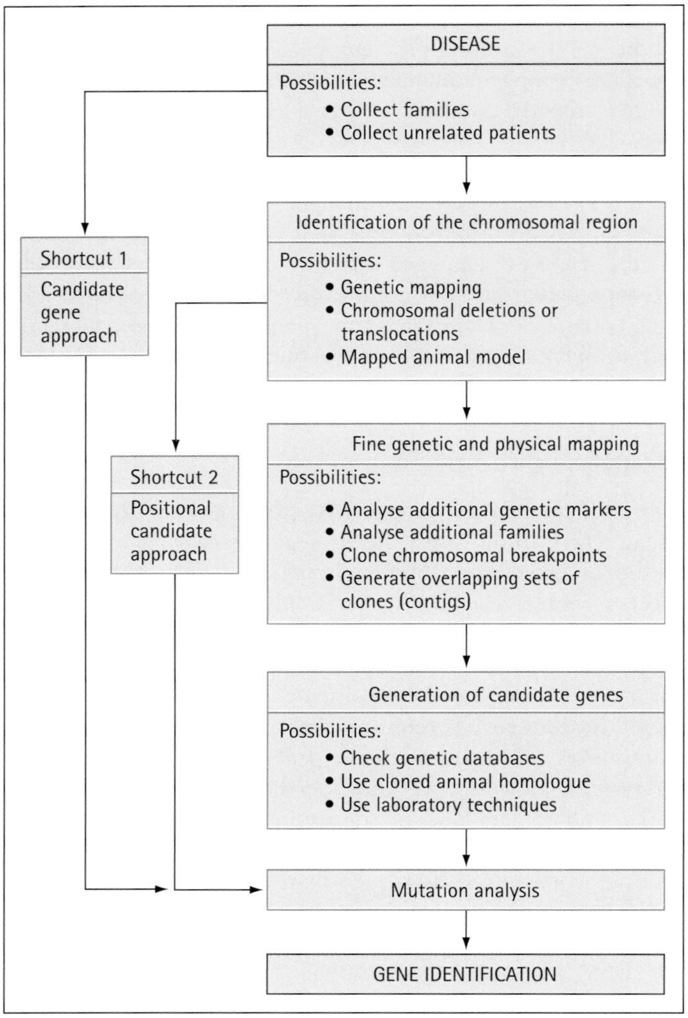

Figure 4.3 Identification of a gene for a monogenic disease.

identified as candidates through comparison with the *Splotch* and *microphthalmia* mouse mutants.

If no obvious candidate gene can be identified, there are two options – test other known genes, even though they have no features making them obvious candidates, or try to isolate novel genes from the candidate region. In our present state of knowledge, predicting which of several genes is the best candidate for a disease is very largely guesswork, so every known gene within the candidate region will probably be examined at least briefly. If none seems promising, then novel genes must be sought. It is important to get some idea of the magnitude of this task. The human genome contains 3×10^9 base pairs of DNA. An average chromosome contains over 100 million base pairs (100 Mb). The best linkage data will not define an interval of less than 1 MB, and 2–10 Mb is more usual. Humans probably have about 80 000 genes, so the average density is about 20–30 genes per Mb. Only a few per cent of any stretch of DNA actually code for protein. Worse, genes in all higher organisms are split into sections (exons) scattered, often quite thinly, among non-coding DNA (introns). When a messenger RNA is made from the gene, all the introns are cut out and degraded, and the exons spliced together. Some genes have over 100 exons. It seems a very strange way for organisms to function, and it certainly makes life hard for gene cloners. They have somehow to identify exons scattered thinly and apparently randomly across a sea of irrelevant DNA, usually with no clue as to the nature of the exons. Until recently, positional cloning (finding unknown genes from a given chromosomal region) was a truly formidable undertaking, involving many years of hard work, often by large collaborations between several laboratories. Nowadays, the Human Genome Project has provided tools to make the task rather easier, in the form of ready-made cloned DNA fragments covering each chromosomal region. There are many ways of searching such cloned DNA fragments for unknown genes. The most obvious is to sequence the clone and use a computer to look for gene-like sequences. This approach identified the *EYA1* gene that underlies the branchio-oto-renal syndrome. An alternative is cDNA library screening: checking the clone for matches to the messenger RNA extracted from a suitable tissue (ideally, the organ of Corti for hearing loss). A third option is exon trapping, which uses special cloning systems to try to mimic the way in which living organisms are able to pick out the thinly scattered exons from large stretches of DNA. None of these approaches is perfect or guaranteed to succeed, and laboratories usually try a combination of methods.

Once a candidate gene has been identified by any of these methods, mutations must be sought in a panel of affected patients. Again, a variety of methods are available, none perfect or guaranteed to succeed. If necessary, all such changes could be identified by sequencing, but sequencing a 10-kb gene in 20 patients can be a lot of work, especially if it is only one of 10 equally good (or poor) candidate genes. Quicker methods are available that detect a reasonable proportion of all changes in a

THE HUMAN GENOME PROJECT

This 15-year project, which started in 1990, aims to determine the complete sequence of the human genome. Before the actual sequencing could start, detailed genetic and physical maps of the human genome needed to be constructed. The genetic map currently includes more than 20 000 genetic markers, many of them ordered in high-resolution genetic maps. The physical map consists of overlapping pieces of DNA (contigs), cloned in yeast (yeast artificial chromosomes or YACs) and bacteria (bacterial artificial chromosomes or BACs). The complete human genome is covered with YAC contigs, and a significant fraction is cloned in BACs that are actually being sequenced. A first draft of the sequence with many inaccuracies and gaps was finished in February 2001. The researchers hope to have the complete 3 billion nucleotides sequenced 2 years ahead of schedule, by 2003.

panel of samples, and these allow rapid but imperfect screening of a candidate gene.

Having found a change, one needs to know whether it is a pathogenic mutation or just a harmless variant. Some changes can be predicted to destroy all functions of the protein product, and these would be convincing candidates for pathogenic mutations. Other changes simply replace one amino acid in the protein by another. It is much harder to assess the impact of such a change. If several different affected families have several different such changes, and if these changes cannot be found on screening a good-sized panel of unaffected people, then probably the changes are pathogenic, and the right gene has been identified. The final proof can only come from some sort of functional test on the protein product of the gene—but in many cases those experiments are not currently possible.

Genetics of auditory disorders

Epidemiology

Approximately 1/1000 children are diagnosed as deaf or hard of hearing in early childhood. In developed countries, more than 50% of these cases are caused by mutations in single genes.[2,3] The mode of inheritance of childhood hearing impairment is autosomal recessive in approximately 80%, autosomal dominant in 15% and X-linked in 2–3%.[2,4]

Hearing impairment with postlingual onset is very frequent: 15–20% of the population is affected with a hearing impairment of more than 25 dB.[2] A majority of cases is found in the elderly population, but genetic factors have also been proven to be important in presbyacusis.[5] Monogenic forms of postlingual hearing impairment also exist, but there are no good estimates for the prevalence. Nearly all published families with monogenic postlingual hearing impairment have an autosomal dominant inheritance pattern.

Syndromic hearing impairment

From a clinical genetic point of view, hereditary hearing impairment is subdivided in syndromic forms, associated with additional clinical abnormalities, and non-syndromic forms. Although less than one-third of all cases of hereditary hearing impairment are syndromic, several hundred different syndromes in which hearing impairment is a symptom have been described. In some of these, hearing impairment is only a minor symtom, or is a secondary effect of another defect (for example, patients with neurofibromatosis type II develop hearing impairment after the formation of a tumour on the acoustical nerve). In other syndromes, however, hearing impairment is a major hallmark, and the responsible gene most likely has an important function in the inner ear, as well as in one or more other tissues that are affected by the syndrome. For a number of syndromic forms of deafness, the responsible gene has been identified. In Table 4.3, the major characteristics of some of the best-known syndromic forms of hearing impairment are given. Certain clinical abnormalities occur frequently in combination with hearing impairment. Examples are pigmentary disturbances, the hallmark of Waardenburg syndrome, and retinitis pigmentosa, a characteristic of Usher syndrome. Waardenburg as well as Usher syndrome are subcategorized further on the basis of additional clinical abnormalities, and different genes are responsible for the different subcategories. Both syndromes are genetically heterogeneous: five different genes are known to be responsible for

Table 4.2 Loci for hearing impairment, classified according to affected frequencies and inheritance pattern.

Inheritance	Low frequencies	Mid-frequencies/All frequencies	High frequencies
Autosomal dominant[a]	*DFNA1* *DFNA6* *DFNA14* *DFNA15*	*DFNA4* *DFNA8/12* *DFNA10* *DFNA11* *DFNA13*	*DFNA2* *DFNA3* *DFNA5* *DFNA7* *DFNA9* *DFNA16* *DFNA17*
Autosomal recessive[b]	None	*DFNB1–B18*	None
X-linked[c]	None	*DFN2* *DFN3* *DFN4*	*DFN6*

[a]The patients from all the families linked to autosomal dominant (*DFNA*) loci have progressive hearing impairment with postlingual onset, with the exception of *DFNA3* and *DFNA8/12*, for which the families have prelingual and stable hearing impairment.
[b]The patients from all recessive (*DFNB*) families have a hearing loss affecting all frequencies, which is prelingual and stable for all loci, except *DFNB3* and *DFNB13*, where the hearing loss is progressive.
[c]X-linked loci *DFN1* and *DFN5* are not mentioned in this table: *DFN1* refers to a syndromic form of deafness, and *DFN5* has been withdrawn.

Table 4.3 Syndromic forms of hearing impairment.

Syndrome	Major additional symptoms	Protein name	Protein class and/or gene function	Reference
Alport	Nephritis	Collagen type IV (different chains)	Extracellular matrix molecule for basement membranes	61,62
Branchio-oto-renal	Branchial anomalies, renal manifestations	EYA1	Transcriptional co-activator	63
Jervell and Lange Nielsen	Cardiac arrhythmia, syncopal episodes	KCNQ1 (KVLQT1) MinK (also called IsK)	Potassium channel subunits	27,64,65
Norrie	Blindness, mental retardation	Norrin	Putative growth factor	66,67
Pendred	Thyroid goitre	Pendrin	Iodide transporter	24
Stickler	Myopia, vitreoretinal degeneration, joint degeneration	Collagen type II (α1 chain)	Extracellular matrix molecule for cartilage	68–70
Treacher Collins	Abnormal craniofacial development	Treacle	Putative nucleolar phosphoprotein	71
Usher (different types)	Retinitis pigmentosa	Myosin VIIa (type 1B) USH2A (type 2A)	Myosin VIIa: motor molecule USH2A: extracellular matrix molecule	19,72
Waardenburg (different types)	Pigmentary abnormalities of hair, iris and skin, dystopia canthorum (type I), upper limb abnormalities (type III), aganglionic megacolon (type IV)	PAX3 (types I and III) MITF (type II) Endothelin 3 Endothelin B receptor SOX10	PAX3, MITF and SOX10: transcription factor with role in migration of neural crest cells during embryonic development Endothelin 3 and endothelin B receptor: vasoactive peptide and receptor that play a role in the development of neural crest-derived enteric neurones	73–78

different types of Waardenburg syndrome, and nine different genes have been localized for Usher syndrome, only two of which have been identified.

Gene localizations for non-syndromic hearing impairment

Non-syndromic congenital deafness is inherited autosomal recessively in a large majority of cases (Table 4.4). When two deaf parents have normally hearing children, a different gene must be responsible for deafness in these parents. Therefore, decades ago, it was deduced from the statistical analysis of deaf–deaf matings that many different genes are responsible for autosomal recessive deafness. This genetic heterogeneity makes it impossible to pool the information from different families, and linkage analysis of the responsible genes must be carried out in separate families. However, most families from the Western world contain only a single affected individual with unrelated parents, which is useless for linkage analysis. For these reasons, it was only in 1994 that the first genes for non-syndromic deafness were localized, when many genes for other frequent autosomal recessive (genetically homogeneous) diseases had already been localized. At this moment, more than 20 genes for non-syndromic recessive deafness have been localized. With a few exceptions, the patients in all these families have profound congenital deafness. Gene localizations for non-syndromic hearing impairment are numbered in the order of discovery, and are given a prefix to denote the inheritance pattern. Loci for autosomal recessive loci for hereditary hearing loss are given the prefix *DFNB*. All the *DFNB* localizations have been carried out on the basis of consanguineous families, originating from ethnically isolated regions, or regions with high consanguinity. The information content of consanguineous families can be very high. For example, a family where the parents are first cousins, and in which there are three affected children, has enough power to find linkage.

An autosomal dominant family with about 10 affected family members is about the minimal size to prove linkage, and

Table 4.4 Genes responsible for non-syndromic hearing impairment.

Protein name	Protein class and/or gene function	Non-syndromic locus (eventual syndrome)	Reference
Diaphanous 1	Regulation of actin polymerization	*DFNA1*	79
Connexin 31	Gap junction protein, forms channels between adjacent cells	*DFNA2*	32
Connexin 26	Gap junction protein, forms channels between adjacent cells	*DFNB1, DFNA3*	30,31
DFNA5	Unknown	*DFNA5*	80
α-Tectorin	Extracellular matrix protein, major structural component of the tectorial membrane	*DFNA8/12*	13
COCH	Putative extracellular matrix protein, specific for cochlea and vestibular apparatus	*DFNA9*	52
Myosin VIIA	Molecular motor protein, moves different macromolecular structures relative to the cytoskeleton of the cell	*DFNB2, DFNA11* (Usher syndrome)	20–22
POU4F3	Transcription factor with role in embryogenesis	*DFNA15*	81
POU3F4	Transcription factor with role in embryogenesis	*DFN3*	18
Myosin XV	Molecular motor protein, moves different macromolecular structures relative to the cytoskeleton of the cell	*DFNB3*	82
Pendrin	Iodide transporter	*DFNB4* (Pendred syndrome)	24
KCNQ4	K^+ ion channel	*DFNA2*	29
Otoferlin	Membrane vesicle trafficking protein	*DFNB9*	83

such families with hearing impairment have been reported in the literature since the 1960s. It is therefore somewhat surprising that the first gene for autosomal dominant hearing impairment was not localized earlier than 1992.[6] As no data about genetic heterogeneity for autosomal dominantly inherited hearing impairment were available from epidemiological studies, it was only through linkage analysis in many additional families that it became clear that dominant hearing impairment is equally genetically heterogeneous as recessive deafness. After the first localization for dominant hearing impairment, more than 20 additional loci have been assigned to different chromosome bands. Dominant loci for non-syndromic hearing impairment are given the prefix *DFNA*.

Non-syndromic hearing impairment: phenotypic characteristics

The patients from all recessive (*DFNB*) families have a hearing loss affecting all frequencies, that is prelingual and stable, except for *DFNB3*[7] and *DFNB13*,[8] where the hearing loss is progressive. The hearing impairment in families with autosomal dominant inheritance patterns is very different from that in the recessive families. In most cases it is progressive, with onset ranging from the first up to the fifth decade. In the beginning, the hearing impairment is limited, and often only certain frequencies are affected (Table 4.2). In some families, the high frequencies are affected first, sometimes progressing to a profound hearing impairment across all frequencies (e.g. some families linked to *DFNA2*[9]), while in other families the low frequencies are spared (e.g. a large Dutch family linked to *DFNA5*[10]). Conversely, the hearing impairment starts in the low frequencies in other families, leading to profound deafness in some (e.g. a large Costa Rican family linked to *DFNA1*[6]), or sparing the high frequencies (families linked to *DFNA6*[11] and *DFNA14*[12]). A few families with autosomal dominant congenital non-progressive hearing impairment have been reported (families linked to *DFNA8* and *DFNA12*), but here the hearing impairment is only moderate to severe.[13]

Although only four different loci for X-linked hearing impairment have been reported, eight different loci have been given a *DFN* prefix denoting X-linked inheritance. The reason for this lies in the fact that one *DFN* locus turned out to be syndromic after more careful clinical analysis (*DFN1*),[14] two localizations have been withdrawn, and three putative localizations have remained unpublished. The phenotype of the X-linked families is variable. Some families have profound congenital hearing impairment (*DFN2*[15] and *DFN4*[16]), while others have progressive postlingual hearing impairment (*DFN6*[17]). Families linked to *DFN3* are characterized by structural abnormalities of the middle and inner ear, including an abnormal communication between cerebrospinal fluid and perilymph.[18] These patients also have fixation of the stapes, giving rise to a conductive hearing impairment in addition to a sensorineural component. When the oval window is penetrated during surgery, a so-called perilymphatic gusher occurs, resulting in complete loss of hearing.

Gene identifications for hereditary hearing impairment

When the currently identified genes for syndromic and non-syndromic hereditary hearing impairment (Tables 4.3 and 4.4) are compared, it is striking that certain categories of genes are present several times. These categories include transcription factors, generally involved in embryonic development, extracellular matrix proteins, unconventional myosins and ion channel/transporter proteins. It is also remarkable that nearly all of these genes are expressed in multiple tissues, but that functional impairment leads to hearing loss as the only phenotype. Possibly, these proteins have several functions, with specific and irreplaceable functions in the inner ear, and redundant functions in other tissues. (Figure 4.4)

One gene can cause syndromic as well as non-syndromic hearing impairment

Two genes, myosin VIIA and pendrin, have been implicated in syndromic as well as non-syndromic hearing impairment. Different mutations in myosin VIIA are responsible for the autosomal recessively inherited Usher syndrome (type 1B),[19] as well as both autosomal dominant and autosomal recessive non-syndromic hearing impairment.[20–22] Myosin VIIA is expressed in the sensory hair cells of the cochlea, as well as the photoreceptor cells in the retina,[23] but it is currently unclear why certain mutations affect both types of cells, while others only affect the hair cells.

Pendred syndrome, a combination of deafness and thyroid abnormalities, is caused by mutations affecting the pendrin protein,[24] which is a chloride–iodide transport molecule.[25] Although this function intuitively associates well with a thyroid defect, the mechanisms leading to hearing impairment are less clear. However, the majority of Pendred patients have been reported to have congenital inner ear malformations, including a Mondini malformation of the cochlea, and enlarged vestibular aqueducts. Enlarged vestibular aqueducts have also been found in the non-syndromic patients with mutations in the Pendred gene. In addition, the thyroid goitre in Pendred patients often develops later in life, and in some Pendred families the same mutation is present in patients with and without goitre, and with and without Mondini malformation. It is now becoming clear that mutations in the gene coding for pendrin are responsible for a wide spectrum of overlapping phenotypes, ranging from non-syndromic hearing impairment with enlarged vestibular aqueducts to classical Pendred syndrome patients with Mondini cochlear malformations and goitre.[26] Most likely, the phenotypic expression of mutations in pendrin is influenced by other as yet unidentified factors, genetic or environmental.

K^+ channels in hearing impairment

The endolymph in the inner ear has a very high K^+ concentration. When the stereocilia of the hair cells in the cochlea are deflected by acoustical vibrations, K^+ enters the hair cells. These ions are recycled to the stria vascularis, where they are actively pumped back into the endolymph. These K^+ ion fluxes play a crucial role in the inner ear, and it is therefore not surprising that many of the genes for hearing impairment encode channels and gap junctions involved in ion transport.

Several mutations in K^+ channels have been implicated in hereditary hearing loss. Homozygotes for mutations in KCNQ1 or KCNE1 cause Jervell and Lange-Nielsen syndrome,[27] a syndromic form of deafness including cardiac arrhythmia. Heterozygotes usually only have the cardiac symptoms, known as long QT syndrome.[28] Mutations in a novel member of the KCNQ K^+ channel family (KCNQ4) cause autosomal non-syndromic dominant hearing loss (*DFNA2*).[29] KCNQ1 is expressed in the stria vascularis, where it passes K^+ ions into the endolymph. KCNQ4 is expressed in the outer hair cells and may be responsible for letting K^+ out of the outer hair cell after stimulation. Another class of molecules that are important in regulating ion fluxes are connexins. Connexins form gap junctions between adjacent cells, through which small molecules can be exchanged. Mutations in connexin 26 are very frequent causes of recessive deafness, and also seem to be a relatively infrequent cause of autosomal dominant hearing impairment.[30,31] Connexin 31 mutations have been found in a few dominant families (*DFNA2*),[32] but whether this gene is a frequent cause of hearing impairment remains to be determined. Both Cx26 and Cx31 are expressed in the supporting cells surrounding the hair cells and in the fibrocytes of the spiral ligament around the stria vascularis.[33] This suggests a role of these gap junctions in the diffusion of K^+ ions from the hair cells to the stria vascularis, completing the circle of K^+ recycling.

Mitochondrial hearing impairment

Mitochondria are important cellular organelles, responsible for energy production. Mitochondria contain a small amount of DNA (16 569 nucleotides in humans) that codes for 36 genes in total. Mutations in mitochondrial genes are usually associated with syndromic disorders, and sensorineural hearing impairment

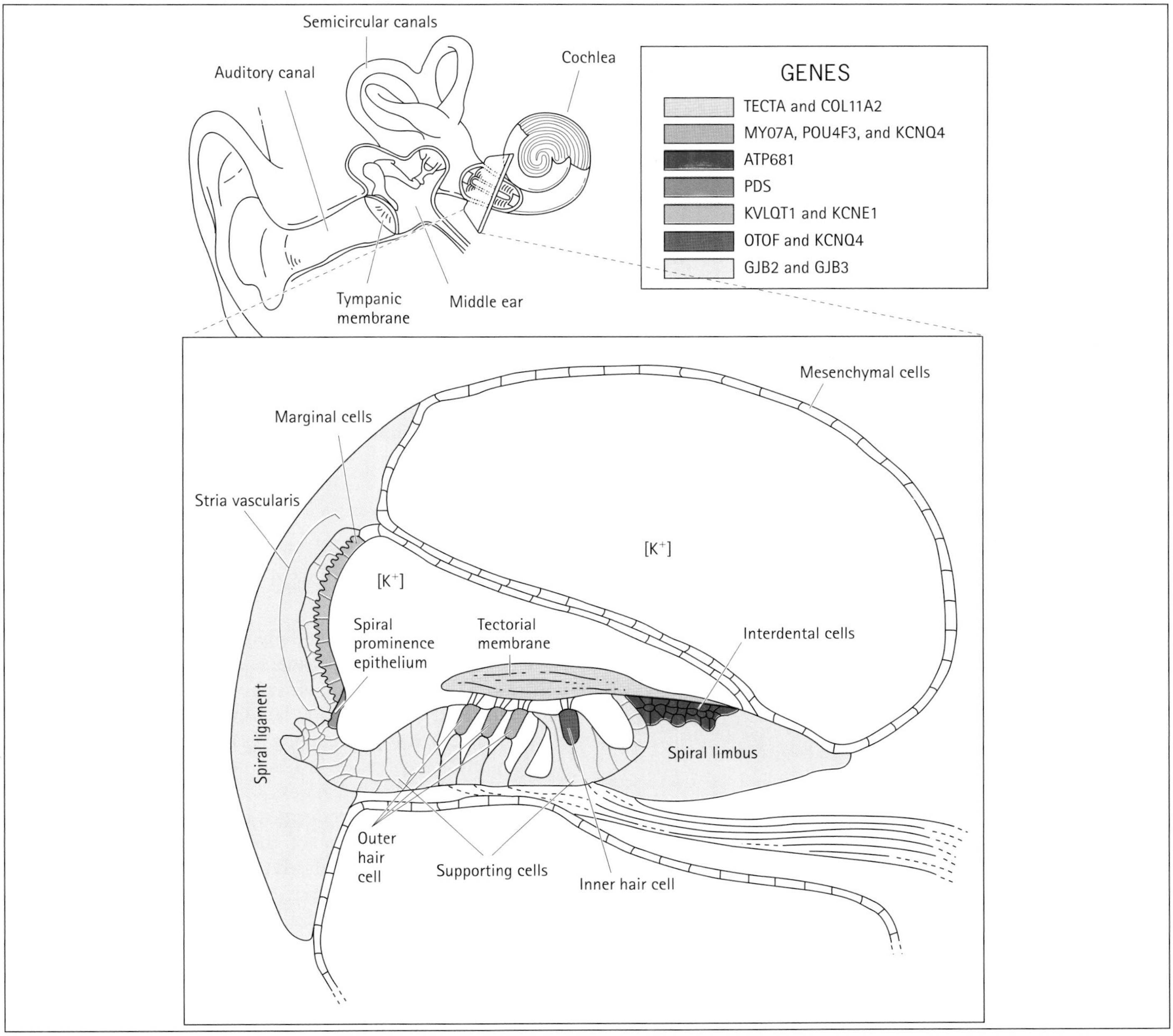

Figure 4.4 Cross-sectional view of the basal turn of the cochlea to illustrate the site of expression of some the genes identified as causing hearing impairment. (From Tekin et al. *Lancet* 2001; **358**: 1082–90 with permission from Elsevier Science Ltd.)

is an accompanying symptom in many of them. Mitochondrial syndromes that include hearing loss are MELAS (mitochondrial encephalomyopathy, lactic acidosis, stroke-like symptoms),[34] MERFF (myoclonus epilepsy with ragged-red fibres),[35,36] PEO (progressive external opthalmoplegia)[37] and Kearns–Sayre syndrome.[37] Also, a combination of diabetes type II and hearing loss has been associated with a mitochondrial mutation.[38] Three mutations give rise to hearing loss as the sole symptom in many patients (Table 4.5). The reason why only the auditory system is affected by these mutations remains unknown.

The first mutation (1555A→G) is found in many pedigrees with non-syndromic deafness and in patients and families with aminoglycoside-induced ototoxic hearing impairment.[39] Apparently this mutation makes individuals susceptible to hearing impairment after treatment with aminoglycosides at concentrations that normally do not affect hearing. Even without exposure to aminoglycosides, many patients with this mutation develop hearing impairment, but it is currently unknown which other factors are involved in the aetiology. Apparently, this mutation is rather frequent in certain regions, such as Spain[40] and Japan.[41]

The two other non-syndromic mitochondrial mutations (7445A→G) and 7472insC) are in some patients associated with palmoplantar keratoderma[42–44] and neurological symptoms[45,46] respectively.

Table 4.5 Mitochondrial mutations leading to hearing impairment as the sole or predominant symptom.

Mitochondrial mutation	Gene	Additional clinical hallmarks	References
1555A→G	12SrRNA	Susceptibility to aminoglycoside ototoxicity	39,41,84
7445A→G	tRNA-ser(UCN)	Palmoplantar keratoderma (thickening of horny layer of the skin of palms and soles)	42–44
7472insC	tRNA-ser(UCN)	Various neurological symptoms	45,46

Otosclerosis

Otosclerosis is a common cause of conductive or mixed hearing impairment, affecting up to 1% of the Caucasian population. The disease has an onset between 10 and 50 years of age, and is characterized by abnormal resorption and redeposition of bone in certain areas of the labyrinthine capsule. These otosclerotic foci invade the oval window and interfere with free motion of the stapes, leading to conductive hearing loss. It is thought that otosclerotic foci can also damage the cochlear endosteum, leading to sensorineural hearing loss. Although the aetiology of otosclerosis is poorly understood and controversial, the finding of many familial cases has indicated that genetic factors are important. Epidemiological studies indicate autosomal dominant inheritance with incomplete penetrance.[47,48] However, large families suitable for genetic linkage analysis seem to be rare, and only a single family that is large enough has been reported. On the basis of this multigenerational family with 16 affected individuals, linkage was found on chromosome 15.[49] Other families were found not to be linked to this locus, suggesting genetic heterogeneity for otosclerosis, but no other locus has been found up to now (G. Van Camp and R. J. H. Smith, unpublished observation).

Vestibular dysfunction

The sensory epithelia of the cochlea, the semicircular canals and the otolith organs are very similar, and it seems logical that a considerable number of inner ear-specific genes exists, with functions in the cochlea as well as in the vestibular system. Mutations in such genes are expected to lead to both hearing and vestibular problems. It is known that vestibular testing is abnormal in 40–80% of deaf individuals.[50,51] However, vestibular testing is seldom reported in genetic papers describing localizations or identifications of deafness genes, and surprisingly little is known about vestibular involvement in most of the currently identified deafness genes. Among the loci for autosomal dominant hearing impairment, the *DFNA9* locus (*COCH* gene) is the only one involving vestibular problems in addition to non-syndromic deafness. Mutations in the COCH gene cause a progressive perceptive hearing impairment accompanied by progressive imbalance and positional vertigo.[52–54] A single mutation in the *COCH* gene (P51S) has been found in more than 130 patients from 10 independent *DFNA9* families from Belgium and The Netherlands, and may be a relatively frequent cause of vestibular dysfunction (G. Van Camp, unpublished observation). It is remarkable that many patients with *COCH* mutations reported vertigo attacks with accompanying hearing loss, tinnitus and/or aural fullness, symptoms characteristic of Menière's disease. In addition, histopathologically confirmed hydrops labyrinthi, considered to be proof of Menière's disease, has been found in patients who were later found to have a *COCH* mutation.[52,55,56]

Molecular diagnostics for hereditary hearing impairment

Molecular diagnostics can be helpful in genetic counselling of patients with hearing impairment. In some cases, DNA diagnostics could be used to determine whether the cause of deafness in a child with normally hearing parents is hereditary or environmental. A parent coming from a family in which a form of adult-onset progressive hearing impairment segregates may request presymptomatic diagnosis for a child. DNA diagnostics in large families can be performed by linkage analysis, even in the absence of knowledge of the disease-causing mutation. Genetic markers can be analysed to determine whether an individual has inherited a certain chromosomal region from his parents, and this can be the basis for a genetic diagnosis. However, a large majority of patients do not come from a large family where linkage analysis is possible. In these cases, DNA diagnostics can only be performed by the analysis of the disease-causing mutation. Many genes responsible for syndromic forms of hearing impairment have been identified. In a patient with a diagnosis of a certain form of syndromic deafness, mutation analysis can be performed in the responsible gene. However, many patients have different mutations, and in most cases mutation analysis of the complete gene has to be carried out to find the responsible mutation. Although molecular diagnostics is in principle possible for many syndromic forms of hearing impairment, it remains expensive.

Molecular diagnostics for non-syndromic hearing impairment is even more difficult. Because of the genetic heterogeneity, the disease-causing mutation could reside in any of a large number of different genes, of which only a small fraction have been identified. For this reason, DNA diagnostics for non-syndromic deafness remained impossible for most patients until recently.

Connexin 26

Mutations in the gene encoding the gap junction protein connexin-26 were shown to cause *DFNB1*. *DNFB1* is estimated to represent up to 50% of all autosomal recessive deafness.[57,58] Subsequent studies have shown that a single mutation, 35delG, accounts for up to 70% of mutant alleles in different ethnic groups.[31,59,60] As the 35delG mutation is easy to detect in the laboratory, this genetic test represents the first genetic test for hereditary deafness that is likely to find widespread use in genetic counselling for the deaf. Despite the enormous genetic heterogeneity of hereditary deafness, the high prevalence of this mutation among the congenitally deaf makes it a test that is useful in individuals from the majority of recessive families in which only a single patient is present.

The future

The sensory epithelia of the inner ear play an important role in hearing and balance by converting stimuli elicited by sound and accelerations into signals to the brain. The understanding of the underlying molecular processes is currently very limited. The identification of the first genes with an important function in the inner ear is contributing a lot to this understanding. These findings are leading to new diagnostic possibilities for hereditary deafness. It is to be expected that a large number of additional genes will be identified over the next decade, and that these findings will further contribute to better insights into the process of hearing. These insights will hopefully lead to future therapies to prevent or even cure certain forms of hearing impairment.

References

1. Strachan T, Read AP. *Human Molecular Genetics* 2nd edn. Oxford: Bios Scientific Publishers, New York: John Wiley, 1999.
2. Morton NE. Genetic epidemiology of hearing impairment. *Ann NY Acad Sci* 1991; **630**: 16–31.
3. Cohen M, Gorlin R. Epidemiology, etiology, and genetic patterns. In: Gorlin R, Toriello H, Cohen M, eds. *Hereditary Hearing Loss and its Syndromes*. Oxford: Oxford University Press, 1995: 9–21.
4. Newton VE. Aetiology of bilateral sensorineural hearing loss in young children. *J Laryngol Otol (Suppl)* 1985; **10**: 1–57.
5. Myers RH, Couropmitree NN, Gates GA. Heritability estimates for age-related hearing loss. *Am J Hum Genet* 1998; **63S**: A217 (abstract).
6. Leon PE, Raventos H, Lynch E, Morrow J, King MC. The gene for an inherited form of deafness maps to chromosome 5q31. *Proc Natl Acad Sci USA* 1992; **89**: 5181–2.
7. Friedman TB, Liang Y, Weber JL et al. A gene for congenital, recessive deafness DFNB3 maps to the pericentromeric region of chromosome 17. *Nat Genet* 1995; **9**: 86–91.
8. Mustapha M, Salem N, Weil D, El-Zir E, Loiselet J, Petit C. Identification of a locus on chromosome 7q31, DFNB14, responsible for prelingual sensorineural non-syndromic deafness. *Eur J Hum Genet* 1998; **6**: 548–51.
9. Van Camp G, Coucke PJ, Kunst H et al. Linkage analysis of progressive hearing loss in five extended families maps the DFNA2 gene to a 1.25-Mb region of chromosome 1p. *Genomics* 1997; **41**: 70–4.
10. Van Camp G, Coucke P, Balemans W et al. Localization of a gene for non-syndromic hearing loss (DFNA5) to chromosome 7p15. *Hum Mol Genet* 1995; **4**: 2159–63.
11. Lesperance MM, Hall JW, Bess FH et al. A gene for autosomal dominant nonsyndromic hereditary hearing impairment maps to 4p16.3. *Hum Mol Genet* 1995; **4**: 1967–72.
12. Van Camp G, Kunst H, Flothmann K et al. A gene for autosomal dominant hearing impairment (DFNA14) maps to a region on chromosome 4p16.3 that does not overlap the DFNA6 locus. *J Med Genet* 1999; **36**: 532–6.
13. Verhoeven K, Van Laer L, Kirschhofer K et al. Mutations in the human tectorin gene cause autosomal dominant non-syndromic hearing impairment. *Nat Genet* 1998; **19**: 60–2.
14. Tranebjaerg L, Schwartz C, Eriksen H et al. A new X linked recessive deafness syndrome with blindness, dystonia, fractures, and mental deficiency is linked to Xq22. *J Med Genet* 1995; **32**: 257–63.
15. Tyson J, Bellman S, Newton V et al. Mapping of DFN2 to Xq22. *Hum Mol Genet 1996;* **5**: 2055–60.
16. Lalwani AK, Brister JR, Fex J et al. A new nonsyndromic X-linked sensorineural hearing impairment linked to Xp21.2. *Am J Hum Genet* 1994; **55**: 685–94.
17. del Castillo I, Villamar M, Sarduy M et al. A novel locus for non-syndromic sensorineural deafness (DFN6) maps to chromosome Xp22. *Hum Mol Genet* 1996; **5**: 1383–7.
18. de Kok YJ, van der Maarel SM, Bitner-Glindzicz M et al. Association between X-linked mixed deafness and mutations in the POU domain gene POU3F4. *Science* 1995; **267**: 685–8.
19. Weil D, Blanchard S, Kaplan J et al. Defective myosin VIIA gene responsible for Usher syndrome type 1B. *Nature* 1995; **374**: 60–1.
20. Weil D, Kussel P, Blanchard S et al. The autosomal recessive isolated deafness, DFNB2, and the Usher 1B syndrome are allelic defects of the myosin-VIIA gene. *Nat Genet* 1997; **16**: 191–3.
21. Liu XZ, Walsh J, Mburu P et al. Mutations in the myosin VIIA gene cause non-syndromic deafness. *Nat Genet* 1997; **16**: 188–90.
22. Liu XZ, Walsh J, Tamagawa Y et al. Autosomal dominant non-syndromic deafness caused by a mutation in the myosin VIIA gene. *Nat Genet* 1997; **17**: 268–9.
23. Hasson T, Heintzelmann MB, Santos-Sacchi J, Corey DP, Mooseker MS. Expression in cochlea and retina of myosin VIIa, the gene product defective in Usher syndrome type 1B. *Proc Natl Acad Sci USA* 1995; **92**: 9815–19.
24. Everett LA, Glazer B, Beck JC et al. Pendred syndrome is caused by mutations in a putative sulphate transporter gene (PDS). *Nat Genet* 1997; **17**: 411–22.
25. Scott DA, Wang R, Kreman TM, Sheffield VC, Karnishki LP. The Pendred syndrome gene encodes a chloride–iodide transport protein. *Nat Genet* 1999; **21**: 440–3.
26. Usami S, Abe S, Weston MD, Shinkawa H, Van CG, Kimberling WJ. Non-syndromic hearing loss associated with enlarged vestibular aqueduct is caused by PDS mutations. *Hum Genet* 1999; **104**: 188–92.

27. Neyroud N, Tesson F, Denjoy I et al. A novel mutation in the potassium channel gene KVLQT1 causes the Jervell and Lange–Nielsen cardioauditory syndrome. *Nat Genet* 1997; **15**: 186–9.
28. Wang Q, Curran ME, Splawski I et al. Positional cloning of a novel potassium channel gene: KVLQT1 mutations cause cardiac arrhythmias. *Nat Genet* 1996; **12**: 17–23.
29. Kubisch C, Schroeder BC, Friedrich T et al. KCNQ4, a novel potassium channel expressed in sensory outer hair cells, is mutated in dominant deafness. *Cell* 1999; **96**: 437–46.
30. Kelsell DP, Dunlop J, Stevens HP et al. Connexin 26 mutations in hereditary non-syndromic sensorineural deafness. *Nature* 1997; **387**: 80–3.
31. Denoyelle F, Weil D, Maw MA et al. Prelingual deafness: high prevalence of a 30delG mutation in the connexin 26 gene. *Hum Mol Genet* 1997; **6**: 2173–7.
32. Xia JH, Liu CY, Tang BS et al. Mutations in the gene encoding gap junction protein beta-3 associated with autosomal dominant hearing impairment. *Nat Genet* 1998; **20**: 370–3.
33. Kikuchi T, Kimura RS, Paul DL, Adams JC. Gap junctions in the rat cochlea: immunohistochemical and ultrastructural analysis. *Anat Embryol (Berl)* 1995; **191**: 101–18.
34. Goto Y, Nonaka I, Horai S. A mutation in the tRNA(Leu)(UUR) gene associated with the MELAS subgroup of mitochondrial encephalomyopathies. *Nature* 1990; **348**: 651–3.
35. Shoffner JM, Lott MT, Lezza AM, Seibel P, Ballinger SW, Wallace DC. Myoclonic epilepsy and ragged-red fiber disease (MERRF) is associated with a mitochondrial DNA tRNA(Lys) mutation. *Cell* 1990; **61**: 931–7.
36. Zeviani M, Muntoni F, Savarese N et al. A MERRF/MELAS overlap syndrome associated with a new point mutation in the mitochondrial DNA tRNA(Lys) gene. *Eur J Hum Genet* 1993; **1**: 80–7.
37. Moraes CT, DiMauro S, Zeviani M et al. Mitochondrial DNA deletions in progressive external ophthalmoplegia and Kearns–Sayre syndrome. *N Engl J Med* 1989; **320**: 1293–9.
38. van den Ouweland JM, Lemkes HH, Ruitenbeek W et al. Mutation in mitochondrial tRNA(Leu)(UUR) gene in a large pedigree with maternally transmitted type II diabetes mellitus and deafness. *Nat Genet* 1992; **1**: 368–71.
39. Prezant TR, Agapian JV, Bohlman MC et al. Mitochondrial ribosomal RNA mutation associated with both antibiotic-induced and non-syndromic deafness. *Nat Genet* 1993; **4**: 289–94.
40. Estivill X, Govea N, Barcelo E et al. Familial progressive sensorineural deafness is mainly due to the mtDNA A1555G mutation and is enhanced by treatment of aminoglycosides. *Am J Hum Genet* 1998; **62**: 27–35.
41. Usami S, Abe S, Kasai M et al. Genetic and clinical features of sensorineural hearing loss associated with the 1555 mitochondrial mutation. *Laryngoscope* 1997; **107**: 483–90.
42. Reid FM, Vernham GA, Jacobs HT. A novel mitochondrial point mutation in a maternal pedigree with sensorineural deafness. *Hum Mutat* 1994; **3**: 243–7.
43. Fischel-Ghodsian N, Prezant TR, Fournier P, Stewart IA, Maw M. Mitochondrial mutation associated with nonsyndromic deafness. *Am J Otolaryngol* 1995; **16**: 403–8.
44. Sevior KB, Hatamochi A, Stewart IA et al. Mitochondrial A7445G mutation in two pedigrees with palmoplantar keratoderma and deafness. *Am J Med Genet* 1998; **75**: 179–85.
45. Tiranti V, Chariot P, Carella F et al. Maternally inherited hearing loss, ataxia and myoclonus associated with a novel point mutation in mitochondrial tRNASer(UCN) gene. *Hum Mol Genet* 1995; **4**: 1421–7.
46. Verhoeven K, Ensink RJH, Tiranti V et al. Hearing impairment and neurological dysfunction associated with a mutation in the mitochondrial tRNASer(UCN) gene. *Eur J Hum Genet* 1999; **7**: 45–51.
47. Causse JR, Causse JB, Otospongiosis as a genetic disease. Early detection, medical management, and prevention. *Am J Otol* 1984; **5**: 211–23.
48. Ben Arab S, Bonaiti-Pellie C, Belkahia A. A genetic study of otosclerosis in a population living in the north of Tunisia. *Ann Genet* 1993; **36**: 111–16.
49. Tomek MS, Brown MR, Mani SR et al. Localization of a gene for otosclerosis to chromosome 15q25–q26. *Hum Mol Genet* 1998; **7**: 285–90.
50. Arnvig J. Vestibular function in deafness and severe hard of hearing. *Acta Otolaryngol* 1955; **45**: 283–8.
51. Sandberg L, Terkildsen K. Caloric tests in deaf children. *Arch Otolaryngol* 1965; **81**: 352–4.
52. Robertson NG, Lu L, Heller S et al. Mutations in a novel cochlear gene cause DFNA9, a human nonsyndromic deafness with vestibular dysfunction. *Nature Genet* 1998; **20**: 299–303.
53. de Kok YJ, Bom SJ, Brunt TM et al. A Pro51Ser mutation in the COCH gene is associated with late onset autosomal dominant progressive sensorineural hearing loss with vestibular defects. *Hum Mol Genet* 1999; **8**: 361–6.
54. Fransen E, Verstreken M, Verhagen WIM et al. High prevalence of symptoms of Menière's disease in three families with a mutation in the COCH gene. *Hum Mol Genet* 1999; **8**: 1425–9.
55. Khetarpal U, Schuknecht HF, Gacek RR, Holmes LB. Autosomal dominant sensorineural hearing loss. Pedigrees, audiologic findings, and temporal bone findings in two kindreds. *Arch Otolaryngol Head Neck Surg* 1991; **117**: 1032–42.
56. Khetarpal U. Autosomal dominant sensorineural hearing loss. Further temporal bone findings. *Arch Otolaryngol Head Neck Surg* 1993; **119**: 106–8.
57. Maw MA, Allen-Powell DR, Goodey RJ et al. The contribution of the DFNB1 locus to neurosensory deafness in a Caucasian population. *Am J Hum Genet* 1995; **57**: 629–35.
58. Gasparini P, Estivill X, Volpini V et al. Linkage of DFNB1 to non-syndromic neurosensory autosomal-recessive deafness in Mediterranean families. *Eur J Hum Genet* 1997; **5**: 83–8.
59. Estivill X, Fortina P, Surrey S et al. Connexin-26 mutations in sporadic and inherited sensorineural deafness. *Lancet* 1998; **351**: 394–8.
60. Kelley PM, Harris DJ, Comer BC et al. Novel mutations in the connexin 26 gene (GJB2) that cause autosomal recessive (DFNB1) hearing loss. *Am J Hum Genet* 1998; **62**: 792–9.
61. Barker DF, Hostikka SL, Zhou J et al. Identification of mutations in the COL4A5 collagen gene in Alport syndrome. *Science* 1990; **248**: 1224–7.

62. Mochizuki T, Lemmink HH, Mariyama M et al. Identification of mutations in the alpha 3(IV) and alpha 4 (IV) collagen genes in autosomal recessive Alport syndrome. *Nat Genet* 1994; **8**: 77–81.
63. Abdelhak S, Kalatzis V, Heilig R et al. A human homologue of the Drosophila eyes absent gene underlies branchio-oto-renal (BOR) syndrome and identifies a novel gene family. *Nat Genet* 1997; **15**: 157–64.
64. Tyson J, Tranebjaerg L, Bellman S et al. IsK and KvLQT1: mutation in either of the two subunits of the slow component of the delayed rectifier potassium channel can cause Jervell and Lange–Nielsen syndrome. *Hum Mol Genet* 1997; **6**: 2179–85.
65. Schulze-Bahr E, Wang Q, Wedekind H et al. KCNE1 mutations cause Jervell and Lange–Nielsen syndrome. *Nat Genet* 1997; **17**: 267–8.
66. Berger W, Meindl A, van de Pol TJ et al. Isolation of a candidate gene for Norrie disease by positional cloning. *Nat Genet* 1992; **1**: 199–203.
67. Chen ZY, Hendriks RW, Jobling MA et al. Isolation and characterization of a candidate gene for Norrie disease. *Nat Genet* 1992; **1**: 204–8.
68. Vikkula M, Mariman ECM, Lui VCH et al. Autosomal dominant and recessive osteochondrodysplasias associated with the COL11A2 locus. *Cell* 1995; **80**: 431–7.
69. Williams CJ, Ganguly A, Considine E et al. A-2->G transition at the 3′acceptor splice site of IVS17 characterizes the COL2A1 gene mutation in the original Stickler syndrome kindred. *Am J Med Genet* 1996; **63**: 461–7.
70. Richards AJ, Yates JR, Williams R et al. A family with Stickler syndrome type 2 has a mutation in the COL11A1 gene resulting in the substitution of glycine 97 by valine in alpha 1 (XI) collagen. *Hum Mol Genet* 1996; **5**: 1339–43.
71. The Treacher Collins Syndrome Collaborative Group. *Nat Genet* 1996; **12**: 130–6.
72. Eudy JD, Weston MD, Yao S et al. Mutation of a gene encoding a protein with extracellular matrix motifs in Usher syndrome type IIa. *Science* 1998; **280**: 1753–7.
73. Tassabehji M, Read AP, Newton VE et al. Waardenburg's syndrome patients have mutations in the human homologue of the Pax-3 paired box gene. *Nature* 1992; **355**: 635–6.
74. Tassabehji M, Newton VE, Read AP. Waardenburg syndrome type 2 caused by mutations in the human microphthalmia (MITF) gene. *Nat Genet* 1994; **8**: 251–5.
75. Hoth CF, Milunsky A, Kipsky N, Sheffer R, Clarren SK, Baldwin CT. Mutations in the paired domain of the human PAX3 gene cause Klein–Waardenburg syndrome (WS-III) as well as Waardenburg syndrome type I (WS-I). *Am J Hum Genet* 1993; **52**: 455–62.
76. Attie T, Till M, Pelet A et al. Mutation of the endothelin-receptor B gene in Waardenburg–Hirschsprung disease. *Hum Mol Genet* 1995; **4**: 2407–9.
77. Edery P, Attie T, Amiel J et al. Mutation of the endothelin-3 gene in the Waardenburg–Hirschsprung disease (Shah–Waardenburg syndrome). *Nat Genet* 1996; **12**: 442–4.
78. Pingault V, Bondurand N, Kuhlbrodt K et al. SOX10 mutations in patients with Waardenburg–Hirschprung disease. *Nat Genet* 1998; **18**: 171–3.
79. Lynch ED, Lee MK, Morrow JE, Welcsh PL, Leon PE, King MC. Nonsyndromic deafness DFNA1 associated with mutation of a human homolog of the Drosophila gene diaphanous. *Science* 1997; **278**: 1315–18.
80. Van Laer L, Huizing EH, Verstreken M et al. Nonsyndromic hearing impairment is associated with a mutation in DFNA5. *Nat Genet* 1998; **20**: 194–7.
81. Vahava O, Morell R, Lynch ED et al. Mutation in transcription factor *POU4F3* associated with inherited progressive hearing loss in humans. *Science* 1998; **279**: 1950–4.
82. Wang A, Liang Y, Fridell RA et al. Association of unconventional myosin *MYO15* mutations with human nonsyndromic deafness *DFNB3*. *Science* 1998; **280**: 1447–51.
83. Yasunaga S, Grati M, Cohen-Salmon M et al. A mutation in OTOF, encoding otoferlin, a FER-1-like protein, causes DFNB9, a nonsyndromic form of deafness. *Nat Genet* 1999; **21**: 363–9.
84. El-Schahawi M, Lopez DM, Sarrazin AM et al. Two large Spanish pedigrees with nonsyndromic sensorineural deafness and the mtDNA mutation at nt 1555 in the 12s rRNA gene: evidence of heteroplasmy. *Neurology* 1997; **48**: 453–6.

5 Immunology of cochlear and vestibular disorders

Tai-June Yoo, Yoshior Yazawa

Introduction

In the past century of medicine, probably one of the most striking and significant advances has been in the field of immunology. The study and understanding of the immune system responses goes to the very heart of disease production. Intact immunity is fundamental for survival. The immune system distinguishes self from non-self and thereby enables us to survive in a hostile environment. The human immune system has evolved with sophisticated biological capacity through the process of clonal expansion. The ability to distinguish even subtle differences from self and many myriad of antigens is made possible by the rearrangement of genes that encode immunogolulins and T-cell receptors,[1] as well as by the requirement for T cells to recognize antigens in context of the presentation by major histocompatibility complex (MHC) molecules.[2] Modulation of function initiated by antigenic stimulation and cell interaction is facilitated by soluble mediators such as cytokines. The understanding of the immune system provides a framework for understanding physiological immune responses as well as the pathogenesis of immunological disorders (Figure 5.1). Through such understanding, potential targets can be identified for therapeutic modulation of the immune system. The inability to react to self is known as tolerance. The tolerance implies that host lymphocytes are not activated by interaction with host self-tissues. Accordingly, autoimmunity defines a state in which tolerance to self is lost.[3] If such activation by self occurs with sufficient magnitude and for sufficient duration, host tissue damage occurs. The pathogenesis of autoimmunity involves various genetic, immunological and viral factors interacting through complicated mechanisms that are still poorly understood.

Recent evidence suggests that at least immunological disturbances are associated with many causes of auditory dysfunction. There are many autoimmune disorders that could affect hearing. Several diseases are associated with hearing loss, including

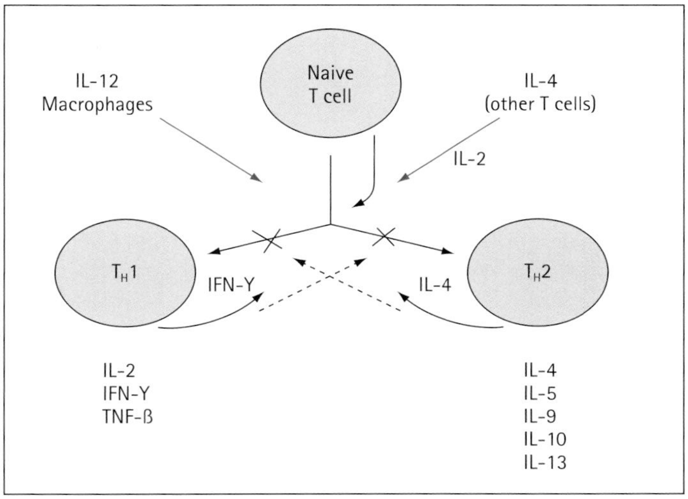

Figure 5.1 Differentiation of T_H1 and T_H2 lymphocytes. Interleukin-12 (IL-12) and interferon gamma (IFN-γ) induce the differentiation of T_H1 cells, and IFN-γ antagonizes the differentiation of T_H2 cells. IL-4 induces the differentiation of T_H2 cells and antagonizes the differentiation of T_H1 cells. The T_H1 cells induce cell-mediated imflammation, and T_H2 cells induce humoral-mediated allergic inflammation. TNF, indicates tumor necrosis factor.

Menière's disease, otosclerosis, autoimmune hearing loss and other forms of sudden hearing loss. These diseases have some immunological manifestations. Several animal models of autoimmune cochlear diseases have been developed. The criteria shown in Table 5.1 determine the relationship of immunological phenomena to disease etiology following the Koch postulate.

An autoimmune response must be regularly associated with disease, a replica of the disease must be inducible in laboratory animals, immunopathological manifestations in the natural and experimental diseases should parallel each other, and immunological illness should be inducible by transfer of serum with

Table 5.1 Criteria for immunological etiology

Autoimmune response associated with disease
Animal model
Immunopathological manifestations uniform in patient and animal model
Lymphocytic transfer of disease from patient to normal individual

lymphocytes from a diseased individual to a normal recipient. Table 5.2 shows clinical criteria for an autoimmune disease, and Tables 5.3 and 5.4 show a list of ear diseases with possible immunological features and autoimmune diseases affecting hearing.

Table 5.2 The clinical criteria for an autoimmune disease[238]

Hyper gammaglobulinemia (1.5 g/dl)
Autoantibody
Immunoglobulin, complement, immune complex etc. in the lesion
Cell infiltration into the lesion
Response to corticosteroid
Combination with other autoimmune diseases

Table 5.3 Ear diseases with immunological features

External ear	Auricular chondritis Relapsing polychondritis
Tympanic membrane	Tympanosclerosis
Eustachian	Autoimmune salpingitis
Middle ear	Otosclerosis Secretory otitis media Necrotizing otitis media Cholesteatoma
Inner ear	Autoimmune sensorineural hearing loss Menière's disease Otosclerosis Cochlear vasculitis Sudden hearing loss
Retrocochlear	Autoimmune central nervous system disease

Table 5.4 Autoimmune diseases affecting hearing

Relapsing polychondritis
Systemic lupus erythematosus
Disseminated vasculitis
Rheumatoid arthritis
Sjögren's syndrome
Systemic sclerosis
Myasthenia gravis
Hashimoto's thyroiditis
Goodpasture's syndrome
Vogt-Koyanagi-Harada syndrome
Cogan's syndrome
Behçet's disease
Sarcoidosis
Wegener's granulomatosis

Historical perspectives

The immune systems was originally implicated as having a role in some idiopathic sensorineural lesions in 1931.[4] Löwenthal[5] has, however, argued that the concept was introduced in 1920.[6]

Cogan's syndrome, interstitial keratitis with audio vestibular disorder progressing to profound hearing loss, was well described in 1945.[7] In 1960, Cody and Williams emphasized that Cogan's syndrome should probably be thought of as part of a systemic disease, not just a disease confined to the eye and cranial nerve.[8] Cody made a clear distinction between the pathology of vascular insufficiencies and that related to vasculitis, implying that Cogan's syndrome was a collagen disease. Treatment included high-dose corticosteroid, and they pointed out that improvement of hearing produced by this drug was lost when the dose was reduced. This pattern came to be seen in many of the other disorders that were referred to as 'vasculitis'. Even at this early stage, the implication was that vasculitis was related to immunological disease and that steroid treatment was indicated.

Lehnardt in 1958 reported cases of bilateral sudden hearing loss, and proposed an etiological hypothesis that the degenerating organ of Corti could induce anticochlear antibody that would react with another intact organ of Corti.[9] Kikuchi[10] reported several cases of hearing loss as 'sympathetic otitis' in which hearing in one ear had been markedly influenced by surgery on the opposite ear. Beickert[11] was the first to publish experimental data concerning autoimmune reactions in the cochlea. He injected anti-guinea pig cochlear antibody, produced in the duck, into the guinea pig. Terayama and Sasaki[12] produced experimental allergic labyrnthitis in the guinea pig by immunization of guinea pig cochlea, emulsified with Freund's adjuvant. They found degenerative changes in the spiral ganglia and stria vascularis, hemorrhages in the scala tympani and disintegration of the organ of Corti. They noted acoustical threshold shifts, although they could not demonstrate any anticochlear antibody. More recently, Schiff and Brown[13] discussed sudden hearing loss as potentially being a result of vasculitis and implied that immune disease was involved. Treatment was instituted with heparin and adrenocorticotropic hormone. Similar investigations were done by Quick,[14] Arnold et al[15] and Weidauer et al.[16]

Credit for the current interest should be directed to McCabe's report on autoimmune sensorineural hearing loss in 1979.[17] He first described a pattern of bilateral SNHL characterized by rapid progression over weeks to months. Hearing loss typically involves both ears, either synchronously or sequentially. Vestibular symptoms were minor or absent. Based on laboratory tests, clinical manifestations, positive immunological tests, and a beneficial treatment response, a clinical entity of autoimmune SNHL was proposed. His reports stimulated clinical research into immune-mediated deafness. Since then, autoimmune activity in patients with idiopathic SNHL has been assessed by the migration inhibition test,[17] enzyme-linked immuno-sorbent test (ELISA),[18] lymphocyte transformation test,[19–21] immunofluorescence microscopy,[21,22] and Western blotting.[23–25] Experimental models of autoimmune SNHL have been developed in a variety of animals by a number of researchers, using type II collagen,[26,27] crude inner tissue extract,[28–31] purified protein Po[32] or tubulin[33] as antigens. Over time, researchers have accumulated considerable evidence indicating the involvement of immune mechanisms in human inner ear disease.

The immune system of the inner ear

Guild reported that the endolymph flows from the cochlear duct to the endolymphatic sac (ES), where it is absorbed and distributed to the numerous perisaccular blood vessels.[34] He defined 22 cell types in the lumen of the ES. This included lymphocytes, whose presence prompted Lim and Silver's[35] proposal that the ES sac acts as a defensive organ in the inner ear. Rask-Andersen and Stahle found immune cells, including lymphocytes and macrophages, in the ES and adjacent tissue of guinea pigs.[36] They also found these in the ES of human Menière's disease patients. A vigorous interaction between lymphocytes and macrophages, similar to that observed in antigen-activated and lymphoid tissue, may occur. This reaction is surrounded by a rich network of lymphatic capillaries and blood vessels. This finding indicates that an immune system is present in the inner ear. Since then, evidence has been accumulating that the inner ear is an immunoreactive organ and is capable of mounting a local immune response.[37,38] The presence and mobilization of macrophages, B cells and T cells in the ES and in the perisaccular space have been reported in a number of species, such as humans,[39] guinea pigs[40] and mice.[41] The study of the distribution and anatomical localization of immunocompetent cells in normal mouse ES, by an immunohistochemical method, showed CD4 cells in the epithelial perisaccular region, whereas CD8 cells were rarely present. Macrophages were present primarily in the lumen of the distal portion of the ES. IgM-bearing cells were seen in the subepithelial lesion. Immunoglobulin-positive cells were occasionally detected in the lumen, and only a few IgA-positive cells were present in the perisaccular region. The EM study of Wackym found that the lumen of ES contained freely floating macrophages with abundant cytoplasmic lysosomes, vacuoles, and phagolysosomes. The lymphocytes are located intraepithelially and within the subepithelial space. In patients with acoustical neuroma, however, a predominance of T-helper cells *vis-à-vis* helper T cells, occasional microphages and granulocytes were observed. Another immunohistochemical study of the extraosseous part of the ES from an autopsy revealed that T-helper cells (CD4 cells) predominate in the ES. CD8 cells are present in small numbers, but B cells as well as macrophages are detected in the lumen and perisaccular region. Langerhans B-cells are present in the lumen and the stroma of the ES and IgA or IgG containing cells in the stroma only, so it seems that the presence of neuroma inverts the relationship between T-helper CD4 and CD8 cells due to chronic antigen stimulation.[42] In histological and immunohistochemical studies of the human inner ear, Arnold et al showed that immunologically active structures were exclusively present in different regions. They found that lymphocytes were situated periepithelially, in some cases arranged in groups, while the epithelium of the ES was infiltrated by lymphocytes, and mast cells and macrophages were found in perisaccular tissue.[21,43]

It was demonstrated that the ES was not originally equipped to possess immunocompetent cells and mount an immune response. Immunocompetent cells distributed in the normal ES might mobilize from the systemic circulation or subsequently develop in the ES in response to antigenic stimuli. Once it has been activated with the inner ear antigenic stimuli, the ES can be the active site of the local immune response of the inner ear.[44]

Ichimiya et al[45] investigated the ES of mice in three different conditions: germ-free(GF), specific pathogenic free (SPF), and conventional (CV). In the ES of GF mice, no immunocompetent cells were found. In the ES of SPF and CV mice, cells positive for IgG, IgA, IgM CD4 cells are present in a much smaller number than in the nasal mucus.[45] Cells positive to Lyt-2 are not seen in the ES of any mice. In the ES of rats that underwent an antigenic challenge in the perilymphatic space after the systemic presensitization B-lymphocyte subsets (positive for IgG, IgA and IgM) were observed in increased numbers, and T-cell subsets were also found 1 week after the perilymphatic challenge.

A number of studies indicate that the inner ear is not an immunoprivileged site,[46] and the ES plays an important role in the immunodefense of the inner ear.[21,36,38,47]

There is considerable evidence supporting the presence of immunoglobulins in the perilymph of humans,[48–50] as well as in experimental animals.[51,52] The immunoglobulins in perilymph have been determined, and they are predominantly IgG, with lesser amounts of IgM and IgA.[43,52,53] There are also secretory pieces found,[54] and IgG_2 in the perilymph of the guinea pig, which should be similar to IgG_1 found in humans.[55–57]

As for the origin of immunoglobulins of the inner ear, the source of the perilymph remains controversial, and the origin of immunoglobulin in the perilymph has not yet been determined.[58,59] However, it was proposed that the protein in the peri lymph, including albumin and immunoglobulin, might come largely from perilymphatic blood vessels rather than from the cerebrospinal fluid (CSF), based on experimental data.[52] There are three probable origins of perilymph immunoglobulins under normal conditions: (1) the filtrate from blood vessels surrounding the perilymphatic space; (2) local production in the inner ear; and (3) from CSF through the cochlear aqueduct and the modiolar space.

It was found that: (1) immune processing occurred within the inner ear, due to a resident population of immunocompetent cells or due to the immunocompetent cells migrating into the inner ear from the systemic circulation; (2) secondary immune response animals developed much higher antibody levels than primary animals; and (3) these responses were independent of the serum or CSF.[37,46] The accumulation of inflammatory cells in the inner ear is seen in reponses such as infection, antigen challenge, or trauma. In eperimental animals, it is found that cells accumulate around and within the spiral modiolar vein (SMV), adjacent to the scala tympani as early as 6h post-stimulation, and then cells began to stream into the scala tympani along the bony canaliculi containing the collecting venules, finally resulting in fibrosis or osteoneogenesis.[60] The blood vessels of the SMV are the initial site through which lymphocytes enter the inner ear.[61] Interleukin-2 (IL-2) is not present in the perilymph in the resting state, but is a component in the inner ear immune responses. The peak rise of IL-2 in the perilymph was at 18h following antigen stimulation, and declined over a 5-day period. This corresponds well with the accumulation of helper T cells and macrophages within the inner ear.[62] Transforming growth factor beta (TGF-β) has also been identified as a mediator in the inner ear immune response. TGF-β is known to be a chemoattractant for monocytes, T cells, and neutrophils, while also increasing levels of IL-1, IL-6, and platelet-derived growth factor (PDGF).[63] It was also demonstrated that there was a weak presence of intercellular adhesion molecule (ICAM-1) on the epithelium of the SMV and collecting venules (cvs) as early as 6h following inoculation of antigen into the scala tympani of animals systemically sensitized to it, reaching a maximum by day 2 and then gradually fading away. The maximum influx of immunocompetent cells into the cochlea was seen between days 3 and 7. By day 28, the inner ear had developed endolymphatic hydrops, but no significant staining with anti-ICAM-1 was observed at that time.[64] Yeo et al[65] found that antigen in the scala tympani could gain access to the lumen of the ES through the perilymph and the perisaccular tissue. In the ES, the antigen may be presented by macrophages to the systemic immune system. In summary, evidence has shown that the inner ear is capable of mounting local immune responses. These could be either normal or autoimmune responses.

Autoimmune inner ear disease

The etiology of many inner ear diseases is unknown. However, some of them, including Menière's disease, otosclerosis, progressive sensorineural hearing loss (PSHL) and sudden deafness, may be of autoimmune origin. In the last two decades, much evidence has been accumulated. These data indicate that the autoantibodies and sensitized lymphocytes in some inner ear diseases may have a key role in the origin or continuation of the diseases.

Clinical features of autoimmune sensorineural hearing loss

McCabe[17] described 18 cases of sensorineural deafness having clinical and laboratory features suggestive of an autoimmune etiology. This condition was characterized by a prolonged period of progressive deafness over weeks or months, rather than hours, days or years. It is usually bilateral or asymmetrical, and the cochlea is always involved. Other features of this disorder are facial paralysis and vestibular dysfunction. Tissue destruction of the tympanic membrane, middle ear, and mastoid may also occur. These patients responded well to high-dose steroid therapy and cyclophosphamide. In total, 42 cases of this disorder were diagnosed in McCabe's series as of January 1982. Two-thirds of the patients had low-grade vestibular symptoms without spells, and the reduction in caloric responses paralleled the hearing loss.

Nine patients subsequently developed other autoimmune disease, e.g. Cogan's syndrome, chronic ulcerative colitis, rheumatoid arthritis, and carotidynia. None of the patients had lupus erythematosus, although nine patients had a positive antinuclear antibody (ANA) titer. Many patients were shown to have an elevated sedimentation rate, and 11 patients demonstrated positive leukocyte migration inhibition assays. Two patients had visible tissue changes and vasculoneogenesis, and one patient had vasculitis. Since then, other reports have described a case of SNHL with positive anti-smooth muscle antibody,[66] two cases of inner ear disease with Cogan's syndrome,[13] and other clinical and immunological observations.[18,67–70]

Menière's disease (MD) as an autoimmune disease[73]

It has been speculated that MD might be an immune-mediated or even autoimmune disease. Experimental evidence to support this hypothesis is as follows: (1) the site of the ES is the site of the immune response of the inner ear and at the same time it is also the site of injury; (2) experimental hydrops can be induced by injection of antigens; (3) the presence of antibodies to inner ear antigens, e.g. type II collagens, 30-kDa protein, c-raf, β-tubulin, 68 kDa protein, presence of lymphocyte blastogenesis, CIC (circulating immune complex) and antiviral antibodies;[267] (4) association of certain D-related (DR) loci with this illness; (5) the temporal bone changes are associated with immunological changes; (6) responses to steroids. These facts suggest that immune processes are involved in the development of Menière's disease (Tables 5.5 and 5.6).

Collagen and autoimmune inner ear disease

Collagens constitute a family of related extracellular matrix proteins assembled in a variety of supramolecular structures to accomplish diverse functions.[74] Nineteen distinct types of collagens have been discovered.[75–77] Type II collagen has been found to be present in the inner ear of various animal species, such as rodents (guinea pig),[78,79] chickens[80] and monkeys[81] (Figure 5.5). It has also been shown by in situ hybridization (ISH) that type I and type II collagen transcripts are coexpressed in almost all cells within the normal otic capsule and membranous cochlea of 16–23-week-old human fetuses.[82–84] Type IV collagen, which is believed to be involved in the pathogenesis of Alport syndrome with progressive renal insufficiency and SNHL,[85] was found to be densely localized around the nerve cells, and the capillary blood vessels of the stria vascularis, and beneath the epithelial cells of the ES in the human[86] and guinea pig inner ear.[87] Type IX collagen is less abundant and is located within the labyrinthine membranes, and within the dense fibers of the tectorial membrane.[88,89]

Collagen has been postulated to be one of the important antigens involved in the pathogenesis of the autoimmune inner ear.[18] Yoo et al were the first to show a raised level of serum antibodies to bovine type II collagen in 5 of 12 patients with otosclerosis.[18] In subsequent studies, the association of antibodies with type II collagen and several inner ear diseases, including Menière's disease, otosclerosis, idiopathic PSNHL and sudden deafness, has been demonstrated by other investigators.[90,91]

Table 5.5 Indirect immunofluorescence test to normal inner ear tissue

Authors	Year	Patients	Inner ear	Positive results (%)	Reference
Elies and Plester	1987	MD ($n = 13$)	Rat and hamster	46	239
Lejeune and Charachon	1991	MD ($n = 12$) + SNHL ($n = 11$)	Human	30	240
Gong	1992	MD ($n = 30$)	Guinea pig	60	241
Salomon et al	1993	MD ($n = 6$) + SNHL ($n = 20$)	Hamster	19	242
Soliman	1996	MD ($n = 50$)	Guinea pig ES	40	243
Alleman et al	1997	MD ($n = 30$)	Human ES	10	244
Soliman	1997	MD ($n = 18$) + SNHL ($n = 28$) + IED (n = 54)	Guinea pig	18	245

MD, Menière's disease; SNHL, sensorineural hearing loss; IED, inner ear disease other than SNHL
ES, endolymphatic sac.

Table 5.6 Immunofluorescent study of the endolymphatic sacs

Authors	Year	Patients	Positive results	Reference
Futaki et al	1988	MD ($n = 16$)	IgG (40%), IgM (20%), IgA (20%), C3 (33%)	246
Yazawa and Kitahara	1989	MD ($n = 21$)	IgG (19%), IgM (10%), IgA (19%)	247
Tomoda et al	1993	MD ($n = 15$)	IgG (50%), IgM (25%), IgA (31%), C3 (39%)	91
Dornhoffer et al	1993	MD ($n = 23$)	IgG (43%)	248

MD, Menière's disease.

Joliat et al[92] found that anti-type II collagen antibodies were present in 12 of 21 (57%) patients, while 13 of 21 (62%) had anti-type IX antibodies detected by Western blot (Table 5.7).

Animal studies strongly suggest that collagen-specific antibodies play a pivotal role in the pathogenesis of some inner ear diseases. Yoo et al[26,27,93,94] reported that type II collagen-induced autoimmune ear disease in animals has histopathological and immunological similarity to human autoimmune ear disease. These animals had spiral ganglion cell degeneration, atrophy of the organ of Corti, arteritis of the cochlea and stria vascularis, and endolymphatic hydrops, with atrophy of the surface epithelium of the endolymphatic duct. In addition, some animals showed otospongiosis-like changes of the bone of the external meatus and otic capsule. Hearing loss and vestibular dysfunction were found in some of these animals as well. Several similar experiments were carried out by other groups to develop SNHL and vestibular dysfunction in various species[96–98] (Table 5.8; Figure 5.2).

Direct infusion of monoclonal antibody against CB11 peptide in the cochlea also produced endolymphatic hydrops. The results support the idea that the appearance of endolymphatic hydrops is due to immunological reactions induced by CB11 antibodies in the cochlea. They also suggested that direct injury to the inner ear by CB11 monoclonal antibodies causes increased hearing thresholds. Therefore, the results of this study suggest that type II collagen autoimmunity is responsible for the production of hearing loss associated with endolymphatic hydrops. Matsuoka et al were succesful in producing ear lesions in more than 80% of animal studies (Figure 5.3).[99]

The transfer of the collagen type II-induced autoimmune inner ear disease from the immunized rats to normal recipients through the transfer of serum was demonstrated by Yoo et al.[100]

Table 5.7 Antibody titers against various collagens

			Rate of positive serum antibodies (%)				
Authors	Year	Patients	Anti-type II	Anti-type V	Anti-type IX	Anti-laminin	Reference
Yoo et al	1982	MD ($n = 50$)	41.7				18
Klein et al	1989	MD ($n = 12$)				14	123
Helfgott et al	1991	MD ($n = 12$)	8.3				90
Joliat et al	1992	MD ($n = 6$) + IED ($n = 15$)	57		62		92
Tomoda et al	1993	MD ($n = 18$)	28				91
Herdman et al	1993	MD ($n = 37$)	5.4~8.1				266
Fattori et al	1994	MD ($n = 45$)	15.5	6.6		11.1	119
Yoshino	1994	MD ($n = 29$)	38				257

MD, Menière's disease; IED, inner ear disease other than SNHL.

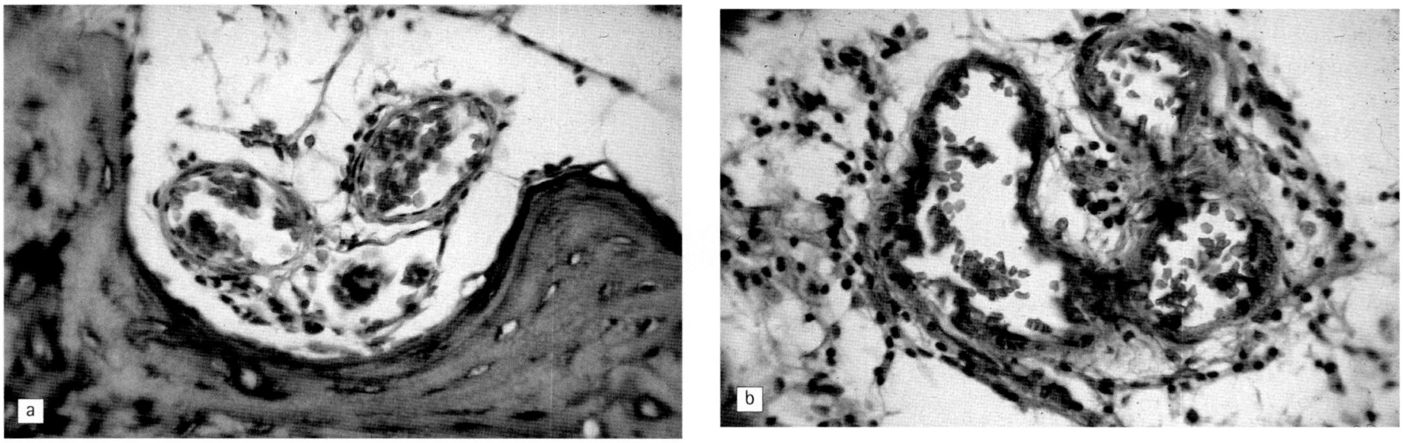

Figure 5.2 (a) Cochlear arteries and veins from normal rats. (b) Inflamed cochlear artery in autoimmune SNHL in rat. Vessel walls are thickened and fibrotic. H&E, ×240; micrograph ×3840.

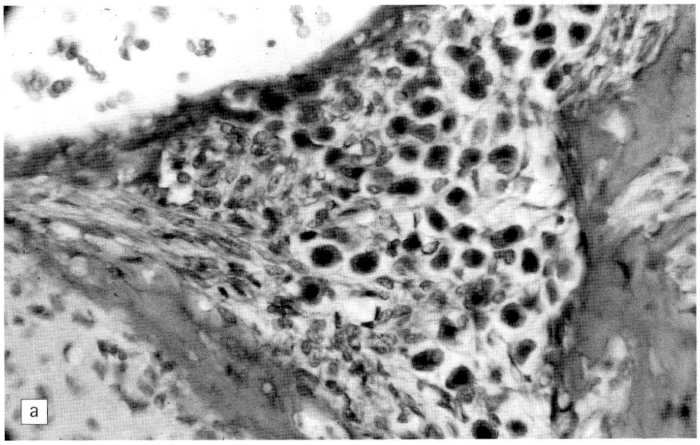

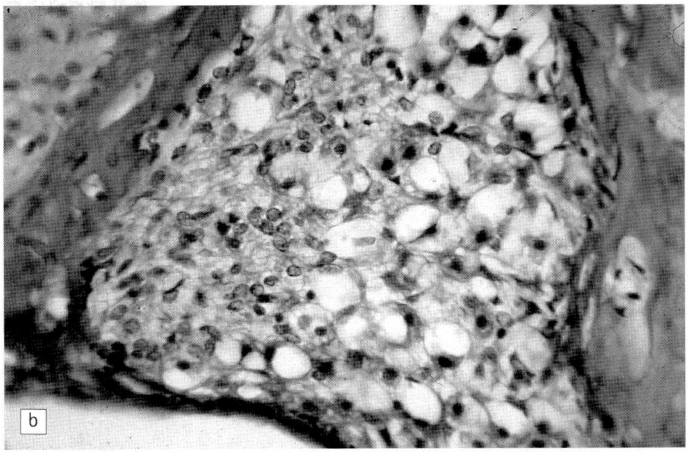

Figure 5.3 (a) Spiral ganglion from normal rat. (b) Degenerated spiral ganglion in ear with autoimmune SNHL. Neurones show vacuolate degeneration in which cell bodies are swollen, cytoplasm is clear, and nuclei are pyknotic and displaced towards two axonal poles of cells. Nerve fibers show a slight decrease in number. ×2304

Table 5.8 Collagen-induced ear diseases

Sensorineural hearing loss
Vestibular dysfunction
Spiral ganglion degeneration
Atrophy of organ of Corti
Cochlear vasculitis
Salpingitis and chondritis
Otospongiosis-like lesion
Endolymphatic hydrops

In addition, the effects of anti-inflammatory drugs, Solumedrol (methyl prednisolene, steroid) and Arthrocin (non-steroid), on collagen-induced autoimmune inner ear disease were also studied. Sudo and Yoo[101] found, by examining the histopathological changes and levels of circulating antibody, that the therapy was beneficial to animals whether the drugs were administered alone or in combination. Fewer lesions were observed in animals given either drug alone, although animals treated with steroid alone showed the least amount of inner ear damage. The involvement of ear structures in autoimmune responses to collagen type II has been investigated in several related rodent models. Collagen type II-induced ear lesions in Lewis rats and guinea pigs were first reported by Yoo et al.[26] However, Harris et al[102] did not observe these phenomena. The immune response depends on MHC restriction. Thus the explanation of the negative data of Harris et al must be related to proper strains and species, state of health of the experimental animal, MHC restrictions, and the intensity and duration of the immune response used to produce ear lesions. Harris used a different strain of experimental animal. Soliman re-examined these controversial results in 1990 and demonstrated impaired hearing thresholds and morphological changes, including endolymphatic hydrops, slight vasculitis of the cochlear artery, and slight degeneration of the spiral ganglion cells, in the guinea pig. These findings support the original observation of Yoo.[94] Huang et al[95] reproduced collagen type II-induced bone resorption in the temporal bone and salpingitis in rats, which also supported Yoo's findings, in contrast to the negative report by Bretlau et al.[103] Bretlau's group used type II collagen as an immunizing antigen in powder form instead of solution. Cruz et al[98] also reproduced spiral ganglion degeneration in guinea pigs with collagen type II immunization. These animals had an increase of latency in wave one. Tomoda et al[104,105] reproduced the collagen type II-induced autoimmune ear disease in the guinea pig in separate experiments.

The arguments against collagen autoimmunity in the inner ear were solely based on the above two experiments. However, this model has been repeatedly produced by other investigators in a number of different species, including rats, mice[253] (Figure 5.4), guinea pigs and non-human primates.

Non-human primate model

Macaca fascicularis and *Macaca mulatta* were injected with purified bovine type II collagen. The injected monkeys developed ear disease, polyarthritis and imbalance. Electrocochleography and brainstem-evoked potential studies showed some shift of the action potential threshold and a decrease in the amplitude, which indicate hearing loss. Histological examination of the inner ear showed vacuolated degeneration of the spiral ganglion, degeneration of the organ of Corti, crista ampullare, and cochlear vasculitis. Histological examination of the involved joints showed a thickening of the synovial membrane with infiltration by a large number of mononuclear cells and giant cells. These results show that type II collagen autoimmunity could induce hearing loss and imbalance in non-human primates.[106]

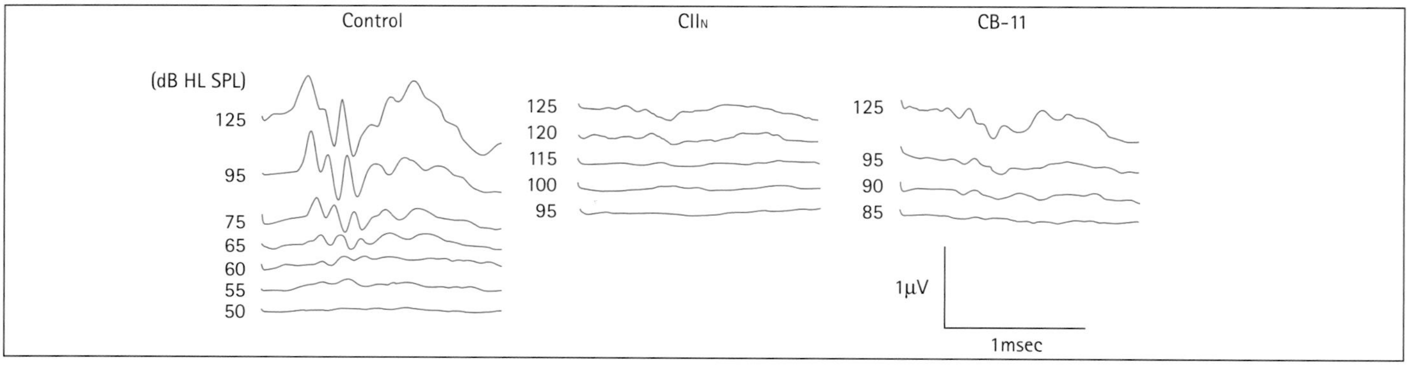

Figure 5.4 Comparison of auditory brainstem evoked response (ABR) records between control, chicken type II collagen (CIIn)-immunized and cyanogen bromide peptide 11 (CB-11)-immunized mice (4-month follow-up). Control animals showed good response at the intensity of acoustical stimuli or 60dBSPL. Note the elevation of threshold and the decrease of ABRs in the immunized mice. The latencies of ABR in immunized mice were slightly delayed (×100). (Adapted from Takeda et al. *Am J Otol* 1996; **17**: 69–75.[253])

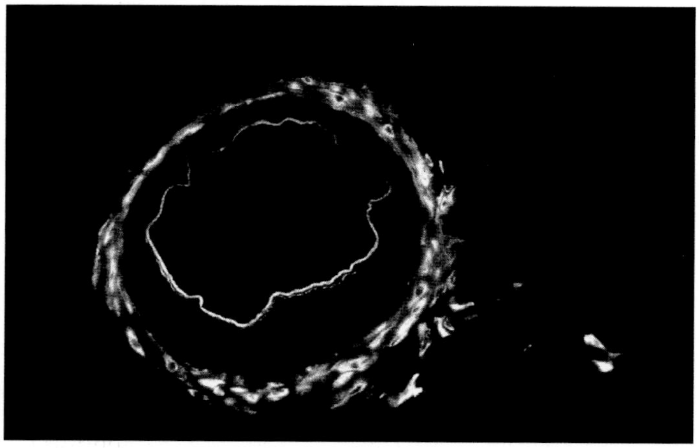

Figure 5.5 Immunofluorescence micrograph shows the presence of type II collagen in the semi-circular canal and labyrinth membrane of rat.[78,79]

Autoantibodies in sera of patients with inner ear disease

Numerous studies have attempted to identify disease-specific circulating antibodies that bind to the inner ear or to purified inner ear antigens. Harris and Sharp[23] used the extracts from the bovine inner ear to study the serum of 54 patients with PSNHL and 14 normal controls by immunoblotting. Nineteen of the patient group (34%) showed a single or double band migrating at 68 kDa, compared with 7% in the controls. In subsequent publications, several similar results were reported.[106–108] Moreover, the 68 kDa protein was found to be ubiquitously present in other bovine organs, especially kidney.[109,110]

The 68-kDa antigens identified by PSNHL sera and by anti-heat shock protein 70 monoclonal antibodies (mAb) copurify on ion exchange and adenosine triphosphate affinity chromatography, and comigrate on one- and two-dimensional (2D) gel electrophoresis. Billings et al[111] have recently provided some tentative evidence linking the 68-kDa protein with the 70-kDa heat shock protein. This is intriguing, since antibodies against heat shock proteins have been associated with a number of autoimmune diseases.[112,113] Antibodies to this particular heat shock protein, hsp 70, have only been found in Lyme disease and ulcerative colitis.[114] However, whether the antibodies against hsp 70 play a primary etiological role in autoimmune inner ear disease or occur as a secondary epiphenomenon, is not yet clear. The exact relationship between hsp 70 and autoimmune inner ear disease remains to be clarified.

A number of other proteins in the extract of bovine inner ear tissue were also reported to have some reactivity with sera from patients with inner ear disease.[107,108,115] These inner ear proteins included non-organ-specific antigens with molecular masses of 62, 55, 50 and 47 kDa and inner ear-specific antigens with molecular masses of 220, 60, 58, 35, 33, and 32 kDa. The 200-, 60- and 58-kDa proteins were also found in the bovine kidney. However, the clinical significance of these proteins remains unknown. Some of them could not distinguish between patients with inner ear disease and controls[110] (Tables 5.9 and 5.10).

30-kDa protein and type IX collagens

Joliat et al[92] used sera fronm 21 patients with inner ear disease to probe Western blots of purified human collagens II and IX and cochlear protein extract. Anti-type II collagen antibodies were detected in 57% of patients, anti-type IX antibodies in 62% of patients. A 30-kDa protein band was found by sodium dodecylsulfate (SDS)–polyacrylamide gel electrophoresis (PAGE) of human cochlear tissue extract. In their series of patients, only three patients with Menière's disease had an antibody binding to this protein on Western blot. They did not draw any conclusion regarding the character of the 30-kDa protein or its role in Menière's disease.

Swine ear antigen

Using swine inner ear Western blot, Veldman et al[116] investigated sera from 76 patients with rapidly progressive PSNHL ($n = 15$) and sudden deafness ($n = 31$), and with other etiolo-

Table 5.9 Results of Western blot immunoassay reported by investigators

Authors	Year	Patients	Inner ear extract	Molecular mass (kDa) of proteins and positive rate	Reference
Harris and Sharp	1990	SNHL (*n* = 54)	Bovine inner ear	68 (35%)	23
Joliat et al	1992	MD (*n* = 6) + IED (*n* = 15)	Human inner ear	30 (62%)	92
Veldman et al	1993	SNHL + IED (*n* = 76)	Swine temporal bone	27, 45, 50, 68 (73%)	116
Yamanobe and Harris	1993	SNHL + IED (*n* = 13)	Bovine inner ear	32, 33–35, 58, 60, 220	107
Moscicki et al	1994	SNHL (*n* = 72)	Bovine inner ear	68 (58%)	110
Gottschlich et al	1995	MD (*n* = 50)	Bovine inner ear	33–35 (18%), 68 (30%)	249
Cao et al	1995	IED (*n* = 82)	Guinea pig inner ear	30, 58 (39%)	25
Rauch et al	1995	MD (*n* = 30)	Bovine inner ear	hsp 70 (47%)	250
Billings et al	1995	SNHL	Bovine kidney	68 = hsp 70	111
Shin et al	1997	MD (*n* = 60)	Bovine kidney	68, hsp 70 (22%)	251
Suzuki et al	1997	MD + IED (*n* = 45)	Guinea pig inner ear	28 (20%), 30 (4%)	141
Atlas et al	1998	MD (*n* = 36)	Bovine temporal bone	42–45 (22%), 68 (56%)	252

MD, Menière's disease; SNHL, sensorineural hearing loss, IED, inner ear disease other than SNHL.

gies of hearing loss ($n = 30$). Seventy-three per cent of the patients with rapidly progressive PSNHL had antibodies to 27-, 45-, 50- and 68-kDa protein. Sixty-five per cent had antibodies to 27-, 45-, 50- and 80-kDa protein. All the antigenic epitopes detected on Western blots were not specific to the cochlea. The antigenic epitopes were also found in other organs, including cranial nerves, kidney and brain.

Correlation between antibody and steroid treatment response

In prospective studies examining the effectiveness of prednisone in patients with idiopathic PSNHL, patients who had antibodies against the 68-kDa bovine inner ear protein or type II collagen responded more frequently than those who did not have these antibodies.[90,110]

Veldman et al[116] analyzed the correlation between antibodies to swine to inner ear protein and the outcome of immunosuppressive treatment in 46 patients with PSNHL and sudden deafness. A positive treatment response was not only observed in patients with a positive, but also in patients with a negative Western blot profile. The overall response to therapy was effective in only 50% of the cases. In patients with sudden deafness, steroid therapy was more effective than no treatment, regardless of the Western blot results. Spontaneous recovery occurred in 50% of the cases, but only in those with a positive test.

Non-specific autoantibodies

A non-specific autoantibody screening was performed in 59 patients with Menière's disease.[117] Twenty-seven (45.8%) of 59 patients with Menière's disease had at least one serum autoantibody, compared with eight (27.6%) of the 29 controls ($p < 0.02$); 23.7% of the patients had two or more autoantibodies, compared with 6.9% of the controls ($p < 0.1$). The most common autoantibodies found were antinuclear antibody in 17 patients, antithyroglobulin antibody in 9 patients, and anti-smooth muscle antibody in 9 patients. Evans et al[118] reported that 73 (48.7%) of 150 patients with Menière's disease had one autoantibody, and 9.3% of patients had two or more autoantibodies. The commonest autoantibody was antinuclear antibody (23.3%); thyroid microsomal antibody occurred in 17%, and smooth muscle antibody in 13%, but no matched data of normal controls were available from their study. In another series of 45 patients with Menière's disease, antinuclear antibodies were not detectable.[119] In patients with PSNHL, the incidence of antinuclear (24%) and antithyroid (41%) antibodies was high, compared with controls. These autoantibodies were nearly absent in patients with sudden deafness[120] (Table 5.11).

Viral antibodies

Antibodies to herpes simplex virus 1 (HSV-1) protein were tested in patients with Menière's disease by ELISA and immunoblotting.[121] Twenty of 21 patients had antibodies to HSV-1. The authors concluded that there was viral reactivation in these patients (Table 5.12).

Table 5.10 Summary of the sources and applications of inner ear antigens

Authors	Date	Source of antigens	Inner ear tissues used	Application of antigens	Reference
Terayama and Sasaki	1964	Guinea pig	Total	AI	12
McCabe	1979	Human	Total	LTT, MIT	17
Yoo et al	1983/84	Bovine/chicken	Pure form	E/AI	18, 27
Harada et al	1984	Rabbit	Lateral wall	AI	28
Hughes et al	1984	Human	Total	LTT, MIT	163
Arnold et al	1985	Human	Total	LTT	21
Harris	1987	Cow	Total	AI	29
Soliman	1989	Guinea pig	Total	AI	30
Zanetti et al	1989	Laminin	Pure form	E	122
Harris and Sharp	1990	Cow	Total	IB	23
Orozco et al	1990	Chick, guinea pig	Total	AI	31
Joliat et al	1992	Human	Total	IB	92
Joliat et al	1992	Type II collagen	Pure form	IB	92
Veldman et al	1993	Swine	Total	IB	116
Yamanobe and Harris	1993	Cow	Total and various parts	IB	107
Cao et al	1994	Guinea pig	Total and various parts	IB	24
Moscicki et al	1994	Cow	Total	IB	110
Takeda et al	1996	CB-11 peptide		AI	253
Carey et al	1998	Guinea pig 68 kDa		IB	125
Tanaka et al	1999	Tubulin (bovine)	Pure form	E	142
Cheng et al	1999	C-raf	Recombinant	E	136
Du and Tau	1999	Tubulin (bovine)	Pure form	AI	254
Matsuoka et al	1999	P0 (bovine)	Pure form	AI	32

AI, animal immunization for experimental autoimmune inner ear disease; E, ELISA; LTT, lymphocyte transformation test; MIT, migration inhibition test; IB, immunoblotting; R, recombinant.

Laminin antibodies

The sera of 413 patients with inner ear disease were examined for ELISA binding to mouse laminin. Anti-laminin antibody reaction was detected in patients with SNHL (68%), tinnitus (60%), sudden deafness (46%), and Menière's disease (14%), and in normal individuals (8%).[122,123] In patients with chronic infectious disease, anti-laminin reactions were observed with almost the same frequency as in patients with SNHL. Immunochemical studies showed that antibody reactivity with laminin results from the Gal alpha 1–3 Gal epitope present in N-linked oligosaccharides of mouse laminin.[123] Although laminin is extensively distributed throughout the inner ear, e.g. in the areas surrounding the spiral ganglion cells and nerve fibers, the capillary vessels in the stria vascularis, and an area beneath the epithelium of the ES,[87] no reaction was observed in the patients with human laminin, which lacks this epitope.[123] These findings

Table 5.11 Results of non-specific laboratory tests

			Positive rate (%)										
Authors	Year	Patients	IgG	IgA	IgM	C1q	C3	CH50	OKT4/OKT8	Anti-DNA	Anti-nuclear	References
Xenellis et al	1986	MD ($n = 52$)	21	2	38	54	17					192
Brookes	1986	MD ($n = 36$)	44.4	2.8	86.1							117
Williams et al	1987	MD ($n = 25$)	12	24	48							255
Evans et al	1988	MD ($n = 110$)	11	23	17		↑					118
Fattori et al	1991	MD ($n = 40$)	15	10	2.5				0			256
Tomoda et al	1993	MD ($n = 26$)	35	4	27				38			91
Yoshino	1994	MD ($n = 29$)	38				24			3.4		257
Gutierrez et al	1994	MD ($n = 40$)	↑		↑			↓				258
Yazawa and Susuki	1996	bil-MD ($n = 36$)	14	11	11		0	61	63	0	17	259

MD, Menière's disease; bil-MD, bilateral MD; C1q and C3, complements; CH50, hemolytic complement level; OKT4/OKT8, ratio of subpopulations of T4 and T8 lymphocytes; ↑, increase; ↓, decrease.

Table 5.12 Serum antibody titer against various viruses reported by investigators

Authors	Year	Patients	Positive results	Reference
Williams et al	1987	MD ($n = 25$)	HSV-1 (60%), VZV (68%), CMV (56%), mumps (24%), rubella (48%), rubeola (32%)	255
Bergstrom et al	1992	MD ($n = 21$)	HSV-1 (95%)	121
Tomoda et al	1993	MD ($n = 18$)	HSV (22%), CMV (11%)	91
Calenoff et al	1995	MD ($n = 10$)	HSV-1 (70%), HSV-2 (70%), CMV (80%), EBV (60%)	260
Arnold and Niedermeyer	1997	MD ($n = 7$)	Perilymph HSV	261

MD, Menière's disease; SNHL, sensorineural hearing loss; HSV, herpes simplex virus; CMV, cytomegalovirus; VZV, varicella zoster virus; EBV, Epstein–Barr virus.

suggest that antibodies against the carbohydrate structures might be stimulated by a persisting infectious process, and certain of inner ear diseases might have a chronic infectious etiology.[123]

68-kDa protein, a 70 hsp and KHRI-3 protein as autoantigens

This 68-kDa protein was later identified as a 70-kDa heat shock protein (hsp 70),[124] although the 68-kDa inner ear antigen from Carey's group is not hsp 70.[125] The 68-kDa protein binds supporting cells in the organ of Corti, while 70 hsp antibody does not bind any site in the inner ear.[126] Patient's sera still bound 68-kDa bovine inner ear antigen after sera was extensively absorbed with bovine hsp 70 (J. P. Harris, personal communication). We were unable to show recombinant human hsp 70 binding autoimmune inner ear disease sera when we used commercial recombinant hsp 70 (T. J. Yoo, unpublished observation). Trune et al were not able to induce hearing loss with hsp 70 in experimental animals,[127] and nor did the Harris group when they immunized the guinea pig with hsp 70 (R. D. Rauch, personal communication). Rauch was not able to induce hearing loss in rats by hsp 70 immunization, though he identified the hsp 70 epitope for Menière's disease.[128]

It has been shown that hsp 70 is not the target of KHRI-3, an antibody which binds 68-kDa protein from guinea pig inner ear membrane, because when proteins were precipitated from inner ear extract by KHRI-3 and western blotted, nothing in the immunoprecipitate reacted with anti-hsp 70 antibodies.

Using guinea pig inner ear tissue as the antigenic substrate and either Western blot or immunofluorescence (IF) or both, sera from 73 patients suspected of having autoimmune hearing loss from inner ear antibodies were tested. Thirty-seven of 73 (51%) had antibody to a 68–70-kDa protein by Western blot. Sera positive by IF stained supporting cells with a staining pattern like that previously observed with the KHRI-3 monoclonal antibody. There was concordance between Western blot and IF assays. Of 36 patients tested by both assays, 29 of 31 (94%) who were positive in Western blot were also positive by IF, three were negative by both tests and two each were positive by one assay but negative by the other. Absorption of patient sera with human inner ear tissue removed antibody reactivity to the guinea pig supporting cell staining, indicating that the antigen detected by the autoantibody is also present in the human inner ear. Sera from three patients positive in both assays also stained a 68–70-kDa inner ear protein immunoprecipitated by the KHRI-3 monoclonal antibody, indicating that the monoclonal and human antibodies recognize the same antigen. The results support the hypothesis that patients with autoimmune SNHL produce autoantibodies to an inner ear supporting cell antigen that is phylogenetically conserved and defined by the murine monoclonal antibody KHRI-3. Since KHRI-3 can induce hearing loss after infusion into the inner ear it is likely that autoantibodies with the same antigenic target are also pathogenic in humans. The serum levels of antibody against hsp 70 in both normal controls and patients with SNHL are identical in the two groups.[125,126]

Thus the role of hsp 70 in Menière's disease is not yet clear because of the consistently low or no binding activity with human heat shock proteins to Menière's disease patients' sera.

P0 protein as autoantigen

Cao et al have shown that patients with SNHL or Menière's disease have antibodies againt a 30-kDa protein extract from the inner ear of guinea pigs.[24,25] They have identified this 30-kDa protein as myelin protein P0 derived from the acoustical nerve and spiral ganglion. Myelin protein P0 is expressed in Schwann cells of the peripheral nervous system (PNS), but not in the mammalian central nervous system (CNS).[129] Myelin protein P0 accounts for 50–60% of the peripheral myelin proteins and plays an important role in the compaction of myelin by means of homophilic interaction.[130–132] This protein is a cell adhesion molecule of the immunoglobulin supergene family.[129] Few inter-species amino acid variations were seen among the P0 sequences from several kinds of species. Mutation of the P0 protein gene, located on chromosome 1q21–23, may lead to Charcot–Marie–Tooth disease type 1B.[133] Charcot–Marie–Tooth disease has been reported to be associated with hearing loss.[134,135]

A 30-kDa protein from human inner ear extracted proteins has been defined as reacting with sera from Menière's patients.[92] It is not clear whether this 30-kDa protein reported is the same as the P0 protein or not.

In order to study autoimmune hearing loss, an animal model of hearing loss was developed by immunizing mice with P0 protein. The brainstem auditory-evoked potential (BAEP) studies were done on P0-sensitized mice. Two P0-sensitized mice showed haunched posture, poor coat, loss of body weight, and abnormal walking with a waddling gait. About 25% of the P0-sensitized mice developed hearing loss. In the BAEP study, peak latencies of waves I, III and V and the interpeak latency I–III were prolonged in the P0-sensitized hearing loss group of mice. Hearing thresholds were elevated in this group of mice in comparison with the control mice. Inflammatory cell infiltration was observed in the cochlear nerve region, and a reduced number of spiral ganglion cells was also detected. The results suggest that P0-sensitized mice are useful models for studying autoimmune inflammation of the peripheral portion of the auditory system[32] (Figure 5.6).

Raf-1 protein as an autoantigen in Menière's disease

Sera from Menière's disease patients contain antibody against proteins from guinea pig inner ear extracted protein. It has been found that a 28-kDa protein from the guinea pig inner ear membrane fraction strongly reacts with the sera from Menière's disease patients.[136] This 28-kDa protein appeared in the membranous fraction (containing basement membrane, organ of Corti, stria vascularis, spiral ligament, and vestibular epithelium), but not in the neural part (containing the spiral ganglion and cochlear nerve in the modiolus and the vestibular nerve in the temporal bone) of the inner ear. It was purified and identified as the Raf-1 protein.[136]

The extracted proteins from the membranous fraction of the inner ear were electrophoresed on a 12% SDS-PAGE gel and transferred immediately to polyvinylidene difluoride (PVDF) membrane. The N-terminal sequencing was determined by classical automated Edman degradation. Nineteen amino acids were obtained (IVQQFGFQRRASDDGKLTQ). A protein data bank search showed that this sequence corresponds to residues 42–59 of human Raf-1 protein. Raf-1 protein is a serine–threonine-specific protein kinase (PK) which functions in a signal transduction pathway(s) between cell membrane and nucleus.[137] In our 113 patients with Menière's disease, we found that 46% were positive to the antigens. However, only 2 of 26

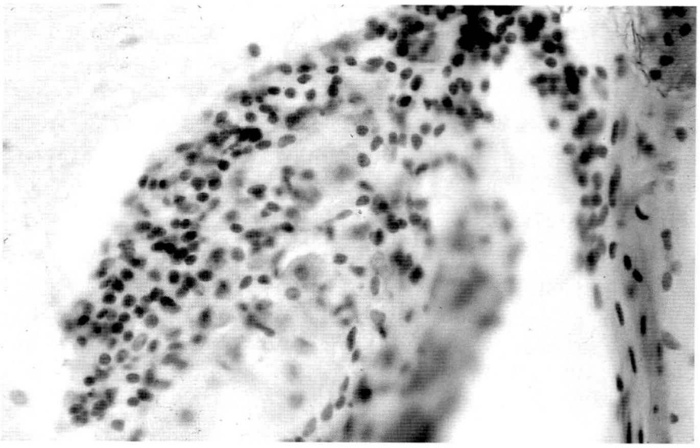

Figure 5.6 Cellular infiltration in cochlear nerve of P0 immunized mice. Mononuclear cell infiltration was observed in the cochlear nerve region in the P0 protein immunized mouse.

PSNHL patients showed positive reactivity to recombinant glutathione-S-transferase (GST) Raf-1 protein. These results suggest that Raf antibodies have a much higher rate of expression in Menière's disease than in the PSNHL. It is also possible that this 28-kDa protein is a new protein which is highly similar to Raf-1 protein.

C-raf immunization of mice produced systemic autoimmune diseases. Three of seven mice which were immunized subcutaneously at the base of the tail, with 100 μg of c-Raf in complete Freund's adjuvant (CFA) with 300 ng of pertussis vaccine with one booster injection 7 days after first immunization developed a hunched posture, loss of body weight, severe skin lesion, lymphadenopathy, splenomegaly, (10 times that of control), and hyperimmunoglobulinemia. When blood from 40 systemic lupus erythematosis (SLE) patients was tested, about 26% of patients with SLE also showed antibody against c-Raf, thus suggesting the role of c-Raf in autoimmune diseases.

The Raf-1 protein belongs to the Raf protein family. Three members have been described: Raf-1, A-Raf and B-Raf. Raf is a tissue non-specific protein and plays a key role in a kinase cascade that regulates cell proliferation, differentiation, and development.[138,139] This phosphorylated map kinase kinase (MEK) activates mytogen-activated protein (MAP) kinase and leads to gene expression and DNA synthesis.[139]

Raf-1 protein is highly conserved in mouse, rat, chicken, *Xenopus laevis*, *Drosophila melanogaster*, and *Caenorhabditis elegans*. The Raf-1 protein is a 74-kDa protein including three conserved regions (CR). CR1 (approximately 53–200 amino acids) and CR-2 (a short sequence in the N-terminal half) are considered to be critical for regulating Raf-1 activity. The mutation of these regions activates the oncogenic potential of Raf-1.[140]

An important convergence point involved in the signal transduction pathways of many different growth factors, hormones, and cytokines is a family of 41–44-kDa serine/threonine kinases collectively called either MAPKs (for mitogen-activated protein kinases) or ERKs (for extracellular regulated kinases). MAPK is activated by sequential phosphorylation on both tyrosine and threonine residues by either the dual serine/threonine kinases MEK (MAPK kinase) alone or by MEK in conjunction with an as yet undescribed kinase. The serine/threonine kinases Raf and Mekk (MAPK kinases) phosphorylate and activate MEK, in turn, during intracellular signaling. Activation of MAPK is directly regulated by a specific MAPK phosphatase and is indirectly regulated by protein kinase A activation, which results in inhibition of Raf activity in mammalian cells. Raf-1 is required for activation of c-Jun via phosphorylation in the transactivation domain.[139]

In our study, we observed that the sera from the inner ear disease patients have antibodies which reacted with 25-kDa and 46-kDa, 52-kDa, 67-kDa, and 79-kDa protein.[141] The results in that study suggested that 52-kDa and 67-kDa proteins are not tissue-specific proteins. This 67-kDa protein does not correspond to the hsp 70 protein.

These results, from our observation and from other laboratories, suggest that multiple antigens are involved in the immunopathology of autoimmune inner ear disease. All three of the study proteins (hsp 70, myelin P0, and Raf-1 proteins) are non-tissue-specific proteins, and are therefore not specific to inner ear tissue. It is of interest to investigate how these non-tissue-specific proteins are involved in autoimmune inner ear disease. Several questions need to be addressed. If this 28-kDa protein is a degraded Raf-1 protein, what is its biological function? Why is this 28-kDa protein observed only in the membranous part of the inner ear tissue, given the fact that Raf-1 is a non-specific protein? How does this immune mechanism target the 28-kDa protein? Does the mutation of this protein break down tolerance or does the immune response to a virus then induce a loss of tolerance to this protein? Clearly, more studies are required to answer these questions (Figure 5.7)

β-Tubulin as an autoantigen for autoimmune inner ear disease

A 52-kDa protein was extracted from the guinea pig inner ear membranous and neural fraction and was identified as β-tubulin in microsequence. It was also identified as the β-tubulin DNA sequence when the cDNA library screening was carried out using a guinea pig cDNA library and the sera of patients with Menière's disease.[142] The antibody to tubulin is elevated in Menière's disease. Sixty-seven of 113 (59%) of Menière's disease patients' sera recognized anti-tubulin antibody using the

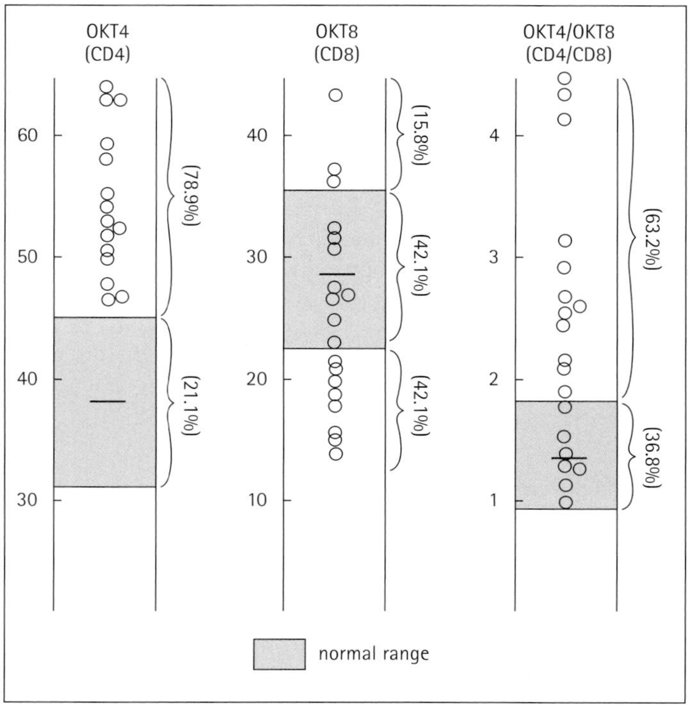

Figure 5.7 T-lymphocyte subpopulations (OKT4, OKT8, OKT4/OKT8) in 19 patients with bilateral Menière's disease indicating a significant raise of the ratio (63%).

ELISA method. In addition, it is elevated in the sera of patients with chronic demyelinating polyneuropathy syndrome.[143]

β-Tubulin is a major intracellular protein involved in the microtubules, prominent structures in the sensory and supporting cells of the organ of Corti in the inner ear. Based on studies of other cell types, it is thought that the functions of microtubules include movement of subcellular organelles,[144] establishment of cell polarity,[145] maintaining cell shape[146] and providing structural support.[147] The determination of cell polarity and shape and the permanence of structures containing microtubules are related to their dynamic properties.[148] Dynamic properties may be determined by the biochemical composition of tubulin.[149,150] Furthermore, immunohistological studies of guinea pig organ of Corti using monoclonal anti-tubulin antibody showed that it is stained in the hair cells, supporting cells, spiral limb, neural pathways of cochlear nerve, and spiral ganglions.

Circulating immune complexes and complement in autoimmune inner ear disease

Circulating immune complexes (CICs) are believed to be involved in the pathogenetic mechanisms in autoimmune inner ear disease. In 1984 Veldman et al reported a 14-year-old girl with SNHL and raised values of CIC.[151] In this case, they believed that the inner ear was involved as one of the target organs in autoimmune disease. Brookes described significantly raised levels of CIC in 26 patients with PSNHL or sudden deafness.[117] He speculated that CICs formed by bacterial antibodies or antibodies to human tissues reached the stria vascularis and reacted with complement in the development of inflammation or cochlear ischemia in the inner ear, resulting in inner ear disease. In 1986, he demonstrated a raised CIC level in 36 (54.5%) of 66 patients with Menière's disease by the polyethylene glycol (PEG) precipitation test.[117] Hsu et al[152] and Derebery et al[153] also reported a raised CIC level in patients with Menière's disease. Plasma exchange to reduce the levels of CIC has been shown to improve auditory thresholds in some cases of SNHL[154] (Table 5.13). Brookes[117] reported that C3c and C1q levels in Menière's disease were significantly raised when compared with the same parameters in controls. Significantly raised IgM complexes and C1q component have also been described in patients with Menière's disease.[118]

The small fragments, C3a and C5a, released during the activation of the complement are sometimes called anaphylatoxin (AT).[155] The pathology of inner ear damage caused by AT was investigated in Hartley strain and C4-deficient guinea pigs.[156] The biological activity of C3a and C5a was found to be strong but of short duration. The resulting ear damage might be reversible, while the damage caused by continuously activated C4a, including atrophy of the stria vascularis, degeneration and sloughing of the cochlear neurones, and stretching of Reissner's membrane, is thought to be irreversible.

Lymphocyte trafficking in the inner ear

Lymphocyte trafficking in the inner ear has been well reviewed with respect to the processes of extravasation, homing of lymphocytes and lymphocyte recruitment signals to the inner ear.[157] The inner ear system follows the general mechanism of the process of extravasation: rolling, tight adherence to a single location on the vessel wall, flattening of cells against the endothelium, and penetration of the vessel wall through intraepithelial cell junctions. At each step, these processes are mediated by cytokines and cytokine receptors as well as cell surface molecules and specific receptors for the ligands: interleukins, chemokines, selectins and adhesion molecules.

T-cell epitope specificity and T-cell receptor usage were investigated in a type II collagen-induced autoimmune ear disease model. An immune response directed against type II collagen (CII) had been reported in several autoimmune ear diseases including the animal models of collagen-induced arthritis (CIA) and collagen-induced autoimmune ear disease (CIAED). We found that T cells from CII-immunized DBA/1-lac mice could transfer auricular chondritis to naive mice. The T cells from CII-immunized H-2r and H-2q mice recognized different

Table 5.13 Circulating immune complex in Menière's disease.

Authors	Year	Patients	Positive rate (%)	Reference
Brookes	1986	MD ($n=66$)	55	117
Evans et al	1988	MD ($n=110$)	↑ ($p<0.001$)	118
Hsu et al	1990	MD ($n=59$)	32	152
Derebery et al	1991	MD ($n=30$)	96	153
Tomoda et al	1993	MD ($n=10$)	40	91
Yoshino	1994	MD ($n=29$)	21	257
Gutierrez et al	1994	MD ($n=40$)	↑ ($p<0.001$)	258

MD, Menière's disease.

epitopes from the CB11 peptide of CII. The CII-specific T cells from H-2q background mice recognize peptide residues p121–147 (P1) but do not respond to residues p211–247 (P2). The T cells of H-2r mice immunized with CII respond better to P2 than to P1. By altering certain amino acids within these epitopes, the response of CII-specific TCR (T-cell receptor) to antigen has been increased or abolished. Our results suggest that the lysine residues at positions 129, 141 and 147 in P1, and the argine residue at position 227 and the glutamic acid at position 230 in P2, might play an important role in the trimolecular interaction. Ten clonally distinct T-cell hybridomas specific for CII have been established from H-2r B10.RIII mice, and the β chains of their TCR have been analyzed. Three subfamilies, $V_{\beta}1$, $V_{\beta}6$, and $V_{\beta}8$, were utilized with dominant expression of $V_{\beta}8$ (60%). This is quite similar to the pattern found in CII-induced arthritis in H-2q mice. This preferential use of $V_{\beta}8$ in CIAED implies that immunotherapy may make it possible to control this autoimmune disease, even in an MHC-diverse situation.[158]

Lymphocyte subsets in autoimmune inner ear disease

The analysis of peripheral lymphocyte subsets was used to assess immune status in a variety of diseases. In 1985, Yoo et al demonstrated that 50% of patients with SNHL had an elevated CD4/CD8 ratio.[159] In another study, Mayot et al found a severe depletion in $CD3^+$ and $CD4^+$ peripheral lymphocytes in patients with sudden deafness, and a marked decrease of $CD8^+$ lymphocytes in patients with sudden deafness and PSNHL.[120] $CD57^+$ cells were significantly increased, while $LFA1^+$ cells were decreased, in both groups. The data showed that different immunological abnormalities appear to be involved in the development of sudden deafness and PSNHL.[120] (Figure 5.8).

Kanzaki et al[160] reported that abnormalities in one or more lymphocyte markers were found in 7 of the 14 patients with 'steroid-responsive SNHL', including 6 of the 11 (54.5%) patients with 'steroid-responsive SNHL' and 1 of the 3 (33%) patients with bilateral idiopathic PSNHL. The CD4/CD8 ratio was less than 0.5 in one patient (7%) and greater than 2 in 6 patients (43%). Suppressor T cells inhibit helper T cells, cytotoxic T cells, and B cells, and play an important role in the adjustment of antibody production and cellular immunity. Some types of suppressor T cells are believed to maintain self-tolerance by inhibiting the immune response to autoantibodies. Therefore, a decrease in suppressor T cells may be related to the production of autoantibodies. However, elevated levels of suppressor T cells are probably due to viral infection resulting in a decrease in immune function.[160,161] In Menière's disease, Tomoda et al[91] showed a significant elevation of the CD4/CD8 ratio and a decrease of CD8 cells in 7 of 18 patients (38%), whereas Fattori et al[119] reported that the total number of lymphocytes, and $CD4^+$ and $CD8^+$ cells, and the $CD4^+/CD8^+$ ratio, were in the normal range in a series of 45 patients with Menière's disease.

Cell-mediated immune response assays

Antigen-specific cellular immune tests used in autoimmune inner ear disease include the migration inhibition test (MIT)[17,162] and the lymphocyte transformation test (LTT).[19,163,164] McCabe was the first to use the MIT in autoimmune inner ear disease.[17] Although he found the MIT to be useful, and it was a standard test for cell-mediated immunity

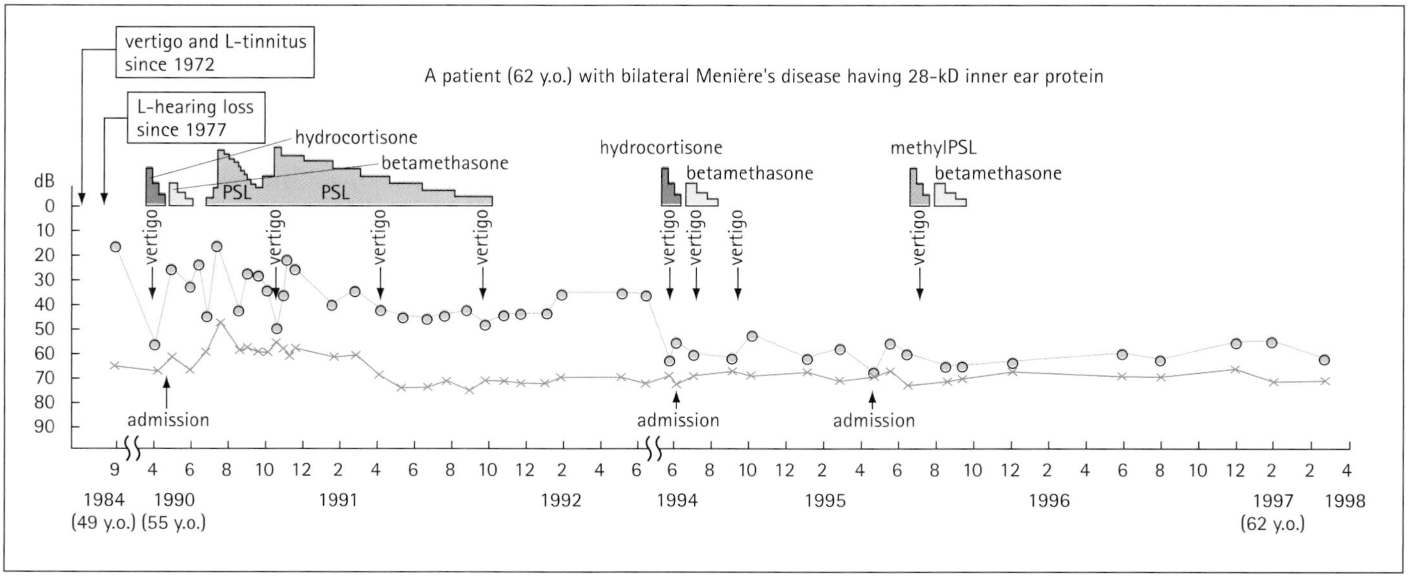

Figure 5.8 A course of hearing threshold of a patient with bilateral Menière's disease having 28-kDa protein. His hearing responded to steroid with 60 dB in his right ear and 70 dB in his left.

(CMI) in the past, it has not been widely applied because of its inherent technical difficulty. Nonetheless, we have used it for several years and found it to be very useful. Hughes et al first reported the preliminary results of LTT in patients with idiopathic PSNHL,[19] and they have since employed the LTT to diagnose autoimmune inner ear disease. The LTT is based on the interaction of the receptors of specifically sensitized T lymphocytes with inner ear antigens and the initiation of cellular activation of the reactive cells in vitro. This response can be detected by measuring proliferation of the T cells. Inner ear tissue, collected from patients during labyrinthine surgery, was used as antigen. It was found that approximately 19% of patients with suspected autoimmune inner ear disease gave positive results.[165] Nevertheless, Harris and Sharp compared the results of LTT in 26 patients with inner ear disease and 19 controls. They found no significant difference between the patient and control groups[23] (Table 5.14). Berger et al described results of LTT using type II collagen as the antigen in 68 patients with PSNHL and 68 healthy volunteers. Thirty-four patients showed a strong stimulation in the LTT, in contrast to only four volunteers in the control group, two of whom had a history of rheumatoid arthritis.[166]

Inner ear involvement in autoimmune inner ear disease

Inner ear involvement in association with other autoimmune diseases has been reported in cases of Cogan's syndrome,[167–169] giant cell vasculitis polyarteritis nodosa,[170–172] relapsing polychondritis,[173,174] systemic lupus erythematosus,[175] Vogt–Koyanagi–Harada syndrome,[176] Sjögren's syndrome,[177] Wegener's disease,[178,179] sarcoidosis,[180,181] hypersensitivity vasculitis[182] and Behçet's disease.[183–187] In some cases, where immune complexes have been strongly implicated, the injury or dysfunction of the inner ear may be merely the result of coincidental injury. Inflammatory bowel disease, rheumatoid arthritis, myasthenia gravis and acute disseminated vasculitis are also associated with hearing loss (Table 5.15).

The audiovestibular involvement in these autoimmune diseases manifests a wide spectrum of symptoms with the variety of: (1) unilaterality or bilaterality; (2) characteristics of onset; (3) ratio of auditory versus vestibular involvement; (4) rate of progress; and (5) response to therapy.[188]

HLA antigens in autoimmune inner ear disease

The MHC, a well-defined system in humans known as human leukocyte antigen (HLA), is a set of loci on the short arm of chromosome 6. The human MHC is very large (about 3500 kb) and is organized as follows: (1) class II genes (HLA-DP, HLA-DQ, HLA-DR); (2) complement genes (class III); (3) heat shock protein and cytokine (TNF, LT, and LT-β) genes, and class I genes (HLA-B, HLA-C, and HLA-A)[189] (Table 5.16). While the external and middle ear can be involved, as in relapsing polychondritis and Wegener's granulomatosis, more severe inner ear disease can also occur, most often in the systemic diseases of polyarteritis nodosa and Cogan's syndrome. Less commonly, hearing loss due to inner ear disease can occur in relapsing polychondritis, Vogt–Koyanagi–Harada syndrome, giant cell arteritis, Takasayu's disease, hypersensitivity vasculitis involving small vessels, sarcoidosis, SLE and endolymphatic hydrops. The findings are not constant, but the sensory organs are degenerated.

HLA plays an important role in the control of cellular interactions responsible for immune responses. MHC-encoded class I and class II molecules bind foreign protein antigens and form complexes that are recognized by antigen-specific T lymphocytes. Class I-associated antigens are recognized by CD8 cytolytic T lymphocytes (CTLs), whereas class II-associated antigens are recognized by CD4 helper T cells. Therefore, it is conceivable that the susceptibility to many supposedly autoimmune diseases is influenced by the inheritance of the HLA genes. In an extensive review, Tiwari and Terasaki[190,191] reported that more than 3000 diseases are associated with the HLA system.

It is believed that autoimmunity is associated with the pathogenesis of some of the previously ill-defined inner ear diseases, including PSNHL, sudden deafness, Menière's disease and otosclerosis. By the HLA serological typing method, using panels of antibodies to identify different alleles, several

Table 5.14 Lymphocyte transformation test (LTT).

Authors	Year	Patients	Positive results: number of patients (%)	Reference
Hughes et al	1983	MD (*n* = 10)	1 (10)	19
Hughes et al	1985	MD (*n* = 12) + IED (*n* = 16)	24 (86)	262
Lejenne et al	1992	MD (*n* = 4) + SNHL (*n* = 12)	MD (0), SNHL (25)	263
Salomon et al	1993	MD + SNHL (*n* = 14)	3 (21)	242

MD, Menière's disease; SNHL; sensorineural hearing loss, IED, inner ear disease other than SNHL.

Table 5.15 Rate of other complicated autoimmune diseases.

Authors	Year	Patients	Total positive rate (%)	Cogan's syndrome (%)	RA (%)	RP (%)	SLE (%)	Hashimoto(%)	Aortitis (%)	Sjogren's syndrome (%)	Reference
Hughes et al.	1987	MD ($n = 27$) + SNHL ($n = 25$)	29.0	13.5	7.7		1.9	1.9	3.8		264
Derebery et al.	1991	MD ($n = 30$)	10.0					6.7	3.3		153
Tomoda et al.	1993	MD ($n = 30$)	13.3	3.3	6.6	3.3					91
Yazawa and Suzuki	1996	bil-MD ($n = 36$)	8.3						2.7	5.6	259

MD, Menière's disease, bil-MD, bilateral MD, SNHL, sensorineural hearing loss; RA, rheumatoid arthritis, RP, relapsing polychondritis, SLE, systemic lupus erythematosus.

attempts have been made to correlate HLA phenotypes and inner ear diseases.[192–194] These studies have shown that inner ear disease susceptibility is associated with the MHC, although the exact nature of the association remains controversial.

In 1986, HLA-A, -B, and -C typing was carried out serologically in 41 patients with Menière's disease by Xenellis et al.[192] Seventy-five per cent of the patients were found to have HLA-Cw7. The association remained significant after correction was made for the number of antigens ($p = 0.035$). The frequencies of HLA-A1 and B8 were also increased but were not significant after corrections. Bowman and Nelson[193] also reported that a significant increase of Cw7 occurred in 51% of patients with autoimmune SNHL compared to 21% of 627 matched controls (RR = 3.95). The possibility of weaker associations with the presence of Cw4 and B35 and the absence of DR4, was demonstrated. However, in another study, HLA-DR4 was distinctly increased in patients with hearing loss (RR = 2.8), Menière's disease (RR = 3.64) and neuronitis vestibularis (RR = 3.12).[195]

Bernstein et al studied the HLA phenotype of 111 patients with inner ear disease.[194] These individuals included 32 patients with Menière's disease, 49 patients with otosclerosis, 14 patients with strial presbyacusis, and 16 patients with SNHL. An increased frequency of Cw7 was not observed in these patients. DR2 may be significantly decreased in patients with SNHL and is present at very low levels in patients with Menière's disease. There was a significant increase in the B8/DR3 and particularly the A1/B8/DR3 haplotypes in these patients. This is intriguing, since a number of autoimmune diseases, including Addison's disease, Sjögren's syndrome, myasthenia gravis, insulin-dependent diabetes, coeliac disease and SLE, are associated with the haplotype B8/DR3.[196–199] Bernstein et al also investigated the autoantibodies to bovine or chick type II collagen in a small sample of patients with ($n = 11$) and without ($n = 11$) the B8/DR3 haplotype.[194] The number of patients with antibodies to type II collagen was significantly greater among patients with B8/DR3 than among patients without this haplotype.

In a Japanese population, Matsuki et al[200] investigated serologically the frequencies of HLA-A, -B, -C, -DR and -DQ in 40 patients with severe unilateral SNHL in childhood. Only HLA-Bw54 showed a significant increase after the correction of the P value (RR = 3.62).

HLA class III complement phenotypes were determined in 39 families with at least one child suffering from moderate or severe bilateral SNHL by serological methods. Steuer et al[201] found that there was a significant difference between the patients and healthy German individuals in the frequencies of the following HLA class III alleles: duplicated C4A (C4"DA"), silent C4A (C4A*Q0), C4B*3, duplicated heavy C4 β chain (C4β"DHH"), and silent C4 β chain (C4β*Q0).

HLA class I, II and III phenotypes were investigated in patients with inner ear disease in different populations by serological typing. Certain HLA class I, II and III alleles were found to be associated with inner ear disease.

Table 5.16 Results of HLA in various inner ear diseases.

Authors	Year	Patients	Positive results	Reference
Xenellis et al.	1986	MD ($n = 41$)	HLA-CW7 (75%)	192
Bowman and Nelson	1987	IED	HLA-DR4 ↓	193
Bernstein et al	1992	SNHL	HLA-A1/B8/DR3 ↑	194
Koyama et al	1993	MD ($n = 20$)	DRB1*1602 subtype of HLA-DR2 ↑	265
Cao et al	1996	SNHL ($n = 34$)	DRB1*0301, ↑ DRB3*0101 ↑	203
			DQB1*0201, ↑ DPB1*0401 ↑	

MD, Menière's disease; SNHL, sensorineural hearing loss; IED, inner ear disease other than SNHL.

In a Korean population, Jung et al[202] undertook genotyping for HLA-DR by PCR-reverse dot hybridization and SSCP (single strand conformation polymorphism) analysis in 40 patients with Menière's disease and in 201 healthy controls. Also, to evaluate immunological abnormalities, antibody to CII was measured by the ELISA method. The level of anti-CII in serum of Menière's disease patients was elevated significantly compared with control serum (0.05). There was no significantly elevated HLA-DR antigen in Menière's disease patients. Only DR13 was significantly decreased in the Menière's disease group. ($p = 0.05$). However, in cases seropositive to the CII group, the frequency of HLA-DR4 was significantly elevated ($p = 0.05$) and that of HLA-DR7 and -14 was decreased compared with control group. The results were comparable to those of the study of rheumatoid arthritis in Korea, suggesting a similar pathogenesis. In summary it can be suggested that specific HLA class II gene products are responsible for the susceptibility to Menière's disease and also for an ethnic variation in the pathogenesis of Menière's disease.

Cao et al found the following on the relevant HLA-DR alleles in patients with idiopathic PSNHL in the Belgian population:[203] DR B1*0301 (increased), DR B3*0101 (increased), DQ B1*0201 (increased), DB1*0301 (decreased), and DP B1*0401 (increased).

Animal models for otoimmunological study

In 1961, Beickert carried out the first study on animals to examine the possibility of autoimmunity with regard to the inner ear.[11] He demonstrated lesions within the cochlea of guinea pigs immunized with inner ear antigen. Terayama and Sasaki immunized guinea pigs with isologous cochlear tissue in Freund's adjuvant, and were also able to produce lesions within the cochlea and alterations in Preye's reflex.[12] However, such observations were essentially ignored at that time. In 1983, Yoo et al reported the development of an animal model of CII-induced autoimmune hearing loss and vestibular dysfunction in rats[26] and guinea pigs.[27] Since then, a large number of animal models have been developed by immunization with a variety of antigens. The animal model of autoimmune inner ear disease induced by CII has already been mentioned above.

To investigate an immunological basis for Menière's disease, Harada et al immunized two groups of guinea pigs with rabbit stria vascularis homogenate.[28] Histological lesions were not observed in the inner ear of guines pigs with a genetic deficit of complement C4, while some normal guinea pigs developed cochlear hydrops. This study suggests the necessity of the integrity of the complement system for obtaining immune-mediated lesions in the inner ear. Harris developed an animal model of autoimmune inner ear dysfunction in guinea pigs immunized with fresh bovine cochlear antigen in Freund's adjuvant.[29] In the experimental group, anticochlear antibodies were detected in the sera, and 32% of the ears tested showed significant hearing loss. Histological injury was characterized by spiral ganglion cell degeneration, perivascular infiltration by plasma cells, edema, and hemorrhage. In 1989, Soliman used a crude inner ear antigen from pigmented guinea pig and developed an animal model of autoimmune inner ear disease in Hartley guinea pigs.[30] The animals demonstrated endolymphatic hydrops, vasculitis, mild cellular infiltration of the ES and occasional spiral ganglion degeneration. Threshold shift was seen in 20% of the tested ears. Subsequent similar studies were reported by others.[204,205]

In another study eight guinea pigs and four mice were immunized with chick and guinea pig cochlear tissue.[31] Hearing loss of 20 dB or greater occurred in eight animals. ELISA demonstrated antibodies to cochlear antigens in the sera of all test animals. Immunocytochemistry revealed immunostaining of hair cells, stereocilia in Corti's organ and saccule. Endolymphatic hydrops, and degeneration of Corti's organ, were observed in these animals.

Tubulin-immunized mice also showed hearing loss and degeneration of the spiral ganglion. The inner ear undergoes apoptosis.[33] Gloddek et al investigated the capacity of sensitized lymphocytes to transfer an adoptive labyrinthitis in naive animals without antigenic stimulation.[207] They demonstrated that lymphocytes of donor animals with labyrinthitis, induced by immunization with keyhole limpet hemocyanin (KLH), were capable of transferring this organ-specific disease to naive recipient animals. Most of the labeled cells were observed in the apical turn of the cochlea in the experimental groups. The deleterious effects of these lymphocytes were shown morphologically by the loss of outer hair cells, and physiologically by the inability to record otoacoustical emissions and the decreased average level of the emissions after cell transfer. The authors proposed that, in humans, lymphocytes become sensitized as a result of exposure to sequestered protein during infection, trauma or operation on the inner ear. These cells recirculate as 'memory' lymphocytes, reach the intact contralateral cochlea, and give rise to an immune response.

Pathology of the inner ear in a systematic autoimmune strain of mice

Inner ear involvement has been investigated in autoimmune strains of mice, such as C3H/lpr,[208,209] MRL-lpr/lpr,[210,211] and NZB/kl[212,213] mice. The inner ears of C3H/pr mice before and after the onset of autoimmune disease were examined. The stria vascularis from older C3H/lpr mice after systemic autoimmune disease onset showed considerable intercellular edema around the strial capillaris and thickening of the capillary basement membrane, compared to controls. Immunoreactivity for IgG was seen in the vessels of the cochlea, particularly in the stria vascularis and bony capsule. These observations suggest that the perivascular abnormalities may result in the stria dysfunction and hearing loss seen in autoimmune disease in human.[208,209,214]

Kusakari et al[210] reported that the auditory brainstem response (ABR) threshold of 20-week-old MPL/lpr mice was significantly higher than that of BALB/c mice at the same age ($p = 0.01$). The inner ears of 20-week-old MRL/lpr mice showed degeneration of intermediate cells, widened intercellular spaces, and IgG deposition on the basement membrane of the stria vascularis, as well as the basal infolding of strial marginal cells. Ruchenstein et al[211] found significant pathology of the basal and middle turns of the cochlea in MRL/lpr mice at early stages of systemic disease. Outer and inner hair cell degeneration, strial edema degeneration, and cellular infiltrate in the tunnel of Corti were also seen.

In NZB/kl mice, spontaneous elevation of the ABR threshold with age was discovered. Pathological changes in the inner ears of NZB/kl mice with a high ABR threshold are confined to the stria vascularis, including marked thickening of the capillary basement membrane and vacuolar degeneration of the intermediate cells. Circular or granular IgM deposits and some IgG deposits were found in the stria vascularis. Deposits of immune complexes (mainly IgM) may cause strial damage and result in the ABR threshold elevation.[212,213,215]

Immunotherapy for autoimmune inner ear disease

The mainstay of treatment for autoimmune inner ear disease is anti-inflammatory drugs, particularly corticosteroids. Treatment with corticosteroids diminishes the production of inflammatory mediators and dampens cellular reactions involved in immune responses. The anti-inflammatory and immunosuppressive properties of corticosteroids are related to at least four major effects: (1) a profound influence on the distribution and trafficking of leukocytes; (2) alteration of the functional properties of individual cells of the immune system, e.g. inhibition of T-cell proliferation; (3) an influence on the synthesis and secretion of soluble mediators that serve as signals between immune cells; and (4) an effect on microvascular permeability. The efficacy of corticosteroids has been shown in many clinical studies.[17,90,93,110,116,216] McCabe recommended that treatment should combine high-dose steroids and cyclophosphamide.[17,268] Initially, intravenous cyclophosphamide 5 mg/kg per day is given for 2 weeks, followed by a rest period of 2 weeks, and then a final 2 weeks of infusions. Dexamethasone 16 mg/day is given orally for 2 months, followed by tapering to 2–4 mg over 2 months. Steroids are continued for 6–24 months, depending on symptoms. Hughes et al recommended high-dose, short-term steroids (prednisone, 1 mg/kg/day).[216] If possible, 1 month of therapy should be followed by a 3-week tapering dosage. In selected cases, many months of low-dose therapy are necessary. Cytotoxic drugs such as cyclophosphamide, methotrexate and nitrogen mustard are recommended, if there is no response to steroids within 6–8 weeks.

Plasmapheresis has been used to reduce circulating levels of antibodies or immune complexes in patients with myasthenia gravis, Eaton–Lambert syndrome, Goodpasture's syndrome, hyperviscosity and Guillain–Barré syndrome.[217–219] Blood taken from the patients is centrifuged, the cells are saved, and the plasma is removed. Cells are resuspended in albumin, fresh normal plasma, or albumin in saline, and returned to the patients. The ill-effects of autoantibodies may be reduced by 65% by removing approximately 2500 ml of plasma. Luetje used plasmapheresis to treat patients with autoimmune inner ear disease.[220] Improved auditory function occurred in six of the eight patients. Three of the six no longer required immunosuppressant medication.

In some autoimmune diseases, antagonists against proinflammatory cytokines, such as IL-1 and TNF, and agents that block leukocyte emigration into tissue, are being tested for anti-inflammatory effects. Immunosuppressive drugs like cyclosporin A and FK 506 are also used to block T-cell activation.[221,222]

On the other hand, many experimental therapies are being attempted. Monoclonal antibodies against surface antigens (e.g. CD3) or the T-cell receptor can be used to deplete or modulate lymphocytes in experimental autoimmune diseases.[223,224] Immunoconjugates of IL-2 and toxins may bind to activated T cells that express high-affinity IL-2 receptors and kill these cells.[225,226] Induction of immune tolerance, e.g. by oral administration of antigens that cause autoimmunity or peptide competition, may be an effective way to prevent autoimmune disease.[227] Their application to clinical disease remains to be further investigated.

Future prospects

Some of the events involved in the autoimmune response to the inner ear and the reasons for their occurrence have been presented. This is the beginning of understanding that an autoimmune response in the auditory system does indeed exist. The knowledge in this field is very limited and brings together research in immunology, audiology, pathology, molecular biology and neuroscience. The rational approach to the problems of autoimmune ear diseases would be the development of better diagnostic tools and therapeutic measures. The development of specific laboratory tests requires the understanding of the etiopathogenesis of disorders and, specifically, further characterizing the autoantigens involved. At present, the medical treatment for these disorders is mostly non-specific and has many undesirable side-effects. Further understanding of the autoimmunity of the auditory system is an essential element for developing specific treatment modalities for better management of patients with this problem. One of the feasible approaches is oral tolerance.

Oral tolerization to antigen has long been recognized as an effective method to induce tolerance. The following sequence of events occurs in oral tolerance: entry of protein into the intestinal tract; passage of protein or peptides through gut epithelium; induction of regulatory T cells; transit of the regulatory T cells into the bloodstream and lymphatic system; and eventual repositioning of reactive cells at the site of autoimmune reaction or within the mucosal epithelium (e.g. inner ear tissue in Menière's disease).[227]

This method has been successfully applied in autoimmune diseases such as experimental allergic encephalomyelitis (EAE),[228–232] collagen-induced arthritis (CIA),[233–235] uveitis, and type I diabetes mellitus.[66,206] It has been suspected that oral tolerance induces IL-4, IL-10 and TGF-β (these are cytokines involved in immune responses) and simultaneously suppresses or inhibits the TH1 (a T-helper cell) cellular response in these autoimmune diseases.[227] This shifting balance of TH1 response to TH2 response reduces the autoimmunity. A trial of TGF-β treatment alone did not totally reverse autoimmune diseases. These results suggest that TGF-β is not the only factor involved in tolerance in these diseases. Although the detailed immune mechanism in oral tolerance is not clear, this treatment has been applied to autoimmune disease patients. Both active suppression and clonal anergy or clonal deletion have been suggested as mechanisms of oral tolerance.[227]

While low-dose antigen treatment induces an active suppression mechanism, high-dose antigen selects clonal anergy. The complexity of treating autoimmune disease might be increasing, and there seems to be some potential to obtain results different from those predicted from animals or in vitro. Obviously, in addition to TGF-β, other factor(s) play(s) a pivotal role in tolerance.[236] In humans, bovine myelin basic protein (MBP) was given orally in a blinded study that included 30 patients with multiple sclerosis.[237] The oral MBP reduced the number of T cells reactive to MBP and was not associated with measurable toxicity.[68] The pilot study suggested some improvement in multiple sclerosis, but clinical efficacy could not be established, due to the small sample size.[68,237] Type II collagens were also used in rheumatoid arthritis, and many other antigens are used in clinical trials. Thus, identifying the autoantigens in autoimmune hearing loss is the first step towards this rational therapy. Recently, delivering protein molecules that could inhibit local inflammation in the ear tissues is being attempted using T cell mediated gene therapy.[269]

References

1. Davis MM. T cell receptor gene diversity and selection. *Annu Rev Biochem* 1990; **59:** 475–96.
2. Germain RN. MHC-dependent antigen processing and peptide presentation: providing ligands for T lymphocyte activation. *Cell* 1994; **76:** 286–99.
3. Steinman L. Autoimmune disease. *Sci Am* 1993; **269:** 106–14.
4. Masugi M, Tomizuka Y. Über die speizifisch zytotoxischen Veränderungen der Niere und ser Leber durch das spezifische Antiserum (Nephrotoxin und Hepatoxin:). *Trans Jap Pathol Soc* 1931: **21:** 329–41.
5. Löwental Z. Djordje Joannovic, Forerunner of the idea of autoaggression in the pathogenesis of disease. *Proc 21st Int Congr Hist Med*, Siena 1968: 1455–62.
6. Joannovic D. Zur Wirkung fermentativ gewonnener spaltungsprodukte aus Geweben und Bakterien. *Wein Klin Wschr* 1920; **70:** 1410–11.
7. Cogan DG. Syndrome of nonsyphilitic interstitial keratitis and vestibuloauditory symptoms. *Arch Ophthalmol* 1945; **33:** 144.
8. Cody DT, Williams HL. Cogan's syndrome. *Laryngoscope* 1960; **70:** 447–78.
9. Lehnhardt E. Plotzliche horstorungen aufbeiden seiten gleichzeitig oder nacheinander, aufgetreten. *Z Laryngol Rhinol Otol* 1958; **37:** 1.
10. Kikuchi M. On the 'sympathetic otitis'. *Zibi Rinsyo Kyoto* 1959; **52:** 600.
11. Beickert VP. Zur Frage der empfindungs Schwerhorigkeit under Autoallergie. *Z Laryngol Rhinol Otol* 1961; **40:** 837–42.
12. Terayama Y, Sasaki U. Studies on experimental allergic (isoimmune) labyrinthitis in guinea pigs. *Acta Oto-laryngol* 1964; **58:** 49–64.
13. Schiff M, Brown B. Hormones and sudden deafness. *Laryngoscope* 1974; **84:** 1959–81.
14. Quick CA. Antigenic cause of hearing loss. *Otolaryngol Clin North Am* 1975; **8:** 385.

15. Arnold W, Weidauer H, Seelig HP. Experimentellerbeweis einer gemeinsamen Anti-genizitat zwischen Innenohr und Niere. *Arch Otorhinolaryngol* 1976; **212:** 99.
16. Weidauer HM, Arnold W, Seelig HP. Nachweis von Bassalmembranantikorpern in Inner-ohr bei experimenteller Masugi-nephritis. *Z Laryngol Rhinol Otol* 1977; **56:** 500.
17. McCabe BF. Autoimmune sensorineural hearing loss. *Ann Otorhinolaryngol* 1979; **88:** 585–9.
18. Yoo TJ, Kang AH, Stuart JM, Tomoda K, Townes AS, Dixit S. Type II collagen autoimmunity in otosclerosis and Menière's disease. *Science* 1982; **217:** 1153–5.
19. Hughes GB, Kinney SE, Barna BP, Calabrese LH, Hamid M. Autoimmune reactivity in Menière's disease: preliminary report. *Laryngoscope* 1983; **43:** 410–17.
20. Hughes GB, Barna BP, Kinney SE, Calabrese LH, Nalepa NL. Predictive value of laboratory test in 'autoimmune' inner ear disease: preliminary report. *Laryngoscope* 1986; **96:** 502–5.
21. Arnold W, Pfatz R, Altermatt H-J. Evidence of serum antibodies against inner ear tissue in the blood of patients with certain sensorineural hearing disorder. *Acta Otolaryngol (Stockh)* 1985; **99:** 437–44.
22. Plester D, Soliman AM. Autoimmune hearing loss. *Am J Otol* 1989; **10:** 188–92.
23. Harris JP, Sharp PA. Inner ear autoantibodies in patients with rapidly progressive sensorineural hearing loss. *Laryngoscope* 1990; **100:** 516–24.
24. Cao MY, Tomasi J-P, Gersdorff M, Deggouj N. Detection of guinea pig inner ear antigens by sera from patients with inner ear disease. In: Mogi G, Veldman JE, Kawauchi H, eds. *Immunobiology in Otology, Rhinology and Laryngology*. Amsterdam/New York: Kluger Publications, 1994: 263–8.
25. Cao MY, Gersdorff M, Deggouj N, Warny M, Tomasi J-P. Detection of inner ear disease autoantibodies by immunoblotting. *Mol Cell Biochem* 1995; **146:** 157–63.
26. Yoo TJ, Tomoda K, Stuart JM, Cremer MA,Townes AS, Kang AH. Type II collagen induced autoimmune sensorineural hearing loss and vestibular dysfunction in rats. *Ann Otorhinolaryngol* 1983; **92:** 267–71.
27. Yoo TJ, Yazawa Y, Tomoda K, Floyd R. Type II collagen-induced autoimmune endolymphatic hydrops in guinea pig. *Science* 1983; **222:** 65–7.
28. Harada T, Matsunaga T, Hong K, Inoue K. Endolymphatic hydrops and III type allergic reaction. *Acta Otolaryngol (Stockh)* 1984; **97:** 450–9.
29. Harris JP. Experimental autoimmune sensorineural hearing loss. *Laryngoscope* 1987; **97:** 63–76.
30. Soliman AM. Experimental autoimmune inner ear disease. *Laryngoscope* 1989; **99:** 188–93.
31. Orozco CR, Niparko JK, Richardson BC, Dolan DF, Ptok MU, Altschuler RAN. Experimental model of immune-mediated hearing loss using cross-species immunization. *Laryngoscope* 1990; **100:** 941–7.
32. Matsuoka M, Cheng KC, Yoo TJ. Autoimmune hearing loss in mice induced by myelin P0 protein, *Ann Otol Rhinol Laryngol* 1999; **8:** 255–64.
33. Du X, Mora R, Barbiera M, Yoo TJ. Tunnel-positive staining in the mouse inner ear caused by tubulin immunization is not apoptosis. *Oto-Rhino-Laryngol* (accepted for publication)
34. Guild SR. Observations upon the structure and normal contents of the ductus and saccus endolymphatic in the guinea pig (*Cavia cobaya*). *Am J Anat* 1927; **39:** 1–4.
35. Lim D, Silver P. The endolymphatic duct system. A light and electron microscopic investigation. In: Pulec J, ed. *Barany Society Meeting*, Los Angeles, 1974: 390.
36. Rask-Andersen H, Stahle J. Immunodefence of the inner ear lymphocyte–macrophage interaction in the endolymphatic sac. *Acta Otolaryngol (Stockh)* 1980; **89:** 283–94.
37. Harris JP. Immunology of the inner ear: evidence of local antibody production. *Ann Otol Rhinol Laryngol* 1984; **93:** 157–62.
38. Tomiyama S, Harris JP. The endolymphatic sac: its importance in inner ear immune responses. *Laryngoscope* 1986; **96:** 685–91.
39. Wackym PA, Friberg U, Linthicum FH Jr. Bui HT, Rask-Andersen H. Human endolymphatic sac: morphologic evidence of immunologic function. *Ann Otol Rhinol Laryngol* 1987; **96:** 276–81.
40. Yamane H, Nakai Y, Sugiyama M, Konishi K, Takahashi K. The occurrence of IgG in the endolymphatic sac of the guinea pig. *Arch Otorhinolaryngol* 1987; **243:** 370–3.
41. Takahashi M, Harris JP. Anatomic distribution and localization of immunocompetent cells in normal mouse endolymphatic sac. *Acta Otolaryngol (Stockh)* 1988; **106:** 409–16.
42. Alternatt HJ, Gebbers Jo, Muller C, Arnold W, Laissue JA. Human endolymphatic sac: evidence for a role in inner ear defense. *ORL J Otolaryngol Relat Spec* 1990; **52:** 143–8.
43. Arnold W. Immunohistochemical investigation of the human inner ear: limitation and prospects. *Acta Otolaryngol (Stockh)* 1998; **105:** 392–7.
44. Kawauchi H, Ichimiya I, Kaneda N, Mogi G. Distribution of immunocompetent cells in the endolymphatic sac. *Ann Otol Rhinol Laryngol* 1992; **101**(suppl 157): 39–47.
45. Ichimiya I, Kawauchi H, Fujiyoshi T, Tanaka T, Mogi G. Distribution of immunocompetent cells in normal mucosa: comparisons among germ-free, specific-pathogen-free, and conventional mice. *Ann Otol Rhinol Laryngol* 1991; **100:** 638–42.
46. Harris JP. Immunology of the inner ear: response of the inner ear to antigen challenge. *Otolaryngol Head Neck Surg* 1983; **91:** 17–23.
47. Tomiyama S, Harris JP. The role of the endolymphatic sac in the inner ear immunology. *Acta Otolaryngol (Stockh)* 1987; **103:** 182–8.
48. Chevance LG, Galli A, Jeanmarie MJ. Immuno-electrophoretic study of the human perilymph. *Acta Otolaryngol (Stockh)* 1960; **52:** 41–6.
49. Fritsch JH, Jolliff CR. Protein components of human perilymph: I. Preliminary study. *Ann Otol Rhinol Laryngol* 1966; **75:** 1070–6.
50. Palva T, Raunio V. Disc electrophoretic studies of human perilymph. *Ann Otol Rhinol Laryngol* 1967; **76:** 23–36.
51. Suzuki Y. Immunological studies on inner ear fluid under the influence of acute middle ear inflammation, *Jpn J Otol* 1977; **80:** 52–60.
52. Mogi G, Lim D, Watanabe N. Immunologic study on the inner ear: immunoglobulins in perilymph. *Arch Otolaryngol* 1982; **108:** 270–5.

53. Arnold W, Altermatt H-J, Arnold R, Gebbers IO, Laissue J. Somatostatin(-like) immunoreactive cells in the human inner ear and endolymphatic sac. *Arch Otolaryngol* 1986; **112:** 934–7.
54. Arnold W, Altermatt H-J, Gebbers IO, Laissue J. Secretory immunoglobulins A in the human endolymphatic sac. An immunohistochemical study. *ORL* 1984; **46:** 286–8.
55. Davis BJ. Disk electrophoresis: II. Method and application to human serum protein. *Ann NY Acad Sci* 1964; **121:** 404–27.
56. Vaerman JP, Heremans JF. IgA system of the guinea pig. *J Immunol* 1972; **108:** 637–48.
57. Goodman JW, Wang AC. Immunoglobulin. Structure and diversity. In: Fudenberg HH, Stites DP, Caldwell JL et al eds. *Basic and Clinical Immunology*, 2nd edn. Altos, Ca: Los Lange Medical Publication, 1978: 23–8.
58. Altmann F, Waltner JG. The circulation of the labyrinthine fluids. *Ann Otol Rhinol Laryngol* 1974; **56:** 684–708.
59. Kellerhals B. Perilymph production and cochlear blood flow. *Acta Otolaryngol (Stockh)* 1979; **87:** 370–4.
60. Harris JP, Fukuda S, Keithly EM. Spiral modiolar vein: its importance in inner ear inflammation. *Acta Otolaryngol* 1990; **110:** 357–65.
61. Gloddek B, Ryan AF, Harris JP. Homing of lymphocytes to the inner ear. *Acta Otolaryngol (Stockh)* 1991; **111:** 1051–9.
62. Gloddek B, Harris JP. Role of lymphokines in the immune response of the inner ear. *Acta Otolaryngol (Stockh)* 1989; **108:** 68–75.
63. Yeo SW, Ryan AF. Transformation growth factor-beta (TGF-β) mRNA expression in the rat cochlea during experimental immune labyrinthitis. In: Mogi G, Veldman J, Harris J, eds. *Immunobiology in Otorhinolaryngology*. Am-stelveen: Kluger, 1994: 181–8.
64. Suzuki M, Harris JP. Expression of intercellular adhesion molecule-1 during inner ear inflammation. *Ann Otol Rhinol Laryngol* 1995; **104:** 69–75.
65. Yeo SW, Gottschlich S, Harris JP, Keithley EM. Antigen diffusion from the perilymphatic space of the cochlea. *Laryngoscope* 1995; **105:** 623–8.
66. Wilson RLK, Stewart IA. Autoimmune sensorineural deafness: case report. *NZ Med J* 1981; **697:** 414–15.
67. Arnold W, Phfaltz CR, Altermatt HJ. Evidence of serum antibodies against inner ear tissue in the blood of patients with certain sensorineural hearing disorders. *Acta Otolaryngol* 1985; **99:** 437–44.
68. Edstrom S, Vahine A. Immunological findings in a case of Cogan's syndrome. *Acta Otolaryngol (Stockh)* 1976; **82:** 212.
69. Elies W. Immunolgische Befunde bei cochleovestibulären Strörungen. *Allergologie* 1983; **6:** 357.
70. Hughes GB, Kinney SE, Barna BP, Calabrese LH. Practical versus theoretical management of autoimmune inner ear disease. *Laryngoscope* 1984; **94:** 758–66.
71. Veldman JE, Roard JJ, O'Conner AF, Shea JJ. Autoimmunity and inner ear disorders: an immune-complex mediated sensorineural hearing loss. *Laryngoscope* 1984; **94:** 501–7.
72. Yoo TJ, Floyd R, Ishibe T, Shea JJ, Bowman C. Immunologic testing of certain ear disease. *Am J Otol* 1985; **6:** 96–100.
73. Yoo TJ. Etiopathogenesis of Menière's disease: a hypothesis. *Ann Otol Rhinol Laryngol* 1984; **93**(suppl 113): 6–12.
74. Vuorio E, de Crombrugghe B. The family of collagen genes. *Annu Rev Biochem* 1990; **59:** 837–72.
75. Kucharz EJ. *The Collagens: Biochemistry and Pathophysiology*. Berlin: Springer-Verlag, 1992: 233–43.
76. Rehn M, Hintikka E, Pihlajaniemi T. Primary structure of the α1 chain of mouse type XVIII collagen, partial structure of the corresponding gene, and comparison of the α1 (XVIII) chain with its homologue, the α1 (XV) collagen chain. *J Biol Chem* 1994; **269:** 13929–35.
77. Myers JC, Yang HY, D'Ippolito JA, Presente A, Miller MK, Dion AS. The triple-helical region of human type XIX collagen consists of multiple collagenous subdomains and exhibits limited sequence homology to α1 (XVI). *J Biol Chem* 1994; **269:** 18549–57.
78. Yoo TJ, Tomoda K. Type II collagen distribution in rodents. *Laryngoscope* 1988; **88:** 1255–60.
79. Ishibe T, Cremer MA, Yoo TJ. Type II collagen distribution in the ear of the guinea pig foetus. *Ann Otol Rhinol Laryngol* 1989; **95:** 176–80.
80. Ishibe T, Choe IS, Yoo TJ. Type II collagen distribution in the ear of developing chick embryo. *Laryngoscope* 1989; **99:** 547–53.
81. Ishibe T, Yoo TJ. Type II collagen distribution in the monkey ear. *Am J Otol* 1990; **11:** 33–8.
82. Khetarpal U, Morton CC. COL1A2 and COL2A1 expression in temporal bone of lethal osteogenesis imperfecta. *Arch Otolaryngol Head Neck Surg* 1993; **119:** 1305–14.
83. Khetarpal U, Robertson NG, Yoo TJ, Morton CC. Expression and localization of COL2A1 mRNA and type II collagen in human fetal cochlea. *Hear Res* 1994; **79:** 59–73.
84. Robertson NG, Khetarpal U, Gutierrez-Espeleta GA, Bieber FR, Morton CC. Isolation of novel and known genes from a human fetal cochlear cDNA library using subtractive hybridization and differential screening. *Genomics* 1994; **23:** 42–50.
85. Van den Heuvel LP, Savage CO, Wong M et al. The glomerular basement membrane defect in Alport-type hereditary nephritis: absence of cationic antigenic components. *Nephrol Dial Transplant* 1989; **4:** 770–5.
86. Kleppel MM, Santi PA, Cameron JD, Wieslander J, Michael AF. Human tissue distribution of novel basement membrane collagen. *Am J Pathol* 1989; **134:** 813–25.
87. Takahashi M, Hokunan K. Localization of type IV and laminin in the guinea pig inner ear. *Ann Otol Rhino Laryngol* 1992; **101**(suppl 157): 58–62.
88. Ye XJ, Terato K, Nakatani H, Cremer M, Yoo TJ. Monoclonal antibodies against bovine type IX collagen (LMW fragment): production, characterization and use for immunohistochemical localization studies. *J Histochem Cytochem* 1991; **39:** 265–71.
89. Slepecky NB, Cefarratri LK, Yoo TJ. Type II and type IX collagen form heterotypic fibers in the tectorial membrane of the inner ear. *Matrix* 1992; **11:** 80–6.
90. Helfgot SM, Moscicski RA, San Martin J et al. Correlation between antibodies to type II collagen and treatment outcome in bilateral progressive sensorineural hearing loss. *Lancet* 1991; **337:** 387–9.
91. Tomoda K, Suzuka Y, Iwai H, Yamashita T, Kumazawa T.

Menière's disease and autoimmunity: clinical study and survey. *Acta Otolaryngol Suppl* 1993; **500:** 31–4.
92. Joliat T, Seyer J, Berstein J et al. Antibodies against a 30 kilodal ton cochlear protein and type II and IX collagens in the serum of patients with inner ear disease. *Ann Otol Rhinol Laryngol* 1992; **101:** 1000–6.
93. Yoo TJ, Yazawa Y, Floyd R, Tomoda K. Antibody activity in perilymph from rats with type II collagen-induced autoimmune inner ear disease. *Ann Otol Rhinol Laryngol* 1984; **93**(suppl 113): 1–2.
94. Yoo TJ, Tomoda K, Hernandez AD. Type II collagen-induced autoimmune inner ear lesions in guinea pigs. *Ann Otol Rhinol Laryngol* 1984; **94**(suppl 113): 3–5.
95. Huang CC, Yi ZX, Abramson M. Type II collagen-induced otospongiosis-like lesion in rats. *Am J Otolaryngol* 1986; **7:** 258–66.
96. Ohashi T, Tomoda K, Yoshie N. Electrocochlographic changes in endolymphatic hydrops induced by type II collagen immunization through the styloid foramen. *Ann Otol Rhinol Laryngol* 1989; **98:** 556–662.
97. Soliman AM. Type II collagen induced inner ear disease: critical evaluation of the guinea pig model. *Am J Otol* 1990; **11:** 27–32.
98. Cruz OL, Miniti A, Cossermelli W, Oliveira RM. Autoimmune sensorineural hearing loss; a preliminary experimental study. *Am J Otol* 1990; **11:** 342–6.
99. Matsuoka H, Kwon SS, Yazawa Y, Yoo TJ. Production of endolymphatic hydrops induced by directly infusion monoclonal antibody against type II collagen CB11 peptide. *Proc 4th International Symposium on Menière's Disease*, Paris, France, April 11–14, 1999. The Hague: Kugler, 2000: 205–14.
100. Yoo TJ, Floyd RA, Kitano H. Animal model of autoimmune ear disease. In: Bernstein JM, Ogra PL, eds. *Immunology of the Ear*. New York: Raven Press, 1987: 463–80.
101. Sudo N, Yoo TJ. Effect of anti-inflammatory drugs on collagen induced autoimmune inner ear disease. *Ann Otol Rhinol Laryngol* 1988; **97:** 153–8.
102. Harris JP, Woolf NK, Ryan AF. A reexamination of experimental type II collagen autoimmunity: middle and inner ear morphology and function. *Ann Otol Rhinol Laryngol* 1986; **95:** 176–80.
103. Bretlau P, Balle V, Causse JB, Horstev-Petersen K, Sorensen CH, Solvsteen M. Is otosclerosis an autoimmune disease? In: Veldman JE *Histophysiology and Tumor Immunology in Otolaryngology* Amsterdam: Kugler, 1987: 201–6.
104. Tomoda K, Maeda N, Yamawaki T, Yamashita T, Kumazawa T, Ohashi T. Immunologically induced experimental hydrops: its mechanisms and pathology. In: Nadal JB, ed. *2nd International Symposium on Menière's Disease*, Amsterdam/Berkley/Milan: Kluger 1989: 165–72.
105. Tomoda K, Yamawaki T, Yamashita T, Kimazawa T. Inner ear immunology and the changes of charge barrier. *Ear Res (Jpn)* 1989; **21:** 275–76.
106. Yoo TJ, Stuart JM, Takeda T et al. Induction of type II collagen autoimmune arthritis and ear disease in monkeys. *NY Acad Sci* 1985; **475:** 341–2.
107. Yamanobe S, Harris JP. Inner ear-specific autoantibodies. *Laryngoscope* 1993; **103:** 319–25.
108. Kosaka K, Yamanobe S, Tomiyama S, Yagi T. Inner ear autoantibodies in patients with sensorineural hearing loss. *Acta Otolaryngol (Stockh)* 1995; **519**(suppl): 176–7.
109. Yamanobe S, Harris JP. Extractions of inner ear antigens for studies in inner ear autoimmunity. *Ann Otol Rhinol Laryngol* 1993; **102:** 22–7.
110. Moscicki RA, Martin JES, Uuintero CH, Rauch SD, Nadol JB Jr, Bloch KJ. Serum antibody to inner ear proteins in patients with progressive hearing loss, correlation with disease activity and response to corticosteroid treatment. *JAMA* 1994; **272:** 611–16.
111. Billings PB, Keithley EM, Harris JP. Evidence linking the 68 Kilodalton antigen identified in progressive sensorineural hearing loss patient sera with heat shock protein 70. *Ann Otol Rhinol Laryngol* 1995; **104:** 181–8.
112. Winfield JB, Jarjour W. Stress proteins, autoimmunity, and autoimmune disease. *Curr Top Microbiol Immunol* 1991; **167:** 161–89.
113. Winfield JB, Jarjour W. Do stress proteins play a role in arthritis and autoimmunity? *Immunol Rev* 1991; **121:** 193–220.
114. Jarjour WN, Jeffries BD, Davis JS 4th, Welch WJ, Mimura T, Winfield JB. Autoantibodies to human stress proteins: a survey of various rheumatic and other inflammatory diseases. *Arthritis Rheum* 1991; **34:** 1133–8.
115. Rauch SD, Sanmartin J, Moscicki RA. Bovine temporal bones as a source of inner ear antigen. *Ann Otol Rhinol Laryngol* 1992; **101:** 688–90.
116. Veldman JE, Hanada T, Meeuwsen F. Diagnostic and therapeutic dilemmas in rapidly progressive sensorineural hearing loss and sudden deafness. *Acta Otolaryngol* 1993; **113:** 303–6.
117. Brookes GB. Circulating immune complexes in Menière's disease. *Arch Otolaryngol Head Neck Surg* 1986; **112:** 536–40.
118. Evans KL, Baldwin DL, Bainbridge D, Morrison AW. Immune status in patients with Menière's disease. *Arch Otorhinolaryngol* 1988; **245:** 287–92.
119. Fattori B, Ghilardi P, Casani A, Migliorini P, Riente L. Menière's disease: role of antibodies against basement membrane antigens. *Laryngoscope* 1994; **104:** 1290–4.
120. Mayot D, Béné MC, Dron K, Perrin C, Faure GC. Immunologic alterations in patients with sensorineural hearing disorders. *Clin Immunol Immunopathol* 1993; **68:** 41–5.
121. Bergstrom T, Edsteom S, Tjellstrom A, Vahlne A. Menière's disease and antibody reactivity to herpes simplex virus type 1 polypeptides. *Am J Otolaryngol* 1992; **13:** 295–300.
122. Zanetti FR, Plester D, Klein R, Bursa-Zanetti Z, Berg PA. Anti-laminin antibodies in inner ear disease: a potential marker for infection and post infection processes. *Arch Otorhinolaryngol* 1989; **246:** 100–4.
123. Klein R, Timpl R, Zanetti FR, Plester D, Berg PA. High antibody levels against mouse laminin with specificity for galactosyl-(alpha 1–3) galactose in patients with inner ear diseases. *Ann Otol Rhinol Laryngol* 1989; **98:** 537–42.
124. Billings PB, Keithley EM, Harris JP. Evidence linking the 68 kilodalton antigen identified in progressive sensorineural hearing loss patient sera with heat shock protein 70. *Ann Otol Rhinol Laryngol* 1995; **104:** 181–8.
125. Michael D, Ramakrishnan A, Nair TS et al. Human autoantibodies and monoclonal antibody KHRI-3 bind to a

phylogenetically conserved inner-ear supporting cell antigen. *Ann NY Acad Sci* 1998; **830:** 253–65.

126. Ramakrishnam A, Arts HA, Telian S, Carey TE. Assessing human sera for antibodies to the KHR1–3 inner ear antigen and HSP-70 protein. ARO abstract 637.
127. Trune DR, Kempton RB, Mitchell CR, Hefeneiden SH. Failure of elevated heat shock protein 70 antibodies to alter cochlear function in mice. *Hear Res* 1998; **116:** 65–70.
128. Bloch DB, Gutierrez JE, Guerriero V, Rauch SD. Antibodies in idiopathic, progressive, bilateral sensorineural hearing loss (IPB-SNHL) recognize an epitope in the carboxy region of bovine HSP 70. ARO Abstract 774.
129. Hayasaka K, Nanao K, Tahara M et al. Isolation and sequence determination of cDNA encoding the major structural protein of human peripheral myelin. *Biochem Biophys Res Commun* 1991; **180:** 515–18.
130. Greenfield S, Brostoff S, Eylar EH, Morell P. Protein composition of myelin of the peripheral nervous system. *J Neurochem* 1973; **20:** 1207–16.
131. Lemke G, Axel R. Isolation and sequence of a cDNA encoding the major structural protein of peripheral myelin. *Cell* 1985; **40:** 501–8.
132. You KH, Hsieh CL, Hayes C, Stahl N, Francke U, Popko B. DNA sequence, genomic organization, and chromosomal localization of the mouse peripheral myelin protein zero gene: identification of polymorphic alleles. *Genomics* 1991; **9**: 751–7.
133. Kulkens T, Bolhuis PA, Wolterman RA et al. Deletion of the serine 34 codon from the major peripheral myelin protein P0 gene in Charcot–Marie–Tooth disease type 1B. *Nature Genet* 1993; **5**(1): 35–9.
134. Satya-Murti S, Cacace AT, Hanson PA. Abnormal auditory evoked potentials in hereditary motor-sensory neuropathy. *Ann Neurol* 1979; **5:** 445–8.
135. Gadith N, Gordon CR, Bleich N, Pratt H. Three modality evoked potentials in Charcot–Marie–Tooth disease (HMSN-1). *Brain Dev* 1991; **13:** 91–4.
136. Cheng KC, Lee KM, Kwon SS et al. Proto-oncogene Raf-1 as an autoantigen in Menière's disease. *Ann Otol Rhinol Laryngol* 2000; **109**: 1093–8.
137. le Guelle R, le Guelle K, Paris J, Phillipe M. Nucleotide sequences of *Xenopus* C-Raf coding region. *Nucleic Acids Res* 1988; **16:** 10357.
138. Egan SE, Weinberg RA. The pathway to signal achievement. *Nature (Lond)* 1993; **365:** 781–3.
139. Blenis J. Signal transduction via the MAP kinases: proceed at your own RSK. *Proc Natl Acad Sci USA* 1993; **90:** 5889–92.
140. Stanton VP Jr, Nickils DW, Laudano AP, Cooper GM. Definition of the human raf amino-terminal regulatory region by deletion mutagenesis. *Mol Cell Biol* 1989; **9:** 639–47.
141. Suzuki M, Krug MS, Cheng KC, Yazawa Y, Bernstein J, Yoo TJ. Antibodies against inner ear protein in the sera of patients with inner ear disease. *ORL* 1997; **59:** 10–17.
142. Tanaka H, Kwon SS, Krug M, Suzuki M, Yazawa Y, Shea J. The β-tubulin as an autoantigen for Menière's disease. In: *Menière's Disease Symposium*, Paris, France, April 11–14, 1999. The Hague: Kugler, 2000.
143. Connolly AM, Keeling RM, Mehta S et al. Serum IgM monoclonal antibody binding to the 301 to 304 amino acid epitope of beta tubulin: clinical association with slowly progressive demyelinating polyneuropathy. *Neurology* 1997; **48:** 243–8.
144. Araki N, Ohono J, Lee T, Takashima Y, Ogawa K. Nematolysosomes (elongated lysosomes) in rat hepatocytes: their distribution, microtubule dependence, and role in endocytic transport pathways. *Exp Cell Res* 1993; **204:** 181–91.
145. Hyde GJ, Hardman AR. Microtubules regulate the generation of polarity in zoospores of *Phytophthora cunnamomi*. *Eur J Cell Biol* 1993; **62:** 75–85.
146. Bulinski JC, Gundersen GG. Stabilization and posttranslation modification of microtubules during cellular morphogenesis. *BioEssays* 1991; **13:** 285–93.
147. Deanin GG, Preston SF, Gordon MW. Carboxyl terminal tyrosine metabolism of alpha-tubulin and changes in cell shape: Chinese hamster ovary cells. *Biochem Biophys Res Commun* 1981; **100:** 1642–50.
148. Schukze E, Kirschner M. Dynamic and stable microtubule population in cells. *J Cell Biol* 1987; **4:** 277–90.
149. Tannenbaum J, Slepecky NB. Localization of microtubules containing posttranslationally modified tubulin in cochlear epithelial cells during development of cell motility and the cytoskeleton. *Cell Motil Cytoskeleton* 1997; **38**: 146–62.
150. Gunderson GG, Khawaja S, Bulinski JC. Postpolymerization detyrosination of alpha-tubulin. A mechanism of subcellular differentiation of microtubules. *J Cell Biol* 1987; **105:** 251–64.
151. Veldman JE, Roord JJ, O'Conner AF, Shea JJ. Autoimmunity and inner ear disorder: an immune-complex mediated sensorineural hearing loss. *Laryngoscope* 1984; **94:** 501–7.
152. Hsu L, Zhu XN, Zhao XN. Immunoglobulin E and circulating immune complexes in endolymphatic hydrops. *Ann Otol Rhinol Laryngol* 1990; **99:** 535–8.
153. Derebery MJ, Rao VS, Siglock TJ, Linthicum FH, Nelson RA. Menière's disease: an immune complex-mediated illness? *Laryngoscope* 1991; **101:** 225–9.
154. Brooks GB, Newland AC. Plasma exchange in the treatment of immune complex-associated sensorineural deafness. *J Laryngol Otol* 1986; **100:** 25–33.
155. Brostoff J, Scadding GK, Male D, Roitt IM. Introduction to immune responses. In: Brostoff J, Scadding GK, Male D, Roitt IM, eds. *Clinical Immunology*. London: Gower Medical Publishing, 1991: 1.1–1.8.
156. Harada T, Sano M, Matsunaga T. The effect of anaphylatoxin component on inner ear damage. *Acta Otolaryngol (Stockh)* 1992; **112:** 265–71.
157. Ryan AF, Gloddek B, Harris JP. Lymphocyte trafficking to the inner ear. *Ann NY Acad Sci* 1997; **830:** 253–65.
158. Yoo TJ, Lee MK, Min YS et al. Epitope specificity and T-cell receptor usage in type II collagen induced autoimmune ear disease. *Cell Immunol* 1994; **157:** 249–62.
159. Yoo TJ, Floyd RA, Ishibe T, Shea JJ, Bowmn C. Immunologic testing of certain ear disease. *Am J Otol* 1985; **6:** 96–100.

160. Kanzaki J, Inoue Y, O-Uchi T. Immunological findings of serological test in steroid-responsive sensorineural hearing loss. *Acta Otolaryngol (Stockh)* 1994; Suppl 514: 66–9.
161. Ikeda K, Kobayashi T, Takasaka T, Itoh Z, Suzuki H, Kusakari J, Takasaka T. Immunological abnormality of the serological tests in bilateral sensorineural hearing loss. *ORL J Otorhinolaryngol Relat* 1989; **51:** 268–75.
162. McCabe BF, McCormick KJ. Test for autoimmune disease in otology. *Am J Otol* 1984; **5:** 447–9.
163. Hughes GB, Kinney SE, Barna BP, Calabrese LH. Practical versus theoretical management of autoimmune inner ear disease. *Laryngoscope* 1984; **94:** 758–67.
164. Hughes GB, Barna BP. Autoimmune inner ear disease: fact or fantasy? *Adv Otorhinolaryngol* 1991; **46:** 82–91.
165. Hughes GB, Fairchild RL, Barna BP. Laboratory diagnosis of immune inner ear disease. In: Mogi G, Veldman JE, Kawauchi H, eds. *Immunobiology in Otolaryngology–Progress of a Decade*. Amsterdam: Kluger Publications, 1994: 231–5.
166. Berger P, Hillman M, Tabak M, Vollrath M. The lymphocyte transformation test with type II collagen as a diagnostic tool of autoimmune sensorineural hearing loss. *Laryngoscope* 1991; **101:** 895–9.
167. Smith JL. Cogan's syndrome. *Laryngoscope* 1970; **80:** 121–32.
168. McDonald TJ, Vollertssen RS, Young BR. Cogan's syndrome: audiovestibular involvement and prognosis in 18 patients. *Laryngoscope* 1985; **95:** 650–4.
169. Schuknecht HF, Nadol JB Jr. Temporal bone pathology in a case of Cogan's syndrome. *Laryngoscope* 1994; **104:** 1135–42.
170. Peitersen E, Carlsen BH. Hearing impairment as the initial sign of polyarteritis nodosa. *Acta Otolaryngol (Stockh)* 1966; **61:** 189–95.
171. Gussen R. Polyarteritis nodosa and deafness. A human temporal bone study. *Arch Otolaryngol* 1977; **217:** 263–71.
172. Wolf M, Kronenberg J, Engelberg S, Leventon G. Rapidly progressive hearing loss as a symptom of polyarteritis nodosa. *Am J Otolaryngol* 1987; **8:** 105–8.
173. Cody DTR, Sone DA. Relapsing polychondritis: audiovestibular manifestation. *Laryngoscope* 1971; **81:** 1208–22.
174. Damiani JM, Levine HL. Relapsing polychondritis: report of ten cases. *Laryngoscope* 1979; **89:** 929–46.
175. Caldarelli DD, Rejowski JE, Corey JP. Sensorineural hearing loss in lupus erythematosus. *Am J Otol* 1986; **7:** 210–13.
176. Stephens SDG, Luxon L, Hinchcliffe R. Immunological disorders and auditory lesions. *Audiol* 1982; **21:** 128–48.
177. Doig JA, Whaley K, Dick WC, Nuki G, Williamson J, Buchanan WW. Otolaryngological aspects of Sjogren's syndrome. *BMJ* 1971; **4:** 460–3.
178. MacCaffrey TV, MacDonald TJ, Facer GW, Deremee R. Otologic manifestation of Wegener's granulomatosis. *Otolaryngol Head Neck Surg* 1980; **88:** 586–93.
179. Okamura H, Ohtani I, Anzai T. The hearing loss in Wegener's granulomatosis: relationship between hearing loss and serum ANCA. *Auris Nasus Laeynx* 1992; **19:** 1–6.
180. Kane K. Deafness in sarcoidosis. *J Laryngol Otol* 1976; **90:** 531–7.
181. Babin RW, Liu C, Aschenbrener C. Histopathology of neurosensory deafness in sarcoidosis. *Ann Otol Rhinol Laryngol* 1984; **93:** 389–93.
182. Campbell SM, Montanaro A, Bardana EJ. Head and neck manifestation of autoimmune disease. *Am J Otolaryngol* 1983; **4:** 187–216.
183. Brama I, Fainaru M. Inner ear involvement in Behçet's disease. *Arch Otolaryngol* 1980; **106:** 215–17.
184. Gemignani G, Berrettini S, Bruschini P et al. Hearing and vestibular disturbances in Behçet's syndrome. *Ann Otol Rhino Laryngol* 1991; **100:** 459–63.
185. Elidan J, Levi H, Cohen E, Ben Ezra D. Effect of cyclosporine A on the hearing loss in Behçet's disease. *Ann Otol Rhinol Laryngol* 1991; **100:** 464–8.
186. Igarashi Y, Watanabe Y, Aso S. A case of Behçet's disease with otologic symptoms. *ORL J Otorhinolaryngol Relat Spec* 1994; **56:** 295–8.
187. Soylu L, Aydogan B, Soylu M, Özsahinoglu C. Hearing loss in Behçet's disease. *Ann Otol Rhinol Laryngol* 1995; **104:** 864–7.
188. Schuknecht HF. The inner ear in autoimmune disease. In: McCabe BF, Veldman JE, Mogi G, eds, *Immunobiology in Otology, Rhinology and Laryngology*. Amsterdam: Kluger Publications, 1992: 95–9.
189. Abbas AK, Lichtman AH, Pober, JS. *Cellular and Molecular Immunology*, 2nd edn. Philadelphia: WB Saunders, 1994: 96–114.
190. Tiwari JT, Terasaki PI. *HLA and Disease Association*. New York: Springer-Verlag, 1985.
191. Tiwari JL, Terasaki PI. The data and statistical analysis. In: *HLA and Disease Association*. New York: Springer-Verlag, 1985: 19–27.
192. Xenellis MD, Morrison AW, MacClowskey D, Festenstein H. HLA antigens in the pathogenesis of Menière's disease. *J Laryngol Otol* 1986; **110:** 21–4.
193. Bowman CA, Nelson RA. Human leukocytic antigens in autoimmune sensorineural hearing loss. *Laryngoscope* 1987; **97:** 7–9.
194. Bernstein JM, Shanahan T, Yoo TJ, Ye XJ. HLA antigens and inner ear disease. In: McCabe BF, Veldman JE, Mogi E, eds. *Immunobiology in Otology, Rhinology and Laryngology*. Kugler New York: Publications, 1992: 3–11.
195. Bumm P, Muller EC, Grim-Muller U, Schlimok G. T-lymphocyte subpopulation and HLA-DR antigens in hearing loss of vestibular neuropathy, Menière's disease and Bell's paralysis. *Laryngorhinotologie* 1991; **70:** 260–6.
196. Lawley TJ, Hall RP, Fauci AS, Katz S, Hamburger MI, Frank MM. Defective Fc-receptor functions associated with the HLA-B8/DRW3 haplotype. *N Engl J Med* 1981; **304:** 185–92.
197. Miyakawa Y, Yamada A, Kosaka K. Defective immune adherence (C3b) receptor on erythrocytes from patients with systemic lupus erythematosus. *Lancet* 1981; **2:** 493–7.
198. Roitt I. Autoimmunity and autoimmune disease. In: Roitt I, Brostoff J, Male D, eds. *Immunology*, 3rd edn. London: Mosby, 1993: 24.1–24.12.
199. Hansen TH, Carreno BM, Sachs DH. The major histocompatibility complex. In: Paul WE, ed. *Fundamental Immunology*, 3rd edn. New York: Raven Press, 1993: 577–628.

200. Matsuki K, Harada T, Juji T, Kanzaku J, Koga K, Toriyama M. Human leukocyte antigen in childhood unilateral deafness. *Arch Otolaryngol Head Neck Surg* 1989; **115:** 46–7.
201. Steuer MK, Gross M, Matthias R, Mauff G. Early onset of sensorineural hearing loss: association studies with major histocompatibility class III (complement) markers. *Am J Otol* 1990; **11:** 326–9.
202. Jung HW, Oh SH, Koo JW et al. A variable association of HLA DR in Korean Menière's patients. *ARO* 2000; Abstract 920, page 265, St. Petersburg Beach, Florida.
203. Cao MY, Thonnard J, Deggouj N et al. HLA class II associated genetic susceptibility in idiopathic progressive sensorineural hearing loss. *Ann Otol Rhinol Laryngol* 1996; **105:** 1–7.
204. Gong S, Wang J. Experimental research of autoimmune inner ear disease. *Chung Hua Erh Pi Yen Hou Ko Tsa Chih* 1995; **30:** 9–12.
205. Liu Y, Guo M, Zhao P. An experimental study on autoimmune sensorineural hearing loss. *Chung Hua Erh Pi Yen Hou Ko Tsa Chih* 1995; **30:** 24–6.
206. Zhang ZJ, Davidson L, Eisenbarth G, Weiner HL. Suppression of diabetes in nonobese diabetic mice by oral administration of porcine insulin. *Proc Natl Acad Sci USA* 1991; **88:** 1025–56.
207. Gloddek B, Gloddek J, Arnold W. Induction of an inner-ear-specific autoreactive T-cell line for the diagnostic evaluation of an autoimmune disease of the inner ear. In: Bernstein J, Faden HS, Henderson D, Ryan AF, Barbara M, Quaranta A, eds. *Immunologic Diseases of the Inner Ear*. Vol. 830. New York: New York Academy of Sciences, 1997: 266–76.
208. Wong ML, Young JS, Nilaver G, Morton JL, Trune DR. Cochlear IgG in C3H/1pr autoimmune strain mouse. *Hear Res* 1992; **59:** 93–100.
209. McMmenomey SO, Russel NJ, Morton JL, Trune DR. Stria vascularis ultrastructural pathology in the C3H/1pr autoimmune strain mouse: a potential mechanism for immune related hearing loss. *Otolaryngol Head Neck Surg* 1992; **106:** 288–95.
210. Kusakari C, Hozawa K, Koike S, Kyogoku M, Takasaka T. MRL/MP-1pr/1pr mouse as a model of immune-induced sensorineural hearing loss. *Ann Otol Rhinol Laryngol* 1992; **101**(suppl 157): 82–6.
211. Ruchenstein MJ, Mount RJ, Harrison RV. The MRL-1pr/1pr mouse: a potential model of autoimmune inner ear disease. *Acta Otolaryngol (Stockh)* 1993; **113:** 160–5.
212. Nariuchi H, Sone M, Tago C, Kurata T, Saito K. Mechanisms of hearing disturbance in an autoimmune model mouse NZB/Kl. *Acta Otolaryngol (Stockh)* 1994; Suppl **514:** 127–313.
213. Sone M, Nariuchi H, Saito K, Yanagita N. A substrain of NZB mouse as an animal model of autoimmune inner ear disease. *Hear Res* 1995; **83:** 26–36.
214. Trune DR, Craven JP, Morton JI, Mitchell C. Autoimmune disease and cochlear pathology in the C3H/1pr strain mouse. *Hear Res* 1989; **38:** 57–66.
215. Tago C, Yanagita N. Cochlear and renal pathology in the autoimmune strain mouse. *Ann Otol Rhinol Laryngol* 1992; **101**(Suppl 157): 87–91.
216. Hughes GB, Barna BP, Kinney SE, Calabrese LH, Koo A, Nalepa NJ. Immune inner ear disease: 1990 report. *Trans Am Otol Soc* **78:** 86–91.
217. Hartung H-P, Reiners K, Toyka KV, Pollard JD. Guillain–Barré syndrome and CIDP. In: Hohlfeld R, ed. *Immunology of Neuromuscular Disease*. Dordrecht: Kluwer Academic Publishers, 1994: 33–104.
218. Hamblin TJ. Plasmapheresis. In: Brostoff J, Scadding GK, Male D, Roitt IM, eds. *Clinical Immunology*. London: Gower Medical Publishing, 1991: 29.1–29.11.
219. Hamblin TJ, Muft GJ. Severe deafness in systemic lupus erythematosis: its immediate relief by plasma exchange. *BMJ* 1982; **284:** 1374.
220. Luetje CM. Theoretical and practical implication for plasmapheresis in autoimmune inner ear disease. *Laryngoscope* 1989; **99:** 1137–46.
221. Tomason AW. FK-506 enters the clinic (new). *Immunol Today* 1990; **11:** 35–6.
222. Wekerle H, Hohlfeld R. Principles of therapeutic approaches to autoimmunity. In: Rose NR, Mackay IR, eds. *The Autoimmune Disease* II. San Diego: Academic Press Inc, 1992: 387–430.
223. Hohlfeld R, Toyka KV. Strategies for the modulation of neuroimmunological disease at the level of autoreactive T-lymphocytes. *J Neuroimmunol* 1985; **9:** 193–204.
224. Wraith DC, McDevitt HQ, Steinman L, Acha-Orbea H. T cell recognition as the target for immune intervention in autoimmune disease. *Cell* 1989; **57:** 709–15.
225. Vitetta ES, Fulton RJ, May RD, Till M, Uhr JW. Redesigning nature's poisons to create anti-tumor reagents. *Science* 1987; **238:** 1098–104.
226. Olsnes S, Sandvig K, Petersen OW, Van Deurs B. Immunotoxin–entry into cells and mechanism of action. *Immunol Today* 1989; **10:** 291–5.
227. Weiner HL, Mayer L. Oral tolerance. *Ann NY Acad Sci* 1996; **778**.
228. Higgins PJ, Weiner HL. Suppression of experimental autoimmune encephalomyelitis by oral administration of myelin basic protein and its fragments. *J Immunol* 1998; **140:** 440.
229. Bitar DM, Whitacre CC. Suppression of experimental autoimmune encephalomyelitis by oral administration of myelin basic protein. *Cell Immunol* 1988; **112:** 364.
230. Whitacre CC, Fuller KA, Gienapp IE. Oral tolerance in experimental autoimmune encephalomyelitis (EAE): evidence for clonal anergy. *FASEB J* 1991; **5:** A1678.
231. Brod SA, Al-Sabbagh A, Sobel A, Hafter RA, Weiner HL. Suppression of experimental autoimmune encephalomyelitis by oral administration of myelin antigens IV. Suppression of chronic relapsing disease in the Lewis rat and strain 13 guinea pig. *Ann Neurol* 1991; **29:** 615.
232. Lider OL, Santos MB, Weiner HL. Suppression of experimental autoimmune encephalomyelitis by oral administration of myelin basic protein; II suppression of disease and in vitro immune response is mediated by antigen-specific CD8+ T lymphocytes. *J Immunol* 1991; **142:** 748.
233. Thompson HSG, Stains NA. Gastric administration of type II collagen delays the onset and severity of collagen-induced arthritis in rats. *Clin Exp Immunol* 1985; **64:** 581.

234. Nagler-Anderson C, Bober LA, Robinson ME, Siskind GW, Thorbecke GJ. Suppression of type II collagen-induced arthritis by intragastric administration of soluble type II collagen. *Proc Natl Acad Sci USA* 1986; **83:** 7443.
235. Zhang Z, Lee CS, Lider O, Wiener HL. Suppression of adjuvant arthritis in Lewis rats by oral administration of type II collagen. *J Immunol* 1990; **145:** 2489–93.
236. Friedman A, Weiner HL. Induction of anergy and/or active suppression in oral tolerance is determined by frequency of feeding and antigen dosage. *Proc Natl Acad Sci USA* 1994; **91:** 6688–92.
237. Weiner HL, Mackin GA, Matsui M et al. Double-blind pilot trial of oral tolerization with myelin antigens in multiple sclerosis. *Science* 1993; **259:** 1321–4.
238. Mackay IR, Burnet FM. *Autoimmune Disease*. Springfield: Charles C Thomas Publications, 1963.
239. Elies W, Plester D. Immunological findings in various sensorineural hearing disorders. In: Veldman JE, McCabe BF, eds. *Otoimmunology*. Amsterdam: Kluger Publications, 1987: 157–61.
240. Lejeune JM, Charachon R. Value of immunobiological tests in Menière's disease and in rapidly progressive sensorineural deafness. *Rev Laryngol Otol Rhinol Bord* 1991; **112:** 127–31.
241. Gong S. Establishment of immunofluorescence for testing serum antibodies against inner ear tissues and its clinical application. *Chung Hua Erh Pi Yen Hou Ko Tsa Chih* 1992; **27:** 138–40.
242. Salomon P, Charachon R, Lejeune JM. Indirect immunofluorescence in the investigation of rapidly progressive sensorineural hearing loss and Menière's disease. *Acta Otolaryngol (Stockh)* 1993; **113:** 318–20.
243. Soliman AM. A subpopulation of Menière's patients produce antibodies that bind to endolymphatic sac antigens. *Am J Otol* 1996; **17:** 76–80.
244. Alleman AM, Dornhoffer JL, Arenberg IK, Walker PD. Demonstration of autoantibodies to the endolymphatic sac in Menière's disease. *Laryngoscope* 1997; **107:** 211–15.
245. Soliman AM. Autoantibodies in inner ear disease. *Acta Otolaryngol (Stockh)* 1997; **117:** 501–4.
246. Futaki T, Nagao Y, Kikuchi S. Immunohistochemical analysis of the lateral wall of the endolymphatic sac in Menière's patients. *Adv Otorhinolaryngol* 1988; **42:** 129–34.
247. Yazawa Y, Kitahara M. Immunofluorescent study of the endolymphatic sac in Menière's disease. *Acta Otolaryngol (Stockh) Suppl* 1989; **468:** 71–6.
248. Dornhoffer JL, Waner M, Arenberg IK, Montague D. Immunoperoxidase study of the endolymphatic sac in Menière's disease. *Laryngoscope* 1993; **103:** 1027–34.
249. Gottschlich S, Billings PB, Keithley EM, Weisman MH, Harris JP. Assessment of serum antibodies in patients with rapidly progressive sensorineural hearing loss and Menière's disease. *Laryngoscope* 1995; **105:** 1347–52.
250. Rauch SD, San Martin JE, Moscicki RA, Bloch KJ. Serum antibodies against heat shock protein 70 in Menière's disease. *Am J Otol* 1995; **16:** 648–52.
251. Shin SO, Billings PB, Keithley EM, Harris JP. Comparison of anti-heat shock protein 70 (anti-hsp 70) and anti-68-kDa inner ear protein in the sera of patients with Menière's disease. *Laryngoscope* 1997; **107:** 222–7.
252. Atlas MD, Chai F, Boscato L. Menière's disease. Evidence of an immune process. *Am J Otol* 1998; **19:** 628–31.
253. Takeda T, Sudo N, Kitano H, Yoo TJ, Type II collagen induced autoimmune ear disease in mice. *Am J Otol* 1996; **17**: 69–75.
254. Du X, Yoo TJ. Mouse hearing loss and pathologic changes in inner ear induced by tubulin. *ARO* Abstract 928, page 267, St. Petersburg Beach, Florida.
255. Williams LL, Lowery HW, Shannon BT. Evidence of persistent viral infection in Menière's disease. *Arch Otolaryngol Head Neck Surg* 1987; **113:** 397–400.
256. Fattori B, Ghilardi PL, Casani A. Immunological aspects of Menière's disease. *Rev Laryngol Otol Rhinol Bord* 1991; **112:** 117–19.
257. Yoshino K. Serum antibodies to type II collagen and immune complex in cases of Menière's disease. *Nippon Jibiinkoka Gakkai Kaiho* 1994; **97:** 887–97.
258. Gutierrez F, Moreno PM, Sainz M. Relationship between immune complex and total hemolytic complement in endolymphatic hydrops. *Laryngoscope* 1994; **104:** 1495–8.
259. Yazawa Y, Suzuki M. Immunological findings in bilateral Menière's disease. *Otol Jpn* 1996; **6:** 157–62.
260. Calenoff E, Zhao JC, Derlacki EL et al. Patients with Menière's disease possess IgE reacting with herpes family viruses. *Arch Otolaryngol Head Neck Surg* 1995; **121:** 861–4.
261. Arnold W, Niedermeyer HP. Herpes simplex virus antibodies in the perilymph of patients with Menière's disease. *Arch Otolaryngol Head Neck Surg* 1997; **123:** 53–6.
262. Hughes GB, Kinney SE, Hamid MA, Barna BP, Calabrese LH. Autoimmune vestibular dysfunction: preliminary report. *Laryngoscope* 1985; **95:** 893–7.
263. Lejeune JM, Charachon R. New immunobiological tests in the investigation of Menière's disease and sensorineural hearing loss. *Acta Otolaryngol (Stockh)* 1992; **11:** 174–9.
264. Hughes GB, Kinney SE, Barna BP, Calabrese LH. Autoimmune inner ear disease. Laboratory tests and audio-vestibular treatment responses. In: Veldman JE, McCabe BF, eds. *Otoimmunology*. Amsterdam: Kluger Publications, 1987: 149–55.
265. Koyama S, Mitsuishi Y, Bibee K, Watanabe I, Terasaki PI. HLA associations with Menière's disease. *Acta Otolaryngol (Stockh)* 1993; **113:** 575–8.
266. Herdman R, Morgan K, Holt PL, Ramsden RT. Type II collagen autoimmunity and Menière's disease. *J Larygol Otol* 1993; **107**: 994–8.
267. Yoo TJ, Sener O, Kwon SS et al. Presence of autoantibodies in the sera of Menière's disease. *Ann Otol Rhinol Larygol* 2001; **110**: 425–9.
268. McCabe BF. Autoimmune inner ear disease: Therapy. *Am J Otol* 1989; **10:** 196–7.
269. Conference Programme abstract: Yoo TJ. Molecular basis of immunity of cochlea. Presented at Autoimmunity of Cochlea 2002 Update: Biology of Hearing and Hearing Loss in Autoimmune Disease, 1–2 November 2002, Genoa, Italy.

6 The epidemiology of hearing and balance disorders

Adrian Davis, Padma Moorjani

Scope

Epidemiology is defined as 'the study of how often diseases occur in different groups of people and why'. The epidemiology of hearing and balance disorders is important for at least three reasons: (1) it shows the scale of need in terms of the prevalence of hearing impairment imbalance, disability and handicap; (2) it shows those factors that are responsible for the deterioration of hearing and balance; and (3) it shows how effective services (health and other public services) are at meeting the need. In the current healthcare system, both purchases and providers need to use epidemiological studies in order to provide optimal services to the current client groups, and to forecast the trends in distribution in order to plan future provision.

The major aim of this chapter is to show that hearing disorders constitute a major disability and handicap, and have been under-reported, underestimated in terms of their burden on society, and traditionally under-supplied with appropriate health services to ameliorate that burden through improving quality of life. This will be discussed first for the adult population and then for children.

Introduction

Deafness is the most frequent sensory impairment in humans, with significant social and psychological implications. It is estimated that approximately 20% of those over 18 suffer from some form of hearing impairment,[1] and about 840 children per year are born in the UK with a significant permanent hearing impairment likely to affect their own and their family's quality of life. There are three major disorders that arise from auditory- or labyrinthine-based pathology: hearing impairment, tinnitus, and vestibular dysfunction. While the first of these has been documented by some systematic population studies[1–4] and also by investigation of the elderly in nursing-home or residential settings,[5–8] tinnitus has been relatively under-documented,[9] and vestibular dysfunction rarely documented.[10] The consequence of our lack of knowledge concerning the extent of those who could benefit from rehabilitation for their disorder is a lack of prioritization of services for these people at a primary and secondary level of healthcare. Hearing impairment and tinnitus are not visible to society, and their effects are therefore under-recognized. However, the effects are there and suffered by those relatives and carers who try to communicate with the hearing-impaired or tinnitus sufferer on a regular basis. In addition to this chronic breakdown in communication facility, when there is an exacerbation of the disorders by an accompanied vestibular dysfunction or lack of orientation, the effects may indirectly manifest in a greater number of accidents requiring emergency treatment or surgery and hospitalization.[11] The impact of hearing impairment in children and their families is also considerable and wide-ranging, and changes over time through its impact on the child's development. The greatest impact of hearing impairment on the child is on the acquisition of language and development of communication, which in turn can lead to poor literacy skills.[12]

The data that are presented are taken from studies that the MRC Institute of Hearing Research has undertaken.[1,2,13–16] The studies that are reported here have been informed by investigations done at other centres and these will be referred to.

Terminology, definitions and methodology

The terminology and definitions used here are taken from the Audiological, Epidemiological and Genetic Definitions agreed by the European Union study group on the genetics of hearing impairment.[17] There is a major conceptual distinction between the prevalence of hearing disorders and the incidence of hearing disorders. This requires emphasis.

> The prevalence of hearing impairment is the total number of instances of a specified degree and type of hearing impairment, e.g. an average air conduction hearing threshold in the better ear (over the frequencies 0.5, 1, 2 and 4 kHz) that is equal to or greater than 25 dBHL, in a given population at a specific time.

Prevalence is often used to denote prevalence rate, i.e. the percentage (or proportion) of the given population who have the defined characteristic.

> The incidence of the defined degree of hearing impairment is the number of new cases of the defined condition occurring in the given population (it is not the number of new cases consulting), per unit time period, e.g. a year. Too often, the term incidence is used when prevalence is meant!

A second emphasis here is the need for population studies of hearing disorders. A population study is the study of a whole collection of units from which a sample may be drawn. Usually, the population is a collection of individual people, but it could also be households, hearing aid clinics or hospitals. For instance, if we study a random sample of 1000 adults taken from the populations of adults aged 70–80 years, and we determine that 603 of this sample reach our criterion for hearing impairment (e.g. as stated above), then the prevalence (or prevalence rate) would be 60.3%. We would try to quantify the accuracy of that prevalence rate by calculating the confidence interval[18] for the given sample. For the sample used in Davis,[1] the 95% confidence interval for the estimated prevalence rate of 60.3% was 52.9–67.3%, using a stratified random sample of 272 people aged 71–80. This means that in 100 replications of the work conducted on this population, with the same sample size and sampling method, we would expect 95 of the replications to have a prevalence estimate falling in the range 52.9–67.3%.

It is useful to distinguish between the concepts of pathology, impairment, disability and handicap.[19–21]

> **Pathology** should be considered to be an abnormality of structure, e.g. the middle ear, the cochlea, or the stria vascularis.
>
> An **impairment** is a defect or abnormality of function of the auditory system which is normally measured by psychoacoustical or physiological function, e.g. pure tone hearing threshold, otoacoustical emission, or brainstem response threshold to clicks.
>
> **Disability** is often a consequence of impairment and is the problem(s) that a person experiences and/or reports in basic tasks, e.g. difficulty communicating in a noisy environment, or knowing who is speaking in a group conversation. Handicap arises from the disadvantage resulting from an impairment or disability that limits or even prevents a person from fulfilling a 'normal' role for that person, e.g. social isolation, or extra effort in communicating.

An indicator of handicap may be obtained by using a questionnaire to measure an individual's quality of life.

In talking and writing about hearing disorders it is often useful to distinguish between two types of hearing impairment, sensorineural and conductive. The majority of permanent impairments are sensorineural, i.e. they are related to disease/deformity of the cochlea or cochlear nerve. In these individuals, there is no 'air–bone gap' (over the average thresholds for the frequencies 0.5, 1 and 2 kHz). It is suggested that if the difference between the air conduction and the bone conduction average thresholds is less than 15 dB, and the average hearing impairment on the ear is 25 dBHL or greater (over the frequencies 0.5, 1, 2 and 4 kHz), then an individual can be presumed to have a sensorineural pathology, whereas if the air–bone gap is 15 dB or greater, the individual has a significant conductive pathology contributing to the impairment. This is a working definition rather than a prescriptive one, because the extent to which the middle ear might be involved in any impairment depends on a number of factors, of which the air–bone gap is only one. Of course, the pathology is important, because conductive impairments may be more amenable to surgical intervention to ameliorate the pathology and reduce the impairment. On the other hand, sensorineural impairments of a mild-to-severe type are not amenable to surgical intervention, and the intervention of choice is rehabilitation centred around the use of a personal hearing aid, which aims to reduce the disability (and hopefully handicap) and increase the quality of life. Profound or total hearing impairment may be amenable to intervention using cochlear implants.[22]

In considering healthcare provision (e.g. interventions through which patients or their families benefit) as well as the concepts given above, there is a need to distinguish three further concepts, those of need, demand for services and supply of services. Furthermore, we should not accept that everyone

> **HEALTHCARE PROVISIONS**
> - Need.
> - Demand for services.
> - Supply of services.

who demands a service actually needs it, or that all services that are provided actually benefit those in need![10] A pragmatic definition of need[23] used here is the ability of groups in the population to benefit from intervention (usually health, social or educational). Thus those with a substantial conductive impairment may have a need for surgery to improve the middle ear's conduction of sound, those with annoying tinnitus may have a need for tinnitus counselling, those with a sensorineural hearing impairment may have a need for rehabilitative training using a personal hearing aid, and the whole population may have a need to be screened around birth for sensorineural hearing impairment; the list could be extended very easily. Providers of healthcare have to enter into dialogue with society (usually through those who purchase health care) to decide the priority given to the hearing health care needs of the population. The major input into these priority decisions should be the epidemiology (i.e. distribution and determinants) of hearing disorders, which will be modified by the national and local realities, such as the configuration of present services and the cost-effectiveness of the different services provided. The rest of this chapter concentrates on the general epidemiological data.[1,16]

Prevalence of hearing disorders in adults

Figure 6.1 shows the broad extent of hearing impairment and reported hearing disability in the adult population (aged 18 and over) in the UK. From this, we see that almost one in three of UK adults has at least a mild hearing impairment in one ear, with one in five showing a bilateral hearing impairment. One in four people report that they have great difficulty hearing what is said in a background of noise, with 1 in 10 reporting that they have prolonged spontaneous tinnitus.[24] At a moderate degree of hearing impairment, in the better ear, about 7% of the adult population are impaired.[1] This represents a substantial number of people in the UK who may have a need for some associated services, i.e. who may benefit from the provision of hearing services. Supplying those services is a substantial public health problem, serious enough to warrant considerable debate. This is discussed by several authors,[25–27] and revolves around the criteria for whether the population could benefit from intervention and the criteria by which any benefit is cost-effective. Obviously, hearing disability and handicap are the major targets of rehabilitation, both present and future. However, the extent of hearing impairment is the best predictor of need that can be

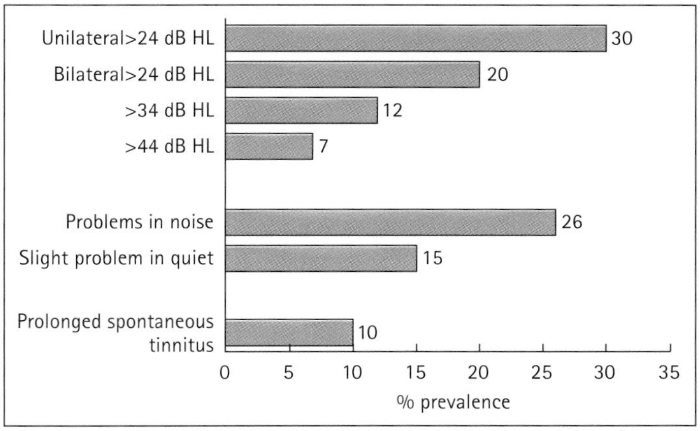

Figure 6.1 The prevalence of hearing impairment at different degrees of severity of hearing disability as shown by finding it 'very difficult' to hear what someone says if there is a background of noise and also by having at least a slight difficulty hearing in quiet. The prevalence of tinnitus that is not only after loud sounds and which lasts for 5 min or more (PST, prolonged spontaneous tinnitus) is also shown.

assessed quantitatively. Both aspects will be presented in this chapter. Some authors[26,27] think that the low threshold for provision of a hearing aid should be set at about 25 dB HL, in the better ear, measured as an average over the frequencies 0.5, 1, 2 and 4 kHz. Other authors[25] consider more complex schemes, and higher thresholds, but the differences are actually quite small operationally and relate mainly to the degree of impairment in the better ear.

Using the lower threshold definition, the prevalence in the adult population (age 18 and over) of a hearing impairment in the better ear of 25 dB HL or greater is 20%. Taking more severe criteria, 12% and 7% are the prevalences for impairments of 35 dB HL or greater and 45 dB HL or greater. The pattern of hearing impairment does change with age,[10] with the higher frequencies being more susceptible to ageing (and noise).

Figure 6.2 shows the prevalence of hearing impairment as a function of age group (see Davis[1] for the confidence intervals and a more detailed description). The data are derived from the National Study of Hearing in the 18–80 age group and from a number of studies for the over 80s.[26,28,29] These do not disagree too much with the estimates made by Soucek and Michaels[30] and by Tolson et al.[8] The estimates up to the 71–80 age group are reasonably accurate in terms of their relatively bias-free derivation. Those for the over-80s have been derived from 862 people using a variety of testing procedures, and are thus more open to criticism. Gatehouse and Davis[31] suggest that at least some of the prevalence in the elderly may be due to central response-based processes rather than peripheral perceptual processing (i.e. it takes a stronger signal for an elderly person to give a response). For public health purposes, this makes very little difference until differential rehabilitation is considered. In any case, it is unlikely that a response bias would make over 10 dB of difference to the hearing thresholds in the over-80s.

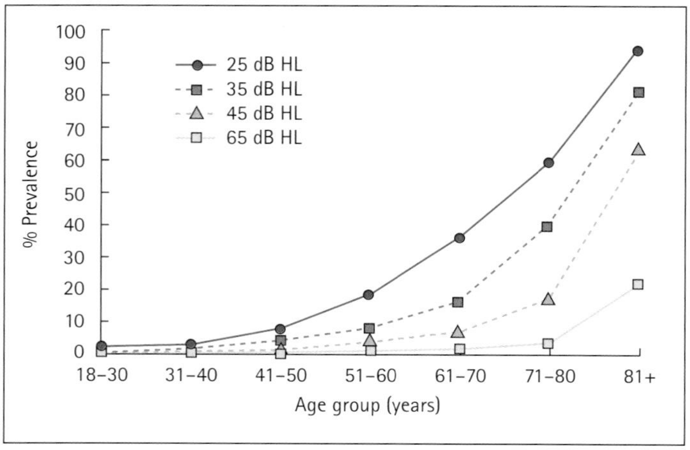

Figure 6.2 The prevalence (%) of different degrees of hearing impairment as a function of age in the Great Britain population.

The major effects on the prevalence of hearing impairment are shown in Davis.[2] By far the most important was age group, with occupational group and occupational noise exposure having major effects throughout the severity range. In terms of gender, at mild–moderate impairments, men have a higher prevalence at 25 dB HL (odds ratio 1.4:1). The effect of age group, as seen in Figure 6.2, is very large and dominates any other factor. Thus, almost one in five people aged 51–60 have a hearing impairment in the better ear, and one in five of the over-80s has a severe hearing impairment which will render speech almost inaudible without amplification. At least 80% of the over-80s would benefit from a hearing aid, if they could use one, and 40% of the population aged 71–80 would benefit likewise. The problem of hearing impairment in the elderly is thus a major issue in terms of the numbers of people involved. The UK National Study of Disability estimated that hearing disability was the third most prevalent disability, and the figures from the National Study of Hearing show that it is in fact the most prevalent disability in the aged (see Davis[2] for a discussion of this difference) and should be given a greater priority than at present. While there is no doubt that hearing impairment and disability are major chronic problems for the population at present,[1] with probably 8.759 million people in the UK with a hearing impairment as described above, the situation may deteriorate due to demographic changes in the population.[10,32] Figure 6.3 shows an extract of the predictions for the number of people with hearing impairment in the UK, USA, developed countries and developing countries in 1995 and 2015.

Figure 6.3 is derived from the National Study of Hearing in Great Britain by convolving the age and sex distribution of different countries (in 5-year bands) with the prevalence of hearing impairment. The increase seen in the overall prevalence is therefore due to the structure of the population alone and assumes no change in aetiology or risk factors over the time period. However, as most of the people who will be contributing to the statistics are already in middle age, they have had their most dangerous time for noxious exposure. There will probably be a more rapid growth in those with hearing problems in the less developed countries as life-expectancy increases over the next 20 years. However, it is noticeable that the proportion of people who have hearing problems is greater in the more developed countries, where life-expectancy is already high. Another key factor for health/hearing services planning is that the expected number of hearing-impaired people in the UK will rise by over 20% in the next 20 years. Using the data for Great Britain, of 8.580 million hearing-impaired people in 1994, 2.131 million were aged 18–60, 4.486 million were aged 61–80 years and 1.963 million were aged over 80. At ≥45 dB HL, there were 0.471 million, 1.132 million and 1.337 million, and at ≥65 dB HL, there were 0.136 million, 0.294 million and 0.469 million respectively for the 18–60, 61–80 and over-80 age groups.[1] Thus, as the severity criterion increases, there is a larger proportion of the very elderly in the hearing-impaired group. Figure 6.4 shows the prevalence of reported hearing disability in the population[1] in the 1980s. The question 'How well can you hear someone talking to you when that person is sitting on your left/right hand side in a quiet room' was used, with responses 'No, slight, moderate and great difficulty' and an

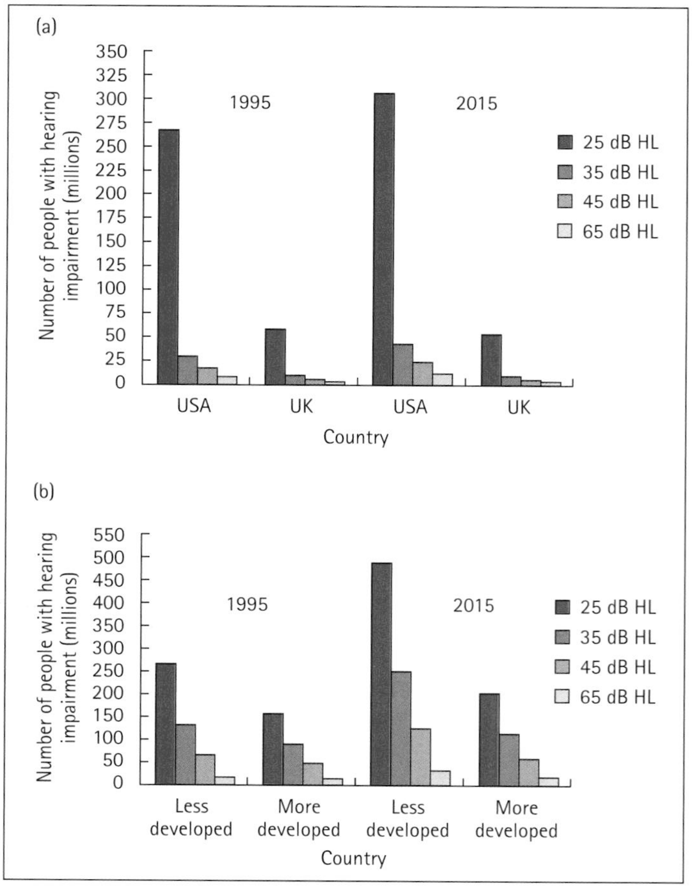

Figure 6.3 Predictions for the number of people with hearing impairment as a function of country and severity of hearing impairment using the 1994 revision of the UN projected world populations in 1995 and 2015. (a) USA and UK; (b) Less and more developed countries.

option for 'Cannot hear at all'. A response of slight difficulty in an ear relates to a median hearing impairment of about 35 dB HL, moderate and worse to 50 dB HL, and great and worse to 75 dB HL (averaged over 0.5, 1, 2 and 4 kHz). Figure 6.4 shows that, at all degrees of reported hearing disability, there is an increase with age. Thus, at 61–70 years, about 15% report difficulty with the better ear, about 25% at 71–80, and 40% for the over-80s. Comparing the reported hearing disability with the measured hearing impairment, it is noticeable that far fewer people have a reported better-ear hearing disability compared to a measured hearing impairment. Furthermore, the ratio of reported problem to measured impairment is not constant across age, showing fair correspondence up to 50 years and then progressive discrepancies. Thus older people are far less likely to report a hearing disability for a given level of hearing impairment. However, it could be argued that they are less likely to benefit from rehabilitation unless they recognize that problem.

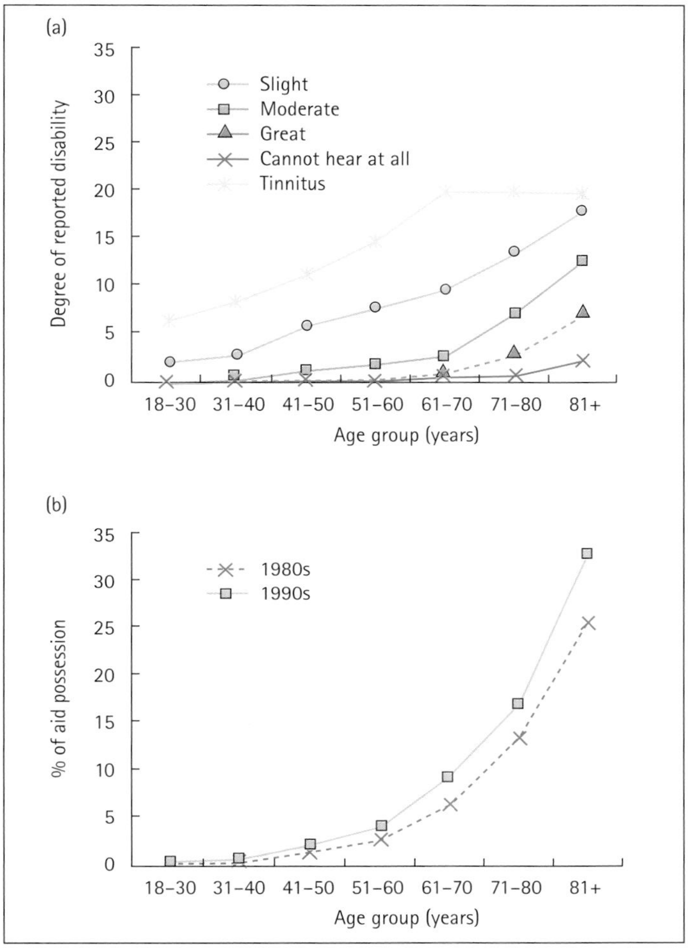

Figure 6.4 Prevalence (%) of different degrees of (a) reported hearing disability, tinnitus and (b) hearing aid possession as a function of age in the Great Britain population.

Figure 6.4 also reports the prevalence of tinnitus that lasts for 5 min or more and not only after loud sounds, adjusted for the proportion of the sample who did not complete all three parts of the question (this was particularly so in the elderly). It is noticeable that the prevalence of tinnitus increases with age until 60 years, when it reaches a peak of one in five people. The factors that influence tinnitus report are systematically explored in Davis et al.[26] Davis and Roberts[11] explore the quality of life implications for those with prolonged spontaneous tinnitus and/or a reported hearing disability. They examined the scores on the SF-36 and showed that both reported hearing disability and tinnitus affect the scores on the SF-36 in a differential way, with severe tinnitus giving the largest deficits, particularly in terms of vitality, social function and mental health. Using the 1990s sample, the largest effect of reported hearing disability was concerned with the social function score (Figure 6.5).

The terms 'hearing difficulty' and 'disability/handicap' were obtained from the subject and situation specific hearing questionnaire devised by Gatehouse[31] and the factor effect shown here is for a shift in 10% of the scores on this questionnaire that only uses items that are relevant to individual patients/hearing aid users. Figure 6.5 shows that the effect of a slight reported hearing disability is a deficit in 6 points of the social function score (range 0–100%), and that a moderate reported disability gives a deficit of 14% with about 30 points for a great disability (using the question in Figure 6.4). However, those who use

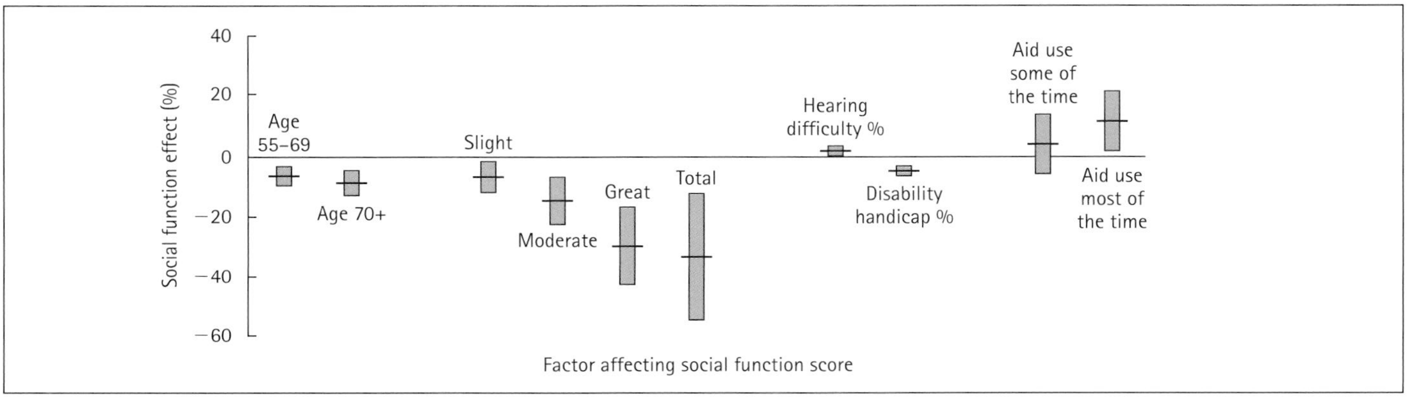

Figure 6.5 The effect (with confidence interval) of age, hearing disability, difficulty handicap and hearing aid use on the social function score of the SF-36 using a general linear model to estimate the effects.

their hearing aids most or all of the time do get this deficit from the hearing disability offset by up to 12%. Those who only use the hearing aid some of the time do not get a significant benefit. This may be for a number of reasons including the fact that there needs to be a reasonable amount of time to adapt to the input from the aid (cognitive plasticity). Also there were significant beneficial effects of 'using a hearing aid most or all of the time' for body pain and mental health scores.

Vestibular dysfunction

Balance disorders include complaints of disequilibrium, vertigo, dizziness, unsteadiness, light-headedness and a wide variety of more unusual symptoms, such as 'difficulty with the legs', 'muzzy-headedness' and feeling 'spaced out'. Moreover, dysfunction in almost any organ can give rise to symptoms of dysequilibrium because of the complex system of balance in Man, which relies upon vision, labyrinthine activity and proprioceptive input. Thus, patients with similar symptoms may present to a range of different medical departments. Thus, frequency and prevelance data for balance disorders are difficult to define and there is a paucity of such data in the medical literature.

Nonetheless, each year, five out of every thousand patients consult their general practitioner, because of symptoms that are classified as vertigo, and a further 10 in a thousand are seen for dizziness or giddiness.[33] One in four patients in a community study of working age adults reported disabling dizziness,[34] and by late middle age this figure begins to increase.[35] By the age of 65 years, 30 per cent of people have experienced episodes of dizziness[36] and by 80 years, two thirds of women and one third of men have suffered episodes of vertigo.[37] Hobson and Pemberton[38] reported that the incidence of vertigo rises with advancing age, and runs roughly parallel with deafness. In younger age groups, few population studies are available, but there are reports of the frequency of various specific conditions, but these are open to criticism in that they usually reflect the referral pattern of the unit reporting the condition, rather than true population-based figures.

Notwithstanding the limitations, the available data may provide some information on the frequency of specific disorders across the broad spectrum of balance disorders.

- Vestibular neuronitis is one of the most frequent causes of vertigo, with an occurrence rate of 4:100,000 population in Japan,[39] and five per cent of patients in a dedicated dizziness unit.[40]
- Between one and two children per thousand are born annually, in the UK, with a sensorineural hearing loss. It is now well recognized that vestibular abnormalities are more common than previously appreciated in congenital hearing loss.[41] Moreover, specific syndromes such as Usher syndrome,[42,43] Pendred syndrome[44] and the CHARGE syndrome have all been associated with vestibular failure.
- Migraine-associated vertigo is now well recognized, and a large carefully designed epidemiological study by Stewart and co-workers[45] identified that nearly 18 per cent of females and 16 per cent of males aged between 12 and 80 years, in the United States, met the case definition for migraine headache. Interestingly, it was noted that prevalence varied inversely with household income, so that more than 40% of women aged between 35 and 40 years, who lived in households with an annual income of less than $10,000 had migrainous headaches, whereas the prevalence was closer to 25% if the income was greater than $30,000. Vertigo has been reported to be present in 42 per cent of patients experiencing migraine headaches with aura,[46] and in the seminal work on this subject,[47] 26.5 per cent of 200 unselected migraine patients experienced vertigo, in association with their migraine, compared with no patients in the tension headache group.
- Benign paroxysmal positional vertigo is the most common cause of vertigo seen in otology departments, and may be associated with many different labyrinthine pathologies, although, most commonly, it is idiopathic. Females outnumber males by a ratio of 1.6 to 1, combining all diagnostic categories of the condition, but the ratio rises to 2 to 1 if only idiopathic and miscellaneous groups are considered.[48]
- Head injuries are a hazard of everyday life in the developed world, with sports and bicycle accidents in the young, industrial and traffic accidents during middle age, and falls in the elderly. The incidence of dizziness has been reported to be as low as 14 per cent in non-hospitalized patients,[49] but in another large series, an incidence of 25–90 per cent has been reported.[50,51] The significance of these figures lies in the annual incidence of minor head injury of between 131 and 511 per 100,000 population in civilised countries.[52]

The economic pressure on health resources, the economic impact on absenteeism from work, and the social impact of imbalance, with accompanying psychological symptoms, emphasize the need for further work on the epidemiology of vestibular disorders.

In this context, a recent UK survey (personal communication) of the prevalence of ear, nose and throat (ENT) symptoms was conducted in 1998 as the first strand of the Health Technology Assessment Project, entitled 'Acceptability, Benefit & Costs of Early Screening for Hearing Disability', the broad aim of which is to investigate screening of people aged 55–74 in order to predict the potential ability to benefit from a hearing aid. A postal questionnaire was sent to 26 100 randomly selected households in targeted areas of England, Scotland and Wales. Everybody over the age of 14 was asked to give details of the occurrence of hearing, balance, throat and nose problems and the disabling effects of these problems. Questionnaires were returned from 34 362 individuals (a response rate of 60.5%). Three questions were asked about the experience of vestibular problems: attacks of dizziness in which things seem to spin around you; unsteadiness, lightheadedness or feeling faint; and attacks of dizziness in which you seem to move.

Overall, 22.2% of responders reported attacks of dizziness in which things spun around them (and 6.9% of responders reported symptoms within the last year)(Table 6.1); 30.2% reported unsteadiness, lightheadedness or feeling faint (6.7% reported experiencing symptoms in the last year)(Table 6.2); and 14.8% of people who responded reported attacks of dizziness in which they seemed to move (3.3% of responders reported symptoms within the last year)(Table 6.3).

The prevalence of all three vestibular problems increased with age, and women reported more symptoms than men.

People were also asked whether they had been to their general practitioner (GP) or had been referred to a hospital about any vestibular problems. Consultations for balance and dizziness increased with age, particularly for respondents aged 81 and over visiting their GP about dizziness problems. The general consultation pattern for vestibular problems by reported hearing difficulty was an increase with worsening hearing in the better ear, particularly for hospital referrals. The patterns for reported tinnitus were similar (Table 6.6).

Table 6.1 The prevalence of self-reported dizziness as a function of age ($n = 31\,085$), gender ($n = 31\,643$) and occupational group ($n = 31\,409$): attacks of dizziness in which things spin around you.

Age group (years)	Prevalence (%)	Gender/ Occupational group	Prevalence (%)
14–30	17.6	Male	16.4
31–40	19.9	Female	27.7
41–50	23.1		
51–60	24.8		
61–70	25.4	Non-manual	21.7
71–80	27.2	Manual	20.4
81+	32.2	Other*	24.4

* Other = housewife/student/unemployed.

Prevalence of hearing impairment in children

This section is concerned only with permanent childhood hearing impairment (PCHI) and not with fluctuating impairments due to otitis media with effusion (OME or glue ear; for a description of the epidemiology of OME see Haggard and Hughes[53]). A major study of PCHI was conducted in the Trent Region of the UK. This region has about 4.8 million people and a typical distribution of ethnic minorities as well as occupational groups. Fortnum et al[16] report the prevalence of hearing impairment shown in Table 6.4, which presents data on the prevalence rate per 100 000 live births for all impairments ≥40 dB HL (i.e. including acquired, progressive and late-onset losses) and for congenital losses alone (i.e. equivalent to incidence) for four degrees of severity of impairment, ≥40 dB HL, 40–69 dB HL (moderate), 70–94 dB HL (severe) and ≥95 dB HL (profound). The confidence intervals have been calculated according to the logistic distribution model, because of the very low values of the prevalences.

The prevalence of all PCHI ≥40 dB HL is 133 per 100 000, and for congenital impairments only is 112 per 100 000. The prevalence of profound impairments that are congenital is of the order of 1 in 4 000 births.

For congenital impairments, the incidence is equivalent to the prevalence. However, there are a number of children, 21 per 100 000, who have either a progressive or an acquired hearing impairment. By the age of about 5 years, the proportion of

Table 6.2 The prevalence of self-reported dizziness as a function of age ($n = 31\,023$), gender ($n = 31\,570$) and occupational group ($n = 31\,343$): unsteadiness, lightheadedness or feeling faint.

Age group (years)	Prevalence (%)	Gender/ Occupational group	Prevalence (%)
14–30	27.9	Male	22.4
31–40	31.0	Female	37.5
41–50	31.6		
51–60	31.1	Non-manual	31.3
61–70	29.6	Manual	26.0
71–80	30.5	Other	32.4
81+	39.2		

Table 6.3 The prevalence of self-reported dizziness as a function of age ($n = 30\,944$), gender ($n = 31\,492$) and occupational group ($n = 31\,266$): attacks of dizziness in which you seem to move.

Age group (years)	Prevalence (%)	Gender/ Occupational group	Prevalence (%)
14–30	12.3	Male	11.1
31–40	14.7	Female	18.5
41–50	16.0		
51–60	15.9	Non-manual	14.0
61–70	15.9	Manual	14.4
71–80	15.6	Other	16.3
81+	20.4		

Table 6.4 Prevalence per 100 000 live births of permanent hearing impairment ⩾40 dB HL, for birth cohorts from 1985 to 1990, for all impairments, for congenital impairments only, for three degrees of severity of congenital impairment (moderate, 40–69 dB HL; severe, 71–95 dB HL; and profound, ⩾95 dB HL), and for congenital sensorineural impairments.

Impairment type and severity	Prevalence per 100 000	95% confidence interval
All		
≥40 dB HL	133	122–146
Congenital		
≥40 dB HL	112	101–123
40–69 dB HL	64	56–73
70–94 dB HL	23	19–28
≥95 dB HL	24	20–30

profoundly hearing impaired who have acquired impairments, mostly through meningitis, is about 20%. The proportion of children with a progressive hearing impairment is not known very accurately, and may be up to 15–25% of those who have a PCHI at the age of 5 years;[54] however, the present study finds only about 10% of PCHI to be progressive.

Aetiology of childhood hearing impairments and major risk factors

The major aspect concerning the aetiology of congenital PCHI is that there are a considerable number of cases with no ascribed aetiology (43%). The major proportion of children who do have an aetiology comprises the approximately 39% who have been given a genetic aetiology. Of those with a genetic aetiology, the dominant genetic inheritance is only about 6%, and children with a stated syndrome comprise about 30%.

There were three major risk factors associated with the hearing impairments. The first and most important was the history of staying in the neonatal intensive care unit (NICU) (26%). The second was a family history of hearing impairment (after excluding those who had an NICU history) (23%), and the third the presence of a craniofacial abnormality noticeable at birth (after excluding those with an NICU or a family history) (4%). Altogether, just over 50% of those with PCHI had a risk factor that might be used as the basis of a targeted screen.[13,15,55] Others have found a higher proportion,[14] so this may be something that varies over districts/regions/countries.

Service indicators for PCHI

Very few studies have looked at the overall benefit derived from finding children with congenital hearing impairments and undertaking a programme of habilitation. The major focus over the last 20 years has been on reducing the age of identification and hearing aid fitting. The National Deaf Children's Society (NDCS) quality standard guidelines[56] apply to children with bilateral ≥50 dB HL average hearing impairment (0.5, 1, 2 and 4 kHz) and suggest that 40% of the children with PCHI should be identified by 6 months of age and 80% by 12 months of age.[56] In the current study, only 14% (95% confidence interval 8–18%) were identified by the age of 6 months and only 42% by the age of 12 months.

Table 6.5 shows the distribution of ages for significant events in the rehabilitative chain: referral, confirmation of the hearing impairment and age at hearing aid fitting. For overall severities, the age at referral was 10 months at the median, with 30% having an age at referral of less than 8 months and 10% having an age at referral of 2 months. It can be seen that the severe and profound impairments are referred earlier and 'diagnosed' earlier than moderate impairments, where the median age at referral is 18 months, and age at hearing aid fitting is 43 months. The data are reasonably encouraging, but regarding the higher percentiles, there are still 30% of children with hearing impairments who have not been referred before about 23 months, and a similar number who are almost 4 years of age before they are fitted with a hearing aid. The delays between referral and fitting are indicative of the long time it takes for some children to be 'diagnosed'. Some of these delays are inevitable. However, many children are kept without amplification while a conductive impairment is ruled out, and inevitably this leads to considerable delays that could be reduced substantially by having a hearing aid while waiting for the operation.[16] The age at referral reflects the service realities that during 1985–90 the targeted neonatal screening services in the region were starting up and that the mainstay for identifying children with permanent childhood hearing impairment was the health visitor distraction test (HVDT). The performance of these tests is discussed elsewhere,[57,58] with the yield coming from the HVDT being much lower than expected and the sensitivity being very dependent on the severity of the hearing impairment.[16] The more systematic use of neonatal hearing screening may substantially improve the age at referral, 'diagnosis' and fitting of hearing aids to those with congenital PCHI. Children with other substantial risk factors, e.g. parental anxiety concerning language development or meningitis, should seek a diagnostic appointment at the first opportunity.[59]

Summary and implications for service provision

The public health priority of hearing impairments and tinnitus in adults should be substantially higher than at present, because hearing disorders comprise the most prevalent chronic impairment in the population, with over 8 million people in the UK (i.e. about 20%) having an impairment. The major factor

Table 6.5 The mean and selected percentiles of the distribution of the age (months) of referral, confirmation of hearing impairment ('diagnosis') and hearing aid fitting, as a function of severity of the hearing impairment, for birth cohorts between 1985 and 1990 who have a congenital hearing impairment.[16]

Age at key points in identification and rehabilitation	Severity group	Mean	Percentiles 10	30	Median	70	90
Age at referral	Overall	19	2	8	10	23	47
Age at 'diagnosis'	Overall	26	5	11	17	37	59
Age at aid fitting	Overall	32	9	16	27	44	63
Age at referral	40–69 dB HL	25	3	9	18	39	55
Age at referral	70–94 dB HL	13	3	7	9	12	34
Age at referral	95+ dB HL	9	1	5	8	10	19
Age at 'diagnosis'	40–69 dB HL	35	9	16	35	46	65
Age at 'diagnosis'	70–94 dB HL	17	3	8	11	19	42
Age at 'diagnosis'	95+ dB HL	11	3	7	10	13	21
Age at aid fitting	40–69 dB HL	42	14	29	43	51	70
Age at aid fitting	70–94 dB HL	24	8	14	18	29	50
Age at aid fitting	95+ dB HL	14	6	9	12	17	24

associated with this high prevalence is age, with noise being the major preventable factor, especially in young people. Because age is the major factor, the whole population prevalence of hearing impairments will increase over the next 20 years by up to 20%, due to the demographics of the population.[23]

Early identification of chronic, but progressive, impairment is not currently being achieved, even for those with substantial impairments, by the mainly reactive hearing services, and hence provision of services substantially lags behind need. Furthermore, the service is not inspiring people to use their hearing aids as only about 40–50% are used for most of the time.

The implications of this global epidemiology are that in the UK, and almost certainly in every developed country, there is a substantial underprovision of services for hearing-disabled people. This could be met by the use of a proactive screening service.[13,28,60] People with hearing disability and tinnitus have a significantly worse quality of life,[11] which can be ameliorated by

Table 6.6 Consultations concerning dizziness problems as a function of age-group (n=31,044), hearing ability (n=31,404), tinnitus report (n=31,578) and gender (n=31,598)

Age	Age group (years) 14–30	31–40	41–50	51–60	61–70	71–80	81+
Visit GP (6.7%)	4.3	5.7	6.1	7.2	8.6	10.8	17.9
Referred to hospital (1.4%)	0.8	0.9	1.2	1.8	1.8	2.1	3.2
Reported hearing difficulty	**Better ear reported hearing difficulty in quiet:** None	Slight	Moderate	Great	Cannot hear		
Visit GP (6.7%)	5.8	12.8	17.4	19.5	11.5		
Referred to hospital (1.4%)	1.1	3.2	4.7	6.0	6.6		
Tinnitus	**Tinnitus for over 5 minutes:** None	Some of the time	Most of the time				
Visit GP (6.7%)	4.9	15.2	14.8				
Referred to hospital (1.4%)	0.9	3.0	5.7				
Gender	Male	Female					
Visit GP (6.7%)	4.5	8.9					
Referred to hospital (1.4%)	1.3	1.5					

the appropriate use of rehabilitation such as the use of a hearing aid for most of the time.[61]

For children, the public health priority stems, on the one hand, from the high burden that the condition confers on a relatively small number of the population (about 700–800 children per year in England), with a prevalence of 112 per 100 000 births for the congenital hearing impaired with average thresholds of 40 dB HL or greater, and on the other, from the very high cost of interventions, e.g. cochlear implants and educational training for the profoundly impaired, who comprise 24 per 100 000 births.

We are still considerably in the dark with respect to the full story of the aetiology of hearing impairments in children; however three risk factors (NICU history, family history of childhood deafness and craniofacial abnormalities) cover over 50% of the population of congenitally hearing-impaired children. There are very few children with rubella as an aetiology (<5%), and so the main scope for prevention may be in understanding why children with an NICU history develop hearing impairment. The understanding of genetic impairments should also be a major priority.

In terms of service development, the wider use of neonatal screening to identify and habilitate hearing-impaired children with the least delay should be given urgent public health attention.

While both adult and child epidemiology support systematic screening of the population for congenital and then later acquired hearing impairment, the precondition for this screening to be successful is that an appropriately staffed and cost-effective service is available for those who do not pass the screen.

Acknowledgements

We would like to thank Vicki Owen for help with the statistics.

References

1. Davis AC. *Hearing Impairment in Adults*. London: Whurr, 1995.
2. Davis AC. The prevalence of hearing impairment and reported hearing disability among adults in Great Britain. *Int J Epidemiol* 1989; **18:** 911–17.
3. Salomon G. Hearing problems and the elderly. *Dan Med Bull* 1986; **33**(suppl): 1–22.
4. Brooks D. *Adult Auditory Rehabilitation*. London: Chapman & Hall, 1989.
5. Alpiner JG Audiological problems of the aged. *Geriatrics* 1963; **18:** 19–27.
6. Martin D, Peckford B. Hearing impairment in homes for the elderly. *Social Work Service* 1978; **17:** 52–62.
7. Schow RL, Norbonne MA. *Introduction to Aural Rehabilitation*, 2nd edn. Pro. Ed., 1989. Texas.
8. Tolson D, McIntosh J, Swan IRC. Hearing impairment in elderly hospital residents. *Br J Nursing* 1992; **1**(14): 705–10.
9. Reich GE, Vernon JA (eds). *Proceedings of the Fifth International Tinnitus Seminar*. Portland: American Tinnitus Association, 1995.
10. Davis AC. Epidemiology. In: Stephens SDG, ed. *Scott-Brown's Otolaryngology* 6th edn, Vol. 2, Ch. 5, *Adult Audiology*. Oxford: Butterworth-Heineman, 1997, pp. 4–38.
11. Davis AC, Roberts H. Tinnitus and health status: SF-36 profile and accident prevalence. In: Reich GE, Vernon JA (eds) *Proceedings of the Fifth International Tinnitus Seminar*. Portland: American Tinnitus Association, 1996, pp. 257–65.
12. Bench R Bamford J. *The Spoken Language of Hearing Impaired Children*. London: Academic Press, 1979.
13. Davis AC, Wood S. The epidemiology of childhood hearing impairment: factors relevant to planning of services. *Br J Audiol* 1992; **26**(2): 77–91.
14. Davis AC, Parving A. Towards appropriate epidemiological data on childhood hearing disability: a comparative European study of birth cohorts 1982–88. *J Audiol Med* 1994; **3:** 35–47.
15. Davis A, Wood S, Rowe S, Webb H, Healey R. Risk factors for hearing disorders: epidemiological evidence of change over time in the UK. *J Am Acad Audiol* 1995; **6:** 365–70.
16. Fortnum HM, Davis A, Butler A, Stevens J. *Health Service Implications of Changes in Aetiology and Referral Patterns of Hearing-impaired Children in Trent 1985–93*. Report for Research and Development Trent RHA. MRC Institute of Hearing Research, 1996.
17. Stephens D, Davis A, Read A. *Audiological, Epidemiological and Genetic Definitions*. In: Martini A, Mazzoli M, Stephens D, Read A (eds). *Definitions, Protocols & Guidelines in Genetic Hearing Impairment*. London: Whurr, 2001.
18. Gardner MJ, Altman DG. *Statistics with Confidence*. London: British Medical Journal, 1989.
19. World Health Organisation. *World Health Organisation International Classification of Impairments, Disabilities and Handicap*. WHO: Geneva, 1980.
20. Davis AC. Hearing disorders in the population: first phase findings of the MRC national study of hearing. In: Lutman ME, Haggard MP (eds). *Hearing Science and Hearing Disorders*. London: Academic Press, 1983.
21. Stephens D, Hetu R. Impairment, disability and handicap in audiology: towards a consensus. *Audiology* 1991; **30:** 185–200.
22. Summerfield AQ, Marshall DH. *Cochlear Implantation in the UK 1990–1994: A Report by the MRC Institute of Hearing Research of the Evaluation of the National Cochlear Implant Programme*. London: HMSO, 1995.
23. Doyal L, Gough I. *A Theory of Human Need*. Basingstoke: MacMillan Education, 1991.
24. Coles RRA, Smith P, Davis AC. The relationship between noise induced hearing loss and tinnitus and its management. In: Berglund B and Lundvall T (eds). *Noise as a Public Health Problem*. Stockholm: Swedish Council for Building Research, 1990, pp. 87–112.
25. Haggard MP, Gatehouse SG. Candidature for hearing aids: justification for the concept and a two-part audiometric criterion. *Br J Audiol* 1993; **27:** 303–18.

26. Davis A, Stephens D, Rayment A, Thomas K. Hearing impairments in middle age: the acceptability, benefit and cost detection (ABCD). *Br J Audiol* 1992; **26:** 1–14.
27. Stephens SDG, Callaghan DE, Hogan S, Meredith R, Rayment A, Davis AC. Hearing disability in people 50–65: effectiveness and acceptability of early rehabilitative intervention. *BMJ* 1990; **300:** 508–11.
28. Davis AC, Thornton ARD. The impact of age on hearing impairment: some epidemiological evidence. In: Jenson JH, ed. *Proceedings of 14th Danavox Symposium. Presbyacusis and Other Age-related Aspects*. Copenhagen: Danavox Jubilee Foundation, 1990, pp. 69–89.
29. Hart FS. *The Hearing of Residents in Homes for the Elderly—South Glamorgan* (Report). University of Wales, Cardiff, 1980.
30. Soucek S, Michaels L. *Hearing Loss in the Elderly*. London: Springer-Verlag, 1987.
31. Gatehouse SG, Davis AC. Clinical pure-tone vs three-inferred forced choice thresholds: effects of hearing level and age. *Audiology* 1992; **31:** 30–44.
32. Davis AC. Epidemiological profile of hearing impairments: the scale and nature of the problem with special reference to the elderly. *Acta Otolaryngol (Stockh) Suppl* 1991: **476:** 23–31.
33. Royal College of General Practitioners and Office of Population Census and Surveys [RCGP/OPCS] *Morbidity Statistics from General Practice*. London: HMSO, 1986.
34. Yardley L, Owen N. Nazareth I et al. Prevalence and presentation of dizziness in a general practice community sample of working age. *Br J Gen Pract* 1998; **148**: 1131–5.
35. Sixt E, Landahl S. Postural disturbances in a 75-year-old population: I. Prevalence and functional consequences. *Age Ageing* 1987; **16**: 393–8.
36. Roydhouse N. Vertigo and its treatment. *Drugs* 1974; **7**: 297–309.
37. Sheldon JH. *The Social Medicine of Old Age*. London: Oxford University Press, 1948.
38. Hobson W and Pemberton J. *The Health of the Elderly at Home*. London: Butterworths, 1955.
39. Sekitani T, Imate Y, Noguchi T et al. Vestibular neuronitis: epidemiological survey by questionnaire in Japan. *Acta Otolaryngol* 1993; Suppl **503**: 9–12.
40. Brandt T. *Vertigo*. London: Springer-Verlag, 1999.
41. Huygen PLM, Verhagen WIM. Peripheral vestibular and vestibulo-cochlear dysfunction in hereditary disorders. *J Vestibular Research* 1994; **4**: 81–104.
42. Smith RJH et al. Localization of two genes of an Usher syndrome type I to chromosome 11. *Genomics* 1992; **14**: 995–1002.
43. Smith RJH et al (1995) Clinical and genetic heterogeneity within the Acadian Usher population. *Am J Med Genet* 1995; **43**: 964–9.
44. Luxon LM, Cohen M, Coffey R, Trembath R, Reardon W. Neuro-otological findings in Pendred Syndrome. *Int J Audiology* 2002 (in press).
45. Stewart WF, Lipton RB et al. Prevalence of migraine headache in the United States: relation to age, income, race, and other sociodemographic factors. *JAMA* 1992; **267**: 64–9.
46. Kuritzky A, Ziegler DK, Hassanein R. Vertigo, motion sickness and migraine. *Headache* 1981; **21**: 227–31.
47. Kayan A, Hood JD. Neuro-otological manifestations of migraine. *Brain* 1984; **107**: 1123–42.
48. Baloh RW. Benign positional vertigo. In: RW Baloh and GM Halmagyi, eds. *Disorders of the Vestibular System*. New York/Oxford: Oxford University Press, 1996; Chapter 26.
49. Coonley-Hoganson R, Sachs N, Desai BT, Whitman S. Sequelae associated with head injuries in patients who were not hospitalized: a follow-up survey. *Neurosurgery* 1984; **14**: 315–17.
50. Linthicum FH, Rand CW. Neuro-otological observations in concussion of the brain. *Arch Otolaryngol* 1931; **13**: 785–821.
51. Müller R, Naumann B. Early ambulation and psychotherapy for treatment of closed head injury. *Arch Neurol Psychiatry* 1956; **76**: 597–607.
52. Wrightson P.Management of disability and rehabilitation services after mild head injury. In: HS Levin, HM Eisenberg, AL Benton, eds. *Mild Head Injury*. New York, Oxford University Press, 1989; 245–56.
53. Haggard MP, Hughes EG. *Screening Children's Hearing*. London: HMSO, 1991.
54. Stevens J, Webb H. Targeted hearing screening in neonates—comparison of follow-up with neonatal results. *Audiens (BACDA Newsletter)* 4 April 1995.
55. Sutton G, Rowe S. Risk factors for childhood sensorineural hearing loss in the Oxford Region. *Br J Audiol* 1997; **31:** 39–54.
56. National Deaf Children's Society. *Quality Standards in Paediatric Audiology*, Vol. 1. London: NDCS, 1994.
57. Wood S, Davis AC, McCromick B. Changing performance of the health visitor distraction test when targeted neonatal screening is introduced into a health district. *Br J Audiol* 1997; **31:** 35–61.
58. Lutman ME, Davis AC, Fortnum HM, Wood S. Field sensitivity of targeted neonatal hearing screening by transient otoacoustic emissions. *Ear Hear* 1997; **18:** 265–76.
59. NDCS. *Quality Standards in Paediatric Audiology*, Vol. 2. London: NDCS, 1996.
60. Cochrane AL. *Effectiveness and Efficiency. Random Reflections on Health Services*. London: The Nuffield Provincial Trust, 1971.
61. Davis A. The epidemiology of hearing in an ageing population. In: M & J Pathey (eds). *Principles and Practice of Geriatric Medicine*, John Wiley and Sons Ltd, 1998, pp. 1087–92.

7 Radiology of auditory and vestibular disease

Jan W Casselman

Introduction

In this chapter, the radiological findings in patients with sensorineural hearing loss (SNHL) and vertigo or abnormal findings at vestibular testing will be discussed. In these patients, the imaging is focused on the inner ear, internal auditory canal (IAC), cerebellopontine angle (CPA) and auditory and vestibular nuclei and central pathways. The possibilities of studing these structures with conventional X-ray methods are limited. In the early 1980s computed tomography (CT) enabled us for the first time to study the bony labyrinth, IAC, CPA and brainstem in more detail. However, the advent of magnetic resonance (MR) in the early 1990s made it possible to evaluate the membranous labyrinth, to see small structures and lesions in the IAC and CPA, and to localize the auditory and vestibular nuclei and pathways in the brainstem. Therefore, MR became the method of choice to study patients with SNHL and/or vestibular disease.

Normal anatomy

High-resolution CT (HRCT) can demonstrate the bony labyrinth and IAC in detail. New software programs and the advent of the helical-CT technique made it possible to make better three-dimensional (3D) reconstructions (surface reconstructions, volume rendering reconstructions), multiplanar reconstructions, and virtual images.[1] The relations of the different foramina on the surfaces of the temporal bone can be evaluated on these surface reconstructions, while the foramina of the semicircular canals, the vestibular aqueduct and the oval and round window in the vestibule can be seen on virtual images of the vestibule. Virtual images can also show the falciform crest, Bill's bar and the foramina for the four nerve branches near the fundus of the IAC (Figure 7.1).

The ability of MR imaging to define soft-tissue structures and fluid-containing structures is well known. However, the advent of new gradient-echo T2-weighted sequences led to the imaging of many structures that were previously not visible.[2–5]

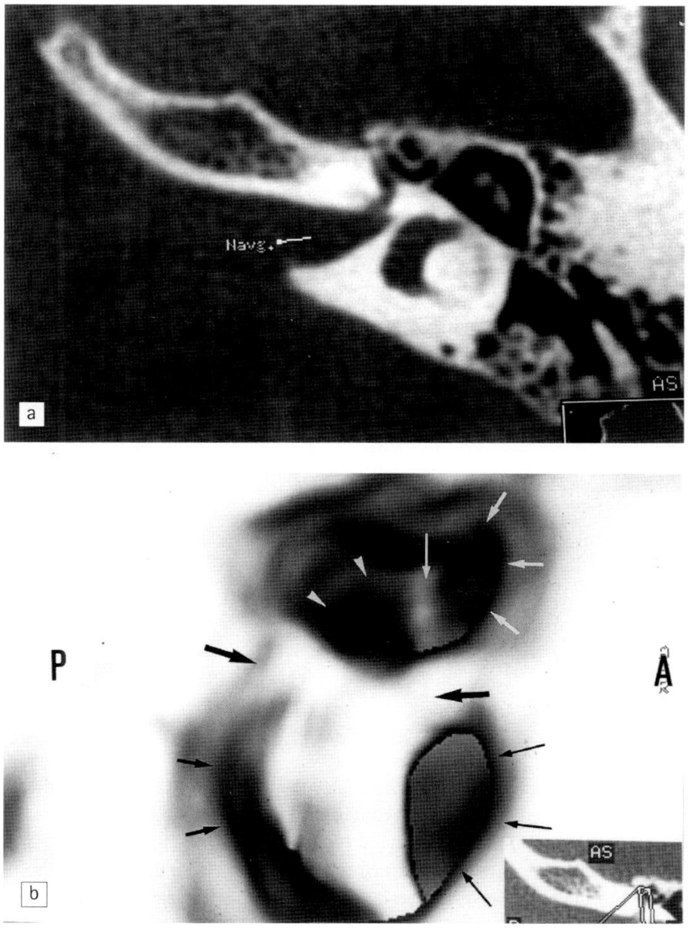

Figure 7.1 Virtual imaging of the internal auditory canal (IAC). Axial CT image through the IAC (a) and virtual image (b) made by using a series of axial CT images. (a) The point in the IAC corresponds with the site where the viewer is situated. The white line shows the direction in which the viewer is looking. (b) The falciform crest (large black arrows) and Bill's bar (long white arrow) can be recognized on this image. At the fundus, the foramen for the facial nerve (small white arrows), cochlear nerve (long black arrows), inferior vestibular (small black arrows) and superior vestibular nerve (arrowheads) can be distinguished. A, anterior, P, posterior.

With this sequence, the cochlear branch, inferior vestibular branch and superior vestibular branch of the vestibulocochlear nerve and the facial nerve can be distinguished from one another in the IAC, and even the posterior ampullar nerve can sometimes be seen (Figure 7.2). The scala tympani and vestibuli can be separated inside the different turns of the cochlea, the utricular nerve can be seen in the vestibule, and the vascular loop (often the anterior inferior cerebellar artery (AICA)) can be followed in the CPA and/or IAC. The semicircular ducts and their ampullae, and the fluid in the endolymphatic sac and duct, can all be seen on these images.

The auditory and vestibular nuclei cannot be visualized but their location can be deduced when the adjacent myelinated structures are demonstrated.[6] This is best achieved when selective T2-weighted spin-echo images of the brainstem are made (Figure 7.3).

The same sequence is used to study the auditory and vestibular pathways, and, in particular, the medial longitudinal fasciculus (MLF) can easily be seen on these images. Finally, the auditory cortex can be evaluated on coronal thin T2-weighted images through the temporal lobes.

MR technique

Several sequences are needed to exclude all possible disease in patients with SNHL and/or vestibular disorders (see Table 7.1 for the parameters of these sequences).

T2-weighted brain study

A routine axial T2-weighted brain study is 'mandatory' in all patients with SNHL, vertigo and tinnitus. It is not always easy for the clinicians to distinguish a central cause from a peripheral cause of SNHL or vertigo. Therefore, central pathology, such as multiple sclerosis or infarctions, must always be excluded.

Unenhanced T1-weighted images

These images are needed to detect spontaneous hyperintensities inside the membranous labyrinth, IAC or CPA. These hyperintensities can be seen in cases of tumour (schwannomas), fat (lipoma), blood (trauma, cholesterol granuloma, vascular malformation) or fluid with a high protein concentration.[7] Slice

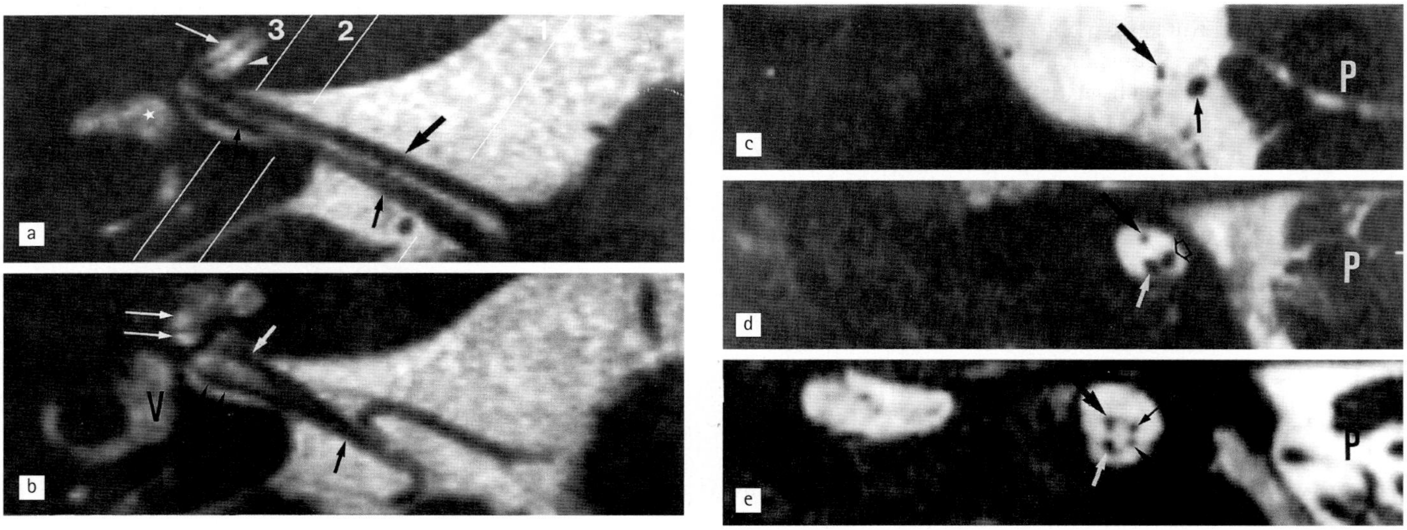

Figure 7.2 Normal anatomy of the cerebellopontine angle (CPA), internal auditory canal (IAC) and membranous labyrinth. Axial 3DFT-CISS (three-dimensional Fourier transformation constructive interference in steady state) image through the upper (a) and lower part (b) of the IAC, and parasagittal reconstructions through the CPA (c), porus (d) and deep part of the IAC (e).

(a) The facial nerve (large black arrow) can be followed from the brainstem to the fundus of the IAC. The vestibulocochlear nerve (small black arrow) can be seen parallel to the facial nerve and becomes the superior vestibular branch of the vestibulocochlear nerve (long black arrow) in the IAC. Scala vestibuli and scala media of the cochlea (white arrow), scala tympani (arrowhead). ★, ampulla of the lateral semicircular duct.

(b) The nerves are bifurcating in the lower part of the IAC. The cochlear branch of the vestibulocochlear nerve is seen anteriorly (small white arrow), and the inferior vestibular branch is seen posteriorly (arrowheads). Main trunk of the vestibulocochlear nerve (black arrow), cochlea (long white arrows). V, vestibule.

(c) Parasagittal reconstruction through the CPA along line 1. The vestibulocochlear nerve (small black arrow) and facial nerve (large black arrow) can be seen in the CPA. At this site, the vestibulocochlear nerve is always 1.5–2 times larger than the facial nerve.

(d) Parasagittal reconstruction through the porus of the IAC along line 2. The facial nerve can be seen high and anteriorly in the IAC (large black arrow). The vestibulocochlear nerve has divided in a cochlear branch (white arrow) and common vestibular nerve (open arrow).

(e) Parasagittal reconstruction through the deep part of the IAC along line 3. The facial nerve is seen high and anterior in the IAC (large black arrow). The three branches of the vestibulocochlear nerve can now be seen separately: the cochlear branch (white arrow), the inferior vestibular nerve (arrowhead), the superior vestibular nerve (long black arrow). P, posterior fossa.

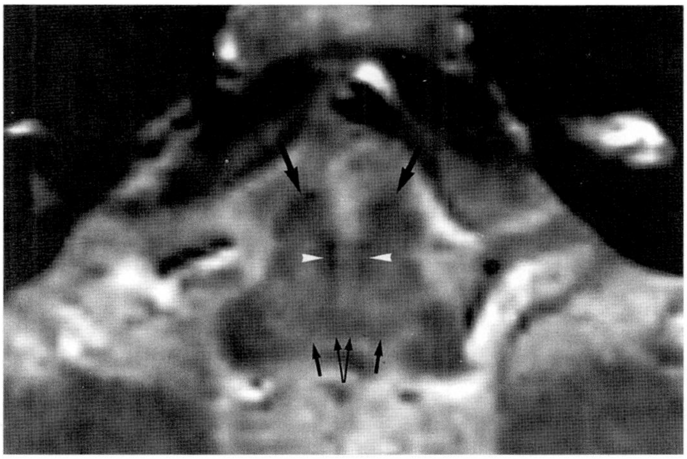

Figure 7.3 Cochlear nucleus. Axial T2-weighted spin-echo image with long repetition time through the upper medulla. The myelinated structures, like the corticospinal tracts (large black arrows), medial lemniscus (arrowheads), and medial longitudinal fasciculus (long black arrows), are used as reference structures. The cochlear nuclei (small black arrows) are situated lateral to the medial longitudinal fasciculus at this level.

thickness should never exceed 3 mm, and 2-mm-thin slices are state of the art. The use of 1-mm slices can add information, and slices of this thickness are routinely used in our institution in the follow-up of acoustic schwannomas (volume measurements) and to evaluate all segments of the facial nerve. For this purpose, we use a 3DFT-MPRAGE sequence.

Gadolinium-enhanced T1-weighted images

Several studies have shown that gadolinium-enhanced T1-weighted images are the most sensitive images to detect pathology in the membranous labyrinth, IAC and CPA. Therefore, the use of a Gd-enhanced T1-weighted sequence is mandatory.[8]

T1-weighted images with fat saturation

This sequence is used in patients who have undergone a translabyrinthine or retrosigmoid resection of an acoustic schwannoma. On these images, tumour recurrence or remnants can be distinguished from the fat, used to close the surgical access route. This sequence is also valuable in the differentiation between subtle enhancement along the walls of the IAC and fatty marrow inside the walls of the IAC.

T2-weighted gradient-echo or fast spin-echo imaging

Gradient-echo or fast spin-echo images are required to evaluate the very small structures and to detect certain pathologies in the CPA, IAC and membranous labyrinth. Good gradient-echo images must be very thin and must provide high contrast between the cerebrospinal fluid (CSF), intralabyrinthine fluid, nerves, and bone. This sequence is mainly used to check the three branches of the vestibulocochlear nerve and the facial nerve in the IAC, to check if the membranous labyrinth is normal and to exclude loss of fluid inside the membranous labyrinth (due to fibrosis or tumour). These images must be very thin and have a very high in-plane resolution (Table 7.1).[2–5,9]

Vascular 'time-of-flight' sequence

This sequence can be used to study vascular loops, vascular malformations or vascular tumours in and around the temporal bone, and is mandatory in patients presenting with pulsatile tinnitus. On these sequences, the vessels have high signal intensity, whereas the nerves remain low in signal intensity. They are used prior to (showing only the arteries) and after (showing arteries and veins) the intravenous administration of Gd.[10]

T2-weighted imaging of brainstem and auditory cortex

In patients with SNHL and/or vertigo, the cochlear and vestibular nuclei, trapezoid body, lateral lemniscus, inferior colliculus, MLF etc. must be checked. A heavily T2-weighted sequence with high resolution and thin slices is used for this purpose. The myelinated structures are easily seen on these images, and the location of the nuclei and structures belonging to the vestibular and auditory pathways can be presumed once the positions of the adjacent myelinated structures are seen. In special cases, very small structures must be evaluated in detail (e.g. MLF), and then an even longer, very sensitive, T2-weighted sequence is used.

Figure 7.4 shows which sequences should be used in cases of SNHL, vertigo and tinnitus. The most important clinical symptoms, SNHL, vertigo or tinnitus, will influence the choice of the sequences. Moreover, different sequences will be used for a central SNHL or vertigo than for a peripheral SNHL or vertigo. It is, however, an illusion to think that peripheral and central SNHL or vertigo can always be distinguished from one another in an easy way.

Lesions involving the membranous and bony labyrinth

Similar lesions can involve the anterior (cochlea) and posterior (vestibule, semicircular canals) labyrinth and can therefore cause SNHL and/or vertigo.[11] The possibilities of visualizing these lesions on CT and MR are discussed here.

Labyrinthitis

Labyrinthitis accounts for 50% of the labyrinthine pathology found in patients presenting with vertigo, and for more than

Table 7.1 Sequence parameters

	TR (ms)	TE (ms)	FA	Specific parameters	Thickness (mm)	Gap (mm)	Matrix	FOV–Rect. FOV	Pixel size	No. of acquisitions	Acquisition time
Routine T1 SE	490	20	90°	Gap = 0	2	0	160 × 256	230–3/4	0.9 × 0.9	4	5 m 17 s
3DFT-MPRAGE	11.6	4.9	12°		1	0	192 × 256	240–3/4	0.94 × 0.94	1	6 m 24 s
3DFT-CISS	12.25	5.9	70°	Slab = 32.2 mm Oversampling 100%	0.7	0	192 × 256	95–8/8	0.49 × 0.37	1	7 m 14 s
Turbo MRA 3DFT-FISP	35	6.4	15°	Slab = 96 mm	0.75	0	160 × 512	230–6/8	1.08 × 0.45	1	6 m 0 s
Routine T2 sequence	1900	12/80	62°	No. of slices = 19	4	0.4	157 × 256	230–6/8	1.1 × 0.9	2	10 min
Special T2 sequence	4000	20/80	75°	No. of slices = 30	4	0.4	128 × 256	230–4/8	0.9 × 0.9	2	17 min

FA, Flip angle; FOV, field of view; MRA, magnetic resonance angiography; Rect. FOV, rectangular field of view; SE, spin-echo; TE, echo time; TR, repetition time; 3DFT-CISS, 3D Fourier transformation constructive interference in steady state; 3DFT-FISP, 3D Fourier transformation fast imaging with steady precession; 3DFT-MPRAGE, 3D Turbo fast low angle shot with magnetization prepared gradient-echo imaging.

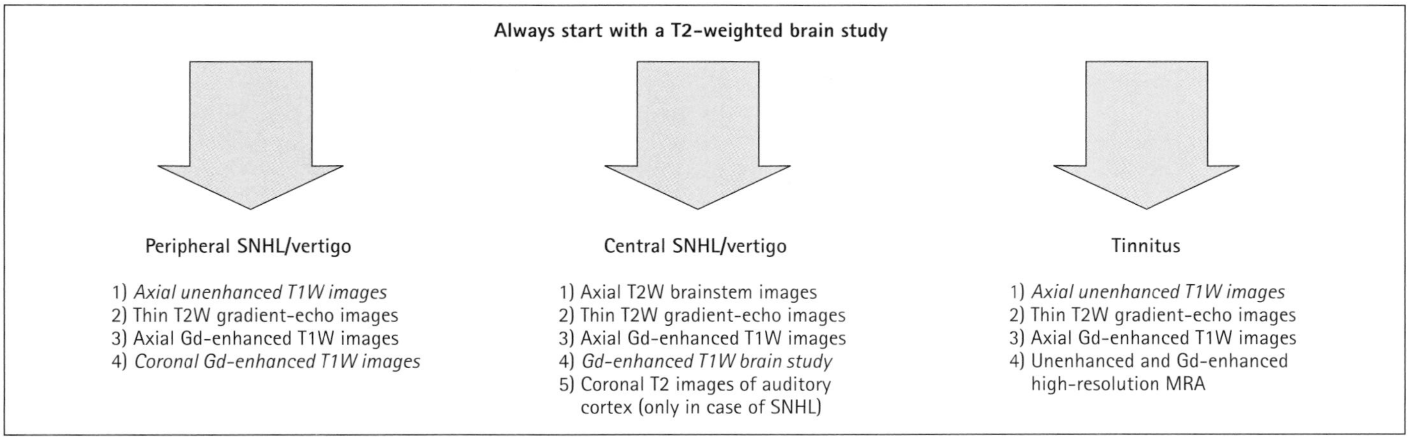

Figure 7.4 Sequences to be used in SNHL, vertigo and tinnitus. Sequences in italics can be omitted to save time, while other sequences are necessary. Gd, gadolinium; MRA, magnetic resonance angiography; SNHL, sensorineural hearing loss; T1W, T1-weighted, T2W, T2-weighted.

50% of the pathology found in patients presenting with SNHL. Several types of labyrinthitis can be distinguished (Tables 7.2–7.4).

Acute labyrinthitis

Acute labyrinthitis can only be recognized on MR. It is characterized by an intralabyrinthine enhancement following intravenous Gd injection.[12] In cases of acute labyrinthitis, the 'blood–labyrinth' barrier is ruptured and Gd leaks from the vessels into the intralabyrinthine fluid. Most often both the anterior and posterior labyrinth enhance, and the edges of the enhancement are not sharp (Figure 7.5). It is obvious that this pathology is best seen on the Gd-enhanced T1-weighted images. However, T2-weighted gradient-echo images (3DFT-CISS) are needed to exclude enhancing tumoral pathology inside the labyrinth. In cases of labyrinthitis, the intralabyrinthine fluid is mixed with Gd and can still be seen as high-signal fluid on the gradient-echo images. However, when a tumour is present inside the labyrinth, the tumour will replace the intralabyrinthine fluid, and the high signal intensity of the fluid will disappear on the gradient-echo image. Therefore, an additional T2-weighted gradient-echo sequence is needed to distinguish these two entities when an enhancement is seen in the membranous labyrinth. Unfortunately, the labyrinthine enhancement is not always present in cases of labyrinthitis. Probably there is an enhancement threshold, explaining why in cases of moderate labyrinthitis, no enhancement is visible. Sometimes the labyrinthitis can be haemorrhagic, and then a spontaneous hyperintensity can be seen inside the membranous labyrinth on the unenhanced T1-weighted images.

Table 7.2 Labyrinthitis

Acute labyrinthitis	Intralabyrinthine enhancement => seen on Gd-enhanced T1W images Intralabyrinthine haemorrhage => seen on unenhanced T1W images	
Chronic labyrinthitis	Fibrotic obliteration of the membranous labyrinth => seen on gradient-echo T2W images Calcification or ossification of the membranous labyrinth => best seen on CT	
Causes	Viral	Herpes *Haemophilus influenzae* Mumps Rubella (German measles)
	Bacterial	*Pneumococcus* *Meningococcus*
	Autoimmune	Cogan's syndrome Sarcoidosis Polychondritis Wegener's disease Lupus erythematosus

Table 7.3 Causes of intralabyrinthine enhancement in order of frequency (results of a study performed by the European Society of Head and Neck Radiology*—114 cases)

Pathology	Frequency (%)
Labyrinthitis (acute, chronic, autoimmune)	47.4
Intralabyrinthine schwannomas	27.2
Postoperative fibrosis	6.1
Otosclerosis	4.4
Tumours invading the membranous labyrinth Meningioma Glomus jugulare Cholesteatoma Ductal carcinoma of parotid gland	3.5
Metastases	3.5
Others Sarcoidosis Pachymeningitis Psoriasis Wegener Gamma knife treatment Alport syndrome Undefined mass	7.9

Casselman JW, Marsot-Dupuch K, Hermans R, Gayet Delacroix M, Manfrè L, Krikke AD, Kösling S, Etorre GC, Appel B, Phelps PD, Majoie CB. Presented at *International Congress of Head and Neck Radiology*, Strasbourg, France, October 15–18, 1997.

Viral labyrinthitis

This can only be recognized in the acute phase, when intralabyrinthine enhancement is seen. Herpes, *Haemophilus influenzae* infections and rubella are the most frequent causes. Most frequently, the enhancement is rather weak and does not persist for a very long time. However, as mentioned above, this enhancement can be absent in less severe cases. Normally, no inflammatory tissue or fibrosis is present in the labyrinth in cases of viral labyrinthitis; this explains why the intralabyrinthine fluid remains visible on the T2-weighted gradient-echo images.

Bacterial labyrinthitis (e.g. *Pneumococcus, Meningococcus*)

A bacterial infection can reach the labyrinth through a fistula between the middle and inner ear (e.g. fistula caused by a cholesteatoma, malformation of a window, post-osteitis) or along the meninges in the cochlear aqueduct into the perilymphatic space. In acute bacterial labyrinthitis, enhancement is again seen inside the membranous labyrinth. The enhancement

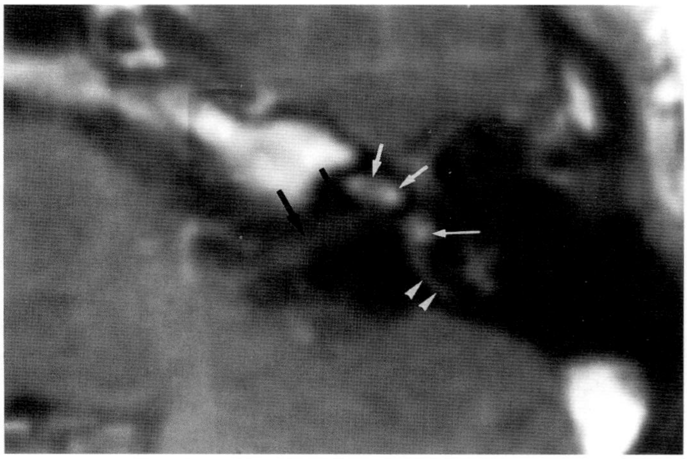

Figure 7.5 Acute viral labyrinthitis in a patient presenting with sudden hearing loss and vertigo. Axial Gd-enhanced T1-weighted spin-echo image through the left inner ear. Enhancement can be seen in the cochlea (small white arrows) and in the vestibule (long white arrow). The edges of the enhancing area are not sharp. Note normal common crus (arrowheads) and neurovascular bundle in the IAC (black arrows). The gradient-echo T2 images (3DFT-CISS) images showed normal fluid inside the membranous labyrinth (not shown).

is strong and can persist for a very long time (several months to more than a year). However, inflammatory tissue and fibrous tissue are often formed very quickly and replace the normal intralabyrinthine fluid. This can be recognized as regions with decreased signal intensity on the T2-weighted gradient-echo images. This is the first phase of chronic labyrinthitis, and in this phase the Gd enhancement is subtle or is no longer present. In a later stage, the inflammatory tissue or fibrous tissue can eventually calcify or ossify (labyrinthitis ossificans).[13] It is not possible to distinguish fibrous and calcified obliterations on gradient-echo MR only. An additional CT is needed to distinguish fibrous (obliteration on MR, normal CT) and calcified (obliteration on MR, intralabyrinthine calcifications on CT) obliterations. The detection of calcifications and/or fibrous obliteration inside the membranous labyrinth is, of course, essential in the preoperative assessment of cochlear implant candidates. As mentioned above, only a combined CT–MR evaluation provides the surgeon with all the necessary information. Moreover, unlike CT, MR is often capable of showing whether a single scala is still open and can be used for cochlear implantation (Figure 7.6).

Autoimmune labyrinthitis

Pathology inside the membranous labyrinth was described in five patients with Cogan's syndrome.[14] They all had vertigo and SNHL. These patients also presented with nonsyphilitic interstitial keratitis. The aetiology is still debated but ischaemia and vasculitis are mentioned as possible causes. In these patients, new bone formation and/or calcifications can be found inside the membranous labyrinth (best seen on CT). However, acidophilic coagulum, cellular debris, connective tissue and hypertrophy of the stria vascularis are more frequent and replace the normal intralabyrinthine fluid (only visible on T2-weighted gradient-

Table 7.4 Preferred imaging techniques—membranous and bony labyrinth

Pathology	Imaging technique
Acute labyrinthitis	Intralabyrinthine enhancement => Gd-enhanced T1 images Intralabyrinthine blood => unenhanced T1 images
Chronic labyrinthitis	Labyrinthitis ossificans => CT Fibrous obliteration => gradient-echo T2 images Note: cochlear implant candidates: CT and gradient-echo T2 images
Congenital malformations	CT first choice T2-weighted gradient-echo images add information in selective cases and when presence of normal cochlear nerve must be checked
Postoperative obliteration	T2-weighted gradient-echo images (fibrosis) and unenhanced (blood) and Gd-enhanced (recent fibrosis) T1-weighted images
Intralabyrinthine schwannomas	Gd-enhanced T1-weighted images and T2-weighted gradient-echo images
Tumours growing in labyrinth	Destruction of bony labyrinth => CT Involvement of membranous labyrinth => gradient-echo T2 images and Gd-enhanced T1-weighted images Characterization of lesions => spin-echo T1, Gd T1 and T2 images
Bony labyrinth lesions	CT
Trauma of labyrinth	First CT to exclude fracture MR when clinical findings cannot be explained by CT: unenhanced T1 images (blood) and gradient-echo T2 images (obliterations by clot or fibrosis)

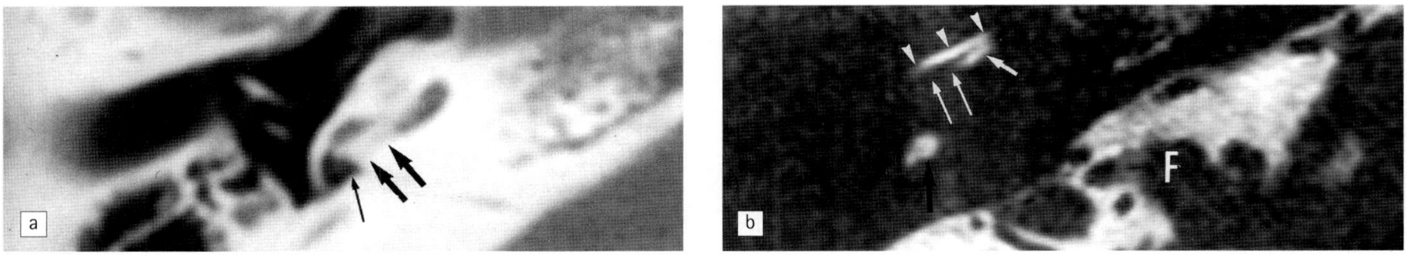

Figure 7.6 Labyrinthitis ossificans in a cochlear implant candidate. Axial CT (a) and 3DFT-CISS image (b) through the right inner ear.
(a) The posterior part of the basal turn of the cochlea is calcified (large black arrows). Note round window (long black arrow).
(b) MR shows loss of the high-signal-intensity fluid in the posterior part of the scala tympani (long white arrows). Only MR showed clearly that the scala vestibula/scala media compartment was not involved (arrowheads) and could still be used for cochlear implantation. Note normal fluid in the ampulla of the posterior semicircular duct (black arrow) and anterior part of the scala tympani (white arrow). F, floccule.

echo images). Moreover, in the acute phase, enhancement on the contrast-enhanced T1-weighted images could be seen in one of the patients, probably representing leakage through the abnormal labyrinthine membrane (vasculitis affecting the stria vascularis). Enhancement inside the membranous labyrinth has also been noticed in relapsing polychondritis, and similar findings have been seen in patients with BBS disease, Wegener's disease and lupus erythematosus.

Congenital malformations

Congenital malformations of the cochlea and vestibular system are frequently found in patients with SNHL and vertigo, and accounted for 25% of the labyrinthine pathology found in a series of patients presenting with vertigo. A congenital malformation will only be found on CT and/or MR in 20% of the patients presenting with congenital hearing loss. These malformations can be detected on CT, but patients presenting with SNHL and/or vertigo are today best first examined on MR. Therefore, the MR technique must include the thin T2-weighted gradient-echo images (3DFT-CISS), as this pathology can be overlooked on the other MR sequences.[15]

Large vestibular aqueduct/duct–sac

The most frequent congenital malformation is a large vestibular aqueduct (CT) or large vestibular duct and sac (MR). The patients present with SNHL, often triggered by minor traumata, and vertigo and loss of equilibrium. In one-third of these patients both SNHL and vertigo are present. The vestibular aqueduct or sac is considered to be large when its diameter is larger than 1.5 mm or when it is greater than the diameter of the posterior semicircular canal or duct.[16, 17] This enlargement occurs bilaterally in more than 50% of the cases. A large vestibular aqueduct is often found in patients with a 'gusher' ear. An enlargement of the scala vestibuli/scala media in comparison with the scala tympani can also be detected on MR in some of these patients (Figure 7.7). This probably indicates that the hydrops of the scala vestibuli/scala tympani compartment already existed during embryologyical development when the bony structures still could be deformed.[18]

Malformations of the semicircular canals (ducts)

Semicircular canals or ducts with an abnormal shape, or increased or decreased diameter, or which are partially absent, can be detected on CT and on T2-weighted gradient-echo images. The lateral semicircular canal or duct is most frequently involved. This is explained by the fact that this is the last structure formed during embryology. These patients often have abnormal findings at vestibular testing. The most frequent malformation is, however, a saccular semicircular canal confluent with an enlarged vestibule. The term 'LCVD' (lateral semicircular canal–vestibule dysplasia) is used when this occurs as a sole radiographically detectable anomaly.[19] Aplasia of all semicircular canals is nearly always associated with a 'CHARGE' (Coloboma, Heart disease, Atresia of choanae, Retarded mental development, Genital hypoplasia, Ear abnormalities–deafness) association.

Malformations of the cochlea

These malformations are often associated with severe congenital SNHL. Aplasia of the complete temporal bone (Michel's syndrome—aplasia of the bony and membranous labyrinth and IAC), aplasia of the cochlea, common cavity formation (cochlea and vestibule form one cavity), dysplasia (severe malformation of the cochlea) and hypoplasia of the cochlea (cochlea is small, number of turns can be reduced) and less severe malformations (Mondini malformation) can all be detected on CT and MR.[20] Jackler et al demonstrated that the severity of these cochlear malformations corresponded with the time when the embryological development was interrupted.[19] However, sometimes only subtle signs can be seen on MR. For instance, the inter- and intrascalar defects inside the cochlea, described by Mondini, can now be recognized in vivo on high-resolution MR and support the diagnosis of a Mondini malformation (Figure 7.8).

Gusher ear

Abnormal connections can exist between the subarachnoid spaces and the perilymphatic space in patients with congenital inner ear malformations. These patients can present with recurrent meningitis, progressive fluctuating hearing loss, tinnitus

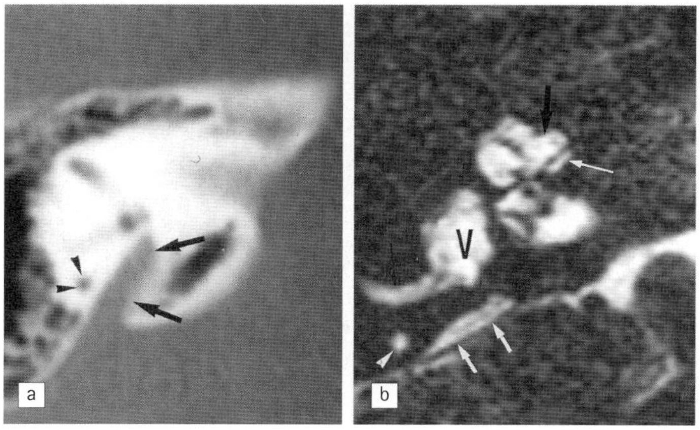

Figure 7.7 Large vestibular aqueduct in a patient with SNHL. Axial CT image (a) and 3DFT-CISS image (b) through the right inner ear.
(a) The enlarged vestibular aqueduct can be seen (large black arrows) and is clearly larger in diameter than the posterior semicircular canal (arrowheads).
(b) The enlarged endolymphatic sac (small white arrows) can be seen, and its diameter is wider than the diameter of the posterior semicircular duct (arrowhead). Note the enlargement of the scala vestibuli/scala media compartment (black arrow), which is much larger than the scala tympani compartment (long white arrow). In normal circumstances, both compartments have the same size (see also Figure 7.2). V, vestibule.

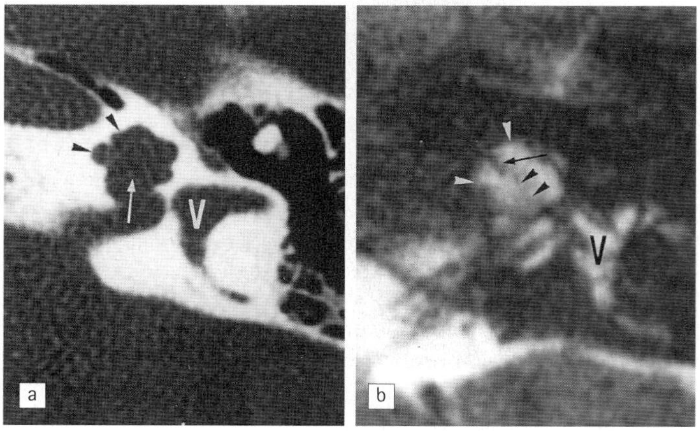

Figure 7.8 Mondini malformation. Axial CT (a) and 3DFT-CISS image (b) through the left inner ear.
(a) The different turns of the cochlea can still be seen (arrowheads) but the modiolus and bony plate between the cochlea and internal auditory canal are absent (white arrow). V, vestibule.
(b) Normal fluid can be seen in the basal and second turn of the cochlea (white arrowheads). However, the separation between the two turns is incomplete (black arrowheads), and only a part of the bony wall (black arrow) can be recognized. V, vestibule.

and/or vertigo. The pressure of the CSF is transmitted to the cochlea and causes a perilymphatic hydrops. When these patients are operated on (e.g. stapedectomy), the intralabyrinthine fluid gushes out of the cochlea and results in deafness.[21] Therefore, the radiologist must warn the surgeon if he detects signs indicating the presence of a 'Gusher ear' (Figure 7.9). The most important imaging signs are:

- absence of bone structure between the cochlea and fundus of the IAC
- enlargement of the labyrinthine segment of the facial nerve canal
- convex angle anteriorly between the labyrinthine and tympanic segment of the facial nerve canal.
- large vestibular aqueduct/duct and sac
- cochlear dysplasia.

Miscellaneous

Abnormalities of the oval window, round window, facial nerve canal and carotid artery and its canal can be detected on CT. Absent, closed or malformed oval and/or round windows can be the cause of the hearing loss.

Postoperative labyrinth obliteration

The intralabyrinthine fluid can be replaced by fibrous tissue after an intervention. When a translabyrinthine resection of a

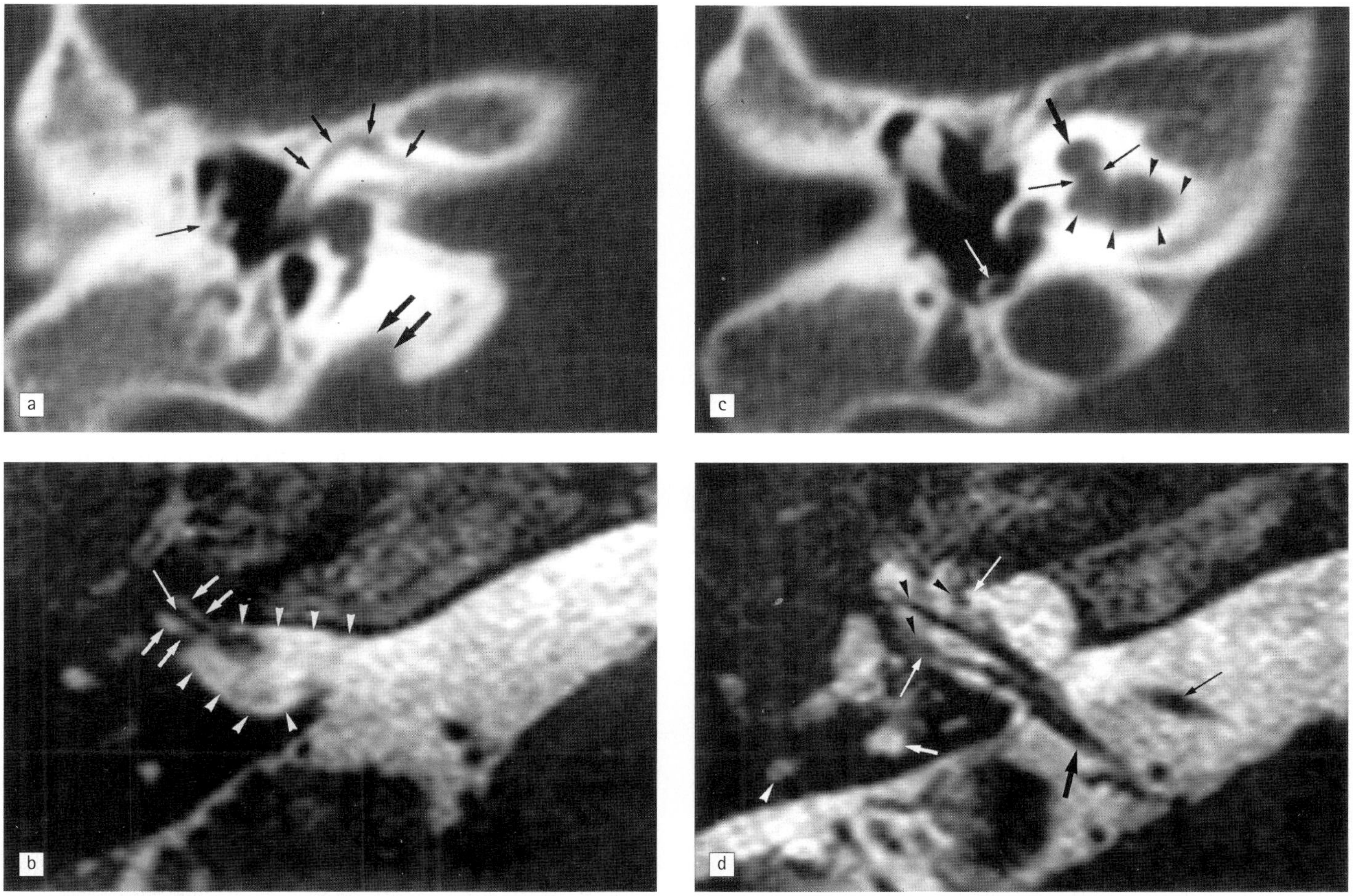

Figure 7.9 Gusher ear. Axial CT and 3DFT-CISS images at the level of the right facial nerve (a, b) and at the level of the right cochlea (c, d).
(a) The angle between the labyrinthine and tympanic portion of the facial nerve canal has an anterior convexity (small black arrows). The vestibular aqueduct is enlarged (large black arrows). These are two findings which are frequently seen in patients with a 'gusher ear'. Note that the ossicles are fixed to the lateral wall of the tympanic cavity (long black arrow).
(b) Fluid (small white arrows) can be seen between the facial nerve (long white arrow) and the walls of the labyrinthine segment of the facial nerve canal. In normal circumstances, fluid can never be seen in this segment of the facial nerve canal. Note IAC (arrowheads).
(c) The cochlea is dysplastic (large black arrow) and there is no bony separation (long black arrows) between the cochlea and the IAC. Note abnormal position of the mastoid segment of the facial nerve canal in the middle ear cavity (white arrow), and IAC (arrowheads).
(d) The absence of the bony wall between the dysplastic cochlea and IAC can again be seen (long white arrows) and several branches of the vestibulocochlear nerve (black arrowheads) can be followed in the dysplastic cochlea. Note facial nerve (small black arrow), common trunk of the vestibulocochlear nerve (large black arrow), large endolymphatic duct (small white arrow), and posterior semicircular duct (white arrowhead).

schwannoma is performed, the remaining parts of the membranous labyrinth which have not been destroyed can lose their fluid and become obliterated. These obliterations also occur when surgery is performed in the vicinity of the membranous labyrinth (Figure 7.10). This can, for instance, be seen in the cochlea after surgery in the region of the geniculate ganglion of the facial nerve. On MR a spontaneous hyperintensity on the unenhanced T1-weighted images can sometimes be seen in the membranous labyrinth, representing blood. Later on the hyperintensity will disappear and fibrous tissue or fibrosis will replace the intralabyrinthine fluid, only visible on T2-weighted gradient-echo images. This will, of course, cause SNHL or vertigo/abnormal findings at vestibular testing when the cochlear or vestibular structures are respectively involved. Even an acute labyrinthitis can be caused by surgery.

Intralabyrinthine schwannomas

Nearly all intralabyrinthine tumours are schwannomas. They can only be visualized on MR, are slightly hyperintense compared to normal CSF or intralabyrinthine fluid on the unenhanced T1-weighted images, and enhance strongly after intravenous Gd administration.[22] Schwannomas are the second most frequent cause of an intralabyrinthine enhancement. (The edges of these enhancements are sharp, and most often the schwannoma only occupies one compartment of the labyrinth, the cochlea, or the vestibule/semicircular canals.) Schwannomas can be distinguished from acute labyrinthitis on thin T2-weighted gradient-echo (3DFT-CISS) images. In cases of schwannoma the high-signal-intensity (white) intralabyrinthine fluid will be replaced by the low-signal-intensity (grey) of the tumour, which is not the case in acute labyrinthitis[8] (Figure 7.11). Patients present with progressive SNHL or vertigo/abnormal findings at vestibular testing.

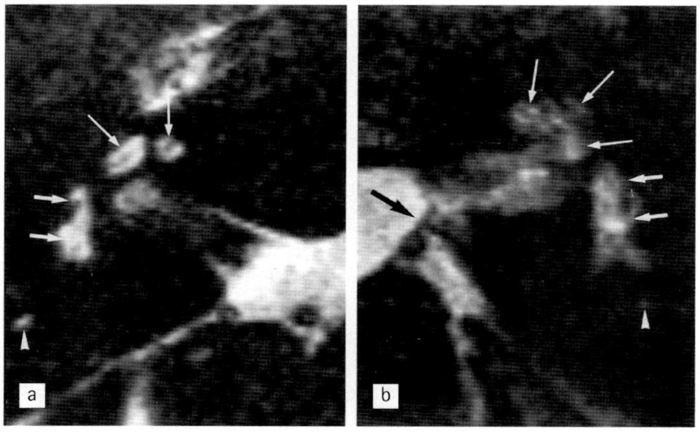

Figure 7.10 Postoperative obliteration of the membranous labyrinth. Patient with hearing loss on the left side and abnormal findings at vestibular testing. Axial 3DFT-CISS images through the normal right (a) and obliterated left (b) inner ear.
(a) Normal high-signal-intensity fluid can be seen in the cochlea (long white arrows), vestibule (small white arrows) and posterior semicircular canal (arrowhead).
(b) The normal high signal intensity of fluid is replaced by low-signal-intensity fibrosis in the left cochlea (long white arrows), and vestibule (small white arrows), and the signal nearly completely disappears in the posterior semicircular duct (arrowhead). Note postoperative changes in the CPA (large black arrow).

Schwannomas in the vestibule originate in the fibres of the vestibular nerves. Branches of these nerves reach the ampullae of the semicircular canals (the superior vestibular nerve reaches the superior and lateral semicircular canal, and the inferior vestibular nerve reaches the posterior semicircular canal), and therefore larger schwannomas will eventually grow into these ampullae. Schwannomas in the vestibule are frequently found in patients with neurofibromatosis type II.[23] In other patients, schwannomas seem to be more frequent in the cochlea (Figure 7.12). Intracochlear schwannomas will only cause vertigo when they block the normal communication between cochlea and vestibule. Intralabyrinthine schwannomas can also grow back into the IAC and can then cause vertigo, because they involve the superior or inferior branch of the vestibulocochlear nerve. Growth of these schwannomas cannot be predicted, and even after several years of no or slow growth, the schwannoma can suddenly grow very quickly and surprise both radiologist and clinician. Nevertheless, a follow-up examination every 6 months during the first 2 years and every year thereafter is a relatively safe way to follow these patients and helps to ascertain the growth rate of the lesion. Today, removal of the intralabyrinthine schwannoma is performed for two reasons. First, when no hearing is left in the involved ear, removal eliminates the chance of sudden growth, which could cause other damage (facial nerve etc.). Second, the tinnitus, which is often associated with cochlear schwannomas, can disappear when the schwannoma is removed.

Tumours invading the membranous labyrinth

Tumours originating in the middle ear (e.g. cholesteatomas), IAC (e.g. metastases, schwannomas)[24] or pneumatization cells of the temporal bone (e.g. cholesterol granulomas) can invade the cochlea, vestibule or semicircular canals/ducts. The bone destruction can be seen on CT but the tumour itself and its characteristics are better or can only be evaluated on MR. High signal intensity of the lesion on unenhanced T1- and T2-weighted spin-echo images corresponds with blood, which is typically found in cholesterol granulomas. Strong Gd enhancement can be seen in metastases. However, only thin T2-weighted gradient-echo images can be used to find the fistula between the lesion and the membranous labyrinth and are able to confirm the replacement of the intralabyrinthine fluid by an invasive tumour. CT, of course, remains the best technique to demonstrate erosions of the lateral semicircular canal and other parts of the bony labyrinth in patients with middle ear cholesteatoma. The coronal plane is the ideal plane to demonstrate lateral semicircular canal fistulas. However, MR can detect whether the underlying membranous labyrinth is involved (loss of high signal of the underlying intralabyrinthine

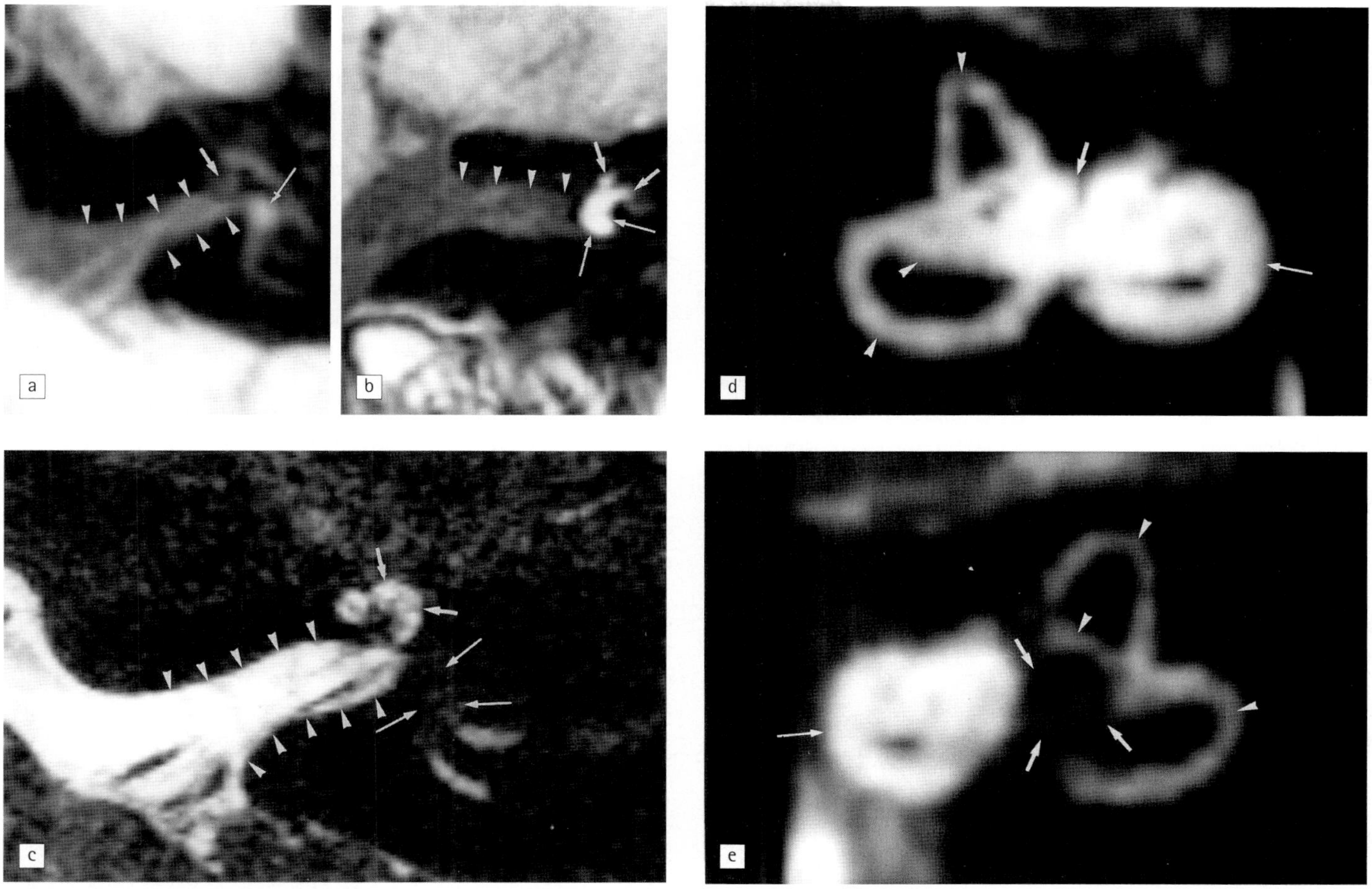

Figure 7.11 Schwannoma in the vestibule in a young woman presenting with vertigo and subtle SNHL. Axial unenhanced T1-weighted image (a), coronal Gd-enhanced image (b) and axial 3DFT-CISS image (c) of the left inner ear, and 3DFT-CISS reconstructions of the right (d) and left (e) inner ear.

(a) The schwannoma can be seen in the vestibule as a region of increased signal intensity (long white arrow) in comparison with the fluid in the rest of the membranous labyrinth. Note cochlea (small white arrow), and IAC (arrowheads).

(b) The schwannoma enhances strongly and is situated in the vestibule (long white arrows) but extends into the lateral and superior semicircular ducts (small white arrows). Note IAC (arrowheads).

(c) The schwannoma replaces the normal high-signal-intensity intralabyrinthine fluid (long white arrows). Normal fluid can be seen in the cochlea (small white arrows). Note IAC (arrowheads).

(d) 3DFT-CISS reconstruction of the right membranous labyrinth with normal high signal intensity in the cochlea (long white arrow), vestibule (small white arrow) and semicircular ducts (arrowheads).

(e) 3DFT-CISS reconstruction of the left membranous labyrinth showing the hypointense schwannoma in the vestibule (small white arrows). Normal high-signal-intensity intralabyrinthine fluid can be seen in the cochlea (long white arrow) and semicircular ducts (arrowheads).

fluid), often predicting severe or total hearing loss following surgery. Other lesions invading the labyrinth are glomus jugulare tumours, rhabdomyosarcomas, spinocellular tumours and adenoid cystic carcinomas originating high in the head and neck region, histiocytosis X, etc. (Figure 7.13). Lipomas can also be found inside the membranous labyrinth.[25] Finally, endolymphatic sac tumours (EST) can cause a hydrops of the labyrinth. These patients can present with (fluctuating) SNHL and vertigo or balance disorders. ESTs occur frequently in patients with von Hippel–Lindau disease. On CT, a defect of the bone is found in the region of the endolymphatic sac and vestibular aqueduct. On MR, the lesions can have both a high (blood) and low (cystic) signal intensity on T1-weighted images. The regions containing blood will also have a high signal on T2-weighted images, and the tumour can also have solid parts which enhance strongly after Gd administration. They can eventually invade the facial nerve canal, the CPA, IAC, and jugular foramen, and can extend into the middle ear cavity.[26]

Bony labyrinth lesions

Paget's disease, fibrous dysplasia, osteopetrosis and otosclerosis can cause vertigo, tinnitus and SNHL.[27, 28] These abnormalities of the bony labyrinth are best studied on CT. Thin T2-weighted gradient-echo images (3DFT-CISS) are needed to recognize compression of and involvement of the membranous labyrinth.

Only these images can detect the loss of intralabyrinthine fluid in these patients.

Demineralization of the bony labyrinth with a fluffy cotton wool appearance of surrounding bone can be seen in Paget's disease. The hearing loss can be explained by the elongation of the neurovascular bundle in the IAC, and the involvement of the bony labyrinth or craniocervical junction.

Enlarged dense bone with an 'hourglass' appearance is seen in fibrous dysplasia, and the bony changes can narrow the IAC or can encase the aqueducts or membranous labyrinth.[8] The bone abnormalities in fibrous dysplasia vary considerably and high signal intensity on T2-weighted spin-echo images and unenhanced T1-weighted images and strong enhancement after Gd administration indicate active fibrous dysplasia.

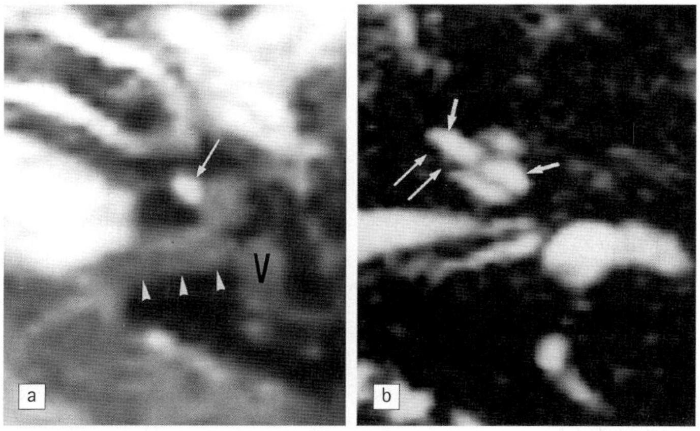

Figure 7.12 Schwannoma in the basal turn of the cochlea. Patient presenting with severe SNHL, especially at the high frequencies. Axial Gd-enhanced T1-weighted image (a) and 3DFT-CISS image (b) through the left inner ear.
(a) An enhancing lesion can be seen in the anterior part of the basal turn (long white arrow). Note internal auditory canal (arrowheads). V, vestibule.
(b) The lesion can be seen as a hypointense area in the anterior part of the basal turn. Moreover, MR shows that the schwannoma is completely situated in the scala tympani (long white arrows) and that the scala vestibuli is open (small white arrows).

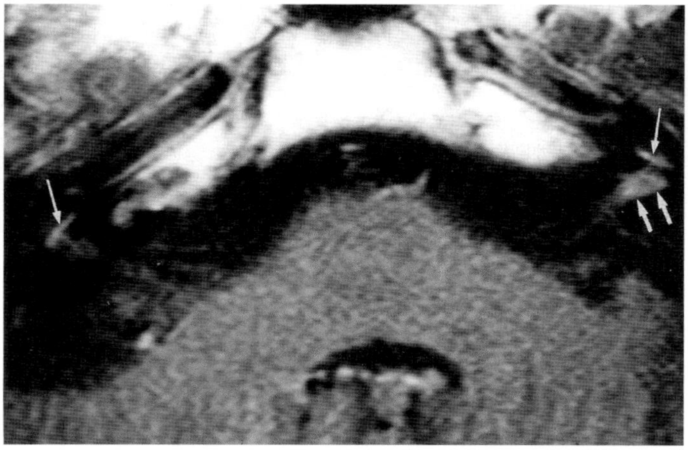

Figure 7.13 Metastases from a lung carcinoma in the left and right cochlea and left IAC. Patient with bilateral SNHL and vertigo. Axial Gd-enhanced T1-weighted image through both inner ears. Enhancement can be seen in the right and left basal turn of the cochlea (long white arrows). Enhancement (metastases) can also be seen deep in the left IAC (short white arrows).

Thick dense bone with a narrow medullary space is seen in osteopetrosis. The neurovascular bundle can be compressed by the narrowed IAC. Dense bone can be seen on CT, and the bone has a hypointense signal on MR.

In fenestral otosclerosis spongy decalcified foci of bone or otosclerotic plaques can involve the anterior and, less frequently, the posterior oval window region, the annular ligament or footplate of the stapes (thickened footplate) and the round window. In these patients, a conductive hearing loss (CHL) is also present. In retrofenestral otosclerosis, the bone around the cochlea is primarily involved and SNHL is the dominant symptom. On CT, hypodense regions are found around the cochlea, vestibule, semicircular canal and IAC. These lesions have a signal intensity similar to the signal intensity of the membranous labyrinth on T1-weighted images and have a high signal intensity on T2-weighted images. The borders of the labyrinth become unsharp on MR images when these lesions are present. Active lesions enhance after intravenous Gd administration (Figure 7.14).

These lesions can be difficult to recognize on MR, but otosclerosis lesions often have intermediate signal intensity on the unenhanced T1-weighted images and can enhance after Gd administration (active lesions).

Focal or lytic lesions can sometimes be found in patients with SNHL, vertigo or tinnitus. Focal lesions can be caused by

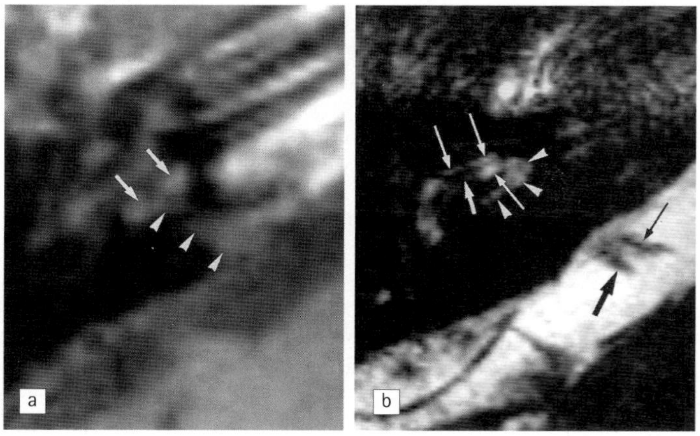

Figure 7.14 Bilateral otosclerosis in patient with mixed hearing loss. Axial Gd-enhanced T1-weighted spin-echo image (a) and 3DFT-CISS image (b) through the right inner ear.
(a) Enhancement can be seen in and around the basal turn of the cochlea (arrows). These lesions correspond with active otospongiosis/otosclerosis lesions. Note neurovascular bundle in the IAC (arrowheads).
(b) Normal high-signal-intensity intralabyrinthine fluid can still be seen in the complete scala vestibuli/scala media and anterior part of the scala tympani of the basal turn of the cochlea (long white arrows). The otosclerosis has, however, caused obliteration of the posterior part of the scala tympani (small white arrow). High signal changes can also be seen in the surrounding bony labyrinth (arrowheads). Note: facial nerve (long black arrow), and common vestibulocochlear nerve (large black arrow).

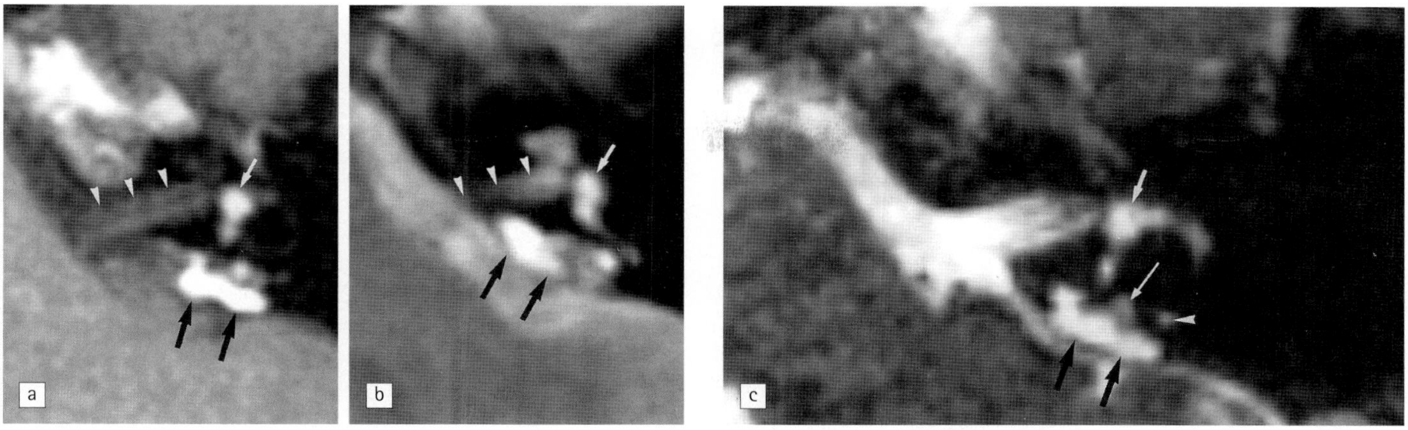

Figure 7.15 Cholesterol granuloma with fistula towards the inner ear. Young woman presenting with vertigo and subtle loss of the low frequencies. Axial unenhanced T1-weighted spin-echo images (a), T2-weighted spin-echo images (b) and 3DFT-CISS images (c) through the left inner ear.
(a) A high-signal-intensity lesion (black arrows) can be seen in the bone behind the IAC. The abnormal high signal intensity can also be seen in the vestibule (white arrow). Note nerves in the IAC (arrowheads). On CT (not shown) only a lytic ovoid lesion could be found behind the IAC.
(b) The high-signal-intensity lesion (black arrows) can still be seen on the T2-weighted image, proving that we are dealing with blood/cholesterol granuloma and not fat. The cholesterol granuloma can again be seen in the vestibule (small white arrow). Note fluid in the IAC (arrowheads).
(c) The lesion (black arrows) can be followed to the posterior semicircular duct (arrowhead). At this site, the fistula between the lesion and the posterior semicircular canal can be seen (long white arrow). The cholesterol granuloma followed this fistula and eventually ended up in the vestibule (small white arrow). These findings were confirmed during surgery.

mucocoeles, cholesterol granulomas, congenital cholesteatomas and chondromas. Cholesterol granulomas have a typical high signal intensity on T1 and T2-weighted images (Figure 7.15). Chondromas have a very high signal intensity on T2-weighted images and enhance strongly. Congenital cholesteatomas (epidermoid tumour) have a low signal intensity on T1-weighted images and do not enhance.

More diffuse lytic lesions are caused by metastases, histiocytosis, osteomyelitis/apicitis and granulomatosis (e.g. TB, syphilis).

Temporal bone trauma

CT is unparalleled in the demonstration of fractures involving the bony labyrinth, explaining the SNHL or vertigo, and is also the best technique to detect a pneumolabyrinth[29] (Figure 7.16). Fractures or lesions of the round or oval window can cause vertigo, very often disappearing in a couple of weeks. Vertigo will more frequently be found in patients with fractures of the bony labyrinth. SNHL is, of course, more frequent when the fracture involves the cochlea. Concussion of the labyrinth in the absence of a fracture can only be seen as high signal intensity on unenhanced T1-weighted images. In the presence of a fracture, blood can again be recognized on MR (Figure 7.17), and loss of intralabyrinthine fluid and fibrosis formation can be seen on the T2-weighted gradient-echo images.

A perilymph fistula can result in vertigo associated with fluctuating SNHL. They can develop spontaneously or can be caused by trauma/barotrauma. These fistulas result from a tear either in the round window membrane or in the ligamentous attachment of the stapedial footplate. CT findings are often negative in these patients, and the haemorrhages resulting from these tears are too small to be detected on unenhanced MR images. The subsequent inflammatory changes that develop following the occurrence of the tear can, however, result in intralabyrinthine enhancement, which is visible on Gd-enhanced

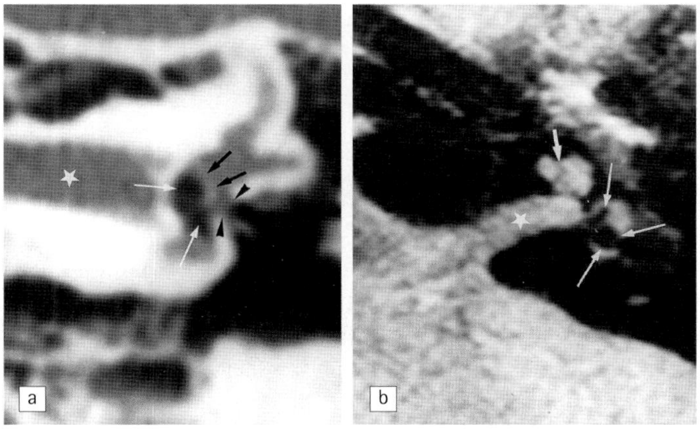

Figure 7.16 Pneumolabyrinth. Patient suffering from severe vertigo attacks, following trauma (cotton bud entered middle ear cavity due to a fall). Coronal CT (a) and axial unenhanced gradient-echo T1-weighted image (b).
(a) Air can be seen inside the vestibule (white arrows). The stapes is displaced inside the vestibule (black arrows). Therefore, a fistula must exist at the level of the oval window (arrowheads) causing the pneumolabyrinth and the vertigo attacks. ★, IAC.
(b) Low-signal-intensity regions (long white arrows) can be seen inside the vestibule. It is impossible to distinguish low signal intensity caused by air, calcifications or displaced ossicles (stapes) on MR images. Only CT can distinguish these entities. Note normal intralabyrinthine fluid in the cochlea (small white arrow). ★, IAC.

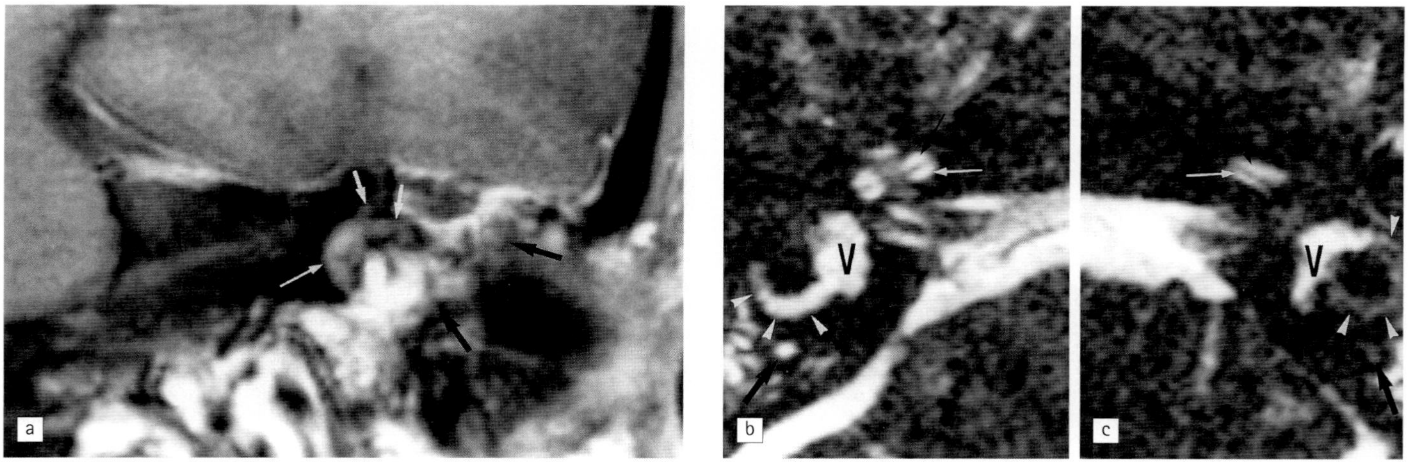

Figure 7.17 Post-traumatic labyrinthine concussion. Patient presenting with hearing loss following a trauma. CT of the temporal bone showed only obliteration of the middle ear cavity. Coronal T1-weighted image through the left inner ear (a) and axial 3DFT-CISS image through the right (b) and left (c) inner ear.
(a) High-signal-intensity fluid, blood, can be seen in the middle ear cavity (black arrows). The vestibule (long white arrow) and posterior and lateral semicircular ducts (small white arrows) are also filled with high-signal-intensity blood. Note nerves in the IAC (arrowheads).
(b) Normal high-signal-intensity fluid can be seen in the scala vestibuli/media (long black arrow) and scala tympani (long white arrow) of the cochlea, the vestibule (V), and the lateral (arrowheads) and posterior (large black arrow) semicircular ducts.
(c) Normal high-signal-intensity fluid can be seen in the scala vestibuli/media (long black arrow) and scala tympani (long white arrow) of the cochlea. The vestibule (V) still contains high-signal-intensity fluid, although the signal on the T1-weighted spin-echo images was high. This corresponds with intralabyrinthine fluid mixed with blood. The lateral (arrowheads) and posterior (large black arrow) semicircular ducts have lost their high signal intensity on the T2-weighted CISS image but have a high signal intensity on the T1-weighted spin-echo image. This corresponds with blood clot formation and the start of fibrosis.

T1-weighted images. Enhancement inside the cochlea or vestibule could, therefore, be a possible indicator of perilymphatic fistulas.[30]

Lesions involving the internal auditory canal

The value of CT in the IAC is limited to the evaluation of the bony walls. MR has almost completely replaced CT in the study of lesions situated inside the IAC (Table 7.5).

Acoustic schwannomas

Acoustic schwannomas are the most frequent lesions found inside the IAC and can cause SNHL, vertigo and tinnitus. They can all be detected on Gd-enhanced T1-weighted images; however, differentiation from neuritis can be difficult. Gradient-echo T2-weighted images are used to distinguish both entities. In cases of schwannoma, a nodular hypointensity will be found in the course of the involved nerve, and a normal or fusiforme thickened nerve will be found in cases of neuritis (Figure 7.18). This applies especially to facial nerve neuritis, as enhancement of the vestibulocochlear nerve (VIIIth nerve neuritis) is rarely seen.

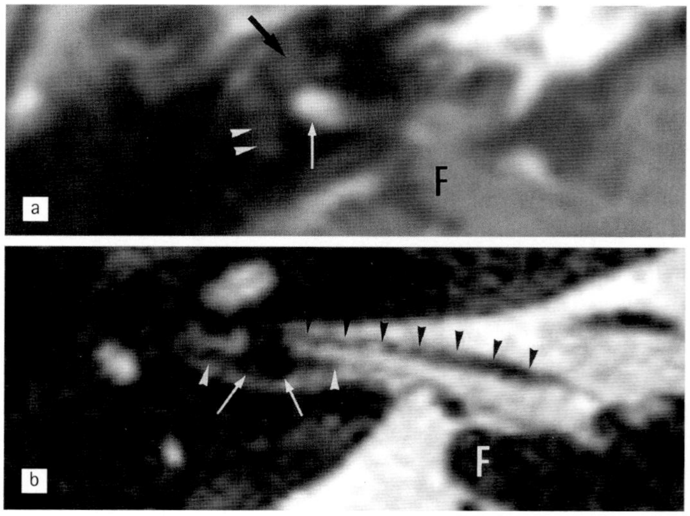

Figure 7.18 Schwannoma of the superior vestibular branch of the VIIIth nerve. Patient presenting with hearing loss and vertigo. Axial Gd-enhanced T1-weighted spin-echo image (a) and 3DFT-CISS image (b) through the right IAC.
(a) A strongly enhancing lesion can be seen deep in the IAC (white arrow). Normal fluid can be seen in the cochlea (black arrow) and vestibule (arrowheads). F, floccule.
(b) The 0.7-mm-thick T2-weighted image shows that the tumour (white arrows) is located in the course of the superior vestibular branch of the VIIIth nerve (white arrowheads). Note facial nerve (black arrowheads). F, floccule.

When the schwannoma is small, one can even determine on which branch (cochlear, inferior vestibular or superior vestibular) of the VIIIth nerve the schwannoma is located. Imaging studies show that vertigo is more frequently correlated with very small and strictly intracanalicular schwannomas. Clinical studies also show that purely intracanalicular acoustical schwannomas result in earlier onset of vestibular symptoms.

Once the diagnosis of a schwannoma is made, the 'growth potential' of the lesion must be assessed. This is best achieved using 1-mm-thick T1-weighted gradient-echo images (e.g. 3DFT-MPRAGE) on which volume measurements are performed. Follow-up studies should be done every 6 months in the first year, and subsequently annually, in case the schwannoma is not growing quickly.

Once it is decided that the schwannoma must be removed, one must find out whether hearing preservation surgery is still possible or not. Imaging plays a key role. First, the presence of fluid between the schwannoma and the fundus of the IAC must be assessed. If fluid is still present, then the surgeon can stay away from the base of the cochlea and a suboccipital or middle cranial fossa approach can be used, so preserving hearing function (Figure 7.19).[31, 32] If no fluid is left, the surgeon has to drill in the cochlear canal, and the patient becomes deaf; therefore, the less invasive translabyrinthine approach is chosen in these patients.

Another important sign is the signal intensity of the CSF between the schwannoma and fundus of the IAC and/or intralabyrinthine fluid. A normal signal intensity of these fluid spaces seems to correlate very well with good results after hearing preservation surgery. However, when the signal intensity of the fluid is decreased, the success of hearing preservation surgery is significantly lower (Figure 7.19).[33]

Neuritis

Neuritis (viral, sarcoid) is the second most frequent pathology found in the IAC in patients presenting with vertigo. However, rarely, an enhancement along the course of the nerve is found on MR in cases of viral neuritis. As already mentioned, a normal or fusiforme thickened nerve can be detected on T2-weighted gradient-echo images.[34]

Tumours (excluding acoustic schwannomas) involving the IAC

Metastases (subarachnoid seeding, melanoma), plasmocytomas, meningiomas, facial nerve schwannomas, arteriovenous malformations, glomus tumours, choristomas, cholesterol granulomas, haemangiomas, congenital cholesteatomas, lipomas, lymphomas, gliomas, carcinomas of the head and neck region, extension of a endolymphatic sac tumour etc. can grow in the IAC or can compress it and can be responsible for the vertigo or SNHL (Figure 7.20).[24,35,36] Most of these tumours are best visualized on Gd-enhanced T1-weighted images. Their extension is also best seen on these images. The extension of these tumours in the CPA is often different from the extension seen in schwannomas. Unlike schwannomas, these tumours (e.g. meningiomas) follow meningeal surfaces and meninges and not the course of the nerve. That is why the nerves sometimes come

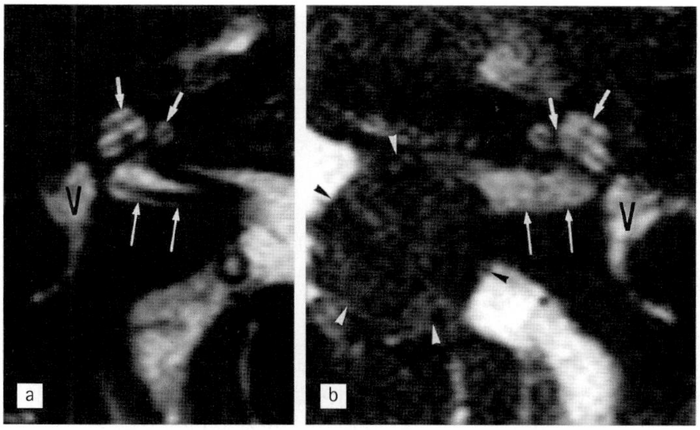

Figure 7.19 Schwannoma of the left CPA. Patient presenting with progressive SNHL on the left side. Axial 3DFT-CISS image through the right (a) and left (b) inner ear.
(a) Normal high-signal-intensity fluid can be seen in the cochlea (small white arrows), the vestibule (V) and the IAC (long white arrows).
(b) A large acoustic schwannoma can be seen in the left CPA (arrowheads). The fluid blocked in the IAC (long white arrows) and the fluid in the cochlea (small white arrows) have a lower signal intensity than the normal fluid in the CPA and vestibule (V). The decrease of the signal intensity in the fluid in the IAC and of the fluid in the cochlea corresponds with worse results when hearing preservation surgery is attempted.

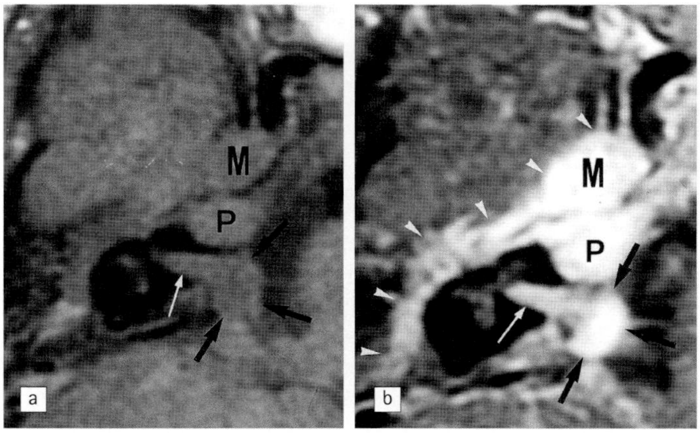

Figure 7.20 Rhabdomyosarcoma involving the IAC. Young child presenting with SNHL. Axial unenhanced (a) and Gd-enhanced (b) T1-weighted spin-echo image.
(a) A tumour can be seen in the CPA (black arrows) and is extending into the IAC (white arrow). Moreover, masses with similar signal intensity are replacing the normal signal intensity of the petrous apex (P) and Meckel's cave (M).
(b) The tumour can be better delineated in the CPA (black arrows) and IAC (white arrow) when Gd is injected. The aggressive nature of the tumour is better seen on the Gd-enhanced images, and the involvement of the tissues around the temporal bone (arrowheads), the petrous apex (P) and Meckel's cave (M) is also better seen on these images. (Courtesy of Dr B. De Foer, St-Augustinus Hospital, Antwerp, Belgium.)

out of these masses in a perpendicular way, making the diagnosis of acoustic schwannoma unlikely.

Unenhanced T1-weighted images and T2-weighted spin-echo images can be used to characterize the lesions, and can, for instance, show the presence of blood in a cholesterol granuloma, involving the IAC.

Congenital cholesteatoma is caused by congenital inclusion of epithelial cells. These slow-growing lesions cause lytic regions in the inner ear; the lesions will not displace the nerves, but will rather follow them. They have a low signal intensity compared to brain tissue on the unenhanced T1-weighted images, and they do not enhance and have a high signal intensity, similar to CSF, on T2-weighted images.

Lipomas have a characteristic high signal intensity on unenhanced T1-weighted images and have a lower signal intensity on T2- or fat suppressed T1-weighted images.[37]

In the case of a small facial schwannoma, thin gradient-echo images can demonstrate the tumour in the course of the VIIth nerve, and the diagnosis also can be made when extension in the facial nerve canal is seen on Gd-enhanced images.

In the case of a haemangioma, a slightly high signal intensity can be seen in the lesion on the unenhanced T1-weighted images, and subtle calcifications are seen on CT. The preoperative differentiation between an acoustic neurinoma and haemangioma is important (but often difficult), because haemangiomas lie adjacent to the (facial or vestibulocochlear) nerve and can be removed without nerve intersection, whereas in schwannomas, the nerve often has to be cut and reconstructed.

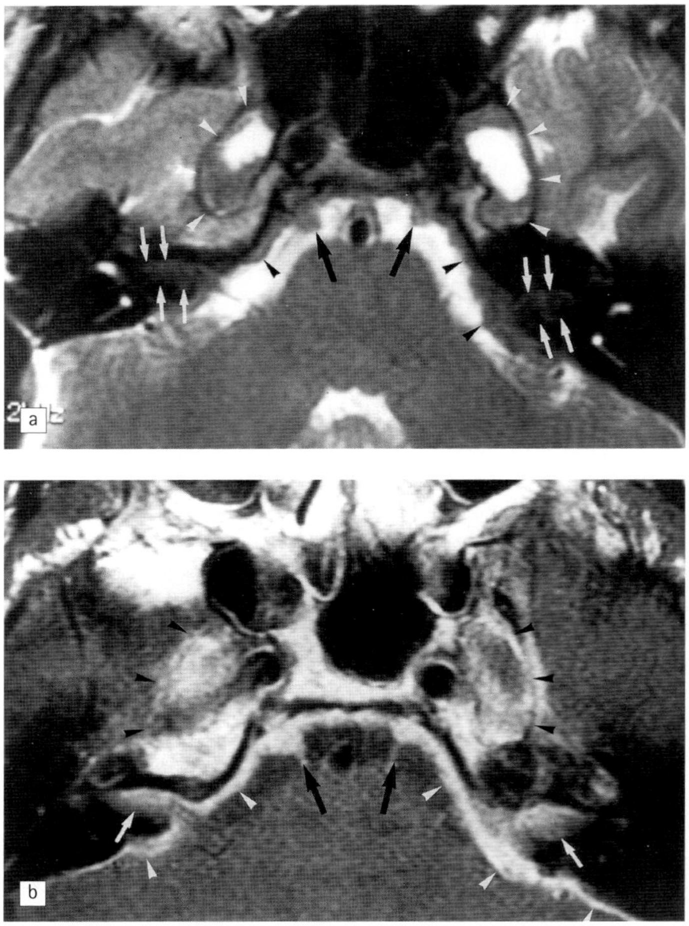

Figure 7.21 Idiopathic pachymeningitis. Young man with progressive and nearly total SNHL. Axial T2-weighted (a) and Gd-enhanced T1-weighted (b) spin-echo images through the posterior fossa and both IACs. Several blood tests excluded viral disease, granulomatous disease etc.
(a) The thickened meninges surround Meckel's cave (white arrowheads), follow the meninges on the medial wall of the temporal bone (black arrowheads) and obliterate the IACs (white arrows). Moreover, the thick meninges follow the cisternal segment of the abducens nerve on both sides (black arrows). The low signal intensity of the thickened meninges is caused by a high concentration of cells, situated close to one another, and with only little space between them (no space for protons).
(b) The thick meninges around Meckel's cave (black arrowheads), on the medial surface of the temporal bone (white arrowheads), along the cisternal segment of the abducens nerve (black arrows) and in the IACs (white arrows) enhance strongly after Gd injection.

Meningitis, postoperative changes

In patients with apicitis or severe meningeal disease (e.g. pachymeningitis), the enhancing meninges can be followed deep in the IAC (Figure 7.21).[38] These findings are a potential explanation for SNHL or the vertigo/abnormal findings at vestibular testing. Sometimes, the thickened meninges completely obliterate the IAC, making the nerves invisible. The cause of the pachymeningits can be infection, venous thrombosis, metastases, liquor hypotension, idiopathic, granulomatosis, etc.

Absence of the vestibular and/or cochlear branches of the VIIIth nerve following surgery can also be depicted on MR and helps to explain SNHL or vertigo in previously operated patients.

Congenital malformations

In patients with congenital deafness or SNHL, the internal auditory canal (IAC) can be absent, very narrow, double, etc. In these patients, the facial nerve canal can leave the IAC, in its middle one-third, or can be completely separated from the IAC and sometimes only a sulcus for the nerve can be found on the roof of the temporal bone. All these malformations can be seen on CT; however, what happens with the nerves in these patients can only be evaluated on MR.

The vestibulocochlear nerve can be hypoplastic or absent in these patients.[39] Two different types can be distinguished on gradient-echo T2-weighted MR images. In 'type 1', the VIIIth nerve is completely absent (three branches of the nerve are absent), and this is often associated with a very narrow IAC, only containing the VIIth nerve. In 'type 2', a common vestibulocochlear nerve is found with absence or hypoplasia of its cochlear branch (Figure 7.22). In 'type 2A', the labyrinth is abnormal, while in 'type 2B' it is normal.

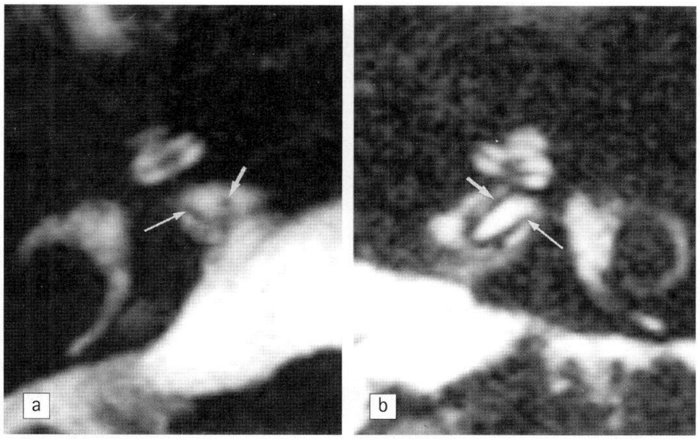

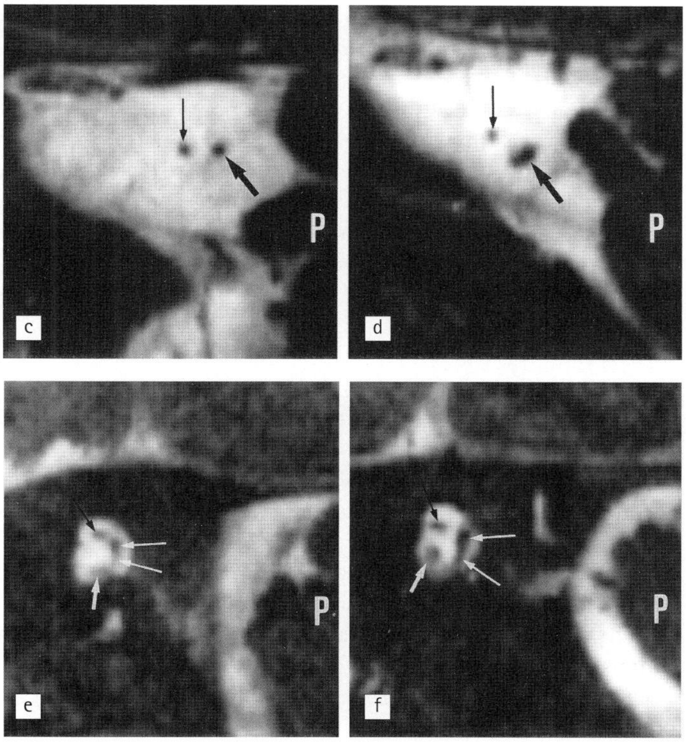

Figure 7.22 Hypoplasia of the vestibulocochlear nerve and its branches. Patient with congenital severe SNHL on the right side, axial T2-weighted 3DFT-CISS images throught the right (a) and left (b) IAC and parasagittal reconstruction through the right (c, e) and left (d, f) CPA and IAC.
(a) A very small cochlear (small white arrow) and inferior vestibular branch (long white arrow) of the VIIIth nerve are seen in the inferior part of the right IAC.
(b) A normal cochlear (small white arrow) and inferior vestibular branch (long white arrow) of the VIIIth nerve can be seen in the left IAC.
(c) The facial nerve (long black arrow) and vestibulocochlear nerve (large black arrow) have a similar size. This proves that the VIIIth nerve is hypoplastic, as normally the VIIIth nerve is 1.5–2 times larger than the facial nerve (see (d)). P, posterior fossa.
(d) The VIIIth nerve (large black arrow) is 1.5–2 times larger than the facial nerve (long black arrow). P, posterior fossa.
(e) Only the facial nerve (black arrow) has a normal size at the level of the IAC. The cochlear branch (small white arrow) and common vestibular branch (long white arrows) of the vestibulocochlear nerve are hypoplastic. Compare with the normal nerves on the left side in (f). P, posterior fossa.
(f) The facial nerve (black arrow), the cochlear branch (small white arrow) and common vestibular branch (long white arrows) of the vestibulocochlear nerve all have a normal size. P, posterior fossa.

Table 7.5 Preferred imaging techniques—internal auditory canal

Pathology	Imaging technique
Schwannoma	Gd-enhanced T1-weighted images Gradient-echo T2-weighted images (CISS) Volume measurement/follow-up: 1-mm-thick T1-weighted gradient-echo images (3DFT-MPRAGE)
Neuritis	Gd-enhanced T1-weighted images Gradient-echo T2 images (CISS)
Tumours (excluding schwannomas) involving the IAC	Unenhanced T1-weighted images Gd-enhanced T1-weighted images T2-weighted spin-echo images CT: to look for fat, calcifications, changes of bony walls
Meningitis, postoperative changes	Gd-enhanced T1-weighted images Gradient-echo T2-weighted images (CISS)
Congenital malformations	Gradient-echo T2-weighted images (CISS) CT (evaluation IAC and facial nerve canal)

One should always check for the presence of a normal cochlear branch in all cochlear implant candidates and in patients with congenital SNHL. In type I, cochlear implant installation is not possible as there is no nerve. In type II, implantation is still possible, as long as the patient has a fluid filled cavity and a single nerve, which is not the facial nerve, that reaches the fluid-filled cavity. Very often this nerve is a so-called 'common nerve' carrying vestibular and cochlear information in its different fibres.

Lesions involving the cerebellopontine angle

Schwannomas of the vestibulocochlear nerve (most frequent lesion in the CPA), meningiomas, cholesterol granulomas and congenital cholesteatomas are discussed above. It is obvious that these lesions can also result in vertigo and SNHL when they appear in the CPA. Other lesions occurring in the CPA[24] and that cause SNHL and/or vertigo are discussed below.

Tumours: schwannomas of other nerves, metastases, epidermoid and dermoid cysts, lipoma etc.

Schwannomas of the Vth and lower cranial nerves (IX, X, XI, XII) can compress the vestibulocochlear nerve and therefore can cause SNHL and vertigo. The best sequence to detect them is the Gd-enhanced T1-weighted sequence (Figure 7.23).

Metastases can be found in the CPA (and IAC) and are again best seen on Gd-enhanced T1-weighted images. They can be nodular or can follow the nerve. Meningeal metastases can be seen as local or more diffuse meningeal enhancements. The MR appearance of a metastasis is atypical. Only a known history of a primary tumour or the presence of multiple lesions helps in the differentiation from other tumours.

Dermoid cysts are rare. They are composed of fat, calcifications and soft tissue elements. The fat is hypodense on CT and has high signal intensity on unenhanced T1-weighted images. The calcifications are hyperdense on CT and are seen as 'signal voids' on MR. The soft tissue parts enhance after Gd administration. In lipoma, the fat characteristics described above can be seen on CT and MR.

Epidermoid cysts are very difficult to detect, as they are isointense with CSF on T1-weighted, proton density and T2- weighted images. They can, however, be seen in a reliable way on T2-weighted gradient-echo images. On these images their signal intensity is much lower than the signal of the CSF (Figure 7.24).

Arachnoid cysts

These are CSF-filled cysts, lined by a thin arachnoid wall. These cysts can compress the nerves or can push them away. They are isointense with CSF on all sequences, but their signal intensity is sometimes slightly higher than that of the signal of CSF on T2-weighted gradient-echo images, because the flow of the free CSF around the brainstem causes a slight decrease in signal intensity. The stationary fluid in the cyst, of course, retains its high signal intensity (Figure 7.25).

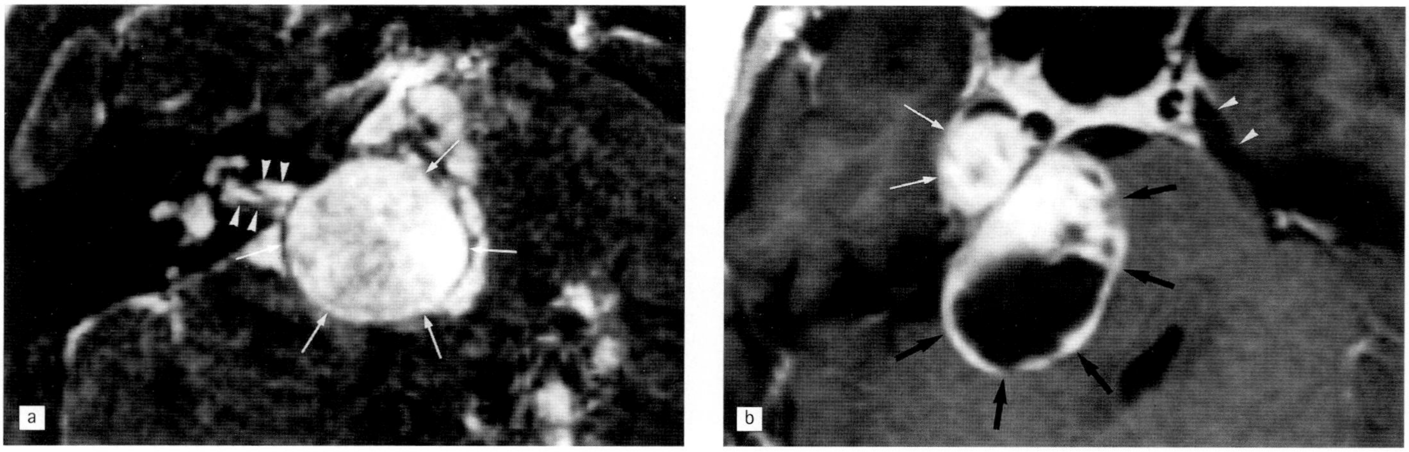

Figure 7.23 Trigeminal nerve schwannoma. Patient presenting with SNHL on the right side. Axial T2-weighted 3DFT-CISS image through the IAC (a) and axial Gd-enhanced T1-weighted image through Meckel's cave (b).

(a) A large tumour is seen in the CPA (long white arrows) and reaches the IAC (arrowheads). The lesion is hyperintense, but some inhomogeneous regions with lower signal intensity can be seen in the posterior part of the lesion. The nerves in the IAC have a perpendicular orientation to the surface of the tumour. However, the tumour is always oriented along the course of the nerves in cases of acoustic schwannoma.

(b) An enhancing dumbbell lesion can be seen at the level of Meckel's cave. A solid component is obliterating Meckel's cave (white arrows) and corresponds with the middle fossa component of the trigeminal schwannoma. A more cystic part extends in the posterior fossa (black arrows) and descends to the level of the IAC (see (a)). Note Meckel's cave on the left side (arrowheads).

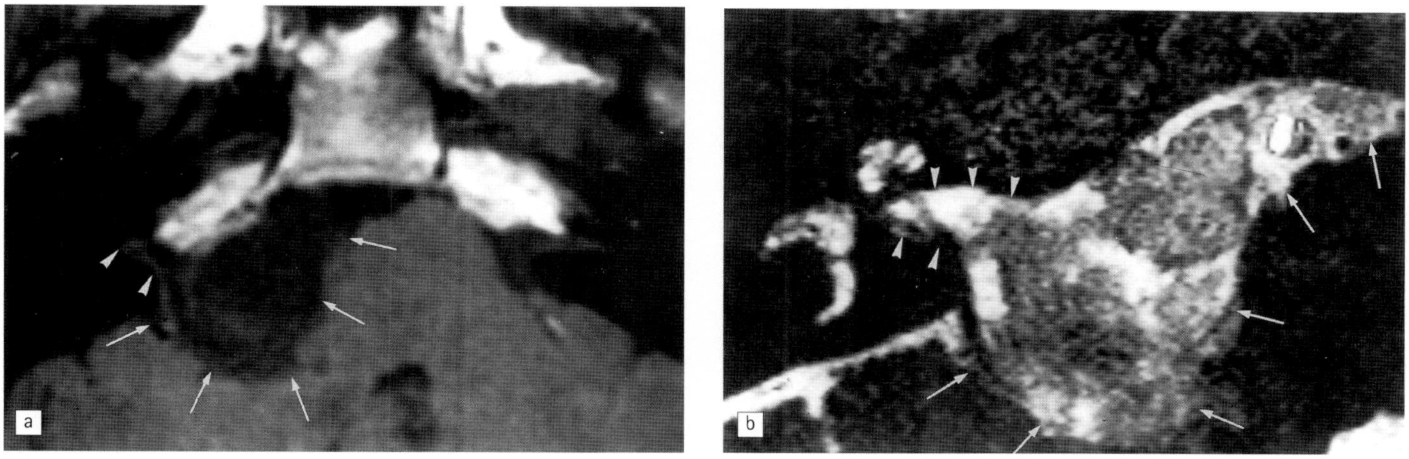

Figure 7.24 Epidermoid tumour in the CPA. Patient presenting with vertigo. Axial unenhanced T1-weighted spin-echo (a) and T2-weighted 3DFT-CISS image through the right CPA.

(a) A large lesion isointense with CSF (also isointense with CSF on the T2-weighted spin-echo image and not enhancing after Gd administration—not shown) can be seen in the right CPA (long white arrows). A subtle internal architecture can be presumed on the T1-weighted image. It is, however, not possible to differentiate a subarachnoidal cyst from an epidermoid tumour on these images. Note IAC (arrowheads).

(b) The T2-weighted 3DFT-CISS images prove that the mass is solid (long white arrows) because the high-signal-intensity fluid of the CPA is replaced by low-signal-intensity solid tissue. Note IAC (arrowheads).

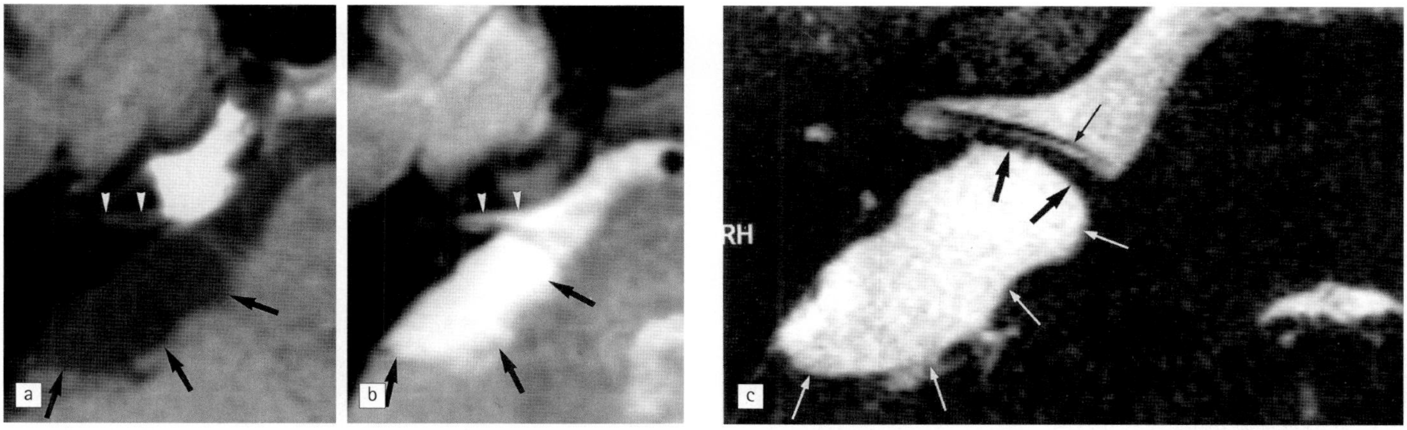

Figure 7.25 Subarachnoid cyst in the right CPA. Patient presenting with SNHL on the right side. Axial T1-weighted (a) and T2-weighted spin-echo image (b) and 3DFT-CISS image (c) through the right CPA.

(a) A space-occupying lesion with low signal intensity, isointense with CSF, can be seen in the right CPA (black arrows). Note IAC (arrowheads).

(b) The lesion remains isointense with CSF on the T2-weighted spin-echo images (black arrows). Note IAC (arrowheads).

(c) The lesion still has a signal intensity isointense with CSF on the 3DFT-CISS images (white arrows), proving that the lesion is cystic. An epidermoid lesion can therefore be excluded. The lesion is displacing the vestibulocochlear nerve anteriorly (large black arrows). Note facial nerve (long black arrow).

Siderosis

Following a severe posterior fossa haemorrhage (surgery, aneurysm, trauma), haemosiderin deposition on the surface of the VIIth and VIIIth nerves can occur. In these patients, the nerves have very low signal intensity on T2-weighted spin-echo or T2 -weighted gradient-echo images. A nodular thickening of the nerves can sometimes be appreciated on the high-resolution and very thin T2-weighted gradient-echo images (CISS) (Figure 7.26).[40]

Neurovascular conflicts

Another frequent indication for imaging is to look for a neurovascular conflict in the CPA causing (fluctuating) SNHL and/vertigo/tinnitus.[41–43]

Both veins and arteries can compress the nerves at their root entry zone (REZ), which is the transition zone from central to peripheral myelin. For the VIIIth nerve, this REZ is situated 10 mm lateral to the site where the nerve leaves the brainstem. At this point, compression of the nerve frequently

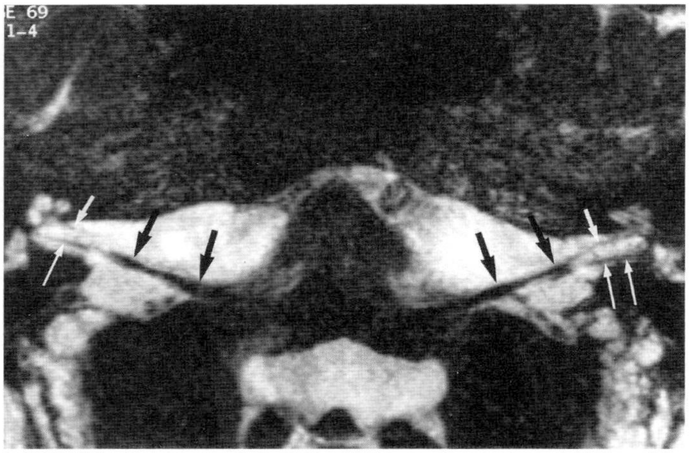

Figure 7.26 Siderosis on the surface of the vestibulocochlear nerve. Patient presenting with post-traumatic severe SNHL, several years after a trauma. Axial 3DFT-CISS image through both CPAs. The vestibulocochlear nerves are thickened and have an irregular diameter (black arrows). This corresponds with changes due to haemosiderin deposition on the nerves, caused by post-traumatic bleeding. The nerves also had a very low signal intensity on the T2-weighted spin-echo images (not shown). The cochlear (small white arrow) and inferior vestibular branches (long white arrows) of the VIIIth nerve are atrophic. This is probably secondary to nerve dysfunction, caused by the siderosis.

results in symptoms. Only MR is able to visualize the nerves and vessels simultaneously (Figure 7.27). Both nerves and vessels can be seen as black structures surrounded by white CSF on the very thin T2-weighted gradient-echo images (3DFT-CISS). Nerves are seen as straight structures, and vessels are winding structures. Excellent multiplanar reconstructions and 3D virtual images can be made using 3DFT-CISS images. High-resolution vascular MR images (3DFT-FISP time-of-flight images) can be used when the vessels and nerves are difficult to distinguish. Only the vessels will have a high signal on these MRA images. Moreover, these MRA images allow us again to make good paracoronal reconstructions (following the course of the nerves). It is very often possible to identify the tortuous, dilated or abnormal vessel, which is compressing the nerve near the REZ, on MR. The vessel can often be identified on the contiguous images or 3D maximum intensity projection (MIP) images. If there is doubt about whether one is dealing with a vein or artery, unenhanced and Gd-enhanced MRA images can give the solution. If it is an artery, the vessels will be seen on both the unenhanced and Gd-enhanced MRA images, whereas a vein will only be seen on the Gd-enhanced MRA sequence. Finally, the chances that the neurovascular conflict is really causing the symptoms increases when the following apply:

- Compression near the REZ (10 mm from the place where the VIIIth nerve leaves the brainstem)
- The vessel is an artery
- The vessel crosses the nerve in a perpendicular way
- The vessel displaces the nerve

Vertebrobasilar dolichoectasia and posterior fossa aneurysm can also cause VIIIth nerve compression and displacement.

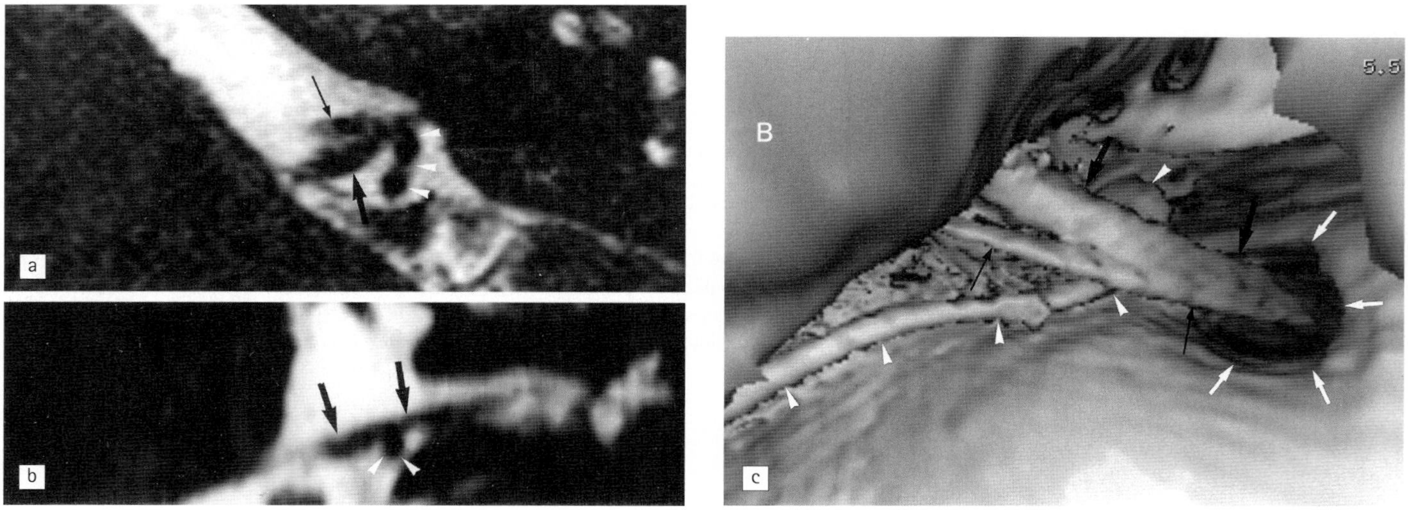

Figure 7.27 Neurovascular conflict. Patient presenting with fluctuating hearing loss and vertigo. Axial T2-weighed 3DFT-CISS image (a) and paracoronal reconstruction (b) through the left CPA and virtual image (c) of the left CPA, viewed from above.

(a) A winding vessel (arrowheads) is crossing the vestibulocochlear nerve (large black arrow) in a perpendicular way at a distance of approximately 10 mm from its emergence from the brainstem. This is the site where the central myelin of the nerve changes into peripheral myelin and where the nerve is most vulnerable. Note facial nerve (long black arrow).

(b) The vessel (arrowheads) is crossing the inferior border of the VIIIth nerve (large black arrows).

(c) The vestibulocochlear nerve (large black arrows) and facial nerve (long black arrows) are crossing the CPA and reach the porus of the IAC (white arrows). The anterior inferior cerebellar artery is crossing the inferior border of the VIIth and VIIIth nerve (arrowheads). B, brainstem.

Petrous bone lesion

Finally, lesions of the petrous bone can become so large that they can displace or compress the nerves in the IAC or CPA. Paget's disease, fibrous dysplasia (Figure 7.28), osteopetrosis and otosclerosis are discussed above. Lesions of the petrous apex, such as cholesterol granuloma, mucocele, epidermoid tumour or primary cholesteatoma, cholesteatoma, cartilaginous tumours, or chordomas, can also cause a conflict with the VIIIth nerve. A more detailed description of these lesions is, however, beyond the scope of this chapter.

Central auditory and vestibular pathways

Tumours, vascular anomalies, haemorrhages, infections or abscesses and demyelination of the brainstem can all involve the cochlear and/or vestibular nuclei and pathways.[44]

The most important structures, which must be checked, are listed in Table 7.6. Lesions involving structures of the auditory or vestibular pathway can cause sudden deafness or vertigo. The deafness will be unilateral when the cochlear nucleus is involved. Bilateral asymmetric SNHL will be found when the lateral lemniscus, inferior colliculus or medial geniculate body are involved. Sounds are perceived, but the interpretation is impaired (auditory agnosia) when the auditory cortex is involved. Lesions in the brain and brainstem at different locations can produce different kinds of vertigo (central vestibular signs) (see Chapter 49).

Infarctions—ischaemia

Infarctions or ischaemic lesions involving structures of the auditory or vestibular pathway can cause sudden deafness or vertigo (Figure 7.29).[45,46] They represent the most frequent brainstem pathology causing deafness or vertigo. The infarctions are most often caused by atheromatosis. Emboli, compression of an artery or dissection (cervical manipulation or trauma) are less frequent causes. Infarctions are best seen on routine T2-weighted spin-echo images and are visible as high-signal-intensity regions. They are only seen on unenhanced T1-weighted images when there is a lot of oedema (low signal) or when they are haemorrhagic (high signal intensity). Enhancement on the Gd-enhanced T1-weighted images is present when the blood–brain barrier is affected. The T2-weighted sequence with a very long TR (repetition time) is used when small lesions in the brainstem are suspected, e.g. vestibular nuclei, MLF, or oculomotor nuclei. The infarctions are again seen as high-signal-intensity regions on these images.

The vertigo and hearing loss can be associated with other neurological signs due to the brainstem involvement. Patients sometimes present with a combination of peripheral and central symptoms when both the posterior inferior cerebellar artery (PICA) and anterior inferior cerebellar artery (AICA) are

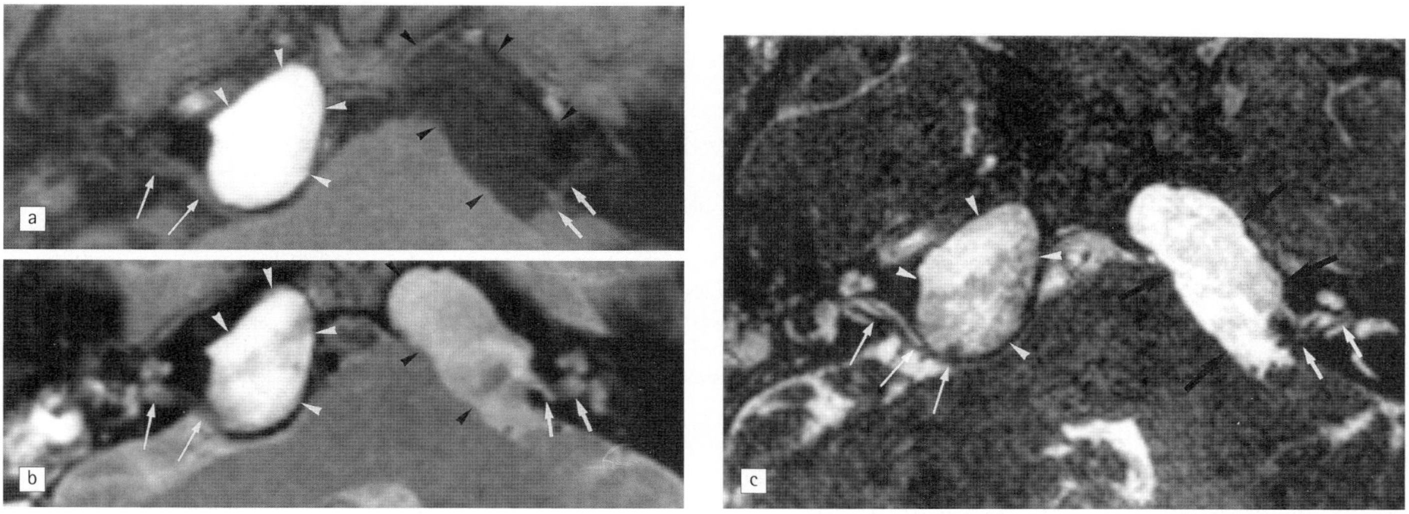

Figure 7.28 Bilateral cholesterol granuloma of the petrous apex. Patient presenting with SNHL. Unenhanced T1-weighted (a) and T2-weighted (b) spin-echo images and 3DFT-CISS image of both temporal bones.

(a) A hyperintense mass is situated in the right petrous apex (white arrowheads) and is displacing the VIIth and VIIIth nerves posteriorly (long white arrows). A similar mass but with low signal intensity is situated in the left petrous apex (black arrowheads) and is also touching the nerves (small white arrows).

(b) The mass in the right petrous apex remains hyperintense (white arrowheads) and is therefore a cholesterol granuloma, containing blood products. The mass on the left side becomes hyperintense on the T2-weighted images (black arrowheads) and is therefore cystic. Previously, the mass on the left side was also a cholesterol granuloma, but the lesion was marsupialized into the mastoid. This caused replacement of the blood products by fluid. The nerves on the right side are displaced posteriorly (long white arrows). Note left IAC (small white arrows).

(c) Both the cholesterol granuloma (white arrowheads) and the drained granuloma (black arrows) have a high signal intensity on the 3DFT-CISS images. The right vestibulocochlear nerve is displaced posteriorly (long white arrows), while the nerves on the left side have a normal position in the IAC (small white arrows).

Table 7.6 Central auditory and vestibular structures to be checked

	Auditory pathway	Vestibular pathway
Brainstem	Cochlear nucleus Trapezoid body (its fibres run through medial lemniscus) Lateral lemniscus Inferior colliculus	Vestibular nucleus MLF and oculomotor nuclei (VOR) Nucleus Praepositus hypoglossus Inferior olive Lateral cuneate nucleus
Supratentorial	Medial geniculate body Planum temporale (auditory cortex) Lobus of Heschl (auditory cortex)	Thalamus Area 2v and 3a (vestibular cortex)
Posterior fossa		Flocculonodular lobe Flocculus Uvula Nodulus Cerebellum

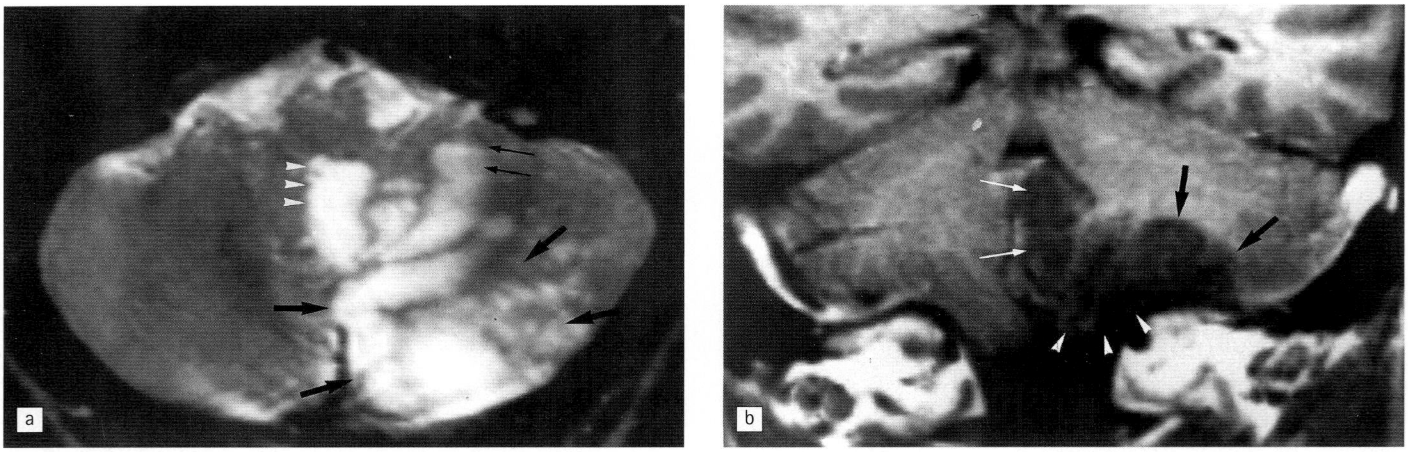

Figure 7.29 Infarction affecting the central vestibular structures. Patient with acute vertigo. Axial T2-weighted spin-echo image (a) and coronal Gd-enhanced T1-weighted spin-echo image (b).
(a) Several high-signal-intensity infarctions are seen in the left cerebellum (large black arrows) and are extending in the region of the left floccule (long black arrows), and in the region of the nodus and uvula of the left cerebellum (arrowheads).
(b) The infarctions in the left cerebellum (black arrows) and in the uvula and nodus of the left cerebellum (white arrows) can again be seen and are hypointense. There is no enhancement and therefore the blood-brain barrier must be intact. The infarctions are causing deviation of the midline structures and therefore the infarctions must be recent (oedema). There is also involvement of the left tonsil (arrowheads).

involved. This is possible because the PICA and AICA supply overlapping territories in the brainstem and cerebellum, and the AICA also supplies the peripheral labyrinth via the internal auditory end artery.

The anterior vestibular branch of the internal auditory artery supplies the superior part of the vestibular labyrinth (only the posterior semicircular canal and utricle are not supplied by this artery), which is very vulnerable to ischaemia. This can result in a vestibular syndrome, which is difficult to distinguish from vestibular neuritis. The AICA further supplies the middle cerebellar peduncle and the anteroinferior cerebellum.

The PICA supplies the paramedian part of the cerebellum with its medial branch and the more lateral part of the cerebellum with its lateral branches. The PICA is responsible for the region towards the transition zone 'cerebellum pons', and lesions in this region will disconnect the vestibular nuclei from the flocculus and vermis.

Today, diffusion imaging on MR enables us to distinguish recent infarctions (already in the first hours after the insult) from old infarctions, so that a 'clinical imaging' correlation can be made in the first hours following the onset of the deafness or vertigo.

Multiple sclerosis

Multiple sclerosis can also cause SNHL and vertigo (Figure 7.30).[47, 48] Vertigo is the first symptom in 5 to 7% of patients with multiple sclerosis. High-signal-intensity lesions can be seen on proton density and T2-weighted spin-echo images or on fluid attenuated inversion recovery images. The lesions enhance when they are active. The cochlear and vestibular nuclei and complete pathways must again be checked on MR.

Tumours

Deafness and vertigo can also be caused by brainstem tumours. Gliomas, fibrillary astrocytomas (Figure 7.31), metastases, lymphoma etc. can all cause deafness and vertigo but very often other brainstem structures are also involved, causing additional symptoms. Fast-growing or fast-appearing tumours like metastases and lymphomas can cause acute deafness. The deafness is more progressive when the tumours are slow-growing.

Miscellaneous

The nuclei and pathways can also be damaged by the following lesions: haemorrhages (traumatic, in tumour, vascular malformation, ischaemic), trauma (Figure 7.32–33) (haemorrhage, contusion, diffuse axonal injury, siderosis), vascular malformation, and inflammation (Figure 7.34). Finally, congenital malformations can be the cause of the hearing loss, e.g. polymicrogyria or pachygyria of the auditory cortex (Figure 7.35).

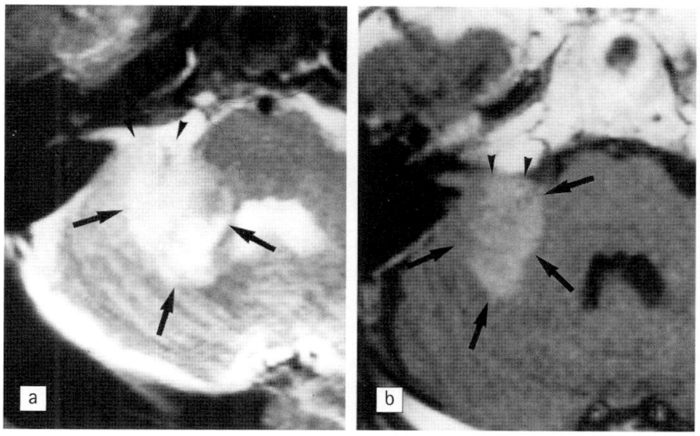

Figure 7.31 Fibrillary astrocytoma. Patient with SNHL on the right side. Axial T2-weighted (a) and Gd-enhanced T1-weighted (b) image through the right CPA.

(a) A large high-signal-intensity tumour is situated between the brainstem and the right cerebellum (black arrows) and obliterates part of the CPA (arrowheads).

(b) The lesion clearly enhances (black arrows) and nearly completely obliterates the CPA (arrowheads).

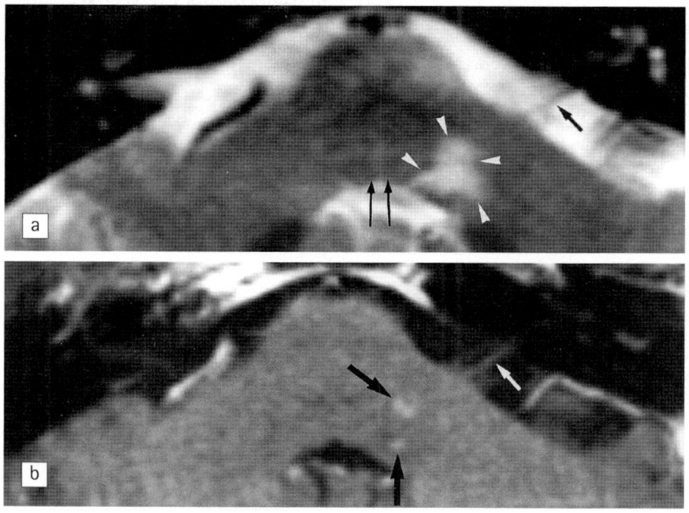

Figure 7.30 Multiple sclerosis, involving the vestibular nucleus. Patient presenting with acute vertigo. Axial T2-weighted (a) and Gd-enhanced T1-weighted (b) spin-echo image through the region of the vestibular nuclei.

(a) A hyperintense lesion can be seen at the site where the left vestibular nucleus is situated (white arrowheads). Note medial longitudinal fasciculus (long black arrows), and vestibulocochlear nerve (small black arrow).

(b) Two small enhancements can be seen in the lesion (black arrows) and therefore this lesion (in a patient with known MS and several other lesions in the brain) is an active one. Note vestibulocochlear nerve (white arrow).

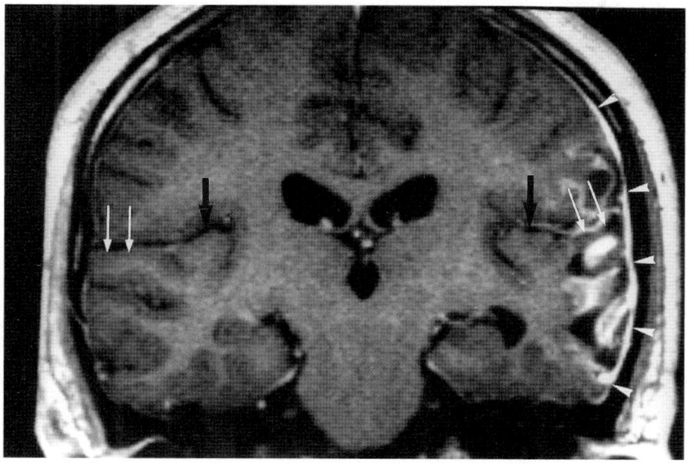

Figure 7.32 Haemorrhagic contusion of the auditory cortex. Patient with hearing loss on the left side due to a trauma. The CT and MR examinations of the temporal bone were negative, and it was difficult to communicate with the patient. Coronal T1-weighted image through the left auditory cortex. High-signal-intensity blood can be seen in the subdural space (arrowheads), and a haemorrhagic contusion is involving the left planum temporale (white arrows). The lobus of Heschl (black arrows), also belonging to the auditory cortex, is still intact.

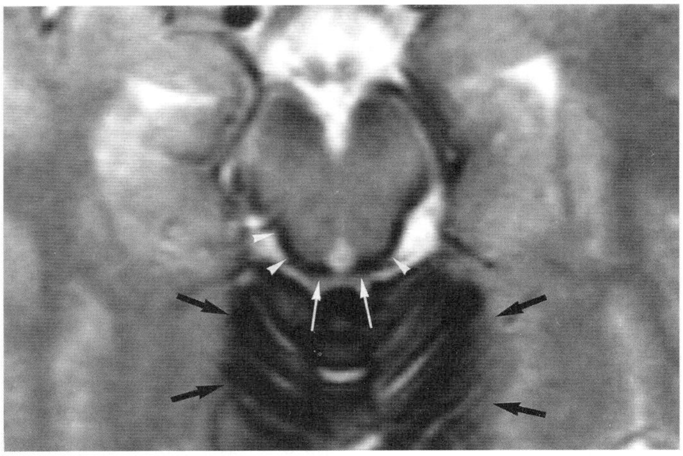

Figure 7.33 Siderosis involving the auditory pathways. Patient with SNHL, status several months after the trauma. Severe bleeding caused by the trauma resulted in significant haemosiderin deposition on the surface of the vermis, cerebellum (black arrows) and on the posterior surface of the brainstem. The auditory pathways are involved at the level of the inferior colliculus (white arrows) and/or lateral or auditory lemniscus (arrowheads).

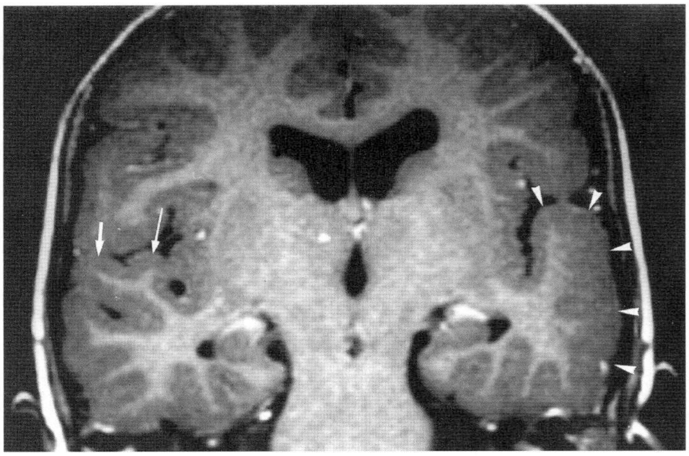

Figure 7.35 Polymicrogyria or pachygyria of the auditory cortex. Cochlear implant candidate, bilateral congenital SNHL. Coronal Gd-enhanced T1-weighted MPRAGE image. The auditory cortex on the left side is abnormal and the different gyri cannot be distinguished from one another (arrowheads). These changes correspond with polymicrogyria or pachygyria. Compare with the normal planum temporale (small white arrow) and lobus of Heschl (long white arrow) on the right side.

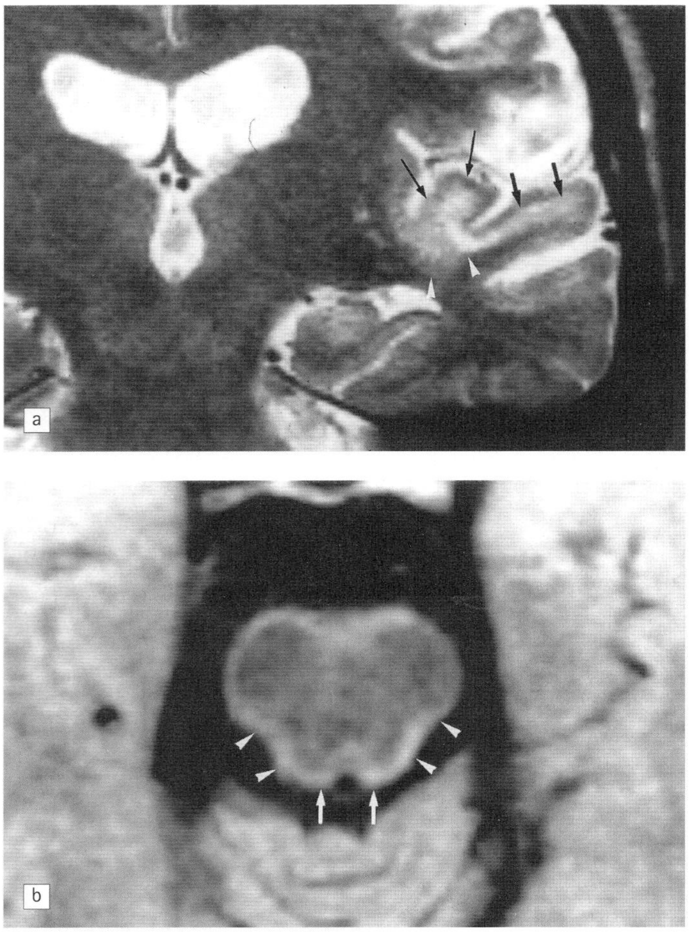

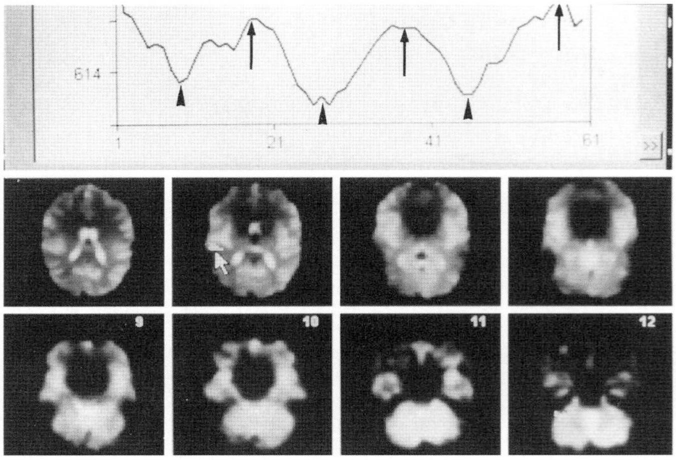

Figure 7.36 Functional MR—normal example. Echo planar imaging (EPI) images during 'noise' stimulation. The stimulation diagram shows the periods without (arrowheads) and with (black arrows) 'noise' stimulation. Activation in the right auditory cortex can be depicted on the second EPI image (white arrow).

Figure 7.34 Rhombencephalitis/encephalitis: young patient with severe SNHL and fast, severe worsening of all functions (intensive care treatment). Coronal T2-weighted image through the auditory cortex (a) and axial proton-density image through the mesencephalon (b).

(a) High-signal-intensity changes can be seen in the white matter tracts going towards the auditory cortex (arrowheads). The signal intensity of the white matter is increased in the lobus of Heschl (long black arrows) and in the planum temporal (short black arrows).

(b) High-signal-intensity changes can be seen in the wall of the brainstem and especially at the level of the inferior colliculus (white arrows) and lateral/auditory lemniscus (arrowheads) on both sides. Both structures belong to the auditory pathways.

Menière's disease

Today, it is not possible to make the diagnosis of Menière's disease using CT or MR. Both techniques confirm that the vestibular aqueduct is frequently smaller than in the normal population, but this is not a reliable sign. The distance between the posterior semicircular canal or duct and the CSF in the posterior fossa is also often very small in patients with Menière's disease. However, this can sometimes also, but less frequently, be seen in the normal population. The value of imaging in patients with Menière's disease is to exclude other pathology mimicking Menière's disease.[49] The most frequent lesions found in these patients are intracanalicular schwannomas, infarctions in the brainstem and/or cerebellum, and obliterations in the membranous labyrinth.

Craniocervical junction

Basilar impression has to be ruled out when vertigo is associated with a palsy of the lower cranial nerves. This can be recognized on the sagittal localizer. The line of Chamberlain (from the hard palate to the posterior border of the foramen magnum) normally passes 5 mm below the upper point of the dens. In case of basilar impression, this line lies more than 5 mm below the upper border of the dens and the tonsils are in a low position, and the brainstem is elongated; syringomyelia can also be present.

Functional MR

The potential of functional MR to study patients with SNHL or cochlear implant candidates is huge. The most frequently used technique today is the 'blood oxygenation level – dependent' (BOLD) technique.[50] This technique depends on small changes in the steady-state level of paramagnetic deoxygenated haemoglobin. These changes become visible when the unstimulated auditory cortex and stimulated auditory cortex are compared. This method is not invasive and has an unlimited repeatability. Stimulation can be achieved using a headphone and noise, but better results are possible when an electrode, placed in the external auditory canal or on the surface of the bony labyrinth, is used.[51] The applications are obvious. Normal activation of the auditory cortex indicates an intact auditory pathway, obviating the need to check the cochlea, IAC, CPA, brainstem and cortex separately. Moreover, in cochlear implant candidates, one can check which ear results in the best activation of the auditory cortex. Of course, this technique is also a tool to perform basic scientific studies on hearing. Today, many of the studies performed are still using normally hearing persons and are done to ameliorate the technique. Large clinical studies in deaf patients or cochlear implant candidates are still lacking.

Tinnitus

Patients with pulsatile tinnitus can today be examined in a non-invasive way with MR.[10, 44, 52] Patients with subjective and non-pulsatile tinnitus can also be examined using MRA, but the yield is much lower. Neurovascular conflicts near the REZ of the facial and vestibulocochlear nerves can best be recognized on gradient-echo T2-weighted images, and were discussed above. These images can also be used to provide the surgeon with virtual images of the conflict in the CPA. Vascular time-of-flight images can be used to identify the vessel causing the conflict or to differentiate between arteries and veins (non-enhanced and Gd-enhanced images).

However, a neurovascular conflict is not the most frequent cause of pulsatile tinnitus. Paragangliomas, dural arteriovenous fistulas, idiopathic venous tinnitus and benign intracranial hypertension are the most frequent causes, and only the first two can be shown on MR. Dural fistulas, causing early venous drainage on the non-enhanced images, can be detected (Figure 7.37). Glomus tumors (Figure 7.38), arteriovenous malformations, aberrant vessels running through the middle ear, high or dehiscent jugular bulbs (Figure 7.39), tortuous carotid arteries near the skull base, fibromuscular dysplasia (Figure 7.40) and carotid dissection (Figure 7.41) can all be detected on both the unenhanced and Gd-enhanced MRA images. Vascularized tumours like meningiomas cause higher arterial and venous flow in their surroundings and therefore can cause tinnitus. This is the reason why tumours in the neighbourhood of the temporal bone must be excluded in these patients. Finally, CT is sometimes necessary to find the cause of the tinnitus. An example is Paget's disease.

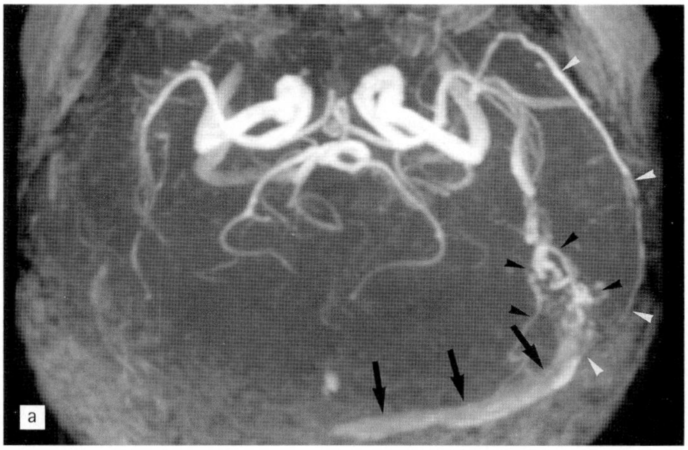

Figure 7.37 Dural fistula. Patient presenting with pulsatile tinnitus on the left side. Unenhanced MR time-of-flight images with 3D reconstruction viewed from above (a), lateral view (b) (on next page).
(a) Early venous drainage can be seen in the transverse and sigmoid sinus (black arrows). Abnormal tortuous vessels coming from the external carotid artery branches (black arrowheads) and the middle meningeal artery territory (white arrowheads) can be seen.

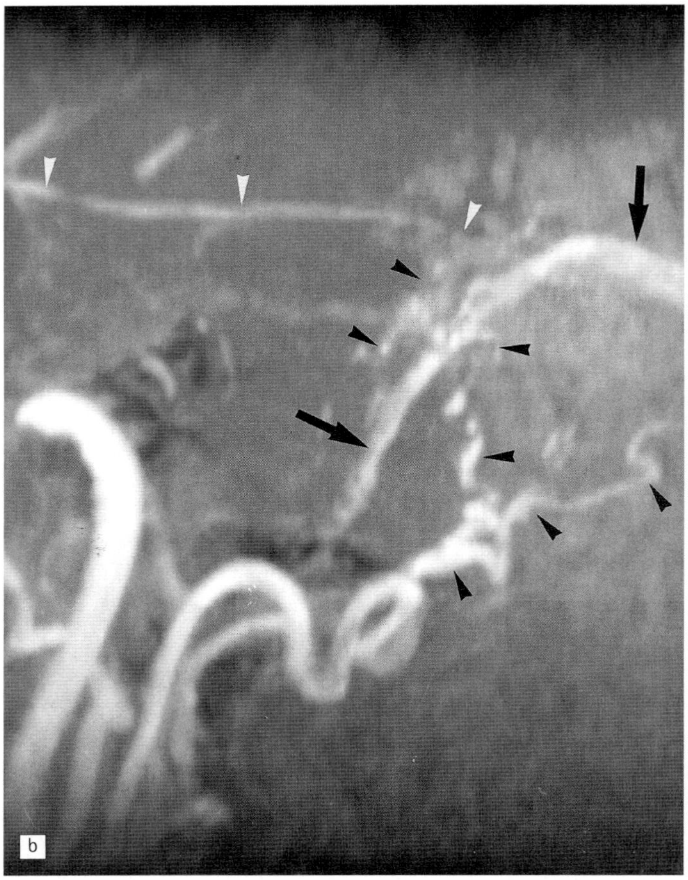

Figure 7.37 (b) The early venous drainage in the transverse and sigmoid sinus (black arrows) can again be recognized, and the tortuous vessels coming from the occipital artery (black arrowheads) and middle meningeal artery (white arrowheads) can be seen.

However, MRA has become the method of first choice and is able to detect many more causes of tinnitus than CT. Angiography is only used to treat patients (embolization) or when the pulsatile tinnitus renders a normal life impossible and MR and CT remain negative. An overview of the possible causes of tinnitus is given in Table 7.7.

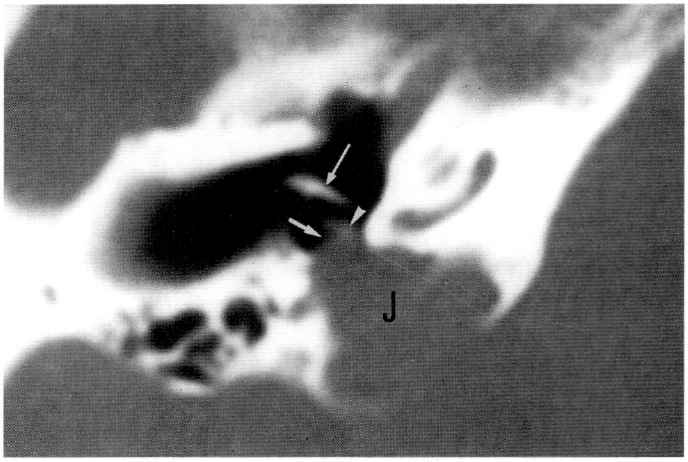

Figure 7.39 Dehiscent jugular bulb. Patient with pulsatile tinnitus on the right side. Axial CT image through the jugular foramen. A large and high jugular bulb (J) can be seen, and there is no bony plate between the jugular bulb and the middle ear cavity. Moreover, the jugular bulb is protruding in the middle ear cavity (small white arrow) and is lying against the stapes (arrowhead). Note umbo of the malleus (long white arrow).

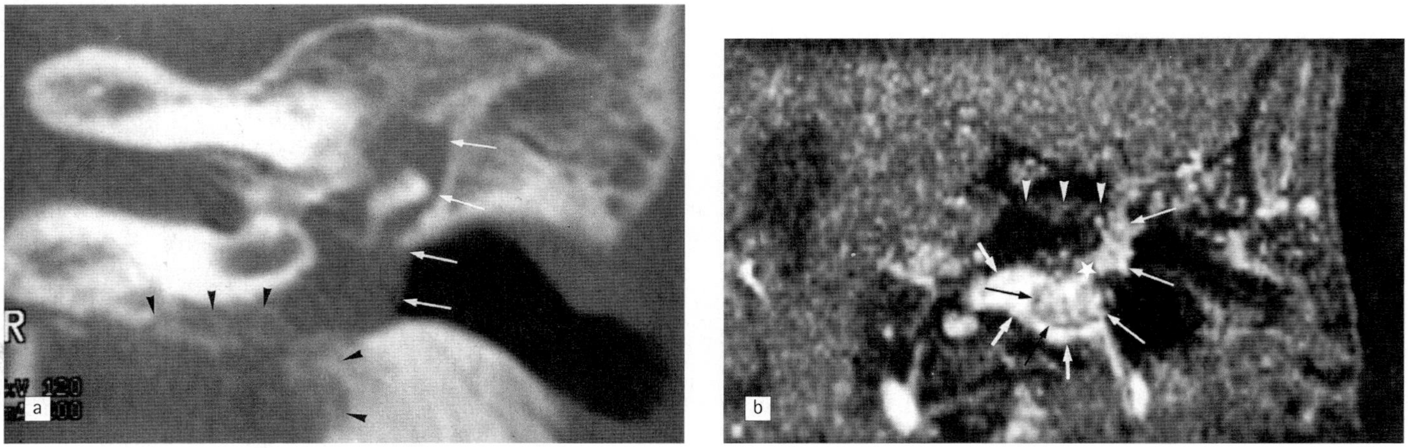

Figure 7.38 Glomus jugulotympanicum. Patient with tinnitus on the left side. Coronal CT image (a) and MRA time-of-flight image, paracoronal reconstruction (b) through the left middle ear and jugular foramen.

(a) The middle ear cavity is completely obliterated (white arrows). The edges of the jugular foramen are unsharp and destroyed, a common finding in glomus tumours (arrowheads).

(b) The MRA image shows the glomus tumor in the middle ear cavity (long white arrows) and in the canal of Jacobson (★). The extension in the jugular foramen (long black arrows) can also be seen, and the compressed and enhancing jugular bulb can be recognized (small white arrows). Note IAC (arrowheads).

Table 7.7 Causes of tinnitus[52]

Arterial causes	Arteriovenous causes	Venous causes
Atherosclerosis	Paraganglioma	Systemic conditions
Fibromuscular dysplasia	Miscellaneous vascular head and neck tumours	Intracranial hypertension
Spontaneous dissection ICA	Paget's disease	Transverse sinus stenosis
Styloid carotid compression	Otosclerosis or spongiosis	Idiopathic venous tinnitus
Petrous carotid aneurysm	Cerebral arteriovenous malformation	Large or exposed jugular bulb or large emissary veins
Aberrant carotid artery	Dural arteriovenous fistula	
Laterally displaced carotid artery Persistent stapedial artery Miscellaneous arterial anomalies	Direct arteriovenous fistula	

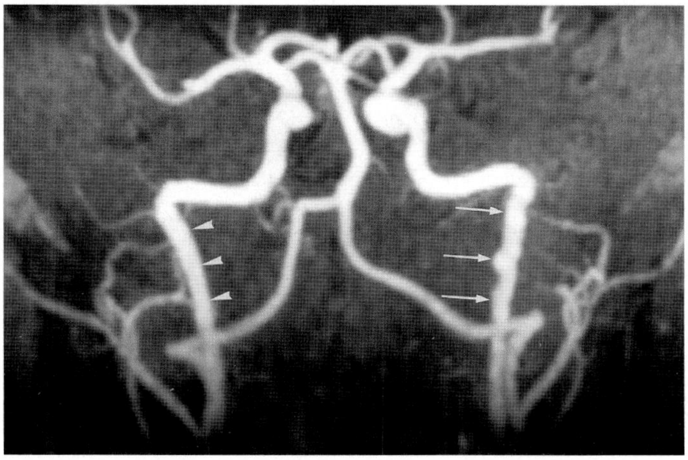

Figure 7.40 Fibromuscular dysplasia of the internal carotid artery. Patient with pulsatile tinnitus on the left side, getting worse during exercise and when the head is turned to the left side. Three-dimensional MRA reconstruction, antero-posterior view. The left internal carotid artery has an inconstant diameter and an irregular wall, compatible with fibromuscular dysplasia (white arrows). Compare with the normal smooth right internal carotid artery (arrowheads).

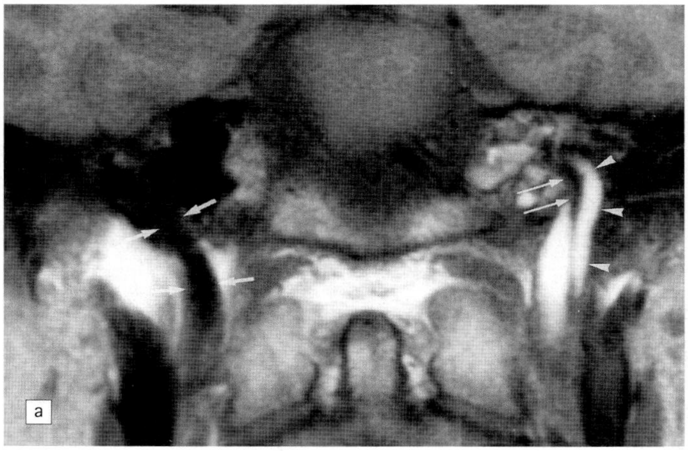

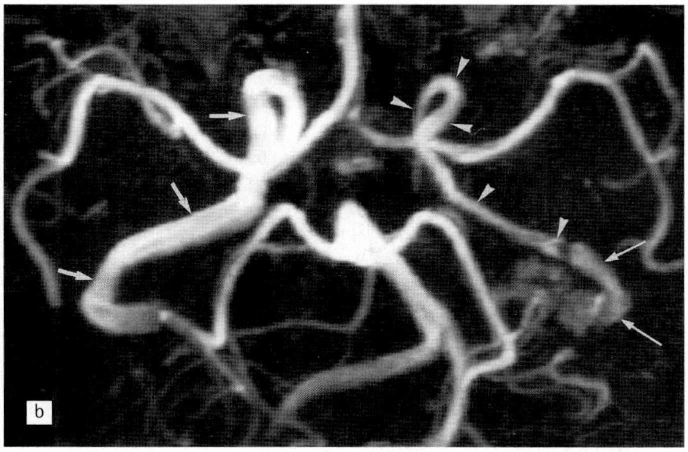

Figure 7.41 Dissection of the internal carotid artery. Patient presenting with a Horner syndrome and pulsatile tinnitus on the left side. Coronal unenhanced T1-weighted image (a) and 3D MRA reconstruction (b), viewed from above.

(a) Methaemoglobin can be seen in the wall of the internal carotid artery, situated just under the skull base (arrowheads). The remaining lumen with a flow void in it can also be seen (long white arrows). Compare with the normal diameter of the right internal carotid artery (small white arrows).

(b) The haematoma in the wall of the left internal carotid artery can be seen (long white arrows). The intracerebral part of the left internal carotid artery is narrowed (arrowheads). Compare with the normal diameter of the right internal carotid artery.

Cochlear implants

CT is needed to evaluate the pneumatization of the mastoid and middle ear cavity prior to surgery. Moreover, CT can be used to exclude the presence of an artery in an abnormal position in the middle ear cavity (e.g. stapedial artery) (Figure 7.42), a dehiscent tympanic portion of the facial nerve canal, abnormal course of the facial nerve in the middle ear cavity, and dehiscent or protruding jugular bulb (Figure 7.39). CT can also detect calcifications inside the cochlea (Figure 7.6) and the presence of a narrowed round window, jeopardizing normal

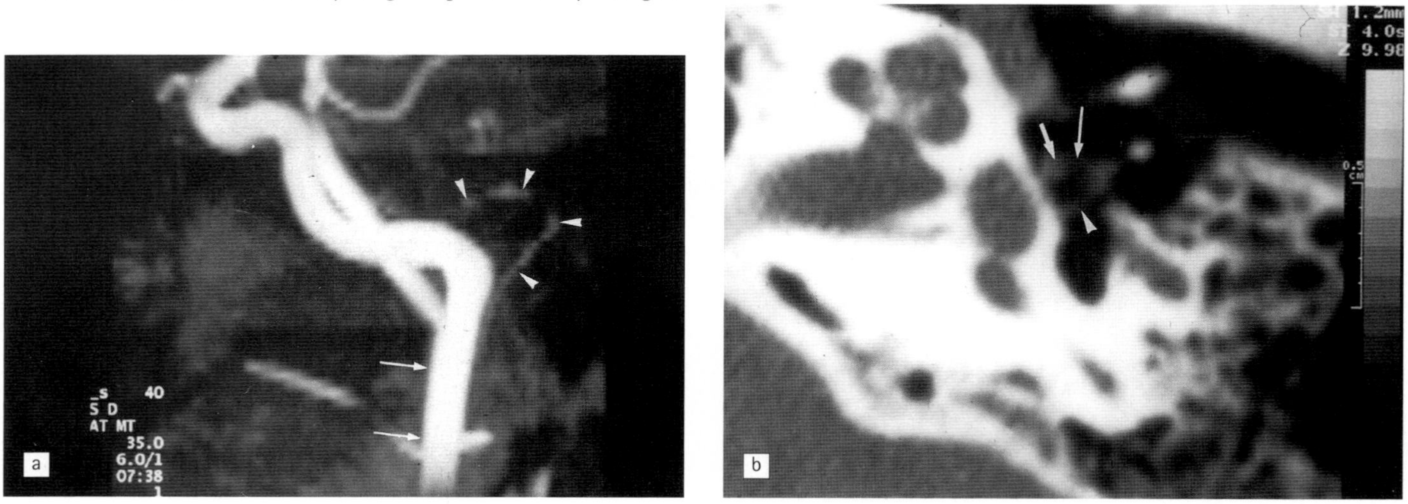

Figure 7.42 Stapedial artery. Patient with pulsatile tinnitus on the left side. Three-dimensional MRA reconstruction, lateral view (a) and axial CT image at the level of the stapes (b).

(a) An abnormal branch (arrowheads) leaves the internal carotid artery in its vertical (temporal bone) segment (white arrows) and has an abnormal course through the middle ear cavity.

(b) The stapedial artery (small white arrow) runs between the crurae of the stapes and is lying against the anterior crus of the stapes (long white arrow). Note posterior crus of the stapes (arrowhead). (Courtesy of Professor F. Veillon, CHRU Strasbourg, France.)

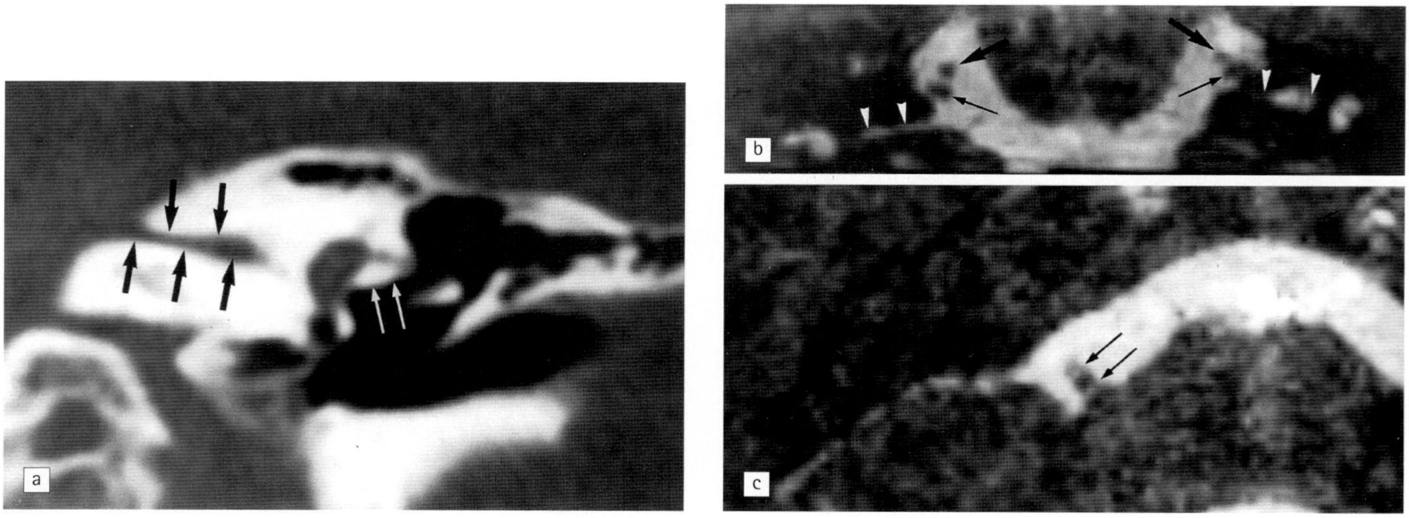

Figure 7.43 Aplasia of the vestibulocochlear nerve with abnormal course of the facial nerve. Bilateral congenital deafness, cochlear implant candidate. Coronal CT image (a) and coronal (b) and axial (c) 3DFT-CISS image through the inner ears.

(a) The left IAC is stenotic (black arrows), and the tympanic segment of the facial nerve canal is not seen in its normal position under the lateral semicircular canal (white arrows). Similar findings were seen on the right side (not shown).

(b) The stenotic IACs are confirmed (arrowheads). No nerves enter the IACs and the facial nerves (long black arrows) can be seen above the level of the IACs and are seen just below the trigeminal nerves (large black arrows).

(c) The vestibulocochlear nerves could not be found on both sides. The right facial nerve leaves the brainstem very high (black arrows). At this level, we see the temporal lobe above the temporal bone. The nerve could be followed to the roof of the temporal bone, where it disappeared between the roof of the temporal bone and the temporal lobe.

cochlear implant installation. The above-mentioned signs of a 'gusher ear' can also be recognized (Figure 7.9). MR is complementary to CT and offers the following possibilities:

- Detection of fibrotic obliteration of the membranous labyrinth
- Detection of enhancement in the cochlea due to infection, recent fibrosis, schwannoma
- Detection of the gusher ear signs
- Detection of a normal or absent or hypoplastic cochlear branch of the vestibulocochlear nerve (Figure 7.22)
- Detection of lesions along the central auditory pathway and in the auditory cortex, or detection of white matter disease which could be life-threatening or could result in important psychomotoric retardation (Figure 7.35).

The real contraindications are absence of a fluid-filled cavity in the temporal bone and absence of a vestibulocochlear nerve (Figure 7.43).

References

1. Alexander AE, Caldemeyer KS, Rigby P. Clinical and surgical application of reformatted high-resolution CT of the temporal bone. *Neuroimaging Clin North Am* 1998; **8:** 31–50.
2. Casselman JW, Kuhweide R, Deimling M et al. Constructive interference in steady state (CISS)-3DFT MR imaging of the inner ear and cerebellopontine angle. *Am J Neuroradiol* 1993; **14:** 47–57.
3. Schmalbrock P, Brogan MA, Chakeres DW et al. Optimization of submillimeter-resolution MR imaging methods for the inner ear. *J Magn Reson Imaging* 1993; **3:** 451–9.
4. Tanioka H, Shirakawa T, Machida T et al. Three-dimensional reconstructed MR imaging of the inner ear. *Radiology* 1991; **178:** 141–4.
5. Tien RD, Felsberg GJ, Macfall J. Three dimensional MR gradient recalled echo imaging of the inner ear: comparison of FID and echo imaging techniques. *Magn Reson Imaging* 1993; **11:** 429–35.
6. Bradley WG. MR of the brain stem: a practical approach. *Radiology* 1991; **179:** 319–32.
7. Weissman JL, Curtin HD, Hirsch BE et al. High signal from the otic labyrinth on unenhanced magnetic resonance imaging. *Am J Neuroradiol* 1992; **13:** 1183–7.
8. Casselman JW, Kuhweide R, Ampe W, Meeus L, Steyaert L. Pathology of the membranous labyrinth: comparison of T1- and T2-weighted and gadolinium-enhanced spin-echo and 3DFT-CISS imaging. *Am J Neuroradiol* 1993; **14:** 59–69.
9. Tien R, Felsberg GJ, Macfall J. Fast spin-echo high resolution MR imaging of the inner ear. *Am J Roentgenol* 1992; **159:** 395–8.
10. Dietz RR, Davis WL, Harnsberger HR, Jacobs JM, Blatter DD. MR imaging and MR angiography in the evaluation of pulsatile tinnitus. *Am J Neuroradiol* 1994; **15:** 890–2.
11. Casselman JW, Kuhweide R, Ampe W et al. Magnetic resonance examination of the inner ear and cerebellopontine angle in patients with vertigo and/or abnormal findings at vestibular testing. *Acta Otolaryngol (Stockh)* 1994; **513**(suppl): 15–27.
12. Mark AS. Contrast-enhanced magnetic resonance imaging of the temporal bone. *Neuroimaging Clin North Am* 1994; **4:** 561–78.
13. Matthews VP, Kuharik MA, Edwards MK, d'Amour PG, Azzarelli B, Dreesen RG. Gd-DTPA enhanced MR imaging of experimental bacterial meningitis evaluation and comparison with CT. *Am J Neuroradiol* 1988; **9:** 1045–50.
14. Casselman JW, Majoor MHJM, Albers F. MR of the inner ear in patients with Cogan syndrome. *Am J Neuroradiol* 1994; **15:** 131–8.
15. Casselman JW, Kuhweide R, Ampe W et al. Inner ear malformations in patients with sensorineural hearing loss detection with gradient-echo (3DFT-CISS) MR imaging. *Neuroradiology* 1996; **38:** 278–86.
16. Jackler RK, De la Cruz A. The large vestibular aqueduct syndrome. *Laryngoscope* 1989; **99:** 1238–43.
17. Hirsch BE, Weisman JL, Curtin HD, Kamerer DB. Magnetic resonance imaging of the large vestibular aqueduct. *Arch Otolaryngol Head Neck Surg* 1992; **118**: 1124–7.
18. Davidson HC, Harnsberger HR, Lemmerling MM, Mancuso AA, White DK, Tong KA, Dahlen RT, Shelton C. MR evaluation of vestibulocochlear anomalies associated with large endolymphatic duct and sac. *Am J Neuroradiol* 1993; **20**: 1435–41.
19. Jackler RK, Luxford WM, House WF. Congenital malformations of the inner ear: a classification based on embryogenesis. *Laryngoscope* 1987; **97:** 2–14.
20. Hasso AN, Casselman JW, Broadwell RA. Temporal bone congenital anomalies. In Som PM, Curtin HD, eds. *Head and Neck Imaging*. St Louis: Mosby-Year Book, 1996; 1351–90.
21. Phelps PD, Reardon W, Pembrey M. X-linked deafness, stapes gushers and a distinctive defect of the inner ear. *Neuroradiology* 1991; **33:** 326–30.
22. Mafee MF, Lachenauer CS, Kumar A, Arnold PM, Buckingham RA, Valvassori GE. CT and MR imaging of intralabyrinthine schwannoma: report of two cases and review of the literature. *Radiology* 1990; **174:** 395–400.
23. Yamamoto M, Hagiwara S, Ide M, Jimbo M, Arai Y, Ono Y. Conservative management of acoustic neurinomas: prospective study of long-term changes in tumor volume and auditory function. *Minim Invasive Neurosurg* 1998; **41:** 86–92.
24. Lo WW, Solti-Bohman LG. Tumors of the temporal bone and the cerebellopontine angle. In Som PM, Bergeron RT, eds. *Head and Neck Imaging*. St Louis: Mosby-Year Book, 1996: 1449–531.
25. Ouallet JC, Marsot-Dupuch K, Kujas M, VanEffenterre R, Tubiana JM. Imaging features of temporal bone tumors in Von Hippel–Lindau disease: tumors with a papillary pattern. *J Neurosurg* 1997; **87:** 445–449.
26. Huang TS. Primary intravestibular lipoma. *Ann Otol Rhinol Laryngol* 1989; **98:** 393–5.
27. Urman ST, Talbot M. Otic capsule dysplasia: clinical and CT findings. *Radiographics* 1990; **10:** 823–38.
28. Swartz JD, Harnsberger HR. The otic capsule and otodystrophies. In: Swartz JD, Harnsberger HR, eds. *Imaging of the Temporal Bone*. New York: Thieme, 1998; 240–317.
29. Veillon F, Baur P, Dasch JC, Braun M, Pharaboz C. Traumatismes de l'os temporal. In: Veillon F, ed. *Imagerie de l'oreille*. Paris, Médecine-Sciences Flammarion, 1991; 243–81.

30. Mark AS, Fitzgerald D. Segmental enhancement of the cochlea on contrast-enhanced MR: correlation with the frequency of hearing loss and possible sign of perilymphatic fistula and autoimmune labyrinthitis. *Am J Neuroradiol* 1993; **14:** 991–6.
31. Casselman JW. Temporal bone imaging. *Neuroimaging Clin North Am* 1996; **6:** 265–89.
32. Dubrulle F, Ernst O, Vincent C, Vaneecloo FM, Lejeune J-P, Lemaitre L. Enhancement of the cochlear fossa in the MR evaluation of vestibular schwannoma: correlation with success at hearing preservation surgery. *Radiology* 2000; **215**: 458–62.
33. Somers T, Casselman J, de Ceulaer G, Govaerts P, Offeciers FE. Prognostic value of MRI findings in hearing preservation surgery for vestibular schwannoma. *Otol Neurotol* 2001; **22**: 87–94.
34. Sartoretti-Schefer S, Kollias S, Wichmann W, Valavanis AS. T2-weighted three-dimensional fast spin-echo MR in inflammatory peripheral facial nerve palsy. *Am J Neuroradiol* 1998; **19:** 491–5.
35. Smith MM, Thompson JE, Castillo M, Carrier D, Mukherji SK, Gilliam D. Choristomas of the seventh and eighth cranial nerves. *Am J Neuroradiol* 1997; **18:** 327–30.
36. Ouallet JC, Marsot-Dupuch K, Kujas M, VanEffenterre R, Tubiana JM. Imaging features of temporal bone tumors in Von Hippel–Lindau disease: tumors with a papillary pattern. *J Neurosurg* 1997; **87:** 445–9.
37. Cohen TI, Powers SK, Williams DW. MR appearance of intracanalicular eighth nerve lipoma. *Am J Neuroradiol* 1992; **13:** 1188–90.
38. Goyal M, Malik A, Mishra NK, Gaikwad SB. Idiopathic hypertrophic pachymeningitis: spectrum of the disease. *Am J Roentgenol* 1997; **169:** 1421–4.
39. Casselman JW, Offeciers FE, Govaerts PJ et al. Aplasia and hypoplasia of the vestibulocochlear nerve: diagnosis with MR imaging. *Radiology* 1997; **202:** 773–81.
40. Bracchi M, Savoiardo M, Triulzi F et al. Superficial siderosis of the CNS: MR diagnosis and clinical findings. *Am J Neuroradiol* 1993; **14:** 227–36.
41. Jannetta PJ. Neurovascular cross-compression in patients with hyperactive dysfunction symptoms of the eighth cranial nerve. *Surg Forum* 1975; **26:** 467–8.
42. Girard N, Poncet M, Chays A et al. Neurovascular compression in the CP angle. *Riv Neuroradiol* 1995; **8:** 981–9.
43. Rousseau GL, Jannetta PJ, Hirsch B, Moller MB, Moller AR. Restoration of useful hearing after microvascular decompression of the cochlear nerve. *Am J Otol* 1993; **14:** 392–7.
44. Swartz JD, Harnsberger HR. Temporal bone vascular anatomy, anomalies, and diseases, emphasizing the clinical–radiological problem of pulsatile tinnitus. In: Swartz JD, Harnsberger HR, eds. *Imaging of the Temporal Bone*. New York: Thieme, 1998; 170–239.
45. Deplanque D, Godefroy O, Guerouaou D, Laureau E, Desaulty A. Sudden bilateral deafness: lateral inferior pontine infarction. *J Neurol Neurosurg Psychiatry* 1998; **64:** 817–18.
46. Praamstra P, Hagoort P, Maassen B, Crul T. Word deafness and auditory cortical function. A case history and hypothesis. *Brain* 1991; **114:** 1197–225.
47. Sasaki O, Ootsuka K, Taguchi K, Kikukawa M. Multiple sclerosis presented acute hearing loss and vertigo *ORL J Otorhinolaryngol Relat Spec* 1994; **56:** 55–9.
48. Schweitzer VG, Shepard N. Sudden hearing loss: an uncommon manifestation of multiple sclerosis. *Otolaryngol Head Neck Surg* 1989; **100:** 327–32.
49. Weissman JL. Imaging in Meniere's disease. *Otolaryngol Clin North Am* 1997; **30:** 1105–16.
50. Kim SG, Ugurbil K. Comparison of blood oxygenation and cerebral blood flow effects in fMRI: estimation of relative oxygen consumption change. *Magn Reson Med* 1997; **38:** 59–65.
51. Millen SJ, Haughton VM, Yetkin Z. Functional magnetic resonance imaging of the central auditory pathway following speech and pure-tone stimuli. *Laryngoscope* 1995; **105:** 1305–10.
52. Lo WWM, Solti-Bohman LG. Vascular tinnitus. In: Som PM, Curtin HD, eds. *Head and Neck Imaging*. St Louis, Mosby-Year Book, 1996; 1535–49.

8 Ethics, law and related matters

Ronald Hinchcliffe

Introduction

The scientist will have it that 'The universe we observe has precisely the properties we should expect if there is, at bottom, no design, no purpose, no evil and no good, nothing but blind, pitiless indifference ... DNA neither cares nor knows. DNA just is. And we dance to its music.'[1] Nevertheless, here on planet Earth, life-forms have evolved in the form of organisms (animals and plants) and microorganisms.

The biologist will attribute human behaviour and beliefs to genes[2] and memes.[3] Another perspective[4] will see the lives and working practices of humans over planet Earth being determined by a constellation of behavioural controls (normative systems) which are subsumed under the headings: customs, religion, laws, ethics, standards, guidelines, instructions. These controls or recommendations range from laws that say we must not kill other members of our species to the instructions on a packet whose contents are for the preparation of a cup of soup. Failure to obey can affect one's quality of life permanently and to the severest degree, or merely transitorily and minimally, as we sense that the taste of the soup is not what we might have expected. These controls are, indeed, all-pervasive. They govern what I say in this chapter, the paper on which it is printed, on which days it may be read, and even whether it may be read at all.

A previous review[5] on the theme of this chapter approached the matter from the perspective of the English common law. But, as pointed out more than half a century ago, 'Nothing can distort the true picture of conditions and events in this world than to regard one's own country as the centre of the universe, and to view all things solely in their relationship to this fixed point. It is inevitable that such a method of observation should create an entirely false perspective.'[6] This review will seek to remedy the Christian anglocentric bias of the previous review, which nevertheless complements this chapter.

Ethics and law have their origins in customs and religion. It is therefore appropriate to consider first these two precursors.

NORMATIVE SYSTEMS

- Custom
- Religion
- Ethics
- Customary law
- Law

Customs and customary law

Customs

The customs or mores of a society are those patterns of behaviour in a society which have come to be accepted as characteristic of, and accepted within, that society.[4] These unwritten customs and conventions are not dictated by some external agency but result from a slow process of social evolution.[7]

Knowledge of the customs within, and the organization of, societies comes from the reports of anthropologists, sociologists, travellers and others. There is, and always has been, an immense amount of literature on this topic. It ranges, for example, from studies of a pre-literate people in East Africa, the Ik,[8] to studies of a most advanced, culturally and economically, society in Far East Asia, the Japanese.[9] The Ik are reported as 'Man without Law'; Japanese society, although capitalistic and industrialized, runs along different lines to European societies.

Customary law

The basis for customary law is when a judicial authority has established sanctions in respect of one or more custom. Non-legal customs remain social conventions.[4]

Customary law is much more important outside Europe, e.g. in Latin America[10] and in Northern Asia.[11] Traditional Arabian tribal society has preserved in its customary law and practice a very great deal that derives directly from the pre-Islamic period.[12] Nevertheless, *'Adah* (customs – of individuals or groups) and *'Urf* (recurring practices which are acceptable to people of sound nature) are recognized as a subsidiary source of the *Shari'ah* by all Islamic schools of jurisprudence.[13]

The *hiit khoong* code of the Lao in Thailand is in all likelihood of pre-Buddhist origin, though partially influenced by Buddhist thought and morality. The practical purpose of the code is the prevention of social and political conflicts. Harmony and conflict-free social interaction are highly appreciated by the Lao. The *hiit khoong* code is the most important expedient to ensure contant social harmony. The preventive character shows an important difference to Western law conceptions, which accept the conflict as a social reality and which are oriented to solve existing conflicts rather than to prevent them.[14]

Customary law gradually became written down, in Europe at least. In France, for example, this was effected under the authority of the local *seigneurs*, and later under royal ordinance, e.g. the *Ordonnance de Montils-les-Tours* of Charles VII in 1453. However, Article 7 of the Act of 21 March 1804 (30 *ventose an* XII), which introduced the *Code civil des Français* (renamed the *Code Napoléon* in 1807), provided that custom was to cease to have effect in matters covered by the Code. Nevertheless, in 1902 the *Cour de Cassation* (the highest court in France) held that a judge must take into account a custom if he is aware of its existence.[15] In Germany, *Gewohnheitsrecht* (customary law) is now a limited source of new law, although it provides the judiciary with an instrument with which they can introduce general principles of law to fill gaps in legislation and to overcome ambiguities in a *Gesetz* (a Statute).[16]

Religion

Religion may be defined as a system of beliefs and practices by means of which a group of people struggle with the ultimate problems of human life.[17]

Hinduism[18,19]

The *Srutis* (1500 to 600 BC) are the ancient sacred texts of Hinduism, the directly revealed scripture. They are the source of all knowledge. They describe principles of morality and behaviour to which everyone must conform in order to live in divine harmony. Only fragments of the *Srutis* remain. To understand fully the teachings of the *Srutis*, one needs to consult the *s(h)astras* or *smr(i)tis* ('memorized tradition'), which are thus secondary to the divine revelations. This second tier comprises four goals for humankind, or pillars on which world order rests, i.e. *dharma*, *artha*, *kama* and *moksha*. *Dharma* encompasses the totality of religion; it specifies the moral norm, which is specific to an individual's social class and stage of life. But other cultures have also sanctioned the stratification of society, and perhaps more so. Early Irish society was hierarchical and inegalitarian. A maxim in an Old Irish law text, *Tecosca Cormaic*, was: *isel cach aithech* (every commoner is low).[20]

Dharma like the Muslim *fikh*, rejects the distinction between religious and legal obligations but is much more all-embracing than *fikh*. In so doing, *dharma* obviates the problems in other cultures of conflicts between law and morality.[21] The concept of 'rights' is alien to *dharma*. *Artha* encompasses the whole range of activities associated with material gain and its protection, extending to the art of government, with concepts reminiscent of those in Machiavelli's *The Prince*,[22] which was to follow much later. *Kama* is concerned with the pursuit of both aesthetic and sensual pleasure. *Moksha* (liberation) is the culmination of *dharma*, *artha* and *kama* when properly followed, i.e. the supreme goal of mortal existence.

Buddhism[23,24]

Buddhism is the tradition of the thinking and practice of Shakyamuni, the Buddha, who lived in India in the 6/5 century BCE. Gautama Buddha's *Ariva-Sacca* (four Noble Truths) relate to the universality of suffering, which is the result of desire and craving. In order to eradicate the suffering, one must follow the threefold path (way, training) of *sila*, *samadhi* and *panna* (*prajna*).[25] *Sila* is the moral code, which comprises the five precepts (*pansil*) of refraining from (1) harming living things, (2) taking that which has not been given to one, (3) excessive sensuality, (4) false and harmful speech, and (5) using intoxicants. The three positive features of *sila* are right speech, right bodily action, and right means of livelihood. *Samadhi* is interpreted variously as concentration,[26] meditation, or even trance.[25] *Prajna* signifies wisdom or, more strictly, apprehending the truth taught by the Buddha,[25] and so perhaps can be interpreted as insight.[26]

Reflecting their belief in Buddhism, the Chinese and Japanese perceive death as a natural part of and an extension of life itself.[27]

Judaism

The *Torah* constitutes the divine teachings of Judaism, a religion which is much older than Christianity or Islam. In its narrowest sense, it refers to the Pentateuch, the first five books of the Hebrew Bible. In its broadest sense, *Torah* encompasses the whole of the Jewish Bible, together with the whole of traditional Jewish lore and law. The *Mishnah* constitutes the first text of rabbinical Judaism; the *Talmud* is the wide-ranging commentary on the *Mishnah*. *Halakhah* refers to the legal material in the *Talmud*. *Aggadah* refers to the non-legal, but ethical, material in rabbinical literature in addition to the *Talmud*.[25,28]

Christianity

With more than a billion followers, Christianity[29] is the most common religion in the world, although in the highly secularized countries of Europe and North America it is often nominal.

Islam

With around a billion followers, Islam[30] is a religion and a way of life based on the commandments of Allah contained in the

Holy Qur'an and the *Sunnah* of the Prophet of Islam, Muhammad (Sallallaho 'Alaihi Wasallam).[31] Unlike Christianity, Islam could never become a private religion of personal conscience and ethics. It is a complete way of life. Even the way in which a glass of water is to be drunk is determined by Islamic religious law.[32]

Shintoism

Shinto[33,34] is a religion that is unique to Japan. Purity of body and soul is a central tenet of Shintoism. Shinto priests will ceremonially cleanse an individual's body and soul (*harai*) to achieve the clean ideal. People will go to the Shinto shrines to pray to the gods, e.g. to avoid disease or seek a cure, or for success in examinations.[35]

Ethics

In general

Ethics is basically concerned with what is good, and what is bad, with what are right courses of action, and what are not. Every culture has developed an ethic of its own. Depending on the social setting, the authority invoked for good conduct is the will of God, the pattern of nature, or the rule of reason. Religions provide various forms of motivation for moral, i.e. ethical, action. Buddhism,[36,37] Christianity,[38–41] Hinduism,[42] Islam,[43] Judaism[44,45] and Shintoism[35] all make contributions. Buddhism teaches us not to harm animals, plants, trees or forests; it is therefore in the forefront of conservation and environmentalism. Its *Path of Life* offers prescriptions for the ethico-spiritual wellbeing of every individual. Moral as well as intellectual perfection is a constituent of the Buddhist *nirvana* (final good).[46] Christian belief makes a crucial difference to an understanding of ethical issues, while at the same time demonstrating some of the weaknesses and confusions of certain popular approaches to them.[47] Several Hindu ethical themes are worthy of the attention of Western philosophers. These include the *Bhagavadgita*, since it is open to various interpretations.[42] Judaism is rooted in the ethical principles of justice and mercy. The *Aggadah* has been referred to as the 'wellspring' of Jewish morality.[28] The *Inaba-no-Shirousagi* (white hare of Inaba) story in the *Kojiki* illustrates the mercy of the Shinto gods to all creatures—comparable to the *Zihi* (benevolence) of Buddhism.[35]

Medical ethics[48]

There are few matters related to health and medical practice that have no ethical implications. The problems range from the use of highly technical procedures, or how the value of these should be assessed, to whether or not resources should be allocated at all to such use or enquiries.[49]

The compassion for all creatures, without discrimination, which Buddhism teaches is an essential component of the medical practitioner's attitude towards his patients.[50] Although beginning from very different religious premises, Buddhism tends to medical ethical conclusions[51] which are broadly similar to those found within mainstream Christianity.[52] Islam also makes a contribution to medical ethics.[53]

A common ethical code for everybody involved in healthcare is desirable, but there are important limitations to the role such a code could play. Such an ethical code could establish important values and describe a common ethical context for healthcare, but it may be of limited use in solving new and complex ethical problems.[54]

It is useful to analyse medical ethical concepts in terms of legal principles and court decisions,[55] but attempts to respond to complex bioethical questions by legislation are difficult and may become controversial.[56]

Related matters

Professional medical ethics

In European civilization, the history of medical ethics goes back to the Hippocratic tradition. The British Medical Association[57] pointed out that, while the ethical systems of other European countries have been codified and incorporated in national civil and criminal law, the UK has proceeded along a different path. The UK's General Medical Council (GMC)[58] has enforced professional standards on the basis of guidance rather than through a codified system. The GMC has the power to restrict or remove a doctor's right to practice if he is found to be guilty of 'serious professional misconduct'.[59]

ETHICS

- Professional
- Doctor–patient
- Research

Partly because of professional solidarity and partly because of the stigma of being a 'whistle-blower', there has been an undoubted reluctance of colleagues to report instances of clinical or research misconduct. The Public Interest Disclosure Act 1998, which took effect from 2 July 1999, has changed this situation in the UK.

Doctor–patient relationship

The basis of the doctor–patient relationship is trust[60] and confidence.[61] The patient has to be given sufficient information for consent to investigation and treatment[62] to be grounded in trust.

Research on human subjects

There are basically two ethical problems in respect of medical research. First, is there valid consent? In this context, consent to an action which is basically wrong cannot change it into a rightful one. Second, do the ends justify the means?[63] To these two basic problems, one should add a third problem: is the confidentiality of the required data safeguarded?

As pointed out by the Council for International Organizations of Medical Sciences,[64] the generalized application of the experimental scientific method by medical research is a product of the present century. Consideration is required both in developed and developing countries as to whether prevailing legal provisions and administrative arrangements ensure that the rights and welfare of subjects involved in research are adequately considered and protected in conformity with the ethical principles prescribed in the Declaration of Helsinki by the 18th World Medical Assembly 1964, as revised by the 48th World Medical Assembly in 1997,[65] or in conformity with other research codes.[66]

In Britain, the Royal College of Physicians of London produced *Guidelines on the Practice of Ethics Committees for Medical Research*.[67] In 1991, the Department of Health produced its own guidelines for local research ethics committees (LRECs).[68] A subsequent Health Service Guidelines document HSG(97)23 introduced a new system for obtaining ethical approval for multicentre research.[69] Multicentre research ethics committees (MRECs) complement the work of existing LRECs. Multicentre research is defined as that which is carried out within five or more LRECs' geographical boundaries.

In the USA, the institutional review boards (IRBs) equate with the British LRECs. The University of Pittsburgh's IRB, for example, maintains a website (Acrobat format) for its guidelines.[70] The US Food and Drug Administration maintains a website[71] for the guidance of IRBs and clinical investigators. The US National Institutes of Health also provides information on bioethics resources on the web.[72]

Of particular relevance to research on human subjects, the US National Library of Medicine provides information at websites on consent,[73] privacy and confidentiality,[74] and clinical trials.[75]

One publication covers every significant ethical issue likely to be faced by researchers and research ethics committees.[76]

Research misconduct

Research misconduct is a topic which is attracting increasing attention.[77] The term covers piracy, plagiarism and fraud.[78]

Medical audit

Medical audit[79,80] encompasses the collection and use of information for effective resource management and improved patient care. Increasingly, computers are becoming an integral part of the clinical audit function.[81] Medical audit is not without ethical considerations,[82] and there are questions as to who audits audit.[83] In making use of clinical audit, one should have in mind its relationship to other forms of quality assurance and knowledge generation.[84] With this in mind, one should not forget the contribution that autopy studies can make.[85]

Medical audit leads on to clinical effectiveness,[86–88] and this leads to clinical governance.[89–92] In association with all this, clinical risk management is of increasing concern.[93,94]

Law

Law has been defined as the enforceable body of rules that governs any society.[95] As the Social Sciences and Humanities Research Council of Canada (SSHRC) points out, the law tends to compel obedience to behavioural norms. Ethics aim to promote high standards of behaviour through an awareness of values, which may develop with practice and which may have to accommodate choice and liability to err. Further, though ethical approaches cannot pre-empt the application of the law, they may well affect its future development or deal with situations beyond the scope of the law.[96]

MAJOR LEGAL SYSTEMS

- Romano-Germanic (civil law)
- English common law
- Socialist law
- Religious
  - *Shari'ah*

Legal systems

Hindu law

The three realms of human activity, *dharma*, *artha* and *kama*, together constitute the custom of Hinduism. Hindu society is expected to live and resolve disputes according to custom. Hence Hindu law is customary law. The *Dharma-S(h)astras*, together with the *Artha-S(h)astras* and *Kama-S(h)astras*, which constitute the commentaries on *dharma*, *artha* and *kama*, are taken as sources for this customary law. The *nibandhas*, which are commentaries on the *dharma-shastras*, are necessary in order to resolve any apparent contradiction in the *dharma-shastras*, which, *inter alia*, include the laws of *Manu*, of *Yajnavalkya* and *Narada*. If there is no rule of law applicable to the case in question, an individual must act, and the judges decide, according to equity, good conscience and justice. The doctrine of precedents has no place in Hindu customary law; a judge (a prince in historical times) must be able in all cases to vary a decision so that it will conform to a more expedient policy at any time in the future.[97–99]

Buddhist law

The influence of law derived from Buddhism has not been comparable to that derived from other religions, such as Islam. It was nevertheless evident in South-East Asia in historical times.[100] In Thailand, Buddhist law codes developed under the influence of Theravada Buddhism from the 13th century. Buddhist law was of special juridical significance in religious and urban centres.[14] A Buddhist theocracy existed in Tibet until 1951, although its excesses were inconsistent with the tenets of the religion it purported to represent.[101] In Bhutan, 12 monastic representatives are elected to the *Tshogdu* (National Assembly) by the Buddhist ecclesiastical bodies.[102] In this way,

Bhutanese law is influenced by Buddhist religion and morality. Article 9 of the Sri Lankan 1972 republican constitution gave pre-eminence to Buddhism.

Jewish law

Jewish Law is founded on the faith that the *Torah* is the word of God. Although it is not primarily a code of law, the *Halakhah* can be equated with Rabbinic jurisprudence.[28] The traditional Jew is bound by codified halakhic decisions.

Islamic law[103]

Every Muslim is under an obligation to model the entirety of his life in accordance with the dictates of the *Qur'an* and *Sunnah*. He therefore must observe at every step the distinction between what is right (*Halal*) and what is wrong (*Haram*). This highlights the need for, and the importance of, a knowledge of the *corpus juris* of Islam, the *Shari'ah*. The *Qur'an* is the first primary source of *Shari'ah*, and the *Sunnah* the second primary source. *Sunnah* needs to be distinguished from *Hadith*; the latter is a narration of the conduct or sayings of the Prophet, whereas Sunnah is the law deduced from such.[13] *Al-Ijma'*, *Al-Quiyas*, *Al-Ijtihad*, *Istishab*, and *Istihsan* constitute secondary sources for the *Shari'ah*. *Al-Ijma'* encompasses the consensus of Islamic juristic opinions; *Al-Qiyas* is the legal principle for deriving a logical conclusion by analogical reasoning; *Al-Ijtihad* is the exercise of reasoning (*Al-Qiyas* is thus a special case of *Al-Ijtihad*); *Istishab* is a presumption in the laws of evidence that a state of affairs known to exist in the past continues to exist until the contrary is proved; a special case is the presumption of innocence until guilt has been proven.[31] As well as coming into play when judgements could be contrary to the public interest, *Istihsan* is similar to the equity of the English common law, in that both are inspired by the principles of fairness and conscience; both authorize a departure from the rule of positive law when its enforcement leads to unfair results; but whereas equity recognizes some superiority of natural law, *Istihsan* recognizes only the superiority of divine revelation.[13] *Usul al-fiqh* embodies the study of the sources of Islamic law and the methodology for its development, i.e. Islamic jurisprudence.[104]

At a time when many Muslim states are moving towards the reintroduction or reinforcement of Islamic law, there is the need for some acquaintanceship with the *Shari'ah*. However, many Islamic states have recently modified their law to meet society's changing values.[105]

Canon law

Canon law is that law which was developed and applied by the Christian church.[106] The ecclesiastical courts in the 12th and 13th centuries exercised considerable control in a number of European countries.[97] This influence declined with the secularization associated with the Reformation. The Vatican City state is now the only one in which canon law now holds sway. The Pope exercises sovereignty there; he has absolute legislative, executive and judicial powers.[102]

English common law

The common law is a uniquely English derivation.[107] Following the end of the Roman occupation in AD 430, England saw invasions by a number of tribes (Angles, Jutes, Saxons and Vikings) from northwestern Europe over the next six centuries. Each brought with them their own customary law. It was William the Conqueror's arrival from Normandy in AD 1066 which resulted in the definition of what these various customary laws had in common: hence the designation of this collated law as the 'common law'.

As well as being uncoded, the common law system is characterized by two other features, i.e. by the method of acquisition of evidence (adversarial, as opposed to the inquisitorial method of civil law systems), and the practice of judicial precedent. It is the latter which gives rise to what is termed case law.

Civil code (Romano-German law)

Civil law countries are those which have a codified law which was based originally on Roman legal principles.[108] Having been at one time part of the Roman Empire or subject to Napoleon's dictates explains the similarities which exist among the civil law countries of contemporary Europe.[15]

Socialist law

Marxist-Leninists saw law as a means of transforming society in the desired direction. Once the ideal of a pure socialist society had been achieved, it would no longer be needed. But the aim of law as being one of 'social engineering' was also perceived by the Harvard jurist Roscoe Pound.[109] Only the conceived end result differed. It has nevertheless been argued that, however ideal the society that socialists envisage, legal institutions would still be necessary to adjudicate conflict between private and public interests.[110]

Geographical entities

State laws

Before the Industrial Revolution, the two principal functions of governments had been to maintain domestic law and order and to make war on the governments and peoples of foreign states. The inhuman conditions of work and life that the Industrial Revolution imposed on a new social class, the workers in mechanized factories, compelled governments to undertake a third function—the provision for social welfare. The first legislation for the protection of factory workers was enacted in Britain in 1802. Between 1883 and 1889, Bismarck extended the social field of governmental action in Germany by securing the passage of legislation that provided insurance against sickness, accidents and incapacitation by old age and other causes. This recognition that governments have a duty to provide for their subjects' welfare was a beneficial ethical advance in the field of politics. The state has now become a welfare organization, besides continuing to be a law-enforcing and a war-making organization, in most of the world's industrialized countries. However, the welfare state is still a controversial issue. The provision of public services for the benefit of the indigent majority of the population required the raising of additional public revenue by steeply graded taxation of the affluent minority. But all states, whatever their ideological colour, have continued to be war-making institutions (with the exception of Costa Rica, which has no Army).[111]

Thus each modern state, e.g. the UK, has developed its social security law,[112] healthcare law,[113] and workers' health and safety law.

Medical law is a rapidly expanding area of law in, for example, Belgium,[114] Canada,[115] Eire,[116] Finland,[115] Greece,[117] New Zealand,[115] the UK[118] and the USA.[115]

With increasing worldwide concern regarding environmental pollution, an ever-increasing number of states have specific environmental laws, but there are different approaches of English, European and international law to environmental pollution control.[119]

With more than 200 states in the world, space does not allow the inclusion of references to the laws of all these countries. A sample of the world's states, in alphabetical order, is considered below.

China

The traditional Chinese concept of law is completely different from that in the West.[97] Confucius (551–479 BC), who was himself a judge, held that the basis of society was not law but ethics and ritual (ways of living). To enact laws was bad policy. The very exactitude which laws establish in social relationships, and the way in which they fix the rights and obligations of each individual, were considered evils. Once individuals think of their 'rights', there is, it was thought, some form of social illness; the only true matter of concern is one's duty to society and to one's fellow men. There is thus some similarity to the ancient principles of Celtic culture, where *firrinys* (truth), *onoir* (honour) and *currym* (duty) were dominant.

When private interests conflict, the Chinese argued that some middle road must be sought which takes into consideration the interests of both parties. One or other social group should act as arbitrator or mediator. Between World Wars I and II, Romano-Germanic codes were adopted to avoid colonization. With the communist takeover in 1949 and the abolition of private property, China was set to implement Soviet-style socialist law. Following the rupture with the USSR, the work of the codification commission came to an end. There was no more mention of socialist legality or humanistic socialism. Both concepts were considered incompatible with true Marxist-Leninist doctrine. With the more recent moves towards capitalism, changes in the law are again taking place.[120–122]

France

The Act of 21 March 1804 (30 *Ventose An* XII) introduced the *Code civil des Français* (renamed the *Code Napoléon* in 1807, and finally the *Code civil* in 1870). Napoleon's codification of the French law was to have a wide impact on the rest of Europe, as a direct result of French military and political power. Thus a number of countries share the common legal heritage not only of Roman law but also of the *Code civil des Français*, e.g. Belgium, Germany, Greece, Italy, Luxembourg, The Netherlands, Québec, Spain and Switzerland.[15,123]

Germany

A more scientific model of the *Code civil* emerged in Germany when the *Bürgerliches Gesetzbuch* (Code of Civil Law) came into force on 1 January 1900. This *Gestzbuch* has influenced the legal systems of Austria, Brazil, Greece, Hungary, Japan, Mexico, Peru, Switzerland and Turkey.[16,124]

The function of the judiciary in the German legal system is to apply the law, not to create it. Thus the doctrine of precedent does not exist; court decisions do not have any effect on future decisions.

India

Section 372 of the 1950 Constitution provided for the continuance of the previous law of India, which was based on the English common law.[125] The Hindu Code Acts 1955–56 largely abolished the shastraic basis of Hindu law and established a more or less uniform law for Hindus of all castes and regions. The current Code applies only to Hindus in India. Outside of the codified law, Hindu law retains its customary and religious base.[98,99]

The aim is to replace eventually all the religion-based laws of Buddhists, Christians, Hindus, Muslims and Parsees with a national secular law which will provide equality of status and opportunity for all individuals and promote the greatest degree of personal freedom consistent with the public good.[126]

Israel

The law of the state of Israel derives from when that land was part of the Ottoman Empire, and then under British rule. Only isolated remnants of Ottoman legislation are in force today. The application of religious laws is covered by the Law of Personal Status (personal, family and succession law). The *qadi* (Islamic judge) decides for Muslims, in accordance with the *Shari'ah*, and the various ecclesiastical courts in respect of the appropriate Christian sect. The Druze also have their own courts. Nevertheless, Jewish law plays an important role in interpreting the law, even in matters outside the jurisdiction of the religious courts. One or two experts in Jewish law sit on the Supreme Court.[127]

Japan

Until Japan was opened up in the mid-19th century, law as such did not exist there. As in China, which had influenced Japan's early history, rules of behaviour (more specifically, rules of propriety), *giri*, governed society. There were no school of law, lawyers or judges in the occidental sense. The whole constellation of *giri* specified the conduct to be observed on all occasions when individuals came into contact with one another. The concept was that of filial relationships based on attentive protection and respectful subordination. Social reprobation was attached to its non-observance. However, following the westernization programme that developed in the 19th century, a legal code based primarily on German law appeared in 1898. After 1945, legal reforms aimed at democratization were introduced at the behest of the USA.[128,129] However, questions have been raised as to whether or not Japanese society has undergone any substantial change behind this facade of westernization. Japanese mystical sentimentalism has rendered the people, basically poetic rather than logical, indifferent to the occidental ideals of human dignity and freedom.[97]

Russia
Prior to the Bolshevik revolution, the Russian social order was dominated by customs and not law. After the revolution, the USSR adopted a socialist legal system.[130] The dissolution of the USSR was followed by a new legal system. The new legal system has its roots in the political and economic origins of *perestroika*.[131]

Turkey
Turkish law exhibits a *mélange* of the laws of various other European countries.[132,133] The Civil Code and the Code of Obligations have been adapted from the corresponding Swiss codes; the Penal Code is based mainly on the Italian Penal Code; the Commercial Code is based on that of Germany. The Code of Civil Procedure is similar to that of Neuchâtel.[102]

UK
It was chance that played a major part and led to the paradox of a collection of feudal laws of continental origin becoming one of the most typical manifestations of English life and thought.[134] The universities have not played the role in the developments of the law of the UK that they have done in the countries of mainland Europe. Consequently, English law stands apart from the mainstream of Western legal culture.[135] Nevertheless, the English common law underpins to some degree or another the operational legal systems that affect more than a billion people on the planet. However, in common with Bhutan, the UK has no written constitution.

USA
It was natural that, after independence, the American colonies should continue with the English common law.

Regional law

In the case of *Costa* v *ENEL* (1964), the European Court of Justice (ECJ) ruled, *inter alia*, 'The transfer by the States from their domestic legal system to the Community legal system of the rights and obligations arising under the Treaty carries with it a permanent limitation of their sovereign rights, against which a subsequent unilateral act incompatible with the concept of the Community cannot prevail.' Thus the ECJ showed that EC provisions which do not specifically mention individuals may still create rights for them. Moreover, the ECJ indicated that the logic of EC law gives it supremacy over the domestic laws of its member states.[136,137]

Evidence, experts and judges

Evidence

A definition of evidence which was approved by a former Chancellor of Monash University[138] was that given in the Indian Evidence Act 1872, which is still in force in India today: 'Facts not otherwise relevant are relevant (1) if they are inconsistent with any fact in issue or relevant fact; (2) if by themselves or in connection with other facts they make the existence or non-existence of any fact in issue or relevant fact highly probably or improbable' (Section 11).

Expert witnesses

The Society of Expert Witnesses[139] has defined an expert as 'anyone with knowledge or experience of a particular field or discipline beyond what is expected of a layman', and an expert witness as 'an *expert* who makes his or her knowledge available to a court (or other judicial or quasi-judicial body)'. The Society of Expert Witnesses is an independent non-profit-making UK body which is run entirely by 'expert witnesses for expert witnesses' (unofficial motto); *Quisque ad praestantium nitens* (each towards excellence striving) (official motto).

Expert witnesses have existed for a long time in legal history. An Old Irish law text, *Bretha Crólige*, states that the sick-maintenance of a woman skilled in handicraft be assessed by three *brithems*: a *brithem* who is knowledgeable about food, a *brithem* competent in legal language, and an evaluating *brithem*.[20] Although the second is clearly a lawyer, the first and third are expert witnesses.

The Australian Federal Court has prepared Guidelines for Expert Witnesses.[140] The Medical Protection Society has provided advice on how to write medico-legal reports.[141]

In the UK, articles by lawyers[142–144] have drawn attention to rules for expert witnesses which follow Lord Woolf's report.[145] *The British Medical Journal* advises doctors to download and study the rules. They may have difficulty in accessing the cited URL (the Lord Chancellor's). It is easier at http://www.davidmarshall.co.uk/cpr.html, where they have been consolidated into a single file (769 kbytes) in Microsoft Word Format.

The lawyers highlight two principal problems, inter-examiner (or inter-expert) variability and financial matters. Inter-expert variability was not a problem when a large and diverse group of individuals and organizations (including representatives of the noise-exposed workers) gave evidence to the Industrial Injuries Advisory Council.[146] None of them were paid. Should we recommend examiners (and experts) to waive their fees? There are historical precedents.[147] In 1687, the College of Physicians and the Society of Apothecaries in London passed a resolution 'that all members of the College, whether fellows, candidates, or licentiates, shou'd give the advice gratis...' But a problem will remain. There appears to be an unbridgeable gap between the common law lawyers and the doctors, scientists and statisticians who are committed to an evidence-based society.[148]

Judgements

Under German law, the *Grundsatz der freien richterlichen Beweiswürdigung* (principle of the unfettered consideration of the evidence) means that there are no legal rules compelling the judge to consider evidence in any particular way and saying what emphasis, if any, should be put on any particular piece of evidence.[16]

Some European jurists have denied 'altogether that judicial law finding was based upon a rational process. The finding of the law according to him [Isay] is an intuitive process directed by certain sentiments and prejudices while the logical argument is substituted as an after-thought for the intuitive process and serves as make-believe towards the other world ... It is an illusion frequent among German exponents of the *Freirechtlehre* that the English judge has that majestic freedom from the fetters of the statute law which the continental judge lacks. In reality the obstacles presented to a progressive development of the law in the English system of precedent are considerably greater than those existing under codes which either contain general clauses or, like the Swiss code, specifically instruct the judge to develop the law in case of need.'[149]

A US judge has arguedly cogently that intuition is involved in judgements.[150] More recently, a psychologist has assessed studies of intuition and concluded that 'cognitive science is now well on the way to resuscitating the idea of the "intelligent unconscious" and along with it, the neglected faculty of intuition'.[151] However, in one case known to the author, a UK judge was unable to intuit the existence of a control group that showed no anamnestic or audiometric differences compared to a group of hazardous noise-exposed claimants.

Judges

It has often been said that the narrow-social-class background of English judges influences them. Eighty years ago, a senior British judge (Lord Justice Scrutton) said 'It is very difficult sometimes to be sure that you have put yourself into a thoroughly impartial position between two disputants, one of your own class and one not of your own class.'[152] However, a study of judicial decisions affecting trade unions does not bear out claims that judges are biased against them, at least not in respect of actions in the civil courts.[153] It has been argued that judges in general (not just English judges) are biased in their approach to certain issues not so much because of their social background but because of the nature of their function, which is seen mainly to preserve the *status quo*.

The considerable inter-judicial variability might be resolved by greater attention to training and selection processes.[154]

Alternative dispute resolution

In general, parties to disputes have become increasingly dissatisfied with litigation as a means of resolving disputes, and look to resolutions other than by litigation. Alternative dispute resolution (ADR) has been develped and implemented to provide such alternatives.[155,156] ADR allows the parties greater control over resolving the issues between them. It encourages problem-solving approaches and provides for more effective settlements. Most importantly, it tends to enhance cooperation and be conducive to the preservation of relationships. Of the various ADR processes, the role of the neutral party in arbitration is to consider the issues and then make a decision which determines the issues and is binding on the parties. However, in mediation, the neutral party does not have any authority to make any decision for the parties, who thus retain full autonomy. Medical mediation is concerned specifically with disputes where there is a medical issue. The contact point is: Tel/Fax: +44 (0) 171 834 3351

ADR is developing rapidly not only in Australasia, Europe and North America, but also in Asia.[157]

DISPUTE RESOLUTION

Consensual procedures

- Negotiation
- Conciliation
- Mediation

Adjudicatory

- Arbitration
- Litigation

Standards and definitions

Standards

There are national, regional and international bodies that develop standards for goods and services to facilitate international trade and exchange. The prefix ISO or IEC means that the standard is an international one (put out by the Interna-

STANDARDS

- Global
  - ISO
  - IEC
- Regional
  - EN
- National
  - ANSI
  - BS
  - DIN
  - IS

tional Organization for Standardization[158] or the International Electrotechnical Commission[159] respectively); an international standard prefixed by EN ('Euronorm') means that the standard has been adopted by Europe; if an international standard is prefixed by BS, it means that the standard has been adopted by the UK and that the British Standards Institution (the national body in the UK dealing with standards)[160] is providing the English language version of that standard; the prefix IS indicates that a standard has been approved by the NSAI (National Standards Authority of Ireland).[161]

The addresses of national standards bodies are available at a website.[162]

Definitions

As with all other branches of Medicine, Audiological Medicine can look to official international documents regarding what things should be called or have been called, and how they can be defined and classified.

TERMINOLOGY

- *Terminologia Anatomica*
- *Index Virum*
- *Approved List of Bacterial Names*
- ICD-10
- ICF
- INN
- ISO 31
- ISO 1000
- IEC 60050

The *Terminologia Anatomica* (TA)[163] has replaced the *Nomina Anatomica* (NA) as the official international list of anatomical terms. Enzyme nomenclature is determined by the Nomenclature Committee of the International Union of Biochemistry and Molecular Biology. An *Approved List of Bacterial Names* (by the Judicial Commission of the International Committee on Systematic Bacteriology) is published by the American Society for Microbiology. The *Index Virum* is the collection of index files that list all the names of virus families, genera and species in the Sixth Report of the ICTV.[177,178]

Bertillon's 1893 Classification of Diseases and Related Health Problems is today's WHO's Tenth Revision of the International Statistical Classification of Diseases and Related Health Problems (ICD-10). ICF (International Classification of Functioning, Disability and Health)[179] is the successor to WHO's ICIDH series the first in which appeared in 1980 as the 'International Classification of Impairments, Disabilities, and Handicaps: A Manual Of Classification Relating To The Consequences of Disease'. It has moved away from the 1980 ICIDH 'consequence of disease' classification to being a 'components of health' classification. This reflects significant developments in the way one thinks about disablement in general. The application of these developments to the field of auditory disorders has also been profound.[180] ICF is a classification of health and health related domains that describe body functions and structures, activities and participation. The domains are classified from body, individual and societal perspectives. Since an individual's functioning and disability occurs in a context, ICF also includes a list of environmental factors. ICF is useful to understand and measure health outcomes. It can be used in clinical settings, health services or surveys at the individual or population level. Thus ICF complements ICD-10.

WHO has published Cumulative List No. 9 of International Nonproprietary Names (INN) for Pharmaceutical Substances.

The International Electrotechnical Commission has produced glossaries. For example, IEC 60050-801 (1994-08) encompasses definitions in acoustics and electroacoustics, and IEC 60050-881 (1983-01) definitions in radiology and radiological physics. The symbols and definitions for officially recognized quantities are given by ISO 31, of which Part 7 covers Acoustics. SI,[181] already endorsed by the IEC and other international science bodies, finds expression in ISO 1000: 1992.

Guidelines

A guideline has been defined as: 'a formal statement about a defined task or function. Examples include clinical practice guidelines, guidelines for the application of preventive screening procedures, and guidelines for the ethical conduct of epidemiologic practice and research.[164] Clinical guidelines have been defined as 'systematically developed statements which assist clinicians and patients in making decisions about appropriate treatment for specific conditions ... Clinical guidelines are produced for one reason, and for one reason only: to improve the quality of care.[165]

There is a whole constellation of guidelines, ranging from *Guidelines for Bias-free Writing*,[166] to *Guidelines for the Assessment of General Damages in Personal Injury*.[167]

There are guidelines for developing clinical guidelines,[168] implementing clinical guidelines,[169] using computers to do so,[170] considering their legality[171] and questioning why clinicians do not use guidelines.[172]

Instructions and manuals

Aside from the guidelines just mentioned, there is an array of what are essentially 'How to do it' books and manuals. These range from how to do audiometry[173] through a step-by-step guide to conducting a clinical audit project[174] to a series of exercises to provide a foundation for clinical governance.[175]

Evidence based medicine

Evidence-based medicine was a logical consequence of two books which were published in 1972, i.e. one by the epidemiologist Cochrane,[182] the other by the philosopher, Popper.[183]

Popper dismissed the value of clinical experience per se: 'The Freudian analysts emphasised that their theories were constantly verified by their 'clinical observations'. As for Adler, I was much impressed by a personal experience. Once, in 1919, I reported to him a case which to me did not seem particularly Adlerian, but which he found no difficulty in analysing in terms of his theory of inferiority feelings, although he had not even seen the child. Slightly shocked, I asked him how he could be so sure. 'Because of my thousandfold experience', he replied; whereupon I could not help saying: 'And with this new case, I suppose, your experience has become a thousand-and-one-fold.' (at p 35).

'Evidence-based medicine de-emphasises intuition, unsystematic clinical experience (it is this that distinguishes the clinical opinion per se to which Popper (1972) objected and the clinical opinion which is sought in modern evidence-based medicine) and pathophysiologic rationale as sufficient grounds for clinical decision making and stresses the examination of evidence from clinical research. Evidence-based medicine requires new skills of the physician, including efficient literature searching ... We will refer to this process as the *critical appraisal exercise*.'[184]

Our otolaryngological colleagues had this to say: 'The term 'evidence-based medicine' has been much used in the health care debate in the 1990s. The concept that everything done in medicine should have proof has been taken up as a mantra not only by politicians but also a considerable body of the medical profession. Indeed, a new journal, *Evidence Based Medicine*, has been introduced in response to this wave of enthusiasm. Those who have been in the profession of medicine, and especially surgery, for any length of time, know that basing every action on previously published proof is virtually impossible. Yet to speak against evidence-based medicine is akin to saying that the king has no clothes (at p 152) ... Our conclusion, therefore, is that on the basis of examination of 5000 articles in leading ENT journals, ENT is not an evidence-based specialty ... the same might be applied to all surgical sub-specialties since there is a fundamental difference between the evaluation of medicines as opposed to surgical procedures.' (at p 156[185])

One of his colleagues responded: 'Whilst it is pertinent to look at the evidence for practice in a particular specialty, there is a danger that if the results are considered unsatisfactory, others might take this to imply that the specialty was inferior to other specialities ... Certainly, the medical specialities are more active in carrying out randomized controlled trials than surgeons, one of the main reasons being that they are required to do this before a drug licence is issued. As yet this is not required for surgical procedures ... What one also wants to known [sic] is how best to arrive at a diagnosis, what the epidemiology of the condition is to understand the natural history and the outcome of the conditions as well as the economics of all aspects ....'[186]

There have been a number of critiques of the methodology of Evidence-based medicine, e.g. by the MRC Biostatistics Unit, which has considered the heterogeneity between study results.[187]

Evidence-based medicine has spawned a plethora of bodies (se Glossary) which follow in the wake of this Zeitgeist.

The Commission for Health Improvement's[188] aim is to improve the quality of patient care in the NHS. CHI will raise standards by:

- assessing every NHS organisation and making its findings public
- investigating when there is serious failure
- checking that the NHS is following national guidelines
- advising the NHS on best practice

Conclusions

It is clear that there is a spectrum of customs, customary law, religions, ethical codes, law and related controls that affect humans. The law in a given state reflects, in many cases, the state's unique and complex history. In Sri Lanka, for example, the one and a half centuries of Dutch rule provided Roman–Dutch Law. This was endorsed by the subsequent British rule, the persistence of which for the next one and a half centuries allowed the infusion of English common law principles. But Sri Lankan law also incorporates the customary law of the Buddhist Sinhalese (*Kandyan law*), the Hindu Tamils (*T(h)esawalamai*) and those of Arab origins, some being pre-Islamic.

Nevertheless, one needs to bear in mind that some societies do not distinguish these various normative systems from one another. The cognosphere of these societies is holistic, culturally bound and embraces competence in day-to-day living. This unitary, grass-roots knowledge, termed indigenous knowledge, can produce conservationist, environmentally sound and socially harmonious practices.[176]

References

1. Dawkins R. *River Out of Eden*. London: Phoenix, 1995.
2. Slater PJB. *Behaviour and Evolution*. Cambridge: Cambridge University Press, 1994.
3. Blackmore S. *The Meme Machine*. Oxford: Oxford University Press, 1999.
4. Allott A. *The Limits of Law*. London: Butterworths, 1980.
5. Hinchcliffe R, Bellman S. Legal and ethical matters. In: Stephens D, ed. *Scott-Brown's Otolaryngology*, 6th edn, Vol. 2, *Adult Audiology*. London: Butterworth-Heinemann, 1997, pp. 2/7/1–2/7/43.
6. Reves E. *The Anatomy of Peace*. London: Penguin, 1947: 13.
7. Hallpike CR. *The Principles of Social Evolution*. Oxford: Clarendon, 1986.

8. Turnbull C. *The Mountain People*. London: Pan, 1974.
9. Nakane C. *Japanese Society*. Harmondsworth, Middlesex: Penguin, 1974.
10. Sieder R. *Customary Law and Democratic Transition in Guatemala*. London: University of London, Institute of Latin American Studies, 1997.
11. Riasanovosky V. *Customary Law of the Nomadic Tribes of Siberia*. London: Curzon, 1997.
12. Serjeant RB. *Customary and Shari'ah Law in Arabian Society*. Aldershot: Ashgate, 1991.
13. Kamali MH. *Principles of Islamic Jurisprudence*. Cambridge: The Islamic Text Society, 1991.
14. Raendchen O, Raendchen J. The Lao Hiit Khoong Code: Traditional Community Rights and Social Values of the Lao. 7th International Conference on Thai Studies, Amsterdam, 4–8 July 1999. In: *Community Rights in Thailand* http://www.pscw.uva.nl/icts7/community.html
15. Dadomo C, Farran S. *The French Legal System*. London: Sweet and Maxwell, 1993.
16. Foster N. *German Law and Legal System (Deutsches Recht und Deutsches Rechtssystem)*. London: Blackstone, 1993.
17. Yinger JM. *Religion, Society and the Individual*. New York: Macmillan, 1957.
18. Chaudhuri NC. *Hinduism*. Oxford: Oxford University Press, 1997.
19. Klostermaier KK. *Hinduism: a Short History*. London: Oneworld, 2000.
20. Kelly F. *A Guide to Early Irish Law*. Dublin: Dublin Institute for Advanced Studies, 1998.
21. Lee S. *Law and Morals*. Oxford: Oxford University Press, 1986.
22. Machiavelli N. *The Prince*. London: Penguin, 1981.
23. Harvey P. *An Introduction to Buddhism*. Cambridge: Cambridge University Press, 1990.
24. Kulananda. *Principles of Buddhism*. London: Harper Collins, 1996.
25. Hinnells JR. *Dictionary of Religions*. Harmondsworth, Middlesex: Penguin, 1986.
26. Buddhadasa Bhikku. *Handbook for Mankind*. Bangkok: Buddhadasa Foundation, 1986.
27. Char DF, Tom KS, Young GC, Murakami T, Ames R. A view of death and dying among the Chinese and Japanese. *Hawaii Med J* 1996; **55**: 286–90.
28. Lewittes M. *Jewish Law*. Northvale, NJ: Jason Aronson, 1994.
29. Labriolle P. *The History and Literature of Christianity*. London: Taylor & Francis, 1997.
30. Waines D. *An Introduction to Islam*. Cambridge: Cambridge University Press, 1995.
31. Doi ARI. *Shari'ah: The Islamic Law*. London: Ta Ha, 1984.
32. Horrie C, Chippindale P. *What is Islam?* London: Virgin, 1994.
33. Muraoka T, Brown DM, Araki JT. *Studies in Shinto Thought*. Westport, CT: Greenwood Press, 1988.
34. Breen J, Teeuwen M. *Shinto in Historical Perspective*. London: Curzon, 2000.
35. Higuchi S, Ogawa T. In: Duncan AS, Dunstan GR, Welbourn RB, eds. *Dictionary of Medical Ethics*. London: Darton, Longman & Todd, 1981: 397–99.
36. Jamgon KLT. *Buddhist Ethics*. Ithaca NY: Snow Lion, 1998.
37. Harvey P. *An Introduction to Buddhist Ethics*. Cambridge: Cambridge University Press, 2000.
38. Gill R. *A Textbook of Christian Ethics*. Edinburgh: T & T Clark, 1995.
39. Pinckaers S. *The Sources of Christian Ethics*. Edinburgh: T & T Clark, 1995.
40. Hoose B. *Christian Ethics*. London: Continuum International, 1998.
41. Porter J. *Moral Action and Christian Ethics*. Cambridge: Cambridge University Press, 1999.
42. Perrett RW. *Hindu Ethics*. Honolulu, HI: University of Hawaii, 1998.
43. Amin SH. *Islamic and Iranian Ethics*. Edinburgh: Royston, 1991.
44. Dorff E, Newman LE. *Contemporary Jewish Ethics and Morality*. Oxford: Oxford University Press, 1995.
45. Sherwin BL. *Jewish Ethics for the Twenty-first Century*. New York, NY: Syracuse University Press, 1999.
46. Keown D. *The Nature of Buddhist Ethics*. London: Macmillan, 1992.
47. Banner M. *Christian Ethics and Contemporary Moral Problems*. Cambridge: Cambridge University Press, 1999.
48. Walton JN. *Report of the Select Committee on Medical Ethics*. London: HMSO, 1994.
49. Duncan AS, Dunstan GR, Welbourn RB (eds). *Dictionary of Medical Ethics*. London: Darton, Longman & Todd, 1981: viii.
50. Rivers J. Buddhism. In: Duncan AS, Dunstan GR, Welbourn RB, eds. *Dictionary of Medical Ethics*. London: Darton, Longman & Todd, 1981: 44–6.
51. Barnes M. Euthanasia: Buddhist principles. *Br Med Bull* 1996; **52**: 369–75.
52. Eijk WJ. Carrying on the healing mission of Christ: medical ethics in the Christian tradition. *Acta Neurochirurg Suppl* 1999; **74**: 53–8.
53. Ali Raja I, Chaudhry MR. Islam and medical ethics. *Acta Neurochirurg Suppl* 1999; **74**: 29–34.
54. Limentani AE. The role of ethical principles in health care and the implications for ethical codes. *J Med Ethics* 1999; **25**: 394–8.
55. Mason JK, Smith AM. *Law and Medical Ethics*. London: Butterworths Law, 1999.
56. Baker R, Strosberg MA, Bynum J. *Legislating Medical Ethics*. Dordrecht: Kluwer, 1995.
57. British Medical Association. *The Handbook of Medical Ethics*. London: BMA, 1984.
58. General Medical Council. http://www.gmc-uk.org
59. General Medical Council. *Facing A Complaint*. London: GMC, 1997.
60. General Medical Council. *Good Medical Practice*. London: GMC, 1998.
61. General Medical Council. *Confidentiality*. London: GMC, 1995.
62. General Medical Council. *Seeking Patients' Consent*. London: GMC, 1998.
63. Pappworth M. Medical ethical committees: a review of their functions. *World Med* 1978; **13**: 199–78.
64. Council for International Organizations of Medical Sciences. *Human Experimentation and Medical Ethics*. Geneva: CIOMS, 1982.
65. Declaration of Helsinki. Recommendations guiding physicians in biomedical research involving human subjects. *JAMA* 1997; **277**: 925–6.

66. International Research Codes of Ethics. *Bull PanAmerican Health Org* 1990; **24**: 604–21.
67. Royal College of Physicians of London. *Guidelines on the Practice of Ethics Committees in Medical Research*. London: Royal College of Physicians of London, 1984.
68. Department of Health. *Local Research Ethics Committees*. HSG(91)5. London: Department of Health, 1991.
69. MRECs. http://dialspace.pipex.com/mrec/
70. http://www.ofres-hs.upmc.edu/irb/irbref/guidelines.pdf
71. Food and Drug Administration. http://www.fda.gov/oc/oha/irb/toc.html (1998 Update).
72. Bioethics Resources on the web (NIH provided). http://www.nih.gov/sigs/bioethics/
73. US NLM. Informed Consent. http://www.nlm.nih.gov/pubs/cbm/hum_exp.html#50
74. US NLM. Privacy and Confidentiality. http://www.nlm.nih.gov/pubs/cbm/hum_exp.html#70
75. US NLM Clinical Trials. http://www.nlm.nih.gov/pubs/cbm/hum_exp.html#140
76. Smith T. *Ethics in Medical Research: a Handbook of Good Practice*. Cambridge: Cambridge University Press, 1999.
77. Nimmo WS. Joint Consensus Conference on Misconduct in Biomedical Research. *Proc R Coll Physicians Edin* 2000; **30**(Suppl 7): 1–26.
78. Royal College of Physicians of London. *Fraud and Misconduct in Medical Research*. London: Royal College of Physicians of London, 1991.
79. Morell C, Harvey G. *The Clinical Audit Handbook*. London: Harcourt, 1999.
80. Sheldon R. *Auditing Clinical Care in Scotland*. London: HMSO, 1994.
81. Kinn S, Siann T. *Computers and Clinical Audit*. London: Hodder & Stoughton Publishers, 1993.
82. British Medical Association. *Ethical Issues in Medical Audit*. London: BMA, 1996.
83. Earnshaw JJ. Auditing audit: the cost of the emperor's new clothes. *Br J Hosp Med* 1997; **58**: 189–92.
84. Kogan M, Redfern S, Kober A, Norman I, Packwood T, Robinson S. *Making Use of Clinical Audit*. Milton Keynes: Open University Press, 1995.
85. Behrendt N, Heegaard S, Fornitz GG. Hospitalsodbuktionen. En vaesentlig faktor i sygehusenes kvalitetssikring. [The hospital autopsy. An important factor in hospital quality assurance.] *Ugeskrift for Laeger* 1999; **161**: 543–7.
86. Houghton G. From audit to effectiveness: an historical evaluation of the changing role of Medical Audit Advisory Groups. *J Eval Clin Prac* 1997; **3**: 245–53.
87. Chambers R. *Clinical Effectiveness Made Easy*. Oxford: Radcliffe Medical Press, 1998.
88. Miles A. *Progress in Clinical Effectiveness*. London: Royal Society of Medicine, 2000.
89. Clinical Governance. Circular: NHS MEL (1998) 7. London: HMSO, 1998.
90. Dewar S. *Clinical Governance Under Construction*. London: King's Fund, 1999.
91. Lugon M. *Clinical Governance: Making It Happen*. London: Royal Society of Medicine, 1999.
92. British Association of Otorhinolaryngologists—Head and Neck Surgeons. *Clinical Governance and the Role of the British Association of Otorhinolaryngologists Head and Neck Surgeons*. London: British Association of Otorhinolaryngologists—Head and Neck Surgeons at the Royal College of Surgeons of England, 2000.
93. Vincent C. *Clinical Risk Management*. London: British Medical Journal, 1996.
94. Wilson J, Tingle J. *Clinical Risk Management*. London: Butterworth-Heinemann, 1997.
95. Martin EA. *A Dictionary of Law*. Oxford: Oxford University Press, 1994.
96. Social Sciences and Humanities Research Council of Canada. http://www.sshrc.ca/english/programinfo/policies/Intro03.htm
97. David R, Jauffret-Spinosi C. *Les Grands Systèmes de Droit Contemporains*. Paris: Dalloz, 1992.
98. Lingat R. *The Classical Law of India*. Oxford: Oxford University Press, 1998.
99. Derrett JDM. *Religion, Law and the State in India*. Oxford: Oxford University Press, 1999.
100. Huxley A. The Reception of Buddhist Law in SE Asia 200 BCE–1860 CE. In: Doucet M, Vanderlinden J, eds. *La Réception des Systèmes Juristiques: Implantation et Destin*. Bruxelles: Bruglant, 1994: 139–237.
101. Epstein I. *Tibet Transformed*. Beijing: New World Press, 1983.
102. Turner B (ed.). *Statesman's Yearbook*. London: Macmillan, 2000.
103. Cotran E, Mallat C. *Yearbook of Islamic and Middle Eastern Law*. Dordrecht: Kluwer, 1997.
104. Ibrahim A. Foreword to Kamali 1991.[13]
105. Coulson NJ. *A History of Islamic Law*. Edinburgh: Edinburgh University Press, 1994.
106. Jones R. *The Canon Law of the Roman Catholic Church and Church of England*. Edinburgh: T & T Clark, 2000.
107. Kynell K von. *Saxon and Medieval Antecedents of the English Common Law*. New York: Edwin Mellen, 1999.
108. Watkin TG. *An Historical Introduction to Modern Civil Law*. Aldershot: Ashgate, 1999.
109. Pound R. A survey of social interests. *57 Harvard Law Review 1*, 1943/4. Cambridge, Mass.
110. Sypnowich C. *The Concept of Socialist Law*. Oxford: Oxford University Press, 1990.
111. Toynbee A. *Mankind and Mother Earth*. Oxford: Oxford University Press, 1976: 583.
112. East R. *Social Security Law*. London: Macmillan, 1999.
113. Montgomery J. Health Care Law. Oxford: Oxford University Press, 1997.
114. Nys H. *Medical Law in Belgium*. Dordrecht: Kluwer, 1998.
115. McLean SAM. *Law Reform and Medical Injury Litigation*. Aldershot: Ashgate, 1995.
116. Tomkin D, Hanafin P. *Irish Medical Law*. London: Sweet & Maxwell, 1995.
117. Koniaris TB, Karlovassitou-Koniari AD. *Medical Law in Greece*. Dordrecht: Kluwer, 1999.

118. Kennedy I, Grubb A. *Principles of Medical Law*. Oxford: Oxford University Press, 1998.
119. Thornton J, Beckwith S. *Environmental Law*. London: Sweet & Maxwell, 1997.
120. Chen J. *Chinese Law*. Dordrecht: Kluwer, 1999.
121. Wang G, Mo J. *Chinese Law*. Dordrecht: Kluwer, 1999.
122. Lin Feng. *Constitutional Law in China*. London: Sweet & Maxwell, 1998.
123. Bell J, Boyron S, Whittaker S. *Principles of French Law*. Oxford: Oxford University Press, 1998.
124. Ebke WF, Finkin MW. *Introduction to German Law*. Dordrecht: Kluwer, 1997.
125. Bhattacharjee AM. *Hindu Law and the Constitution*. New Delhi: Eastern Law House, 1994.
126. Galanter M. *Law and Society in Modern India*. Oxford: Oxford University Press, 1993.
127. Bin-Nun A. *The Law of the State of Israel*. Jerusalem: Rubin Mass, 1972.
128. Fujikura K. *Japanese Law and Legal Theory*. Aldershot: Ashgate, 1995.
129. Oda H. *Japanese Law*. Oxford: Oxford University Press, 1999.
130. Butler WE. *Russian Law*. Oxford: Oxford University Press, 1999.
131. Feldbrugge FJM. *Russian Law*. Dordrecht: Kluwer, 1993.
132. Ansay T, Wallace D. *Introduction to Turkish Law*. Dordrecht: Kluwer, 1996.
133. Ural E. *Handbook of Turkish Law*. London: Milet, 1999.
134. van Caenegem RC. *The Birth of the English Common Law*. Cambridge: Cambridge University Press, 1988.
135. van Caenegem RC. *Judges, Legislators, and Professors*. Cambridge: Cambridge University Press, 1992.
136. Steiner J. *Textbook on EC Law*. London: Blackstone, 1994.
137. Oppenheimer A. *The Relationship Between European Community Law and National Law: the Cases*. Cambridge: Cambridge University Press, 1994.
138. Eggleston R. *Evidence, Proof and Probability*. London: Weidenfeld and Nicolson, 1983.
139. Society of Expert Witnesses. http://www.sew.org.uk/
140. Expert Witnesses, Guidelines re Federal Court of Australia. http://www.fedcourt.gov.au/practice.htm#practiced1.htm
141. Writing Medico-legal Reports. Prepared for members of the Medical Protection Society, 1997. Knight BH, Palmer RN. http://www.mps.org.uk/medical/articles/pum1rep1.htm, http:// www.mps.org.uk/medical/articles/pum1rep2.htm and http:// www.mps.org.uk/medical/articles/pum1rep3.htm
142. Foy J. New court rules for expert witnesses. *ENTNews* 1999; **8**: 28–9.
143. Clement-Evans C. Cenric Clement-Evans comments. *ENTNews* 1999; **8**: 29.
144. Friston M. New rules for expert witnesses: the last shots of the medicolegal hired gun. *BMJ* 1999; **316**: 1365–6.
145. Woolf, Lord. *Access to Justice: Interim Report to the Lord Chancellor on the civil justice system in England and Wales*, July 1996. http://www.law.warwick.ac.uk/woolf/report/
146. Department of Health and Social Security. *Occupational Deafness. Report by the Industrial Injuries Advisory Council in accordance with Section 62 of the National Insurance (Industrial Injuries) Act 1965 on the question whether there are degrees of hearing loss due to noise which satisfy the conditions for prescription under the Act*. Cmnd 5461. London: HMSO, 1973.
147. Gray BK. *A History of English Philanthropy*. New York: Kelley, 1967.
148. Smith AFM. Mad cows and ecstasy: chance and choice in an evidence-based society. *J R Statist Soc A* 1996; **159**: 367–83.
149. Friedmann W. *Legal Theory*. London: Stevens, 1949.
150. Hutcheson JC. The judgement intuitive: the function of the 'Hunch' in judicial decision. *Cornell Law Q* 1929; **14**: 274–88.
151. Claxton G. Investigating human intuition: knowing without knowing why. *Psychologist* 1998; **11**: 217–20.
152. Wedderburn KW. *The Worker and the Law*. Harmondsworth, Middlesex: Penguin, 1965: 20.
153. O'Higgins P, Partington M. Industrial conflict: judicial attitudes. *32 Modern Law Rev* 1969: 53.
154. Council of Europe. *The Training of Judges and Public Prosecutors in Europe*. Strasbourg: Council of Europe Publishing, Council of Europe, 1996.
155. Brown H, Marriott A. *ADR Principles and Practice*. London: Sweet and Maxwell, 1999.
156. York S. *Practical ADR Handbook*. London: Sweet and Maxwell, 1999.
157. Mittal DP. *New Law of Arbitration, ADR and Contract Law in India*. Dordrecht: Kluwer, 1997.
158. International Organization for Standardization. http://www.iso.ch/addresse/membodies.html
159. International Electrotechnical Commission. http://www.iec.ch/
160. British Standards Institution. http://194.74.46.150/bsis/SISO/index.htm
161. National Standards Authority of Ireland. http://www.nsai.ie/
162. Addresses of national standards bodies. http://www.iso.ch/addresse/membodies.html
163. FCAT (Federative Committee on Anatomical Terminology). *Terminologia Anatomica*. Stuttgart: Thieme, 1998.
164. McDonald CJ, Overhage JM. Guidelines you can follow and can trust: an ideal and an example. *JAMA* 1994; **271**: 872–3.
165. National Health Service Executive. *Clinical Guidelines: Using Clinical Guidelines to Improve Patient Care within the NHS*. London: Department of Health, 1996.
166. Schwartz M. *Guidelines for Bias-free Writing*. Bloomington, IN: Indiana University Press, 1995.
167. Judicial Studies Board. *Guidelines for the Assessment of General Damages in Personal Injury*. London: Blackstone, 1998.
168. Grimshaw J, Eccles M. *Clinical Guidelines from Conception to Use*. Oxford: Radcliffe Medical Press, 2000.
169. Humphris D, Littlejohns P. *Implementing Clinical Guidelines: a Practical Guide*. Oxford: Radcliffe Medical Press, 1999.
170. Corb GJ, Liaw Y, Brandt CA, Shiffman RN. An object-oriented framework for the development of computer-based guideline implementations. *Methods Information Med* 1999; **38**: 148–53.
171. Hurwitz B. *Clinical Guidelines and the Law*. Oxford: Radcliffe Medical Press, 1998.

172. Cabana MD, Rand CS, Powe NR et al. Why don't physicians follow clinical practice guidelines? A framework for improvement. *JAMA* 1999; **282**: 1458–65.
173. Arlinger S (ed.). *Manual of Practical Audiometry*. Vol. 1. London: Whurr, 1989.
174. Morell C, Harvey G. *The Clinical Audit Handbook*. London: Harcourt, 1999.
175. Lilley R. *Making Sense of Clinical Governance*. Oxford: Radcliffe Medical Press, 1999.
176. Indigenous Knowledge. http://www.nuffic.nl/ciran/ikdm/1-2/articles/aspects.html.
177. The International Committee on Taxonomy of Viruses. A Perspective on Virus Taxonomy and the Role of the ICTV. http://www.uct.ac.za/microbiology/ictv/ICTV.html
178. *Virus Taxonomy: The Classification and Nomenclature of Viruses.* The Sixth Report of the International Committee on Taxonomy of Viruses. Murphy FA, Fauquet CM, Bishop DHL, Ghabrial SA, Jarvis AW, Martelli GP, Mayo MA, Summers MD. Vienna: Springer-Verlag, 1995.
179. *International Classification of Functioning, Disability and Health.* Geneva: World Health Organization, 2001. http://www3.who.int/icf/icftemplate.cfm?myurl=introduction.html%20&mytitle=Introduction
180. Stephens SDG, Kerr P. Auditory Disablements: An Update. *Audiology* 2000; **19**: 322–332.
181. SI (*Le Sustème International d'Unités*). The International System of Units. National Physical Laboratory. HMSO. 1993. 6th edition *see* ISO 1000: 1992; BS 5555: 1993.
182. Cochrane AL. *Effectiveness and Efficiency: random reflections on health services*. London: Nuffield Provincial Hospitals Trust, 1972.
183. Popper KR. *Conjectures and Refutations*. London: Routledge and Kegan Paul, 1972.
184. Evidence-Based Medicine Working Group. Evidence-Based Medicine: A New Approach to Teaching the Practice of Medicine. *J Am Med Asso* 1992; **420**: 2425.
185. Maran AGD, Molony NC, Armstrong MWJ, Ah-See K. Is there an evidence base for the practice of ENT surgery? *Clin Otolaryngol* 1997; **22**: 152–57.
186. Browning GG. Is there an evidence base for the practice of ENT surgery? *Clin Otolaryngol* 1998; **23**: 1–2.
187. Higgins J, Thompson S, Deeks J, Altman D. Statistical heterogeneity in systematic reviews of clinical trials: a critical appraisal of guidelines and practice. *J Health Serv Res Pol* 2002; **7**: 51–61.
188. Commission for Health Improvement. http://www.chi.nhs.uk/ (accessed 13-10-2002)

Glossary

CHI Commission for Health Improvement
Clinical Outcomes Group A multi-professional committee which advises the Department of Health on how to improve outcomes of clinical care.
Clinical Standards Board Scottish equivalent to *National Institute of Clinical Excellence*.
COG *Clinical Outcomes Group*
National Institute of Clinical Excellence For decision as to whether or not a new drug or interventional procedure will be used by the NHS (England and Wales).
NICE *National Institute of Clinical Excellence*
Safety and Efficacy Register of New Interventional Procedures The body to which all new interventional procedures must be reported (UK).
Scottish Intercollegiate Guidelines Network A collaborative Scottish Development which produces guidelines for the health care specialties; the establishment of each guideline starts with a systematic review à la Cochrane, everything being annotated with a grading of the evidence.
SERNIP *Safety and Efficacy Register of New Interventional Procedures*
SIGN *Scottish Intercollegiate Guidelines Network*

Section **II**

Audiology

9 Development and plasticity of the human auditory system

Rémy Pujol, Mireille Lavigne-Rebillard

Introduction

This chapter specifically describes the anatomy and function of cochlear development in the human, with an emphasis on maturation of sensory cells and their neural connections. Subsequently, the development of the auditory pathways is summarized, focusing on the critical role of a healthy cochlea in building the auditory brain.

Development of the human cochlea

The development of the peripheral auditory organ, the cochlea, is relatively well documented in humans (reviewed in references 1 and 2) as well as in most common experimental small mammals (reviewed in references 1, 3, 4 and 5). A detailed account of this development does, however, remain to be completed. Functional data concerning the earlier stages are still missing, due to obvious difficulties in fetal recordings, while anatomical data from the latter stages are of poor quality, due to the bad preservation of tissues from therapeutic abortions. It is, however, possible to achieve quite good extrapolations from experimental data, due to the remarkable similarity of structure, and to a lesser extent of function, of most mammalian cochleas. It is thus possible to precisely date the onset of human cochlear function on the basis of anatomical data. Similarly, the completion of human cochlear maturation can be mostly estimated from physiological recordings in premature babies.

The human cochlea develops in utero. At 10–12 weeks of gestation, the sensory hair cells differentiate. At 18–20 weeks of gestation, the cochlea starts functioning. At 30–36 weeks, it is mature. At birth, although cochlear development is almost complete, the brain auditory structures are far from mature: the last part of the primary auditory pathway (i.e. the thalamocortical connections) is not believed to be fully developed until postnatal year 4–8. During these first years of life, synapses in the auditory brain are formed, selected, stabilized, and interconnected depending on the type of stimulation they receive from the peripheral organ. Thus a normally functioning cochlea, normally stimulated, is needed.

Anatomy of the developing human cochlea

Embryology and gross morphology

The neural and sensory elements of the inner ear develop from the ectodermal otic placode, which forms in the 23-day-old human embryo, and gives rise to the otocyst.[6] Differentiation of the vestibular and then the cochlear end organs from the otocyst takes place during the second month of pregnancy.

The gross anatomical development of the human cochlea has been precisely described.[7] Complete coiling of the cochlea can be observed at 8–9 weeks of gestation. However, complete formation of the bony capsule is not achieved before the last months of pregnancy.

Anatomy and histology

First signs of differentiation

The first sign of differentiation of the organ of Corti, as observed by scanning and light microscopy (Figure 9.1), is not observed until 9–10 weeks of pregnancy.[2,8,9] As in most common mammals studied,[3,10] development appears to proceed regularly from the base towards the apex. Meanwhile, since a complete serial study of the whole cochlea has never been performed, the possibility cannot be excluded that although development starts in the first turn, it may begin at a certain distance from the basal end and progress toward both extremities.[4] The cochlea in a 9-week-old human fetus is completely coiled[2,9] (Figure 9.1a), but its sensory epithelial surface is totally undifferentiated, i.e. all the cells have microvilli and a kinocilium.[9,11] The tectorial membrane is just beginning to form at this stage (Figure 9.1b).

Hair cell differentiation

Hair cells begin to morphologically differentiate at 11–12 weeks of gestation.[2] About 1 week earlier, nerve fibres are seen entering the undifferentiated epithelium.[11] This indicates that nerve endings interact very early with the differentiation of hair cells. The growing of stereocilia (i.e. ciliogenesis) is the main morphological criterion of hair cell differentiation. It starts around week 12[2,8,9] (Figure 9.2a),[9] and it is characterized by two gradients: a basal-to-apical and an inner hair cell (IHC) to outer hair cell (OHC) gradient. From the beginning, the classical pattern of one row of IHCs and two rows of OHCs can be observed. When they first appear, the bundles of stereocilia are quite similar on both types of hair cells (Figure 9.2a): round with stereocilia of about the same length, a pattern resembling that of auditory hair cells from lower vertebrates.[9]

Then, staircase and V-like arrangements are created (Figure 9.3). On IHCs, the 'V-shaped' arrangement is broad, especially at the base of the cochlea, where stereocilia appear to be almost linearly arranged. The OHC V- or W-pattern is always more recognizable. An adult-like organization of stereocilia is observed in the fetal cochlea around week 22.[2,9]

Bredberg,[12] using surface preparations, first detailed the organization (number and pattern) of human cochlear sensory cells. It would appear that an adult-like pattern is acquired as soon as the 4th month in utero. The numbers of sensory cells in the fetal cochleas are slightly greater than the mean adult values, i.e. 3500 IHCs and 13 000 OHCs.

Transient appearance of supernumerary hair cells (Figure 9.4)

With the exception of the extreme apex, the single row of IHCs and the three rows of OHCs are clearly visible at week 14 along almost the entire length of the cochlea.[2,12] For a couple of weeks, however, IHCs are loosely arranged, with spaces between adjacent cells. This could explain the transitory appearance of extra IHCs at about week 15 or 16 (Figure 9.4), which seems to occur more frequently in the human than in other mammalian cochleas.[13] At OHC level, a transitory overproduction is also clearly seen (Figure 9.4). OHCs are frequently organized in four or even five rows. Again, this pattern is much more frequently encountered in the human[9,14] than in other mammals and it lasts longer than extra IHCs. The transitory extra OHCs have been tentatively correlated with the observation that otoacoustical emissions in human babies present a richer spectrum of peaks than in adults.[15,16] It is interesting to note that the apical coil of the human cochlea displays this supernumerary feature of OHCs even in adulthood, suggesting some 'uncompleted maturation' of the apical cochlea (see below). Both a normal overproduction of OHCs[17] and a drug (retinoic acid)-stimulated overproduction of IHCs and OHCs[18] have been described. Overproduction of hair cells, followed by a down regulation process, seems to be a

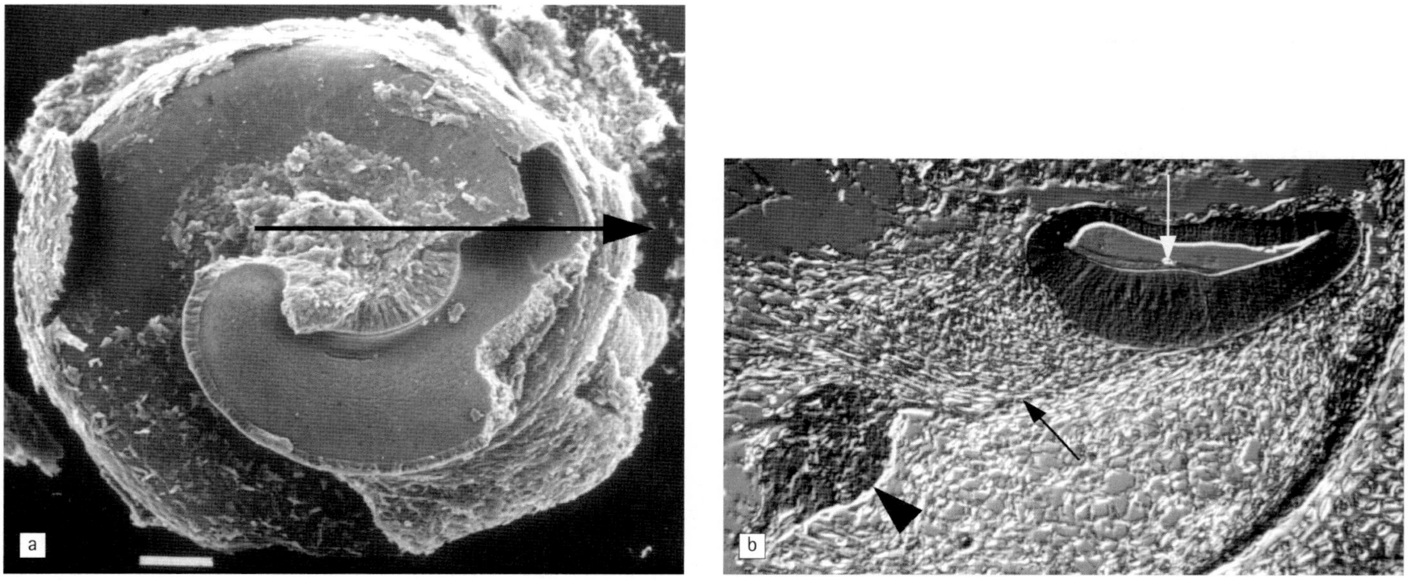

Figure 9.1 Nine to ten weeks of gestation. (a) Scanning EM (bar: 1 mm) showing the complete coiling of the cochlear spiral. The black arrow indicates the plane of section seen in Nomarski optics on the right (bar: 50 µm). (b) The sensory epithelium is not yet differentiated, as only a ridge and some filaments of the nascent tectorial membrane (white arrow) mark its location. However, the spiral ganglion (triangular arrow) is visible and nerve fibres may be tracked (arrow) up to the otocyst.

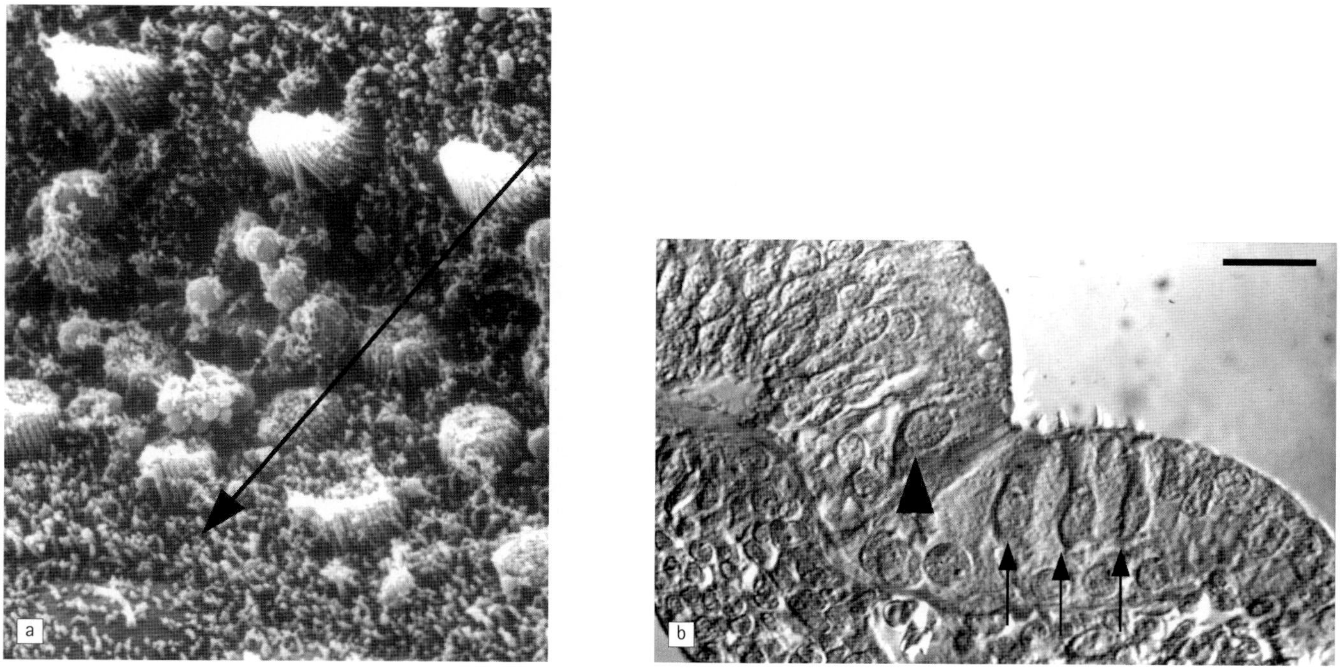

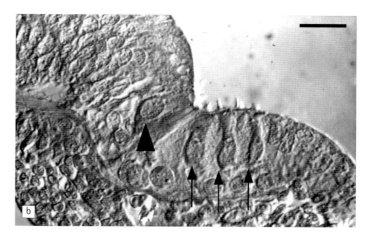

Figure 9.2 Twelve to fourteen weeks of gestation. (a) Scanning EM (bar: 10 μm). The round-shaped bundle of growing stereocilia, jutting out from the surrounding microvilli, appears first on the IHCs and then on OHCs. This is the clearest sign of morphological differentiation of hair cells. (b) Nomarski section along the plane of the black arrow seen on the left (bar: 10 μm). The IHC (triangular arrow), the inner pillar and three OHCs (arrows) are easily recognizable.

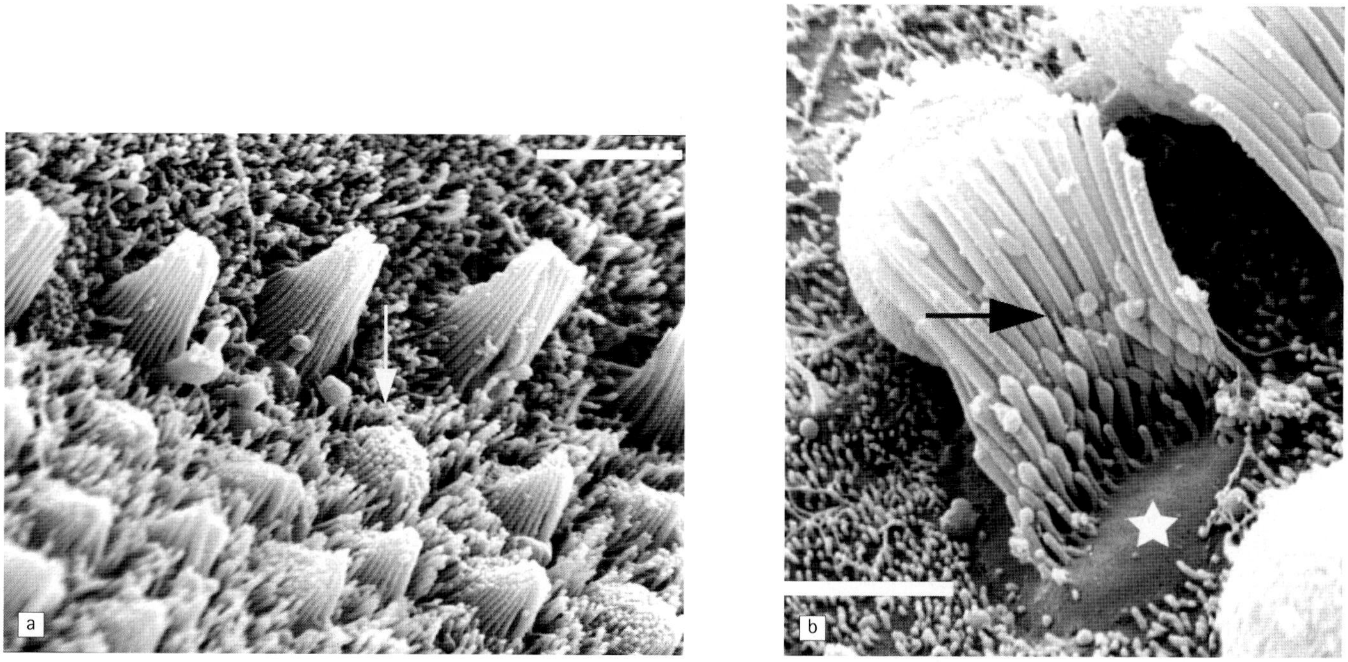

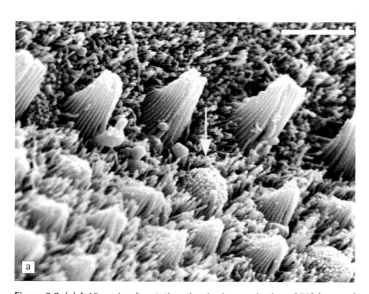

Figure 9.3 (a) A 15 weeks of gestation, the classic organization of IHC (top row) and OHC (bottom rows) stereocilia is recognizable on most of the hair cells. However, some OHCs still display the typical immature round-shaped tuff (white arrow). Note the advanced maturation of IHC stereocilia Bar: 5 μm. (b) At 16 weeks of gestation, the IHC surface shows graded rows of stereocilia, tip links (black arrow) and glabrous (devoid of microvilli) cuticular plate (star). Bar: 3 μm.

'normal' phenomenon during the in vivo development of the human cochlea. Tracking the molecular mechanisms of this phenomenon may appear to be most valuable for the 'regeneration' challenge.

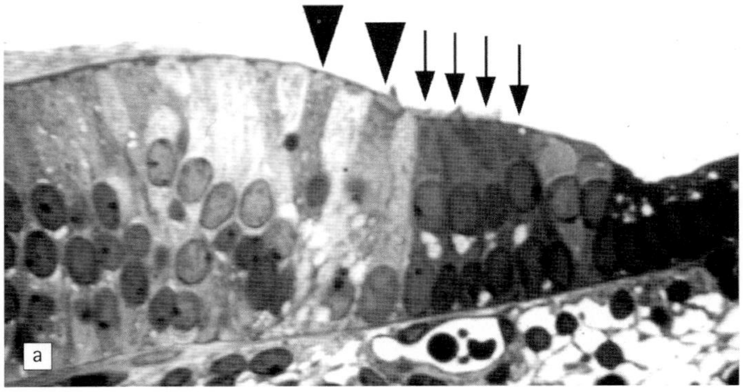

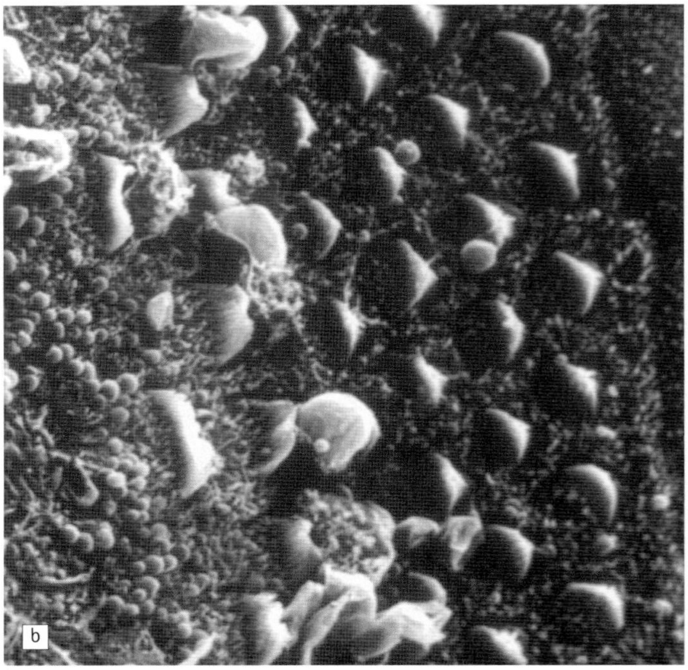

Figure 9.4 Supernumerary hair cells. Frequently, two rows of IHCs (triangular arrows) and four or five rows of OHCs (arrows) are seen in the human developing cochlea between 16 (a, Nomarski) to 18 (b, scanning EM) weeks of gestation.

Stage of onset of cochlear function

At about gestational weeks 18–20, human cochlear morphology (Figure 9.2) is similar to what has been reported experimentally in other mammals at a stage corresponding to the onset of cochlear function.[19] This stage is characterized by an opening of the tunnel of Corti, the formation of Nuel's spaces, and the regression of Kölliker's organ that results in the release of the tectorial membrane. From this stage onwards, the main changes observed at the light microscopic level are an elongation of the outer pillars and OHCs, and a development of neighbouring Deiters' and Hensen's cells.

End of morphological maturation

As stated above, the end of morphological maturation is hard to determine in the human, because of the poorer preservation of tissues as fetal specimens get older. Nevertheless, it seems that by 8 months in utero, the histological development of the human cochlea is completed, apart from the ganglion of Corti, where myelination has not yet been achieved.[19] At this stage, the human organ of Corti resembles what has been described in most adult common laboratory mammals[1,20] (Figure 9.5).

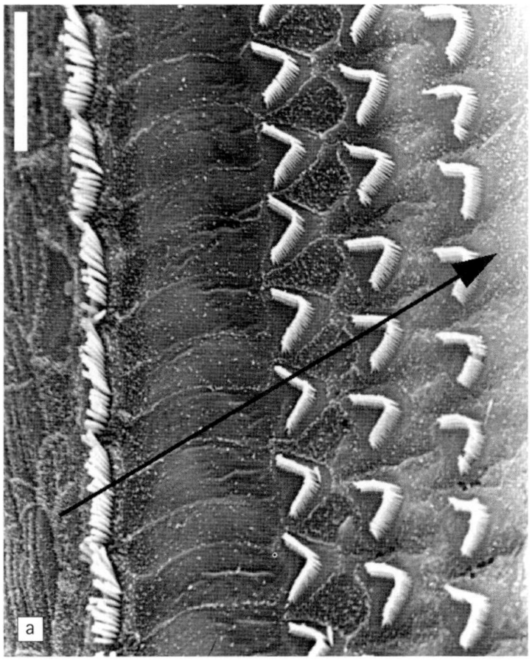

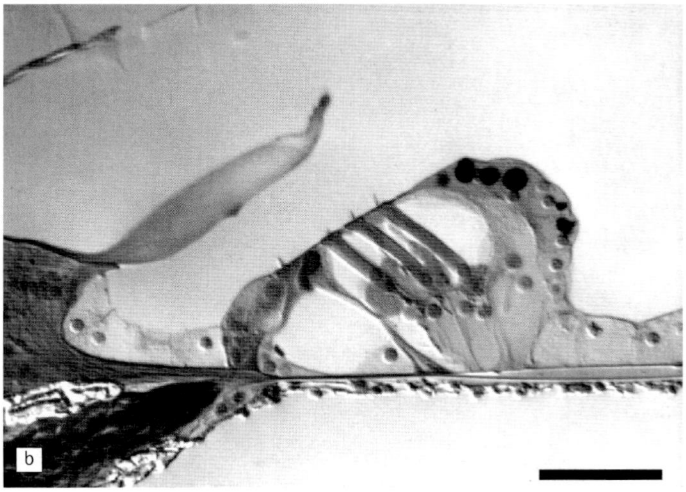

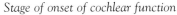

Figure 9.5 End of maturation of the mammalian organ of Corti. This adult stage is reached in human cochlea at around 30 weeks of gestation. (a) Scanning EM from the base of a rat cochlea (courtesy of Marc Lenoir); the black arrow indicates the plane of the right section. (b) Normarski optics. Bars: 12 μm (a) and 20 μm (b).

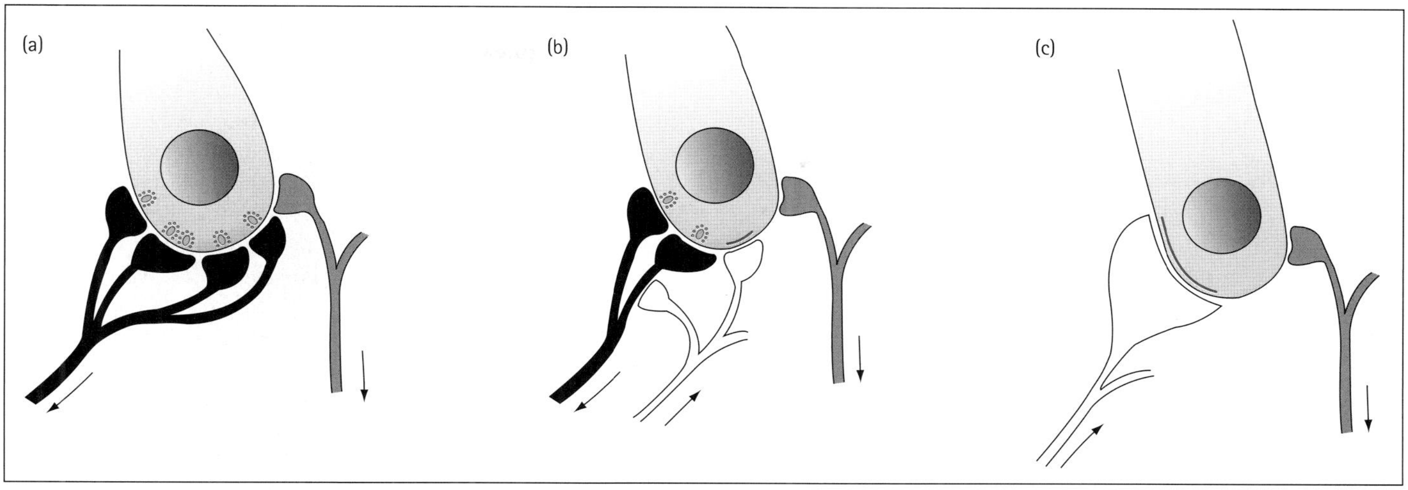

Figure 9.6 (a) The OHC is first exclusively innervated by afferent endings probably belonging to radial (left) and spiral (right) systems. The OHC is a pure sensory cell. Stage 14–16 weeks. (b) Medial efferent endings begin to form synapses with the OHC, while radial afferents retract. The OHC turns into the motile type. Stage 18–20 weeks (at onset of cochlear function). (c) All OHCs in the basal half of the cochlea have lost radial afferents: large medial efferent synapses are now prominent. Stage 26–30 weeks.

Synaptogenesis

IHCs mature earlier than OHCs, and synaptogenesis in both types of cells begins very early.[11] In a 12–13-week-old fetus (i.e. at least 6–8 weeks before the onset of function), classic afferent synapses, with presynaptic bodies surrounded by vesicles, can be first seen at the IHC bases, and then a week later at the OHC bases. The first pattern of IHC innervation is not really different from the eventual adult configuration, apart from the great number of afferent endings due to the branching of dendrites, and the frequent occurrence of direct 'synaptic-like' contacts between efferent endings and the base of the IHC. On the contrary, at this stage, the OHCs are exclusively innervated by afferents (Figure 9.6a). The late stages of synaptogenesis, as described in small experimental mammals,[21] then quite exclusively involve OHCs. Here, together with a drastic modification of cell shape when pear-shaped becomes cylindrical, the development of synapses involves the late arrival of fibres from the medial efferent system, which eventually form synapses directly with the OHC base (Figure 9.6b). This occurs at about the onset of cochlear function, i.e. around week 20 in the human fetus. However, mature efferent–OHC synapses are not found until 1 or 2 months later (Figure 9.6c).

To summarize, in the human as in other mammals, the evolution of the synaptic organization at OHC level seems to follow its physiological evolution. Starting from a typical sensory stage (i.e. a cell just innervated to send auditory messages to the brain), the OHC eventually takes on at the end of maturation specific properties more linked to cochlear micromechanics (i.e. its motile properties are regulated by the efferent system). It appears that this complete OHC development occurs mainly in the basal part of the cochlea (the portion involved in coding high or mid-range frequencies). In the apical part, this development may be incomplete, especially because fewer efferents arrive at this level. The adult apical OHC may well retain some classical sensory properties; at least it seems to be innervated for that purpose.

A similar conclusion thus emerges from the study of two of the major events in the sensory and neural maturation of the cochlea: synaptogenesis and ciliogenesis. Not only do the maturation processes begin at the base, but they do not appear to be completed at the apex. It would appear from our findings that humans have a 'basal' cochlea (with OHCs mechanically very 'active') less extended than in most common laboratory mammals. Conversely, a longer portion of the cochlea bearing 'apical' properties: i.e., with OHCs having a prominent afferent innervation[22] and possibly more classic sensory properties, could have something to do with a better coding of low-frequency tones.

Physiology of the developing human auditory system

If animal physiological data are abundant and strongly correlated with anatomy (reviewed in references 1, 2 and 3), our knowledge about the physiological development of the human cochlea is to a large extent based not on cochlear recordings, but on much more integrated responses such as brainstem auditory-evoked potentials (BAEP) or behavioural responses. This implies that some bias is introduced by the maturation of the brain auditory pathway. Indeed, when the cochlea starts sending auditory messages to the brain (around week 20 of gestation), the maturation of auditory pathways is far from completed (Figures 9.7 and 9.9). Moreover, while the cochlea finishes its maturation during the last trimester of pregnancy, the auditory brain structures are not supposed to end their development until the age of 4–8 years.[1]

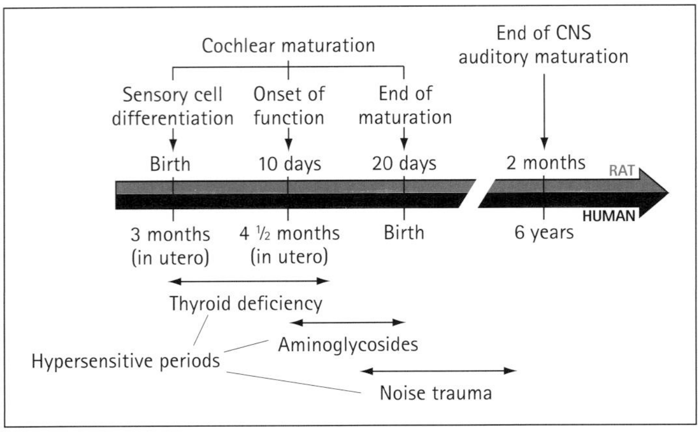

Figure 9.7 Linear development of the cochlea and the auditory brain in both human and rat. The human scale (bottom black line) shows the three main stages of cochlear development (all in utero) and the delayed completion of maturation for the auditory brain (up to 6 or 8 years). Hypersensitive periods are the estimated periods of development when the cochlea has been shown, in the rat, to be particularly affected by thyroid deficiency, exposure to ototoxic drugs, or noise trauma. CNS, central nervous system.

The maturation within the auditory pathways proceeds following a centripetal gradient from the brainstem to the cerebral cortex:[23] this means that primary or basic decoding (frequency, intensity, localization) and reflex responses mature earlier than complex decoding and cognitive aspects of auditory perception.

Onset of cochlear function

The BAEP technique has been used to assess hearing and to measure its maturation in newborn and premature infants.[24] Starr et al[25] succeeded in recording slow cortical-evoked potentials from preterm infants as young as 25 weeks of gestation. Interestingly, the minimum stimulus intensity required to elicit evoked responses was 65 dB SPL. Uziel et al[26] recorded BAEP in three premature infants ranging in gestational age from 30 to 32 weeks, and found the thresholds to be about 40–50 dB SPL.

Despite these late first recordings, the onset of cochlear function in the human fetus can be estimated from the structural development of the cochlea and its correlation with similar studies in experimental mammals (see previous section). By 20 weeks of gestation, the human cochlea has achieved a developmental status comparable to that found in other mammals when the first responses to sound can be readily evoked.[20] At this time, the cochlea has high thresholds and very poor discriminative properties which, together with the environment of the fetal inner ear (fluids in external and middle ear, sound attenuation by maternal tissues, etc.), account for the impossibility of detecting signs of cochlear activity using behavioural or electrophysiological methods until a few weeks later.

End of physiological cochlear development

It is also reasonable to assume from morphological data on the fetal cochlea that the period of development of cochlear potentials is all included within the normal prenatal period. Actually, morphological findings tend to indicate that the development of the human cochlea is achieved by 30 weeks of gestation.

This is confirmed by behavioural and BAEP studies performed in premature infants showing that threshold sensitivity is adult-like at about 35 weeks of gestational age.[25,26] It is likely that, as in other mammals, the development of frequency selectivity is achieved at about the same time. N1 latency, as measured from BAEP, only reaches adult values a few weeks after birth, partly because of the delayed maturation (myelination) of the spiral ganglion and auditory nerve fibres.[24–26]

Otoacoustical emissions, which directly reflect the activity of OHCs, have been used to assess cochlear function in newborns.[15,16,27] It appears that most of the development of this sophisticated cochlear function also occurs prenatally: only subtle changes are observed in the first few weeks after birth.

Critical periods during cochlear development

Many experimental studies have shown that the developing ear is more susceptible than the adult ear to factors arising from external or internal development (reviewed in reference 28). These studies have found periods of increased susceptibility to various factors such as ototoxic antibiotics (reviewed in reference 29), noise exposure (reviewed in reference 30), and thyroid deficiency (reviewed in reference 31). Here, we will just emphasize the main points from these experimental data and their possible implications for human cochlear development. Figure 9.7 gives a schematic representation of the sensitive period of the rat cochlea to hypothyroidism, aminoglycosides, and noise trauma. The corresponding stages of the cochlear development both in rat and human are indicated.

Period of sensitivity to thyroid deficiency

The association of congenital deafness with thyroid deficiency has been reported for years. A detailed experimental study done in rats[31] clearly demonstrates that thyroid deficiency, at a very early stage of cochlear development, results in severe abnormalities in the anatomical and functional maturation of the cochlea. A translation from the rat to the human scale (see Figure 9.7) enables a thyroid hormone-sensitive period in the human fetus cochlea to be scheduled at about the 3rd month of pregnancy.

Period of sensitivity to antibiotic treatment

Above a certain dosage, aminoglycoside antibiotics are well known to have an ototoxic effect on the adult cochlea. However, these drugs have different effects on developing cochleas.[29] Three main results arise from experimental data: (1) the cochlea is affected by aminoglycosides as soon as it begins to function; (2) during the period of its functional maturation, the cochlea is much more sensitive to aminoglycosides than in adulthood—the threshold of ototoxicity can be reached with a 4–5 times lower dose; (3) in the guinea pig, which undergoes in utero cochlear development, this increased susceptibility to aminoglycosides also occurs.

If such a period of sensitivity is to be found in humans, it would be (see Figure 9.7) during the last 5 months of pregnancy, and as a result premature babies would be at higher risk than expected from aminoglycoside antibiotic treatment.

Period of sensitivity to noise trauma

The traumatic effects of intense noise on the adult cochlea have been also extensively studied. In young rodents or cats, during the developmental period, damage has been reported to occur at a level of noise exposure which would not have been traumatic in adulthood.[30] This period of supra-sensitivity to noise trauma has been correlated with the last stage of cochlear development, when the cochlea acquires its exquisite properties of sensitivity and frequency–selectivity. This means that a developing human cochlea is probably more sensitive to noise from 6 months in utero to a few months after birth. Again, premature babies represent a high-risk group, especially if we take into account an overlapping at that time of antibiotic and noise-sensitive periods (see Figure 9.7). These two factors could well combine to increase the deleterious effect, as suggested in animal experiments. Indeed, a harmful combination of noise (non-traumatic by itself) and aminoglycoside treatment (also non-ototoxic by itself) often occurs with premature babies maintained in incubators.

From what we know of the existence and the precise time-course of these sensitive periods in experimental mammals, we must take all precautions in human premature babies to prevent a possible combined effect of the potentially harmful factors that may affect cochlear development. This is a serious matter, even if most of the studies carried out in paediatric ear, nose and throat (ENT) departments do not show clear damage linked with antibiotics, or noise trauma. In fact, damage could well be small and/or limited to a high-frequency range, causing it to be overlooked at the time of treatment.[32] Later, if perceptible hearing impairment develops, a correlation with what happened in the developmental period may prove to be difficult.

What does the human fetus hear?

As stated just above, the human fetus cochlea is both anatomically and functionally capable of coding a sound and sending the message to the brain from about mid-pregnancy onwards. There is also behavioural evidence that the human baby is able to hear in utero.[33–36] The human fetus shows motor responses to acoustical stimuli between 24 and 25 weeks[33] and cardiac responses from 26 weeks on.[34,35] Several studies have quantitatively assessed the sound environment that surrounds the fetus in utero.[36] Maternal tissues may attenuate sounds from the external environment, depending upon the frequency (the higher the frequency, the higher the attenuation). The rather good transmission of low-frequency environmental sounds makes it likely that stimuli of sufficient intensity in this range of frequencies are audible during the 3rd trimester of gestation.

It is nevertheless very difficult to estimate exactly what the human baby hears in utero, as both the external and middle ear are filled with amniotic fluid. In an extrauterine organism, such a status would result in a threshold increase of 30–40 dB. Consequently, any estimation of what the human baby is really capable of hearing is speculative. Recent observations suggest that the fetus is more sensitive to temporal than spatial cues; at least, prenatal auditory learning involves the rhythm or prosody more than frequency selectivity.

Plasticity of the developing auditory system

Plasticity, defined as a change in the functional properties of neurones mainly depending on synaptic remodelling, is a general characteristic of neural structures. The auditory system, like all other sensory systems, is thus susceptible to lesion- and/or use-related plasticity, and this plasticity is much more pronounced during development than in adulthood.

After peripheral deprivation or lesion, as well as after specific training, the auditory brain (especially the cortex) is known to reorganize its structures and functional properties (remapping, for instance, its frequency representation). Even the first synapses in the cochlea (between the IHCs and the auditory nerve) have been shown to regenerate after being wiped out by an excitotoxic injury.[37] Only a brief review of developmental plasticity will be given, and the hot debate about hair cell regeneration will not be included, as it deserves a special chapter.

Developmental plasticity

The development of any specific sensory areas in the brain depends on appropriate stimulations during the developmental period. This has been abundantly documented in the visual system where it is clear that early experience is critical for the acquisition of different properties of vision, such as stereoscopy. Similarly, in the auditory system the cochlea plays a key role during the first years of life in building the adult auditory brain. Therefore, any impairment in the development and functioning of the cochlea will affect the development of the auditory brain.

This can be summarized as follows. Normal maturation of the cochlea, reaching its maximum performance at birth, will slowly (within 4–8 years, depending on the perceptual task) drive a normal auditory brain to the acquisition of its maximum performance (Figure 9.8a).

Conversely, with abnormal or uncompleted maturation of the cochlea, the auditory brain will not receive enough stimulation to fully develop (Figure 9.8b).

The influence of early stimulation (i.e. messages sent by the cochlea) on the auditory cortex neurones is illustrated in Figure 9.9. The same area of the cat auditory cortex is represented at the time before the onset of cochlear function (Figure 9.9a), when pyramidal neurones have few dendritic branches (i.e. few synapses), and at the end of cortical maturation (after months of normal functioning of the cochlea) (Figure 9.9b), when

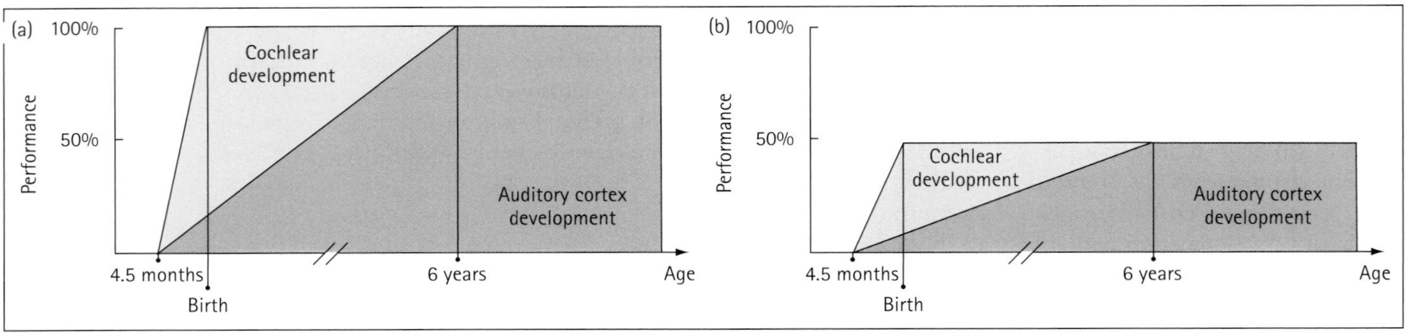

Figure 9.8 (a) Scheme illustrating that a cochlea reaching 100% of performance will enable the auditory brain to reach the same level later on. (b) Scheme illustrating that, with a cochlea reaching over 50% of performance, the auditory brain development will be limited.

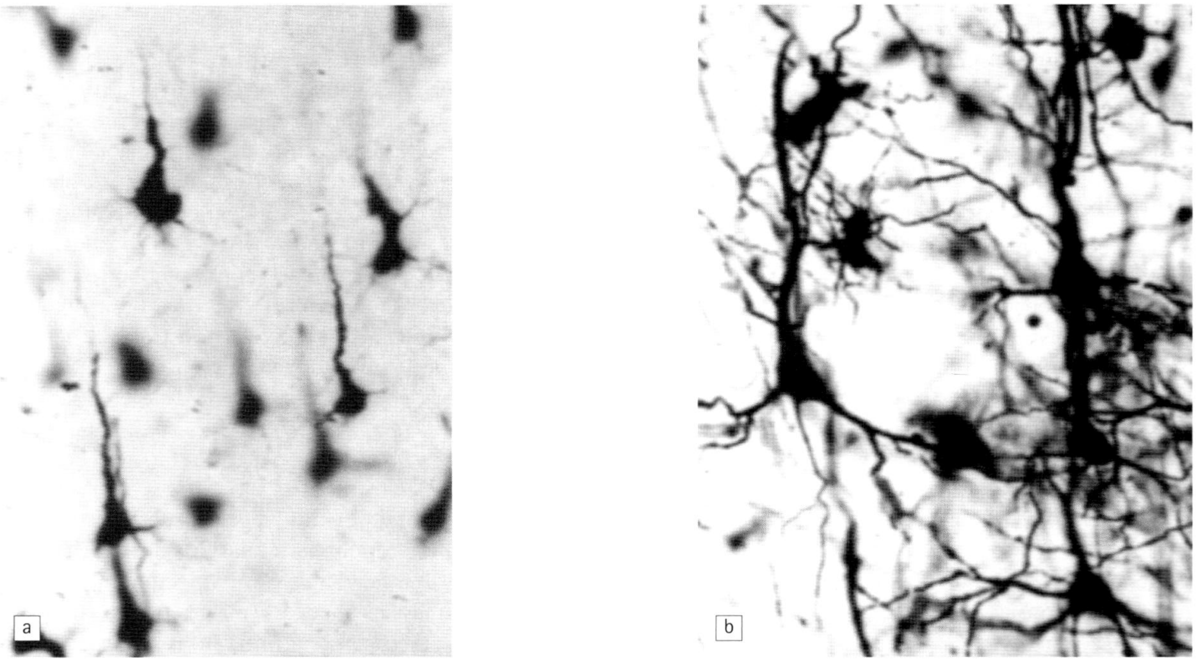

Figure 9.9 (a) Pyramidal cortex auditory neurones in a new born kitten (a stage which corresponds to 16 weeks of gestation in humans). The cochlea has not yet begun to send messages, and dendritic branches (and therefore synapses) are poor. (b) Similar neurones in a 6-month (fully mature) cat auditory cortex (a stage which corresponds to age 6 years in human). Mostly because of messages sent by a normal cochlea, the dendritic branches (and therefore synapses) of pyramidal neurones are very dense.

pyramidal neurones exhibit a profuse dendritic branching (i.e. a lot of synapses). In deaf white cats, where the cochlea is genetically dysfunctional, the neurones in adulthood resemble more those of the immature stage, as they have not received the proper stimulation to form and stabilize their synapses.

These findings are relevant for an early rehabilitation or implantation in infants: anything which can improve the messages sent to the brain during the developmental period, will improve the abilities of the cortical neurones to carry out their perceptual tasks.

It should be mentioned that the brain can be deprived of normal stimulation, not because of cochlear problems, but because of middle ear problems. While the clinical solution is easier, the same care should be taken to detect and cure the problem as early as possible.

Similarly, it could be particularly rewarding to 'feed' the cochlea (and therefore the auditory brain) early in a specific domain, in order to obtain the best perceptual and long-lasting results: this is particularly true for learning a foreign language or music.[38]

Acknowledgements

The authors of this chapter are deeply indebted to their past co-workers, especially to Alain Uziel for the physiological and pathological data in the human, and to Marc Lenoir, who did a lot of reference work in experimental mammals. Illustrations have been realized thanks to Centre Régional d'Imagerie Cellulaire (Université Montpellier 1 / INSERM) and its staff. Thanks also go to George Tate for editing work. Most of the figures are from the educational web site of the Centre 'Promenade around the cochlea' by R. Pujol, S. Blatrix, and T. Pujol. (http://www.iurc.montp.inserm. fr/cric/audition).

References

1. Pujol R, Uziel A. Auditory development peripheral aspects. In: Meisami E, Timiras PS, eds. *Handbook of Human Growth and Developmental Biology*. Vol I. *Neural, Sensory, Motor, and Integrative Development. Part B. Sensory, Motor, and Integrative Development*. Boca Raton: CRC Press, 1988; 109–30.
2. Lavigne-Rebillard M, Pujol R. Auditory hair cells in human fetuses: synaptogenesis and ciliogenesis. *J Electron Microsc Techn* 1990; **15**: 115–22.
3. Rubel EW. Ontogeny of structure and function in vertebrate auditory system. In: Autrum H, Jung R, Loewenstein WR, MacKay DM, Teuber HL eds. *Handbook of Sensory Physiology*, Vol. IX. Berlin: Springer Verlag, 1978.
4. Romand R. *Development of Auditory and Vestibular Systems*. New York: Academic Press, 1983.
5. Pujol R, Lavigne-Rebillard M, Lenoir M. Development of sensory and neural structures in the mammalian cochlea. In: Rubel EW, Popper AN, Fay RR, eds. *Development of the Auditory System, Springer Handbook of Auditory Research*, Vol. XII. New York: Springer, 1997; 146–92.
6. Streeter GL. The development of the scala tympani, scala vestibuli and perioticular cistern in the human embryo. *Am J Anat* 1917; **21**: 299–320.
7. Bast TH, Anson BJ. *The Temporal Bone and Ear*. New York: Charles C. Thomas, 1949.
8. Igarashi Y. Cochlea of the human fetus: a scanning electron microscope study. *Arch Histol Jap* 1980; **43**: 195–209.
9. Lavigne-Rebillard M, Pujol R. Development of auditory hair cell surface in human fetuses: a scanning electron microscopy study. *Anat Embryol* 1986; **174**: 369–77.
10. Pujol R. Morphology, synaptology and electrophysiology of the developing auditory periphery. *Acta Otolaryngol (Stockh)* 1985; Suppl 421: 5–9.
11. Pujol R, Lavigne-Rebillard M. Early stages of innervation and sensory cell differentiation in the human fetal organ of Corti. *Acta Otolaryngol (Stockh)* 1985; Suppl 423: 43–50.
12. Bredberg G. Cellular pattern and nerve supply of the human organ of Corti. *Acta Otolaryngol (Stockh)* 1968; Suppl 236.
13. Kawabata I, Nomura Y. Extra internal hair cells: a scanning electron microscopic study. *Acta Otolaryngol* 1978; **85**: 342–48.
14. Tanaka K, Sakai N, Terayama Y. Organ of Corti in the human fetus. Scanning and transmission electron microscope studies. *Ann Otol Rhinol Laryngol* 1979; **88**: 749–58.
15. Bonfils P, Uziel A, Pujol R. Screening for auditory dysfunction in infants by evoked otoacoustic emissions. *Archiv Otolaryngol Head Neck Surg* 1988; **114**: 887–90.
16. Kemp DT, Ryan S. Otoacoustic emission tests in neonatal screening programmes. *Acta Otolaryngol (Stockh)* 1991; Suppl **482**: 73–84.
17. Abdouh A, Despres G, Romand R. Hair cell overproduction in the developing mammalian cochlea in culture. *Neuroreport* 1993; **5**: 33–6.
18. Kelley MW, Xiao-Mei Xu, Wagner MA, Warchol ME, Corwin JT. The developing organ of Corti contains retinoic acid and forms supernumerary hair cells in response to exogenous retinoic acid in culture. *Development* 1993; **119**: 1041–53.
19. Chiong CM, Burgess BJ, Nadol JB. Postnatal maturation of human spiral ganglion cells: light and electron microscopic observations. *Hear Res* 1993; **67**: 211–19.
20. Pujol R, Hilding D. Anatomy and physiology of the onset of auditory function. *Acta Otolaryngol (Stockh)* 1973; **76**: 1–11.
21. Pujol R. Synaptic plasticity in the developing cochlea. In: Ruben RW, Van de Water TR, Rubel EW, eds. *The Biology of Change in Otolaryngology*. New York: Elsevier, 1986; 47–54.
22. Nadol JB. Serial section reconstruction of the neural poles of the hair cells in the human organ of Corti. II. Outer hair cells. *Laryngoscope* 1983; **93**: 780–91.
23. Pujol R. Development of tone-burst responses along the auditory pathway in the cat. *Acta Otolaryngol (Stockh)* 1972; **74**: 383–91.
24. Schulman-Galambos C, Galambos R. Brainstem auditory evoked responses in premature infants. *J Speech Hear Res* 1975; **18**: 456–65.
25. Starr A, Amlie RN, Martin WH, Sanders S. Development of auditory function in newborn infants revealed by auditory brainstem potentials. *Pediatrics* 1977; **60**: 831–9.
26. Uziel A, Marot M, Germain M. Les potentiels évoqués du nerf auditif et du tronc cérébral chez le nouveau-né et l'enfant. *Rev Laryngol Otol Rhinol* 1980; **101**: 55–9.
27. Morlet T, Collet L, Salle B, Morgon A. Functional maturation of cochlear active mechanisms and of the medial olivocochlear efferent system in humans. *Acta Otolaryngol (Stockh)* 1993; **113**: 271–7.
28. Eggermont JJ, Bock GR. Critical periods in auditory development. *Acta Otolaryngol (Stockh)* 1986; Suppl 429.
29. Pujol R. Periods of sensitivity to antibiotic treatment. *Acta Otolaryngol (Stockh)* 1986; Suppl 429: 29–33.
30. Lenoir M, Pujol R, Bock GR. Critical periods of susceptibility to noise induced hearing loss. In: Salvi R, Henderson RP, Hamernik, Colletti V eds. *Basic and Applied Aspects of Noise Induced Hearing Loss*. New York: Plenum Publishing, 1986, pp. 227–36.
31. Uziel A. Periods of sensitivity to thyroid hormone during the development of the organ of Corti. *Acta Otolaryngol (Stockh)* 1986; Suppl 429: 23–7.
32. Bernard PA. Freedom from ototoxicity in aminoglycoside-treated neonates: a mistaken motion. *Laryngoscope* 1981; **16**: 1985–94.
33. Birnholz JC, Benacerraf BR,. Development of human fetal hearing. *Science* 1983; **222**: 516–18.

34. Sonntag LW, Wallace RF. Changes in the rate of the human fetal heart in response to vibratory stimuli. *Am J Obstet Dis Child* 1936; **51**: 583–9.
35. Read JA, Miller FC. Fetal heart rate acceleration in response to acoustic stimulation as a measure of fetal well-being. *Am J Obstet Gynecol* 1977; **129**: 512–17.
36. Granier-Deferre C, Lecanuet JP, Cohen H, Busnel MC. Feasibility of prenatal hearing tests. *Acta Otolaryngol (Stockh)* 1985; Suppl **421**: 93–101.
37. Puel JL, Safieddine S, Gervais d'Aldin C, Eybalin M, Pujol R. Synaptic regeneration and functional recovery after excitotoxic injury in the guinea pig cochlea. *CR Acad Sci Paris, ser III* 1995; **318**: 67–75.
38. Pantev C, Oostenveld R, Engelien A, Ross B, Roberts LE, Hoke M. Increased auditory cortical representation in musicians. *Nature* 1998; **392**: 811–14.

10 Physiology of the auditory system

Edward F Evans

Introduction: physics and psychophysics

Auditory signals

Sound is any fluctuation of air (or water) pressure which elicits the sensation of hearing. What we perceive as pitch is related to the frequency of the vibrations, and loudness is related to their amplitude.

Frequency is measured in the number of vibrations per second (Hz). The human ear is sensitive to frequencies from about 20 Hz to 20 kHz (Figure 10.1). The note 'A' used for tuning an orchestra is at 440 Hz, in the middle of the piano scale. Frequency is commonly plotted on a logarithmic scale (as in Figure 10.1), which corresponds to the mapping of frequency in the ear (see later) and the piano scale. On this scale, equal distances represent equal ratios of frequency. Thus octaves represent doubling of the frequency.

Sound amplitude is typically measured on a logarithmic scale of the ratios of sound power. Thus: the decibel (dB) = 10 $\log_{10}$ (intensity 1/intensity 2) = 20 $\log_{10}$ (pressure 1/pressure 2).

It is important to remember that the decibel scale is therefore relative rather than absolute, i.e. it refers to ratios of powers or of intensities (same thing). However, it is conventional and convenient to refer any given sound intensity to an internationally accepted reference (known as 0 dB SPL). In pressure terms, this reference is 20 μPa.

On this SPL scale, the human ear can hear from about 0 dB SPL at 4 kHz (see Figure 10.1) up to the threshold of pain around 140 dB SPL (Table 10.1).

The ear has a substantial task to analyse and process complex sounds like speech (Figure 10.2). It has to break down a complex sound into its component frequencies (indicated by degrees of blackness in Figure 10.2), so that they can be separated from other frequency components simultaneously present and their trajectories followed in time. Figure 10.2a indicates the spectogram of the speech sound 'spike', and Figure 10.2b the waveform as recorded by a microphone, both on the same time axis.

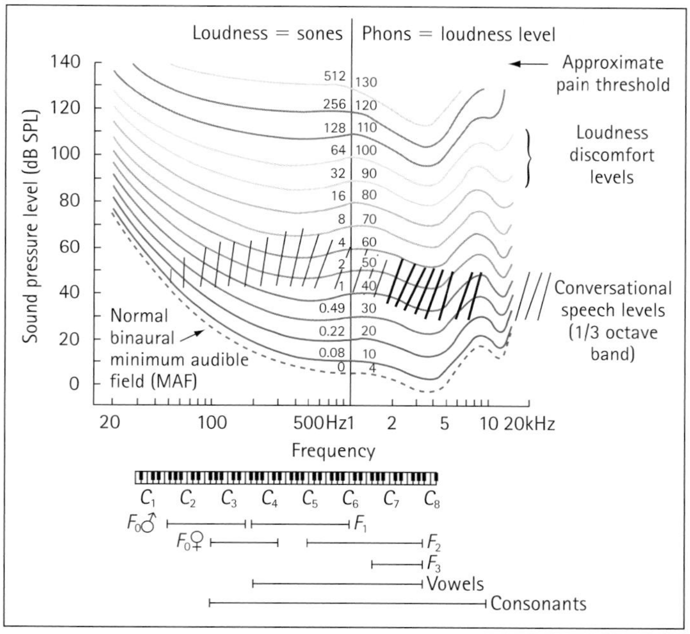

Figure 10.1 Frequency and intensity range of human hearing. Frequency is mapped out on a logarithmic scale (see piano keyboard) and intensity in terms of sound pressure level (dB SPL). The lower dashed line indicates the threshold of hearing of a young adult with normal hearing in the 'free field'. The cross-hatched area indicates conversational speech levels measured in 1/3 octave bands. (Reproduced from Evans EF. In: HB Barlow and JD Mollon, eds. *The Senses*. Cambridge: Cambridge University Press, 1982. Figure 13.3.[1])

This is accomplished by four levels of 'filtering' in the auditory system:

1. Peripheral mechanisms—setting the sensitivity to the auditory modality; outer, middle and inner ears, especially hair cells.
2. Peripheral mechanisms—setting the sensitivity to the frequency range of hearing; outer, middle and inner ears, especially middle ear.
3. Peripheral filtering at the receptor/neural level.

Table 10.1 Relations between sound pressure, power, and level, with typical examples drawn from common situations.

Sound pressure (N/m^2 or Pa)	Power (intensity) (W/m^2)	Sound pressure level (dB SPL, i.e. referred to 20 μPa)	Examples and some effects (approximate only)
200	100	140	Jet engine; over-amplified rock group; threshold for pain
20	1	120	Damage to cochlear hair cells
6.32	10^{-1}	110	Threshold for discomfort
2	10^{-2}	100	Motor cycle engine
			Orchestra playing
6.32×10^{-1}	10^{-3}	90	*fff*
2×10^{-1}	10^{-4}	80	*ff*, busy traffic; shouting
2×10^{-2}	10^{-6}	60	*mf*, normal conversation
2×10^{-3}	10^{-8}	40	*pp*; quiet office
6.32×10^{-4}	10^{-9}	30	*ppp*; soft whisper
2×10^{-4}	10^{-10}	20	Country area at night
2×10^{-5}	10^{-12}	0	Threshold of hearing of young person at 1–5 kHz
6.32×10^{-6}	10^{-13}	−10	Threshold of cat's hearing (1–10 kHz)

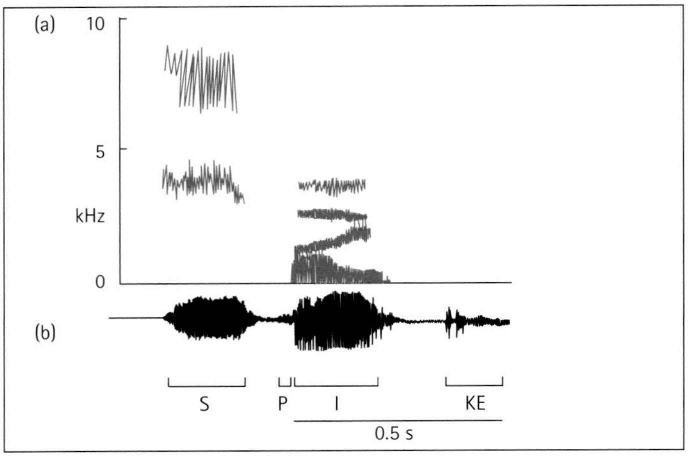

Figure 10.2 Spectrogram and waveform of word 'Spike'. The spectrogram (a) shows in red the frequency analysis with time of the waveform shown in (b). (Reproduced from Evans EF. In: HB Barlow and DJ Mollon, eds. *The Senses*. Cambridge: Cambridge University Press, 1982. Figure 15.8.[1])

4. Central filtering—assessing the significance of complex sounds.

Filters and tuning

A filter is a mechanical, electronic or mathematical device that separates wanted from unwanted signals. Thus a coffee filter separates the wanted liquid from the unwanted coffee grounds. In radio and TV sets, filters are used to separate a wanted channel from unwanted channels. This is accomplished by electronic filters tuned to the frequencies of the channels. The ear operates in a remarkably similar way.

Filters come in a variety of 'flavours': low-pass, high-pass and bandpass (Figure 10.3). A low-pass filter passes low frequencies up to a given cut-off frequency; a high-pass filter passes high frequencies down to the cut-off frequency. A bandpass filter is the sum of two overlapping low- and high-pass filters, so that only a band of frequencies (the pass-band) between two cut-offs is passed. Frequencies outside the pass-band are rejected. In a band pass filter, the centre of the pass-band is called the centre frequency. The width of the filter is the width of the pass-band, otherwise known as its bandwidth. The curve depicting the outline of the pass-band (as in Figure 10.3, middle) is called its tuning curve, and the centre frequency its tuned frequency. Bandpass filters having narrow bandwidths are called sharply tuned, and those with wide bandwidths, broadly tuned.

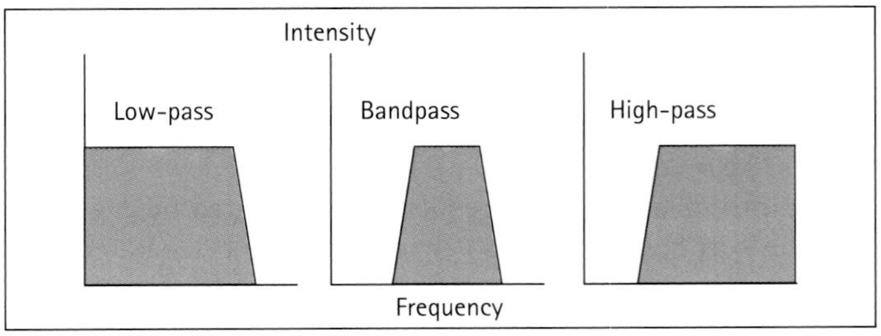

Figure 10.3 Diagrammatic representation of three types of filter showing the energy passed as a function of frequency.

As we will see, the ear acts as if it contains a very large number ('a bank') of narrow bandpass filters, each tuned to a slightly different frequency from its neighbour.

The outer ear

This consists of the pinna or auricle (present only in non-aquatic mammals) and the external auditory meatus.

The pinna and external auditory canal together form a resonator giving a substantial increase in sound pressure at the eardrum of 10–20 dB between 2 and 6 kHz, an important frequency region for communication. Different animals have different dimensions of these structures, and therefore the resonant frequency will be different (typically higher in smaller mammals) but is also matched to the appropriate communication frequency region.

The shape and folds of the pinna, by multiple reflections of sounds, cause minor variations in the amplitude spectrum of the sounds entering the ear, and are utilized in monaural localization.

The outer ear can therefore be regarded as a signal conditioner.

Middle ear

The middle ear acts as an impedance transformer and further modifies the frequency response of the overall ear.

The middle ear (eardrum, ossicles, stapes footplate) converts vibrations from the air to pressure changes inside the fluids of the inner ear. Because the acoustical impedance of the fluids of the inner ear is much higher than that of the air, the middle ear in mammals acts as an impedance transformer. Without this, the efficiency of transmission of energy from the air to the fluids would be very poor. The transformer action is largely determined by the ratio of areas of the eardrum to stapes footplate and partly by the lever ratio (Figure 10.4).

The transmission of vibrations through the middle ear can be controlled to an extent by the middle ear muscles acting on the first and third ossicle. Reflex activation of these muscles is responsible for the middle ear reflex used to reduce sound transmission at very high sound levels for protection.

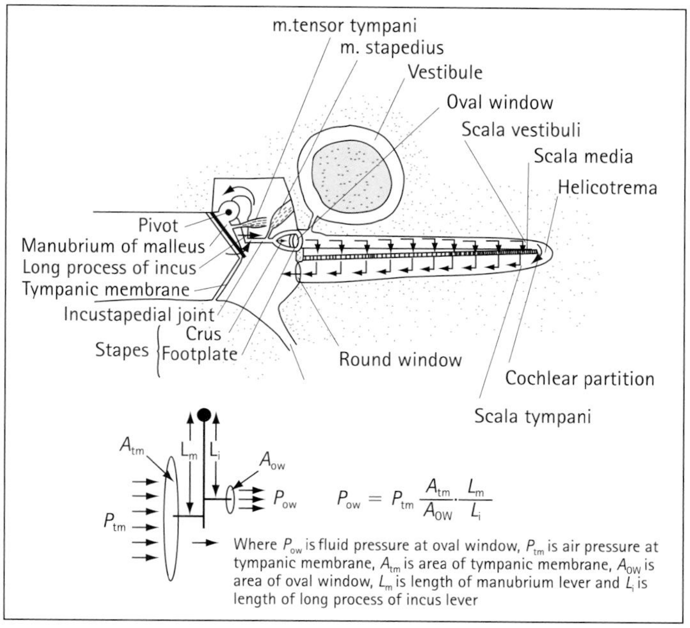

Figure 10.4 Schematic functional diagram of middle ear and uncoiled inner ear, and middle ear transformer. Vibrations of the tympanic membrane are transmitted as rotations of the malleus and incus about the common axis (normal to page, marked with dot). This produces piston-like movements of the stapes footplate in the oval window, with transmission of the pressure changes across the cochlear partition virtually instantaneously throughout the cochlear length. Arrows indicate direction of movements in response to a compression wave. The lower diagram illustrates transformer action of the middle ear by virtue of the large difference in area between the tympanic membrane and oval window, and the (smaller) lever ratio (L_m/L_i). The middle ear muscles are contained in bony canals. The m. stapedius acts sideways on the incustapedial joint to stiffen the ossicular chain. (Reproduced from Evans EF. In: HB Barlow and DJ Mollon, eds. *The Senses*. Cambridge: Cambridge University Press, 1982. Figure 14.4.[1])

Inner ear

Mechanics

Changes in fluid pressure transmitted by the stapes footplate in the oval window into the scala vestibuli (Figure 10.4) are transmitted across the cochlear partition because the round window is able to freely vibrate. These pressure changes across the cochlear partition produce travelling waves (Figure 10.5) along part or all of the length of the basilar membrane of the cochlear

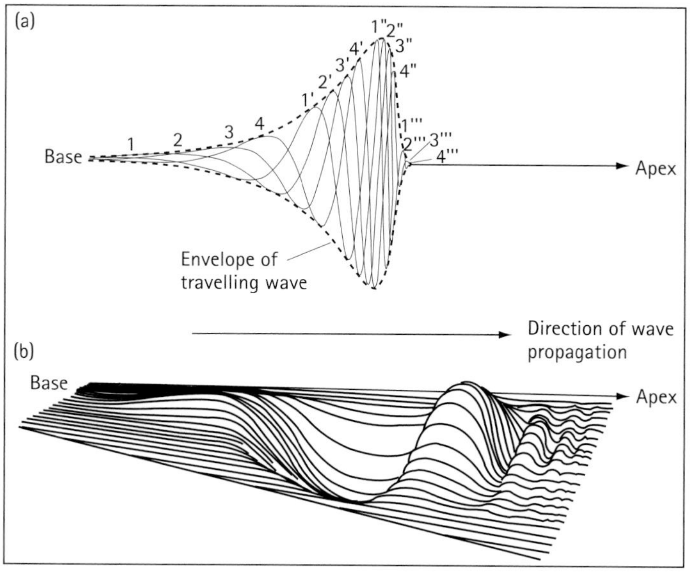

Figure 10.5 Diagrammatic representation of the travelling wave along the basilar membrane. (Reproduced from Evans EF. In: HB Barlow and DJ Mollon, eds. *The Senses*. Cambridge: Cambridge University Press, 1982. Figure 14.8.[1])

partition, depending on the frequency of the sound. This mapping of the maximum amplitude of vibration with frequency is a natural consequence of the changes in width and stiffness of the basilar membrane along its length. For high frequencies, the travelling wave is limited to the basal portion (minimum width and maximum stiffness), whereas for low frequencies, the travelling wave extends throughout the cochlear partition but is maximal at the apex (maximum width and lowest stiffness). Thus, frequency is mapped out along the basilar membrane, low frequencies at the furthest, apical end, to high frequencies at the nearer, basal end. Interestingly, this cochleotopic/tonotopic mapping is according to a logarithmic scale; that is, equal distances represent approximately equal ratios of frequency.

Electrochemical environment of the hair cells

Figure 10.6 shows a simplified electrical schematic of the cochlea. Perilymph in the scala vestibuli and scala tympani consists of normal extracellular fluid rich in sodium and is at body ('earth') potential. In contrast, the fluid filling the scala media (endolymph) is rich in K^+ and is at a relatively high endocochlear potential of about +80 mV. The high K^+ concentration and this high voltage are generated by an energy-requiring K^+ pump located in the stria vascularis. This is the main battery driving current through the cochlear circuit.

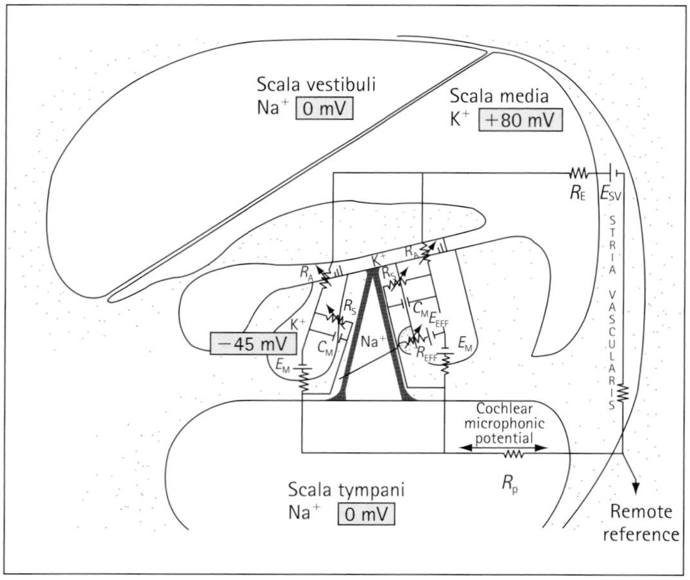

Figure 10.6 Electrical diagram of the cochlea. (Reproduced from Evans EF. In: HB Barlow and DJ Mollon, eds. *The Senses*. Cambridge: Cambridge University Press, 1982. Figure 14.10.[1])

Transduction

Deflections of the hairs on the hair cells in one direction open and in the other direction close relatively non-specific ion channels (probably at the tips of the hairs through which current flows, predominantly carried by the abundant K^+ ions). This current depolarizes the hair cell, producing a receptor potential (Figure 10.7). A low-frequency sinusoidal tone burst as in Figure 10.7 (300 Hz) therefore produces a sinusoidal receptor potential in the hair cell. Much higher frequencies (3 kHz in Figure 10.7) produce mainly a DC (i.e. biased in the depolarizing direction) receptor potential.

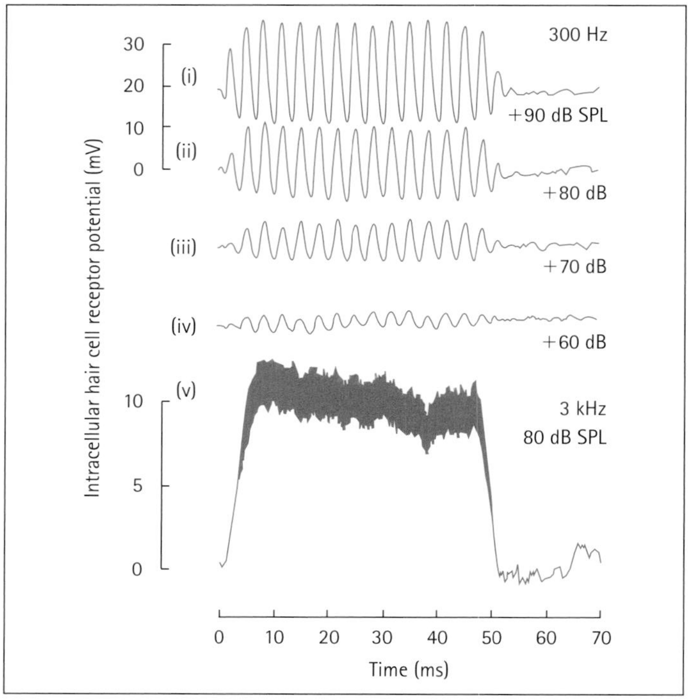

Figure 10.7 Receptor potentials recorded from guinea-pig inner hair cell. (After Russell and Sellick. *J Physiol* 1978: **284**; 261–90[2] and Evans EF. In: HB Barlow and DJ Mollon, eds. *The Senses*. Cambridge: Cambridge University Press, 1982. Figure 14.11.[1])

Because the receptor current corresponding to the potential flows out of the hair cell and across the tissue resistance (R_p in Figure 10.6), a small proportion will be recordable by an external electrode in the tissues around the cochlea, e.g. on the round window as the cochlear microphonic (Figure 10.8). This potential is used clinically, together with the cochlear action potential (CAP), which represents a neural response predominantly from the cochlear nerve.

Inner ear and cochlear nerve

Peripheral tuning at cochlear nerve level

Cochlear nerve fibres respond to tonal stimuli by producing bursts of action potentials (Figure 10.9a). During a tone burst, the discharge rate adapts relatively slowly (Figure 10.9b).

Figure 10.10 shows that this excitatory response is sharply tuned. The frequency–intensity response area is bounded by the

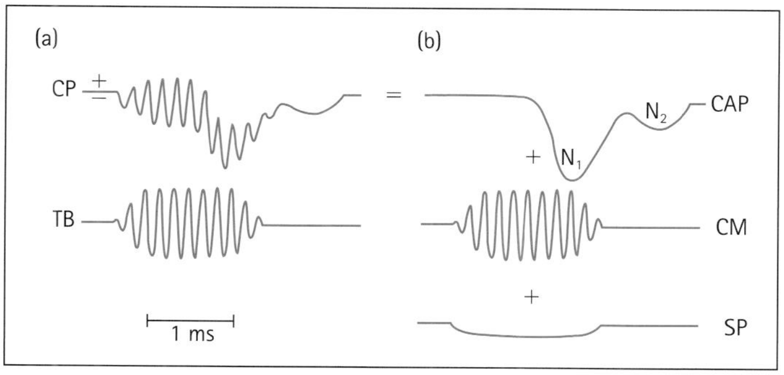

Figure 10.8 Gross cochlear potentials recorded by an electrode on the cochlea. (a) Waveform of cochlear potential (CP) evoked by a short tone burst (TB). (b) This waveform can be analysed into three components: gross cochlear action potential (CAP)—a neural response; the AC cochlear microphonic (CM)—a receptor response; the DC summating potential (SP), probably also a receptor response.(Reproduced from Evans EF. In: HB Barlow and DJ Mollon, eds. *The Senses*. Cambridge: Cambridge University Press, 1982. Figure 14.12.[1])

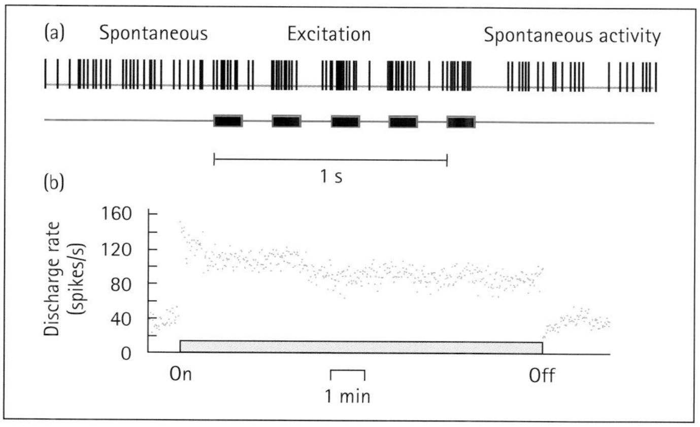

Figure 10.9 Cochlear nerve action potentials: response to tones. (a): recording of action potential spikes in a single nerve fibre of the guinea-pig cochlear nerve in response to five brief tone bursts shown as thickenings on the lower trace. (b): peristimulus time histograms of the discharge rate of a single cat cochlear nerve fibre before, during and immediately following a continuous tone of several minutes' duration. (Reproduced from Evans EF. In: HB Barlow and DJ Mollon, eds. *The Senses*. Cambridge: Cambridge University Press, 1982. Figure 14.14.[1])

frequency threshold ('tuning') curve: the FTC. Figure 10.11 shows families of these curves from cat, guinea pig and squirrel monkey, the curves representing the FTCs of cochlear nerve fibres selected from representative different positions along the cochlea from apex (low frequency) to base (high frequency). The FTCs have comparable shapes across species: at tip frequencies (characteristic frequencies (CFs)) below about 2 kHz, the FTCs are more symmetrical; above about 2 kHz, they are very asymmetrical, with an extended low-frequency 'tail'. These FTCs represent excellent filters which are not easy to mimic in electronic hardware.

If we replot an FTC as a filter function (Figure 10.12), we can estimate its effective or equivalent rectangular bandwidth

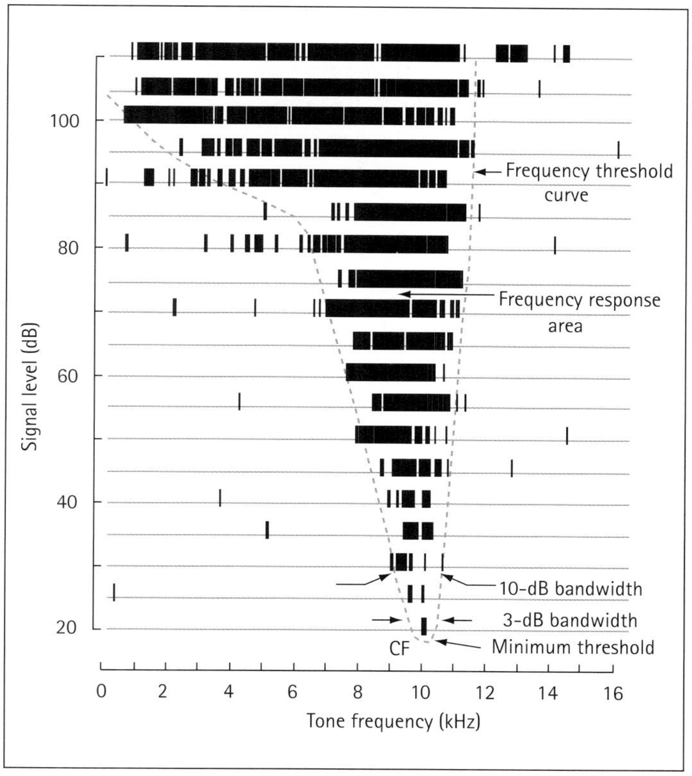

Figure 10.10 Mapping of the frequency-response area of a single cochlear nerve fibre. The action potential spike responses of the nerve fibre are displayed in response to sweeping a continuous tone frequency (horizontally in the Figure), each successive sweep at a higher intensity (vertically). The dashed outline represents the threshold contour: the frequency threshold Curve (FTC); the dark area the frequency response area. (Reproduced from Evans EF. In: HB Barlow and DJ Mollon, eds. *The Senses*. Cambridge: Cambridge University Press, 1982. Figure 14.15.[1])

(ERB) as the width of the rectangular filter having the same area on linear-power, linear-frequency coordinates.

It has recently been shown that this peripheral tuning, as exemplified in the FTCs of cochlear nerve fibres, can account exactly for the psychophysical frequency selectivity in the same species (Figure 10.13). The circles and dotted line represent the bandwidths (ERBs) of cochlear nerve fibres recorded under optimal conditions in the guinea pig; the bracket symbols and continuous line indicate the behavioural ERBs in guinea pigs measured with comb-filtered noise masking, and the crosses similar measurements using band-stop noise masking. Thus our ear's auditory frequency selectivity (our ability to separate a complex sound into its component frequency parts by filtering) is already accomplished at the lowest level of the auditory system, i.e. the cochlea.

Peripheral tuning at basilar membrane and hair cell levels

Figure 10.11b shows the first comparison between basilar membrane (lower curves) and cochlear nerve tuning (upper curves)

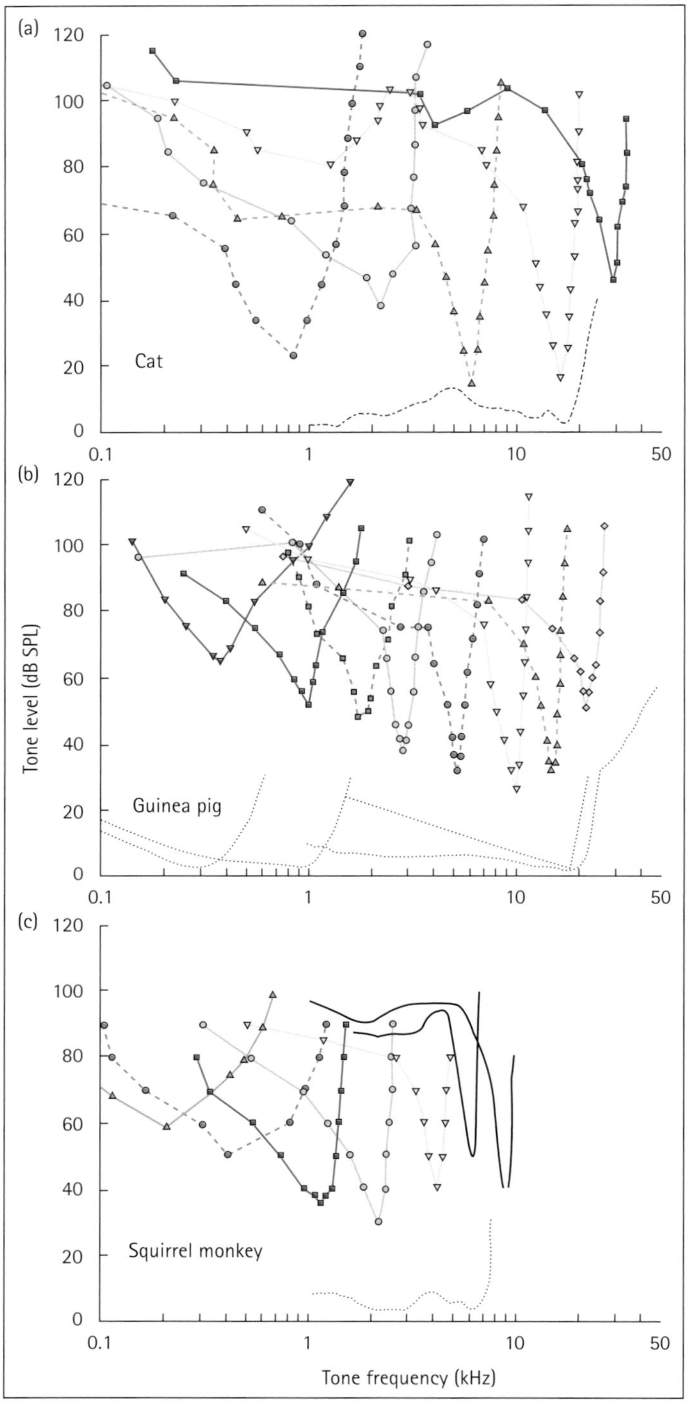

Figure 10.11 Cochlear nerve FTC's for three species. A small number of representative curves are depicted from (a): cat (after Kiang et al. *J Acoust Soc Am* 1967; **42**: 1341-2[3]); (b): guinea-pig (reproduced from Evans EF. *J Physiol* 1972; **226**: 263-87[4]); and (c) squirrel monkey (reproduced from Rose. *J Neurophysiol* 1971; **34**: 685-99.[5]) (Reproduced from Evans EF. In: HB Barlow and DJ Mollon, eds. *The Senses*. Cambridge: Cambridge University Press, 1982. Figure 14.16.[1])

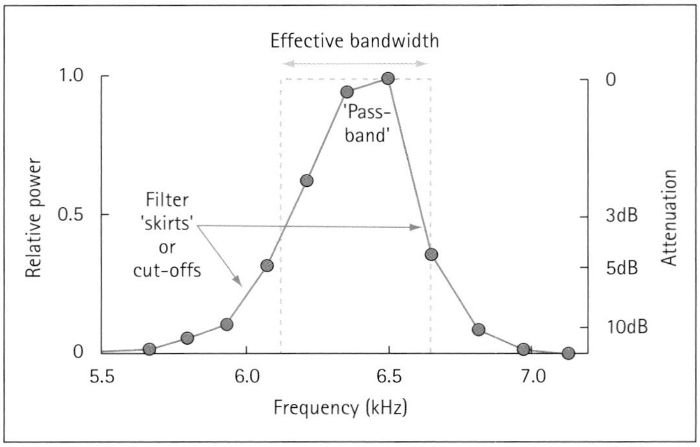

Figure 10.12 Cochlear nerve fibre FTC plotted as a band-pass filter function. The tip of the FTC is plotted upside down compared with Figure 10.11. The red dashed rectangle has the same area as the FTC and is the equivalent rectangular bandwidth (ERB) of the FTC considered as a filter. (Reproduced from Evans EF. In: HB Barlow and DJ Mollon, eds. *The Senses*. Cambridge: Cambridge University Press, 1982. Figure 15.1.[1])

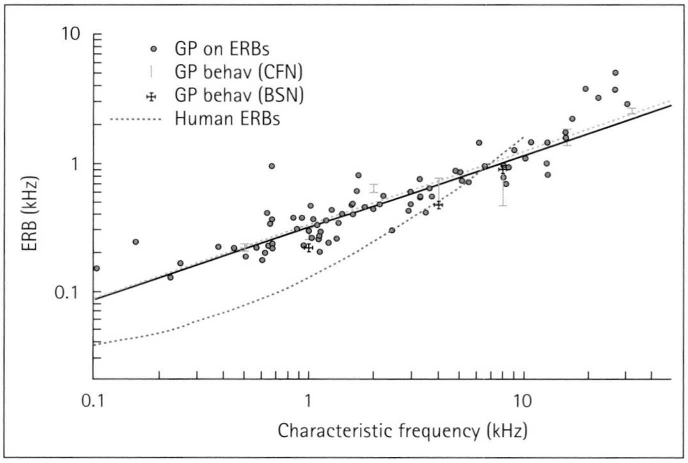

Figure 10.13 Comparison between the physiological and behavioural frequency selectivity in the same species (guinea-pig). All measurements are of ERB's as defined in Figure 10.12: of cochlea nerve fibre FTC's: the circle points; behavioural measurements using comb filtered noise masking: brackets; and using band-stop noise masking: crosses. Regression lines are drawn in black through the physiological data and in red through the behavioural to show the close correspondence. For comparison, human ERB's are shown as the red dashed line. (From Evans EF. *Proc 12th international Conference of the Audio Engineering Society*. New York: A E S. 1983, 11–21. Figure 7.[6])

in the same species—the guinea pig. These early measurements of basilar membrane tuning showed a large discrepancy with the neural tuning. Because we showed that the neural tuning was physiologically vulnerable, i.e. it could be changed from normally sharp to abnormally poorly tuned by lack of oxygen (Figure 10.14), mechanical or drug damage to the cochlea etc., we suggested that there might be two filters acting within the cochlea: a first filter being the poor basilar membrane filter, followed by some sort of additional filtering process to sharpen that up to produce the sharp neural tuning, a process that we called the cochlear 'second filter'. It is now clear that while this

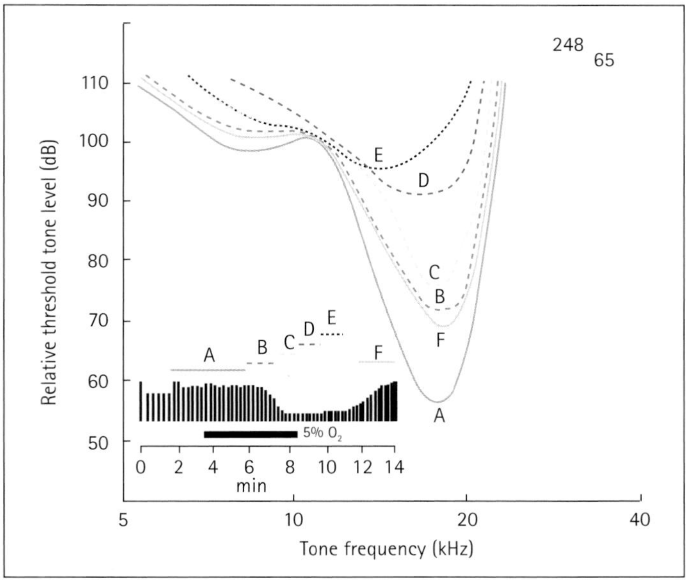

Figure 10.14 Effect of hypoxia on cochlear nerve fibre tuning. A: control curve FTC; B, C, D, E: FTC's obtained from the same fibre during progressive hypoxia (5% oxygen in inspired air); F shows partial recovery after re-oxygenation. From Evans EF. In: Zwicker, Terhardt, eds. *Facts and Models in Hearing*. Springer, Heidelberg: 1974, 118–29.[7])

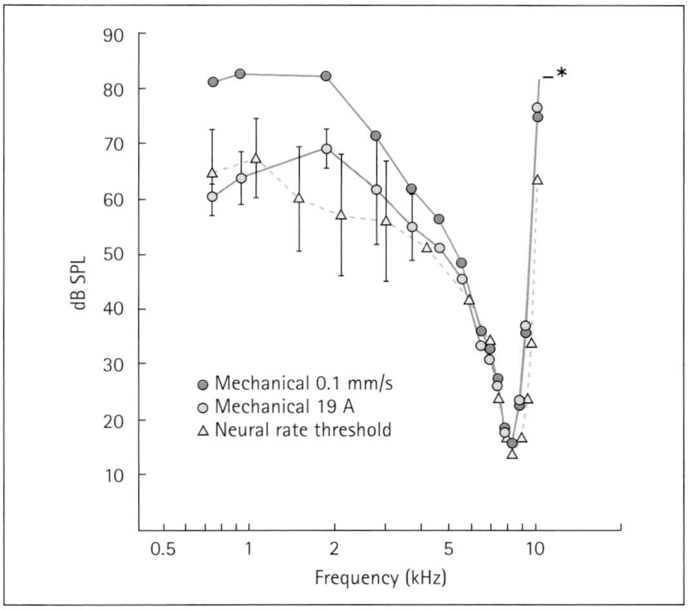

Figure 10.15 Modern basilar membrane tuning curve compared with that of cochlear nerve fibre in chinchilla. (After Robles L et al. *J Acoust Soc Am* 1986; **80**: 1364–74.[8])

serial process remains a good description of cochlear tuning for some animals (e.g. reptiles), for mammals the second filter is not in series with the first, as we originally proposed, but in parallel with it. Measurements of basilar membrane motion in the last 10 years or so under very carefully controlled conditions (so that the function of the cochlea is unaffected by the measurement conditions) have shown the mechanical tuning to be much sharper than the earlier measurements. This is shown in Figure 10.15, taken from the chinchilla.

It is clear that there is a large difference between the early and modern measurements of basilar membrane motion, with regard to tuning. The modern measurements show the basilar membrane to be virtually as sharply tuned as the cochlear nerve. Furthermore, the inner hair cell receptor potential is as sharply tuned as the cochlear nerve fibres (Figure 10.16).

Positive feedback of mechanical energy in the mammalian cochlea

A great deal of research in the last 20 years has led to the suggestion that the relatively poor 'passive' tuning of the basilar membrane is sharpened up by a positive 'feedback' operation involving the outer hair cells (Figure 10.17). We now know that the outer hair cells undergo length changes extremely rapidly in an electrical field. This length change is such that it adds to the incoming vibration pattern on the basilar membrane to reinforce it and therefore enhance its tuning. An analogy for this positive feedback is the 'howl' produced by a microphone too close to its own loudspeaker. Just short of the 'howl', the sensitivity to frequencies in a narrow band is markedly enhanced. It is suggested that this is the case in the cochlea (Figure 10.17). Thus, the chain of events is: vibration of the basilar membrane, bending the stereocilia of the inner and outer hair cells; transduction into receptor potentials; generation of length changes in the outer hair cells;

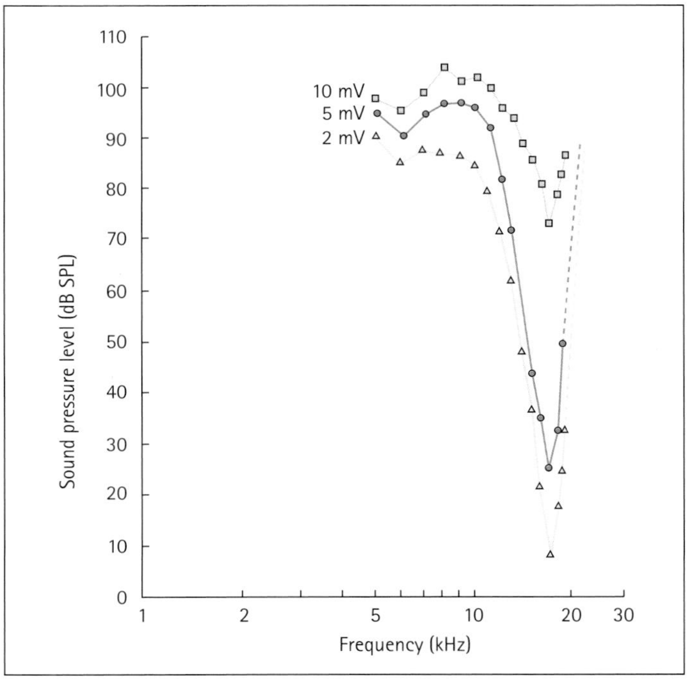

Figure 10.16 Tuning of inner hair cells receptor potential (after Russell and Sellick. *J Physiol* 1978: **284**; 261–90[2] and Evans EF. In: HB Barlow and DJ Mollon, eds. *The Senses*. Cambridge: Cambridge University Press, 1982. Figure 14.11.[1])

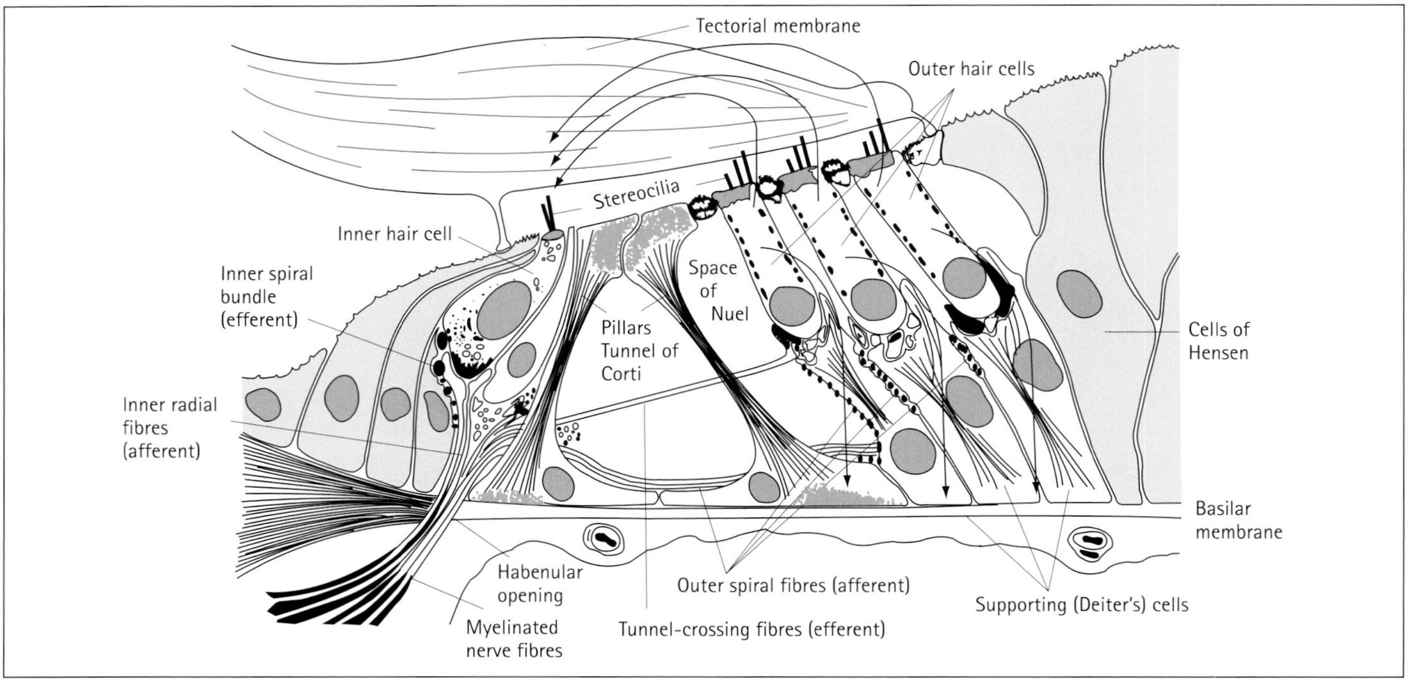

Figure 10.17 Diagrammatic representation of positive feedback of energy from motile OHC to basilar membrane (lower arrows) and inner hair cell region (upper arrows).

mechanical feedback of these changes to the tectorial membrane and basilar membrane; and enhancement of the frequency response (filtering) at that place. The sharp mechanical filtering is therefore reflected in the basilar membrane tuning curve (Figure 10.15) and in the equally sharp tuning of the receptor potential in the inner hair cells (Figure 10.16) leading to equally sharp tuning of the cochlear nerve afferents (Figure 10.11). (The afferent fibres of the cochlear nerve predominantly innervate the inner hair cells.)

Evidence for positive feedback

A mechanism of this kind requires energy in order to effect amplification of the mechanical movements leading to bending of the stereocilia and those fed back from the length changes in the outer hair cells to the same region.

The first evidence for such a mechanism came from the observations of the physiological vulnerability of cochlear tuning (Figure 10.14), namely that reduction in oxygen, blood supply etc. reduced the cochlear tuning to the 'passive' characteristics of the basilar membrane alone.

Next, the observation was made that loss of the outer hair cells through ototoxic antibiotic insult (Figure 10.18) led to loss of tuning in the frequency regions corresponding to the outer hair cell loss, even though the inner hair cells appeared to be relatively normal (under the light microscope at least).

Evidence was then obtained of the mechanical energy generated by the positive feedback process which can actually be recorded by a very sensitive microphone located in the ear canal. These are the otoacoustical emissions (OAEs), either evoked by acoustical stimuli (EOAEs) (e.g. clicks, Figure 10.19), or spontaneous (SOAEs), i.e. continuously emitted without requiring a stimulus trigger.

Finally, there has been the demonstration in vitro and then in vivo of length changes in the outer hair cells only, in response to AC electrical fields.

Control of these processes

The outer hair cells in the mammalian cochlea have very rudimentary afferent terminals, so much so that it is not clear what their function can be. However, there are a large number of very large efferent terminals, i.e. from nerve fibres descending from higher regions of the auditory system (particularly from the region of the superior olivary nucleus, in the olivocochlear bundle (OCB)). These efferents liberate acetylcholine on the outer hair cells, and this produces a change in their mechanical characteristics such that the positive feedback is diminished. This has the effect of reducing the sensitivity of the cochlea and its tuning. Thus, these are capable of being nicely controlled by the higher levels of the auditory system.

Pathophysiology of cochlear hearing loss

If the ear's frequency selectivity is already determined at the cochlear level, and if the tuning of the cochlea is physiologically vulnerable (Figure 10.14), this suggests that in impairment of inner ear function our auditory frequency selectivity will deteriorate, and many investigations have supported this. Thus, deterioration in psychophysical tuning can be used diagnostically, and as an 'early-warning indicator' of impending hearing damage.

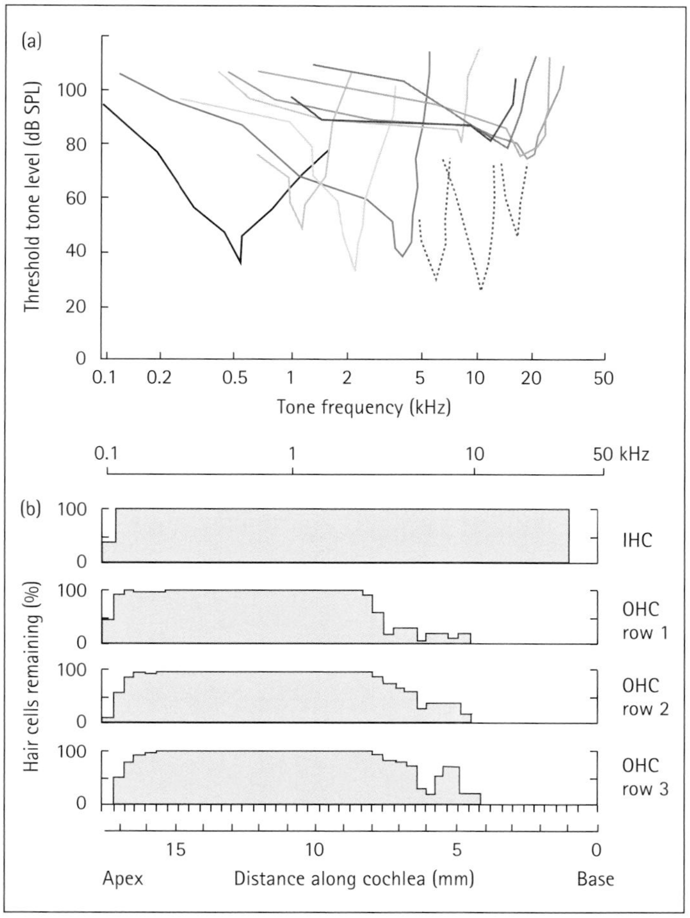

Figure 10.18 Broad cochlear nerve fibre tuning associated with loss of outer hair cells in a guinea-pig ear damaged by long-term injections of kanamycin. (a): the continuous curves indicate FTC's recorded in the ear compared with FTC's expected in an intact ear (black dotted curves). The blunt curves in the right hand half correspond to the loss of outer hair cells in the cochleograms in (b). (Reproduced from Evans EF. In: HB Barlow and DJ Mollon, eds. *The Senses*. Cambridge: Cambridge University Press, 1982. Figure 15.18.[1])

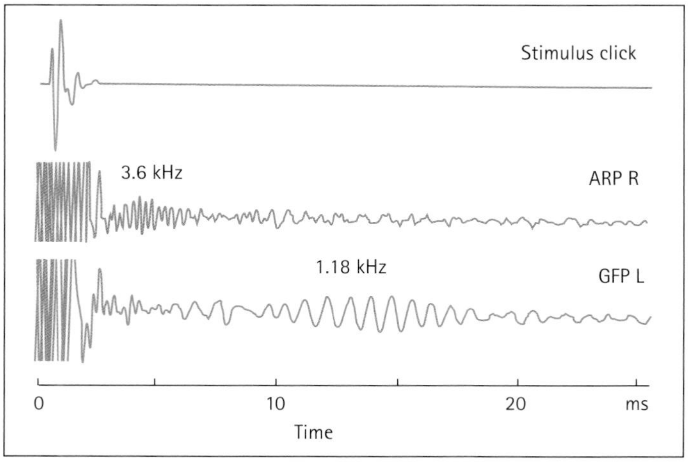

Figure 10.19 Click-evoked Oto-acoustic emissions recorded in two human ears. (After Wilson JP. *Hearing Res* 1980; **2**: 233–52.[9])

Encoding of frequency at cochlear nerve level

Place coding

The peripheral frequency analysis outlined in the previous section allows the component frequencies of complex sounds to be dissected out and represented as peaks of activity in the array of cochlear nerve fibres spanning low to high frequencies (Figure 10.20). This is the 'place' or 'labelled lines' coding of frequency. Deterioration in cochlear tuning will 'blur' this representation (Figure 10.20c), and cause loss of intelligibility, which cannot be compensated for by conventional hearing aids.

There is a problem, however, in seeing how this representation of frequency in terms of the discharge rate of cochlear nerve fibres can work over the wide dynamic range of intensities that we know the ear can process (Figure 10.21). These are the rate-level functions of a number of cochlear nerve fibres in the same animal (cat) showing the transition from spontaneous discharge rate through increase in discharge rate with stimulus level (the dynamic range) to saturation. This shows that the dynamic range of the majority of cochlear nerve fibres is relatively restricted to 20–40 dB, compared with some 120 dB for hearing as a whole. This restricted peripheral dynamic range means that the map of discharge rate activity along position in the cochlear nerve fibre array (Figure 10.22) is going to be blurred out at moderate to high intensities (upper half of Figure 10.22), because of the saturation of the discharge rate.

However, while this is true of the majority of cochlear nerve fibres, it is not true of all. It has been shown (Figure 10.23) that a small minority of cochlear nerve fibres (indicated by the upward arrows) have extended dynamic ranges. These are cochlear nerve fibres having the lowest spontaneous discharge rates. It therefore looks as though there are at least two populations of nerve fibres in the cochlear nerve: a minority population having extended dynamic ranges and extremely low or absent spontaneous discharge rates (3–5%), and the majority of cochlear nerve fibres having relatively restricted dynamic ranges. It is possible, though not very parsimonious, that this minority of cochlear nerve fibres may serve to convey 'place'-encoded information on the spectral (i.e. energy versus frequency) profile of complex sounds.

Time coding

Another possibility is that the frequency of sounds is encoded in the 'time' of occurrence of the action potentials (Figure 10.24). This phase locking of spikes to individual cycles of low-frequency waveforms up to about 5 kHz could enable the brain to extract the intervals between the spikes and from the reciprocal, the frequency. The spectra of speech sounds can be beautifully encoded in this fashion (Figure 10.25) by the degree of synchronization ('phase locking') of the neurones to the speech sound mapped across their characteristic frequency, far more precisely than by the discharge rate profiles of the majority (Figure 10.26, upper half), particularly at the higher sound levels, where saturation blurs out the 'place' representation. (On the other hand, the representation is, as noted above, roughly maintained in the rate profile of the low spontaneous

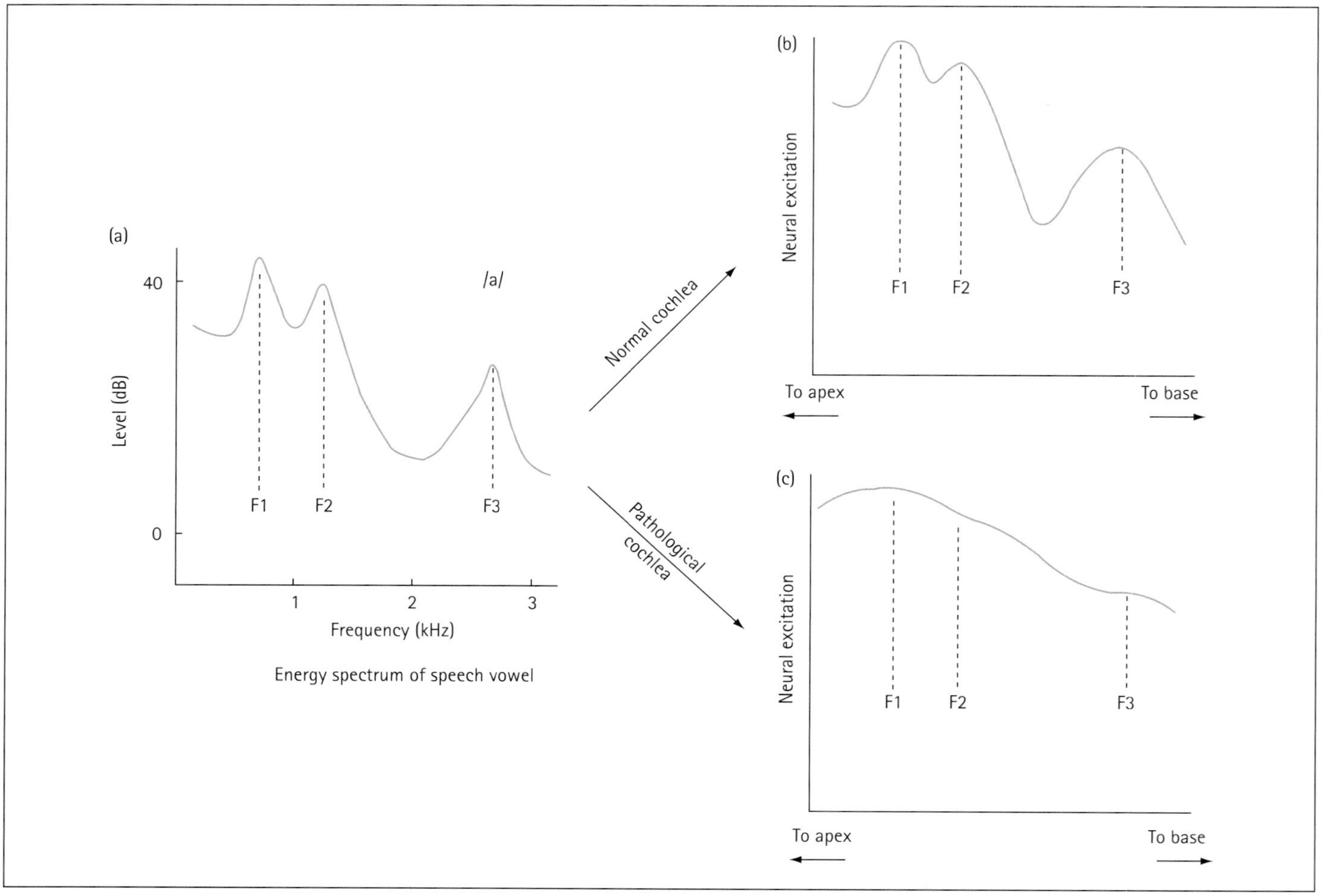

Figure 10.20 Diagrammatic representation of energy spectrum of speech vowel 'ah' (a); and hypothetical representation of cochlear excitation along the normal cochlea (b) and in a pathological cochlea (c). (After Pick and Evans EF. In: Perkins, ed. *High Technology Aids for Disabled People*. London: Butterworths, 1982, Chapter 12.[10])

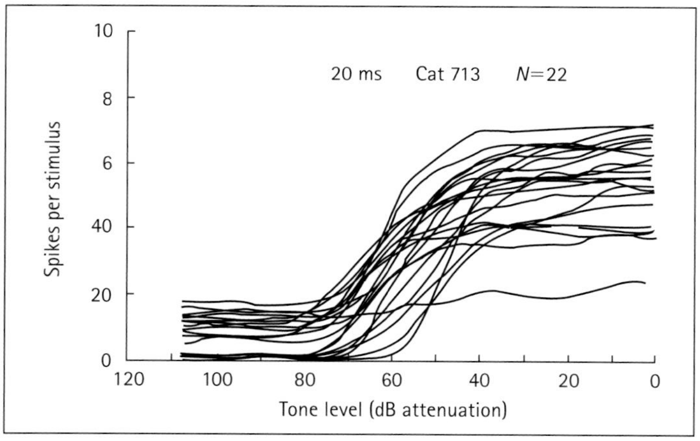

Figure 10.21 Rate-level functions of several cochlear nerve fibres from the cat. (After Palmer and Evans EF. *Exp Brain Res* 1979; **2** (suppl): 19–26.[11])

rate fibres—lower half of Figure 10.26, again mapped out across characteristic frequency.) Thus, Figure 10.25 represents a 'time' map, and Figure 10.26 a 'rate' map. It needs to be noted that both of these are 'place' maps, i.e. maps of synchronization (Figure 10.25) and discharge rate (Figure 10.26) across the cochlear nerve fibre array (characteristic frequency).

What we do not know is whether the higher levels of the brain can make use of these 'time' patterns. Certainly, as far as the pitch of complex sounds is concerned, there is now good evidence that both place and time mechanisms may be involved in pitch: if they occur alone, then a relatively weak pitch is heard; but when the time and place cues occur together and are congruent, then the most salient and most discriminable pitch is heard.

Frequency discrimination

The ability to hear as different one tone presented after another is likely to depend on both 'place' and 'time' mechanisms. As far as 'place' coding is concerned it is likely to be related to the sharp edge between the locus of activity and inactivity as in Figure 10.22, left half for 8 kHz. This sharp edge in turn depends

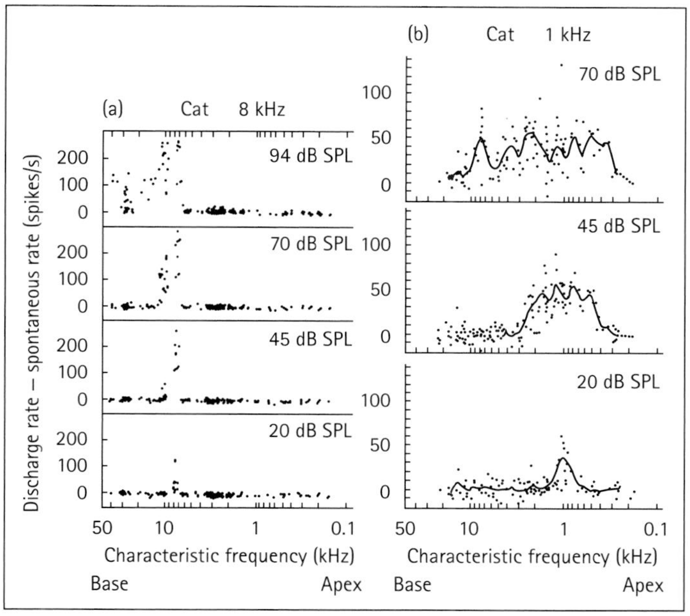

Figure 10.22 Blurring of rate place representation of pure tones at high sound pressure levels. The points show the activity in a population of cochlear nerve fibres in a single ear evoked by a tone of 8 kHz in the left-half and at 1 kHz in the right half. (Reproduced from Evans EF. In: HB Barlow and DJ Mollon, eds. *The Senses*. Cambridge: Cambridge University Press, 1982. Figure 15.5.[1])

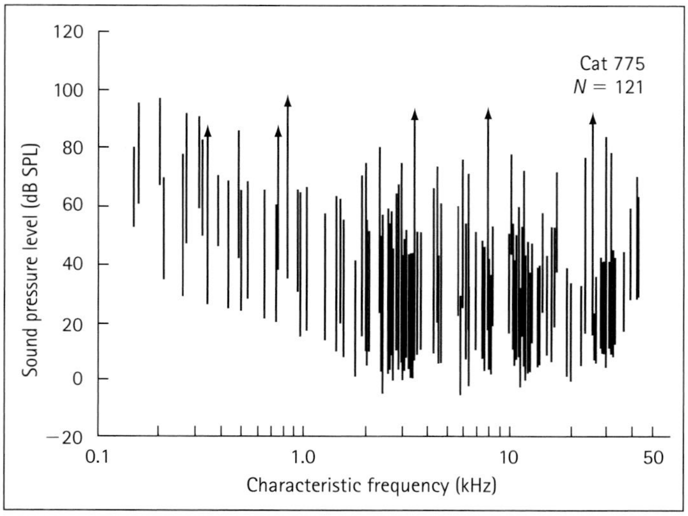

Figure 10.23 Dynamic ranges of over a hundred cochlear nerve fibres in the same ear. Each vertical line represents the dynamic range of a single cochlear nerve fibre plotted at its characteristic frequency. Only the fibres indicated with they arrow symbols are not saturated at the highest levels. (Reproduced from Evans EF. In: HB Barlow and DJ Mollon, eds. *The Senses*. Cambridge: Cambridge University Press, 1982. Figure 15.4.[1])

upon the high-frequency cut-offs of the cochlear nerve fibre tuning curves. Hence, frequency discrimination is far more acute than frequency selectivity—about 50 times better (Figure 10.27).

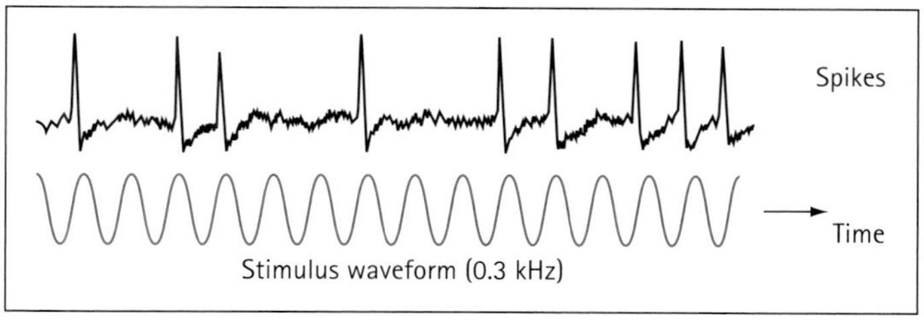

Figure 10.24 Phase-locking of single cochlear nerve fibre spikes to low-frequency sound. (Reproduced from Evans EF. In: HB Barlow and DJ Mollon, eds. *The Senses*. Cambridge: Cambridge University Press, 1982. Figure 14.21.[1])

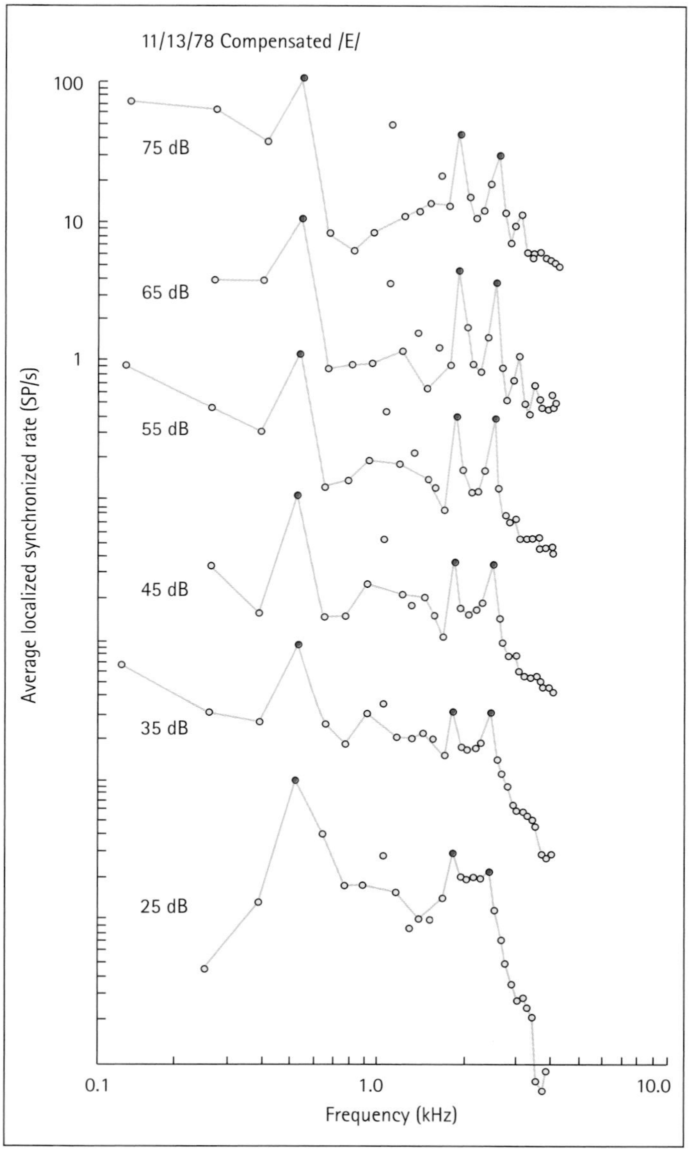

Figure 10.25 Profiles of synchronisation of spike discharges to vowel 'eh' at six intensities. The vowel spectrum is clearly represented even at the highest intensities (top of Figure). (After Young ED and Sachs MB. *J Acoust Soc Am* 1979: **66**: 1381–403.[12])

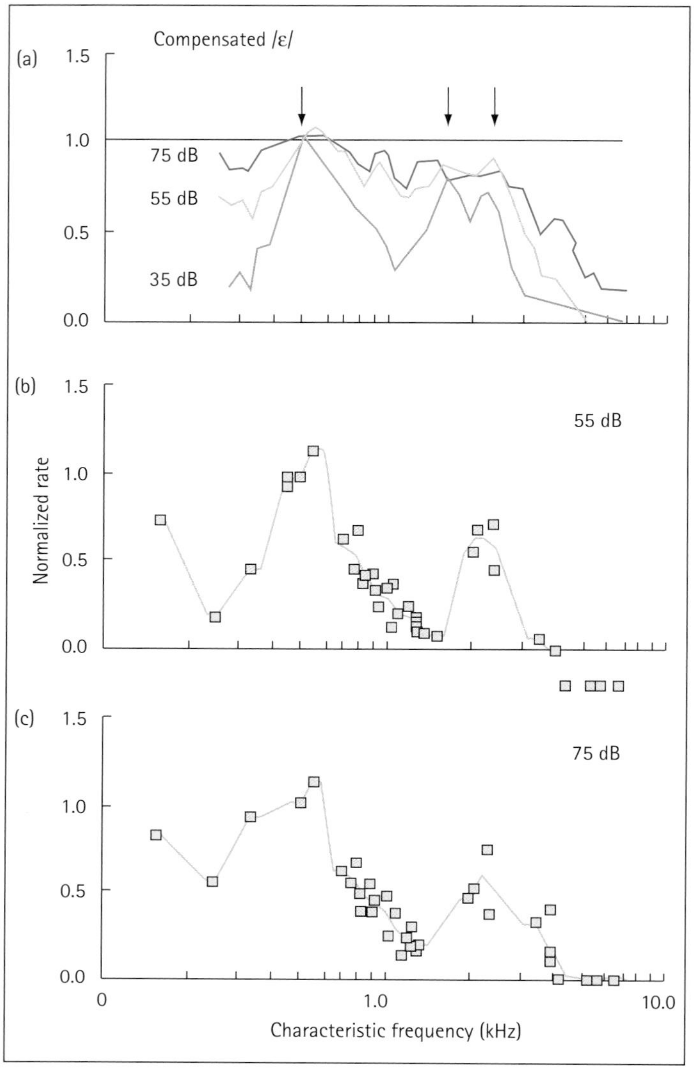

Figure 10.26 Saturation of rate profile corresponding to Figure 10.25 (After Sachs MB and Young ED. *J Acoust Soc Am* 1979; **66**: 470–9.[13])

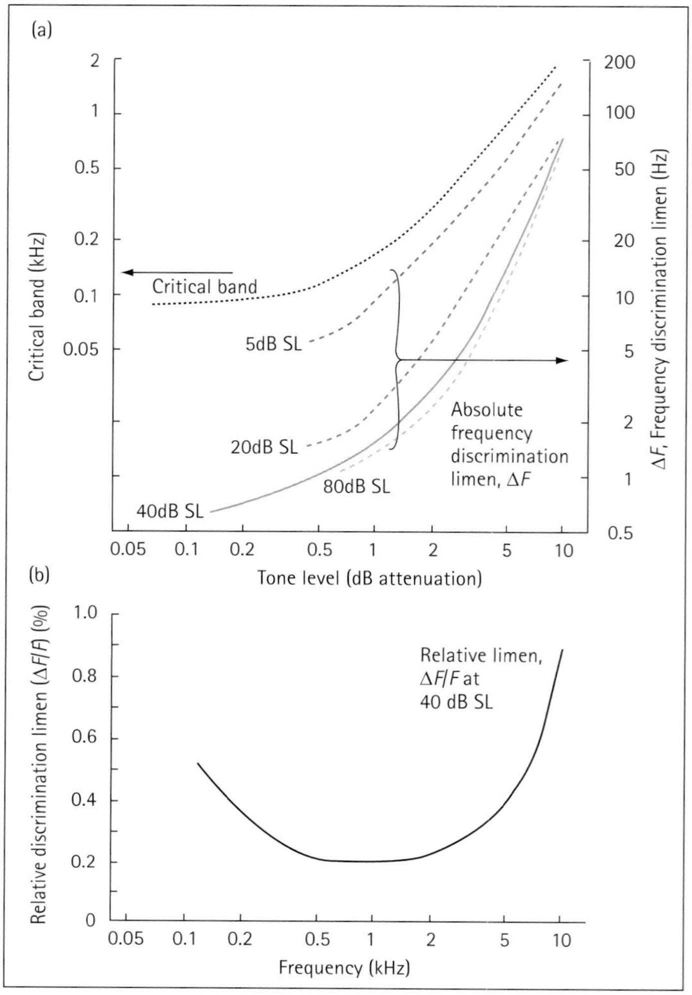

Figure 10.27 Human frequency selectivity (Critical band) and frequency discrimination compared. (Reproduced from Evans EF. In: HB Barlow and DJ Mollon, eds. *The Senses*. Cambridge: Cambridge University Press, 1982. Figure 15.6.[1])

Brainstem and higher mechanisms

Here we see good examples of both serial and parallel processing of auditory information as we ascend the auditory pathways (Figure 10.28).

Information from the cochlea passes via the cochlear nerve to the ipsilateral cochlear nucleus (CN). From here, several pathways pass across to the other side of the brainstem to innervate the superior olivary nucleus (SON) and thence to the inferior colliculus (IC), while some fibres reach the IC directly from the CN. It should be noted that, unlike the superior colliculus in the visual system, the IC is an obligatory station on the auditory pathway in the midbrain. From there, information travels via the medial geniculate nucleus (MGN) in the thalamus and thence to the auditory cortex (AI).

Cochlear nucleus: divergence of anatomy and physiology

The cochlear nucleus consists of three main divisions (Figure 10.29, middle): the more homogeneous anterior and posterior ventral divisons (AVN and PVN), and a more or less laminated and more complex dorsal division (DCN). Each of these divisions has a cochleotopic organization (Figure 10.29, top) and contains a wide variety of cell types, particularly the DCN (Figure 10.29, bottom).

Incoming cochlear nerve fibres branch to supply the many classes of cell types (Figure 10.30), distinguishable by their different anatomical shapes, output connections and physiology. From these different classes of cells, different pathways proceed across the mid-line to project to the SON and/or IC.

A great deal of work is in progress with regard to the 'wiring diagram' of the CN (e.g. Figure 10.31). We still have a long way to go. Of considerable help are newer techniques allowing

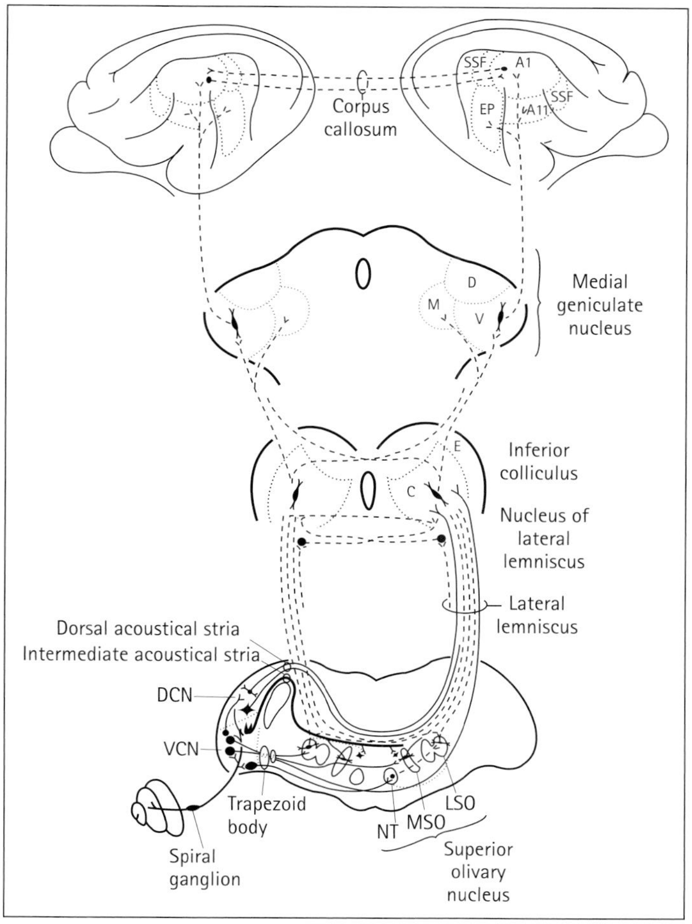

Figure 10.28 Main ascending anatomical pathways of auditory system. Simplified diagram of the ipsilateral and contralateral projections of one cochlea to the left and right auditory cortex in the cat. (Reproduced from Evans EF. In: HB Barlow and DJ Mollon, eds. *The Senses*. Cambridge: Cambridge University Press, 1982. Figure 14.2.[1])

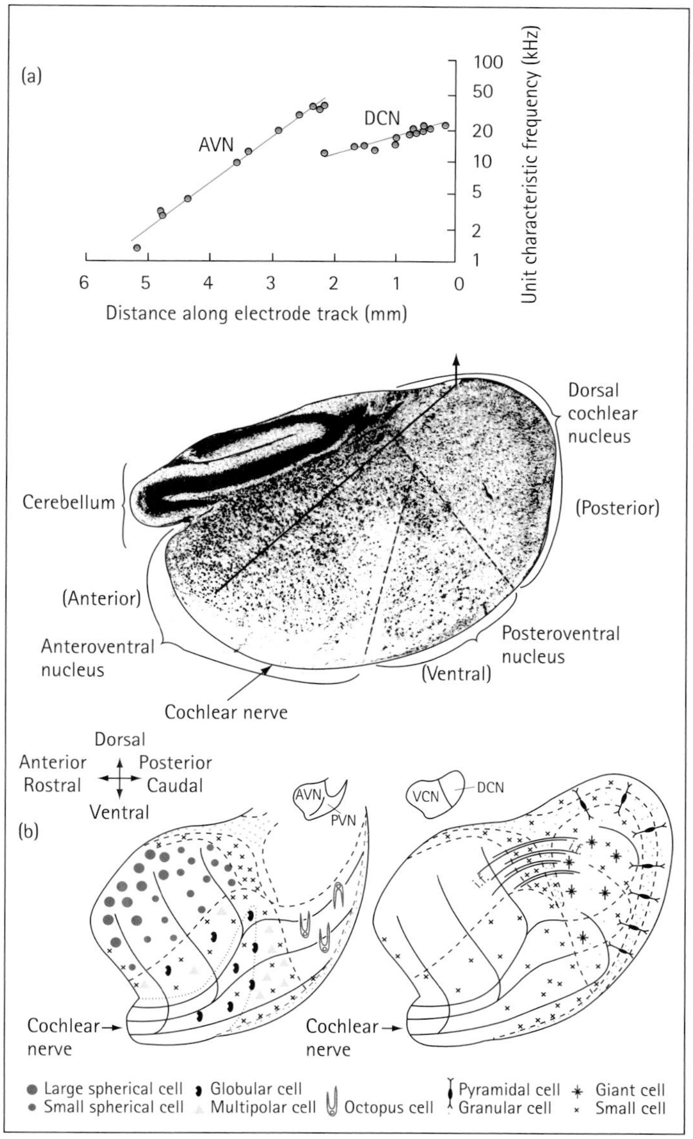

Figure 10.29 Anatomical organisation of cochlear nucleus. (a): cochleotopic organisation of neurone characteristic frequencies along electrode track shown by the arrow in the para-sagittal section in the middle panel. (b): shows examples of the cell types encountered in the section. (Reproduced from Evans EF. In: HB Barlow and DJ Mollon, eds. *The Senses*. Cambridge: Cambridge University Press, 1982. Figure 14.23.[1])

injections of horseradish peroxidase (HRP) to be made from a microelectrode intracellularly into a cell from which physiological recordings have been taken, thus linking structure with function directly.

As would be expected from their morphology (and their connections), the different cell types in the CN show widely different response characteristics (Figure 10.32). Thus CN cells in the simpler AVN have receptive fields and response time-courses (PSTHs) virtually identical to those of cochlear nerve fibres and are therefore termed 'primary-like' (Figure 10.32a). Other cells have a cochlear nerve-like receptive field but a regular firing pattern producing a 'chopper' PSTH (Figure 10.32b). Other cells, particularly in the PVN, have broader receptive fields (Figure 10.32c) and on-set responses.

In the DCN, however, extensive 'lateral' inhibition is found both in the receptive fields and as seen in the complex 'pauser', 'build-up' or 'inhibitory' PSTH's (Figure 10.32d,e,f).

We are now beginning to understand where the inhibition comes from and what its role might be.

Classical 'lateral' inhibition is glycinergic, and can be blocked by strychnine, a specific antagonist of glycine (Figure 10.33). The left-hand receptive field in Figure 10.33a shows the receptive field of a typical type IV DCN cell, where the whiter patches represent the 'lateral' inhibition. After iontophoretic injection of strychnine around the cell recorded from (middle panel of Figure 10.33a), the inhibition disappears and the true extent of the excitatory input to the cell is revealed. By subtraction of these two receptive fields, we obtain the inhibitory receptive field shown in the right panel. This indicates that the inhibition is not just 'lateral' but extends throughout the unit's

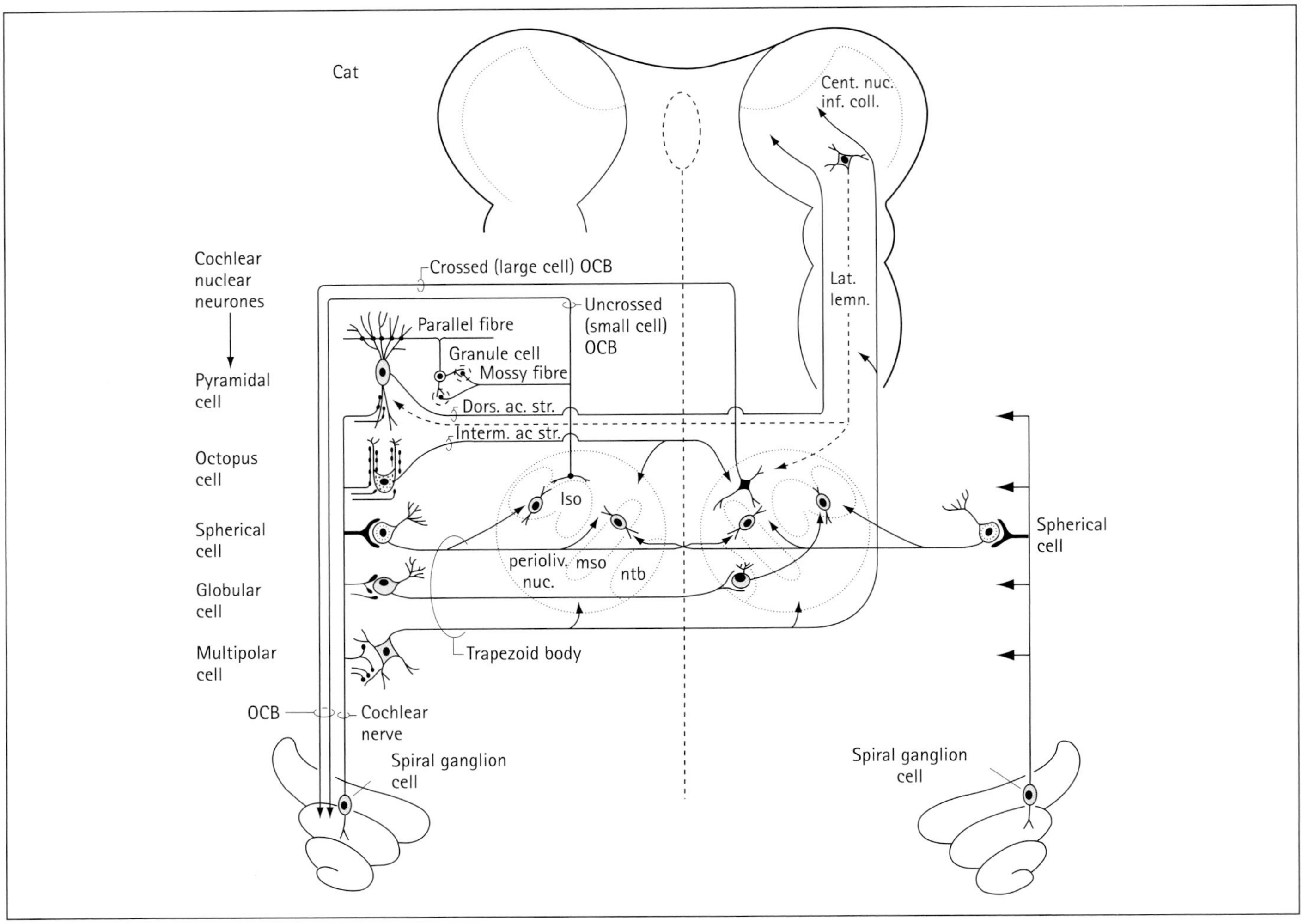

Figure 10.30 Schematic showing projections of cochlear nerve fibres to different cell types within the cochlear nucleus and their out-flow connections. After Osen (personal communication).

receptive field, and is in fact maximal at the receptive field centre. Figure 10.33b also indicates how strychnine blockade of the inhibition converts the complex non-monotonic discharge rate/stimulus level function (left) to the sigmoid function typical of cochlear nerve fibres (right). Figure 10.33c indicates the effect of the inhibition narrowing the excitatory response area and enhancing response contrast. Figure 10.33c plots the discharge rates across frequency when the stimulus level is held constant (at the level shown by the arrow at A in Figure 10.33a). The 'lateral' inhibitory dips are clearly seen on either side of the central excitatory response area in Figure 10.33c, left. After strychnine blockade, the inhibitory dips have virtually disappeared, and the true width of the excitatory response area is revealed. Thus 'lateral' inhibition narrows the response area and greatly increases the response contrast between the receptive field centre (peak) and the edge (surrounding dips), just as in the retina. (The DCN is the homologue of the retina.) Figure 10.33d indicates the time-course of the responses and demonstrates that the strychnine blocks the sustained inhibition with relatively little effect on the transient inhibition, particularly the 'off'-inhibition following the cessation of the stimulus (indicated by the asterisk). Thus off-inhibition must be mediated by another neurotransmitter or process.

Figure 10.34 shows that another inhibitory system, mediated by GABA, performs a quite different function. This sets the 'working point' of the cell by inhibiting the background spontaneous activity. Thus blocking the GABAergic inhibition with bicuculline (right column) increases the background spontaneous activity, thus revealing the inhibition (Figure 10.34a and f).

Superior olivary nucleus: integration of information between the ears

Figure 10.35 shows highly schematically the connections between the outflows of the cochlear nucleus pathways (mainly from the ventral nuclei) and the different subdivisions of the SON. Cells in the medial superior olivary nucleus (MSO) and lateral superior olivary nucleus (LSO) receive inputs from both ears via the CN on each side. The MSO receives excitatory

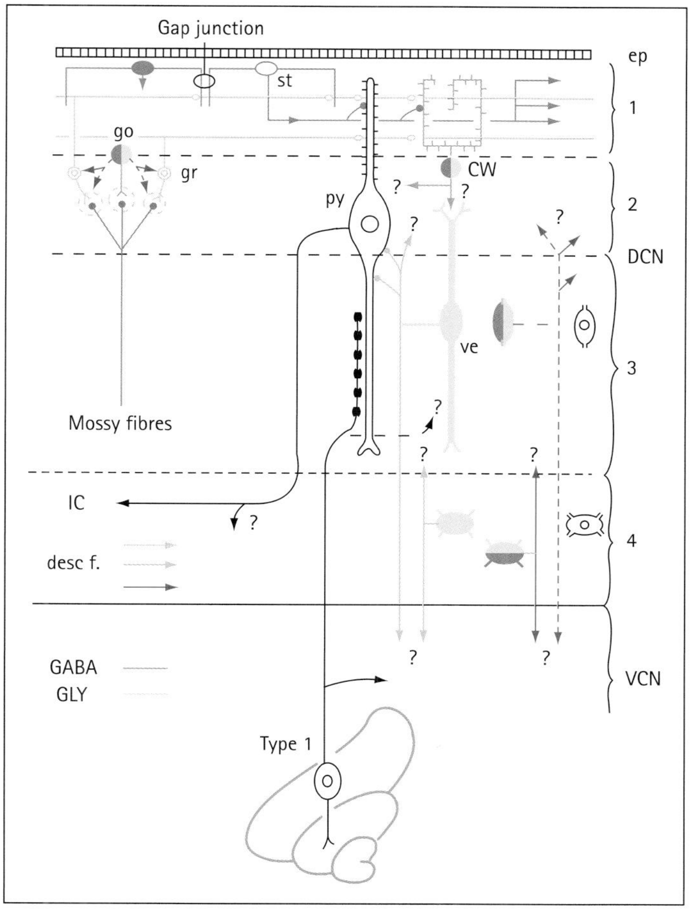

Figure 10.31 Provisional 'wiring diagram' of cochlear nucleus with provisional indications of neuro-transmitter types (dark shading: GABA; light shading: glycine). (After Osen In: *Glycine neurotransmission*. New York: Wiley, 1990: 417–51.[14])

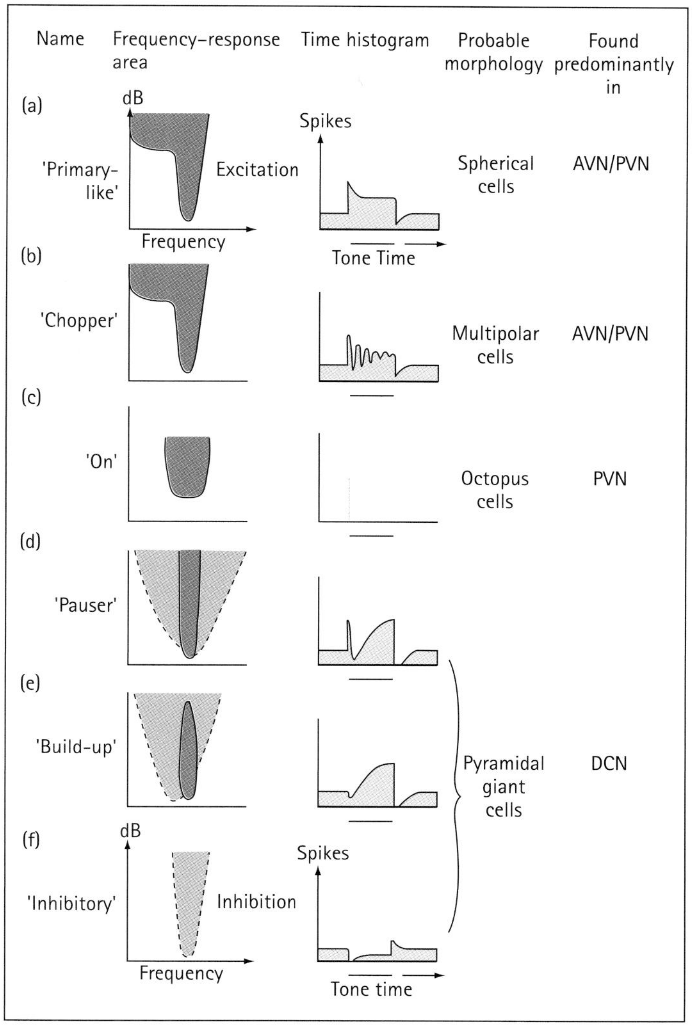

Figure 10.32 Varieties of frequency and time responses in different cochlear nucleus cells. (Reproduced from Evans TE. In: HB Barlow and DJ Mollon, eds. *The Senses*. Cambridge: Cambridge University Press, 1982. Figure 14.24.[1])

inputs from both ears, whereas the LSO receives excitatory inputs from the ipsilateral cochlear nucleus and inhibitory inputs (via an interneurone in the medial nucleus of the trapezoid body (MNTB-NT in Figure 10.28) from the contralateral cochlear nucleus. The so called 'E-E' cells in the MSO are very sensitive to correlated intensities between the two ears. The 'E-I' cells in the LSO, on the other hand, are more sensitive to intensity differences between the two ears. Both nuclei, but particularly the MSO, are sensitive to interaural time delays between the sounds reaching the ears. Some cells have 'critical delays', in other words a maximal response at a particular interaural delay, largely irrespective of the frequency or the level of a tone (Figure 10.36, taken from the inferior colliculus).

The sensitivity of, particularly, 'E-I' cells to interaural intensity differences and time delays means that the probability of discharge of a cell can be shifted by changing either the interaural delay or by the interaural level. One can be traded for the other, and the physiological results are consistent with the human psychophysical data (time–intensity trading).

A more simplified view of the pathways within the brainstem can therefore be given, as in Figure 10.37, where the two major pathways from the cochlear nucleus to the higher levels of the auditory system are emphasized: the ventral pathway involving the SON and chiefly concerned with 'where is it' questions; and the dorsal pathway from the DCN, direct to the IC, and probably concerned with 'what is it' questions or, in cats at least, with the orientation of the ears to the direction of the incoming sound.

Higher auditory centres

Auditory cortex: abstraction of behaviourally useful features from complex stimuli

While the auditory cortex is, in primates, buried in the region of the Sylvian fissure (Figure 10.39b), in the cat, it is conveniently spread out over the surface of the hemisphere (Figure 10.38a). Recordings can be taken from unanaesthetized animals

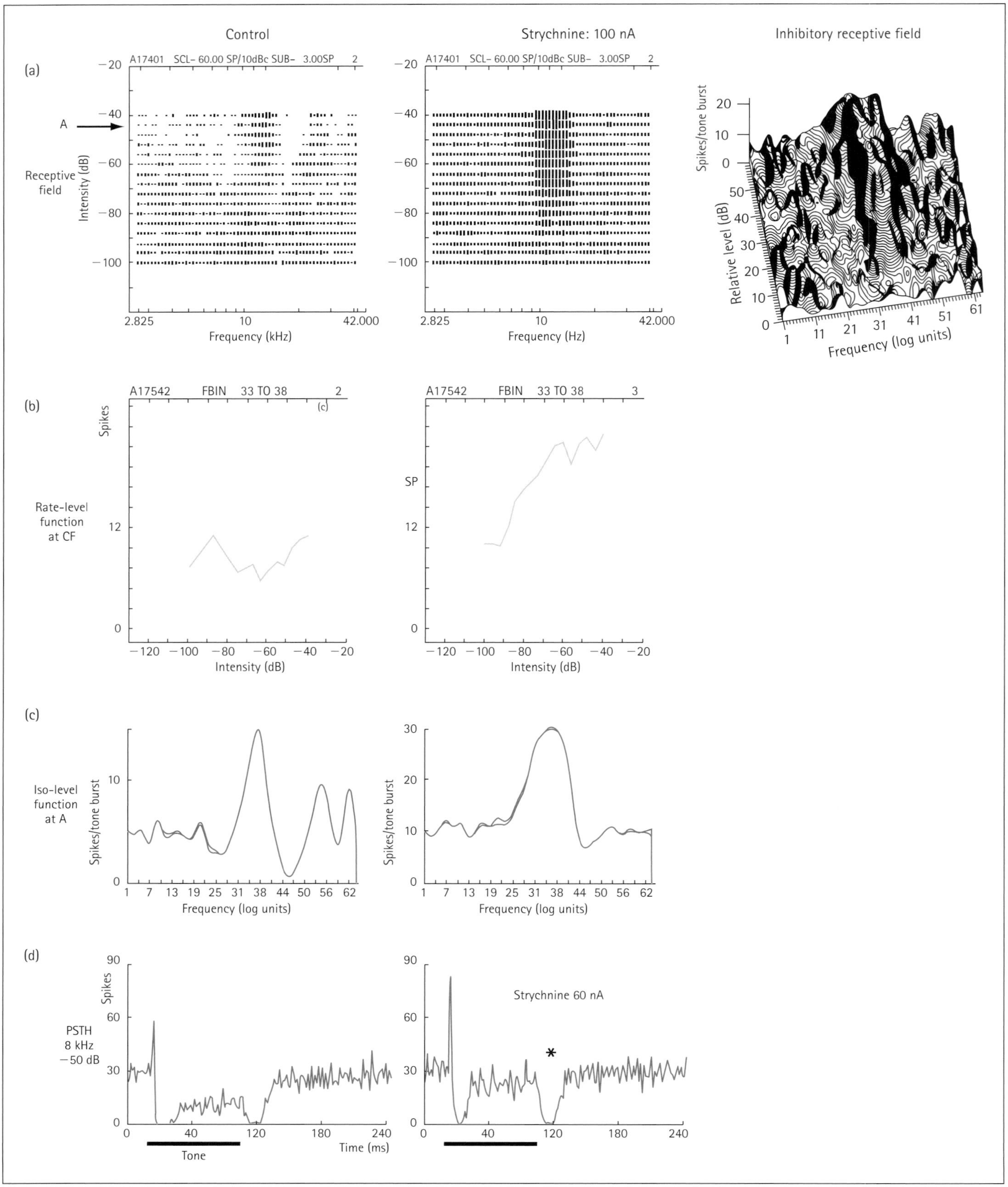

Figure 10.33 Role of 'lateral inhibition' in determining the response properties of dorsal cochlear nucleus (Type IV) cells. (From Evans, 1992. Figure 8.[15])

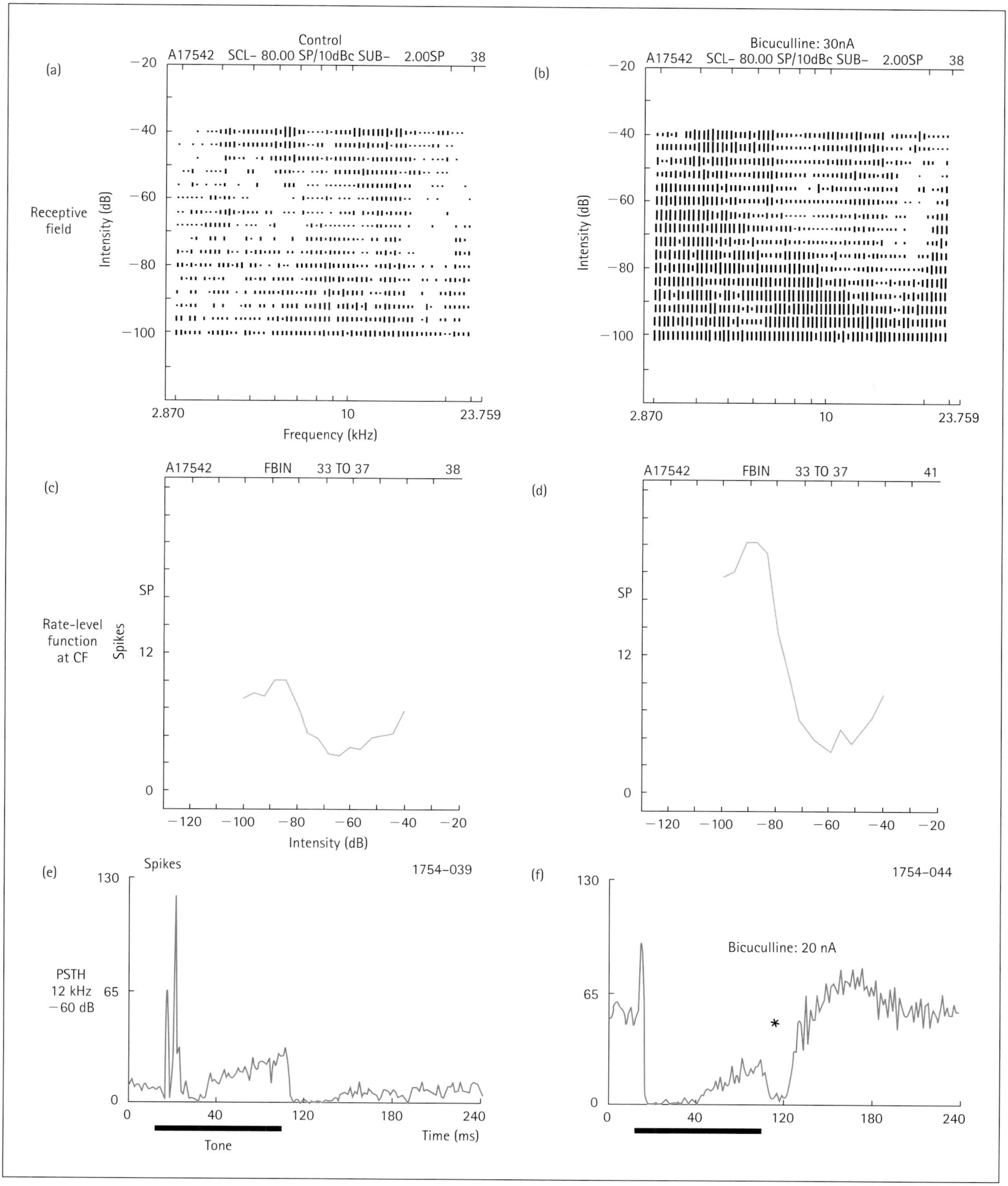

Figure 10.34 Role of GABA- ergic inhibition in cochlear nucleus type IV cell. (After Evans EF and Zhao W. *Prog Brain Res* 1993; 97: 117–26.[16])

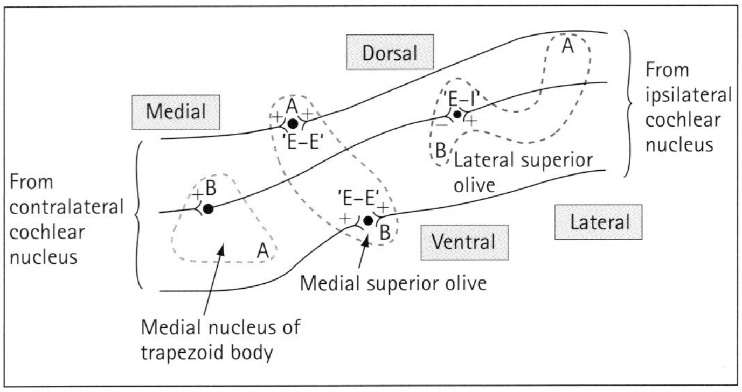

Figure 10.35 Functional anatomy of superior olive. (Reproduced from Evans EF. In: HB Barlow and DJ Mollon, eds. *The Senses*. Cambridge: Cambridge University Press, 1982. Figure 14.26.[1])

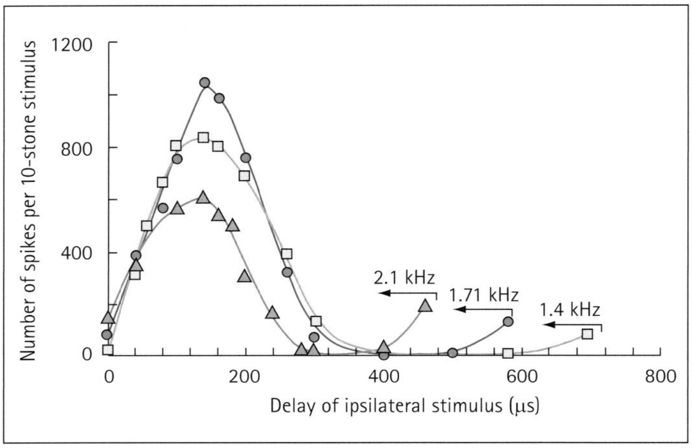

Figure 10.36 'Critical delay' unit in inferior colliculus. (Reproduced from Evans EF. In: HB Barlow and DJ Mollon, eds. *The Senses*. Cambridge: Cambridge University Press, 1982. Figure 14.27.[1])

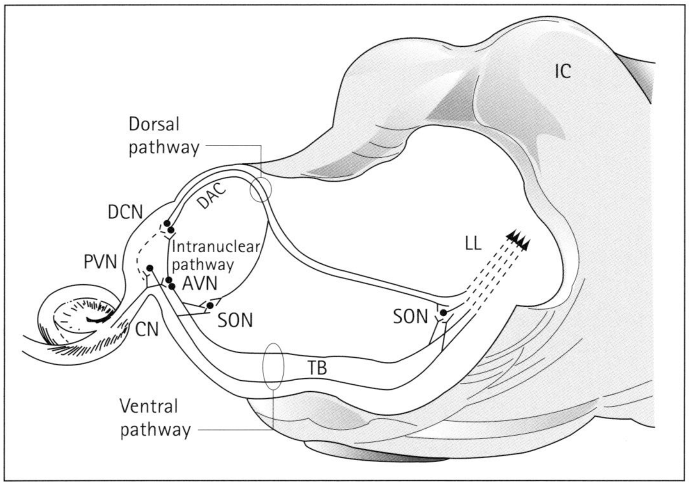

Figure 10.37 Simplified diagram of dorsal and ventral pathways in brain stem of cat. From Evans EF. The cochlear nerve and cochlear nucleus. In: *Handbook of sensory Physiology Vol V/2 Auditory System*. WD Keidel and WD Neff, eds Heidelberg: Springer 1975: 1–108.[17])

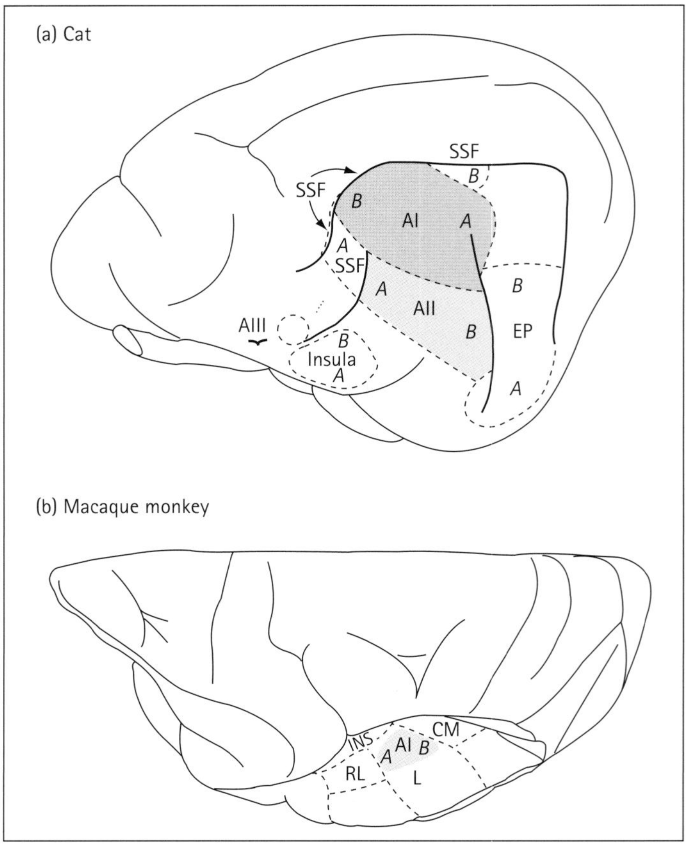

Figure 10.38 Auditory cortex of cat and monkey showing primary (AI) and secondary areas. (Reproduced from Evans EF. In: HB Barlow and DJ Mollon, eds. *The Senses*. Cambridge: Cambridge University Press, 1982. Figure 14.28.[1])

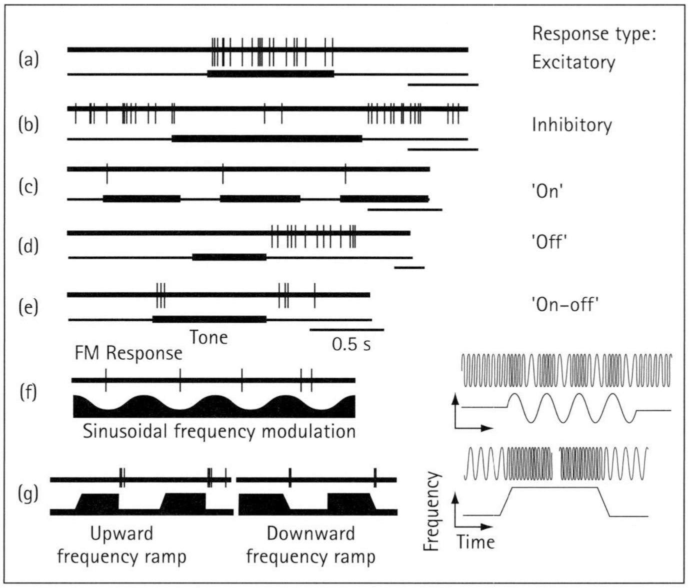

Figure 10.39 Diversity of single unit responses in unanaesthetised primary auditory cortex. (Reproduced from Evans EF. In: HB Barlow and DJ Mollon, eds. *The Senses*. Cambridge: Cambridge University Press, 1982. Figure 14.30.[1])

by means of a permanently implanted chamber into which microelectrodes can be introduced at intervals without any discomfort while recordings are made from the animal in a normally behaving or even sleeping condition. (The brain has no pain receptors.)

There is a striking diversity of response patterns recordable from neurones in the unanaesthetized primary auditory cortex (Figure 10.39). What is even more striking is that, in contrast to the auditory periphery, not all neurones respond to pure tones (Figure 10.40). A small number respond to visual stimuli, most to some sort of auditory stimulus; only about 60%, however, respond to tones. Some 20% respond only to complex sounds, and these are the most effective stimuli for the majority of cells, namely 'backdoor noises'—the noises heard outside the average British backdoor when the pet feline is called in for the night!

Even many of the cortical cells that do respond to pure tones respond only when the pure tones are patterned in time. Many show habituation of response to repeated presentations of the same stimulus. It requires a great deal of ingenuity and patience on the part of the experimenter to obtain consistent responses and to elucidate the optimal stimulus pattern for a given cell.

Of particular interest are the small proportion of cells (about 10%) that respond to tonal stimuli only if their frequency is changing (Figure 10.39f,g). This part of Figure 10.39 shows the excursions in frequency: sinusoidally in (f) and in upward- and downward-going 'ramps' (i.e. linear frequency changes) in (g). These cells that are selective to frequency change are often selective to the direction also. The cell in Figure 10.39f and 10.39g is selective only to downward frequency changes. Some of the cells are selective, in addition, for the rate of frequency change.

Of great interest is the finding that a very small proportion of cortical cells of the squirrel monkey are selective for individual calls of the animal's vocal repertoire. Squirrel monkeys are an intensely social species living in an arboreal environment. They have developed a system of species-specific vocalizations or calls, each of which has a specific significance. Thus, Figure 10.41 shows a cell responding selectively to the 'trill' call, which means 'go away—I'm feeding—leave me alone'.

Cells in the auditory cortex are organized according to their input projection fibres into cochleotopic maps (Figure 10.42), and also into slabs which relate to ear dominance (Figure 10.42).

Thus cells in the cortex can answer questions such as: is the stimulus on, or off? If on, how is it patterned in time? Is the frequency changing? Is it changing up or down? How often is it changing? What is the position of the stimulus in space? Thus, cells in the auditory cortex are less interested in the frequencies and intensities of sound (as in the periphery) than in the patterning of these in time and in space. These cells are therefore capable of acting as feature-selective units, and may be involved in extracting features of behavioural significance from a complex sound. The finding of call-specific neurones in the auditory cortex of the squirrel monkey suggests that there may be in our own brains neurones specifically selective for the acoustical features associated with speech. There is behavioural evidence from studies of auditory perception in infants that there may be a 'critical period' during which acoustical distinctions necessary for correct speech interpretation are established or can be lost by the auditory cortex.

Ablation of the auditory cortex produces specific defects in pattern recognition, e.g. in discriminating frequency change, and in the ability of an animal to localize a sound source in space.

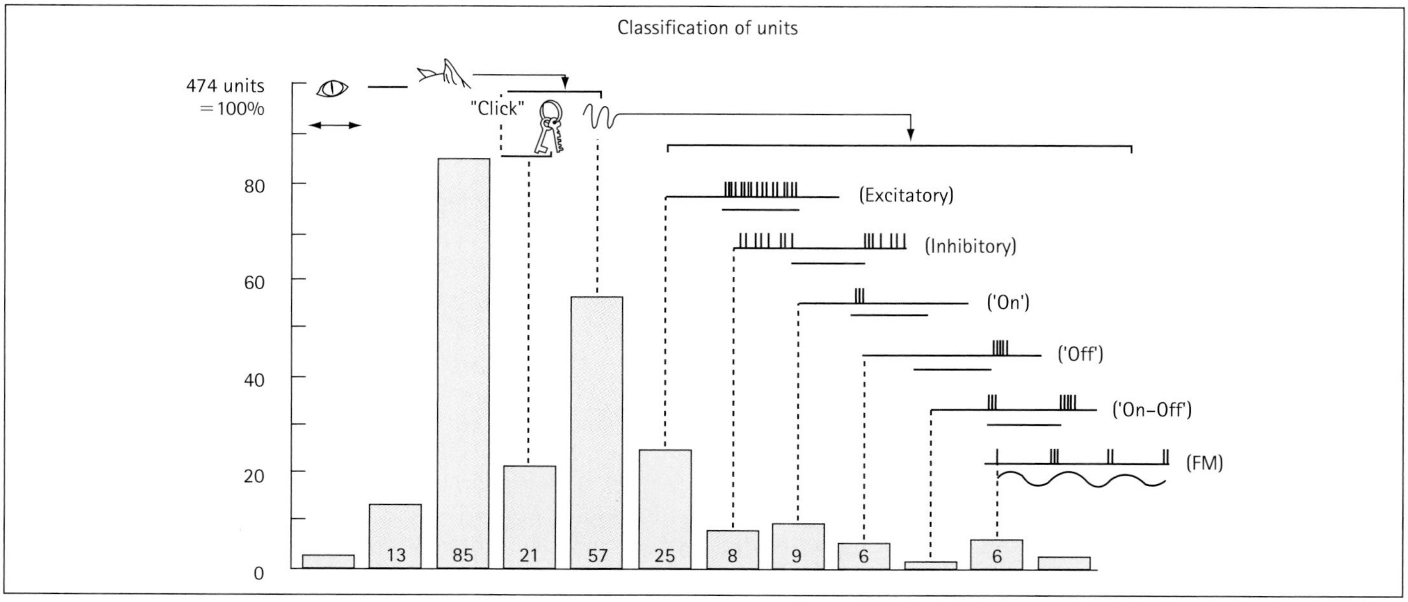

Figure 10.40 Classification of units in unanaesthetised primary auditory cortex. (After Evans EF and Whitfield IC. *J Physiol* 1964; **171**: 476–93.[18])

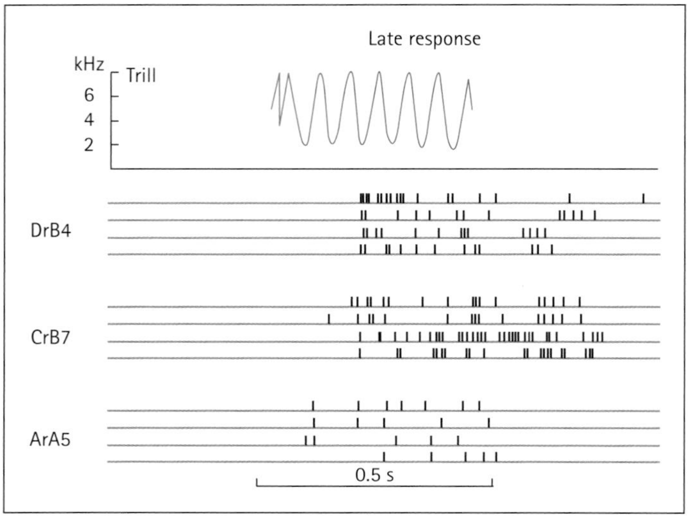

Figure 10.41 Response of three units in squirrel monkey primary auditory cortex to trill vocalisation. (After Winter and Funkenstein. *Proc 3rd Congress in Primatology* Zurich. 2. Basel: Kruger 1971: 24–8.[19])

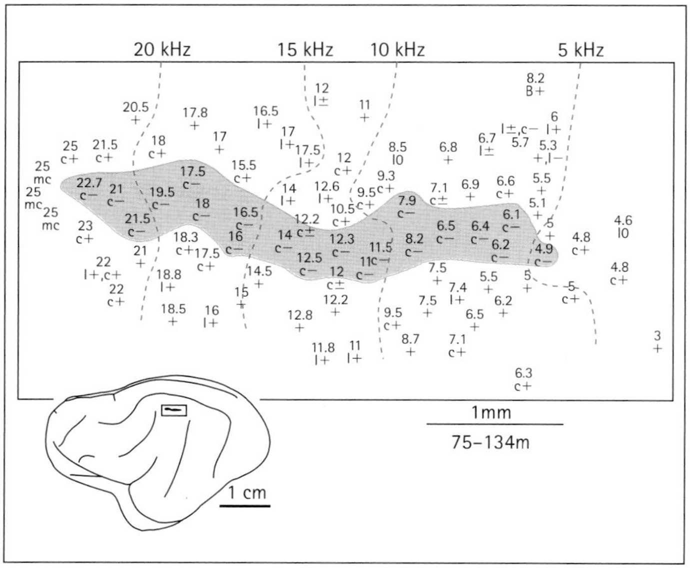

Figure 10.42 Ear dominance slabs in a cat auditory cortex shaded area shows predominant contralateral eye dominance dominance of contralateral ear. (Reproduced from Evans EF. In: HB Barlow and DJ Mollon, eds. *The Senses*. Cambridge: Cambridge University Press, 1982. Figure 14.29.[1] Originally published in Imig and Adrian, *Brain Res* 1977; **138**: 241–57.[20])

Descending control

Running in the opposite direction to the ascending auditory pathway are pathways descending from higher centres and presumably exerting some form of control from the higher to the lower levels of the auditory pathway. The best known of these is the OCB, ending particularly on the outer hair cells in the cochlea, from the contralateral medial part of the periolivary nuclei. Stimulation of these crossed OCB fibres is known to reduce the sensitivity and the tuning of the cochlea, presumably by changing the mechanical properties of the outer hair cells. There is also a predominantly uncrossed projection from the more lateral regions of the olivary nuclei to the inner hair cells, but ending on the primary afferents themselves. The function of these is not yet known.

An obvious use for these descending pathways is to reduce the sensitivity of the auditory system during an animal's own vocalizations. This happens from the level of the middle ear muscles upwards, particularly in bats, so that they may more easily detect the weak echos from their own vocalizations.

References

1. Evans, EF. In: HB Barlow and JD Mollon, eds. *The Senses*. Cambridge: Cambridge University Press, 1982: 239–332.
2. Russell IJ, Sellick PM. Intracellular studies of hair cells in the mammalian cochlea. *J Physiol* 1978: **284**; 261–90.
3. Kiang NYS, Sachs MB, Peake WT. Shapes of tuning curves for single auditory-nerve fibers. *J Acoust Soc Am* 1967; **42**: 1341–2.
4. Evans EF. The frequency response and other properties of single fibres in the guinea-pig cochlear nerve. *J Physiol* 1972; **226**: 263–87.
5. Rose JE, Hind JE, Anderson DJ, Brugge, JF. Some effects of stimulus intensity on response of auditory nerve fibers in the squirrel monkey. *J Neurophysiol* 1971: **34**; 685–99.
6. Evans EF. 1993 *Proc 12th International Conference of the Audio Engineering Society*. New York: A E S, 1993: 11–21.
7. Evans, EF. In: Zwicker E, Terhardt, E eds. *Facts and Models in Hearing*. Heidelberg: Springer, 1974, 118–29.
8. Robles L, Ruggero MA, Nola CR. Basilar membrane mechanics at the base of the chinchilla cochlea. I Input-output functions, tuning curves, and response phases. *J Acoust Soc Am* 1986; **80**: 1364–74.
9. Wilson JP. Evidence for a cochlear origin for acoutic re-emissions threshold fine-structure and total tinnitus. *Hearing Res* 1980; **2**: 233–52.
10. Pick and Evans EF. In: Perkins, ed. *High Technology Aids for Disabled People*. London: Butterworths, 1982, Chapter 12.
11. Palmer AR, Evans EF. On the peripheral coding of individual frequency components of complex sounds at high sound levels. *Exp Brain Res* 1979; Suppl **2**: 19–26.
12. Young ED, Sachs MB. Representation of steady-state vowels in the temporal aspects of the discharge patterns of populations of auditory nerve fibers. *J Acoust Soc Am* 1979: **66**: 1381–403.
13. Sachs MB, Young ED. Encoding steady-state vowels in the auditory nerve: representation in terms of discharge rate. *J Acoust Soc Am* 1979; **662**: 470–9.
14. Osen KK. In: *Glycine Neurotransmission*. New York: Wiley, 1990: 417–51.
15. Evans EF. Auditory processing of complex sounds: an overview. *Phil Trans Roy Soc B* 1992; **336**: 295–306.

16. Evans EF and Zhao W. Varieties of inhibition in the processing and control of processing in the mammalian cochlear nucleus. *Prog Brain Res* 1993; **97**: 117–26.
17. Evans EF. The cochlear nerve and cochlear nucleus. In: WD Keidel and WD Neff, eds. *Handbook of Sensory Physiology Vol V/2 Auditory System*. Heidelberg, Springer, 1975: 1–108.
18. Evans EF and Whitfield IC. Classification of unit responses in the auditory cortex of the unanaesthetised and unrestrained cats. *J Physiol* 1964; **171**: 476–93.
19. Winter P, Funkenstein H. *Proc Third Congress in Primatology* Zurich. 2. Basel: Kruger, 1971: 24–8.
20. Imig TJ and Adrian HO. Binaural columns in the primary field (A1) of cat auditory cortex. *Brain Res* 1977; **138**: 241–57.

Further reading

Evans EF. Auditory processing of complex sounds: an overview. *Phil Trans R Soc* B 1992; **336**: 295–306.

Haggard MP, Evans EF. (ed.) Hearing. *Br Med Bull* 1987; **43**.

Pickles JO. *Introduction to the Physiology of Hearing* 2nd edn. London: Academic Press, 1988: 775–1042.

11 Central auditory anatomy and function

Frank E Musiek, Victoria B Oxholm

Central auditory nervous system: anatomical definition

We define the anatomical limits of the central auditory nervous system (CANS) as beginning at the cochlear nucleus (CN) and ending at the auditory cortex. However, the endpoint of the CANS is unclear, as it might be somewhere in the efferent system or possibly in a non-auditory area of the cerebrum. The endpoint of the CANS may also depend on the types of acoustical stimuli and the task to be completed. Thus, it may be physiologically rather than anatomically determined (Figure 11.1).

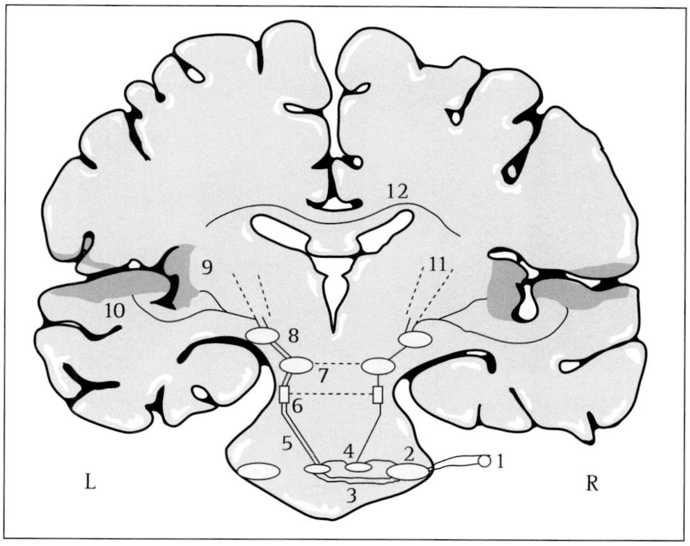

Figure 11.1 Coronal view of the brain with key auditory structures and areas defined. 1, Cochlear nerve; 2, cochlear nucleus; 3, stria (dorsal, intermediate, ventral); 4, superior olivary complex; 5, lateral lemniscus; 6, nuclei of lateral lemniscus; 7, inferior colliculus; 8, medial geniculate bodies; 9, insula (shaded); 10, primary auditory region in temporal and parietal lobes (shaded); 11, internal capsule; 12, corpus callosum.

Cochlear nucleus (CN)

The CN is located in the cerebellopontine angle area, a lateral recess formed at the juncture of the pons, medulla and cerebellum. It consists of three principal sections: the anterior ventral cochlear nucleus (AVCN), the posterior ventral cochlear nucleus (PVCN), and the dorsal CN. Cochlear nerve fibers enter this complex at the junction of the AVCN and PVCN, where each fiber then divides and sends branches to the three individual nuclei[1] (Figures 11.1 and 11.2).

The CN is composed of multiple cell types. Among the most prominent of these are the pyramidal (fusiform), octopus, stellate, spherical (bushy), globular (bushy) and multipolar cells.[2, 3] The pyramidal cells in the cat are at the dorsal fringe of the dorsal CN, the octopus cells are in the PVCN, and the spherical cells are in the AVCN. Globular and multipolar cells are found between the AVCN and PVCN[3,4] (Figures 11.3 and 11.4).

Incoming neural impulses can be modified by these cells in a characteristic manner that provides the basis for coding information by the type of neural activity within the CN. The average response of a particular neural unit over time to a series of short tones presented at the unit's characteristic frequency is shown in post-stimulatory histograms.[5] The principal response patterns include the following: (1) primary-like response, an initial spike preceded by a steady response until the stimulus ceases; (2) the 'chopper' post-stimulatory response, an extremely rapid oscillatory neural response to the stimulus; (3) the onset response, a solitary initial spike at the onset of the stimulus; and (4) the pauser response, similar to the primary-like response but which ends soon after the initial spike and resumes a graded response.[6] An additional pattern, the 'build-up' response, is when the cell fires increasingly throughout the stimulus presentation.[5,6] This correspondence between cell type and response pattern suggests a significant relationship between anatomy (structure) and physiology (function) of the cells within the CN. Post-stimulatory histograms from the CN provide details of the complex processing of auditory information at the CN, such as the precise timing needed for localization and distinguishing interaural time differences.[7] The various cell types also have

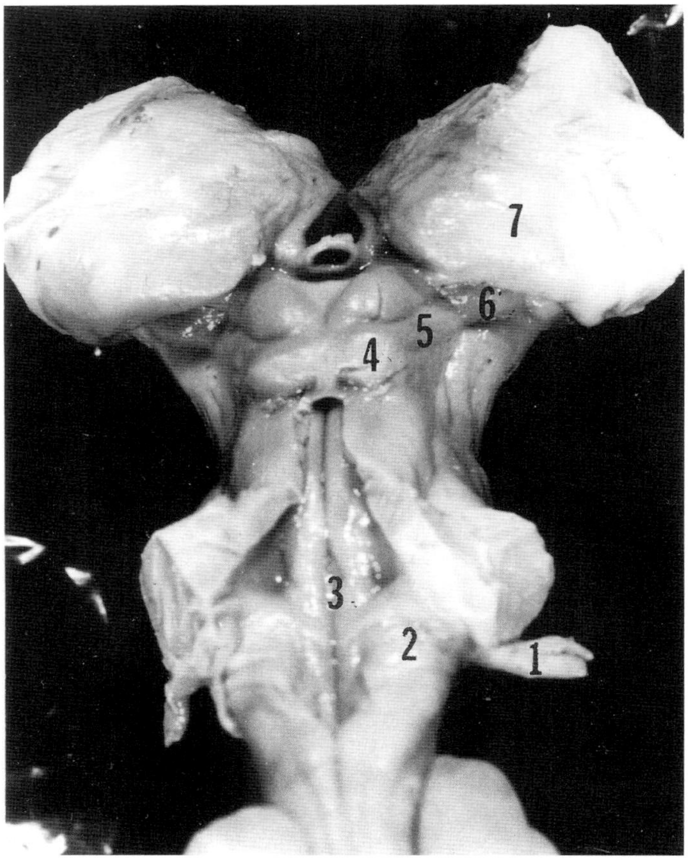

Figure 11.2 Posterior view of the human brainstem (cerebellum and vessels removed). 1, Cochlear nerve (entering cochlear nucleus just below the cerebellar peduncle); 2, cochlear nucleus; 3, fourth ventricle; 4, inferior colliculus; 5, brachium of inferior colliculus; 6, medial geniculate body; 7, thalamus. (Courtesy of W. Mosenthal and F. Musiek.)

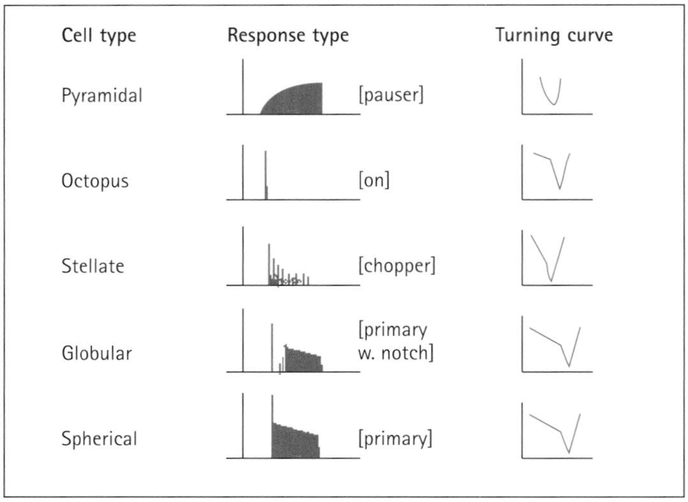

Figure 11.3 Examples of five cell types found in the cochlear nucleus with associated post-stimulatory histogram types and tuning curve configurations.

associated tuning curves; the main difference among the cell types is the shape of their tails (Figures 11.3 and 11.4).

The cochlear nerve enters the brainstem on the lateral posterior aspect of the pontomedullary juncture and projects to the cochlear nuclear complex. Cochlear nerve fibers entering each section of the CN are arranged in a systematic fashion which preserves the frequency organization from the cochlea.[8,9] All three sections of the CN contain this tonotopic organization, with low frequencies represented ventrolaterally and high frequencies represented dorsomedially within each nucleus[8,9] (Figure 11.5a). Some tuning curves derived from AVCN units using tone bursts have a similar shape to those of the cochlear nerve.[7,10] However, some CN fibers produce wider tuning curves than do cochlear nerve fibers.[11] Frequency resolution of acoustical information coming from the cochlear nerve may thus be maintained but not necessarily enhanced by CN units.

The tuberculoventral tract, a fiber pathway thought to be primarily inhibitory in nature, connects the dorsal and ventral portions of the CN (Ortel, personal communication). Three main neural tracts continue from the CN complex to the superior olivary complex (SOC) and higher levels of the CANS.

A large fiber tract called the dorsal acoustical stria emanates from the dorsal CN and continues contralaterally to the SOC, lateral lemniscus (LL),[12] and inferior colliculus (IC).[6] The intermediate acoustical stria originates in the PVCN and communicates with the contralateral lemniscus (ventral nucleus) as well as the central nucleus of the contralateral IC[6] (Figure 11.5b). The ventral acoustical stria, the largest tract, arises from the AVCN and merges with the trapezoid body as it nears the mid-line of the brainstem.[12] The ventral stria extends contralaterally along the LL to the SOC and other nuclear groups. Interestingly, in animal studies for simple detection tasks of tones or noise, performance was not affected by sectioning of the intermediate and dorsal acoustical stria. However, severe deficits were noted with sectioning of the ventral stria.[13]

In addition to these three primary tracts, other fibers project ipsilaterally from each division of the CN. Some of these fibers synapse at the SOC and nuclei of the LL within the pons. Other fibers synapse only at the IC, and bypass completely the SOC and the nuclei of the LL. The contralateral pathways carry the largest number of fibers, even though many neural tracts project both ipsilaterally and contralaterally from the CN.[14]

The CN is a unique brainstem auditory structure, in that its only afferent input is ipsilateral, coming from the cochlea via the cochlear nerve. Consequently, damage to the CN can mimic cochlear nerve dysfunction,[15] as it may only produce ipsilateral pure tone deficits.[16–18] Extra-axial tumors, such as vestibular schwannomas (acoustic neuromas), often affect the CN, due to its posterolateral location on the brainstem surface.[17,19,20]

Tumors situated in this cerebellopontine region can often affect the CN and may produce central auditory deficits. Nevertheless, the cerebellopontine angle is large enough in some cases to accommodate lesions of sizeable mass without compromising neural function.[21,22]

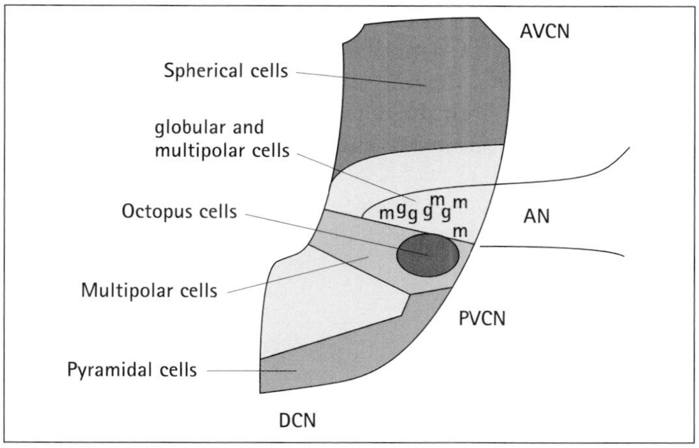

Figure 11.4 Location of cell types in the cochlear nucleus. AVCN, anterior ventral cochlear nucleus; AN, auditory nerve; PVCN, posterior ventral cochlear nucleus; DCN, dorsal cochlear nucleus. (Based on the work of Osen. *J Comp Neurol* 1969; **136**: 453–84.[3])

Superior olivary complex

The SOC is positioned ventral and medial to the CN in the caudal portion of the pons[14] (Figure 11.5a). It consists of numerous groups of nuclei, but this discussion will be limited to the following five: the lateral superior olivary complex (LSO), the medial superior olivary nucleus (MSO), the nucleus of the trapezoid body, and the lateral and medial preolivary nuclei. In humans, evidence suggests that the MSO is the largest of these nuclei.[23] In some animal species, however, the largest and most prominent nucleus is the S-shaped LSO.[24]

Similar to that of the CN, tonotopic organization in the SOC seems to be preserved in all groups of nuclei. The LSO and MSO have been studied most extensively. In the LSO, lower frequencies are represented laterally and the higher frequencies medially following the S-shaped contour of the nucleus, which gives it a unique tonotopic organization.[25] The MSO has a primarily low-frequency representation, while the LSO responds to a broader range of frequencies.[14] The nucleus of the trapezoid body has a tonotopic orientation, with the low frequencies represented laterally and the high frequencies medially.

The tuning curves for the trapezoid body, LSO and MSO are mainly quite sharp, denoting good frequency selectivity.[4] The trapezoid and MSO post-stimulatory responses are primary-like with a notch, whereas the LSO has shown 'chopper' and primary-like-type responses.[4,26]

Within the SOC, the LSO is innervated bilaterally[27] and receives ipsilateral input from the AVCN and contralateral innervation from both the AVCN and PVCN.[28] Both ipsilateral and contralateral inputs from the AVCN are also received in the MSO.[29] Afferent input to the trapezoid body is not fully understood, but a significant contribution seems to arise from the contralateral CN.[27] Innervation of the lateral and the medial preolivary nuclei may come primarily from the ipsilateral AVCN, but this is also unclear and appears to differ among species.[27]

The SOC is a complex relay station in the auditory pathway. It is the first, but not only, place where a variety of ipsilateral and contralateral inputs provide the system with the anatomical foundation for unique functions in binaural listening. Sound localization is determined mainly by interaural time[30] and intensity[31] variations reflected in inputs to the SOC. The SOC has excitatory and inhibitory cells (and also some cells that are both excitatory and inhibitory) which are time (and hence directionally) sensitive. These excitatory and inhibitory responses help clarify directional cues for the higher auditory system.[32] Tasks that necessitate the integration and interpretation of binaurally presented signals depend on the SOC and convergence of neural information from each ear. For example, audiological tests, such as rapidly alternating speech perception and the binaural fusion test (see Chapter 29), rely on binaural integration and the interaction of information in the SOC.[33] Abnormal results are often seen on these tests in

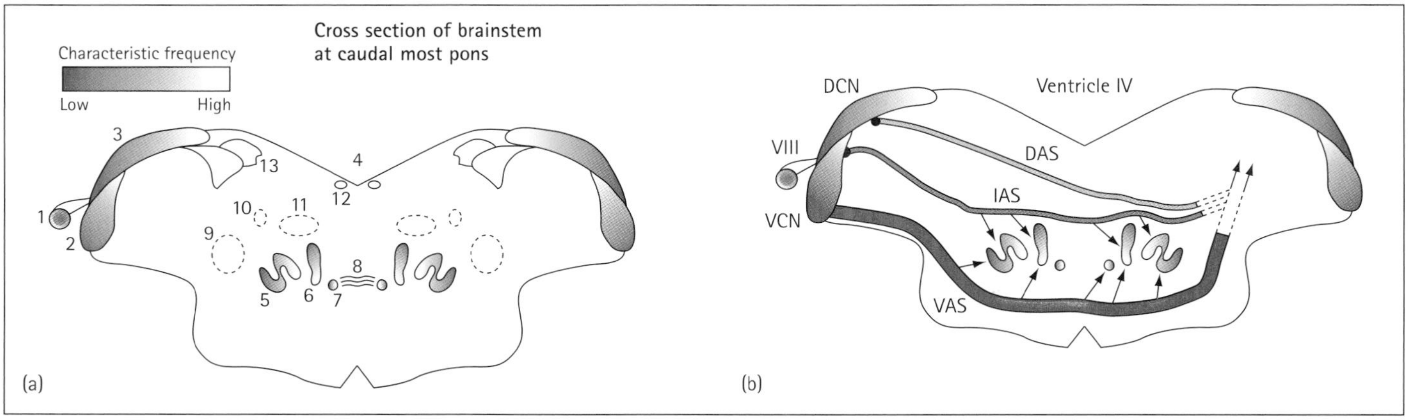

Figure 11.5 (a) Cross-section of the lower pons, focusing on the cochlear nucleus, superior olivary complex and associated structures in this region of the brainstem. (b) The same cross-section as in (a), showing the three acoustical stria coursing from the left cochlear nucleus only. VIII, Cochlear nerve; VCN, ventral cochlear nucleus; DCN, dorsal cochlear nucleus; DAS, dorsal acoustical stria; IAS, intermediate acoustical stria; VAS, ventral acoustical stria. Arrows indicate fibers ascending via the lateral lemnicus.

cases with signal degradation prior to the SOC or SOC pathology.[34] Binaural integration is also necessary for the measurement of masking level differences (MLDs), which are a sensitive index of brainstem integrity.[35] Changing the phase of the stimulus (tones or speech) in the presence of noise results in a change in the ability to detect the signal, which makes temporal cueing at the SOC critical in MLDs. The importance of the SOC in the measurement of MLDs and the fusion of binaural signals is supported by several studies which show that low-brainstem lesions affect MLDs, while lesions in the upper brainstem or auditory cortex do not.[35,36]

The SOC also appears to be an important relay station in the reflex arc of the acoustical stapedius muscle reflex.[37] The reflex is thought to entail both direct and indirect neural pathways,[38] but the neurophysiology of the reflex arc is not entirely understood.[39] The direct reflex arc appears to consist of a three- or four-neurone chain which is activated when a sufficiently intense acoustical stimulus is presented to one or both ears. Neural impulses are conveyed via the cochlear nerve to the AVCN, and then proceed to the ipsilateral MSO and/or facial nerve nucleus. Transverse input seems to arise from the AVCN and travels to the contralateral MSO by way of the trapezoid body. Neurones originating in the MSO region terminate in the motor nucleus of the facial nerve area, from where motor fibers then descend to innervate the stapedius muscle. Consequently, unilateral acoustical stimulation results in bilateral stapedius muscle contractions.[37]

The existence of an indirect pathway for the acoustical reflex has also been postulated. A slower polysynaptic pathway, possibly including the extrapyramidal system of the reticular formation, has been proposed by Borg[37] as this indirect reflex arc. Although all the pathways involved in the neural arc are not specified, significant clinical acoustical reflex data support the existence of this neural pathway.[39]

Lateral lemniscus

The LL is the primary auditory pathway in the brainstem and is composed of both ascending and descending fibers. The ascending portion extends bilaterally from the CN to the IC in the midbrain and contains both crossed and uncrossed fibers from the CN and SOC[40] (Figure 11.1).

Within the LL, there are two main cell groups: the ventral and dorsal nuclei of the lateral lemniscus (NLL), and a minor cell group called the intermediate nucleus of the LL. These nuclei are located posterolaterally in the upper portion of the pons, near the lateral surface of the brainstem.[41] Afferent input to the NLL arises from the dorsal CN on the contralateral side, and from the ventral CN on both sides of the brainstem.[42] Both the ipsilateral and contralateral SOC also provide input to the NLL.[14] The dorsal NLL from either side of the brainstem are interconnected by a fiber tract called the commissure of Probst.[43] Lemniscal fibers may also cross from one side to the other through the pontine reticular formation.[41] Most neurones of the dorsal segment of the LL can be activated binaurally. However, a majority of neurones from the ventral segment can be activated only by contralateral stimulation.[26] As with the CN and the SOC, definite tonotopic organization has been demonstrated for both the dorsal and ventral NLL.[23] However, recent work has questioned the tonotopic arrangement of the LL, and indicated a possible concentric organization.[44] Tuning curves are highly variable, and temporal resolution appears to be markedly decreased at the LL, as compared to more caudal auditory nuclei.[4]

Inferior colliculus

The IC is one of the largest and most identifiable auditory structures of the brainstem.[45] The IC is located on the dorsal surface of the midbrain, approximately 3–3.5 cm rostral to the pontomedullary junction (Figure 11.2).

From the dorsal aspect of the midbrain, the IC is clearly visible as two spherical mounds.[38] Two additional rounded projections, the superior colliculi, can be seen on the dorsal surface of the midbrain, slightly rostral and lateral to the IC.[38]

Two major divisions exist within the IC: the central nucleus—or core—which is composed of purely auditory fibers, and the pericentral nucleus—or belt—which surrounds the central nucleus and consists mainly of somatosensory and auditory fibers.[26]

The majority of auditory fibers from the LL and the lower auditory centers synapse directly or indirectly at the IC.[46] Van Noort[47] found that the IC receives input from the dorsal and ventral CN, lateral and medial superior olivary nuclei, dorsal and ventral nuclei of the LL, and contralateral IC. Other reports[12,26,48] suggest that the lower nuclei provide both contralateral and ipsilateral inputs to the IC. Many interneurones appear to exist in the IC, suggesting the presence of strong neuronal interconnections.[45] The superior colliculi, generally associated with the visual system, also receives input from the auditory system, which is integrated into the reflexes involving the position of the head and eyes.[49]

Many of the functional properties of the IC have been described. As with other brainstem auditory structures, the IC has a high degree of tonotopic organization. In the IC, the high frequencies are ventral and the low frequencies are dorsally positioned.[50]

Moreover, the IC contains a large number of fibers which yield extremely sharp tuning curves, suggesting a high level of frequency resolution.[51] The IC contains many time- and spatial-sensitive neurones[52,53] and neurones sensitive to binaural stimulation.[54] This suggests a role in sound localization.[38] Finally, in considering its neural connections and its position astride the auditory pathways, the IC has been referred to as the obligatory relay nuclear complex in transmitting auditory information to higher levels.[14]

As with the LL, the IC has a commissure that permits neural communication between the left and right IC.[12] A unique feature of the IC is its brachium, a large fiber tract that lies on the dorsolateral surface of the midbrain. This tract projects fibers ipsilaterally to the medial geniculate body (MGB), which is the principal auditory nucleus of the thalamus. Three cell types make up the majority of neural elements in the IC. Disk-shaped cells represent 75–85% of the cells in the central nucleus. Simple and complex stellate cells also exist in the IC.[55] In terms of response properties, the IC has two main types of responses: transient onset and sustained. The transient onset is an increase in response that grows only at the beginning of the stimulus; the sustained response gradually increases for the duration of the stimulus.[56] It is important to know that, in the IC, all the response types described at the CN are present, although apparently to a lesser degree.[57] The temporal resolution of the IC, as with the LL, is less efficient than at the lower brainstem auditory structures.[4] Interestingly, intensity coding at the IC reveals a large number of neurones with non-monotonic functions.[57]

Medial geniculate body

The MGB is located on the inferior dorsolateral surface of the thalamus, just anterior, lateral and slightly rostral to the IC (Figure 11.2). Although the MGB sits in the thalamus and the IC in the midbrain, these structures are located only approximately 1 cm apart. The MGB contains ventral, dorsal and medial divisions.[58] Cells in the ventral division respond primarily to acoustical stimuli, while the other divisions contain neurones that respond to both somatosensory and acoustical stimulation.[26,48] The ventral division appears to be the portion of the MGB that transmits specific discrimination (speech) auditory information to the cerebral cortex.[59,60] The dorsal division projects axons to association areas of the auditory cortex. This division may maintain and direct auditory attention. The medial division may function as a multisensory arousal system.[59]

Afferent inputs to the MGB are primarily uncrossed, arriving from the IC via the branchium. It is possible, however, that some input may come from the contralateral IC and that some lower nuclei may input directly on the MGB.[53] In the cat, crossed inputs from the IC connect to the medial division of the MGB.[58,59]

Tonotopic organization has been reported in the ventral segment of the MGB, with low frequencies represented laterally and high frequencies represented medially. Tuning curves range from broad to sharp, but MGB fibers in general are not as sharply tuned as are those of the IC.[61] As reviewed by Rouiller,[4] the MGB has neurones with response properties that include transient onset, sustained, offset and inhibitory. The MGB also has sharp tuning curves which allow good frequency selectivity. There are both monotonic and non-monotonic neurones for the coding of intensity. Temporal resolution varies across the three regions of the MGB, and the ventral division has the best fidelity (measured by phase locking or synchronization to individual clicks). In general, the temporal resolution of the ventral portion is similar to that of the IC and much poorer than that of the CN.

As with the IC, the MGB has many neurones sensitive to binaural stimulation and interaural intensity differences.[48,61]

Another important structure that closely interacts with the auditory pathway is the reticular formation or reticular activating system. Discussion of this system is beyond the scope of this chapter, but those interested in reviewing the reticular formation are directed to references 62 and 64.

Vascular anatomy of the brainstem

Many auditory dysfunctions of the brainstem and periphery have a vascular basis. For example, vertebrobasilar disease, mini-strokes, vascular spasms, aneurysms and vascular loops have all been shown to affect the auditory system.[21,65,66]

The major blood supply of the brainstem is the basilar artery, which originates from the left and right vertebral arteries, 1–2 mm below the pontomedullary junction on the ventral side of the brainstem (Figure 11.6). At the low- to mid-pons level, the anterior inferior cerebellar artery branches from the basilar artery to supply blood to the CN. The CN may also receive an indirect vascular supply from the posterior inferior cerebellar artery.[67] In many cases, the anterior inferior cerebellar artery gives rise to the internal auditory artery, which supplies the VIIIth nerve, and then branches into three divisions to supply the cochlear and vestibular periphery. The internal auditory artery sometimes branches directly from the basilar artery.[68]

At the mid-pons level, small pontine branches of the basilar artery, perhaps with the circumferential arteries, indirectly supply the SOC and possibly the LL.[25] In addition, a strong possibility exists that the paramedian branches of the artery supply the SOC and LL. The superior cerebellar arteries are located at the rostral pons or midbrain level. Their branches supply the IC

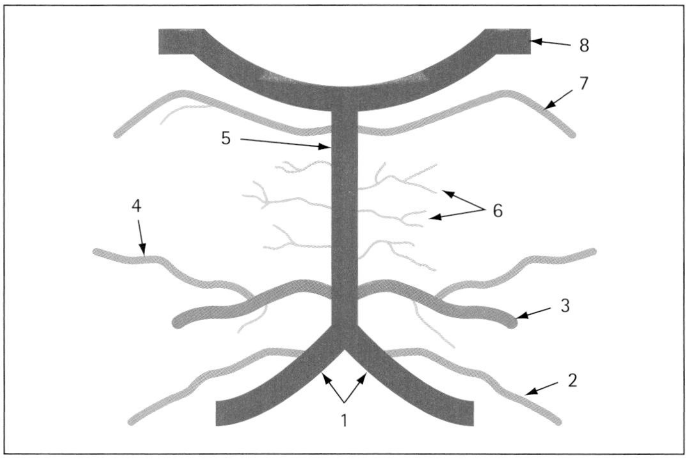

Figure 11.6 Key vessels of the rostral medulla and pons segment of the brainstem. These vessels are located on the ventral side of the pons/medulla. 1, Vertebral arteries; 2, posterior inferior cerebellar artery (PICA); 3, anterior inferior cerebellar artery (AICA); 4, internal auditory artery; 5, basilar artery; 6, pontine arteries; 7, superior cerebellar artery; 8, posterior cerebral artery.

and in some cases the NLL.[64] At the midbrain level, the basilar artery forms the posterior cerebral arteries. Each posterior cerebral artery has circumferential branches that supply the MGB ipsilaterally (Waddington, personal communication).

Significant variability has been shown in the vasculature of the brainstem.[67,69] Because vascular patterns vary among specimens, no one description can encapsulate all vascular patterns. Because most brainstem auditory structures are on the dorsal side of the brainstem, they may receive secondary and tertiary branches of the key arteries mentioned previously.

Key concepts in function

The following section introduces concepts about general auditory anatomy and physiology and reviews them in reference to auditory brainstem structures.

Intensity coding

As sound intensity increases, the firing rate of many of the auditory fibers in the brainstem increases; exceptions to this will be discussed later. Because the range between the threshold and saturation point of any given fiber is much smaller than the range of intensities audible to the human ear, large-intensity increases cannot be encoded by individual nerve fibers.[70] Rather, at high intensities many neurones must interact to achieve accurate coding. The mechanisms of this interaction are poorly understood,[48,71] since most information on intensity coding is based on the study of individual neurones.

Neurones of various brainstem nuclei respond to stimulus intensity in three principal ways.[12,48] One type of response is monotonic, meaning that as the stimulus intensity increases, the firing rate of the neurone(s) increases proportionally. The second type of intensity function is monotonic for low intensities, but, as stimulus intensity increases, the firing rate levels off. The third type of intensity function is non-monotonic. With this type of function, the neuronal firing rate reaches a plateau at a relatively low intensity and sometimes actually decreases as intensity increases, resulting in a rollover phenomenon. For example, some neurones in the IC reach their maximum firing rate 5 dB above their threshold.[12] These three types of intensity coding appear to be common throughout the auditory brainstem, although the extent of each type varies among nuclei groups. On the other hand, most fibers in the CN have monotonic intensity function. The CN fibers have a 30–40-dB dynamic range, and, in this regard, are similar to the cochlear nerve fibers.[4]

One can hypothesize that a high-intensity signal would be coded inappropriately when there is damage to brainstem auditory neurones of the first type (monotonic) but not to the latter two types of neurones. This could result in higher intensities being coded incorrectly, which might result in what is known clinically as the rollover phenomenon.[72]

Aspects of temporal coding

> The CANS is an elegant time-keeper. Physiological measures of latency, phase locking, phase difference and synchronicity are common ways of detailing temporal processing. The latency of brainstem neuronal responses varies, depending on the type of auditory stimulus and the neurone or neurone group analyzed.[12,48] Some neurones react quickly to stimulation, while others have lengthy latency periods. Some neurones respond only upon termination of the stimulus.

Phase locking is another phenomenon related to timing in the auditory system.[26,70] Many auditory neurones appear to lock onto the stimulus according to phase, and fire only when the stimulus waveform reaches a certain point in its cycle. This is particularly evident with low-frequency sounds. Moreover, at lower frequencies certain neurones fire on every cycle, while at higher frequencies they fire only at every third or fifth cycle. This phase relationship is especially apparent in lower auditory brainstem neurones and may have considerable relevance to the mechanisms underlying MLDs.[73] Generally, the firing rates of brainstem auditory neurones are higher than those of cortical nerve fibers for steady-state signals or for periodic signals. The speed with which a neurone can respond to repeated stimuli depends on its refractory period. The refractory period is the time interval between two successive discharges (depolarizations) of a nerve cell. The refractory period depends on the cell metabolism, and dysfunction of metabolic activity will lengthen the refractory period.[74] Phase locking could be viewed as a form of synchronicity, in that responses occur repeatedly in the same time domain. A good example of auditory synchronicity is the auditory brainstem response (ABR). In an ABR, the waves represent synchronous electrical activity.

In reviewing timing of the auditory system, it is necessary to discuss temporal processing. As Phillips[75] conveys, this phrase may mean different things to different people. Clinicians often use the phrase temporal processing to indicate performance on an audiological test that requires some type of timing decision about the stimuli presented. Basic scientists look at various types of temporal processing and how these contribute to other auditory functions. Phillips[75] provides several examples of how timing is key to certain auditory processes. Localization of a sound source requires relative timing of acoustical signal arriving at the two ears. The auditory system has a temporal sensitivity to phase differences (of the signal) which may help us hear in noise. MLD is a good example of phase differential sensitivity. The pitch perception of complex sounds depends on timing (and related coding) of rapidly repeated acoustical events. In addition, sequencing of successive stimuli, masking of signals (existing close in time), discrimination of element duration and time intervals, integration of acoustical energy and pitch changes can all be considered aspects of temporal processing. Even detection, recognition and discrimination processes operate over critical time periods and thus may be considered as having a temporal element.

Frequency coding

The three concepts relevant to our discussion of frequency coding include tonotopicity, frequency discrimination, and physiological tuning curves. The central auditory system is tonotopically arranged, and certain neurones respond best to certain frequencies. This arrangement provides a 'spatial array' of various frequencies to which the system responds. The characteristic frequency is the frequency at which a neurone has its most sensitive threshold to a pure tone stimulus (the frequency that requires the least amount of intensity to raise a neurone's activity just above its spontaneous firing rate). A physiological tuning curve refers to a plot of the intensity level needed to reach the threshold of a nerve cell over a wide range of frequencies. This measure can convey much information about the frequency resolution of a neurone (or group of neurones). Frequency discrimination is the differential sensitivity to various frequencies. This differential measurement can be accomplished psychophysically and is often referred to as a difference limen, which is the smallest frequency difference that can be discerned between two acoustical stimuli. An electrophysiological correlate of the frequency difference limen can be accomplished using the evoked potential mismatched negativity (MMN). Differential sensitivity to intensity and duration of tones can be accomplished in the same way, but is not used in physiological studies on audition as much as the frequency parameter is used.

The auditory brainstem response

In concluding this section on the auditory pathways of the brainstem, it is important to discuss aspects of the ABR (see Chapter 16). The ABR has gained most of its popularity because of its clinical applications, but it has also been a valuable addition to basic science. The ABR has provided a physiological approach to the study of multiple neurone groups and the way in which they interact in the brainstem. This avenue of study is different from the single-neurone studies which have been common in auditory brainstem anatomy and physiology.

The exact origins of some elements of the ABR are uncertain, but research on humans has helped clarify the subject.[70,76] Möller[70] indicated that wave I of the ABR is generated from the lateral aspect of the auditory nerve, whereas wave II originates from the medial aspect. Wave III probably has more than one generator, as do other subsequent waves of the ABR, but the CN is probably the principal source of wave III.[70,76] In a study on patients with multiple sclerosis who underwent detailed magnetic resonance imaging and ABRs, observations indicated that waves I and II were generated peripheral to the rostral ventral acoustical stria.[77] This same study indicated that wave III was generated by the AVCN and rostral ventral stria, with the IV–V complex generated rostrally to these structures. Clinical studies have shown that a mid-line lesion in the low pons which did not affect the cochlear nuclei preserved waves I, II and III and delayed the IV–V wave complex. This lesion appeared to compromise the SOC.[78] Wave IV probably has multiple generator sites as well, but it arises predominantly from the SOC and has a contralateral influence that may be stronger than the ipsilateral contribution. According to Möller[70] and to Wada and Starr,[76] wave V is generated from the LL. Levine et al[77] state that the IV–V complex may be generated by the MSO system, perhaps where it projects contralaterally onto the LL or IC. In a simplified view of the ABR origins, it is plausible that the first five ABR waves may be generated entirely within the cochlear nerve and pons. However, the IC may exert some influence on wave V, and this has been shown in detailed analyses of the ABR.[79]

The typical clinical findings of ABR abnormalities in the ear ipsilateral to a brainstem lesion[80–82] seem to be inconsistent with known neuroanatomy, which shows a majority of the auditory fibers crossing to the contralateral side at the level of the SOC. It is unclear what these ABR findings mean with regard to brainstem pathways and associated physiology. However, it is important to consider these clinical findings in the framework of how the brainstem pathways may function in the pathological situation.

Animal studies by Wada and Starr[76] and our own observations with humans show that the first five waves of the ABR are not affected by specific lesions of the IC, with the exceptions noted earlier. Unfortunately, the ABR may not be a useful tool in evaluating lesions at or above the IC. Powerful clinical tests such as the ABR, MLDs and acoustical reflexes appear to be restricted to detecting lesions below the midbrain level. In cases where lesions of the IC or the MGB (midbrain and thalamic levels) are suspected, other procedures are necessary to detect and define the abnormality.

The cerebrum

Auditory cortex and subcortex

Neurones originating in the MGB and radiating outward to the auditory areas of the brain create the ascending auditory system that proceeds from the thalamic area to the cerebral cortex (Figure 11.7).

The cerebral cortex, the gray matter comprising the brain surface, consists of three principal types of cells: pyramidal, stellate and fusiform. Six cell layers in the cortex can be distinguished by type, density and arrangement of the nerve cells.[64] In the auditory region of the cortex, cells responsive to acoustical stimuli exist in all the layers, with the exception of layer one.[83]

The principal auditory area of the cortex is considered to be Heschl's gyrus, sometimes referred to as the transverse gyrus

Researchers disagree on which areas constitute the auditory cortex. This controversy results from adapting animal models to the human brain, and from disagreement over whether to include 'association' areas as part of the auditory cortex.[84] We believe these association areas are critical to understanding the system, although they also contain some fibers which are not sensitive to auditory stimuli.

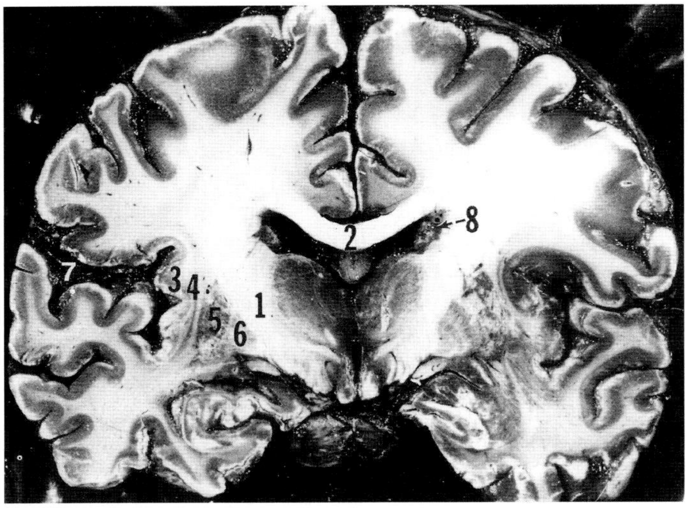

Figure 11.7 Coronal section through a human brain (gray matter stained), emphasizing the subcortical structures. 1, Internal capsule; 2, corpus callosum; 3, insula; 4, external capsule with the claustrum (gray matter strip); 5, putamen; 6, globis pallidus; 7, Sylvian fissure; 8, caudate. (Courtesy of W. Mosenthal and F. Musiek.)

(Figure 11.8). This gyrus is located in the Sylvian fissure, approximately two-thirds posterior on the upper surface of the temporal lobe (supratemporal plane). It courses in a posterior and medial direction. Heschl's gyrus can be defined by the acoustical sulcus at its anterior and transverse sulcus at its posterior fringes. The temporal lobe must be displaced inferiorly or separated from the brain to expose the supratemporal plane to examine Heschl's gyrus.

Campain and Minckler[85] analyzed numerous human brains and concluded that the configuration of Heschl's gyrus differed on the left side compared to the right. In some brains, double gyri were present unilaterally, while in other brains double gyri were present on both sides. Musiek and Reeves[86] studied 29 human brains and reported that the number of Heschl's gyri ranged from one to three per hemisphere, although there was no significant left–right asymmetry in the number of Heschl's gyri within individual brains. The mean length of Heschl's gyrus, however, was found to be larger in the left hemisphere.[86]

The planum temporale is located on the cortical surface from the most posterior aspect of Heschl's gyrus and continuing posteriorly to the endpoint of the Sylvian fissure. In the human

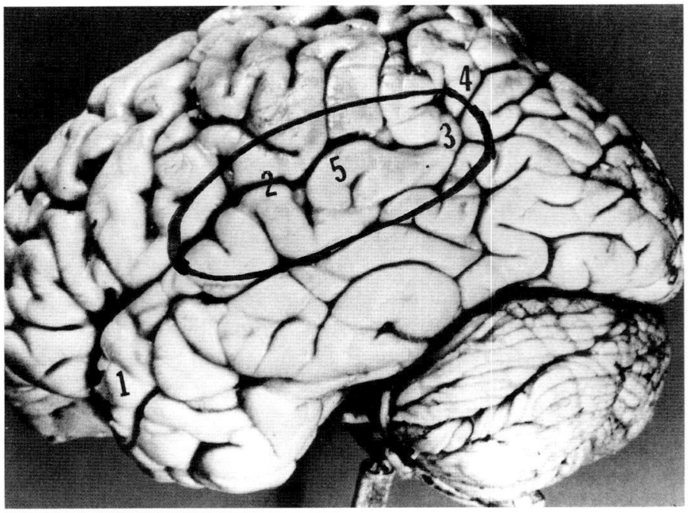

Figure 11.8 Lateral view of the left hemisphere of the brain with the auditory responsive area encircled. 1, Temporal pole; 2, Sylvian fissure; 3, supramarginal gyrus; 4, angular gyrus; 5, superior, posterior temporal gyrus. From Waddington *Atlas of Human Intracranial Anatomy*.[67] Rutland Vt: Academy Books 1984: 79–95. with permission.

brain, the planum temporale was shown to be significantly larger on the left side (3.6 cm) than on the right (2.7 cm) by Geschwind and Levitsky.[87] These researchers thought that the planum temporale may be an anatomical correlate to language (receptive) in humans, since the planum temporale is located in Wernicke's region and in the left hemisphere, which is dominant for speech. Musiek and Reeves[86] supported these earlier findings[87] on the differences in the lengths of the left and right planum temporale. Musiek and Reeves proposed, however, that asymmetries in higher auditory and language function may be related to anatomical differences not only of the planum temporale but also of Heschl's gyrus.

The primary auditory area and a portion of the language area in humans are contained within the Sylvian fissure. Rubens[88] reviewed earlier anatomical work on the Sylvian fissure showing the left Sylvian fissure to be larger than the right. Others have corroborated this finding, including Musiek and Reeves,[86] who found that asymmetry of the Sylvian fissure was correlated with the greater length of the planum temporale on the left side.

Curving around the end of the Sylvian fissure is the supramarginal gyrus, an area responsive to acoustical stimulation.[89] It is located in the approximate Wernicke's area region, along with the angular gyrus, which is situated immediately posterior to the supramarginal gyrus.[87] These constitute a portion of a complex association area that appears to integrate auditory, visual and somesthetic information, making it vital to the visual and somesthetic aspects of language, such as reading and writing.

Also responsive to acoustical stimulation are the inferior portion of the parietal lobe and the inferior aspect of the frontal lobe[89,90] (Figure 11.8). The insula (a portion of the cortex located deep within the Sylvian fissure medial to the middle segment of the temporal gyrus) is yet another acoustically responsive area. It appears that the most posterior aspect of the insula is contiguous with Heschl's gyrus. The only way to observe the insular cortex is by removing the temporal lobe or displacing it inferiorly (Figures 11.9 and 11.10).

The insula contains fibers that respond to somatic, visual and gustatory stimulation. Acoustical stimulation, however, causes the greatest neural activity.[91] The posterior aspect of the insula, the section nearest to Heschl's gyrus, seems to possess the most acoustically sensitive fibers.[91] Located just medial to the insula is a narrow strip of gray matter called the claustrum. The function of the claustrum is not well understood, but it seems to be highly responsive to acoustical stimulation.[14,91]

People with dyslexia have been reported to have anatomical brain irregularities.[92,93]

> The planum temporale, normally significantly longer in the left hemisphere, was found to be symmetrical bilaterally in the brains of dyslexic patients. Furthermore, brains of patients with dyslexia had an unusually large number of cell abnormalities called cerebrocortical microdysgenesias, which are nests of ectopic neurones and glia in the first layer of the cortex. These ectopic areas are often connected with dysplasia of cortical layers (including focal microgyria), sometimes with superficial growths known as brain warts. Up to 26% of normal brains may contain these focal anomalies, but they are usually found in small numbers, often in the right hemisphere. A greater number of anomalies occur in patients with developmental dyslexia, frequently in the left hemisphere in the area of the presylvian cortex.[93]

The findings just mentioned are interesting for two reasons. First, the areas of symmetry versus asymmetry and microdysgenesias appear to involve areas that in humans are mostly considered auditory regions of the cerebrum. Second, the reason for the high incidence of cortical dysplasias in people with learning disorders is unknown. One might speculate that these morphological abnormalities have functional or perhaps dysfunctional correlates. More studies are needed to relate these findings to behavioral consequences.

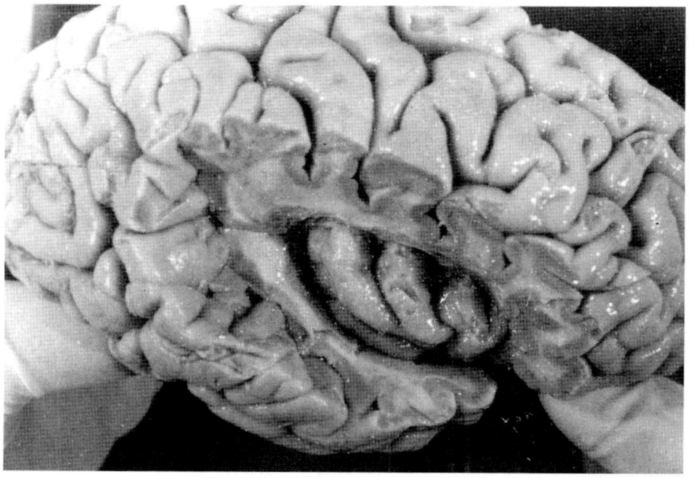

Figure 11.9 Right lateral view of the insula observed after removal of part of the parietal, frontal and temporal lobes. (Courtesy of W. Mosenthal and F. Musiek.)

Thalamocortical connections

Auditory fiber tracts ascending from the MGB to the cortex and other areas of the brain follow multiple routes. One of these groups of fibers provides input to the basal ganglia, which is the large subcortical gray matter structure consisting of the caudate nucleus, putamen and globus pallidus (Figures 11.7 and 11.10). The lenticular process, or nucleus, lies between the internal and external capsules, the white matter neural pathways, and contains the putamen and globus pallidus. In animal studies, the MGB has been shown to transmit fibers that connect with the

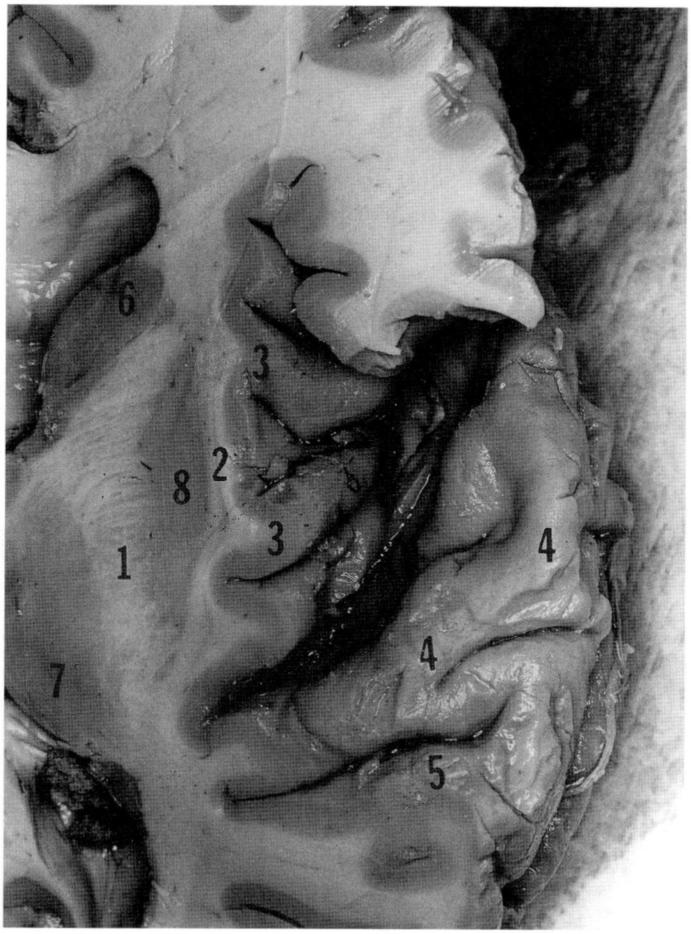

Figure 11.10 Transverse section of the right hemisphere cut along the Sylvian fissure. 1, Internal capsule; 2, external capsule with claustrum coursing through it; 3, insula; 4, Heschl's gyrus; 5, anterior part of the planum temporale (posterior part is cut away); 6, caudate; 7, thalamus; 8, lenticular process (putamen, globis pallidus).

putamen, the caudate nucleus and the amygdaloid body, a small almond-shaped expansion located at the tail of the caudate nucleus.[94]

Two main pathways link the MGB and the cortex besides the aforementioned connections to the basal ganglia. The first pathway follows a sublenticular route through the internal capsule to Heschl's gyrus and contains all auditory fibers emanating from the ventral MGB. The second pathway courses from the MGB through the inferior aspect of the internal capsule, and ultimately under the putamen to the external capsule, and consists of auditory, somatic and possibly visual fibers. Beyond the external capsule, fibers connect to the insula.[21,95] Further connections proceed from the MGB to the auditory cortex and most likely overlap the two pathways discussed here.[96,97] These pathways represent the varied and complex connections of the thalamocortical auditory anatomy.

Interhemispheric connections

The corpus callosum (CC), which is located at the base of the longitudinal fissure, is the primary connection between the left and right hemispheres (Figures 11.1, 11.7 and 11.11).

The CC is covered by the cingulate gyri and forms most of the roof of the lateral ventricles.[98] It consists of long, heavily myelinated axons and is the largest fiber tract in the primate brain. In an adult, the CC is approximately 6.5 cm long from the anterior genu to the posterior splenium, and is approximately 0.5–1 cm thick.[99] The CC seems to be larger in left-handed than in right-handed people, but it has significant morphological variability.[100]

The CC is not exclusively a mid-line structure,[99] as it essentially connects the two cortices and thereby must span much of the intercortical space above the basal ganglia and lateral ventricles. Because it encompasses such a large portion of the cerebrum, it is probable that in many 'cortical' lesions some region of the CC is involved.

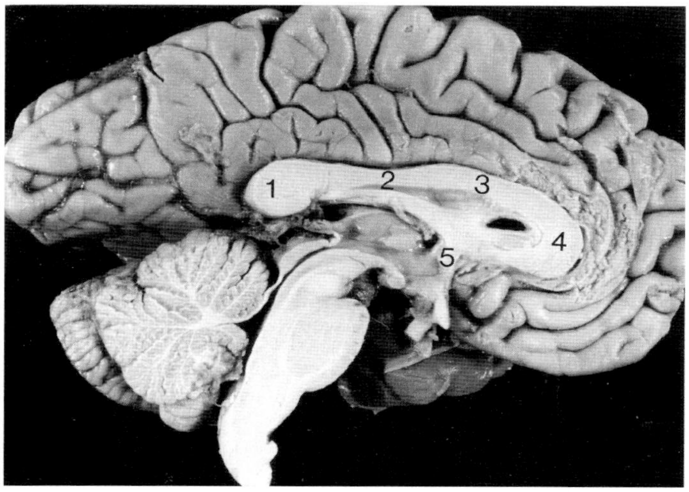

Figure 11.11 Sagittal cut separating the two hemispheres of the brain and sectioning the corpus callosum at its mid-line. The focus is on the corpus callosum. 1, Splenium (visual); 2, sulcus (auditory); 3, trunk or body (somatic and motor); 4, genu (olfactory? frontal lobe fibers), rostrum (olfactory?); 5, anterior commissure. (Courtesy of W. Mosenthal and F. Musiek.)

Homolateral fibers (those which connect to the same locus in each hemisphere) are the primary fibers in the CC. The CC also contains heterolateral fibers, which are those connecting to different loci on each hemisphere.[101] Heterolateral fibers frequently have a longer and less direct route to the opposite side, which may necessitate a longer transfer time than required by their homolateral counterparts. The latency of an evoked potential recorded from one point on the cortex following stimulation of the homolateral point on the other hemisphere is referred to as the transcallosal transfer time (TCTT). The TCTT in humans decreases with age, and minimum values are achieved during teenage years.[102] These findings are consistent with increased myelination of the CC axons.[103] The TCTT varies significantly, from a minimum of 3–6 ms to a maximum of 100 ms, in primates and humans.[104–106] The concept of inhibitory and excitatory neurones in the CC may be substantiated by this variability.

The neural connections of the CC correspond to, and the anatomy subserves, various regions of the cortex. The genu, or anterior region of the CC, contains fibers leading from the anterior insula and the olfactory fibers.[107] The trunk comprises the middle section of the CC, where the frontal and temporal lobes are also represented. The posterior half of the trunk, called the sulcus, is thinner and contains most of the auditory fibers from the temporal lobe and insula. The splenium is the most posterior portion of the CC and contains mostly visual fibers that connect with the occipital cortex.[107]

Just anterior to the splenium in the posterior half of the CC is the auditory area of the CC at the mid-line. Although this information was obtained through primate research,[107] data on humans helped localize the auditory areas of the CC. Baran et al[108] found little or no change in tasks requiring interhemispheric transfer (i.e. dichotic listening or pattern perception) after the sectioning of the anterior half of the CC. However, markedly poorer performance on these auditory tasks was shown in patients with a complete section of the CC.[109]

Lesions along the transcallosal auditory pathway may bring about interhemispheric transfer degradation. Although we have much information about the anatomy of the CC at the mid-line, we know little about the course of the transcallosal auditory pathway. It is thought to begin at the auditory cortex and course posteriorly and superiorly around the lateral ventricles. It then crosses a periventricular area known as the trigone, and courses medially and inferiorly into the CC proper. This information about the transcallosal auditory pathway comes from anatomical and clinical studies.[109]

A recent study demonstrated size differences in the CC for children with attention deficits, as compared with control subjects.[110] The auditory and the genu areas of the CC in the experimental group were smaller than those of the control group.[111]

The vascular anatomy of the CC is simple. The splenium, or posterior fifth, is supplied by branches of the posterior cerebral artery.[64] The remainder of the CC is supplied by the pericallosal artery, a branch of the anterior cerebral artery.[64]

Tonotopic organization

As in the brainstem, distinct tonotopic organization exists in the primary auditory cortex of the primate, with low frequencies represented rostrolaterally and high frequencies represented caudomedially.[112] Using positron emission tomography (PET) to measure changes in cerebral bloodflow, Lauter et al[113] demonstrated a similar pattern in the human brain. Tones of 500 Hz evoked increased activity in the lateral part of Heschl's gyrus, while tones of 4000 Hz resulted in activity in the medial position. Most tonotopic information on the insular cortex has been obtained from studies of cats.[114] In the cat insula, the high-frequency neurones appear to be located in the inferior segment.[114]

In the primary auditory area where cells are sharply tuned, highly definable tonotopic organization and isofrequency strips (contours) can be found.[115] There appear to be 'columns' within the cortex which have similar characteristic frequencies.[83] There also seems to be a spatial component to frequency representation in the auditory cortex; approximately 2 mm is required to encompass the frequency range of one octave. For extremely high frequencies, less space is needed to represent an octave range.[116]

> The tonotopicity of the auditory cortex has the plasticity to change if there is a lack of input at a given frequency range. Schwaber et al[117] demonstrated in primates that if one frequency band of the auditory cortex was deprived of input, after about 3 months that frequency band shifted to the neighboring lower frequency for which there was input and stimulation. In this manner, the cortical tissue remains active and viable, even though its tonotopic arrangement was different. This type of finding has important clinical implications.

Intensity coding

The discharge or firing rate of cortical neurones in primates varies as a function of intensity, and takes two forms: monotonic and non-monotonic.[118] Most neurones in the primary auditory cortex display rate–intensity functions similar to those of the cochlear nerve (i.e. the firing rate is monotonic for increments of approximately 10–40 dB). Intensities greater than 40 dB do not increase firing rates. Many neurones in the auditory cortex are sharply non-monotonic. In some cases, the firing rate may be reduced to a spontaneous level, with a 10-dB increase above the threshold intensity.[48]

Phillips[71] reported similar results with cats, identifying both monotonic and non-monotonic profiles. For some non-monotonic neurones, firing rates decreased precipitously, often to zero, at stimulus levels slightly above threshold. Phillips[71] also found that the introduction of wide-band noise raised the threshold level of the cortical neurones. However, once threshold sensitivity was achieved in noise, the firing rate increased in a manner similar to the unmasked condition, with the intensity profile remaining basically unchanged. With successive increments in the level of the masking noise, the tonal intensity profile is displaced toward progressively higher sound pressure levels. This phenomenon could be a way in which some cortical neurones can provide the auditory system with an improvement in signal-to-noise ratio, perhaps permitting better hearing in noise. One may also hypothesize that if these cortical neurones are damaged, the signal-to-noise ratio is compromised and that hearing in noise may be more difficult.

Animal studies show some cortical neurones to be intensity selective. Certain cells respond only within a given intensity range, but collectively the neurones cover a wide range of intensities. For example, cortical cells may respond maximally, minimally or not at all at a given intensity. When the intensity is changed, different cells may respond at a maximum level, and the previous neurones may respond minimally or not at al.[112]

Temporal factors

Like the brainstem, the auditory cortex responds in various ways to the onset, presence and offset of acoustical stimuli. Abeles and Goldstein[119] found four types of responses of cortical neurones to a 100-ms tone. One type of neurone sustained a response for the duration of the stimulus, although the firing rate was considerably less at the offset of the tone. 'On' neurones responded only to the onset, and 'off' neurones responded only after the tone was terminated. The fourth type responded to both the onset and the offset of the tone, but did not sustain a response during the tone.

Additional information on timing or temporal processing in the auditory cortex can be found in the work of Goldstein et al.[120] These investigators studied cells in the primary auditory area (A1) of rats and found four categories of response to clicks presented at different rates. Approximately 40% of the A1 cells responded to each click at rates of 10–1000/s while 25% of the A1 cells did not respond at all. The third classification of A1 cells showed varying response patterns as the click rate changed. The fourth group of cells responded only to low click rates. Eggermont[121] reported that several studies found click rates of auditory cortex neurones to be approximately 50–100/s or less. He also reported that recording methodology may influence the quantification of the response rates of these neurones. However, it seems that cortical neurones have difficulty following high-rate periodic events.

The coding of transient events by the cortex is related to temporal resolution and is different from coding periodic events. Examples of transient events would be tasks such as click fusion or temporal ordering. For these kinds of tasks, the cortex is temporally sensitive.[75] Only 2–3-ms differences were needed between two clicks to determine in humans that there are two stimuli and not one.[122]

Timing within the auditory cortex plays a critical role in localization abilities. Many neurones in the primary auditory cortex are sensitive to interaural phase and intensity differences.[123] In a soundfield, more cortical units fire to sound stimuli from a contralateral source than from an ipsilateral source.[124,125] This finding provided the basis for the initial clinical work on sound localization.

In 1958, Sanchez-Longo and Forster[126] reported that patients with temporal lobe damage had difficulty in locating sound sources in the soundfield contralateral to the damaged hemisphere. Recently, Moore et al[127] studied the abilities of both normal and brain-damaged subjects to track a fused auditory image as it moved through auditory space. The perceived location of the auditory image, which varies according to the temporal relationship of paired clicks presented one each from matched speakers, is referred to as the precedence effect. Although the normal subjects were able to track the fused auditory image accurately, two subjects with unilateral temporal lobe lesions (one in the right hemisphere, one in the left) exhibited auditory field deficits opposite the damaged hemispheres. Results of these investigations are consistent with other localization and lateralization studies which show contralateral ear effects.[128,129]

Electrical stimulation of the auditory cortex

Various auditory stimulation experiments with humans during neurological procedures were performed by Penfield and coworkers.[130,131] These investigators electrically stimulated areas along the margin of the Sylvian fissure while the patient, under local anesthesia, reported what he or she heard. Numerous patients reported experiencing no auditory sensation during the electrical stimulation. Some patients, however, reported hearing buzzing, ringing, chirping, knocking, humming and rushing sounds when the superior gyrus of the temporal lobe was stimulated. These sounds were directed primarily to the contralateral ear, but sometimes to both ears.

Penfield's patients frequently reported the impression of hearing loss during the electrical stimulation, although they heard and understood spoken words. Furthermore, patients claimed that the pitch and volume of the surgeon's voice varied during the electrical stimulation. A later study[132] reported cases where patients heard music and singing during electrical stimulation of the right auditory cortex. When the left posterosuperior temporal gyrus was stimulated, many patients who responded heard voices shouting and other acoustical phenomena.

Lateralization of function in the auditory cortex

One important issue in central auditory assessment using behavioral tests relates to lateralization of the deficit. It is well known that behavioral testing often indicates deficiencies in the ear contralateral to the damaged hemisphere. The fact that each ear provides more contralateral than ipsilateral input to the cortex may explain this contralateral ear deficit. Solid physiological evidence upholds this theory. Mountcastle[116] reported that contralateral stimulation of cortical neurones ordinarily had a 5–20-dB lower threshold for activation than did ipsilateral stimulation. Celesia[89] also showed that near-field potentials recorded from human auditory cortices during neurosurgery had larger amplitudes with contralateral ear stimulation than with ipsilateral stimulation. Studies of cats have also demonstrated comparable findings which indicate a stronger contralateral representation.[133]

Late auditory evoked potentials recorded with temporal/parietal region electrode placement in humans also revealed variances between contralateral and ipsilateral stimulation. The auditory evoked potentials recorded from contralateral stimulation were generally earlier and of greater amplitude than ipsilateral recordings.[134] However, this may not always be the case, and these findings for far-field evoked potentials are controversial.[133]

Behavioral ablation studies

Ablation experiments have served as the basis for the development of several auditory tests. By monitoring auditory behavior in animals, the effects of partial or total ablation of the auditory cortex have been measured and have been valuable in the localization of function.

> Kryter and Ades,[135] in one of the first studies involving ablation of the cat auditory cortex, found little or no effect on absolute thresholds or differential thresholds for intensity. These findings are consistent with data obtained from humans with brain damage or surgically removed auditory cortices.[136,137] However, some investigators[71,138,139] report that bilateral ablations of the primate auditory cortex result in severe hearing loss for pure tones. Bilaterally ablated animals demonstrated gradual recovery, but many retained some permanent pure tone sensitivity loss, especially in the middle frequencies.[139] Unilateral cortical ablations resulted in hearing loss in the ear contralateral to the lesion and normal hearing in the ipsilateral ear.[138] Permanent residual hearing loss has also been reported in humans with bilateral cortical lesions.[140–142]

Differences among animal species are shown in studies with opossums[143] and ferrets,[144] in which auditory threshold recovery is almost complete after bilateral lesions of the auditory cortex. The effects of auditory cortex ablation on frequency discrimination in animals remain unclear, even after many years of research. Early studies[145,146] reported that frequency discrimination was lost after ablation of the auditory cortex, while later studies[147] contradicted these early findings. These discrepancies may be related to the difficulty of the discrimination tasks, as each study used a different test paradigm to measure pitch perception. The complexity of the tasks, rather than the differences in frequency discrimination, is probably responsible for the discrepant findings.[48]

Lesion effects on frequency discrimination in humans may differ from those in animals. Thompson and Abel[148] showed that patients with temporal lobe lesions have significantly poorer frequency discrimination for tones than do normal control subjects. Patients with lesions of the left temporal lobe yielded a greater deficit than did patients with right temporal lobe lesions (Figure 11.12). Similar results of poor frequency discrimination in patients with central auditory lesions have been noted on a more informal test basis by the authors of this chapter.

Because ablation of the auditory cortex has debatable effects on absolute or differential thresholds for intensity or frequency, more complex tasks were sought to examine the results of cortical ablation. Diamond and Neff[149] used patterned acoustical stimuli to examine the ability of cats to detect differences in frequency patterns after various bilateral cortical ablations. After ablation of primary and association auditory cortices, the cats could no longer discriminate different acoustical patterns, and despite extensive retraining they could not relearn the pattern task. Based on subsequent studies, Neff[150] reported that auditory cortex ablations affected primarily temporal sequencing and not pattern detection or frequency discrimination of the tones comprising patterns. Colavita[151,152] demonstrated in cats that ablation of only the insular–temporal region resulted in the inability to discriminate temporal patterns. The early research of Diamond and Neff influenced Pinheiro in her development of the frequency (pitch) pattern test, a valuable clinical central auditory test in humans.[153–155] Another pattern-perception test, duration patterns, has

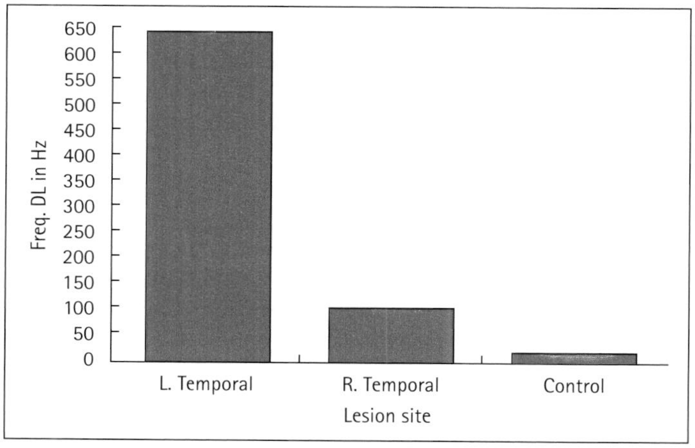

Figure 11.12 Column graph shows the mean difference limen (DL) in hertz obtained from subjects with left and right temporal lobe lesions, as compared to a control group. (Based on the work of Thompson and Abel. *Scan Audiol* 1992; **21**(35): 3–22.[148])

emerged as a potentially valuable clinical tool.[156] Temporal ordering appears to be a critical part of pattern perception, which in turn is affected by lesions of the auditory cortex.

Other studies show that the temporal dimension of hearing is linked to the integrity of the auditory cortex. Gershuni et al[157] demonstrated that a unilateral lesion of the dog's auditory cortex resulted in decreased pure tone sensitivity for short but not long tones in the ear contralateral to the lesion.

In contrast, Cranford[158] showed that cortical lesions had no effect on brief tone thresholds in cats. Cranford[158] also demonstrated that auditory cortex lesions in cats markedly affected the frequency difference limen for short- but not long-duration tones presented to the contralateral ear. Following the animal study, Cranford et al[159] examined brief tone frequency difference limens in seven human subjects with unilateral temporal lobe lesions. Findings with human subjects were essentially the same as those with animals. Brief tone thresholds for subjects with temporal lobe lesions were the same as those of a normal control group, but the brief tone frequency difference limen was markedly poorer for subjects with lesions. The frequency difference limen was poorer for the contralateral ear for stimulus duration under 200 ms.

Auditory stimulation influences on the auditory cortex

The auditory cortex appears to respond to acoustical stimulation and/or auditory training. This statement is associated with a number of important recent studies. One such study was conducted by Recanzone et al[160] on owl monkeys. These animals were trained on a frequency discrimination task. After extensive training, each animal's auditory cortex was tonotopically mapped. The neural substrate matching the frequency of the training was two to eight times larger than the same region in a control group of animals that did not receive training. In addition, these animals' behavioral frequency discrimination improved markedly after training. Other studies, though differently oriented, have also shown changes (reorganization) in the auditory cortex as a result of stimulation and/or training.[161,162] This has changed our view on auditory training, especially its use with auditory processing disorders; for reviews see Chermak and Musiek[163] and Musiek and Berge.[164]

Imaging techniques

Advanced imaging technology has made possible anatomical and physiological inspection of the human brain. This is important, because at the subcortical and cortical levels animal brains are structurally and functionally different from the human brain, and it has been with concern that extrapolations have been made from animal models to humans with regard to brain function related to audition. With imaging techniques, it is possible to measure some functions of hearing in humans. Although it is too soon for these imaging techniques to replace the important animal studies, they have important potential.

Two types of imaging technique will be discussed here: positron emission tomography (PET), and functional magnetic resonance imaging (fMRI).[165] The basis of PET is the decay of radioactive tracers which have been introduced into the body and emit positrons. These positrons undergo transformations that result in the release of photons which are detected by the scanning equipment. The radioactive tracer becomes perfused in the brain, and brain activity results in photon emissions, which are measured. There are two types of PET: one based on regional bloodflow, and one based on glucose metabolism. The bloodflow technique requires inhalation or injection of the radioactive tracer, which has a short half-life of about 2 min. Because the body clears the radioactive substance quickly, repeated tests are possible, but each test is obviously limited by time. The glucose metabolism technique uses fluoro-2-deoxy-D-glucose (FDG), which has a byproduct linked to glucose, which in turn perfuses the brain differentially. The maximum perfusion is where the metabolism is greatest. The time window for measurement is 30–40 min after tracer injection, and multiple scans should not be performed, because of risk to the patient.

The second imaging technique is fMRI. In fMRI, a strong magnetic field is used to align the body's protons, and a brief radio signal is then used to alter the tilt of the aligned protons. The energy released when the protons resume their original positions is measured. Since the blood acquires paramagnetic properties when the body is in a strong magnetic field, bloodflow can be visualized via MRI. Bloodflow is related to blood volume and oxygenation, which are increased when certain areas of the brain are active. Hence, the magnetic susceptibility of the blood changes with increased neural activity, and these changes are reflected in the MRI measurements.[165] With fMRI, no radioactivity is involved and the resolution is greater than that of PET. The noise present during fMRI testing is considerable, and this remains a factor in auditory studies.

There have been many contributions from imaging studies to auditory anatomy and physiology, but we will highlight only a few studies. As mentioned, one early PET study investigated the tonotopic arrangement of Heschl's gyrus.[113] This showed low frequencies (500 Hz) to be anterior and lateral, while the high frequencies (4000 Hz) were posteromedial. Similar tonotopic results have been reported recently for fMRI.[166]

An fMRI study[167] using speech (context, reading passages) and tonal stimuli showed primarily activation at the superior temporal gyrus, with more activity on the left side than on the right. Activity appeared to occur in the insula as well. The regions that were active along the superior temporal gyrus varied. Interestingly, different intensities of the stimuli seemed to have no effect on activation patterns. In an fMRI study on word presentation rates, greater activation was seen on the left side than on the right, with activity increasing from 10 to 90 words/min, and a drop in activity at 130 words/min. The superior temporal gyrus areas, including Heschl's gyrus, planum temporale and a small area immediately anterior to Heschl's gyrus, were activated at high rates of word presentation. The posterior insula also became involved at high rates.[168] In a PET study using words from a song for which pitch judgement of target words was required, the left cortex was more active than the right. Most activity was in the area of Heschl's gyrus, but activity often extended both posteriorly and anteriorly beyond Heschl's gyrus. In this study, the subjects were also asked to imagine performing the task. The auditory regions (though smaller and less intense) were activated for this type of task. This showed a way to activate the auditory cortex without external stimuli.[169]

Auditory cortex vascular anatomy

The middle cerebral artery (MCA) branches directly from the internal capsule at the base of the brain and is the main artery supplying blood to the auditory cortex.[69] The length of the MCA varies. It can be only 2 cm long prior to its diffuse branching,[157] or it can extend the full length of the Sylvian fissure before becoming the angular artery and coursing posteriorly and laterally on the brain surface. Its route fluctuates greatly between species, but it courses primarily in an anterior-to-posterior direction within the Sylvian fissure.[69]

Starting with an anterior view of the MCA, the fronto-opercular artery is the first major branch supplying an auditory region. This artery follows a superior route, supplying the anterior section of the insula. Just posterior to the fronto-opercular artery is the central sulcus artery which supplies the posterior insula and the anterior parietal lobe. Three arteries ascend from the MCA and course over the middle and posterior part of the temporal lobe.[69] These three are the anterior, middle and posterior arteries and they supply the middle and superior temporal gyri. A combination of the MCA and angular artery presumably supplies the primary auditory area, along with the angular gyrus and a portion of the supramarginal gyrus. The posterior parietal artery supplies the remainder of the supramarginal gyrus.

Significant tissue damage to gray and white matter in the temporparietal regions of the brain may be caused by vascular insults involving the MCA. These lesions are devastating to both the morphology and function of the auditory cortex, and are among the most common anomalies affecting this region.

The efferent auditory system

The efferent auditory system probably functions as one unit, but the pathways are often viewed in two sections. The caudal-most part of the system, the olivocochlear bundle (OCB), has been studied, but little is known about the more rostral system. The rostral efferent pathway starts at the auditory cortex and descends to the medial geniculate and the midbrain regions, including the IC. A loop system appears to exist between the cortex and these structures, and fibers descend from the cortex to neurones in the brainstem. The IC also receives efferents from the medial geniculate.[48] The descending connections from the IC to nuclei in the SOC have not been well established. Sahley et al[170] reviewed these connections and stated that connections exist from the IC to the ipsilateral trapezoid body nuclei and preolivary nuclei. There also appear to be widespread bilateral connections from the IC to different areas of the SOC. Some areas of the descending pathway have not been well studied, but a system is known to exist which allows neural communication from the cortex to the cochlea. In this regard, it is known that electrical stimulation of the cortex results in the excitation or inhibition of single units in the lower auditory system.[171] Physiological evidence exists for a descending train of impulses which eventually reaches the cochlea from the cortex.[172]

The OCB is the best-known circuitry of the efferent system. The OCB has two main tracts: the lateral and the medial.[170,173] The lateral tract originates from preolivary cells near the lateral superior olive and is composed mostly of uncrossed, unmyelinated fibers which terminate on the (ipsilateral) dendrites beneath the inner hair cells. These preolivary cells also send projections ipsilaterally to the cochlear nuclei by way of the ventral and dorsal acoustical stria. The medial tract of the OCB is composed of myelinated fibers which originate in preolivary nuclei in the area around the medial superior olive. Most fibers cross to the opposite cochlea, where they connect directly to the outer hair cells. There are also bilateral (mostly contralateral) connections to the CN via both the dorsal and ventral acoustical stria. The lateral and medial OCB fibers, after connecting to various divisions of the CN, course along the vestibular nerves in the internal auditory meatus before terminating at the type I auditory nerve fibers below the inner hair cells and the base of the outer hair cells (see Sahley et al[170] for review).[48,173]

Early physiological studies show that stimulation of the crossed (medial) OCB fibers results in reduced neural response from the cochlea and cochlear nerve.[174] Since then, the suppressive effect of the medial system has been shown in humans. In 1962, Fex[175] showed that acoustical stimulation of the contralateral ear will trigger medial OCB function. By stimulating the contralateral ear in humans, the action potential is reduced in amplitude, as is the amplitude of the transient and distortion product otoacoustic emissions.[176,177] It has also been shown that cutting the vestibular nerves in the internal auditory meatus results in absent suppression of otoacoustical emissions.[178]

Another important aspect related to function of the OCB is hearing in noise. Pickles and Comis[179] showed that the application of atropine (a cholinergic blocker) in the region of the OCB resulted in poorer hearing in noise in animals. Other studies have also shown that the OCB has an important role in hearing in noise.[180–182] The mechanism underlying this facilitation of hearing in noise may be related to the ability of the medial OCB to trigger outer hair cell expansion/contraction, thereby enhancing or damping basilar membrane activity. This, in turn, may limit to low levels cochlear nerve activity for unimportant (noise) stimuli, resulting in a larger dynamic range for the cochlear nerve neurone to respond to other acoustical stimuli (see Sahley et al[170] for review). It is also important to consider that the OCB may sometimes enhance responses, even though data indicate that many of its activities are related to suppression (see below). Evidence shows that when an animal is surrounded by noise and the OCB is triggered (by electrical stimulation or by contralateral noise presented to the ear), a release of the cochlear nerve from noise is accomplished, allowing better overall hearing in noise.

Auditory neurochemistry

Neurochemistry is reviewed as part of the discussion of auditory neuroanatomy and physiology because many known neurotransmitters are associated with the central auditory system. Neurotransmitters are neurochemical agents which convey information across the synapse between nerve cells. The type of synapse and particular neurotransmitters involved may influence many characteristics of auditory function and processing. Research on auditory neurotransmitters frequently has profound clinical implications.

The anatomy of neurotransmission

The synapse is the connecting link between nerve cells, and the main structure in neurotransmission. It involves the synaptic button of the axon, which communicates neurochemically with the dendrites, or in some cases the cell body, of another nerve cell. The neurotransmitters are released by vesicles and permeate the synaptic region to bind to proteins, called receptors, embedded in the adjacent cell membrane. Various events can take place as a result of this transmitter binding. One such event is a change in ion concentrations across the cell membrane, which may induce an alteration in a postsynaptic cell receptor potential. A number of neurotransmitter interactions occurring in a restricted time period will cause the postsynaptic cell to depolarize and fire its own impulse or action potential. An excitatory neurotransmitter is associated with this response.[183]

Hyperpolarization of the postsynaptic cell membrane is caused by inhibitory neurotransmitters making the cells less likely to fire an impulse or more difficult to excite.[183] The synapse can also be influenced by other biochemical actions of the cell, but these will not be discussed.

> Numerous therapeutic drugs are used to influence synaptic activity. Agonists can bind to and activate postsynaptic receptors, mimicking natural neurotransmitters. Antagonists can produce the opposite effect by binding to but not activating the receptor, thus blocking the natural neurotransmitter function.

Afferent auditory neurotransmission

If synaptic activity can be controlled by neurotransmitters, it may be feasible to control the functions that are based on these synaptic interactions. To accomplish this, neurotransmitters must first be localized and identified, keeping in mind that before a chemical can be considered as a neurotransmitter it must meet strict criteria.[183] New information on function and dysfunction of a system may be obtained through the use of agonists and antagonists, once these neurotransmitters have been identified.

It is not known which neurotransmitter operates between the cochlear hair cells and cochlear nerve fibers, but one possibility is glutamate.[184] Glutamate or aspartate is believed to be involved in cochlear nerve-to-CN transmission.[184,185] Within the CN, it is likely that several excitatory neurotransmitters exist, such as aspartate, glutamate and acetylcholine (ACh).[186–188] Inhibitory amino acids found at high levels within the CN are gamma-amino-butyric acid (GABA) and glycine.[189] Gamma-amino-butyric acid and glycine are also both found in the SOC.[190,191] Also located in the SOC are excitatory amino acids, including quisqualate, glutamate and *N*-methyl-D-aspartate (NMDA).[192] Glycine and glutamate are likely neurotransmitters in the IC.[193] Increased activity at the IC level has been shown with both NMDA and aspartate.[194]

Little information exists on auditory cortex transmitters. Evidence shows that ACh and opiate drugs affect auditory cortex activity or evoked potentials, but further research is needed before the neurochemistry of this brain region is understood fully.[195,196]

Efferent auditory neurotransmission

More data are available on efferent neurotransmitters than on afferent neurotransmitters. Neurotransmission within the OCB, for example, has been studied extensively. Both medial and lateral systems are cholinergic, and the lateral system also contains the opioid peptides enkephalin and dynorphin.[197,198] These efferent neurotransmitters can be found in the perilymph of the cochlea. The results of electrical stimulation on the OCB can be mimicked by applying ACh to this region.[199]

Auditory function and neurotransmitters

Several studies have examined neurotransmitter effects on auditory function which are measured electrophysiologically or behaviorally. Cousillas et al[200] found that cochlear nerve activity during sound stimulation was diminished when glutamatergic blockers were perfused through guinea pig cochleas. The application of aspartate, an excitatory amino acid, was also found to increase the spontaneous and acoustically stimulated firing rates of CN fibers. This effect was reversed when an antagonist drug was administered. Homogeneous neural modulating outcomes were shown in a similar study using antagonists and agonists such as glutamate, aspartate and NMDA at the IC level.[194]

The late auditory evoked potential (P2) also showed an increased amplitude after administration of naloxone, an opioid antagonist, in humans. Fentanyl, an opioid agonist, was also found to reduce the P2 amplitude in the same study.[195]

Auditory function of the OCB and neurotransmission have also been studied. The OCB plays a role in enhancing hearing in noise.[179,201] The chemical interaction of the OCB and the hair cells of the cochlea may mediate this role. The fact that outer hair cells can expand and contract might indicate a link to the OCB, since neurotransmitters may control this hair cell function. Regulation of this motor activity may in turn allow the OCB modulation of incoming impulses via the outer hair cells.

In studies on chinchillas, the cochlear nerve action potential was enhanced significantly by injecting the opioid agonist pentazocine.[170,202] Because opioids are found in the (lateral) OCB system, this effect, only noted at intensity levels near threshold, assuredly involves the OCB system.

Summary and conclusions

Knowledge of the structure and function of the CANS is vital to the audiologist. Audiological procedures and related communication increasingly involve the CANS, and without an understanding of the way in which this system works, potential clinical insights will not be realized. The CANS is a complex system in which parallel and sequential processing take place. In the brainstem, there are ipsilateral, contralateral and commissural connections to various auditory nuclei. Auditory neurones in the brainstem are composed of a variety of different cell types, which respond in certain ways (often according to their structure) to alter or preserve the impulse pattern coming into the cell. This same type of processing takes place in the cells of the auditory cortex, but there are fewer cell types in the cortex than in the brainstem. This type of processing may provide a basis for increased information pertaining to complex acoustical stimuli. The brainstem and the cortex are both highly tonotopic and present with a variety of tuning curves. In regard to intensity coding, the majority of cells in the brainstem and cortex have a range of 30–40 dB; however, some have severely reduced dynamic ranges. It is of interest that in a listening situation with background noise some cortical neurones will not respond until the target sound is above the noise floor, with apparently no restriction in their dynamic range.

In the cerebrum, the auditory regions have intrahemispheric and interhemispheric connections to other auditory areas and to sensory, cognitive and motor regions. At the cortical level, seldom does a system function totally independently. This makes for efficient processing of environmental input, but also makes it difficult to design tests to isolate only auditory function. Much scientific study has been devoted to the afferent auditory system, and information on the efferent system is increasingly available. We have known for years that the efferent system – especially the OCB – can affect acoustical input. The OCB appears to play a role in allowing better hearing in noise. In a broader sense, the OCB (and probably the entire efferent system) may have a modulatory effect on peripheral function. Some influences of the OCB can be measured in humans by using otoacoustical emissions and/or evoked potentials.

Contributions to the anatomy and physiology of the CANS have been, and will continue to be, made by careful study of patients with lesions of the auditory system. This kind of study often involves the clinician and clinical tests. The study of patients with structural abnormalities of the auditory system can now be enhanced by the use of PET or fMRI studies. These imaging techniques can provide insight about the locus and degree of function in normal and abnormal states. The use of functional imaging techniques will help solve two major problems in the study of the CANS. One is that now humans can be studied directly, the other is more complex and relevant stimuli such as speech can be used to study associated physiology.

A new area of study of the CANS is its neurochemistry or neuropharmacology. Surprisingly, the neurotransmitters of the OCB are better known than those of the afferent system. Neurotransmission takes place at the synapse of the nerve cell, and synaptic activity is governed largely by the type and amount of the neurotransmitter. Agonists are chemicals that can enhance the neural response and the synapse, while antagonists will shut down the response. Complex synaptic interactions among agonists and antagonists are the basis for complex auditory processing.

New information on the CANS is increasing on all fronts. More data on audition are available from audiologists, pharmacologists, physiologists, anatomists and psychologists. The basic scientists have provided much knowledge that will enhance the diagnosis and treatment of central auditory disorders. However, this basic knowledge can be used to its greatest potential only if the clinician is well versed in the structure and function of the CANS.

References

1. Schuknecht HT. *Pathology of the Ear*. Cambridge: Harvard University Press, 1974.
2. Pfeiffer RR. Classification of response patterns of spike discharges for units in the cochlear nucleus. Tone burst stimulation. *Exp Brain Res* 1966; **1**: 220–35.
3. Osen KK. Cytoarchitecture of the cochlear nuclei in the cat. *J Comp Neurol* 1969; **136**: 453–84.
4. Rouiller EM. Functional organization of the auditory pathways. In: Ehret G, Romand R, eds. *The Central Auditory System*. New York: Oxford University Press, 1997: 3–96.
5. Rhode W. The use of intracellular techniques in the study of the cochlear nucleus. *J Acoust Soc Am* 1985; **78**: 320–7.
6. Kiang NYS. Stimulus representation in the discharge patterns of auditory neurons. In: Tower DB, ed. *The Nervous System*. Vol. 3. *Human Communication and its Disorders*. New York: Raven Press, 1975: 81–96.
7. Rhode W. Physiological–morphological properties of the cochlear nucleus. In: Altschuler R, Bobbin R, Clopton B, Hoffman D, eds. *Neurobiology of Hearing: The Central Auditory System*. New York: Raven Press, 1991: 47–78.
8. Sando I. The anatomical interrelationships of the cochlear nerve fibers. *Acta Otolaryngol* 1965; **59**: 417–36.
9. Webster DB. Projection of the cochlea to cochlear nuclei in Merriam's kangaroo rat. *J Comp Neurol* 1971; **143**: 323–340.
10. Rose JE, Galambos R, Hughes JR. Microelectrode studies of the cochlear nuclei of the cat. *Johns Hopkins Hosp Bull* 1959; **104**: 211–51.
11. Moller AR. Physiology of the ascending auditory pathway with special reference to the auditory brain stem response (ABR). In: Pinheiro ML, Musiek FE, eds. *Assessment of Central Auditory Dysfunction: Foundations and Clinical Correlates*. Baltimore: Williams and Wilkins, 1985: 23–41.
12. Whitfield IC. *The Auditory Pathway*. Baltimore: Williams and Wilkins, 1967.
13. Masterton RB, Granger EM. Role of acoustic striae in hearing contribution of dorsal and intermediate striae to detection of noises and tones. *J Neurophysiol* 1988; **60**: 1841–60.
14. Noback CR. Neuroanatomical correlates of central auditory function. In: Pinheiro ML, Musiek FE, eds. *Assessment of Central Auditory Dysfunction: Foundations and Clinical Correlates*. Baltimore: Williams and Wilkins, 1985: 7–21.
15. Jerger J, Jerger S. Auditory findings in brain stem disorders. *Arch Otolaryngol* 1974; **99**: 342–50.
16. Matkin N, Carhart R. Auditory profiles associated with Rh incompatibility. *Arch Otolaryngol* 1966; **84**: 502–13.
17. Dublin W. *Fundamentals of Sensorineural Auditory Pathology*. Springfield: Charles C. Thomas, 1976.
18. Dublin W. The cochlear nuclei—pathology. *Otolaryngol Head Neck Surg* 1985; **93**: 448–63.
19. Nodar R, Kinney S. The contralateral effects of large tumors on brain stem auditory evoked potentials. *Laryngoscope* 1980; **90**: 1762–8.
20. Musiek FE, Kibbe-Michael K. The ABR wave IV–V abnormalities from the ear opposite large CPA tumors. *Am J Otol* 1986; **7**: 253–7.
21. Musiek FE, Gollegly KM. ABR in eighth nerve and low brain stem lesions. In: Jacobson JT, ed. *The Auditory Brain Stem Response*. San Diego: College-Hill Press, 1985: 181–202.
22. Musiek FE, Kibbe-Michael K, Geurkink N, Josey A, Glasscock M. ABR results in patients with posterior fossa tumors and normal pure tone hearing. *Otolaryngol Head Neck Surg* 1986; **94**: 568–73.
23. Brugge IF, Geisler CE. Auditory mechanisms of the lower brain stem. *Am Rev Neurosci* 1978; **1**: 363–94.
24. Moore JK. The human auditory brainstem: a comparative view. *Hear Res* 1987; **29**: 1–32.
25. Tsuchitani C, Boudreau JC. Single unit analysis of cat superior olive S–segment with tonal stimuli. *J Neurophysiol* 1966; **29**: 684–97.
26. Keidel W, Kallert S, Korth M, Humes L. *The Physiological Basis of Hearing*. New York: Thieme-Stratton, 1983.
27. Strominger NL, Hurwitz JL. Anatomical aspects of the superior olivary complex. *J Comp Neurol* 1976; **170**: 485–97.

28. Warr WB. Fiber degeneration following lesions in the anterior ventral cochlear nucleus of the cat. *Exp Neurol* 1966; **14**: 453–74.
29. Strominger NL, Strominger AL. Ascending brain stem projections of the anteroventral cochlear nucleus in the rhesus monkey. *J Comp Neurol* 1971; **143**: 217–32.
30. Masterson B, Thompson GC, Bechtold JK, Robards MJ. Neuroanatomical basis of binaural phase difference analysis for sound localization: a comparative study. *J Comp Physiol Psychol 1975*; **89**: 379–86.
31. Boudreau JC, Tsuchitani C. Cat superior olive S–segment cell discharge to tonal stimulation. In: Neff WD, ed. *Contributions to Sensory Physiology* Vol. 4. New York: Academic Press, 1970: 143–213.
32. Tsuchitani C, Johnson DH. Binaural cues and signal processing in the superior olivary complex. In: Altschuler RA, Bobbin, RP, Clopton BM, Hoffman DW, eds. *Neurobiology of Hearing: The Central Auditory System*. New York: Raven Press, 1991: 163–93.
33. Tobin H. Binaural interaction tasks. In: Pinheiro ML, Musiek FE, eds. *Assessment of Central Auditory Dysfunction: Foundations and Clinical Correlates*. Baltimore: Williams and Wilkins, 1985: 151–71.
34. Matzker J. Two new methods for the assessment of central auditory functions in cases of brain disease. *Am Otol Rhinol Laryngol* 1959; **68**: 1188–97.
35. Lynn G, Gilroy J, Taylor P, Leiser R. Binaural masking level differences in neurological disorders. *Arch Otolaryngol* 1981; **107**: 357–62.
36. Cullen J, Thompson C. Masking release for speech in subjects with temporal lobe resections. *Arch Otolaryngol* 1974; **100**: 113–16.
37. Borg E. On the organization of the acoustic middle ear reflex. A physiologic and anatomic study. *Brain Res* 1973; **49**: 101–23.
38. Musiek FE, Baran JA. Neuroanatomy, neurophysiology, and central auditory assessment. Part 1: Brain stem. *Ear Hear* 1986; **7**: 207–19.
39. Hall JW III. The acoustic reflex in central auditory dysfunction. In: Pinheiro ML, Musiek FE, eds. *Assessment of Central Auditory Dysfunction: Foundations and Clinical Correlates*. Baltimore: Williams and Wilkins, 1985: 103–30.
40. Goldberg JM, Moore RY. Ascending projections of the lateral lemniscus in the cat and the monkey. *J Comp Neurol* 1967; **129**: 143–55.
41. Ferraro J, Minckler J. The human lateral lemniscus and its nuclei. The human auditory pathways. A quantitative study. *Brain Language* 1977; **4**: 277–94.
42. Jungert S. Auditory pathways in the brain stem. A neurophysiologic study. *Acta Otolaryngol* (Suppl) 1958; **138**.
43. Kudo M. Projections of the nuclei of the lateral lemniscus in the cat. An autoradiographic study. *Brain Res* 1981; **221**: 57–69.
44. Merchan M, Saldana E, Plaza I. Dorsal nucleus of the lateral lemniscus in the rat. Concentric organization and tonotopic projection to the inferior colliculus. *J Comp Neurol* 1994; **342**: 259–78.
45. Oliver DL, Morest DK. The central nucleus of the inferior colliculus in the cat. *J Comp Neurol* 1984; **222**: 237–64.
46. Barnes W, Magoon H, Ranson S. The ascending auditory pathway in the brain stem of the monkey. *J Comp Neurol* 1943; **79**: 129–52.
47. Van Noort J. *The Structure and Connections of the Inferior Colliculus: An Investigation of the Lower Auditory System*. Leiden: Van Corcum, 1969.
48. Pickles JO. *An Introduction to the Physiology of Hearing*. 2nd ed. New York: Academic Press, 1988.
49. Oliver D, Huerta M. Inferior and superior colliculi. In: Webster D, Popper A, Fay R, eds. *The Mammalian Auditory Pathway: Neuroanatomy*. New York: Springer-Verlag, 1992: 168–221.
50. Merzenich MM, Reid MD. Representation of the cochlea within the inferior colliculus of the cat. *Brain Res* 1974; **77**: 397–415.
51. Aitken LM, Webster WR, Veale JL, Crosby DC. Inferior colliculus, I. Comparison of response properties of neurons in central, pericentral, and external nuclei of adult cat. *J Neurophysiol 1975*; **38**: 1196–207.
52. Knudson EI, Konishi M. Space and frequency are represented separately in auditory midbrain of the owl. *Neurophysiology* 1978; **41**: 870–84.
53. Pickles JO. *An Introduction to the Physiology of Hearing*. New York: Academic Press, 1982.
54. Benerento L, Coleman P. Responses of single cells in cat inferior colliculus to binaural click stimuli: combinations of intensity levels, time differences, and intensity differences. *Brain Res 1970*; **17**: 387–405.
55. Oliver DL, Shneiderman A. The anatomy of the inferior colliculus: a cellular basis for integration of monaural and binaural information. In: Altschuler RA, Bobbin RP, Clopton BM, Hoffman DW, eds. *Neurobiology of Hearing: The Central Auditory System*. New York: Raven Press, 1991: 195–222.
56. Moore DR, Irvine DRF. Development of binaural input, response patterns and discharge rate in single units of the cat inferior colliculus. *Exp Brain Res* 1980; **38**: 103–8.
57. Ehret G, Merzenich MM. Complex sound analysis (frequency resolution, filtering and spectral integration) by single units of the inferior colliculus of the cat. *Brain Res Revs* 1988; **13**: 139–63.
58. Morest DK. The neuronal architecture of medial geniculate body of the cat. *J Anat* 1964; **98**: 611–30.
59. Winer JA. The human medial geniculate body. *Hear Res* 1984; **15**: 225–47.
60. Winer JA. The medial geniculate body of the cat. *Adv Anat Embryol Cell Biol* 1985; **86**: 1–98.
61. Aitkin LM, Webster WR. Medial geniculate body of the cat: organization and response to tonal stimuli of neurons in the ventral division. *J Neurophysiol* 1972; **35**: 365–80.
62. Sheperd G. *Neurobiology*. New York: Oxford Press, 1994: 284–555.
63. French J. The reticular formation. *Sci Am* 1957; **66**: 1–8.
64. Carpenter M, Sutin J. *Human Neuroanatomy*. Baltimore: Williams and Wilkins, 1983.
65. Colclasure J, Graham S. Intracranial aneurysm occurring as a sensorineural hearing loss. *Otolaryngol Head Neck Surg* 1981; **89**: 283–7.
66. Moller M, Moller AR. Auditory brain stem evoked responses (ABR) in diagnosis of eighth nerve and brain stem lesions. In: Pinheiro ML, Musiek FE, eds. *Assessment of Central Auditory Dys-*

function: Foundations and Clinical Correlates. Baltimore: Williams and Wilkins, 1985: 43–65.
67. Waddington M. *Atlas of Human Intracranial Anatomy*. Rutland, Vt: Academy Books, 1984: 79–95.
68. Portman M, Sterkers J, Charachon R, Chouard C. *The Internal Auditory Meatus: Anatomy, Pathology, and Surgery*. New York: Churchill Livingstone, 1975.
69. Waddington M. *Atlas of Cerebral Angiography With Anatomic Correlation*. Boston: Little, Brown and Company, 1974.
70. Moller AR. *Auditory Physiology*. New York: Academic Press, 1983.
71. Phillips D. Neural representation of sound amplitude in the auditory cortex: effects of noise masking. *Behav Brain Res* 1990; **37**: 197–214.
72. Jerger J, Jerger S. Diagnostic significance of PB word functions. *Arch Otolaryngol* 1971; **93**: 573–80.
73. Jeffress L, McFadden D. Differences of interaural phase and level of detection and lateralization. *J Acoust Soc Am* 1971; **49**: 1169–79.
74. Tasaki I. Nerve impulses in individual auditory nerve fibers of the guinea pig. *J Neurophysiol* 1954; **17**: 97–122.
75. Phillips D. Central auditory processing: a view from auditory neuroscience. *Am J Otol* 1995; **16**: 338–50.
76. Moller A. *Hearing: its Physiology and Pathophysiology*. San Diego: Academic Press, 2000: 265–342.
77. Levine RA, Gardner JC, Stufflebeam SM et al. Binaural auditory processing in multiple sclerosis subjects. *Hear Res* 1993; **68**: 59–72.
78. Musiek FE, Baran JA, Pinheiro M. *Neuroaudiology: Case Studies*. San Diego: Singular Publishing Group, Inc., 1994.
79. Durrant J, Martin W, Hirsch B, Schwegler J. ABR analysis in a human subject with unilateral extirpation of the inferior colliculus. *Hearing Res* 1994; **72**: 99–107.
80. Oh S, Kuba T, Soyer A, Choi I, Bonikowski F, Viter J. Lateralization of brain stem lesions by brain stem auditory evoked potentials. *Neurology* 1981; **31**: 14–18.
81. Musiek FE, Geurkink N. Auditory brain stem response and central auditory test findings for patients with brain stem lesions. *Laryngoscope* 1982; **92**: 891–900.
82. Chiappa K. *Evoked Potentials in Clinical Medicine*. New York: Raven Press, 1983.
83. Phillips D, Irvine D. Responses of single neurons in physiologically defined area AI of cat cerebral cortex: sensitivity to interaural intensity differences. *Hear Res* 1981; **4**(9): 299–307.
84. Musiek FE. Neuroanatomy, neurophysiology and central auditory assessment. Part II: The cerebrum. *Ear Hear* 1986; **7**: 283–94.
85. Campain R, Minckler J. A note in gross configurations of the human auditory cortex. *Brain Language* 1976; **3**: 318–23.
86. Musiek FE, Reeves AG. Asymmetries of the auditory areas of the cerebrum. *J Am Acad Audiol* 1990; **1**: 240–5.
87. Geschwind N, Levitsky W. Human brain: left–right asymmetries in temporal speech region. *Science* 1968; **161**: 186–7.
88. Rubens A. Anatomical asymmetries of the human cerebral cortex. In: Harnad S, Doty R, Goldstein L, eds. *Lateralization in the Nervous System*. New York: Academic Press, 1976.
89. Celesia G. Organization of auditory cortical areas in man. *Brain* 1976; **99**: 403–14.
90. Galaburda A, Sanides F. Cytoarchitectonic organization of the human auditory cortex. *J Comp Neurol* 1980; **190**: 597–610.
91. Sudakov K, MacLean P, Reeves A, Marino R. Unit study of exteroceptive inputs to the claustrocortex in the awake sitting squirrel monkey. *Brain Res* 1971; **28**: 19–34.
92. Galaburda A, Sherman G, Rosen G, Aboitiz F, Geschwind N. Developmental dyslexia: four consecutive patients with cortical anomalies. *Ann Neurol* 1985; **18**: 222–35.
93. Kaufman W, Galaburda A. Cerebrocortical microdysgenesias in neurologically normal subjects: a histopathological study. *Neurology 1989*; **39**: 238–43.
94. LeDoux J, Sakaguchi A, Reis D. Subcortical efferent projections of the medial geniculate nucleus mediate emotional responses conditioned to acoustic stimuli. *J Neurosci* 1983; **4**: 683–98.
95. Streitfeld B. The fiber connections of the temporal lobe with emphasis on the Rhesus monkey. *Int J Neurosci* 1980; **11**: 51–71.
96. Seltzer B, Pandya D. Afferent cortical connections and architectonics of the superior temporal sulcus and surrounding cortex in Rhesus monkey. *Brain Res* 1978; **149**: 1–24.
97. Jones E, Powell T. An anatomical study of converging sensory pathways within the cerebral cortex of the monkey. *Brain* 1970; **93**: 793–820.
98. Selnes OA. The corpus callosum: some anatomical and functional considerations with special reference to language. *Brain Language* 1974; **1**: 111–39.
99. Musiek FE. Neuroanatomy, neurophysiology, and central auditory assessment: Part III: Corpus callosum and efferent pathways. *Ear Hear* 1986; **7**(6):349–58.
100. Witelson S. Wires of the mind: Anatomical variation in the corpus callosum in relation to hemispheric specialization and integration. In: Lepore F, Ptito M, Jasper H, eds. *Two Hemispheres—One Brain: Functions of the Corpus Callosum*. New York: Alan R. Liss, Inc., 1986: 117–38.
101. Mountcastle V. *Interhemispheric Relations and Cerebral Dominance*. Baltimore: Johns Hopkins Press, 1962.
102. Gazzaniga M, Sperry R. Some functional effects of sectioning the cerebral commissure in man. *Proc Natl Acad Sci USA* 1962; **48**: 1765–9.
103. Yakovlev P, LeCours A. Myelogenetic cycles of regional maturation of the brain. In: Minkowski A, ed. *Regional Development of the Brain in Early Life*. Philadelphia: FA Davis, 1967: 3–70.
104. Chang HT. Cortical response to activity of callosal neurons. *J Neurophysiol* 1953; **16**: 117–31.
105. Bremer F, Brihaye J, Andre-Balisaux G. Physiologie et pathologie du corps calleux. *Arch Suisses Neurol Psychiat* 1956; **78**: 31–2.
106. Salamy A. Commissural transmission: maturational changes in humans. *Science* 1978; **200**: 1409–10.
107. Pandya D, Seltzer B. The topography of commissural fibers. In: Lepore F, Pitito M, Jasper H, eds. *Two Hemispheres—One Brain: Functions of the Corpus Callosum*. New York: Alan R. Liss, Inc., 1986: 47–74.
108. Baran JA, Musiek FE, Reeves AG. Central auditory function following anterior sectioning of the corpus callosum. *Ear Hear* 1986; **7**(6): 359–62.

109. Musiek FE, Kibbe K, Baran J. Neuroaudiological results from split-brain patients. *Semin Hear* 1984; **5**(3): 219–29.
110. Damasio H, Damasio A. Paradoxic ear extension in dichotic listening: Possible anatomic significance. *Neurology* 1979; **25**(4): 644–53.
111. Hynd GW, Semrud-Clikeman M, Lorys AR, Novey ES, Eliopulos D, Lyytinen H. Corpus callosum morphology in attention deficit–hyperactivity disorder: morphometric analysis of MRI. *J Learn Dis* 1991; **24**: 141–6.
112. Merzenich M, Brugge J. Representation of the cochlear partition on the superior emporal plane of the Macaque monkey. *Brain Res* 1973; **50**: 275–96.
113. Lauter J, Herscovitch P, Formby C, Raichle M. Tonotopic organization of human auditory cortex revealed by positron emission tomography. *Hear Res* 1985; **20**: 199–205.
114. Woolsey C. Organization of cortical auditory system: a review and synthesis. In: Rasmussen G, Windell W, eds. *Neuromechanics of the Auditory and Visibility Systems*. Springfield, IL: Charles C. Thomas, 1960: 165–80.
115. Pickles JO. Physiology of the cerebral auditory system. In: Pinheiro M, Musiek F, eds. *Assessment of Central Auditory Dysfunction: Foundations and Clinical Correlates*. Baltimore: Williams and Wilkins, 1985: 67–85.
116. Mountcastle V. Central neural mechanisms in hearing. In: Mountcastle V, ed. *Medical Physiology* Vol 2. St. Louis: CV Mosby Co., 1968: 1296–355.
117. Schwaber M, Garraghty P, Morel A, Kaas J. Neuroplasticity of the adult primate auditory cortex following cochlear hearing loss. *Am J Otol 1994;* **14**(3): 252–8.
118. Pfingst B, O'Conner T. Characteristics of neurons in auditory cortex of monkeys performing a simple auditory task. *J Neurophysiol* 1981; **45**: 16–34.
119. Abeles M, Goldstein M. Responses of a single unit in the primary auditory cortex of the cat to tones and to tone pairs. *Brain Res* 1972; **42**: 337–52.
120. Goldstein M, DeRibaupierre R, Yeni-Komshian G. Cortical coding of periodicity pitch. In: Sachs M, ed. *Physiology of the Auditory System*. Baltimore: National Education Consultants Inc., 1971: 299–306.
121. Eggermont J. Rate and synchronization measures of periodicity coding in cat primary cortex area. *Hear Res* 1991; **56**: 153–67.
122. Lackner JR, Teuber HL. Alterations in auditory fusion thresholds after cerebral injury in man. *Neuropsychologia* 1973; **11**: 409–415.
123. Benson D, Teas D. Single unit study of binaural interaction in the auditory cortex of the chinchilla. *Brain Res* 1976; **103**: 313–338.
124. Evans E. Cortical representation. In: de Reuck A, Knight J, eds. *Hearing Mechanisms in Vertebrates*. London: Churchill Livingstone, 1968: 277–87.
125. Eisenmann L. Neurocoding of sound localization: An electrophysiological study in auditory cortex of the cat using free field stimuli. *Brain Res* 1974; **75**: 203–14.
126. Sanchez-Longo L, Forster F. Clinical significance of impairment of sound localization. *Neurology* 1958; **8**: 118–25.
127. Moore C, Cranford J, Rahn A. Tracking for a 'moving' fused auditory image under conditions that elicit the precedence effect. *J Speech Hear Res* 1990; **33**: 141–8.
128. Pinheiro M, Tobin H. Interaural intensity differences for intracranial lateralization. *J Acoust Soc Am* 1969; **40**: 1482–7.
129. Liden G, Rosenthal V. New developments in diagnostic auditory neurological problems. In: Paparella M, Meyerhoff W, eds. *Sensorineural Hearing Loss, Vertigo and Tinnitus*. Baltimore: Williams and Wilkins, 1981: 273–94.
130. Penfield W, Rasmussen T. *The Cerebral Cortex of Man*. New York: Macmillan and Company, 1950.
131. Penfield W, Roberts L. *Speech and Brain Mechanisms*. Princeton, NJ: Princeton University Press, 1959.
132. Penfield W, Perot P. The brain's record of auditory and visual experience: a final summary and discussion. *Brain 1963;* **86**: 596–695.
133. Donchin E, Kutas M, McCarthy G. Electrocortical indices of hemispheric utilization. In: Harnad S et al, eds. *Lateralization in the Nervous System*. New York: Academic Press, 1976: 339–84.
134. Butler R, Keidel W, Spreng M. An investigation of the human cortical evoked potential under conditions of monaural and binaural stimulation. *Acta Otolaryngol* 1969; **68**: 317–26.
135. Kryter K, Ades H. Studies on the function of the higher acoustic centers in the cat. *Am J Psychol* 1943; **56**: 501–36.
136. Hodgson W. Audiological report of a patient with left hemispherectomy. *J Speech Hear Dis* 1967; **32**: 39–45.
137. Berlin C, Lowe-Bell S, Janetta P, Kline D. Central auditory deficits after temporal lobectomy. *Arch Otolaryngol* 1972; **96**: 4–10.
138. Heffner H, Heffner R. Hearing loss in Japanese Macaques following bilateral auditory cortex lesions. *J Neurophysiol* 1986; **55**: 256–71.
139. Heffner H, Heffner R. Hearing loss in Japanese Macques following bilateral auditory cortex lesions. *J Neurophysiol* 1986; **55**: 256–71.
140. Jerger J, Weikers N, Sharbrough F, Jerger S. Bilateral lesions of the temporal lobe. A case study. *Acta Otolaryngol* 1969; **258**: 1–51.
141. Auerbach S, Allard T, Naeser M, Alexander M, Albert M. Pure word deafness. Analysis of a case with bilateral lesions and a defect at the prephonemic level. *Brain 1982;* **105**: 271–300.
142. Yaqub B, Gascon G, Al-Nosha M, Whitaker H. Pure word deafness (acquired verbal auditory agnosia) in an Arabic-speaking patient. *Brain* 1988; **111**: 457–66.
143. Ravizza R, Masterton R. Contribution of neocortex to sound localization in opossum (*Didelphis virginiana*). *J Neurophysiol* 1972; **35**: 344–56.
144. Kavanagh G, Kelly J. Hearing in the ferret (*Mustela putorius*): effects of primary auditory cortical lesions on thresholds for pure tone detection. *J Neurophysiol* 1988; **60**: 879–88.
145. Allen W. Effect of destroying three localized cerebral cortical areas for sound on correct conditioned differential responses of the dog's foreleg. *Am J Physiol* 1945; **144**: 415–28.
146. Meyer D, Woolsey C. Effects of localized cortical destruction on auditory discriminative conditioning in the cat. *J Neurophysiol* 1952; **15**: 149–62.

147. Cranford J, Igarashi M, Stramler J. Effect of auditory neocortical ablation on pitch perception in the cat. *J Neurophysiol* 1976; **39**: 143–52.
148. Thompson ME, Abel SM. Indices of hearing in patients with central auditory pathology. *Scand Audiol* 1992; **21**(35): 3–22.
149. Diamond I, Neff W. Ablation of temporal cortex and discrimination of auditory patterns. *J Neurophysiol* 1957; **20**: 300–15.
150. Neff W. Neuromechanisms of auditory discrimination. In: Rosenblith W, ed. *Sensory Communication*. New York: John Wiley and Sons, 1961: 259–78.
151. Colavita F. Auditory cortical lesions and visual pattern discrimination in cats. *Brain Res* 1972; **39**: 437–47.
152. Colavita F. Insular–temporal lesions and vibrotactile temporal pattern discrimination in cats. *Psychol Behav* 1974; **12**: 215–18.
153. Musiek FE. Application of central auditory tests: an overview. In: Katz J, ed. *Handbook of Clinical Audiology*. Baltimore: Williams and Wilkins, 1985: 321–36.
154. Pinheiro M, Musiek FE. Sequencing and temporal ordering in the auditory system. In: Pinheiro M, Musiek, eds. *Assessment of Central Auditory Dysfunction: Foundations and Clinical Correlates*. Baltimore: Williams and Wilkins, 1985: 219–38.
155. Musiek FE, Pinheiro M. Frequency patterns in cochlear, brainstem, and cerebral lesions. *Audiology* 1987; **26**: 79–88.
156. Musiek FE, Baran JA, Pinheiro M. Duration pattern recognition in normal subjects and patients with cerebral and cochlear lesions. *Audiology* 1990; **29**: 304–13.
157. Gershuni J, Baru A, Karaseva T. Role of auditory cortex and discrimination of acoustic stimuli. *Neurol Sci Trans* 1967; **1**: 370–2.
158. Cranford J. Detection vs. discrimination of brief tones by cats with auditory cortex lesions. *J Acoust Soc Am* 1979; **65**: 1573–5.
159. Cranford J, Stream R, Rye C, Slade T. Detection vs. discrimination of brief duration tones: findings in patients with temporal lobe damage. *Arch Otolaryngol* 1982; **108**: 350–6.
160. Recanzone G, Schreiner C, Merzenich M. Plasticity in the frequency representation of primary auditory cortex following discrimination training in adult owl monkeys. *J Neurosci* 1993; **13**: 87–103.
161. Hassmannova J, Myslivecek J, Novakova V. Effects of early auditory stimulation on cortical centers. In: Syka J, Aitkin L, eds. *Neuronal Mechanisms of Hearing*. New York: Plenum Press, 1981: 355–9.
162. Knudsen E. Experience shapes sound localization and auditory unit properties during development in the barn owl. In: Edelman G, Gall W, Kowan W, eds. *Auditory Function: Neurobiological Basis of Hearing*. New York: John Wiley & Sons, 1988: 137–52.
163. Chermak GD, Musiek FE. *Central Auditory Processing Disorders*. San Diego: Singular Publishing Group, Inc., 1997.
164. Musiek FE, Berge B. Neuroaudiological aspects of auditory training/stimulation and CAPD. In: Katz J, ed. *Central Auditory Processing Disorders: Mostly Management*. Boston: Allyn and Bacon, 1998: 15–32.
165. Elliott LL. Functional brain imaging and hearing. *J Acoust Soc Am* 1994; **96**(3): 1397–408.
166. Talavage TM, Ledden PJ, Sereno MI, Benson RR, Rosen BR. Preliminary fMRI evidence for tonotopicity in human auditory cortex. Paper presented at the 2nd International Conference on Functional Mapping of The Human Brain, Boston, MA.
167. Millen SJ, Haughton VM, Yetkin Z. Functional magnetic resonance imaging of the central auditory pathway following speech and pure tone stimuli. *Laryngoscope* 1995; **105**: 1305–10.
168. Dhankhar A, Wexler BE, Fulbright RK, Halwes T, Blamire AM, Shulman RG. Functional magnetic resonance imaging assessment of the human brain auditory cortex response to increasing word presentation rates. *J Neurophysiol* 1997; **77**(1): 476–83.
169. Zatorre RJ, Halpern AR, Perry DW, Meyer E, Evans AC. Hearing in the mind's ear: a PET investigation of musical imagery and perception. *J Cognit Neurosci* 1996; **8**(1): 29–46.
170. Sahley TL, Nodar RH, Musiek FE. *Efferent Auditory System: Structure and Function*. San Diego: Singular Publishing Group, Inc., 1997.
171. Ryugo D, Weinberger N. Corticofugal modulation of the medial geniculate body. *Exp Neurol* 1976; **51**: 377–91.
172. Desmedt J. Physiological studies of the efferent recurrent auditory system. In: Keidel W, Neff W, eds. *Handbook of Sensory Physiology*. Vol. 2. Berlin: Springer-Verlag, 1975: 219–46.
173. Warr WB. Efferent components of the auditory system. *Ann Otol Rhinol Laryngol* 1980; **89**(suppl 74): 114–20.
174. Galambos R. Suppression of auditory nerve activity by stimulation of efferent fibers to cochlea. *J Neurophysiol* 1956; **19**: 424–37.
175. Fex J. Auditory activity in centrifugal and centripetal cochlear fibers in cat *Acta Physiol Scand* 1962; **189**(55): 5–68.
176. Folsom RL, Owsley RM. N_1 action potentials in humans. Influence of simultaneous contralateral stimulation. *Acta Otolaryngol* 1987; **103**: 262–5.
177. Collet L. Use of otoacoustic emissions to explore the medial olivocochlear system in humans. *Br J Audiol* 1993; **27**: 155–9.
178. Williams EA, Brookes GB, Prasher DK. Effects of contralateral acoustic stimulation on otoacoustic emissions following vestibular neurectomy. *Scand Audiol* 1993; **22**: 197–203.
179. Pickles JO, Comis SD. Role of centrifugal pathways to cochlear nucleus in detection of signals in noise. *J Neurophysiol* 1973; **29**: 1131–7.
180. Dewson J. Efferent olivocochlear bundle: some relationships to stimulus discrimination in noise. *J Neurophysiol* 1968; **31**: 122–30.
181. Nieder P, Nieder I. Antimasking effect of crossed olivocochlear bundle stimulation with loud clicks in guinea pigs. *Exp Neurol* 1970; **28**: 179–88.
182. Kawase T, Liberman MC. Antimasking effects of the olivocochlear reflex. I. Enhancement of compound action potentials to masked tones. *J Neurophysiol* 1993; **70**(6): 2519–32.
183. Musiek FE, Hoffman D. An introduction to the functional neurochemistry of the auditory system. *Ear Hear* 1990; **11**: 395–402.
184. Bledsoe S, Bobbin R, Puel J. Neurotransmission in the inner ear. In: Jahn A, Santo-Sacchi J, eds. *Physiology of the Ear*. New York: Raven Press, 1988: 385–406.
185. Guth P, Melamed B. Neurotransmission in the auditory system: a primer for pharmacologists. *Annu Rev Pharmacol Toxicol* 1982; **22**: 383–412.
186. Oliver DL, Potashner S, Jones D, Morest D. Selective labeling of

spiroganglion and granule cells with D-aspartate in the auditory system of the cat and guinea pig. *J Neurosci* 1983; **3**: 455–72.
187. Altschuler RA, Wenthold R, Schwartz A et al. Immunocytochemical localization of glutaminase-like immunoreactivity in the auditory nerve. *Brain Res* 1984; **29**: 173–8.
188. Godfrey D, Park J, Dunn J, Ross C. Cholinergic neurotransmission in the cochlear nucleus. In: Drecher D, ed. *Auditory Neurochemistry*. Springfield, IL: Charles C. Thomas, 1985: 163–83.
189. Godfrey D, Carter J, Berger S, Lowry D, Matschinsky F. Quantitative histochemical mapping of candidate transmitter amino acids in the cat cochlear nucleus. *J Histochem Cytochem* 1977; **25**: 417–31.
190. Helfert R, Altschuler R, Wenthold R. GABA and glycine immunoreactivity in the guinea pig superior olivary complex. *Neurosci Abstr* 1987; **13**: 544.
191. Wenthold R, Huie D, Altschuler R, Reeks K. Glycine immunoreactivity localized in the cochlear nucleus and superior olivary complex. *Neuroscience* 1987; **22**: 897–912.
192. Otterson O, Storm-Mathison J. Glutamate- and GABA-containing neurons in the mouse and rat brain, as demonstrated with a new immunocytochemical technique. *J Comp Neurol* 1984; **229**: 374–92.
193. Adams J, Wenthold R. Immunostaining of GABA-ergic and glycinergic inputs to the anteroventral cochlear nucleus. *Neurosci Abstr* 1987; **13**: 1259.
194. Faingold CL, Hoffmann WE, Caspary DM. Effects of excitant amino acids on acoustic responses of inferior colliculus neurons. *Hear Res* 1989; **40**: 127–36.
195. Velasco M, Velasco, F, Castaneda R, Sanchez R. Effect of fentanyl and naloxone on human somatic and auditory-evoked potential components. *Neuropharmacology* 1984; **23**(3): 359–66.
196. McKenna T, Ashe J, Hui G, Weinberger N. Muscarinic agonists modulate spontaneous and evoked unit discharge in auditory cortex of the cat. *Synapse* 1988; **2**: 54–68.
197. Altschuler RA, Fex J. Efferent neurotransmitters. In: Altschuler RA, Hoffman DW, Bobbin RP, eds. *Neurobiology of Hearing: The Cochlea*. New York: Raven Press, 1986: 383–96.
198. Hoffman DW. Opioid mechanisms in the inner ear. In: Altschuler RA, Hoffman DW, Bobbin RP, eds. *Neurobiology of Hearing: The Cochlea*. New York: Raven Press, 1986: 371–82.
199. Bobbin RP, Konishi T. Acetylcholine mimics crossed olivocochlear bundle stimulation. *Nature* 1971; **231**: 222–4.
200. Cousillas H, Cole KS, Johnstone BM. Effect of spider venom on cochlear nerve activity consistent with glutamatergic transmission at hair cell–afferent dendrite synapse. *Hear Res* 1988; **36**: 213–20.
201. Winslow R, Sachs M. Effect of electrical stimulation of the crossed olivocochlear bundle on auditory nerve responses to tones in noise. *J Neurophysiol* 1987; **57**: 1002–21.
202. Sahley TL, Kalish R, Musiek FE, Hoffman D. Effects of opiate drugs on auditory evoked potentials in the chinchilla. *Hear Res* 1991; **55**: 133–42.

12 Acoustics, measurement of sound and calibration

John Stevens

Introduction

This chapter gives an introduction to those aspects of acoustics, sound measurement and calibration that are relevant to clinical audiology. The reader is referred to references 1 and 2 for more comprehensive texts on acoustics and to reference 3 for a more detailed description of those aspects of acoustics found in audiology. In addition, there are many excellent publications from the various professional organizations. The *Journal of the Acoustical Society of America*, *Acustica*, and the *Journal of the Audio Engineering Society* are particularly well respected. Manufacturers of acoustical equipment also produce many good technical publications which can provide an excellent source of practical information. The various standards institutes (see Appendix), national standards laboratories and national institutes of acoustics and vibration research are also very good sources of up-to-date information.

Sound

Nature of sound and wave propagation

Sound is used to describe a mechanical disturbance propagated in a solid or fluid elastic medium, whether audible or not. Frequencies higher than the audible range are described as ultrasonic, and those below the audible range as infrasonic. In this chapter, sound refers only to frequencies in the audible range.

Sound levels within a room

The simplest generator of sound is a point source radiating sounds equally in all directions. However, this situation only exists in practice in a room with no reflections—i.e. an anechoic chamber. Such rooms are difficult and expensive to construct and would not form an acceptable environment in the audiology clinic. Sound field testing in clinical audiology uses sound sources, such as a hand-held stimulator, that can often be considered as point sources. A knowledge of how the sound level from such a source will vary across a typical test room is therefore useful. As the sound propagates from the source, it will initially be in a free-field environment, and will drop off at a rate governed by the inverse square law (6-dB drop for each doubling of distance). However, at greater distances the sound level is affected by reflections from the walls, and the rate of reduction in sound level will reduce. This is illustrated in Figure 12.1. In a typical test room, the relationship between sound level and distance cannot be assumed, and direct measurements of the sound level presented to the subject should be made. This is discussed in more detail under soundfield calibration.

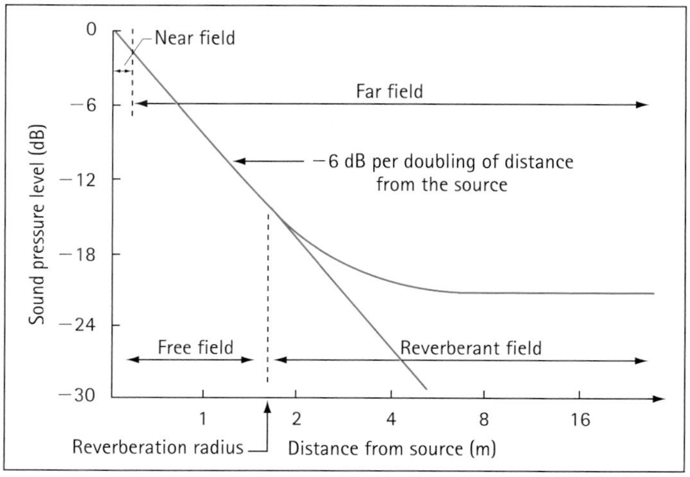

Figure 12.1 Reduction in sound level at a distance from a point source in a room. (Reproduced from Hassel and Zaveri, *Acoustic Noise Measurements* with permission from Bruel and Kjaer.)

> **FOR A TYPICAL TEST ROOM**
>
> - Initial drop of 6 dB for doubling of distance
> - Changing to a more uniform sound level

Measurement of sound

Sound level and decibels

In general, it has been found more practical to measure the level of sound in terms of pressure rather than the power. The international unit for pressure is the pascal, but for sound the decibel is used more in practice. The decibel value for a sound gives the ratio of the measured sound to a reference value. A chart of typical sounds with the sound levels in pascals and decibels is given in Table 12.1. Note that the decibel is a much more practical scale, as the range of values is much less. A second reason for using the decibel is that equal intervals on the decibel scale describe approximately equal increments in perceived loudness, for example, 10 dB describes an approximate doubling in loudness. The loudest sound shown in Table 12.1 still represents a very small perturbation in pressure when compared with the static atmospheric pressure.

Decibel formulae

The equation which is used to calculate the decibel sound pressure level from the value in pascals is given below:

$$\text{Sound pressure level (SPL)} = 20 \log_{10} p/p_0 \,\text{dB SPL}$$

where p is the measured pressure in pascals, and p_0 the reference pressure (see below)

Table 12.1 Some typical sound pressure levels

Sound pressure (μPa)	Sound pressure level (dB re 2×10^{-5} Pa)	
100 000 000	140	
	130	Near to a jet aircraft taking off
	120	
10 000 000	110	
	100	Near a pneumatic drill
1 000 000	90	
	80	Inside a motor car
100 000	70	
	60	General office
10 000	50	
	40	Quiet living room
1000	30	
	20	Quiet countryside
100	10	
20	0	Threshold of hearing

From this formula, it can be seen that 6 dB represents a doubling of sound pressure, and 20 dB represents a 10-fold increase.

It is always important to remember that the decibel value is a relative measure and not an absolute measure. When using a decibel scale, the reference value must be given or implied by the type of decibel scale used, e.g. dB SPL, decibel hearing level (dB HL). It is also important to use only the term sound pressure level and not sound intensity level, as intensity usually refers to power and not pressure.

Reference levels

The internationally agreed reference level for sound pressure is 20 μPa ($20 \times 10^{-6}\,\text{N/m}^2$). The reference point for sound pressure level was chosen to coincide approximately with the threshold of hearing of normal subjects at 1 kHz.

Hearing level scale

In the human ear, the threshold of hearing varies with frequency, as shown in Figure 12.2. For the purpose of pure tone audiometry, a practical scale is required which enables the hearing threshold of an individual to be easily compared with the normal average value. This scale is the hearing level scale measured in decibels. Instead of a fixed value for the reference level, the median normal hearing threshold at each frequency is used. Values for the reference level are given in ISO 389. This is discussed further under audiometric equipment calibration later in this chapter.

Sound pressure level, hearing level and sensation level

The basis of the sound pressure level scale and the hearing level scale have already been outlined. Sound pressure level (dB SPL), as expressed in decibels, is used to measure the physical pressure of sound above the internationally recognised reference value of 20μPa. The hearing level scale (dB HL) is used to express the decibel difference between a measured hearing threshold and the median value for those with normal hearing at a particular audiometric frequency. The term dBnHL (n = normal) may be found which is also used to express the level of a sound in decibels above the threshold in those with normal hearing. In some instances it is useful to use a fourth scale, sensation level (dB SL). This is defined as the level of sound, expressed in decibels, relative to the threshold for that sound for the individual listener. This may be of use where sounds are presented to subjects at a set level above their individual thresholds rather than at a level relative to the threshold for those with normal hearing.

> - Decibels (dB) are a relative measure
> - A reference value is required
> - The hearing level scale uses the median normal threshold as a reference
> - 20 dB is a 10-fold increase in physical sound pressure
> - A doubling of perceived loudness is about 10 dB

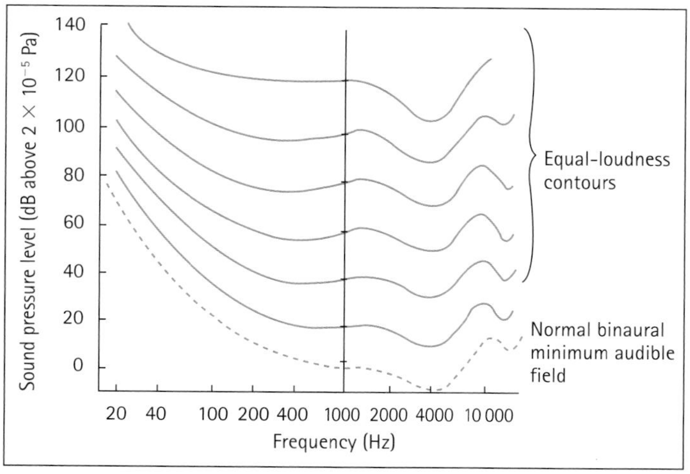

Figure 12.2 Normal equal-loudness contours for pure tones heard binaurally in a free field, from ISO 226. The dashed line shows the minimum audible level.

Frequency weighting

We have noted the use of a frequency correction in the hearing level scale. If it is required to measure the perceived level of sound correctly, some form of frequency weighting will be required in our measuring instrument. Figure 12.2 shows the equal-loudness contours at different sound levels which are used to define the weighting required. Note that the weighting must also vary with sound level, as the curves shown in Figure 12.2 are not the same at each sound level.

Many weighting standards have been produced. The principal one in international use is called the 'A' weighting scale (defined in IEC 60651). The 'A' weighting curve corresponds approximately to the equal-loudness contour passing through 40 dB SPL at 1 kHz (Figure 12.3). Sound measurement equipment often provides other weightings, such as B and C, relating to equal-loudness contours passing through 70 and 100 dB SPL at 1 kHz, and which are intended for use when sounds with a mean sound pressure level around these values are being recorded. However, in the majority of cases, the 'A' weighting is used. Levels measured using the 'A' weighting should always be

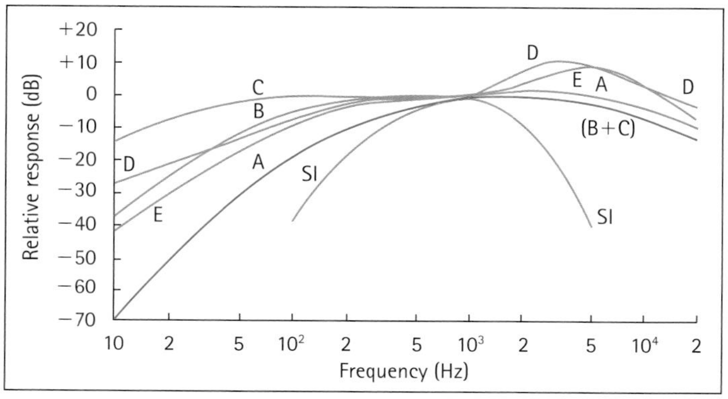

Figure 12.3 The internationally standardized weighting curves for sound level meters and suggested E and SI weighting. (Reproduced from Hassel and Zaveri, *Acoustic Noise Measurements* with permission from Bruel and Kjaer.)

suffixed thus: 23 dBA SPL. Similarly, any other weighting curve used should be included in the unit description.

Temporal integration

If the duration of a sound is less than about 200 ms, then its perceived loudness is less than when the sound is heard continuously. In the assessment of hearing, it is particularly important to be aware of this, as many stimuli used in behavioural testing and electrophysiological testing are of short duration. This will be dealt with in more detail under calibration.

- Weighting is required to simulate the variation in threshold with frequency
- Different weighting is required at different sound levels
- In practice, most measurements are made with A weighting
- The loudness of a sound is less when its duration is below about 200 ms

Frequency analysis

A very useful method of analysing sounds is to consider the frequency content. This is particularly the case when the frequency content of a stimulus is required or when analysing otoacoustic emissions. The analysis calculates the energy at each frequency and plots this against frequency to give a frequency spectrum. Long pure tones with a slow rise time, as used in pure tone audiometry, will have narrow spectra, and short transient sounds, such as those used in electric response audiometry, will have broader spectra. The determination of the spectrum of a stimulus as perceived by the cochlea is a complex subject and is outside the scope of this chapter.

Statistical analysis

Most environmental sounds vary in amplitude and frequency content with time. It is therefore necessary to carry out a statistical analysis in order to adequately describe the sound. For example, it might be specified that the noise level in a hospital ward should not exceed 40 dBA SPL for more than 10% of the time during the working day. A recording of the sound throughout a typical working day and an analysis of the time at each sound level would be required to determine whether the specification had been met. Similar methods need to be employed in the measurement of industrial and other noise that may be the cause of hearing loss.

Summary

Sound is a mechanical disturbance propagated in a solid or fluid elastic medium.

Sound is normally measured in terms of pressure rather than power. A decibel scale is preferred. This is a relative scale with a reference approximating to the threshold of human hearing at 1 kHz.

The threshold of hearing varies with frequency. The hearing level scale, used for pure tone audiometry, uses the median normal hearing threshold at each frequency as its reference.

As decibels give only a relative value, the reference value must always be indicated in the unit description, e.g. dB SPL or dB HL, but not just dB.

The effect of frequency and temporal integration needs to be taken into account when measuring the sound pressure level.

Frequency and statistical analysis over time are two useful methods of analysing sound.

Standards and calibration

Introduction

Calibration of audiometric equipment is essential for safe and accurate working practices in an audiology clinic. National and international bodies cooperate very closely to bring together scientific data to establish and maintain standards that can be used to design and calibrate audiometric equipment. The International Electrotechnical Commission (IEC) and the International Organization for Standardization provide most of the international standards used in audiology. In the UK, these standards are also provided by the British Standards Institution (BSI), and the American National Standards Institution also provides a range of standards. A list of those standards most frequently used in audiology is given in the Appendix.

For any professional involved in acoustical measurements and calibration, it is essential to be familiar with the relevant standards. They are being continuously updated. It is therefore important, when putting these standards into practice, that the most up-to-date information is used, and any laboratory should ensure that it is notified of revisions as they appear.

Standards usually refer to measurements made under highly specified conditions. In audiological practice, clinical measurements can be subject to many factors which introduce errors, and the professional audiologist should be aware of this. Examples of such errors are assumptions made about ear canal volume for insert earphones, the effect of coupling force when carrying out bone conduction audiometry, measuring sounds that are only just above the background noise, and not understanding the limitations of the sound level meter.

- The IEC and ISO are the main international sources of standards for audiology
- A knowledge of the relevant standards affecting clinical practice is required
- There are many factors which if not understood can result in incorrect measures

Equipment for sound level measurement

Sound level meters

The purpose of a sound level meter is to measure the sound pressure level of the incident sound and provide an appropriate analysis. A diagram showing the main elements of a sound level meter is given in Figure 12.4.

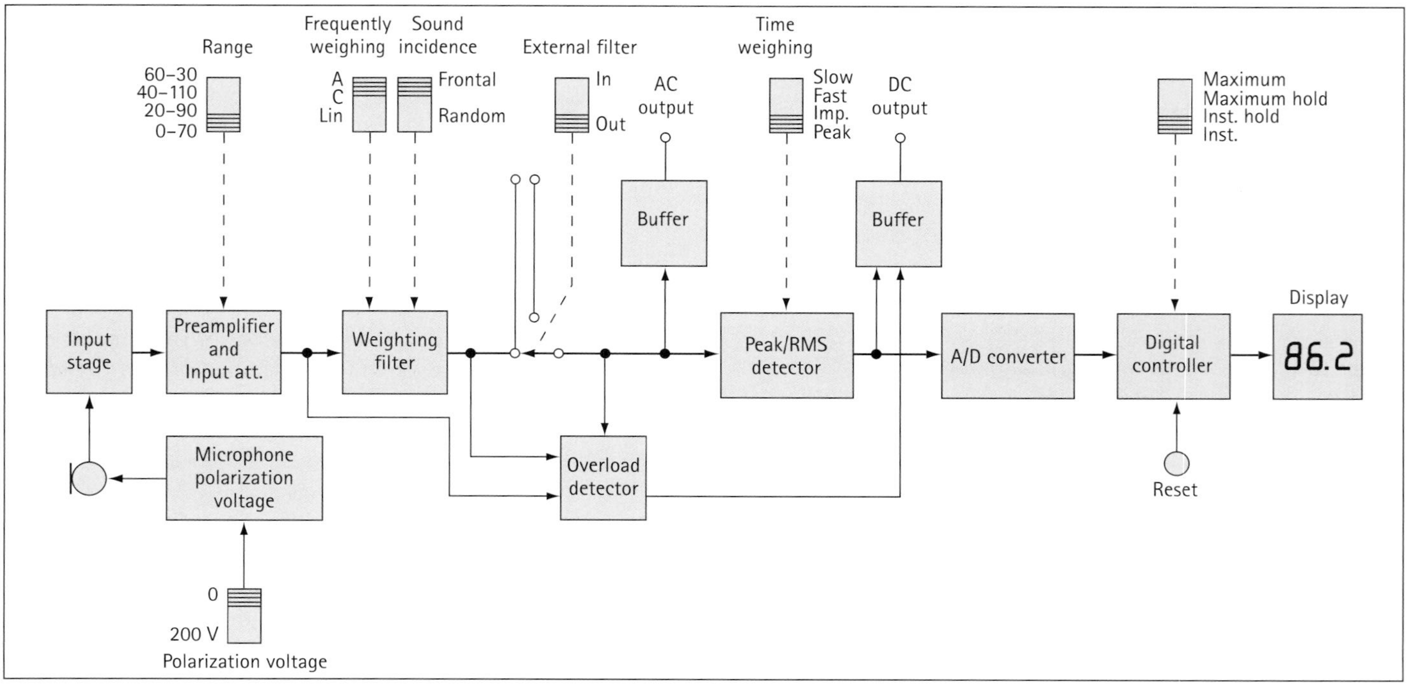

Figure 12.4 Block diagram of a typical sound level meter. (Reproduced from Hassel and Zaveri, *Acoustic Noise Measurement* with permission from Bruel and Kjaer.) Imp. = Impulse; Inst. = Instantaneous; Att. = Attenuation.

The most critical element of a sound level meter is the microphone. A microphone is a device which converts sound energy into electrical energy. Most high-grade sound level meters use a condenser microphone. These microphones have high sensitivity and low distortion, but are expensive and prone to damage. For some low-cost sound level meters, an electret microphone is used. Their major advantage is their extreme ruggedness; they are resistant to shock, vibration, humidity, and other adverse environments. This type of microphone is commonly used in hearing aids.

Free-field and pressure microphones

When using a sound level meter, it is important to ensure that the correct type of microphone is being used. Microphones are generally designed to work in a free field or in a closed cavity (pressure type), e.g. in a coupler. An example of the use of the former would be in soundfield testing, and of the latter in the calibration of an audiometer using a coupler. The sensitivity at high frequencies is particularly affected by the wrong choice of microphone. Expert advice should be sought when selecting which microphone to use.

Filters and weighting

The need to use frequency weighting in some sound level measurements was noted earlier. Most sound level meters offer one or more of A, B, C and D weightings. A 'linear' setting is also usually present on higher-grade sound level meters to enable unweighted sound pressure levels to be measured.

It was also noted that it can be useful to carry out a frequency analysis of the sound. The higher grades of sound level meter incorporate octave and one-third-octave filters to measure the sound level in each frequency band. This is now often done by digital signal processing within the sound level meter, allowing a near-continuous spectrum to be displayed.

- The most crucial component of a sound level meter is the microphone
- Different microphones are required for free-field and coupler measurements
- The correct frequency weighting should be selected

Amplitude measures—root mean square and peak

Sound waves may be sinusoidal in nature (such as a pure tone) or they may have a more complex morphology. The amplitude of a pure tone could be described by its peak-to-peak value. In practice, the root mean square (RMS) value has been chosen as the normal value that is displayed. Figure 12.5 compares the peak, peak-to-peak and RMS values for a pure tone. The sound levels of more complex waveforms are more difficult to describe by a single parameter. For a transient sound, the peak value may be a better measure; for example in sound-field audiometry, a short stimulus such as a drum beat may be best measured in terms of its peak or peak-to-peak value. More information on this is given under soundfield calibration.

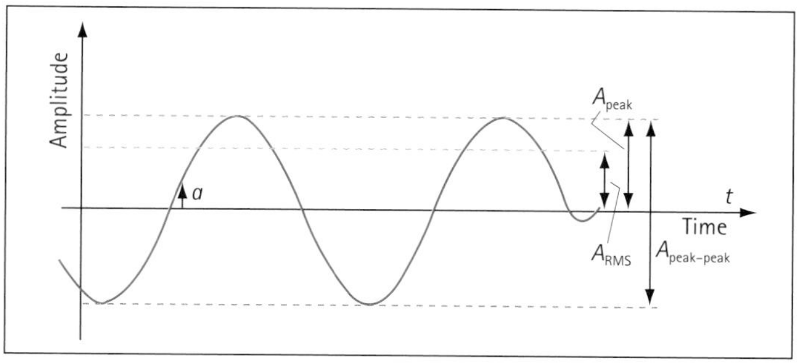

Figure 12.5 Sinusoidal signal (pure tone) showing various measures of signal amplitude. (Reproduced from Hassel and Zaveri, *Acoustic Noise Measurements* with permission from Bruel and Kjaer.)

Time weighting

Sound level meters incorporate a fast or slow time constant. The fast time constant (0.125 s) allows rapidly fluctuating sound levels to be monitored, while the slow time constant (1 s) smooths out rapid fluctuations. It was noted earlier that for sounds of less than about 200 ms in duration, the perceived level will be reduced due to the effect known as temporal integration. For example, a sound of duration 20 ms will be perceived at about −10 dB, compared to the same sound if it were continuous.

On higher-grade sound level meters, an impulse scale is often available which is intended to give a closer reading to the perceived level for short-duration sounds. However, for any short-duration sounds used in clinical testing, calibration should not rely on such meter settings (see sections on sound-field calibration and ERA calibration).

Display

Sound level meters can have either an analogue or a digital display. The former has the advantage that rapidly changing sound levels can be more easily followed. More complex meters have the advantage of a dual display. The choice will depend on the use of the sound level meter. In the clinic, an analogue display may be found to be quicker and easier to read, whereas in calibration work a digital display may be more useful.

The electrical signal corresponding to the sound signal is available on most sound level meters to enable more complex analysis of the sound to be carried out by external equipment such as a frequency analyser. Many sound level meters now also incorporate a digital output for connection to computers to enable sound level measurements to be stored on a computer for later analysis.

Calibration of sound level meters

Regular calibration of sound level meters is essential. A calibrated sound source is used which is placed over the microphone. A typical calibrator contains a miniature loudspeaker, the output level and frequency of which are controlled within fine limits by a built-in electronic circuit. A typical example operates at 1.0 kHz at 94 dB SPL, which corresponds (conveniently) to a sound pressure of 1 Pa. This device permits calibrations to within about ±0.3 dB to be obtained.

The pistonphone is the most accurate calibrator of this type, permitting accuracies of about ±0.15 dB. However, it should be noted that both the sound source and pistonphone only calibrate at a single frequency and level. If the sound level meter lost sensitivity at frequencies other than that tested, this would go unnoticed and errors would result.

- The root mean square (RMS) is normally used to measure sound levels
- For transient sounds, the peak or peak-to-peak measure may be better
- Slow and fast settings change the time constant on the sound level meter
- The sound level can be displayed in analogue or digital form
- The pistonphone is the most accurate calibrator for sound level meters

Standards for sound level meters

The IEC Publication 60651 consolidates a number of preceding standards. This divides the performance into several classes, in descending order of sophistication and precision:

- Type 0 laboratory reference grade
- Type 1 precision grade
- Type 2 general field application
- Type 3 noise survey application

Other noise-measuring instruments

In addition to the sound level meter, other noise-measuring devices exist. One of the most important of these for routine noise survey and monitoring purposes is the personal sound exposure meter, often called the noise dose meter. This is a small instrument designed to measure personal exposure to noise in, for example, industrial situations.

The microphone of the device is simply clipped on the lapel or mounted in an alternative position close to the ear, in order to receive approximately the same noise as the wearer's ear. These meters measure the average noise dose, which takes into account both the sound level and its duration. Occupational safety regulations define a maximum allowable noise exposure for a normal working period. In most countries, 85 dBA SPL or 90 dBA SPL is the defined equivalent continuous level for an 8-h day. Higher levels are permitted if a corresponding shorter exposure time occurs.

Summary

International standards for the construction and calibration of audiometric equipment exist. Regular calibration of audiometric equipment using these standards is essential for safe working practice.

A sound level meter enables sound to be measured and analysed by converting sound into an electrical signal.

Sound level meters enable both frequency and time weighting to be applied to the sound signal and for the result to be displayed in several ways. A knowledge of the effects of different settings and choice of microphone is essential before using a sound level meter.

Sound level meters are built to international standards and need regular calibration.

Specialized noise-measuring instruments are available to simplify the measurement of personal noise exposure.

Audiometric equipment and calibration

Audiometers

Figure 12.6 shows the main components of a pure tone audiometer. Standards have been produced for both screening and diagnostic audiometers (IEC 60645). Modern audiometers are very stable in both the level of output and frequency of the test tone. However, faults still occur, particularly in the leads, earphones and bone conduction transducers. It is important, therefore, in clinical practice to have a protocol to ensure regular calibration and the identification of faults.

Practitioners should carry out a daily subjective check of the output level from the audiometer at different test frequencies and listen for the presence of unwanted sounds, which may give a false threshold. They should be familiar with their own hearing threshold and have this checked regularly, so that they can interpret the results of their daily check accurately.

At regular intervals, a full laboratory calibration should be carried out. In the laboratory calibration, the main parameters that define the sound presented to the subject are checked. Essentially, the objective of the procedure is to determine whether the audiometer meets the specifications given in IEC 60645. An example of one of the specifications is the characteristic of the attenuator, which must be linear, such that the difference between the actual and measured sound levels at adjacent settings (normally 5 dB) is within ±1 dB. The output of the audiometer is compared to that given in the relevant part of ISO 389 (Appendix).

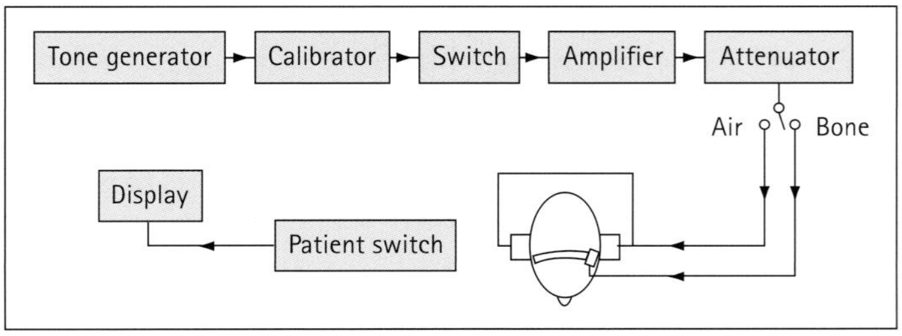

Figure 12.6 Block diagram of a pure tone audiometer.

Artificial ears and couplers

The sound that emanates from the earphone of an audiometer is measured by placing the earphone on an artificial ear. This is a device that is designed to mimic the acoustical characteristics of the ear. Two types are in common use: that designed to IEC 60318-3 (based on the 6-ml-volume NBS 9A coupler defined by the National Bureau of Standards in Washington) and that designed to IEC 60318-1, which is a more accurate representation of the ear and allows a wider range of earphones to be calibrated. A version of the former of these is shown in Figure 12.7. The reference equivalent threshold sound pressure levels (RETSPLs) used for the calibration for each earphone and coupler combination are given in ISO 389-1.

Mechanical coupler (artificial mastoid)

The force produced by the bone conductor used for bone conduction audiometry is measured by placing the bone conductor on an artificial mastoid defined in IEC 60373. This simulates the compliance of the skin and soft tissues covering the mastoid. An artificial mastoid built to this standard is shown in Figure 12.8. The standard reference equivalent threshold force levels over the frequency range 250 Hz to 8 kHz are defined in ISO 389-3.

Couplers for insert phones and hearing aids

Two couplers have been defined for the measurement of hearing aids. Both are intended to represent the ear when occluded by an earmould and fitted with either an insert- or postaural-type earphone. The oldest and most basic is the '2cc' coupler (Figure 12.9) as defined in IEC 60126. This does not represent the response of the occluded ear well, particularly at low and high frequencies, and it is therefore of limited application. However, because of its simplicity, it is still the standard coupler used in commercially available hearing aid test equipment. An improved device, the occluded ear simulator, is defined in IEC 60711 and closely reproduces the physical characteristics of the average human ear. This permits the accurate measurement of the performance of insert earphones and postaural hearing aids fitted with tubes. The performance of 'in-the-ear' aids can also be measured.

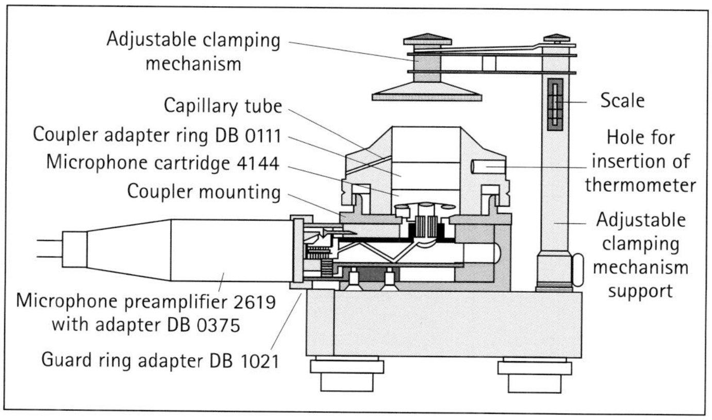

Figure 12.7 Cross-section of the NBS9A acoustic coupler (equivalent to IEC 60318-3) used for earphone calibration. (Reproduced from Hassel and Zaveri, *Acoustic Noise Measurements* with permission from Bruel and Kjaer.)

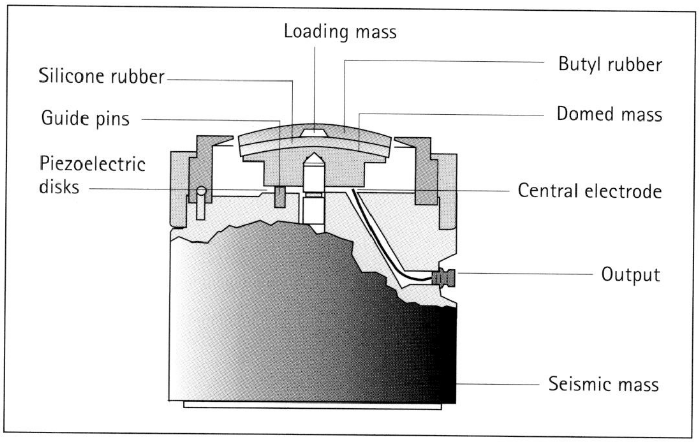

Figure 12.8 Cutaway view of the most important parts of the artificial mastoid (to IEC 60373). (Reproduced from Hassel and Zaveri, *Acoustic Noise Measurements* with permission from Bruel and Kjaer.)

- Modern audiometers are very stable
- Faults still occur with mechanical components, e.g. leads
- A daily subjective check is important
- Regular laboratory calibration is required
- Special couplers exist to measure the output from earphones and bone conductors
- Two couplers are available for measuring hearing aid output

Equipment for speech audiometry

Historically, speech audiometry was implemented by recording the material on a tape recorder and playing it back through an audiometer to control the sound level. Digital methods of recording are now readily available, and the material for speech audiometry is slowly becoming available in a digital format. This gives the considerable advantages of a much higher-quality signal and random access to each stimulus. A compact disk is often the chosen source for routine speech audiometry, whereas a computer might be the source for a more complex speech test.

Speech audiometry calibration

The calibration of speech audiometers which use recorded material is difficult, due to the problem of defining the sound level of speech. The difficulty is complicated by the fact that different sets of 'standard' word lists are available. In practice, the reference threshold of each word list must be determined locally from speech audiograms carried out on normal subjects. The reader is referred to Martin[4] for more details. The move to the use of digitally recorded material should ensure

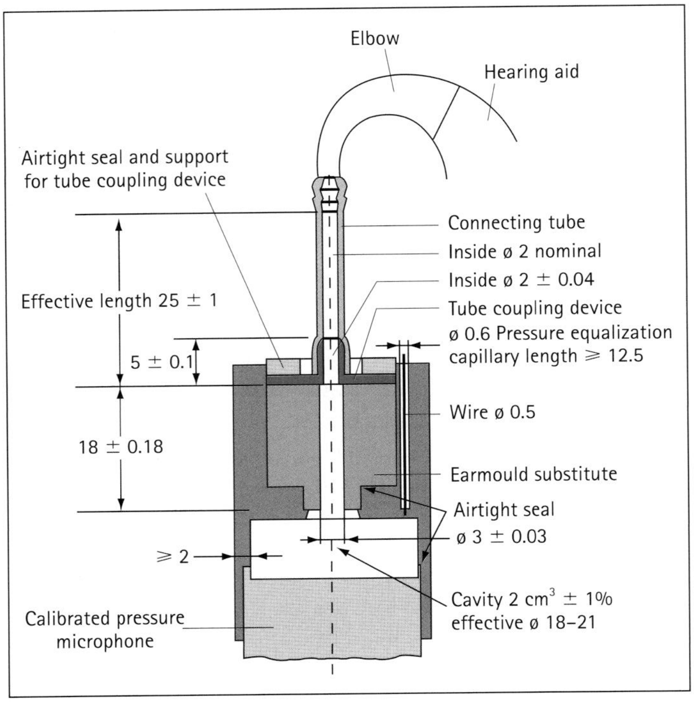

Figure 12.9 Cross-section of a '2cc' coupler to IEC 60126. All measurements are in mm. (Reproduced from Hassel and Zaveri, *Acoustic Noise Measurements* with permission from Bruel and Kjaer.)

that speech material is of higher quality and there will be greater comparability across centres using it for audiological assessment.

Acoustical impedance meters

Acoustical impedance or otoadmittance meters represent the second most commonly used instrument in diagnostic testing. The basic components of an acoustical impedance meter are shown in Figure 12.10. The specification for their design is given in IEC 61027. In the majority of basic instruments, the measurement is made at one frequency, usually about 220 Hz.

The more complex instruments allow the separate components of admittance (reciprocal of impedance) to be measured at more than one frequency. These find application in the diagnosis of such conditions as otosclerosis and in the measurement of admittance in the neonate.

It is possible to carry out daily checks on otoadmittance instruments by the use of test cavities whose volumes cover the range of admittance values found (using units of equivalent volume). In addition, the operator can measure his own tympanogram and reflex thresholds to check whether there is any change which might indicate a fault with the instrument. However, at regular intervals, the equipment should be given a full laboratory calibration against the IEC 61027 standard and the manufacturer's specification. Included in the calibration should be: a check of the pressure system against a calibrated pressure meter; a check on admittance values for a range of test cavity sizes; and a check on the stimulus generator for acoustical reflex testing using the standards for pure tone audiometers.

- Speech material should be held in digital format
- Reference threshold for speech audiometry requires calibration on normal subjects
- Acoustical impedance meters should be calibrated against the IEC 61027 standard
- Regular checks can be made by using test cavaties and the operator's own tympanogram

Calibration of sound generators for soundfield testing

In many audiometric test situations, it is desirable to use a stimulus presented in the soundfield rather than by earphones. This is particularly the case in paediatric audiology, where earphones may not be tolerated. However, this presents a problem with calibration, as it is more difficult to specify the test conditions. For example, there are many different types of sound generator being used, and the geometrical relationship to subject and room acoustics can affect the level of sound that reaches the ear under test.

One method of checking the sound delivered by a soundfield stimulator is by presenting the sound again to a sound level meter. The value obtained is fairly repeatable if the procedure is carried out carefully, and the meter will give a reasonably accurate value in dBA SPL if the sound is continuous, with little fluctuation in level. However, most sound level meters can only measure accurately in dBA SPL down to a level of 35–40 dBA SPL. In addition, many sounds used in soundfield testing are transient in nature, and a sound level meter will not give a correct reading.

Ideally, a value referenced to the threshold of hearing is required. For warble tones and narrow band noise, standards are now available to enable sound field testing to be set up accu-

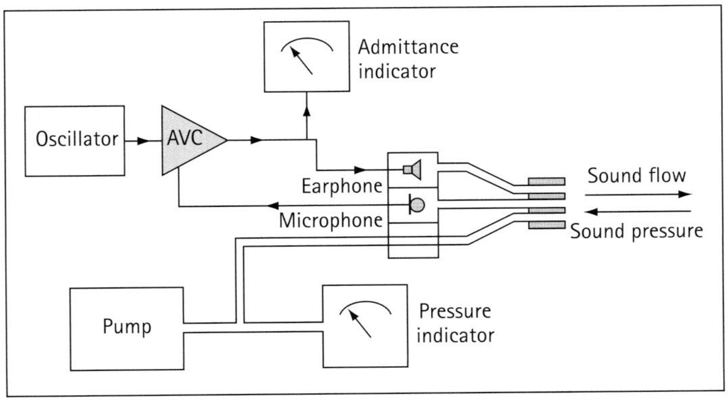

Figure 12.10 Schematic diagram of an acoustical impedance meter. AVC, automatic volume control.

rately, giving values referenced to the normal threshold of hearing (ISO 8253–2 and ISO 389–7, see Appendix). The solution to this is to carry out a study on normally hearing subjects to obtain the RETSPL for each stimulus used. A room quiet enough to hear the sounds over the range of normal human hearing thresholds is required. Such conditions are difficult to achieve in normal clinical rooms. This is discussed later under audiometric test environment. The scale used for the stimuli is dB relative to normal hearing level (dBnHL).

Electric response audiometry calibration

The stimuli used in electric response audiometry (ERA) vary with the type of test being carried out. Click and tone burst stimuli of varying length are the two most common of these. The procedure for establishing an RETSPL again requires the measurement of threshold for each stimulus in a group of normally hearing subjects. Suitable couplers to measure the sound output from the earphone are those to IEC 60318-1 and IEC 60318-3.

The procedure for establishing the RETSPL for soundfield and ERA stimuli is time-consuming, and it is sensible to exchange information on this between audiology centres to avoid duplication of effort.

The recorded waveform on ERA equipment is scaled in amplitude against time. Both of these variables need to be calibrated to ensure that clinical results are accurately reported. Internal calibration sources are often provided to allow a check to be made of the recording system.

- Most sound level meters cannot measure very quiet sounds accurately
- Transient sounds are also difficult to measure
- A calibration on normal subjects should be carried out
- Calibration data should be shared to reduce costs

Audiometric test environment

Many of the general principles described in the previous section apply to audiometric test rooms. The environment must be sufficiently quiet for the test signal to be heard and, for soundfield tests, to enable the sound to be presented at an accurate level without reverberation. Standards have been produced for the maximum permissable ambient noise levels for audiometric test rooms. Two examples are ISO 8253-2 and ANSI S3.1. The ANSI standard specifies maximum levels that will produce negligible masking (<2 dB) of pure tones presented at the RETSPL as specified in ISO 389. The low sound levels required can be difficult to achieve, particularly where the audiometric test room is located in a busy hospital or near to roads with a high traffic density. In many cases, it is necessary to use a double sound-insulated room, i.e. a room within a room, the inner one of which is mounted on flexible supports, and has no rigid structural contact with the outer room. It is very important to carry out a full noise survey and to use these data together with those provided by manufacturers of audiometric test rooms in order to determine whether the desired ambient noise levels will be achieved within the test room.

As well as achieving acceptable ambient noise level within the test room, it is important to ensure that the room has adequate temperature control, ventilation, lighting and power supply. The additional sound insulation provides very high levels of thermal insulation, and it may be necessary to provide cooling within the ventilation system. Most ventilation equipment is too noisy to be used for audiometric test rooms without the addition of silencer ducts. For both temperature and ventilation control, a careful engineering design procedure is required to ensure that the correct environment will be provided.

Electrophysiological testing has now become routine in clinical audiology. The electrical potentials are often less than one microvolt, and recordings can be subject to artefacts from electrical and magnetic field sources such as power cables, lift motors and fluorescent lights. Artefacts can usually be avoided by location of the test room away from magnetic sources of interference and by the provision of a metal screen lining to the test room, which is earthed. The latter will greatly attenuate any electrical fields that are present. Finally, care should be taken that no significant electrical or magnetic fields are then introduced into the room. For example, lighting should be screened or short filament lamps should be used, power cables should be screened or be in screened trunking, and the patient should be kept well away from the test equipment. Where testing has to take place outside a specially designed test room, e.g. in a neonatal intensive care unit or in the operating theatre, sources of artefact are more difficult to control. Expert advice should be sought.

- Environmental sound levels for audiometric rooms can be specified
- A careful engineering design procedure is required to ensure the correct environment
- For ERA, electrical interference from power cables and lighting must be controlled

Summary

A daily subjective check and a regular laboratory calibration to the international standards should be carried out on all audiometers to ensure accurate hearing measurements.

Specialized couplers have been developed to calibrate earphones and bone conductors used in audiometry.

Couplers have also been developed for the measurement of hearing aid performance and the output of insert earphones.

Speech test material is calibrated by reference to the thresholds of a group of normal subjects.

Acoustical impedance meters should also be subject to regular calibration.

Sound sources used for soundfield testing and electrical response audiometry can only be properly calibrated by carrying out measurements on a group of normally hearing subjects. There are important limitations if the calibration of the sound stimulus is carried out by a sound level meter alone.

Standards now exist for the specification of the audiometric test environment to enable tests to be carried out down to threshold in normal subjects. Of equal importance to sound insulation is the control of temperature and lighting.

References

1. Hall DE. *Basic Acoustics*. Krieger US, 1993.
2. Kinsler LE, Frey AR, Coppens AB, Sanders JV. *Fundamentals and Acoustics*, 3rd edn. New York: John Wiley, 1983.
3. Stevens JC. Acoustics. In: Stephens D, ed. *Adult Audiology* Vol. 2 of *Scott-Brown's Otolaryngology*. Butterworth Heinemann, 1997.
4. Martin M. *Speech Audiometry*. London: Whurr, 1987.

Further reading and useful organizations

National Physical Laboratory, UK. http://www.npl.co.uk

Harris CM. *Handbook of Acoustical Measurements and Noise Control*. McGraw, 1991.

Hassall JR, Zaveri K. *Acoustic Noise Measurements*, 5th edn. Copenhagen: Bruel and Kjaer, 1988.

Haughton PM. *Acoustics for Audiologists*. London: Elsevier/Academic Press, 2002.

Rossing TD. *The Science of Sound*. New York: Addison Wesley, 1989.

Appendix: Selection of standards relevant to audiology (contact standards organizations for latest information)

International Organization for Standardization, Geneva, Switzerland: http://www.iso.ch/

ISO 226: 1987	Acoustics—Normal equal loudness level contours.
ISO 389	Acoustics—Reference zero for the calibration of audiometric equipment:
	389-1: 1989—Reference equivalent threshold sound pressure levels for pure tones and supra-aural earphones.
	389-2: 1994—Reference equivalent threshold sound pressure levels for pure tones and insert earphones.
	389-3: 1994—Reference equivalent threshold force levels for pure tones and bone vibrators.
	389-4: 1994—Reference levels for narrow band masking noise.
	389-5: 1998—Reference equivalent threshold sound pressure levels for pure tones in the frequency range 8 kHz to 16 kHz.
	389-7: 1996—Reference threshold of hearing under free-field and diffuse field listening conditions.
ISO TR 4870:1991	Acoustics—The construction and calibration of speech intelligibility tests.
ISO 6189:1983	Acoustics—Pure tone air conduction threshold audiometry for hearing conversation purposes.
ISO 7029:1984	Acoustics—Threshold of hearing by air conduction as a function of age and sex for otologically normal persons.
ISO 8253	Acoustics—Audiometric test methods:
	8253-1: 1989—Basic pure tone air and bone conduction threshold audiometry.
	8253-2: 1992—Sound field audiometry with pure tone and narrow-band test signals.
	8253-3: 1996—Speech audiometry.

International Electrotechnical Commission, Geneva, Switzerland: http://www.iec.ch/

IEC 60118	Hearing aids:
60118-0: 1983	Measurement of electroacoustical characteristics (2nd edition).
60118-1: 1983	Hearing aids with induction pick-up coil input (2nd edition).
60118-2: 1983	Hearing aids with automatic gain control circuits (2nd edition) (+AMD 1: 1993).
60118-3: 1983	Hearing aid equipment not entirely worn on the listener (2nd edition).
60118-4: 1981	Magnetic field strength in audio-frequency induction loops for hearing aid purposes.
60118-5: 1983	Nipples for insert earphones.
60118-6: 1999	Characteristics of electrical input circuits for hearing aids.

60118-7: 1983	Measurements of performance characteristics of hearing aids for quality inspection or delivery purposes.
60118-8: 1983	Methods of measurement of performance characteristics of hearing aids under simulated *in situ* working conditions.
60118-9: 1985	Methods of measurement of characteristics of hearing aids with bone vibrator output.
60118-10: 1986	Guide to hearing aid standards.
60118-11: 1983	Symbols and other markings on hearing aids and related equipment.
60118-12: 1996	Dimensions of electrical connection systems.
IEC 60126: 1973	Reference coupler for the measurement of hearing aids using earphones coupled to the ear by means of ear inserts (2nd edition). (Will become IEC 60318-5.)
IEC 61260: 1995	Octave band and fractional octave band filters.
IEC 60318	Electroacoustics: simulators of the human head and ear. 60318-1: 1998—Ear simulator for the calibration of supra-aural earphones. 60318-2: 1998—An interim acoustic coupler for the calibration of audiometric earphones in the extended high frequency range. 60318-3: 1998—Acoustic coupler for the calibration of supra-aural earphones used in audiometry.
IEC 60373: 1990	Mechanical coupler for measurements on bone vibrators (2nd edition). (Will become IEC 60318-6.)
IEC 60645	Audiometers 60645-1: 1992—Pure-tone audiometers (+ Corrigendum: 1992). 60645-2: 1993—Equipment for speech audiometry. 60645-3: 1994—Audiometric test signals of short duration for audiometric and neuro-otological purposes. 60645-4: 1994—Equipment for extended high frequency audiometry.
IEC 60651: 1979	Sound level meters
IEC 60711: 1981	Occluded-ear simulator for the measurement of earphones coupled to the ear by ear inserts. (Will become IEC 60318-4.)
IEC 60942: 1997	Sound calibrators
IEC 60959: 1990	Provisional head and torso simulator for acoustic measurements on air conduction hearing aids. (Will become IEC 60318-7.)
IEC 61027: 1991	Instruments for the measurement of aural acoustic impedance/admittance.

British Standards Institution, London, UK: http://www.bsi-global.com

BS EN ISO 389:	Equivalent to ISO 389.
BS 3383: 1988	Equivalent to ISO 226: 1987.
BS 4009: 1991	Equivalent to IEC 60373.
BS 6083	Equivalent to IEC 60118-0 to 60118-11.
BS 6111: 1981 [1988]	Equivalent to IEC 60126.
BS 6310: 1982	Equivalent to IEC 60711.
BS 6655: 1986	Equivalent to ISO 6189:1983.
BS 6951: 1988	Equivalent to ISO 7209:1984.
BS EN ISO 8253-1: 1998	Equivalent to ISO 8253-1:1989.
BS EN ISO 8253-2: 1998	Equivalent to ISO 8253-2:1992.
BS EN ISO 8253-3: 1998	Equivalent to ISO 8253-3:1996.
BS EN 60318	Equivalent to IEC 60318.
BS EN 60645	Equivalent to IEC 60645.
BS EN 61027: 1993	Equivalent to IEC 61027.

American National Standards, Washington, USA: http://www.ansi.org/

ANSI S1.4-1997	Specification for sound level meters.
ANSI S1.40-1984 (R 1997)	Specifications for acoustical calibrators.
ANSI S3.1-1991	Maximum permissible ambient noise levels for audiometric test rooms.
ANSI S3.5-1997 (R 1986)	Methods for the calculation of the articulation index.

ANSI S3.6-1996	Specification for audiometers.
ANSI S3.7-1995 (R 1986)	Method for coupler calibration of earphones.
ANSI S3.13-1987	Mechanical coupler for measurement of bone vibrators.
ANSI S3.22-1996	Specification of hearing aid characteristics.
ANSI S3.25-1989	Occluded ear simulator.
ANSI S3.36-1985 (R 1990)	Specification for a manikin for simulated *in situ* airborne acoustic measurements.
ANSI S3.39-1987	Specifications for instruments to measure aural acoustic impedance and admittance (aural acoustic immittance).
ANSI S3.35-1985 (R 1997)	Methods of measurement of performance characteristics of hearing aids under simulated in situ working conditions.

13 The threshold of hearing

Ronald Hinchcliffe

Introduction

It was inevitable that attempts should have been made to quantify what has been variously termed the acuity or sensitivity of an individual's hearing. Essentially, it is answering the question of how quiet a sound a particular individual can hear. The answer can be provided in its simplest form by asking him (or her) whether or not they can hear a pin drop, a whisper, a conversational voice or a shout. These questions can be supplemented at this zero level of technology by determining at what distance a forced whisper or conversational voice may be heard. Minimum technology, e.g. tuning forks, can provide the means to measure this ability with greater precision. A higher level of technology using electroacoustical equipment is claimed to provide even greater precision by what has come to be termed audiometry (Figure 13.1).

Apart from the level of technology that is employed, methods for measuring hearing sensitivity may vary according to:

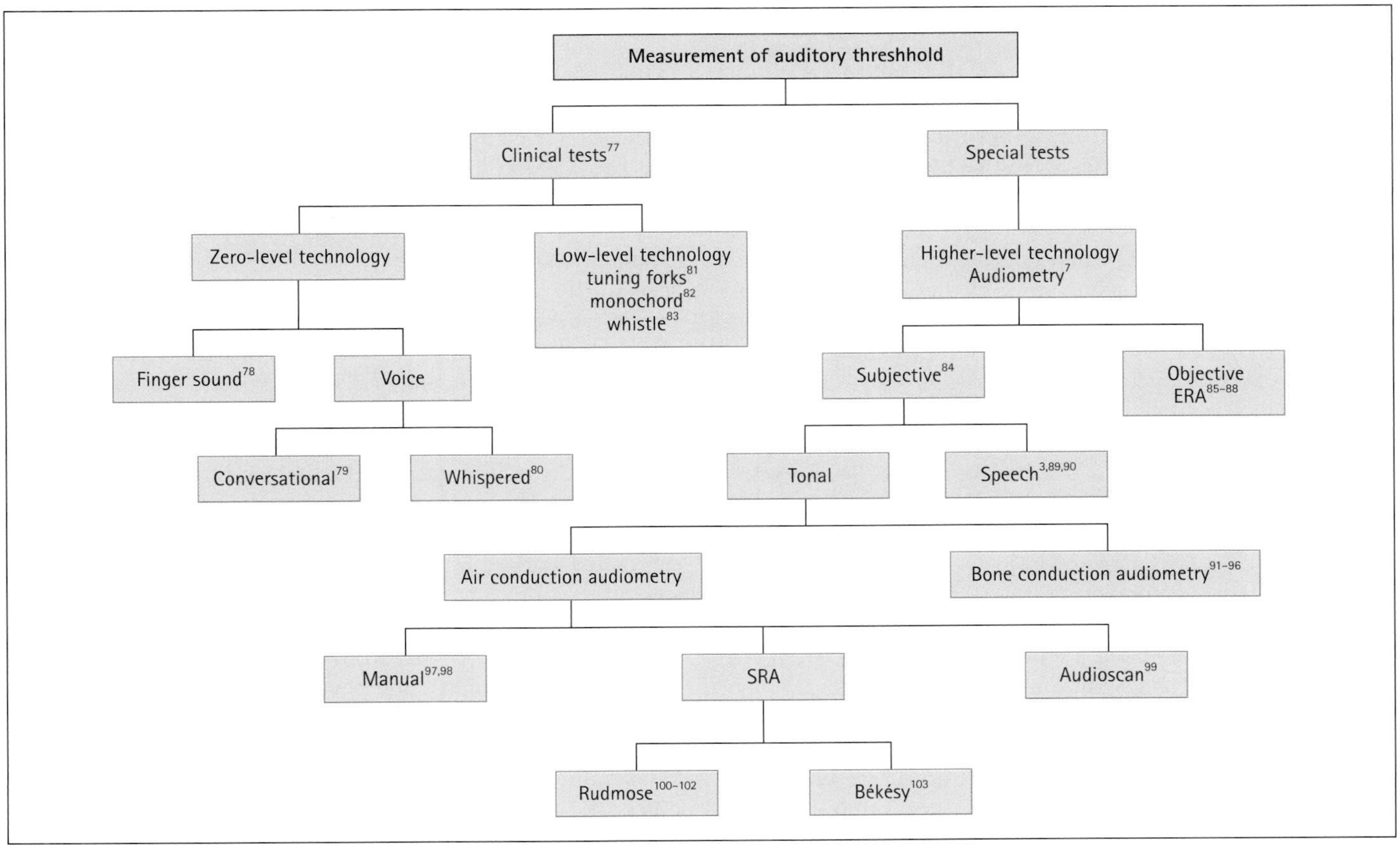

Figure 13.1 SRA, self-recording audiometry.

- the type of test material, e.g. pure tones,[1] noise[2] or speech[3]
- the primary acoustical path, i.e. by air conduction (AC) or bone conduction (BC)
- the mode of coupling of the acoustical source to the individual, i.e. free-field (soundfield) or close coupling (by means of earphones)[4]
- whether it is monoaural or binaural stimulation[5]
- the psychophysical procedure for measuring the threshold, i.e. method of adjustment, method of limits, method of constant stimuli[5]

For the past 100 years, the most widely employed methods for measuring hearing sensitivity have been those using pure tones, almost exclusively by earphone listening.[1,6,7]

In the UK, the Royal Air Force (RAF) conducted the major study ('a thousand ears of subjects between the ages of 18 and 23 years')[8] that was to form the basis for a series of national and international standards (the first was BS 2497:1954; currently BS EN ISO 389–1:2000). Care was taken in selecting the subjects (all men) to ensure that all were clinically otologically normal and able to hear a forced whisper at a distance of 20 feet. Only subjects who had shown an ability to undergo audiometry successfully (using a commercial 5-dB-step audiometer) were accepted. The subjects were then tested at seven frequencies over the range 256–8192 Hz with purpose-designed equipment which had attenuator settings in multiples of 2 dB. The Standard Telephones and Cables type 4026 earphones (probably the best earphones ever produced) were calibrated by the National Physical Laboratory (NPL) on their '3 c-c, Artificial Ear'.[9] The data analysis was restricted to thresholds within a 20-dB band centred on the value of maximum occurrence so that the results would be representative only of subjects with 'normal good hearing'. A quantization error (QE) of 1 dB was not allowed for. The study was such that it was able to detect differences of less than 1 dB between the thresholds of the various skill groups who provided the subjects. A better threshold was demonstrated only for wireless operators and attributed to 'their being accustomed to listening to keyed tones'. Paradoxically, poorer hearing in those who were exposed to potentially hazardous occupational noise levels could not be demonstrated. This was attributed to 'the short time of employment in the trades concerned' (the average age of the whole group was 19.7 years). The RAF did not measure thresholds at 6 kHz. Appreciable unexplained variability had already been noted by that time. Moreover, clinicians had noted that those who have hearing impairment only at very high frequencies (≥6 kHz) do not report speech communication problems.[10] Furthermore, it was argued that if a shift in threshold at 6 kHz had become meaningful and significant, a detectable shift at one or other frequency on either side of 6 kHz would have appeared.

A parallel study by the NPL[9] on 99 otologically normal subjects (45 men, 54 women) extended the upper age limit to 25 years and tested over a broader frequency range (80 Hz to 15 kHz, including 6 kHz). The NPL did not employ separate pretest audiometry, but immediately prior to the 2-dB-step threshold measurement the threshold was determined 'by varying the intensity in 5-dB steps'. The NPL allowed the force of application of the headband to 'range from 350 to 500, averaging about 450 [equivalent to 4.41 N]' (the RAF kept the force constant at 383 g (equivalent to 3.76 N)). The standard (BS 2497:1954) to which these studies gave rise provided for an 'application of the standard earphone to human ears with a force of the order of 500 g weight [equivalent to 4.9 N]'. BS 2497:1992 (technically equivalent to ISO 389: 1991) stated that 'a headband shall be provided to hold the earphone on the human pinna [auricle] with a static force of 4.5 N ± 0.5 N'.

> Standardization
>
> - IEC 60645
> - ISO 389
> - ISO 8253
>
> Calibration

The stringent clinical exclusion criteria, equipment, testing procedure, calibration system and data processing employed by the NPL were identical to those employed by the RAF.

Over the six frequencies (0.5, 1, 2, 3, 4 and 8 kHz), the mean threshold difference between the two studies was 0.0 dB; for the mode it was +0.5 dB.

A subsequent Medical Research Council/Royal Navy (MRC/RN) study[11,12] showed that the thresholds for young men in the RN were essentially the same (after allowing for the QE) as those for their colleagues in the RAF.

The RAF/NPL thresholds were nearer to the best weighted means of a number of laboratory studies of auditory threshold,[4] but around 10 dB lower (more sensitive) than the then US Standard (ASA Z24.5-1951), which was based on a population survey.[13] It was therefore suggested that there existed both laboratory and field 'norms'. An MRC survey of a general rural population with a high yield showed this not to be the case, provided that a correction of 2.5 dB was made for the audiometer's 5-dB attenuator step and 1.5 dB for the learning effect.[14] This accounts for the 4-dB difference between other population studies and the International Reference Zero for audiometers. In retrospect, the use of a 2.5-dB correction for QE represented an overcorrection by 1 dB, since neither the NPL nor the RAF subtracted 1 dB from their data in respect of the use of a 2-dB-step attenuator.

As a result of further work in a number of laboratories,[15–18] the standard reference zero for the calibration of pure tone AC audiometers has undergone several changes over the years. Concern has centred on the frequency of 6 kHz[19] and the TDH 39 earphone.[16,20]

Paralleling studies on the AC threshold, there have been a number of laboratory studies on the BC threshold.[21–25] Consequently, the standard reference zero for the calibration of pure tone BC audiometers (currently BS ISO 389-3:1994) has also undergone changes over the years. BS 6950:1988 (ISO 7566-1987) typically yielded BC thresholds that were about 3–4 dB less acute averaged over 1, 2 and 3 kHz as compared with BS 2497, Part 4: 1972, and about 5–8 dB less acute at 1 kHz in particular, depending on the date of manufacture of the mechanical coupler used for calibration.[26]

Factors influencing the measured threshold

Apart from disorders of the auditory system, a considerable number of factors, including sources of error, have now been identified (Figure 13.2).

At the outset, it is important to know to what standard an audiometer has been calibrated. Moreover, one needs to know how long before and how long after any threshold measurement the calibration had been performed. In the UK, the audiometer should be calibrated by a United Kingdom Accreditation Service (UKAS)-approved laboratory[27] to provide a National Accreditation of Measurement and Sampling (UK) (NAMAS) certificate. The audiometer should be used according to a set procedure (BS EN ISO 8253-1:1998).

SOURCES OF ERROR IN THRESHOLD MEASUREMENTS

- Calibration errors
- Ambient noise
- Earphone placement
- External acoustical meatus collapse
- Personal equations

Change in threshold with age

Ageing processes, of which there are many,[28,29] produce a variety of effects on auditory functioning.[30] A diminution in auditory sensitivity with increasing age is the one effect which

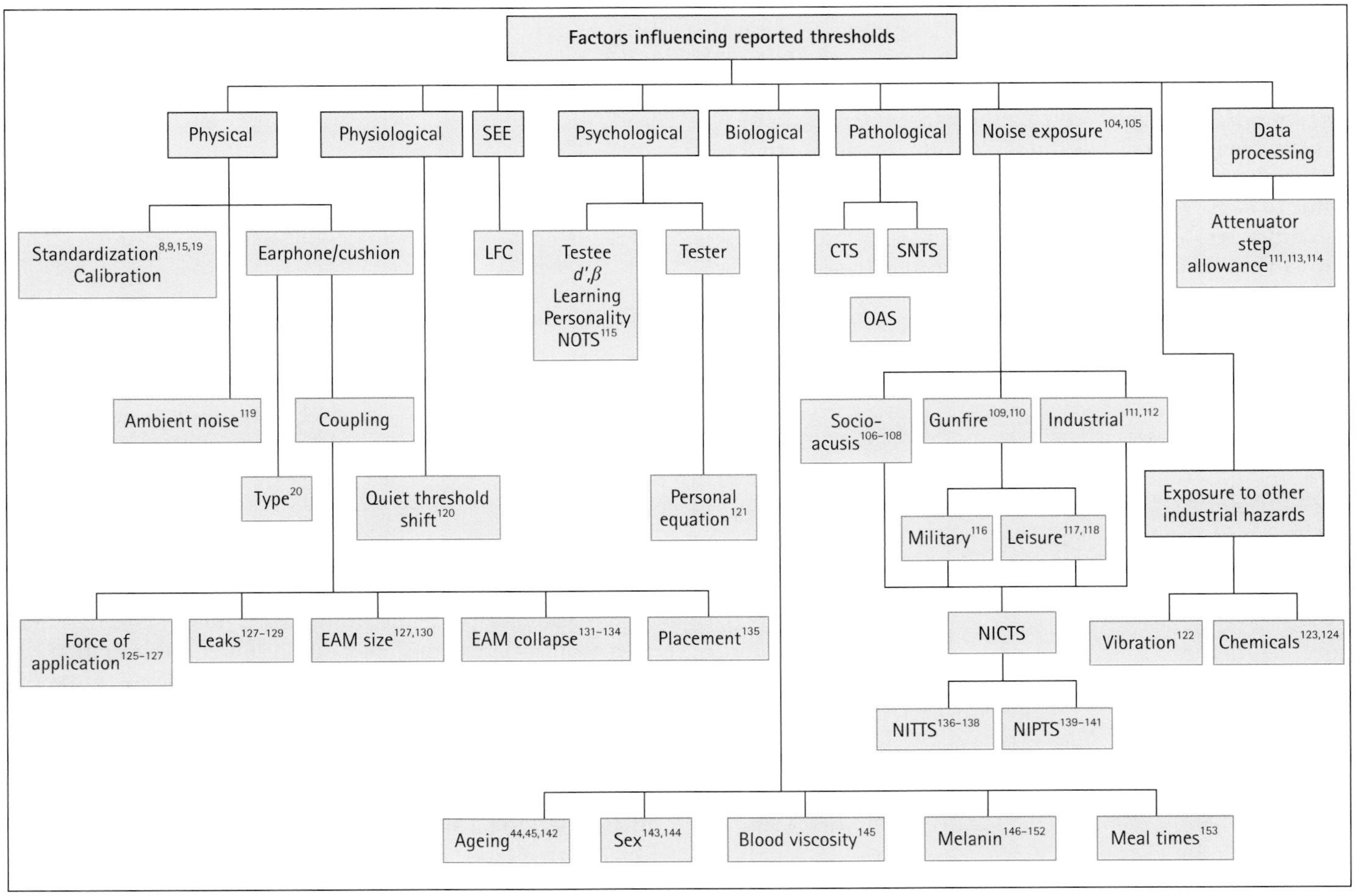

Figure 13.2 Factors affecting measured threshold of hearing. LFC, L-factor complex; CTS, conductive threshold shift; OAS, otological abnormality score; SNTS, sensorineural threshold shift; NICTS, noise-induced compound threshold shift; NITTS, noise-induced temporary threshold shift; NIPTS, noise-induced permanent threshold shift; EAM, external acoustical meatus; SEE, socio-economic-environmental.

dominates all others and which may indeed underlie most other changes.

Despite the plethora of ageing processes, there appear to be systematic changes in the threshold of hearing with increasing age. This may well be because the basic biological process is apoptosis.[31–34] The mathematical expressions used to describe these changes have been exponential functions,[35,36] power functions,[37–39] or polynomials, specifically a second-degree polynomial (parabola).[40] Deviations in the 'oldest old'[41] may well appear because these are what epidemiologists refer to as 'survivor populations'. The latter will be different in different communities.

The parabolic and two of the power function formulations indicate that young adults have the most sensitive hearing, becoming poorer on either side of that peak. This is consistent with measurements of the hearing of young children.[42] However, 16-year-old males[43] have better hearing than 18-year-old males, although the parents of these younger teenagers were 'mostly middle socioeconomic status'. The apparently poorer sensitivity in young children may be due to secondary factors which have masked the basic exponential decay that characterizes apoptotic processes.

Threshold measurements made by the MRC on a random sample of a rural population[44] provided the core of an NPL analysis of epidemiological data in general[45] that was to establish ISO 7029. Figures 13.3–13.5 show that the ISO 7029's values for changes in auditory threshold with age can be fitted very well with exponential equations. This applies equally to those who are more 'susceptible' to ageing processes.

Since ISO 7029 is yoked to the standard reference zero for the calibration of pure tone AC audiometers (currently BS EN ISO 389–1:2000), it will change every time that that standard changes. When the zero-offset effect is taken into account, it would appear that the changes in thresholds with age have remained stationary, in the UK at least, over a period of 30 years.[46]

Epidemiological studies in Jamaica[47] and in Nigeria[48] indicate that melanoderms may have slower deteriorations in thresholds with increasing age than do leucoderms. However, even leucoderms may show differences from one country to another.[49]

Since ISO 389 refers to a point (or series of points) on a function(s) which is defined by ISO 7029, it would have seemed more logical to have defined ISO 389 in terms of the threshold which corresponds to 16 years, 18 years or any other age instead of vice versa.

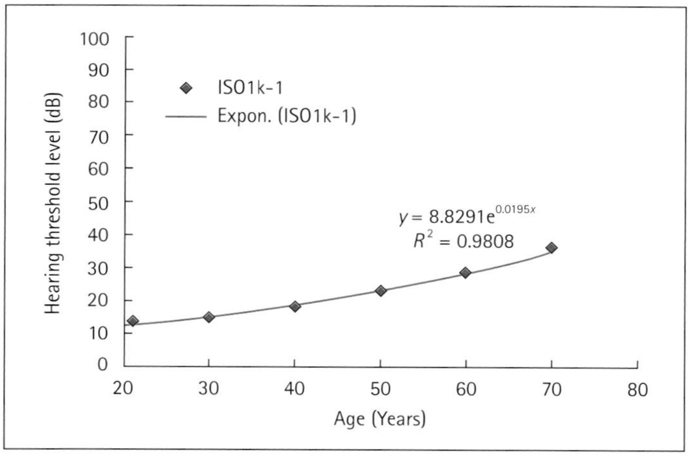

Figure 13.3 Change with age in the 1%ile ('highly susceptible' to ageing) thresholds of hearing at 1 kHz as given by ISO 7029 for men (ISO1k-1); trend line (exponential) fitted. Thus the 'normal' ageing of hearing acuity can be considered as an exponential decay process.

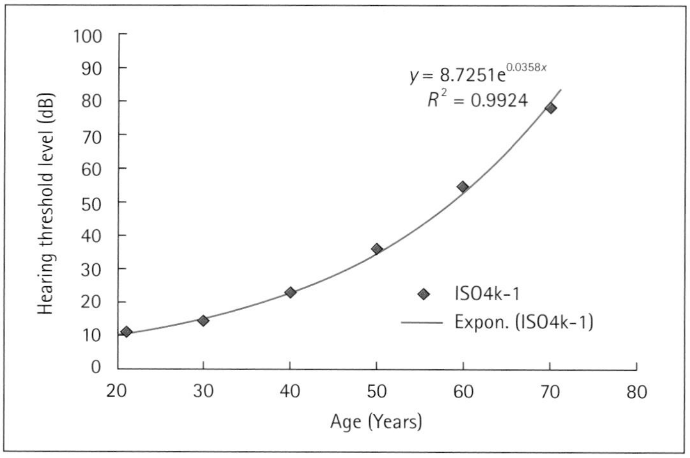

Figure 13.4 Change with age in the 1%ile ('highly susceptible' to ageing) thresholds of hearing at 4 kHz as given by ISO 7029 for men (ISO4k-1); trend line (exponential) fitted. Thus the 'normal' ageing of hearing acuity can be considered as an exponential decay process.

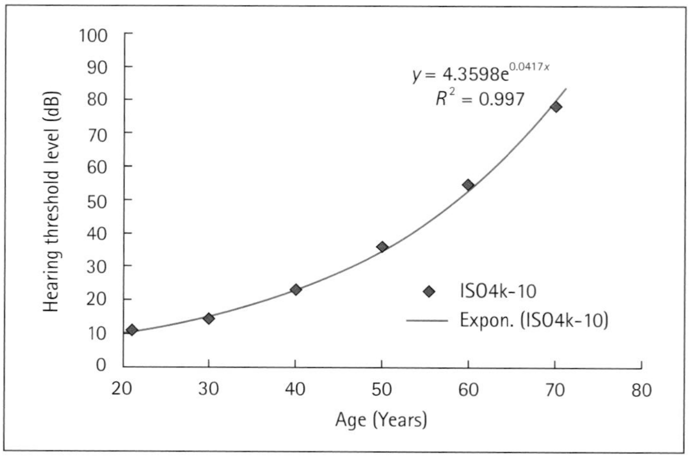

Figure 13.5 Change with age in the 10%ile ('susceptible' to ageing) thresholds of hearing at 4 kHz as given by ISO 7029 for men (ISO4k-10); trend line (exponential) fitted.

Threshold analysis in practice: an example for guidance

An ability to assess threshold of hearing is particularly important in the matter of chronic noise trauma to hearing (occupational noise-induced hearing loss, ONIHL). The condition is characteristically not only asymptomatic but also asemeionic.[50] Moreover, if symptoms are present they are non-specific.[51] The audiogram in cases of alleged or proven chronic noise trauma therefore assumes a particular importance. The English common law appears to have endorsed, at least in the countries of the British Isles, the dictum 'Every decibel counts'.[52] The medical examiner in these countries therefore needs to be able to conduct a more critical analysis of thresholds of hearing than would be required in clinical practice.

INFORMATION REQUIRED FOR THRESHOLD ANALYSIS

- Sex
- Age
- AC Threshold
- BC Threshold
- Cortical electrical response audiometry thresholds

Medical examinations conducted during the course of litigation provide audiometric data that have been acquired in a milieu that is different to that of healthcare practice. Questions arise regarding the appropriateness of comparative data. This has rested primarily on what might be termed the numerical descriptors of historical controls. The epidemiologist would rightly regard these with suspicion. There is a requirement to compare 'like with like'.[53] In the course of 20 years of litigation in the UK in this field, the lawyers have provided us (unwittingly, it would appear) with only one example to which one could apply the principles of evidenced-based medicine. This is in respect of what will be referred to as Factory 'X'.

Broadly speaking, some of the workers in Factory 'X' had been assemblers and had not been exposed to equivalent continuous sound levels in excess of 90 dB(A). 'The limit for continuous exposure to a reasonably steady sound for 8 hours in any one day is that the sound level should not exceed 90 dB(A).'[54] Others had been press operators with exposure to noise levels of, typically, 96 dB(A) (Figure 13.6).

The essential information on the six workers on whom this analysis is based is set out in Table 13.1.

Each of three medical examiners (MX-1, MX-2 and MX-3) had examined the ears clinically and obtained both AC and BC manual audiograms as well as tympanograms on each claimant. MX-2 had examined the acoustical stapedius reflexes also on each of the six.

All the medical examiners' audiograms were obtained over a 3.4-year period after the first audiogram on 30 July 1988. During

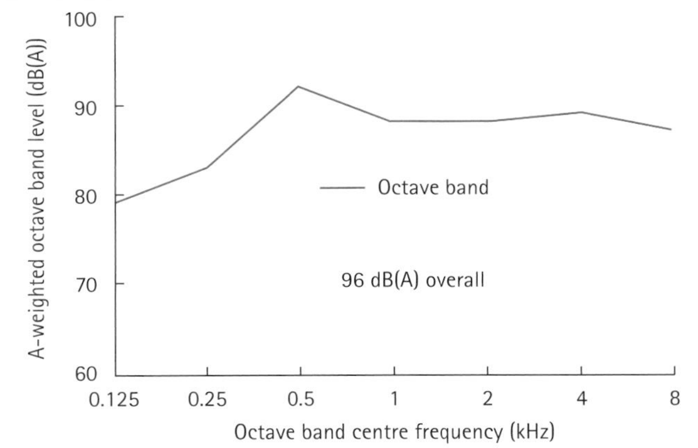

	125 Hz	250 Hz	500 Hz	1 kHz	2 kHz	4 kHz	8 kHz
Octave band	79	83	92	88	88	89	87 db(A)

Figure 13.6 A-weighted octave band noise spectrum of forge press impact noise.[104]

that period, one would ideally have hoped to have found something like the following in a UK examiner's report: 'All audiograms were obtained with a clinical audiometer (make and model) fulfilling the requirements of BS 5966:1980 and calibrated according to BS 2497:1988. The audiometer was fitted with (make and model) earphones with (type) cushions and a (?standard) headband. The reference zero for the bone conduction calibration was that of BS 6950:1988. The headband provided to hold the bone vibrator in position exerted a static force of (giving a value in the range 5.4 ± 0 5 N). The measurements were performed in a sound-insulated booth whose ambient sound levels were lower than those specified in ISO/DIS 8253:1984, thus fulfilling the criteria for threshold measurements at 0 dB HL. The frequency and methods of calibrating (including daily biological calibration) also conformed to that standard.' In the absence of such information, one can only presume (hopefully) that those standards had been adhered to. MX-3 had provided no such information for any of his six reports. MX-1 had stated on each occasion that the 'results were obtained in a quiet room using a diagnostic audiometer recently calibrated to BS 5966.' (Presumably, what he intended to say was 'an audiometer fulfilling the requirements of BS 5966:1980 and calibrated to BS 2497:1988'.) In all cases, MX-2 stated that the audiometric examination 'was performed by an experienced audiological technician in the purposely adapted audiological facilities ... using regularly maintained and calibrated equipment after (duration that claimant had not been exposed to potentially hazardous noise specified) free from noise.'

Each claimant had also been tested in a centre specializing in auditory measurement (CSAM), where cortical electrical response audiometry (CERA) was performed and a fourth air conduction audiogram obtained. Békésy audiometry was not performed on any occasion.

Having regard to the number of tests conducted and the frequencies tested, more than 600 measurements had thus been performed. These data form the basis for this analysis.

Table 13.1 Data on six claimants, three of whom (F65, M56, F35) had been exposed to noise levels of 96 dB (A) and were subject to a court hearing, and three of whom (F44, F42, M36) had been exposed to noise levels not exceeding 90 dB(A) and were not subject to a court hearing; the latter three served as controls.

ID	Sex	Age at I[a]	Age at II[b]	Age at III[c]	Age at IV[d]	L_{eq}[e]	T[f]	TNIL[g]
F65	F	23.4	24.2	26.2	26.3	96	1.5	97.8
M56	M	32.4	33.2	35.1	35.3	96	5.0	103.0
F35	F	53.4	54.5	56.0	56.3	96	5.0	103.0
F44	F	44.1	45.3	46.6	47.2	84		
F42	F	45.9	46.6	48.5	48.7	84		
M36	M	52.1	53.0	55.4	55.5	90		

It may well be said that even this control group was exposed to L_{eq}s in excess of the 71 dB(A) which a Health and Safety Executive (UK) report[154] indicates is the level at which noise starts to become hazardous. A gradient should nevertheless be discernible in the L_{eq}/hearing sensitivity (acuity) relationship. All six workers lived in the same geographical area, were exposed to the same economic, environmental and social factors, and the same factory conditions (apart from the level of noise exposure). None of the claimants were albinos or melanoderms, factors which might have influenced the hearing.[146–152] All were also (at least initially) pursuing an action for damage to their hearing. All six had been examined by the same three medical examiners (MX-1, MX-2 and MX-3), in the same sequence and separated by about the same intervals of time. Each examiner had examined each subject in the same place and, it would appear, with the same equipment. The only difference was that the average age of the first group was 37.6 years, and that of the second group 48.6 years (a difference of 11 years); the age range of the total group was 30 years. For the audiometric analyses, age corrections could be (and were) made to measured hearing threshold levels using ISO 7029-1984. Age adjustments were made to take into account the various times of the hearing tests. During the court hearing, Counsel for the three plaintiffs announced that the claimants were an unselected group (or words to that effect). There was therefore no reason to suspect any sampling bias.

[a]Age when examined by first medical examiner.

[b]Age when examined by second medical examiner.

[c]Age when examined by third medical examiner.

[d]Age when tested in centre specializing in auditory measurements.

[e]Equivalent continuous sound level of factory noise to which they were exposed.

[f]Duration in years for which worker was exposed to that noise.

[g]Total noise immission level for corresponding worker.

Based on the CSAM's pure tone audiograms, none of the six would have been considered to be deaf,[55] or to have a disabling hearing impairment,[56] a material impairment,[57] or a hearing loss.[58] None reached the threshold of hearing inability[59] or the 'handicap' level of the British Standard (BS 5330). All had normal hearing threshold levels[54] at all frequencies in both ears, except for one man (M36) and one woman (F65) who had one frequency in one or other ear where the age-corrected threshold exceeded 20 dB HTL. (The age-corrected level was 24.1 dB at 8 kHz in the right ear, and 24.7 dB at 6 kHz in the left ear of the man; and 29.2 dB at 6 kHz in the left ear of the woman.)

Figure 13.7 indicates that there was some degree or other of non-organic threshold shift (NOTS). This did not appear to be systematic (Figures 13.8 and 13.9).

There was no difference in thresholds between the 96-dB(A) exposed group and a control group (Figure 13.10).

The age-adjusted CERA thresholds for the two groups straddled the thresholds for young UK manual workers (Figure 13.13).

MX-2 reported that one of the six claimants was 'an inconsistent audiological subject' and another was 'slightly inconsistent'; in the report of a third claimant, there appeared the words 'suggests the hearing loss in the low tones which appears rather severe may be a little better …'. After age adjustments and comparison with the manual pure tone thresholds obtained by CSAM (and so confirmed as genuine), these three 'suspicious' responders had consistently poorer thresholds at all frequencies tested than the non-suspicious responders. The four frequency average (FFA) difference was 6.7 dB. Neither MX-1 nor MX-3 (nor their technicians) noted anything untoward in the audiometric responses of any of the claimants. Nevertheless, their threshold data showed the same separation when the analysis was performed on the basis of MX-2's classification. The accuracy of the measurements performed by MX-2's technician was supported by comparison with the manual pure tone audiometric thresholds obtained by the CSAM audiometer operator. The mean FFA (age-adjusted) of the non-suspicious responders as measured by MX-2's technician was 1.04 dB with respect to the

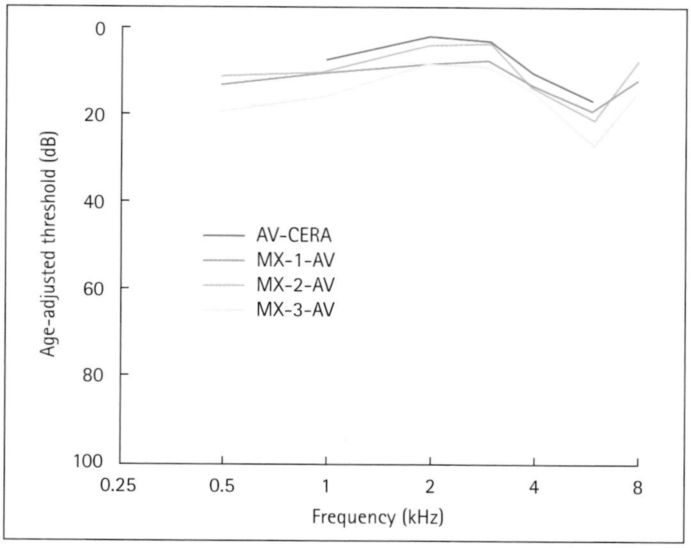

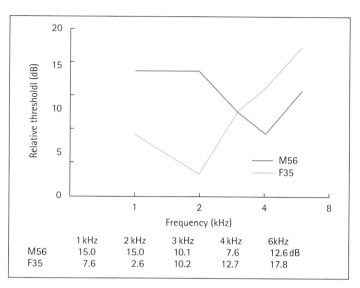

Figure 13.7 Interexaminer variability. The mean thresholds for the six ears of the noise-exposed group which apply to the three medical examiners are shown together with the mean CERA thresholds for comparison. All three examiners report thresholds which are consistently poorer than the CERA thresholds, and to varying degrees. All thresholds have been age-adjusted (appropriate to sex) using ISO 7029.

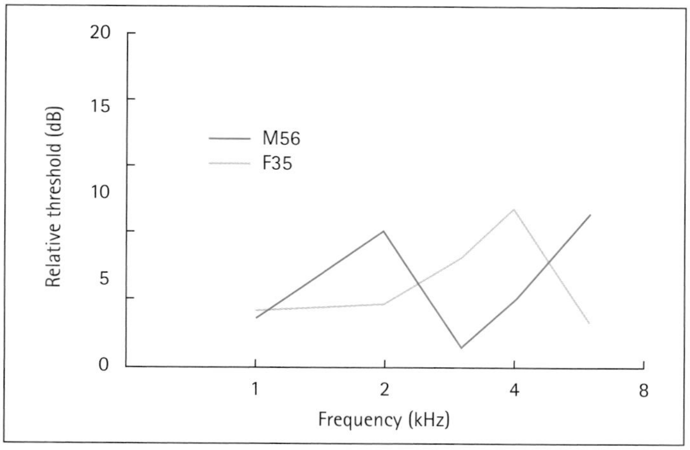

Figure 13.8 Hearing thresholds of two claimants (M56 and F35) reported by MX-1 expressed with respect to thresholds recorded by CERA; thresholds reported by MX-1 were adjusted (using ISO 7029) to the age when CERA was performed. Although all differences are positive, there does not appear to be any systematic trend; these age-adjusted thresholds are the average levels for the two ears.

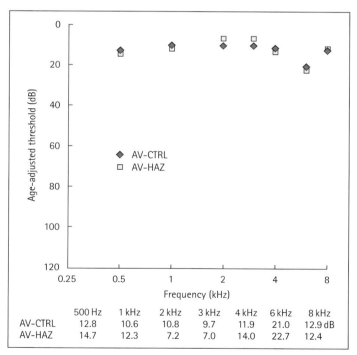

mean CSAM threshold. The latter would have been about (CERA was not conducted at 500 Hz) −1.35 dB with respect to the corresponding CERA threshold. Hence the MX-2 technician's measurements were 0.31 dB (FFA) better than CERA. On this basis, it could well be argued that the MX-2 technician provided the most accurate threshold measurements in the entire case.

The NOTS theme is developed in Figures 13.12–13.16. The term 'non-organic' does not necessarily imply that such

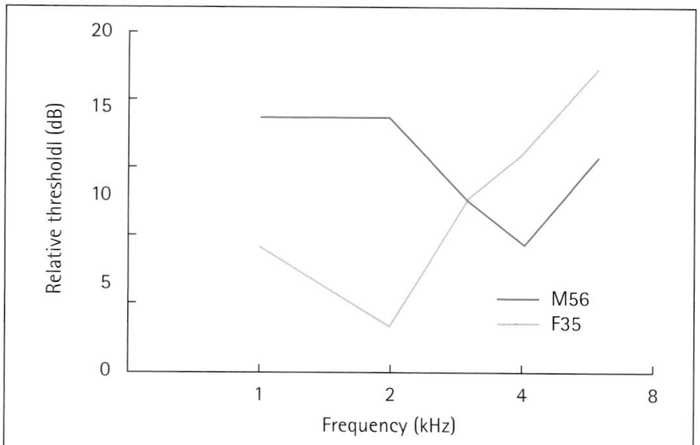

	1 kHz	2 kHz	3 kHz	4 kHz	6kHz
M56	15.0	15.0	10.1	7.6	12.6 dB
F35	7.6	2.6	10.2	12.7	17.8

Figure 13.9 Hearing thresholds of two claimants (M56 and F35) reported by MX-3 expressed with respect to thresholds recorded by CERA; thresholds reported by MX-3 were adjusted (using ISO 7029) to the age when CERA was performed. Although all differences are positive, there does not appear to be any systematic trend; these age-adjusted thresholds are the average levels of the two ears.

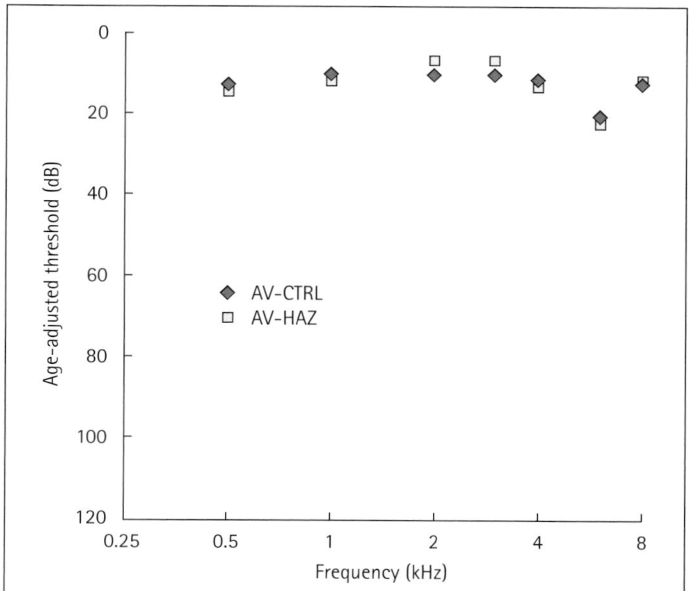

	500 Hz	1 kHz	2 kHz	3 kHz	4 kHz	6 kHz	8 kHz
AV-CTRL	12.8	10.6	10.8	9.7	11.9	21.0	12.9 dB
AV-HAZ	14.7	12.3	7.2	7.0	14.0	22.7	12.4

Figure 13.10 The mean manually determined AC hearing threshold levels (HTLs) (after the fiftieth centile ISO 7029 values for the age appropriate to the sex had been subtracted) for both ears of three factory workers who had been exposed to potentially hazardous noise levels (AV-HAZ), and for both ears of three factory workers who had been exposed to noise levels which were not considered to be hazardous (AV-CTRL); there was one man and two women in each group; these thresholds are the means for those measured by three examiners, i.e. three audiograms on each ear.

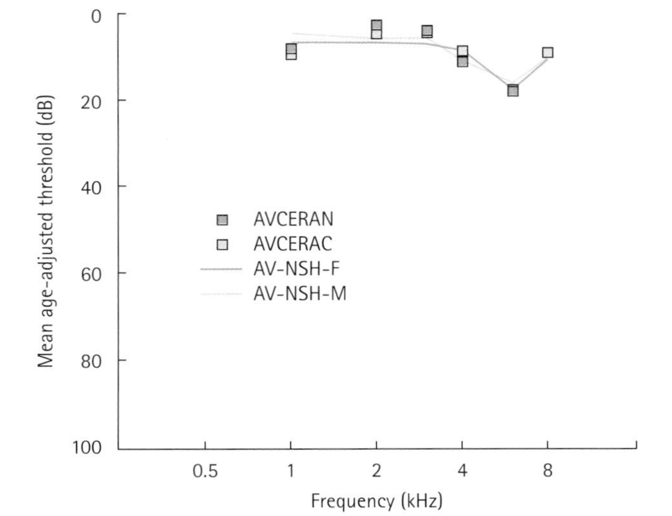

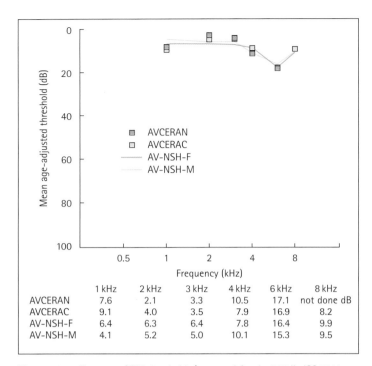

	1 kHz	2 kHz	3 kHz	4 kHz	6 kHz	8 kHz
AVCERAN	7.6	2.1	3.3	10.5	17.1	not done dB
AVCERAC	9.1	4.0	3.5	7.9	16.9	8.2
AV-NSH-F	6.4	6.3	6.4	7.8	16.4	9.9
AV-NSH-M	4.1	5.2	5.0	10.1	15.3	9.5

Figure 13.11 The mean CERA thresholds (corrected for the 50%ile ISO 7029 values which relate to the appropriate sex and age) for both ears of three workers in factory 'X' who had been exposed to 96 dB(A) for a period of $1\frac{1}{2}$–5 years (AVCERAN). Comparison with thresholds for three other workers in the same factory whose noise exposure was not considered to be potentially hazardous (AVCERAC). AV-NSH-F = mean HTLs for 18–30-year-old manual female workers with no previous hazardous noise exposure and with no audiometric evidence for middle ear malfunction (Table 538 in reference 142); AV-NSH-M = mean HTLs for 18–30-year-old manual male workers with no previous hazardous noise exposure and with no audiometric evidence for middle ear malfunction (Table 540 in reference 143). In each case, the mean is the average value for the two ears. Adjusting the claimants' mean threshold for the 2.45 dB element of conductive threshold shift and the gunfire element at 4 kHz (see later) would show the claimants to have a better basic sensorineural hearing sensitivity than their counterparts in the general population of the UK.

threshold shifts (TS) are due entirely to conscious exaggeration on the part of the subject. They could well be due to factors in the domain of the audiometer operator. The ephemeral nature of the 6-kHz notch suggests that poor placement of the earphone or undetected external acoustical meatus (EAM) collapse might be responsible.

Figure 13.17 points to gunfire as a factor influencing thresholds at 4 kHz.

Figures 13.18 and 13.19 show that hazardous occupational noise exposure cannot be implicated in any TS.

Nine of the 12 ears had clinical (structural and/or functional) or acoustical impedance evidence for some degree or other of conductive hearing impairment. Support for a conductive component was forthcoming from an analysis of the air–bone gap (ABG) (Figures 13.20 and 13.21). The authenticity of the ABG might well be questioned on the grounds that the AC threshold has already been shown to be contaminated with NOTS. However, it is likely that all the biases

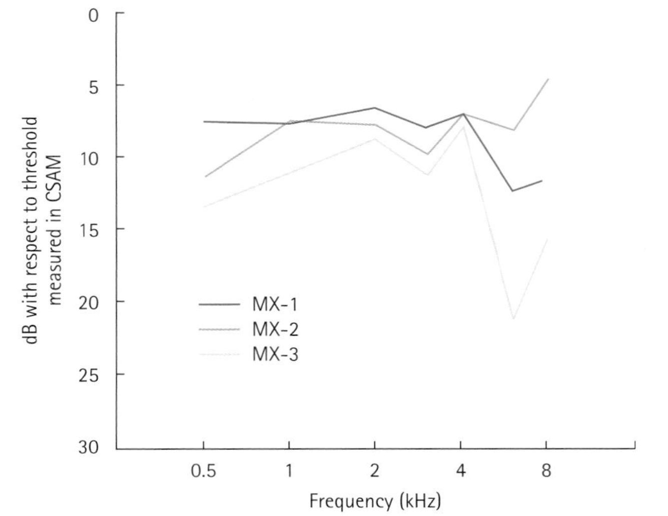

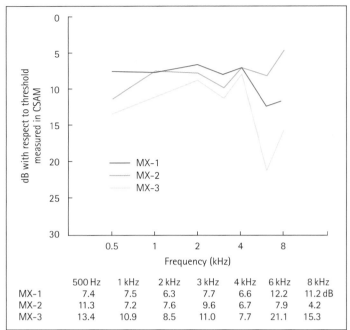

	500 Hz	1 kHz	2 kHz	3 kHz	4 kHz	6 kHz	8 kHz
MX-1	7.4	7.5	6.3	7.7	6.6	12.2	11.2 dB
MX-2	11.3	7.2	7.6	9.6	6.7	7.9	4.2
MX-3	13.4	10.9	8.5	11.0	7.7	21.1	15.3

Figure 13.12 Factory 'X': mean auditory thresholds for the 'suspicious' audiometric responders for each medical examiner with respect to thresholds for that group reported by a CSAM using manual audiometry with confirmation that these were genuine by CERA. 'Suspicious' categorization based on report by MX-2 of some inconsistency. The enhancement of the 6-kHz notching is not what one would expect if these non-organic shifts were to be attributed to the subject latching onto equal-loudness contours; 6-kHz notch enhancement must therefore reside in the examination (? external auditory meatus collapse). The values have been corrected for age differences between the time when seen by the medical examiner and the CSAM.

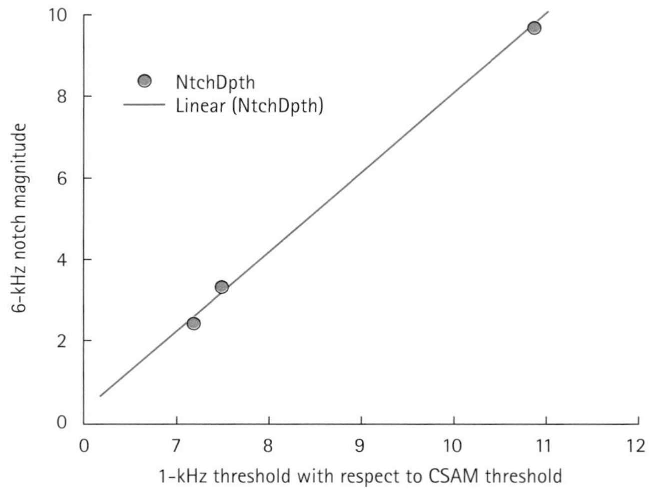

Figure 13.13 Factory 'X': notch magnitude as a function of overall auditory sensitivity (using the threshold at 1 kHz as an indicant) for the three claimants in 'the 'suspicious responding' group (averages for the two ears). This picture of increasing notch magnitude as a function of overall auditory sensitivity is not what one would expect if the 6-kHz thresholds were also being influenced primarily by exaggeration on the part of the claimants.

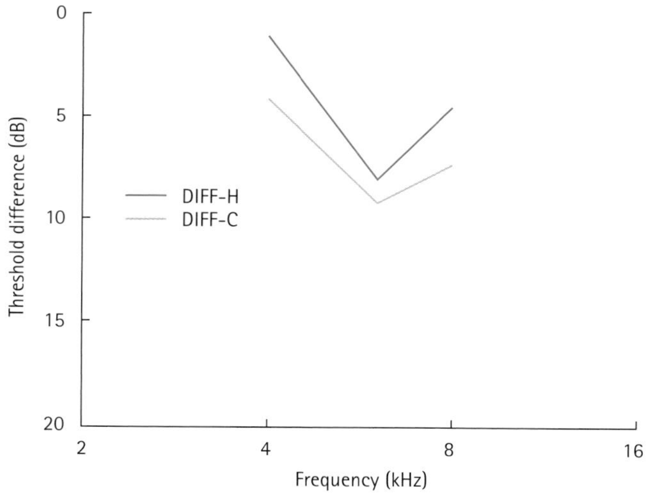

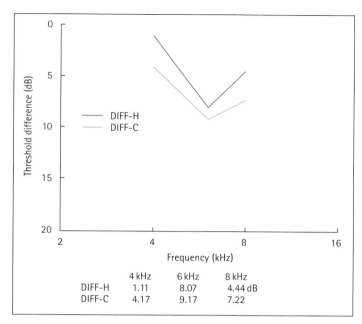

	4 kHz	6 kHz	8 kHz
DIFF-H	1.11	8.07	4.44 dB
DIFF-C	4.17	9.17	7.22

Figure 13.14 The graphical presentation concentrates on the area of interest, i.e. 6 kHz. DIFF-H = Difference between the means of the HLs which had been reported by the three medical examiners (at mean age 37.6 years) and the means of the levels reported by a CSAM (at mean age of 39.3 years). (Data for the workers who had been exposed to equivalent continuous sound levels of 96 dB(A).) DIFF-C = Difference between the means of the HLs which had been reported by the three medical examiners (at mean age of 48.6 years) and the means of the levels reported by a CSAM (at mean age of 50.5 years). (Data for the workers who had been exposed to equivalent continuous sound levels of less than 90 dB(A).) The similarity of the effect (improvement in threshold) in the two groups would oppose an attribution to a resolution of an occupational noise-induced temporary threshold shift. One or other worker in each group had had some weapons noise exposure, but this had not been for the last 10 years. Thus an attribution of the 6-kHz notching to a resolution of a weapons noise-induced temporary threshold shift cannot be countenanced either.

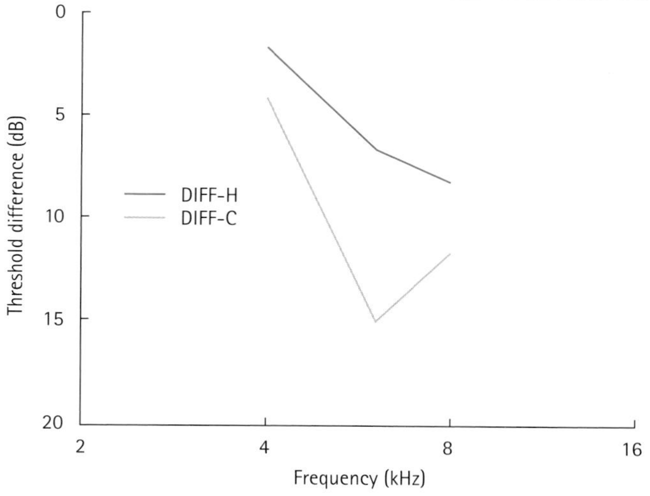

	4 kHz	6 kHz	8 kHz
DIFF-H	1.67	6.67	8.33 dB
DIFF-C	4.17	15.00	11.67

Figure 13.15 This graphical presentation concentrates on the area of interest, i.e. 6 kHz. Change (a deterioration in threshold) from the second (MX2) to the third (MX3) examiner. DIFF-H = Difference between the means of HLs which had been reported by MX-2 (at mean age of group 37.3 years) and MX-3 1.8 years later. (Data for the workers who had been exposed to equivalent continuous sound levels of 96 dB(A).) DIFF-C = Difference between the means of HLs which had been reported by MX-2 (at mean age of group 48.3 years) and MX-3 1.9 years later. (Data for the workers who had been exposed to equivalent and continuous sound levels of less than 90 dB(A).) The greater effect in the control group would oppose attributing the growth of the 6 kHz notching to the development or progression of an occupational noise-induced threshold shift. Moreover, all three workers who had previously been exposed to 96 dB(A) were wearing hearing protection over the period when examined by MX-2 and MX-3. One or other worker in each group had had some weapons noise exposure, but this had not been for at least 10 years. The effect is not of a pattern which would be attributed to exaggeration by the claimants. The effect must lie in the domain of the examiners (hence the classification in Figure 13.16).

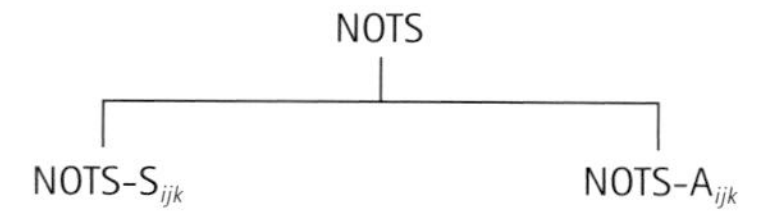

Figure 13.16 Classification of NOTS. NOTS-S_{ijk} denotes NOTS associated with subject *i* at frequency *j* on test *k*; similarly, NOTS-A_{ijk} denotes NOTS associated with audiometrician *i* at frequency *j* on test *k*. Separation of these various components is difficult, but Békésy audiometry can help in detecting and demonstrating NOTS-S.

arising in the domain of the tester and of the testee which had affected the AC measurements would have affected the BC measurements also. The technician would have been the same and the BC test would most likely have been conducted immediately after the AC test.

THRESHOLD COMPONENTS

- Age-associated threshold shift
- Non-organic threshold shift
- Conductive threshold shift
- Sensorineural threshold shift
  - Nosoacusis
  - Noise-induced compound threshold shift
    - Noise-induced permanent threshold shift
      - Socioacusis
      - Gunfire
      - Occupational
- Quantization error
- L-factor complex

This analysis produces an apportionment of threshold which is shown in Table 13.2.

Note that this approach to the analysis is an extension of that adopted by the NPL in analysing thresholds within the normal range.[19] The analysis does not depend on the

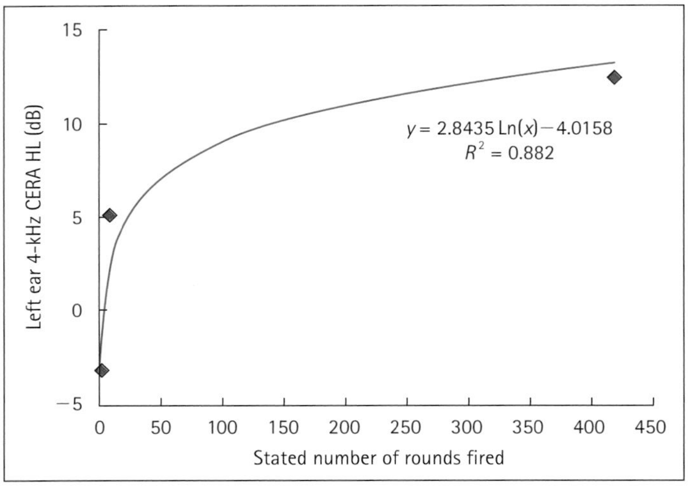

Figure 13.17 Factory 'X'. Correlation between threshold reported for CERA at 4 kHz in the left ear and number of rounds of ammunition fired. Data are for the three workers ('A', 'B' and 'C') among the six who had fired guns. 'A' had fired 3 times, 'B' 9 times, and 'C' 420 times; all had fired from the right shoulder. 'A' and 'B' had also both been exposed to potentially hazardous factory noise with an equivalent continuous sound level of 96 dB(A) for 5 years. All CERA thresholds had been adjusted using ISO 7029 for age-associated TS appropriate to the sex.

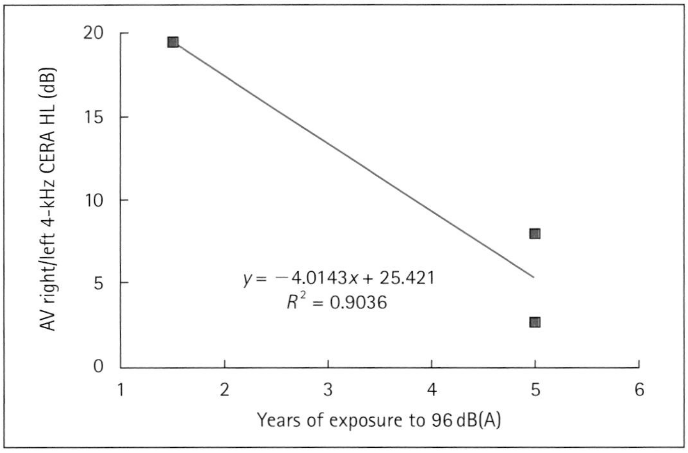

Figure 13.18 Factory 'X'. Correlation between threshold reported for CERA at 4 kHz (average for the two ears) and number of years of exposure to an equivalent continuous sound level of 96 dB(A). Data are for three workers ('D', 'B' and 'C') who had been exposed to this sound level. HTLs for 'B' and 'C', who had been exposed for 5 years, have been adjusted for the use of firearms using a regression equation derived from the data. The interpretation of this graph is that the longer the exposure to this potentially hazardous noise, the better the hearing. This graph therefore fails to confirm the positive gradient that would be needed to implicate industrial noise and exposure as a factor influencing HTL in this group. The thresholds had been adjusted for the use of firearms by 'B' and 'C', both of whom had been exposed to 96 dB(A) of noise for 5 years.

Table 13.2 Composition of measured FFA (500 Hz, 1 kHz, 2 kHz and 4 kHz) threshold of the Factor 'X' workers.

Factor	How determined	Magnitude
NOTS	PTA-CERA	6.24 dB
AATS	ISO 7029	6.19
QE	Half of audiometer attenuator step	2.50
CTS	AC−BC	2.40
Gunfire	Regression equation	0.60
ONITS	Residual TS	0.00
LFC	Residual TS	0.00
Overall threshold		17.93

The calculated threshold shift (17.93 dB) agrees well with the measured threshold shift of 17.87 dB; NOTS, non-organic threshold shift; AATS, age-associated threshold shift; CTS, conductive threshold shift; QE, quantization error; ONITS, occupational noise-induced threshold shift; PTA, manual pure tone audiogram; CERA, cortical evoked response audiogram; ISO 7029, International Specification for the threshold of hearing by air conduction as a function of age and sex for otologically normal persons; AC, air conduction threshold of hearing; BC, bone conduction threshold of hearing; TS, threshold shift; LFC, L-factor complex[73] refers to the aggregate of all the social, economic and environmental factors which affect the threshold of hearing,[142,155] it may have a value anywhere in the range 0–6.[156]

application, or even the validity, of any formula. It does not depend on the validity of the noise immission level (NIL) or other principle or of how noise-induced threshold shifts and age-associated threshold shift interact. It generates its own model.

It may well be pointed out that a clinician's diagnosis is a pattern-recognition exercise.[60–62] One would therefore have expected the examiners to have noted that the audiometric pictures which they obtained were those of EAM collapse (Figure 13.22). None had commented on this and asked their technicians to repeat the audiogram with a stent in place. We shall therefore never know to what extent the apparent impairment of high-frequency hearing with its 6 kHz notching can be attributed to this artefact. It may be pointed out that we have already accounted for the measured thresholds (Table 13.2). There is nothing more to explain. However, any EAM collapse would have been accommodated under NOTS-A in that table. But CERA thresholds are also not immune from being affected by EAM collapse.

The finding that three out of six claimants were exaggerating is consistent with US reports that '25–40% of claims for deafness have a significant amount of NOHL in them'.[63] An even higher proportion would be expected if the amount might not be considered to be 'significant' for the individual and the NOTS not sufficient to amount to an NOHL. Medical examiners need to be more vigilant in detecting spurious thresholds; this is particularly so when one considers that there is a 0.6 probability that there is no 'underlying organic element' in these cases.[63]

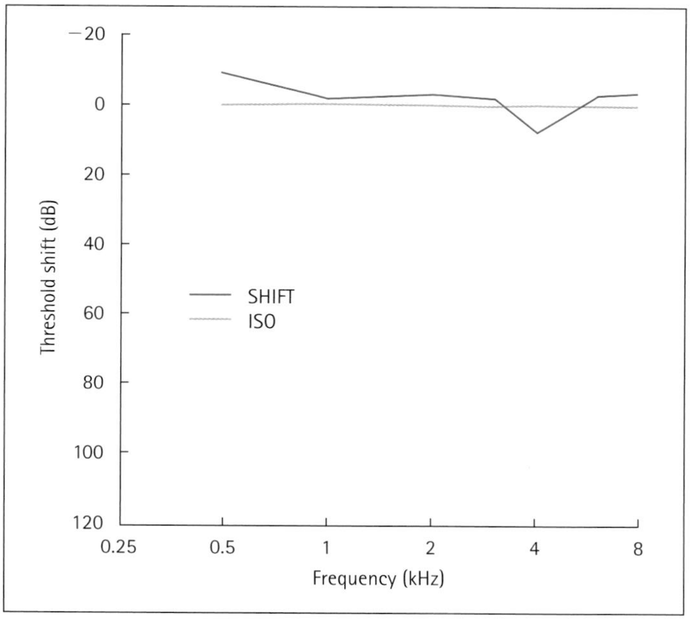

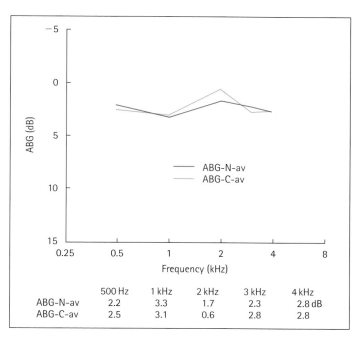

Figure 13.19 F65: shift in manually determined AC threshold from 24.6 years of age to 26.3 years of age (averages for the right and left ears). The threshold at 24.6 years of age was the mean for three manually determined AC HTLs recorded by three experienced examiners. The manually determined AC HTLs at 26.3 years of age were obtained on the same day as CERA was done. ISO indicates the shift in the 50th centile of ISO 7029 between 24.6 and 26.3 years of age. The data indicate that, over the 1.7-year period from the ages of 24.6 years to 26.3 years, there had been a deterioration, averaged for the two ears, of 7.5 dB at 4 kHz and 2.5 dB at 6 kHz (or more if we take into account what appears to have been a baseline shift of 2 dB). This pattern is consistent with the course of occupational noise-induced damage to hearing. However, F65 said that earmuffs had been worn over the period in question, beginning 2 months prior to the first examination, when a normal non-notched audiogram had been recorded on one side (occupational noise-induced damage to hearing affects both ears). The expected real-world sound attenuation for earmuffs is 20 dB. The equivalent continuous sound level applying to the period in question would therefore have been (96 − 20) = 76 dB(A). Redundancy had occurred 7 weeks prior to the third examination.

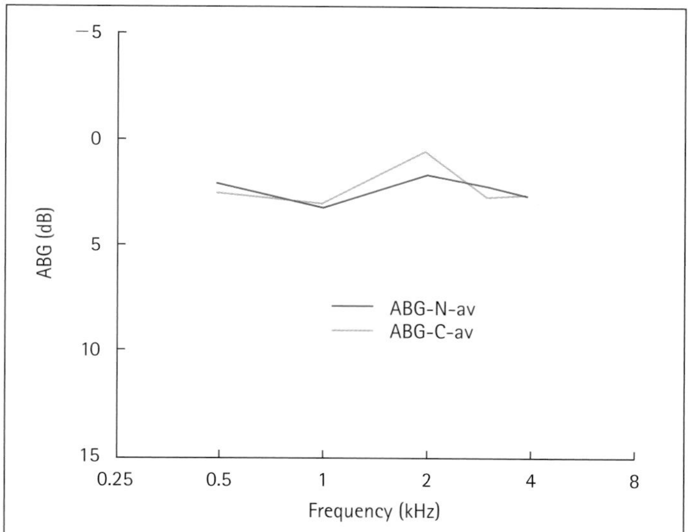

	500 Hz	1 kHz	2 kHz	3 kHz	4 kHz
ABG-N-av	2.2	3.3	1.7	2.3	2.8 dB
ABG-C-av	2.5	3.1	0.6	2.8	2.8

Figure 13.20 Mean ABGs of the manually determined air and bone conduction HTLs for both ears of the three unselected noise-exposed claimants (ABG-N-av) and of the three control subjects (ABG-C-av) (three audiograms done on each ear of each factory worker); the average ABG for the noise-exposed claimants is 2.5 dB, and for the controls 2.4 dB. These conductive TSs reflect the residua of childhood middle ear disease, so that they would have been there before adult employments. The effect of the 2.5 dB on the 96 dB(A) noise exposure would be to reduce the effective level to 93.5 dB(A).

Békésy audiometry or CERA may not be available to the examiner to validate manual pure tone audiometric thresholds. There are, however, tests which can be performed with manual audiometers to verify thresholds[64,65] or even used as the method of choice for manual audiometry.[66] If medical examiners find that they have a poor detection rate for NOTS, they should employ these tests routinely.

Six-kilohertz notches have many causes.[67] Medical examiners need to bear this in mind. They should avoid using TDH39 earphones; if they have already done so, the earphones should be calibrated using an artificial ear complying with IEC 60318-1 instead of using an IEC 60318-3 coupler.

The analysis shows that the measurement of BC thresholds is important. Care needs to be exercised in doing so. The Rinne is too insensitive a test, particularly with the 512-Hz tuning fork[68,69] used to analyse thresholds which are within the range or normality. Only one examiner had used the more sensitive Bing test,[69,70] and then not consistently.

In some factories, as here, gunfire exposure may be more important than factory noise exposure.[10]

One might have expected $1\frac{1}{2}$ of the 3 cases to have had an occupational noise-induced permanent threshold shift.[71] Zero out of three is not significantly different from $1\frac{1}{2}$ out of 3.

This analysis serves as a cautionary tale for medical examiners in the UK, lest they fall for the logical fallacy of *post hoc, ergo propter hoc*. Science is not an extension of common sense; much is counter-intuitive and unexpected.[72]

The lawyers withdrew the controls. The claims of F65, M56 and F35 were heard in court. The judge accepted the evidence of MX-1 and MX-3 that these three claimants suffered noise-induced hearing loss as a result of their exposure to the 96-dB(A) industrial noise. He castigated those who said otherwise. This is a salutary lesson for all who would dare sail into the unchartable and shark-infested waters of litigation.

Formulae

As well as the formulae which have been mentioned above in respect of age changes in threshold, a number of other formulae have appeared which incorporate the effects of noise and other

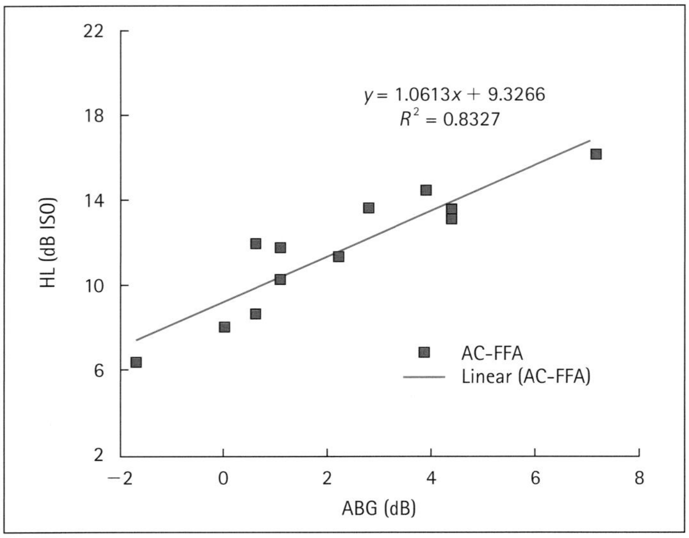

Figure 13.21 Dependence of AC threshold on ABG; ABG is the mean air–bone gap (the AC threshold less the BC threshold) in decibels over the frequencies 0.5, 1 and 2 kHz; AC-FFA is the four frequency (0.5, 1, 2 and 4 kHz) average HTL corrected for the ageing factor usig ISO 7029. Data are from the manual AC and BC audiograms obtained by three medical examiners on the ears of the six factory workers. This analysis shows that, after accounting for ageing effects, 83% of the variation in the workers' overall hearing acuity (sensitivity) is accounted for by the magnitude of the ABG, i.e. factors related to middle ear malfunction. At zero ABG, the equation gives an FFA AC HTL of 9.33 dB. Correction of this value for NOTS (6.24 dB), QE (2.50 dB) and gunfire (0.60 dB) gives an FFA of −0.01 dB (BS EN ISO 389). The overall hearing sensitivity of the six workers can therefore be explained without recourse to postulating the influence of other factors, such as occupational noise-induced damage to hearing.

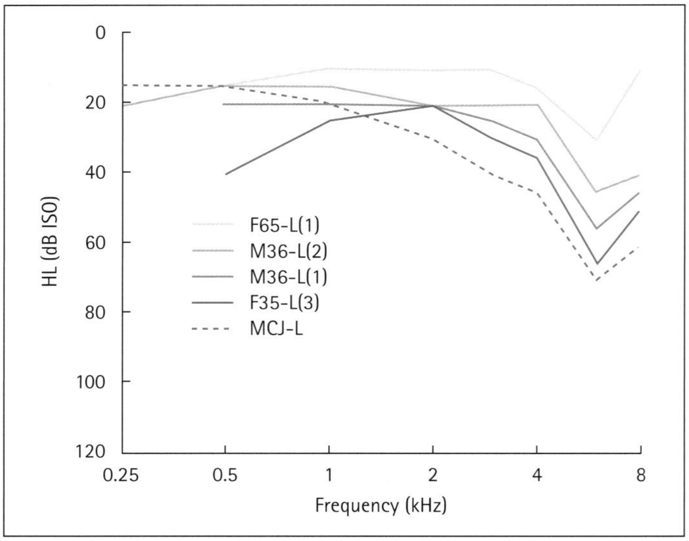

Figure 13.22 Manually determined AC thresholds for the left ears of F65, M36, M36 and F35 as reported by MX-1, MX-2, MX-1 and MX-3, respectively, compared to the similarly determined thresholds for the left ear of a 19-year-old man (MCJ) who had a spurious hearing loss due to close of the EAM occasioned by the pressure of the audiometer earphone on the auricle.[133] This phenomenon is not an all-or-none effect. It exists in varying degrees which exhibit a family of curves to which these audiograms appear to conform. The audiograms were not repeated with a tubular insert in place,[132,133] or the thresholds re-determined with soundfield audiometry.[135] It will therefore never be known to what extent the phenomenon contributed to the TS reported by these examiners. In the current analysis, it would have been included in the category of NOTS-A_{ijk} (Figure 13.16). By the time these factory workers were tested, the phenomenon had been known to British otology for over half a century.[131] BC threshold measurements are insufficiently accurate at 6 kHz to be helpful in the detection of meatal collapse. The above pattern 'mimics the type of impairment often associated with small-arms noise. The left ear is more affected than the right in a man who fires from the right shoulder, and maximum effect at 6000 Hz is usual with this type of noise'.[133] This is in contrast to ONIHL, where the maximum effect is at 4 kHz.[141] Both M36 and F35 had fired guns. It might therefore just as well be claimed that the 6 kHz notching in those cases was attributable to gunfire exposure.

factors.[73] The bearing that these have on the medical examiner's report has been discussed previously.[74]

Audiometry

The special tests employed to measure the threshold of hearing in clinical practice are referred to collectively as *audiometry*.[1,7,84] The electro-acoustic instruments used for this purpose are termed *audiometers*.

In a number of papers Stephens[6,157,158] has traced the development of audiometers since Hughes'[159] invention in 1879.

Around a hundred years ago audiometers were being introduced not only into the UK but also into other countries.[157,160,161]

The first audiometer was enthusiastically accepted by the doctor who should be considered to have been the first audiological physician.[162] Otology in the USA was later to be enthusiastic about the Western Electric 1A audiometer.[163] However, even later, Otology in the UK was less than enthusiastic: 'They [the earphones of audiometers] have the following disadvantages: ... They exert different degrees of pressure on the cartilage, and if this is excessive the tragus may be displaced so that the full sound does not reach the meatus [now referred to as 'external acoustic meatus collapse', or just 'canal collapse', and a recognised source of spurious high tone audiometric notches, e.g. Coles,[133] Mahoney and Luxon.[164]]. If the pressure is insufficient there may be a leakage of sound and an inaccurate result in testing' [since confirmed: Erber[127] (at p 15). The report concluded: 'As oscillometers, the present audiometers are scientifically accurate. It is in their application to clinical otology that they have failed, in that results obtained differ from those obtained from tuning forks. The results of testing by tuning forks have been for many years, and still are, the standard in otology, and until audiometers give results directly comparable with them, they cannot be accepted as a standard means of testing. New methods must evolve from existing knowledge, and the Committee considers that future methods of testing must be based on the old-established tests by tuning forks' (at p 15).[131]

This report has neither been revoked nor amended. No other report has dealt with the clinical examination of hearing in such detail. The committee had been advised by an eminent physicist (Sir William Bragg*).

There was no official acceptance of audiometers in the UK until a 1947 Medical Research Council report.[165]

The data obtained by audiometric testing are usually presented graphically as *audiograms*. Such graphs were constructed initially, as one would expect from engineers and scientists, with the horizontal axis setting out the frequency and the vertical axis setting out the signal sound intensity[166] or pressure.[167] Both co-ordinates were on a logarithmic scale.Until the mid 20th century it was held that the subjective magnitude of a sensation varied as the logarithm of the physical magnitude of that stimulus (Weber-Fechner Law).[5] This scientific graphic presentation[168, 169] can reflect different audiometric patterns in different disorders just as well as the present convention.

The explanation for the change in audiogram format is given by Davis and Silverman: 'When the famous Western Electric Company 2A audiometer was designed in the Bell Telephone Laboratories in the early 1920s, a basic decision was made concerning the reference zero level. An obvious choice fom the engineering point of view would have been the dyne per square centimeter [the *pascal* is now the unit for pressure], the same for all frequencies...However, the otological consultant to the project, Dr Edmund P. Fowler, saw the new instrument as a *diagnostic tool* for the otologist, and wished to emphasize the *deviation from normal* of each subject. He believed, probably quite correctly, that this form of presentation of the results would promote the acceptance and general use of the electric audiometer by otologists. Dr. Fowler's counsel prevailed, and the intensity dial of the audiometer was labeled 'hearing loss' meaning 'decibels less sensitive than normal.' The format of the audiogram was devised with the reference zero level represented as a straight horizontal line near the top of the sheet and hearing loss (poorer hearing) plotted downwards.' ([76]at pp 194–5). This decision was the source of problems and misunderstandings ever since. Metrologists saw this 'reference zero level' concept as providing the major problem for pure tone audiometry. 'The problems of pure-tone audiometry can be conveniently grouped into three distinct phases. The first and most fundamental of these is the determination of the absolute threshold of hearing for normal listeners. The second is the transfer of this information to the dials of practical audiometers, which we refer to as the realization of the audiometric zero. Finally there is the actual technique of hearing loss measurement, which is principally though not exclusively to be thought of in terms of clinical application...The importance of an internationally agreed set of standard values for the normal threshold of hearing, as a step towards interchangeability of clinical information, is widely recognised, and the task of formulating such a standard has been undertaken by the Acoustics Committee of the International Organization for Standardization (ISO).[170] But towards the end of his life this leading British audiological scientist was coming round to the belief that the article of faith that he had enunciated forty years previously 'The first and most fundamental of these is the determination of the absolute threshold of hearing for normal listeners' was indeed a quest for the Holy Grail of 'pure and unsullied hearing.'

Controversy continues regarding the level of 'normal' auditory sensitivity. Gradenigo had conducted an early study of hearing sensitivity.[171] Licklider[172] conjectured that having the subject hold the earphone to his ear may have accounted for relative poorer sensitivities in some earlier surveys of hearing. The act of holding the earphone to the ear produces a measurable amount of low-frequency noise in the external acoustic meatus.[173] Yet even laboratory based studies are subject to disagreements. There are claims that Standards based on the 1952 British work[8,9] are too stringent. But previous studies by Békésy[174] in Budapest and by Waetzmann and Keibs[175] in Breslau [now Wroclaw, Poland] had indicated even more sensitive hearing. This merely serves to emphasize the importance of having appropriate controls whenever any studies involving the threshold of hearing are conducted. There are a plethora of factors influencing measured auditory thresholds.[68,176]

The biophysical bases for audiometry are clarified by Haughton.[177]

Manual audiometry

The instruments that we have mentioned so far have been *manual audiometers*. They are 'manual' in the sense that the selection and presentation of test tones to the subject is made by the operator (sometimes referred to as the 'audiometrician'). They are also 'manual' in the sense that the recognition of responses, noting at which stimulus levels these occur and transferring this information to the audiogram blank is also made by the operator.

Manual air conduction audiometry

The instruments that we have mentioned so far have also been manual audiometers *with earphone listening*.

It is termed 'with earphone listening' because the test tones are delivered from the audiometer to the ears by means of earphones. The alternative method would be 'with loudspeaker listening' (sound field listening). The latter condition would be more akin to natural conditions and would be free from those problems listed previously which arise from the use of earphones. It is often said that audiometry took the path it did towards the use of earphone listening because one had less control over a signal in a sound field than from an earphone. A more likely explanation is that the audiometric evolution followed the technological one. Hughes' invention was a

*Nobel Prizewinner, formerly Professor of Physics, London, and subsequently President of the Royal Society.

logical development after Alexander Graham Bell's invention of the telephone three years previously, i.e. in 1876. Moreover, a suitable transducer to permit sound field listening was not available until later (in the 20th century), when CW Rice and EW Kelley invented the electrodynamic loudspeaker.[178] There is now a standard (ISO 389–7:1996) for the reference zero for the calibration of audiometric equipment used for measuring the threshold of hearing under free-field and diffuse-field listening conditions. However even had the technological evolution been otherwise it is unlikely that we would now have had 'audiometry with sound field listening' in clinical practice because of the size and cost of equipping with sound treated testing chambers.

Matters relevant to manual air conduction audiometry with earphone listening have been discussed earlier in this chapter. But here we should say something about the problem of cross-hearing, i.e. the ear not under test responding to test sounds.

A hundred years ago Bárány invented his noise box to demonstrate cases of unilateral deafness.[179] Clinicians must therefore have been aware of the problem of cross-hearing and of the need to apply masking noise to the ear not being tested for a much longer period of time. With the advent of audiometers the problem and its solution needed to be addressed again.[180,181] The basis of the problem has been well set out in a recent textbook on 'Adult Audiology': 'It is natural to assume that, when sound is presented to the earphone on the left ear, it is the sensitivity of the left ear which is being measured; likewise for the right ear. Unfortunately, this assumption does not hold true under all circumstances because the earphone also transmits a certain amount of energy into the skull as a vibration, albeit at a much lower level than the acoustic signal. The vibration energy travels through the skull almost equally to both cochleae.[84] The risk of cross-hearing is governed by the contralateral cochlear sensitivity. If this is normal then a sound level in the test earphone of as little as 40 dB HL may be sufficient to be heard in that contralateral ear, i.e. ear not being tested. The level is frequency dependent and there is considerable inter-subject variability. If there appears to be a risk of cross-hearing then the problem is managed (but not necessarily always solved) by reducing temporarily the hearing sensitivity of the non-test ear. This is accomplished by delivering an audible noise (termed a masking noise) through either a supra-aural or an insert earphone to that contralateral ear. The threshold for that contralateral cochlea is elevated in proportion to the level of the masking noise. The exercise of determining an ear's threshold of hearing at increasing levels of contralateral masking noise is termed a *graduated masking* (or *plateau-seeking*) procedure. The results appear as a zig-zag curve when plotted graphically. The segment of the curve which appears as a plateau corresponds to the true threshold of hearing for the tested ear.

Studies of the masking of one pure tone by another[182] and of pure tones by noise[183] contributed to understanding the scientific basis of the masking phenomenon. A unifying concept was provided by Fletcher's[184] *critical band*. This is derived from two assumptions: (1) the only frequencies in a given noise which are important for masking lie within a narrow band of the noise (hence the term 'critical band'), (2) when a tone is just audible in the given noise, the total energy in the critical band is equal to the energy of the tone. Subsequent experimental work indicated that the critical band of noise needs to be about 4 dB more intense than the pure tone.[185]

There is sometimes a problem of spurious audiograms, more so with medico-legal cases. One may need to address the problem of exaggeration by the testee or by the tester. A number of tests are available to clarify the situation.[186,187] These include tests using manual audiometry,[63–66] aural acoustic immittance,[188,189] Békésy audiometry (see later), CERA,[87,88] evoked otoacoustic emissions[190] and speech audiometry.[63]

Exaggeration by the tester can be detected by Békésy audiometry. The tester can have no influence on the response or the transcription of thresholds.

Manual bone conduction audiometry

The first bone conduction audiometer was developed by Gradenigo in 1892.[191] The principles and practice of bone conduction audiometry have been set out by Hood,[91,192] Lutman[84] and others.

With bone conduction audiometry the stimulus to the cochlea is delivered by vibrational energy transmitted through the skull from a transducer (termed a vibrator) that has been placed on the head. The mode of excitation of the cochlear sound receptors is the same whether the sound stimulus is delivered by air conduction or by bone conduction.[193]

The simplistic interpretation of thresholds of hearing measured by bone conduction audiometry is that these reflect hearing sensitivity, which is not contaminated by any external or middle ear lesion. Having 'by passed' the aural sound transmission mechanism they reflect solely the function of the cochlea and its nerve, i.e. the sensorineural sensitivity. Alas, this is not the case (see below). Disorders of the external and middle ear may affect measured bone conduction thresholds to varying degrees and in various ways. Nevertheless the difference between an ear's air conduction threshold and its bone conduction threshold, termed the air-bone gap (ABG), is used as a measure of the degree of conductive threshold shift, i.e. the impairment of the aural sound transmission mechanism. This is of course where the measured air conduction threshold is poorer than the bone conduction threshold. Excluding minor separations attributable to mensurational uncertainties, the converse relationship (bone conduction poorer than air conduction) indicates that the measured thresholds are spurious.

The complex bases of bone conduction audiometry have been elucidated principally through the experimental studies of Békésy,[193–195] Bárány,[196–198] Allen and Fernandez,[199] and Tonndorf.[200,201] Athough there were earlier experimental studies on the biophysics of the tympano-ossicular mechanism by von Helmholtz.[202]

Three different mechanisms are involved when the ear is being stimulated by bone conduction, i.e. inertial bone conduction, compressional bone conduction and a bone conduction pathway that reaches the cochlea via the air in the external acoustic meatus.

Inertial bone conduction arises mainly when the bone conducted sound is of a frequency which is less than 800 Hz. In this situation the skull moves as a rigid body. Because of inertial forces ossicular movements do not follow skull movements. Consequently there is a relative sinusoidal movement of the stapes base in the round window thereby providing an acoustic stimulus to the cochlea.

Compressional bone conduction occurs when the skull is stimulated with bone conducted sounds above its resonant frequency (between 800 Hz and 1 kHz). With these frequencies the skull no longer moves as a rigid body but undergoes alternate compressions and expansions. These vibration patterns also involve the osseous labyrinth thereby providing another acoustic stimulus to the cochlea.

The third mode of bone conducted stimulation arises when the skull bones transmit the vibrations to the air in the external acoustic meatus.

This complexity of the biophysical basis for bone conduction stimulation contributes to the variance of bone conduction threshold measurements. Moreover, and most importantly, it denies bone conduction audiometry any claim to be a 'pure' measure of sensorineural (cochlear and auditory pathway) sensitivity. Hearing sensitivity to both higher[203] and lower frequency bone conducted sound can be affected by outer and middle ear disorders.

There are a number of factors, which influence bone conduction threshold measurements. Vibrator placement[204] has been the subject of a number of studies. Data relating to placing the vibrator on the vertex[197] and on the frontal bone[205–208] are also available.

Increase in vibrator surface area improves bone conduction thresholds for frequencies greater than 2 kHz.[209,210] The application force of the vibrator influences measured bone conduction thresholds.[211–214]

As mentioned earlier, erroneous bone conduction threshold measurements may arise as a result of air-borne radiation from bone-conduction transducers.[92–96] This artefact occurs when measuring bone conduction thresholds at 3 kHz and 4 kHz. To nullify the effect when testing at these frequencies the insertion of an earplug into the external acoustic meatus of the test ear has been recommended. But this means that the resulting bone conduction audiogram for that ear is in part an absolute bone conduction threshold, and in part a relative bone conduction threshold (see later). It is assumed that the occlusion effect is negligible at these two frequencies. It would be preferable to measure full bone conduction thresholds twice, on one occasion the relative bone conduction thresholds, on the other occasion the absolute bone conduction thresholds. This would then constitute the Aubry and Giraud method (see later) of bone conduction threshold measurements.

Artefacts may arise due to tactile sensation, especially at low frequencies.[215]

The problem that dominates bone conduction threshold measurements is that of cross-hearing, i.e. the ear not under test responding to test sounds. The cross-hearing problem is greater for bone conduction threshold measurements than for air conduction threshold measurements because transmission losses across the skull are effectively zero. A vibrator positioned anywhere on the head is effectively stimulating both cochleae simultaneously.[84,92,192] It follows that all bone conduction measurements should be made using graduated masking procedures. However, in clinical practice (especially when the testee is a claimant) useful information can be gained by first determining the bone conduction thresholds without masking. The testee is also asked to say, when responding to a test tone, where he hears the sound. Békésy attached great importance to this response in determining which cochlea was responding. Correlating this information with that derived from measured unmasked and masked air conduction and bone conduction thresholds can give a reasonable indication of the actual aural and cochlear sensitivities. Neither cochlea can be more sensitive than the unmasked bone conduction thresholds. The cochlear sensitivity on one or other side cannot be poorer than the aural sensitivity, i.e. air conduction threshold, on the corresponding side.

Alternative bone conduction methods are available to counteract the problem of cross-hearing.[216–219]

In spite of all these precautions bone conduction threshold measurements have limited accuracy.[26]

The occlusion phenomenon is less exploited than it should be in bone conduction audiometry. Depending on the stimulus frequency and the condition of the auditory mechanism, bone conduction thresholds may be modified by occluding the external acoustic meatus. As well as being elicited by a threshold method the phenomenon can be elicited by a loudness comparison method. The latter was described by Wheatstone in 1827.[220] The test is usually attributed to Bing[221] who reported the use of this occlusion phenomenon for the diagnosis of disorders of hearing. The phenomenon was however first described by Koyter over 400 years ago.[222] It is due primarily to the elimination of the normal high-pass filter effect produced by the unoccluded external acoustic meatus.[200] A quantitative expression of the occlusion phenomenon can be obtained by bone conduction audiometry. It is, of course, the difference between Aubry and Giraud's[223] COA (conduction osseuse absolue) curve and their COR (conduction osseuse relative) curve [Clinicians will recognise that the former corresponds to Pomeroy's test,[224] the value of which was stressed by Hallpike,[225] and the latter to the Schwabach test[226]]. Previous studies by Kelley and Reger[227] had shown that this shift was of the order of 20 dB for frequencies below 1 kHz. An 'occlusion index' has been used to quantify the phenomenon.[228] The index is the sum of the differences between the absolute and the relative bone conduction thresholds at 250 Hz, 500 Hz, 1 kHz and 2 kHz. The value of the index ranged from 0 dB to 60 dB, normal ears giving an average value of 34 dB. As well as the test being negative in conductive hearing losses, the test was negative in the majority of 28 ears with Menière's disease. The response to the test was associated with the activity of the disorder. During periods of remission, the test became positive, i.e. normal. A possible explanation is that a dilated saccule (or other part of the membranous labyrinth) splints the stapes base. Bone conduction measurements with the meatus occluded are as reproducible as those with the meatus open.[229] One source of variability is the force of an applied occluding device. For example, the magnitude of the effect is a function of the force of application of an occluding earphone.[230]

Although an old instrument (stemming from the 19th century) the manual pure-tone audiometer has been, and still is, the workhorse for the measurement of the threshold of hearing in clinical practice. However, it is not being used to its full potential. For all those who contemplate using the instrument, or even are already doing so, perusing the publications mentioned here should reap dividends.

Arlinger has provided manuals of practical audiometry[7] which should be of help to those needing to perform audiometric testing themselves.

International Standards that apply to manual pure tone audiometry are given at the end of this chapter.

Self-recording (Békésy and Rudmose) audiometry

A technological advance on manual pure tone audiometry was reported by Békésy in 1947,[231] the year in which he moved from the Royal Institute of Technology in Stockholm to Harvard University.

The applications of SRA (automatic, self-recording audiometry) to medical practice and research occurred in the first instance in the country in which he developed the instrument and in the country which then received him. Lundborg[232] reported results obtained on individuals with tumours of the nerve of hearing. The Harvard[137] and the Iowa[233,234] schools showed the value of the instrument both in research and in clinical medicine.

The use of both sweep and fixed frequencies and both continuous and intermittent test tones and for both threshold and most comfortable loudness tracking provides an eminently successful battery of Békésy audiometric tests for the investigation of sensorineural hearing disorders.[235]

What is a Békésy audiometer?

'An audiometer is described, in which the intensity of the tone increases continuously so long as a signal button is pressed and decreases automatically when the button is released [subsequent audiometers provided the opposite arrangement, i.e. pressing the button produces a progressive decrease in the sound level of the signal; releasing the button allows the sound level to progressively increase]. The subject controlling the button thus is able to let the intensity of the tone fluctuate between just above and just below threshold[231] (at p 411) ... The subject determines his own threshold [hence the description of this type of audiometry as *self-recording audiometry*] by pressing the button until the tone is perceived, then releasing the button until the tone disappears, pressing the button again till the tone reappears etc, etc. In this way the tone oscillates around the threshold of the subject the whole time ... A motor M_1 causes a continuous change in the frequency of the audio generator. The whole range between 100 and 10000 c.p.s. is covered in 15 minutes. On the same shaft as the frequency control is a drum supporting a paper on which the intensity of the sound at each frequency is recorded by a stylus. The audio frequency generator works into a potentiometer which covers a range of 140 db and supplies the telephone receiver.'[231] (at p 412).

This instrument thus differs from the conventional, manual audiometer in that the sound level is under the control of the subject. But even this control may be overridden by the operator.

It is outside the scope of this review to consider the various commercially available products which enable the practitioner to conduct Békésy audiometry. However, the Grason-Stadler Company of the USA produced Békésy audiometers based on Scott Reger's machines.[233] Currently the author use a Grason Stadler GSI instrument which incorporates Telephonics TDH-50 earphones.

What has Békésy audiometry had to offer?

In clinical practice

A threshold audiogram

(a) air conduction

'In order to give the normal audiogram the appearance of a straight line at zero level, a suitable filter circuit is inserted between the attenuator and the receiver. This filter circuit attenuates the frequencies between 1000 and 3000 especially much ...[231] (at p 413) ... If one wants a completely straight and horizontal line for the normal audiogram it may be suitable to compensate for small residual differences left by the electric equalizing circuit by means of a mechanical arrangement, the drum carrying the audiogam paper being shifted along the db axis by means of a guiding profile on the same shaft of the drum.'[231] (at p 422) [the curvilinear absolute threshold of hearing was indeed corrected mechanically on the earlier commercially available Békésy audiometers.]

As with manual pure tone audiometry, Békésy audiometry provides information on the threshold pattern, which constitutes the basic information that a clinician requires of audiometry as a diagnostic aid.

(b) bone conduction
'... in bone conduction measurements, it is necessary to change the intensity of the noise masking the not investigated ear in proportion to the intensity of the test tone [so he anticipated the arguments for a graduated masking procedure]. This can easily be done in the described audiometer. The result is an arrangement which with certainty prevents the masking noise to interfere with the hearing of the ear under investigation, while at the same time it always is sufficiently strong.'[231] (at p 411).

The importance of the technique for masking the non-test ear in the various Békésy audiometric procedures has been stressed by Priede and Coles.[236]

Authentication of recorded thresholds

'In order to control if the real auditory threshold is observed or not it is possible to use an extra attenuation of 10 db which is periodically inserted in the circuit. If one lets the recording paper make a corresponding movement automatically, a normal audiogram keeps its straight course, with the exception of one larger spike at each change in attenuation (at p 420) ... In malingering and dissimulation, where the real threshold is not observed, the subject is unable to follow the intensity changes and a typical curve is obtained ... the periodic 10 db shifts are easily distinguished.'[231] (at p 422).

Jerger and Herer[237] subsequently reported that a particular Békésy audiometric pattern (Type V) pointed to a *nonorganic hearing loss*. It was characterised by better thresholds for continuous (sustained) than for intermittent (pulsed) test tones. Rinteleman and Carhart[238] suggested that this pattern arose because of the higher sound pressure levels that are required for pulsed (compared to sustained) test tones to achieve equal loudness with the Békésy audiometer. Out of a group of 30 former military personnel with otherwise diagnosed nonorganic hearing loss, Stein[239] observed that 17 had Type V Békésy audiograms and a further nine had unclassifiable patterns.

An *increased tracking width* is also indicative of a nonorganic hearing loss.[240]

A number of reports from the Iowa school[241–243] demonstrated the possibility of conducting and quantifying the *Stenger test* using Békésy audiometry.

Other refinements in Békésy testing[244–246] showed how different procedures could increase the detection of nonorganic hearing loss.

Loudness functions

'The new audiograms besides giving a graph representing the absolute intensity as a function of frequency also show how the difference limen for intensity changes with frequency. This gives additional data for the differential diagnosis between perceptive and conductive lesions. In normal ears, the difference limen increases somewhat between 100 and 1000 c.p.s. and then keeps constant to about 4000 c.p.s. Above this frequency it drops again and reaches the original value at 10000 c.p.s. This relation between difference limen and frequency agrees with the well-known Kingsbury curves of equal loudness [i.e. equal loudness contours]. (at pp 418, 419) ... The method is equivalent to the *recruitment test* of Fowler but permits isolated investigation of one ear. It is of special value when the perceptive lesion does not affect the whole frequency region to the same extent, because in this case the difference limen changes between different regions of the same audiogram.'[231] (at p 420).

Lundborg[232] showed that the tracking width (sometimes referred to as the amplitude or extent of the Békésy audiometric excursions) was reduced in patients with various types of sensorineural hearing losses (acoustic trauma, Ménière's disease, retrocochlear lesions). He considered this pattern to be characteristic of cochlear, and not retrocochlear, sensorineural hearing losses and so consistent with the observations of Dix and her colleagues.[247] They had shown that the phenomenon of loudness recruitment, as demonstrated by the alternate binaural loudness balance test of Fowler [248, 249], was characteristic of cochlear lesions. Thus Lundborg supported Békésy's interpretation of reduced tracking width, i.e. it was an index of loudness recruitment. However, others[250] suggest that this phenomenon reflects rapid abnormal auditory adaptation, i.e. occurring in milliseconds, yet still arising from cochlear events.

Bilger[251] confirmed the significance of the tracking width, i.e. relating these to cochlear malfunction, for fixed frequency continuous test tones.

Most comfortable loudness levels are also of diagnostic value.[252–254] Reductions in the size of the excursions of the tracked threshold for most comfortable loudness levels are indicative of cochlear disorders.

The most comfortable loudness level which has been tracked with a glide tone is a convenient way of recording a particular equal loudness contour. It is thus similar to the equal loudness contours, which Reger[255] obtained by monaural bi-frequency loudness matches. When plotted on a threshold audiogram equal loudness contours provide evidence for *loudness recruitment*[255] which, as Hirsh[5] showed, is particularly convincing in respect of the phenomenon being associated with high tone notches.

The *threshold of uncomfortable loudness*[256] can also be used as a measure of loudness recruitment, as exploited by Hood and Poole[257] in their loudness discomfort level. Békésy audiometry provides a convenient means of recording the threshold of uncomfortable loudness.[258]

One should bear in mind that most comfortable (and threshold of uncomfortable) loudness level contours are not identical to equal loudness contours.[259]

Abnormal auditory adaptation

'It is necessary to avoid sounds which are appreciably louder than the threshold, since they cause fatigue phenomena which may interfere with correct threshold determinations.'[231] (at p 411). Békésy was clearly aware of perstimulatory adaptation/fatigue but did not grasp the full extent of these phenomena since he used only sustained (continuous) test tones. Moreover, fixed frequency test tones do not appear to have been used in the testing of patients. Such a signal mode appears to have been used only for assessing reproducibility of recorded thresholds and to investigate the effect of various test parameters.

Reger and Kos[234] showed that the drift of a tracked fixed frequency threshold for a steady state, i.e. continuous, test tone was associated with retrocochlear lesions. This drift of a continuous test tone could occur in the presence of normal thresholds for pulsed test tones, as Kos[260] showed for a patient with a pinealoma. The phenomenon of what came to be termed *abnormal auditory adaptation* emerged as a feature of tumours of the nerve of hearing.[261]

The influence of *tracking direction* on the recorded threshold was demonstrated by Rose.[262] Sweep frequency tracings using both continuous and pulsed test tones were each tracked in an ascending mode from 100 Hz to 10 kHz and in a descending mode from 10 kHz to 100 Hz. There was no effect on pulsed test tones but a downward sweep for continuous test tones accentuated the separation between the continuous and pulsed tracings. Harbert and Young[263] pointed out that the relationship of continuous and pulsed audiograms to one another was essentially the same whether they are obtained in an ascending or descending mode unless abnormal auditory adaptation is present. The reverse sweep threshold is always the poorer when differences are observed between ascending and descending continuous test tone thresholds and this is associated with retrocochlear lesions.[264]

An additional, and diagnostically important, factor is that both fixed frequency[265,266] and sweep frequency Békésy tracings are affected by both ipsilateral and contralateral *masking noise* at low-intensity levels even when there is no question of cross-hearing. The application of contralateral masking noise accentuates the detection of abnormal auditory adaptation, and increases its magnitude if present.

Use of the Collet effect[267] has demonstrated a link between *otoacoustic emission* behaviour and abnormal auditory adaptation.[268] This study should herald a better approach to understanding the various types (there is not one, but a number of, types of abnormal auditory adaptation) of this phenomenon which can be recorded by Békésy audiometry.

Abnormal auditory adaptation may be evident on most comfortable loudness tracking when it is absent on threshold tracking. Orchik and colleagues[269] described two such cases (surgically confirmed vestibulocochlear schwannomas). Thus most comfortable loudness level tracking provides evidence for both loudness recruitment and abnormal auditory adaptation.[270]

Tinnitus studies

Békésy audiometry is eminently suitable for the investigation of tinnitus. The results of pitch and loudness matching studies can be conveniently recorded. A particular method can be used to determine personal loudness functions as a necessary preliminary to expressing the subjective magnitude of tinnitus in terms of personal loudness units.[271]

Categorisation of patterns

'In pathological cases three different types of audiograms were observed ... In the top curve [first type] ... there is no great change in difference limen with frequency ... In the lower curve [second type] ... there is a sharp decrease in the amplitude of the intensity oscillations, »spikes», the difference limen drops at the higher frequencies. The top curve was obtained in a case where from other reasons a diagnosis of conductive lesion was made. The lower curve similarly was diagnosed as a perceptive lesion (p 419) ... The third type of pathological curve ... large spikes at irregular intervals indicate the presence of tinnitus, which disturbs the observations.'[231] (at p 420).

Jerger's classification of Békésy audiometric patterns for diagnostic purposes[272] has been extended by Jerger and Herer,[237] Harden and Kiessling[273] and others.

In addition to considering audiometric patterns, the subject's perception of the test tone also has diagnostic significance. Sørensen[74] reported that some patients noticed a change in the sound of a continuous test tone from a tonal to an atonal quality. The bilateral occurrence of this phenomenon, termed 'tone perversion', has been reported in association with disorders involving the pons.[275]

In occupational medicine

Discrete frequency SRA

The Rudmose audiometer[276] is an automated pulsed fixed frequency audiometer designed for hearing conservation programmes in industry. Consequent on their systematic studies, McCommons and Hodge[277] recommended pulsed test tones in industrial and military hearing conservation programmes.

Studies in British industry concluded that the 'use of occupational health nurses with self-recording audiometers is a satisfactory method of audiometric screening in hearing conservation programmes.'[278] The British Armed Services have also confirmed the value of self-recording audiometry in hearing conservation programmes.[279]

However, a study in the USA[280] found differences of the order of 10 dB between thresholds measured by self-recording audiometry and those measured by manual audiometry, the latter being the more acute. The phenomenon was related to a claims environment.

Sweep frequency SRA

Swedish studies demonstrated the superiority of sweep frequency self-recording audiometry over manual audiometry for hearing conservation programmes in industry.[281] Sweep-frequency methods, using whatever equipment, are more sensitive than fixed frequency methods for detecting the notches on the threshold of hearing that provide the first evidence for noise damage to hearing.[282] Békésy audiometry is eminently suitable for the early detection of noise damage to hearing.[283]

Forensic purposes

The arguments for using sweep frequency self-recording audiometry (vis-à-vis manual audiometry) for medicolegal work are:

- Virtual elimination of bias attributable to the audiometrician
- The unambiguous nature of the subject's response. If necessary, sweep frequency SRA can be backed up by fixed frequency SRA, e.g. if there is uncertainty about the threshold measured by sweep frequency testing.
- The provision of a permanent record without possibility of transcription errors.
- There is a visible indication of the quality of the subject's test performance
- Sweep frequency SRA has the advantage that it can detect incipient, or other noise-induced, notches when discrete frequency audiometry, whether manual or self-recording, has failed to do so.
- The use of continuous test tone sweep frequency audiometry, in addition to pulsed test tone sweep frequency audiometry, considerably enhances the possibility of detecting spurious thresholds.
- Diagnostic sweep frequency SRA also has a much greater facility of picking up hearing losses due to conditions other than noise damage to the ear.

Full acceptance of double sweep SRA could well rid us of the scourge of multiple audiometry. Many claimants say 'Why do I have to have yet another test?' Yes 'Why?'

Other auditory investigations

Gauz and his colleagues extended the frequency range of conventional Békésy audiometry up to 16 kHz or 20 kHz.[284]

Albers[285] reported the use of Békésy techniques in the measurement of binaural diplacusis. The Békésy technique can also be used to measure and record monaural frequency discrimination.[286] Domico[287] has used Békésy audiometry to study aural harmonic distortion thresholds.

John and his colleagues[288] showed low frequency shifts of the Békésy audiogram were associated with raised intracranial pressure.

Over thirty years ago there were reports that sweep frequency Békésy audiometry could detect the normal hearing carriers of genes for sensorineural hearing disorders.[289] This has been confirmed in respect of X-linked hearing loss.[290] Others have either failed to detect carriers using sweep frequency Békésy audiometry[291] or found it less sensitive than another sweep frequency method†.[292] These findings may have been due to the use of a pulsed instead of a continuous test tone. The optimum parameters of the test tones for carrier detection have yet to be defined. Nevertheless, even those workers who have used interrupted glide tones have found Békésy audiometry a useful adjunct to the Audioscan. A possible carrier may have a hearing loss due to a factor (or factors) other than the gene under investigation. In such cases the Audioscan takes too long, the subject becomes fatigued and spurious results ensue. Because of its pre-constrained test duration, Békésy audiometry presents no such problems.[293]

Because of the ability to track thresholds over short periods of time, self-recording audiometry provides a convenient tool for both human and animal research. In particular, it is useful in tracking the temporary changes in threshold in experimental studies of the effects of noise.[137, 220]

† Meyer-Bisch's (1990) Audioscan.

Stability, specificity and sensitivity of recorded measures

Studies of these features can be grouped broadly into those which have been concerned with the factors influencing measured thresholds, and those which have been concerned with the factors influencing other patterns of response. The first group has thus centred around the use of Rudmose audiometry because of its employment in hearing conservation programmes with the need to detect deviations from some reference threshold which has been derived from the individual or from some outside source. The second group has centred around the use of Békésy audiometry because of employing patterns of response in the diagnosis of auditory disorders.

Measurements of the threshold of hearing

From the mid-fifties studies were conducted to relate thresholds of hearing measured by self-recording audiometry to manual audiometry.[12,101,102,104,281,295,296] The differences reported were probably primarily attributable to inter-tester variability influencing the manual audiometric measurements and to the failure in some instances to take into account Leijon's[114] quantization error in respect of manual audiometer attenuation steps.

McCommons and Hodge[277] conducted two studies to determine the parameters affecting the sensitivity and variability of fixed frequency self-recorded thresholds. The first study was concerned with the effects of varying period, duty cycle and frequency on threshold measurements obtained using pulsed test tones in order to derive an 'optimal' pulsed test tone. The 'optimal' tone was found to have a period of 500 ms, a duty cycle of at least 50% but probably no greater than 60% and an attenuation rate of at least 4, but not to exceed 5 dB.s-1, The second study compared thresholds taken with the 'optimized' pulsed test tone to those obtained with continuous test tones. Pulsed test tones were found to yield superior threshold measurements both in terms of greater sensitivity and less intratest variability. Continuous tone thresholds were susceptible to changes in attenuation rate; pulsed tone thresholds were not. The authors considered that 'the primary advantage of the pulsing tone is greater feedback that has the effect of making the S's task easier. This, in turn, makes him better able to make or delay his response, whichever is appropriate.'

For young normal adults, Jokinen[297] found that, for experienced listeners, manually determined thresholds were superimposed on continuous fixed frequency thresholds, but, for inexperienced listeners, the manual thresholds were poorer than the continuous thresholds.

The 'Notes on Occupational Deafness' issued by the British Department of Health and Social Security (1974) state, with regard to audiometry, 'There is an initial learning period which leads to improvements of from 1 to 15 dB with manually operated audiometry. A proportion of persons have difficulty with self-recording audiometry and may show learning effects of up to 30dB.'[54] This statement must apply to claimants. It is not my experience. In the 1960s MRC/NPL survey of noise and hearing in British industry the subjects were tested by Rudmose self-recording audiometry. 'The mean audiogram level (average HTL across 6 frequencies, i.e. 0.5, 1, 2, 3, 4 and 6 kHz) repeated on average to within ± 3 dB ... Positive and negative shifts were nearly equal in frequency of occurrence indicating that the principal cause was a random process, and this is attributed mainly to subjective uncertainty of the threshold.'[298]

Knight studied *learning effects* on sixteen normally hearing adults.[299] The subjects were tested by Rudmose audiometry twice daily for five consecutive days. There was an improvement of the order of 1 dB from the first to the second test each day. After the ten complete audiometric tests there had been a mean improvement of about 3 dB, which improvement appeared to be continuing. The learning effect appears to be frequency dependent, being maximum around 1 kHz and falling off on either side of that, becoming negative at 4 kHz.[115] The effect was slightly greater with introverts than with extraverts.

There have been occasions when the greater sensitivity of sweep frequency Békésy audiometry in detecting high tone notches has been questioned. These have been when the Békésy audiometer has 'missed' a 6 kHz notch that has been picked up with manual audiometry. In most, if not all, cases this has been because the manual audiometer has been equipped with Telephonics TDH-39 earphones, which have been calibrated (following correct procedures) according to ISO 389 on an IEC 303 coupler. The Békésy audiometer has been equipped with Telephonics TDH-50 earphones. The common occurrence of 6 kHz notches is an artefact arising from a particular interaction between the IEC 303 coupler and the TDH-39, but not the TDH-50, earphone.[20]

Sweep frequency Békésy audiometry may, however, miss high tone notches at higher attenuation rates (and therefore higher sweep speeds) that it would otherwise detect at lower rates.

Measurements of other responses

At a given frequency, the *tracking width* is primarily determined by the attenuation rate, for continuous test tones increasing from 4 to 9 dB for a 1 $dB.s^{-1}$ rate to 10 to 30 dB for a 4 $dB.s^{-1}$ rate.[300] Using an attenuation rate of 2.1 $dB.s^{-1}$, Jokinen[297] observed that for both continuous or pulsed fixed frequency test tones, the width is greater for low than for higher frequencies, falling by about 30% over the range from 125 Hz to 8 kHz. Stephens[115] confirmed this slight frequency dependence for pulsed fixed frequency test tones, the width falling from mean values of 6.5 dB at 250 Hz to 6 dB at 8 kHz. Tracking width is influenced both by reaction time[301] and by personality factors.[302]

Earlier failures[232,303] to observe *abnormal auditory adaptation* in retrocochlear lesions may well have been attributable to using instruments where the attenuation changed in steps of 1 dB or more.[272] A silent interval of less than 20 ms between successive short tones was sufficient to maintain a stable horizontal trace in a patient who would exhibit abnormal auditory adaptation on continuous stimulation. Jerger's instrument featured 25 mB attenuation changes, i.e. a virtually continuous attenuation change.

Classification of Békésy audiograms according to the Jerger method shows little inter-observer variation.[304] The poor performance of Békésy audiometry in studies using clinical decision analysis [305] is almost certainly attributable to including Békésy audiograms which have been obtained without reverse glide tones, contralateral noise application and suprathreshold recordings.

Hopkinson's report[306] that 48% of her 52 patients with conductive hearing loss showed Type V Jerger patterns points to the need, as she states, to define more precisely the criteria for this pattern class. Quantification of the continuous-pulsed threshold separation would appear to be one approach.

Factors influencing the *threshold of uncomfortable loudness* (TUL) have been studied at the National Physical Laboratory. Stephens[258] found that the mean pulsed fixed frequency TUL for 25 naïve, normally hearing adults was 105.7 dB HL, the corresponding value for a continuous fixed frequency test tone was 101.4 dB HL and for conventional 5-dB step manual audiometry, 93.4 dB HL. The TUL is influenced by both test anxiety and failure avoidance motivation.[258,307]

Influence of age

Younger

'I am testing five to seven year old children. I tested a four year old the other day who had a swing of only 20 about the threshold as a mean ...' (Reger in discussion of communication by Reger and Kos.[234]

One in twelve children show better thresholds for continuous test tones than for pulsed test tones, but this tendency decreases with age.[308]

Price and Falck[309] stated that it is possible to obtain clinically useful information with Békésy audiometry from 98% of all subjects with a mental age of 7 years or more.

Older

Using *fixed frequency* test tones, Jokinen[297] reported that '... switch button manipulation caused no difficulties even at advanced age: 12 of the subjects were over 70 and 2 over 80 years, and their performance' was comparable to younger age groups. In young normal adults the 'continuous and pulsed tone tracings were overlapping ... but in old age the pulsed tone tracing was clearly better than the steady tone threshold.' The attenuation rate was 2.1 $dB.s^{-1}$ in 25 mB steps; the tone pulse had a rise and fall time of 25 ms and a duty cycle of 50%.

Using *sweep frequency* test tones changing at 5 $dB.s^{-1}$ in 25 mB steps, Harbert and colleagues [310] had reported that for older people the *tracking width* was relatively constant as a function of frequency for pulsed test tones, but showed a steady decrease with increasing frequency for continuous test tones. There was no separation between continuous and pulsed test tone thresholds for younger adults but for older people there was a separation (pulsed better) which became greater with increasing frequency, attaining an average difference of 5 dB at 8 kHz.

Other sources of variance

Rarely it has been observed during the course of hearing surveys that the subject has been responding to individual pulses instead of the 'quietest sound' that he could hear. On one occasion out of many thousands of tests a non-response was observed to be due to the patient pressing the retaining screw of the signalling switch instead of the button proper. Both of these observations point to the need for all self-recorded audiograms to be monitored by experienced staff.

Computerised statistical analyses; taxonometry

A variety of schemes for grouping threshold configurations has been proposed since Guild[311] published his method for classifying manual pure tone audiograms. Concomitant with the recent surge of interest in genetical auditory disorders there has been a corresponding upsurge of interest in these configurations.[312] But 'pure tone audiometry may be insufficient'.[313] Moreover, the classification of threshold configurations remains at the best an intuitive, *Gestalt* approach.

These considerations therefore lead us not only to considering sweep frequency Békésy audiometry but also to a more sophisticated numerical approach in line with Sokal and Sneath's taxonometric one.[314] Following this line, Job and his colleagues[315] have applied a Hotelling principal component analysis[316] to the threshold configurations of Békésy audiograms. Three components were extracted and explained 70% of the total variance. The first component reflected the degree of hearing loss. The second and third reflected the different configurations (asymmetry, shape). The use of cluster analysis[317] produced four main classes: normal, attributable to firearms, associated with 'skin-diving and pressure problems', and attributable to 'heterogeneous pathologic problems with no apparent correlation to the army context.'[318] The authors used a form of discriminant analysis[319,320] to 'correctly' classify 93% of configurations. Özdamar and his colleagues[321] reported a dynamic Bayesian procedure, which was applied to the behavioural testing of the hearing of young children. The method depends on using an already accepted classification of audiometric configurations. It could be adapted to classifying Békésy audiograms.

The classification of audiograms is a pattern recognition exercise. This leads to considering signal analysis techniques which treat the audiogram as a stochastic waveform. Consequently, Chalabi and Soucková[322] pointed to the type of mathematical analysis needed to classify the threshold patterns of sweep frequency Békésy audiograms. The approach is to discard the notion of dividing any one audiogram into a number of principal segments where a classification procedure is carried out separately on each segment. Instead an audiogram is considered as a singleton within in its own stochastic nature. The problem is to determine an optimal mathematical strategy for discriminating between the different classes of audiograms in order to attach a statistical significance to each audiogram as being either a member of any one single class, the *n*th stage of a progressive condition, or the *n*th degree of severity of a condition existing in varying degrees of severity. The mathematical strategies used orthogonal transformation based on the Karhunen-Loève expansion. The optimal orthogonal expansion basis functions were Chebyshev polynomials. The audiograms were smoothed using cubic spline interpolation. The analysis used orthogonal Householder transformation, Gauss-Markov theory, and Sturm-Liouville differential equation properties.

This signal statistical approach to classifying Békésy audiograms could be applied to both fixed and sweep frequency and both threshold and suprathreshold trackings following both pulsed and continuous test tone stimulation, as well their separations. Nor should tracking width be forgotten.

The production of a Windows software application[318] for the analysis and classification of Békésy audiograms brings these exercises nearer to clinic usage.

It is both inevitable and desirable that the next generation of Békésy type audiometers will make full use of technological developments, especially in computer science, that have emerged and progressed in the past half century. There will be greater control over stimulus parameters to maximise the value of each of various tests. A randomisation facility would dispose of the 'predictability' of the stimuli in current Békésy audiometers. On line analysis of a number of subject responses will provide an immediate printout (or display on a monitor) for the clinician, occupational hygienist or research worker. To meet the constraints of clinical practice, algorithms will maximise the information to be derived in a given time-window. This customising facility could annul the main argument (speed) for using manual audiometry. All this will of course bring us into another programme of standardisation.

Conclusions

A large repertoire of methods for the examination of the threshold of hearing is available. Different tests can demonstrate different features of auditory sensitivity, and each with a different diagnostic value. Practical advice is given on analysing threshold data in order to avoid the many pitfalls. As the data presented in respect of the Factory 'X' litigation show it is imperative that medical examiners, at least in the UK, use controls drawn from their own contemporaneous and situation-specific clinical and audiometric experience.

Computerisation of audiometric testing, which began more than a quarter of a century ago[323] and has continued but slowly[324,325] should now flourish. Current developments in the mathematical and statistical sciences will now be able to exploit more fully the examination of the various features of thresholds of hearing using all audiometric techniques.

Acknowledgements

I am indebted to all who have read the manuscript for this chapter and provided most helpful and constructive comments.

No funding was either obtained or solicited for the data analyses in this chapter or for writing the chapter.

References

1. Bunch CC. *Clinical Audiometry*. St Louis: Mosby, 1943.
2. Hinchcliffe R. Threshold of hearing for random noise. *J Speech Hear Res* 1961; **4**: 3–9.
3. Martin M. *Speech Audiometry*, 2nd edn. London: Whurr, 1997.
4. Sivian LJ, White SD. On minimum audible sound fields. *J Acoust Soc Am* 1933; **4**: 288–321.
5. Hirsh IJ. *The Measurement of Hearing*. New York: McGraw-Hill, 1952.
6. Stephens SDG. David Edward Hughes and his audiometer. *J Laryngol Otol* 1979; **93**: 1–6.
7. Arlinger S (ed.). *Manual of Practical Audiometry*. London: Whurr, 1990 (Vol. 1), 1991 (Vol. 2).
8. Wheeler LJ, Dickson EDD. The determination of the threshold of hearing. *J Laryngol Otol* 1952; **66**: 379–95.
9. Dadson RS, King JH. A determination of the normal threshold of hearing and its relation to the standardization of audiometers. *J Laryngol Otol* 1952; **66**: 366–78.
10. Dobie RA. *Medical-Legal Evaluation of Hearing Loss*. New York: Van Nostrand Reinhold, 1993.
11. Knight JJ, Coles RRA. Determination of the hearing threshold levels of naval recruits in terms of British and American standards. *J Acoust Soc Am* 1960; **32**: 800–4.
12. Knight JJ. Normal hearing threshold determined by manual and self-recording techniques. *J Acoust Soc Am* 1966; **39**: 1184–5.
13. US Public Health Service. *National Health Survey, Bulletins in the Hearing Study Series*. Washington: USPHS, 1938.
14. Hinchcliffe R. The threshold of hearing of a random sample rural population. *Acta Otolaryngol (Stockh)* 1959; **50**: 411–22.
15. Whittle LS, Robinson DW. British normal threshold of hearing. *Nature* 1961; **189**: 617–18.
16. Whittle LS, Delany ME. Equivalent threshold sound-pressure levels for the TDH39/MX41-AR earphone. *J Acoust Soc Am* 1966; **39**: 1187–8.
17. Weissler PG. International standard reference zero for audiometers. *J Acoust Soc Am* 1968; **44**: 264–75.
18. Robinson DW. *A Proposal for Audiometric Zero Referred to the IEC Artificial Ear*. Acoustics Report Ac 65. Teddington: National Physical Laboratory, 1978.
19. Robinson DW, Shipton MS, Hinchcliffe R. Audiometric zero for air conduction. *Audiology* 1981; **20**: 409–431.
20. Lutman ME, Qasem HYN. A source of audiometric notches at 6 kHz. In: Prasher D, Luxon LM eds. *Advances in Noise Research Series*, Vol. 1. London: Whurr, 1997, pp. 170–6.
21. Dirks DD, Lybarger SF, Olsen WO, Billings BL. Bone conduction calibration—present status. *J Speech Hear Disord* 1979; **44**: 143–55.
22. Robinson DW, Shipton MS. A standard determination of paired air and bone conduction thresholds under different masking noise conditions. *Audiology* 1982; **21**: 61–82.
23. Haughton PM, Pardoe K. Normal pure tone thresholds for hearing by bone conduction. *Br J Audiol* 1981; **15**: 113–21.
24. Richter U, Brinkmann K. Threshold of hearing by bone conduction—a contribution to international standardization. *Scand Audiol* 1981; **10**: 235–7.
25. Brinkmann K, Richter U. Determination of the normal threshold of hearing by bone conduction using different types of bone vibrators. *Audiol Acoust* 1983; **22**: 62–85, 114–22.
26. Coles RRA, Lutman ME, Robinson DW. The limited accuracy of bone conduction audiometry: its significance in medicolegal assessments. *J Laryngol Otol* 1991; **105**: 518–21.
27. http://www.ukas.org.
28. Schuknecht HF. *Pathology of the Ear*. Cambridge, Massachusetts: Harvard University Press, 1974.
29. Hinchcliffe R. The age function of hearing—aspects of the epidemiology. *Acta Otolaryngol* 1991; Suppl 476: 7–11.
30. Willott JF. *Aging and the Auditory System*. London: Whurr, 1991.
31. Kerr JFR, Wyllie AH, Currie AR. Apoptosis: a basic biological phenomenon with wide-ranging implications in tissue kinetics. *Br J Cancer* 1972; **26**: 239–57.
32. Wyllie AH, Kerr JFR, Currie AR. Cell death: the significance of apoptosis. *Int Rev Cytol* 1980; **68**: 251–306.
33. Raff M. Why are your cells waiting to kill themselves? *MRC News* 1995; 28–30.
34. Usami S-I, Takumi Y, Fujita S, Shinkawa H, Hosokawa M. Cell death in the inner ear associated with aging is apoptosis? *Brain Res* 1997; **747**: 147–50.
35. Beasley WC. The general problem of deafness in the population. *Laryngoscope* 1940; **50**: 856–905.
36. Hinchcliffe R. The pattern of the threshold of perception for hearing and other special senses as a function of age. *Gerontologia* 1958; **2**: 311–20.
37. Glorig A, Nixon J. Hearing loss as a function of age. *Laryngoscope* 1962; **72**: 1596–610.
38. Spoor A. Presbycusis values in relation to noise induced hearing loss. *Int Audiol* 1967; **6**: 48–57.

39. Robinson DW, Sutton GJ. Age effect in hearing—a comparative analysis of published threshold data. *Audiology* 1979; **18**: 320–34.
40. Pearson JCG. Prediction of presbycusis. *J Soc Occup Med* 1977; **27**: 125–33.
41. Rosenhall U, Jonsson R, Davis A, Parving A. Hearing in the 'oldest old' a cross-sectional collaborative study from three European countries. *J Audiol Med* 2000; **9**: 43–52.
42. Delany ME, Whittle LS, Knox EC. A note on the use of self-recording audiometry with children. *J Laryngol Otol* 1966; **80**: 1135–43.
43. Roche AF, Siervogel RM, Himes JH, Johnson DL. Longitudinal study of human hearing: its relationship to noise and other factors. AMRL-TR-76-110, 1976.
44. Hinchcliffe R. The threshold of hearing as a function of age. *Acustica* 1959; **9**: 303–8.
45. Robinson DW, Sutton GJ. Age effect in hearing—a comparative analysis of published threshold data. *Audiology* 1979; **18**: 320–34.
46. Hinchcliffe R. Hypoacousies et bourdonnements: une perspective globale. *Rev Laryngol* 1993; **114**: 93–101.
47. Hinchcliffe R, Jones WI. Hearing levels of a suburban Jamaican population. *Int Audiol* 1968; **7**: 239–58.
48. Hinchcliffe R, Osuntokun BO, Adeuja AOG. Hearing levels in Nigerian ataxic neuropathy. *Audiology* 1972; **11**: 218–30.
49. Karlsmose B, Lauritzen T, Engberg M, Parving A. A five-year longitudinal study of hearing in a Danish rural population aged 31–50 years. *Br J Audiol* 2000; **34**: 42–55.
50. Atherley GRC. The extent and severity of occupational deafness among men employed as drop forgers. In: Taylor W, ed. *Disorders of Auditory Function*. London: Academic Press, 1973: 159–66.
51. Department of Health and Society Security. *Occupational Deafness*. Report by the Industrial Injuries Advisory Council in accordance with Section 62 of the National Insurance (Industrial Injuries) Act 1965 on the question whether there are degrees of hearing loss due to noise which satisfy the conditions for prescription under the Act. Cmnd 5461. London: HMSO, 1973.
52. Merluzzi F, Hinchcliffe R. Threshold of subjective auditory handicap. *Audiology* 1973; **12**: 65–9.
53. Armitage P. *Statistical Methods in Medical Research*. Oxford: Blackwell, 1973.
54. Department of Health and Social Security. *Notes on Occupational Deafness ND1*. London: HMSO, 1974.
55. World Health Organization. *International Classification of Impairments, Disabilities, and Handicaps—A Manual of Classification Relating to the Consequences of Disease*. Geneva: WHO, 1980.
56. World Health Organization. *Conclusions and Recommendations of First Informal Consultation on Future Programme Developments for the Prevention of Deafness and Hearing Impairment*. Geneva: WHO, 1997.
57. US Department of Labor—Occupational Safety and Health Administration. Occupational noise exposure: hearing conservation amendment. *Fed Reg* 1981; **46**(11): 4078–179.
58. British Society of Audiology. Descriptions for pure-tone audiograms. *Br J Audiol* 1988; **22**: 123.
59. Robinson DW, Wilkins PA, Thyer NJ, Lawes JF. *Auditory Impairment and the Onset of Disability and Handicap in Noise-induced Hearing Loss*. ISVR Technical Report No. 126. Southampton: University of Southampton, 1984.
60. Abernathy CM, Hamm RM. *Surgical Intuition*. Philadelphia, PA: Hanley and Belfus, 1994.
61. Abernathy CM, Hamm RM. *Surgical Scripts*. Philadelphia, PA: Hanley and Belfus, 1994.
62. Dunea G. Diagnosing trees and men. *BMJ* 1997; **315**: 434.
63. Coles RRA, Priede VM. Nonorganic overlay in noise-induced hearing loss. *Proc R Soc Med* 1971; **64**: 194–9.
64. Harris DA. Rapid and simple technique for detection of non-organic hearing loss. *Arch Otolaryngol* 1958; **68**: 758–60.
65. Kerr AG, Gillespie WJ, Easton JM. Deafness: a simple test for malingering. *Br J Audiol* 1975; **9**: 24–6.
66. Cooper J, Lightfoot G. A modified pure-tone audiometric technique for medico-legal assessment. *Br J Audiol* 2000; **34**: 37–46.
67. Luxon LM. The clinical diagnosis of noise-induced hearing loss. In Prasher D, Luxon LM, eds. *Advances in Noise Research Series*, Vol. 1. London: Whurr, 1998, pp. 83–113.
68. Hinchcliffe R, Littler TS. The detection and measurement of conductive deafness. *J Laryngol Otol* 1961; **75**: 201–15.
69. Golabek W, Stephens SDG. Some tuning fork tests revisited. *Clin Otolaryngol* 1980; **4**: 421–30.
70. Sheehy JL, Gardner G, Hambley WM. Tuning fork tests in modern otology. *Arch Otolaryngol* 1971; **94**: 132–8.
71. Dobie RA, Archer RJ. Results of otologic referrals in an industrial hearing conservation program. *Otolaryngol Head Neck Surg* 1981; **89**: 294–301.
72. Wolpert L. *The Unnatural Nature of Science*. London: Faber and Faber, 1992.
73. Hinchcliffe R. Hearing threshold level and its component parts. In: Rossi G, ed. *Proceedings of the International Advanced Research Workshop: 1975–1995: Man and Environmental Noise Twenty Years After*. Turin: Minerva Medica, 1995.
74. Hinchcliffe R. Effects of noise on hearing—aspects of assessment: guidelines for giving advice to expert witnesses. *J Audiol Med* 2000; **9**: 1–18.
75. DHSS. *Occupational Deafness*. Cmnd 5461. London: HMSO, 1973: para. 31.
76. Davis H, Silverman SR. *Hearing and Deafness*. New York: Holt, Rinehart and Winston, 1978.
77. Hinchcliffe R. Clinical tests of auditory function in the adult and in the schoolchild. In: Beagley HA ed. *Audiology and Audiological Medicine*, Vol. 1. Oxford: Oxford University Press, 1981: 320–64.
78. Klingon GH, Bontecou DC. Localisation in auditory space. *Neurology* 1966; **16**: 879–86.
79. Sϕhoel T. Acute suppurative otitis media in children 0–10 years of age. *Acta Otolaryngol* 1956; **46**: 422–38.
80. King PF. Some imperfections of the free-field voice tests. *J Laryngol Otol* 1953; **67**: 358–64.
81. Feldmann H. Die Geschichte der Stimmgabel. Teil II: Die Entwicklung der klassischen Versuche nach Weber, Rinne und Schwabach. *Laryngorhinootol* 1997; **76**: 318–26.
82. Schulze FA. Monochord zur Bestimmung der oberem Hörgrenze und der Perzeptionsfähigkeit des Ohres für sehr hohe Töne. *Z Ohrenheilkunde* 1908; **56**: 17–173.

83. Burckhardt-Merian A. Vergleichende Ergebnisse verschiedenartiger Hörprüfung. *Arch Ohren Nasen Kehlkopfheilkunde* 1885; **22**: 177–94.
84. Lutman ME. Diagnostic audiometry. In: Stephens D, ed. *Scott-Brown's Otolaryngology*, 6th edn, Vol. 2 *Adult Audiology*. London: Butterworth-Heinemann, 1997: 2/12/1–2/18/31.
85. Beagley HA. The role of electrophysiological tests in the diagnosis of nonorganic hearing loss. *Audiology* 1973; **12**: 470–80.
86. Sayers BMcA, Beagley HA, Ross AJ. Auditory evoked potentials of cortical origin. In: HA Beagley, ed. *Auditory Investigation: The Scientific and Technological Basis*. Oxford: Clarendon Press, 1979, pp. 489–506.
87. Coles RRA, Mason SM. The results of cortical electric response audiometry in medicolegal investigations. *Br J Audiol* 1984; **18**: 71–8.
88. Prasher D, Mula M, Luxon LM. Cortical evoked potential criteria in the objective assessment of auditory threshold: a comparison of noise induced hearing loss with Menière's disease. *J Laryngol Otol* 1993; **107**: 780–6.
89. Knight JJ, Littler TS. The technique of speech audiometry and a simple speech audiometer with masking generator for clinical use. *J Laryngol Otol* 1953; **67**: 248–65.
90. Priede VM, Coles RRA. Speech discrimination tests in investigation of sensorineural hearing loss. *J Laryngol Otol* 1976; **90**: 1081–92.
91. Hood JD. Principles and practice of bone conduction audiometry. *Laryngoscope* 1960; **70**: 1211–28.
92. Lightfoot GR. Air-borne radiation from bone-conduction transducers. *Br J Audiol* 1979; **13**: 53–6.
93. Bell I, Goodsell S, Thornton ARD. A brief communication on bone conduction artefacts. *Br J Audiol* 1980; **14**: 73–5.
94. Shipton MS, John AJ, Robinson DW. Air-radiated sound from bone vibration transducers and its implications for bone conduction audiometry. *Br J Audiol* 1980; **13**: 53–6.
95. Lightfoot GR, Hughes JB. Bone conduction errors at high frequencies: implications for clinical and medico-legal practice. *J Laryngol Otol* 1993; **107**: 305–8.
96. Harkrider AW, Martin FN. Quantifying air-conducted acoustic radiation from the bone-conduction vibrator. *J Am Acad Audiol* 1998; **9**: 410–16.
97. Anon. Recommended procedures for pure-tone audiometry using a manually operated instrument. *Br J Audiol* 1981; **15**: 213–16.
98. Anon. Recommendations for masking in pure tone audiometry. *Br J Audiol* 1986; **20**: 307–14.
99. Meyer-Bisch C. Audioscan: a high definition audiometry technique based on constant-level frequency sweeps—a new method with new hearing indicators. *Audiology* 1996; **35**: 63–72.
100. McMurray RF, Rudmose W. An automatic audiometer for industrial medicine. *Noise Control* 1956; **2**: 33–6.
101. Rice CG, Coles RRA. Normal threshold of hearing for pure tones by earphone listening with a self-recording audiometric technique. *J Acoust Soc Am* 1966; **39**: 1185–7.
102. Robinson DW, Whittle LS. A comparison of self-recording and manual audiometry: some systematic effects shown by unpractised subjects. *J Sound Vibration* 1973; **26**: 41–62.
103. Hinchcliffe R. György Békésy (1899–1972) 50 years of Békésy audiometry (1947–97). *J Audiol Med* 1999; **8**: 72–91.
104. Kryter KD. *The Handbook of Hearing and the Effects of Noise*. San Diego: Academic Press, 1994.
105. Alberti PW. Noise and the ear. In: Stephens D, ed. *Scott-Brown's Otolaryngology*, 6th edn. Vol. 2 *Adult Audiology*. London: Butterworth-Heinemann, 1997: 2/11/1–2/11/34.
106. Glorig A. *Noise and Your Ear*. New York: Grune and Stratton, 1958.
107. Davis AC, Fortnum HM, Coles RRA, Haggard MP, Lutman ME. *Damage to Hearing Arising from Leisure Noise: A Review of the Literature*. London: HSE, 1985.
108. Clark WW. Noise exposure from leisure activities: a review. *J Acoust Soc Am* 1991; **90**: 175–81.
109. Coles RRA, Garinther GR, Hodge DC, Rice CG. Hazardous exposure to impulse noise. *J Acoust Soc Am* 1968; **43**: 336–43.
110. Hinchcliffe R. Noise hazards to the general population: hearing surveys reassessed. *J Audiol Med* 1999; **8**: 113–21.
111. Robinson DW (ed.). *Occupational Hearing Loss*. London: Academic Press, 1971.
112. Sataloff RT, Sataloff J. *Occupational Hearing Loss*. New York: Dekker, 1993.
113. Steinberg JC, Montgomery HC, Gardner MB. Results of the World's Fair Hearing Tests. *J Acoust Soc Am* 1940; **12**: 291–301.
114. Leijon A. Quantization error in clinical pure-tone audiometry. *Scand Audiol* 1992; **21**: 103–8.
115. Stephens SDG. Some individual factors influencing audiometric performance. In: Robinson DW, ed. *Occupational Hearing Loss*. London: Academic Press, 1971: 109–20.
116. Dancer A, Buck K, Parmentier G, Hamer YP. The specific problems of noise in military life. In: Prasher D, Luxon LM eds. *Advances in Noise Research Series*, Vol. 1. London: Whurr, 1998: 139–56.
117. Coles RRA, Rice CG. Auditory hazards of sports guns. *Laryngoscope* 1966; **76**: 1728–31.
118. Prosser S, Tartari MC, Arslan E. Hearing loss in sports hunters exposed to occupational noise. *Br J Audiol* 1988; **22**: 85–91.
119. Berry BF. *Ambient Noise Limits for Audiometry*. NPL Acoustics Report Ac 60 (2nd). Teddington: National Physical Laboratory, 1973.
120. Bryan ME, Parbrook HD, Tempest W. A note on quiet threshold shift in the absence of noise. *J Sound Vibration* 1965; **2**: 147–9.
121. Fearn RW, Hanson DR. Audiometric zero for air conduction using manual audiometry. *Br J Audiol* 1983; **17**: 87–90.
122. Pyykko I, Starck J, Farkkila M, Hoikkala M, Kohonen Ol, Nurminen M. Hand–arm vibration in the aetiology of hearing loss in lumberjacks. *Br J Indust Med* 1981; **38**: 281–9.
123. Morata TC, Engel T, Durao A et al. Hearing loss from combined exposures among petroleum refinery workers. *Scand Audiol* 1997; **26**: 141–9.
124. Morata TC, Fiorini AC, Fischer FM et al. Toluene-induced hearing loss among rotogravure printing workers. *Scand J Work Environment Health* 1997; **23**: 289–98.
125. Burkhard MD, Corliss ELR. The response of earphones in ears and couplers. *J Acoust Soc Am* 1954; **26**: 679–85.

126. Delany ME. The acoustical impedance of human ears. *J Sound Vibration* 1964; **1**: 455–67.
127. Erber NP. Variables that influence sound pressures generated in the ear canal by an audiometric earphone. *J Acoust Soc Am* 1968; **44**: 555–62.
128. Ithell AH. The measurement of the acoustical input impedance of human ears. *Acustica* 1963; **13**: 140–5.
129. Ithell AH. A determination of the acoustical input impedance characteristics of human ears. *Acustica* 1963; **13**: 311–14.
130. Zwislocki J. Some measurements of the impedance at the eardrum. *J Acoust Soc Am* 1957; **29**: 349–56.
131. Royal Society of Medicine. *Report of the Committee appointed by the Section of Otology for the Consideration of Hearing Tests*. London: Longmans Green, 1932.
132. Ventry IM, Chaiklin JB, Boyle WF. Collapse of the ear canal during audiometry. *Arch Otolaryngol* 1961; **73**: 727–31.
133. Coles RRA. External meatus closure by audiometer earphone. *J Speech Hear Disord* 1967; **32**: 296–7.
134. Chaiklin JB, McClellan ME. Audiometric management of collapsible ear canals. *Arch Otolaryngol* 1971; **93**: 397–407.
135. Hickling S. Studies on the reliability of auditory threshold values. *J Auditory Res* 1966; **6**: 39–46.
136. Chamberlain D. Occupational deafness: audiometric observations on aural fatigue and recovery. *Arch Otolaryngol* 1942; **35**: 595–602.
137. Hirsh IJ, Ward WD. Recovery of the auditory threshold after strong acoustic stimulation. *J Acoust Soc Am* 1952; **24**: 131–41.
138. Atherley GRC. Monday morning auditory threshold in weavers. *Br J Indust Med* 1964; **21**: 150–4.
139. Gallo R, Glorig A. Permanent threshold shift changes produced by noise exposure and aging. *Am Indust Hygiene Assoc J* 1964; **25**: 237–45.
140. Burns W, Robinson DW. *Hearing and Noise in Industry*. London: HMSO, 1970.
141. Robinson DW. Characteristics of noise-induced hearing loss. In Henderson D, Hamernik RP, Dosanjh DS, Mills JH eds. *Effects of Noise on Hearing*. New York: Raven, 1976: 383–94.
142. Davis A. *Hearing in Adults*. London: Whurr, 1995.
143. Ward WD, Glorig A, Sklar DL. Susceptibility and sex. *J Acoust Soc Am* 1959; **31**: 1138.
144. Jerger J, Chmiel R, Stach B, Spretnjak M. Gender affects audiometric shape in presbyacusis. *J Am Acad Audiol* 1993; **4**: 42–9.
145. Gatehouse S, Lowe GDO. Whole blood viscosity and red cell filterability as factors in sensorineural hearing impairments in the elderly. *Acta Otolaryngol (Stockh)* 1991; Suppl. 476: 37–43.
146. Tota G, Bocci G. L'importanza del colore dell'iride nella valutazione della resistenza dell'udito all'affaticamento. *Riv Otoneurooftalmol* 1967; **43**: 183–92.
147. Hood JD, Poole JP, Freedman L. The influence of eye colour upon temporary threshold shift. *Audiology* 1976; **15**: 449–64.
148. Carter NL. Eye colour and susceptibility to noise-induced permanent threshold shift. *Audiology* 1980; **19**: 86–93.
149. Royster LH, Driscoll DP, Thomas WG, Royster JD. Age effect hearing levels for a black nonindustrial noise exposed population (ninep). *Am Indust Hygiene Assoc J* 1980; **41**: 113–19.
150. Royster LH, Royster JD, Thomas WG. Representative hearing levels by race and sex in North Carolina industry. *J Acoust Soc Am* 1980; **68**: 551–66.
151. Thomas GB, Williams CE, Hoger JM. Some nonauditory correlates of the hearing threshold levels of an aviation noise-exposed population. *Aviation Space Environ Med* 1981; **52**: 531–6.
152. Barrenas M-L. *Pigmentation and Noise-induced Hearing Loss*. Göteborg: Sahlgren's University Hospital, 1996.
153. Laird DA. Acuity of hearing. *Science*. 1935; **82**: 152–3.
154. Robinson DW, Lawton BW, Rice CG. *Occupational Hearing Loss from Low-level Noise*. HSE Contract Research Report No. 68/1994. Southampton: Institute of Sound and Vibration Research, University of Southampton, 1994.
155. Lutman ME, Spencer HS. Occupational noise and demographic factors in hearing. *Acta Otolaryngol (Stockh)* 1991; Suppl. 476: 74–84.
156. Robinson DW, Lawton BW. Concept of the notional person in the assessment of hearing disability. *Br J Audiol* 1996; **30**: 45–54.
157. Stephens SDG. Audiometers from Hughes to modern times. *Br J Audiol* 1979; **13**: 17–23.
158. Stephens SDG. The British medical profession and the first audiometers. *J Laryngol Otol* 1981; **95**: 1223–35.
159. Hughes DE. On an induction-current balance and experimental researches made therewith. *Proc Royal Soc London* 1879; **29**: 56–65.
160. Gradenigo G. Ueber ein neues elektrisches Akumetermodell[1]. *Archiv für Ohren-, Nasen- und Kehlkopfheilkunde* 1890; **30**: 240–5.
161. Urbanschitsch V. Zwei neue Hörmessapparate[2]. *Monatschift für Ohrenheilkunde* 1914; **48**: 561–8.
162. Richardson BW. Some researches with Professor Hughes' new instrument for the measurement of hearing; the audiometer. *Proc Royal Soc London* 1879; **29**: 65–70.
163. Phillips WC. *Diseases of the Ear, Nose and Throat*. 6th edition. Philadelphia: Davis, 1922.
164. Mahoney CF, Luxon LM. Misdiagnosis of hearing loss due to ear canal collapse: a report of two cases. *J Laryngol Otol* 1996; **110**: 561–6.
165. Medical Research Council. *Hearing Aids and Audiometers*. Committee on Electro-acoustics, Medical Research Council. Special Report Series No. 261. London: HMSO, 1947.
166. Beatty RT. *Hearing in Man and Animals*. London: Bell and Sons, 1932.
167. Békésy G von, Rosenblith. The mechanical properties of the ear. Ch 27 in SS Stevens (Ed). *Handbook of Experimental Psychology*. New York: John Wiley, 1951. pp 1075–115.
168. Waetzmann E. Ein erb-biologisches Problem am menschlichen Gehörorgan[3]. *Nachrichtung Gesellschaft Wissenschaft Göttingen* 1935; **1**: 157–61.
169. Waetzmann E. Ueber Symmetrie- und Erblichkeitsfragen am menschlichen Gehörorgan[4]. *Akustiche Zeitung* 1936; **1**: 155–9.

[1] Concerning a new electrical acoumeter [audiometer].
[2] Two new audiometers.
[3] Heredity and the organ of hearing in man.
[4] Questions of symmetry and heredity in the human auditory organ.

170. Robinson DW. Variability in the Realization of the Audiometric Zero. *Ann Occupational Hygiene* 1960; **2**: 107–26.
171. Gradenigo G. Studien und Vorschläge zur Messung der Hörschärfe[5]. *Archiv für Ohrenheilkunde* 1912; 87: 123–33.
172. Licklider JCR. Basic correlates of the auditory stimulus. Ch 25 in SS Stevens (Ed). *Handbook of Experimental Psychology*. New York: John Wiley, 1951. pp 985–1039.
173. Brogden WJ, Miller GA. Physiological noise generated under earphone cushions. *J Acoustic Soc Am* 1947; **19**: 620–3.
174. Békésy G von. Ueber die Hörschwelle und Fühlgrenze langsamer sinusförmiger Luftdruckschwankungen[6]. *Annalen die Physik* 1936; **26**: 554–66.
175. Waetzmann E, Keibs, L. Hörschwellenbestimmungen mit dem Thermophon und Messungen am Trommelfell[7]. *Annalen die Physik* 1936; **26**: 141–4.
176. Stephens SDG. Clinical Audiometry. Ch. 15 in HA Beagley (Ed) *Audiology and Audiological Medicine*. Volume 2. Oxford: OUP, 1981. pp 365–90.
177. Haughton PM. *Acoustics for Audiologists*. New York: Academic Press, 2002.
178. Wimberly M. An Application of Electromagnetics: The Loudspeaker http://ece.gmu.edu/~pceperle/st3/ece305~1.htm (accessed 10 October 2002)
179. Bárány R. Lärmapparat zum Nachweis der einseitegen Taubheit[8]. *Verhandlung Deutsche Otologische Gesellschaft* 1908; 84–5.
180. Aubry M, Giraud JC. Le problème de l'assourdissement dans l'examen de l'audition[9]. *Annales d'Oto-Laryngologie* 1939; **4**: 333–48.
181. Studebaker GA. Clinical masking of air- and bone-conducted stimuli. *J Speech Hear Disord* 1963; 29: 23–35.
182. Wegel RL, Lane CE. The auditory masking of one pure tone by another and its probable relation to the dynamics of the inner ear. *Phys Rev* 1924; **23**: 268–85.
183. Hawkins JE Jr, Stevens SS. The masking of pure tones and of speech by noise. *J Acoustic Soc Am* 1950; **22**: 6–13.
184. Fletcher H. Auditory patterns. *Rev Modern Phys* 1940; **12**: 47–65.
185. Scharf B. Critical bands. In: JV Tobias (Ed). *Foundations of Modern Auditory Theory*. Volume 1. New York: Academic Press, 1970. Pp 157–202.
186. Chaiklin JB, Ventry IM. The efficiency of audiometric measures used to identify functional hearing loss. *J Auditory Res* 1965; **5**: 196–211.
187. Haughton PM, Lewsley A, Wilson M,D Williams RG. A Forced-Choice Procedure to Detect Feigned or Exaggerated Hearing Loss. *BrJ Audiol* 1979; **13**: 135–8
188. Niemeyer W, Sesterhenn G. Calculating the hearing threshold from the stapedius reflex threshold for different sound stimuli. *Audiology* 1974; **13**: 421–7.
189. Jerger J, Burney P, Maudlin L, Crump B. Predicting hearing loss from the acoustic reflex. *J Speech Hearing Disord* 1974; **96**: 513–23.
190. Kemp DT. Evidence for mechanical nonlinearity and frequency selective wave amplification in the cochlea. *Arch Oto-Rhino-Laryngol* 1979; **224**: 37–45.
191. Stephens D, Orzan E. Pioneers of audiological medicine: Giuseppe Gradenigo (1857–1926). *J Audiol Med* 1997; **6**: 59–61.
192. Hood JD. The principles and practice of bone conduction audiometry. *J Royal Soc Med* 1957; **50**: 689–97.
193. Békésy G von. Zur theorie des Hörens bei der Schallaufnahme durch Knochenleitung[10]. *Annalen die Physik* 1932; **13**: 111–36.
194. Békésy G von. Ueber die Schallausbreitung bei Knochenleitung[11]. *Zeitschrift für Hals- Nas, -Ohrenheilkunde* 1941; **47**: 430–42.
195. Békésy G von. Vibration of the head in a sound field and its role in hearing by bone conduction. *J Acoustic Soc Am* 1948; **20**: 749–60.
196. Bárány E. Ueber die Bedeutung der Knochenleitung für das hören von Luftschall[12]. *Acta oto-laryngol* 1935; **22**: 229–33.
197. Bárány E. A contribution to the physiology of bone conduction. *Acta oto-laryngol* 1938, Supplement 26, pp 1–223.
198. Bárány E. New points of view on the problem of bone conduction. *Acta oto-laryngol* 1940; **28**: 393–9.
199. Allen GW, Fernandez C. The mechanism of bone conduction. *Ann Otology, Rhinol Laryngol* 1960; **69**: 5–29.
200. Tonndorf J, Campbell RA, Bernstein L, Reneau JP. Quantitative evaluation of bone conduction components in cats. *Acta oto-laryngol* 1966; Supplement 213 pp 10–38.
201. Tonndorf J. Bone conduction. Ch 2 in Keidel WD, Neff W (Eds) *Handbook of Sensory Physiology* Vol 3 Berlin: Springer, 1976.
202. von Helmholtz H. Ueber die Mechanik der Gehörknöchelchen und des Trommelfels[13]. *Pflügers Archiv füf gesampte Physiologie* 1868; **1**: 1–60.
203. Carhart R. Clinical application of bone conduction. *Arch Oto-laryngol* 1950; **51**: 798–807.
204. Watson PB, Gengel RW, Hirsh IJ. Effects of vibrator types and their placement on bone-conduction threshold measurements. *J Acoustic Soc Am* 1967; **41**: 788–92.
205. Békésy G von. Ueber die piezoelektrische Messung der absoluten Hörschwelle bei Knochenleitung[14]. *Akustiche Zeitung* 1939; **4**: 113–25;
206. Link R, Zwislocki J. Audiometrische Knockenleitungsuntersuchungen[15]. *Zeitschrift für Ohrenheilkunde* 1951; **160**: 347–57.

[5] Studies [on] and proposals [for] the measurement of hearing sensitivity.
[6] Concerning the thresholds of hearing and feeling for slow sinusoidal pressure variations.
[7] The determination of auditory thresholds by means of the thermophone; impedance measurements on the tympanic membrane.
[8] A noise device for proving unilateral deafness.
[9] The problem of masking (the contralateral ear) in the examination of hearing.
[10] The theory of hearing applied to sound perception through bone conduction.
[11] On the transmission of sound by bone conduction.
[12] The significance of bone conduction for air conduction.
[13] The mechanics of the auditory ossicles and the eardrum
[14] Determination of the absolute threshold for bone conduction by piezoelectric measurements.
[15] Audiometric investigation of bone conduction.

207. Hart C, Naunton R. Frontal bone conduction tests in clinical audiometry. *Laryngoscope* 1961; **71**: 24–9.
208. Dirks D, Malmquist C. Comparison of frontal and mastoid bone conduction thresholds in various conduction lesions. *J Speech Hearing Res* 1969; **12**: 725–46.
209. Watson NA. Limits of audition for bone-conduction. *J Acoustic Soc Am* 1938; **9**: 294–300.
210. Nilo ER. The relation of vibrator surface area and static application force to the vibrator-to-head coupling. *J Speech Hearing Res* 1968; **11**: 805–10.
211. Békésy G von. Ueber die piezoelektrische Messung der absoluten Hörschwelle bei Knochenleitung[16]. *Akustiche Zeitung* 1939; **4**: 113–25.
212. Harris JD, Haines HL, Myers CK. A helmet-held bone conduction vibrator. *Laryngoscope* 1953; 998–1007.
213. König E. Les variations de la conduction osseuse en fonction de la force de pression exercée sur la vibrateur[17]. *Proceedings of the 2nd Congress of the International Society of Audiology*, Paris, 1955.
214. Whittle LS. A determination of the normal threshold of hearing by bone conduction. *J Sound Vibration* 1965; **2**: 227–48.
215. Boothroyd A, Cawkwell S. Vibrotactile thresholds in pure tone audiometry. *Acta oto-laryngol* 1970; **69**; 381–7.
216. Rainville MJ. Nouvelle méthode d'assourdissement pour le revelé des courbes de conduction osseuse[18]. *Journal français d'otorhino-laryngologie* 1955; **4**: 851–8.
217. Jerger J, Tillman T. A new method for the clinical determination of sensorineural acuity level. (SAL). *Arch Otolaryngol* 1960; **71**: 948–53.
218. Lightfoot C. The M-R test of bone conduction. *Laryngoscope* 1960; **70**; 1552–9.
219. Tillman T. The assessment of sensorineural acuity. In: B Graham (Ed). *Sensorineural hearing processes and disorder*. Boston: Little, Brown and Co., 1967.
220. Wheatstone C. Experiments in audition. *Quarterly Journal of Science, Literature and Arts* 1827 pp 67–72.
221. Bing A. Ein neuer Stimmgabelversuch[19]. *Wiener medizinisch Blatt* 1891; **14**: 637–8.
222. Koyter (or Coiter) *De Auditus Instrumento*. Groningen, 1572.
223. Aubry M, Giraud JC. Etude de la conduction osseuse[20]. *Presse médicale* 1939; **47**: 653–5.
224. Pomeroy OD. *Diagnosis and treatment of diseases of the ear*. New York: Appleton, 1883. at p 337.
225. Hallpike CS. Suggested graphic method of representing the tuning fork tests. *J Laryngol Otol* 1927; **32**: 322–7.

[16] Determination of the absolute threshold for bone conduction by piezoelectric measurements.
[17] Variations in bone conduction as a function of the force applied to the vibrator.
[18] New method of masking for the determination of bone conduction curves.
[19] A new tuning fork test.
[20] A study of bone conduction.

226. Schwabach P. Ueber den Werth des Rinne'schen Versuches für die Diagnostik des Gehörkrankheiten[21]. *Zeitschrift für Ohrenheilkunde* 1885; **14**: 61–148.
227. Kelley NH, Reger SN. The effect of binaural occlusion of the external auditory meati on the sensitivity of the normal ear for bone conducted sound. *J Exp Psych* 1937; **21**: 211–17.
228. Sullivan JA, Gotlieb CC, Hodges WE. Shifts of bone conduction threshold on occlusion of the external ear canal. *Laryngoscope* 1947; **57**: 690–703.
229. Dirks D, Swindeman J. The variability of occluded and unoccluded bone conduction thresholds. *J Speech Hearing Res* 1967; **10**: 232–49.
230. Hodgson WR, Tillman T. Reliability of bone conduction occlusion effects in normals. *J Auditory Res* 1966; **6**: 141–53.
231. Békésy G von. A new audiometer. *Acta oto-laryngol (Stockholm)* 1947; **35**: 411.
232. Lundborg T. Diagnostic problems concerning acoustic neuromas. *Acta oto-laryngol (Stockholm) Supplement* 1952; **99**, 1–110.
233. Reger SN. A clinical and research version of the Békésy audiometer. *Laryngoscope* 1952; **62**: 1333–51.
234. Reger SN, Kos CM. Clinical measurements and implications of recruitment. *Ann Otol, Rhinol Laryngol* 1952; **61**: 810–23.
235. Hinchcliffe R. Examen otoneurologique pour le diagnostic des neurinomes acoustiques. *Acta oto-rhino-laryngologica belgica* 1971; **25**: 770–83.
236. Priede VM, Coles RRA. Masking of the non-test ear in tone decay, Békésy audiometry, and SISI tests. *J Laryngol Otol* 1975; **89**: 227–36.
237. Jerger J, Herer G. An unexpected dividend in Békésy audiometry. *J Speech Hearing Disord* 1961; **26**: 390–1.
238. Rintelman WF, Carhart R. Loudness tracking by normal hearers via Békésy audiometer. *J Speech Hearing Res* 1964; **7**: 79–93.
239. Stein L. Some observations on type V Békésy tracings. *J Speech Hearing Res* 1963; **6**: 339–48.
240. Istre CO, Burton M. Automatic audiometry for detecting malingering. *Arch Otolaryngol* 1969; **90**: 326–32.
241. Reger SN, Reneau J, Watson JE. Quantitative evaluation of the Stenger test. *Int Audiol.* 1963; **2**: 144–7.
242. Cheesman AD, Stephens SDG. A new method for the detection of functional hearing loss. *Charing Cross Hospital Gazette* 1965; **63**: vii–xi.
243. Watson JE, Voots RJ. Clinical application of the Reger modification of the Stenger test. *Int Audiol.* 1965; **4**: 149–53.
244. Hood WH, Campbell RA, Hutton CL. An evaluation of the Békésy ascending descending gap. *J Speech Hearing Res* 1964; **7**: 123–32.
245. Hattler KW. Lengthened-off time: a self-recording screening device for nonorganicity. *J Speech Hearing Disord* 1970; **35**: 113–22.
246. Chaiklin JB. A descending LOT-Békésy screening test for functional hearing loss. *J Speech Hearing Disord* 1990; **55**: 67–74.

[21] Concerning the worth of Rinne's tests for the diagnosis of hearing disorders.

247. Dix MR, Hallpike CS, Hood JD. Observations upon the loudness recruitment phenomenon, with especial reference to the differential diagnosis of disorders of the internal ear and VIII nerve. *Proceedings of the Royal Society of Medicine* 1948; **41**: 516–26.
248. Fowler EP. A method for the early detection of otosclerosis. *Arch Otolaryngol* 1936; **24**: 731–41.
249. Fowler EP. The diagnosis of diseases of the neural mechanism of hearing by the aid of sounds well above threshold. *Trans Am Otol Soc* 1937; **27**: 207–19.
250. Harbert F,D Young IM. Threshold auditory adaptation. *J Auditory Res* 1962; **2**: 229–46.
251. Bilger RC. Some parameters of fixed frequency Békésy audiometry. *J Speech Hearing Res* 1965; **8**: 85–95.
252. Melnick W. Comfort level and loudness matching for continuous and interrupted signals. *J Speech Hearing Res* 1967; **10**: 99–109.
253. Jerger J, Jerger S. Diagnostic value of Békésy comfortable loudness tracings. *Arch Otolaryngol*1974; **99**: 351–60.
254. Dancer JE. Excursion size of Békésy tracings of continuous and interrupted tones at threshold and at most comfortable loudness in cochlear-impaired ears. *J Auditory Res* 1983; **23**: 72–6.
255. Reger SN. Differences in loudness response of the normal and hard-of-hearing ear at intensity levels slightly above the threshold. *Ann Otol, Rhinol Laryngol* 1936; **45**: 1029–39.
256. Watson NA. Certain fundamental principles in prescribing and fitting hearing aids. *Laryngoscope* 1944; **54**: 531–8.
257. Hood JD, Poole JP. Tolerable limit of loudness: its clinical and physiological significance. *J Acoustic Soc Am*1966; **40**: 47–53.
258. Stephens SDG. Studies on the uncomfortable loudness level. *Sound* 1970; **4**: 20–5.
259. Tsuiki T, Sakamoto S, Homma T, Numakura M, Aizawa H, Ishimoda M. Loudness Tracking for Supra-threshold Levels. *Proceedings of Xth Annual Congress of Japan Audiological Society, Kyoto* 19–20 October 1965; pp 7–10.
260. Kos CM. Auditory function as related to a complaint of dizziness. *Laryngoscope* 1955; **65**: 711–21.
261. McLay K. The place of the Békésy audiometer in clinical audiometry. *J Laryngol Otol* 1959; **73**: 460–5.
262. Rose DE. Some effects and case histories of reversed frequency sweep in Békésy audiometry. *J Auditory Res* 1962; **2**: 267–78.
263. Harbert F, Young IM. Clinical application of Békésy audiometry. *Laryngoscope* 1968; **78**: 487–97.
264. Karja J, Palva A. Reverse frequency-sweep Békésy audiometry. *Acta oto-laryngol* 263 (suppl), 1970; pp 225–8.
265. Dirks DD, Norris JD. Shifts in auditory thresholds produced by ipsilateral and contralateral maskers at low-intensity levels. *J Acoustic Soc Am* 1966; **40**: 12–19.
266. Blegvad B. Contralateral masking and Békésy audiometry in normal listeners. *Acta oto-laryngol* 1967; **64**: 157–65.
267. Collet L, Kemp DT, Veuillet E, Duclaux R, Moulin A, Morgon A. Effect of contralateral auditory stimuli on active cochlear micromechanical properties in human subjects. *Hearing Res* 1990; **43**: 251–62.
268. Ryan S, Kemp DT, Hinchcliffe R. The influence of contralateral stimulation on click-evoked otoacoustic emissions. *Br J Audiol* 1991; **25**: 391–7.
269. Orchik DJ, Dunckel DC, Culbertson MC. Békésy comfortable loudness: supportive case studies. *J Speech Hearing Disord* 1977; **42**: 126–9.
270. Bolla I, Baldo D, Bottazzi D, Collini M. Audiometria automatica sopraliminare nelle ipoacusie neurosensorali. *Ateneo Parmense - Acta Bio-Medica* 1980; **51**: 453–9
271. Hinchcliffe R, Chambers C. Loudness of tinnitus: an approach to measurement. *Adv Oto-Rhino-Laryngol* 1983; **29**: 163–73.
272. Jerger J. Békésy audiometry in analysis of auditory disorders. *J Speech Hearing Res* 1960; **3**: 275–87.
273. Harden T, Kiessling J. Zur Interpretation von Békésy-Audiogrammen. *Arch Oto-Rhino-Laryngol* 1979; **222**: 265–71.
274. Sørensen H. Clinical application of continuous threshold recordings. *Acta oto-laryngol* 1962; **54**: 403–22.
275. Parker W, Decker RL, Richards NG. Auditory function and lesions of the pons. *Arch Otolaryngol* 1968; **87**: 228–40.
276. Rudmose W. Ch.2 Automatic audiometry. In: *Modern Developments in Audiology* J Jerger (Ed). New York: Academic Press, 1963.
277. McCommons RB, Hodge DC. Comparison of Continuous and Pulsed Tones for Determining Békésy Threshold Measurements. *J Acoustic Soc Am*1969; **45**: 1499–1503.
278. Pelmear PL,D Hughes BJ. Self-recording audiometry in industry. *Br J ind Med* 1974; **31**: 304–9.
279. Frampton MC, Counter RT. A comparison of self recording audiometry in naval establishments and clinical audiometry in a hospital setting. *J Royal Naval Med Serv* 1989; **75**: 99–104.
280. Gosztonyi RE, Vassallo RA, Sataloff J. Audiometric reliability in industry. *Arch Env Health* 1971; **22**: 113–18.
281. Erlandsson B, Hakånson H, Ivarsson A, Nilsson P. Comparison of the Hearing Threshold Measured by Manual Pure-Tone and by Self-Recording (Békésy) Audiometry. *Audiology* 1979; **18**: 414–29.
282. Plomp R. Hearing Losses induced by small arms. *Int Audiol* 1967; **6**: 31–6.
283. West PDB, Evans EF. Early detection of hearing damage in young listeners resulting from exposure to amplified music. *Br J Audiol* 1990; **24**: 89–103.
284. Gauz MT,D Smith MM. High-frequency Békésy audiometry. VI Pulsed vs. continuous signals. *J Auditory Res* 1987; **27**: 37–52.
285. Albers GD. Diplacusimetry. *Proceedings of VIII International Congress of Otolaryngology* Tokyo 1965. Amsterdam: Excerpta Medica, 1966. p 401.
286. Grisanti G. An automatic test for frequency discrimination. *Br J Audiol* 1987; **21**: 233–7.
287. Domico WD. Békésy-tracked aural harmonic distortion thresholds and uncomfortable loudness levels. *Ear & Hearing* 1985; **6**: 260–5.
288. John PY, Kacker SK, Tandon PN. Békésy audiometry in evaluation of hearing in cases of raised intracranial pressure. *Acta oto-laryngol* 1979; **87**: 441–4.
289. Anderson H, Wedenberg E. Audiometric identification of normal hearing carriers of genes for deafness. *Acta oto-laryngol* 1968; **65**: 535–54.

290. Parving A. Reliability of Békésy threshold tracing in identification of carriers of genes for an X-linked disease with deafness. *Acta oto-laryngol* 1978; **85**: 40–4.
291. Cohen M, Francis M, Luxon LM, Bellman S, Coffey R, Pembrey M. Dips on Bekesy or audioscan fail to identify carriers of autosomal recessive non-syndromic hearing loss. *Acta Oto-Laryngol* 1996; **116**: 521–7.
292. Meredith R, Stephens D, Sirimanna T, Meyer-Bisch C, Reardon W. Audiometric detection of carriers of Usher's syndrome type II. *J Audiol Med* 1992; **1**: 11–19.
293. Stephens SDG. Personal communication, 1999.
294. Hood JD. Hearing acuity and susceptibility to noise induced hearing loss. *Br J Audiol* 1987; **21**: 175–81.
295. Corso JF. Effect of testing methods on hearing thresholds. *Arch Otolaryngol* 1955; **63**: 78–91.
296. Burns W, Hinchcliffe R. Comparison of the Auditory Threshold as Measured by Individual Pure Tone and by Békésy audiometry. *J Acoustic Soc Am* 1957; **29**: 1274–7.
297. Jokinen K. Presbyacusis. *Acta oto-laryngol* 1969; **68**: 327–35.
298. Robinson DW. Audiometric configurations and repeatability in noise-induced hearing loss. *ISVR Technical Report No. 123*. Southampton: Institute of Sound and Vibration Research, University of Southampton, 1984.
299. Delany ME. Some sources of Variance in the Determination of Hearing Level. In *Occupational Hearing Loss* DW Robinson (Ed) London: Academic Press, 1971. pp 97–108.
300. Epstein A. Variables involved in automatic audiometry. *Ann Otol,, Rhinol Laryngol* 1960; **69**: 137–41.
301. Suzuki T, Kubota K. Normal width in tracing on Békésy audiograms. *J Auditory Res* 1966; **6**: 91–6.
302. Shepherd DC, Goldstein R. Intrasubject variability in amplitude of Békésy tracings. *J Speech Hearing Res* 1968; **11**: 523–5.
303. Palva T. Recruitment tests at low sensation levels. *Laryngoscope* 1956; **66**: 1519–40.
304. Granitz DW, Byers VW. Typing of Békésy audiograms. *Audiology* 1976; **15**: 215–21.
305. Turner RG, Shepard NT, Frazer GL. Clinical performance of audiological and related diagnostic tests. *Ear & Hearing* 1984; **5**: 187–94.
306. Hopkinson NT. Type V Békésy audiograms: specification and clinical utility. *J Speech Hearing Disord* 1965; **30**: 243–51.
307. Stephens SDG, Anderson CMB. Experimental studies on the uncomfortable loudness level. *J Speech Hearing Res* 1971; **14**: 262–70.
308. Stark EW. Jerger types in fixed frequency Békésy audiometry with normal and hypacusic children. *J Auditory Res* 1966; **6**: 135–40.
309. Price LL, Falck VT. Békésy audiometry *J Speech Hearing Res* 1963; **6**: 129–33.
310. Harbert F, Young IM, Menduke H. Audiologic findings in presbycusis. *J Auditory Res* 1966; **6**: 297–312.
311. Guild S. A method of classifying audiograms. *Laryngoscope* 1932; **42**: 821–36.
312. Gorlin RJ, Toriello HV, Cohen MM. *Hereditary hearing loss and its syndromes*. Oxford: OUP, 1995.
313. Martini A, Milani M, Rosignoli M, Mazzoli M, Prosser S. Audiometric Patterns of Genetic Non-syndromal Sensorineural Hearing Loss. *Audiology* 1997; **36**: 228–36.
314. Sokal RR, Sneath PHA. *Principles of Numerical Taxonomy*. San Francisco, CA: Freeman, 1963.
315. Job A, Delplace F, Anvers P, Gorzerino P, Grateau P, Picard J. Analyze automatique d'audiogramme visant à la surveillance épidémiologique de cohortes exposées aux bruits impulsifs. *Revue d'Epidémiologie et de Santé Publique* 1993; **41**: 407–15.
316. Hotelling H. Analysis of a complex of statistical variables into principal components. *J ed Psycd* 1933; **24**: 498–520.
317. Gower JC, Ross GJS. Minimum spanning trees and single linkage cluster analysis. *J Royal Stat Soc* 1969; C 18.
318. Job A, Buland F, Maumet L, Picard J. Windows software application for Békésy audiogram analysis and hearing research. *Computer Methods & Programs in Biomedicine* 1996; **49**: 95–103.
319. Romeder JM. *Méthodes et Programmes pour l'Analyse Discriminante*. Paris: Dunod, 1973.
320. Robert C. *Analyse desciptive multivariée: application à l'intelligence artificielle*. Paris: Flammarion, 1989.
321. Özdamar Ö, Eilers RE, Miskiel E, Widen J. Classification of audiograms by sequential testing using a dynamic Bayesian procedure. *J Acoustic Soc Am* 1990; **88**: 2171–9.
322. Chalabi Z, Souckova S. Pattern analysis of Békésy audiograms. *J Acoustic Soc Am* 1985; **77**: 1185–91.
323. Wood TJ, Wittich WW, Mahassey RB. Computerised pure-tone audiometric procedures. *J Speech Hearing Res* 1973; **16**: 676–94.
324. Harris JD. A Comparison of Computerized Audiometry by ANSI, Bekesy fixed frequency, and Modified ISO Procedures in an Industrial Hearing Conservation Program. *J Auditory Res* 1980; **20**: 143–67.
325. Lutman ME. Microcomputer-controlled psychoacoustics in clinical audiology. *Br J Audiol* 1983; **17**: 109–14.

Glossary

(Abstracted with permission from Hinchcliffe R, Luxon LM, Williams RG. *Readings for the Medical Examiner Assessing Cases of Occupational Noise-induced Hearing Loss*, Vol. I of Luxon LM, ed. *Noise and Hearing*. London: Whurr, 2001.)

abiotrophy Tissue degeneration with loss or disturbance of function, particularly in diseases of genetic origin.

accreditation A formal recognition of competence; accreditation is granted when measurement competence is demonstrated in all of the laboratory's technical practices (UKAS).

acuity Sharpness, acuteness, as in *auditory acuity*.

air–bone gap The separation between the hearing threshold levels measured by air conduction and by bone conduction audiometry expressed as the degree to which the air conduction hearing threshold level exceeds the corresponding bone conduction hearing threshold level; having regard to degrees of uncertainty, the value, if positive, would indicate a conductive (middle ear) impairment of hearing, and, if negative, a non-organic component in the measured threshold of hearing.

air conduction audiometry *Audiometry*, invariably using *earphones*, whereby the test sounds are sent through the normal air conduction pathway of hearing, i.e. through the air-containing outer and middle ears. The method is used to determine an individual's threshold of hearing by air conduction; the results are portrayed graphically as an air conduction *audiogram*.

apoptosis Biologically programmed cell death (the molecular biological basis of ageing).

artificial ear A piece of equipment used to calibrate air conduction audiometers; the device is designed to simulate the physical properties (specifically, the *acoustic impedance* of the ear) of the average normal adult human ear which are relevant to measuring hearing by earphone listening; the specification for such a device is given in IEC 318 (referred to as an *ear simulator* in IEC 60318-1 (1998-07)).

artificial mastoid A piece of equipment used to calibrate bone conduction audiometers; specifically, it is designed to simulate the relevant physical properties of the firm prominence of the adult human head behind the *auricle* for the purpose of calibrating a *bone vibrator*.

audiogram A chart which portrays in graphic form the results of *audiometry*.

audiometer An electroacoustical instrument for the measurement of hearing.

audiometric picture The constellation of audiometric abnormalities which either characterizes a hearing disorder or characterizes a particular individual's hearing disorder; for occupational noise damage to hearing, there is 'a characteristic pattern on the audiogram showing typically the greatest loss at the 4,000 Hz frequency.'[75]

audiometry The measurement of hearing using electroacoustical equipment.

auditory acuity A term to denote sharpness of hearing; used to refer to the hearing threshold level or more broadly to also cover other auditory functions, e.g. frequency and intensity discriminations; broadly synonymous with *auditory sensitivity*.

auditory sensitivity A term to denote hearing sensitivity without any commitment as to whether or not the hearing is within the range of normality or outside it, and, if the latter, whether it is better or poorer, and, if the latter, whether it amounts to an *impairment* (material or otherwise) or a *hearing loss* and whether or not it results in one or more inabilities, disabilities or handicaps; broadly synonymous with *auditory acuity*.

auricle The soft flange-like structure on either side of the head which, being the only visible part of the ear, is generally recognized as 'the ear' (syn. *pinna*).

β (Greek letter beta) Response criterion; a measure derived from signal detection theory.

Békésy audiometer An automatic (self) recording audiometer which is able to conduct sweep frequency audiometry, i.e. to test a subject's hearing using a continuously variable test tone (glide tone).

bone conduction audiometry *Audiometry* using a *bone vibrator* in lieu of *earphones* in order to send the test sounds through the solid structures of the head to the cochlea of the internal ear; the aim is to bypass the normal air conduction pathway of hearing so that any obstruction to the passage of sound therein is circumvented.

calibration A test procedure applied to a piece of equipment to ensure that it conforms to a particular *standard*.

conductive threshold shift That shift in the auditory threshold which is to be attributed to sound attenuation through the outer and middle ear and which is measured by the *air–bone gap*; it may or may not be of sufficient degree to amount to a conductive hearing loss.

d′ Detectability index; a measure derived from signal detection theory; ROC curves show the probability of a true positive response versus a false-positive response for a signal, sound or other.

deafness Total hearing loss.

decibel The unit used for expressing the physical magnitude of sounds.

decibel scale A logarithmic ratio scale used to quantify the magnitude of a sound level; since it is a ratio scale, there is a reference sound level; a sound which has a (sound) level of 0 dB is one whose pressure (in pascals) is numerically equivalent to that of the reference zero; consequently, there are many 0 dB levels (not one), depending on the reference level used; the decibel scale is thus unlike the arithmetically linear scales that are used, for example, to measure length and mass, where each scale has one zero value only.

disabling hearing impairment (1) In adults should be defined as a permanent unaided hearing threshold level of 41 dB or greater; (2) in children under the age of 15 years should be defined as a permanent unaided hearing threshold level for the better ear of 31 dB or greater. For both children and adults, the 'hearing threshold level' is to be taken as the better ear average hearing threshold level for the four frequencies: 0.5, 1, 2 and 4 kHz.[56]

EUROMET A cooperative organization linking the national metrological organizations in the EU and EFTA states and the European Commission; the participating metrology institutes intend to collaborate in EUROMET, with the objective of promoting the coordination of metrological activities and services with the purpose of achieving higher efficiency.

FFA Four frequency average (the average of the hearing threshold levels at 0.5, 1, 2 and 4 kHz); used by the Medical Research Council as an index of hearing ability.

frequency An attribute of a periodic quantity being the repetition rate of the cycles; unit is the hertz (Hz).

hearing level For a specified frequency of pure tone and testing system, the sound pressure level (essentially the physical magnitude of the sound) (in the case of air conduction audiometers) or vibratory force level (essentially the physical magnitude of the vibration) (in the case of bone conduction audiometers) or the *tone* relative to that of a reference zero (as defined by an International or National Standard). It is the dial setting of an audiometer if the instrument has been properly calibrated. Expressed in decibels, i.e. as dB HL.

hearing loss An impairment of hearing that exceeds a criterial level; no units, but may be qualified, in terms of severity, as 'mild', 'severe' etc. Neither the term 'hearing loss' nor the term 'hearing gain' should be used to describe hearing which is, respectively, greater than, or less than, the average hearing threshold level, just as the terms 'height loss' or 'height gain' would not be used to describe the height of someone who was less than, or greater than, average height unless it had been shown that a loss or a gain in height had occurred, e.g. by serial measurements. Criteria for defining a 'hearing loss' of an individual ear: an ear with a 'mild hearing loss' (the minimum severity of a hearing loss) needs to show an audiometric threshold of 20 dB to 40 dB HL averaged over the five frequencies 250 Hz, 500 Hz, 1000 Hz, 2000 Hz and 4000 Hz; but 'average hearing losses of less than 20 dB do not necessarily imply normal hearing'.[58]

hearing status A description of the degree to which the hearing of an individual functions normally with respect to accepted criteria (analogous to health status).

hearing threshold level For a particular *ear*, and a given frequency and test system, it is an individual's threshold of hearing (i.e. the quietest sound that the individual can hear) as determined in a stated manner and expressed by the system's indicated 'hearing level' value. Expressed in decibels, i.e. as dB HTL.

hearing threshold shift The change in the threshold of hearing for a given frequency (or group of frequencies) over a particular period of time; expressed in decibels.

IEC International Electrotechnical Commission, the international body (based in Geneva) that deals with standards in the field of electrical technology; a prefix to a standard to denote that it is one of that organization.

IHR Institute of Hearing Research (the MRC unit for research on hearing; epidemiology forms a strong component in its research programme).

International Organization for Standardization The international body (based in Geneva) including standards groups from many countries which develops standards for goods and services to facilitate international trade and exchange.

ISO International Organization for Standardization; a prefix to a standard to denote that it is one of that organization.

L_{Aeq} Equivalent continuous A-weighted sound pressure level (in dB with respect to 20 μPa).

L-factor complex A term used at the 1995 International Advanced Research Workshop on Man and Environmental Noise to cover the various factors affecting hearing threshold levels which are subsumed under the term socio-economic factor (hence *L(ibra)*-factor); the term serves to emphasize the multifactorial nature of such a factor and avoids implicating any strictly 'social' or 'economic' factor.

manual audiometer A pure tone audiometer where selecting the 'loudness' and pitch of a test tone (signal) is done manually, as is the presentation of the signal, and the recording of the subject's responses to it.

mastoid process The bony prominence of the skull which underlies the mastoid prominence.

mastoid prominence The firm projection of the head behind the auricle which covers the bony *mastoid process* and on which a bone vibrator is placed.

mean The arithmetic mean (colloquially termed the 'average') is the sum of all the observations divided by the number of observations. In hearing surveys, the difference between "mean" and "median" hearing level can be significant. The mean, however, ... gives a better description of the sample when supplemented with standard deviations. Mean HTLs are particularly sensitive to clinical rejection criteria.

median The middle point when a series of measurements is ranked in ascending or descending order.

mode The most frequently occurring value in a distribution.

MRC Medical Research Council (the main UK government body for the promotion of medical and related biological research).

NAMAS National Accreditation of Measurement and Sampling (UK). NAMAS accreditation is granted by UKAS. Certificates bearing the NAMAS logo are widely accepted in the UK and throughout the world. There are multilateral agreements recognizing the equivalence of accreditation.

National Measurement System The technical and organizational infrastructure within the UK which ensures that everyone can have confidence in the measurements that are made in support of research and development, manufacturing, commerce, health and safety; responsibility of NMSPU.

NMSPU National Measurement System Policy Unit: that part of the DTI (UK) which has responsibility for the integrity and efficient functioning of the National Measurement System.

National Physical Laboratory (UK) The focus of the National Measurement System with responsibility for developing, maintaining and disseminating measurement standards for most physical quantities; all activities in the NPL, excluding those accredited by UKAS, are operated to a certified ISO 9001:1994 quality system standard; accredits calibration services to EN 4500/ISO Guide 25.

noise immission level A measure of noise exposure that takes into account both the level of the noise and the time to which an individual has been exposed to such a noise, combining these two factors into a single value which is expressed in dB (NI); employs equal energy principle (3-dB change for halving or doubling the time component) to trade these two factors one with the other. Basis of NPL Ac 61 model.

noise-induced compound threshold shift Inclusive of both noise-induced temporary threshold shift and noise-induced permanent threshold shift.

non-organic hearing loss A hearing loss which is not to be attributed to a disorder of the subject's auditory system.

non-organic threshold shift (NOTS) A threshold shift which is not to be attributed to a disorder of the subject's auditory system and which may or may not be of sufficient degree to amount to a hearing loss.

normal threshold of hearing 'A term which should be avoided because of its medical and medicolegal implications.'[76] There is no single normal threshold of hearing; there are indeed a number of normal thresholds of normal hearing.

NOTS-S NOTS residing in the domain of the subject (testee).

NOTS-E NOTS residing in the domain of the examiner (tester) or examination.

NSH National Study of Hearing (the principal epidemiological programme of the IHR).

ONITS Occupational noise-induced threshold shift, i.e. a shift in the threshold of hearing which may or may not amount to an occupational noise-induced hearing loss.

presbyacusis A diagnostic term applied by clinicians to explain the difficulties in hearing of older people; strictly speaking, such a term should be used only after a medical examination has shown no cause for a patient's hearing difficulties apart from an age-related permanent threshold shift which is of sufficient degree to constitute a hearing loss.

pure tone audiometer An audiometer which uses pure tones to measure a subject's ability to hear, in particular, the quietest sounds that he can detect (threshold of hearing).

reference zero A point on a scale of measurement to which all other measurements on that scale are referred; there will thus be values (at least in theory) both above (denoted as '+' values) and below (denoted as '−' values) that point; values other than zero do not necessarily denote values that are abnormal, since the reference zero itself does not predicate a range of normality, let alone what is that range.

reference zero, standard A reference zero which has been set by one or other national or international standards institute, e.g. the British Standards Institution, the International Organization for Standardization; specifications exist for a standard reference zero for the calibration of pure tone air (BS EN ISO 389-1:2000) and bone (BS ISO 389-3:1994) conduction audiometers.

Rudmose audiometer An automatic recording audiometer which tests a subject's hearing using a fixed-frequency test tone only (used in industrial hearing conservation programmes).

sensorineural threshold shift A shift in the threshold of hearing due to disorder of the auditory nervous system (inclusive of cochlea) which may or may not be of sufficient magnitude to be termed a sensorineural hearing loss.

SI The international abbreviation for *Le Système International d'Unités*.

socioacusis Non-industrial noise-induced threshold shifts.

threshold shift, noise-induced permanent The term that has been used for some 40 years or more by workers in the field of noise-induced damage to hearing to designate the permanent noise component in a threshold of hearing that would be attributable to noise damage.

traceability The ability to trace back any calibration to the primary standard.

United Kingdom Accreditation Service UK national body responsible for assessing and accrediting the competence of organizations in the fields of calibration, measurement, testing, inspection and the certification of systems, personnel and products. UKAS-accredited calibration laboratories represent the main focus for traceable calibration in the UK, acting as local guarantors of measurement quality.

United States of America Standards Institute Name of the national standards body of the USA from 1966 until October 1969, when renamed American National Standards Institute.

Appendix

Some standards relating to measurements of the threshold of hearing

IEC 60318-1:1998
Electroacoustics—Simulators of human head and ear—Part 1: Ear simulator for the calibration of supra-aural earphones.

IEC 60318-2:1998
Electroacoustics—Simulators of human head and ear—Part 2: An interim acoustic coupler for the calibration of audiometric earphones in the extended high-frequency range.

IEC 60318-3:1998
Electroacoustics—Simulators of human head and ear—Part 3: Acoustic coupler for the calibration of supra-aural earphones used in audiometry (formerly IEC 303).

IEC 60645-1:1992
Audiometers—Part 1: Pure-tone audiometers.

Specifies general requirements for audiometers and particular requirements for pure tone audiometers designed for use in determining hearing threshold levels in comparison with the standard reference threshold level by means of psycho-acoustical test methods.

IEC 60645-1 Corr. 1 (1993-02)
Audiometers—Part 1: Pure-tone audiometers.

IEC 60645-2:1993 Audiometers. Part 2: Equipment for speech audiometry.

Specifies requirements for audiometers designed to present speech sounds to a subject in a standardized manner, e.g. for the measurement of speech recognition.

IEC 60645-4:1994
Audiometers—Part 4: Equipment for extended high-frequency audiometry.

Specifies requirements for audiometric equipment designed for use in pure tone audiometry in the frequency range from 8000 Hz to 16 000 Hz, in addition to those that are applicable and specified in IEC 60645-1.

IEC 61027:1991
Instruments for the measurement of aural acoustic impedance/admittance.

Covers instruments designed primarily for the measurement of modulus of acoustical impedance/admittance in the human external acoustical meatus using a probe tone of 226 Hz. Defines the characteristics to be specified by the manufacturer, lays down performance specifications for four types of instrument, and specifies the facilities to be provided on three of these types. Methods of test to be used for approval testing rather than routine calibration are also specified.

BS 6950:1988 specified a standard reference zero for the calibration of pure tone bone conduction audiometers (superseded by BS ISO 389-3:1994).

BS EN ISO 389-1:2000 (formerly BS 2497: 1992) Acoustics. Reference zero for the calibration of autiometric equipment – Part 1: Reference equivalent threshold sound pressure levels for pure tones and supra-aural earphones.

Specifies reference equivalent threshold sound pressure levels for Beyer DT 48 and telephonics TDH 39 earphones in a coupler complying with IEC 60318-3:1998 together with other supra-aural earphones, meeting stated requirements, in an artificial ear complying with IEC 60318-1:1998. Note that the term 'normal' which appeared in the title of the first British Standard, i.e. BS 2497:1954, was subsequently deleted. The original samples (i.e. not random samples of the general population.) (Royal Air Ford; National Physical Laboratory) on which the standard was based provided *modal* values for a *clinically otologically normal* population; the individual subjects, having had a prior screening audiogram, were tested with a precision 2-dB step audiometer [Note that this standard is one to which *audiometers* should conform, not individuals].

BS ISO 389-3:1999—Acoustics. Reference zero for the calibration of audiometric equipment. Reference equivalent threshold force levels for pure tones and bone vibrators (specifies a standard reference zero for the calibration of pure tone *bone* conduction audiometers).

BS ISO 389-4:1999—Acoustics. Reference zero for the calibration of audiometric equipment. Reference levels for narrow-band masking noise.

BS ISO 389-5:2001—Acoustics. Reference zero for the calibration of audiometric equipment. Reference equivalent threshold sound pressure levels for pure tones in the frequency range 8 kHz to 16 kHz.

BS EN ISO 389-7:1998—Acoustics. Reference zero for the calibration of audiometric equipment. Reference threshold of hearing under free-field and diffuse-field listening conditions.

BS EN ISO 8253-1:1998—Acoustics. Audiometric test methods. Basic pure tone air and bone conduction threshold audiometry.

The standard dealing with methods for performing audiometry; it also covers methods (biological and physical) and frequency of calibrations as well as standards for maximum permissible ambient noise levels for audiometric test rooms.

BS EN ISO 8253-2:1998—Acoustics. Audiometric test methods. Soundfield audiometry with pure tone and narrow-band test signals.

Specifies test signal characteristics and procedures for determining hearing threshold levels in the range 125–12 500 Hz.

BS EN ISO 8253-3:1998—Acoustics. Audiometric test methods. Speech audiometry.

ISO 6189-1983: the International Standard specification for pure tone air conduction audiometry for hearing conservation purposes: '0 Introduction. This International Standard lays down requirements and procedures for conducting pure tone air conduction audiometry when it is deemed by the responsible authority to monitor the hearing of subjects exposed to noise at work ... Methods of conducting audiometric tests with manual and automatic recording fixed frequency [i.e. for the Rudmose audiometer which is used in industry, not the sweep frequency Békésy audiometer which is used for clinical diagnostic purposes] audiometers are presented in this International Standard ... 2 Field of Application ... The specifications in this International Standard are not intended for clinical purpose [i.e. for the Rudmose audiometer] ... 8.2 Determination of hearing threshold levels in automatic recording audiometry ... Average the peaks and (the) valleys of the tracing ... This mean value, rounded up to the nearest whole number in decibels, is taken as the hearing threshold level at that frequency and that ear ... 9.2 Comparison of Audiograms ... To compare audiograms which have been recorded by automatic recording and manual audiometry, 3 dB should be added to the hearing threshold levels determined by means of automatic recording audiometers.'

ISO 7029-1984—International Specification for the threshold of hearing by air conduction as a function of age and sex for otologically normal persons [of course, this cannot be so, since the data reflect the effects of ageing (as the standard intends)].

The web sites for various International and National Standards bodies are shown in Tables 13.3 and 13.4.

Table 13.3: Some International Standards bodies and their websites

STANDARDS BODY	ABBREV	WEBSITE
Comité Européen de Normalisation (European Committee for Standardisation)	CEN	http://www.cenorm.be/ http://www.cenorm.be/catweb/
Comité Européen de Normalisation Eléctrotechnique	CENELEC	http://www.cenelec.org/
European Telecommunications Standardization Institute	ETSI	http://www.etsi.org/
International Electrotechnical Commission	IEC	http://www.iec.ch/
International Organization for Standardization	ISO	http://www.iso.ch/

Table 13.4: Some National Standards bodies and their websites. Others are given at the World Standards Services Network website: http://www.wssn.net/WSSN/script-cache/links_national.htm. All CEN (*Comité Européen de Normalisation*) members are listed here and denoted by an asterisk.

COUNTRY	STANDARDS BODY	ABBREV	WEBSITE
Australia	Standards Australia International Ltd	SA	http://www.standards.com.au/catalogue/script/search.asp
Austria*	*Österreichisches Normungsinstitut*	ON	http://www.on-norm.at
Belgium*	*Institut Belge de Normalisation/Belgisch Instituut voor Normalisatie*	IBN/BIN	http://www.ibn.be
Canada	Standards Council of Canada - Conseil canadien des normes	SCC	http://www.scc.ca/
Czech Republic*	Czech Standards Institute	CSNI	http://www.csni.cz
Denmark*	*Dansk Standard*	DS	http://www.ds.dk
Finland*	*Suomen Standardisoimisliitto r.y.*	SFS	http://www.sfs.fi
France*	*l'Association française de normalisation.*	AFNOR	http://www.afnor.fr
Germany*	*Deutsches Institut für Normung e.V.*	DIN	http://www.din.de
Greece*	Hellenic Organization for Standardization	ELOT	http://www.elot.gr
Iceland*	*Stadlarad Islands* (Icelandic Standards)	IST	http://www.stadlar.is
India	Bureau of Indian Standards	BIS	http://www.bis.org.in/

Table 13.4: continued.

COUNTRY	STANDARDS BODY	ABBREV	WEBSITE
Indonesia	*Badan Standardisasi Nasional*	BSN	http://www.bsn.go.id/
Iran	Institute of Standards and Industrial Research of Iran	ISIRI	http://www.isiri.org/
Ireland*	National Standards Authority of Ireland	NSAI	http://www.nsai.ie
Israel	The Standards Institution of Israel	SII	http://www.sii.org.il/
Italy*	*Ente Nazionale Italiano di Unificazione*	UNI	http://www.uni.com
Japan	Japan Industrial Standards Committee	JISC	http://www.jisc.go.jp/
Luxembourg*	*Service de l'Energie de l'Etat Organisme Luxembourgeois de Normalisation*	SEE	http://www.see.lu
Malta*	Malta Standards Authority	MSA	http://www.msa.org.mt
Netherlands*	*Nederlands Normalisatie-instituut*	NEN	http://www.nen.nl/
New Zealand	Standards New Zealand	SNZ	http://www.standards.co.nz/
Norway*	*Norges Standardiseringsforbund*	NSF	http://www.standard.no/nsf
Peru	*Instituto Nacional de Defensa de la Competencia y de la Protección de la Propiedad Intelectual*	INDECOPI	http://www.indecopi.gob.pe/
Portugal*	*Instituto Português da Qualidade*	IPQ	http://www.ipq.pt
Russia	State Committee of the Russian Federation for Standardization, Metrology and Certification	GOST-R	http://www.gost.ru/sls/gost.nsf
South Africa	South African Bureau of Standards	SABS	http://www.sabs.co.za/
Spain*	*Asociación Española de Normalización y Certificación*	AENOR	http://www.aenor.es
Sweden*	Swedish Standards Institute	SIS	http://www.sis.se
Switzerland*	*Schweizerische Normen-Vereinigung* (Swiss Association for Standardization)	SNV	http://www.snv.ch
Thailand	Thai Industrial Standards Institute	TISI	http://www.tisi.go.th/
Turkey	*Türk Standardlari Enstitüsü*	TSE	http://www.tse.org.tr/
UK*	British Standards Institution	BSI	http://www.bsi-global.com
USA	American National Standards Institute	ANSI	http://www.ansi.org/

14 Psychoacoustical auditory tests

Joseph W Hall

Psychoacoustics is the study of the psychological correlates of the physical parameters of sound. Perhaps the simplest psychoacoustical measurement deals with the determination of the lowest level of sound that can be detected reliably in a quiet setting (the auditory detection threshold). This measurement is the cornerstone of clinical audiological assessment and is considered in some detail elsewhere in this book, along with other auditory measures that are valuable in clinical diagnosis. In addition to providing diagnostic information, psychoacoustical testing can furnish information about the basic nature of hearing and hearing impairment. For example, psychoacoustical measurements can be performed to indicate the extent to which the ear can hear a target sound in the presence of a competing sound, and the effect that hearing loss has on that ability. Such knowledge can contribute to the understanding of the disability associated with hearing loss, and may suggest possible strategies for mitigating the effects of hearing loss (perhaps through design of hearing aid hardware/software). This chapter focuses on the psychoacoustical study of the nature of hearing impairment. In this chapter, the main focus is on hearing loss of cochlear origin. In most cases of sensorineural hearing loss, the main site of lesion is usually assumed to be in the cochlea (outer hair cells, inner hair cells, or both outer and inner hair cells), rather than the cochlear nerve itself. A more thorough treatment of this subject matter can be found in Moore.[1]

Basic measures related to the coding of sound level

Loudness and the dynamic range of hearing

Figure 14.1 depicts what might be termed the dynamic range of hearing, describing the limits between the audibility threshold (extremely soft)[2] and the discomfort/pain threshold (extremely loud).[3] Notable characteristics are the range of frequencies to which the healthy human ear is sensitive (approximately 20 Hz to 20 kHz), the pronounced sensitivity in the 3-kHz frequency range, and the enormous range of intensity values encoded by the ear. The main psychological correlates of frequency and intensity are pitch and loudness, respectively. An interesting question is how loudness relates to the range of intensities shown in Figure 14.1. One way of addressing this question is to ask listeners to rate the loudness of sounds of various intensities. An example of this type of method is the loudness growth in 1/2 octave bands,[4] where sounds are rated categorically as very soft, soft, OK, loud, very loud or too loud; this is depicted in Figure 14.2. This figure shows typical data from a normal ear and an ear with a moderate hearing loss of cochlear origin.[5] One way of characterizing the hearing loss is in terms of a reduction of the dynamic range of intensity. As seen in Figure 14.2, the upper bound of the range in the hearing-impaired ear is similar to normal, but the hearing-impaired ear is insensitive to sound at the

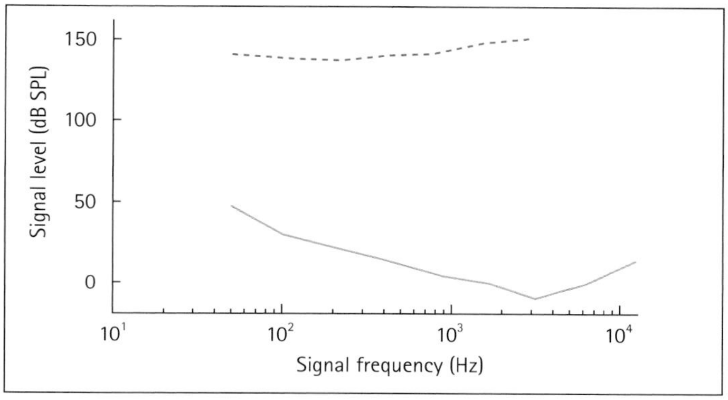

Figure 14.1 The lower, solid line refers to the lowest level of sound that can be detected in the free field as a function of sound frequency. The upper, dotted curve refers to the threshold of pain.

> A defining characteristic of cochlear hearing loss is the reduced dynamic range between auditory threshold and loudness discomfort. The steep growth of loudness is referred to as loudness recruitment.

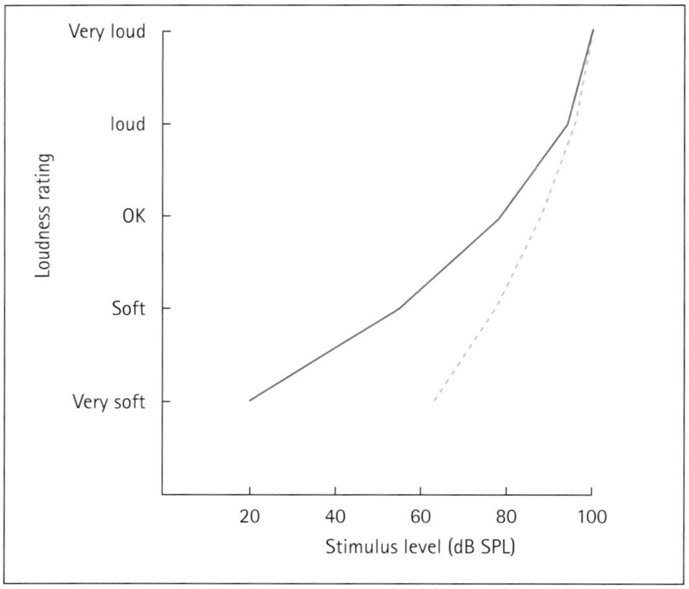

Figure 14.2 Examples of the type of loudness growth functions that are obtained for normal ears (solid line) and ears with moderate sensorineural hearing loss (dotted line).

lower intensity values. One of the hallmarks of cochlear hearing loss concerns the relationship between this reduced dynamic range and the growth of loudness with increasing intensity. The finding is that the ear experiences a change from soft to loud over a relatively small range of intensities. This steep growth of loudness is referred to as loudness recruitment.[6–8]

Intensity discrimination

One of the most basic measures of hearing is the ability to discriminate a small change in the intensity of a sound. One test of intensity discrimination, the Short Increment Sensitivity Index,[9–11] was used at one time in audiology to differentiate cochlear from retrocochlear (e.g. vestibular schwannoma) hearing loss. In this test, the sensitivity to 1-dB intensity modulations is determined for a sinusoidal carrier presented 20 dB above threshold (20-dB sensation level). Patients having a primarily cochlear site of lesion are generally quite sensitive to such increments, whereas patients with vestibular schwannomas are not. This test is no longer used widely, because it has been replaced by electrophysiological and imaging tests with greater diagnostic utility.

> Generally, intensity discrimination is substantially poorer in cases of vestibular schwannoma than in cases of cochlear hearing loss or normal hearing. Intensity discrimination can be poorer than normal in cochlear-impaired listeners, depending upon aetiology.

Differences in intensity discrimination between normally hearing listeners and listeners with cochlear impairment have been studied for a number of years. Two basic methodologies have been used (Figure 14.3). One involves an intensity increment being imposed upon a carrier, and is sometimes referred to as the loudness modulation method. This is similar to the method used in the Short Increment Sensitivity Index. The other method involves the presentation of temporally discrete stimulus presentations that differ in intensity, and is sometimes referred to as the loudness memory method. Difference in intensity discrimination between normal and impaired ears depends critically upon whether stimuli are presented at the same sensation level (SL) or at the same sound pressure level (SPL). When stimuli are presented at matched, low SL (e.g. 20 dB SL), listeners with cochlear hearing loss generally show better performance. Under such circumstances, the SPL is higher for the hearing-impaired ear. When stimuli are presented at matched, high SPL (e.g. 85–90 dB SPL), large differences in intensity discrimination between normal and impaired ears are generally not seen.[12–14] However, a study by Fastl and Schorn[15] indicated that intensity discrimination may vary significantly among aetiologies of cochlear-related hearing loss. For example, they found relatively poor performance in listeners with Menière's disease.

Intensity discrimination reflects very basic auditory abilities, and the practical implications of poor intensity discrimination are not completely clear. One possibility relates to the differentiation and recognition of complex sounds based upon subtle across-frequency differences in intensity (spectral shape processing). If the ability to code intensity cues is reduced, the processing of certain complex environmental sounds could be compromised.

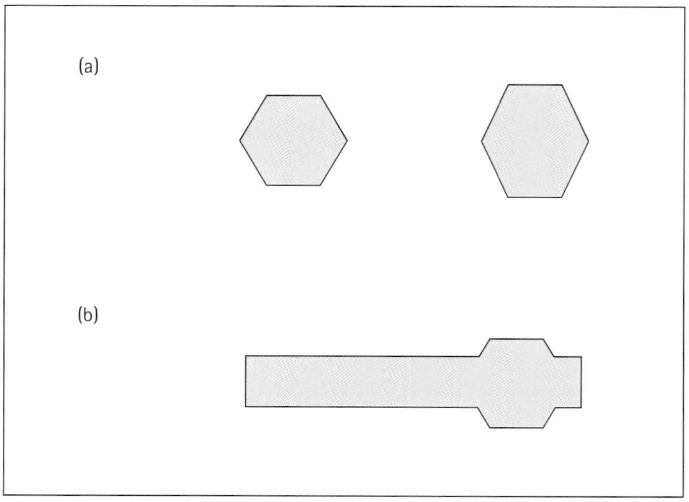

Figure 14.3 Time–amplitude representations of the types of stimuli used in (a) the loudness memory and (b) the loudness modulation methods of intensity discrimination.

Basic measures related to frequency coding

Frequency resolution

The mapping of frequency to a place on the basilar membrane is one of the bases of the frequency selectivity of the ear. One result of this process is that simultaneously present sounds from different spectral regions will not interfere with or mask each other substantially, because they are associated with activity in frequency-specific, quasi-independent neural populations. Although several different psychoacoustical methods reveal the frequency-selective nature of the ear, perhaps the method that is subject to the fewest problems in interpretation is the notched noise method.[16] In this method, the detection threshold of a pure tone signal in masking noise is determined as a function of the width of a spectral notch (band-stop region) in the vicinity of the signal frequency (Figure 14.4). Techniques have been developed[17–19] for deriving auditory filter bandwidths and shapes using this technique. In ears with normal hearing, the threshold of the signal improves steeply as the width of the notch increases, a finding consistent with a high degree of frequency selectivity. In contrast, many cases of cochlear hearing loss are associated with only a gradual improvement with increasing notch width, consistent with poor frequency selectivity.[20–22] Cochlear hearing losses often indicate abnormally asymmetrical auditory filter shapes, with a disproportionate amount of low-frequency energy being present at the auditory filter output.[20]

A second psychoacoustical measure of frequency selectivity, the psychophysical tuning curve (PTC),[23–25] is worthy of mention, partly because of its conceptual similarity to the physiological tuning curve. In the physiological tuning curve, the lowest level of stimulation that results in an increase in the spontaneous rate of an cochlear nerve neurone is determined as a function of the frequency of stimulation. The best frequency of the neurone is associated with the lowest sound level, with frequencies diverging from this frequency requiring progressively higher intensities to alter the spontaneous rate of the neural firing. The steepness of the resulting V-shaped function summarizes the frequency selectivity of the neurone. In the PTC, the threshold for a target tone of a given frequency is first determined (Figure 14.5). Then, the level of the target tone is maintained at approximately 10 dB SL, and the level of a narrow band of noise required to mask the target tone is determined as a function of the centre frequency of the narrow band of noise. The resulting 'tuning curve' is similar in shape to that for the physiological tuning curve, with progressively higher masking energy required as the frequencies of the masking and target stimuli diverge. In agreement with the notched noise results, hearing-impaired ears show broader PTC functions with raised tips, and sometimes 'W' shapes instead of the normal 'V' shape.[26,27] The practical implications of reduced frequency resolution may include poor hearing in noise and poor ability to discriminate/recognize sounds based upon spectral shape differences (e.g. certain speech sounds).

> Cochlear hearing impairment is often associated with a reduced ability to process a particular frequency region in a complex sound. This may limit the ability of listeners with cochlear hearing impairment to code the spectral variations that provide cues for the understanding of speech.

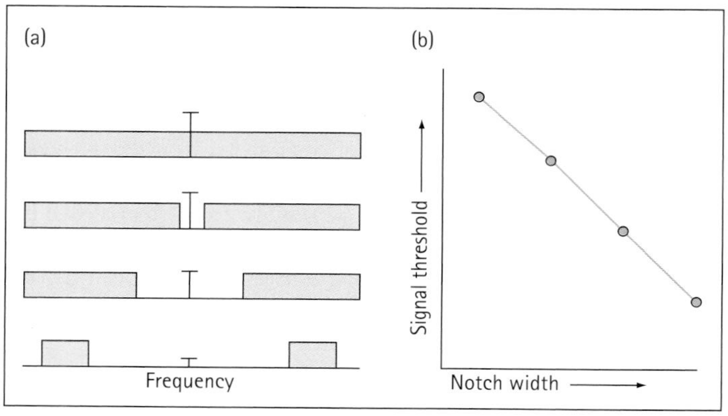

Figure 14.4 Schematic representations of the stimuli (a) and masked signal thresholds (b) associated with the notched noise method of measuring frequency resolution.

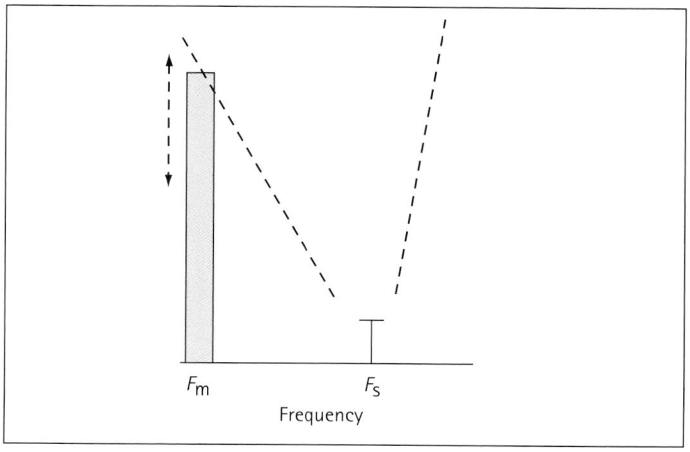

Figure 14.5 Schematic representation of the psychophysical tuning curve method of measuring frequency resolution. The signal has a constant frequency, and its level is held at approximately 10 dB SL. The level of a narrow-band noise masker that just masks the signal is then determined as a function of masker frequency. The dotted line represents the finding that greater masker level is required as the frequencies of the signal and masker diverge.

Frequency discrimination

Frequency discrimination refers to the ability to report that two sequentially presented pure tones differ in frequency. Listeners usually hear this frequency difference as a change in pitch. The two cues that are thought to contribute to frequency discrimination are related to the place of cochlear activation (and subsequent tonotopic neural coding) and the phase-locked neural coding of stimulus fine structure periodicity. The coding of temporal fine structure has a low-pass characteristic, as neural phase locking diminishes above 1–2 kHz,[28] so the respective roles of temporal and place cues may vary importantly as a function of stimulus frequency. In normal ears, frequency discrimination is remarkably good, with frequency difference limens on the order of 0.5%.[29,30] Frequency discrimination is often diminished in listeners with hearing loss of cochlear origin, both at low and high frequencies.[31–33] Some of this reduction in frequency discrimination can probably be attributed to the broader cochlear tuning (poor frequency resolution) that often occurs in cochlear loss. It has also been speculated that there may be a reduced phase-locking ability in cochlear hearing loss. A reduction in phase locking would then be associated with relatively poor frequency discrimination performance in middle to low frequencies. Some studies have suggested that the detection of low rates of frequency modulation depends upon neural phase locking at low and middle signal frequencies.[34] Lacher-Fougere and Demany[35] found relatively poor detection at low-rate frequency modulation in listeners with cochlear hearing loss. They interpreted this as possibly indicating poor phase locking with cochlear hearing loss, particularly for hearing losses greater than 50 dB. Physiological evidence concerning the question of phase locking in hearing losses of cochlear origin is equivocal at this point,[36,37] and it is uncertain what mechanism might underlie such a condition in cochlear-based hearing loss.

It is again somewhat problematic to delineate precisely the practical implications of poor frequency discrimination. One possible implication relates to the fact that many speech sounds are characterized by frequency transitions that provide information for speech identification. Poor ability to encode differences in frequency and changes in frequency value may therefore be associated with reduced speech-understanding abilities.

Basic measures related to temporal coding

Temporal resolution

Temporal resolution refers to the ability of the ear to follow rapid transitions in the amplitude envelope of a stimulus. Temporal resolution in hearing-impaired listeners has most often been investigated using either the gap detection method or the temporal modulation transfer function (TMTF) method. Gap detection refers to the ability to detect a short silent gap in an otherwise continuous signal.[38–41] With the TMTF method,[42,43] temporal resolution is characterized in terms of the steepness with which sensitivity to the presence of amplitude modulation falls off as the modulation frequency is increased. The stimuli used in the gap and TMTF methods are represented in Figure 14.6. Such measures in the normal ear indicate relatively precise temporal coding and suggest a time constant of 1–3 ms. Although many listeners with cochlear hearing loss also show relatively precise temporal resolution, some show markedly poor performance.[44–47] In interpreting results from these experiments, care must be taken to ensure that the results of hearing-impaired listeners are not critically limited because all or part of the stimulus is below or near the threshold of hearing. When this factor is taken into account, results usually indicate time constants that are near the normal range, with an occasional hearing-impaired listener showing abnormally prolonged time constants. Because some aspects of speech perception depend upon the coding of rapid acoustical transitions,[48,49] it is possible that reduced temporal resolution may contribute to poor speech recognition in hearing-impaired listeners.

> Measures of temporal resolution often indicate similar time constants for normal and cochlear-impaired listeners. However, some cochlear-impaired listeners show increased time constants that may contribute to overall hearing disability in individual cases.

Temporal summation

Temporal summation is a term that is used to describe the function relating signal duration to detection threshold (Figure 14.7). In the normal ear, it is found that as the signal duration increases (up to durations of 200–400 ms), the signal intensity necessary for detection decreases. As an approximation, it is found that the signal intensity at threshold reduces by 3 dB for every doubling of duration. Although this would be consistent with an interpretation of a simple integration of intensity over a relatively long temporal interval of 200–400 ms, it is probably not appropriate to conceptualize the temporal summation phenomenon in this way. For one thing, the relatively small time constant indicated by temporal resolution studies would suggest that a long summation time is not obligatory. In a similar vein, a study by Viemeister and Wakefield[50] indicated that the temporal summation of sound can be somewhat ‘selective’. This study showed that the energy from two short signals separated in time by a masking appeared to be integrated without a concomitant integration of the intervening masking noise. This suggests that some aspects of temporal summation might be viewed as a combination of information obtained through multiple, sequential samples.

A number of studies have indicated that temporal summation is often substantially reduced in cases of hearing loss of cochlear origin, and at one point in the history of audiology,

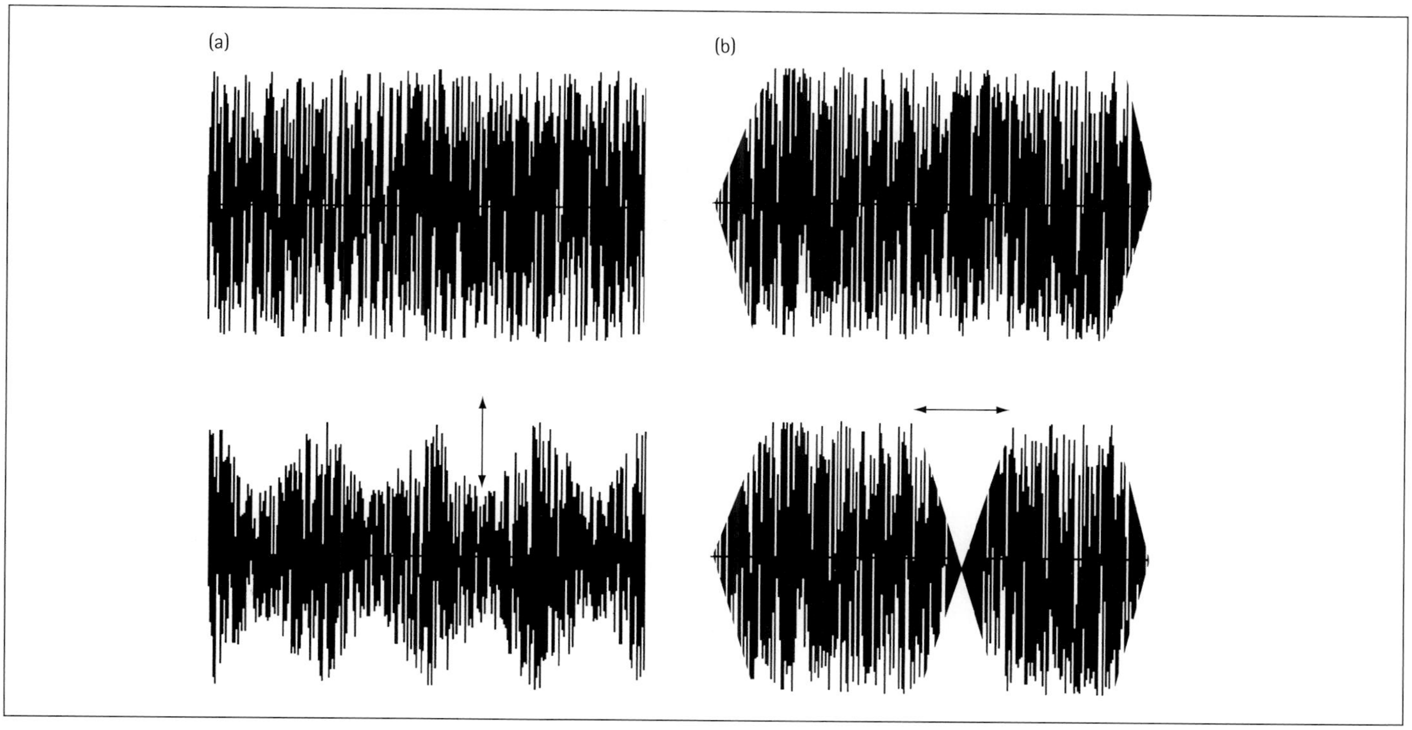

Figure 14.6 Representation of the stimuli used in the TMTF (a) and gap detection (b) measures of temporal resolution. In the TMTF, the listener must be able to differentiate an unmodulated noise (top) from a modulated noise (bottom). The arrow represents the fact that the depth of modulation is the manipulated parameter. The modulation detection threshold is obtained as a function of the rate of modulation. In gap detection, the listener must be able to differentiate an uninterrupted noise (top) from a noise having a temporal gap (bottom). The arrow represents the fact that the gap duration is the manipulated parameter. The gap detection threshold is the shortest gap that can just be detected.

measures of temporal summation were used in diagnostic site-of-lesion tests.[51–53] Although several hypotheses have been put forward to explain this reduction in temporal summation (see Moore[1] for a discussion), none would presently appear to account entirely satisfactorily for the effect found with cochlear hearing loss.

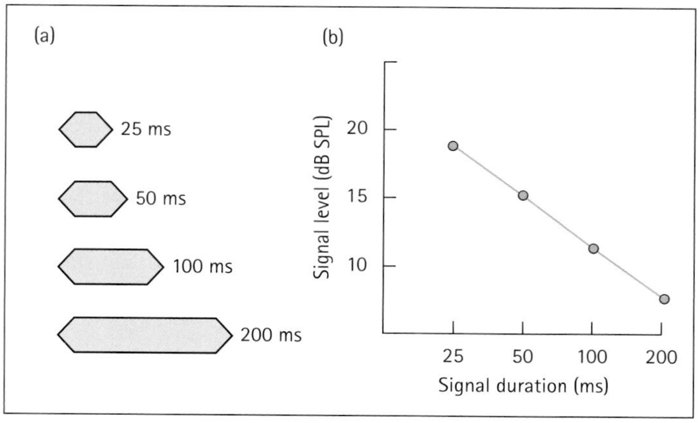

Figure 14.7 Schematic representation of the stimuli (a) and threshold data (b) associated with the temporal summation paradigm. Signal detection threshold is determined as a function of the duration of the signal.

Manifestations of abnormality in cochlear amplification

Whereas the main function of inner hair cells is to transduce mechanical energy into signals carried by the cochlear nerve, a primary role of the outer hair cells of the cochlea appears to be to provide frequency-specific amplification.[54] This process results in relatively low auditory thresholds and fine frequency selectivity, and the associated intensity input–output function is non-linear and compressive. One way of conceptualizing this compressive function is in terms of a saturating amplification wherein progressively less amplification is applied as intensity increases.[55] Unfortunately, outer hair cells are vulnerable to damage, and impaired outer hair cell function probably

> It is likely that most cases of elevated thresholds in cochlear hearing loss can be understood in terms of reduced frequency-specific amplification associated with the outer hair cells. This reduced amplification probably has wide-ranging implications for hearing, including frequency resolution, loudness recruitment, and other basic hearing abilities.

accounts for much of the poor sensitivity and frequency selectivity associated with mild-to-moderate cochlear hearing losses.[56,57] It has been hypothesized that other psychoacoustical findings in cochlear-impaired listeners (including some considered above) can also be attributed to abnormalities in cochlear amplification. For example, reduction or elimination of cochlear amplification would diminish the compressive nature of the intensity input–output function, potentially accounting for the steeper growth of loudness (loudness recruitment) often found in cochlear hearing loss. Moore[1] has also pointed out that the abnormal cochlear amplifier associated with outer hair cell damage may also account for aspects of reduced temporal resolution and reduced temporal summation.

Binaural hearing

Because the two ears are in different spatial locations and are separated by the head, they often receive substantially different acoustical signals. For example, a sound located on a listener's right side will reach the right ear of the listener approximately 600 μs before it reaches the left ear. In addition, the higher frequencies of the sound will be attenuated by the 'head shadow', resulting in a more intense sound in the right ear. These binaural differences of time and amplitude constitute cues that aid in the spatial analysis of auditory sources in the environment (Figure 14.8). Perhaps the two most prominent benefits related to binaural hearing are sound source localization and enhanced perception of signals in noise.

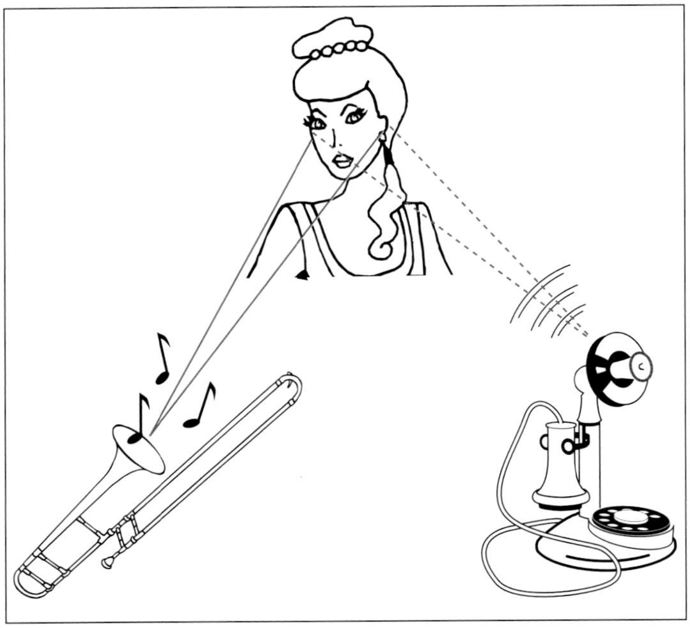

Figure 14.8 Schematic representation of binaural cues that aid in the localization of sound. The cues include time-of-arrival differences between the ears, and interaural differences in intensity due to the head shadow.

Sound localization

Measures of localization ability indicate that cochlear hearing loss is often associated with poor sound localization ability.[58–62] As might be expected, poor localization ability is particularly likely to occur in cases of asymmetrical hearing loss. However, poor localization is not uncommon even when hearing loss is relatively symmetrical and stimulation occurs well above threshold.[63] Although measures of sound localization are valuable in that they provide direct evidence of the highly practical ability to localize sound sources in the free field, they do not always provide clear interpretations of the particular cues that are utilized by the listener. Therefore, several studies have been performed using headphones to investigate the effect of hearing loss on particular types of binaural hearing ability.

Interaural time and intensity discrimination

In headphone testing, it is relatively easy to manipulate interaural time and amplitude cues separately and examine the sensitivity to each. Measurement of the sensitivity to interaural time disparities in low-frequency sounds indicates particularly acute sensitivity in the normal ear. For example, classical studies show that interaural time differences as small as 10–20 μs can be detected for stimuli up to frequencies of approximately 1.0–1.5 kHz.[64,65] For pure tone signal frequencies higher than this, sensitivity to interaural time differences in the ongoing stimulus fine structure is poor or absent in the human ear. However, if the stimulus has a relatively low-frequency temporal envelope (as occurs with amplitude modulation, or with a narrow-band noise stimulus), interaural time differences in the envelope can support relatively acute interaural time discrimination even for high-frequency stimuli.[66,67] Interestingly, interaural time discrimination is often poor in listeners with hearing loss of cochlear origin.[68–71] Because interaural time discrimination depends ultimately upon binaural neural analysis, the mechanism underlying poor performance in listeners with hearing loss of cochlear origin is not entirely obvious. One possibility is that some forms of cochlear hearing loss may affect the precision of phase locking to stimulus periodicity. As noted above, this argument has also been applied to the finding that the detection of frequency modulation at low modulation frequencies is often poor in cases of cochlear hearing loss.

> Binaural hearing is often poor in cases of cochlear hearing loss. It is currently a challenge to determine whether binaural processing deficits may be related to basic peripheral processes such as neural phase locking.

Interaural intensity discrimination is also sometimes poorer in listeners with cochlear hearing loss than in listeners with normal hearing.[71] However, there are instances where listeners with cochlear hearing loss show normal interaural intensity discrimination,[70] and it is probably the case that interaural time discrimination is more deleteriously affected than interaural intensity discrimination in cases of cochlear hearing loss.

Detection in noise

The masking-level difference (MLD)[72] refers to a paradigm in which the masked detection threshold for a signal is determined as a function of the relative interaural differences of the signal and masker. The MLD depends upon the ability of the auditory system to process relatively subtle interaural difference cues of time and intensity. Whereas the anatomical stage of processing most critical for the MLD has its locus in the auditory brainstem, the MLD also hinges upon more peripheral auditory processing. The most common MLD conditions are referred to as NoSo (noise and signal both presented interaurally in phase) and NoSπ (noise presented interaurally in phase, but signal presented 180° out of phase, Figure 14.9). In normally hearing listeners, the threshold for the NoSπ condition is approximately 15 dB better than that for the NoSo condition, reflecting the sensitivity of the auditory system to the small interaural differences that are introduced when the Sπ signal is presented in the No noise. Several studies have indicated that this binaural advantage is often reduced in listeners with cochlear hearing loss.[69,73,74] MLDs are particularly likely to be reduced in cases of asymmetrical hearing loss, but reduced MLDs are not uncommon in cases of symmetrical loss.

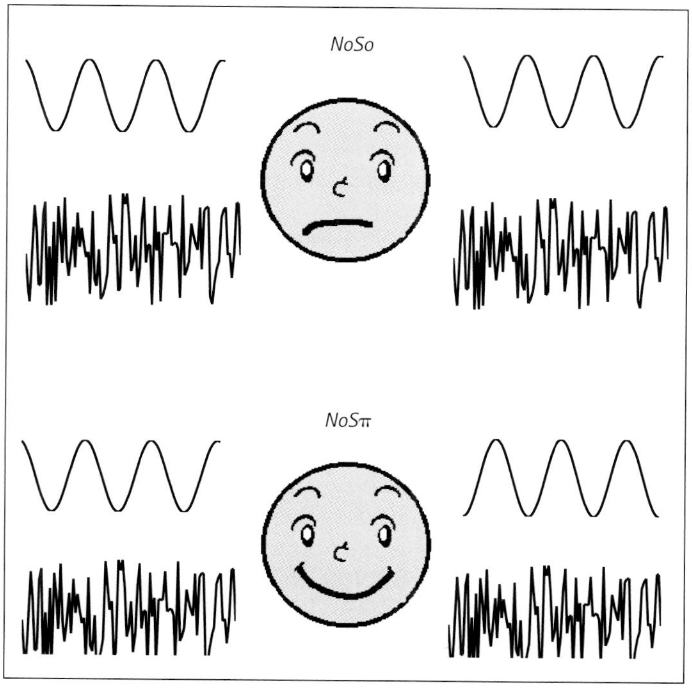

Figure 14.9 Schematic representation of stimuli used in typical MLD experiment. In the NoSo condition (top), both the masking noise and the sinusoidal signal have exactly the same phase relation between the two ears, and detection is relatively poor. In the NoSπ condition (bottom), the masking noise has exactly the same phase relation between the two ears, but the sinusoidal signal is interarally phase inverted. Here, signal detection improves substantially.

As suggested above, poor sensitivity to interaural differences of time and intensity and reduced MLDs indicate the likelihood of reduced binaural hearing performance in real environments. This could take the form of a reduced ability to localize sounds and detect and recognize desired signals when they occur at low signal-to-noise ratios in spatially complex backgrounds.

Conductive hearing loss

Conductive hearing loss is often considered in terms of a simple attenuation of sound. In this sense, performance in an ear with conductive hearing loss would be expected to be similar to that in a normal ear stimulated at a lower level. Therefore, it is not surprising that basic measures of temporal[75] and frequency[76] resolution indicate normal performance in conductive hearing loss for stimuli presented at appropriate sensation levels. The situation for binaural hearing is less straightforward. If the conductive loss is different in the two ears, the associated attenuation will be asymmetrical. This asymmetry could reduce the efficiency of binaural hearing. Colburn and Hausler[77] also showed that another possible source of poor binaural hearing in conductive impairment is related to bone conduction. For sound delivery over headphones, both the air conduction route and the bone conduction route are relevant. In the normal ear, the bone-conducted sound is generally better than 40–50 dB down relative to air-conducted sound. In such a case, the bone-conducted sound probably does not have a material effect on the composite sound. This may not be the case when a conductive loss is present. Here, the bone-conducted sound may be lower than the air-conducted sound by, for example, 10 dB. In such a case, the bone-conducted sound could have a material effect on the composite waveform, and could appreciably affect the interaural difference cues. Therefore, in cases of conductive hearing loss, MLDs could be substantially reduced because of this factor.

Several studies that have investigated binaural hearing in conductively impaired listeners have found that, in many subjects, binaural hearing is rather poor.[59–61,78,79] Perhaps of greater interest, binaural hearing does not always return to normal immediately following corrective middle ear surgery. For example, it has been shown that binaural hearing may remain abnormal for up to 1–2 years following the restoration of a normal audiogram, both in adults[78,80,81] and in children.[82–84] It has been speculated that some of the difficulties in the binaural hearing

> Binaural hearing is often surprisingly poor in cases of conductive hearing loss, and can remain poor for some time after corrective surgery. Slow recovery after corrective surgery may be related to alterations in the efficiency of the neural processing of binaural difference cues.

of conductively impaired listeners may be related to alterations in the efficiency of the neural processing of binaural difference cues.[82]

Vestibular schwannoma

Although vestibular schwannoma is rare in comparison to other forms of auditory disease, the condition has received considerable attention in the audiological literature because of the importance of differentiating cochlear from retrocochlear sites of lesion. Several psychoacoustical findings have been noted in cases of vestibular schwannoma. One is abnormal adaptation, wherein a tone presented above detection threshold rapidly fades into inaudibility.[85] Another typical finding pertains to loudness growth. Whereas loudness recruitment occurs typically in cases of cochlear site of lesion, this phenomenon is less common in cases of schwannoma.[86] Acoustical neuroma is also associated with poor performance in the binaural MLD task.[73,87] It is thought that the reduced MLD may be related to an inability to code temporal fine structure cues when an vestibular schwannoma is present. This type of processing problem may also underlie the very poor speech perception performance often found in patients with vestibular schwannomas.[88,89]

Summary

The most obvious, and usually the most significant, characteristic of hearing loss of cochlear origin is a reduction in sensitivity to the presence of sound. This loss of sensitivity, in and of itself, results in serious problems in communication. The focus of this chapter has been on a compounding of this problem due to degradations in the auditory processes that underlie our abilities to analyse the subtle spectral, temporal and spatial features of suprathreshold sounds. The literature indicates that such suprathreshold analyses are often compromised in hearing loss of cochlear origin.

Abnormalities in auditory processes related to frequency, temporal and spatial analyses probably contribute significantly to the disability that hearing-impaired listeners face when trying to hear desired signals in complex auditory backgrounds.

References

1. Moore BCJ. *Perceptual Consequences of Cochlear Damage*. Oxford: Oxford University Press, 1995: 232.
2. Sivian LJ, White SD. On minimum audible sound fields. *J Acoust Soc Am* 1933; **4**: 288–321.
3. Bekesy GV. *Experiments in Hearing*. New York: McGraw-Hill, 1960.
4. Allen JB, Hall JL, Jeng PS. Loudness growth in 1/2-octave bands (LGOB)—a procedure for the assessment of loudness. *J Acoust Soc Am* 1990; **88**: 745–53.
5. Hall JW, Grose JH, Hatch DR. Temporal analysis and stimulus fluctuation in listeners with normal and impaired hearing. *J Speech Hear Res* 1998; **41**: 340–54.
6. Reger SN. Differences in loudness response of the normal and hard-of-hearing ear at intensity levels slightly above the threshold. *Ann Otol* 1936; **45**: 1029–39.
7. Fowler EP. A method for the early detection of otosclerosis. *Arch Otolaryngol* 1936; **24**: 731–41.
8. Hallpike CS. The loudness recruitment phenomenon: its clinical significance and neurological basis. *Proc R Soc Med* 1965; **58**: 190–6.
9. Jerger J. The SISI test. *Int Audiol* 1962; **1**: 246–7.
10. Buus S, Florentine M, Redden RB. The SISI test: a review. Part I. *Audiology* 1982; **21**: 273–93.
11. Buus S, Florentine M, Redden RB. The SISI test: a review. Part II. *Audiology* 1982; **21** 365–85.
12. Turner CW, Zwislocki JJ, Filion PR. Intensity discrimination determined with two paradigms in normal and hearing-impaired subjects. *J Acoust Soc Am* 1989; **86**: 109–15.
13. Schroder AC, Viemeister NF, Neslon DA. Intensity discrimination in normal-hearing and hearing-impaired listeners. *J Acoust Soc Am* 1994; **96**: 2683–93.
14. Glasberg B, Moore B. Psychoacoustics abilities of subjects with unilateral and bilateral cochlear hearing impairments and their relationship to the ability to understand speech. *Scand Audiol Suppl* 1989; **32**: 1–25.
15. Fastl H, Schorn K. Discrimination of level differences by hearing impaired patients. *Audiology* 1981; **20**: 488–502.
16. Patterson RD. Auditory filter shapes derived with noise stimuli. *J Acoust Soc Am* 1976; **59**: 640–54.
17. Patterson RD, Nimmo-Smith I, Weber DL, Milroy R. The deterioration of hearing with age: frequency selectivity, the critical ratio, the audiogram, and speech threshold. *J Acoust Soc Am* 1982; **72**: 1788–803.
18. Glasberg BR, Moore BCJ, Patterson RD, Nimmo-Smith I. Dynamic range and asymmetry of the auditory filter. *J Acoust Soc Am* 1984; **76**: 419–27.
19. Glasberg BR, Moore BCJ. Derivation of auditory filter shapes from notched-noise data. *Hear Res* 1990; **47**: 103–38.
20. Tyler RS, Hall JW, Glasberg BR, Moore BCJ, Patterson RD. Auditory filter asymmetry in the hearing impaired. *J Acoust Soc Am* 1984; **76**: 1363–76.
21. Hall JW, Grose JH. Spectro-temporal analysis and cochlear hearing impairment: effects of frequency selectivity, temporal resolution, signal frequency and rate of modulation. *J Acoust Soc Am* 1989; **85**: 2550–62.
22. Glasberg BR, Moore BCJ. Auditory filter shapes in subjects with unilateral and bilateral cochlear impairments. *J Acoust Soc Am* 1986; **79**: 1020–33.
23. Zwicker EB. On the pscyhophysical equivalent of tuning curves. In: Zwicker E, Terhardt E, eds. *Facts and Models in Hearing*. Berlin: Springer-Verlag, 1974.
24. Moore BCJ. Psychophysical tuning curves measured in simultaneous and forward masking. *J Acoust Soc Am* 1978; **63**: 524–32.

25. Moore BCJ, Glasberg BR, Roberts B. Refining the measurements of psychophysical tuning curves. *J Acoust Soc Am* 1984; **76**: 1057–66.
26. Zwicker E, Schorn K. Psychoacoustical tuning curves in audiology. *Audiology* 1978; **17**: 120–40.
27. Tyler RS, Wood EJ, Fernandes M. Frequency resolution and hearing loss. *Br J Audiol* 1982; **16**: 45–63.
28. Rose JE, Brugge JF, Anderson DJ, Hind JE. Patterns of activity in single auditory nerve fibres of the squirrel monkey. In: Reuck AVSD, Knight J, eds. *Hearing Mechanisms in Vertebrates*. London: Churchill, 1968: 144–57.
29. Wier CC, Jesteadt W, Green DM. Frequency discrimination as a function of frequency and sensation level. *J Acoust Soc Am* 1977; **61**: 178–84.
30. Shower EG, Biddulph R. Differential pitch sensitivity of the ear. *J Acoust Soc Am* 1931; **2**: 275–87.
31. Formby C. Frequency and rate discrimination by Meniere patients. *Audiology* 1986; **25**: 10–18.
32. Hall JW, Wood EJ. Stimulus duration and frequency discrimination for normal-hearing and hearing-impaired subjects. *J Speech Hear Res* 1984; **27**: 252–6.
33. Freyman RL, Nelson DA. Frequency discrimination as a function of signal frequency and level in normal-hearing and hearing-impaired listeners. *J Speech Hear Res* 1991; **34**: 1371–86.
34. Moore BC, Sek A. Detection of frequency modulation at low modulation rates: evidence for a mechanism based on phase locking. *J Acoust Soc Am* 1996; **100**: 2320–31.
35. Lacher-Fougere S, Demany L. Modulation detection by normal and hearing-impaired listeners. *Audiology* 1998; **37**: 109–21.
36. Woolf NK, Ryan AF, Bone RC. Neural phase-locking properties in the absence of cochlear outer hair cells. *Hear Res* 1981; **4**: 335–46.
37. Harrison RV, Evans EF. Some aspects of temporal coding by single cochlear fibres from regions of cochlear hair cell degeneration in the guinea pig. *Arch Otorhinolaryngol* 1979; **224**: 71–8.
38. Plomp R. Rate of decay of auditory sensation. *J Acoust Soc Am* 1964; **36**: 277–82.
39. Eddins DA, Hall JW, Grose JH. The detection of temporal gaps as a function of frequency region and absolute noise bandwidth. *J Acoust Soc Am* 1992; **91**: 1069–77.
40. Shailer MJ, Moore BCJ. Detection of temporal gaps in bandlimited noise: effects of variations in bandwidth and signal-to-masker ratio. *J Acoust Soc Am* 1985; **77**: 635–9.
41. Grose JH. Gap detection in multiple narrow bands of noise as a function of spectral configuration. *J Acoust Soc Am* 1991; **90**: 3061–8.
42. Viemeister NF. Temporal modulation transfer functions based upon modulation thresholds. *J Acoust Soc Am* 1979; **66**: 1364–80.
43. Eddins DA. Amplitude modulation detection of narrow-band noise: effects of absolute bandwidth and frequency region. *J Acoust Soc Am* 1993; **93**: 470–9.
44. Bacon SP, Viemeister NF. Temporal modulation transfer functions in normal-hearing and hearing-impaired subjects. *Audiology* 1985; **24**: 117–34.
45. Buus S, Florentine M. Gap detection in normal and impaired listeners: the effect of level and frequency. In: Michelsen A, ed. *Time Resolution in Auditory Systems*. New York: Springer-Verlag, 1985: 159–79.
46. Moore BCJ, Glasberg BR, Donaldson E, McPherson T, Plack CJ. Detection of temporal gaps in sinusoids by normally hearing and hearing-impaired subjects. *J Acoust Soc Am* 1989; **85**: 1266–75.
47. Hall JW, Grose JH. The relation between gap detection, loudness and loudness growth in noise-masked normal-hearing listeners. *J Acoust Soc Am* 1997; **101**: 1044–9.
48. van Wieringen A, Pols LCW. Frequency and duration discrimination of short first-formant speechlike transitions. *J Acoust Soc Am* 1994; **95**: 502–11.
49. Tyler RS, Summerfield AQ, Wood EJ, Fernandes MA. Psychoacoustic and phonetic temporal processing in normal and hearing-impaired listeners. *J Acoust Soc Am* 1982; **72**: 740–52.
50. Viemeister NF, Wakefield GH. Temporal integration and multiple looks. *J Acoust Soc Am* 1991; **90**: 858–65.
51. Sanders JW, Honig EA. Brief tone audiometry. Results in normal and impaired ears. *Arch Otolaryngol* 1967; **85**: 640–7.
52. Pedersen CB. Brief tone audiometry in patients with acoustic trauma. *Acta Otolaryngol* 1973; **75**: 332–3.
53. Olsen WO, Rose DE, Noffsinger D. Brief-tone audiometry with normal, cochlear, and eighth nerve tumor patients. *Arch Otolaryngol* 1974; **99**: 185–9.
54. Patuzzi R. Cochlear micromechanics and macromechanics. In: Dallos P, Popper AN, Fay RR, eds. *The Cochlea*. New York: Springer, 1996; 186–257.
55. Yates GK. Basilar membrane nonlinearity and its influence on auditory nerve rate-intensity functions. *Hear Res* 1990; **50**: 145–62.
56. Ryan A, McGee TJ. Development of hearing loss in kanamycin treated chinchillas. *Ann Otol Rhinol Laryngol* 1977; **86**: 176–82.
57. Patuzzi RB, Yates GK, Johnstone BM. Outer hair cell receptor current and sensorineural hearing loss. *Hear Res* 1989; **42**: 47–72.
58. Abel S, Birt B, McClean J. Sound localization: value in localizing lesions of the auditory pathway. *Can J Otol* 1978; **7**: 132–40.
59. Hausler R, Marr EM, Colburn HS. Sound localization with impaired hearing. *J Acoust Soc Am* 1979; **65**: S133.
60. Jonkees L, van der Veer R. Directional hearing capacity in hearing disorders. *Acta Otolaryngol* 1957; **48**: 465–74.
61. Nordlund B. Directional audiometry. *Acta Otolaryngol* 1964; **57**: 1–18.
62. Roser D. Directional hearing in persons with hearing disorders. *J Laryngol Rhinol* 1965; **45**: 423–40.

63. Hausler R, Colburn HS, Marr E. Sound localization in subjects with impaired hearing. *Acta Otolaryngol* 1983; Suppl 400: 1–62.
64. Klump RG, Eady HR. Some measurement of interaural time difference thresholds. *J Acoust Soc Am* 1956; **28**: 859–60.
65. Zwislocki J, Feldman RS. Just noticeable differences in dichotic phase. *J Acoust Soc Am* 1956; **28**: 860–4.
66. Henning GB. Detectability of interaural delay in high-frequency complex waveforms. *J Acoust Soc Am* 1974; **55**: 84–90.
67. McFadden D, Pasanen EG. Lateralization at high frequencies based on interaural time differences. *J Acoust Soc Am* 1976; **59**: 634–9.
68. Smoski WJ, Trahiotis C. Discrimination of interaural temporal disparities by normal-hearing listeners and listeners with high-frequency sensori-neural hearing loss. *J Acoust Soc Am* 1986; **79**: 1541–7.
69. Hall JW, Tyler RS, Fernandes MA. Factors influencing the masking level difference in cochlear hearing-impaired and normal-hearing listeners. *J Speech Hear Res* 1984; **27**: 145–54.
70. Hawkins DB, Wightman FL. Interaural time discrimination ability of listeners with sensori-neural hearing loss. *Audiology* 1980; **19**: 495–507.
71. Gabriel KJ, Koehnke J, Colburn HS. Frequency dependence of binaural performance in listeners with impaired binaural hearing. *J Acoust Soc Am* 1992; **91**: 336–47.
72. Hirsh IJ. Binaural summation and interaural inhibition as a function of the level of the masking noise. *J Acoust Soc Am* 1948; **20**: 205–13.
73. Olsen W, Noffsinger D. Masking level differences for cochlear and brainstem lesions. *Ann Otol Rhinol Laryngol* 1976; **85**: 1–6.
74. Jerger J, Brown D, Smith S. Effect of peripheral hearing loss on the MLD. *Arch Otolaryngol* 1984; **110**: 290–6.
75. Zwicker E, Schorn K. Temporal resolution in hard of hearing patients. *Audiology* 1982; **21**: 474–92.
76. Florentine M, Buus S, Scharf B, Zwicker E. Frequency selectivity in normal-hearing and hearing-impaired observers. *J Speech Hear Res* 1980; **23**: 643–69.
77. Colburn HS, Hausler R. Note on the modeling of binaural interaction in impaired auditory systems. In: Brink GVD, Bilsen FA, eds. *Physical Physiological and Behavioral Studies in Hearing*. Delft: Delft University, 1980: 491–503.
78. Hall JW, Derlacki EL. Effect of conductive hearing loss and middle ear surgery on binaural hearing. *Ann Otol Rhinol Laryngol* 1986; **95**: 525–30.
79. Quaranta A, Cervellera G. Masking level differences in normal and pathological ears. *Audiology* 1974; **13**: 428–31.
80. Hall JW, Grose JH, Pillsbury HC. Predicting binaural hearing after stapedectomy from pre-surgery results. *Arch Otolaryngol Head Neck Surg* 1990; **116**: 946–50.
81. Magliulo G, Gagliardi M, Muscatello M, Natale A. Masking level difference before and after surgery. *Br J Audiol* 1990; **24**: 117–21.
82. Hall JW, Grose JH, Pillsbury HC. Long-term effects of chronic otitis media on binaural hearing in children. *Arch Otolaryngol Head Neck Surg* 1995; **121**: 847–52.
83. Moore DR, Hutchings ME, Meyer SE. Binaural masking level differences in children with a history of otitis media. *Audiology* 1991; **30**: 91–101.
84. Pillsbury HC, Grose JH, Hall JW. Otitis media with effusion in children: binaural hearing before and after corrective surgery. *Arch Otolaryngol Head Neck Surg* 1991; **117**: 718–23.
85. Jerger J, Jerger S. A simplified tone decay test. *Arch Otolaryngol* 1975; **102**: 403–7.
86. Fowler EP. Some attributes of 'loudness recruitment' and 'loudness decruitment'. *Trans Am Otol Soc* 1965; **53**: 78–84.
87. Noffsinger D, Martinez CD, Schaefer AB. Auditory brainstem responses and masking level differences from persons with brainstem lesion. *Scan Audiol* 1982; **15**: 81–93.
88. Jerger J, Neely JG, Jerger S. Speech, impedance, and auditory brainstem response audiometry in brainstem tumors. Importance of a multiple-test strategy. *Arch Otolaryngol* 1980; **106**: 218–23.
89. Bess FH, Josey AF, Humes LE. Performance intensity functions in cochlear and eighth nerve disorders. *Am J Otol* 1979; **1**: 27–31.

15 Otoacoustic emissions

Borka Ceranic

Otoacoustic emissions (OAEs) are weak signals that can be recorded in the ear canal and are considered to reflect cochlear activity. OAEs were demonstrated and recorded for the first time by Kemp in 1978[1] and led to a revolutionary change in hearing research and clinical audiology, as our understanding of how the cochlea processes sound has fundamentally altered.

Introduction

Historical background

The basic understanding that the cochlea converts sound waves into nerve impulses, which are transmitted into the brain, has existed for more than 200 years. Throughout this period, a number of theories on how the cochlea processes sound were proposed. The auditory theory, established by the eminent telephone engineer von Békésy,[2] following a series of experiments in the early 1940s, assumed the rise of the travelling wave in a mechanically passive and linear system, which delivered sound energy of different frequencies to different parts of the cochlea. However, this passive, anterograde travelling wave, in a viscous environment, would lead to energy loss and degradation of the cochlear travelling wave, which would inevitably lead to loss of sensitivity and frequency resolution of the cochlea. This theory was challenged by Gold,[3] who proposed a theoretical model in which he anticipated active involvement of the cochlea in a positive, self-enforced system, which compensated for the energy loss of sound propagation through the high damping inner ear fluids. However, at that time, his views were not seriously considered. Only with Kemp's discovery of OAEs was there direct proof that the cochlea is capable not only of forward propagation of the travelling wave, but also of retrograde transmission of sound. The cochlea was shown to represent an active, highly non-linear system, able to overcome the damping of the travelling wave and enable sound amplification and sharp frequency tuning.

Cochlear micromechanics and generation of OAEs

Kemp has proposed that OAEs are emitted from the cochlea as a byproduct of an active, non-linear, biomechanical, feedback process from the outer hair cells (OHCs) to the basilar membrane. This process improves low-level sensitivity and sharpness of tuning, by enhancing the vibration of a narrow region of the cochlear partition. The concept of sound emission from the cochlea implies a transmission mechanism to propagate the sound out of the cochlea. According to Kemp,[4] this retrograde energy transmission in the cochlea could be due to some form of 'localized perturbation', possibly as a result of discontinuities in OHC arrangements, resulting in modification of the propagation of the forward travelling wave.

Research over the past two decades has provided the evidence that OAE generation is related to active, fast and slow, physiologically vulnerable, motility of the OHCs,[5,6] through the contraction of the actinomyosin complex in the cytoskeleton of the OHCs. Thus, the OHCs have the capacity to act as peripheral effector cells. This has been demonstrated by efferently induced OHC motility following electrical[5,7] or chemical (γ-aminobutyric acid – one of the main neurotransmitters of the efferent auditory system) stimulation.[8] The fast contractions[5] are phase-locked to the stimulating sound and follow sound-driven passive vibrations of the cochlear partition. They stimulate the actinomyosin network of the OHCs, acting to oppose viscous damping in the cochlea and to enhance the oscillations of the cochlear partition and, thus, the mechanical stimulation of the IHCs. The slow, tonic contractions of the OHCs[6] can alter the stiffness of the cochlear partition in a sharply restricted area, modifying the envelope of the travelling wave. These slow contractions result from the activity of the efferent system (see below), known as electromechanical transduction (electromotility), and have an important role in setting the position of the basilar membrane. These active oscillations of the OHCs are responsible for the generation of OAEs.

The vibrations of the stapes footplate in the oval window, driven by sound pressure waves, cause a dynamic displacement of the cochlear partition in the shape of a travelling wave. Since the walls of the endolymphatic duct (scala media) are flexible, the travelling waves are transmitted to the scala tympani, and the wave-like distortion of the endolymphatic duct causes Reissner's membrane and the basilar membrane to swing from one side to the other, i.e. towards the scala tympani and the scala vestibuli, alternately. The amplitude of the travelling wave has a clearly defined maximum. The site at which maximal displacement of the endolymphatic duct occurs is the 'characteristic' for the frequency of sound: high frequencies have their maximum reception near the stapes, while low frequencies are situated towards the apex. The velocity of the travelling waves and their wavelength gradually decrease with increasing distance from the oval window. Among the reasons for this attenuation, besides the damping properties of the liquid-filled scalae, is that towards the apex, the basilar membrane gradually becomes wider (increased mass) and less rigid (reduced stiffness). This hydrodynamic mechanism, initially thought to be a passive response to the propagating sound, was extensively investigated and described by von Békésy.[2] Sound-driven passive mechanical movements of the basilar membrane and OHCs are accompanied by additional induction of active, fast, mechanical movements of the OHCs and subsequent slow movements, thus creating a highly non-linear and saturating positive feedback system. The OHC fast motility, which enhances the basilar membrane motion (near-hearing threshold amplification by ≈40 dB), is linearly correlated with the intensity of sound stimuli.[9] However, with an increase in sound pressure level, the cochlea is capable of correcting undesirable (high) shifts of the basilar membrane by the slow OHC movements, leading to a reduction of the passive displacement, and non-linear compression of cochlear dynamics (attenuation).[9,10] Thus, the OHCs act as controlled mechano-amplifiers within the cochlea and feed amplified mechanical oscillations to the inner hair cells (IHCs), which are directly involved in the transformation of mechanical energy into neural activity.

The OHCs' activity is controlled by the positive feedback mechanism, involving the efferent olivocochlear (OC) system (Figure 15.1), which was first described by Rasmusen.[11] The fibres of the OC system originate from the superior olivary complex, in the medulla oblongata, which consists of medial and lateral nuclei.

The fibres from the lateral nucleus are arranged in the predominantly uncrossed, lateral OC bundle which projects to the afferent fibres of the IHCs. The fibres from the medial nucleus are arranged in the mainly crossed, medial OC bundle, which travels along the vestibular nerve and projects directly onto the OHCs. The medial efferent OC (MOC) system is considered to be inhibitory[12] and responsible for the control of OHC motility (cochlear micromechanics). This effect is consistent with the results of a number of studies in which stimulation of the efferents in the silent condition has been employed. However, when efferents are activated in noisy background, they exhibit an enhancement of the transient stimulus.[13,14]

With the introduction of OAEs, the MOC system has been extensively investigated. However, very little is known about the lateral OC system. It is believed that it plays an important role in the firing of cochlear neurones, and therefore may have a protective role against excessive noise and/or excitotoxicity.[15]

The OC system is only a part of the auditory efferent system and has multisynaptic connections with the upper parts of the auditory system.

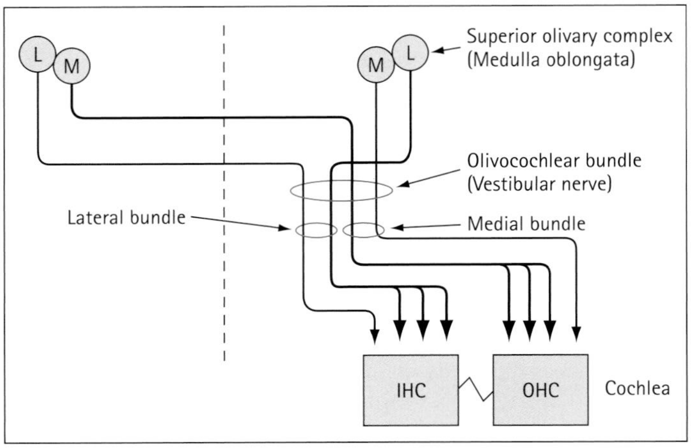

Figure 15.1 Schematic diagram of the olivocochlear efferent system.

The first recording of OAEs in 1978 revolutionized clinical audiology and hearing research. OAEs have supported the existence of active mechanical amplification of sound in the cochlea and retrograde propagation of the travelling wave, with a small 'leakage' of sound energy from these active processes, which can be recorded in the ear canal.

The active processes in the cochlea are the result of contractile properties of the OHCs, thus creating the basis for the generation of OAEs. The sound vibrations that produce active and passive fast oscillations of the OHCs at the same time activate the medial OC system. This leads to the slow tonic contraction of the OHCs, creating the forces to oppose the displacement of the cochlear partition, i.e. a suppressive effect on the OHCs.

Classification and recording of OAEs

Classes of OAEs

OAEs can be recorded in the ear canal in the absence of acoustical stimulation, as spontaneous OAEs (SOAEs), or can be evoked by acoustical stimuli. Evoked OAEs are divided into different categories, according to the type of stimuli: transient evoked OAEs (TEOAEs), distortion product OAEs (DPOAEs), and stimulus frequency (SFOAE) OAEs. SOAEs, TEOAEs and DPOAEs are commonly used in clinical practice and will be described in this chapter in more detail.

SFOAEs are the signals generated by the cochlea at the same frequency as the stimulating continuous tone, but they are difficult to measure and the instrumentation is complex. Therefore, a recording system for SFOAEs is not commercially available.

Recording of OAEs

A standard recording setup (Figure 15.2) includes the stimulus generator, stimulus delivery system (including probe), signal averager and signal display system.[16] A probe, which is inserted into the ear canal, contains the transducer, which delivers the stimulus. The stimulus generates a travelling wave, a part of which is reflected and described as the 'cochlear echo'. The 'cochlear echo' radiates out and is recorded using a sensitive microphone, which is also contained in the probe.

It is of importance to stress that only a fraction of the reflected energy can be recorded in the ear canal, partly due to loss through the retrograde transmission via the middle ear. The influence of middle ear function on OAEs is very well documented.[17] Therefore, when OAE responses are evaluated, the middle ear function must be taken into account.

SOAEs

SOAEs represent a unique class of OAEs, since they can be recorded in the absence of any acoustical stimulation.[18] They result from the process of enhancing the vibration of a narrow region of the cochlear partition, feeding energy back into the mechanical system. The excess of acoustical energy from that feedback process is radiated out of the cochlea, and a small amount of that energy may be recorded in the ear canal.

SOAEs can be recorded in two ways. In one, the sound pressure level in the ear canal is recorded by a sensitive microphone placed in the ear canal with no stimulus applied, and the signal is averaged in the frequency domain. In the other (used in the ILO88 system), SOAEs are synchronized by acoustical stimuli (clicks), using averaging in the time domain. This method allows the detection of sustained oscillations following stimulus (click)-evoked OAEs.

Studies applying these two methods have shown, generally, good correspondence of obtained SOAEs.[19,20] With the synchronizing method, SOAEs exhibit lower levels (≈10 dB less) and more peaks (? better sensitivity in recording of SOAEs) than those obtained by direct recording; the reasons for this are yet to be clarified.

Figure 15.3 shows a standard default screen with SOAEs using the ILO88 Otodynamics equipment.

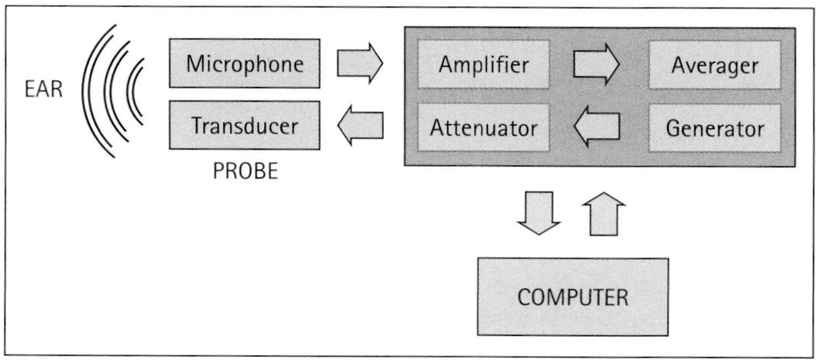

Figure 15.2 A schematic view of a standard setup for recording of OAEs.

TEOAEs

TEOAEs are recorded in response to the transient stimuli and show a delay (latency) with respect to the onset of the acoustical stimulus. The click is the most commonly used stimulus, because it has energy over a broad frequency range. Similar to the travelling wave, click-evoked OAEs also demonstrate frequency dispersion, with the shortest latency being for the high, and the longest for the low, frequencies (about 4 ms for 5 kHz; 20 ms for 0.5 kHz).

TEOAEs exhibit 'compressive' non-linearity, i.e. 'compressive' growth of the TEOAE amplitude as a function of the stimulus intensity. The maximal gain occurs at lower sound levels (around hearing threshold level) and gradually reduces with an increase in sound intensity, before reaching saturation level, after which a further increase in sound intensity does not lead to an increase in TEOAE amplitude.[1]

TEOAEs can be recorded using different techniques, as follows.

Differential non-linear technique (ILO88 system, Otodynamics)
This technique has been in widespread clinical use since the commercial availability of the hardware and software (1988). The stimulus presentation, data recording, averaging and spectrum analysis have been described by Kemp et al.[16] The stimuli are clicks (bandwidth ≈5 kHz), with a duration of 80 µs, presented at a repetition rate of 50/s, with a peak reception level at around 80 dB SPL. They are presented in the non-linear differential mode: four clicks, with three clicks at the same level and polarity, and a fourth click three times greater in level and reverse polarity, and with a 10-dB increase in amplitude. This

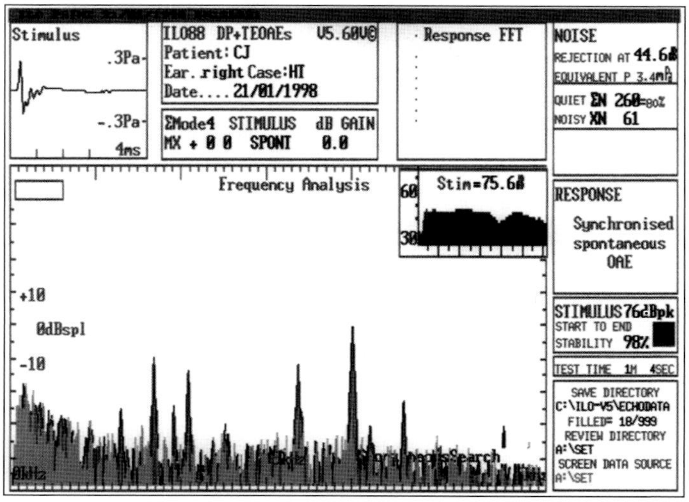

Figure 15.3 Spontaneous OAEs in a normal subject with a multiple frequency component spectrum.

paradigm cancels the linear portion of the stimulus and response, including the meatal and middle ear echoes, so that non-linear cochlear emissions can be extracted. The responses from the cochlea are recorded and averaged alternately in two separate buffers (A and B) using a synchronous time-domain averaging technique. The waveforms present in the buffers A and B are compared, and their high cross-correlation (reproducibility) suggests the presence of the cochlear response. The post-stimulus analysis time is 2.5–20 ms. The fast Fourier transformation (FFT) spectrum analysis of averaged waveforms is automatically performed and plotted against the averaged random noise in the ear canal. A typical screen of a normal adult is displayed in Figure 15.4.

The recording of TEOAEs using maximum length sequence (MLS) technique

This technique[21] has been developed specifically to improve the quality and duration of TEOAE recording in less than optimal conditions (e.g. a noisy child). It applies MLS, which represents a quasi-random train of clicks and silences, with a higher click stimulus rate (up to 5000 clicks/s, in contrast to the conventional 50 clicks/s), and the subsequent overlapped responses are subjected to the process of recovery.

This technique, as well as the deconvolution method,[22] although not used in routine clinical practice, heralds further developments in OAE recording technology.

DPOAEs

DPOAEs or 'combination tones', can be defined as acoustical energy resulting from the non-linear interaction of two simultaneously applied pure tones, which partially overlap the vibration fields in the cochlea. The continuous tones, known as the primaries f_1 and f_2 (the frequency $f_2 < f_1$), are most commonly presented with equal levels (in dB SPL) at the eardrum (or with the level of f_2 slightly less than f_1) at closely-spaced frequencies, with the optimal f_2/f_1 ratio about 1.22.[23] DPOAEs consist of new frequencies which are not represented in the primaries, and in humans, the strongest DPOAE is at the frequency described by the expression $2f_1 - f_2$.

The most frequently used application is the DPOAE-gram, obtained by cycling through the preset stimulus frequency sequence, with the fixed ratio f_1/f_2, and building a plot of DPOAE levels as a function of the frequency (Figure 15.5). Another method is the input–output measure of DPOAE, which presents signals at several levels for a specific frequency and provides information, such as detection threshold, growth function, or maximum output level.

There are several commercially available recording technologies, one of which is the ILO92 Otodynamics system.

All OAEs can be divided into two classes: spontaneous and evoked. Spontaneous OAEs are continuous narrowband signals emitted by the cochlea in the absence of any stimulation. They can be recorded directly from the ear canal using a sensitive microphone or using a synchronizing click (the latter method is used in the ILO88 Otodynamics system). Evoked OAEs are recorded following stimulation by different stimuli: TEOAEs can be evoked by transient impulses, such as clicks or tone bursts, and DPOAEs can be evoked by two continuous tones, f_1 and f_2, at the two closely spaced frequencies, delivered into the ear canal.

A standard recording setup includes the stimulus generator, stimulus delivery system (including probe), signal averager and signal display system.

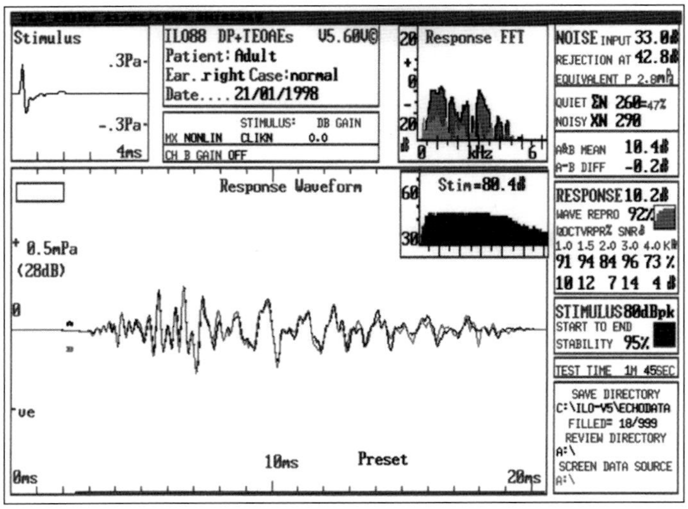

Figure 15.4 TEOAEs, recorded with non-linear click stimuli of 80.4 dB SPL, from a normal subject, showing in the response window two alternate (A and B) recorded time waveforms and the FFT with the frequency spectrum of the response.

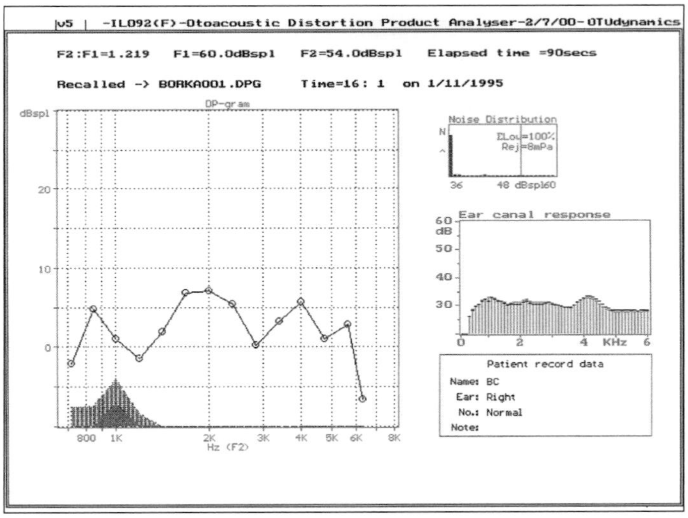

Figure 15.5 DPOAE-gram recorded from a normal subject. Amplitude of the distortion product (dB SPL) is illustrated as a function of frequency (f_2).

Characteristics of OAEs in normal subjects and their clinical relevance

General properties of OAEs

1. OAEs are physiological, bio-acoustical energy and are the consequence of active sound processing in the cochlea. However, OAEs are not only the result of cochlear activity, but also reflect the transmission of sound through the middle ear and the resonant characteristics of the sealed ear canal.
2. All classes of OAEs exhibit a saturating type of non-linearity with stimulus level, and above 40 dB SL they become relatively insignificant. OAEs themselves rarely exceed 30 dB SPL. The non-linear property of OAEs (which reflects non-linear behaviour of the OHCs, as described above) provides the basis for distinguishing OAEs from the passive, linear response of the cochlea to sound.
3. OAEs exhibit periodicity in their microstructure. The phenomenon of local periodicity, the presence of the 'peaks' and 'valleys', has been observed in the frequency spectra of SOAEs,[18,24,25] SFOAEs, TEOAEs[26,27] and DPOAEs.[28] A possible source of the periodicity is in the 'cochlear resonances', the places where OAE peaks are most likely to occur,[24] resulting from the recirculation and partial reflection of the acoustical stimulus energy, between the place of characteristic frequency and the oval window.
4. OAEs are highly reproducible, with temporal and spectral properties unique for each individual, being commonly described as 'fingerprints' of the inner ear.

SOAEs

Characteristics in normal subjects

SOAEs can be recorded in 30–50% (~30% males and ~50% females) of individuals with normal hearing, and the prevalence of SOAEs in individuals above the age 50 is markedly reduced.[29] It has been recognized that the detection of SOAEs depends on the sensitivity of the recording system, and that technological advances may increase the number of subjects with recordable SOAEs. A study by Penner and Zhang[30] demonstrated that the detection of SOAEs (62% for males and 83% for females) could be increased by suitably tailored spectral analyses.

In addition to gender variation, there have also been reports of racial differences, SOAEs being more common in black than white populations,[31] and a laterality effect, with SOAEs being more commonly recorded in right ears.[32–34] The latter authors reported that right ears are 13% more likely to have SOAEs than left ears, and that the occurrence of multiple SOAEs is much more prevalent in females than in males. A genetic contribution to the expression of SOAEs is thought to be significant.[35]

In the normal population, SOAEs show intra-session, as well as inter-session, short-term (few hours) and long-term (4 months) frequency stability, with physiological variations, being typically less than 1%, but rarely exceeding 2%.[36–41] The amplitude of SOAEs, however, may vary over a much wider range (more than 10 dB SPL).[42,43]

Although SOAEs are the signals generated by the inner ear, they are not audible to the subjects who possess them. In some rare cases of high-amplitude SOAEs, they can be heard by another person – e.g. at 1 m distance.[29] It has been hypothesized that continuous emissions do not produce an auditory perception, because of adaptation. Perception occurs only in non-adaptive situations,[44–47] which can be simulated in experimental conditions, such as changing the impedance of the middle ear, which may cause a change in the frequency spectrum of SOAEs, making them audible to the subject.[18,45,48]

Clinical relevance of SOAEs

SOAEs have been extensively investigated in the normal population, but their clinical significance still remains unclear. They could be an expression of the cochlear integrity, as their presence is associated with functionally intact OHCs and exquisite hearing sensitivity, with audiometric thresholds, according to most authors, better than 15 dB HL but less than 20 dB HL at homologous frequencies.[49,50] Furthermore, it has been demonstrated that individuals with recordable SOAEs have better psychophysical thresholds than those without.[51] It is widely accepted that SOAEs are sensitive (vulnerable) to alterations in the cochlear status: for example, physiological degeneration, i.e. ageing, leads to their loss.[52] Furthermore, SOAEs are subject to small but systematic alterations during physiological, e.g. circadian,[37,39] or menstrual,[39–41] cycles, in the form of systematic frequency shifts, which are thought to be governed by daily variation in the secretion of melatonin by the pineal gland, and, in females, by monthly variations linked to the pituitary–gonadal axis. However, the possibility of SOAE fluctuation as a result of circulatory changes cannot be excluded. The observation of fluctuation suggests that SOAEs may not only be an expression of the cochlear status, but could also be influenced by higher levels of auditory and/or other central nervous system structures. Such an effect may be mediated through efferently induced mechanisms of electromechanical transduction,[6] which may alter the gain in the feedback loop of a cochlear amplifier, and, thus, the SOAE frequency spectrum.

Kemp[24] suggested that SOAEs might result from some areas of localized damage in the cochlea that could interfere with normal active feedback mechanisms. Furthermore, Ruggero et al.[53] demonstrated that SOAEs could be generated from the segment of the organ of Corti, where there is a sharp transition between relatively normal OHCs and an adjacent damaged area. SOAEs were also reported at the frequencies that correspond to the abnormalities on the audiogram.[48] In experiments with chinchillas, SOAEs have been induced by traumatic noise exposure,[54,55] and there is evidence that they may interfere with auditory function: it has been observed that the presence of strong SOAEs degrades the ability of the neurone to respond to sound.[55] However, there are insufficient data to explain the significance of these 'pathological' SOAEs, and their clinical relevance remains unclear.

The discovery of the existence of SOAEs led to the expectation that they might be an objective correlate of tinnitus, and the relationship between tinnitus and SOAEs has therefore been studied extensively.[56] Although, in general, attempts to attribute tinnitus to SOAEs have been disappointing, there are some patients with convincing evidence of a close correspondence between tinnitus and SOAEs.[46,47,57–63] According to Penner,[58] the 95% confidence limits for the prevalence of SOAE-related tinnitus among members of a self-help group were 1% and 9.5%. The effect of aspirin, which in these subjects (with SOAE-related tinnitus) abolishes tinnitus and SOAEs simultaneously, has been explored.[60,63,64]

However, in view of aspirin ototoxicity, this treatment has not been considered appropriate.

SOAEs can be recorded in 40–70% of individuals with normal hearing and their prevalence depends on the sensitivity of the recording system. SOAEs display high frequency stability on repeated measurements; however, systematic physiological variations, although small, have been observed. They are associated with exquisite hearing sensitivity – they correspond to the best audiometric frequencies, with homologous audiometric frequency better than 15 dB HL. Although SOAEs have been extensively investigated in normal subjects, their physiological significance, and therefore their clinical relevance, remains unclear.

TEOAEs

Characteristics in normal subjects and clinical relevance

Since TEOAEs are invariably associated with functioning OHCs, they can be recorded in all subjects with normal hearing:[29] OAEs are present in 96–100% of normally hearing ears, and absent if hearing loss is greater than 25–35 dB HL. Therefore, the presence of TEOAE responses is a reliable indicator of global cochlear (OHC) structural integrity (from 0.5 to 5 kHz), although the best responses are recorded in the 1–2-kHz range, where the reverse-transfer function of the middle ear is most effective.[65] Their absence suggests at least a 25-dB loss due to either middle ear or cochlear lesions. In general, TEOAEs cannot be elicited if the hearing loss is greater than 35 dB HL.[66,67]

TEOAE responses have been shown to have excellent test–retest and within-ear stability, and a measurement error with variability of amplitude of less than 1 dB,[68–70] as shown in Figure 15.6. However, TEOAEs have demonstrated considerable between-ear variability.[1,71]

A major limitation of TEOAEs is that the emitted responses of the OHC activity are small-amplitude signals, with a limited dynamic range before response saturation, and are further compromised before measurement by the necessary reverse transmission through the middle ear.

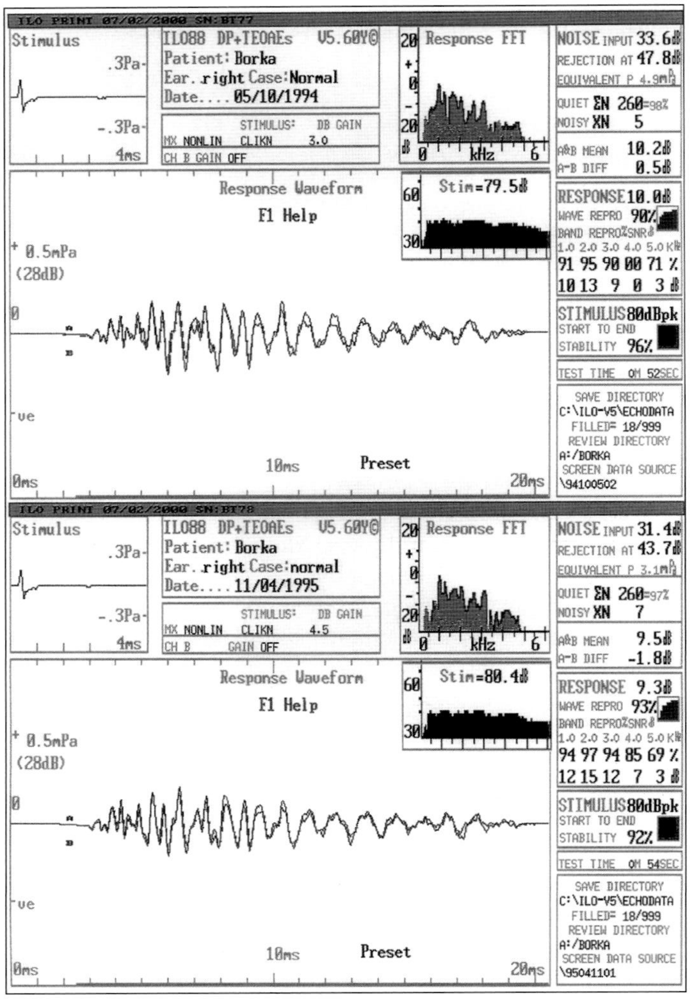

Figure 15.6 TEOAE responses recorded from the right ear of a normal subject over a period of 1 year (1994–95), demonstrating a high reproducibility of the response amplitude (< ± 1 dB) and power spectra.

Characteristics of TEOAEs in subjects with hearing loss

In the impaired cochlea, as judged by sensorineural hearing loss, the prevalence and amplitude of TEOAEs decrease and the detection threshold increases.[66] In subjects with a history of noise exposure, TEOAEs exhibit a reduction/absence of the response amplitude in the regions where the audiometric thresholds are unaffected.[72,73] Therefore, by recording OAEs, a subclinical cochlear lesion may be detected, and this is in agreement with the finding that up to 30% of the OHC population may be damaged prior to audiometric evidence, in the quarter-octave audiometry from 0.125 to 16 kHz.[74]

It has been demonstrated that, in addition to the lower amplitudes and 'worse' non-linearity thresholds, the spectra of TOAEs in ears with noise-induced hearing loss are narrow in comparison with those with normal hearing.[75] This confirms that, although the TEOAE frequency spectrum is not a direct measure of hearing sensitivity, frequency band parameters can indicate whether hearing sensitivity at a homologous audiometric frequency is normal or abnormal (< or >20 dB HL)[16,76] and, therefore, can be useful in the detection of frequency-specific subclinical cochlear (OHC) lesions.

The aetiology of the cochlear impairment may also be of relevance: TEOAEs can vary in amplitude and spectral composition in cases with a similar configuration of hearing loss of different aetiology. This has been demonstrated for noise-induced hearing loss,[49] where the prevalence and spectral peaks of TEOAEs showed significant reduction in comparison with ears with similar audiometric patterns caused by other factors. In patients with Menière's disease,[77] the amplitudes of TEOAEs were significantly lower and contained fewer spectral peaks in comparison with results obtained from a database. These results illustrate that changes in TEOAE responses may represent an expression of the degree and variety of the pathological processes in the cochlea.

> TEOAEs can be recorded in practically all normal subjects (prevalence 96–100%). They are absent if hearing loss is greater than 25–30 dB. TEOAEs exhibit excellent test–retest, intra-individual stability (± 1 dB) and are therefore often referred to as cochlear 'fingerprints'. However, they show considerable inter-subject variability.

DPOAEs

Like TEOAEs, DPOAEs are generated by normally functioning OHCs, and can be recorded, essentially, in all normally hearing subjects.

The advantages of DPOAEs over TEOAEs are as follows:

1. DPOAEs are more frequency specific.[78]
2. DPOAEs have better responses at high frequencies (up to 6–8 kHz) than TEOAEs, where, due to time-gating and cut-off in the first 2.5–3 ms, the responses are recorded up to 5 kHz.
3. DPOAEs are less sensitive to hearing loss and can be recorded in ears with hearing loss up to 45 dB HL,[67] because a continuous stimulus level provides a more intense stimulus than the mean level used in standard TEOAE recording.

Characteristics (2) and (3) enable DPOAEs to be used as a sensitive method for site-of-lesion testing to track the pattern of OHC lesions.[79]

DPOAEs have some practical disadvantages:

1. Lower-frequency responses are easily contaminated by noise, because the DPOAE response is frequency shifted downwards from the test frequencies by 2/3 octave. Additionally, the noise rejection system cannot be applied in DPOAE recording.
2. Longer duration of the test.

> DPOAEs have similar characteristics to TEOAEs. They are more frequency specific, and, due to the difference in recording techniques, they provide responses at higher frequencies than TEOAEs and can be recorded when audiometric thresholds are elevated up to 45 dB HL.

Clinical applications of OAEs

> **CLINICAL APPLICATIONS OF SOAES**
>
> - *evaluation of cochlear (OHC) integrity*
> - *intra-subject monitoring of cochlear status*
> - *indicators of cochlear functional state ('overactivity')*
> - *assessment of patients with tinnitus*

To date, SOAEs have been used very little in clinical practice, partly due to the purely defined physiological significance, and partly because they are not recordable in all normal subjects. Nevertheless, there are several possible clinical applications of SOAEs, limited to those subjects in whom they are recordable:

1. Recordable SOAEs are indicators of structural integrity of the cochlea (OHCs) and exquisite hearing sensitivity in the frequency region in which they occur.
2. SOAEs can be used for intra-subject monitoring of the cochlear status as the most vulnerable product (e.g. to ototoxicity, noise, or hypoxia) of the active processes in the cochlea.[64,80]
3. SOAE presence may suggest the 'overactivity' of the cochlea , with an 'excess' of acoustical energy from the positive feedback loop, and, therefore, may reflect the functional status of the cochlea, as well as of the higher levels in the auditory system: SOAEs may result from altered feedback control mechanisms, but a clinical application as an indicator of pathology has yet to be investigated.
4. SOAEs in patients with tinnitus — in some cases, SOAEs may explain tinnitus. A set of criteria for establishing a relationship between tinnitus and SOAEs has been proposed by Penner and Burns:[81]

   (a) correlation of tinnitus pitch with SOAE frequency
   (b) suppression of SOAEs making tinnitus inaudible
   (c) masking of tinnitus abolishing SOAEs
   (d) frequency-specific isomasking contours of tinnitus.

> **CLINICAL APPLICATIONS OF TEOAES**
>
> - *evaluation of cochlear (OHC) integrity*
> - *neonatal hearing screening*
> - *intra-subject monitoring in cochlear status*
> - *differential diagnosis of cochlear and retrocochlear lesions*

All of these criteria should be met if tinnitus is to be directly related to the presence of SOAEs. It may also be possible that the finding of frequency-variable SOAEs (as opposed to the frequency-stable SOAEs) is of relevance to the perception of tinnitus, as they are more commonly observed in patients with tinnitus than in normal subjects.[82]

Among all the classes of OAEs, TEOAEs are the most commonly used in clinical practice. Their extensive use is facilitated by the non-invasiveness of the method and the speed at which they can be recorded (≤60 s per ear).

1. Evaluation of cochlear (OHC) integrity

As TEOAEs are invariably associated with structurally intact OHCs, their presence indicates normal cochlear (OHC) function. Furthermore, the absence of TEOAEs in subjects with normal audiometric thresholds and normal middle ear function is an indication of an early, subclinical, cochlear lesion.[73,83]

TEOAEs also display, besides a global cochlear response, frequency specificity.[84] The narrowing of the TEOAE spectrum may suggest localized OHC damage (e.g. absence of high-frequency responses in noise-induced hearing loss).[75]

As an objective test, TEOAE recording is invaluable for screening of hearing, to separate ears with normal hearing from those with hearing loss,[86] e.g. in difficult-to-test patients, or non-organic hearing loss.

2. Neonatal hearing screening

This is one of the most frequent applications of TEOAEs, and OAEs in general,[86–88] for the detection of peripheral auditory lesions. At present, this programme primarily targets neonates and infants at risk for hearing loss, but universal neonatal hearing screening programmes may become the rule (see Chapter 20).

3. Intra-subject monitoring of changes in cochlear status

This application is a result of the high intra-subject stability of TEOAEs. TEOAEs can be applied in monitoring the effects of excessive noise exposure, ototoxicity, anaesthesia, or cochlear function during vestibular Schwannoma surgery.[67,73,89] They can be also used in monitoring the changes in cochlear status in Menière's disease.[90,91]

4. Differential diagnosis of cochlear and retrocochlear lesions

TEOAEs and other OAEs are the products of cochlear (OHC) activity, and their generation is independent of the afferent and efferent innervations.[92] Therefore, if TEOAEs are recorded in subjects with moderate or severe sensorineural hearing loss, this would strongly suggest a retrocochlear lesion,[93,94] providing that functional hearing loss has been excluded. This application is limited to those patients with recordable TEOAEs. No conclusion can be drawn if TEOAEs are absent: the abnormality could be anywhere within the auditory system.

DPOAEs

The clinical applications of DPOAEs are similar to those for TEOAEs, with the advantages and disadvantages explained in the previous section.

The application of OAEs in assessing the MOC system

Characteristics of the MOC system

The discovery of the existence of OAEs has allowed examination of the function of the MOC system in humans, which innervates the OHCs. It has been demonstrated that in normal subjects contralateral acoustical stimulation of the MOC system can alter the frequency and reduce the amplitude of SOAEs,[95,96] and reduce the amplitude and shift the phase of TEOAEs[97,98] (Figure 15.7) and DPOAEs.[99] This implies an inhibitory function of the MOC system. There is a suggestion that the MOC system may exhibit a laterality effect, with a greater effect in the right than the left ear in right-handers.[33,100]

The magnitude of the suppressive effect on OAE responses during efferent MOC stimulation depends on the intensity of both contra- and ipsilateral stimuli. The MOC system can be activated by low-level contralateral acoustical stimulation (e.g. 30–40 dB SPL) and the suppressive effect increases with more intense contralateral stimulation.[97,98] However, the suppressibility of the OAE response evoked by lower levels of ipsilateral stimulation, e.g. 50–60 dB SPL, is greater than the suppressibility of those responses evoked by higher-intensity stimuli.[99,101] This property is consistent with a physiological role in the amplification of low-intensity sounds. At high ipsilateral stimulus levels, a loss of contralateral effect has been observed. This

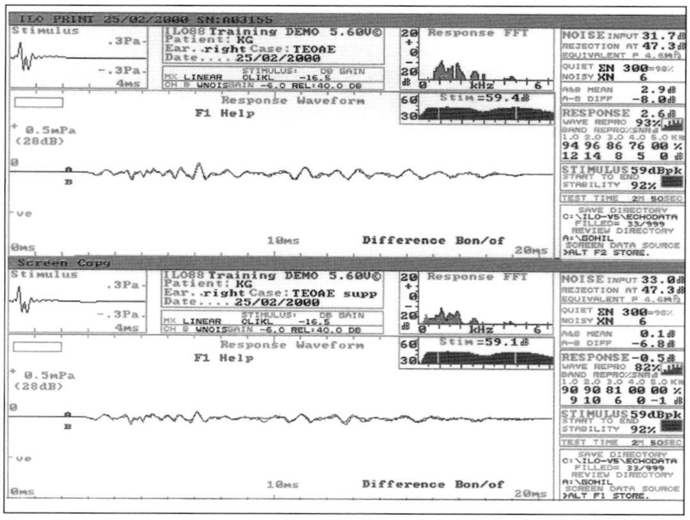

Figure 15.7 TEOAEs in a normal subject, recorded without (upper trace) and with (lower trace) the application of contralateral white noise, with *respective* average response amplitudes of 2.6 dB SPL and −0.5 dB SPL, thus indicating a 3.1-dB suppressive effect.

'compressive' growth function can be attributed to the MOC system, implying a role in defining the dynamic range of cochlear activity. With the ability to modulate the activity of the OHCs, the MOC system appears to be responsible for automatic gain control, adaptation and homeostasis of the cochlea.

Confounding effects of the stapedius acoustical reflex and 'cross-talk'

It is of importance to note that the stapedius reflex (SR) also attenuates acoustical stimuli. Therefore, the SR may have a synergistic effect with the MOC system. This interaction is supported by the findings of the particularly strong suppressive effect of the MOC system in patients with no SR[99] and the reduction in SR thresholds after surgical section of the OCB (olivocochlear bundle) in rabbits.[102] However, the contribution of the SR to the MOC suppressive effect is diminished by the application of contralateral acoustical stimulation at the level necessary to produce this effect, which is considerably lower than the intensity of sound which triggers the SR.

Acoustical 'cross-talk' is another factor with a potential confounding effect on the MOC reflex. However, experimental evidence, based on testing MOC activity in unilaterally deaf subjects (absent suppression), does not support any significant effect of 'cross-talk' on the suppressive effect produced by low-level, contralateral acoustical stimulation.[97]

Clinical applications of the MOC suppression test

The suppressive effect of the MOC system can be demonstrated by recording OAEs (in clinical use, mainly TEOAEs) under contralateral acoustical stimulation. The MOC suppression test provides general information on the structural integrity of the MOC reflex arc, and a glimpse into the modulation of cochlear mechanics by its stimulation.

Although clinical applications of this test are still being developed, it may be useful in the evaluation of the pathological states in which an abnormality of the MOC system may exist, including the following.

Vestibular nerve section

Vestibular nerve section due to the anatomical proximity of the vestibular nerve and the MOC bundle is also accompanied by the section of the MOC bundle, resulting in the absence of an MOC suppressive effect.[103,104]

Central nervous system pathology

This may cause a lesion of the MOC arc, with a subsequently absent/reduced suppressive MOC effect.[103,105–107] This test could contribute to neuro-otological topographic diagnosis, in identification of a lesion up to the brainstem level (superior olivary complex).

Tinnitus/hyperacusis

The alteration of the MOC effect, predominantly reduced functioning, has been observed in patients with tinnitus and hyperacusis,[103,107–115] suggesting that the MOC system may play a role in dysfunction of the auditory system.

Summary

All classes of OAEs provide information on the cochlea, but with the application of different technologies for response measurement, they complement each other. All OAEs are indicators of OHC structural integrity, with SOAEs being the most sensitive, followed by TEOAEs and then DPOAEs. TEOAEs are more appropriate for assessment of global cochlear function, while DPOAEs provide more frequency-specific responses. As OAEs show remarkable intra-subject stability, they can be used as a sensitive tool for intra-subject monitoring of changes in OHC status. The important applications of OAEs are in the evaluation of peripheral auditory function in difficult-to-test subjects (e.g. children, or mentally retarded patients) and retrocochlear lesions, and particularly in neonatal hearing screening. OAEs can also be applied in exploring the MOC system.

In clinical audiology, OAEs should be applied and interpreted in conjunction with other tests.

References

1. Kemp DT. Stimulated acoustic emissions from within the human auditory system. *J Acoust Soc Am* 1978; **64**: 1386–91.
2. von Békésy G. *Experiments on Hearing*. New York: McGraw-Hill, 1960.
3. Gold T. Hearing II. The physical basis for the action of the cochlea. *Proc R Soc Lond B* 1948; **135**: 492–8.
4. Kemp DT. Otoacoustic emissions, travelling waves and cochlear mechanisms. *Hear Res* 1986; **22**: 95–104.
5. Brownell WE, Bader CR, Bertrand D, de Ribaupierre Y. Evoked mechanical responses of isolated cochlear outer hair cells. *Science* 1985; **227**: 194–6.
6. Zenner HP. Motile responses in outer hair cells. *Hear Res* 1986; **22**: 83–90.
7. Nuttall AL, Ren T. Electromotile hearing: evidence from basilar membrane motion and otoacoustic emissions. *Hear Res* 1995; **92**: 170–7.
8. Plinkert PK, Gitter AH, Möhler H, Zenner HP. Structure, pharmacology and function of $GABA_A$ receptors in cochlear outer hair cells. *Eur Arch Otorhinolaryngol* 1993; **250**: 351–7.
9. LePage EL. Frequency-dependent self-induced bias of the basilar membrane and its potential for controlling sensitivity and tuning in the mammalian cochlea. *J Acoust Soc Am* 1987; **82**: 1539–54.
10. LePage EL. Functional role of the olivo-cochlear bundle: a motor unit control system in the mammalian cochlea. *Hear Res* 1989; **30**: 177–98.
11. Rasmussen G. The olivary peduncle and other fibre projections of the superior olivary complex. *J Comp Neurol* 1946; **84**: 141–219.
12. Wiederhold ML. Physiology of the olivocochlear system. In: Altschuler R, Bobin R, Hoffman D, eds. *Neurobiology of Hearing, The Cochlea*. New York: Raven Press, 1986; 349–70.

13. Dolan DF, Nuttall AL. Cochlear whole-nerve responses altered by electrical stimulation of the inferior colliculus, *Soc Neurosci Abstr* 1988; **14**: 650.
14. Kawase T, Delgutte B, Liberman MC. Antimasking effects of the olivocochlear reflex. II. Enhancement of auditory-nerve response to masked tones. *J Neurophysiol* 1993; **70**: 2533–49.
15. Pujol R. Lateral and medial efferents: a double neurochemical mechanism to protect and regulate inner and outer hair cell function in the cochlea. *Br J Audiol* 1994; **28**: 185–91.
16. Kemp DT, Ryan S, Bray P. A guide to effective use of otoacoustic emissions. *Ear Hear* 1990; **11**: 93–105.
17. Margolis RH, Trine MB. Influence of middle ear-disease on otoacoustic emissions. In: Robinette MS, Glattke TJ, eds. *Otoacoustic Emissions: Clinical Applications*. New York: Thieme, 1997: 130–50.
18. Kemp DT. Evidence of mechanical nonlinearity and frequency selective wave amplification in the cochlea. *Arch Otolaryngol Laryngol* 1979; **224**: 37–45.
19. Gobsch H, Tietze G. Interrelation of spontaneous and evoked otoacoustic emissions. *Hear Res* 1993; **69**: 176–81.
20. Smurzynski J, Probst R. Error in the calculation of synchronised spontaneous otoacoustic emissions frequencies measured with the ILO88 system. *J Acoust Soc Am* 1996; **100**: 2555–6.
21. Thornton ARD. Clicked-evoked otoacoustic emissions: new techniques and applications. *Br J Audiol* 1993; **27**: 109–15.
22. Grandori F, Ravazzani P. Deconvolution of otoacoustic emissions and response nonlinearity. In: Grandori F, Cianfrone D, Kemp DT, eds. *Cochlear Mechanisms and Otoacoustic Emissions*. Basel: Karger, 1990: 99–109.
23. Harris FP, Lonsbury-Martin BL, Stagner BB, Coats AC, Martin GK. Acoustic distortion products in humans: systematic changes in amplitude as a function of f_2/f_1 ratio. *J Acoust Soc Am* 1989; **85**: 220–9.
24. Kemp DT. Physiologically active cochlear micromechanisms—one source of tinnitus. In: Evered D, Lawrenson G, eds. *Tinnitus. CIBA Foundation Symposium* 85. London: Pitman Books Ltd, 1981: 54–81.
25. Schloth E. Relation between spectral composition of spontaneous otoacoustic emissions and fine-structure of threshold in quiet. *Acustica* 1983; **53**: 250–6.
26. Zwicker E. A hardware cochlear nonlinear processing model with active feedback. *J Acoust Soc Am* 1986; **80**: 146–53.
27. Zweig G, Shera CA. The origin of periodicity in the spectrum of evoked otoacoustic emissions. *J Acoust Soc Am* 1995; **94**: 2018–47.
28. He N, Schmiedt RA. Fine structure of the $2f_1 - 2f_2$ acoustic distortion product: changes with primary level. *J Acoust Soc Am* 1993; **94**: 2659–69.
29. Probst R, Lonsbury-Martin BL, Martin GK. A review of otoacoustic emissions. *J Acoust Soc Am* 1991; **89**: 2027–67.
30. Penner MJ, Zhang T. Prevalence of spontaneous otoacoustic emissions in adults revisited. *Hear Res* 1997; **103**: 20–34.
31. Whitehead ML, Kamal N, Lonsbury-Martin BL, Martin GK. Spontaneous otoacoustic emissions in different racial groups. *Scand Audiol* 1993; **23**: 3–10.
32. Bilger RC, Matties ML, Hammel DT. Genetic implications of gender differences in the prevalence of spontaneous acoustic emissions, *J Speech Hear Res* 1990; **33**: 418–32.
33. McFadden D. A speculation about the parallel ear asymmetries and sex differences in hearing sensation and otoacoustic emissions. *Hear Res* 1993; **68**: 143–51.
34. Penner MJ, Glotzbach L, Huang T. Spontaneous otoacoustic emissions: measurement and data. *Hear Res* 1993; **68**: 229–37.
35. McFadden D, Loehlin JC. On the heritability of otoacoustic emissions: a twin study. *Hear Res* 1995; **85**: 181–98.
36. Strickland E, Burns EM, Tubis A, Jones K. Long-term stability and familial aspects of spontaneous otoacoustic emissions. *J Acoust Soc Am* 1984; **75** (suppl 7): S82.
37. Wit HP. Diurnal cycle for spontaneous otoacoustic emission frequency. *Hear Res* 1985; **18**: 197–9.
38. Whitehead ML. Slow variation of the amplitude and frequency of spontaneous otoacoustic emissions. *Hear Res* 1991; **53**: 269–80.
39. Bell A. Circadian and menstrual rhythms in frequency variations of spontaneous otoacoustic emissions from human ears. *Hear Res* 1992; **58**: 91–100.
40. Haggerty HS, Lusted HS, Morton SC. Statistical quantification of 24-hour and monthly variabilities of spontaneous otoacoustic emission frequency in humans. *Hear Res* 1993; **70**: 31–49.
41. Penner MJ. Frequency variation of spontaneous otoacoustic emissions during a naturally occurring menstrual cycle, amenorrhea, and oral contraception: a brief report. *Ear Hear* 1995; **16**: 428–32.
42. Wit HP. Amplitude fluctuations of spontaneous otoacoustic emissions caused by internal and externally applied noise. *Prog Brain Res* 1993; **97**: 59–65.
43. van Dijk P, Wit HP. Amplitude and frequency variations of spontaneous otoacoustic emissions. *J Acoust Soc Am* 1990; **88**: 1779–93.
44. Penner MJ, Brauth S, Hood L. Temporal cause of the masking of tinnitus as a basis for inferring its origin. *J Speech Hear Res* 1981; **24**: 257–61.
45. Schloth E, Zwicker E. Mechanical and acoustical influence on spontaneous acoustic emissions. *Hear Res* 1983; **11**: 285–93.
46. Penner MJ. Audible and annoying spontaneous otoacoustic emissions. *Arch Otolaryngol Head Neck Surg* 1988; **114**: 150–3.
47. Burns EM, Keefe DH. Intermittent tinnitus resulting from unstable otoacoustic emissions In: Aran JM, Dauman R, eds. *Tinnitus 91. Proceedings of the IV International Tinnitus Seminar, Bordeaux*. Amsterdam: Kugler Publications, 1992: 89–93.
48. Wilson JP, Sutton GJ. Acoustic correlates of tonal tinnitus. In: Evered D, Lawrenson G eds. *Tinnitus (CIBA Foundation Symposium)*. London: Pitman Books Ltd, 1981: 82–107.
49. Probst R, Lonsbury-Martin BL, Martin GK, Coats AC. Otoacoustic emissions in ears with hearing loss. *Am J Otolaryngol* 1987; **8**: 73–80.
50. Bonfils P. Spontaneous otoacoustic emissions: clinical interest. *Laryngoscope* 1989; **99**: 752–6.
51. McFadden D, Mishra. On the relation between hearing sensitivity and otoacoustic emissions. *Hear Res* 1993; **17**: 208–13.
52. Moulin A, Collet L, Veuillet E, Morgon A. Interrelations between transiently evoked otoacoustic emissions, spontaneous otoacoustic

emissions and acoustic distortion products in normally hearing subjects. *Hear Res* 1993; **65**: 216–33.

53. Ruggero M, Rich N, Freyman R. Spontaneous and impulsively evoked otoacoustic emissions: indicators of cochlear pathology? *Hear Res* 1983; **10**: 285–93.
54. Zurek PM, Clark WW. Spontaneous narrowband acoustic signals emitted by chinchilla ears after noise exposure. *J Acoust Soc Am* 1981; **70**: 446–50.
55. Powers NL, Salvi RJ, Wang J, Spongr V, Chun Xiao Qui. Elevation of auditory thresholds by spontaneous cochlear oscillation, *Nature* 1995; **375**: 585–7.
56. Ceranic JB, Prasher DK, Luxon LM. Tinnitus and otoacoustic emissions. *Clin Otolaryngol* 1995; **20**: 192–200.
57. Penner MJ. Empirical tests demonstrating two coexisting sources of tinnitus: a case study. *J Speech Hear Res* 1989; **32**: 458–62.
58. Penner MJ. An estimate of the prevalence of tinnitus caused by spontaneous otoacoustic emission. *Arch Otolaryngol Head Neck Surg* 1990; **116**: 418–23.
59. Plinkert PK, Gitter AH, Zenner HP. Tinnitus associated with spontaneous acoustic emission. *Acta Otolaryngol* 1990; **110**: 342–7.
60. Penner MJ, Coles RR. Indication for aspirin as a palliative for tinnitus caused by spontaneous acoustic emissions: a case study. *Br J Audiol* 1992; **26**: 92–6.
61. Baskill JL, Coles RRA. Current studies on spontaneous emissions and tinnitus. In: Aran JM, Dauman R, eds. *Tinnitus 91. Proceedings of the IV International Tinnitus Seminar*, Bordeaux. Amsterdam: Kugler Publications, 1992: 79–83.
62. Baskill JL, Coles RA. A two year study of SOAEs in tinnitus. In: Reich GE, Vernon JA, eds. *Proceedings of the V International Tinnitus Seminar 1995*, Portland, Oregon. Oregon: American Tinnitus Association, 1996: 31–7.
63. Baskill JL, Coles RA. Pharmacological suppressive treatment for SOAE-tinnitus. In: Reich GE, Vernon JA, eds. *Proceedings of the V International Tinnitus Seminar 1995*, Portland, Oregon. Oregon: American Tinnitus Association, 1996: 195–9.
64. McFadden D, Plattsmier HS. Aspirin abolishes spontaneous acoustic emissions. *J Acoust Soc Am* 1984; **76**: 443–7.
65. Kemp DT. Towards the model for the origin of cochlear echos. *Hear Res* 1980; **2**: 533–48.
66. Bonfils P, Uziel A. Clinical application of evoked otoacoustic emissions: results in normally hearing and hearing-impaired subjects. *Ann Otol Rhinol Laryngol* 1989; **98**: 326–31.
67. Probst R, Harris FP. Transiently evoked and distortion product otoacoustic emissions. *Arch Otolaryngol Head Neck Surg* 1993; **119**: 858–60.
68. Harris FB, Probst R, Wenger R. Repeatability of transiently evoked otoacoustic emissions in normal-hearing humans. *Audiology* 1990; **30**: 135–41.
69. Franklin DJ, McCoy MJ, Martin GK, Lonsbury-Martin BL. Test/retest reliability of distortion-product and transiently evoked otoacoustic emissions. *Ear Hear* 1992; **13**: 417–29.
70. Engdahl B, Arnesen AR, Mair IWS. Reproducibility and short-term variability of transient evoked otoacoustic emissions. *Scand Audiol* 1993; **23**: 99–104.
71. Robinette MB. Clinical observation of transient evoked otoacoustic emissions in adults. *Semin Hear* 1992; **13**: 23–36.
72. Prasher D, Luxon L, Mula M. The role of oto-acoustic emissions in the evaluation of noise-induced hearing loss. In: Grandori F, eds. *Advances in Otoacoustic Emissions: Fundamentals and Clinical Application*, Vol 1. Brussels: Commission of the European Communities, 1994: 74–84.
73. Hotz MA, Probst R, Harris FP, Hauser R. Monitoring of the effect of noise exposure using transiently evoked otoacoustic emissions. *Acta Otolaryngol* 1993; **113**: 478–82.
74. Bohne B, Clark WW. Growth of hearing loss and cochlear lesion with increasing duration of noise exposure. In: Hamernik RP, Henderson D, Salvi R eds. *New Perspectives on Noise-induced Hearing Loss*. New York: Raven Press, 1982: 283–300.
75. Reshef I, Attias J, Furst M. Characteristics of click-evoked otoacoustic emissions in ears with normal hearing and with noise-induced hearing loss. *Br J Audiol* 1993; **27**: 387–95.
76. Hurley RM, Musiek FE. Effectiveness of transient-evoked otoacoustic emissions (TEOAE) in predicting hearing level. *J Am Acad Audiol* 1994; **5**: 195–203.
77. Harris FP, Probst R. Transiently evoked emissions in patients with Menière's disease. *Acta Otolaryngol* 1992; **112**: 36–44.
78. Avan P, Bonfils P. Frequency specificity of human distortion product otoacoustic emissions. *Audiology* 1993; **32**: 12–26.
79. Lonsbury-Martin BL, McCoy MJ, Whitehead ML, Martin GK. Clinical testing of distortion product otoacoustic emissions. *Ear Hear* 1993; **1**: 11–22.
80. Norton SJ, Mott JB, Champlin CA. Behavior of spontaneous otoacoustic emissions following intense acoustic stimulation. *Hear Res* 1989; **38**: 243–58.
81. Penner MJ, Burns E. Five empirical tests for relation between spontaneous acoustic emissions and tinnitus. In: Feldmann H, ed. *Proceedings of the III International Tinnitus Seminar*, Münster. Karlsruhe: Harsh Verlag, 1987: 82–5.
82. Ceranic B, Prasher DK, Luxon LM. Presence of tinnitus indicated by variable spontaneous otoacoustic emissions. *Audiol Neuro-Otol* 1998; **3**: 332–44.
83. Ceranic JB, Prasher DK, Upcott J, Luxon LM. Changes in cochlear mechanics due to impulse noise. In: Schoonhoven R, Kapteyn TS, de Laat JAPM, eds. *Proceedings of the European Conference on Audiology*. Leiden: Nederlandse Vereniging voor Audiologie 1995: 89–95.
84. Ueda H. Do click-evoked otoacoustic emissions have frequency specificity? *J Acoust Soc Am* 1999; **105**: 306–10.
85. Harrison WA, Norton SJ. Characteristics of transient evoked otoacoustic emissions in normal-hearing and hearing-impaired children. *Ear Hear* 1999; **20**: 75–86.
86. Kemp D, Ryan S. The use of transient evoked otoacoustic emissions in neonatal screening programs. *Semin Hear* 1993; **14**: 30–45.
87. White KR, Vohr BR, Maxon AB, Behrens TR, McPherson MG, Mauk GW. Screening all newborns for hearing loss using transient otoacoustic emissions. *Int J Paediatr Otolaryngol* 1994; **29**: 203–17.
88. Culpepper NB. Neonatal screening via evoked otoacoustic emissions. In: Robinette MS, Glattke TJ, eds. *Otoacoustic Emissions: Clinical Applications*. New York: Thieme, 1997; 233–70.

89. Cane MA, O'Donoghue GM, Lutman ME. The feasibility of using otocoustic emissions to monitor cochlear function during acoustic neuroma surgery. *Scand Audiol* 1992; **21**: 173–6.
90. Uziel A, Bonfils P. Assessment of endolymphatic cochlear hydrops by means of evoked acoustic emissions. In: Nadol JB Jr, ed. *Menière's Disease*. Amsterdam: Kugler and Ghedini Publications, 1989: 379–83.
91. Haginomori S, Makimoto K, Araki M, Kawakami M, Takahashi H. Effect of lidocaine injection on EOAE in patients with tinnitus. *Acta Otolayngol* 1995; **115**: 488–92.
92. Norton S. Cochlear function and otoacoustic emissions. *Semin Hear* 1992; **13**: 1–14.
93. Robinette MB. Otoacoustic emissions in cochlear vs. retrocochlear auditory dysfunction. *Hear J* 1992; **45**: 32–4.
94. Stach BA, Westerberg BD, Robertson JB Jr. Auditory disorder in central nervous system miliary tuberculosis. *J Am Acad Audiol* 1998; **9**: 305–10.
95. Mott JB, Norton SJ, Neely ST, Warr WB. Changes in spontaneous otoacoustic emissions produced by acoustic stimulation of the contralateral ear. *Hear Res* 1989: **38**: 229–42.
96. Harrison WA, Burns EM. Effects of contralateral acoustic stimulation on spontaneous otoacoustic emissions. *J Acoust Soc Am* 1993; **94**: 2649–58.
97. Collet L, Kemp DT, Veuillet E, Duclaux R, Moulin A, Morgon A. Effect of contralateral auditory stimuli on active cochlear micromechanical properties in human subjects. *Hear Res* 1990; **43**: 251– 62.
98. Ryan S, Kemp DT, Hinchcliffe R. The influence of contralateral acoustic stimulation on click-evoked otoacoustic emissions in humans. *Br J Audiol* 1991; **25**: 391–7.
99. Moulin A, Collet L, Duclaux R. Contralateral auditory stimulation alters acoustic distortion products in humans. *Hear Res* 1993; **65**: 193–210.
100. Khalfa S, Micheyl C, Veuillet N, Collet L. Peripheral auditory lateralisation assessment using TEOAEs. *Hear Res* 1998; **121**: 29–34.
101. Veuillet E, Duverdy-Bertholon F, Collet L. Effect of contralateral acoustic stimulation on the growth of click-evoked otoacoustic emissions. *Hear Res* 1996; **93**: 128–35.
102. Borg E. Efferent inhibition of afferent acoustic activity in the unanesthetised rabbit. *Exp Neurol* 1971; **31**: 301–12.
103. Collet L, Veuillet E, Bene J, Morgon A. The effects of contralateral white noise on click-evoked emissions in normal and sensorineural ears: towards an exploration of the medial olivocochlear system. *Audiology* 1992; **31**: 1–7.
104. Williams EA, Brookes GB, Prasher DK. Effects of contralateral acoustic stimulation on otoacoustic emissions following vestibular neurectomy. *Scand Audiol* 1993; **22**: 197–203.
105. Collet L. Use of otoacoustic emissions to explore the medial olivocochlear system. *Br J Audiol* 1993; **27**: 155–9.
106. Prasher D, Ryan S, Luxon L. Contralateral suppression of transiently evoked otoacoustic emissions and neuro-otology. *Br J Audiol* 1994; **28**: 247–54.
107. Ceranic B, Prasher DK, Raglan E, Luxon LM. Tinnitus after head injury: Evidence from otoacoustic emissions. *J Neurol Neurosurg Psychiatry* 1998; **65**: 523–9.
108. Veuillet E, Collet L, Disant F, Morgon A. Tinnitus and medial cochlear efferent system. In: Aran JM, Dauman R, eds. *Tinnitus 91. Proceedings of the IV International Tinnitus Seminar*, Bordeaux. Amsterdam: Kugler Publications, 1992: 205–9.
109. Chéry-Croze S, Collet L, Morgon A. Medial olivocochlear system and tinnitus. *Acta Otolaryngol* 1993; **113**: 285–90.
110. Chéry-Croze S, Moulin A, Collet L, Morgon A. Is the test of medial efferent system function a relevant investigation in tinnitus? *Br J Audiol* 1994; **28**: 13–25.
111. Chéry-Croze S, Truy E, Morgon A. Contralateral suppression of of transiently evoked otoacoustic emissions in tinnitus. *Br J Audiol* 1994; **28**: 255–66.
112. Graham RL, Hazell JW. Contralateral suppression of transient evoked otoacoustic emissions: intra-individual variability in tinnitus and normal subjects. *Br J Audiol*, 1994; **29**: 235–45.
113. Attias J, Bresloff I, Furman V. The influence of the efferent auditory system on otoacoustic emissions in noise induced tinnitus: clinical relevance. *Acta Otolaryngol* 1996; **116**: 534–9.
114. Zhao F, Meredith R, Özçaglar H, Stephens SDG. Transient evoked otoacoustic emissions with contralateral stimulation in King-Kopetzky syndrome. *J Audiol Med* 1996; **6**: 36–44.
115. Duchamp C, Morgon A, Chéry-Croze S. Tinnitus sufferers without hearing loss. In: Reich GE, Vernon JA, eds. *Proceedings of the V International Tinnitus Seminar 1995*, Portland, Oregon. Oregon: American Tinnitus Association, 1996: 266–9.

16 Human auditory electrophysiology

Hillel Pratt

Introduction

Brief historical review

Recording the electrical responses of the auditory system of humans has followed the development of physiological recordings from animals and the development of technology for non-invasive signal acquisition. Five years after the cochlear microphonic potentials from animals were first reported,[1] they were recorded from the round window of humans through a perforation in the tympanic membrane.[2] Ten years after the human electroencephalogram (EEG) was first reported,[3] changes in the EEG that were evoked by auditory stimulation were described.[4,5] Auditory evoked potentials from animal cortex were reported 3 years later,[6] and after the first description of signal averaging for recording evoked potentials[7] and its implementation in the average-response computer,[8] middle-latency cortical responses were recorded from the scalp of humans in response to clicks.[9] Longer-latency 'vertex potentials' were described soon after,[10] as was the P_{300} evoked potential associated with cognitive processing of auditory stimuli.[11,12] The electrical response of the cochlea, the electrocochleogram, recorded from the round window was developed for clinical use around that time, and the response components were identified as containing cochlear microphonics[13] and the cochlear nerve compound action potential.[14] Evaluation of inner ear function when the tympanic membrane was not perforated was performed using transtympanic needle-electrode recording from the promontory.[15,16] Moving even farther from the cochlea, and using signal averaging over a large number of repetitions, the feline cochlear action potential was recorded from the auricle, and was found to be followed by additional components which were attributed to brainstem activity.[17] Three years later, the human cochlear nerve and brainstem evoked potentials were first described as such,[18] and their audiological[19] and neurological[20,21] applications came soon after. In the quarter century that followed, auditory brainstem evoked potentials reigned supreme in the field of auditory neurophysiology, and a variety of uses for diagnostics, monitoring and basic research have been described in thousands of publications.

Outline of relevant factors

Human auditory electrophysiology includes non-invasive recording of cochlear potentials and of neural activity along the auditory pathway. Such recordings belong to a class of electrophysiology called 'evoked potentials', or 'event-related potentials', defined as changes in voltage ('potentials') that occur at a particular time before, during or after ('related') a change in the physical world and/or some psychological process ('event') that gave rise to ('evoked') these voltage changes.[22] Evoked potentials are classified according to the event that evoked them: when evoked by a stimulus in the physical world outside the brain, they are called 'exogenous', and when evoked by a psychological process within the brain, they are termed 'endogenous'. Typically, exogenous evoked potentials are determined by the physical properties of the evoking stimulus, while endogenous evoked potentials reflect the psychological significance of the stimulus. Because of the nature of information processing in sensory systems, exogenous components of evoked potentials tend to be earlier (usually < 100 ms) than endogenous components (typically > 100 ms).

Classification of auditory evoked potentials is based on their latencies and on their generators. The major classes of auditory evoked potentials are thus the short-latency cochlear and brainstem potentials, the middle-latency thalamocortical potentials, the long-latency cortical potentials, and the late cognitive potentials. In addition to stimulus parameters (in exogenous potentials), and stimulus context (in endogenous potentials), the potentials are affected by subject and acquisition factors.

Stimulus factors affecting exogenous auditory evoked potentials include stimulus type (click, tone burst, speech), frequency, duration, intensity, presentation rate, acoustical polarity (condensation, rarefaction), type of transducer and mode of presentation (speakers in free field, earphones, monaural, binaural). Endogenous evoked potentials are affected by the stimulus context. Such factors as attending to the stimulus, task-relevance of the stimulus, or semantic congruity in case of a verbal stimulus, could affect the potentials recorded.

Acquisition factors that may affect the potentials include type and placement of the electrodes used for recording, the amplification and filtering performed on the potentials, the time window about the stimulus (analysis time) dedicated to the recording, and the type and degree of processing used to enhance the electrical signal above background electrical noise.

Non-pathological and pathological subject factors

The clinical utility of electrophysiological responses depends on the abilities to detect changes in the responses and to determine whether these changes exceed the normative range and cannot be attributed to non-pathological factors affecting the subject's responses. Non-pathological factors include the subject's age, body temperature and state of arousal, the effects of drugs, muscle tension and, to a lesser degree, gender. Pathological factors affecting auditory evoked potentials include conductive hearing loss, cochlear hearing loss, cochlear nerve pathology, auditory brainstem dysfunction, cortical dysfunction and cognitive impairments.

Determination of a pathological change, therefore, depends on good control and documentation of non-pathological subject factors, and well-defined limits of the normal variability of evoked potentials measures. The variety of factors that may affect electrophysiological responses necessitates incorporating into their evaluation as much information as possible on the subject's state, to rule out non-pathological factors.

Correlation with other audiological tests

When properly acquired and analysed, auditory evoked potentials are a sensitive tool to assess the functional integrity of their generators. These generators are each involved in a particular stage of transduction, transmission and processing that together contribute to the process of hearing. Auditory evoked potentials are therefore sensitive indices of the functions of specific stages that comprise hearing, but they do not reflect hearing. Evoked potentials reflect the auditory sensitivity and neurophysiological integrity of neuronal assemblies, whereas hearing involves the conscious appreciation and discrimination of the auditory stimulus at the end of its processing.

It is therefore not surprising that electrophysiological tests vary in their correlations with other audiological tests. Such correlations depend on the aspect of hearing evaluated by the audiological test, and on the involvement of the evoked potentials' generators in that aspect of hearing. The main contributions of evoked potentials to patient evaluation stem from their direct measurement of neural function, independent of subject report or cooperation, and their sensitivity to the functional integrity of specific generators along the auditory pathway. They thus provide an objective tool for assessing auditory sensitivity at specific levels of the pathway, and allow localization of functional lesions.

Research underpinning subject

The advent of human auditory neurophysiology has followed the development of auditory neurophysiology in animal models and the technological advances that allowed its non-invasive implementation in humans. This pattern of development is still under way, with the major developments in the field drawing from basic auditory research and then being implemented in the clinical setting using new techniques for signal acquisition and processing.

The primary challenge in human auditory electrophysiology is estimation of auditory function, objectively and non-invasively, and the definition of site of lesion. The research and development directions have thus included: the development of stimulus types and recording procedures that are frequency specific, allowing estimation of the audiogram; signal-processing procedures that improve estimation of the intracranial sources of the surface-recorded potentials; signal-processing techniques that estimate the likelihood of a signal in a noisy recording; and stimulus and recording techniques that allow the recording of potentials at very high stimulus rates to save recording time.

Technique and procedures

The recording from the scalp of intracranial electrical activity generated by the nervous system amounts to recording potentials in a volume conductor. Volume conductor theory[23,24] predicts that charged membranes, such as those of living cells, generate potentials which are recordable at any point within, or on the surface of, the conducting medium. In addition to the electrical properties of the medium between the electrode and the generator membrane, the magnitude of the potential is determined by the membrane potential and the solid angle which the membrane occupies about the recording electrode. This solid angle is, in turn, larger near the membrane and is decreased by the squared distance of the recording electrode from the membrane and the cosine of the angle by which the membrane tilts relative to the recording electrode (Figure 16.1). In general, an electrode in a volume conductor records a potential that is determined by the potential difference across the membrane at the source, by the size of the membrane, by its distance and by its orientation relative to the electrode.

When bio-electrical events are recorded, the potential recorded can be predicted from the summed contributions of all generator membranes in the volume conductor. It can be shown that only charged membranes associated with active cells (i.e. cells undergoing a change in membrane potential) but not uniformly charged cells (at rest, or depolarized over the entire membrane) contribute to the potential recorded in a volume

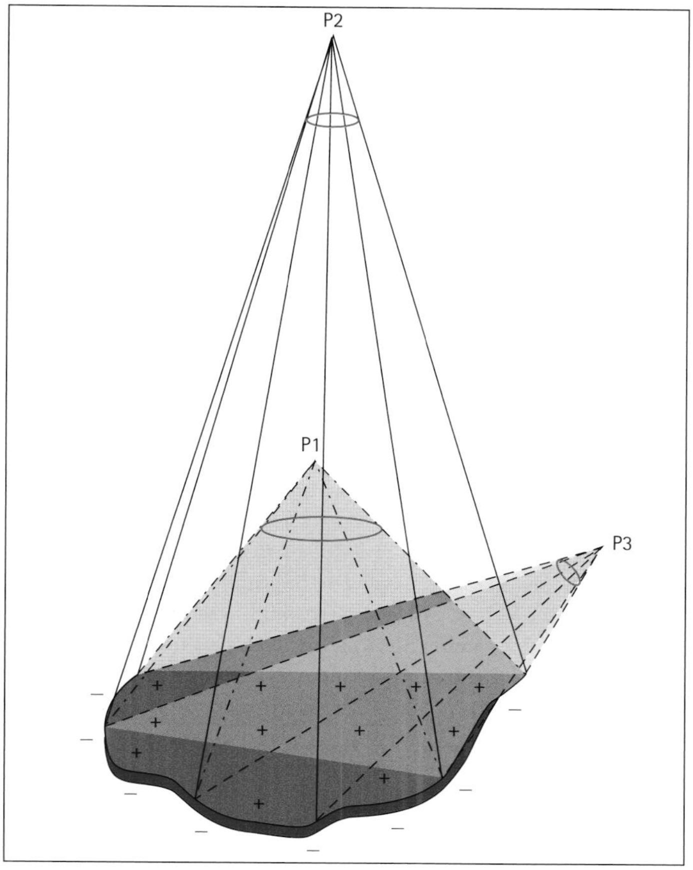

Figure 16.1 Solid angles that a charged membrane occupies from three positions in a volume conductor. From position P1, which is close and vertically above the membrane, the solid angle is larger than from P3, which is close but diagonally positioned to the membrane, and from P2, which is farther away.

conductor. The recording electrode is not selective with regard to the sources of the potentials, and all potentials summate at the electrode and contribute to the potential that is recorded. Consequently, an electrode on the scalp records any electrical activity occurring within the volume conductor—auditory or other. Thus, in auditory electrophysiology, in addition to the specific potential of interest which is generated in the auditory system ('signal'), other types of activity which are not of interest ('noise') summate at the electrode. Noise includes activity from the auditory system that is not the subject of study, activity from other sensory systems, ongoing background EEG, electrical activity from the heart (ECG), electrical activity from skeletal muscles (EMG), potential changes due to eye movements (EOG), and slow potentials associated with conductivity changes of the skin (GSR). In addition to these noises of biological origin within the body, there are external sources of electrical noise, such as the alternating current of the electrical supply lines (50/60 Hz), electromagnetic radiation from the stimulus transducer (stimulus artefact), radio signals, instrumentation noise and discharge of static electricity. The challenge of auditory electrophysiology is to increase the signal and decrease the noise, i.e. to improve signal-to-noise ratio (SNR).

Improving SNR includes signal enhancement as well as noise reduction. Increasing the signal is achieved by placing the electrodes at optimal positions for recording the activity of interest, and by using a stimulus that activates a large number of neural elements synchronously. Noise reduction is obtained by minimizing irrelevant sensory stimuli, by isolating the subject in a quiet and dimly illuminated examination area. Keeping the subject relaxed and comfortable minimizes myogenic noise and eye-movement artefacts. Electrically shielding the transducers and recording system minimizes stimulus artefact and electrical pickup from external instrumentation, radio and power supply sources of noise.

The interface of the recording system with the subject comprises the electrodes and their attachment to the skin (Figure 16.2). Proper attachment of electrodes to the subject is therefore crucial. The quality of attachment is assessed by the impedance of the contact of the electrode, usually measured between pairs of electrodes on the subject. Typical electrode impedance when contact is good is in the range 2–5 kΩ. Because input impedance of the differential amplifier is in the megaOhm range, electrode impedance has little effect on the input to the amplifier. However, electrode impedance determines the voltage recorded as a result of the local currents induced in the electrode by both bio-electrical events in the volume conductor and external electrical artefacts. According to Ohm's law, therefore, higher impedance at the electrode will lead to increased noise voltages resulting from a given induced current.

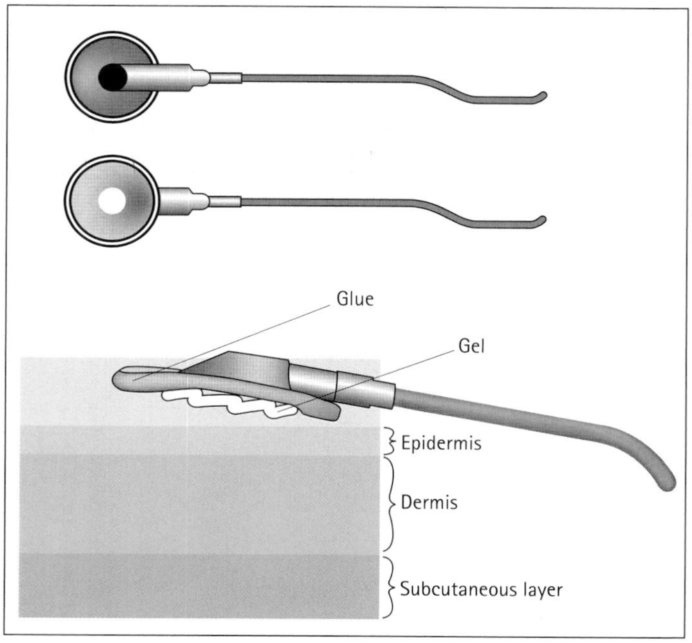

Figure 16.2 Typical surface electrodes for evoked potential recording (top) and their attachment to the skin (bottom). The electrodes comprise a concave metal disk (typically 9 mm in diameter) with a hole in its centre to allow access to the skin after the electrode is attached by glue or tape to the skin. The electrode is filled with conducting gel or paste that improves contact with the surface of the skin.

In addition, if the impedance of the electrodes is not the same across recording sites, the noise levels picked up by different electrodes will not be the same, reducing the benefit of differential amplification (see below). It is thus important to secure low and similar impedances across all electrodes.

The initial stage of the recording system is a differential amplifier, which amplifies and filters the potential difference between pairs of recording electrodes. The amplification is in the order of a few hundred thousand, and serves to bring the potentials from the electrodes to a magnitude of a few volts, which can then be further processed by the recording system. The potential difference between the non-inverting (positive) and the inverting (negative) electrodes is amplified within a prescribed bandpass. In addition, a third input to the amplifier, from the ground electrode on the subject, serves as the common reference which otherwise does not contribute to the output. Electrical activity that is recorded similarly by the inverting and non-inverting electrodes will be diminished by the subtraction of the differential. Thus, differential recording rejects activity that is common to both inputs (common mode rejection), and augments activity that is of opposite phase at the inverting and non-inverting amplifier inputs (Figure 16.3). If the recording electrodes are placed so that the signal of interest is recorded with opposite polarity at the two differential inputs, the signal will be enhanced by the subtraction of inputs. At the same time, noise common to both inputs will be diminished, and SNR will thus be markedly improved. If the impedances of the inverting and non-inverting electrodes are not the same, the noise levels picked up by them will be different, and their difference will not be zero, reducing the benefits from differential amplification. It is thus important to keep electrode impedance low and similar across inputs.

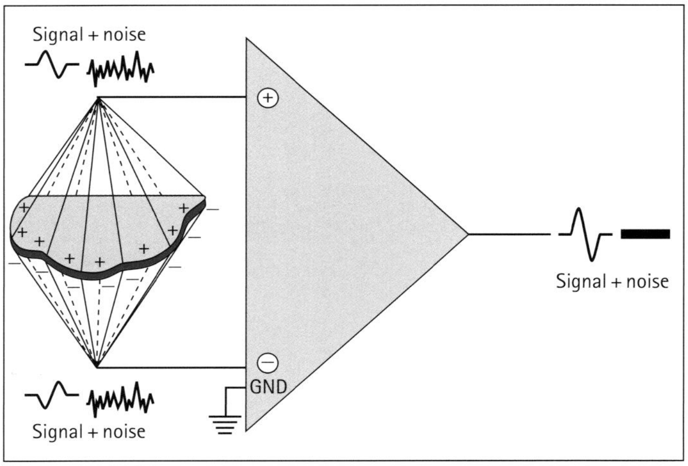

Figure 16.3 Differential recording of a noise-contaminated signal from an active membrane. By placing the recording electrodes so that the signal of interest is recorded with opposite polarity at the two differential inputs, the signal will be enhanced by the subtraction of inputs. At the same time, noise common to both inputs will be diminished, and SNR will thus be markedly improved.

Because the output of the differential amplifier reflects the difference between two inputs, the waveform obtained should be treated with caution: if the two inputs were not in phase, the output waveform may be distorted. In addition, the output reflects the difference between inputs, and the specific contribution of each input cannot be determined from this difference: a positive peak in the output of a differential amplifier can reflect a positive peak in the non-inverting input, a negative peak in the inverting input, a larger positive peak in the non-inverting than in the inverting input, or any combination that will yield positivity in the difference waveform (Figure 16.4).

Filtering the signals through the amplifier can also improve SNR by allowing frequencies (bandpass) that make up the signal and rejecting frequencies that contribute to the noise, above (low-pass) and below (high-pass) that band (Figure 16.5). For example, when recording compound action potentials ascending the auditory pathway, their waveform power spectrum includes a major frequency band around a few hundred to a thousand hertz, while the ongoing EEG has most of its energy below 30 Hz. Allowing through only activity above (high-pass) 30 Hz will diminish the EEG noise, and thus improve SNR. On the high-frequency end, limiting frequencies

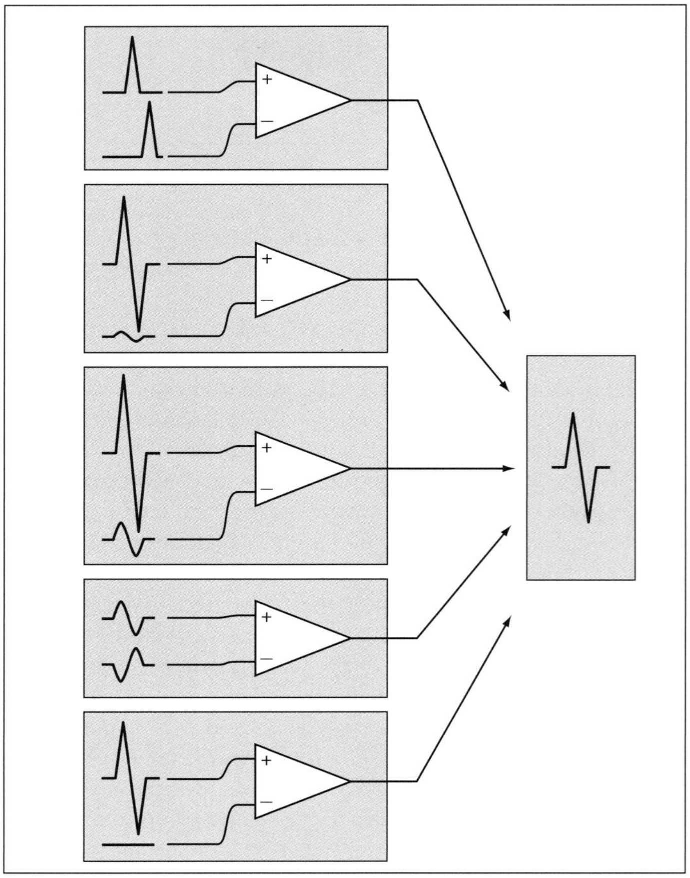

Figure 16.4 Ambiguity of determining the inputs that contributed to a given differential recording waveform. All input waveform pairs to the differential amplifiers on the left result in the same output waveform depicted on the right.

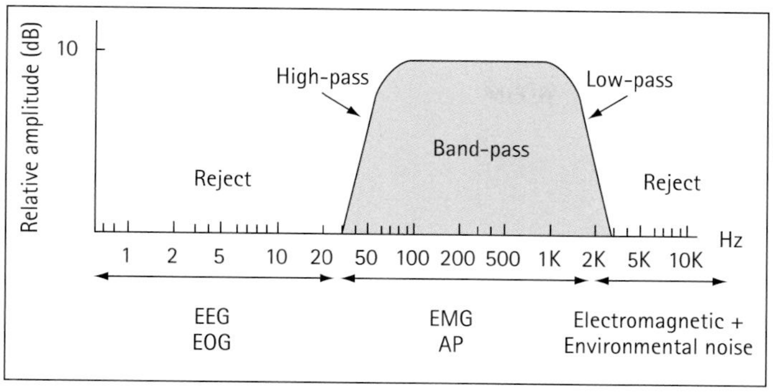

Figure 16.5 Filtering signals by allowing frequencies (bandpass) that make up the signal and rejecting frequencies which contribute to the noise, above (low-pass) and below (high-pass) the bandpass. In this example of recording compound action potentials, their waveform power spectrum includes a major frequency band around a few hundred to a thousand Hertz, while the ongoing EEG has most of its energy below 20 Hz. Allowing through only activity above (high-pass) 30 Hz and below (low-pass) 3000 Hz creates a bandpass of 30–3000 Hz, which will augment the contribution of compound action potentials relative to EEG and environmental noise.

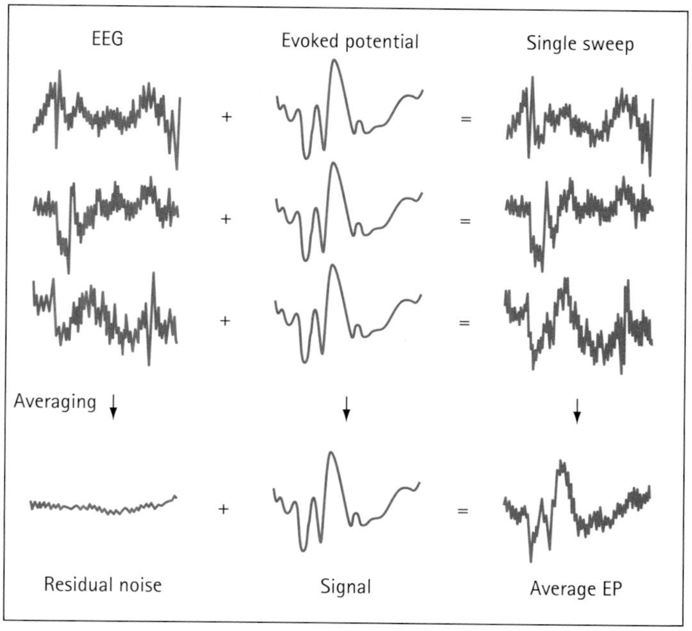

Figure 16.6 Diminishing random noise and enhancing SNR by averaging. Random EEG diminishes with averaging, while a constant signal, such as an evoked potential, persists. In practice, single sweeps of electrical activity following a stimulus (right column) consist of the evoked potential (centre column), which is the same following all stimulus repetitions, and EEG noise (left column), which is random. The averaged waveform (bottom row, right) consists of the evoked potentials and some residual noise.

beyond the upper limit of biological signals will reduce electromagnetic environmental noise. Thus a bandpass of 30–3000 Hz will augment the contribution of compound action potentials relative to EEG and environmental noise.

Differential amplification and filtering improve SNR but not sufficiently for identification of the small electrophysiological signal embedded in the background noise associated with surface electrodes. The procedure most commonly used in evoked potentials to separate small signals from the noise in which they are embedded is averaging. Improvement of SNR by averaging is based on the assumption that the signal is time-locked to the stimulus, i.e. always occurs with the same delay after the stimulus, in contrast to noise that is random. Thus, whenever a stimulus is presented, at a given point in time following the stimulus, the signal will always contribute the same potential to the recording, whereas noise will randomly vary in its contribution. Because the average of random noise is zero, and the average of a repetitive constant is the constant, averaging many repetitions of mixed random noise and a constant signal will not affect the signal but will diminish the noise, improving SNR (Figure 16.6). In practice, signal averaging is conducted digitally by first converting the analog output of the differential amplifier to discrete digital representation (analog-to-digital (A/D), conversion) at each point in time following the presentation of the stimulus (Figure 16.7). Thus, the continuous voltage change from the electrodes is converted to a series ('sweep') of numbers, each of which is stored in the computer's memory ('address'). The numbers comprising a sweep are proportional to the magnitude and polarity of the potential at each point in time during the sweep. This A/D conversion is repeated with repeated stimulation, and corresponding points in time across stimulus presentations are averaged, resulting in an averaged sweep. With a truly random noise, the residual noise in the averaged sweep decreases with the square root of the number of sweeps included in the average. The practical implication of this relationship is that in order to improve SNR by a factor of 2, the number of sweeps that must be averaged has to increase four-fold.

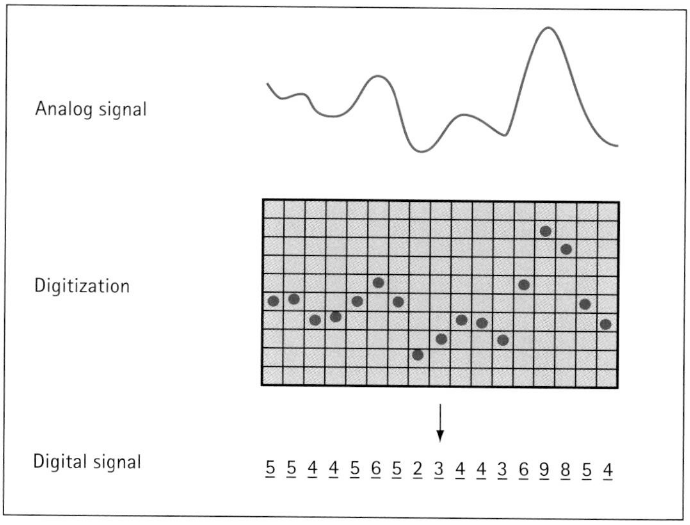

Figure 16.7 Analog-to-digital (A/D) conversion (digitization) of a signal. The continuous analog signal (top) is converted (middle) to a series of discrete numbers (bottom) representing the voltage at discrete points in time.

The rate at which the analog output of the differential amplifier is converted to discrete digital representations ('sampling rate') will determine the temporal resolution of the process. In order to detect a given frequency in the signal, the sampling rate must be at least twice that frequency (Nyquist frequency), but preferably four times the signal frequency (Figure 16.8). In order to detect low frequencies in the waveform, the sweep duration must include at least a quarter of the period of the detected frequency. In order to detect a very small signal in large noise, the digital representation of the noise with the signal should be different from noise alone (Figure 16.9). In other words, the amplitude resolution of the A/D converter should be fine enough to distinguish the small signal. A/D amplitude resolution is characterized by the power of 2 (bits) that describes the number of intermediate values that its full range includes. Thus, for example, a 12-bit A/D converter can divide its full range of input voltage (typically ± 5 V, i.e. 10 V) into 4096 (2^{12}) intermediate values, i.e. a resolution of about 2.5 mV.

Sporadic, very high amplitude noise may not be sufficiently diminished by averaging and may thus remain as residual noise in the averaged waveform. To avoid such residual noise, averaging often includes scanning the sweeps before they are included in the average, and rejection of sweeps with high-amplitude noise. This procedure ('artefact rejection') improves the SNR enhancement of averaging. Because SNR enhancement with averaging assumes that the latency of the signal is constant across sweeps, any deviation from this assumption will result in signal distortion. Thus, if during the averaging process the timing of the signal is not constant, but drifts in time or jitters, amplitude, waveform and even latency of the signal may be distorted. Factors that might affect the latency of the potential of interest must therefore be as constant as possible during signal acquisition. Conversely, electrical signals that are artefactual, but constant in their timing across sweeps, such as stimulus artefacts, will be enhanced by averaging, sometimes obscuring the physiological response of interest. Such artefacts must be treated by shielding against them and alternating their polarity, when appropriate, so that their average is zero.

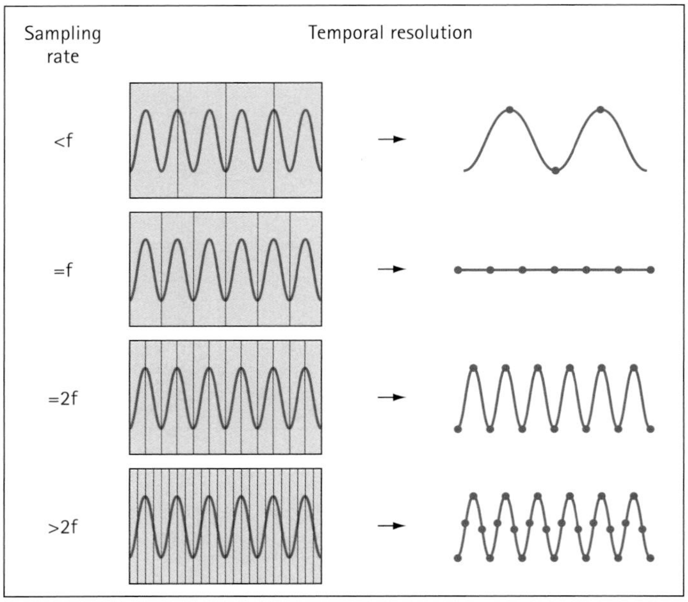

Figure 16.8 The effect of sampling rate (temporal resolution) on the reconstructed digital waveform. Sampling rates lower than twice the signal frequency (top two rows) result in waveform distortions (aliasing). Aliasing may manifest in frequencies that were not part of the signal (top row) or non-detected frequencies (second row from top). The minimum sampling rate for detecting a signal is twice the signal frequency (third row), but for more accurate waveform reconstruction, higher sampling rates should be used (bottom row).

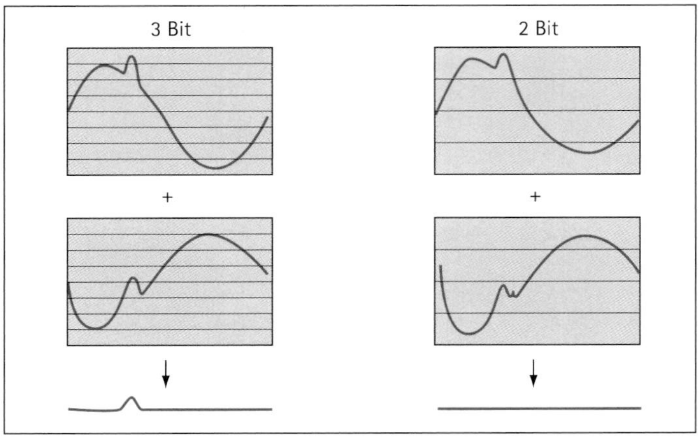

Figure 16.9 The effect of amplitude resolution of the A/D conversion on the detection of small signals embedded in large noise. With a low amplitude resolution (right column), the small signal does not contribute to the digitized sweep, and therefore goes undetected after averaging. When amplitude resolution is such that the digital representation of the single sweep is affected by the presence of the small signal (left column), the signal is detected after averaging.

The final product of the recording system is a series of averaged numbers representing the average voltage at specific stimulus-related points in time. These numbers represent the averaged waveform of voltage fluctuations as a function of time. The waveform can be displayed, plotted, and stored digitally for further processing (Figure 16.10) to extract quantitative measures of the electrical activity evoked by the stimulus.

Waveform analysis typically includes amplitudes and latencies of specific peaks, or differences between peaks (Figure 16.11) and troughs in the waveform, or more advanced signal-processing procedures that quantify specific attributes of the response.

Description

General description of auditory evoked potentials

Auditory evoked potentials span activity from the full length of the auditory pathway, from cochlear hair cells to cerebral cortex, as well as activity associated with cognitive processing of

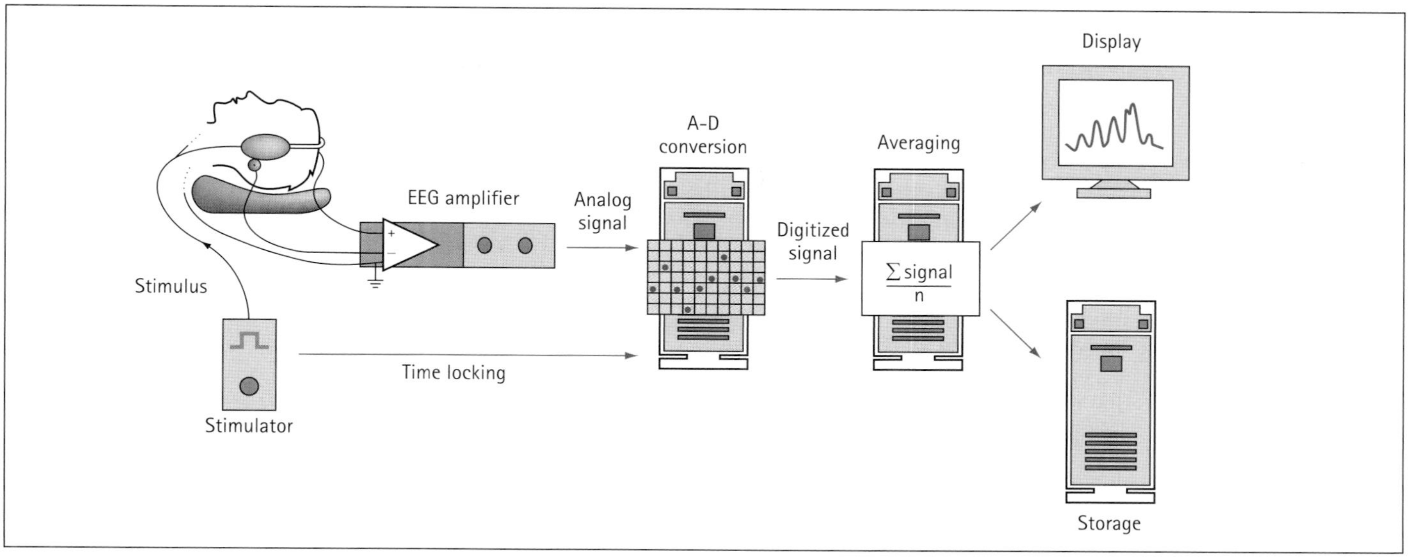

Figure 16.10 Data flow through a typical evoked potential recording setup, from subject to stored waveform. A stimulus-related time-locking pulse triggers the sampling and averaging of the signal from the subject, and the averaged waveform is displayed as a voltage–time plot and stored digitally for further analysis.

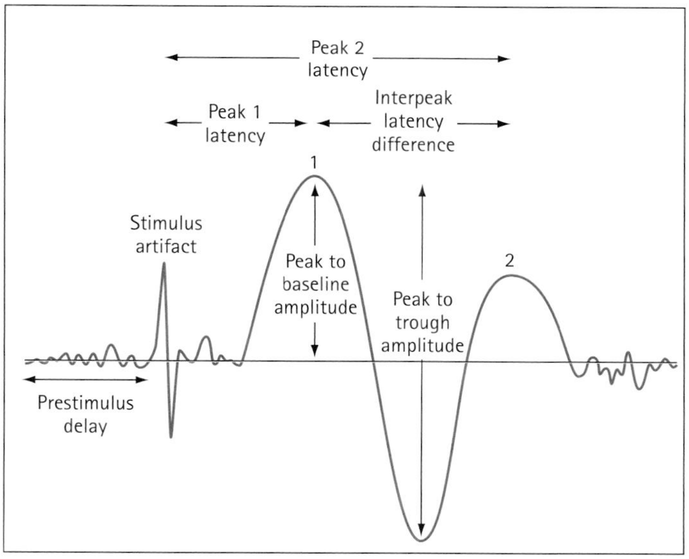

Figure 16.11 Commonly derived amplitude and latency measures, as measured from a schematic waveform with two peaks. Latency measures include latencies of each peak, measured from stimulus onset, as well as the interpeak latency difference. Amplitude measures include the voltage difference between the peak and baseline (defined as the average voltage in the pre-stimulus period) and between the peak and the following trough.

auditory stimuli. The methods described above separate auditory potentials that are time-locked to the stimulus from background noise. However, the recording electrodes are non-selective in terms of the potentials they record, and any stimulus-related activity along the auditory pathway will summate and contribute to the potential at a given electrode. In order to record selectively from a given level along the auditory pathway, specific attributes of the activity at that level must be utilized. The timing and waveform of activity vary between different levels of the auditory system, and the orientations and positions of the generators vary along the pathway. Therefore, electrode locations, filter settings and analysis times can be set to selectively record activity from a specific generator along the auditory pathway. The following section is an overview of the evoked potentials generated along the auditory pathway and recorded from the surface, highlighting the parameters that determine their selective recording.

Cochlear potentials

Cochlear potentials from humans can be recorded with the largest amplitudes, using an electrode that is inserted as close as possible to the inner ear. In this procedure, 'electrocochleography', if the tympanic membrane is intact, a needle electrode is inserted through the tympanic membrane, and placed on the promontory in the middle ear. In the case of a perforation, a ball electrode can be used, and the electrode is then placed on to the round window. This procedure should be performed under microscope, and local anaesthetic may be applied to the tympanic membrane to ensure patient comfort. In the case of children, or difficult-to-test adults, the procedure is performed under general anaesthesia. Transtympanic electrocochleography should be performed with all the precautions of a surgical procedure.

As this technique represents a near-field recording, transtympanically recorded cochlear potentials are 20 times larger in amplitude than those recorded non-invasively from an electrode in the ear canal, and 10 times greater than those recorded from the tympanic membrane. Cochlear potentials that can be recorded non-invasively from humans include the cochlear microphonic potentials, the summating potential, and the compound action potential of the cochlear nerve. These potentials are most readily recorded in the electrocochleogram (ECOG), which can be recorded from the ear canal using an electrode resting on the tympanic membrane.[25] The electrode (Figure 16.12, bottom) is constructed from 5-cm-long medical-grade silicon tubing (approximately 2 mm outer diameter and 1.5 mm inner diameter) into which a Teflon-insulated silver or copper wire (0.2 mm diameter) is inserted with foam rubber 2 × 2 × 5 mm tied to one of its bared ends, protruding by about 1 mm from the end of the tubing. The foam rubber is saturated with conducting gel for improved contact with the tympanic membrane. The other bared end of the insulated wire, protruding from the other end of the tubing, is connected to the amplifier input. Before the tympanic membrane electrode is placed, the integrity of the tympanic membrane must be verified otoscopically and the ear canal thoroughly cleansed of deposits to ensure good electrical contact of the electrode. Once in place, the electrode is stabilized by placing a compressed-foam earplug through which a sound delivery tube enables stimulus presentation. When the foam earplug expands, it secures the electrode and sound delivery tube in the ear canal (Figure 16.12, top).

When the tympanic membrane electrode is non-inverting, and an inverting silver disk electrode is placed on the contralateral mastoid or earlobe, the cochlear compound action potential in response to alternating-polarity, high-intensity clicks is recorded as a major negative peak of a few microvolts, called N_1 or AP for action potential, at approximately 1.5 ms after stimulus onset at the eardrum, followed by a minor negativity called N_2, at about 2.5 ms (Figure 16.13). The summating potential (SP), preceding N_1 as a negative step-like deflection from baseline, is recordable with alternating-polarity stimuli, but when all stimuli are of the same polarity, it is obscured by

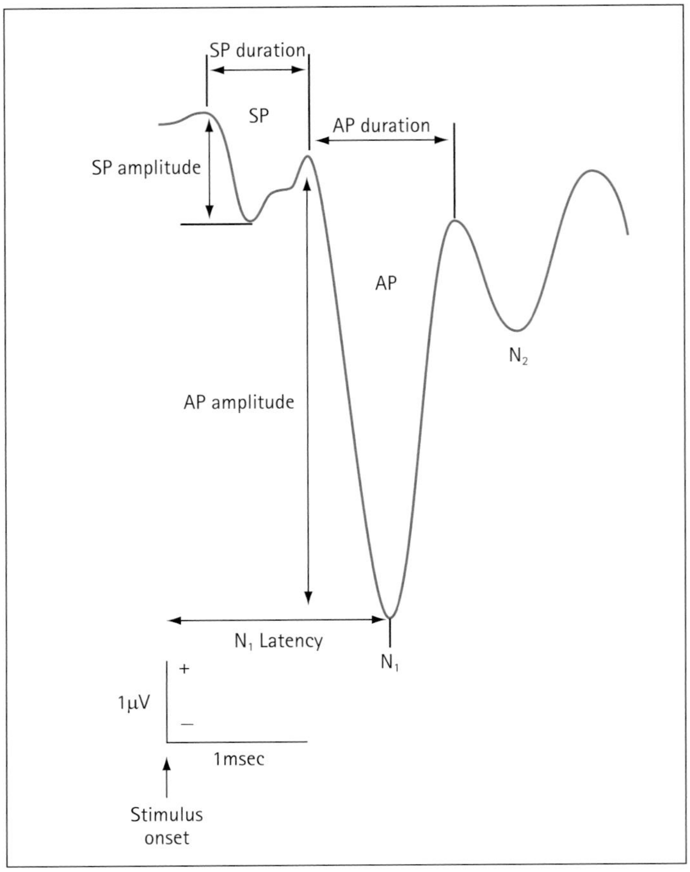

Figure 16.13 Major components and the measures derived from an electrocochleogram in response to alternating-polarity clicks. The step-like negative deflection from baseline at the beginning of the record is the summating potential (SP), which is followed by the cochlear compound action potential (AP), recorded as a major negative peak, also known as N_1. N_1 is followed by a minor negativity called N_2.

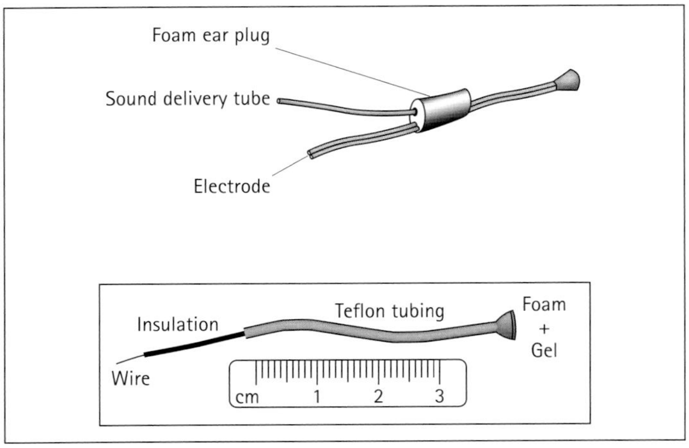

Figure 16.12 Tympanic membrane recording electrode for electrocochleography. Its components are included in the inset at the bottom, and a schematic drawing of the electrode in place is shown on top. Once in place, the electrode is stabilized by placing a compressed-foam earplug through which a sound delivery tube enables stimulus presentation. When the foam earplug expands, it secures the electrode and sound delivery tube in the ear canal with the electrode tip leaning against the tympanic membrane.

the cochlear microphonics (CM). The electrocochleogram is affected by auditory sensitivity in the range 1000–4000 Hz and is independent of the subject's state of arousal or the effects of drugs.

In routine clinical application, a typical recording bandpass is 3–3000 Hz, stimulus rate is around 10/s, and the number of responses averaged for each trace is between 1000 and 2000. To avoid waveform distortions and to enhance latency resolution, sampling rate should not be lower than 20 kHz (50 μs/address or less). Important measures derived from the waveform (Figure 16.13) include N_1 latency (from stimulus onset) and amplitude (between the transition from SP to N_1 and the negative peak of N_1), as well as SP duration (between its onset and transition to N_1) and amplitude (between SP onset and its most negative point).

Cochlear potentials can also be recorded from the ear canal, using a ball-tipped wire secured against the canal wall, or from the mastoid or earlobe, using a standard surface disk electrode, referenced to a disk electrode on the contralateral earlobe or mastoid. The amplitude of cochlear potentials decreases when recorded farther from the cochlea, due to distance, but also due to the more pronounced attenuation by the intervening tissues of high than of low frequencies. Consequently, it is recommended that for surface recording of CM, a 1000-Hz tone burst be used rather than the higher-frequency click. The longer duration of such a burst necessitates a larger temporal separation between stimulus artefact and CM, which is typically achieved using a 66-cm sound delivery tube (2-ms acoustical delay) and a tone burst of one period (1-ms duration). The diameter of the sound delivery tube should be large (1–2 cm) to avoid acoustical distortion of the lower-frequency tone burst. Therefore, for mastoid or earlobe recording of CM with surface electrodes, the sound delivery system includes a headset coupled to the transducer with a relatively long sound delivery tube (Figure 16.14). When only CM are recorded, stimulus rate can be increased to 90/s without any effect on CM, which, having no refractory period, are thus enhanced relative to the neural potentials, which are diminished at high stimulus rates.

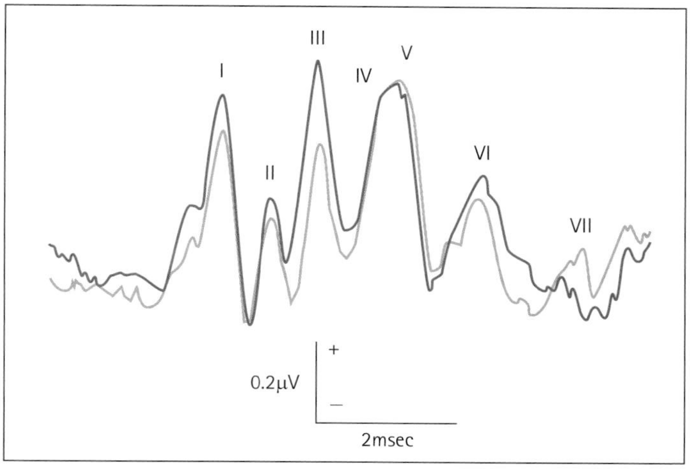

Figure 16.15 Auditory brainstem responses (ABR) to alternating-polarity clicks, differentially recorded between vertex and the mastoid ipsilateral to the stimulated ear. Two replications of the recording from the same subject are superimposed to assess reproducibility.

Auditory brainstem responses

Auditory brainstem evoked responses (ABRs) are optimally recorded from the scalp by disk or cup electrodes in response to high-intensity clicks presented at a rate of about 10/s. Potential differences between an electrode on the top of the head (C_z or F_z according to the 10–20 system[26]) and in the vicinity of the stimulated ear (mastoid or earlobe) are amplified in a bandpass of about 30–3000 Hz, and averaged across a few thousand sweeps of 10–15 ms. To avoid waveform distortions and to enhance latency resolution, sampling rate should not be lower than 20 kHz (50 μs/address, or less). Under such stimulus and recording conditions, the normal waveform includes a series of 5–7 voltage oscillations, approximately 1 ms apart, during the first 6–10 ms after stimulus onset (Figure 16.15). Amplitudes of the components are in the order of tenths of a microvolt, and, like the electrocochleogram, components are affected by auditory sensitivity in the range 1000–4000 Hz and are independent of the subject's state of arousal or the effects of drugs. Components are labelled by Roman numerals, beginning with the vertex positive peak at approximately 1.5 ms after stimulus onset, which is followed by a prominent negative trough. Peak I and its associated trough (I′) are followed by four fast oscillations, II, III, IV and V, about 1 ms apart, which appear to be superimposed on a slow rising positivity (the 'pedestal'), with peak V typically identified as the most positive in the complex. The components following V exhibit such large inter-subject variability, as well as large within-subject session-to-session variability, that they are not used in clinical diagnosis.

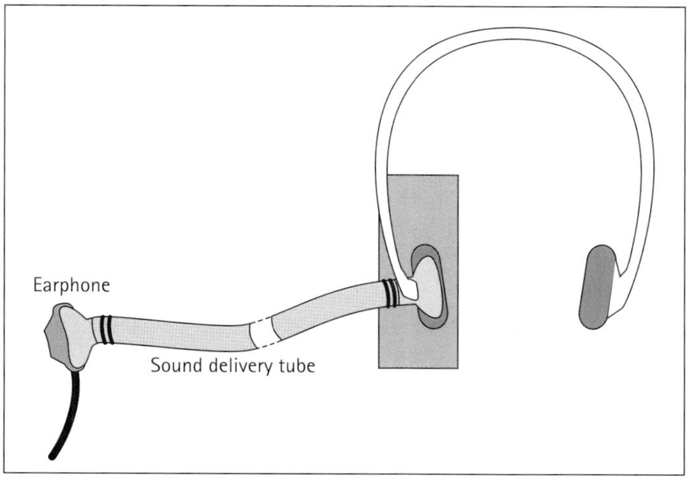

Figure 16.14 Sound delivery system for mastoid or earlobe recording of CM by surface electrodes. The system includes a headset coupled to the transducer with a relatively long sound delivery tube that delays the arrival of sound at the ear, temporally separating it from stimulus artefact.

The generators of ABRs have been the subject of much research and controversy and are still not entirely agreed upon. However, for clinical purposes, the following relationships between ABR peaks and neuroanatomy suffice. The first peak in the sequence, peak I, is the only one on which there is general agreement regarding its generator. This peak is the only one to survive section of the cochlear nerve central to the internal auditory canal, placing its generator in the cochlea. It is synchronous with N_1 of the electrocochleogram, is affected by masking, reverses polarity around the mastoid, and does not change polarity with stimulus polarity, indicating its neural origin within the cochlea.

The generators of the second peak, II, are among the most controversial. Correlations with intracranial recordings in humans, intraoperatively,[27,28] and from experimental animals[29] indicate that it is synchronous with proximal cochlear nerve activity. However, it does not reverse polarity around the mastoid and it is not entirely obliterated with cochlear nerve section. Some attribute it to overlapping activity from the cochlear nerve and from the cochlear nucleus.[30] Others suggest that it is generated by the electrical field distortions due to the changing geometry and conductance of the volume conductor, as the nerve passes through the internal auditory canal and through the posterior fossa prior to its merging into the brainstem.[31] Regardless of the fine details, there is general agreement that peak II is generated in the vicinity of the cochlear nerve's entry into the brainstem.

Peak III is generally agreed to be generated in the brainstem, but there is disagreement on the exact generator set, because intracranial recordings from humans and correlations with animal experiments have not been conclusive. Suggested generators span the lower brainstem between the cochlear nucleus, through the trapezoid body to the superior olivary complex. Because the anatomical distance between these structures is small, for practical clinical purposes the generators may be attributed to the lower pons.

The fourth component is not always identified in human subjects, and it is generally absent in animals. When identified, peak IV is usually partially merged with V, creating a bifid IV–V complex. It is generally agreed that the fourth peak of animals corresponds to the human V. The exact generators of this complex are still under debate, but all evidence points to the upper pons, between the superior olivary complex, through the lateral lemniscus, with a possible contribution from the inferior colliculus. For clinical purposes, the IV–V complex can be attributed to the upper pons and its junction with the midbrain.

ABR measures include measuring the lowest stimulus intensity at which a response is detected (detection threshold). Neuro-otological measures of ABRs include peak latencies and amplitudes, as well as interpeak latency differences and amplitude ratios (Table 16.1). In general, peak latencies measure the time lapse between stimulus onset and the time of highest synchronous activity in the generator set of the measured component. With auditory evoked potentials, this time includes sound conduction from the transducer (typically an earphone or speaker), mechanical transmission through the middle and inner ear, receptor transduction and cochlear nerve activation, and transmission along the auditory pathway to the generators of the surface-recorded activity. Peak latencies are therefore affected by all these processes, which should all be taken into consideration when interpreting latency data. The multitude of factors contributing to peak latency has led to the definition of interpeak latency difference measures. By deriving the difference in latency between two peaks, factors affecting the latency of both peaks are negated, and the latency measure gains in specificity. Thus, for example, the V–I interpeak latency difference reflects central transmission time from the cochlea to the ponto–midbrain junction, and is usually unaffected by more peripheral factors such as conductive hearing loss. With ABRs, the most widely used interpeak latency differences are V–I, III–I and V–III, reflecting transmission along the auditory pathway between cochlea and ponto–midbrain junction, between cochlea and pontomedullary junction, and along the pons, respectively.

The functionally intact auditory pathway is typically symmetrical, with equal transmission times in response to left-ear and to right-ear stimulation. Thus, a significant interaural difference in respective measures, in response to left- and right-ear stimulation, may be indicative of a unilateral functional abnormality. Peak amplitudes are affected by a variety of recording factors, such as electrode impedance, the precise location of the electrodes relative to the generators of the potentials, and the effective stimulus intensity reaching the inner ear. Amplitude measures, therefore, exhibit very large variability across subjects as well as between sessions with the same subject. Amplitude ratios between peaks in the same record quantify the amount of synchronous activity at different levels of the pathway, cancelling out sources of variance that are common to both peaks, such as electrode impedance and relative positions of electrodes and generators. The most widely used amplitude ratio is that between peaks V and I, reflecting the amount of synchronous activity at the upper pons normalized by the cochlear output that evoked it.

Table 16.1 Typical adult normative upper limits for measurements of BAEP in response to 10/s, 70-dB HL clicks.

		Mean	Upper limit	Interaural difference
Absolute	I	1.75	2.2	0.3
latencies	II	2.8	3.3	0.4
	III	3.9	4.5	0.4
	IV	5.1	5.9	0.6
	V	5.7	6.4	0.5
Interpeak	V–I	4.0	4.5	0.5
latency	III–I	2.1	2.5	0.5
difference	V–III	1.9	2.4	0.5
Amplitude ratio	V/I	1.3	0.5	Lower limit

Values are representative of three typical values and should not be used as norms for any particular setting. The norms for each laboratory should be calculated based on records from subjects recorded on the same system in the same setting. Neonates and children may have different normative values. Latency measures are in milliseconds. Interaural differences are in the same units as their monaural counterparts in the same line, amplitude ratios are in decimal fractions.

ABRs are affected by a variety of non-pathological factors, including the subject's age, body temperature and gender, and stimulus factors such as frequency composition, intensity, presentation rate and envelope. Because ABRs reflect the synchronous firing of neural elements distributed along the auditory pathway that summates on the scalp, the more synchronous their activation, the larger the peak amplitudes. Fast-rising stimulus envelopes result in more synchronous neural activation. Because high-frequency stimuli have a fast rise time, they are more effective in synchronous neural activation.

Moreover, because high frequencies are represented in the more basal portions of the cochlea, where longitudinal mechanical coupling along the basilar membrane is more pronounced, the responses across a wider frequency range are synchronous. The mechanical travelling wave reaches the basal cochlea earlier, and therefore potentials evoked by high frequencies have shorter latencies. In summary, high-frequency stimuli and stimulus envelopes with a steep rise time evoke ABRs with larger amplitudes and shorter latencies. Increasing stimulus intensity results in earlier activation of nerve fibres, usually because the cochlear postsynaptic potentials rise higher and faster, and reach threshold earlier. Thus, ABR peak latencies shorten with increasing stimulus intensity (Figure 16.16). With increasing stimulus rate, synaptic efficacy is reduced, typically because recycling of the transmitter cannot keep up with the rate of its depletion. Thus the synaptic potentials are smaller, resulting in longer delays until the next neural level reaches threshold. Thus, because of the cumulative effect along the chain of synapses leading to successive generators of ABRs, peak latencies are progressively prolonged with increasing stimulus rate, with the later peaks' latencies more affected by high rates than the earlier peaks. As a result, interpeak latency differences are prolonged with increasing stimulus rate.

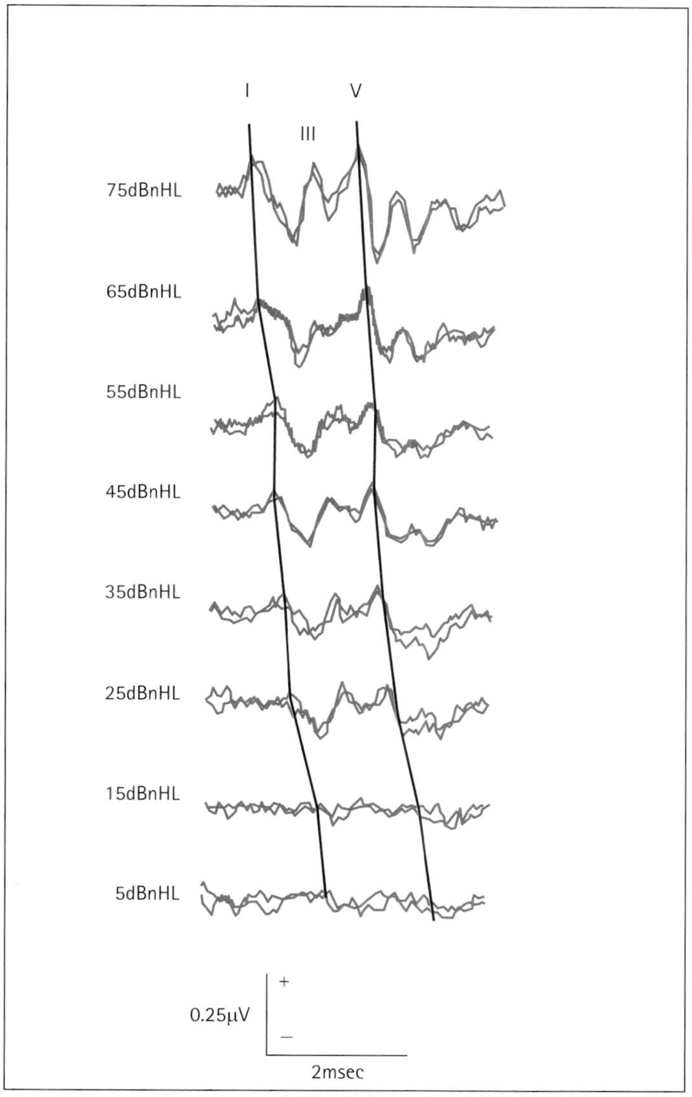

Figure 16.16 ABRs from a young infant to alternating-polarity clicks presented over a 70-dB intensity range. Note the parallel prolongation of peak latencies with decreasing intensity down to near-threshold levels, and the preservation of the V–I interpeak latency difference. Also note the typical neonatal waveform, with only a rudimentary peak II.

The effect of age may be divided into two periods: maturation and adulthood. During maturation, which can be followed in premature neonates, through full-term babies and up to 2 years of age, significant changes in component amplitudes, latency and interpeak latency differences take place. In premature neonates, ABRs are not detectable before 26 weeks of conceptional age. After 26 weeks, components II, IV and VI are not well defined, and peak latencies and interpeak latency differences are prolonged. Interpeak latency differences shorten with maturation at a rate of 0.1–0.2 ms/week until week 40, and at a slower rate until the age of 2 years, when they reach adult values. During childhood, the definition of components II, IV and VI improves. Peak amplitudes are typically larger than in adults, particularly component I, which is often larger than V, leading to an amplitude ratio between V and I which is typically larger than 1 in adults, but smaller than 1 in children. Consequently, the V/I amplitude ratio must be used with caution, taking into account the profound effects of age on this measure. During adulthood, the age-related changes in amplitude and latency measures are so small as to not warrant age-adjusted norms in clinical use. The effects of increasing stimulus rate on interpeak latency differences are large in neonates, decrease during childhood and reach stable adult values at adolescence.

The effect of lowering body temperature on ABRs is prolongation of peak latencies such that peak V latency increases by 0.2 ms/°C down to a core temperature of 27°C. Below 27°C, component definition becomes difficult. Some effects of drugs and alcohol, as well as circadian rhythms, on ABR measures have been attributed to changes in body temperature.

The effect of gender on ABRs is apparent only in adults, where latencies and interpeak latency differences are shorter and amplitudes are larger in women. Attempts have been made to relate these differences to gender differences in body and brain size and/or to differences in body temperature, water content and adipose tissue. The differences are small and well within normal ranges for each gender, but some insist on separate normative adult data for men and women.

Auditory thalamocortical evoked potentials

Auditory thalamocortical potentials are also called auditory middle-latency evoked potentials (AMEPs) and are optimally recorded from the scalp by disk or cup electrodes in response to high-intensity clicks or tone pips presented at a rate of about 10/s or less. Potential differences between an electrode on the top of the head (C_z, C_3 or C_4 according to the 10–20 system[26] and in the vicinity of the stimulated ear (mastoid or earlobe) or lower neck are amplified in a bandpass of about 10–3000 Hz, and averaged across 1000 sweeps of 60–100 ms. To avoid waveform distortions and to enhance latency resolution, sampling rate should not be lower than 5 kHz (200 μs/address, or less). Under such stimulus and recording conditions, the normal waveform includes a series of about three voltage oscillations, between 10 and 50 ms after stimulus onset (Figure 16.17, top). Amplitudes of the components are in the order of a microvolt or two, and components are affected by auditory sensitivity to the stimulus used to evoke them. Unlike the ECOG and ABRs, AMEPs are affected by the subject's state of arousal and by some drugs. Components are labelled according to their polarity (P for positive, N for negative), with a numerical or alphabetical subscript denoting their sequential order, beginning with the vertex negative–positive peaks at approximately 10 ms after stimulus onset (N_0, P_0), followed by a negative–positive trough-peak (N_a, P_a) at about 15 and 25 ms, and another (N_b, P_b) at about 35 and 50 ms.

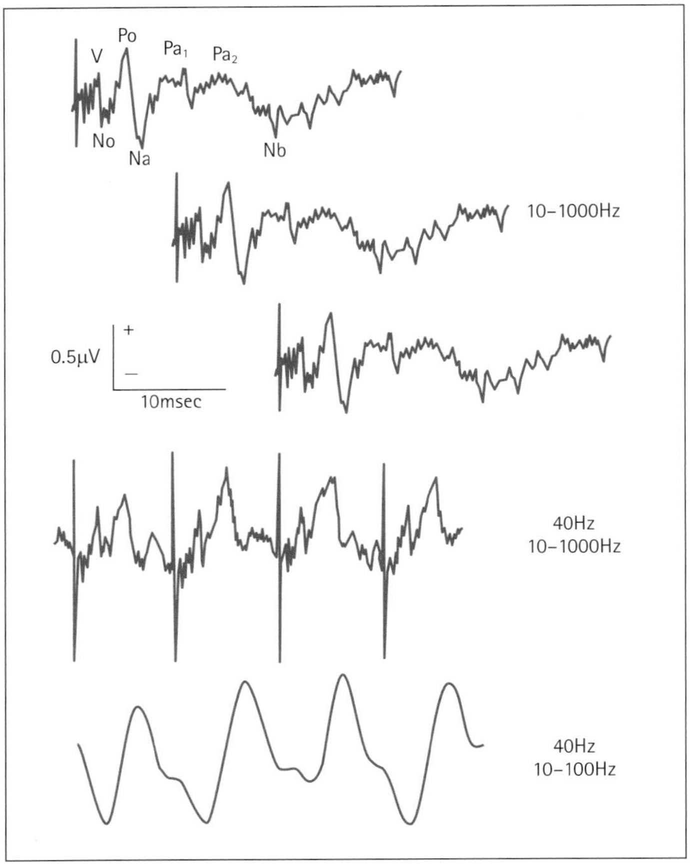

Figure 16.17 Auditory middle latency evoked potentials (AMEPs) recorded from the vertex in response to clicks presented at a rate of 10/s (top trace) and 40/s (bottom trace). When stimuli are presented at intervals of 25 ms (i.e. at a rate of 40/s), the AMEPs evoked by one stimulus are not over when the AMEPs evoked by the next stimulus are evoked. The top three traces show AMEPs that are replicated with a 25-ms delay, which, when summated (fourth trace from the top), yield a composite waveform which oscillates at 40/s. When the higher frequencies of this composite waveform are filtered out (bottom trace), a sinusoidal waveform of 40 Hz is obtained.

AMEPs are generally accepted to be of thalamocortical origin, with contributions from the extralemniscal reticular formation. The relative contributions of these generators differ according to the recording electrodes' positions. P_a is a composite of two major contributions (Figure 16.17, top), reflecting more of the primary auditory cortex when recorded over temporoparietal areas (e.g. C_3, C_4), while subcortical levels are optimally recorded over the midline (C_z).

Because the major peaks of AMEPs are approximately 25 ms apart, stimulation (with clicks or tone pips) at a rate of 40/s (Figure 16.17, middle) results in summation of non-corresponding components to consecutive stimuli (e.g. P_0 from one stimulus with P_a to the preceding stimulus, 25 ms earlier, and P_b of the stimulus before that, 25 ms earlier yet), creating a periodic sinusoidal waveform (Figure 16.17, bottom) of 40 Hz.[32] At other stimulus rates, the components do not summate and the waveform does not attain a smooth sinusoidal 'steady state', as opposed to the 'transient response' obtained with slow stimulus rates that do not superimpose components across consecutive stimuli. This steady-state sinusoidal variant of AMEPs is also called 'the 40-Hz response', but the exact stimulus rate at which constructive summation of components occurs varies. In adults, constructive summation to a sinusoid occurs between 37 and 40 Hz, and in very young children it may be closer to 20 Hz. The recording bandpass for the 40-Hz response can be narrow and around 40 Hz: for clinical use, it is set to about 10–100 Hz. Averaging about 1000 sweeps will usually suffice to produce a clean sinusoidal waveform, with amplitudes of 1–2 μV from normal awake subjects. The generators of the 40-Hz response are ambiguous, because of the temporal overlap of components from a variety of subcortical and cortical generators. The differential effect of stimulus rate on these generators adds to the ambiguity in their relationship to the generators of AMEPs with slower stimulus rates. Suspected generators include extralemniscal brainstem, thalamus, and possibly some contribution from auditory cortex.

AMEP measures include the stimulus intensity at which a response is just detected (detection threshold), for both the 40-Hz steady-state response and the transient response with a slower stimulus rate, as well as peak latencies of the transient response. Amplitudes are too variable to be clinically useful.

Unlike ABRs and the ECOG, AMEPs are affected by the subject's state of arousal and by sedation and anaesthetic drugs. The subject's age and stimulus rate interact to produce a marked effect on the potentials of young children.

Auditory cortical and cognitive potentials

Auditory cortical potentials are also called auditory long-latency (or late) evoked potentials (ALEPs), and they span the transition from exogenous to endogenous components. ALEPs are optimally recorded from the scalp by disk or cup electrodes in response to a variety of stimuli, from clicks or tone pips, to more complex sounds including speech and music, presented at a rate of less than 1/s. ALEPs are optimally recorded in response to tone pips with envelopes having relatively long (about 25 ms) rise–fall times and plateaus (about 50 ms). The potential differences between an electrode on the top of the head (F_z, C_z, or P_z according to the 10–20 system[26]) and one on the lower surface of the head (mastoids, lower neck or chin), are amplified in a bandpass of about 1–100 Hz, and averaged across 50–100 sweeps of 500–1000 ms. To avoid waveform distortions and to keep a reasonable latency resolution, sampling rate should not be lower than 250 Hz (4 ms/address, or less).

The normal ALEP waveform (Figure 16.18, bottom) includes two voltage fluctuations, between 60 and 200 ms after stimulus onset, which are exogenous and therefore dependent on stimulus parameters and auditory sensitivity. These components are followed by later components (Figure 16.18, top) which are endogenous and vary with the task relevance and with the context of the stimulus, rather than with its physical characteristics. Amplitudes of the components are in the order of a few microvolts, and are markedly affected by the task that the subject performs and the subject's state of arousal. Components are labelled according to their polarity (P for positive, N for negative) with Arabic numerical subscripts denoting their sequential order or average latency in milliseconds (e.g. N_1 or N_{100} for the first vertex-negative peak at approximately 100 ms after stimulus onset). The initial scalp positive peak (P_1 or P_{60}) is followed by a negative–positive (N_1, P_2) complex at about 100 and 160 ms, which is maximal in amplitude at the vertex,

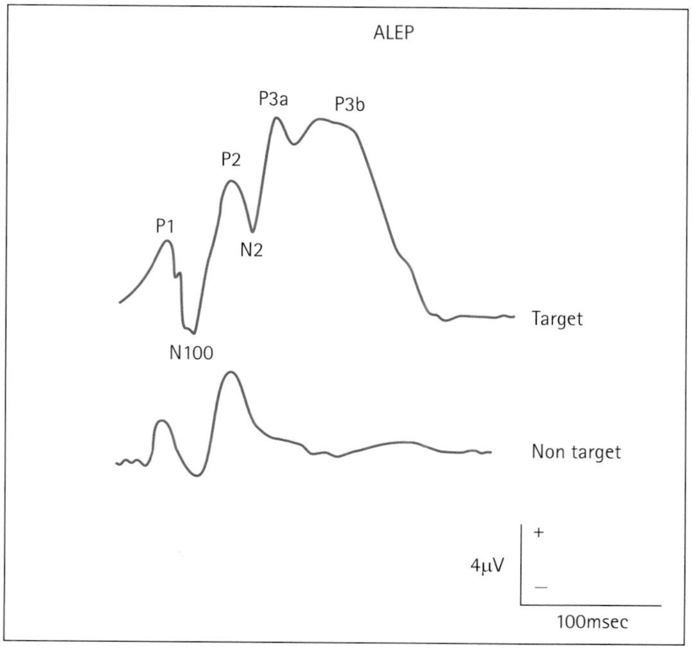

Figure 16.18 Auditory long-latency evoked potentials (ALEPs) recorded from the vertex in response to frequent, non-target stimuli (bottom) and to rare, target stimuli (top). The initial, mostly exogenous P_1, N_1 and P_2 components are evoked by both types of stimuli, while the later, endogenous N_2 and P_3 complexes are evident only in response to the target stimuli.

and is therefore also called the 'vertex potential'. The vertex potential is primarily exogenous but also has a number of endogenous traits, many of them simultaneously contributing to N_1.[33]

Negative contributions to N_1 include a slow negativity beginning about 70 ms after an attended stimulus, peaking about 30 ms later and then slowly resolving back to baseline. This negativity can be isolated from the exogenous components that it overlaps by subtracting the potentials to unattended stimuli from those to the physically identical stimuli when they are being attended to. This slow endogenous negativity is called 'processing negativity'[34] or 'negative difference' (N_d), and is assumed to reflect selective attention.[35] Another endogenous negative component overlapping the vertex potential is the mismatch negativity (MMN), beginning at about 100 ms after onset of a deviant stimulus. It can be isolated from the other components on which it is superimposed by subtracting the response to the rare, deviant stimuli from that to the common, repetitive stimuli of a train of stimuli in which the deviants are randomly presented. The MMN can be recorded even if stimuli are all unattended or even not perceived.[36] The MMN is larger in response to more deviant stimuli, and its scalp distribution is compatible with generators in the primary auditory cortex.

Following the vertex potential, the components are endogenous and vary with the context and relevance of the stimuli, rather than their physical characteristics. The negative–positive endogenous components at 200 ms (N_2 or N_{200}) and 300–700 ms (P_3 or P_{300}), which have been associated with the discrimination of a rare, task-relevant target stimulus, are called the N_{200}–P_{300} complex.[11,37–39] The most widely used paradigm to obtain the P_{300} is the 'oddball' paradigm, in which the subject discriminates unexpected or infrequent 'target' stimuli from more frequent 'non-target' stimuli among which the targets are randomly distributed. P_{300} has been shown to include two distinct components: P_{3a}, which is frontally distributed on the scalp, shorter in latency, and is associated with the detection of the mismatch between the rare and frequent background stimuli (the 'orienting response'); and P_{3b}, which is parietally distributed on the scalp, longer in latency, and associated with active discrimination of the task-relevant target stimuli.[40] The P_{300} component is affected by the subject's age and vigilance, as well as by task difficulty. Children presented with infrequent stimuli in the 'oddball' paradigm show a large, frontally distributed negativity at about 700 ms, followed by a late positivity at 1300 ms,[41] and a late, parietal P_{300} which decreases in latency to reach a minimum in the early teens and then increases throughout adulthood at a rate of 1–2 ms/year.[42,43] The juvenile frontal negativity is diminished with development and is replaced by P_{300} by the age of 10, or adolescence at the latest. Decreased vigilance is associated with a decrease in the amplitude of P_{300} while decreased task difficulty (e.g. easier discriminability of targets from non-targets) manifests in shorter latencies of P_{300}.[44,45]

The N_{400}, a late negativity following the vertex potential and P_{300}, has been associated with semantic processing of verbal material.[46] The paradigm most commonly used to elicit N_{400} includes presenting the subject with sentences in which the last word is semantically incongruous with the preceding sentence. The N_{400} to the semantically anomalous word has an onset latency of about 200 ms, peaking at about 400 ms, even when the word is longer. This suggests that words do not need to be fully heard before their semantic appropriateness is recognized. N_{400} is larger over the right hemisphere's temporal region,[47] consistent with that area's role in understanding the context of narratives, in interpreting metaphors and in appreciating humour. N_{400} is smaller in response to the presentation of single words that are members of an established semantic category,[48] or when presented after semantically related words. N_{400} is larger in response to words that are unpredictable or non-words.[49]

ALEPs are generally accepted to be of cortical origin, but the precise generators are unclear. The primary auditory cortex probably contributes to components N_1 and P_2 but, in general, the long-latency components are generated by multiple generators that are simultaneously activated. Thus, for example, the P_{300} component has been associated with widespread brain activity, including activity in two systems: one related to P_{3a} and orientation of attention, centred in paralimbic and fronto-parietocingular cortex; and the second related to P_{3b} and cognitive contextual integration, involving inferotemporal, perirhinal and ventrolateral prefrontal cortices and the hippocampus.[50] The relative contributions of these multiple generators may vary with tasks and the specific strategy that the subject uses in the task, and thus the scalp distributions of endogenous components may change. It is therefore advisable to add scalp distribution to the measures of latency and amplitude, particularly when ALEPs are studied.

Discussion of normal/abnormal

The purpose of all clinical measures is to determine whether the subject falls within or outside the normal variability of the healthy population. The definition of normalcy is therefore critical for the clinical use of any measure, including measures of auditory evoked potentials. Most normal evoked potential measures have a Gaussian, bell-shaped distribution, and standard deviations can therefore be used to limit normal ranges. The normal range should include at least 98% of the normal population, and therefore the normal limit most often used is 2.5 standard deviations from the normal mean, which includes 98.8% of normals. A stricter upper limit of 3 standard deviations includes 99.7% of the normal values, while the laxer 2 standard deviations limit includes 95.4%. When measures do not exhibit a symmetrical normal distribution, other limits of normalcy are more appropriate. Amplitude measures typically show a steeper decline in the prevalence of low amplitudes than in that of high amplitudes. In such cases, using the most extreme value of normals as the limit may be more appropriate than more elaborate statistical descriptors of the non-Gaussian distribution. A normative database from 30–40 subjects is usually sufficient to determine stable and representative normal limits.

Relevance in diagnosis

ECoG is used to monitor cochlear function intraoperatively, to assist in the diagnosis of Menière's disease, and to enhance the detection of the cochlear microphonics and compound action potential. The sensitivity and specificity of the SP/N_1 amplitude ratio, or SP duration, for cochlear pathology, particularly in Menière's disease, have been controversial.[51–58] The conflicting results regarding Menière's disease are partially due to differences in electrode placements (transtympanic or ear canal), in the normative variability, and in criteria for abnormality of ECoG. Another clinical use of ECoG includes measuring the latency of the cochlear action potential for the determination of central auditory transmission time when ABR peak I is unreliable due to a peripheral hearing loss. ECoG is also used in intraoperative monitoring when cochlear function is at risk.

ABRs represent a useful adjunct to clinical diagnosis as indicators of the auditory sensitivity of the cochlea and brainstem, as well as of the functional integrity of the auditory pathway between the cochlea and the upper pons. Auditory sensitivity is estimated by noting the lowest sound level at which the components are detected. Typically, clicks (which are the optimal stimulus for evoking the potentials) are used, and then detection threshold for ABRs correlates with the audiometric threshold at 3–4 kHz within 5–10 dB (Figure 16.16). More frequency-specific stimuli may be used to assess auditory sensitivity at other frequencies. The appropriate stimulus must present a compromise between abrupt onset and short duration, optimal for evoking neural responses, and long duration, which ensures frequency specificity. Such stimuli are pure tones gated by a smoothing window such as Hanning or Blackman, or more simply by an envelope that includes two periods during onset and offset and one period at full intensity.[59] When frequency-specific stimuli are used, the most prominent component of ABRs is a slow negativity following peak V, at about 10 ms,[60] otherwise called SN_{10} (slow negativity at 10 ms). This slow negativity, or the preceding peak V, can be detected down to about 10–15 dB above the subject's hearing threshold for the stimulus used to evoke SN_{10}.

In addition to comparison of the patient's ABR measures to the norms, clinical application of ABRs involves noting missing peaks that are always detected in normals. Such absence may indicate a lesion at the level activating the generators of the missing component. Detection of abnormality does not define the pathological process causing the impairment, but merely demonstrates a functional impairment at the affected level. Different pathological processes may have the same manifestation in ABRs, and the same disease process may manifest at different levels of the pathway.

ABRs with all of the components present, but at longer latencies than appropriate for the stimulus intensity that was used, may indicate a peripheral hearing loss. The hearing loss may be conductive, resulting in a lower stimulus level reaching the inner ear, or a sensorineural loss affecting the high frequencies. ABRs with prolonged peak I latency but normal latencies of the subsequent peaks are also compatible with high-frequency sensorineural hearing loss. It is thus essential to identify peak I in order to define peripheral impairments and differentiate them from central ones. When ABRs fail to reveal peak I, ECoG may be used to determine the latency of the cochlear action potential.

Once a peripheral hearing loss has been ruled out or accounted for, central auditory function can be assessed using interpeak latency differences. A prolonged III–I indicates slowed conduction between the cochlear nerve and the lower pons. When V–III is longer than normal, slowed transmission between the lower pons and midbrain is indicated. When peak I is not defined, the transmission to the lower pons cannot be assessed. The V/I amplitude ratio is the only amplitude measure that may be clinically helpful, and then only when used with great caution. This measure is affected by the subject's age, by hearing loss and by stimulus intensity, and is therefore susceptible to non-neurological biases. A genuine abnormality of this measure indicates impaired transmission central to the lower pons.

Interaural differences in ABRs indicate an impairment that is more severe on one side. With peripheral lesions, findings are more abnormal in response to stimulation of the ear on the affected side. Surprisingly, this is often true for central lesions as well, in contrast to the mostly contralateral representation in the central pathway. However, there are many exceptions to this tendency, and, as a rule, caution should be used in determining the side of a central lesion based on ABRs. The above ABEP measures reflect impaired transmission along the auditory nerve and brainstem, and best correlate with conduction blocks and slowing as occurs in white matter lesions resulting from fibre discontinuity, compression and demyelination.

The effects of increasing stimulus rate have been suggested to be more sensitive to grey matter lesions such as brainstem nuclear lesions and synaptic efficacy impairments. The effects of increasing stimulus rate are assessed by subtracting the respective measure's value (e.g. V–I interpeak latency difference) in response to slow-rate stimulation (e.g. 10/s clicks) from its counterpart in response to a higher rate (e.g. 55/s. The measures thus derived subtract sources of inter-subject variability common to slow and fast stimulus rates, and are thus highly specific to the effect of increased stimulus rate. These measures have been found to be abnormal in brainstem nuclear viral infections, mild vascular impairments, renal failure and a variety of metabolic abnormalities that may not affect ABRs to slow rates.

AMEPs' clinical uses include frequency-specific threshold estimates in older children and adults, assessment of central auditory function above the level of the brainstem, and resolution of discrepancies between pure tone audiograms and ABR findings in older children and adults. Clinical application of AMEPs entails caution and is limited because of the uncertainty regarding the response generators, the unreliable recording of both transient and steady-state responses in young children and in sleeping adults. The susceptibility of both variants of AMEP to the subject's state of arousal and the effects of drugs may alter the detection threshold in audiometric uses. These effects may also alter the contribution of cortical generators to the waveform in neuro-otological uses. When the appropriate precautions are taken, AMEPs can contribute to the evaluation of the functional integrity of the auditory system.

With the above-listed precautions, AMEPs can be reliably recorded in response to tone pips of mid-range frequencies; hence their utility in frequency-specific threshold estimation in awake older children and adults. For assessment of cortical lesions, temporoparietal recordings should be used, to enhance the contributions of auditory cortex to the waveform. In such records, marked asymmetry between the waveforms recorded from the two sides of the scalp is compatible with a lesion on the side with the absent or smaller response. The AMEPs recorded from the vertex may be insensitive to unilateral cortical lesions. Detection of lesions above the level of the midbrain may help resolve discrepancies between behavioural audiometry (which may be impaired) and ABR findings (which may be normal). Another type of discrepancy may result from impaired synchrony along the auditory pathway, anywhere from the auditory nerve (e.g. auditory neuropathy) to the midbrain (e.g. multiple sclerosis). In such cases, ABRs, which reflect highly synchronous activity, may be absent, while AMEPs, which, thanks to the longer duration of their components, are less sensitive to synchrony, will be present. Because of their longer latency, and hence temporal separation from stimulus artefact, AMEPs have been used to objectively assess the efficacy of cochlear implants.[61]

ALEPs' clinical utility is determined by their relationship to higher brain function and cognitive aspects of hearing, and by their inter- and intra-subject variabilities, which render their sensitivity and specificity lower than those of the earlier potentials. The P_{300} component has been shown to be delayed in demented patients,[62] and smaller in amplitude,[63] and abnormal in scalp distribution,[64] in schizophrenic patients. However, these statistical differences are not always clinically significant in individual cases, because of the overlap of P_{300} measures between patients and controls. Improved diagnostic value of P_{300} may be achieved by adjusting the discrimination task to the patient's specific cognitive impairment.[65] In the context of hearing, cognitive components may be used to assess higher-level auditory processing such as discrimination and speech perception,[66] but such applications are not widely accepted and are still in the experimental stage.

Acknowledgement

Graphics work for the figures of this chapter by Naomi Bleich is gratefully acknowledged.

References

1. Wever E, Bray C. Action currents in the auditory nerve in response to acoustic stimulation. *Proc Natl Acad Sci USA* 1930; **16:** 344–50.

2. Fromm B, Nylen C-O, Zotterman Y. Studies in the mechanism of the Wever and Bray effect. *Acta Otolaryngol* 1935; **22:** 477–86.
3. Berger H. Uber das Elektrenkephalogramm des Menschen. *Arch Psychiatrie Nervenkrankh* 1929; **87:** 527–70.
4. Davis PA. Effects of acoustic stimuli on the waking human brain. *J Neurophysiol* 1939; **2:** 494–9.
5. Davis H, Davis PA, Loomis AL, Harvey EN, Hobart G. Electrical reactions of the human brain to auditory stimulation during sleep. *J Neurophysiol* 1939; **2:** 500–14.
6. Woolsey CN, Walzl EM. Topical projection of nerve fibers from local regions of the cochlea to the cerebral cortex of the cat. *Bull Johns Hopkins Hosp* 1942; **71:** 315–44.
7. Dawson GD. A summation technique for detecting small signals in a large irregular background. *J Physiol* 1951; **115:** 2–3.
8. Clark WA Jr. Average response computer (ARC-1). *Q Rep Electronics* 1958; 114–17.
9. Geisler CD, Frishkopf LS, Rosenblith WA. Extracranial responses to acoustic clicks in man. *Science* 1958; **128:** 1210–11.
10. Davis H, Yoshie N. Human evoked cortical responses to auditory stimuli. *Physiologist* 1963; **6:** 164.
11. Davis H. Enhancement of evoked cortical potentials in humans related to a task requiring a decision. *Science* 1964; **145:** 182–3.
12. Sutton S, Braren M, Zubin J, John ER. Evoked potential correlates of stimulus uncertainty. *Science* 1965; **150:** 1187–8.
13. Ruben RJ, Knickerbocker GG, Sekula J, Nager GT, Bordley JE. Cochlear microphonics in man. *Laryngoscope* 1959; **69:** 665–71.
14. Ruben RJ, Sekula J, Bordley J. Human cochlear response to sound stimuli. *Ann Otol Rhinol Laryngol* 1960; **69:** 459–76.
15. Yoshie N, Ohashi T, Suzuki T. Non-surgical recording of auditory nerve action potentials in man. *Laryngoscope* 1967; **77:** 76–85.
16. Aran J-M, Portmann C, Delaunay J, Pelerin J, Lenoir J. L'electro-Cochleogramme: methodes et premiers resultats chez l'enfant. *Rev Laryngol* 1969; **90:** 615.
17. Sohmer H, Feinmesser M. Cochlear action potentials recorded from the external ear in man. *Ann Otol Rhinol Laryngol* 1967; **76:** 427–38.
18. Jewett DL, Romano MN, Williston JS. Human auditory evoked potentials: possible brainstem components detected on the scalp. *Science* 1970; **167:** 1517–18.
19. Sohmer H, Feinmesser M. Routine use of electrocochleography (cochlear audiometry) in human subjects. *Audiology* 1973; **12:** 167–73.
20. Sohmer H, Feinmesser M, Szabo G. Sources of electrocochleographic responses as studied in patients with brain damage. *Electroencephalogr Clin Neurophysiol* 1974; **37:** 663–9.
21. Starr A, Achor LJ. Auditory brainstem responses in neurological disease. *Arch Neurol* 1975; **32:** 761–8.
22. Picton TW. Introduction. In: Picton TW, ed. *Human Event-Related Potentials. Handbook of Electroencephalography and Clinical Neurophysiology*, Vol. 3. Amsterdam: Elsevier, 1988: 1–5.
23. Plonsey R, Fleming DG. *Bioelectric Phenomena*. New York: McGraw-Hill, 1969; 202–75.
24. Nunez PL, Katznelson RD. *Electric Fields of the Brain. The Neurophysics of EEG*. New York: Oxford University Press, 1981: 42–175.
25. Stypulkowski P, Staller S. Clinical evaluation of a new EcoG recording electrode. *Ear Hear* 1987; **8:** 304–10.
26. Jasper HH. The ten twenty electrode system of the international federation. *Electroencephalogr Clin Neurophysiol* 1958; **10:** 371–5.
27. Hashimoto I, Ishiyama Y, Yoshimoto T, Nemoto S. Brainstem auditory evoked potentials recorded directly from human brainstem and thalamus. *Brain* 1981; **104:** 841–59.
28. Moller AR, Jannetta PJ, Sekhar LN. Contributions from the auditory nerve to the brainstem auditory evoked potentials (BAEPs): results of intracranial recording in man. *Electroencephalogr Clin Neurophysiol* 1988; **71:** 198–211.
29. Starr A, Zaaroor M. Eighth nerve contributions to cat auditory brainstem responses (ABR). *Hear Res* 1990; **48:** 151–60.
30. Zaaroor M, Starr A. Auditory brain-stem evoked potentials in cat after kainic acid induced neuronal loss. II. Cochlear nucleus. *Electroencephalogr Clin Neurophysiol* 1991; **80:** 436–45.
31. Martin WH, Pratt H, Schwegler JW. The origin of the human auditory brain-stem response wave II. *Electroencephalogr Clin Neurophysiol* 1995; **96:** 357–70.
32. Galambos R, Makeig S, Talmachoff PJ. A 40-Hz auditory potential recorded from the human scalp. *Proc Natl Acad Sci USA* 1981; **78:** 2643–7.
33. Naatanen R, Picton TW. The N_1 wave of the human electric and magnetic response to sound. *Psychophysiology* 1986; **24:** 375–425.
34. Naatanen R. Processing negativity: an evoked potential reflection of selective attention. *Psychol Bull* 1982; **92:** 605–40.
35. Hansen JC, Hillyard SA. Endogenous brain potentials associated with selective auditory attention. *Electroencephalogr Clin Neurophysiol* 1980; **49:** 277–90.
36. Naatanen R, Simpson M, Loveless NE. Stimulus deviance and evoked potentials. *Biol Psychol* 1982; **14:** 53–98.
37. Squires KC, Wickens C, Squires NK, Donchin E. The effect of stimulus sequence on the waveform of the cortical event-related potential. *Science* 1976; **193:** 1142–6.
38. Duncan-Johnson CC, Donchin E. On quantifying surprise: the variation of event-related potentials with subjective probability. *Psychophysiology* 1977; **14:** 456–67.
39. Courchesne E, Hillyard SA, Courchesne RY. P3 waves to the discrimination of targets in homogeneous and heterogeneous stimulus sequences. *Psychophysiology* 1977; **14:** 590–7.

40. Squires NK, Squires KC, Hillyard SA. Two varieties of long-latency positive waves evoked by unpredictable auditory stimuli in man. *Electroencephalogr Clin Neurophysiol* 1975; **38:** 387–401.
41. Courchesne E. Neurophysiological correlates of cognitive development: changes in long-latency event-related potentials from childhood to adulthood. *Electroencephalogr Clin Neurophysiol* 1978; **45:** 468–82.
42. Goodin D, Squires K, Henderson B, Starr A. Age related variations in evoked potentials to auditory stimuli in normal human subjects. *Electroencephalogr Clin Neurophysiol* 1978; **44:** 447–58.
43. Picton TW, Stuss DT, Champagne SC, Nelson RF. The effects of age on human event-related potentials. *Psychophysiology* 1984; **21:** 312–25.
44. Ritter W, Simson R, Vaughan HG. Auditory cortex potentials and reaction time in auditory discrimination. *Electroencephalogr Clin Neurophysiol* 1972; **33:** 547–55.
45. McCarthy G, Donchin E. A metric for thought: a comparison of P_{300} latency and reaction time. *Science* 1981; **21:** 77–80.
46. McCallum WC, Farmer SF, Pocock PV. The effects of physical and semantic incongruities on auditory event-related potentials. *Electroencephalogr Clin Neurophysiol* 1984; **59:** 477–88.
47. Kutas M, Hillyard SA. Brain potentials during reading reflect word expectancy and semantic association. *Nature* 1984; **307:** 161–3.
48. Polich J, Vanasse L, Donchin E. Category expectancy and the N200. *Psychophysiology* 1981; **18:** 142.
49. Bentin S, McCarthy G, Wood CC. Event-related potentials, lexical decision and semantic priming. *Electroencephalogr Clin Neurophysiol* 1985; **60:** 343–55.
50. Halgren E, Marinkovic K, Chauval P. Generators of the late cognitive potentials in auditory and visual oddball tasks. *Electroencephalogr Clin Neurophysiol* 1998; **106:** 156–64.
51. Yoshie N. Electrocochleographic study of Menière's disease: pathological pattern of the cochlear nerve compound action potential in man. In: Ruben RJ, Elberling C, Salomon G, eds. *Electrocochleography*. Baltimore: University Park Press, 1976; 353–86.
52. Eggermont JJ. Summating potentials in electrocochleography: relation to hearing disorders. In: Ruben RJ, Elberling C, Salomon G, eds. *Electrocochleography*. Baltimore: University Park Press, 1976; 67–87.
53. Coats AC. The summating potential and Menière's disease: I. Summating potential amplitude in Menière's and non Menière's ears. *Arch Otolaryngol* 1981; **107:** 199–208.
54. Goin D, Staller S, Asher D, Mischke RE. Summating potential in Menière's disease. *Laryngoscope* 1982; **92:** 1383–9.
55. Gibson W, Prasher D, Kilkenny G. Diagnostic significance of transtympanic electrocochleography in Menière's disease. *Ans Otol Rhinol Laryngol* 1983; **92:** 155–9.
56. Podoshin L, Ben-David Y, Pratt H, Fradis M, Feiglin H. Noninvasive recordings of cochlear evoked potentials in Menière's disease. *Arch Otolaryngol Head Neck Surg* 1986; **112:** 827–9.
57. Staller SS. Electrocochleography in the diagnosis and management of Menière's disease. *Semin Hear* 1986; **7:** 267–78.
58. Dauman R, Aran J-M, Savage R, Portmann M. Clinical significance of the summating potential in Menière's disease. *Am J Otol* 1988; **9:** 31–8.
59. Davis H, Hirsh SK, Popelka GR, Formby C. Frequency sensitivity and thresholds of brief stimuli suitable for electric response audiometry. *Audiology* 1984; **23:** 59–74.
60. Davis H, Hirsh SK. A slow brainstem response for low-frequency audiometry. *Audiology* 1979; **18:** 445–61.
61. Kileny PR, Kemink JL. Electrically evoked middle-latency auditory potentials in cochlear implant candidates. *Arch Otolaryngol Head Neck Surg* 1987; **113:** 1072–7.
62. Goodin DS, Squires KC, Starr A. Long latency event-related components of the auditory evoked potential in dementia. *Brain* 1978; **101:** 635–48.
63. Shagass C, Straumanis JJ, Roemer RA, Amadeo M. Evoked potentials of schizophrenics in several sensory modalities. *Biol Psychiatry* 1977; **12:** 221–35.
64. Morstyn R, Duffy FH, McCarley RW. Altered P_{300} topography in schizophrenia. *Arch Gen Psychiatry* 1983; **40:** 729–34.
65. Attias J, Huberman M, Kott E, Pratt H. Improved detection of auditory P_3 abnormality in dementia using a variety of stimuli. *Acta Neurol Scand* 1995; **92:** 96–101.
66. Attias Y, Pratt H. Auditory event related potentials during lexical categorization in the oddball paradigm. *Brain Language* 1992; **43:** 230–9.

17 Measurements of inner ear fluid pressure and clinical applications

Robert Marchbanks

Introduction

We are beginning to understand how the intracranial (cerebral) fluid interacts with fluid within the labyrinth, and several international scientific meetings have addressed this topic. It is now recognized that even small elevations in intracranial pressure may have adverse effects on the ear. This has been shown to be a cause of tinnitus, vertigo and hearing loss. Permanent damage to the ear can also result, as shown by Weider and Saunders,[1,2] who provided clinical evidence showing that sustained elevation of the intracranial pressure can result in recurrent perilymphatic fistula.

The audiovestibular symptoms associated with intracranial hypertension also form the basis for the diagnosis of classical Menière's disease or Menière's-like disorders. Correct differential diagnosis depends on identifying the underlying signs and symptoms of intracranial hypertension; however, this is seldom possible even by those experienced in neurology. The situation is even more complex, since we know that in many cases intracranial hypertension will occur without the expected pressure-specific headache and without papilloedema. It is evident that such patients are referred to the otolaryngological clinic but will not be cross-referred to neurology for appropriate treatment.

The commercially available 'TMD cerebral and cochlear fluid pressure (CCFP) analyser' now provides a valuable means for monitoring the treatment of intracranial pressure-related conditions.[3] The tympanic membrane displacement measurement (TMD) technique has been used in combination with detailed studies of the symptomatology to identify patients with raised intracranial pressure. The relationship between changes in the intracranial pressure and the symptoms can be investigated using repeat TMD measurements. This technique is especially valuable for monitoring the effectiveness of treatments in terms of changes in intracranial pressure, and can be used to reduce the number of repeat lumbar punctures or surgical intracranial pressure measurements made.

Furthermore, pathological intra-aural pressure waves can be seen in many patients. These are presumed to reflect pressure waves of intracranial origin and are clearly visible with the TMD system. I believe we are seeing a new beginning to our understanding of certain neurological and audiological disorders, and that this will be at the forefront of research over the next decade.

INTRACRANIAL HYPERTENSION

Associated frequently with an unknown pathology that results in raised intracranial (cerebral) pressure. In its idiopathic form it is often referred to as benign intracranial hypertension (BIH) or pseudo-tumour cerebri. The use of 'benign' is understood to be a misnomer as this condition can cause irreversible damage to the eye, optic nerve and also the ear, as recently shown.

DIFFICULT (IMPOSSIBLE) TO DIAGNOSE BY SYMPTOMS ALONE

- Headaches — can be severe but often mild or not present at all.
- Neurological symptoms — not present or minor.
- Papilloedema — only present in less than 20% of cases and then only if you look!
- Chronic fatigue — too non-specific.

Also:-

- The adult form is different from the paediatric form.

Historical review

The principle of measuring cerebral and cochlear fluid pressure depends on qualifying movements of the tympanic membrane on contraction of the stapedial muscle. When we acoustically stimulate the stapedial reflex, the movement of the tympanic membrane (TM) will be in one of three configurations—inward, outward or inward/outward.[4–7] When I first measured this in 1975, it appeared rather anomalous that a muscle acting in one direction could result in these three distinctly different displacements. By 1978, I had developed the TMD technique, which was sufficiently sensitive to show an even more puzzling property of the stapedial reflex, in that the TM displacement could be outward, then bi-directional, and then inward, in the same ear! An easy way of mediating the displacement configuration was by changing the posture of the subject from sitting to supine (Figure 17.1). In 1978, I hypothesized that these different displacements were due to the changing resting position of the stapes footplate within the oval window as brought about by changing perilymphatic fluid pressure (Figure 17.2). Around the same time, other independent work by Brask and Casselbrant et al similarly proposed that the TM displacement on contraction of the stapedial muscle was cochlear pressure dependent.[8,9] The mechanics proposed by these researchers differed in detail; nevertheless, the idea of a means for measuring cochlear fluid pressure was born. The mechanism is a combination of a rocking motion about the anterior or the posterior portion of the ligament and a piston-like in–out motion. This mechanism has been mathematically modelled[10] and simulated using temporal bone preparations.[11]

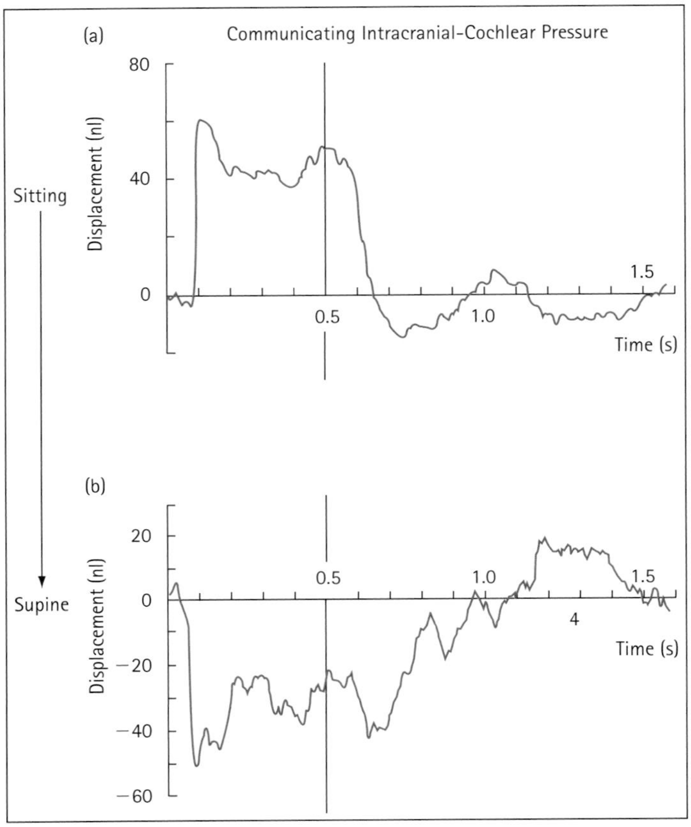

Figure 17.1 The change in TMD configuration with posture for stimulation of the acoustic stapedial reflex with a 500 ms, 1000 Hz tone set at 20 dB above the reflex threshold. (a) An average of 10 TMD records for sitting, (b) An average of 10 TMD records for supine.

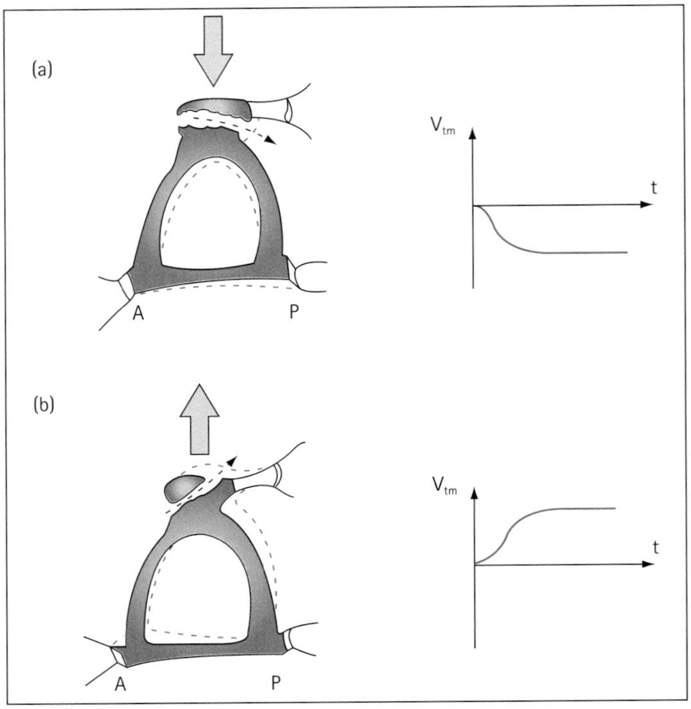

Figure 17.2 Schematic showing the method by which cochlear (perilymphatic) pressure can be measured using the TMD system on acoustic stimulation of the stapedial muscle (1000 kHz, 500 ms, nominally 20 dB above acoustical reflex threshold). (a) In the case of raised perilymphatic pressure, there is freedom of motion only in the inward direction. There is a rotation about the anterior portion of the ligament, so for high pressure, there is an inward movement of the tympanic membrane. (b) Conversely in cases of lower than normal pressure (hypotension), the footplate will sit in towards the cochlea, so on stimulation of the stapedial muscle there is only freedom of movement in the outward direction and corresponding outward motion of the tympanic membrane.

The TMD measurement technique

> The TMD technique indirectly measures perilymphatic pressure in terms of the resting position of the stapes footplate.

The TMD measurement technique is so called because it measures movement of the TM in terms of volume displacement. It comprises a headset onto which is mounted an air-flow sensor which measures the amount of air pushed from the ear canal or drawn into the ear canal when the TM moves (Figure

17.3). By this method, volume displacements of the TM as small as a nanolitre (1×10^{-9} l) can be resolved.

The TMD technique provides a measure of perilymphatic pressure by indirectly assessing the resting position of the stapes footplate, and it is this resting position which is pressure sensitive. The resting position of the stapes footplate is assessed by stimulating the acoustical reflex with a pure tone of 1000 Hz of 500 ms and, more recently, 300 ms. The TMD technique should be used in conjunction with standard tympanometry and acoustical impedance acoustical reflex threshold measurements to first confirm the normality of middle ear function.

Proving the technique

A method was required by which the proposed TMD cochlear pressure measurement method could be proven. It was clearly not possible to attempt to correlate reflex TM displacement with direct measures of perilymphatic pressure in normal human subjects. An alternative could be to use direct measurements of intracranial pressure; however, this depended on the intracranial and perilymphatic fluids being interconnected.

Prior to 1980, the cochlear aqueduct was considered to provide an effective route for pressure transfer between the intracranial fluid and perilymph in certain mammals such as the cat and guinea pig; however, there was much doubt about the patency of this aqueduct in humans. In humans the cochlear aqueduct is known to be narrow, with connective tissue running throughout its length. In 1978, a histological study by Wlodyka[12] demonstrated that, in most humans, the cochlear aqueduct was patent and that patency decreased with age (Figure 17.4).

Figure 17.5 shows the results from the very first patient whom we tested with confirmed raised intracranial fluid pressure. This patient had a condition called benign intracranial hypertension (BIH); lumbar puncture confirmed that the pressure was a high 300 mm of saline, and on stimulation of the stapedial muscle, an inward motion of the TM occurred as predicted. The patient was fitted with a lumbar–peritoneal shunt, which returned the pressure to normal, and a complete reversal of the tympanic displacement, from an inward displacement to an outward displacement, was observed. Proof that intracranial-to-cochlear pressure transfer existed in humans was therefore provided and we published this in the form of three case studies.[13]

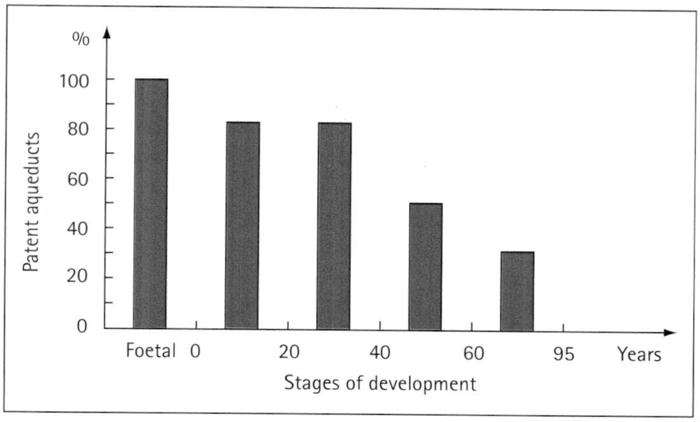

Figure 17.4 Age dependency of cochlear aqueduct patency according to a histological study by Wlodyka. (Adapted from Wlodyka. *Ann Otolaryngol* 1978; 87: 22–7.[12])

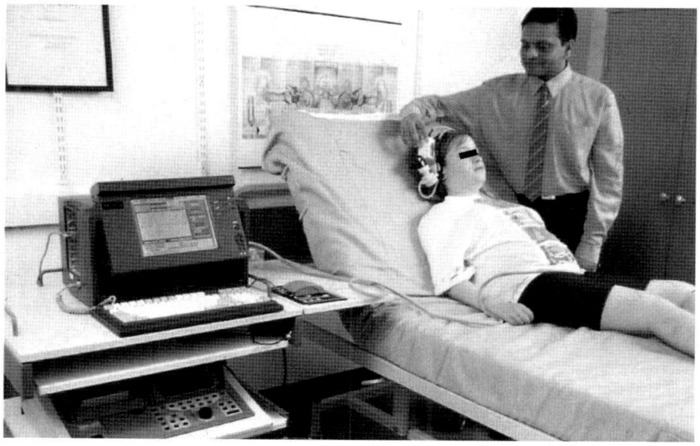

Figure 17.3 The commercially available MMS-11 Cerebral and Cochlear Fluid Pressure Analyser (www.marchbanks.co.uk).

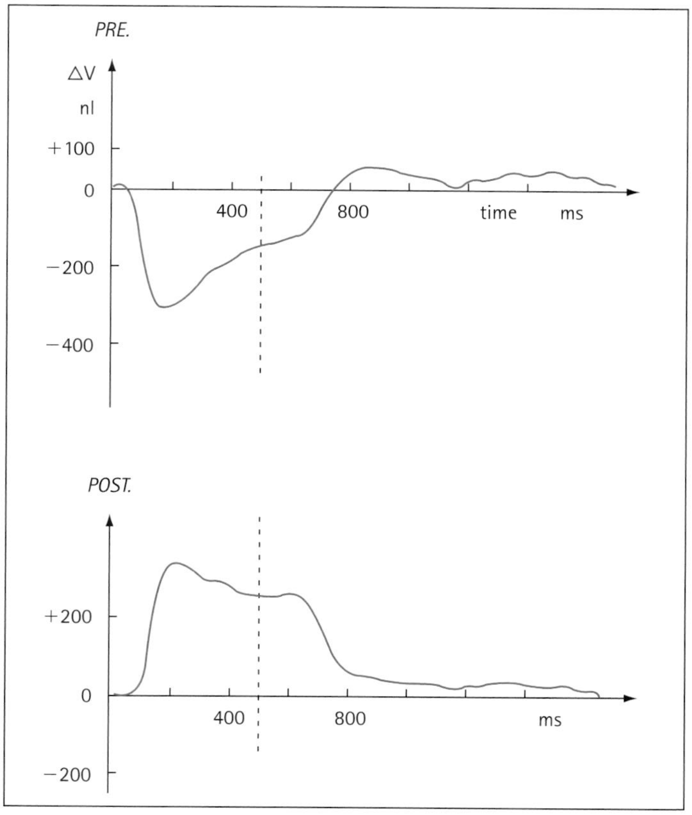

Figure 17.5 The first Benign Intracranial Hypertension (BIH) patient tested with the TMD technique. This clearly shows a change from an inward tympanic displacement to an outward displacement as the high cerebrospinal fluid pressure is reduced to normal.

TMD measurements in patients undergoing direct intracranial pressure monitoring confirm that in cases of low or normal intracranial pressure, there is an outward motion of the TM. In cases of normal pressure it is either outward or bi-directional, inward followed by outwards; and in cases of high pressure, there is an inward motion of the TM. The displacement is quantified by measuring the area under the curve, V_m (Figure 17.6).

Comparison of CCFP analyser measurements with direct intracranial pressure measurements

The relationship between reflex TM displacement and intracranial pressure was first published in 1990.[14] This work was later performed under more controlled conditions by restricting measurements to direct intraventricular pressure monitoring (Figure 17.7).[15] In this study, 77 comparative measurements were undertaken on patients with intracranial hypotension, normal pressure and hypertension. A correlation of greater than 0.9 was found between TMD and direct intraventricular pressure measurements. Further work is necessary to understand why some subjects demonstrate a very clear and well-behaved TMD–intracranial pressure relationship, whereas in others anomalies exist. The answer is likely to be found in anatomical differences, including varying cochlear aqueduct patency, as discussed later.

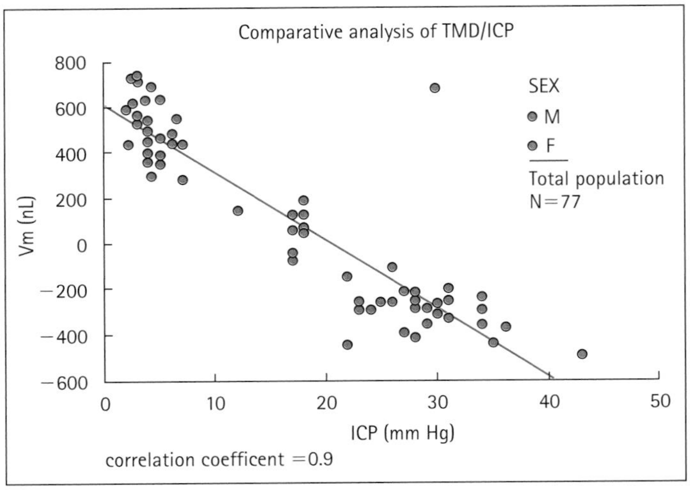

Figure 17.7 Relationship between direct intraventricular intracranial pressure measurements in millimetres of mercury on the *x*-axis, and tympanic membrane displacement (TMD) expressed as a mean displacement, V_m, on the *y*-axis.

Clinical measurements of cochlear and intracranial pressure

The idea of measuring intracranial pressure through the ear is not new. In 1985, Krast proposed that acoustical impedance could be used to monitor intracranial pressure fluctuations.[16] More recently, papers have been published on the effects of intracranial pressure on auditory evoked potentials at high pressures and on otoacoustical emissions, although it is questionable whether these methods are suitable as a means for non-invasive intracranial pressure measurement.[17,18] The success of the CCFP analyser using TMD measurements can be measured in terms of its clinical use for non-invasive measurement of intracranial pressure.[13,14,19–21] The neurological and neurosurgical applications of the CCFP analyser are of paramount importance to audiology. These allow the technique to be perfected on a patient population with known intracranial hypertension or hypotension, and also provide the opportunity to study in detail the auditory and vestibular symptomatology of intracranial pressure problems.

The relationship between intracranial pressure and stapedial reflex-induced TM displacement also holds across animal species. Figure 17.8 demonstrates that TMD correlates with direct intracranial pressure recordings in the cat.[22]

The TMD test has been used as a non-invasive measure of intracranial pressure for over 15 years.[23,24] The cochlear aqueduct provides communication between the intracranial and cochlear fluids, and the patency of this route is assessed by per-

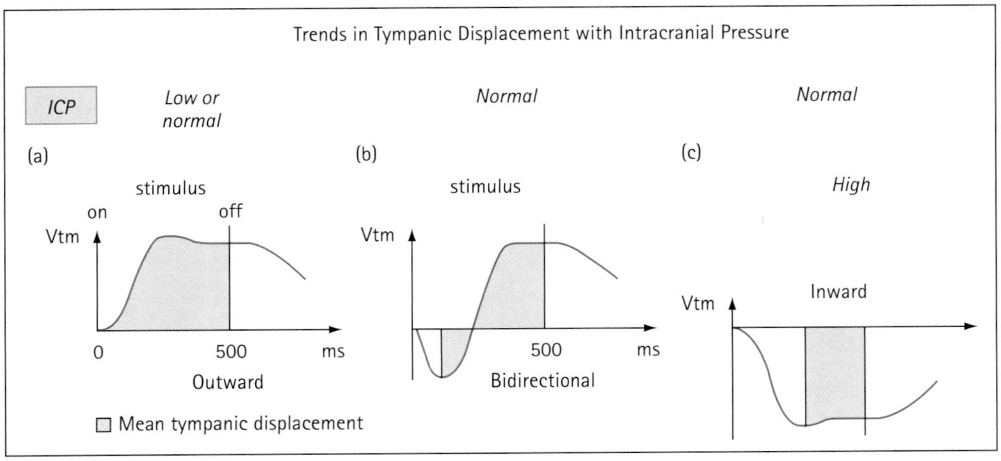

Figure 17.6 Tympanic membrane displacement is quantified in terms of the mean volume displacement, V_m, by measuring the hashed area under the curve for: (a) an outward TMD in the case of normal or low intracranial pressure (hypotension); (b) a bi-directional in the case of normal intracranial pressure and (c) an inward displacement in the case of raised intracranial pressure (hypertension).

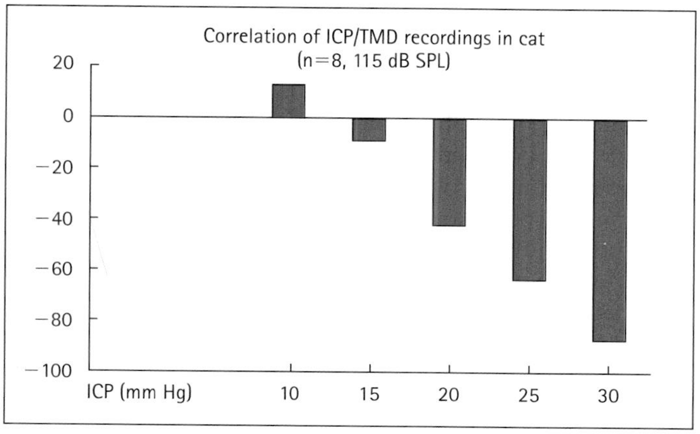

Figure 17.8 Tympanic membrane displacement with direct intracranial pressure (ICP) recordings in the cat.

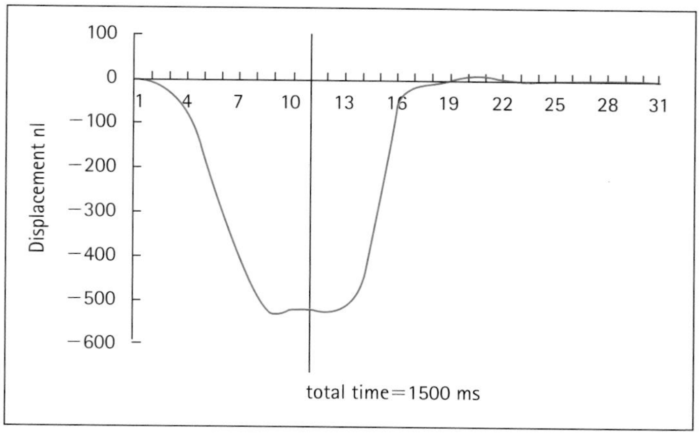

Figure 17.9 Inward tympanic membrane displacement as typically found with raised intracranial/cochlear pressure, i.e. intracranial hypertension.

forming the TMD test with the patient in the sitting posture, and then repeating it with the patient in the supine position.[25–27] There is a relative increase in the intracranial pressure in the supine position, and a more inward TMD is observed if there is free communication between the intracranial and cochlear fluids. In this instance, we assume a patent cochlear aqueduct, although of course we have only demonstrated that connectivity exists by some route. Testing in normal subjects shows that stable TMD results are obtained throughout the day and after exercise.[28] These normative data also demonstrate large intersubject differences; nevertheless, the correlation of test results within one individual is high. From this, we conclude that the TMD test gives the optimum results when testing for pressure changes within the same individual, such as changes which may occur with symptoms or treatment.

Clinical assessment of cochlear and intracranial pressure

The Southampton clinical trials allow criteria to be set for differentiating abnormal cochlear and intracranial pressure in the clinic.[15]

High pressure—intracranial/perilymphatic hypertension

A mean TM displacement, V_m, more negative than −200 nl is indicative of a hypertensive condition, i.e. where an intracranial pressure greater than 15 mmHg (20 cm saline) is considered to exist.[15]

The Southampton studies give a sensitivity of 83% and a specificity of 100%, and a positive predictive value of 100% and a negative predicted value of 29%, for detecting raised pressure by this criterion (Figure 17.9).

Low pressure—intracranial/perilymphatic hypotension

For low pressure, the Southampton clinical trials give a TMD range of 263–717 nl, with a mean of 431 nl for mean displacement, V_m (Figure 17.10). My experience is that if 263 nl is taken as the lower limit, then there will be an unacceptably high false-positive rate. I usually take 400 nl to be the upper limit for normal pressure; however, this assumption needs to be tested by addressing the problems associated with obtaining a sufficiently large sample of TMD measurements on patients with normal intracranial pressures.

Normal intracranial/perilymphatic pressure

The typical trace for normal pressure is bi-directional and is shown in Figure 17.11. Small inward and small outward traces which are not classified as high or low pressure are also within the normal range.

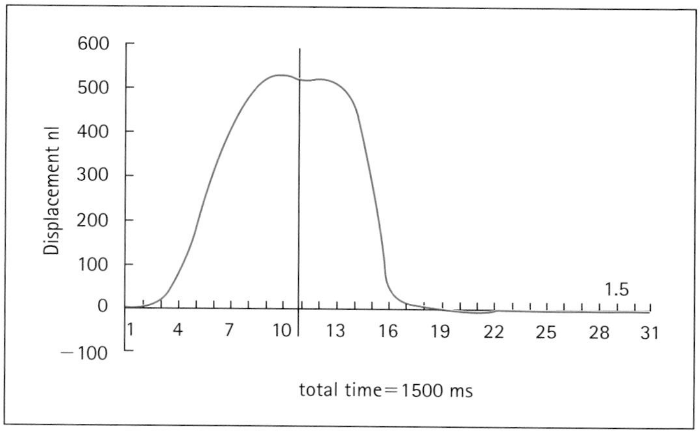

Figure 17.10 Outward tympanic membrane displacement as typically found with low intracranial/cochlear pressure, i.e. intracranial hypotension.

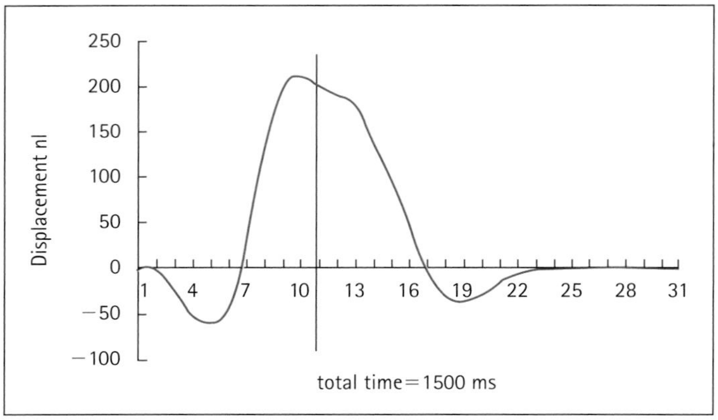

Figure 17.11 Bi-directional tympanic membrane displacement as typically found with normal intracranial/cochlear pressure,

The above findings are from a clinical trial where we compared TMD with intraventricular pressure measurements. Further trials are currently investigating the relationship with lumbar puncture pressure. The findings should be similar but not exactly the same.

Measurement of intra-aural pressure waves

The TMD technique is also used to investigate infrasound emitted from the ear, i.e. intra-aural pressure waves. Components of this infra-sound include cardiovascular and respiratory pressure waves. Each of these components provides information on the normality or otherwise of the ear and the cerebral-to-cochlear pressure coupling. It is evident that some of these pressure waves come directly from the intracranial fluid.

The intracranial pressure is changing on a second-to-second basis. Superimposed on the baseline intracranial pressure are periodic changes due to cardiovascular activity and respiration, and, over longer periods, there is a diurnal rhythm and a monthly cycle in females, as demonstrated in Figure 17.12.[7,29,30]

> Intracranial pressure waves of cardiovascular and respiratory origins can be linked to imbalance, low frequency or pulsatile tinnitus.

Intra-aural pressure waves of cardiovascular origin can be clearly seen in most ears. This activity is transmitted to the intracranial fluid and the ear via the arteries, with a fundamental frequency of 1–2 Hz, which corresponds to a heart rate of 60–120 beats/min. The significance of intra-aural cardiovascular activity was reported by Andreasson et al in 1978 and was also researched by myself.[7,29,31,32] Interest in intra-aural cardiovascular activity arises from the fact that externally applied low-frequency sound and infrasound produce nystagmus and sensations of falling forwards.[33–37] It is hypothesized that internally generated cardiovascular infrasound may also be linked to some forms of peripheral balance problems, and low-frequency or pulsatile tinnitus, which is experienced by patients with intracranial hypertension and other pressure problems.[38–40]

The amplitude of intra-aural cardiovascular activity has been studied using the TMD analyser (Figure 17.13).[7,41] The intracranial cardiovascular pressure wave is known to increase with increasing intracranial pressure, due to reduced mechanical compliance of the cerebrospinal fluid system. That is, as the cerebrospinal system becomes stiffer with increasing total volume, a given increase of the cerebral blood volume produces a correspondingly larger intracranial pressure change (Figure 17.14).[42,43] The TMD technique has been used to study this effect in patients undergoing repeated lumbar puncture. Figure 17.15 shows the increase in cardiovascular TMD and the relationship between amplitude and lumbar pressure.

The intra-aural cardiovascular amplitude has been observed in relation to body posture, intracochlear fluid pressure, middle ear compliance and pressure, and cerebral-to-labyrinth fluid pressure transfer.[41] The main positive findings were definite changes in amplitude with body posture, and a highly significant relationship with peak compliance of the middle ear ($P = 0.001$).

Categorization of the intra-aural pressure waves is in its infancy; nevertheless, distinct pressure wave characteristics can

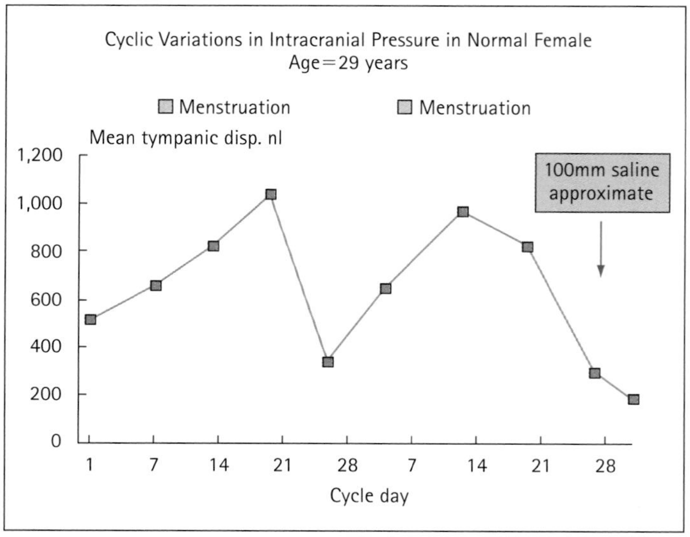

Figure 17.12 Test results from a normal female showing the change in intracranial pressure, which was measured in terms of tympanic membrane displacement throughout the menstrual cycle. Upwards represents a decrease in intracranial pressure and downward an increase in intracranial pressure. Changing from the sitting to the lying position produces at least 100 ml of saline pressure change, as shown by the length of the vertical downward facing arrow (right). There is clearly a substantial pressure change occurring within this subject.

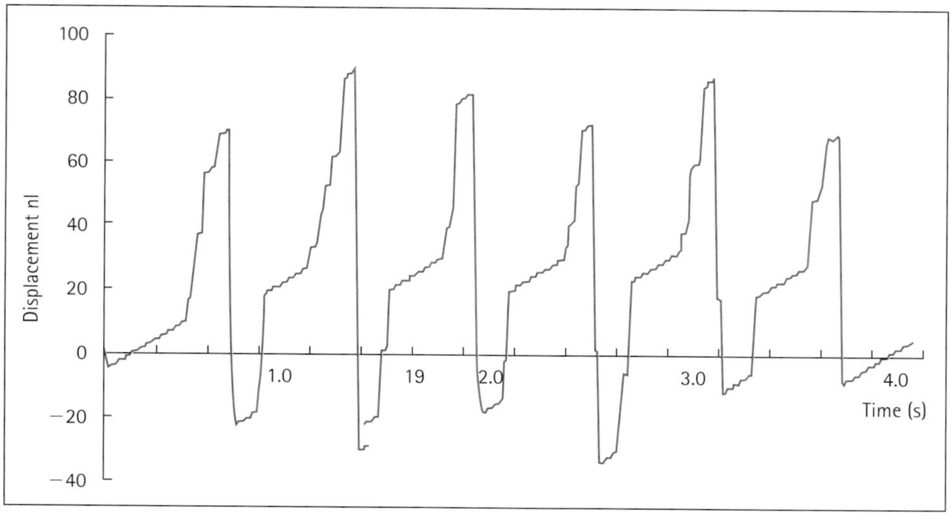

Figure 17.13 Intra-aural cardiovascular pressure waves.

be seen, and these are shown in Figure 17.16.[44] Some of these intra-aural pressure waves have only been observed in patients with intracranial abnormalities, and they are presumed to reflect pressure waves of intracranial origin. In many cases, the wave amplitude is grossly abnormal, and the waves only appear in the sitting position.[44] This is a new research area that I am sure will be of major importance for helping us to understand the underlying pathophysiology of neurological and audiological disorders.

The hydromechanics of the cochlea

A knowledge of the hydromechanical interactions between the intracranial and intralabyrinthine fluids is important to our understanding of the normal physiology and pathophysiology of

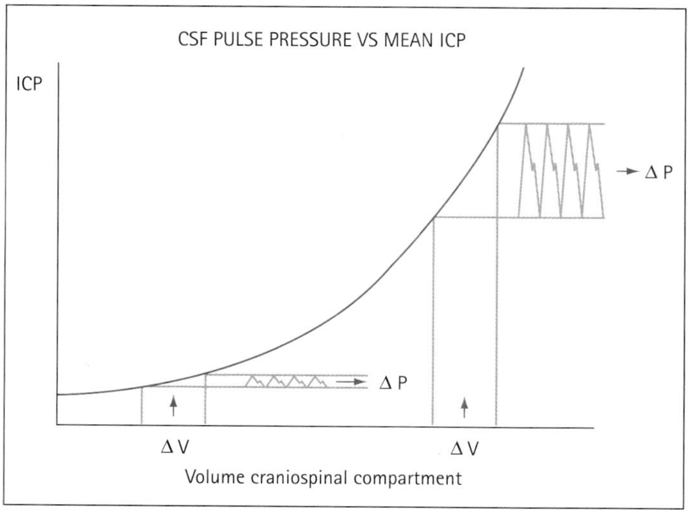

Figure 17.14 Changing amplitude of the cerebrospinal (CSF) cardiovascular pressure wave with increasing intracranial pressure (ICP). The amplitude increases as the CSF compliance reduces with increasing ICP.

the labyrinth. In the normal labyrinth, a homeostasis exists between the intracranial fluid, the perilymph and the endolymph. The nature of this homeostasis will change according to intracranial fluid pressure or blockage of one or more of the interconnecting pathways. Several clinical studies have shown that paroxysmal vertigo, tinnitus and fluctuating hearing loss may be present and reversible in patients with intracranial hypertension.[45–47]

There are two fluids within the cochlea, the endolymph and the perilymph. It is the perilymph which interfaces with the footplate, and it is the pressure of this fluid that is assessed by the CCFP analyser and the TMD technique. Both fluids are 'referenced' to the same pressure, and this pressure is that of the intracranial fluid. The cochlear aqueduct is the main fluid communication route between the intracranial and perilymphatic fluids; it runs from the subarachnoid space and enters the cochlea in a niche just near the round window (Figure 17.17). The endolymph indirectly communicates with the intracranial fluids via the endolymphatic sac and maintains homeostasis with the perilymphatic pressure across the Reissner's and other intralabyrinthine membranes.[48] Perivascular or perineural routes between the intracranial and labyrinthine spaces may also provide a means of communication, but these may only be significant in cases of extremely raised intracranial pressure or certain malformations. Experiments on the cat have demonstrated that labyrinthine pressure mirrors that of the cerebrospinal fluid and that no change in labyrinthine pressure can be measured if the cochlear and vestibular aqueducts are sealed.[49,50]

Wlodyka studied the cochlear aqueduct in over 100 temporal bone preparations. At birth the cochlear aqueduct is open, but it seals off throughout life, so at the age of 20–39 there is an 80% chance that a connection exists.[12] Later in life, it decreases to 40%, and at the age of 60 the chance is only 20%. We can replicate this work using the CCFP analyser with TMD measurements and by inducing increases in the intracranial pressure by changing the posture of the person from sitting to supine. Using this method, there is good agreement between

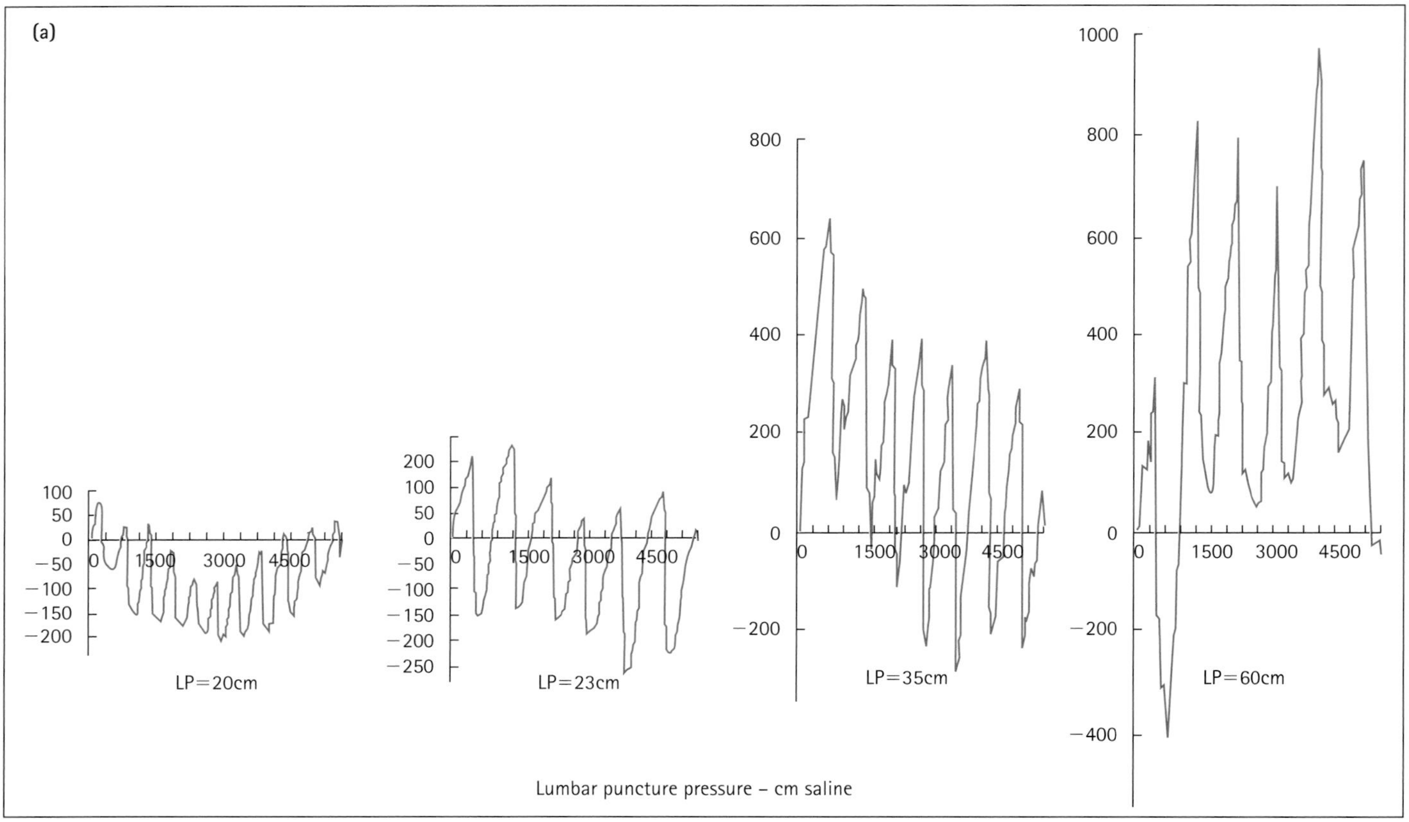

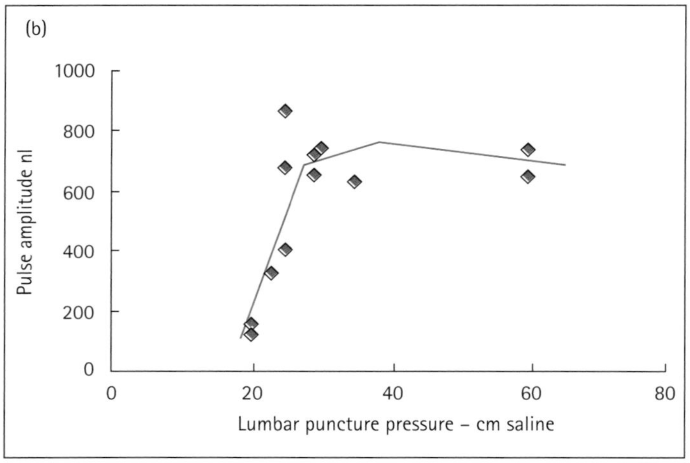

Figure 17.15 Actual TMD test results obtained immediately before repeated lumbar puncture over a period of several months. The patient was a 15-year old male with Benign Intracranial Hypertension (BIH), i.e. Pseudo Tumor Cerebri. Repeated lumbar punctures where undertaken to drain cerebrospinal fluid and/or to monitor treatment. (a) These are examples of the amplitude of the intra-aural cardiovascular pressure wave increasing with increasing lumbar opening pressure (cm of saline). (b) A plot of the intra-aural cardiovascular pulse amplitude versus lumbar puncture opening pressure.

the Wlodyka histological findings and those of Philips and Marchbanks,[25] who used the TMD technique to provide a functional measure of intracranial–labyrinthine pressure transfer in different age groups (Figure 17.18).

Clinical studies demonstrate that imbalance, paroxysmal vertigo, tinnitus and fluctuating hearing loss may be present and reversible in patients with intracranial hypertension.

Importance of the intracranial–labyrinthine impedance mismatch

The equilibrium state that exists between the intracranial and labyrinthine fluids is in a perpetual state of flux (Figure 17.19). The cochlear aqueduct acts as a low-pass filter to intracranial pressure changes and attenuates frequency components above its cut-off frequency. Long-period intracranial pressure waves should be transmitted to the labyrinth without obstruction. The transmission of pressure waves with short periods will depend on the mechanical properties of the cochlear aqueduct and cochlear windows, as demonstrated in Figure 17.20.

Since the cochlear windows are the principal source of labyrinthine compliance, the compliance of these windows is of key importance to the hydromechanical impedance mismatch between the two systems. Since the compliance of the cochlear windows will in turn depend on the middle ear pressure, a mechanism exists whereby middle ear pressure may influence the physiology of the labyrinth and perhaps provide a link between middle ear problems and associated vestibular dysfunction.

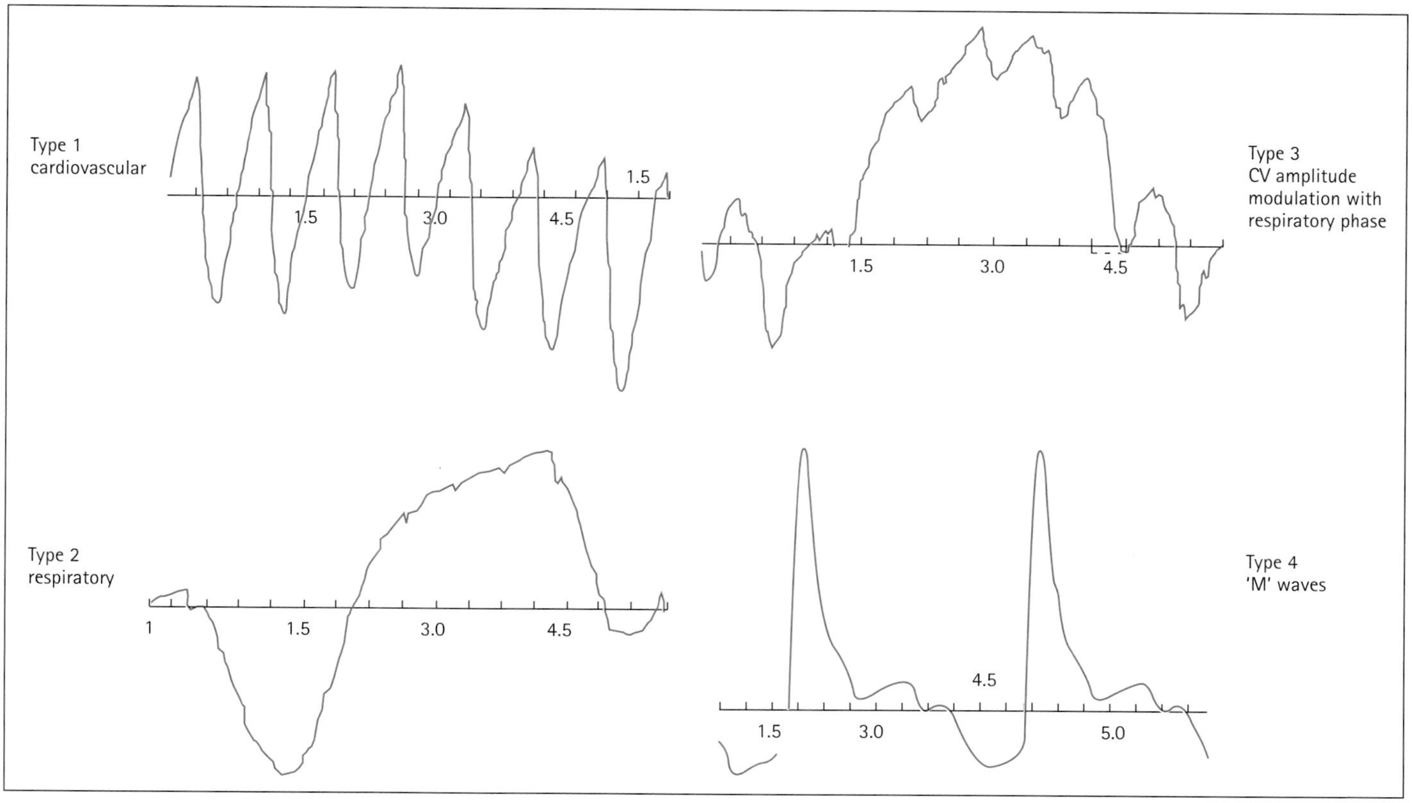

Figure 17.16 Classification of intra-aural pressure waves into four types.

Relatively large and rapid changes in intracranial pressure can result from everyday events such as coughing.[51] The intracranial–labyrinth impedance mismatch is important in limiting the amount of mechanical stress, and therefore possible intralabyrinthine damage, that may occur for a given intracranial pressure change.

A narrow cochlear aqueduct and compliant cochlear windows should reduce the risk of pressure-related structural

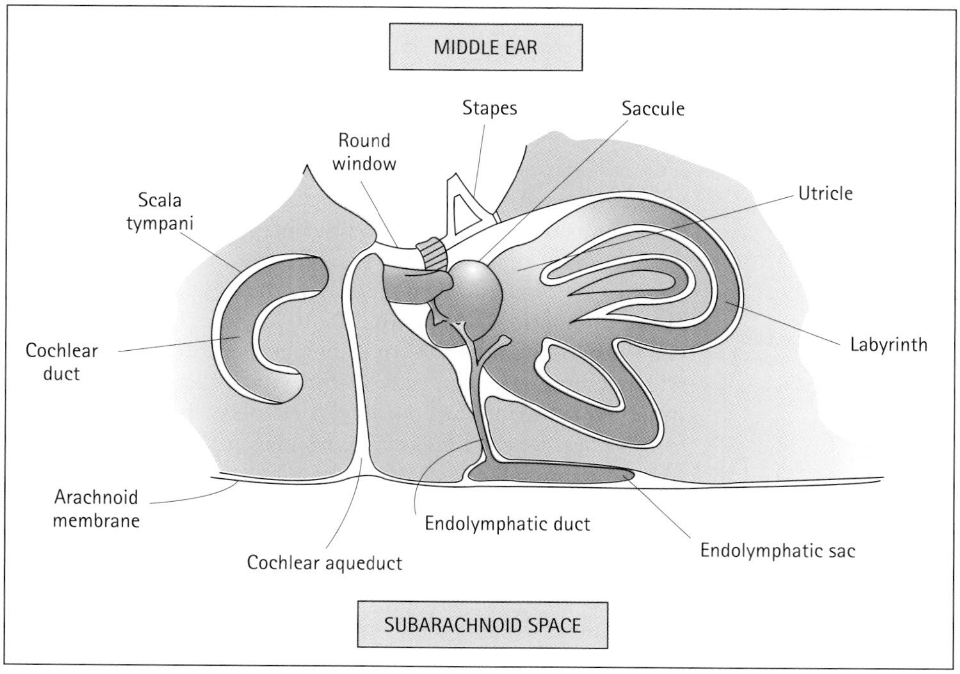

Figure 17.17 Schematic of the cochlea showing the pressure communication routes between the intracranial fluid and the inner ear.

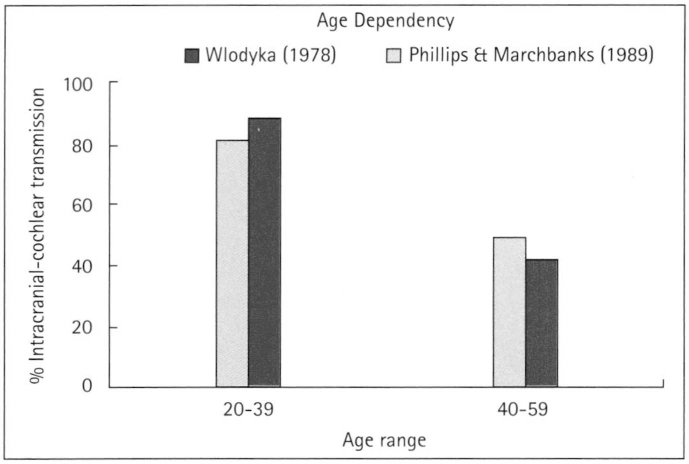

Figure 17.18 A comparison of age related histological measurement of cochlear aqueduct patency[12] with functional patency assessment using TMD measurements and induced changes in intracranial pressure with posture. (Adapted from Phillips and Marchbanks. *Br J Audiol* 1989; **23**: 279–84.[25])

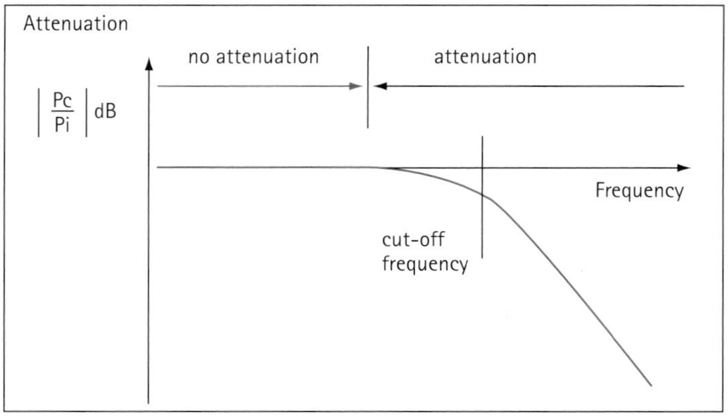

Figure 17.20 A simple model of the cochlear aqueduct considers it in terms of a low pass filter. This allows low frequency intracranial pressure waves to pass to the cochlear with little or no attenuation and high frequency pressure waves to be attenuated. An example of a high frequency intracranial pressure wave may be an impulsive pressure change with couching or sneezing where the filter characteristics afford the cochlea protection from mechanical damage.

damage, such as perilymphatic fistulae (Figure 17.21). In practice, this should mean that the risk of damage will be increased by any process that reduces the compliance of one or both of the cochlear windows, such as extremes of middle ear pressure resulting from Eustachian tube dysfunction combined with barometric pressure changes. Clinically, this may be seen in terms of perilymphatic fistulae resulting from barotrauma. The susceptibility to damage should also increase in cases where the baseline intracranial pressure is abnormal, such as with intracranial hypertension. Weider and Saunders provide a number of clinical examples of this in patients with a predisposition to recurrent perilymphatic fistulae and who were found to have chronic raised intracranial pressure, i.e. pseudotumor cerebri (BIH).[1,2] Treatment for the intracranial hypertension reduced the occurrence of perilymphatic fistulae.

A review of this topic would not be complete without acknowledging the extensive investigations undertaken and the significant contributions made by other researchers, including

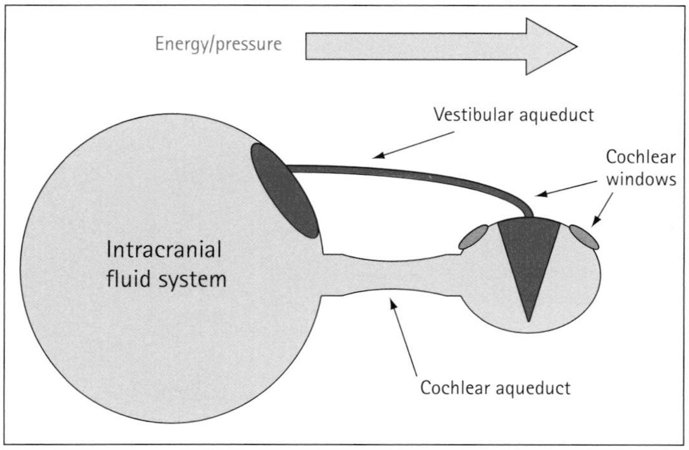

Figure 17.19 Schematic showing intracranial/labyrinthine fluid interactions.

Böhmer and research groups in Sweden.[9,11,48,50] Carlborg et al conclude that 'the cochlear aqueduct patency is the single most important factor with respect to the pressure transfer from the cerebrospinal fluid to the perilymph'. The work of this group indicates that the characteristics of the cochlear aqueduct are likely to be quite complex. In particular, animal studies show that a patent aqueduct allows faster pressure equilibration between the intracranial and cochlear fluids in the case of reduced intracranial pressure compared with an increased pressure. This seems to suggest an easier flow of fluid towards the cochlea than towards the cerebrospinal compartment.[52] Whether the same situation exists in humans needs to be established, and the TMD technique is likely to play a role in this research. If this asymmetry of intracranial–cochlear pressure exchange exists, then the perpetually changing intracranial pressure should theoretically create pressure differentials between the intracranial fluids, perilymph and endolymph. Are these pressure differentials important in the pathogenesis of endolymphatic hydrops, or are they merely incidental to the physiology of the inner ear? It is clear that we are only at the beginning of our understanding of intralabyrinthine fluid interactions.

In 1999, I published a set of hypotheses which relate to the above interactions (Appendix 1).[53] Clearly, as hypotheses these are merely statements of what may be possible, and only time will tell how relevant these are to our understanding of the inner ear system. What our work has shown is that we can no longer consider the inner ear hydromechanics in isolation from the intracranial fluid system or the middle ear.

The clinical perspective

The clinical findings from patients with known intracranial hypertension clearly demonstrate interaction with the vestibu-

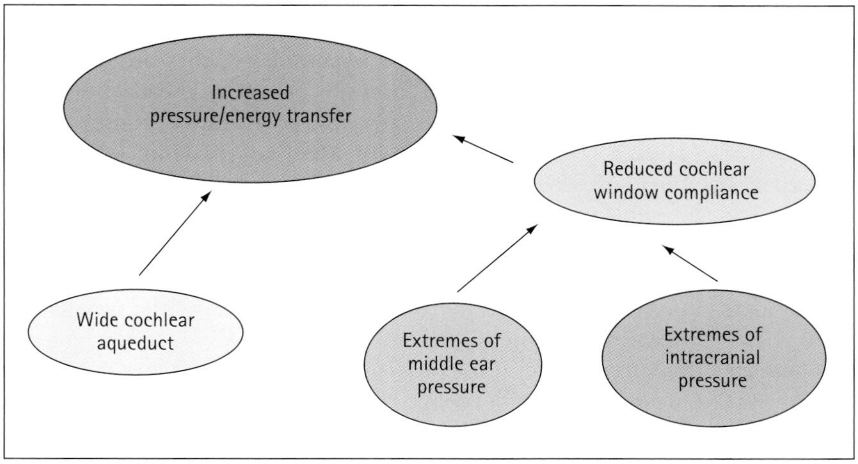

Figure 17.21 Schematic of theoretical factors which increase the likelihood of intracranial pressure waves transferring to the labyrinth with little or no attenuation. These factors therefore increase the potential of mechanical damage to the inner ear.

lar system at a peripheral level. A priori, it is reasonable to assume that the intracranial cardiovascular pulse and other intracranial activity do directly stimulate the vestibular system. A number of centres have independently proposed these interactions with the vestibular system, and the site of interaction is hypothesized to be the saccule or utricle.[39,40] Further support comes from research showing that low-frequency pressure waves entering the labyrinth through the cochlear windows cause a vestibular response.[35–37] It is also found that a middle ear overpressure may cause vertigo in otologically normal ears.[54,55] It is difficult to explain this phenomenon in terms other than the effect of cochlear window compliance on intracranial–labyrinthine impedance mismatch as discussed earlier, and this should clearly be the subject of future research.

Likewise, are these intracranial pressure waves being perceived as internally generated sounds? Adult patients suffering from BIH commonly report having a low-frequency tinnitus. This is often reported as a 'rushing', 'water' or 'wind-like' noise, and some patients reported the tinnitus as having characteristics which are synchronous with their heartbeat—'sounds like a steam train' or 'I can hear my pulse and it gets worse with physical activity'. It seems likely that some people perceived the low frequencies associated with the intracranial cardiovascular pulse. Are the higher-frequency components due to fluid turbulence as the intracranial pressure wave traverses regions of narrowing within the cochlear aqueduct? This may explain why adults with intracranial hypertension frequently report tinnitus, whereas children and adolescents rarely do—in children, we expect the cochlear aqueduct to be wider and therefore favour laminar rather than turbulent fluid flow. Otoacoustical emissions are found to be intracranial–cochlear pressure dependent.[17] Are otoacoustical emissions being modulated on a second-to-second basis by intracranial pressure waves and can this be perceived by some as tinnitus? At present, we can only speculate, and only research will tell us which aspects of intracranial–labyrinthine hydrodynamics are important and which can be ignored.

Audiovestibular dysfunction, tinnitus and hearing loss

Understanding the associations between intracranial pressure and audiovestibular dysfunction is of key importance for correct diagnosis of certain audiovestibular disorders. The clinical aspects of this and the interactions between the intracranial and labyrinthine fluids are of interest to researchers worldwide. These have been the topic of three international meetings and two books.[56,57]

An early study was undertaken at Southampton, where a group of 34 patients with confirmed BIH were seen over a period of 6 years.[38] In 29 patients, an open connection between the intracranial and perilymphatic fluids could be demonstrated using the CCFP analyser. Of these patients, 16 (55%) complained of tinnitus and 11 (38%) suffered from vertigo. Unilateral tinnitus was reported by 6 (21%), and it was bilateral in 10 (34%) cases. Tinnitus of a low-frequency nature with pulsatile characteristics was reported by 9 (31.0%) patients. When present, vertigo was principally objective in nature, as opposed to general imbalance, which occurred with most patients. However, subsequent clinical trials on a wider population showed that general imbalance is the most common feature, and vertigo will only occasionally occur and, in particular, in less than the 38% reported in the above paper. For example, my patients sometimes report the need to 'sight' a distant object to walk towards when outside, as otherwise they will deviate or even stumble 'sideways'.

Sismanis commented that the most common aetiologies for pulsatile tinnitus are idiopathic intracranial hypertension (BIH pseudotumour cerebri), glomus tumours, and carotid atherosclerosis.[58] He considers that atherosclerotic carotid artery disease is the most common cause of pulsatile tinnitus in patients older than 50 years of age, especially when associated risk factors for atherosclerosis exist—such as hypertension, angina, hyperlipidaemia, diabetes mellitus, and smoking. The aetiology in younger females is more likely to be ideopathic intracranial hypertension. We can broaden pulsatile tinnitus to include the tinnitus with low-frequency characteristics, as described above.

Hearing loss with intracranial hypertension has been reported by a number of researchers, including Ernst et al, and if the loss exists it appears to be a combination of conductive and sensorineural.[59] Figure 17.22 shows a typical low-frequency hearing loss from a Southampton patient with BIH. Similar low-frequency and also fluctuating hearing losses have been found by Sismanis, and the loss will reduce or completely recover when cerebrospinal fluid is removed at the time of lumbar puncture.[60] Most patients do not have such a marked hearing loss, and in many cases no hearing loss exists or is perhaps subclinical.

The pathophysiology underlying the hearing loss is unclear. A conductive component should be expected, since increased perilymphatic pressure will reduce the compliance of the round and oval windows. Other postulates for the hearing loss include a masking effect of the low-frequency tinnitus and even endolymphatic hydrops, which has been proposed by Walsted in her studies of hearing loss in cases of intracranial hypotension.[61,62]

Problems using symptoms to differentiate intracranial hypertension and Menière's-like disorders

It is evident that the otolaryngological symptoms associated with intracranial hypertension may be confused with those of Menière's-like disorders.

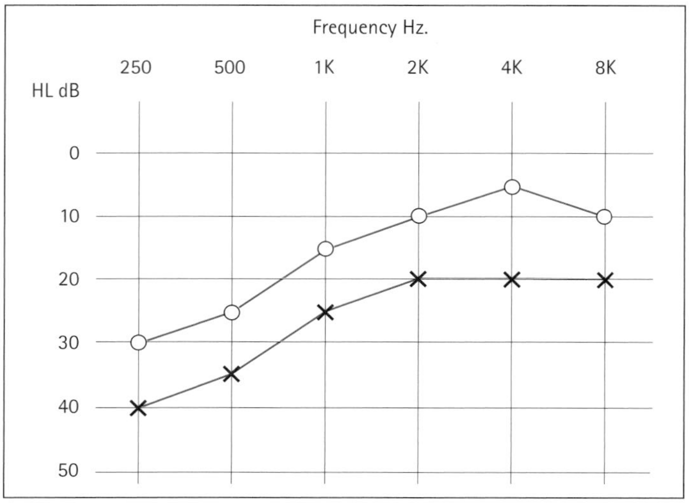

Figure 17.22 The audiogram for a 35-year old patient with intracranial hypertension, which shows a mild low frequency hearing loss.

Furthermore, although headaches are the most common symptom found with intracranial hypertension, they are not infrequently absent, mild or non-specific. Also, headaches often accompany vertiginous episodes or tinnitus. Rassekh and Harker reported that 22% of Menière's patients suffer from migraine, and this increases to 81% for those with so-called vestibular Menière's.[63]

Visual problems and papilloedema are further important pointers to underlying intracranial hypertension.[64] However, in one of the few otolaryngological clinics where BIH is regularly diagnosed, Sismanis found that only 4/20 (20%) patients reported actual visual problems.[60] It is also recognized that the absence of papilloedema may not be taken to indicate the absence of raised intracranial pressure.[65] It is reported that clinically significant changes in the fundus which are recognizable as papilloedema are only apparent in a minority of patients (5–10%) with raised intracranial pressure, and then only after a prolonged period of several days or even weeks.[65]

This may leave the otolaryngological symptoms of intracranial hypertension as the main reason for referrals from the general practitioner to the specialist consultant. Round and Keane studied a series of patients with confirmed intracranial hypertension.[47] They concluded that, in some patients, symptoms such as joint pain, neck stiffness and tinnitus may be better indications of increased intracranial pressure than the usually accepted headache or visual obscurities. Wang et al presented the results from a case–control study in a headache centre of idiopathic intracranial hypertension without papilloedema.[66]

Of all the neurological and audiological symptoms, they found that pulsatile tinnitus was the strongest indicator for idiopathic intracranial hypertension without papilloedema and, furthermore, that pulsatile tinnitus was associated with the prognosis in terms of a poor outcome.

Milhorat et al, in their study of 364 symptomatic patients with Chiari I malformation, provided an intriguing insight into the underlying aetiology in some cases of idiopathic intracranial hypertension and perhaps in some cases of Menière's-like disease.[67] Of the 364 patients tested, a total of 269 patients (74%) experienced otoneurological disturbances which included one or more of the following symptoms: dizziness including vertigo, peripheral vestibular dysfunction and disequilibrium, pressure in the ears, tinnitus, low-frequency hearing loss or hyperacusis, vertigo, and oscillopsia. In their opinion, a significant proportion of their patients had a diagnosis which was fully consistent with Menière's disease and endolymphatic hydrops. They considered this to suggest that Chiari I malformation alters the cerebrospinal fluid hydromechanics in such a manner as to cause disturbances of the cerbrospinal fluid–perilymph dynamics.

Undiagnosed intracranial hypertension

The actual prevalence of undiagnosed intracranial hypertension existing in general medical practice or the otolaryngological clinic is as yet unknown. The generally accepted low incidence of 1 case of BIH per 100 000 population per year cited by Wall and George cannot be taken as representative of undiagnosed intracranial hypertension, which is likely to be significantly more common in certain groups of the population, for a number of reasons.[68] First, the condition mostly affects women within the age range of 14–45, and there will be a cohort of women patients in whom the condition is never correctly diagnosed. Second, the diagnosis of BIH largely depends on a referral for papilloedema. However, as described above, for each patient with papilloedema there could be 10 or more patients with intracranial hypertension without papilloedema. Added to this, unless the visual condition is progressive, detection of papilloedema may be a lucky event dependent on a visit to a vigilant optician—of the first 10 patients seen in the latest BIH series at Southampton, half have been referred to neurology from opticians. Self-referral by the patient is also highly unlikely, because papilloedema normally goes unnoticed unless a significant visual deficit has developed.

It is now recognized that the misdiagnosis of intracranial hypertension is not just occurring in otolaryngology. Studies have shown that patients with intracranial hypertension are being referred to headache clinics, and the condition is being missed because of one of the key symptoms, papilloedema, is absent.[66] In a study conducted at the Houston Headache Clinic, all patients with refractory chronic daily headache underwent lumbar puncture, even though they did not have papilloedema. Of the 85 patients, 12 (14%) were found to have raised cerebrospinal fluid pressure.[69] Considering the difficulty of diagnosing ideopathic intracranial hypertension by symptoms alone, undiagnosed instances of this condition may be fairly common, particularly in specific patient populations such as women in the age range of 15–45 years.[70]

> The existence of a cohort of mostly female patients with undiagnosed intracranial hypertension has a cost implication for the health service and is also a 'quality of life' issue for the individual.

It should be remembered that, besides the symptoms described above, intracranial hypertension is normally associated with a general feeling of malaise and dulling of memory. These are disabling conditions and are often described by the patient as 'not feeling in this world' or 'feeling in a constant daze'. These symptoms alone may be so severe as to be incapacitating and to make it impossible for patients to continue with their occupation.

Current Southampton research aims to more clearly define the characteristics of the tinnitus, vertigo, aural fullness and hearing loss found with intracranial hypertension (Figure 17.23). This allows questionnaires and an 'at-risk profile' to be developed to help identify patients with intracranial hypertension and to allow cross-referral to neurology.

Low-frequency tinnitus of a pulsatile and/or 'whooshing' 'sea-like' nature appears to be the key symptom for diagnosing intracranial hypertension, and in many cases may be the only defining symptom. If present, gentle compression of the internal jugular vein will often reduce the intensity of the tinnitus or even cause a complete cessation. Likewise, in cases of unilateral tinnitus, turning the head to the ipsilateral side will often reduce or abolish the tinnitus.

The value of the TMD technique in finding undiagnosed intracranial hypertension

The TMD technique is used to screen for raised or low cochlear fluid pressure (Figure 17.24). The technique can be used to establish whether or not there is an open connection between the intracranial fluids and the cochlear fluids. We do this simply by changing the posture of the person, which induces a change in intracranial pressure (Figure 17.1). If there is a corresponding change in cochlear pressure, it is assumed that a fluid connection exists. In this instance, a raised cochlear fluid pressure implies a raised intracranial fluid pressure. The next step is to use the technique to establish associations between periods of low or high intracranial pressures and the audiovestibular symptomatology and neurological symptomatology. Finally, the technique is used to monitor the success of any treatment in terms of controlling the intracranial pressure.[38] It is appropriate both for surgical treatments such as cerebrospinal shunts and for drug treatments such as steroids or diuretics. Since patients with treated intracranial hypertension remain 'at risk' of further occurrences, the TMD technique is also proving valuable for providing pressure assessments with long-term patient reviews.

Treatment

Patients with intracranial hypertension typically report immediate relief from the tinnitus on lumbar puncture. Long-term treatments include dietary management in terms of weight loss, if appropriate, and restricted salt intake. Medication includes diuretics such as acetazolamide, often in combination with a 1-week course of a steroid such as prednisolone. If this fails, then surgical treatments have been used for treating the audiovestibular symptomatology, and include cerebrospinal fluid drainage by either repeated lumbar puncture or

Predominantly female: at least 4:1, (female/male) ratio. The patient may be 20% or more overweight.

Typical age range: 18–45 years

Likely to be suffering from a low-frequency tinnitus which will be described as *'hum'*, *'roaring'*, *'whooshing'* or perhaps *'sea-like'*, with occasionally characteristics which are synchronous with the heart beat. About 60% of patients will report tinnitus, and of these about 60–70% (36–42% of total) will be of a low-frequency type. In cases of unilateral tinnitus, gentle compression of the internal jugular vein will often result in a reduction in the intensity of the tinnitus or even a complete cessation. Likewise turning the head to the ipsilateral side will often reduce the tinnitus.

Most patients will report a mild imbalance or 'unsteadiness on their feet'. About 40% of those with tinnitus will be suffering some form of objective vertigo. This will be described as episodes when the 'room appears to move' and this can last for several minutes and sometimes hours. This is often not fully developed rotary vertigo. The feeling is often associated with nausea, but only infrequently vomiting.

The patient will be suffering from a malaise which will often be associated with a 'deterioration in memory', 'mental slowing' or 'dulling of mind'. The patient will commonly report headaches; however, in most cases these headaches will be mild, (sometimes described as a *'dull'* headache). The headache may be associated with a pressure or fullness sensations in the head, ears or behind the eyes.

If investigated, papilloedema will only probably be found in less than 10% of cases. Interestingly, although visual deficits are often found, these or visual disturbances frequently go unreported by the patient. If these occur, they may include *'greying'* or *'tunnelling'* which may occur – as with other symptoms – with change of posture and subsequently last for several minutes.

Low-frequency and/or fluctuating hearing losses are also symptoms, but only rarely are significant enough to be noticed by patients.

The most distinguishing associations of intracranial hypertension are probably *'female'* and *'low-frequency and/or pulsatile tinnitus'*. Nevertheless, if this latter symptom alone was taken for a clinical screen for this condition, then we would probably miss over 50% of the patients.

Figure 17.23 A typical profile for sub-clinical intracranial hypertension.

lumbar–peritoneal shunts.[1,66,71] As our understanding of intracranial–inner fluid interactions improves, we are beginning to see the advent of new surgical treatments such as the posterior fossa cochlear aqueduct occlusion procedure, which appears to relieve certain forms of tinnitus and vertigo.[2]

TMD measurements and Menière's disease

The TMD analyser allows a fuller understanding of audiovestibular manifestations and consequences of intracranial hyper/hypotension. This in turn allows for the differential diagnosis of Menière's-like diseases of the labyrinth from those in which a combination of tinnitus, vertigo and hearing loss is symptomatic of abnormal intracranial pressure and of a retrocochlear disorder.[38,71]

Use of the TMD technique on Menière's patients with the classical triad of symptoms appears to show normal perilymphatic pressure.[27,72,73] There may, however, be exceptions. Using the same technique, Ernst et al have observed marked changes in pressure in a patient during a Menière's attack, and other studies suggest that there may be differences with the Menière's patient compared with the normal subject.[72,74–78] Some of these differences appear to be associated with the pressure transfer between the intracranial and cochlear fluids.

Currently, the principle use of the TMD technique with Menière's patients is to indirectly support the diagnosis in terms of eliminating the possibility of intracranial hypertension as being the underlying cause for the symptoms.[38] In the future, direct diagnostic TMD tests may be possible.[77,78]

Other applications of non-invasive intracranial pressure assessment

There are several other interesting applications for non-invasive intracranial pressure assessment. For example, research indicates that raised pressure is a factor in patients with X-linked progressive mixed deafness syndrome in association with perilymphatic gusher during stapes surgery.[79]

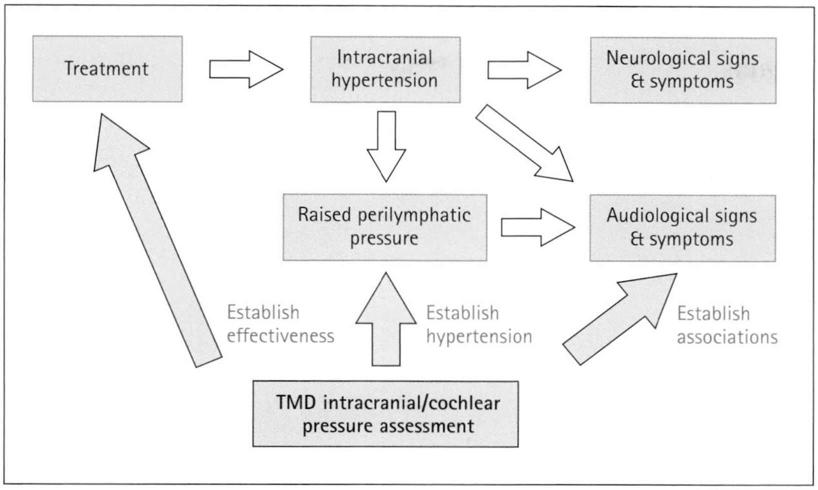

Figure 17.24 Clinical use of the TMD technique for cerebral and cochlear pressure assessment.

Intraventricular shunt assessment

The clinical signs and symptoms associated with abnormal intracranial pressure in patients with hydrocephalus and/or cerebrospinal shunts are often subtle and hard to diagnose. The difficulties of diagnosing shunt disorders are even greater in children, who are unable to describe symptoms clearly. Prior to the development of the TMD test, clinicians relied on the clinical history, presenting symptoms and pumping the shunt chamber. CT scanning and MR imaging have not proved conclusive for detecting shunt disorders.[80] The integrity of the shunt system and intracranial pressure status are, therefore, often unknown unless invasive measurements are carried out. Intermittent shunt blockages in a child, in particular, could go undetected for months or years, but may nevertheless affect the social and educational welfare of the child.

Studies with the TMD test in hydrocephalus and shunted patients have shown that TMD results vary with symptoms of shunt dysfunction and pre- and post-shunt revision surgery.[15,81–83] The test has also been useful in tracking intracranial pressure changes with fluctuating symptoms over periods of days or weeks.[84]

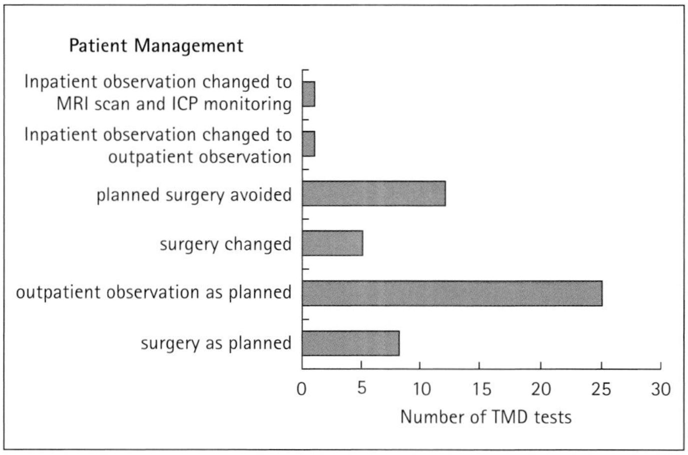

Figure 17.25 Intraventricular shunt assessment: a comparison of the proposed patient management before TMD testing with actual management after TMD testing.

Overall, TMD was 93% accurate, and conventional clinical assessment was 66% accurate. Additionally, the TMD test gave useful information where clinical suspicions were unclear. Figure 17.25 shows a comparison of proposed patient management before TMD testing with actual management after TMD testing. The key benefits of TMD testing include: long-term management of a hydrocephalic patient, monitoring shunt function and shunt revision, and differentiating raised from low intracranial pressure.[85]

Currently, the TMD technique is not a replacement for the invasive pressure measurement methods, but it is complementary and has a number of important advantages. One advantage is that measurements can be made as often as required and these can normally be undertaken on an outpatient basis. Another important advantage is that it is possible to differentiate patients with intracranial hypotension from those with hypertension. These conditions have similar symptom profiles, such as headaches, and it can be very difficult, looking at symptoms alone, to determine whether a person is suffering from low pressure or high pressure, or indeed whether their pressure is normal and they are suffering headaches for other reasons. A typical pressure history for a patient with hydrocephalus is shown in Figure 17.26.

Another cost benefit of the CCFP analyser and the TMD technique is in reducing the need for inpatient observations and allowing earlier than usual surgical intervention or hospital discharge.

Altitude and aerospace applications

Other applications of the TMD technique include the following:

- The investigation of changes in intracranial fluid with altitude. The objective of this study, which was undertaken on

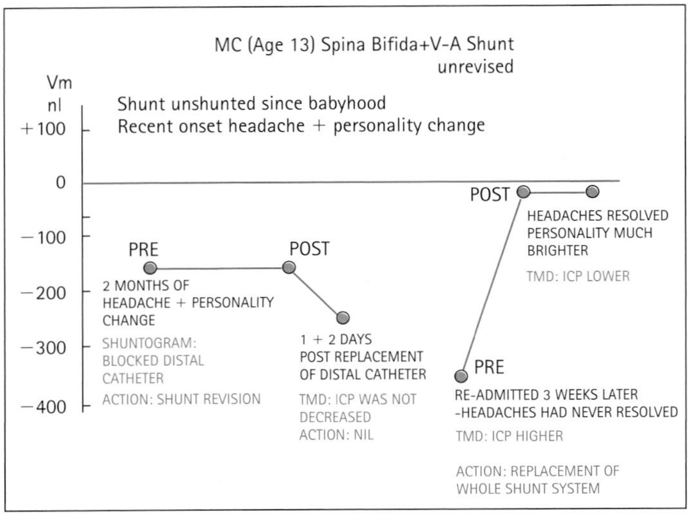

Figure 17.26 A typical TMD pressure history for a patient with hydrocephalus

Mount Everest, was to see whether there is any relationship between intracranial pressure and acute mountain sickness. No change was found in this respect, perhaps due to the lack of subjects; however, a relationship existed between the non-invasive measure of intracranial pressure and hypoxia.[86]

- Measuring changes in intracranial pressure with 'g' force on a centrifuge. A feasibility study at the Farnborough School of Aviation Medicine demonstrated that these measurements are a practical proposition (Figure 17.27).

The future of TMD measurements in space

The CCFP analyser and TMD technique now form part of a NASA programme to monitor changes in intracranial pressure and intra-aural pressure waves in astronauts during space shuttle missions. The objectives are to assess in-flight hypertensive intracranial pressure changes and the relationship with the symptomatology of space sickness. Further objectives are to monitor recovery from in-flight intracranial hypertension through immediate post-flight tests. Associations between the intracranial pressure and in-flight and post-flight headaches and vestibular dysfunction will be investigated.

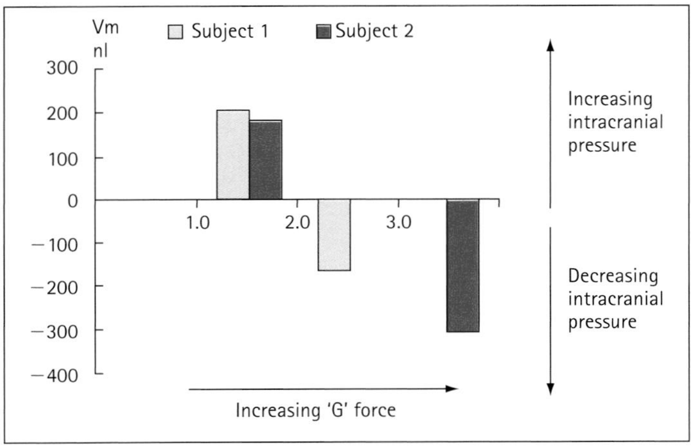

Figure 17.27 Changes in intracranial pressure expressed in terms of TMD (nl) with increasing *g* force on a centrifuge at the Farnborough School of Aviation Medicine.

Acknowledgements

I wish to thank 'Defeating Deafness', Hearing Research Trust for supporting this research.

Appendix 1: Principles of static and dynamic interactions between the middle ear, intracranial and intralabyrinthine fluids

On consideration of research into the intracranial–labyrinthine–middle ear mechanics and clinical research findings, I have proposed the following theorems:-

Theorem 1

Given a patent cochlear aqueduct, the intracranial pressure will always provide the reference pressure for the endolymph and perilymph within the limits set by:

- dynamics properties of the cochlear aqueduct
- resting tension of the Reissner's membrane.

Theorem 2

Given a patent cochlear aqueduct, pressure waves of intracranial origin will be transmitted to the labyrinth in a manner dependent on the:

- hydromechanical properties of the cochlear aqueduct
- mechanical properties of the cochlear windows
- middle ear pressure and any tension applied to the oval window via the ossicles.

Theorem 3

Direct stimulation of the vestibular system and manifestations of tinnitus can occur due to intra-aural amplitude and phase variations in transmitted intracranial pressure activity brought about by:

- raised intracranial pressure
- changes in the compliance of the cochlear windows such as those secondary to changes in middle ear pressure.

Theorem 4

Intracranial–labyrinthine fluid impedance mismatch is important in limiting the degree of mechanical stress and therefore possible labyrinthine structural damage which may occur for given pressure pulses of intracranial or middle ear origins.

Theorem 5

Differential pressures may exist between the cerebral fluid, endolymph and perilymph due to:

- the existence in some cases of a finite opening pressure across the lumen of the cochlear and vestibular aqueducts
- non-linear hydromechanical properties of the cochlear and vestibular aqueducts which allow pressure waves of intracranial origin to pass more readily to the labyrinth in one direction compared to the other direction.

Theorem 6

In consideration of the non-linear properties of the cochlear and vestibular aqueducts (Theorem 5), the perpetual pressure fluctuations within the cerebral fluid of cardiovascular and respiratory origins may produce sustainable pressure differences between the cerebral, endolymphatic and perilymphatic fluids which are important to:

- normal labyrinthine physiology and fluid homeostasis
- the pathogenesis of conditions such as endolymphatic hydrops.

Theorem 7

The physiology and pathophysiology of the labyrinth will be dependent on changes in and interactions occurring between the mean intracranial pressure, and pressure waves of cardiovascular and respiratory origins, and also:

- the substantial pressure increases which occur with intracranial plateau waves
- airway flow restrictions and nasal obstruction.

References

1. Weider DJ, Saunders RL, Musiek FE. Repair of a cerebrospinal fluid perilymphatic fistula primary through the middle ear and secondarily by occluding the cochlear aqueduct. *Otolaryngol Head Neck Surg* 1991; **105**: 35–9.
2. Weider DJ, Saunders RL. Recurrent perilymphatic fistula as the initial and prime symptom of pseudotumour cerebri: diagnosis and management with lumbar–peritoneal shunt—Report of three cases. In: Ernst A, Marchbanks R, Samii R (eds). *Intracranial and Intralabyrinthine Fluids: Basic Aspect and Clinical Applications*. Berlin, Heidelberg: Springer Verlag, 1996.
3. Marchbanks RJ. *MMS-10 Tympanic Displacement Analyser in Research and Clinical Practice: The Users Handbook*. Lymington: Marchbanks Measurement Systems Ltd, 1993.
4. Moller AR. Effect of tympanic muscle activity on measurement of the ear drum, acoustic impedance and cochlear microphonics. *Acta Otolaryngol* 1964; **58**: 525–9.
5. Casselbrant M, Ingelstedt S, Ivarsson A. Volume displacement of the tympanic membrane at stapedial reflex activity in different postures. *Acta Otolaryngol* 1977; **85**: 1–9.
6. Yonowitz A, Harris JD. Ear drum displacement following stapedius muscle contraction. *Acta Otolaryngol* 1976; **81**: 1–7.
7. Marchbanks RJ. A study of tympanic membrane displacement. PhD, Brunel University, 1980.
8. Brask T. Extratympanic manometry in man. *Scand Audiol Suppl* 1978; 7.
9. Casselbrant M, Ingelstedt S, Ivarsson A. Volume displacement of the tympanic membrane in the sitting position as a function of middle ear muscle activity. *Acta Otolaryngol* 1977; **84**: 402–13.
10. Tweed JJ. Development of a model of stapes motion during contraction of the stapedius muscle. MSc Dissertation, Institute of Sound and Vibration Research, Southampton University, 1985.
11. Densert O, Ivarsson A, Pedersen K. The influence of perilymphatic pressure on the displacement of the tympanic membrane. *Acta Otolaryngol* 1977; **84**: 220–6.
12. Wlodyka J. Studies on cochlear aqueduct patency. *Ann Otolaryngol* 1978, **87**: 22–7.
13. Marchbanks RJ, Reid A, Martin AM, Brightwell AP, Bateman D. The effect of raised intracranial pressure on intracochlear fluid pressure: three case studies. *Br J Audiol* 1987; **21**: 127–30.
14. Reid A, Marchbanks RJ, Burge DM et al. The relationship between intracranial pressure and tympanic membrane displacement. *Br J Audiol* 1990; **24**: 123–9.
15. Samuel M, Marchbanks RJ, Burge DM. Tympanic membrane displacement test in regular assessment in eight children with shunted hydrocephalus. *J Neurosurg* 1998; **88**: 983–95.
16. Krast R. A new method for noninvasive measurement of short term cerebrospinal fluid pressure changes in humans. *J Neurol* 1985; **232**: 260–1.
17. Avan P, Buki B, Lemaire JJ, Dordain M, Chazal J. Otoacoustic emissions: a new tool for monitoring intracranial pressure. In: Ernst A, Marchbanks R, Samii M (eds). *Intracranial and Intralabyrinthine Fluids: Basic Aspect and Clinical Applications*. Springer Verlag, 1996.
18. Froehlich P, Ferber C, Remond J et al. Lack of association between transiently evoked otoacoustic emission amplitude and experimentation linked-factors (repeat acoustic stimulation, cerebrospinal fluid pressure, supine and sitting positions, alertness level). *Hear Res* 1994; **75**: 184–90.
19. Marchbanks RJ. Implications of measuring intracranial pressure: emerging technology provides new challenges for audiological practice. *Hear Instrum* 1991; **42**(9): 30–1.
20. Banister K, Chambers I, Mendelow D. Clinical evaluation of the MMS-10 Tympanic Membrane Displacement Analyser in the non-invasive assessment of raised intracranial pressure. In: *Pro-*

ceedings of the 11th International Symposium of Intracranial Pressure, Cambridge 2000: 226.
21. Flynn S, Marchbanks RJ, Burge D. The application of the tympanic membrane displacement (TMD) test as part of the clinical service for hydrocephalus patients. In: Reid A, Marchbanks R (eds). *Intracranial and Inner Ear Physiology and Pathophysiology*. Whurr Publishers, 1998.
22. Wunderlich K, Brinker T, Ernst A. The correlation of tympanic membrane displacement measurements to direct intracranial pressure recordings in cat. In: Ernst A, Marchbanks R, Samii M (eds). *Intracranial and Intralabyrinthine Fluids: Basic Aspect and Clinical Applications*. Berlin, Heidelberg: Springer Verlag, 1996.
23. Reid A, Marchbanks RJ, Bateman D, Martin AM, Brightwell AP, Pickard J. Mean intracranial pressure monitoring by a non-invasive audiological technique—a pilot study. *J Neurol Neurosurg Psychiatry* 1989; **52**: 610–12.
24. Moss SM, Marchbanks RJ, Reid A, Burge D, Martin AM. Comparison of intracranial pressure between spina bifida patients and normal subjects using non-invasive pressure assessment technique. *Kinderchirurg* 1989; **44**: (suppl I): 29–30.
25. Phillips AJ, Marchbanks RJ. Effects of posture and age on tympanic membrane displacement. *Br J Audiol* 1989; **23**: 279–84.
26. Murthy G, Marchbanks RJ, Watenpaugh DE, Meyer U, Eliashberg N, Hargens AR. Increased intracranial pressure in humans during simulated microgravity. *Physiologist* 1992; 35(1 Suppl) S-184–5.
27. Rosingh HJ, Wit HP, Albers FWJ. Perilymphatic pressure dynamics following posture change in patients with Meniere's disease and in normal hearing subjects. *Acta Otolaryngol Stockh* 1998; **118**(1): 1–5.
28. Rosingh HJ, Wit HP, Albers FWJ. Non-invasive perilymphatic pressure measurement in normal hearing subjects using the MMS-10 Tympanic Displacement Analyser. *Acta Otolaryngol (Stockh)* 1996; **116**: 382–7.
29. Marchbanks RJ, Reid A. Cochlear and cerebral fluid pressure: their interrelationships and control mechanisms. *Br J Audiol* 1990; **24**: 179–87.
30. Sørensen PS, Hammer M, Gjerris F, Lundberg J. 24-hour cerebrospinal fluid levels of vasopressin in hydrocephalic patients. *Regul Pept* 1985, **10**: 115–26.
31. Andreasson L, Harris S, Ivarsson A. Pulse volume recordings in outer ear canal in pulse synchronous tinnitus. *Acta Otolaryngol* 1978; **86**: 241–7.
32. Marchbanks RJ. Measurement of tympanic membrane displacement arising from aural cardiovascular activity, swallowing and intra-aural muscle reflex. *Acta Otolaryngol (Stockh)* 1984; **98**: 119–29.
33. Evans MJ, Bryan ME, Tempest W. Clinical application of low frequency sound. *Sound* 1971; **5**: 47–51.
34. Erlich MA, Lawson W. The incidence and significance of the Tullio phenomenon in man. *Otolaryngol Head Neck Surg* 1980; **88**: 630–5.
35. Kacker SK, Hinchcliffe R. Unusual Tullio phenomena. *J Laryngol* 1970; **84**: 155–66.
36. Hill Britton B. Vestibular responses to pressure variations: a review. *Otolaryngol, Head Neck Surg* 1986; **4**: 516–22.
37. Parker DE, von Gierke HE, Reschke M. Studies of acoustical stimulation of the vestibular system. *Aerospace Med* 1968; **39**: 1321–25.
38. Marchbanks, RJ. Why monitor perilymphatic pressure in Menière's disease? *Acta Otolaryngol (Stockh) Suppl* 1996; **526**: 27–9.
39. Marchbanks RJ. Hydromechanical interactions of the intracranial and intralabyrinthine fluids: In: Ernst A, Marchbanks R, Samii M. (eds). *Intracranial and Intralabyrinthine Fluids: Basic Aspect and Clinical Applications*. Berlin, Heidelberg: Springer Verlag, 1996.
40. Epley JM. Aberrant coupling of otolithic receptors: manifestations and assessment. In: Kaufman Arenberg I (ed). *Dizziness and Balance Disorders*. Amsterdam: Kugler Publications. 1993: 183–99.
41. Hughes M, Marchbanks RJ. Characteristics of infrasonic otoacoustics emissions generated by the cardiovascular system. In: Reid A, Marchbanks R (eds). *Intracranial and Inner Ear Physiology and Pathophysiology*. London: Whurr Publishers, 1998.
42. Davson H, Welch K, Segal MB. *The Physiology and Pathophysiology of the Cerebrospinal Fluid*. Edinburgh: Churchill Livingstone, 1987.
43. Avezaat CJJ, Van Eijndhoven JHM, Wyper DJ. Cerebrospinal fluid pulse pressure and intracranial volume–pressure relationship. *J Neurol Neurosurg Psychiatry* 1997; **42**: 687–700.
44. Marchbanks, RJ. Aberrant intra-aural pressure waves: exciting developments in TMD research. *Br Society of Audiology Annual Conference*, Winchester 2001, abstracts, p. 14.
45. Sismanis A. Otologic manifestations of benign intracranial hypertension syndrome: diagnosis and management. *Laryngoscope* 1987; **97**: 1–17.
46. Tandon PN, Sinha A, Kacker RK, Saxena RK, Singh K. Auditory function in raised intracranial pressure. *J Neurol Sci* 1973; **18**: 455–67.
47. Round R, Keane JR. The minor symptoms of increased intracranial pressure: 101 patients with benign intracranial hypertension. *Neurology* 1998; **38(9)**: 1461–4.
48. Böhmer A. Hydrostatic pressure in the inner ear fluid compartments and its effects on inner ear pressure. *Acta Otolaryngol (Stockh)* Suppl 1993; **507**: 1–24.
49. Beentjes BIJ. The cochlear aqueduct and the pressure of the cerebrospinal and endolabyrinthine fluid *Acta Otolaryngol* 1972; **17**: 112–20.
50. Carlborg BIR, Konrádsson KS, Carlborg AH, Farmer JC, Densert O. Pressure transfer between the perilymph and the cerebrospinal fluid compartments in cats. *Am J Otol* 1992; **13**: 41–8.
51. Marchbanks RJ, Reid A. Cochlear and cerebrospinal fluid pressure: their interrelationships and control mechanisms. *Br J Audiol* 1990; **24**: 179–87.
52. Carlborg B, Densert O, Densert B. Functional patency of the cochlear aquaeduct. *Ann Otol Rhinol Laryngol* 1982; **91**: 202–15.
53. Marchbanks RJ. Principles of static and dynamic interactions between the middle ear, intracranial and intralabyrinthine fluids. First presented in entirety at the Irish Society of Audiology Meeting, Mater Hospital, Dublin, November 1999.
54. Ingelstedt A, Ivarsson A, Tjernström Ö. Vertigo due to relative overpressure in the middle ear. *Acta Otolaryngol (Stockh)* 1974; **78**: 1–14.
55. Tjernström Ö. Further studies on alternobaric vertigo. *Acta Otolaryngol (Stockh)* 1974; **78**: 221–31.

56. Ernst A, Marchbanks R, Samii M (eds.). *Intracranial and Intralabyrinthine Fluids: Basic Aspect and Clinical Applications*. Berlin, Heidelberg: Springer Verlag, 1996.
57. Reid A, Marchbanks R (eds.). *Intracranial and Inner ear physiology and pathophysiology*. London: Whurr Publishers, 1998.
58. Sismanis A. Pulsatile tinnitus. *Neurologist* 1998; **4**(2): 66–76.
59. Ernst A. Diagnostics of perilymphatic hypertension. In: Ernst A, Marchbanks R, Samii M (eds). *Intracranial and Intralabyrinthine Fluids: Basic Aspect and Clinical Applications*. Berlin, Heidelberg: Springer Verlag, 1996.
60. Sismanis A. Otologic manifestations of benign intracranial hypertension syndrome: diagnosis and management. *Laryngoscope* 1987; **97**: 1–17.
61. Walsted A, Salomon G, Thomsen J, Tos M. Hearing decrease after loss of cerebrospinal fluid. A new hydrops model? *Acta Otolaryngol (Stockh)* 1991; **111**: 468–76.
62. Walsted A, Nielsen OA, Borum P. Hearing loss after neurosurgery. The influence of low cerebrospinal fluid pressure. *J Laryngol Otol* 1994; **108**: 637–41.
63. Rassekh CH, Harker LA. The prevalence of migraine in Menière's disease. *Laryngoscope* 1992; **102**(2): 135–8.
64. Pickard JD. Which patients with benign intracranial hypertension can we help? In: Warlow CP, Garfield JF (eds.). *More Dilemmas in the Management of the Neurological Patients*. Edinburgh: Churchill-Livingston; 1987: 156–70.
65. Eifert B, Steffen H, Ascoff A, Kolling GH. Papilledema in cases of acute elevated intracranial pressure. In: Ernst A, Marchbanks R, Samii M (eds). *Intracranial and Intralabyrinthine Fluids: Basic Aspect and Clinical Applications*. Berlin, Heidelberg: Springer Verlag, 1996: 223–5.
66. Wang SJ, Silberstein SD, Patterson S, Young WB. Idiopathic intracranial hypertension without papilledema. *Neurology* 1998; **51**: 245–9.
67. Milhorat TH, Chou MW, Trinidad EM et al. Chiari I malformation redefined: clinical and radiographical findings for 364 symptomatic patients. *Neurosurgery* 1999; **44**(5): 1005–17.
68. Wall M, George D. Idiopathic intracranial hypertension, a prospective study of 50 patients. *Brain* 1991; **114**: 155–64.
69. Mathew NT, Ravishankar K, Sanin LC. Coexistence of migraine and idiopathic intracranial hypertension without papilledema. *Neurology* 1996; **46**: 1226–1230.
70. Reid A, Cottingham CA, Marchbanks RJ. The prevalence of perilymphatic hypertension in subjects with tinnitus: a pilot study. *J Scand Audiol* 1993; **22**: 61–3.
71. Weider DJ, Musiek FE. Recurrent perilymphatic fistula in patients with possible patent cochlear aqueduct: role for cochlear aqueduct blockage—report of five cases. In: Reid A, Marchbanks R (eds.) *Intracranial and Inner Ear Physiology and Pathophysiology*. London: Whurr Publishers, 1998.
72. Gosepath K, Maurer J, Pelster H, Thews O, Mann W. Pressure relation between intracranial and intracochlear fluids in patients with disease of the inner ear. *Laryngorhinootology*. 1995; **74**: 145–9.
73. Rosingh HJ, Wit HP, Albers FWJ. Non-invasive perilymphatic pressure measurements in patients with Meniere's disease. *Acta Otolaryngol* 1996; **21**: 335–8.
74. Ernst A, Issing PR, Bohndorf M. The non-invasive assessment of intracochlear pressure—II: Findings in patients suffering from Menière's disease, fluctuating deep tone hearing and peripheral–vestibular attacks of vertigo. *Laryngorhinootology*. 1995; **74**(1): 13–20.
75. Marchbanks RJ, Martin AM. Infra-sonic measurement of human intra-cochlear hydrodynamics: variations with age, sex and audiovestibular pathology. ISVR Technical Report 148 Southampton: Institute of Sound and Vibration Research, Southampton University, 1986: 10–20.
76. Ernst A, Bohndorf M, Lenarz T. The non-invasive assessment of intracochlear pressure—III: Case reports on patients suffering from intracochlear hypertension and hypotension. *Laryngorhinootology*. 1995; **74**(1): 150–4.
77. Bouccara D, Ferrary E, El-Garem H, Couloigner V, Coudert C, Sterkers O. Inner ear pressure in Meniere's disease and fluctuating hearing loss determined by tympanic membrane displacement analysis. *Audiology*. 1998; **37(5)**: 255–61.
78. Konrádsson KS, Nielsen LH, Carlborg BIR, Borgkvist B. Pressure transfer between intracranial and cochlear fluids in patients with Meniere's disease. *Laryngoscope* 2000; **110**: 264–8.
79. Ernst A, Snik A, Mylanus I, Cremers C. Noninvasive assessment of the intralabyrinthine pressure: a new technique applied to patients with X-linked progressive mixed deafness syndrome with perilymphatic gusher during stapes surgery. *Arch Otolaryngol Head Neck Surg* 1995; **121**: 926–929.
80. Watkins L, Hayward R, Andar U, Harkness W. The diagnosis of blocked cerebrospinal fluid shunts: a prospective study of a paediatric neurological unit. *Child Nervous System* 1994; **10**(2): 87–90.
81. Moss SM, Marchbanks RJ, Burge DM. Non-invasive assessment of ventricular shunt function using the tympanic membrane displacement measurement technique. *Z Kinderchirurg* 1990; **45**(Suppl I): 26–8.
82. Samuel M, Marchbanks RJ, Burge DM. Tympanic membrane displacement test in regular assessment of children with shunted hydrocephalus. *Eur J Pediatr Surg* 1996; **I**(suppl) 47–51.
83. Samuel M, Marchbanks RJ, Burge DM. Quantitative assessment of intracranial pressure by the tympanic membrane displacement audiometric technique in children with shunted hydrocephalus. *Eur J Pediatr Surg* 1998; **8**: 1–9.
84. Moss SM, Marchbanks RJ, Burge DM. Long term assessment of intracranial pressure using the tympanic membrane displacement measurement technique. *Eur J Paediatr Surg* 1991; Supp I: 25–6.
85. Burge D, Flynn S, Marchbanks R. Assessment of the clinical value of the tympanic membrane displacement (TMD) test in children with shunted hydrocephalus. In: Ernst A, Marchbanks R, Samii M (eds.). *Intracranial and Intralabyrinthine Fluids: Basic Aspect and Clinical Applications*. Berlin, Heidelberg: Springer Verlag, 1996.
86. Wright AD, Imray CHE, Morrissey MSC, Marchbanks RJ, Bradwell AR. Intracranial pressure at high altitude and acute mountain sickness. *Clin Sci* 1995; **89**: 201–4.

18 The auditory processing of speech

Andrew Faulkner

Aims

The aims of this chapter are

- to outline the fundamental acoustic structures that convey meaning in speech and the wide variability in the acoustic realization of speech sounds that auditory processing of speech has to contend with;
- to give an overview of the auditory processing of speech by both people with normal hearing and those who are significantly affected by hearing impairment.

Introductory remarks

Speech is generated by coordinated motor activity that produces a stream of acoustic information to represent a meaningful message. The task of speech reception is to analyse this acoustic information stream so as to decode the talker's message, isolating it, if necessary, from other acoustic information (or noise). Visual cues from the movements of the speech articulators, and from facial expressions and gestures, also contribute. The extraction of meaning from speech is a complex and incompletely understood process. The decoding of speech ultimately entails the identification of meaning in terms of words, syntactic structure, and other linguistic aspects. In audiology, however, the primary interest lies in the impact of damage to the auditory periphery on the decoding of speech, and the effects that this has on speech intelligibility. As Figure 18.1 shows, with more severe degrees of hearing loss, these effects are substantial.

It is conceptually convenient to consider the reception of speech in terms of the decoding of auditory information provided by the peripheral analysis of the acoustic input. Within this acoustic input, we can imagine segments of information that each broadly correspond to individual speech sounds. These segments are known as phonemes. This is not to assume that speech perception necessitates the isolation and decoding of each such segment. Rather, a partial decoding of phoneme segments is generally sufficient, given the high predictability of spoken messages, which allows imperfectly identified segments

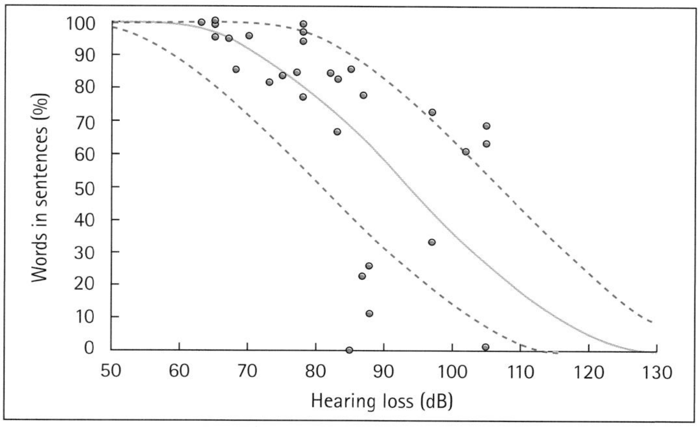

Figure 18.1 The impact of hearing impairment on speech recognition. The figure represents the number of words that can be recognized from simple sentences in the quiet by hearing-impaired adults using hearing aids. The solid curve shows the mean performance as a function of average hearing loss (at 500, 1000 and 2000 Hz). The dashed lines show the expected statistical variation about the mean. Circles are scores from individual subjects. (After Boothroyd. *Acta oto-laryngologica* 1990; **469** (Suppl 1): 166–71.[1]).

to be filled in by the listener. Where hearing impairment develops after the process of language development is essentially complete (at around age 5), it is essentially only peripheral auditory analysis that is affected by hearing impairment, this analysis being a prerequisite for the phonemic decoding of speech (Figure 18.2). However, in children whose hearing is severely impaired during or prior to the completion of language development, the auditory processing of speech is further hampered. This arises from the lack of a completely developed mental representation of the language-specific mappings between auditory patterns of speech and meaningful linguistic elements.

The acoustic basis of speech: source–filter model

The patterns of sound that we recognize as speech are generated by two distinct component processes: the generation of an

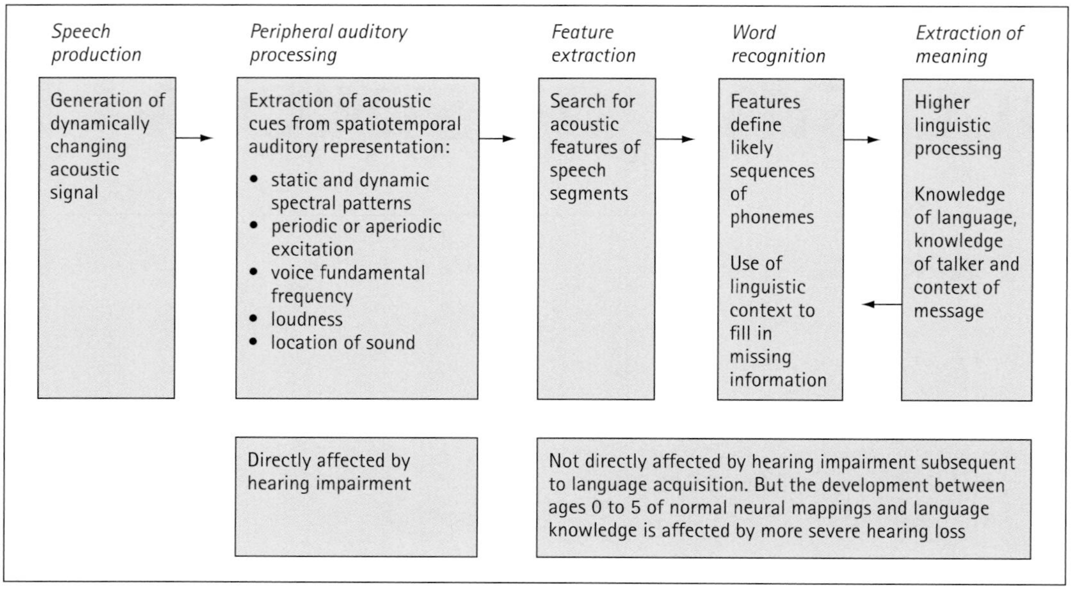

Figure 18.2 Stages of auditory speech processing.

acoustic source, and the modulation of this source by changes in the configuration of the vocal tract.

There are two mechanisms that provide the acoustic excitation of speech. The primary source is due to quasi-periodic opening and closing of the vocal folds within the glottis, as for example, in the production of a vowel sound (see Figure 18.3).

Laryngeal (voiced) excitation

Here, air flow from the lungs is modulated by the opening and closing of the vocal folds, and enters the vocal tract bearing pressure variations whose frequency is directly controlled by the frequency of vocal fold closure. This quasi-periodic source is often termed 'voice', and speech sounds formed with this excitation are classified as 'voiced'.

The sound of the laryngeal source, if it could be heard, would not be recognized as speech, but as a buzzing tone. The generation of speech depends also on the shaping of the source by the vocal tract, which acts as a complex acoustic filter. The oral part of the vocal tract exhibits a series of resonant frequencies known as formants. These resonances determine the frequency components of the source that are allowed to pass into the air, while the remaining frequency components of the exci-

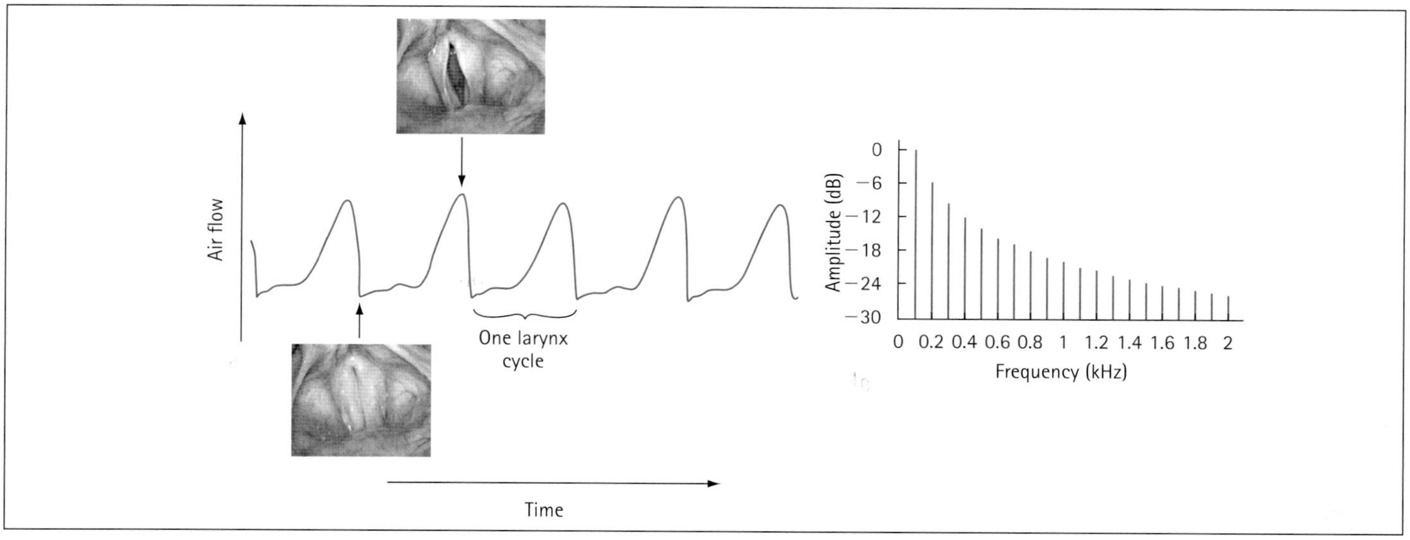

Figure 18.3 The left panel shows a schematic air flow wave from six cycles of vocal fold closure. Here the frequency of the wave is 100 Hz, i.e. each larynx cycle lasts 10 ms. Air flow is at its minimum at the point of vocal fold closure, and at its maximum when the vocal folds are fully open. The right panel shows the frequency components of the spectrum of this wave up to 2000 Hz. Components exist at the overall, or fundamental, frequency of 100 Hz, and at each harmonic frequency. The components above 100 Hz are all integral multiples of the fundamental frequency. As is typical for the periodic acoustic source of speech for normal levels of speech effort, the level of the components declines by about 6 dB for each octave (doubling of frequency). There will also be weaker higher-frequency harmonics present beyond those shown here.

tation source are partially absorbed within the vocal tract. This process of shaping the speech spectrum from that of the voiced source is described by a source and filter model, which is illustrated in Figure 18.4.

The voiced source is not constant. Changes in vocal effort affect both the intensity of the source and its spectrum; the higher harmonics show a higher relative intensity as vocal effort increases. Changes in the rate of vibration of the vocal folds provide the basis for our perception of changes in the pitch of the voice, which is one important element in the perception of spoken messages. Raised pitch can mark important information, and rising pitch in English is often used to indicate that a sentence is intended as a question rather than a statement. The range of vocal fold vibration frequency varies with age and sex, and also between individuals (Table 18.1). The vocal fold vibration rate is termed voice fundamental frequency, which can be abbreviated as F_0.

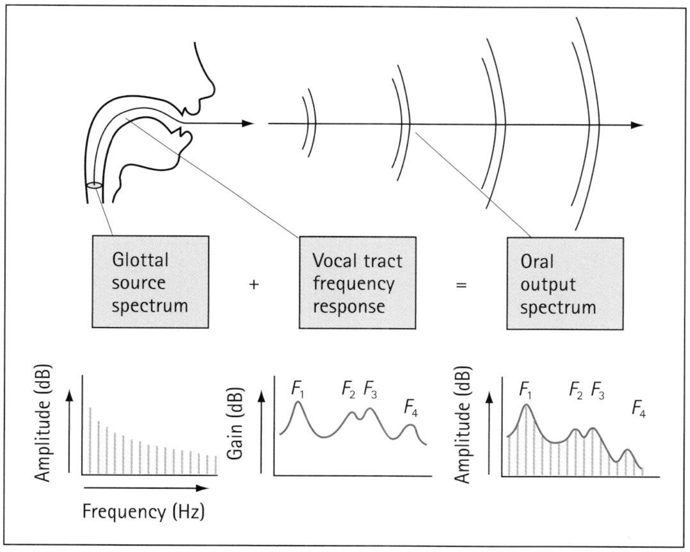

Figure 18.4 The source–filter model for the production of a vowel. The three spectra shown here represent: on the left, a typical spectrum for the voiced source generated by vocal fold vibration; in the centre, a frequency response arising from the resonances of the vocal tract; and to the right, the resulting speech spectrum. The speech spectrum results from applying the frequency-dependent gain of the vocal tract to the glottal source. Here, four vocal tract resonances or formants are shown (F_1 to F_4, covering a frequency range up to about 4000 Hz).

Table 18.1 Typical voice fundamental frequency ranges.[2]

Talker	Typical frequency range (Hz)
Adult male	85–155
Adult female	165–255
Child (age 10)	208–259
Infant (12 months)	247–410

Aperiodic ('voiceless') excitation

A second acoustic source in speech production arises when the vocal tract is configured to form a narrow constriction, as when the tongue is placed close to the roof of the mouth to produce the sound of the first consonant in 'she' (Figure 18.5). Here, air is forced to rush through a constriction in the vocal tract. For a sufficiently small constriction and sufficiently high rate of air flow, turbulence develops in the flow, generating random noise with substantial high-frequency energy. Much as with voiced excitation, the vocal tract shape modifies the spectrum of this noise, depending on the location of the constriction in the vocal tract. The resonances of the cavity between

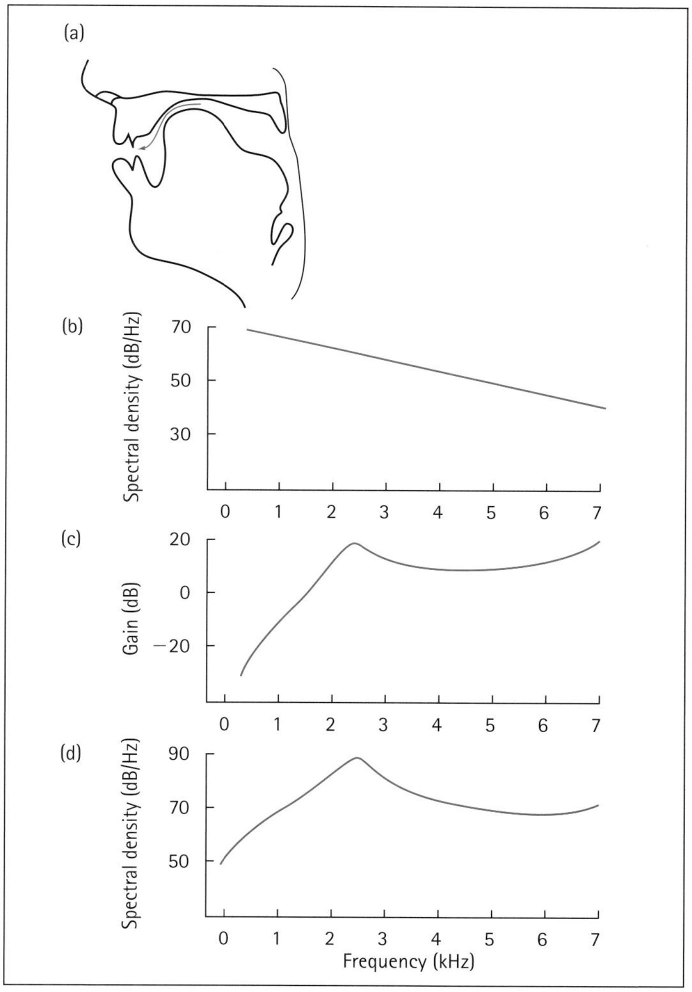

Figure 18.5 Production of voiceless fricative /ʃ/ as in 'she'. The vocal tract configuration is shown in (a). The tongue is placed close to the roof of the mouth between the alveolar ridge and the soft palate. Air flowing from the lungs is forced through the narrow passages here and also further forward around the teeth, leading to turbulent air flow that generates noise. The spectrum of this noise source is shown in (b). In (c) is shown the vocal tract response, with one resonance at about 2.2 kHz, and another around 7 kHz. As in vowel production, the speech spectrum (d) is the result of the source spectrum being modified by the vocal tract response. (After Rosen and Howell. *Signals and Systems for Speech and Hearing*. London: Academic Press, 1991.[3])

the constriction and the lips primarily determine the prominent frequencies of the sound.

Patterns in spectral shape

The configuration of the articulating elements, the tongue, the lips, and the velar flap (which acts to open or close the nasal passages), controls the spectral shape of speech. It is the first three formants that change most significantly with changes of the position of the articulators. The values of these formants depend on vocal tract length as well as its configuration. The typical length of the vocal tract, from vocal folds to lips, is 14 cm for women and 17 cm for men, and increases with age in children, with length at age 5 typically being 11 cm. Shorter vocal tracts result in proportionally higher formant values for a given vocal tract configuration. The nasal tract, when open, adds a further low-frequency resonance, the nasal formant.

Vowel production

Vowels are characterized by a slowly changing and open vocal tract configuration compared to the more rapid articulations in the production of consonants. Hence, vowels show a slowly changing formant structure. The vocal tract configurations for three typical vowels, and the consequent speech spectra, are shown in Figure 18.6. Because of individual differences in vocal tract size, there are rather wide variations in the spectra of the same vowel produced by different talkers, as is shown in Figure 18.7. The English vowel system makes use only of oral tract resonances, with the velar flap normally being closed. Some languages, e.g. French, also make use of the nasal tract in the production of some 'nasalized' vowels.

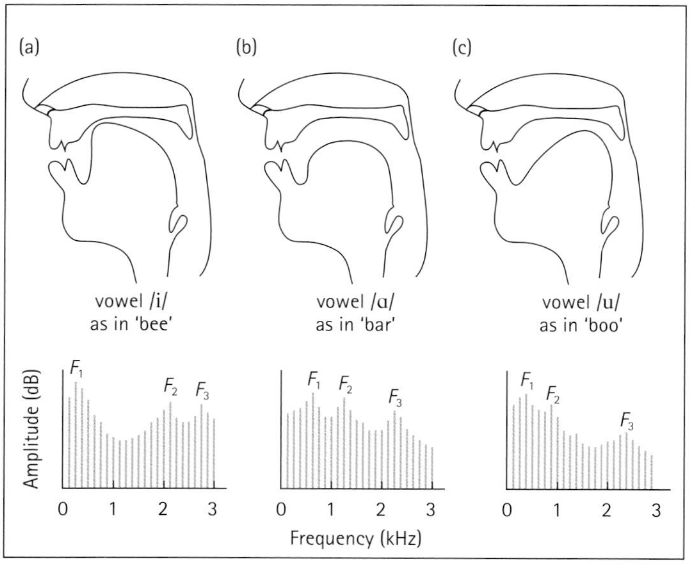

Figure 18.6 Vocal tract configurations and spectra for three English vowels. Shown in (a) is the vowel in the word 'bee'. The tongue is in a high position towards the front of the mouth. The effect is that the lowest resonance, F_1, is relatively low in frequency, while the next resonance, F_2, is relatively high. Shown in (b) is the vowel in the word 'bar'. Here the tongue stays low and has a middle, rather than front or back position. F_1 is higher than for the vowel in 'bee', while F_2 is much lower. Finally, in (c) is shown the vowel in 'boo'. The tongue is high and has a back position in the mouth. Both F_1 and F_2 are relatively low here. Notice that F_1 and F_2 provide the main cues to vowel identity, while F_3 has similar values in all three vowels. The absolute values of the formants will be higher for a woman than for a man, and higher still for a child. However, the relative values of the formants are determined by the vocal tract shape, and are unaffected by vocal tract length. The nasal tract is closed in all these vowels and is not shown.

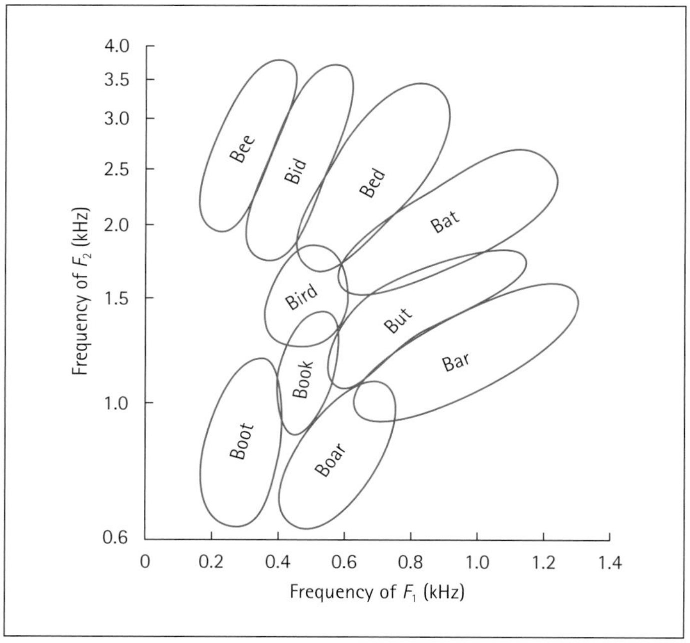

Figure 18.7 Each ellipse covers the range of typical values of F_1 and F_2 for vowels in a sample of American English words. The enclosed areas show the range of these formant frequencies from a sample of 33 adult male, 28 adult female and 15 child talkers. Note that there is considerable variability, but only small areas of overlap. The higher extreme values of F_1 and F_2 are attributable to the child talkers. (Redrawn from Peterson and Barney. *J. Acoust Soc Am* 1952; **24**: 175–84.[4])

Consonant production

Consonants involve relatively rapid movements of the articulators. All consonants involve a short closure or constriction of the vocal tract, lasting for around 100–200 ms, at a characteristic oral location. Consonants can be classified in terms of three articulatory features, place of articulation, voicing, and manner of articulation, which are sufficient to uniquely specify consonant identity. The consonants of English are shown classified in this way in Table 18.2.

Place of articulation

The place of articulation of a consonant refers to the location of the oral closure or constriction. Places of articulation that commonly occur in English consonants are set out in Table 18.3.

Table 18.2 The 24 consonants of standard British English. Example words are shown for each sound. The affricate consonants are essentially formed from a plosive followed by a fricative, e.g. /t/ followed by /ʃ/, as the phonetic notation suggests.

Manner	Voicing	Place (from front to back)							
		Bilabial	*Labiodental*	*Dental*	*Alveolar*	*Palatoalveolar*	*Palatal*	*Velar*	*Pharyngeal*
Plosive	+	b (*b*y)			d (*d*ip)			g (*g*ap)	
(obstruent)	−	p (*p*ie)			t (*t*ip)			k (*c*ap)	
Nasal stop	+	m (*m*y)			n (*n*ip)			ŋ (si*ng*)	
Fricative	+		v (*v*at)	ð (*th*is)	z (*z*ip)		ʒ (trea*s*ure)		
	−		f (*f*at)	θ (*th*in)	s (*s*ip)		ʃ (*sh*ip)		h (*h*ip)
Affricate	+						dʒ (*j*u*dg*e)		
	−						tʃ (*ch*op)		
Approximant	+	w (*w*ar)			l (*l*awn)	y (*y*awn)	r (*r*aw)		

Table 18.3 Places of articulation of English consonants.

Place of articulation	Site of closure or constriction
Bilabial	Upper and lower lip
Labiodental	Upper incisors and lower lip
Dental	Tongue tip and upper incisors
Alveolar	Tongue tip and alveolar ridge
Palatoalveolar	Tongue tip between alveolar ridge and palate
Palatal	Tongue and soft palate
Velar	Tongue and velum
Pharyngeal	Constriction in the pharynx

Voicing and manner of articulation

All consonants are classified as either voiced (+ voicing in Table 18.2) or voiceless. Voiceless consonants are, throughout their duration, produced with only aperiodic voiceless excitation. Voiced consonants involve primarily voiced excitation. Manner of articulation refers to the nature of the oral closure. This may be complete, as in the plosive consonants, or partial, as in the fricative and approximant manners. For the nasal manner, the oral tract is closed as for a plosive, but the nasal tract is opened by the raising of the velar flap. The patterning of voiced and voiceless excitation, and silence in the absence of excitation, play an important part in distinguishing consonants that differ in voicing and in manner of articulation. Further acoustic cues that distinguish between plosive, nasal and approximant manners within the voiced consonants come from different characteristic patterns of vocal tract resonance associated with articulatory configuration during closure or constriction. Figure 18.8 shows spectrograms illustrating the acoustic differences that are associated with voicing and manner classes for six English alveolar consonants when these are produced between two vowels.

As the spectrogram shown in Figure 18.9 illustrates, speech is not delivered to the listener as a presegmented sequence of phonemes. The acoustic patterns in running speech are largely continuous. It is by no means clear that speech perception requires the listener to isolate each phonemic segment from the input. Rather, it may be that perceptual features of a sequence of phonemes are used to identify syllables or words.

Perceptual cues to the identity of the sounds making up the sequence are mostly contained in the dynamic changes in the acoustic signal. There are few invariant acoustic cues to the identity of consonants. Consonant manner and voicing features are broadly independent of context, and are conveyed by relatively gross temporal and spectral features. However, the cues to consonant place of articulation are more subtle, and are primarily carried in the context-dependent dynamic acoustic pattern of the transitions between consonants and surrounding vowels. Even in the case of isolated consonant–vowel sounds, the cues that identify consonants are context-dependent. Figure 18.10 illustrates the context-dependent acoustic cues that distinguish the place of articulation of the voiced plosive consonants of English when followed by a vowel. While the acoustic characteristics of the vocal tract at the time of the consonant closure are closely tied to place of articulation, there is typically little or no acoustic energy generated at this time. This is due to the onset of voiced excitation in typical English productions of these voiced stops commencing 20–40 ms after the release of the closure. It is not until voicing begins that the formant resonances become audible, and at this point, the vocal tract configuration is already changing towards that required for the following vowel.

These context-dependent cues to consonant place of articulation represent the variability of acoustic cues within a single talker. Since talkers vary in vocal tract size, the typical formant frequencies for vowels and also the starting values of the second formant for the different voiced plosives will also vary between talkers. The task of identifying plosive place of articulation thus

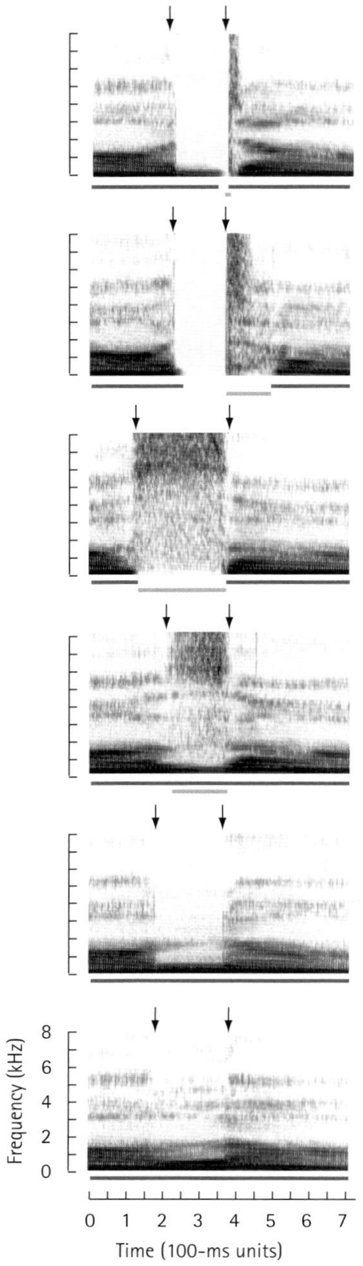

Voiced stop /ɑdɑ/: Voiced excitation continues after the closure, although acoustic energy is low in level, since the mouth is closed. At release, there is a very brief burst of voiceless excitation as air pressure is released, and voicing resumes shortly after the release

Voiceless stop /ɑtɑ/: Voicing ceases at closure, and does not resume until around 80 ms after the release. From the release point until voicing commences, there is voiceless excitation

Voiceless fricative /ɑsɑ/: Voicing stops at the formation of the constriction, and resumes when the constriction is released. During the constriction, only voiceless excitation occurs

Voiced fricative /ɑzɑ/: Voicing continues through the constriction. Air flow through the constriction leads to voiceless excitation simultaneous with voicing

Voiced nasal stop /ɑnɑ/: Voicing continues through the oral closure. During the oral closure the nasal tract is opened at the velum. There is primarily low-frequency energy during the oral closure, reflecting the characteristic resonances of the nasal tract

Voiced approximant /ɑlɑ/: Voicing is continuous. The oral tract is not completely closed; rather, the tip of the tongue contacts only the central region of the alveolar ridge. Unlike /n/, vowel-like formant patterns are evident during the partial closure

Figure 18.8 Acoustic correlates of manner and voicing for six consonants having an alveolar place of articulation. Each spectrogram shows an alveolar consonant and the spectral transitions from a preceding vowel and into a following vowel. The level of grey in each spectrogram represents the amplitude on frequency and time coordinates. The vowel in each case is /ɑ/ as in 'bar'. These are more or less typical examples of slowly articulated speech. The presence of voiced and voiceless excitation is indicated by raised and lowered bars (respectively) under each spectrogram. The arrows at the top of each panel indicate the points in time at which the oral closure or constriction begins and ends.

involves dealing with this between-talker variability as well as the vowel-dependent variability in formant transitions.

> The perception of speech depends on the extraction of dynamic patterns of spectral and temporal information from the acoustical input. While speech perception is assisted by the application of contextual linguistic information, and, in some situations, by visible speech cues from the talker's face, auditory processing has a key role and is the primary aspect of speech perception that is influenced by postlingual hearing impairment.

Auditory processing of speech

> Perceptual cues to the identity of vowels, and to manner and voicing features of consonants, are relatively robust and also relatively invariant for a given talker. However, cues to the place of articulation of consonants depend strongly on the surrounding speech sounds, and are often relatively weak and hard for hearing-impaired listeners to discern. Variations of vocal tract size between talkers lead additionally to substantial between-talker variability of the spectral features of speech.

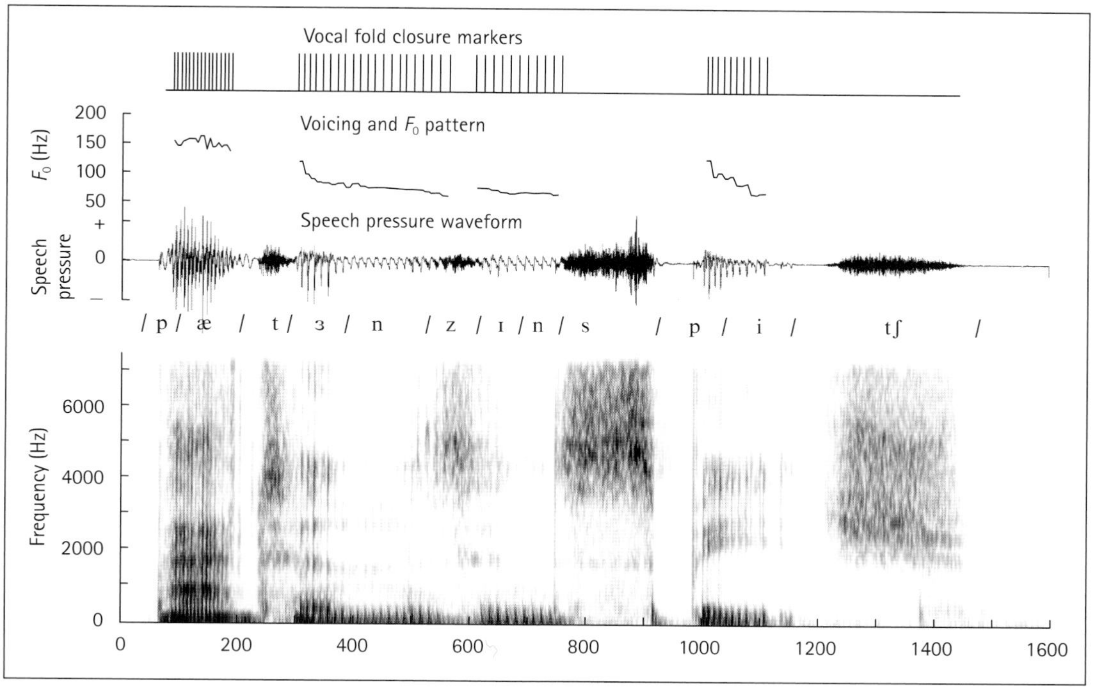

Figure 18.9 Spectrogram showing the phrase 'patterns in speech'. The top panel marks the instants in time of larynx closure. Repeated larynx vibration produces voicing, as shown in the second panel. The rate of larynx closure determines fundamental frequency, which leads to a perception of pitch that changes through the phrase. Syllables that are accented or stressed show a raised pitch except where speech is voiced. Here the initial syllable of 'patterns' and the word 'speech' are accented. The phonetic annotation /pætɜnz//ɪn//spitʃ/ shows the sequence of sounds located in time with the associated acoustic information. The more rapid acoustic changes occur for the consonants.

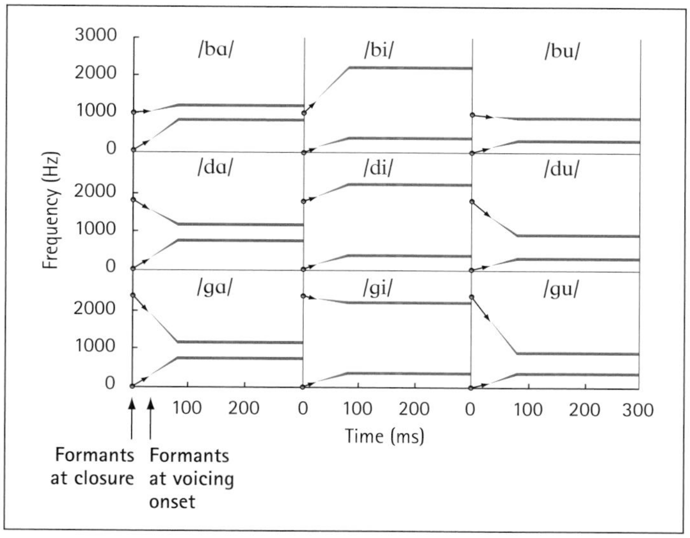

Figure 18.10 Schematic spectrograms showing first (F_1) and second (F_2) formant resonances and their transitions from the initial consonants /bdg/ into the vowels /ɑiu/. Formant values during closure are shown at 0 ms. F_1 always starts at a low frequency, because the oral tract is initially closed. The starting frequency of F_2 depends on the place of the oral closure. The bilabial closure of /b/ results in a low initial F_2. The closure between the tongue and the alveolar ridge in /d/ leads to a mid initial F_2, while the tongue-to-velum contact in /g/ leads to a relatively high initial F_2. Both F_1 and F_2 move during the transition to the formant values characteristic of the following vowel. Because voiced excitation typically begins 20 ms or more after the release of the closure, the starting frequency of F_2 is rarely prominent in speech. Hence the listener must derive cues to place of closure from the audible context-dependent form of the F_2 transition after voicing onset.

The frequency analysis and neural transduction processes of the auditory periphery lead to a spatiotemporal neural representation of the speech spectrum. This encodes the energy across frequency tonotopically as a result of cochlear filtering. Within each neural frequency channel, the time pattern of nerve firing also preserves temporal features of the acoustic signal up to rates of 1000–1500 Hz. The spectral shape of a vowel will thus be represented in terms of the distribution of neural activity across the tonotopically organized auditory nerve bundles. The fundamental frequency of the vowel, and the frequency of harmonic components of a vowel within the F_1 region, will also be represented temporally in the rate of firing (Figure 18.11).

The spatiotemporal encoding performed by the human peripheral auditory system is exquisitely well adapted to extract information from a world of multiple sound sources. In the real world, the task of auditory processing is far more complex than simply to transmit to the brain a representation of the acoustic cues to the sounds of speech. We rarely listen to speech in the absence of any other sound. Hence, auditory processing must also segregate the acoustic components that are produced by multiple sounds.

Hearing impairment limits access to the full range of auditory speech information, both from limited audibility, and because of the reduction in auditory frequency resolution that is associated with cochlear hearing loss.

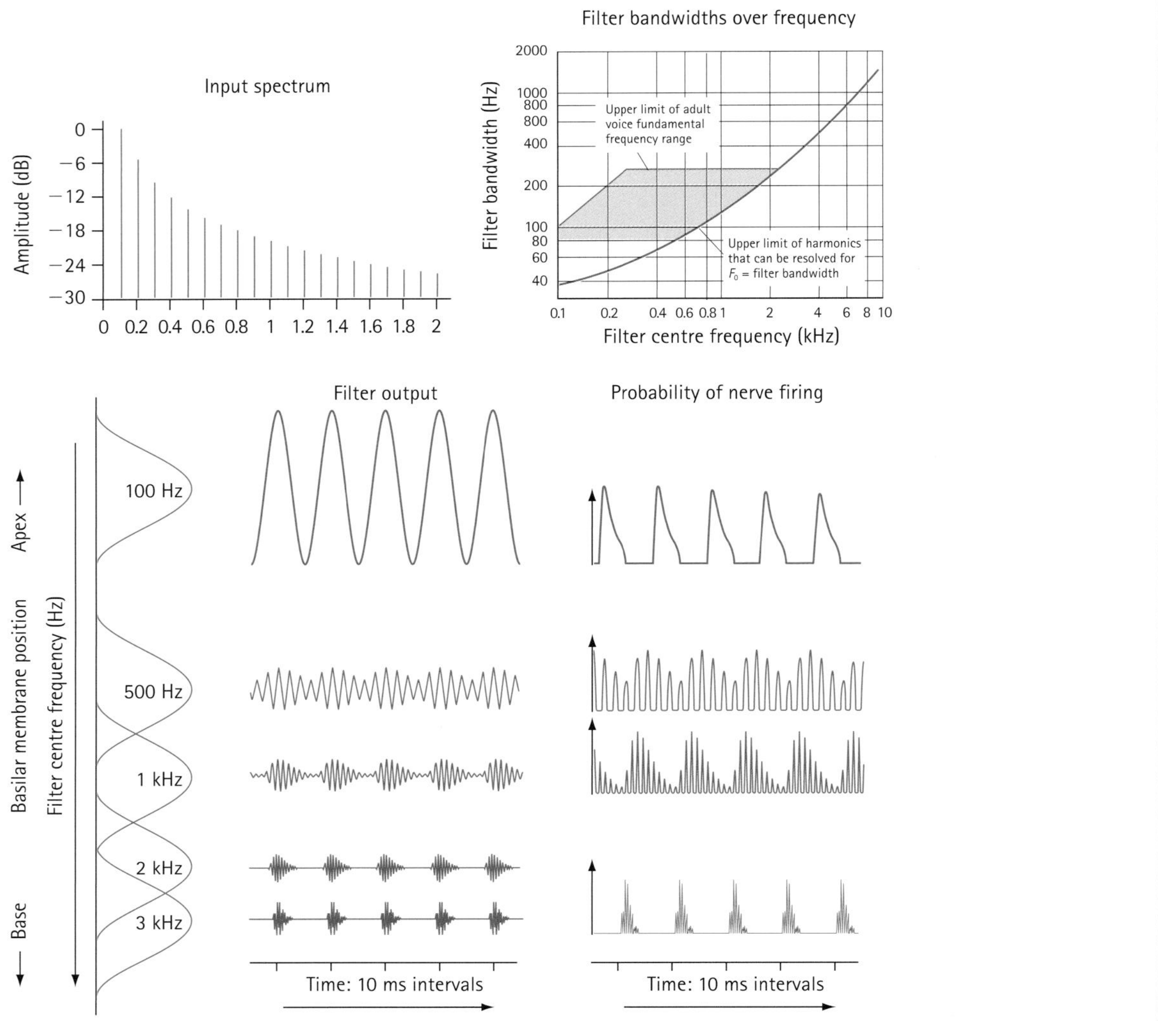

Figure 18.11 Temporal and spatial auditory analysis. The figure shows the responses of selected auditory filter channels to a periodic signal with a 100 Hz fundamental frequency. The input spectrum is shown at top left. The top right panels shows the normal auditory filter bandwidth as a function of filter centre frequency as estimated from a formula given by Moore and Glasberg.[7] The shaded area of this graph shows the range of harmonic components that will be resolved by auditory frequency analysis (as referred to the center frequency axis) over the voice fundamental frequency range (as referred to the bandwidth axis).

The lower part of the figure shows on the left the output waveforms of auditory filters centred at 100, 500, 1000, 2000 and 3000 Hz. To the right are representations of the time-varying probability of firing in the auditory nerve for the corresponding filter outputs (the neural response at 2 kHz is omitted for clarity). These were calculated from a computational model of transduction on the inner hair-cell (Meddis, Hewitt and Shackleton).[8]

The output level of each filter provides a spatial representation of the spectrum in terms of level across frequency. Because the filter bandwidths are approximately proportional to filter centre frequency, at higher centre frequencies the 100 Hz spacing between harmonics becomes small compared to filter bandwidth. Here the filter at 100 Hz shows a response that is dominated by a single harmonic, and this periodicity is very clearly preserved in the neural response. At 1000 Hz and above, the filters respond to several harmonics within their bandwidth, and the temporal pattern of the filter output and the neural response is strongly linked to the fundamental frequency. The response at 500 Hz is intermediate, with the periodicity of the 5th harmonic at 500 Hz being the major component, while modulation at the fundamental frequency is also evident.

The spatial aspect of auditory coding of frequency derives from the dependence of nerve firing rate on the level of the output of each auditory filter. Firing rate will be relatively low in frequency channels that are remote from harmonic components of the input, and relatively high in channels tuned to frequencies near to those of the harmonic components. The encoding of level by firing rate is, however, limited by saturation of neural firing rate, so that this spatial coding will break down at very high input levels.

The temporal properties of the outputs of each filter are preserved in the timing pattern of auditory nerve activity. This is possible because auditory nerve responses tend to be synchronized to peaks of one polarity in the output waveform of the auditory filter, even when the rate of firing is saturated. The timing of neural activity in the 100 Hz channel will represent the 10 ms period of the signal. The neural activity in the 500 Hz channel is dominated by the 2 ms period of the harmonic at 500 Hz. Up to rates of 1000–1500 Hz, nerve activity is able encode the fine temporal structure of the filter output, which is determined primarily by the harmonic of the signal nearest to the filter centre frequency. In the higher frequency channels, for example at 3 kHz, the neural responses are dominated by the 10 ms periodicity of the complex filter output, both because of the interaction of harmonics in the 3 kHz filter and because the periodicity of the individual interacting components is higher than the maximum rate at which the auditory nerve can fire.

Effects of hearing loss on peripheral auditory processing

> The spatiotemporal representation of acoustic input that is provided by the peripheral auditory system is remarkably well adapted to providing an auditory representation of speech information, even in the presence of noise and competing speech inputs.

In cochlear hearing impairment, peripheral auditory processing is affected in several ways. Most obvious is the loss of sensitivity as reflected in the pure tone audiogram. Accompanying this sensitivity loss are two other aspects of impairment. One is a reduced dynamic range, so that even with amplification, the range of sound intensities that can be heard is reduced. Speech has a dynamic range of around 50 dB. In more severe hearing loss, the auditory dynamic range is often reduced to less than that of speech. As a result, the full range of speech levels can only be audible if a hearing aid compresses the range of speech levels. Figure 18.12 illustrates the dynamic range of speech in relation to audibility and the frequency regions of speech where audibility is of the greatest importance.

Auditory frequency analysis is at least as significant as audibility for the processing of speech in everyday situations. In cochlear hearing impairments, the acuity of this analysis is significantly reduced. For frequencies where hearing loss is severe, the sharpness of auditory frequency analysis can be reduced by a factor of two or three,[5] and where the loss is profound, this capability can be completely lost.[6] The normal ear has the use of some 25 auditory frequency channels over the frequency range up to 5 kHz, where the bulk of speech information lies. These filters are rather sharply tuned at lower frequencies, and become broader as frequency increases (Figure 18.11). This degree of auditory frequency analysis allows the ear to resolve the spectral structures of speech that are associated with the first few formants. It also permits representations of the temporal details within each frequency channel of the acoustic input. For voiced speech, the temporal information conveyed depends on the relationship between the filter frequency and the voice fundamental frequency. Lower-frequency harmonic components of voiced speech in the quiet will be individually resolved, and the temporal details will represent the frequency of the harmonic component. Higher-frequency harmonic components will lie at frequencies where the filter bandwidth is broad compared to the fundamental frequency, and hence two or more harmonic components will pass through the filter. In this case, the temporal details will tend to follow the fundamental frequency.

The importance of auditory frequency resolution in speech perception

Understanding speech from one talker in the presence of a fairly constant background noise, e.g. from office machinery, or engine and road noise in a moving vehicle, makes considerable demands on auditory frequency resolution. The auditory filtering of the normal ear is able to preserve important spectral features of speech in the presence of noise. With the broader filters associated with cochlear hearing loss, this ability is markedly impaired (Figure 18.13).

Impaired auditory filtering in itself has relatively modest effects on the perception of speech in ideal quiet conditions. However, it does lead to difficulties in the perception of consonants, where the relatively subtle spectral cues to place of articulation become obscured, as do the frequencies of closely spaced vowel formants. Impaired frequency resolution leads to

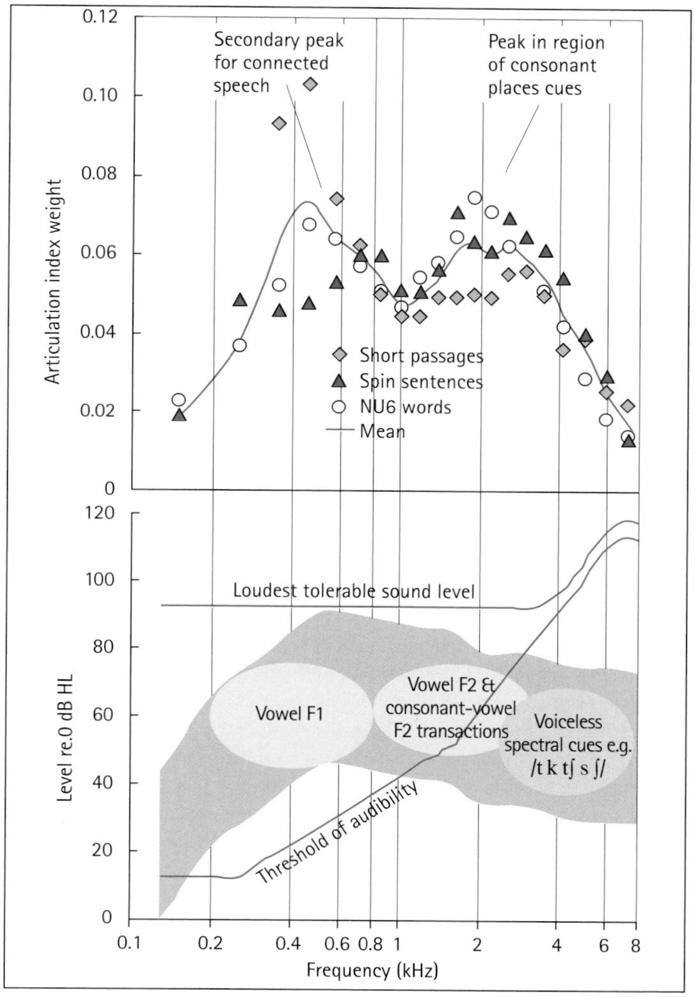

Figure 18.12 The shaded area in the lower panel represents the dynamic range of speech over frequency. Levels are shown relative to the normal threshold of hearing. The area between the two curves in the lower panel represents the range of audible levels over frequency for a typical sloping hearing loss. The portion of the shaded area within this is the audible part of the dynamic range of speech given this hearing loss and without a hearing aid. One important objective of fitting a hearing aid is to adjust the gain and compression over frequency so as to maximize the audibility of speech over the widest possible frequency range. The upper panel shows weightings derived from Articulation Index theory. These 'frequency importance functions' indicate the relative importance of the audibility of different frequency regions of speech for intelligibility. The symbols represent different types of speech materials (NU6 words, SPIN sentences and prose passages: ANSI).[9] At frequencies of high importance, it is especially helpful to maximize the audibility of the full dynamic range of speech.

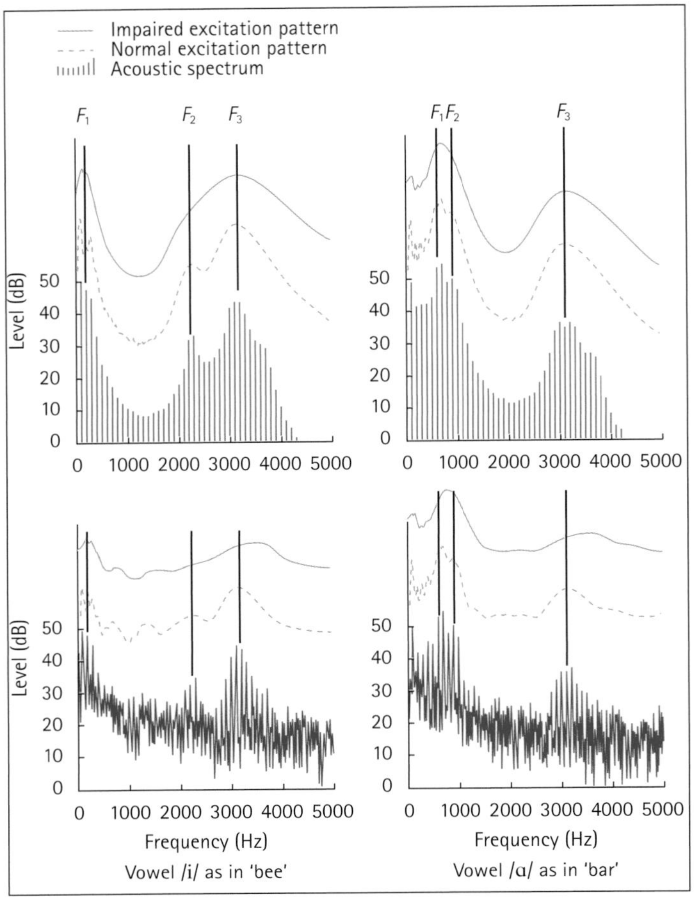

Figure 18.13 Acoustic spectra and auditory excitation patterns of two vowels in quiet and in noise. Excitation patterns are shown for the auditory filtering of normal hearing and for filtering with auditory filters three times broader than normal, such as might result from a severe hearing loss across all frequencies. The excitation pattern shows the output of a series of auditory filters, plotted against filter centre frequency. It shows the auditory representation of the spectrum on the basis of the spatial cochlear representation of level against frequency. The upper two panels represent the vowel in quiet; in the lower panels, the speech level is only 6 dB above that of the background noise. In quiet, the excitation pattern from normal filtering can be seen to resolve the lower harmonics of each vowel, and all three formants. The broader filters lead to an excitation pattern in quiet that blurs together closely spaced formants (F_2 and F_3 in /i/, and F_1 and F_2 in /ɑ/. In noise, the formants are still discernible from the normal excitation pattern, but with broadened filters, the higher formants are becoming obscured.

markedly greater disruption by noise than that seen with normal filtering. Several studies have examined the effects of noise and the reduction of spectral information that is a consequence of broader auditory filters (Figure 18.14).

> Impaired frequency resolution has pronounced effects on the ability to process speech in the presence of other sounds, and also leads to difficulties in the perception of the more subtle and rapid spectral cues to consonant place of articulation.

Speech-like background noise

It is when background sounds have acoustic features similar to speech, or when the background sounds are themselves speech, that the full power of auditory processing comes into its own. Here, slowly changing characteristics of a sound source, such as the pitch of a talker's voice, or the direction from which the voice comes, are key features that allow the listener to attach the acoustic components of the desired source to a single perceptual object.

The role of pitch in the segregation of multiple acoustic sources can be illustrated by the identification of two simultaneously heard vowels.[10] The spatiotemporal auditory representation of sound allows components that are evident in the auditory representation to be associated together by virtue of shared temporal characteristics. Here, auditory processing is able to group together harmonics that share a common fundamental frequency. When two simultaneous vowels are produced with differing fundamental frequencies, they are heard as two distinct sounds with differing pitches, and at least one, and often both vowels can be identified. When two simultaneous vowels share the same fundamental frequency, a single sound is heard, and neither vowel can be identified (Figure 18.15).

Speech-processing prostheses

Hearing aids of the future are likely to incorporate far more intelligent processing than current aids. Most hearing aids of today are essentially amplifiers, with the degree of amplification, and perhaps the compression of the signal, controlled over frequency. These aids can compensate for loss of sensitivity, and can accommodate the wide dynamic range of sounds to the limited range of sound levels that are audible for many impaired listeners. This can achieve a goal of maximizing the audibility of speech. But ensuring audibility over the widest possible range of frequency and intensity does not always ensure that speech information can be analysed; such prostheses cannot compensate for the impairment of frequency-analysing ability that accompanies more severe hearing loss.

Research efforts have been directed at hearing aids that provide analysis within the prosthesis itself, so that the signal delivered to the impaired ear makes fewer demands on auditory processing. A number of approaches have been explored. All have the aim of selecting the desired information, that which carries cues to the wanted spoken message, and thus eliminating other sound that would interfere with the impaired listener's perception. One of the major difficulties in such developments is to determine a heuristic or algorithm that can identify the desired information in real environments. This area of research has so far proved to have a rather low yield in the development of improved commercial hearing aids. A comprehensive review of this area in 1991 concluded that, despite many varied attempts, the conventional hearing aid was likely to be the most effective prosthesis for the foreseeable future.[11] There has not been dramatic progress since then. However, our increasing

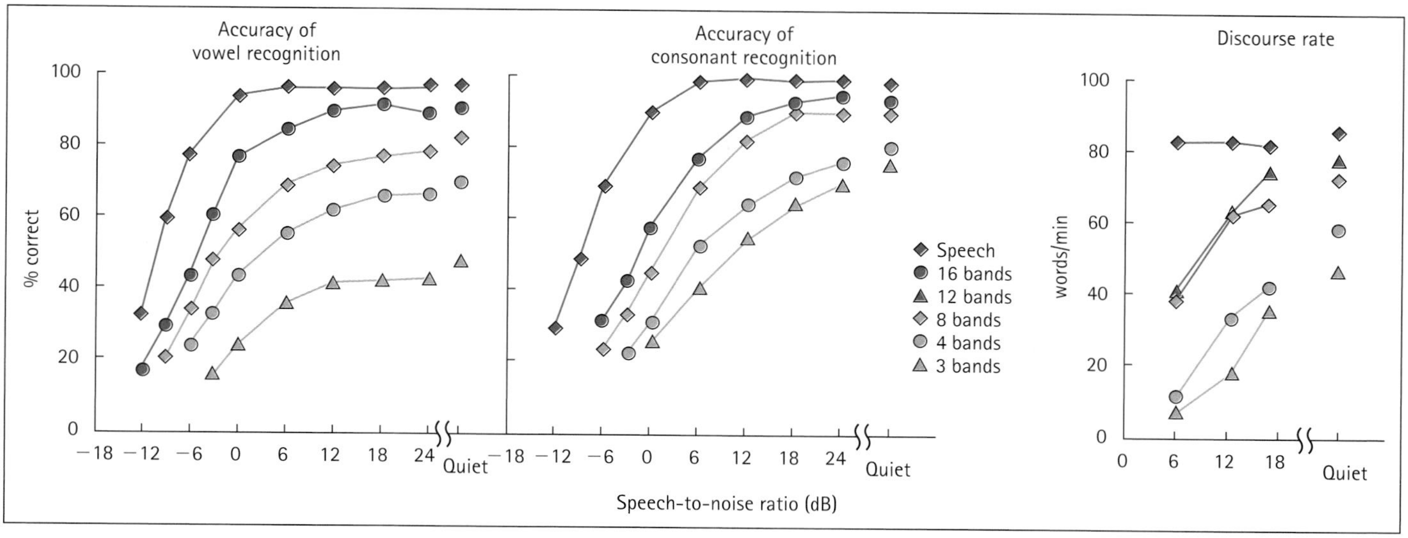

Figure 18.14 Effects of reduced spectral resolution and speech-to-noise ratio on speech perception. All of these data are from studies in normally hearing listeners in conditions that simulate the limited spectral resolution of a cochlear implant. Here spectral resolution is reduced by presenting speech spectra processed through a small number of filter bands covering the speech frequency range. Within each band, all spectral detail is lost, and only the changes over time in speech level averaged over the whole of a given band are presented to the listener. The data here are for the identification of vowels and consonants,[14] and for a task requiring the listener to repeat back correctly connected speech, and which measures rate of communication.[15] One remarkable aspect of these data is the relatively good perception that is possible in quiet with only a small number of filter bands; the normal ear has approximately 25 auditory filter bands in the frequency range up to 5 kHz. Increasing levels of background noise lead to poorer scores. With reduced spectral resolution, levels of noise that would be innocuous for unprocessed speech have severe effects on perception.

understanding of the human auditory processing of speech can be expected to lead to more sophisticated and 'human-like' processing methods.

Directional aids

Directional hearing aids make use of single or multiple microphones to selectively reduce the level of all sounds that do not come from a selected location. The aid user can select the desired sound source by head movement, most naturally by turning to face the source of the sound he wishes to listen to.

Noise-cancelling aids

These incorporate signal processing designed first to determine the characteristics of lower-level continuous sound, on the assumption that this is background noise. The second processing stage shapes the frequency response of a filter to reduce the levels of those frequencies that predominate in this background. When the wanted signal has a sufficiently different spectrum to the continuous background, the signal-to-noise ratio can be significantly enhanced.

Speech-enhancing aids

A related approach to that used in noise-cancelling aids aims to enhance frequency regions where wanted information is assumed to lie. For example, Simpson et al[12] described a form of processing modelled on the auditory frequency analysis of the ear. Here the processing involves analysis of the input through a series of filter bands. Spectral peaks in the signal are identified from the output of these filters. Then, frequency regions where spectral peaks are absent are reduced in level. This can give significant, although relatively small, advantages in intelligibility for speech in noise.[13]

Pattern-extracting aids

A more radical and forward-looking approach would be to identify acoustic features that are known to be important. Rather than filter the signal to reduce noise, a noise-free signal could be synthesized that contains only the selected information. It is well beyond the capability of current computer speech recognition methods to recognize all of the auditory cues required to support the perception of speech. It has, however, proved possible to apply this approach to the special case of auditory–visual speech perception. Here, visible speech-reading information from the talker's lips and face provides cues that are highly correlated with the spectral speech cues that are in accessible to listeners with more extreme hearing losses. Speech reading can be substantially supported by minimal auditory information, representing invisible components of speech such as the presence of voicing and the pitch of the voice. Noise-resistant speech analysis methods are available that can detect voicing and measure the pitch of speech. By generating a simple acoustic tone containing this information, an experimental prosthesis has been shown to be more effective for the audiovisual perception of speech in noise than a simple amplifying aid for some profoundly hearing impaired persons.[16]

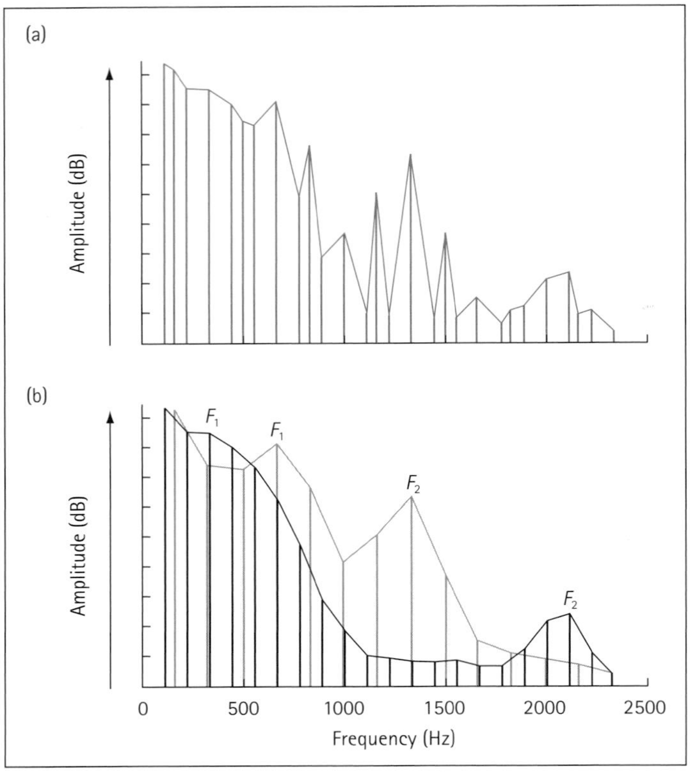

Figure 18.15 (a) shows the spectral components present when two simplified vowel sounds are present together. The two vowels are /i/, with a fundamental frequency of 110 Hz, and /ɑ/ with a 165-Hz fundamental frequency. The line drawn across the top of the higher-level spectral peaks represents the overall shape or 'envelope' of the spectrum. This spectral envelope cannot be readily recognized as the sum of two vowels; the two lower peaks could indicate a /u/ vowel, for example. In (b) the harmonic components are segregated by fundamental frequency (note that at some frequencies, 330, 660, 990 and higher multiples of 330 Hz, harmonics of both vowels exist at the same frequency, and cannot be segregated in this way). The grey and black spectral envelopes, derived from the segregated harmonics, indicate clearly the characteristic formant peaks of the /i/ and /ɑ/ vowels. It appears that it is the ability of the auditory system to derive pitch information from the temporal responses to different components of these two sounds across frequency that is crucial to the segregation of vowels according to pitch. The reader should note that this figure does not represent the spectral resolution limits of the ear. As is shown in Figure 18.13, the normal ear is able to resolve only the lower harmonics of a typical vowel, and an impaired ear will show still more limited spectral resolution.

Future developments

Digital technology in hearing aids brings with it the possibility of processing that is enormously more sophisticated than that possible in analogue hearing aids. The application of processing methods based on an understanding of normal auditory processing, and of cues essential in speech perception, has great potential for providing prostheses that do much more than maximize audibility. Advances in our understanding of normal perceptual processes are still required to achieve this goal, and this will remain a vital area of research. In parallel, miniature signal processor units that can fit in a hearing aid are becoming increasingly powerful and may in the near future be capable of performing 'auditory' processing similar to that carried out by the human auditory periphery.

Acknowledgements

The author wishes to thank Laryngograph Ltd for permission to reproduce stroboscopic images of the vocal folds, and Stuart Rosen for helpful suggestions on the manuscript.

References

1. Boothroyd A. Signal processing for the profoundly deaf. *Acta Oto-laryngol (Stockh)* 1990; Suppl 469: 166–71.
2. Baken RJ. *Clinical Measurement of Speech and Voice*. London: Taylor & Francis, 1987.
3. Rosen S, Howell P. *Signals and Systems for Speech and Hearing*. London: Academic Press, 1991.
4. Peterson GE, Barney HL. Control methods used in a study of vowels. *J Acoust Soc Am* 1952; **24**: 175–84.
5. Moore BCJ. *Cochlear Hearing Loss*. London: Whurr, 1998.
6. Faulkner A, Rosen S, Moore BCJ. Residual frequency selectivity in the profoundly hearing impaired listener. *Br J Audiol* 1990; **24**: 381–92.
7. Moore BCJ, Glasberg BR. Suggested formulae for calculating auditory-filter bandwidths and excitation patterns. *J Acoust Soc Am* 1983; **74**: 750–3.
8. Meddis R, Hewitt MJ, Shackleton TM. Implementation details of a computational model of the inner hair-cell auditory-nerve synapse. *J Acoustic Soc Am* 1990; **87**: 1813–16.
9. ANSI. Draft ANSI standard for calculation of the Speech Intelligibility Index 1511 formerly the Articulation Index (A1) Accredited Standards Committee S3, Bioacoustics.
10. Assman PF, Summerfield Q. Modeling the perception of concurrent vowels: vowels with different fundamental frequencies. *J Acoust Soc Am* 1990; **88**: 680–97.
11. Watson CS. Speech-perception aids for hearing-impaired people—current status and needed research. *J Acoust Soc Am* 1991; **90**: 637–85.
12. Simpson AM, Moore BCJ, Glasberg BR. Spectral enhancement to improve the intelligibility of speech in noise for hearing-impaired listeners. *Acta Oto-laryngol (Stockh)*, 1990: Suppl. 469; 101–7.
13. Baer T, Moore BCJ, Gatehouse S. Spectral contrast enhancement of speech in noise for listeners with sensorineural hearing impairment—effects on intelligibility, quality, and response-times. *J Rehabil Res Dev* 1993; **30**: 49–72.
14. Fu Q-J, Shannon RV, Wang X. Effects of noise and spectral resolution on vowel and consonant recognition: acoustic and electric hearing. *J Acoust Soc Am* 1998; **104**: 3586–96.
15. Faulkner A, Rosen S, Wilkinson L. Effects of the number of channels and speech-to-noise ratio on rate of connected discourse tracking through a simulated cochlear implant speech processor. *Ear Hear* 2001; **22**: 431–8.

16. Faulkner A, van Son N, Beijk C. The TIDE project OSCAR. *Scand Audiol* 1997; **26**(suppl 47): 38–44.

Further Reading

Moore BCJ. *Cochlear Hearing Loss*. London: Whurr, 1998.

Pickett JM. *The Acoustics of Speech Communication: Fundamentals, Speech Perception Theory, and Technology*. Boston: Allyn and Bacon, 1999.

Plant G, Spens KE (eds). *Profound Deafness and Speech Communication*. London: Whurr, 1995.

Tyler RS (ed.). *Cochlear Implants: Audiological Foundations*. San Diego: Singular Publishing Group, 1993.

19 Speech and language development in normally hearing and hearing-impaired children

Emily A Tobey, Beth Morchower Douek

Introduction

One of the first questions you will be asked by a parent whose child has been newly diagnosed with a hearing impairment is, 'Will my child be able to learn to talk or will my child need to learn sign language or another means of communicating?' The objectives of this chapter are to provide a broad review of the processes involved in the development of normal speech and language and to highlight how these processes are influenced by the presence of a hearing impairment. The chapter is designed to provide you with information to recognize the speech and language patterns of a child with a hearing impairment, give you strategies to enhance the development of speech and language skills, and provide advice you may give parents of children with hearing impairments to involve them in developing the speech and language of their child.

Parental concern regarding the future communication status of their child with a hearing impairment must be addressed by professionals. Professionals should be prepared to discuss different modes of communication and their outcomes on oral communication. In addition, it will be important for professionals to recognize the patterns of development in speech and language for children with hearing impairment and provide suggestions to allow parents to enhance the opportunities for their child to develop language and oral speech skills. The following sections will review key aspects associated with the development of oral language skills in children with hearing impairments.

Early identification and later language development

Several investigators[1] suggest that there is a critical or sensitive period when children are best able to learn language. The actual length of this critical period is controversial. Some individuals believe that the critical period starts at birth, and other individuals argue it starts some time within the first year of life. The conclusion of a critical period also is controversial, with some individuals suggesting that the period ends at a young age and other individuals suggesting that the period extends into puberty. A growing body of literature suggests that early and appropriate management of a hearing loss via conventional hearing aids or assistive sensory devices, such as cochlear implants, tactile aids, or frequency modulated (FM) systems, is essential if young children are to maximize their potential for developing language and communication skills during this critical period.

Available evidence suggests that early identification and amplification positively impacts on later language development.[2] As shown in Figure 19.1, children with normal cognitive abilities whose hearing losses are identified by 6 months of age demonstrate significantly higher language abilities at 30 and 36 months of age than children whose hearing losses are identified after 6 months of age.[2] By 36 months of age, children whose hearing losses are not identified until after 6 months of age

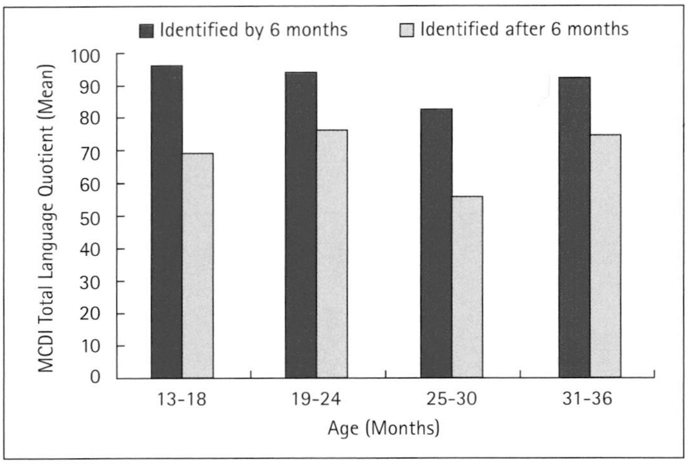

Figure 19.1 Mean language quotients for children identified with a hearing loss before 6 months of age and after 6 months of age are shown when the children are tested at older chronological ages. Language scores are significantly higher in children who are identified with a hearing loss and habilitated during the first 6 months of age than for children identified between 6 months and 1 year, suggesting that early identification and treatment of a hearing loss has a positive impact on language. (Adapted from Yoshinaga-Itano et al. *Pediatrics* 1998; **120**(5): 1161–71.[2])

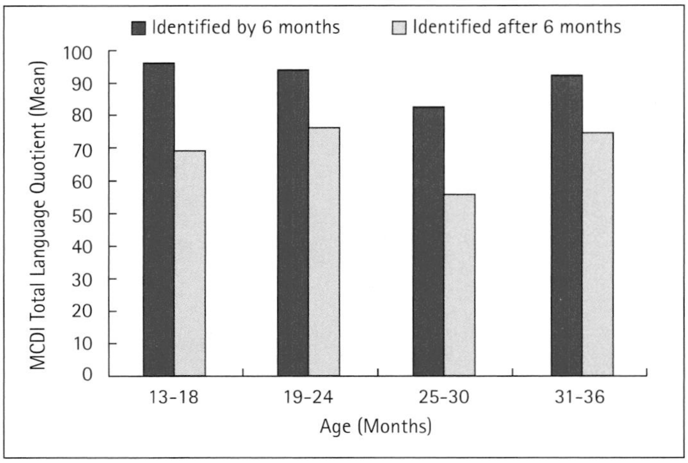

Figure 19.2 Mean language quotients for children identified with a hearing loss before 6 months of age and after 6 months of age are shown for children with differing degrees of hearing loss. It can be seen that significantly higher language scores are observed for children who are identified within the first 6 months of life, regardless of the amount of loss experienced by the children. Differences in language performance are particularly evident for children who experience severe or profound hearing impairments. (Adapted from Yoshinaga-Itano et al. *Pediatrics* 1998; **120**(5): 1161–71.[2])

show significant gaps between their cognitive and language abilities.[2] A cognitive–linguistic gap may affect later academic performance, since several studies demonstrate discrepancies between academic performance and verbal intelligence scores in hearing-impaired children whose hearing losses are not detected early.[2] Figure 19.2 shows that even a mild hearing loss is a concern; children identified within the first 6 months of age demonstrate better language performance than children identified after 6 months, regardless of the severity level of hearing loss. Collectively, these findings suggest that the cognitive–linguistic gaps seen in children of elementary school age with hearing losses may originate within the first year of life. Moreover, it appears that the size of the gap may be significantly reduced if identification and amplification occur in the first 6 months of life.

Parental reports may be used to assist in the early detection of hearing loss. Table 19.1 provides examples of questions which may be asked to help determine how well young children are communicating and whether they are meeting important communication milestones. Failure to reach these milestones by the months indicated requires referral to ensure that the infant or young child does not have a hearing impairment which would adversely influence his ability to develop effective communication skills. It also requires follow-up to ensure that, if a hearing loss is detected, a child will receive the appropriate amplification as early as possible.

In addition to the age of identification and amplification, it appears that the severity of the hearing impairment also affects the development of speech and language. However, although many articles are available which describe the abnormal behaviors of profoundly hearing-impaired children, there are far fewer articles discussing the characteristics of children with mild, moderate or severe hearing losses. Therefore, this chapter primarily refers to findings from studies which examine the development of children with profound hearing losses. To understand how hearing impairment influences the development of oral speech and language, normal development of communication throughout childhood must be considered.

What is meant by communication?

Communication may take many forms, and human communication is particularly inventive. Even normally hearing individuals convey important ideas from one person to another person in many different ways by using facial gestures, gestures of the body, and oral speech. Generally speaking, the role of a speaker is to generate an idea, determine the appropriate linguistic properties needed to convey the idea to a listener, marshal the requisite physiological entities to produce specific changes to the air-filled cavities of the vocal tract, and produce an acoustical output. In addition, the speaker may accentuate the message with facial or body gestures. The listener, in turn, receives the visual and acoustical signals by transforming them into physiological signals which may be interpreted by the brain to render the original idea intended by the speaker.

When children acquire a language, they acquire the ability to take an idea that is internal and private to them and make it external for others to share. Language has three components: form, content, and use.[3] Language form refers to the shapes of words and sentences – the way language sounds when it is spoken – or the way it looks in sign languages or gestures. Content

Table 19.1 Key milestones of communication during the first year of life: a guide for doctors

Age (months)	Question
1	When did your baby first startle to a sound?
1.5	When did your baby smile at you when you talked or played with them?
3	When did your baby start cooing and producing long vowels?
4	When did your baby turn to you when you spoke to them?
5	When did your baby start saying [goo, ah, goo]?
5	When did your baby give you a raspberry?
5	When did your baby start squealing and growling while talking?
11	When did your baby start saying [dadadad] or [mamamam]?

describes what the words and sentences mean, and use of language refers to how we influence the thoughts and actions of other people. The uses of language are numerous and include: sending and receiving information, influencing the thoughts and actions of other people, and providing instructions regarding how to accomplish something.

Language may be expressed and received in many different ways. These are referred to as modes, or forms of communication when talking about the expression of language in individuals with hearing losses. Modes of communication fall into two broad categories: those which emphasize gestures/signs, and those which emphasize oral speech. Although these two broad classifications are most commonly used, each of the classifications has several different ways in which language may be expressed, as shown in Table 19.2.

Expression and reception of language through signs or gestures may involve formal sign languages, such as American Sign Language (ASL) or French Sign Language (FSL). Different countries and languages have different formal sign languages. In such instances, the formal sign language has vocabulary and grammatical features which are unique to it and do not follow the rules associated with the vocabulary and grammar of the spoken language. Conversely, simultaneous communication or total communication refers to a spoken language accompanied by signs presented in the spoken word order. In some instances, speech may be emphasized in the message and in other instances, the sign may be emphasized. In the USA, these modes are referred to as manual coding of English, and may include a variety of methods, including the Rochester method, Seeing Essential English, and Signing Exact English.

Communication modes which focus more on conveying language via listening and speaking are referred to as oral methods. There are several different modes of communicating via listening and talking. Individuals who express and receive language concepts via an auditory–verbal mode of communication are encouraged to listen and speak. Lipreading is not emphasized, in order to encourage a reliance on listening. Auditory–oral modes of communication differ from auditory–verbal modes by encouraging lipreading, as well as listening and speaking, in order to convey language. Cued speech refers to a method of conveying language by speaking accompanied by hand signals near the face intended to aid in lipreading. The hand gestures provide cues regarding aspects of the oral signal which are not visible, e.g., when a sound is voiced (involving laryngeal vibration) versus unvoiced (not involving laryngeal vibration).

Table 19.2 Modes of communication for children with hearing impairments

Auditory–verbal	Child taught to maximize and rely on the use of residual hearing. No additional gestural system used. Reading lips not taught.
Auditory–oral	Child taught to use residual hearing with visual cues such as lip reading.
Cued speech	A gestural system used to emphasize the oral movements involved in speech production.
Total communication	Both sign language and speech are used in parallel.
Sign language	Primary mode of communication is sign language without oral speech.

Parents will need to make decisions regarding how they wish to convey language to their child with a hearing loss and how the child will convey language to them. This important decision may be guided by professionals. In the USA, 41.1% of deaf children are addressed using auditory methods, 56.1% of deaf children are addressed with simultaneous communication methods (speaking and signing), 1.9% of deaf children are addressed primarily with formal sign languages, and 0.5% of deaf children are addressed using cued speech. Distributions of communication modes differ in different countries and languages. The remainder of this chapter will focus on the spoken language of children using either auditory methods or simultaneous communication methods, since it appears that the majority of children with hearing losses may use these modes.

Speech and language patterns during infancy

Normally hearing babies undergo several stages of speech-like development, as shown in Table 19.3.[4–7] During the first 2 months of life, babies produce 'comfort sounds'. These sounds appear to be the precursors to vowel production. Between 2 and 3 months, infants enter a 'gooing' stage. During this stage, they learn to articulate in the back of the mouth and, therefore, acquire a repertoire of vowel-like and 'g-like' sounds. Between 4 and 6 months, babies begin the 'expansion' stage, when they produce growls, yells, whispers, squeals, and isolated vowel-like sounds. Well-formed syllables appear between 7 and 10 months during the 'canonical babbling' stage. During this stage, the use of reduplicated sequences such as [mamamama] or [dadadada] begins. Reduplicated babbling is particularly important, since it signals the first use of adult-like syllables, paving the way for a child to develop his first words.

Early communicative efforts of profoundly hearing-impaired or deaf infants parallel those of normally hearing infants in several stages; however, deaf babies do not achieve the reduplicated or canonical babbling stage at the same time as normal babies. As shown in Figure 19.3, deaf babies do not approach the canonical babbling period until at least 11 months and some individuals do not obtain reduplicated syllables until 2.5 years of age or later.[4] Thus, all professionals should suspect that a baby may be deaf or have a significant hearing impairment if the parents report that their child is not trying to say vocal sequences like [mamama] or [dadada] by 11 months of age.

Early amplification appears to positively affect the development of canonical babbling in infants with hearing impairments, as shown in Figure 19.4. Placing hearing aids on young infants with hearing impairments increases the likelihood that they will begin the canonical babbling stage at an earlier age than if they remain unaided.[4] Although these children still remain at risk for further delays in their communication development, early amplification increases the likelihood of achieving the reduplicated sequences necessary to build the foundation of early words.

Speech and language patterns post-infancy

Speech and language developmental milestones after infancy are often described in terms of the following subcomponents: pragmatics, semantics, syntax, suprasegmentals, morphology, and phonology. These important language components are shown in Table 19.4. Pragmatics refers to the use of verbal and non-verbal language for a purpose or intention. Semantics examines the use of words to create a shared meaning at the level of a word, phrase, sentence, paragraph, or conversation.

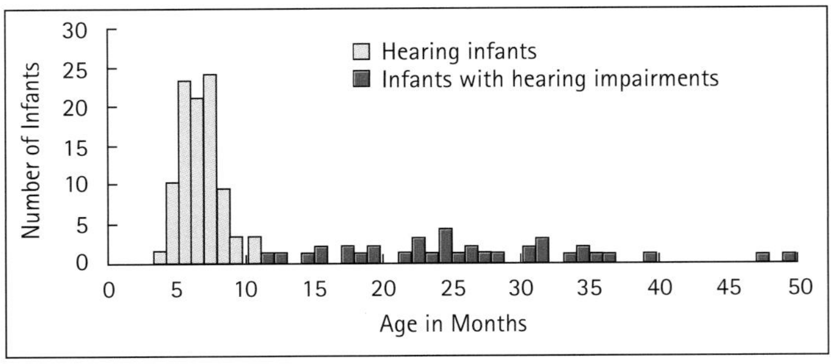

Figure 19.3 The number of infants who begin canonical babbling at various ages. It is important to note that all of the normally hearing babies initiate canonical babbling between 4 and 10 months of age; however, deaf babies do not begin to produce canonical babbling until 11 months of age. Indeed, many deaf babies do not begin to produce canonical babbling until 2 or 3 years of life. (Adapted from Eilers and Oller. J Paediatrics 1994; **124**(2): 199–203.[4])

Table 19.3 Key milestones of communication during the first year of life: a guide for parents

Age (months)	Communication activity
0–2 months: *Phonation Stage*	Baby should produce 'comfort' sounds and coo with normal sounding vocalizations. A few utterances may sound 'vowel-like'.
2–3 months: *Gooing Stage*	Baby should produce 'vowel-like' sounds and some 'consonant-like' sounds made in the back of the mouth.
4–6 months: *Expansion Stage*	Baby produces a variety of sounds including raspberries (labial trills), squeals, growls, yells, whispers, isolated vowel-like syllables.
7–10 months: *Canonical Stage*	Baby will say [bababa], [dadada], [mamama] or other reduplicated syllabic sequences.
11–12 months: *Variegated Babbling*	Baby will produce gibberish speech with a wide variety of sounds and sequences.

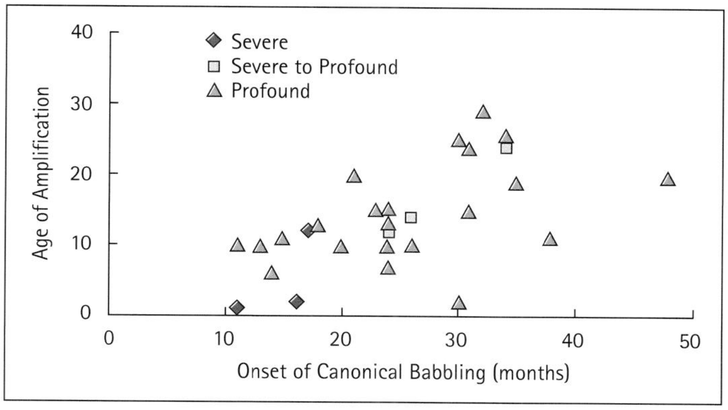

Figure 19.4 The age of amplification following the identification of a hearing loss is also important for speech behaviors. Babies who receive their hearing aids at early ages begin to produce canonical babbling at earlier ages, regardless of the severity of the hearing loss. (Adapted from Eilers and Oller. *J Paediatrics* 1994; **124**(2): 199–203.[4])

Syntax deals with the order or arrangement of words in phrases and sentences. Suprasegmentals include the variations in volume, pitch and stress across phrases and sentences. Morphology represents the smallest parts of words that carry meaning. Phonology is the study of sound structures and rules governing the pronunciation of words in a language. Each of these components is discussed below with regard to the development of children with and without hearing impairments.

Pragmatics

Young children with normal hearing use both verbal and non-verbal language with the intention to communicate before they have fully developed all sub-components of language. Speech–language pathologists refer to these behaviors as pragmatics, or the social use of language. Pragmatic behaviors include: making and maintaining eye contact, sharing visual attention, taking turns communicating, responding to communication, requesting or asking for an object, repeating words or phrases, and negating (denying or resisting a statement, request, or question). Pragmatic behaviors do not require vocalizations: for example, a young child may reach for a mother's hand and lead her to the refrigerator if it wants a drink of juice or milk, or an adult may indicate difficulty in comprehension by means of arm postures and head turning.

Communicative intent, as represented by pragmatic behaviors, marks the beginning of a transition to the use of symbolic language. Therefore, preverbal communicative behaviors may provide important information about the communicative abilities of young infants and children with hearing losses.[8–12] Typically, early pragmatic behaviors are measured by engaging the parent and child in a play situation. Activities are video recorded and transcribed to determine how the children take turns in communicating, maintaining eye contact, and responding to communication attempts from the parents.[2,13] Pragmatic behaviors are observed early in a child's communicative life and lead the way for the development of other language processes.

Table 19.4 Language components

Component	Definition
Phonology	The sounds of a language
Morphology	The meaningful component of language
Syntax	The grammar of a language
Semantics	The meaning of language
Pragmatics	The social use of language

Both normally hearing and hearing-impaired children appear to move from non-communicative vocal behaviors to intentional (communicative) gestures or behaviors, and finally to vocal behaviors with communicative intent.[14,15] As they move from non-communicative behaviors into communication with intent, young children, including those with hearing losses, appear to develop spontaneous non-verbal requests for information or objects.[2,16,17] Young children learn to non-verbally acknowledge or protest requests from others, e.g., by shaking their head 'no'. At later ages, children use symbolic representations of actions or objects. Such symbolic representations are demonstrated when children pretend they are drinking, sleeping or hammering.[13] Finally, children will use verbal communicative intents to gain attention or actions from others. Children with hearing impairments who do not have intelligible verbal behaviors typically pair their unintelligible verbalizations with non-verbal behaviors to increase the likelihood of successful communication. Figure 19.5 illustrates the various stages of preverbal to verbal behaviors commonly observed in

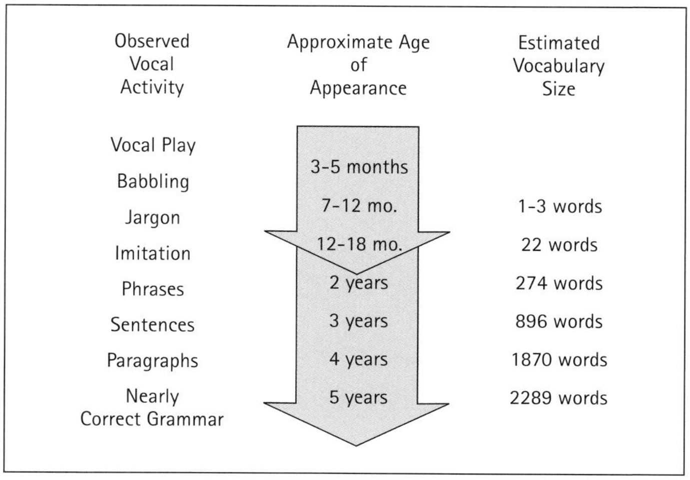

Figure 19.5 Development of communication involves many activities which develop at different time periods. The left-hand column details the various types of vocal behavior which occur in communication development. The center column indicates the approximate ages at which these behaviors occur in normally hearing children. The right-hand column indicates the growth in vocabulary size in speakers of English associated with the changes in chronological age.

young infants and toddlers. It can be seen that, as young children expand their communicative intention behaviors, they learn to take turns communicating, increase their conversational skills, and develop paralinguistic and extralinguistic aspects of communication. Examples of the types of behaviors that parents can watch for which indicate pragmatic development in children are shown in Table 19.5. Children with hearing impairments, however, often fail to master these skills as fully or as quickly as children with normal hearing. However, when young children with hearing impairments receive intervention, pragmatic behaviors may be the first linguistic behaviors to show measurable improvement. Parents should be encouraged to watch for these important stages of language development and to enhance the development of these stages by responding to their child's intentions and providing language models.

Children with hearing impairments typically produce fewer meaningful communication acts than children with normal hearing.[18] Such observations suggest that hearing-impaired children lag significantly behind their normally hearing peers, not only in the types of communicative functions they use, but also in the frequency with which they use the functions. The order of emergence for key communicative functions appears to be similar between normally hearing and hearing-impaired children. Thus, parents of hearing-impaired children may enhance the development of communication by encouraging verbal and non-verbal pragmatic behaviors.

Syntax and semantics

Two language subcomponents examine the roles of words or vocabulary. The order or arrangement of words in a phrase or sentences is called syntax. Syntax examines the relationships of meaning within a sentence and across a series of sentences. Semantics refers to the meaning in language. Language meaning or semantics occurs at many levels, within words themselves, or across phrases, sentences, paragraphs, or conversations. As children develop, their use of syntax and semantics increases in complexity, allowing them to express their ideas using novel forms. A progression of vocal behaviors occurs developmentally, leading to the advanced use of language and speech. Children with hearing impairments may exhibit both syntactical and semantic delays in their verbal language. Despite these delays, children with profound hearing impairments may spontaneously develop gestural systems which contain syntactic and semantic elements by inventing special signs to represent meaningful items in their environment.

Suprasegmentals

Suprasegmentals are the melodic modulations of speech carried across entire phrases. Children produce suprasegmentals by varying the duration, pitch and loudness of syllables. Suprasegmentals vary widely in their use and significance across languages. Typically, suprasegmentals develop without instruction and are used to express emotion, change stress patterns or provide emphasis. Abnormal suprasegmentals are observed for children with hearing impairments when the children are unable to carefully control their pitch, loudness, and durations. Children with hearing losses may demonstrate excessively high pitches, very loud or soft speech, and long durations. Poor suprasegmental productions contribute to the reduced speech intelligibility commonly observed in children with hearing losses.

Table 19.5 Key examples of pragmatic communication behaviors: a guide for parents

Paralinguistic behaviors
Your child should use pitch and loudness variations to gain your attention.
Your child should have an ease of vocalizations.
Extralinguistic behaviors
Your child should closely watch your face when you engage in conversation.
Your child should remain close to you when you engage in conversation.
Linguistic behaviors
Your child should comment, request, warn, assert, promise, direct and acknowledge you during comversation.
Your child should learn to initiate and maintain a conversation.
Your child should learn to take a turn during talking.
Your child should learn how to repair a conversation by repeating or rewording.
Your child should learn to use pronouns and other parts of speech.

Morphology

Another feature of language commonly examined in young children is morphology. A morpheme is the smallest unit of speech that carries meaning. In some instances, the root or base word is held constant and additional morphemes are added to create plurality or verb tenses. In English, for example, the morpheme 's' can be added to change a word to its plural form. In other instances, new words are constructed by adding additional word parts to a base word: for example, the morpheme 'fine' can be modified by adding the morpheme 're' to form 'refine'. This can be further altered by adding the morpheme 'ment' to from 'refinement'. Children with hearing impairments often produce morpheme errors, such as leaving the endings off the end of a word, which makes it difficult to tell what tense (past, present, or future) they are intending to use.

Phonology

Phonology is the study of sound structures and the rules governing the pronunciation of words in a language. Between the ages of 2 and 6 years, children with normal hearing acquire the sounds of speech (phonemes) and use them to make the meaningful contrasts necessary to form different words. Typically, vowels are achieved between the ages of 2 and 4 years, while the acquisition of consonants extends through later ages. Young children learn to produce consonants accurately in the initial positions of words first, and later learn to produce consonants accurately in the middle and at the end of words. Nasal (i.e. m, n) and oral (i.e. p, t, k, b, d, g) consonants are among the first consonants correctly produced by children. Fricatives or sibilants (i.e. s, z, sh, zh) tend to appear around 5 years of age. The correct use of consonant combinations also occurs when children are 5 and 6 years of age. Examples of the age of acquisition for English consonant sounds are shown in Table 19.6.

A study by Miskiel et al investigated sound acquisition in young preschoolers with normal hearing.[19] Data from this study indicated that the overall ability of young children with normal hearing to correctly imitate sounds increased from 3 to 5 years of age. Generally speaking, the normally hearing children were most accurate at repeating sounds that varied in duration, pitch, or loudness. Vowels and single, simple consonants were the next most accurately imitated sounds, while consonant blends (i.e. multiple consonants) in initial and final positions were the least accurately imitated sounds. Thus, children gradually acquire the motor and linguistic skills necessary to correctly produce the consonants and vowels of their language over a critical period that spans several years.

The variety of consonant sounds produced by normally hearing children increases as their sound repertoires increase; however, young children with profound hearing impairments tend to either maintain or reduce the number of consonants that they use as they get older. Children with profound hearing impairments frequently produce vowels and consonants with a number of errors.[20–24] Substitutions of one sound for another, omissions of sounds, distortions of sound and reduction of multiple consonants to a single consonant are commonly observed.[25–27] Sounds made in the front of the mouth, which are more visible, are used more frequently than sounds made in the back of the mouth, which are not as visible. Errors associated with laryngeal voicing also contribute to the abnormal patterns; sometimes children with hearing losses substitute voiced sounds for voiceless sounds, and at other times they make the opposite mistakes. Children with profound hearing losses also appear to have difficulty in regulating air flow. This leads them to make errors such as substitutions of nasal for oral consonants. Studies also show that they produce vowels in the back of the mouth more accurately than in the front of the mouth.[27,28] Children with profound hearing losses also make frequent errors on vowels produced high in the mouth, suggesting difficulties with tongue positioning.

Children with severe or profound hearing losses who receive training that relies on listening and talking demonstrate similar speech patterns to other profoundly hearing-impaired children. They tend to produce consonants in initial positions in words more accurately than sounds in final positions.[29] Geffner[30] noted that the phonological system for children with profound hearing losses is governed by features related to intensity, visibility and frequency, as demonstrated in Table 19.7. In

Table 19.6 Earliest appearance of consonant sounds correctly produced in 75% of 208 children

Consonant sounds	Age of appearance in initial position of words (years)	Age of appearance in final position of words (years)
p	2	4
b	2	3
t	2	3
d	2	4
k	3	4
g	3	4
m	2	3
n	2	3
ng	–	3
h	2	–
s	5	5
z	5	3
f	3	3
v	5	5
sh	5	5
l	4	4
r	5	4
w	2	–
j	4	6
ch	5	4

Adapted from: Powers MH. Functional disorders of articulation/symptomatology and etiology. In Travis LE (ed.) *Handbook of Speech Pathology and Audiology*. Englewood Cliffs, NJ: Prentice-Hall, 1971.

Table 19.7 Source structure based on acoustic cues of English

Acoustic cue	Sounds
Greater intensity	Vowels
Less intensity	Consonants
Low frequency	Vowels
High frequency	Consonants
High visibility	Sounds made with lips and teeth
Low visibility	Sounds made in the back of the mouth

this model of sound structure, children with hearing losses distinguish sounds by relying on differences in their loudness, where they are made in the mouth, and how often they are used in a given language. She suggests that vowels are produced more accurately because of their intensity and visibility cues. Sounds made with the lips are more visible than sounds made with the soft palate, and contribute to the accuracy of some consonants.

Speech intelligibility

Accuracy of sound production appears to be related to overall speech intelligibility.[31–36] The more complex the sound or word structures are, as in combinations of multiple consonants or polysyllabic words, the less understandable is a speaker with a profound hearing loss.[37] Poor production of consonant glides (i.e. l, r, w) and affricatives (i.e. ch) also appears to contribute to low speech intelligibility scores.[38] Degree of hearing loss also appears to influence overall speech intelligibility: the more severe the hearing loss, the less intelligible is a speaker.[27,38–41]

Measures of speech intelligibility offer special challenges to parents and doctors, as shown in Table 19.8. Several studies indicate that a listener who is familiar with the speech of a child with a hearing loss tends to judge that child's speech as more intelligible than a listener who is unfamiliar with the child.[26,27,37,42] Parents are more likely to understand their child speaking than a stranger or a less familiar listener. Another factor that appears to influence overall speech intelligibility is the length of the sentences.[37] Speech intelligibility is rated more accurately if longer sentences rather than shorter sentences are used; thus, children who are older and use longer sentences are usually rated more intelligible than younger children who use shorter sentences. The context of the sentence also plays an important role. Listeners are able to guess what an unintelligible speaker is saying if the sentence provides sufficient context. In assessing speech intelligibility, it is important to recognize that tests do not always provide a complete picture. For example, many tests of speech intelligibility require that a child listen and repeat a sentence or read and say a sentence out loud.

Table 19.8 Factors influencing speech intelligibility

Factor	Examples
High context vs low context	Key word may be guessed in 'The flag is *red*, white and blue'. Key word may NOT be guessed ' The *fat* baby is crying'.
Short sentence vs long sentence	It is easier to understand longer sentences because additional words provide context. When speaker intelligibility is an issue, it may be easier to understand 'The flag is red, white and blue'. than 'Keep quiet'.
Familiar listener vs unfamiliar listener	A familiar listener may be more likely to understand a speaker than an unfamiliar listener. For example, a child's mother may understand that 'Dede wa baba' means that Jeffery wants his blanket. An unfamiliar listener may interpret this as 'dedewababa' a totally meaningless utterance.

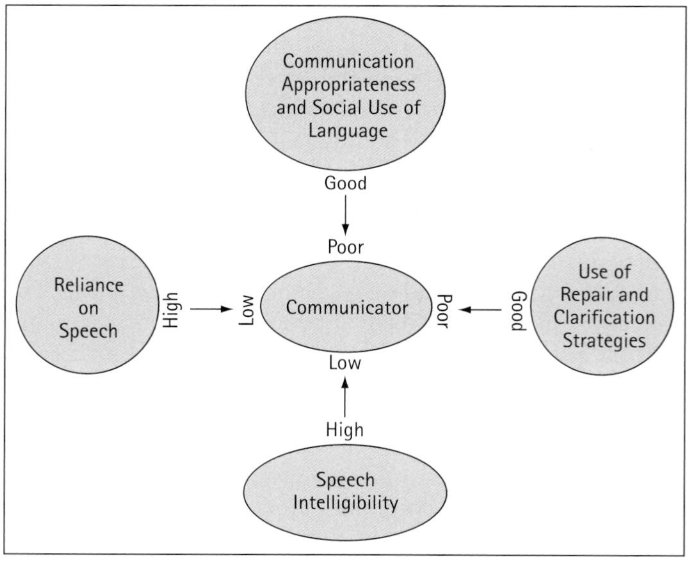

Figure 19.6 Several central factors contribute to the overall communication skills of a child. These factors include how much a child relies on speech for communication, how appropriate is a child's social use of language, how intelligible is a child's speech to another individual, and how well a child clarifies and repairs a situation when communication breaks down. (Adapted from Kent. In: Kasser and Grey, eds. *Enhancing Children's Communication.* Baltimore MD: Paul 4 Brooks 1993: 233–9.[43])

Such procedures may underestimate overall speech intelligibility, since the child may have difficulty hearing the stimulus sentence or may not be able to read.

As Figure 19.6 illustrates, speech intelligibility is related to overall oral communication skills in children with hearing losses. Children who experience high levels of intelligibility are rarely poor oral communicators.[43] Poor oral communicators appear to rely less on spoken speech than good oral communicators. With poor oral communicators, listeners often need to implement communication repair strategies such as requesting clarification. When children with hearing losses fail to use appropriate oral communication and repair strategies, they reduce their success in social use of language. Overall speech intelligibility may be a key limiting factor, and thus must be addressed directly. This should be done through specific intervention designed to improve the intelligibility deficits within the overall framework of the child's social use of language.[43]

Expressive and receptive spoken language in children with hearing impairments

The consequence of poor use of oral language in children with hearing losses has been documented in several studies.[36,44,57] Children with hearing losses are delayed in expressive vocabulary, syntax, and morphological skills.[58] Combining signing with spoken language does not appear to significantly improve spontaneous or imitated expressive language.[56,59] Although there is considerable individual variation in language performance, children with hearing losses tend to be delayed in their verbal skills, academic achievement, and social development.[57] These studies highlight the importance of providing children with hearing losses with good language models and encouraging the children to use spoken and gestural language even if it is not understood by listeners all of the time.

Hearing loss also appears to influence reading and writing skills. In the USA, the average reading level of 18-year-old adolescents with profound hearing losses ranges between third- and fourth-grade levels.[60] Literacy development appears to be related to at least three factors: severity of the hearing loss, early intervention, and spoken language skills. Geers and Moog[61] reported profoundly hearing-impaired high-school seniors who had been enrolled in either oral or mainstream high schools had reading levels commensurate with those of their peers. They concluded that the high levels of reading abilities in these children were related to their good use of residual hearing, early amplification, and strong oral language abilities, specifically vocabulary, grammar and conversational skills. Many investigators have proposed that the development of reading skills in individuals with profound hearing losses may be directly linked to the development of early communication skills. Extra efforts will be needed to fully develop reading and writing skills in children with hearing impairments, particularly if the hearing impairment is not identified early. Parents should be encouraged to serve as 'coaches' for their children in developing these important skills. For example, parents should be encouraged to provide quiet times where books or toys serve as the focus of developing communication skills in their children who have hearing impairments.

Effects of assistive sensory devices on speech and language development in children with hearing impairments

As discussed earlier, early identification and intervention is important for children with hearing impairments. Technical intervention may be achieved by conventional hearing aids, FM devices, tactile aids or multichannel cochlear implants. Several studies have examined the speech and language development in children with hearing impairments using such devices.[20,24,62–71] In addition to early detection and amplification, these studies have identified several variables that influence speech and language performance, including the type of assistive sensory device used, the length of assistive device use, and the mode of communication.

Initial studies compared the speech and language performance in children with hearing impairments who used either conventional hearing aids, tactile aids, or cochlear implants.[24,39,40,66–68,70–76] In some of the earliest studies, Osberger et al[74] examined speech samples from children who used single-channel cochlear implants, multichannel cochlear implants or tactile aids. Comparisons of speech inventories before device use and following 1 year of experience with the devices indicated that the greatest number of speech sounds were produced by the children using multichannel cochlear implants, although all devices appear to influence sound emergence to some extent.

Geers and co-workers[66,69–71,76,77] also conducted a carefully controlled study examining the speech and language development in children using different types of devices when the children were enrolled in an auditory–oral educational program. In this study, children were matched on variables such as chronological age, age of hearing loss identification, intelligence quotient, family support, and hearing profiles. Performance over a 3-year time period demonstrated significant improvements in performance for children using cochlear implants relative to children using either tactile or conventional hearing aids on many measures of speech production and perception. Receptive language scores were also significantly higher for the children with cochlear implants than for the children who used only conventional hearing aids or tactile aids. These results were particularly interesting when the rate of receptive language of the cochlear-implanted children was compared to norms collected on other hearing-impaired children. The cochlear implant children demonstrated scores that progressed from slightly above average to the 86th percentile in only a 3-year time period. Accuracy of sound production also reflected differences across the three devices. Children with cochlear implants had higher percentage-correct sounds than the children using hearing aids or tactile aids.[67] Three examples of speech production measures acquired in children with hearing aids, tactile aids and cochlear implants are shown in Figure 19.7. The left-hand panel demonstrates the accuracy of sound production for vowels which are visible (produced in the front of the mouth), the middle panel illustrates the accuracy for producing fricative consonants, such as 's', and the right-hand panel depicts the accuracy of consonants produced in the back of the mouth, which are not visible. The important point to notice is that all three groups at the beginning of the study, before children received their cochlear implant or tactile aid, had similar performance. Experience with the devices over time demonstrated more accurate performance for the cochlear-implanted children, although all children demonstrated benefit from their auditory–oral education.

Language acquisition studies continue to suggest that children with cochlear implants outpace children with comparable hearing losses who use other types of assistive listening device. Miyamoto and co-workers[78–80] found that prelingually deaf children using cochlear implants equaled or exceeded normal language growth as shown on the Reynell Developmental Language Scales. Comparisons of language-age equivalent scores at 6 and 15 months postoperatively exceeded predicted language scores determined from pre-implant performance, suggesting that faster rates of language acquisition occurred post-implantation. In addition, differences in scores between the predicted and acquired language equivalent scores were greater at 15 months than at 6 months postoperatively, suggesting that significant gains were made in language performance. Tomblin et al[81] tracked 29 children with cochlear implants and found syntax scores post-implant which were 20 points higher and greater than one standard deviation higher than in children using hearing aids. Later analyses revealed that performance was related to years of experience with a cochlear implant rather than chronological age, per se. These data provide further evidence that information provided by a cochlear implant assists young children in acquiring oral language skills.

Length of experience of using a cochlear implant appears to be an important variable in examining how language is acquired in these children. More than half of the children exceeded the 95% prediction interval for their syntactic performance after only 2 years of experience. These data suggest that children will demonstrate rapid and significant changes in language development in the very early years of cochlear implant use and that failures to observe such language increases may signal that additional efforts should be directed towards a given child. Figure 19.8 illustrates another approach for examining language acquisition in cochlear-implanted children.[82] The diagonal line across the graph indicates the language growth that might be expected from a normally hearing child. This line indicates that as a child increases in chronological age, a concomitant increase in expressive language age occurs. The lowest line indicates the rate of expressive language gains found in profoundly hearing-impaired children who use hearing aids. The slope of this line indicates that these children fail to demonstrate expressive language gains comparable to those of normally hearing children. The gap between the performance

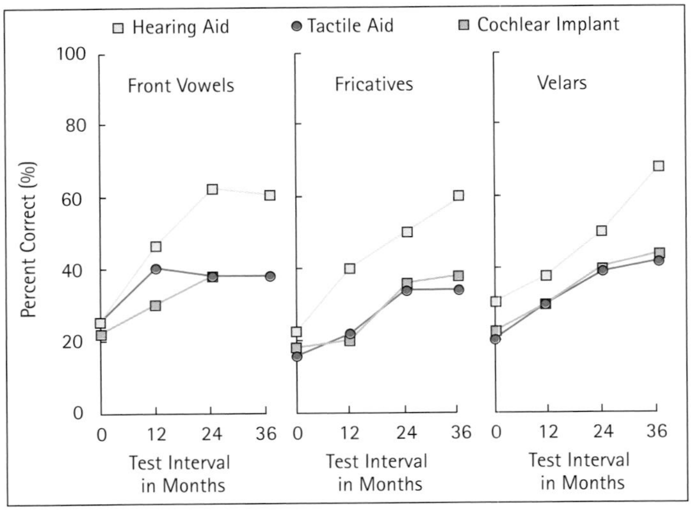

Figure 19.7 Accuracy of sound production is shown for three different groups of children with hearing losses using different types of sensory aid devices (hearing aids, tactile aids, and cochlear implants). All the children show improvement in the accuracy of their sound production over time; however, the greatest gains are seen for the children with cochlear implants. Examples of sound production for vowels are shown in the left-hand panel, fricatives (such as 's') are shown in the middle panel, and velar consonants (sounds made in the back of the mouth, such as 'g') are shown in the right panel. (Adapted from Tobey et al. *Volta Rev* 1994; **96**(5): 109–31.[67])

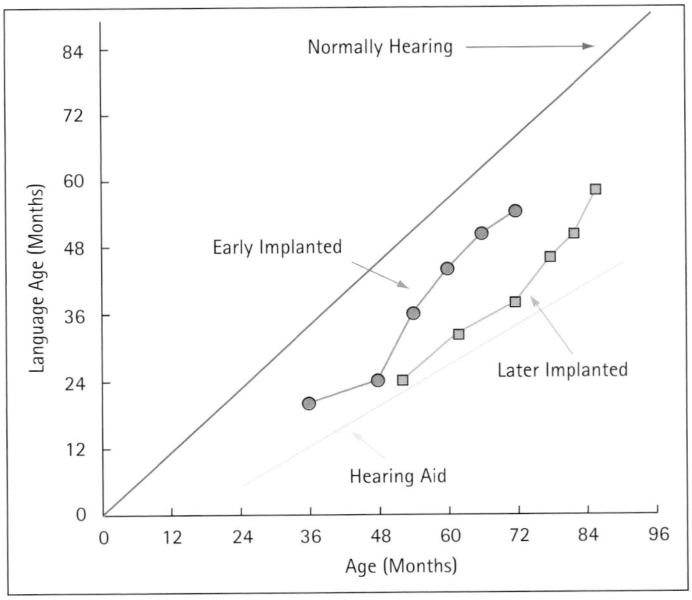

Figure 19.8 Expressive language scores achieved at various chronological ages in normally hearing and hearing-impaired children. The diagonal line refers to the predicted change in expressive language age for normally hearing children of various ages. Data are also given for children with hearing aids and cochlear implants. Note that expressive language scores are routinely higher for children who receive their cochlear implants at early ages relative to children who receive their implants at later ages. (Adapted from Svirsky. *Psychological Science* 2000; **11**(2): 153–8.[82])

levels increases over time, with significant differences in performance clearly evident. Note that the slopes of the performance for the cochlear-implanted children are similar to the slope of the normally hearing children, indicating that the cochlear-implanted children are making language gains comparable to language gains made by the normally hearing children. Moreover, the gap in performance between normally hearing children and cochlear-implanted children does not increase over time. These data suggest that cochlear implants provide valuable information that children may use to develop expressive language skills.

Techniques for enhancing oral communication in children with hearing losses

Several curricula have been developed to enhance the acquisition of auditory, speech and language skills in children using cochlear implants. Each of these curricula may be adapted for children with a range of hearing losses and different assistive sensory aids. Each of the curricula develops auditory skills through detection, discrimination and identification tasks. Children are taught to detect when a sound is present or absent. Discrimination training concentrates on teaching children to determine if sounds are similar or different. Identification tasks work on expanding sounds and words that a child understands. Speech production is incorporated as a necessary ingredient for associating speaking and listening. Thus, children learn to monitor and adjust their own speech. As skills increase, stimuli are varied and increased in complexity, thus facilitating language development. Information on reference textbooks and curricula which develop communication skills are given in the Appendix.

One of the earliest stages involves training young children to be aware of sound and to be responsive to the voices of members of their families. As young children become aware of sound, they will begin to recognize sounds that they produce and to explore how to vary these sounds. As children begin to associate sound with meaningful acts, they will turn and respond when their name is called. Children will also begin to listen to more complex sentences and begin to use oral language to express their ideas. These steps of receptive and expressive language acquisition occur for normally hearing children and serve as the model for training young hearing-impaired children to acquire language skills.

Parents should be encouraged to work on communication skills daily with their child. Time should be set aside each day for activities designed to encourage communication. Examples of activities which facilitate language development include playing with age-appropriate toys, looking at and reading books, taking walks and talking about what one sees on the walks, playing make-believe games, or participating in household activities (e.g. making cookies or decorating a cake). Parents must expect their child to communicate and participate in activities designed to facilitate communication. Several techniques may be used to stimulate language.[83] One method is to describe a sequence of events using language that is more complex than what their child typically uses. Using more complex language provides a model for a child to follow and encourages them to associate more advanced vocabulary and sounds. Parents also may engage in 'self-talk', where the adults provide a running commentary on the event or situation they are sharing with the child. In other situations, parents may provide parallel talk by allowing the child to lead an activity and simply commenting on the activity. Such comments provide structure and language for the child's activity. As children continue to develop communication skills, parents may engage in modeling and expansion techniques to further increase exposure to language. Modeling and expanding on the child's message reinforce what the child has said, demonstrate that the child's message was understood, and introduce new language structures. Parental involvement must continue as children enter school, in order to ensure facilitation of language and communication skills within the academic environment.

Summary

This chapter has reviewed key aspects of speech and language development in normally hearing and hearing-impaired children. Early identification and treatment of hearing loss is important, since evidence suggests that delaying identification until after 6 months of age may result in reduced language abilities. It is important to facilitate language development and communication skills, regardless of the mode of communication used. Parents are ideal facilitators for developing communication skills, and should be guided by professionals to be major contributors in facilitating communication.

References

1. Lenneberg EH. *Biological Foundations of Language* New York: Wiley, 1967.
2. Yoshinaga-Itano C, Sedey A, Coulter B, Mehl A. Language of early- and later-identified children with hearing loss. *Pediatrics* 1998; **120**(5): 1161–71.
3. Bloom L, Lahey P. *Language Development and Language Disorders*. New York: Wiley, 1978.
4. Eilers RE, Oller DK. Infant vocalizations and the early diagnosis of severe hearing impairment. *J Pediatrics* 1994; **124**(2): 199–203.
5. Eilers RE, Cobo-Lewis AB, Vergara KC, Oller DK, Friedman KE. A longitudinal evaluation of the speech perception capabilities of children using multichannel tactile vocoders. *J Speech Hear Res* 1996; **39**(3): 518–33.
6. Kusko CW. Language and linguistic development. *Otolaryngology Clinics of North America* 1985; **18**(2): 315–22.

7. Eilers RE, Gavin WJ, Oller DK. Cross linguistic perception in infancy: early effects of linguistic experience. *J Child Language* 1982; **9**(2): 289–302.
8. Tait M, Lutman ME. The predictive value of measures of preverbal communicative behaviors in young deaf children with cochlear implants. *Ear Hear* 1997; **18**(6): 472–8.
9. Lutman ME, Tait DM. Early communicative behavior in young children receiving cochlear implants: factor analysis of turn-taking and gaze orientation. *Ann Otol Rhinol Laryngol Suppl* 1995; **166**: 397–99.
10. Tait DM, Wood DJ. From communication to speech in deaf children. *Child Language Teaching Ther* 1987; **3**(1): 1–17.
11. Tait M, Lutman ME. Comparison of early communicative behavior in young children with cochlear implants and with hearing aids. *Ear Hear* 1994; **15**(5): 352–61.
12. Tait M. Making and monitoring progress in the pre-school years. *J Br Assoc Teachers Deaf* 1987; **11**(5): 143–53.
13. Yoshinaga-Itano C, Stredler-Brown A. Learning to communicate: babies with hearing impairments make their needs known. *Volta Rev* 1992; **94**(2): 107–129.
14. Robinshaw HM. Acquisition of speech, pre- and post-cochlear implantation: longitudinal studies of a congenitally deaf infant. *Eur J Disord Commun* 1996; **31**(2): 121–39.
15. Robinshaw HM. The pattern of development from non-communicative behaviour to language by hearing impaired and hearing infants. *Br J Audiol* 1996; **30**(2): 177–98.
16. Apuzzo ML, Yoshinaga-Itano C. Early identification of infants with significant hearing loss and the Minnesota Child Development Inventory. *Semin Hear* 1995; **16**(2): 124–39.
17. Yoshinaga-Itano C. Efficacy of early identification and early intervention. *Semin Hear* 1995; **16**(2): 115–23.
18. Nicholas JG, Geers AE. Communication of oral deaf and normally hearing children at 36 months of age. *J Speech Language Hear Res* 1997; **40**(6): 1314–27.
19. Miskiel LW, Carney AE, Johnson CJ, Carney E. An analysis of phonetic level evaluation: age and task factors. *Language Speech Hear Services Schools* 1994; **25**: 165–73.
20. Tobey E. Auditory feedback delivered by electrical stimulation from a cochlear implant and speech production. In: Bell-Berti F, Raphael L, eds. *Producing Speech: Contemporary Issues for Katherine Safford Harris*. New York: American Institute of Physics, 1995: 455–69.
21. Tobey EA. Speech production considerations in the management of children receiving cochlear implants. *Semin Hear* 1986; **7**(4): 407–22.
22. Tobey EA. *Stop Consonant Perception and Production in Cochlear Implant Users–Grant Application*, 1989.
23. McGarr NS, Lofqvist A. Laryngeal kinematics in voiceless obstruents produced by hearing-impaired speakers. *J Speech Hear Res* 1988; **31**(2): 234–9.
24. Geers AE, Moog JS. Assessing the benefits of cochlear implants in an oral education program. *Adv Otorhinolaryngol* 1995; **50**: 119–24.
25. McGarr NS, Lofqvist A. Obstruent production by hearing-impaired speakers: interarticulator timing and acoustics. *J Acoust Soc Am* 1982; **72**(1): 34–42.
26. Hanson VL, McGarr NS. Rhyme generation by deaf adults. *J Speech Hear Res* 1989; **32**: 2–11.
27. Osberger MJ, McGarr N. Speech production characteristics of the hearing impaired. In: Lass N, ed. *Speech and Language: Advances in Basic Research and Practice*. New York: Academic Press, 1982: 221–283.
28. Tye-Murray N, Kirk KI. Vowel and dipthong production by young users of cochlear implants the relationship between the phonetic level evaluation and spontaneous speech. *J Speech Hear Res* 1993; **36**(3): 488–502.
29. Abraham S. Using a phonological framework to describe speech errors of orally trained, hearing-impaired school-agers. *J Speech Hear Disord* 1989; **54**: 600–9.
30. Geffner D. Feature characteristics of spontaneous speech production in young deaf children. *J Commun Disord* 1980; **13**(6): 443–54.
31. Miyamoto RT, Kirk KI, Robbins AM, Todd S, Riley A, Pisoni DB. Speech perception and speech intelligibility in children with multichannel cochlear implants. *Adv Otorhinolaryngol* 1997; **52**: 198–203.
32. Kvam MH, Bredal UJ. Do we understand the speech of deaf adolecents? An evaluation and comparison of the intelligibility in two similar research projects from 1979 and 1995. *Logoped Phoniatr Vocol* 2000; **25**(2): 87–92.
33. Klimacka L, Patterson A, Patterson R. Listening to deaf speech: does experience count? *Int J Lang Commun Disord* 2001; **36**(Suppl): 210–5.
34. Monsen RB. A usable test for the speech intelligibility of deaf talkers. *Am Annal Deaf* 1981; **126**(7): 845–52.
35. Monsen RB. Toward measuring how well hearing-impaired children speak. *J Speech Hear Res* 1978; **21**(2): 197–219.
36. Monsen RB. The oral speech intelligibility of hearing-impaired talkers. *J Speech Hear Disord* 1983; **48**(3): 286–96.
37. McGarr N. The intelligibility of deaf speech to experienced and inexperienced listeners. *J Speech Hear Res* 1983; **26**: 451–8.
38. Osberger MJ, Robbins AM, Todd S, Riley A. Speech intelligibility of children with cochlear implants. *Volta Rev* 1994; **96**(5): 169–80.
39. Osberger MJ, Maso M, Sam LK. Speech intelligibility of children with cochlear implants, tactile aids, or hearing aids. *J Speech Hear Res* 1993; **36**(1): 186–203.
40. Osberger MJ. Speech intelligibility in the hearing impaired: research and clinical implications. In: Kent R, ed. *Intelligibility in Speech Disorders*. Amsterdam: John Benjamins, 1992: 233–64.
41. Elfenbein JL, Hardin-Jones MA, Davis JM. Oral communication skills of children who are hard of hearing. *J Speech Hear Res* 1994; **37**(1): 216–26.
42. McGarr NS. The effect of context on the intelligibility of hearing and deaf children's speech. *Language Speech* 1981; **24**(Pt 3): 255–64.
43. Kent RD. Speech intelligibility and communicative competence in children. In: Kaiser AP, Gray DB, eds. *Enhancing Children's Communication*. Baltimore, MD: Paul H. Brooks, 1993: 233–9.
44. Bouvet D. The speech of the deaf child: the role of sign language in the process of language acquisition by the deaf child; La Parole

de l'enfant sourd: l'apport de la langue des signes dans le processus d'appropriation du langage par l'enfant sourd. *Langage l'Homme* 1982; **48**: 47–52.
45. Arnold P. Teaching English to hearing-impaired children. *J Br Assoc Teachers Deaf* 1989; **13**(4): 100–9.
46. Bernstein J, Boyce S, Bush MA et al. Studies of speech production and speech discrimination by children and by the hearing-impaired. *RLE Prog Rep* 1979; **121**: 112–13.
47. Cavallazzi G, De Filippis A. Severe hearing loss in early childhood: results of reeducation methods; La surdite profonde dans la premiere enfance: resultats des methodes de reeducation. *Acta Otol Rhinol Laryngol Belg* 1974; **28**(1): 83–90.
48. Bakkum MJ, Plomp R, Pols LW. Objective analysis versus subjective assessment of vowels pronounced by deaf and normal-hearing children. *J Acoust Soc Am* 1995; **98**(2Pt 1): 745–62.
49. Dagenais PA, Critz-Crosby P, Fletcher SG, McCutcheon MJ. Comparing abilities of children with profound hearing impairments to learn consonants using electropalatography or traditional aural–oral techniques. *J Speech Hear Res* 1994; **37**(3): 687–99.
50. Geers AE, Schick B. Acquisition of spoken and signed English by hearing-impaired children of hearing-impaired or hearing parents. *J Speech Hear Disord* 1988; **53**(2): 136–43.
51. Gallaway C, Aplin DY, Newton VE, Hostler ME. The GMC project: some linguistic and cognitive characteristics of a population of hearing-impaired children. *Br J Audiol* 1990; **24**(1): 17–27.
52. Geers AE, Moog JS. Predicting spoken language acquisition of profoundly hearing-impaired children. *J Speech Hear Disord* 1987; **52**(1): 84–94.
53. Geers A, Moog J. Spoken language results: vocabulary, syntax, and communication. *Volta Rev* 1994; **96**(5): 131–48.
54. Geers AE, Lagati S. Recent studies that show the validity of the oral method in teaching hearing-impaired children; Una ricerca recente che mette in evidenza la validita del metodo orale nell'insegnamento dei bambini audiolesi. *Effeta* 1989; **82**(5): 84–7.
55. Geers A, Moog J, Schick B. Acquisition of spoken and signed English by profoundly deaf children. *J Speech Hear Disord* 1984; **49**(4): 378–88.
56. Geers AE, Moog JS. Syntactic maturity of spontaneous speech and elicited imitations of hearing-impaired children. *J Speech Hear Disord* 1978; **43**(3): 380–91.
57. Davis JM, Elfenbein J, Schum R, Bentler RA. Effects of mild and moderate hearing impairments on language, educational, and psychosocial behavior of children. *J Speech Hear Disord* 1986; **51**(1): 53–62.
58. Moeller MP, Osberger MJ, Eccarius M et al. Receptive language skills/expressive language skills/academic skills/visual processing, short-term memory, and visual–motor coordination skills. *ASHA Monogr* 1986; **23**: 41–83.
59. Brentari D, Wolk SJ. The relative effects of three expressive methods upon the speech intelligibility of profoundly deaf speakers. *Commun Disord* 1986; **19**(3): 209–18.
60. LaSasso CJ, Mobley RT. National survey of reading instruction for deaf or hard-of-hearing students in the US. *Volta Rev* 1997; **99**(1): 31–58.
61. Geers EA, Moog JS. Speech perception and production skills of students with impaired hearing from oral and total communication education settings. *J Speech Hear Res* 1992; **35**(6): 1384–93.
62. Serry T, Blamey P, Grogan M. Phoneme acquisition in the first 4 years of implant use. *Am J Otol* 1997; **18**(6 Suppl): S122–4.
63. Tye-Murray N, Spencer L, Bedia EG, Woodworth G. Differences in children's sound production when speaking with a cochlear implant turned on and turned off. *J Speech Hear Res* 1996; **39**(3): 604–10.
64. Miyamoto RT, Kirk KI, Svirsky MA Sehgal ST. Communication skills in pediatric cochlear implant recipients. *Acta Otolaryngol* 1999; **119**(2): 219–24.
65. Waltzman SP, Cohen NLM, Pivak LP, et al. Improvement in speech perception and production abilities in children using a multichannel cochlear implant. *Laryngoscope* 1990; **100**(3): 240–3.
66. Boothroyd A, Geers AE, Moog JS. Practical implications of cochlear implants in children [published erratum appears in *Ear Hear* 1991; **12**(6): 442]. *Ear Hear* 1991; **12**(4 Suppl): 81S–9S.
67. Tobey EA, Geers A, Brenner C. Speech production results: speech feature acquisition. *Volta Rev* 1994; **96**(5): 109–31.
68. Tobey EA, Geers AE. Speech production benefits of cochlear implants. *Adv Otorhinolaryngol* 1995; **50**: 146–53.
69. Geers AE. Comparing implants with hearing aids in profoundly deaf children. *Otolaryngol Head Neck Surg* 1997; **117**(3 Pt 1): 150–4.
70. Geers AE, Tobey EA. Longitudinal comparison of the benefits of cochlear implants and tactile aids in a controlled educational setting. *Ann Otol Rhinol Laryngol Suppl* 1995; **166**: 328–9.
71. Geers AE, Moog JS. Evaluating the benefits of cochlear implants in an educational setting. *Am J Otol* 1991; **12**(Suppl): 116–25.
72. Osberger MJ. Audiological rehabilitation with cochlear implants and tactile aids. *ASHA* 1990; **32**(4): 43–8.
73. Carney AE, Osberger MJ, Carney E, Robbins AM, Renshaw J, Miyamoto RT. A comparison of speech discrimination with cochlear implants and tactile aids. *J Acoust Soc Am* 1993; **94**(4): 2036–49.
74. Osberger MJ, Robbins AM, Berry SW, Todd SL, Hesketh LJ, Sedey A. Analysis of the spontaneous speech samples of children with cochlear implants or tactile aids. *Am J Otol* 1991; **12**(suppl): 151–64.
75. Geers A, Moog J. Effectiveness of Cochlear Implants and Tactile Aids for Deaf Children: The Sensory Aids Study at the Central Institute for the Deaf. *Volta Rev* 1994; **96**(5): 109–31.
76. Geers AE. Speech and language evaluation in aided and implanted children. *Scand Audiol Suppl* 1997; **46**: 72–5.
77. Moog JS, Geers AE. Impact of the cochlear implant on the educational setting. *Adv Otorhinolaryngol* 1995; **50**: 174–6.
78. Carney AE, Kienle M, Miyamoto RT. Speech perception with a single-channel cochlear implant: a comparison with a single-channel tactile device. *J Speech Hear Res* 1990; **33**: 229–37.
79. Miyamoto RT, Svirsky MA, Robbins AM. Enhancement of expressive language in prelingually deaf children with cochlear implants. *Acta Otolaryngol* 1997; **117**(2): 154–7.
80. Robbins AM, Osberger MJ, Miyamoto RT, Kessler KS. Language development in young children with cochlear implants. *Adv Otorhinolaryngol* 1995; **50**: 160–6.

81. Tomblin J, Spencer L, Flock S, Tyler R, Gantz B. A comparison of language achievement in children with cochlear implants and children using hearing aids. *J Speech Language Hear Res* 1999; **42**(2): 497–509.
82. Svirsky. *Language development in early implanted, prelingually deaf children*. Paper presented at Iowa Conference on Implantable Prostheses, *Psychological Science* 2000; **11**(2): 153–8.
83. Tye-Murray N. *Let's Converse: A 'How-to' Guide to Develop and Expand Conversational Skills of Children and Teenagers Who Are Hearing Impaired*. Washington, DC: Alexander Graham Bell Association for the Deaf, 1994.

Appendix: resource for professionals working with children with hearing losses

Curricula for training communication skills

Koch ME. *Bringing Sound to Life: Principles and Practices of Cochlear Implant Rehabilitation*. Timonium, Maryland: The Advisory Board Foundation, York Press, 1999.

Moog JS, Biedenstein JJ, Davidson LS. *SPICE: Speech Perception Instructional Curriculum and Evaluation*. St Louis, Missouri: Central Institute for the Deaf, 1995.

Vergara KC, Miskiel LW. *CHATS: The Miami Cochlear Implant, Auditory and Tactile Skills Curriculum*. Miami, Florida: Intelligent Hearing Systems, 1994.

Wayner D, Abrhamson JE, Casterton J. *Learning to Hear Again with a Cochlear Implant. Better Communication and Cochlear Implants: A User's Guide*. Washington, DC: Alexander Graham Bell Association for the Deaf, 1995.

Examples of resource materials

Deconde Johnson C, Benson P, Seaton J. *Educational Audiology Handbook*. San Diego, CA: Singular Publishing Group, Inc. 1997.

Estabrooks W. *Cochlear Implants for Kids*. Washington DC: Alexander Graham Bell Association for the Deaf, 1998.

Hull R. *Aural Rehabilitation Serving Children and Adults*, 3rd edn. San Diego, CA: Singular Publishing Group, Inc. 1997.

Luterman D. *Counseling Persons with Communication Disorders and Their Families*, 3rd edn. Austin, TX: Pro-Ed, 1996.

McAnally P, Rose S, Quigley S. *Language Learning Practices with Deaf Children* 2nd edn. Austin, TX: Pro-Ed, 1994.

Nevins ME, Chute PM. *Children with Cochlear Implants in Educational Settings*. Washington DC: Alexander Graham Bell Association for the Deaf, 1996.

Tye-Murray N. *Children with Cochlear Implants: A Handbook for Parents, Teachers, and Speech and Hearing Professionals*. Washington DC: Alexander Graham Bell Association for the Deaf, 1992.

Tye-Murray N. *Let's Converse: A 'How-To' Guide to Develop and Expand Conversational Skills of Children and Teenagers who are Hearing-Impaired.'* Washington, DC: Alexander Graham Bell Association for the Deaf, 1994.

Tye-Murray N. *Foundations of Aural Rehabilitation: Children, Adults, and their Family Members*. Washington, DC: Alexander Graham Bell Association for the Deaf, 1998.

Section III

Auditory disorders and their management

20 Screening programs for hearing loss

Karl R White

The need for identifying hearing loss during the first few months of life was advocated in Great Britain more than 50 years ago, when Ewing and Ewing noted 'an urgent need to study further and more critically methods of testing hearing in young children . . . During this first year the existence of deafness needs to be ascertained . . . Training needs to be begun at the earliest age that the diagnosis of deafness can be established.'[1]

Since that time, a variety of procedures have been tried to identify babies with congenital hearing loss during the first few months of life. The latest approach, being advocated by many in Europe and the USA, is the measurement of otoacoustical emissions (OAE) or automated auditory brainstem response (AABR) for hearing screening for all newborns prior to the time they are discharged from the hospital. Such universal newborn hearing screening (UNHS) has been recommended by such influential groups as the National Institutes of Health[2] and the American Academy of Pediatrics[3] in the USA and 1998 European Consensus Development Conference attended by representatives from most western European countries.[4]

> All hearing impaired infants should be identified and treatment initiated by 6 months of age . . . The consensus panel recommends screening of all newborns . . . for hearing impairment prior to discharge.[2]

> The American Academy of Pediatrics . . . endorses the goal of universal detection of hearing loss in infants before 3 months of age . . . [which] requires universal screening of all infants.[3]

> Identification by screening at or shortly after birth has the potential to improve quality of life and opportunities for those affected . . . Implementation of neonatal screening programs should not be delayed.[4]

Given such positive support from authoritative groups, it is not surprising that the implementation of universal newborn hearing screening programs continues to grow. For example, more than two thirds of all babies born in the USA are now screened for hearing loss prior to hospital discharge, and there has been a dramatic growth in the number of birthing hospitals with UNHS programs (Figures 20.1 and 20.2).

Not everyone is convinced that UNHS is feasible, effective, or beneficial. For example, even though they recognize

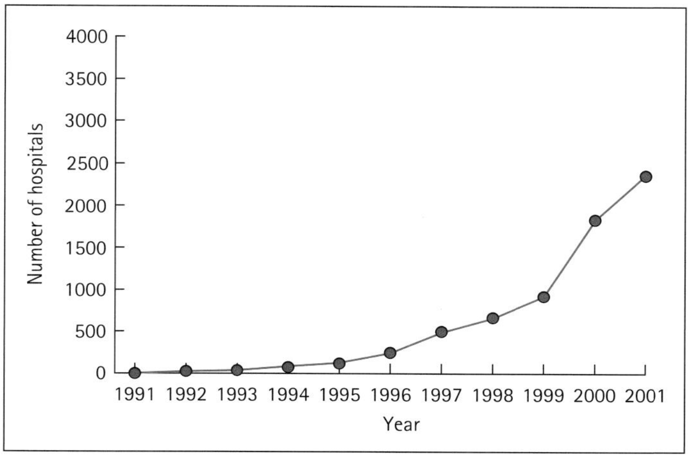

Figure 20.1 Number of hospitals in the USA with universal newborn hearing screening programs. (Adapted from Hyde et al. *J Am Acad Audiol* 1990; 1: 59–66.[28])

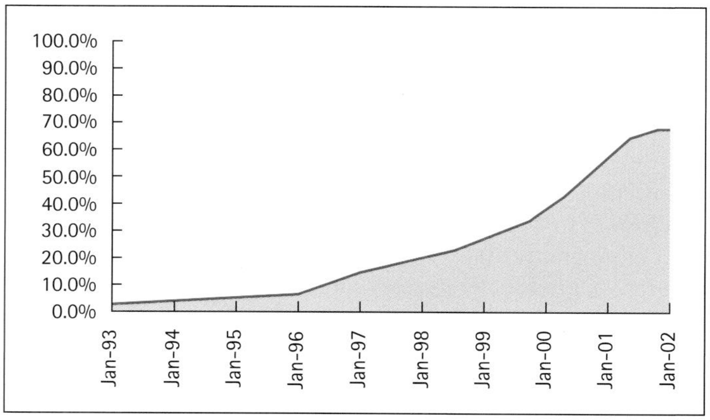

Figure 20.2 Percentage of newborns in the USA screened for hearing prior to hospital discharge.

that 'congenital hearing loss is a serious health problem associated with developmental delay in speech and language function', the 1996 recommendations of the prestigious US Preventive Services Task Force concluded that 'there is little evidence to support the use of routine, universal screening for all neonates'.[5] Similarly, a 1999 article in *Pediatrics* concluded:[6]

> universal newborn hearing screening in our present state of knowledge is not necessarily the only, or the best, or the most cost-effective way to achieve [early identification of hearing loss], and more importantly, that the benefits of universal newborn hearing screening may be outweighed by its risks.[6]

The rapid growth of UNHS programs over the last 5 years, juxtaposed with the concerns about the effectiveness and value of UNHS programs, emphasizes the need to examine whether hospital-based UNHS programs should become the standard of care throughout the world. This chapter will summarize the evidence related to the following issues:

- Are there a sufficient number of babies with congenital hearing loss to justify UNHS?
- How accurate and efficient are various newborn hearing screening techniques?
- Are there negative 'side-effects' for families?
- Are there positive benefits associated with early identification of hearing loss?

Prevalence of congenital hearing loss

The prevalence of permanent congenital hearing loss (PCHL) depends on the definition. For example, Figure 20.3 shows the results of nine different studies[7–15] to determine the number of children with bilateral PCHL in cohorts ranging in size from 30 000 to over 4 million children. Not surprisingly, the prevalence of bilateral PCHL is substantially higher when milder hearing loss is included. If the analysis is limited to children with 50-dB or greater bilateral loss, the prevalence is about 1/1000. However, when children with 30-dB bilateral losses are included, the prevalence is more than 2.0/1000.

Each of the studies in Figure 20.2 only included children with bilateral hearing losses. If children with unilateral losses had been included, the prevalence would increase by one-third to one-half, as shown by the data in Table 20.1.[16–18] Taken together, these data suggest that we should expect to find 3 or 4 children per 1000 with PCHL from well-run, hospital-based, UNHS programs. As shown in Table 20.2, this is what is being reported in published reports of large-scale UNHS programs.[19–26]

It is important to note that the numbers reported from the retrospective studies listed in Table 20.1 could have included children with acquired, instead of congenital, hearing losses. It is often assumed that there are about as many infants and toddlers with acquired losses as with congenital losses. However, geographical areas with long-established UNHS programs in

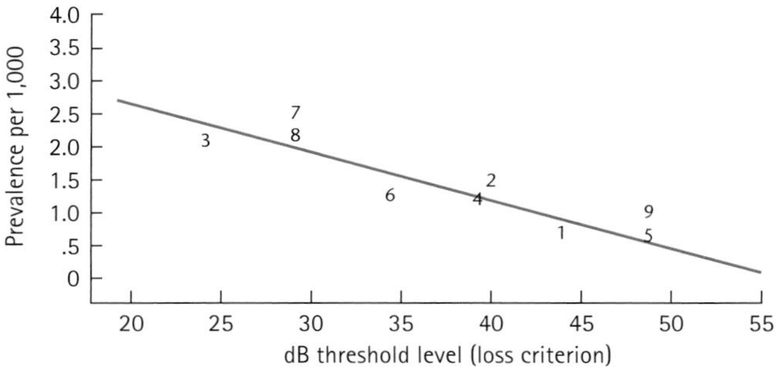

Study/subject ages sample size/prevalence per 1,000; Loss threshold

1. Barr[7]; 1980; 2–5 year olds (*n* = 65,000); 0.9 per 1000; 45 dB HL
2. Feinmesser et al[8]; 1986; infants born between 1967 and 1978 (*n* = 62,000); 1.7 per 1,000; 40 dB HL
3. Fitzland[9]; 1985; 6-month-olds (mean) (*n* =30,890); 1.9 per 1,000; 25 dB HL
4. Kankkunen[10]; 1982; 6-year-olds (*n* =31,280); 1.3 per 1,000; 40 dB HL
5. Martin[11]; 1982; 8-year-olds (*n* =4,126,268); 0.9 per 1,000; 50 dB HL
6. Parving[12]; 1985; 8-year-old (median) (*n* = 82,265); 1.4 per 1,000; 35 dB HL
7. Sehlin et al[13]; 1990; 2–12-year-olds (*n* = 63,463); 2.4 per 1,000; 30 dB HL
8. Sorri & Rantakallio[14]; 1985; 15-year-olds (*n* = 11.780); 2.1 per 1,000; 30 dB HL
9. Davis & Wood[15]; 1992; 2–6 year-olds (*n* = 29,317); 1.1 per 1,000; 50 dB HL

Figure 20.3 Reported prevalence rates of sensorineural and mixed hearing losses.

Table 20.1 Percentage of sensorineural hearing losses which are unilateral.

Author (year)	Number of hearing impaired children in sample	% Unilateral
Kinney (1953)[16]	1307	48%
Brookhauser et al (1991)[17]	1829	37%
Watkin et al (1990)[18]	171	35%

Table 20.2 Prevalence of PCHL in published reports of UNHS programs with large samples.

Location	Number screened	Prevalence per 1000	Hospital-based screening method
Rhode Island[19]	3,300	4.0	OAE
Rhode Island[20]	52,695	2.1	OAE
Colorado[21]	41,796	2.6	AABR
Wessex[22]	7,593	2.6	OAE
Texas[23]	54,228	2.1	OAE & AABR
New York[24]	43,004	1.9	OAE & AABR
Hawaii[25]	9,605	4.2	OAE
New Jersey[26]	15,749	3.3	ABR

the USA, where tens of thousands of infants have now been screened, are finding very few children with acquired losses. For example, in Rhode Island, Hawaii, and Colorado, hundreds of children have now been identified with PCHL. These programs have been operating long enough that there are thousands of 7-, 8- and 9-year-olds who were screened as infants. If acquired hearing loss were as frequent as is often assumed, we should now be discovering dozens of children with acquired losses as they enter school. In fact, very few of such children have been identified.[27] A more reasonable hypothesis is that many children who were previously thought to have acquired losses really had congenital mild or moderate PCHL, which may have been progressive. As infants, they had enough hearing to babble, acquire some speech, or turn to loud noises. Later, because of delayed speech, hearing loss was diagnosed and it was assumed that it was an acquired loss. In fact, many of these cases probably represented mild or moderate progressive congenital losses.

Accuracy of newborn hearing screening methods

THE FOLLOWING FIVE METHODS HAVE BEEN USED FREQUENTLY TO DETECT HEARING LOSS IN INFANTS AND YOUNG CHILDREN

- Behavioral evaluations at 7–9 months
- Auditory brainstem response (ABR)
- High-risk indicators
- Otoacoustical emissions
- Automated ABR

How much is known about the accuracy of those methods? Even though the terms 'sensitivity' and 'specificity' are often used with regard to these techniques, there are no population-based studies of universal newborn hearing screening where there are sufficiently large sample sizes and sufficently good follow-up to definitively establish the sensitivity and specificity of any of these techniques. Most studies which refer to sensitivity and specificity have used very small sample sizes, have focused only on high-risk babies, or have not followed all of the babies who passed the screening test to determine their true hearing status. A frequent problem is that studies that have allegedly examined the sensitivity and specificity of a particular screening technique have really only compared one screening technique with another screening technique. Thus, data are not available to definitively establish the sensitivity and specificity of any of the techniques. As summarized below, however, information is available that provides reasonably good evidence about the accuracy of each of these screening techniques.

Auditory brainstem response (ABR)

Many different studies have examined the use of ABR to detected hearing losses among young children. For example; Hyde et al[28] evaluated 713 high-risk babies who were screened with ABR prior to hospital discharge, and then were assessed by diagnosticians who did not know the screening results when the children were an average of almost 4 years old (Figure 20.4). The behaviorally confirmed hearing status was compared to the results of the hearing screening test. For this high-risk population, the sensitivity and specificity were 98% and 96% when the ABR screening threshold was set at 40 dB HL, and 100% and 91% when the ABR screening threshold level was set at 30 dB HL. Additional data about the accuracy of ABR as a hearing screening tool were reported by Barsky-Firkser and Sun,[26] who screened more than 5000 newborns over a 3-year period. An average of 3.3 infants per 1000 were identified with a congenital hearing loss and referred to intervention programs. In spite of abundant evidence about the accuracy of ABR as a screening tool for hearing loss in young children,[29] it is seldom advocated for UNHS programs, because it is relatively expensive.

High-risk indicators

Until the early 1990s, the most frequent method used in the USA to identify hearing loss in very young children was based on the high-risk indicators recommended by the Joint Committee on Infant Hearing (JCIH).[30] About 10% of all

ABR screen (40 dBHL)	Hearing status: Impaired	Hearing status: Normal
Refer	44	57
Pass	1	1265

Sensitivity = 98%
Specificity = 96%

ABR screen (30 dBHL)	Hearing status: Impaired	Hearing status: Normal
Refer	45	125
Pass	0	1197

Sensitivity = 100%
Specificity = 91%

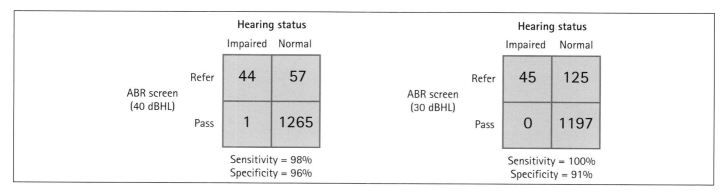

Figure 20.4 Accuracy of ABR for UNHS. NB: Results based on 1367 cases with reliable ABR and puretone results. (Adapted from Hyde et al. *J Am Acad Audiol* 1990; 1: 59–66.[28])

children born will exhibit one or more of these indicators, including family history of congenital hearing loss, very low birthweight, congenital malformations of the head and neck, and hyperbilirubinemia. The JCIH recommendation was that infants with one of these risk indicators be screened for hearing loss using ABR. The rationale for this approach was that by focusing on a subset of the population which was at higher risk, hospitals could afford to use ABR because a smaller number of children would require testing.

Very few hospitals are currently using this approach, for two reasons. First, as shown in Figure 20.5, even though children with risk factors are more likely to have hearing loss, only about half of all children with congenital hearing loss will exhibit one or more of these indicators.[8,18,31–33] Thus, even if a high-risk-based screening program were to work perfectly, about half of all children with PCHL would be missed.

More importantly, high-risk-based screening programs have found it difficult to get parents to return for the diagnostic evaluations. For example, Mahoney and Eichwald[11] reported the results of a high-risk based screening program over a 7-year period (1978–84). During that time, the JCIH indicators were incorporated into the legally required birth certificate, so they were reported for every child. The program included computerized mailings and follow-up, free diagnostic assessments at regional offices, and/or a mobile van that went to parents' homes. As summarized in Figure 20.6, only about one-third of parents whose children had a high-risk indicator ever made an appointment for a diagnostic evaluation, and only about three-quarters of those parents completed the evaluation. Only 0.36 children per 1000 were identified with sensorineural hearing loss. Other high-risk-indicator-based programs experienced similar difficulties, and such programs have very low sensitivity and specificity.

Behavioral evaluations at 7–9 months of age

Another alternative for early identification of hearing loss that has been used extensively in Western Europe is to do behavioral assessments of children when they are 7–9 months old.[35–37] Most of these programs include hearing screening as a part of the work done by home visitors who are already making routine visits as a part of the well-child healthcare system. The data on the success of such home-based behavioral screening programs are very disappointing. For example, Watkin et al. did a retrospective analysis of over 55 000 children in one geographical district in England.[18] For each of the 171 2–15-year-old children who had a hearing loss, a determination was made of whether the child was first identified through a home visitor or school-age screening program, a parent, or someone else, such as a doctor or teacher. Of the 39 children with severe/profound bilateral losses, only 44% were identified based on the behavioral evaluation during the home visit. For children with mild moderate bilateral losses and children with unilateral losses, the behavioral evaluation identified only 25% and less than 10%, respectively. Thus, even with home visitors who were specifically trained to do behavioral assessments in a home setting, most of the young children with hearing loss are missed.

Otoacoustic emissions (OAE)

A more recent addition to the repertoire of newborn hearing screening tools is the use of otoacoustical emissions. Numerous small-scale studies have demonstrated that otoacoustical emissions have a very high rate of agreement with ABR.[38–41] The first large-scale evaluation of otoacoustical emissions in a UNHS program was the Rhode Island Hearing Assessment Program (RIHAP) conducted between 1990 and 1994.[42] Of the first cohort of 1850 infants from well-baby and special-care nurseries, 11 were identified with sensorineural hearing loss. Based on the ABR screening done with all infants as a part of

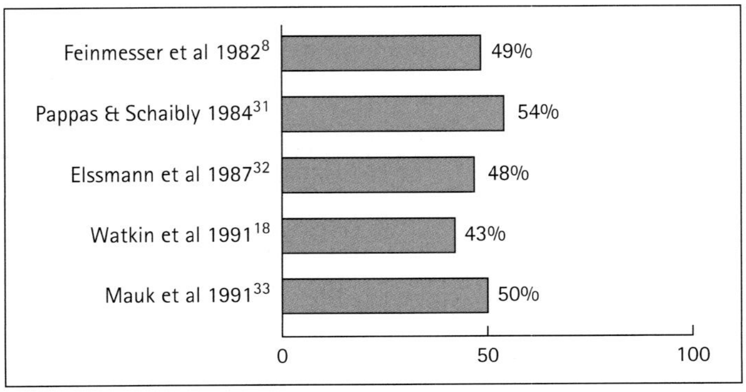

Figure 20.5 Percentage of hearing-impaired children who were high risk as infants.

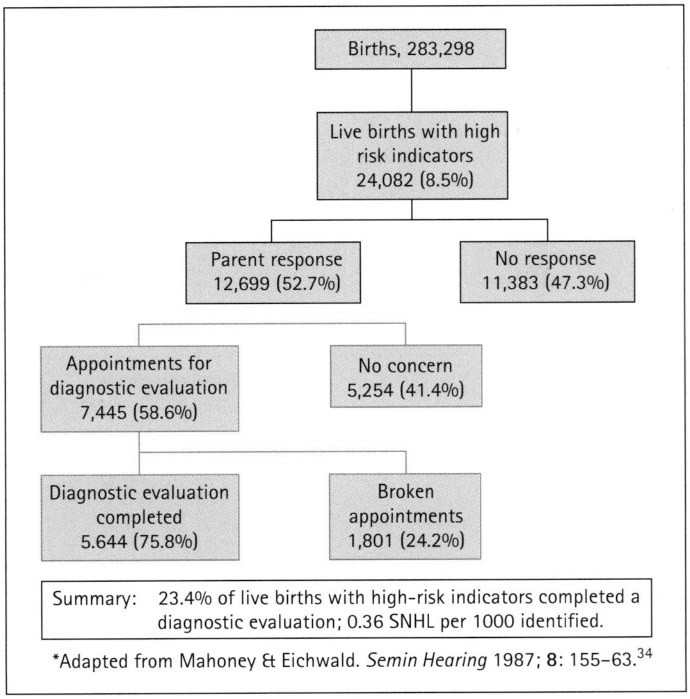

Figure 20.6 Results of birth certificate-based high-risk registry to identify hearing loss in Utah (1978–84).

the study, there was very high agreement betwen otoacoustical emissions screening and ABR. Furthermore, four of the babies would have been missed if screening had only been done with high-risk infants or with babies in the NICU. A summary of the results of OAE screening compared to hearing status (based on the generous assumption that babies who passed the initial screening have normal hearing) is shown in Figure 20.7.[19] Since the Rhode Island study, many others have demonstrated the feasibility and accuracy of using otoacoustical emissions in UNHS programs.[19,20,22–25] Although follow-up studies have not been done which enable the determination of sensitivity, it is clear from the data in Table 20.2 that many infants are being identified based on the use of otoacoustical emissions.

Automated auditory brainstem response (AABR)

Another widely used technique for UNHS programs is AABR. Although several such units are now available, the most widely used is the Algo manufactured by Natus Medical. In addition to the data reported earlier in Table 20.2 from the Colorado study, there are numerous smaller studies which have examined the accuracy of the Algo equipment. For example, Hermann et al[43]

OAE Screen	Hearing status: Impaired	Hearing status: Normal
Refer	11	79
Pass	0	1643

Sensitivity = 100%
Specificity = 95%

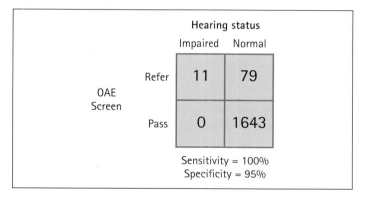

Figure 20.7 Accuracy of OAE two-stage screen. NB: Analysis is based on heads. Infants initially screened but lost to follow-up or rescreen because of parent refusal, lost contact, or repeated broken appointments (> 3) are not included. (From White et al. *Int J Paediatric Otorhinolaryngol* 1994; **29**: 203–17.[19])

AABR screen	Conventional ABR: Refer	Conventional ABR: Pass
Refer	101	38
Pass	2	1046

Sensitivity = 96%
Specificity = 98%

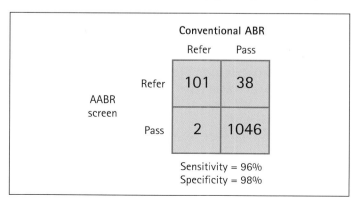

Figure 20.8 Accuracy of AABR: summary of four studies. (Adapted from Hermann et al. *Am J Audiol* 1995; **4**: 6–14.[43])

summarized the results of four studies[43–46] which compared the screening results of AABR with conventional ABR. Although this is not a true test of sensitivity, because the comparison is to another screening technique, based on what is known about the accuracy of ABR,[28,29] the results of Hermann's analysis shown in Figure 20.8 provide convincing evidence that AABR is an accurate tool for newborn hearing screening.

Summary: accuracy of screening techniques

It is important to note that newborn hearing screening equipment continues to evolve rapidly and is becoming less expensive, faster, and more accurate. The last 5 years have seen dramatic changes in both AABR and OAE equipment, and it is safe to predict that similar advances will happen during the next five years.

Although many articles refer to the sensitivity of various newborn hearing screening methods, definitive information about the sensitivity compared to behaviorally confirmed congenital PCHL is not available for any of the methods. This is because studies reporting sensitivity have assumed that all babies who pass the initial screen have normal hearing, have only followed a small percentage of the babies who passed the initial screen, have compared one screening technique with another screening technique to derive sensitivity figures, or were based on samples of only high-risk babies or unacceptably small samples.

The lack of data on sensitivity with behaviorally confirmed PCHL for ABR, OAE and AABR is a concern, but understandable given the high expense of following all children who pass the initial screening with behavioral evaluations and the fact that other data provide good evidence that most children with congenital PCHL are being identified in these screening programs. Rigorous studies of sensitivity/specificity for universal newborn hearing screening programs using these techniques would certainly be useful, but very expensive to conduct.

Even though definitive studies of sensitivity are not available, there is substantial evidence for the accuracy of several of the techniques, as described below.

Accuracy of ABR

There is good evidence that ABR is effective in identifying PCHL in newborns as long as it is used appropriately. Reports of sensitivity for identifying hearing loss among small samples of high risk infants are very good (97–100%), and there is at least one study in which ABR was used successfully in a universal newborn hearing screening programme.[26] Because of the expense and time involved in doing ABR, it is generally not considered a tool for universal newborn hearing screening programmes, but is used in some cases to screen high-risk infants.

Accuracy of high-risk indicators followed by ABR

Until the early 1990s, the most frequent technique for early identification of congenital PCHL in the USA was to identify children who exhibited one of the high-risk indicators specified by the JCIH, or to target all children in the neonatal intensive care unit (since a large percentage of these will have one of the JCIH high-risk indicators), and to screen those children with ABR. By targeting screening to this approximately 10% subset of the population, it was possible to keep the cost of screening lower and still identify a substantial number of children. However, because approximately half of the children with congenital PCHL do not exhibit any of the risk indicators, many children are missed when using this technique. Furthermore, programs have experienced substantial difficulty in getting families of children with high-risk indicators to come back for diagnostic evaluations, and consequently, the sensitivity of such programs is very low. If the presence of a high-risk indicator is considered to be a positive screen, the specificity is also very low. With the advent of new screening techniques (OAE and AABR), most high-risk-based early hearing detection programs in the United States have been discontinued.

Accuracy of behavioral evaluation at 7–9 months of age

Such programs are used primarily in countries where a home health visitor program is already in place. However, some people have generalized from this model and suggested that such techniques could be used to do screening as a part of well-baby care at the doctor's office. Data from well-established programs which rely on behavioral evaluations at 7–9 months indicate unacceptably low sensitivity. Such programs report missing more than half of the children with bilateral sensorineural hearing loss and even higher numbers of children with mild to moderate and unilateral losses.

Accuracy of OAE

Reported agreement between OAE and ABR testing is high, but there are no studies with operational UNHS programs in which the sensitivity related to behaviorally confirmed hearing loss can be determined. Early reports of OAE-based newborn hearing screening programs had unacceptably high referral rates for inpatient screening (> 25%). Numerous, more recent, reports, however, report inpatient referral rates of 2–8%.[20–24] There are now hundreds of hospital-based UNHS programs using OAEs. These programs report identifying 2–4 PCHL children per 1000 (programs unable to track a substantial number of referred children are at the lower end of that range, and programs with the most successful follow-up are near the upper range).

Accuracy of AABR

Hundreds of hospital-based UNHS programs are using AABR to identify children with congenital PCHL. Although there are no data on the sensitivity of this technique with behaviorally confirmed PCHL, the vast majority of reports which have examined the agreement between AABR and ABR find very high agreement (sensitivity and specificity greater than 95%). AABR-based programs report identifying 2–4 PCHL children per 1000 with referral rates of 2–4% at discharge.

Effects of newborn hearing screening on families

A number of people have raised concerns about whether UNHS programs may have negative psychological and emotional impact on the infant's family.[47–49] For example, it has been suggested that parents of children who have false-positive screening results may experience unacceptable levels of parental stress, fear and anxiety, and damage to the infant–mother bond. The concerns about hearing screening are based, in part, on the literature concerning the psychological effects of screening for other disorders. For example, shortly after screening for phenylketonuria (PKU) became widespread in the USA, Rothenburg and Sills[50] observed a number of families whose babies had false-positive results suffering from what they called PKU anxiety syndrome, a 'chronic anxiety, ranging in degree from mild, periodic bouts to acute anxiety hysteria'.

More substantial and convincing empirical studies of other newborn screening techniques have corroborated these observations. For example, in their study of the psychological effects of screening for congenital hypothyroidism, Bodegård et al[51] found that the majority of parents whose children had false-positive results reported shock, sleep disturbances, and infant feeding problems. Similarly, Tluczek et al[52] found that most parents reported reacting with anxiety, shock, denial, depression and anger in response to their infants' false-positive test for cystic fibrosis (CF).

Because there is evidence that neonatal screening for diseases, such as PKU, CF, and hyperthyroidism, can have both initial and long-term adverse psychological effects on some families, critics of newborn hearing screening programs[6,47–49] have raised questions about whether newborn hearing screening could be having similar effects. Several studies investigating adverse psychological effects of infant hearing screening suggest that the assumption that hearing screening will result in similar adverse psychological effects is unfounded.

For example, in interviews with 26 couples whose children had been screened for hearing impairment, Magnuson and Hergils[53] found that all of the couples had a positive attitude towards the screening and that all would do the test again if they had another child. Similarly, Vohr et al[54] questioned 157 mothers from Rhode Island at the time of the initial screening and found that the vast majority of the mothers (88%) reported that they felt little or no stress. An evaluation of Ohio's infant hearing screening program[55] found that the majority of parents whose children were screened thought that the screening process was excellent.

Similarly, Watkin et al[56] found that only 2 of the 57 (3.5%) mothers whose children were retested after failing a screen prior to hospital discharge were very worried. They also did not find a significant difference in anxiety (as measured by Spielberger's State-Trait Anxiety Inventory) between the retest group and a control group. Even in light of the possibility of additional stress and anxiety resulting from rescreening, most parents recognize the importance of the rescreening process. When Barringer and Mauk[57] asked parents whether the additional anxiety that they were experiencing would be outweighed by the benefits of early detection, 84.9% said yes.

Parents whose children's hearing loss was not detected very early also recognize the importance of infant hearing screening. A 1995 study[42] questioned 208 children and young adults with hearing loss and their parents about the need for neonatal hearing screening. Only 28% of the parents reported that they were reasonably satisfied with the age at which their child's hearing loss was confirmed, and 80% would have welcomed neonatal screening had it been available, even when the child had only mild or unilateral loss.

Contrary to the findings of screening programs for diseases, such as for PKU, CF, and hypothyroidism, which have found long-term negative effects,[50–52] research on hearing screening suggests that additional stress and anxiety resulting from rescreening may be only temporary. For example, Magnuson and Hergils[53] found that, although parents reported increased anxiety if their child was referred for rescreening, the anxiety dissipated when parents were informed and developed a plan for the future. Also, the anxiety appears to have had little or no long-term negative effects on the children or their parents. Of the 26 couples, only one reported that they were still anxious after their child's hearing loss was detected and that this anxiety might have had a negative influence on the child.

In summary, critics of UNHS have argued that negative effects for families, such as increased levels of anxiety, fear, and stress, may outweigh the benefits of UNHS. These conclusions appear to be based, in large part, on a literature that may not be relevant to newborn hearing screening. It appears that families' reactions to screening for diseases, such as CF and PKU, are more intense than reactions to screening for a hearing loss. The studies conducted so far have not found serious negative effects for families participating in UNHS.

Effects of earlier identification and intervention

A key question about UNHS is whether babies who are identified earlier do better than those who are identified later. For obvious reasons, it is not practical to identify hearing-impaired children early and randomly assign them to receive intervention or not. Thus, there are no prospective clinical trials which can be used to address this question. There are a number of retrospective studies, however, in which children have been categorized into groups who were identified early or identified later, matched on relevant variables, and assessed on developmental outcomes and success in school-related areas. All of this research can be criticized because there is potential for selection bias, most studies do not include long-term follow-up, sample sizes are generally quite small, and, in some of the studies, the types of outcome assessed were somewhat subjective.

In spite of those weaknesses, the evidence is quite convincing that there are benefits associated with earlier identification and intervention. For example, a study reported by Yoshinaga-Itano et al[59] compared the language abilities of 46 children with bilateral hearing loss identified before 6 months of age with those of 63 similar children identified after 6 months of age. Language abilities were measured by parent report using a cross-sectional assessment design in which children were categorized into four different age groups. As can be seen in Figure 20.9, the 23 children assessed when they were 13–18 months old already showed a clear advantage for the earlier-identified group. This advantage for the earlier-identified group becomes larger for the 28 children assessed when they were 19–24 months of age, larger still for the 31 children assessed when they were 25–30 months of age, and even larger for the 27 children assessed when they were 31–36 months of age. Other studies by this group have shown similar results.[60–63]

Another study conducted by Watkins[66] also supports the conclusion that earlier intervention is more beneficial. The design for this study is stronger, because all of the children were assessed at the same time, sample sizes were larger for each group, and there was more extensive matching and statistical adjustment for potential confounding variables. However, the 'earlier' group was substantially older than in the Yoshinaga-Itano studies. In the Watkins study, there were three groups of 23 children who had been matched or the scores were statistically adjusted for a variety of variables, including severity of hearing loss, age, presence of other handicap, age of mother, SES indicators, and number of childhood middle ear infections. The first group received an average of 9 months of home intervention, beginning at 21 months of

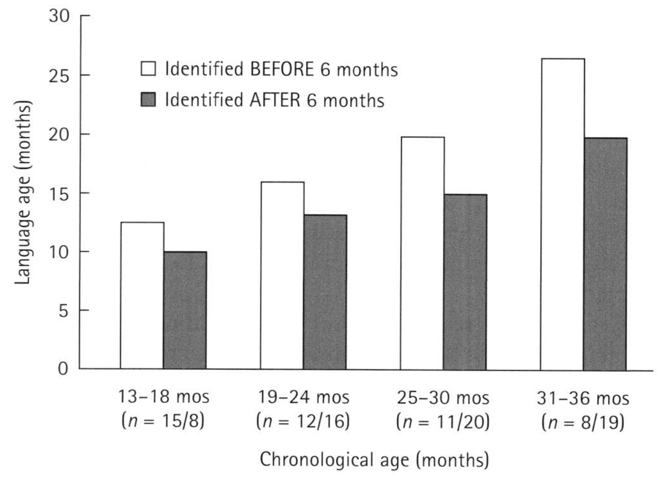

Figure 20.9 Language comprehensive scores for hearing-impaired children identified before and after 6 months of age. (Adapted from Yoshinaga-Itano et al. *The effect of early identification on the development of deaf and hard-of hearing infants and toddlers.*[59])

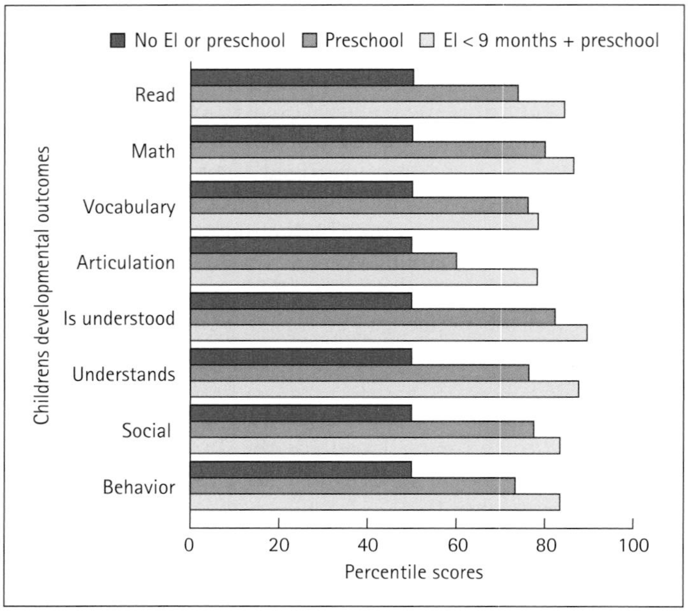

Figure 20.10 Effects of earlier intervention for children with hearing loss. (Adapted from Watkins. *Work Scope of the Early Intervention Research Institute.* Logan, Utah: Utah State University, 1983.[66])

age, and then received preschool intervention until they were enrolled in public school. The second group of children received no home intervention, but began a preschool intervention program at 36 months of age. The third group received no home intervention or preschool intervention.

A wide variety of measures were collected by trained diagnosticians who were unaware of the group to which the children belonged. As shown in Figure 20.10, it is clear that those who received both home-based intervention and preschool intervention did substantially better than those who received only preschool intervention or did not receive any intervention prior to beginning public school. The effects for reading, arithmetic, vocabulary, articulation, percentage of the child's communication understood by non-family members, percentage of non-family communication understood by the child, social adjustment and behavior show that children who received the most intensive early intervention perform 20–45 percentile points higher than children who do not receive such intervention.

Even though results of randomized clinical trials are not available to address the question of whether earlier intervention is better than later intervention for children with hearing loss, the consistency of findings from a number of quasi-experimental studies provides consistent and convincing evidence about the benefits of earlier intervention. As more and more children are identified at earlier ages, it is expected that more data about the benefits of early intervention will become available.

Conclusion

Much of the recent expansion in UNHS programs can be traced to the recommendation in 1993 by the United States National Institutes of Health that all babies be screened for hearing loss prior to hospital discharge.[2] The controversy caused by this recommendation[47] is not surprising in light of how little evidence existed at the time regarding the feasibility and effectiveness of UNHS programs. Since then, dozens of studies have been reported, and thousands of successful UNHS programs are operating in many countries of the world. The data and experiences of these programs now provide convincing evidence that UNHS programs can be operated with existing technology effectively, cost-effeciently, and successfully. As a result of such programs, infants with congenital hearing loss are being identified younger than ever before.

Clearly, there are important challenges that must still be addressed, but many of the concerns people had in the mid-1990s about UNHS programs have been resolved. Although more research would be helpful, there is a growing body of evidence demonstrating substantial benefits associated with earlier identification and services and an absence of significant negative effects for families. It is important to continue to systematically collect data that will lead to further improvements, but it is just as important to build on the knowledge that has accumulated over the last decade to ensure that babies with congenital hearing loss are identified and provided with appropriate services during the first few months of life.

References

1. Ewing IR, Ewing AWG. The ascertainment of deafness in infancy and early childhood. *J Laryngol Otol* 1944; **59**: 309–33.
2. National Institutes of Health. *Early Identification of Hearing Impairment in Infants and Young Children* NIH consensus statement. United States Department of Health & Human Services Publications, 1993: Vol. 11.
3. Erenberg A, Lemons J, Sia C et al. Newborn and infant hearing loss: detection and intervention. American Academy of Pediatrics Task Force on Newborn and Infant Hearing, 1998–1999. *Pediatrics* 1999; **103**: 527–30.
4. Grandori F. The European Consensus Development Conference on Neonatal Hearing Screening. *Arch Otolaryngol Head Neck Surgery* 1999; **125**: 118.
5. US Preventive Services Task Force Guide to Clinical Preventive Services. *Screening for hearing impairment.* Baltimore: Williams & Wilkins, 1996; pp. 393–405.
6. Paradise JL. Universal newborn hearing screening: should we leap before we look? *Pediatrics* 1999; **103**: 670–2.
7. Barr B. Early detection of hearing impairment. In: Taylor IG, Markides A, eds. *Disorders of Auditory Function*, Vol. III. New York: Academic Press, 1980; Vol. III. New York: Academic Press, pp. 33–42.
8. Feinmesser M, Tell L, Levi H. Etiology of childhood deafness with reference to the group of unknown cause. *Audiology* 1986; **25**: 65–9.

9. Fitzaland RE. Identification of hearing loss in newborns: results of eight years' experience with a high risk hearing register. *The Volta Review* 1985; **87**: 195–203.
10. Kankkunen A. Preschool children with impaired hearing. *Acta Otolaryngolica Suppl* 1982; **391**: 1–124.
11. Martin JAM. Atiological factors relating to childhood deafness in the European community. *Audiology* 1982; **21**: 149–58.
12. Parving A. Hearing disorders in childhood, some procedures for detection, identification and diagnostic evaluation. *Int J Pediatr Otorhinolaryngol* 1985; **9**: 31–57.
13. Sehlin P, Holmgren G, Zakrisson J. Incidence, prevalence and etiology of hearing impairment in children in the county of Vasterbotten, Sweden. *Scand Audiol* 1990; **19**: 193–200.
14. Sorri M, Rantakallio P. Prevalence of hearing loss at the age of 15 in a birth cohort of 12,000 children from northern Finland. *Scand Audiol* 1985; **14**: 203–7.
15. Davis AC, Wood S. The epidemiology of childhood hearing impairment: factors relevant to planning of services. *B J Audiol* 1992; **26**: 77–90.
16. Kinney C. Hearing impairments in children. *Laryngoscope* 1953; **63**: 220–6.
17. Brookhouser PE, Worthington DW, Kelly WJ. Unilateral hearing loss in children. *Laryngoscope* 1991; **101**: 1264–72.
18. Watkin PM, Baldwin M, Laoide S. Parental suspicion and identification of hearing impairment. *Arch Dis Child* 1990; **65**: 846–50.
19. White KR, Vohr BR, Maxon AB et al. Screening all newborns for hearing loss using transient evoked otoacoustic emissions. *Int J Pediatr Otorhinolaryngol* 1994; **29**: 203–17.
20. Vohr BR, Carty LM, Moore PE, Letourneau K. The Rhode Island Hearing Assessment Program: experience with statewide hearing screening (1993–1996). *J Pediatric* 1998; **133**: 353–7.
21. Mehl AL, Thomson V. Newborn hearing screening: the great omission. *Pediatrics* 1998; **101**: E4.
22. Wessex Universal Neonatal Hearing Screening Trial Group. Controlled trial of universal neonatal screening for early identification of permanent childhood hearing impairment. *Lancet* 1998; **352**: 1957–64.
23. Finitzo T, Albright K, O'Neal J. The newborn with hearing loss: detection in the nursery. *Pediatrics*. 1998; **102**: 1452–60.
24. Prieve BA, Stevens F. The New York State Universal Newborn Hearing Screening Demonstration Project: Introduction and Overview. *Ear Hear* 2000; **21**: 85–91.
25. Johnson JL, Kuntz NL, Sia CC et al. Newborn hearing screening in Hawaii. *Hawaii Med J* 1997; **56**: 352–5.
26. Barsky-Firkser L, Sun S. Universal newborn hearing screenings: a three-year experience. *Pediatrics* 1997; **99**: E4.
27. Personal communication with Y Weirather, B Vohr, and V Thomson. 1999.
28. Hyde ML, Riko K, Malizia K. Audiometric accuracy of the click ABR in infants at risk for hearing loss. *J Am Acad Audiol* 1990; **1**: 59–66.
29. Murray A, Javel E, Watson C. Prognostic validity of auditory brainstem evoked response screening in newborn infants. *Am J Otolaryngol* 1985; **6**: 120–31.
30. Joint Committee on Infant Hearing 2000 Position Statement: Principles and guidelines for early hearing detection and intervention programs. *Am J Audiology*. 2000; **9**: 9–29.
31. Pappas DB, Schaibly M. A two-year diagnostic report on bilateral sensorineural hearing loss in infants and children. *Am J Otol* 1984; **5**: 339–42.
32. Elssmann SF, Matkin ND, Sabo MP. Early identification of congenital sensorineural hearing impairment. *Hear J* 1987; **40**: 13–17.
33. Mauk GW, White KR, Mortensen LB, Behrens TR. The effectiveness of screening programs based on high-risk characteristics in early identification of hearing impairment. *Ear Hear* 1991; **12**: 312–19.
34. Mahoney TM, Eichwald JG. The 'ups and downs' of high-risk hearing screening: the Utah statewide program. *Semin Hear* 1987; **8**: 155–63.
35. McClelland RJ, Watson DR, Lawless V et al. Reliability and effectiveness of screening for hearing loss in high-risk neonates. *BMJ* 1992; **304**: 806–9.
36. Haggard MP. Hearing screening in children—state of the art(s). *Arch Dis Child* 1990; **65**: 1193–8.
37. Scanlon PE, Bamford JM. Early identification of hearing loss: screening and surveillance methods. *Arch Dis Child* 1990; **65**: 479–85.
38. Bonfils P, Uziel A, Pujol R. Screening for auditory dysfunction in infants by evoked oto-acoustic emissions. *Arch Otolaryngol Head Neck Surg* 1988; **114**: 887–90.
39. Stevens JC, Webb HD, Hutchinson J et al. Click evoked oto-acoustic emissions compared with brainstem electric response. *Arch Dis Child* 1989; **64**: 1105–11.
40. Stevens JC, Webb HD, Hutchinson J et al. Click evoked oto-acoustic emissions in neonatal screening. *Ear Hear* 1990; **11**: 128–33.
41. Plinkert PK, Sesterhenn G, Arold R, Zenner HP. Evaluation of otoacoustic emissions in high-risk infants by using an easy and rapid objective auditory screening method. *Eur Arch Otorhinolaryngol* 1990; **247**: 356–60.
42. White KR, Behrens TR, eds. The Rhode Island Hearing Assessment Project: Implications for universal newborn hearing screening. *Semin Hear* 1993; **14**(1).
43. Herrmann BS, Thornton AR, Joseph JM. Automated infant hearing screening using the ABR: Development and validation. *Am J Audiol* 1995; **4**: 6–14.
44. Hall JW, Kileny PR, Ruth RA, Kripal JP. Newborn auditory screening with ALGO-1 vs. conventional auditory brainstem response. *Asha* 1987; **29**: 120.
45. Jacobson JT, Jacobson CA, Spahr RC. Automated and conventional ABR screening techniques in high-risk infants. *J Am Acad Audiol* 1990; **1**: 187–95.
46. Von Wedel H, Schauseil-Zipf U, Doring WH. Horscreening bei Neugeborenen and Sauglingen. *Laryngol Rhinol Otol* 1988; **67**: 307–11.
47. Bess FH, Paradise JL. Universal screening for infant hearing impairment: not simple, not risk-free, not necessarily beneficial, and not presently justified. *Pediatrics* 1994; **93**: 330–4.

48. Luterman D, Kurtzer-White E. Identifying hearing loss: parents' needs. *Am J Audiology*. 1999; **8**: 13–18.
49. Tharpe AM, Clayton EW. Newborn hearing screening: issues in legal liability and quality assurance. *Am J Audiol* 1997; **6**: 5–12.
50. Rothenberg MB, Sills EM. Latrogenesis: the PKU anxiety syndrome. *J Am Acad Child Psychiatry* 1968; **7**: 689–92.
51. Bodegård G, Fyrö K, Larsson A. Psychological reactions in families with a newborn who has a falsely positive screening test for congenital hypothyroidism. *Acta Paediatr Scand Suppl* 1983; **304**: 1–2.
52. Tluczek A, Mischier EH, Farrell PM et al. Parents' knowledge of neonatal screening and response to false-positive cystic fibrosis testing. *Dev Behav Pediatrics* 1992; **13**: 181–6.
53. Magnuson M, Hergils L. The parent's view on hearing screening in newborns. *Scand Audiol* 1999; **28**: 47–56.
54. Vohr BR, Letourneau KS, McDermott C. Maternal worry about neonatal hearing screening. *J Perinatol* 2001; **21**: 15–20.
55. White KR, Shalala M. *A sound beginning: Ohio's Infant Hearing Screening and Assessment Program*. National Center for Hearing Assessment and Management, Utah State University, Logan, Utah. 1998.
56. Watkin PM, Baldwin M, Dixon R, Beckman A. Maternal anxiety and attitudes to universal neonatal hearing screening. *Br J Audiol* 1998; **32**: 27–37.
57. Barringer DG, Mauk GW. Survey of parents perceptions regarding hospital-based newborn hearing screening. *Audiol Today* 1997; **9**: 18–19.
58. Watkin PM, Beckman A, Baldwin M. The views of parents of hearing impaired children on the need for neonatal hearing screening. *Br J Audiol* 1995; **29**: 259–62.
59. Yoshinaga-Itano C, Sedey A, Apuzzo M et al. *The effect of early identification on the development of deaf and hard-of-hearing infants and toddlers*. Paper presented at the Joint Committee on Infant Hearing Meeting, Austin, TX. July 1996.
60. Yoshinaga-Itano C, Coulter DK, Thomson V. The Colorado Newborn Hearing Screening Project: Effects on speech and language development for children with hearing loss. *J Perinatol* 2000; **20**(suppl 8): S132–S137.
61. Yoshinaga-Itano C, Sedey AL, Coulter DK, Mehl AL. Language of early- and later-identified children with hearing loss. *Pediatrics* 1998; **102**: 1161–71.
62. Apuzzo ML, Yoshinaga-Itano C. Early identification of infants with significant hearing loss and the Minnesota child development inventory. *Seminars in Hearing*. 1995; **16**: 124–39.
63. Yoshinaga-Itano C, Sedey AL, Coulter DK, Mehl AL. Language of early- and later-identified children with hearing loss. *Pediatrics* 1998; **102**: 1161–71.
64. Calderon R, Naidu S. Further support of the benefits of early identification and intervention with children with hearing loss. *Volta Rev* 2000; **100**: 53–84.
65. Moeller MP. Early intervention and language development in children who are deaf and hard of hearing. *Pediatrics* 2000; **106**: E43.
66. Watkins S. Final Report: *1982–83 Work scope of the Early Intervention Research Institute*. Logan, Utah: Utah State University. 198

21 Clinical and audiometric assessment of hearing

Rosalyn A Davies

An accurate assessment of hearing is best made using both otological and audiological information. This is because of the complex inter-relationship between structure and function in the auditory system—one aspect cannot be considered without the other. Hearing impairment implies a lesion somewhere in the auditory pathway: the sound wave arrives at the pinna, is conducted through the middle ear, is transduced into electrical energy in the inner ear, is relayed through the brainstem and finally projected to the auditory cortex. Occasionally there may also be a psychological component to the hearing loss, which only rarely is the entire basis of the hearing loss.

Thus the aim of this chapter is to describe the clinical assessment of hearing, referring both to the structure of the auditory system (the otological perspective) and to the functional aspects as assessed by auditory testing (the audiological perspective).

The anamnesis

The history of auditory symptoms should be used to guide the examination.

HEARING LOSS

- Date of onset.
- Gradual or sudden.
- Progressive, stable or fluctuating.
- Unilateral or bilateral.

ASSOCIATED SYMPTOMS

- Aural fullness, discharge, pain, vertigo.
- Tinnitus (pitch, pulsatile or clicking).
- Diplacusis, hyperacusis, distortion.
- Any difficulties in localizing sound.
- Past medical history: noise exposure (occupational, social or gunfire), ear/head trauma, use of ototoxic drugs, allergies, previous surgery to ear(s), infections (mumps, measles, meningitis), cardiovascular risk factors.
- Birth and neonatal history
- Family history: family pedigree, syndromal or non-syndromal hearing loss.

It is also important to ask about more general points, e.g. the effect of the hearing loss on the patient, the social situation of the patient and any past attempts at rehabilitation, i.e. assistive listening devices and communication training.

Clinical examination

From the moment the patient steps through the door, information can be collected about the patient's hearing status. Do they communicate easily? Do they have to face the examiner to hear them? Are there any general medical or neurological features that can be picked up from observation, e.g. tremor or abnormal gait?

In general, the medical examination will be guided by the anamnesis. It should include:

- appearance of the facies: xanthelasma, plethora, syndromal features (see below)
- tenderness of the superficial temporal and facial arteries
- auscultation of the supraclavicular fossae and carotid arteries in the neck
- blood pressure measurement
- evidence of thyroid dysfunction, i.e. exophthalmos, tremor, enlargement of the thyroid in the neck
- assessment of the patient's affect, intellectual performance and memory capabilities (important for assessing the patient's ability to understand the diagnosis and its implications and to follow a rehabilitative programme)
- assessment of central language functions.

Neurological examination will again be guided by the anamnesis.

CRANIAL NERVE EXAMINATION

- Olfactory (I): sense of smell as tested using aromatic substances such as oil of cloves, peppermint
- Optic nerve (II): pupil size and ipsilateral and consensual reactivity to light and accommodation; examination of fundi; visual acuity tested using Snellen charts; assessment of visual fields
- Oculomotor (III), trochlear (IV) and abducens (VI): assessment of full range and conjugacy of eye movements, identification of ptosis
- Trigeminal (V): ipsilateral and consensual corneal reflexes, facial sensation to light touch, pinprick and temperature, assessment of jaw muscles
- Facial (VII): facial asymmetry and assessment of muscles of facial expression, including orbicularis oculi; assessment of taste using sugar, salt, quinine and acid
- Cochleovestibular (VIII): tested using Rinne and Weber tuning fork tests; vestibular component tested using caloric stimulation
- Glossopharyngeal (IX) and vagus (X): observation of palatal movement and symmetry; swallowing and eliciting gag reflex
- Accessory (XI): movement of head to right and left against resistance; shrugging shoulders
- Hypoglossal (XII): observing the tongue at rest and then protruded, looking for fasciculation and asymmetry.

If central nervous system (CNS) dysfunction is suspected, a full CNS examination will be helpful and should include assessment of power, sensation, coordination and reflexes in all four limbs in addition to the cranial nerve examination.

Clinical speech tests

These tests, using the human voice over a range of intensities, can be used to give an estimation of auditory threshold and help to detect non-organic hearing loss. Three intensities of the human voice are used to assess hearing: a whisper, a conversational voice and a loud voice. It is useful for testers to calibrate themselves against a sound level meter as they learn to use speech tests:

- Whispered voice (WV)—this should be a forced whisper, i.e. the loudest whisper that the tester can produce. The vocal chords should be abducted throughout.
- Conversational voice (CV)—the intensity used when conversing in a quiet room.
- Loud voice (LV)—the loudest shout that the tester can produce.

Swan[1] determined the equivalent pure tone audiometric thresholds for a range of voice tests delivered by two otologists to 101 patients, showing a mean of WV at 60 cm of 51 dBA, a mean of CV at 60 cm of 73 dBA, and a mean of LV at 60 cm of 92 dBA. Browning et al[2] evaluated the sensitivity and specificity of a whispered voice test at 60 cm for detection of a speech frequency impairment greater than 30 dB as 96% and 91% respectively.

The tester should position himself to one side of the patient in such a way that visual clues are excluded, and that he is standing either at 15 cm or 60 cm from the test ear. 60 cm is arm's length and allows the tester to mask the non-test ear throughout testing. Masking is achieved by tragal rubbing, i.e. occlusion of the external auditory meatus by fingertip pressure on the tragus and gentle rubbing, to produce broadband noise, or the use of a Bárány noise box (but only when the test stimulus is delivered using a loud voice). The stimulus typically used is a series of three numbers, e.g. 3–6–2. A positive test is correct identification of >50% of the numbers presented.

Speech tests are limited and not a substitute for audiometry. They have a role in estimating auditory thresholds and are valuable in the identification of non-organic hearing loss and where the patient cannot be relied on to give accurate pure tone audiometric thresholds e.g. the mentally handicapped. It should be remembered when diagnosing a non-organic hearing loss that exaggeration of a mild hearing loss is more common than a total non-organic hearing loss. Other methods of estimating auditory thresholds, e.g. finger friction tests, are now largely obsolete because of the difficulties of standardizing the stimulus.

Clinical examination of the ear

Careful inspection of the ear is essential. It includes examination of the auricle (pinna), the external auditory meatus and the middle ear as far as can be assessed by the examination of the tympanic membrane (TM). The TM offers a window into the middle ear cleft and is affected by most of the changes that can take place in the middle ear.

Before the otologist can proceed further with the evaluation, two common problems must be ruled out, both of which can cause spurious conductive hearing loss.

Presence of a collapsing external acoustic meatus

The pressure of a test earphone can be sufficient to produce a valve-like closing of the external acoustic meatus, such that a conductive hearing loss can be simulated (Figure 21.1). This can occur as a result of loss of the elasticity of the cartilage. To determine if a collapse is likely to occur during testing, pressure should be exerted on the auricle, pressing it in towards the head. If the opening of the meatus closes, a device should be entered into the opening to prevent it collapsing when the test earphone is in place, e.g. a piece of small-diameter tubing or an impedance probe tip. Alternatively, an MC41 ear cushion may be used.

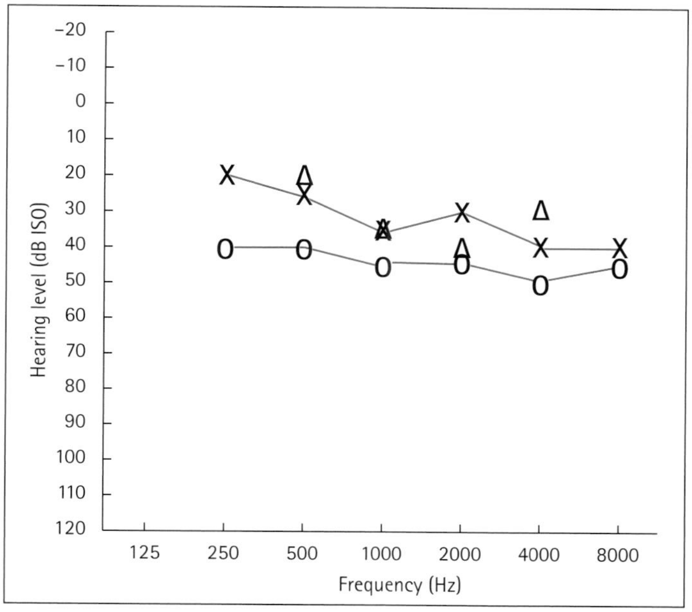

Figure 21.1 Pure tone audiometry: collapsed external auditory meatus. By comparison with left-ear thresholds, the auditory thresholds from the right ear are raised by an average of 12.5 dB as a result of a collapsed auditory meatus.

Presence of obstructing wax (cerumen) or debris

A large amount of hardened wax in the external acoustic meatus may become impacted and lead to a conductive hearing loss (Figure 21.2). If impacted, the wax must be removed carefully without causing pain to the patient. Hard lumps can be removed using the Jobson Horne probe or a Cawthorne wax hook. Material can be removed with forceps, e.g. Tilley's dressing forceps (large blades) or smaller forceps, although they tend to tear the debris, making it more difficult to remove. Cotton wool may be twisted onto the carrier end of the Jobson Horne probe to mop out wet material. A sterile swab may be used to sample infected material for fungal and bacteria culture and for antibiotic sensitivity.

An alternative method for removing wax is by syringing.

If the wax seems very hard, it can be softened over a period of a week using warm olive oil drops administered nightly. Alternatively, 5% sodium bicarbonate drops may be used, or a ceruminolytic preparation, which is available commercially.

ABSOLUTE CONTRADICTIONS TO SYRINGING

- in the presence of an infection
- when the ear is known to have a perforation
- if, from the history, the ear is suspected to have a vulnerable tympanic membrane.

The method of syringing is as follows (Figure 21.3):

- Ask the patient to sit in a chair and protect them with a plastic cape and towel.
- Ask the patient to hold a kidney dish receiver on the shoulder.
- Draw up a solution of sterile water at 37°C in a metal or rubber syringe (any variation from this temperature will cause the patient to experience vertigo).
- Draw the pinna upwards and backwards.
- Place the nozzle a few millimetres into the canal, pointing it upwards and backwards.
- Direct the stream along the roof of the canal between the skin and wax.

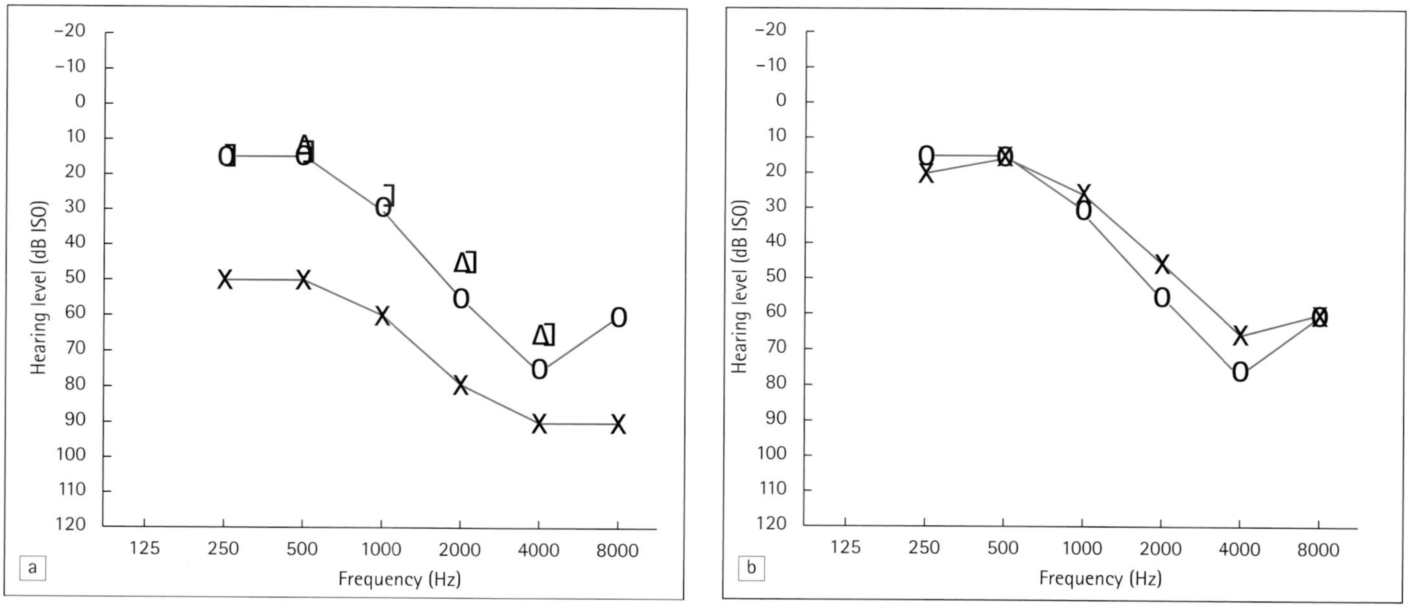

Figure 21.2 Pure tone audiometry. (a) Impacted wax, before removal: by comparison with the right ear, auditory thresholds are raised on the left by an average of 24 dB. (b) Impacted wax, after removal: following wax removal, auditory thresholds have improved on the left by an average of 32 dB.

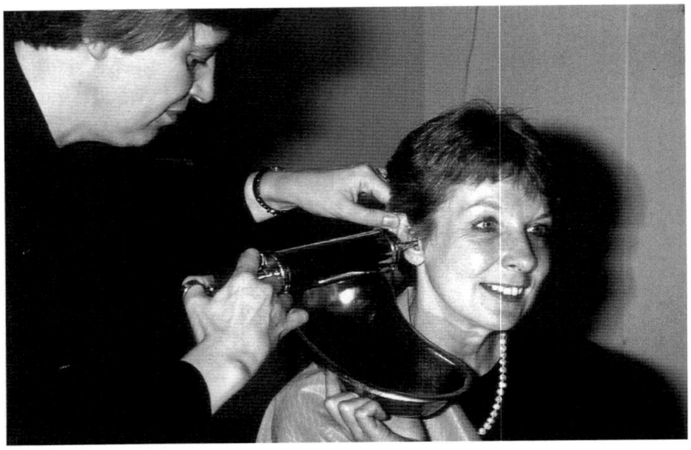

Figure 21.3 Ear syringing (see text).

Syringing should not be painful, and must be stopped if the patient complains of pain. Dedicated syringing machines are available to deliver mechanically a stream of water at body temperature.

The external ear

The auricle

The auricle (Figure 21.4) is essentially vestigial, contributing only to the collection of sound, slightly enhancing the efficacy of the ear, and to conducting the sound towards the TM and the middle ear .

The pinna and postaural area should be inspected for signs of inflammation, trauma (specifically looking for evidence of a surgical operation, e.g. a postaural incision or an end-aural incision between the tragus and rest of helix), or haematoma auris following a blow to the ear, and importantly, deformities.

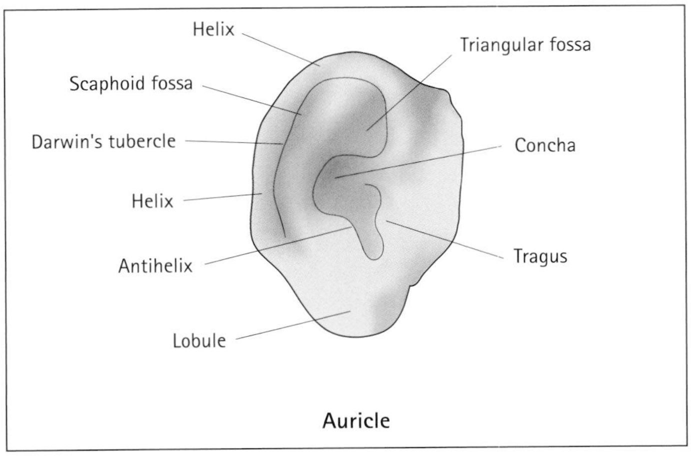

Figure 21.4 Auricle.

Congenital

Most developmental deformities are fairly obvious, but must be carefully identified because of the likely associated findings of middle and inner ear abnormalities and consequent hearing impairment (see below).

- **Anotia:** the absence of an auricle. It may be completely absent or there may be rudimentary tubercles. The external auditory meatus is likely to be absent.
- **Microtia:** a smaller than normal and probably misshapen auricle. The external auditory meatus is likely to be absent and there are often abnormalities of the ossicular chain. Three types exist: grade 1—malformed pinna, but with most of the features; grade 2—rudimentary pinna with cylindrical bar of tissue curved at the cranial end; grade 3—more severe with only a malformed nodule present.
- **Macrotia:** an excessively large auricle, often with no other associated abnormalities of structure or function.
- **Polyotia:** very rarely found; a typical abnormality would be two auricles facing each other on one side of the head.
- **Synotia and melotia:** misplaced auricle; synotia is when it is placed posteriorly in the cervical part of the neck, and melotia when it is placed anteriorly.
- **Abnormalities of the helix:** a cat's ear describes a downward-folded auricle; a cup ear is a hollow ear; a Mozart ear has an enlarged antihelix continuous with the helix.
- **Pre-auricular appendages:** may represent accessory and rudimentary auricles and are found in 1.5% of the population. Normally found anterior to the tragus, the auricular appendage contains cartilage which extends medially.
- **Fistula auris:** a small blind pit seen commonly anterior to the tragus (i.e. pre-auricular sinus Figure 21.5). It results from incomplete fusion of the auricular tubercles. It can become infected.

Acquired

- **Haematoma:** may follow a blow on the ear and is commonly found in boxers and rugby players. Bleeding occurs between the cartilage and covering layers of perichondrium. The whole auricle may become involved, appearing as a bluish shapeless mass. If left untreated, the cartilage necroses and the auricle becomes a shrivelled appendage—a cauliflower ear.
- **Acute dermatitis:** may occur as an extension of the meatal infection in otitis externa. The oedematous red auricle desquamates, with the copious production of serous fluid—'weeping eczema'.
- **Chondrodermatitis chronicus helicus:** most often occurs in elderly males, presenting with a nodular and exquisitely tender swelling of the helix which may be ulcerated.
- **Squamous cell** and **basal cell carcinomas** may be sited on the auricle, tending to occur on the upper edge, and examination will require a search for associated lymphadenopathy.

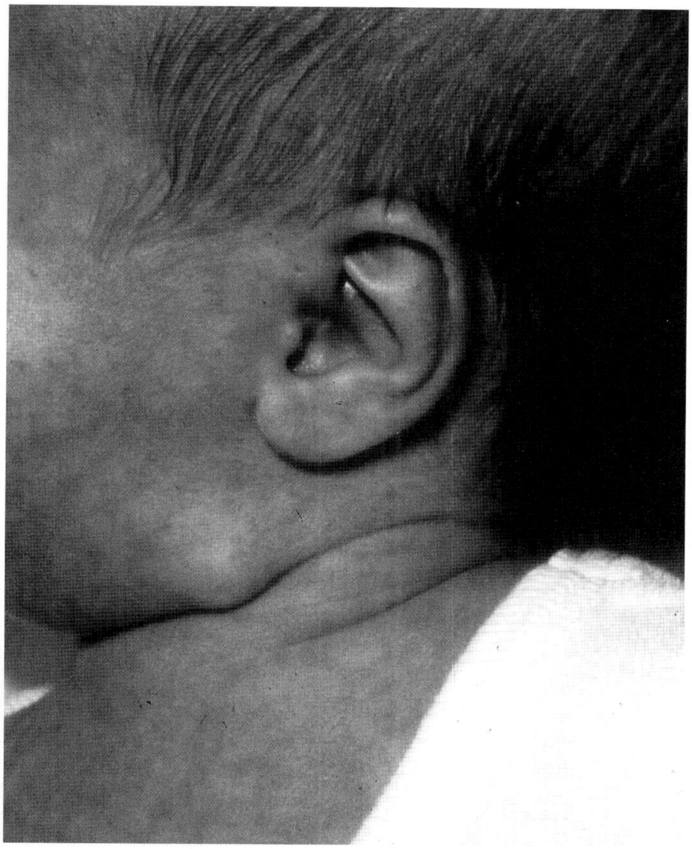

Figure 21.5 Pre-auricular sinus and branchial cyst in a baby with branchio-oto-renal syndrome. (Courtesy of Dr Tony Sirimanna.)

External acoustic meatus

Congenital

- **Narrowed external acoustic meatus (EAM):** a patent EAM, but narrowed along the whole length. May require microsuction to prevent occlusion by keratin.
- **Stenosed EAM:** the EAM is narrowed at the junction of the cartilaginous and bony part of the EAM. It can be bi- or unilateral, can be familial, and can be associated with other abnormalities.
- **Atretic EAM:** this is closed over with a membranous and/or bony wall across the canal. It is caused by a failure of the ectodermal cord to canalize and is frequently associated with other abnormalities, being found in 1–2/100 000 births. One in four are bilateral. Atretic EAMs are graded according to severity:
  (a) Grade 1 (mild)—part of the external canal is present, the TM is present, but may be smaller than normal. The middle ear cavity is of a normal or slightly reduced size.
  (b) Grade 2 (moderate)—the external canal is completely absent, the TM is diminished and the ossicles deformed. The atretic plate is partly or completely ossified.
  (c) Grade 3 (severe)—the external ear canal is completely absent, the middle ear cavity is markedly smaller and the atretic plate completely ossified.

Audiometry and immittance testing on these children, if possible, has prognostic value for hearing improvement as far as surgery is concerned and the following tests are recommended: pure tone audiometry, tympanometry, and stapedial reflex testing. Radiological investigation needs to be pursued if atresia is identified. The prospect of improving the likely associated conductive deafness with surgical intervention is very dependent on the size and shape of the middle ear cavity, which can best be assessed by CT scanning. Ideally base CT scans and coronal 2-mm sections should be performed. Phelps and Lloyd[3] recommend that all neonates with atretic meati should be imaged before the baby is discharged following birth. This is for reasons of ease of investigation and to identify any surgically correctable associated abnormalities early.

For example, where unilateral atresia is found associated with a deformity of the pinna, often a normally formed mastoid is seen and there is good pneumatization of the middle ear. This again has implications for the surgical prognosis. An air-containing middle ear is likely to be associated with a good surgical outcome, whereas if the middle ear is filled with undifferentiated embryological mesenchyme, indistinguishable from glue on imaging, then surgical results are poor. This is because of persistence of tubal dysfunction and the possibility of thin bony septa dividing the middle ear into several different compartments, all of which may not have been identified by the surgeon.

Additionally, with the dramatic developments in localizing and identifying genes responsible for both syndromal and non-syndromal hearing impairment, the diagnostic protocol for abnormalities of the outer and middle ear should include clinical genetics assessment.[4]

Acquired

- **Otitis externa:** bacterial infection of the skin of the EAM resulting in tissue oedema and swelling so as to obstruct the canal and produce a conductive hearing loss. The most common bacterial infections are those with *Staphylococcus*, *Pseudomonas aeruginosa* and diphtheroids; fungal infections include *Aspergillus niger* and *Candida albicans*, and the vesicular eruptions of *Herpes zoster* virus may also be seen in the distribution of the auriculotemporal division of the trigeminal nerve in the Ramsay Hunt syndrome.
- **Furunculosis:** infection of the hair follicles with *Staphylococcus* is limited to the outer part of the meatus.
- **Foreign body obstruction:** examples are small objects, such as beads or pips, inserted into the EAM often by young children. Other foreign bodies include insects such as the common fly, which on entering the EAM may produce an irritation due to the flapping of its wings.
- **Osteoma:** discrete, rounded, white excrescences of bone. Can be confused with cholesteatoma.

- **Exostoses,** or small osteomata, are quite common and usually bilateral. They are often found in people who swim or dive regularly and are thought to be due to prolonged exposure to cold water. They are hard and smooth, covered with canal skin, hard to palpation, and exquisitely sensitive.
- **Hyperostosis:** A diffuse bony narrowing of the canal.

Tympanic membrane and middle ear

Examination of the tympanic membrane and middle ear

Inspection of the ear may be carried out either with the use of an otoscope, or with a head-worn light source whereby the hands are free to remove wax or discharge. Alternatively, the light source can be a separate lamp with the light reflected by a head-worn mirror and directed coaxially to the line of vision and down the hand-held speculum.

A binocular microscope for inspection and manipulation of the ear canal is also an essential tool for inspection of the ear canal. It is used optimally with the patient lying on a couch, but can also be used with the patient sitting close to horizontal. The objective should have a focal length of between 200 and 250 mm, and the range of magnification should be between 6× and 25×. A Seigle's (or pneumatic) speculum with clear glass is a valuable adjunct to the microscope, as it allows assessment of the mobility of the TM.

The largest speculum that can be comfortably fitted into the canal should be chosen and introduced carefully into the canal, with the pinna held between the thumb and forefinger of the examiner's hand and gently retracted backwards to straighten out the curve in the cartilaginous meatus. The speculum should then be directed around the complete circumference of the canal, looking for debris or foreign bodies, inflammation, and in particular defects of the posterior or attic wall. To identify the TM the floor of the meatus should be followed, as it makes a sharp angle with the TM.

The magnifying lens of the Siegle's speculum can be fitted into the speculum and the bulb squeezed to raise intrameatal pressure, and then relaxed, sucking the membrane outwards. In the presence of a middle ear effusion, the membrane is immobile; however, a very flaccid TM may have been sucked back onto the middle ear mucosa, and lowering the pressure may suck it out again, allowing a retraction pocket to be distinguished from a perforation. Alternatively, the Valsalva manoeuvre (which is the standard method of auto-inflation of the ear) can be employed to raise middle ear pressure and to observe these changes: the patient is asked to pinch the nostrils between the forefinger and thumb and then, with lips closed, blow out their cheeks while trying to blow down the nose. If successful, the patient will experience a sensation of fullness in the ears.

Fistula sign

This sign is elicited in those patients where there is a transmission of air pressure changes from the external auditory meatus via a fistula to the labyrinth causing endolymph movement and resulting in nystagmus. Raised pressure causes a conjugate deviation of the eyes towards the opposite ear, and with maintenance of pressure, a corrective fast eye movement will be introduced and the nystagmus will beat towards the affected ear. The direction of nystagmus will depend on where the fistula has developed, but most commonly, the site is the horizontal semicircular canal, and the nystagmus is horizontal; if in the anterior canal, the nystagmus is torsional and toward the affected ear, and if in the posterior canal, it is vertical.

The pressure may be raised by finger pressure on the tragus, but more accurately by tympanometry to induce a precise increase in pressure. This sign should be sought in all dizzy patients and particularly in those with chronic middle ear disease. False negative signs may be found when cholesteatomatous disease is well advanced and the labyrinth has become unresponsive. Hennebert's sign is a positive fistula sign in the presence of an intact TM, and is classically attributed to syphilitic otitis.

The tympanic membrane

The standard landmarks and features of the TM should be identified: i.e. the central portion and the handle of the malleus, which are the most consistent features; distinction between the pars flaccida and the pars tensa of the drum; and identification of the long process of the incus and the stapedius tendon, which may be visible in transparent membranes.

Perforations

Those of the pars tensa are classified as marginal or central, according to whether the rim of the tympanic membrane forms part of the circumference of the perforation. Defects of the epitympanic recess are described as attic perforations and qualified as small or large (Figure 21.6). The position of the perforation is then defined as anterior, inferior or posterior if it is marginal. Very large central perforations are described as subtotal, and very large marginal perforations as total.

Colour

Normally, the TM has the appearance of mother of pearl. The light reflex is found anteroinferiorly, where reflection of the

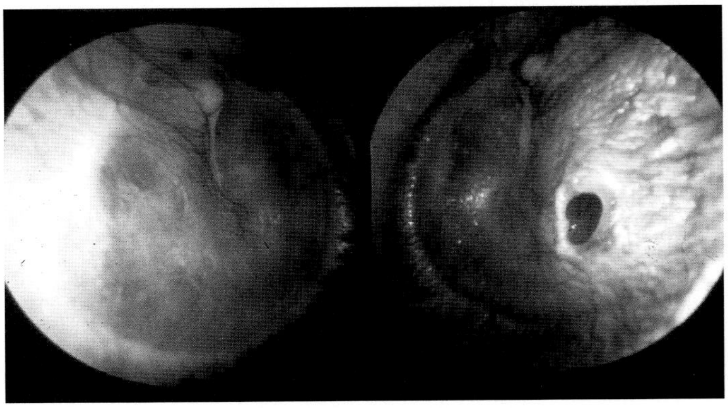

Figure 21.6 Small central perforation of the left tympanic membrane. (Courtesy of Mr Gerald Brookes.)

examining light occurs. Where the membrane is thickened, the reflex may be lost. Hyaline degeneration may occur when the middle layer of fibrous tissue undergoes hyaline degeneration, and may become impregnated with deposits of calcium, i.e. tympanosclerosis (Figure 21.7).

Position of the membrane

Retraction of the membrane may result when there is a chronic lowering of pressure in the middle ear, such as is seen when there is chronic obstruction of the Eustachian tube. The handle of the malleus is drawn inward, and there is retraction of the TM towards the medial wall of the middle ear. In severe cases, the membrane is stretched around the long process of the incus and head of the stapes. At worst, the membrane is plastered against the promontory. A fluid level may be visible if secretory otitis media has resulted from the reduction of middle ear pressure. If air bubbles are seen, middle ear fluid is confirmed.

The TM may bulge outwards into the meatus as a result of raised middle ear pressure. This increased middle ear pressure may be due to acute suppurative otitis media (the bulge showing the pus) when the colour is a bright cherry red. A yellow nipple may be a sign that the membrane is about to give way. Alternatively, if the colour is normal, the bulge is due to alteration in raised air pressure in the middle ear alone. If the TM has been weakened by loss of the connective tissue middle layer by repeated large pressure changes in the middle ear, e.g. in wind instrument players, or where a perforation has healed over, the bulge may be restricted.

Abnormalities of the tympanic membrane and middle ear

Congenital

In general, the following abnormalities can occur:

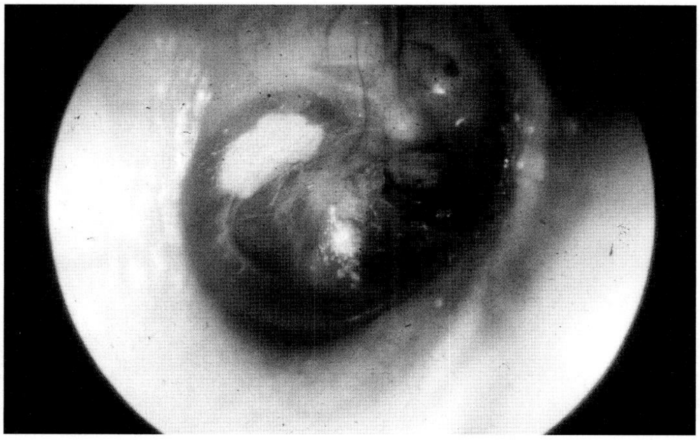

Figure 21.7 A right tympanic membrane showing a patch of tympanosclerosis posteriorly. (Courtesy of Institute of Laryngology and Otology, London.)

- fused malleus and incus
- incus fixed to posterior bony annulus
- congenital stapes fixation (+grossly deformed stapes)
- absent stapedius tendon
- uncovered VIIth nerve
- aberrant VIIth nerve
- partial bony plate formation.

The clinical signs of common syndromes and conigental presentations are outlined in detail in the Overview section beginning p. 366 in this chapter.

Audiological abnormalities may include the following:

- audiometry—air–bone gaps of <60 dB
- tympanometry—flattened tympanogram
- stapedius reflexes—absent.

Note that the hearing loss depends on the degree of abnormality of ossicular transmission.

Acquired

Acute otitis media

Acute otitis media (Figure 21.8) is frequently associated with upper respiratory tract infections. The most common causative organisms are *pneumococcus*, *Haemophilus influenzae* and *Moraxella catarrhalis*, and all can be treated with amoxycillin (paediatric dose: 125 mg three times daily; or 750 mg twice daily for adults for 2 days).[5] There is an exudative phase with an associated conductive hearing loss, and a recovery phase when

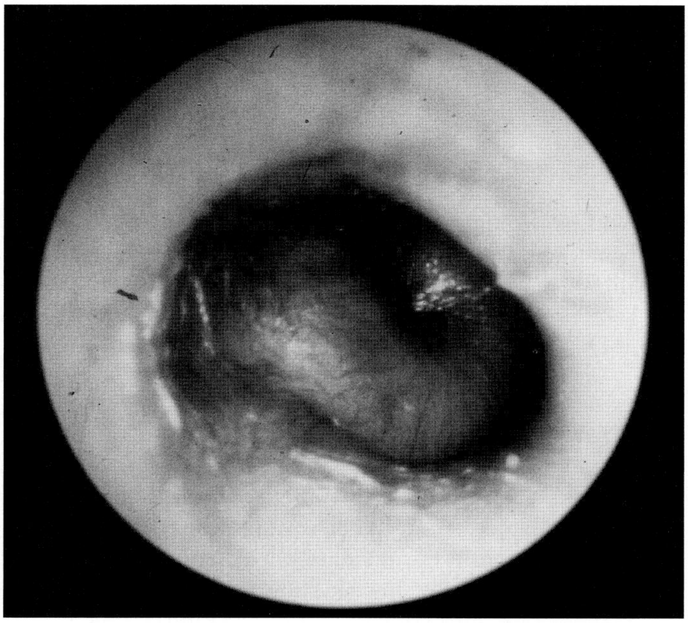

Figure 21.8 Swollen, hyperaemic tympanic membrane in a patient with acute otitis media. (Courtesy of Mr Gerald Brookes.)

the middle ear becomes well ventilated again. On occasion, resolution is not complete and the conductive loss may persist.

- Pure tone audiogram: may be normal or may show conductive hearing loss.
- Tympanometry: negative middle ear pressure, may be abnormal even with normal pure tone audiogram.

Chronic otitis media

Acute otitis media can lead to chronic otitis media (COM), and in association with COM a variety of other pathologies can be seen: TM perforation, incus necrosis, myringostapediopexy, malleus head fixation and cholesteatoma and tubo-tympanic disease.

Perforation

The drum can be destroyed in some cases of long-standing low-grade infection, or in incompletely treated acute otitis media. The size and location of the perforation determines the degree of conductive hearing loss. A large perforation, in general, is associated with a greater loss of sound pressure, but even a small perforation sited over the round window can produce a severe loss. If the perforation is associated with dislocation of the ossicular chain, when the advancing sound front strikes the mobile stapes directly, the loss is approximately 30–40 dB.

Ossicular abnormalities

The ossicular chain may be damaged in long-standing infection, with the lenticular process and lower half of the long process of the incus being most frequently involved. Even with an intact drum, a discontinuous ossicular chain can lead to a 60-dB loss.

The drum remnant may occasionally attach itself to the stapes head, leading to a myringostapedopexy. The hearing loss may be negligible, despite a very damaged drum. Alternatively, the malleus head may fix to the attic wall, producing a clinical picture similar to otosclerosis.

Tympanosclerosis

Tympanosclerosis is not infrequently found with long-standing infection, and indicates hyaline degeneration of the TM and impregnation with calcium. Large masses of tympanosclerosis may grow anywhere, producing fixation of the malleus, incus and stapes. A large conductive loss may be seen despite an intact TM.

Cholesteatoma

Cholesteatoma is a cyst lined with squamous epithelium which can arise in ears undergoing long periods of negative middle ear pressure and recurring middle ear infection. Cholesteatomatous cysts are likely to begin in the attic of the ear and extend into the mastoid antrum. They are filled with cast-off epithelial cell debris and slowly increase in size. They can erode the bone with which they come into contact and produce intracranial complications by eroding through the dura of the middle or posterior fosssa, through the lateral sinus or into the lateral semicircular canal (Figure 21.9). The facial nerve may be eroded in the middle ear or mastoid.

Cholesteatoma can be diagnosed from an attic or marginal ('unsafe') perforation, chronic foul-smelling discharge from the ear and keratin debris in the pars flaccida area on otoscopic examination. Cholesteatoma is potentially serious, and requires surgical removal. Cholesteatoma in the attic area may be removed by atticotomy, but usually mastoid tympanoplasty is required. Even following surgery, the patient must be followed for many years to be certain there is no recurrence of the cyst.

Tubo-tympanic disease

Chronic active otitis media unassociated with cholesteatoma is known as tubo-tympanic disease, it is characterized by recurrent infections rather than persistent infections, and by odourless and profuse mucoid discharge rather than offensive discharge. A central TM perforation and a break in the ossicular chain or malleus fixation are regarded as 'safe' and unlikely to be associated with cholesteatoma. A variety of bacterial species have been cultured from chronically draining ears: *Pseudomonas aeruginosa*, *Streptococcus*, *Escherichia coli* and *Staphylococcus aureus*, with Gram-negative organisms predominating. Management includes periodic cleaning of the ear to remove keratin debris and the use of antibiotic steroid drops. If the ear becomes dry with this treatment, the patient may be suitable for myringoplasty or ossiculoplasty to repair the drum and ossicular chain. Otherwise, mastoid tympanoplasty may be required to remove chronic infection from mastoid air cells.

Polyp formation

Polyp formation may occur in chronic otitis media with perforation, when the mucosa hypertrophies and polypoid changes occur. They are identified by their soft shiny appearance, covered with mucosa.

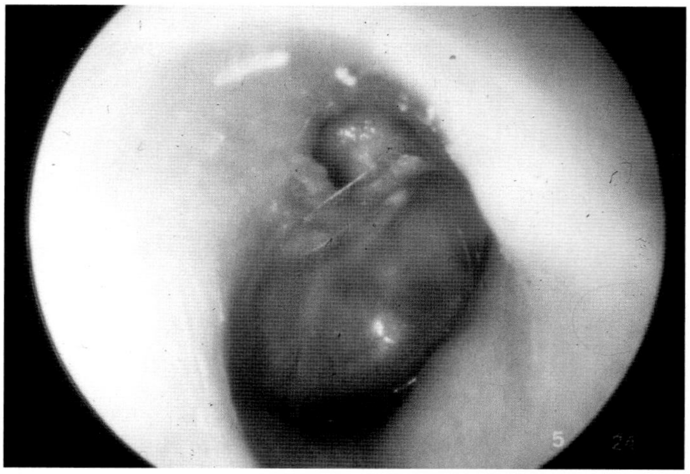

Figure 21.9 Attic defect in the right ear of a patient (Courtesy of Institute of Laryngology and Otology, London.)

Otitis media with effusion (OME)

OME is recognized by the presence of an air–fluid level in the middle ear or a bluish discoloration of the TM, and lack of compliance of the drum as tested by pneumo-otoscopy or tympanometry. It is the most common cause of conductive hearing loss in children (see Chapter 23). In the adult, the presence of OME must initiate a search for neoplastic obstruction of the nasopharyngeal end of the Eustachian tube by indirect or direct nasopharyngoscopy and radiological imaging of the nasopharynx.

In children, the search should be for a medically treatable cause of Eustachian tube dysfunction, e.g. allergy, adenoidal hypertrophy, or craniofacial abnormalities. Palatal abnormalities, particularly cleft palate, may be associated with OME because of the compromised mechanism for opening and closing the Eustachian tubes. These children may require long-term otological management of recurrent OME (Figure 21.10).

Management, in general, includes a trial of decongestants, auto-inflation through a modified Valsalva manoeuvre (or Politzer bag) or, eventually, myringotomy and insertion of a ventilating tube (normally in place for 8–12 months). For children with recurrent OME, myringotomy may be combined with adenoidectomy. Aural amplification in children with recurrent OME is now being evaluated.[6]

Other effusions include blood (i.e. haemotympanum) or cerebrospinal fluid within the middle ear space. Haemotympanum following head injury suggests a basal skull fracture, but haemotympanum may also result from barotrauma, e.g. scuba diving.

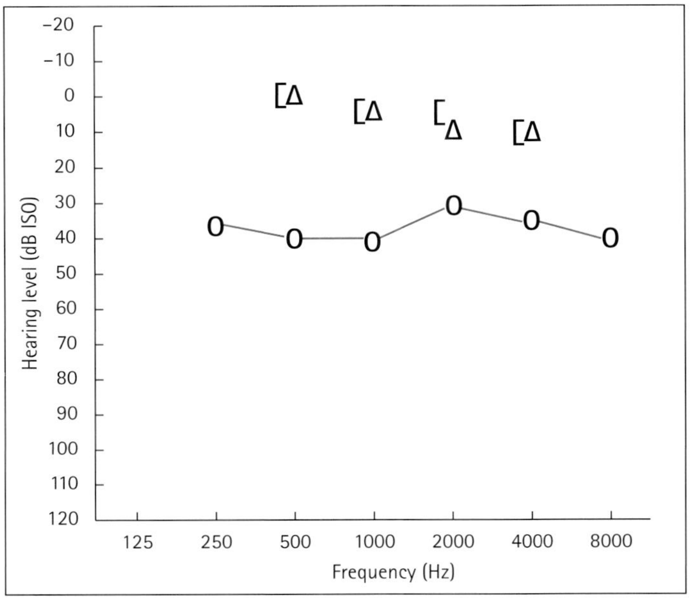

Figure 21.10 Pure tone audiometry in a 6-year-old with serous otitis media with effusion, showing an air–bone gap of between 25 and 40 dB.

Otosclerosis

Typically, in the early osteoblastic phase of this autosomal dominantly inherited condition, the appearance of the tympanic membrane is of hyperaemia of the malleus i.e. Schwartze's sign.

- Pure tone audiometry: typically a conductive hearing loss is seen early in the condition with a reduced air–bone gap at 2 kHz,[7] but later a sensorineural loss may be seen as well.
- Tympanometry: low tympanic compliance peak.

Head/ear trauma

A variety of outer and middle ear abnormalities can arise as a result of head trauma. If bloody otorrhoea is identified, there is a possibility that a longitudinal fracture of the petrous temporal bone has occurred and there has been perforation of the TM and possible dislocation of the ossicular chain. Audiometry is mandatory.[8]

- Pure tone audiometry: may identify a conductive hearing loss, but a variety of configurations of sensorineural hearing loss may also be seen associated with labyrinthine concussion. A total hearing loss is suggestive of a transverse fracture of the petrous temporal bone.
- Radiology: skull X-ray and CT scanning to exclude a temporal bone fracture.

Glomus tumours

A glomus tympanicum tumour may be identified as a vascular mass behind the tympanic membrane (also described as the 'setting sun' sign), and the patient may describe pulsatile tinnitus.

- Pure tone audiometry: may identify a conductive hearing loss.
- Tympanometry: may identify a pulsatile tympanogram.
- Radiology: erosion of the middle ear cavity by space-occupying lesion.

The clinical value of tuning fork tests

Tuning fork tests have been traditionally used to distinguish conductive from sensorineural hearing loss and identify functional hearing loss. With the advent of pure tone audiometry, only a few have withstood the test of time and are still used clinically. A full account of the history of tuning fork tests has been given by Hinchcliffe.[9]

They rely on two general principles: (1) that the inner ear is more is more sensitive to sound conducted by air than by bone; and (2) in a pure conductive hearing loss, the affected ear is subject to less environmental noise and is more sensitive to bone-conducted sound.

The most commonly used tuning forks are those tuned to 256 and 512 Hz, lower frequencies than 256 Hz producing a vibrotactile stimulus which causes misleading thresholds. The 256 Hz tuning fork has been shown in clinical practice to distinguish air–bone gaps more effectively than the 512–Hz fork.[10] In general, when carrying out tuning fork tests:

- They should be performed in a quiet room.
- The prong should be struck against a hard but elastic mass, e.g. a rubber pad, as otherwise overtones may be produced.
- The fork should be struck two-thirds of the way along its tines, to minimize distortion products.

Differentiation of conductive and sensorineural impairment

Rinne's tuning fork test

Heinrich Rinne described his eponymous tuning fork test in 1855.[11,12] The following is the loudness comparison method (Figure 21.11):

- The fork is struck and held with the tines perpendicular to the long axis of the EAM, with the closest tine within 1 cm of the entrance to the meatus.
- The patient is asked to report if he can hear the sound.
- The fork is then immediately transferred behind the ear, with the base soundly pressed to the bone overlying the mastoid.
- The patient is asked which sound is louder: that 'in front of the ear' or that 'behind the ear'.
- If the sound in front of the ear is reported as louder (i.e. air-conducted (or AC) sound) than that behind the ear (i.e. bone-conducted (or BC) sound), the Rinne test is described as being positive. The test is described as negative if the sound in front of the ear is reported as quieter.

Positive test (AC > BC)

In an ear with a normal conductive mechanism, air-conducted sound will be perceived as louder than bone-conducted sound. A positive test indicates either a normal hearing ear or an ear with a sensorineural hearing loss.

Negative test (AC < BC)

If, however, the test is negative, this indicates a significant conductive component to the hearing loss, i.e. of >15 dB HL. A false negative Rinne can occur if there is a severe sensorineural hearing loss in the tested ear. In this situation, the bone conduction stimulus is heard in the non-tested ear because of transcranial transmission and will be louder than the air conduction stimulus. Masking of the non-affected ear can be carried out using a Barany noise box (this emits white noise and raises the threshold of hearing such that intracranial transmission of the bone-conducted sound cannot be heard). Results should, however, be interpreted with caution, as the loudness of sound heard by bone conduction is very dependent on the pressure with which the fork is held against the bone.

In the threshold comparison method, the fork is pressed against the bone over the mastoid and the patient is asked to say when the tone disappears. When this occurs, the fork is immediately placed in front of the ear and the patient is asked if they can still hear the tone. If not, this would suggest that there is a conductive hearing component to the hearing loss.

The Rinne is best used as a test for a significant conductive component to the hearing loss. It has a high specificity but a low sensitivity,[13] with the sensitivity not reaching 90% until the air–bone gap exceeded 30 dB in a typical series.[14] The crossover point at which the Rinne test is likely to become negative is at an air–bone gap of around 18 dB.

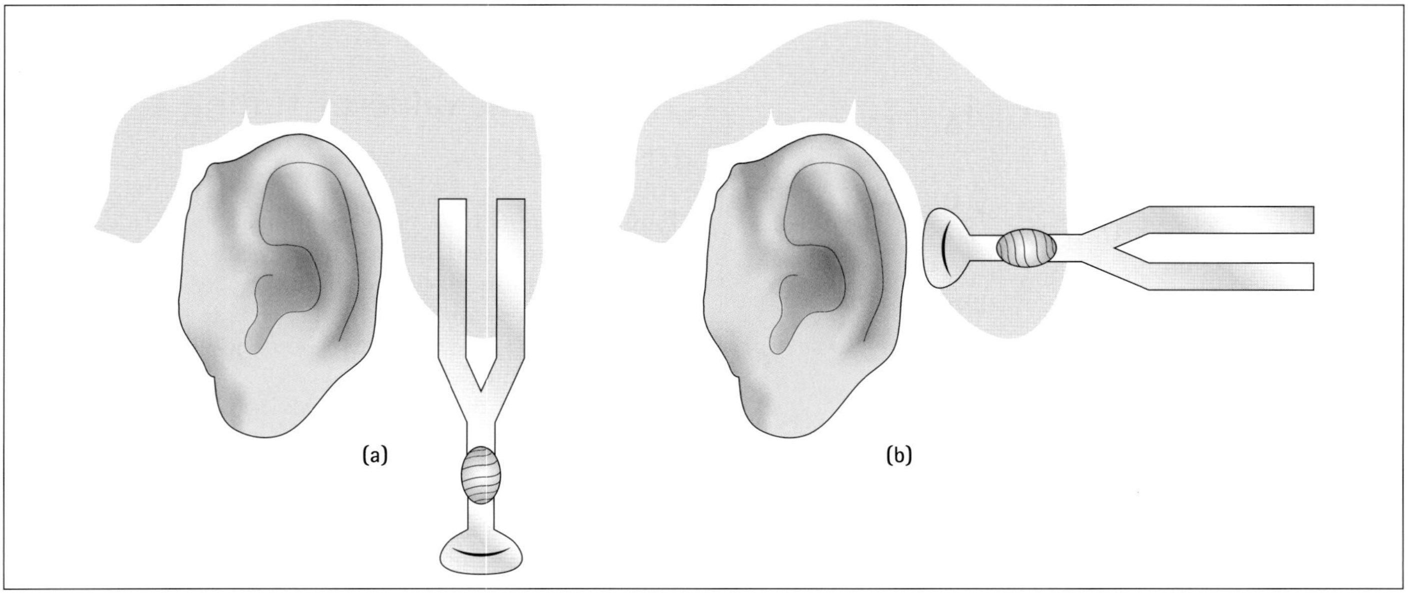

Figure 21.11 Rinne's tuning fork test (see text). (a) The tuning fork is held 1 cm away from the orifice of the external auditory meatus until the sound has disappeared. (b) The tuning fork is then applied to the mastoid process behind the ear, and the patient is asked to say if he can still hear the sound.

Weber's tuning fork test

The Weber test is used in conjunction with the Rinne test and is of most use in patients with unilateral hearing loss. The aim is to identify the better-hearing cochlea.

Ernst Weber described the test in 1834:[15]

- The 512 Hz tuning fork is struck and placed to the head in the mid-line (vertex or forehead).
- The patient is asked whether the sound is heard better in one ear or equally in both ears.

In a normally hearing patient, the tone is heard centrally. Otherwise, the tone is heard on the side of the better-hearing cochlea, except if there is a conductive component to the hearing loss, in which case the tone may be heard in the poorer-hearing ear.

The results need to be interpreted with caution and only in conjunction with the remaining battery of hearing tests. This test is best reserved for cases of unilateral hearing impairment.

Tuning fork tests can also be used to identify a cochlear component to a hearing loss:

- A vibrating tuning fork is presented to one ear.
- The patient is asked if the musical note sounds the same in the two ears.

Dysacusis is present if the patient describes the sound as being distorted or rough; diplacusis describes the phenomenon when a patient hears a single tone as two different pitches. It may be monaural or binaural, i.e. the two different pitches are heard as if coming from the same ear or from the two ears separately, respectively. Both these phenomena are features of cochlear hearing loss and are not uncommon in Menière's disease. They can also be heard in noise-induced temporary threshold shift.

Identification of non-organic hearing loss

Clinical suspicion is probably the strongest pointer to further investigation for a non-organic hearing loss. Throughout the examination, the clinician needs to be making an assessment as to whether the history and the hearing behaviour of the patient are compatible. Quite often, normal conversation can be achieved with a patient with a non-organic hearing loss, but as soon as voice tests or subjective hearing tests are carried out, thresholds are exaggerated. However, most patients with non-organic hearing loss do have some degree of hearing loss, and this must be borne in mind.

Stenger test

The aim of the Stenger test is to identify patients who feign a unilateral hearing loss. If pure tones of the same frequency but of different intensities are presented simultaneously to each ear, the normal subject will only be aware of the louder stimulus.

- Two tuning fork tests of the same frequency are presented simultaneously, one to each ear of the patient.
- The fork presented to the 'deaf' ear is held close to the ear, while the other fork is held at a distance from the other ear.

In a patient with a genuine hearing loss, the patient will hear the fork in the good ear. However, the patient with a non-organic hearing loss will only be aware of the fork in the 'deaf' ear and will therefore deny the fork. When the test is performed as a tuning fork test, it can be difficult to judge the relative intensity of the two forks. For this reason, it is better that the test is performed with an audiometer, where the exact intensities of the stimuli are known and can be varied.

Diagnostic test procedures

Pure tone audiometry

Accurate air and bone conduction audiometry (carefully masked where necessary) shows the existence and extent of hearing loss and allows determination of whether the loss is conductive or sensorineural or both. It requires the cooperation of the subject and, as such, is a subjective estimate of hearing threshold. If the patient is unwilling or unable to cooperate with pure tone audiometry, additional electrophysiological investigation will be necessary to provide objective measures of threshold.

The technique involves measurement of the threshold of hearing, i.e. the lowest intensity at which a sound can still just be heard. There are two methods which can be used: manual audiometry and self-recording audiometry. As a psychoacoustical measurement, the results of audiometry may be biased by particular methods of conducting the test, and so a well-defined procedure must be adopted.

Manual audiometry

An audiometer consists of a pure tone oscillator which may be set to one of several frequencies; a stepped attenuator to adjust the level of the signal according to a calibrated scale over a range from −10 dB to +90 dB hearing level; an amplifier; earphones (and, for bone conduction, a vibrator) and a power supply. The British Standard BS 5966[16] specifies the characteristics for these instruments.

A quiet test environment is required to obtain the subject's true threshold. Audiometric booths are specifically designed to eliminate external noise, particularly sound at low noise levels. The International Standardization Organization 6189[17] gives limiting noise levels for threshold measurements down to −10 dB HTL.

The threshold of hearing for a pure tone at a particular frequency is defined as the lowest level of the tone which still can be heard on at least 50% of its presentations. This level is influenced by the manner in which the level of tones is presented; that is, in manual audiometry with 5-dB steps, the apparent threshold is lower if approached from above (descending threshold) than if approached from below (ascending threshold). The reference intensity level, which is designated 0 dB at each frequency, is the mean value of the minimal audible intensity of pure tones in a group of healthy, normally hearing young male adults and corresponds to sound pressure levels set by the International Standards Organization.[17]

Table 21.1 indicates the loudness of different intensities of sound in terms of everyday sounds and as magnitudes of amplification of sound pressure levels.

Testing at the frequencies 250, 500 1000, 2000, 4000 and 8000 Hz is recommended. Where abnormalities are detected adjacent additional frequencies may also be tested, i.e. 1500, 3000 and 6000 Hz. The frequency to be tested first should be 1000 Hz, as this is often the easiest frequency for the subject to hear; one should then progress to the higher frequencies in ascending order before dropping to the lower frequencies and then retesting at 1000 Hz. A disparity of greater than 5 dB suggests that further repeats are necessary. It is important that the subject is instructed to respond to even the faintest sound, by pressing the button for the duration of the sound. A recommended protocol has been described.[18] Figure 21.12 shows the pure tone audiometry of a patient with mixed hearing loss.

Table 21.1 Decibel levels of sounds

Decibels	Sound	Magnitudes of amplification
140 dB	Jet engine	100 000 000 000 000
120 dB	Propeller aircraft	1 000 000 000 000
100 dB	Rock drill	10 000 000 000
90 dB	Heavy vehicle	1 000 000 000
70 dB	Private car	10 000 000
60 dB	Conversation	1 000 000
30 dB	Soft music	1 000
10 dB	Leaf rustle	10
0 dB	Barely audible	1

The results of measurement should be plotted on an audiogram chart in standard format:

- X = left air conduction
- O = right air-conduction
- Δ = unmasked bone conduction (identify on which mastoid the bone conductor was used)
- [= right masked bone conduction
-] = left masked bone conduction

Self-recording audiometry (see Chapter .....)
Most of the considerations applicable to manual audiometry are applicable to self-recording audiometry. However, the subject has a different task. The Rudemose self-recording audiometer uses a regularly pulsed tone (between 2 and 2.5 pulses/s) as the stimulus, and the apparatus automatically changes from one frequency to another and from one ear to the other according to a preset programme. The level of the signal is controlled by the subject, who has a press-button which he depresses when he can hear the pulsing tone. When the button is pressed, the stimulus is altered at a preset rate to reduce the signal level until the subject ceases to press the button because the pulsed tone has become inaudible. The attenuator drive is then automatically reversed and the level increases at a similar rate until the subject presses the button again.

The subject thereby causes the signal level to bracket his threshold, and the audiometer plots this tracking with time on an audiogram chart. Thus the threshold may be determined from the chart for each frequency, and a permanent record is produced. Figure 21.13 demonstrates self-recording audiometry.

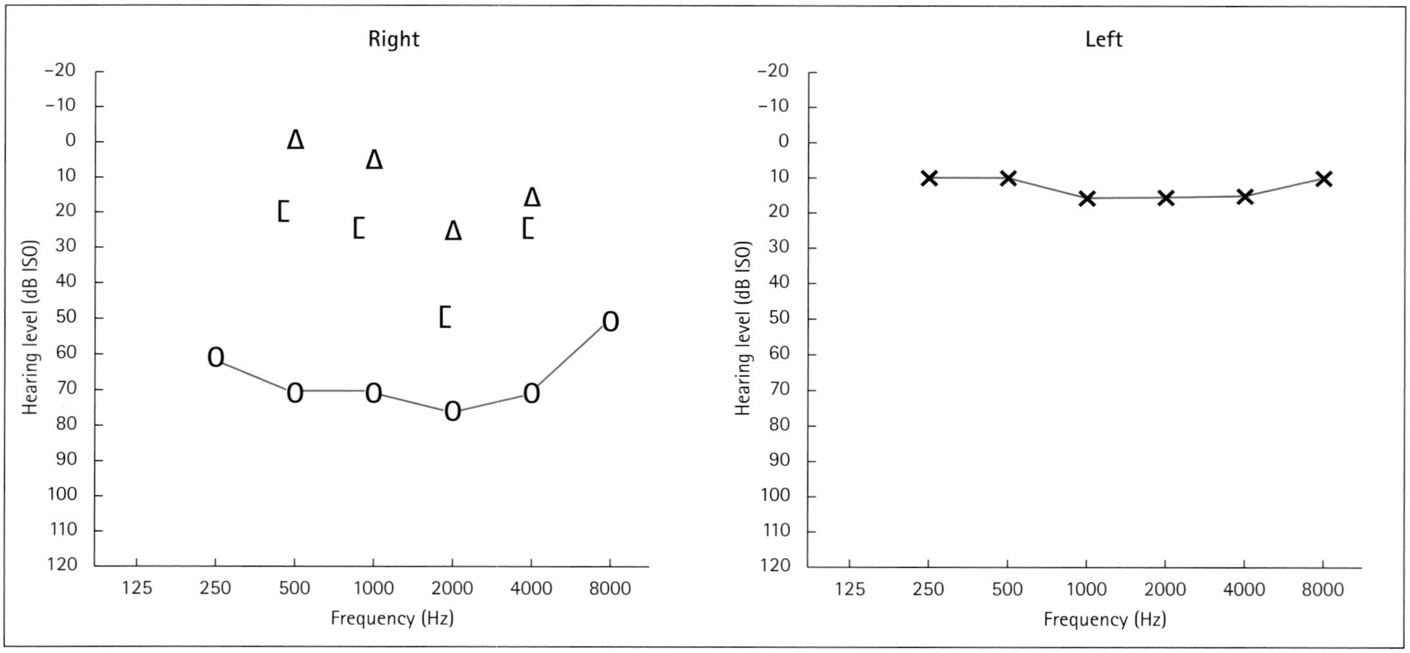

Figure 21.12 Pure tone audiometry from a patient with otosclerosis affecting the right ear and showing a mixed hearing loss with an air–bone gap varying between 25 and 50 dB on this side.

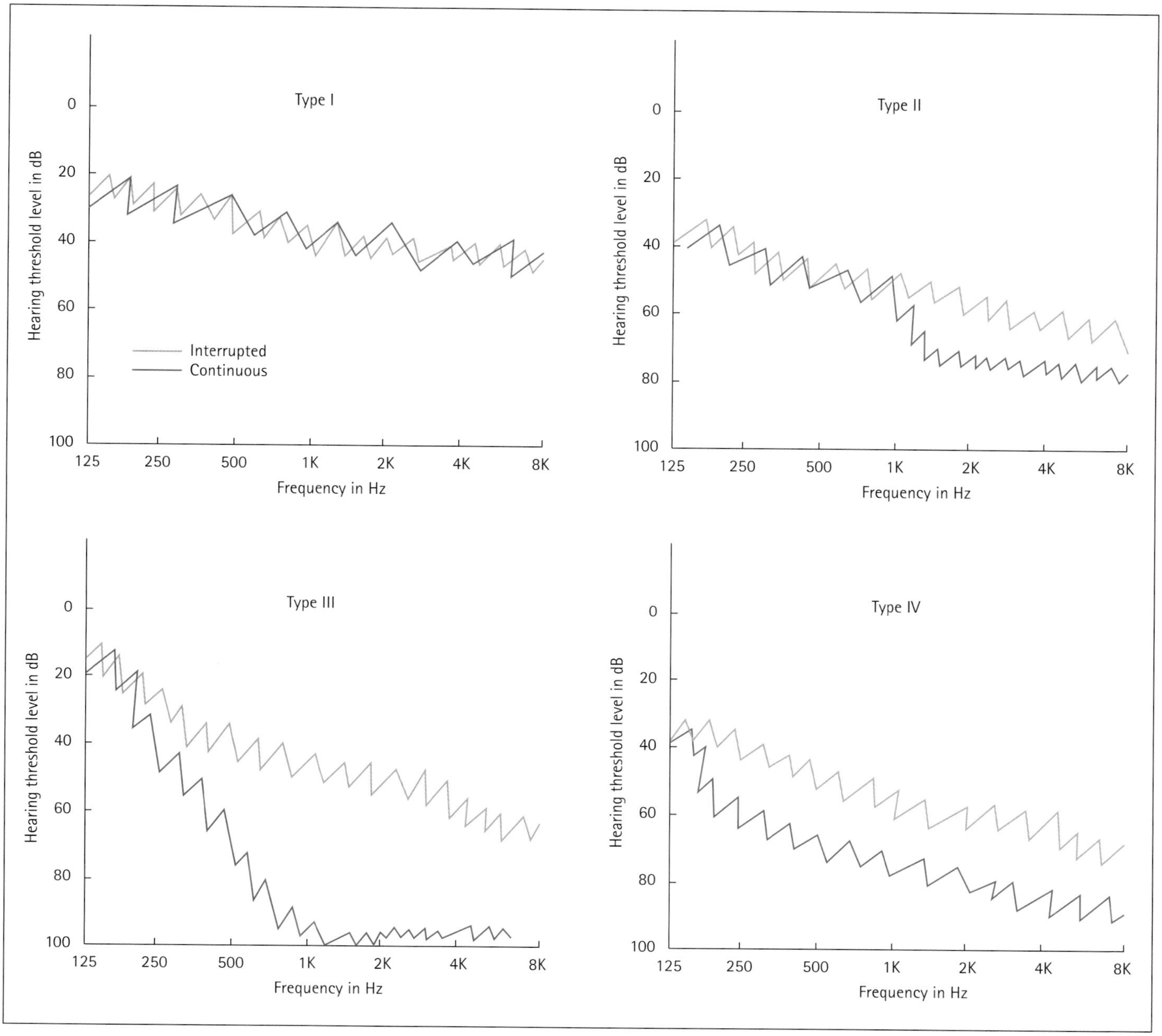

Figure 21.13 Self-recording audiometry. Dotted line, interrupted tone; continuous line, continuous tone. Type I: expected primarily from normal ears or those with a conductive hearing loss. Type II: typical of a cochlear loss. Type III and type IV: possible presentations of patient with retrocochlear loss or sudden hearing loss. (Adapted from Békésy. *Acta oto-laryngol* 1947; **35**: 411–22.[40])

Masking

The amount of sound lost in crossing the head, the transcranial transmission loss, varies from person to person: for air-conducted sound, the range of attenuation is 40–85 dB, and for bone conduction it is 5–15 dB. Masking is the noise applied to the non-test ear to ensure that the threshold obtained using pure tone audiometry is from the test ear and not from the non-test ear. In air conduction audiometry, the masking noise is presented through the earphone opposite to the one providing the test tones. In bone conduction audiometry, the usual procedure is to deliver the masking noise via an insert earphone.

Narrow bands of noise (⅓ to ½ octave wide) centred on the frequency of the test tone are most effective, but wide-band noise can be used.

Masking (Figure 21.14) is used to establish the pure tone threshold in the following situations.

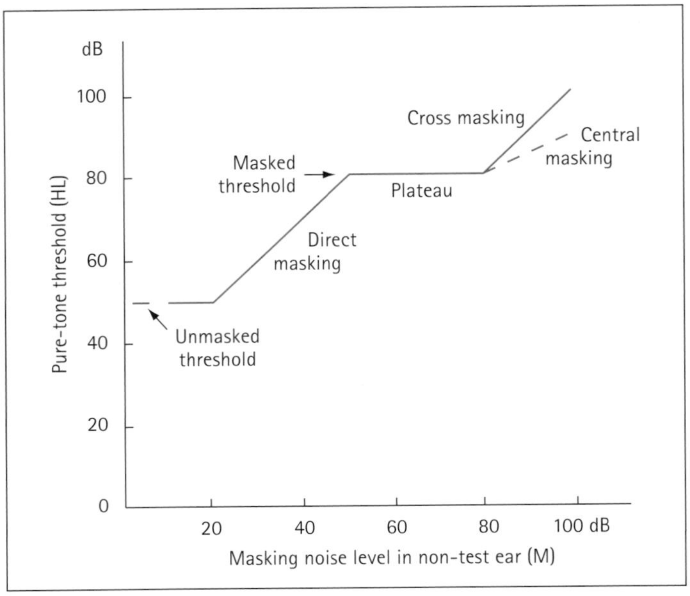

Figure 21.14 Masking chart (see text).

- **Air conduction:** (a) the difference between the left and right non-masked air conduction thresholds is 40 dB or more; (b) the air conduction threshold is 40 dB or more worse than the non-masked binaural threshold.
- **Bone conduction:** the air-conduction threshold is 10 dB or more worse than the non-masked bone conduction threshold at two or more adjacent frequencies.

The 'shadowing' technique of determining the true auditory threshold is the most commonly used masking technique. Starting from a low noise level, the unmasked threshold is elevated dB for dB, by masking noise in the non-test ear. Beyond a certain level, further additions of masking noise to the non-test ear cause no further dB for dB elevation in threshold, and the test ear must then be able to hear the tone. The level of the test tone at this plateau is the true, masked threshold of the test ear.

Acoustic immitance measurement

Measurement of the acoustical immitance of the ear, or tympanometry, is a technique for obtaining information about the state of the middle ear as a function of ear canal pressure. The graph produced is an expression of how the immitance of the ear is altered when the external ear canal is pressurized above (positive pressure) and below (negative pressure) atmospheric pressure.

Aural impedance represents the difficulty encountered by acoustical energy as it is transmitted through the ear. The reciprocal of impedance is admittance, which represents the ease of energy flow through the system. Stiffness is the characteristic of the ear which maintains its shape and brings about restoration after a force has been applied. Compliance of the auditory system is the reciprocal of stiffness and represents the mobility of the middle ear system. Stiffness is the major contributor to the impedance of the auditory system, and compliance measurements can justifiably be used as a close approximation to impedance.

Aural immittance has an important clinical use in identifying high-impedance middle ear abnormalities, i.e. otitis media and otosclerosis, and low-impedance abnormalities such as ossicular interruption.

Advantages of tympanometry

- Objective—requires no behavioural response.
- Non-invasive.
- Well tolerated and quick.
- Inexpensive.

Principles of acoustic immittance measurements

A variable-intensity, low-frequency, pure tone (usually 220 or 226 Hz, but can also be 660 or 678 Hz), generated by a miniature sound source, is delivered to the EAM by means of a flexible tube connected to one of three orifices in a probe tip assembly. The other two components fitting into the probe are (1) a tube connected to a pump which alters the ear pressure in the EAM, measuring the pressure manometrically; and (2) a tube which transmits sound waves from the EAM to a microphone for transduction to electrical activity. The electrical signal is amplified and rectified to direct current and represents the sound pressure level. It is compared with a reference voltage delivered by the impedance meter and the comparison registered on a balance meter (Figure 21.15).

The probe assembly is inserted into the EAM to make an airtight seal.

Middle ear pressure

In normal ears, the middle ear pressure will range from +50 to −50 mmH_2O (or +50 to −100 mmH_2O for children).

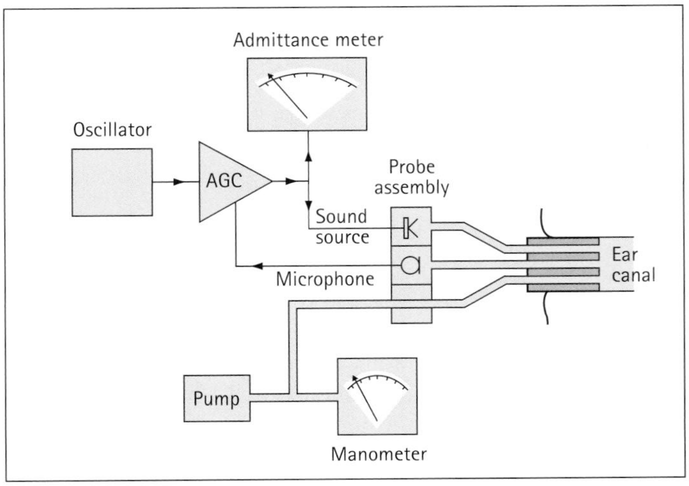

Figure 21.15 Principle of the aural admittance meter (see text).

Middle ear compliance

With the EAM pressure at middle ear pressure (MEP), the measured compliance is primarily that of the air in the external meatus plus that of the middle ear structures. If the EAM air pressure is increased considerably above MEP, e.g. MEP + 200 mmH_2O, the compliance of the middle ear structures becomes very small in comparison to the compliance of the air in the EAM, and the measured compliance is approximately equal to that of the air in the EAM. If this value is subtracted from the maximum compliance obtained with EAM pressure equal to MEP, this difference will be approximately equal to the compliance of the middle ear (MEC).

In normal ears measured in this way, the MEC shows large variations, depending on the physical quality of the TM, the degree of pneumatization of the temporal bone, and many other factors. Normal values range from 0.3 to 1.5 ml of equivalent air volume.

The tympanogram

The tympanogram is obtained by varying the external meatus pressure from −600 to +200 daPa (decapascal) (or mmH_2O). In the past, the procedure was carried out manually, measuring the compliance at a few specific pressures, but for speed, and production of a plot of an entire tympanogram, the recordings are now made automatically. This can also give hard copy evidence of rhythmic fluctuation in compliance due to conditions such as a patulous Eustachian tube, glomus tumour or tensor tympani myoclonus.

Purpose of acoustic immittance

- Method for objective determination of middle ear pressure.
- Measurement of 'static' acoustic impedance.
- Tympanometric shapes.

Middle ear pressure

If the Eustachian tube fails to ventilate the middle ear adequately, negative air pressure develops in the air spaces of the temporal bone. This is thought to happen as a result of:

- gases diffusing from the air into the cells because of the unequal concentration of gases in the air and in the middle ear tissues[19]
- the movement of fluid by cilia out of the closed Eustachian tube, thereby increasing the effective middle ear volume and leading to a negative MEP.[20]

The early proponents of middle ear tympanometry[21] suggested that the tympanometric peak pressure occurs when the difference between the different sides of the eardrum is zero. When the tympanometric peak pressure is negative, the MEP must be negative as well. However, the tympanometric peak pressure is not exactly equal to MEP, for several reasons:

- *Instrumental lag*: the automatic gain control systems used to keep the probe sound pressure level constant in the EAM as the air pressure is varied may not be able to keep up with the rapid immitance changes encountered when recording tympanograms with high pressure peaks, causing the peak to be reduced and shifted on the pressure axis.
- *Hysteresis*: this is the displacement of the pressure peak in the direction of the pressure sweep, that is, when the sweep is from positive to negative, the displacement is in a negative direction and vice versa.
- *MEP changes*: there is a change in MEP as a result of movement of the TM during tympanometry which is normally <30 daPa, but can be much greater in inflammatory middle ear conditions, the direction of the error always being an overestimate of the MEP. Nonetheless, although the tympanic peak pressure is not a measure of MEP, it is an important indicator of the pressure status of the middle ear.

Static acoustical immittance at the tympanic membrane

Measurement of acoustical immittance is in the plane of the probe tip rather than at the surface of the TM, and thus includes the effects of the ear canal as well as the middle ear transmission system. A mathematical correction needs to be applied to the immittance measurements to calculate the acoustical immittance attributable to the ear canal volume. Quantitative measurement requires frequent calibration, with corrections made for elevation and atmospheric pressure.

Static acoustical immittance measurements are controversial. This is in part due to the overlap in static immittance values between normal and pathological middle ears.[22] Many of the published data have been obtained with instruments that measure only the magnitude of the acoustical immittance vector with one low-frequency probe tone. When instruments measuring both components of acoustic impedance or admittance have been used, investigators have found static acoustical immittance measurements to be useful in the differential diagnosis of middle ear pathologies, i.e. distinguishing otosclerosis from normal middle ears, and evaluating progress in patients who have undergone stapedectomy.[23,24] Several factors influence static acoustical immittance:

- Instruments without automatic gain control circuits require a manual balancing procedure to make measurements in absolute physical units.
- Measurement of static immittance at the tympanic peak with specification of the tympanic peak pressure is the optimum method for reporting the immittance at the TM.
- The best pressure for estimating ear canal volume is the one that results in the minimum admittance (maximum impedance). Measurement at −400 daPa provides the best average estimate of ear canal volume.
- Low-frequency probe tone may not be optimal for the differential diagnosis of some middle ear pathologies; that is, middle ear disease may shift the resonant frequency of the middle ear transmission system. A probe tone frequency close to the resonant frequency of the normal human middle ear, i.e. 800–1200 Hz, may provide the maximum information in the detection of pathologies such as ossicular discontinuity.

- Most instruments measure only the magnitude of the admittance vector, although the acoustical admittance and impedance are complex issues requiring two values for their complete description. Measurement of the two immittance components facilitates both the evaluation of tympanometric shape and the calculation of static immittance.
- Guidelines are available for calculating static immittance based on available data and clinical efficiency.[25]

Tympanometric shapes

The most commonly used classification system was introduced by Liden[26] and modified by Jerger.[22] (Figure 21.16):

- Type A is a normal tympanogram—the peak immittance is at or near 0 daPa. This type is consistent with a normal, air-filled middle ear.
- Type A_D is a tympanogram with an unusually high peak pressure, e.g. a flaccid tympanic membrane or ossicular discontinuity.
- Type A_S is a tympanogram with a reduced pressure peak, as can be found with ossicular fixation and some forms of otitis media.
- Type B shows a flat pressure peak. This can be found with middle ear effusions or other space-occupying lesions of the middle ear. Alternative explanations for this shape include impacted wax or poor placement of the immittance probe against the ear wall canal.
- Type C has a negative peak pressure and indicates negative middle ear pressure.
- Type D shows sharp notching characteristic of scarred eardrums or hypermobile TM.
- Type E is characterized by broad smooth notching and is most commonly found in cases of partial or complete ossicular discontinuity.

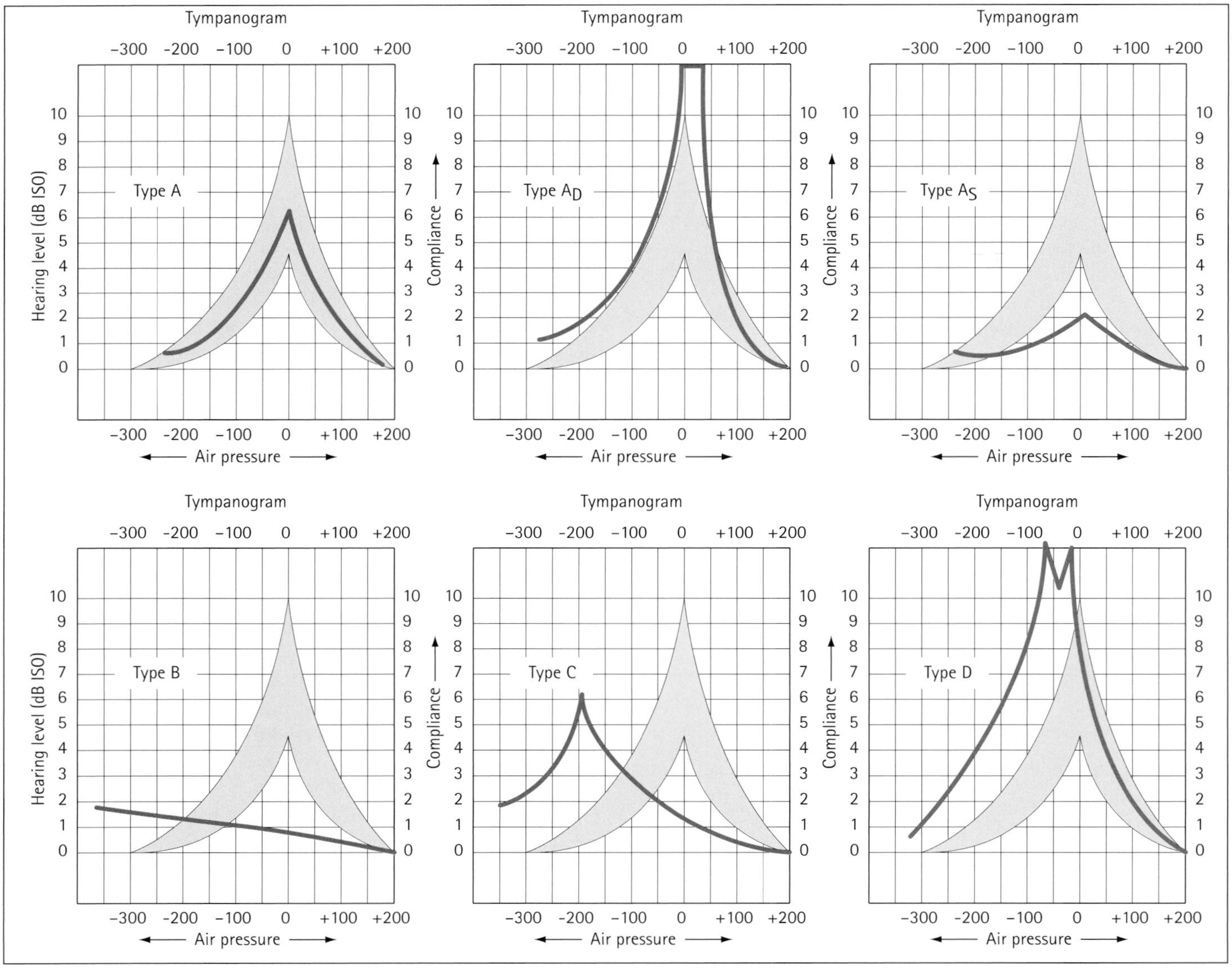

Figure 21.16 Liden-Jerger classification of tympanogram shapes. (After Feldman. In Feldman and Wilbur, eds. *Acoustic Impedance and Admittance—the Measurement of Middle Ear Function*. Baltimore: Williams and Williams, 1985: 423–37.[27])

Feldman[27] described an analytical approach to tympanometric shapes based on three features (Figure 21.17):

- Tympanometric peak pressure: normal, negative, positive or absent.
- Amplitude: normal, increased or decreased.
- Shape: normal, flat, peaked or notched.

Vanhuyse et al[28] developed a conceptual model for understanding all tympanograms, based on assumptions about the nature of acoustical resistance and reactance tympanograms, which predicts the measured conductance, susceptance and admittance tympanograms. The model assumes a basic understanding of the principles of acoustic immittance.[29]

High-impedance abnormalities

Middle ear conditions that produce abnormally high acoustical impedance results may have the following tympanograms: normal single peaks with reduced amplitude; abnormal tympanometric shapes; or flat tympanograms. Some examples are as follows.

Perforated tympanic membrane

- Flat tympanogram.
- Volume estimate of >2.5 ml for adults (may be as high as 4.5 ml in patients with no evidence of disease of the middle ear mucosa).

Patients with larger middle ear volumes tend to have better long-term surgical results than patients with smaller volumes.

Middle ear effusion

- High impedance.
- Flat tympanogram.
- May be positive or negative tympanometric peak (has low gradient).
- Tympanic peak amplitude inversely correlated with amount of middle ear effusion.

Retracted tympanic membrane

- Rounded tympanograms.
- May have increased ear canal volume.

Ossicular fixation

- Shallow tympanic peak.
- Middle ear pressure around 0 daPa.

Dual lesions

- The more lateral pathology generally dominates the tympanometric findings.

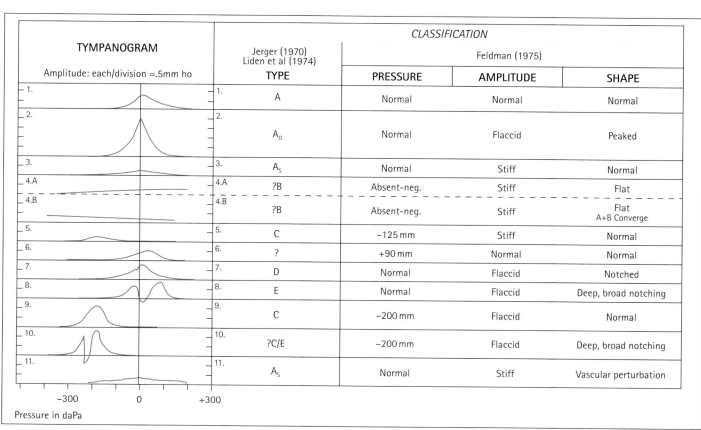

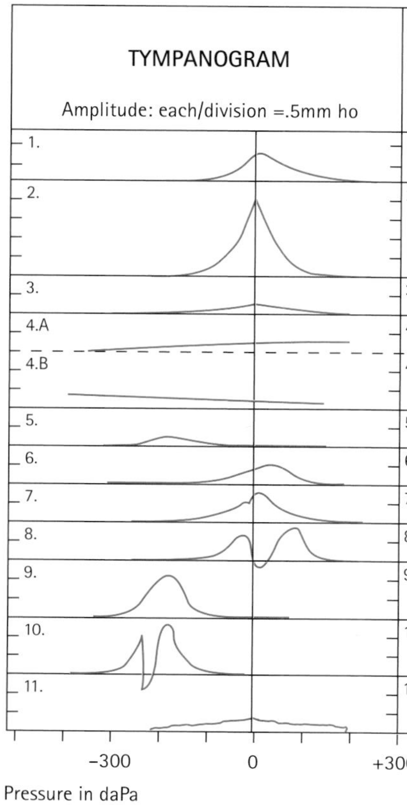

	Jerger (1970) Liden et al (1974)	CLASSIFICATION Feldman (1975)		
	TYPE	PRESSURE	AMPLITUDE	SHAPE
1.	A	Normal	Normal	Normal
2.	A_D	Normal	Flaccid	Peaked
3.	A_S	Normal	Stiff	Normal
4.A	?B	Absent-neg.	Stiff	Flat
4.B	?B	Absent-neg.	Stiff	Flat A+B Converge
5.	C	−125 mm	Stiff	Normal
6.	?	+90 mm	Normal	Normal
7.	D	Normal	Flaccid	Notched
8.	E	Normal	Flaccid	Deep, broad notching
9.	C	−200 mm	Flaccid	Normal
10.	?C/E	−200 mm	Flaccid	Deep, broad notching
11.	A_S	Normal	Stiff	Vascular perturbation

Figure 21.17 Feldman's descriptive analysis of tympanometric shapes. (From Feldman. *Audiology* 1977; **16**: 294–306.[41])

Low-impedance abnormalities

Two types of middle ear pathology result in abnormally low impedance at the TM—thin atrophic TMs and ossicular disruptions.

Thin, atrophic tympanic membranes

During the healing of a tympanic perforation (i.e. secondary to traumatic injury, necrosis, rupture from raised middle ear pressure and barotrauma), there may be incomplete regeneration of the connective tissue layer of the TM, producing a region of the membrane that is thin and flaccid. These scars do not cause measurable hearing loss but do produce distinctive abnormalities:

- low static immittance values
- high tympanic pressure peak
- may have deep susceptance notch.

Ossicular disruption

This may follow trauma or be associated with congenital defects, e.g. osteogenesis imperfecta. It lowers the primary resonant frequency of the middle ear.

- Low static impedance measurements.
- High tympanic pressure peak.

Summary

In conclusion, a full clinical assessment of hearing requires both an understanding of the underlying process of audition and the ways in which patho-physiological mechanisms can impact on this, as well as a comprehensive knowledge of the clinical methods available to detect hearing. In this way, structural abnormalities can be married to functional abnormalities and a full diagnosis made, allowing appropriate treatment/rehabilitation to be initiated. Currently available methodology dictates that, at a minimum, investigation of a patient with hearing loss requires pure tone audiometry, and that frequently this will need to be supplemented by other tests from the audiological test battery. Nonetheless, much can be learnt by a thorough clinical appraisal of the patient as described in the preceding pages, before proceeding to both audiological and actiological investigations.

Overview of developmental anomalies

A very brief description of the embryonic phase of the development in utero of the outer and middle ears is given for a fuller appreciation of the anatomy of the human ear and associated abnormalities.

During early embryonic life, the mesenchyme surrounding the primitive foregut and pharynx differentiates into a maxillary and mandibular swelling on each side of the mid-line just above and below the buccopharyngeal membrane. This membrane then breaks down and and a cavity is formed which will become the nasal and buccal cavities. In the mesenchyme surrounding the pharynx, five parallel thickenings develop as bands that surround the pharynx. These are the branchial arches, which are numbered 1 to 5 caudorostrally. On the external surface, a groove develops between each branchial arch and this is matched by a cleft on the inner pharyngeal surface.

Occasionally, there is a failure of this system and the different branchial arch defects can occur as sinuses when a cleft or groove fails to regress, or less commonly as fistulae when the ectodermal–endodermal junction breaks down. The first pharyngeal pouch expands to become the Eustachian tube, middle ear and mastoid antrum. The endoderm lying against the ectoderm of the first pharyngeal pouch is the precursor of the middle ear. The ossicles develop from the outer ends of the first arch (Meckel's) and the second arch (Reichert's) cartilages, which lie above and below the first pharyngeal pouches. The external ear canal develops from the small cartilaginous tubercles that surround the first pharyngeal groove (Fig. 21.18).

Congenital hearing loss can be associated with a variety of syndromes. Because of the specific clustering of characteristic features, a short synopsis of the different syndromes is given here with particular reference to the type of hearing loss seen, the underlying pathomechanism where known, and with guidance for the appropriate tools for further investigation. Accurate characterization of syndromal hearing loss has great importance for further management, which may in some cases be surgical, as well as for aural rehabilitation, and also for prognosis and genetic counselling.

Most attempts at classification are incomplete because of the limited understanding of the pathogenesis of many of these conditions, but, for simplicity, syndromes have been classified here as follows:

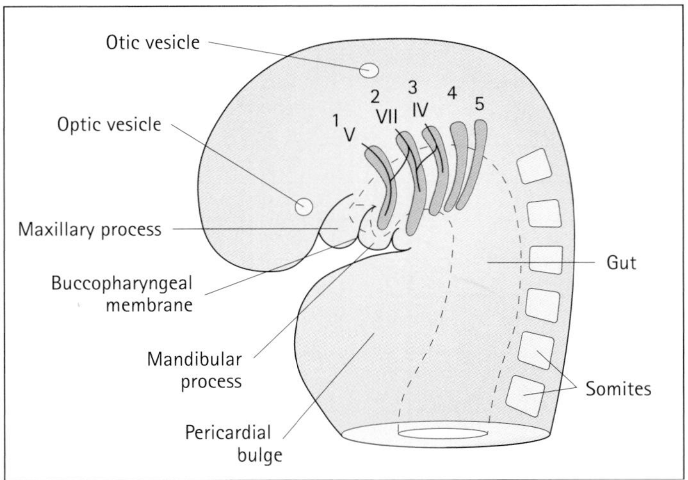

Figure 21.18 Schematic diagram of 16–28-somite embryo. (From Wright, with permission. In: Ludman and Wright, eds. *Diseases of the Ear*. London: Arnold 1998: 3–31.[42])

- Otocraniofacial (ear, face and skull).
- Otocervical (ear, face and shoulder).
- Otoskeletal (bone dysplasias).
- Chromosomal abnormalities.
- Miscellaneous.

Otocraniofacial syndromes

These syndromes comprise anomalies of the first and second branchial arch derivatives.

Craniofacial microsomia

Hemifacial microsomia is the commonest of these syndromes, with 1/3500 live births. In this condition, there is under-development of one half of the face, with mandibular and maxillary hypoplasia, macrostromia, microtia and atresia of the external auditory meatus (EAM). A suggested pathomechanism is embryonic haematoma formation. Only 20% of all patients have bilateral abnormalities, and when present these are asymmetrical.

Where these findings are seen in association with abnormalities of the eye and vertebral column, this is known as 'Goldenhar's syndrome' or oculoauriculovertebral dysplasia (Figure 21.19). Temporal bone studies in Goldenhar's syndrome have been reported by Mafee and Valvasorri[30] among others. The following features were reported by Phelps and Lloyd[3] in a study of the examination of 61 affected temporal bones, including CT studies.

External ear: Pinna—deformity ranging from complete absence to only one lobule present in some cases.
EAM—normal to complete atresia, low anterior position, gross descent of tegmen.

Middle ear: Middle ear cavity—very small with poor pneumatization.
Ossicles—frequently absent, otherwise abnormal in size, shape and situation, sometimes fused.
VIIth nerve—partial palsies in some.
± Patulous Eustachian tube.
± Cleft palate.

Inner ear: Cochlea—normal function.
Vestibular end organ—lateral semicircular canal commonly dysplastic.

Mandibulofacial dysotosis

Possible pathomechanisms include deficient neural crest cell migration into the first and second branchial arches.[31]

The syndrome known as Treacher Collins syndrome (Figure 21.20) is inherited with an autosomal dominant pattern of variable expressivity. The facies are very characteristic:

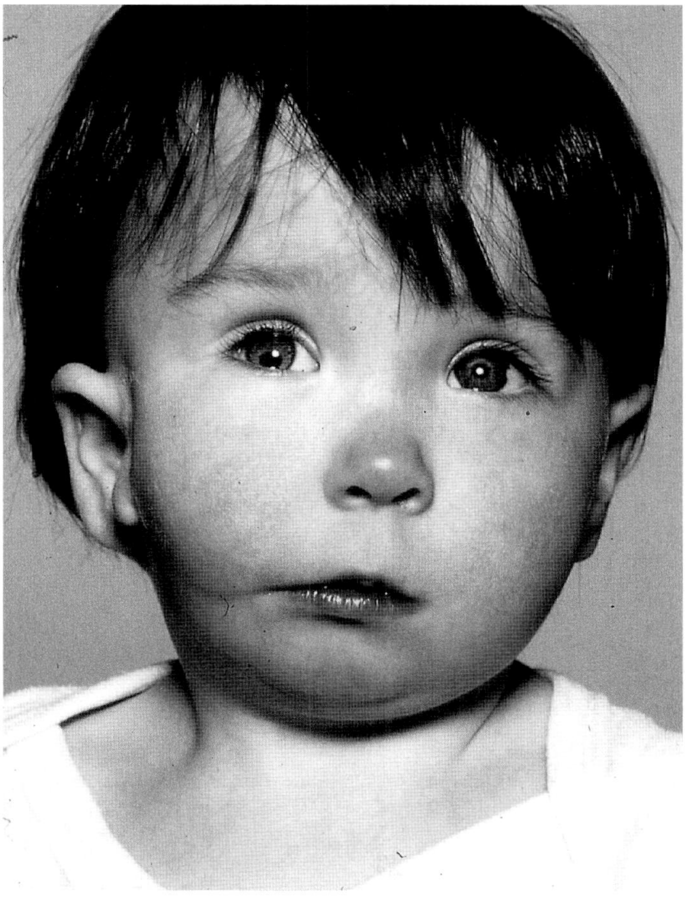

Figure 21.19 Craniofacial microsomia—Goldenhar's syndrome (with permission from Professor Dafydd Stephens).

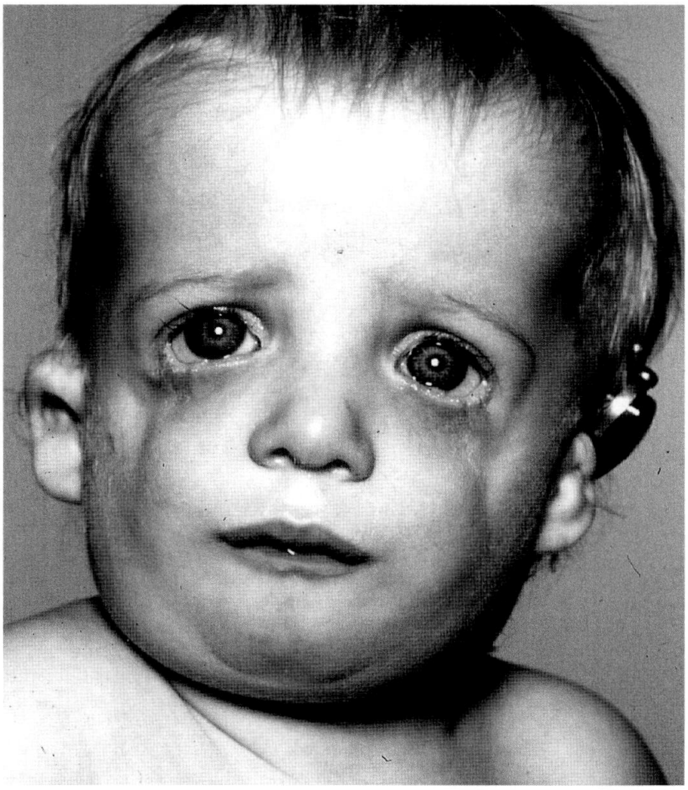

Figure 21.20 Mandibulofacial dysostosis–Treacher Collins syndrome (with permission from Dafydd Stephens).

- antimongoloid slanting of the palpebral fissures
- malar and mandibular bone hypoplasia with or without cleft palate
- coloboma of the lower eyelid in 75%.

External ear: Pinna—always malformed, often hypoplastic and cupped, pre-auricular tags and sinuses seen. Abnormalities tend to be bilateral and symmetrical. EAM—atresia, microtia common.
Middle ear: Mastoid—deficient and unpneumatized. Ossicles—abnormalities common.
Internal ear: Cochlea—normal function. Vestibular end organ—dysplastic semicircular lateral canal.

- Pure tone audiometry: conductive hearing loss.
- Radiology: a thorough radiological assessment is required because of the wide range of severity of ear lesions.

Pierre–Robin
This syndrome is thought to result from arrested development of the first and second branchial arch derivatives and is characterized by the following:

- micrognathia
- glossoptosis
- cleft palate.

Outer ear: Pinnae—low slung, may also be deformed. EAMs—may be atretic.
Middle ear: Ossicles—may be deformed.

Craniofacial dysostoses
These conditions are characterized by premature closure of skull sutures, which leads to a sagittal shortening of the skull base. Otopathology is less frequent than in the mandibulofacial dysostoses. There are four craniofacial dysostosis syndromes associated with deafness which have an autosomal dominant pattern of inheritance.

Acrocephalosyndactyly 1: Apert's syndrome

- Turret skull as a result of irregular craniostenosis.
- Facial asymmetry.
- Hypertelorism.
- Dental malocclusion.
- High arched palate.
- Syndactyly and partial webbing of fingers.
- Mental retardation.

External ear: Pinna—normal. EAM—normal.
Middle ear: Middle ear cavity—filled with gelatinous fluid. Ossicles—fixation of stapes, may be deformed and ankylosed.
Inner ear: Dilated horizontal lateral semicircular canal.

- Pure tone audiometry: conductive deafness.[32]
- Tympanometry: decreased compliance—no drum movement, no ossicular movement.

Acrocephalosyndactyly 2: Pfeiffer syndrome
This is very similar to Apert's syndrome, and may be a milder variant.

Acrocephalosyndactyly 3: Saethre–Chotzen syndrome
A minor degree of hearing loss has been reported.

Crouzon's syndrome
This is the commonest of the craniofacial dysostoses, and the abnormalities are confined to the cranium and the face.

- beak nose
- hypertelorism
- hypoplastic maxillae
- mandibular prognathism
- proptosis.

Outer ear: EAMs—atretic.
Middle ear: Eustachian tube dysfunction. Otitis media with effusion. Ossicles—may be fused with fixation of the stapes.

- Pure tone audiometry: conductive hearing loss.
- CT scanning: tilting of the petrous pyramids, poorly pneumatized mastoids.

Cryptophthalmos
This condition is identified when the skin of the forehead completely covers one or both eyes. It is associated with multiple congenital abnormalities:[31]

- urogenital system abnormalities
- syndactyly of the fingers
- abnormalities of the nose (50%)
- meningoencephalocoele (10%).

Outer ear: Pinnae—small and poorly modelled (30%). EAM—narrowed and atretic.
Middle ear: Ossicles—may be malformed.

- Pure tone audiometry: conductive hearing loss.

Waardenberg's syndrome (Figure 21.21)
This syndrome is inherited in an autosomal dominant fashion. It is characterized by:

- hypoplasia of the base of the nose
- lateral displacement of the middle canthi
- underdeveloped orbits
- heterochromia iridium
- white forelock.

Inner ear: Organ of Corti—absent. Vestibular end organ—anomalies, e.g. aplasia of the semicircular canal. VIIIth nerve—spiral ganglion atrophied.

- Pure tone audiometry: sensorineural hearing loss
- Vestibular function: abnormal—more common than hearing loss.

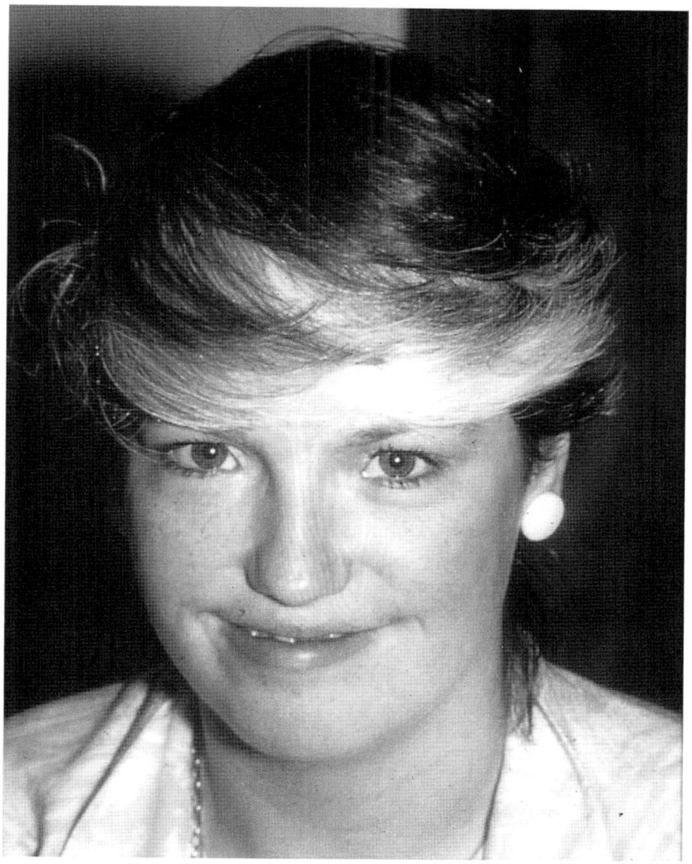

Figure 21.21 Patient with Waardenburg's syndrome demonstrating the typical white forelock seen in this syndrome. (Courtesy of Dr Maria Bitner-Glindzicz, Institute of Child Health, London, UK.)

Familial mixed deafness with branchial arch defects—earpits deafness syndrome

This is an autosomal dominant disorder, which may be associated with lacrimal duct aplasia and urinary tract abnormalities, i.e. branchio-oto-renal syndrome (see Figure 21.5).

Outer ear: Pinnae—auricular deformities, pre-auricular pits and sinuses, branchial fistulae/ clefts/ cysts.
EAM—atresia (75%).
Middle ear: Ossicles—minor abnormalities, mainly of stapes, with fixation.
Inner ear: Dysplastic lateral semi-circular canal
Cochlear hypoplasia

- Pure tone audiometry: conductive or mixed hearing loss.
- Distortion of base of skull and petrous pyramids.
- Internal auditory meatus slants upwards and backwards.
- Small cochlea (decreased number of turns—but not a Mondini-type deformity).

Otocervical syndromes

Klippel–Feil syndrome

Inheritance of this condition is autosomal dominant. It is typified by:

- characteristic fusion of several cervical vertebrae
- high-arched or cleft palate
- severe sensorineural deafness.

Middle ear: Ossicles—stapes gusher, incudostapedial junction abnormalities.
Inner ear: Cochlea—Mondini type defects.
Internal acoustic meatus—narrow

- Sensorineural and conductive hearing losses.
- Internal ear dysplasia with deficiencies of central bony spiral.

Wildervanke's syndrome (cervical oculoacousticus) is an association of Klippel–Feil syndrome with deafness and Duane's syndrome (limited abduction and adduction of the eye with retraction when lateral deviation of the eyes is attempted, due to fibrous displacement of the appropriate rectus muscles).

Cleidocranial dysostosis

- Dominant pattern of inheritance.
- Variable deficiency/absence of the clavicles.
- Abnormalities of the skull.

Outer ear: EAM—atresia.
Middle ear: Ossicles—ossicular chain malformations.

Otofacial-cervical syndrome

- Dominant pattern of inheritance.
- Narrowing and flattening of the face.
- Cervical and shoulder abnormalities.

External ear: Pinna—always deformed.

- Conductive hearing loss.

Sprengel's syndrome

This is a dominantly inherited syndrome with an association of hearing loss with a high, malformed and malrotated atresia of the shoulder capsule. It is often associated with narrow middle ear and absent stapes.

Otoskeletal syndromes

The main disorders of bone affecting ears are otosclerosis, fibrous dysplasia and Paget's disease, and tend to present in adult life,[33] Generalized bone dysplasia commonly manifests with Eustachian tube obstruction and otitis media. Sensorineural hearing loss may occur as a result of compression of the middle ear structure by fibrous dysplasia.

Osteogenesis imperfecta

This is an inborn error of osteoblasts or osteoclasts. There is an incidence of 20–60% of associated otopathology and hearing loss.[34] Only one-third present with a complete syndrome:

- large skull
- bowing of legs
- multiple fractures of the long bones
- laxity of ligaments
- atrophic skin
- blue sclera
- abnormal tooth dentine.

Two forms of the disease are recognized: the lethal form (present at birth), and the tarda form, which has a dominant mode of inheritance.

Middle ear: Ossicles—stapedial crura are often fragile, while footplate is heavy, but not significantly fixed.

- Pure tone audiometry, conductive deafness predominantly, but mixed and pure sensorineural hearing loss also.
- Deficient ossification; changes in otic capsule indistinguishable from those of labyrinthine otospongiosis. Appearances of 'cochlea within a cochlea', i.e. thick demineralized bone replacing the otic capsule but sparing the modiolus.

Osteopetroses

These comprise a group of uncommon disorders characterised by increased skeletal density and abnormalities of bone modelling and associated with hearing loss: Albers-Schonberg disease, Van Buchem's disease, Gorlin–Hart syndrome and Engelman's disease. Typically, the skull base and calvaria are involved, resulting in cranial nerve palsies, i.e. optic nerve and audiovestibular nerve as well as the mandibular portion of the trigeminal and facial nerve. Recurrent facial nerve palsies are not uncommon.

Outer ear: EAM—narrowed.
Middle ear: Encroachment of the bony walls of the attic on the ossicles.
Narrowing of the oval and round windows.
Inner ear: Interior auditory meatus: bony constriction.

- Pure tone audiometry: conductive hearing loss, sensorineural hearing loss.
- Tympanometry: low impedance
- Generalized sclerosis and expasion of the petrous pyramid.
- Narrowing of the interior auditory meatus. Increased bulk of ossicles.

Kniest syndrome

- Autosomal dominant inheritance.
- Round, flat mid-face.
- Short neck.
- Waddling gait.
- Club feet.
- Basilar impression of skull/cleft palate (in 50%).
- Shallow orbits with myopia, retinal detatchment and cataracts.
- Conductive or mixed type hearing loss.
- Tilting and shortening of petrous pyramids and squat thickened ossicles.

Mohr syndrome (orofacial digital syndrome type II)

NB: In the much commoner orofacial digital syndrome type I, hearing is normal.

- Polydactyly.
- Metaphyseal irregularity and flaring.
- Hypoplasia of the mandible, cleft lip and lobulated tongue.
- Conductive hearing loss.
- Malformed ossicles.

Other dysplasias with ossicular abnormalities and conductive deafness include otopalatodigital syndrome, multiple synostosis, Cockayne syndrome and achondroplasia.

Chromosome abnormalities with ear malformations

Autosomal trisomy

13–15 or Trisomy D

- Cardiac abnormalities.
- Neurological abnormalities.
- Cleft palate and lip.

Outer ear: Pinnae—low-set and deformed.
Inner ear: Cochlea and semicircular canal abnormalities.

18 or Trisomy E

The majority are non-familial and chromosomal deletions. The long-arm and ring types (18g and 18r) are associated with structural deformities of the ear.

- cardiac abnormalities
- elfin face
- ptosis, corneal opacities and glaucoma
- mental deficiency.

Outer ear: EAM—atresia.
Middle ear: Ossicles—ossicular abnormalities.

21 Trisomy

Chronic otitis media is a common feature of Down's syndrome. Comprehensive audiological assessment[35] identified 64% of patients with hearing loss, of which 83% had conductive hearing loss. Of these, middle ear effusion or TM perforation accounted for only 60%, with the remainder being due to congenital anomalies of the auditory ossicles, especially the stapes.

Middle ear: Ossicles—fixation and superstructure deformity of the stapes.

Dehiscence of the Eustachiuan tube.
Middle ear cavity—erosive lesions caused by cholesteatoma.

- Pure tone audiometry: conductive hearing loss, sensorineural high-frequency loss.

Sex trisomy—Turner's syndrome

- Webbing of the neck.
- Multiple eye abnormalities.
- Micrognathia.
- Infertile.

Outer ear: Low-set pinna.
Middle ear: Middle ear cleft—abnormal orientation with frequent otitis media.
Ossicles—fixation of the stapes.

Ear abnormalities with endocrine disorders

Pendred syndrome
This has a recessive mode of inheritance. There is a partial block in the synthesis of thyroxine.

- Goitre—presenting in puberty.
- Positive perchlorate test, but euthyroid.
- Congenital sensorineural deafness.
- Severe sensorineural hearing loss.
- Mondini type defects of the cochlea with deficiency of the modiolus.[36]
- Widened vestibular aqueduct (WVA) and/or hypoplastic semicircular canals.

Drug-induced ear malformations

Thalidomide embryopathy:
Ten per cent of the patients affected in utero by thalidomide, administered between 1959 and 1962, have ear lesions:[37]

- bilateral, severe
- external, middle and inner ears involved
- partial or complete, unilateral or bilateral facial palsy.

Phelps[38] found that all but one of 19 cases of VIth and VIIth nerve palsies (Moebius syndrome) accompanying congenital ear deformities were born within the thalidomide era.

- Complete absence of tympanic bone, middle ear cavity flattened, distorted and opaque due to glue-like mesenchyme.

Note that there is an operative finding of hyperplastic ossicular mass.

Miscellaneous

Neurofibromatosis—von Recklinghausen's disease

This syndrome with neurocutaneous manifestations follows an autosomal dominant transmission (see Chapter 4).

CHARGE association

Pagon and coworkers[38] applied the acronym CHARGE to an association of congenital defects:

- coloboma
- heart disease
- atresia of the nasal choanae,
- retarded development
- central nervous system abnormalities
- genital hypoplasia
- ear anomalies.

To be classified as the CHARGE syndrome, patients must have choanal atresia and coloboma and a total of at least four of seven of the attributes.

- Sensorineural hearing loss—mild to moderate.
- Absence of semicircular canals. Oval window may be absent.

References

1. Swan IRC. Clinical aspects of hearing aid provision. MD thesis, University of Glasgow, 1984.
2. Browning GG, Swan IRC, Chew KK. Clinical role of informal tests of hearing. *J Laryngol Otol* 1989; **1033**: 7–11.
3. Phelps PD, Lloyd GAS. Syndromes with congenital hearing loss. In: Phelps PD, Lloyd GAS, eds. *Diagnostic Imaging of the Ear*, 2nd edn. London: Springer-Verlag, 1990: 67–93.
4. Calzolari F, Garani G, Sensi A, Martini A. Clinical and radiological evaluation in children with microtia. *Br J Radiol* 1999; **33**: 303–12.
5. Anon. Tackling antimicrobial resistance. *Drug Ther Bull* 1999; **37**: 9–16.
6. Ahmmed AK, Curley JA, Newton VE, Muhkerjce D. Hearing aids versus ventilation tubes in persistent otitis media with effusion: a survey of clinical practice. *J Laryngol Otol* 2001; **115**: 274–9.
7. Carhart R. Clinical application of bone conduction audiometry. *Arch Otolaryngol* 1950; **51**: 798–807.
8. Davies RA, Luxon LM. Dizziness following head injury—a neuro-otological study. *J. Neurol* 1995; **242**: 222–30.
9. Hinchcliffe R. The clinical examination of aural function. In: Stephens SDG, ed. *Scott-Brown's Otolaryngology*, 5th edn, Vol 2. London: Butterworths, 1987: 203–43.
10. Stankiewicz JA, Mowry HJ. Clinical accuracy of tuning fork tests. *Laryngoscope* 1979; **89**: 1956–63.
11. Rinne HA. Beitrage zur Physiologie des menschlichen Ohres. *Vjschr Prakt Heilkunde Med Fak Prag* 1855; **12**: 71–123.
12. Huizing EH. The early descriptions of the so-called tuning fork tests of Weber and Rinne, Schwabach and Bing. II. The 'Rinne Test' and its first description by Polansky. *J Otorhinolaryngol Borderlands* 1975; **35**: 278–82.
13. Browning GG, Swan IRC. Sensitivity and specificity of the Rinne tuning fork test. *BMJ* 1988; 297: 1381–2.
14. Capper JWR, Slack RWT, Maw AR. Tuning fork test in children (an evaluation of their usefulness). *J Laryngol Otol* 1987; **1011**: 780–3.

15. Weber EH. De pulse, resoptione, auditu et tactu. In: *De Utilitate Cochleae in Organo Auditus*. Leipzig; 1834: 25–44.
16. British Standards Institution. *Specification for Audiometers*. BS 5966. 1980.
17. International Standards Organization. *Limiting Noise Levels for Threshold Measurements Down to –10 dB HTL*. ISO 6189, ISO, 1983.
18. Anon. Recommended procedures for pure-tone audiometry using a manually operated instrument. *Br J Audiology* 1981; **15**(3): 213–16.
19. Ingelstedt S, Jonson B. Mechanisms of gas exchange in the normal middle ear. *Acta Otolaryngol (Suppl)* 1966; **224**: 452–61.
20. Hilding AC. Summary of some known facts concerning the common cold. *Ann Otol Rhinol Laryngol* 1944; **53**: 444–60.
21. Terkildsen K, Thomsen KA. The influence of pressure variations on the impedance of the human eardrum. *J Laryngol Otol* 1959; **73**: 409–18.
22. Jerger J. Clinical experience with impedance audiometry. *Arch Otolaryngol* 1970; **92**: 311–24.
23. Burke K, Nilges T. A comparison of three middle ear impedance norms as predictors of otosclerosis. *J Audiol Res* 1970; **10**: 52–8.
24. Margolis RH, Osguthorpe JD, Popelka GR. The effects of experimentally-produced middle-ear lesions on tympanometry in cats. *Acta Otolaryngol* 1978; **86**: 428–36.
25. Margolis RH, Shanks JE. Tympanometry. In: Katz J, ed. *Handbook of Clinical Audiology*, 3rd edn. Baltimore: Williams and Wilkins, 1985: 438–75.
26. Liden G. The scope and application of current audiometric tests. *J Laryngol Otol* 1969; **83**: 507–20.
27. Feldman AS. Tympanometry—procedures, interpretation and variables. In: Feldman AS, Wilbur LA, eds. *Acoustic Impedance and Admittance—the Measurement of Middle Ear Function*. Baltimore: Williams and Wilkins, 1976; 103–55.
28. Vanhuyse VJ, Creten WL, Van Camp KJ. On the W-notching of tympanograms. *Scand Audiol* 1975; **4**: 45–50.
29. Wiley TL, Block MG. Overview and basic principles of acoustic immittance measurements. In: Katz J, ed. *Handbook of Clinical Audiology*, 3rd edn. Baltimore: Williams and Wilkins, 1985: 423–37.
30. Mafee MF, Valvassori GE. Radiology of the craniofacial anomalies. *Otolaryngol Clin North Am* 1981; **14**: 939–88.
31. Poswillo PD. The pathogenesis of the Treacher Collins syndrome (mandibulo-facial dysostosis). *Br J Oral Surg* 1975; **13**: 1–26.
32. Konigsmark B, Gorlin RJ. *Genetic and Metabolic Deafness. Apert Syndrome 194*. Philadelphia: WB Saunders Co., 1976.
33. Booth JR. Medical management of sensorineural hearing loss. *J Laryngol Otol* 1982; **96**: 773–95.
34. Bergstrom LA. Osteogenesis imperfecta: otologic and maxillofacial aspects. *Laryngoscope* 1977; **87/9**(2 suppl 6).
35. Balkany TJ, Mischke RE, Downs MP, Jafek BW. Ossicular abnormalities in Down's syndrome. *Otolaryngol Head Neck Surg* 1979; **87:** 372–84.
36. Phelps PD, Coffey RA, Trembath RC et al. Radiological malformations of the ear in Pendred syndrome. *Clin Radiol* 1998; **53:** 268–73.
37. Phelps PD, Roland PE. Thalidomide and cranial nerve abnormalities. *BMJ* 1977; ii: 1672.
38. Phelps PD. Congenital lesions of the inner ear, demonstrated by tomography. *Arch Otolaryngol* 1974; **100:** 11–18.
39. Pagon RA, Graham JM, Zonana J, Young SL. Coloboma, congenital heart disease and choanal atresia with multiple abnormalities. CHARGE association. *J Paediatrics* 1981; **99:** 223–7.
40. Békésy GV. A new audiometer. *Acta Otolaryngol* 1947; **35:** 411–22.
41. Feldman AS. Diagnostic applications and interpretation of tympanometry and the acoustic reflex. *Audiology* 1977; **16:** 294–306.
42. Wright A. Anatomy and development of the ear and hearing. In: Ludman H, Wright A, eds. *Diseases of the Ear*. London: Arnold, 1998: 3–31.

22 Assessment of hearing-impaired children

Agnete Parving

Introduction

Within audiological medicine, hearing impairment (HI) in children is defined as a sign or symptom (in older children) resulting from any damaging factor(s) affecting the hearing organ, in the periphery and/or in the central auditory pathways. This implies that the assessment of the hearing-impaired child consists of two major steps: identification and/or confirmation of the HI, including determination of both the hearing thresholds and the site of the lesion (i.e. classification) by means of current test procedures; and evaluation of the causative factor(s) of the hearing disorder, based on an appropriate protocol with respect to the individual child.[1]

Clinical examination

Before any assessment of the hearing level, a physical examination is necessary, including history-taking (anamnesis) and clinical examination, in this context focusing on the ears, including meticulous otoscopy, and preferably also an examination of the nose and throat. In most cases, a complete physical evaluation is appropriate.

Most parents give highly valuable information on their child concerning the general development and behaviour. In order to obtain relevant specific information concerning a child suspected or detected (by hearing screening) as being hearing impaired, questions should be asked about any hearing-impaired family members and the cause of any identified HI, about delivery and the condition of the child at birth, including progress during the neonatal period. Information on the necessity for admission to a NICU is especially important, and also information on the progress there. The infant/child history should concentrate on: ear diseases, such as otitis media (recurrent, acute, or chronic), previous meningitis, and/or encephalitis, severe head injuries, and completion of any vaccination programme(s); and the child's behaviour and reaction to sounds in daily life, speech and language development, and psychomotor development, with information on important developmental milestones (i.e. sitting, standing, walking, etc.). It should be noted that, in infancy, continuous babbling after the age of 6–8 months is especially important and may preclude the presence of severe/profound hearing loss in an infant. The social situation of the child and information on its daily care (i.e. nursery, kindergarten) is important. In general, the parents should be asked explicitly about the relevant information at the clinical examination, or they should complete a questionnaire before the examination, with the responses confirmed by dialogue at the appointment in the clinic.

> The physical examination should note specific features of the child, such as low-set ears, ear pits and fistulas, cranial morphology and malformations, not only in the head and neck region, but also elsewhere. The otoscopic findings should be noted, and a drawing of the tympanic membrane may give valuable information concerning abnormal findings. In some cases, records on a child from other physicians, e.g. paediatricians, geneticists, ear, nose and throat (ENT) physicians, ophthalmologists, and neurologists, are available, and these should be consulted, as the assessment of the hearing-impaired child often requires an interdisciplinary team approach.

Determination of the hearing level

Psychometric procedures

Until the age of 6 months, formal behavioural testing of a child is so difficult that electrophysiological procedures, such as auditory brainstem evoked response audiometry (ABR), is preferred for threshold determination. Until the child is able to cooperate in pure tone audiometry (at around 3–4 years of age), various types of behavioural audiometry can be performed, indicating HI graded according to various scales, such as mild, moderate, severe, and profound, as shown in Table 22.1.[3] Other descriptors may be used and should be defined, as no uniform worldwide accepted criteria for description of the degree of hearing level exist.

AUDIOMETRIC THRESHOLD TESTS IN CHILDREN

0–6 months	Otoacoustic emissions Auditory brainstem evoked responses
6 months–2/3 years	Behavioural observational audiometry/distraction testing
6 months–3 years	Conditioned orientation reflex audiometry Visual reinformcement audiometry

Objective tests for difficult test children;

- Otoacoustic emissions
- Auditory brainstem responses
- Electrocochleography (rare)

The hearing level can be determined by behavioural observation audiometry (BOA),[4] conditioned orientation reflex audiometry (COR),[5,6] and visual reinforcement audiometry (VRA).[7,8] The BOA includes stimulation with different sound sources, with a more or less well-defined frequency content, and a relatively well-defined stimulus intensity, which may be varied by distance and force applied to provide the sound. In general, the specificity and sensitivity of this testing are poor, with a high proportion (approximately 10%) of false negatives (i.e. false recognition of normal or better hearing) as the worst outcome for the child. However, it should be noted that the sensitivity/specificity is highly dependent on the experience of the tester, and also on the condition of the child. Thus, this testing procedure may offer valuable information on the hearing level in a child who is uncooperative with pure tone audiometry due to age, but in infants suffering from, for example, mental retardation or autistic behaviour, it should be considered highly unreliable.

The distraction test, which was first described by Ewing and Ewing in 1944,[9] is a specific form of BOA, often used by health visitors as a screening test at the age of 6–7 months.[9,10] The distraction test or modifications of the distraction test are widely used also for hearing level assessment in non-cooperative children up to the age of 2–3 years. The COR and VRA are important techniques, resulting in fairly reliable auditory hearing levels between the ages of 6 months and 3 years, with no major differences between the two techniques.[7] The principle in VRA is to visually reward and reinforce a head turn to locate a frequency-specific sound. On turning to locate the sound source, the child receives a visual reward, e.g. light on a toy. This principle has recently been used for hearing threshold determination in infants, giving reliable air and bone conduction thresholds.[11]

The final assessment of hearing ability in children depends on the psychoacoustical determination of hearing thresholds by means of pure tone audiometry. From the ages of 2–3 years up to 6 years, pure tone auditory thresholds for at least three frequencies may be obtained by play-conditioning techniques. These comprise a variety of motivational games, ranging from peep shows through ring-towers to finger-raising techniques.[12]

It is well known that the behavioural thresholds improve in children with increasing age, and it has been argued that younger children have poorer auditory sensitivity than older children. However, several explanations for the apparent age-related differences in auditory sensitivity may be considered: difficulties in concentrating; learning effects; poor fitting of ear-

Table 22.1 Hearing impairment graded according to various scales (descriptors) such as mild, moderate, severe and profound HI according to the HEAR Project and WHO

HEAR[2]		WHO[3]	
Grade of impairment	Hearing level (dB HL)[a]	Grade of impairment	Hearing level (dB HL)[a]
Normal	<20	None	≤25
Mild	20–39	Slight	26–40
Moderate	40–69	Moderate	41–60
Severe	70–94	Severe	61–80
Profound	≥95	Profound	≥81

[a] Better ear pure tone average across the frequencies 0.5, 1, 2 and 4 kHz.

phones; middle ear effusion in younger children; varying test procedures for threshold determination with poor test–retest reliability; and a true difference in auditory sensitivity as a function of age, owing to developmental changes. Moreover, a trend towards better mean auditory thresholds and less variation in thresholds has been reported in girls, which may be ascribed to an earlier maturation of the auditory system in females. In contrast, tests on normal children, in whom thresholds were obtained by a forced choice adaptive procedure, revealed no systematic differences in thresholds as a function of age, and no significant differences from thresholds in adults were present.[13] From studies using electrocochleography (ECoG) for hearing threshold determination where the true cochlear sensitivity is assessed, only minor differences between the psychoacoustical hearing threshold and the threshold obtained by ECoG have been found.[1,14]

Thus it can be stated that hearing thresholds in young children depend on the measurement procedure, and, if this is optimal, the thresholds indicate the true hearing sensitivity.

In uncooperative children, various electrophysiological methods can be used for hearing threshold determination. Among these techniques, ABR is usually preferred, due to its non-invasive nature, and a high hearing threshold diagnostic sensitivity/specificity. In addition, the method can be used for the evaluation of paediatric neurological disorders, but, due to abnormalities in the EEG caused by the neurological disease, hearing threshold identification by ABR may be difficult or impossible. In such children, otoacoustical emissions (OAEs) may be helpful in the identification of a hearing level/threshold. At present, OAEs are predominantly used for neonatal hearing screening. However, it may be expected that the recording of both transient and distortion product OAEs will be more frequently implemented as a test procedure for hearing sensitivity in the clinic, as OAEs are useful in the confirmation and classification of HI, not least in combination with ABR[15,16] (see Chapters 15 and 16).

> Besides determination of hearing thresholds, assessment of speech recognition in children is important.

Procedures independent of speech and language production ability have been developed, whereby the perception of specific speech features in both normally hearing and hearing-impaired infants can be discriminated.[17,18] Some tests—or modifications of tests—use target words or real objects to measure speech recognition in 2–4-year-old children;[19–21] in older children, word recognition tests or word recognition scores as part of a play situation can be used.[21] In general, the older the child, the better is the opportunity to perform speech recognition tasks, giving important information on the hearing capacity and also having the potential to distinguish between peripheral and central auditory disorders.

Classification of the hearing loss, i.e. topical site of lesion

In combination with otoscopy, impedance audiometry indicating middle ear pressure and compliance is essential in children showing a high prevalence of recurrent or chronic otitis media with effusion (OME), at least under the age of 5.[22] The method has a diagnostic sensitivity/specificity of >90%, which is even higher in combination with tympanic membrane movement examination. The HI diagnosed in OME is typically moderate and conductive, and may in chronic or recurrent OME result in adverse effects on speech and language development.[23,24] In children with an existing permanent HI, OME may cause further deterioration in hearing sensitivity, a condition that should be treated vigorously.

Recording of stapedial reflexes, ipsi- and/or contralateral thresholds, gives important information in relation to the classification of an HI in children, and the interpretation and diagnostic validity are similar to the findings in adults (see Chapter 14). It should, however, be noted that impedance audiometry is dependent on the cooperation of the child, and thus may be difficult or impossible to perform in young children and infants.

Valuable information on the site-of-lesion diagnosis may be obtained by electrophysiological procedures (Chapter 16). Besides threshold determination, ECoG gives information on a conductive component by a parallel shift in the input/output latency function and may also differentiate between a pre- or postsynaptic lesion.[25] As ABR is a non-invasive technique, which also offers a differentiation between conductive, sensorineural and mixed hearing loss in children, this recording method is preferable and will, in combination with the recording of evoked otoacoustic emissions, indicate a cochlear or retrocochlear lesion. Recordings of longer-latency responses are necessary when non-organic or central auditory lesions in children are suspected (see Chapter 16).

Additional tests for site of lesion diagnostic purposes are available, and can be performed in children as well as in adults. However, the majority of auditory testing requires some cooperation by the subject which, in children, results in limitations.

Vestibular investigation

Owing to the close anatomical relationship between the cochlea and the vestibular system, hearing-impaired children should undergo vestibular examination, including caloric testing. However, the majority of young children (i.e. ≤4 years of age) cannot cooperate with a caloric test, but questions (preferably to the mother) concerning milestones for sitting, standing and walking give essential information on the vestibular system in a young child. About 30% of hearing-impaired children are clumsy and uncoordinated, which points towards involvement of also the vestibular system, giving important information on the aetiology of the hearing disorder. In older children complete vestibular testing, based on an appropriate test protocol, can be performed.[26]

Assessment of the causative factor(s)

Whenever the identification and classification of HI in a child has been established, efforts should be directed towards finding the causative factor(s). This challenge demands interdisciplinary cooperation, on the basis of which valuable information can be offered to the physician who is in charge of the surveillance programme of the hearing-impaired child, e.g. an audiological physician, paediatrician, ENT physician, or other clinician, depending on the variety of paediatric hearing services available throughout the world. It should be mentioned that although audiological methods may be insufficient for an aetiological diagnosis, they provide supplementary information, both because of their potential to establish the site of the lesion, and because of specific patterns relating to the cause(s) of the HI.[1,27]

The aetiological evaluation of a hearing-impaired child is an ongoing process, and should be based on a protocol performed systematically (Table 22.2). As the aetiology of HI in childhood may differ as a function of country or local area,[28] the protocol for aetiological evaluation should reflect the causative factors in the specific geographical region. Although no regional surveys directed towards the aetiological evaluation have been performed, numerous data on the aetiology of hearing disorders in children have been reported from various countries and areas within the last 20 years.[27,29–43] In Table 22.3, the proportions of various factors causing permanent HI in some cohort studies are shown. It should be noted that the proportions indicated represent different cohorts, varying hearing level definitions, and some uncertainties in the categories as the various authors use different categorization systems.

Table 22.2 Protocol for routine diagnostic evaluation

1. Thorough clinical examination
2. Hearing threshold determination (including parents, siblings)
3. Classification of the HI (i.e. site of lesion)
4. Vestibular testing
5. Ophthalmological assessment
6. CT/MRI scanning
7. Blood testing: e.g
   Viral antibodies (rubella, CMV, HIV and others)
   Bacterial antibodies (syphilis, toxoplasmosis, others)
   Thyroid function (T3, T4, thyroid-stimulating hormone, others)
   Cytogenetic testing (chromosomal abnormalities)
8. Urine analysis
9. Electrocardiogram
10. Mutation analysis in connexin 26

Specific tests:
Perchlorate discharge test

Thus, it is important to understand that major differences in the inclusion criteria, definition of samples, age of the children, and definition of hearing levels are often present in studies concerning the aetiology of permanent HI in children, and preclude comparative analyses and aggregation of data. However, it can adequately be stated that in children with permanent HI, inheritance comprises the major proportion (about 50%), and that this nosology should be further subdivided into non-syndromal and syndromal genetic HI, and described according to the mode of transmission of the mutant gene in question (i.e. autosomal dominant/recessive, X-linked or mitochondrial).[44] A varying proportion of 18–41% of unknown cause is also indicated in the various samples (Table 22.2), reflecting important quality aspects of the available services and surveillance programmes offered.[28] The rapid development within the field of molecular genetics may, in the future, provide clinicians with additional valuable information, which will probably result in a reduction of the proportion of unknown cause and in improved counselling and, thus, in prevention of genetic HI.[45]

In surveillance programmes, a constant clinical awareness of the factor(s) causing a HI may yield additional or new information on diseases causing HI in children. Through such awareness, a relationship between fetal infections and congenital HI has been demonstrated (see below), and a relationship between HI and fetal alcohol syndrome has been reported.[46] The ototoxic and teratogenic effects of drugs have long been established,[47–49] and noise exposure even from infant toys[50] or from the general environment may represent a hazard to the hearing of children. In fact, fetal noise exposure has been suggested as a causative factor,[51] however, the supportive evidence is scarce and fairly speculative.

Some causes of HI relating to specific examination procedures, which should be part of a protocol, are mentioned below.

HI caused by fetal infections

Since 1944, fetal rubella infection has been recognized as a causative factor in congenital HI,[52,53] and the risk of defects has been demonstrated to be very high, predominantly affecting the eyes, ears, and heart.[54] Among samples of hearing-impaired children, it has previously been estimated that approximately 15–30% of cases can be ascribed to fetal rubella infection,[27,55–57] and a reduction in the proportion of children with congenital HI has been found after introduction of rubella vaccination (Table 22.2).[58,59] In countries where rubella vaccination does not form part of the child health surveillance programme fetal rubella infection still results in a high proportion of congenital HI.[60] The causative diagnosis may be obtained from additional information in the clinical record, but ultimately depends on the demonstration of IgM or IgG rubella antibodies (before 6 months of age). However, as IgG rubella antibodies are present in approximately 5–10% of children aged 6 months to 4 years, due to postnatal infection,[61] the detection of IgG rubella antibodies in the individual child cannot be conclusive, but may be

Table 22.3 Proportion of some factors causing permanent HI in children reported in various cohort studies

	Parving[27] 1993 (%)	France and Stephens[29] 1995 (%)	Fortnum and Davis[39] 1997 (%)	Mäki-Torkko et al[41] 1998 (%)	Billings and Kenna[42] 1999 (%)
Inheritance	46	50	40	46	25
Fetal infections	5	3	3	0.9	1.4
Craniofacial malformations	3	–	1	6	–
Perinatal complications	9	1	7	8	19
Meningitis/encephalitis	3	8	5	0.9	6
Chronic otitis media	12	2	1	–	24
Ototoxic drugs	–	–	–	0.9	–
Trauma	–	–	–	–	–
Various	–	–	2	–	–
Unknown cause	20	31	41	38	25

used to estimate a retrospective diagnosis. Thus, serological testing indicating the presence of rubella antibodies may support a diagnosis of HI caused by congenital rubella.[62]

Another important viral fetal infection causing congenital HI is cytomegalovirus (CMV) infection.[63–65] The diagnosis of congenital CMV infection cannot be made on clinical grounds alone, and must be based on isolation of the virus from fresh urine or tissue during the first week of life, with a variety of serological tests available to detect CMV and thus document the presence of the infection. It is likely that many cases of congenital HI due to CMV infection remain undiagnosed, due to the limited period during which a proper diagnosis can be made.[63] However, the potential to establish CMV as the causative factor of HI may be improved by the introduction of universal neonatal hearing screening.

A causal relationship between fetal infection with human immunodeficiency virus (HIV) and HI may exist, and as the virus is neurotropic, a central auditory dysfunction may be the result.[66–68] In this context, it should also be mentioned that a permanent HI in HIV-infected subjects may be caused by other infectious agents or by sequelae of encephalitis/meningitis.

Apart from viral infections, other infections, e.g. toxoplasmosis and syphilis, may cause congenital HI, and when these infections are suspected, appropriate serological testing should take place.[49]

Ophthalmological investigation

In the individual child, the detection of rubella antibodies may support the diagnosis of rubella embryopathy, but supplementary diagnostic information should be obtained by ophthalmological examination. Thereby, the visual acuity can be assessed, which is of utmost importance for the further rehabilitation and training of a hearing-impaired child. The most frequent ophthalmological manifestation of fetal rubella infection—and many other fetal infections—is retinopathy, which occurs with an incidence of 20–50%. The retinal changes are characteristically located in the macular area or fundus periphery, mainly taking the form of a fine or coarse pepper and salt configuration. The retinal changes are highly specific for fetal viral infections and are not seen in normal children. It should be noted that the retinal changes found in rubella embryopathy should be distinguished from retinitis pigmentosa developing as part of Usher's syndrome.

> Ophthalmological examination should be part of a routine evaluation protocol in hearing-impaired children, because it offers important information on the visual acuity and on the differential diagnosis of a large number of syndromes which involve both the aural and visual systems.[69]

Genetic factors

In children with congenital or acquired HI, genetic factors are most prevalent (Table 22.2). Although a thorough family history may raise suspicion of a genetic factor causing the HI, the protocol directed towards aetiological assessment should also include audiometric testing of the parents/siblings and, if possible, of other family members. In autosomal dominant inheritance, traditional audiometry is often sufficient; however, a carrier state in recessive inherited HI may be revealed only by specific test procedures.

Thus, unusual dips in the threshold tracings have been demonstrated in Békésy audiograms from heterozygote carriers of recessive deafness, and in addition elevated acoustical reflex thresholds have been found.[70,71] However, the sensitivity of the method is poor in relation to the identification of carriers of genetic HI,[72,73] but more recent studies based on the Audio scan have shown a higher reliability,[74–76] and the method may prove useful in appropriate samples. In addition, heterozygote carriers may be revealed by the recording of distortion product otoacoustical emissions, having a significantly lower amplitude than in controls.[77,78] In combination with DNA analysis, various mutations in carriers may be identified, and the assessment of recessive non-syndromal inherited HI in children be improved. Thus, mutations in the gene (*GJB2*) encoding the connexin 26 molecule, which is a component of gap junctions, i.e. links allowing small molecules to pass between cells, have been found in non-syndromal recessive inherited HI[79–83] and been reported with a high prevalence of 0.58–4.03% in various populations.[82] In this context, it should be mentioned that connexin 26 has also been linked to dominantly inherited HI.[84]

Thus, a combination of acoustic carrier testing and developments within molecular genetics, with the identification of gene loci, positional cloning, and assessment of the biological function of the mutant gene, may in the future improve the assessment of inherited HI in children.

Imaging of the inner ear

Modern imaging techniques offer valuable information concerning malformations of the inner ear in hearing-impaired children.[85] (See Chapter 6) Although a malformation of the inner ear does not allow assessment of the aetiology, it should form part of the evaluation protocol, as it offers supplementary information. It is, however, important to inform both the child and the parents that the imaging of the inner ears cannot cure or improve the HI, which is sometimes anticipated, due to the radiation.

Table 22.2 lists the minimum requirements for a routine diagnostic evaluation of a hearing-impaired child. In this context, it should be emphasized that no false expectations concerning improvements in a permanent HI should emerge from the evaluation protocol in any of the examined subjects or the family. Specific tests, such as the perchlorate discharge test, should be performed when suspicion of Pendred syndrome is raised, and testing for mutations in connexin 26 should be performed routinely as part of an aetiological assesment.

Concluding comments

The assessment of a hearing-impaired child is a long-term, ongoing process, which should be performed as part of a surveillance program. Audiological as well as non-audiological test procedures are of importance for the aetiological diagnostic evaluation. An examination protocol should be performed, appropriately tailored to the individual child, and can only be realized by means of broad interdisciplinary cooperation, preferably established as diagnostic assessment teams. By these means the aetiology of HI in the individual child can be identified, also providing precise epidemiological data on the distribution of various aetiological categories of HI in well-defined samples. Thereby, primary prevention of permanent HI in children can be achieved, which is the ultimate goal of the assessment of the hearing-impaired child.

References

1. Parving A. Hearing disorders in childhood, some procedures for detection, identification and diagnostic evaluation. *Int J Pediatr Otorhinol* 1985; **9**: 31–57.
2. Luxon L, Moller C. HEAR: European workgroup on genetics of hearing impairment. *Infoletter* 1996; **2**: November.
3. WHO International classification of impairments, disabilities, and handicaps. Geneva: World Health Organization; 1980.
4. Thompson G, Weber BA. Responses of infants and young children to behavioural observation audiometry (BOA). *J Speech Disord* 1974; **39**: 140–7.
5. Suzuki T, Ogiba Y. Conditioned orientation reflex audiometry. A new technique for pure tone audiometry in young children under 3 years of age. *Arch Otolaryngol* 1961; **84**: 84–90.
6. Johansson RK, Salmivalli A. Arousing effect of sounds for testing infants' hearing ability. *Audiology* 1983; **22**: 417–20.
7. Liden G, Kankkunen A. Visual reinforcement audiometry. *Acta Otolaryngol* 1969; **67**: 281–92.
8. Widen JE, Folsom RC, Cone-Wesson B, Carty L, Dunnell JJ, Koebsell K, Levi A, Mancl L, Ohlrich B, Trouba S, et al. Identification of neonatal hearing impairment: Hearing status at 8 to 12 months corrected age using a visual reinforcement audiometry protocol. *Ear & Hear* 2000; **21**: 471–85.
9. Ewing IR, Ewing AWG. The ascertainment of deafness in infancy and early childhood. *J Laryngol Otol* 1944; **59**: 309–38.
10. McCormick B. *The Medical Practitioner's Guide to Paediatric Audiology*. Cambridge: Cambridge University Press, 1995.
11. Gravel JS, Traquina DN. Experience with the audiologic assessment of infants and toddlers. *Int J Pediatr Otorhinolaryngol* 1992; **23**: 59–71.
12. Hodgson WR. Evaluation of infants and young children. In: Katz DR, ed. *Handbook of Clinical Audiology*, 4th edn. Baltimore: Williams & Wilkins, 1994: 465–76.
13. Yost AW. A forced-choice adaptive procedure for measuring auditory thresholds in children. *Behav Res Meth Instrument* 1978; **10**: 671–7.
14. Parving A, Elberling C, Salomon G. ECoG and psychoacoustic tests compared in identification of hearing loss in young children. *Audiology* 1981; **20**: 365–81.
15. Bonfils P, Uziel A. Clinical applications of evoked acoustic emissions: results in normally hearing and hearing-impaired subjects. *Ann Otol Rhinol Laryngol* 1989; **98**: 326–31.

16. Sun X-M, Jung MD, Kim DO, Randolph KJ. Distortion product otoacoustic emission test of sensorineural hearing loss in humans: comparison of unequal- and equal-level stimuli. *Ann Otol Rhinol Laryngol* 1996; **105**: 982–90.
17. Kuhl PK. Perceptual constancy for speech sound categories in early infancy. In: Yeni-Komshian G, Kavanagh J, Fergusson C, eds. *Child Phonology: Perception and Production*. New York: Academic Press, 1980: 41–66.
18. Kuhl PK, Williams KA, Lacerda F, Stevens KN, Lindblom B. Linguistic experience alters phonetic perception in infants by six months of age. *Science* 1992; **255**: 606–8.
19. Dawson PW, Nott PE, Clark GM, Cowan RSC. A modification of play audiometry to assess speech discrimination ability in severe to profoundly deaf 2–4 year old children. *Ear Hear* 1998; **19**: 371–84.
20. Osberger MJ, Miyamoto RT, Zimmerman-Phillips S et al. Independent evaluation with speech perception abilities of children with a Nucleus 22 channel cochlear implant system. *Ear Hear* 1991; **12**(suppl): 66–84.
21. Robbins AM, Kirk KI. Speech perception assessment and performance in paediatric cochlear implant users. Semin Hear 1996; **17**: 353–66.
22. Bluestone CD. Epidemiology and pathogenesis of chronic suppurative otitis media: implications for prevention and treatment. *Int J Pediatr Otorhinolaryngol* 1998; **42**: 207–33.
23. Chalmers D, Stewart E, Silva P, Mulvena A. Otitis media with effusion in children—the Dunedin Study. *Clin Dev Med* 1989; **108**: 1–108.
24. Gravel JS, Wallace IF, Ruben RJ. Auditory consequences of early mild hearing loss associated with otitis media. *Acta Otolaryngol* (Stockh) 1996; **116**: 219–21.
25. Salomon G, Elberling C. Estimation of inner ear function and conductive hearing loss based on electrocochleography. *Adv Audiol* 1989; **5**: 46–55.
26. Luxon L, Moller C. HEAR: European workgroup on genetics of hearing impairment. Infoletter. 1996.
27. Parving A. Hearing disability in childhood—a cross-sectional and longitudinal investigation of causative factors. *Int J Pediatr Otorhinolaryngol* 1993; **27**: 101–11.
28. Parving A. Factors causing hearing impairment: some perspectives from Europe. *J Am Acad Audiol* 1995; **6**: 387–95.
29. France EA, Stephens SDG. All Wales audiology and genetic service for hearing impaired young adults. *J Audiol Med* 1995; **4**: 67–84.
30. Parving A, France EA, Stephens SDG. Factors causing hearing impairment in identical birth-cohorts in Denmark and Wales. *J Audiol Med* 1996; **5**:67–72.
31. Kankkunen A. Pre-school children with impaired hearing. *Acta Otolaryngol* 1982; **391**(suppl): 59–99.
32. Newton WE. Aetiology of bilateral sensorineural hearing loss in young children. *J Otolaryngol* 1985; **10**(suppl): 1–57.
33. Hirsch A. Hearing loss and associated handicaps in pre-school children. *Scand Audiol* 1988; **30**: 61–4.
34. Lenzi A, Zaghis A. Incidence of genetic factors in the causation of deafness in childhood. *Scand Audiol* 1988; **30**: 37–41.
35. Davidson J, Hyde ML, Alberti PW. Epidemiology of hearing impairment in childhood. *Scand Audiol* 1988; **30**(suppl): 13–20.
36. Dias O, Andrea M. Childhood deafness in Portugal—aetiological factors and diagnosis of hearing loss. *Int J Pediatr Otorhinolaryngol* 1990; **18**: 247–55.
37. van Rijn PM, Cremers CWRJ. Causes of childhood deafness at a Dutch school for the hearing impaired. *Ann Otol Rhinol Laryngol* 1991; **100**: 903–8.
38. Vanniasegaram I, Tungland OP, Bellmann S. A five year review of children with deafness in a multi-ethnic community. *J Audiol Med* 1993; **2**: 9–19.
39. Fortnum H, Davis A. Epidemiology of permanent childhood hearing impairment in Trent Region 1985–1993. *Br J Audiol* 1997; **31**:409–46.
40. McPherson B, Swart SM. Childhood hearing loss in sub-Saharan Africa: a review and recommendations. *J Pediatr Otorhinol* 1997; **40**:1–18.
41. Mäki-Torkko EM, Lindholm PK, Väyrynen MRH, Leisti JT, Sorri MJ. Epidemiology of moderate to profound childhood hearing impairments in northern Finland. Any changes in ten years? Scand Audiol 1998; **27**: 95–103.
42. Billings KR, Kenna MA. Causes of pediatric sensorineural hearing loss. *Arch Otolaryngol Head Neck Surg* 1999; **125**: 517–21.
43. Streppel M, Richling F, Roth B, Walger M, von Wedel H, Echel E. Epidemiology and aetiology of acquired hearing disorders in childhood in the Cologne area. *J Pediatr Otorhinol* 1998; **44**: 235–43.
44. Parving A, Newton V. Guidelines for description of inherited hearing loss. *J Audiol Med* 1995; **2**: ii–v.
45. Resendes BL, Williamson RE, Morton CC. Review article: At the speed of sound: gene discovery in the auditory system. *Am J Hum Genet* 2001; **69**: 923–35.
46. Church MW, Gerkin KP. Hearing disorders in children with foetal alcohol syndrome: findings from case reports. *Paediatrics* 1988; **82/2**: 147–54.
47. Barr B. Teratogenic hearing loss. *Audiology* 1982; **21**: 111–17.
48. Gerber SE, Epstein L, Mencher L. Recent changes in the aetiology of hearing disorders: perinatal drug exposure. *J Am Acad Audiol* 1995; **6**: 371–7.
49. Strasnick B, Jacobson JT. Teratogenic hearing loss. *J Am Acad Audiol* 1995; **6**: 28–38.
50. Jerger J. Hazardous toys. *J Am Acad Audiol* 1994; **5**: 76.
51. Lalande NM, Hétu R, Lampers J. Is occupational noise exposure during pregnancy a risk factor of damage to the auditory system of the foetus? *Am J Ind Med* 1986; **10**: 427–35.
52. Swan C, Torstevin AL, Moore B, Maj H, Black GHB. Congenital defects in infants following infectious diseases during pregnancy. *Med J Austr* 1943; **2**: 201–10.
53. Gregg NMA. Further observations on congenital defects in infants following maternal rubella. *Trans Ophthal Soc Aust* 1944; **4**: 119–31.
54. Miller GW, Cradock-Watson JE, Pollock TM. Consequences of confirmed maternal rubella at successive stages of pregnancy. *Lancet* 1982; **1**: 781–4.
55. Barr B. Early identification of hearing impairment. In: Taylor IG, Markides A, eds. *Disorders of Auditory Function*, III. London: Academic Press, 1980: 33–42.

56. Martin JAM, Bentzen O, Colley JRT et al. Childhood deafness in the European community. *Scand Audiol* 1981; **10**: 165–74.
57. Taylor IG. The prevention of congenital sensorineural deafness. In: Taylor IG, Markiedes A, eds. *Disorders of auditory function*, III. London: Academic Press, 1980: 25–31.
58. Upfold LJ. Children with hearing AIDS in the 1980s: aetiologies and severity of impairment. *Ear Hear* 1988; **9/2**: 75–80.
59. Davis A, Wood S, Healy R, Webb H, Rowe S. Risk factors for hearing disorders: Epidemiological evidence of change over time in the UK. *J Am Acad Audiol* 1995; **6**: 365–70.
60. Prasansuk S. Incidence/prevalence of sensorineural hearing impairment in Thailand and South East Asia. *Audiology* 2000; **39**: 207–11.
61. Peckham GS, Martin JAM, Marshall WS, Dudgeon JA. Congenital rubella deafness: a preventable disease. *Lancet* 1979; **1**: 258–61.
62. Parving A, Vejtorp M, Møller K, Jensen JH. Congenital hearing loss and rubella infection. *Acta Otolaryngol* 1980; **90**: 262–6.
63. Reynolds DW, Stagno S, Stubbs KG et al. Inapparent congenital cytomegalovirus infection with elevated cord IgM levels. Cause and relationship with auditory and mental deficiency. *N Engl J Med* 1974; **290**: 291–6.
64. Stagno S, Reynolds DW, Ana CS, Darle AJ. Auditory and visual defects resulting from symptomatic and sub-clinical congenital cytomegalovirus and toxoplasmal infections. *Pediatrics* 1977; **59**: 669–77.
65. Dahle AJ, Fowler KB, Wright JD, Boppana SB, Britt WJ, Pass RF. Longitudinal investigation of hearing disorders in children with congenital cytomegalovirus. *J Am Acad Audiol* 2000; **11**: 283–90.
66. Real R, Thomas M, Gerwins JM. Sudden hearing loss and acquired immunodeficiency syndrome. *Otolaryngol Head Neck Surg* 1987; **97**: 409–12.
67. Birchall MA, White RG, French PD, Cockbanes Z, Smith SJM. Auditory function in patients infected with the human immunodeficiency virus. *Clin Otolaryngol* 1992; **17**: 117–21.
68. Madriz JJ, Herrera G. Human immune deficiency virus and acquired immune deficiency syndrome age related hearing disorders. *J Am Acad Audiol* 1995; **6**: 358–64.
69. Gorlin RJ. Genetic hearing loss with no associated abnormalities. In Gorlin RJ, Toriello HV, Cohen MM, eds. *Hereditary Hearing Loss and its Syndromes*. New York: Oxford University Press, 1995; pp. 43–61.
70. Andersen H, Wedenberg E. Audiometric identification of normal hearing carriers of genes for deafness. *Acta Otolaryngol* 1968; **65**: 535–54.
71. Andersen H, Wedenberg E. Identification of normal hearing carriers of genes for deafness. *Acta Otolaryngol* 1976; **82**: 245–8.
72. Parving A. Reliability of Békèsy threshold tracing in identification of carriers of genes for an X-linked disease with deafness. *Acta Otolaryngol* 1978; **85**: 40–4.
73. Parving A, Schwartz M. Audiometric tests in gene carriers of Norrie's disease. *Int J Pediatr Otorhinolaryngol* 1991; **21**: 103–11.
74. Meredith R, Stephens D, Sirimanna T, Meyer-Bisch C, Reardon W. Audiometric detection of carriers of Usher's syndrome type II. *J Audiol Med* 1992; **1**: 11–19.
75. Meyer-Bisch C. Audioscan: a high-definition audiometry technique based on constant-level frequency sweeps—a new method with new hearing indicators. *Audiology* 1996; **35**: 63–72.
76. Laroche C, Hétu R. A study of the reliability of automatic audiometry by the frequency scanning method (Audioscan). *Audiology* 1997; **36**: 1–18.
77. Cohen M, Francis M, Coffey R, Pembrey ME, Luxon LM. Abnormal audiograms and elevated acoustic reflex thresholds in obligate carriers of autosomal recessive non-syndromic hearing loss. *Acta Otolaryngol* 1997; **117**: 337–42.
78. Liu XZ, Newton VE. Distortion product emissions in normal-hearing and low-frequency hearing loss carriers of genes for Waardenburg's syndrome. *Ann Otol Rhinol Laryngol* 1997; **106**: 220–5.
79. Morrell RJ, Kim HJ, Hood LJ et al. Mutations in the Connexin 26 gene (GJB2) among ashkenazi jews with nonsyndromic recessive deafness. *N Engl J Med* 1998; **359**: 1500–5.
80. Kelsell DP, Ldunlop J, Stevens HP et al. Connexin 26 mutations in hereditary non-syndromic sensorineural deafness. *Nature* 1997; **387**: 80–3.
81. Zelante L, Gasparini P, Estivill X et al. Connexin 26 mutations associated with the most common form of a non-syndromic neurosensory autosomal recessive deafness (DFNB1) in Mediterraneans. *Hum Mol Genet* 1997; **6**: 1605–9.
82. Kenna MA, Wu B-L, Cotanche DA, Korf BR, Rehm HL. Connexin 26 studies in patients with sensorineural hearing loss. *Arch Otolaryngol Head Neck Surg* 2001; **127**: 1037–42.
83. Estivill X, Foritna P, Surrey S et al. Connexin 26 mutations in sporadic and inherited sensorineural deafness. *Lancet* 1998; **351**: 394–8.
84. Denoyelle F, Lina-Granade G, Plauchu H et al. Connexin 26 gene linked to a dominant deafness. *Nature* 1998; **393**: 319–20.
85. Harcourt JP, Lennox P, Phips PD, Brooks GB. CT-screening for temporal bone abnormalities in idiopathic bilateral sensorineural hearing loss. *J Laryngol Otol* 1997; **111**: 117–21.

23 Otitis media with effusion in children (Glue ear)

Ewa Raglan

Introduction

Otitis media with effusion (OME) is a very common recurrent condition in children, being most prevalent in children below the age of 2 years, and becoming less frequent and of shorter duration with increasing age.[1] It frequently follows an episode of acute otitis media (AOM) or an upper respiratory tract infection. The duration of the effusion varies, but it resolves spontaneously in most children. In 40–56% of children, resolution occurs within 2 weeks,[2] in 60–94% it will resolve within 3 months,[3–5] but in approximately 10% it persists for more than one year.[6] There is some evidence that the duration of OME effusion may be longer in younger children.[7]

Cases of OME peak around the age of 2 and 5 years and they occur most commonly in winter, with the lowest prevalence in summer.[3, 8]

Figure 23.1 shows the combined results of the prevalence of OME with 95% confidence limits in selected studies.[9] Around the age of 2 years the prevalence is about 20%, then it falls off to peak again to about 15% at the age of 5, the age of school entry, when there is more contact with other children.

There are a number of reasons including anatomical, functional (position of Eustachian tube impeding drainage of middle ear effusion (MEE) caused by inflammation)[10,11] and immunological factors (development of protective antibodies to invading bacteria),[12] for the increased prevalence of OME below 2 years of age. In some young infants, OME may be asymptomatic.[2]

Children who suffer a first episode of AOM at an early age are at a much greater risk of developing chronic OME.[2,13]

The early onset of OME is related to the early onset of AOM, which, in turn, may be the result of a combination of an innate predisposition (differences in anatomy/function of Eustachian tube) and decreased ability to produce antibodies against common bacterial/viral pathogens. The latter factor is associated with specific risk factors, including a shorter duration of breast feeding,[14] feeding in a supine position,[15] Owen et al,[16] and attendance at a nursery, with increased exposure to various upper respiratory tract pathogens.[17,18]

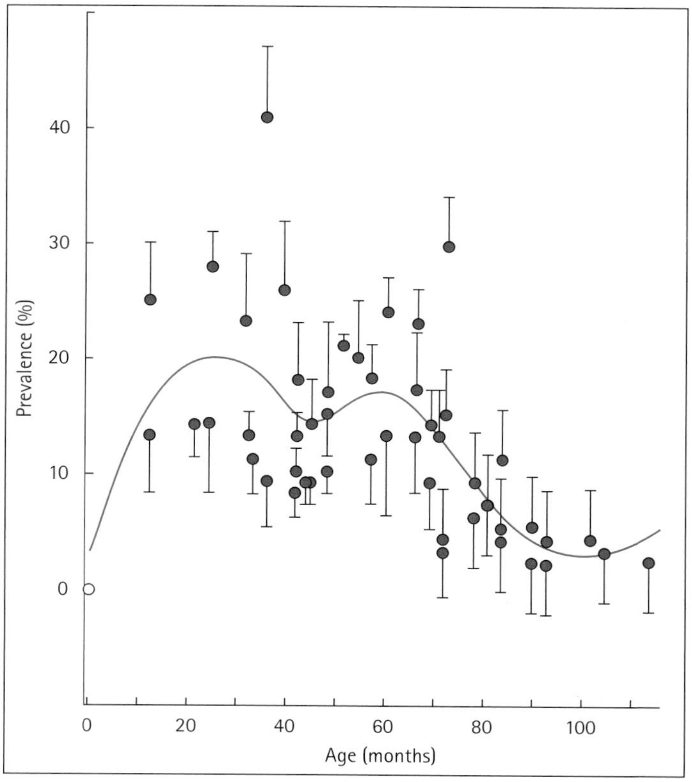

Figure 23.1 Combined results of selected studies on the prevalence of OME with 95% confidence limit. (From Zielhuis et al. *Clin Otolaryngol* 1990; **15**: 283–8.[9])

Diagnosis

Otitis media reflects inflammation of the middle ear system. The terminology of the condition has been defined by the 4th Research Conference on Recent Advances in Otitis Media,[19] and clinical criteria are used as the basis for classification.

TYPES OF OTITIS MEDIA

- Acute suppurative otitis media.
- Otitis media with effusion.
- Chronic suppurative otitis media.

Acute suppurative otitis media (AOM)

This condition presents as sudden, short infection of the middle ear, characterized by otalgia, hearing impairment and an opaque, red, pink or yellow looking drum, which is often bulging. The child may, additionally, have non-specific symptoms such as irritability, headache, apathy, anorexia, vomiting, diarrhoea and fever. The typical otoscopic picture (Figure 23.2)[20] and poor drum mobility on tympanometry will reveal the diagnosis.

Otitis media with effusion (OME)

This condition is characterized by the presence of an effusion in the middle ear cleft, which may be asymptomatic or, if the condition becomes chronic, may present with a hearing impairment or secondary sequelae such as tinnitus, dizziness, imbalance, speech, language and developmental delay or behavioural problems. The tympanic membrane may be opaque and

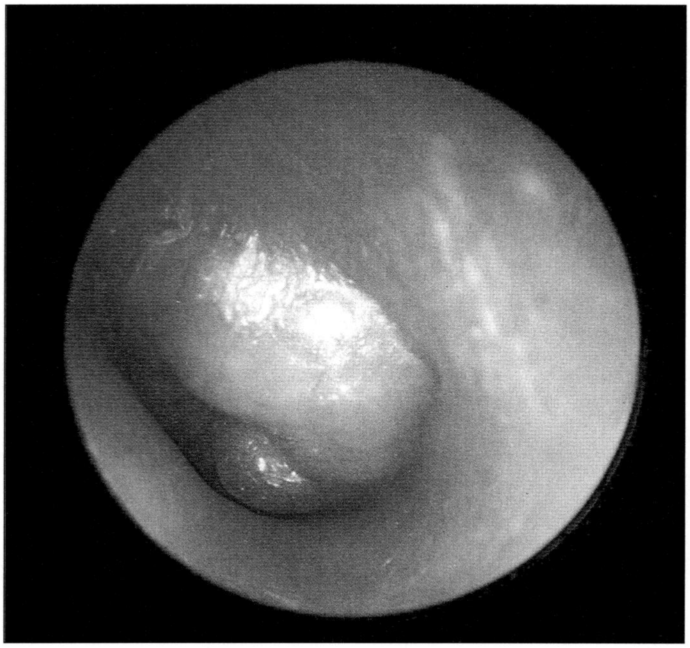

Figure 23.2 Acute otitis media. There is redness of the drum and, laterally, a bulging large segment of the drum, filled with mucopurulent exudates. (From Hawke and McCombe. *Diseases of the Ear Pocket Atlas*. Austin TX: Manticore Communications Inc, 1995.[20])

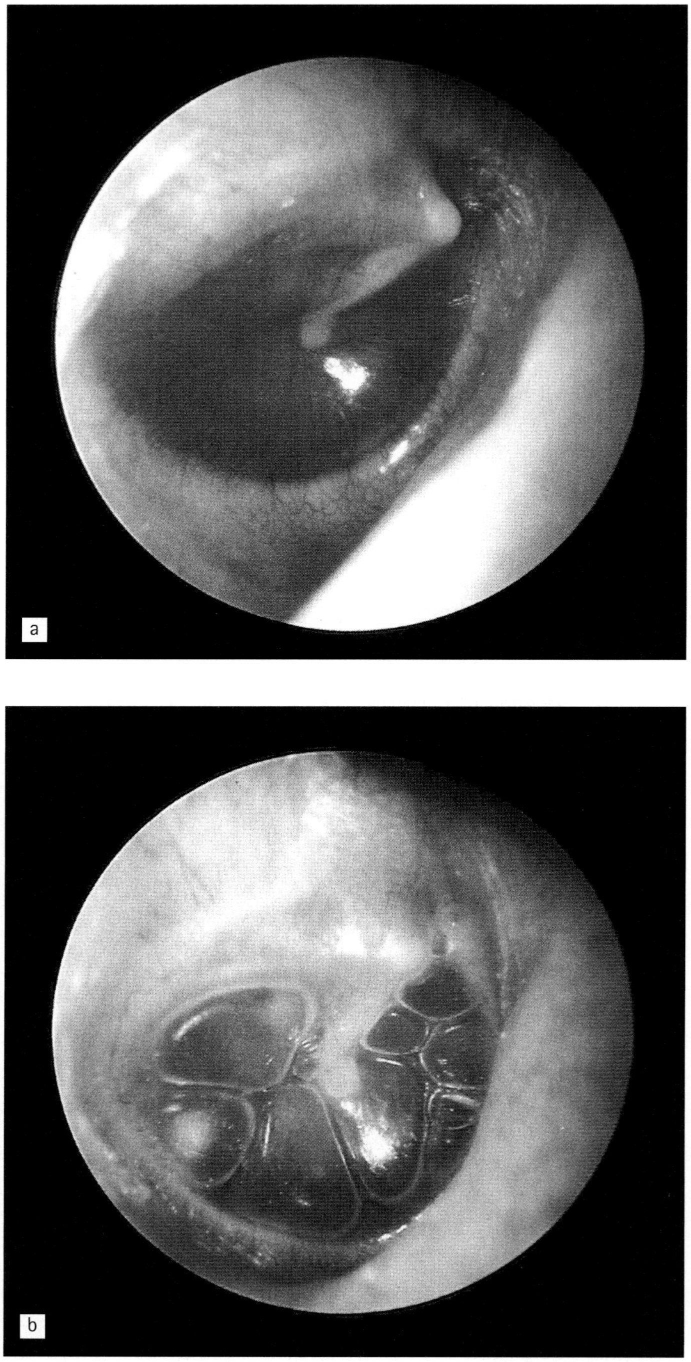

Figure 23.3 Secretory otitis media (a) with effusion (Glue ear). Dull appearance of the tympanic membrane, indicative of the presence of fluid in the middle ear, retraction of the drum is shown by a more horizontal position of the handle of the malleus. (b) Presence of serous fluid in the ear. (From Hawke and McCombe. *Diseases of the Ear Pocket Atlas*. Austin TX: Manticore Communications Inc, 1995.[20])

retracted, with reduced mobility, or the presence of fluid bubbles, behind the drum (Figure 23.3a,b),[20] may be observed. The effusion may be serous or mucoid (thick and sticky and referred to as 'glue ear') or a combination of both.[21,22] The distinction between acute and chronic is based on the duration of the effusion: less than 3 months will denote an acute condition, whereas more than 3 months is regarded as chronic.[21]

Chronic suppurative otitis media

This condition is characterized by chronic purulent discharge, through a perforated tympanic membrane. The pathological drum may be in a neutral or retracted position, discoloured (usually opaque) and with no mobility. (Figure 23.4).[20]

Diagnosis of the specific condition is made by otoscopy and confirmed by tympanometry, with audiometric evidence of a conductive hearing impairment. A type B tympanogram, indicative of poor middle ear compliance, would be found in otitis media, or when a middle ear effusion is present. A type C tympanogram, with a rising curve, indicative of negative middle ear pressure will be found in early cases of OME (Figure 23.5).[23, 24]

Audiometric testing demonstrates a conductive hearing loss, and may be bilateral or unilateral. In early cases of OME, the loss may be present only at low frequencies (0.5 and 1.0kHz), while in advanced cases of longer duration, the loss may span the whole range of frequencies leading to a pantonal moderate degree of hearing impairment (Figure 23.6).[25] In such cases, the correction of the conductive component by treatment of the glue ear allows the evaluation of the possibility of an underlying sensorineural hearing component.

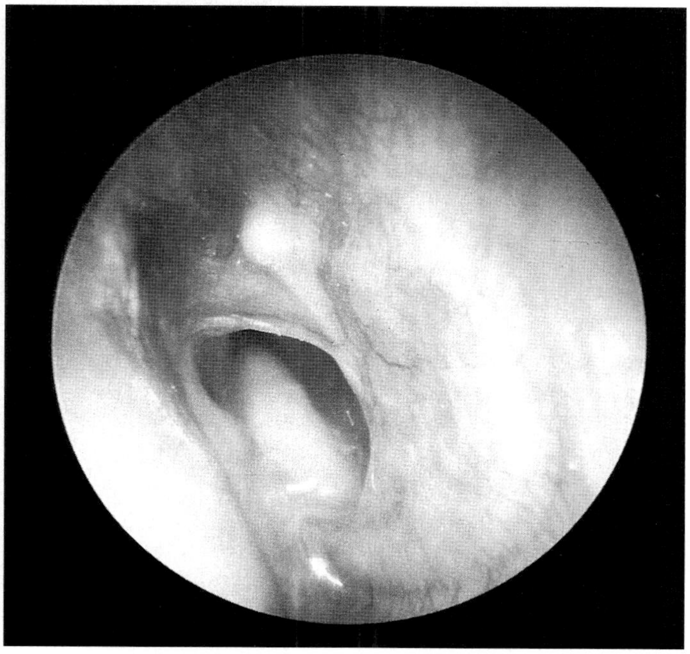

Figure 23.4 Chronic suppurative otitis media. Perforation of the tympanic membrane with granulomatous edges and mucopurulent discharge. (From Hawke and McCombe. *Diseases of the Ear Pocket Atlas*. Austin TX: Manticore Communications Inc, 1995.[20])

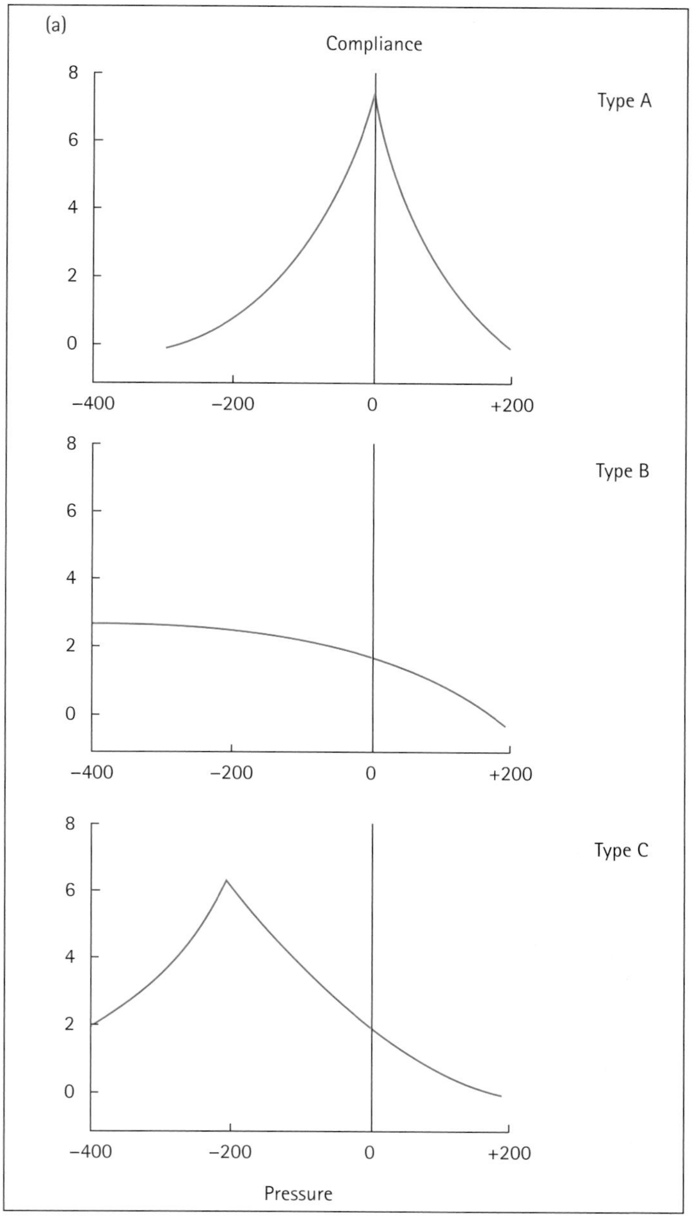

Figure 23.5 Classification of shapes of tympanograms, Type A – normal middle ear pressure. Type B – presence of ME effusion. Type C - rising curve indicative of presence of negative pressure in the ME cleft. (From Browning, ed. *Clinical Otology and Audilogy* 2nd Edition. Oxford: Butterworth Heinemann, 1998: 185–90[24] with further details in Jerger et al. *Arch Otolaryngol* 1974; **99**: 165–71.[23])

Pathophysiology/aetiology

A number of factors leading to the development of OME have been postulated, and it is possible that in any individual case all the different mechanisms may be involved.

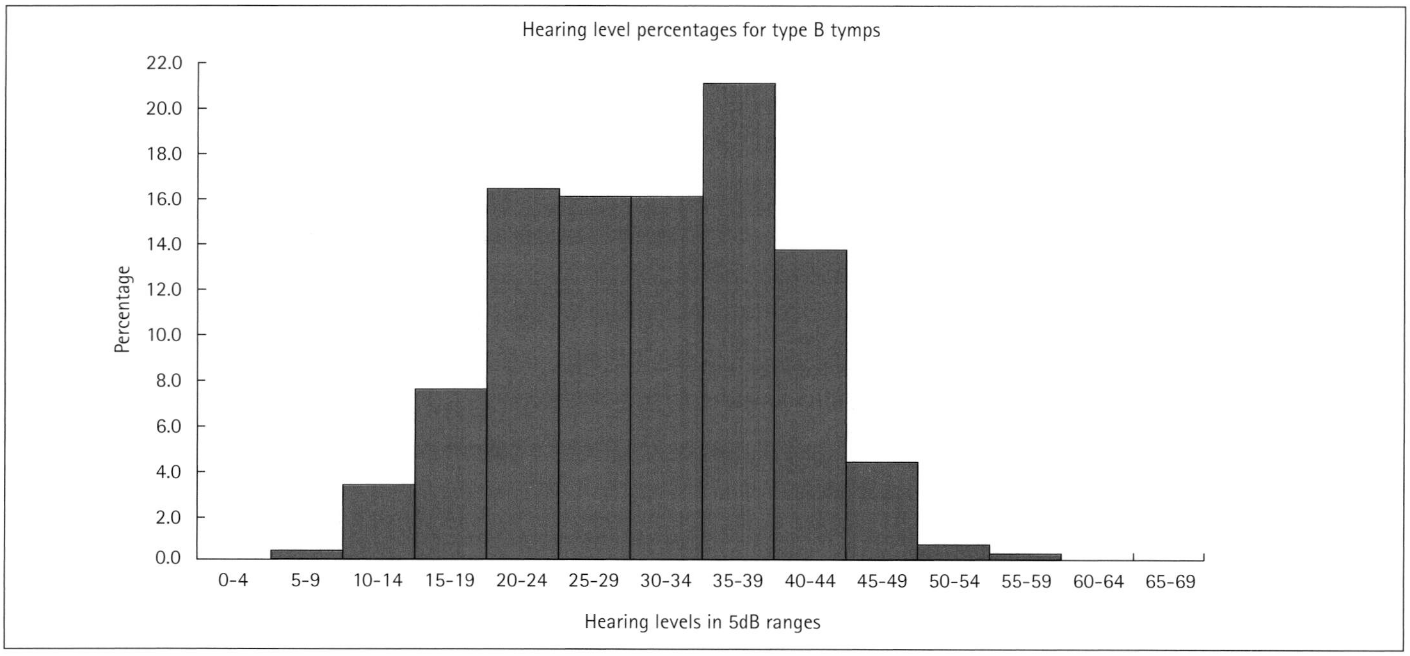

Figure 23.6 Histogram of hearing level (pure tone average/0.5, 1 and 2 kHz) in children's ears with OME confirmed by Type B tympanogram.

> **FACTORS ASSOCIATED WITH THE DEVELOPMENT OF OME**
>
> - Eustachian tube dysfunction/occlusion[26]
> - Unresolved infection with continued inflammation, in the nasopharynx/middle ear (cleft)
> - Allergy
> - Immature or impaired immunological systems in infants
> - Craniofacial abnormalities
> - Social factors such as passive smoking, lack of breast feeding and attendance at nursery.[27]

Eustachian tube dysfunction/occlusion

The Eustachian tube is the part of the middle ear system positioned between the nasopharynx and the middle ear cavity, and mastoid air cells system. The entire surface is covered by mucous membrane. The Eustachian tube in infancy and childhood differs from that of an adult, in that it is more horizontal and shorter, about 18mm long[10] compared with 31–38mm in the adult.[11] In addition, the ostium lies in the lower part of the nasopharynx and the isthmus is narrower (Figure 23.7).[28]

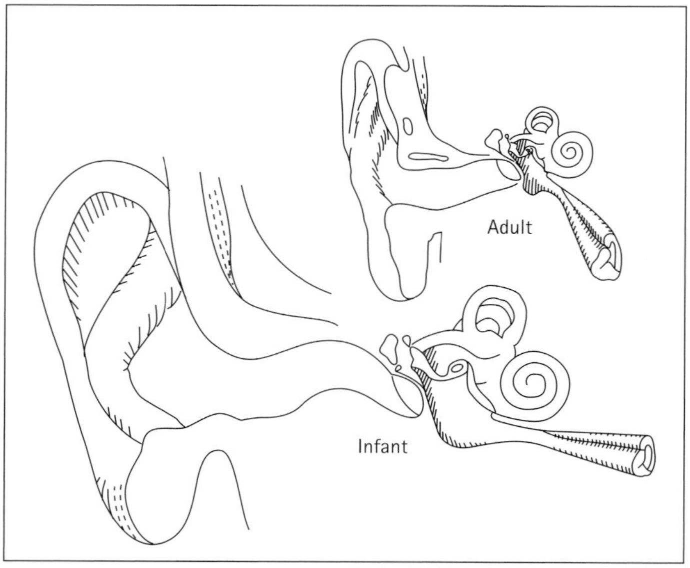

Figure 23.7 Diagram showing the difference in position and configuration of eustachain tubes in infants and adults. (From Bluestone and Klein. In: Wu, ed. *Otitis Media in Infants and Children* 2nd ed. Philadelphia: Saunders Co, 2001: 58–78.[28])

The Eustachian tube allows equalisation of the pressure in the middle ear with atmospheric pressure, enabling free movement of the tympanic membrane. The Eustachian tube can become blocked internally by swelling of the mucous membrane due to the infection (upper respiratory tract infection) or allergy, or externally by compression due to enlarged adenoids. The air in the middle ear cavity is then absorbed into the blood vessels of the mucous membrane, causing a reduction of middle ear pressure, leading to retraction and restriction of movement of the tympanic membrane.

The anatomical configuration of the Eustachian tube in the infant allows for easy access to the middle ear from the nasopharynx predisposing to more frequent episodes of glue ear. Gross negative pressure, within the middle ear cleft, may lead to aspiration of secretions from the nasopharynx, with the development of acute bacterial otitis media.

Nasopharyngeal infection

Nasopharyngeal infection may spread along the mucous membrane of the Eustachian tube into the middle ear cleft.[29] An effusion in the middle ear may also result from incomplete resolution of an acute middle ear infection.[30]

Allergy

The role of allergy in the formation of OME has been postulated for many years.[31–34] However, the mechanism of its association has remained unclear,[35] but more recently, it has been proposed that the middle ear mucosa may be functioning as a target organ. Allergy may lead to inflammatory swelling of the mucosal lining of the Eustachian tube, or bacteria and allergens may be aspirated from the nasopharynx into middle ear space.[36–38]

Immunological status

It has been observed that children with a defective or immature immunological status have a higher incidence of OME,[39] and Sigurdardottir et al reported that children aged 3 years or above, with chronic middle ear effusion, may have a functional antibody deficiency to Streptococcus pneumoniae.[40]

Craniofacial abnormalities

Nearly all infants with unrepaired cleft palate present with MEE,[41] but surgical repair of the cleft improves Eustachian tube function and, thus, diminishes the occurrence of MEE.[42]

In children with Down's syndrome, Eustachian tube position is such that it facilitates access of secretions from the nasopharynx into the middle ear cleft, resulting in chronic MEE.[43]

Genetics

Epidemiological and anatomical information suggests that the predisposition to chronic MEE may be of genetic origin. The pneumatisation of mastoid air cells linked causally to otitis media was found to be greater in monozygotic than dizygotic twins.[44] Moreover, the position of the Eustachian tube leading to an increased incidence of MEE may also be genetically determined.[45]

Social and environmental factors

Children's attendance at nursery leads to an increased occurrence of repeated upper respiratory tract infections and, hence, persistent OME. Rassmussen[46] and Casselbrant and co-workers[47] found that first-born children were less affected by MEE during the first 2 years of life, than were their siblings.

A strong positive association between MEE and passive smoking has been recognised by some[48–49] but not other researchers.[50] A metabolite of nicotine (cotinine), which serves as a marker of passive smoking, has been measured in the saliva of children aged 6–7 years and its value correlated with tympanometric findings of middle ear status. Abnormal tympanograms, and the number of smokers in a house correlated with increased cotinine concentrations.[51]

In a further study, children in a nursery, who were shown to have elevated cotinine concentration, demonstrated a higher rate of both new and longer episodes of MEE.[52]

SEQUELAE OF OME

- Functional.
- Structural.

Chronic OME may lead to a range of functional sequelae, which broadly can be subdivided into those associated with vestibular dysfunction, leading to imbalance, and those associated with auditory dysfunction, leading to speech and language impairments, with subsequent communication and behaviour problems.

FUNCTIONAL SEQUELAE OF OME

- Hearing impairment.
- Speech & language delay.
- Behavioural problems.
- Balance dysfunction.

Hearing, speech, language development and behaviour

OME, especially of prolonged duration or recurrent nature may lead to long lasting or fluctuating hearing impairment, which in turn may have consequences upon speech and language development, with secondary communication and behaviour difficulties. The complexity of this relationship depends upon the degree and duration of the impairment and the child's stage of development, at the time of the condition. Early history of OME leading to hearing impairment in the first and second year of life may result in a delay in expressive more than repetitive development.[53]

A young child, in the early critical period for language development, requires acute hearing to be able to distinguish the important auditory signals of speech and to filter speech signals from the background noise.[54] The presence of middle ear effusion, resulting in a conductive hearing impairment of various degrees and of various duration impairs the perfect acquisition of sounds and semantic, syntactic, and pragmatic rules of language. Instead, the received signal is partial or incomplete, which leads to false coding in a child's language database. Moreover, the child's interaction with the care-giver may be diminished because of the effects of the chronic condition. These impairments may lead to the child's withdrawal, lack of interest and concentration, frustration or clinging behaviour.

At a later stage, during school, the child may present with problems in listening in background noise, poor academic achievement, and attention and behavioural problems. Withdrawal, in a school setting, leads to the report that 'the child is in a world of his own', day dreaming and, thus, attracting less attention from the teacher and consequently, falling behind academically.

A child with hearing impairment due to OME will frequently ignore the attenuated auditory input, and this is exacerbated situations where he has to listen against background noise. The child, who does not have a well established auditory base for language, struggles when addressed by further fluctuating hearing impairment, because he is not able to refer to an established language code when further auditory messages are incomplete.[54]

A younger child, in this situation, with a history of conductive hearing loss, who has not developed a language database, is unable to use contextual cues or previous experience to decipher a new auditory message. He will frequently ask for the question to be repeated and will mishear or provide an incorrect reply. He will also ask for the volume of the television to be increased and he may shout or be reported to lip read. He may manifest learning difficulties such as slowness to learn, inattention and poor concentration. Additionally, he may have poor pronunciation or, indeed, may not be understood by strangers, as his words may be incomplete.[55]

It has been shown in human and animal studies of prolonged MEE[56] that the attenuated or delayed auditory inputs[57] lead to impairment of binaural hearing and of other elements of central auditory processing, such as temporal resolution and sensitivity to short tones in the presence of background noise,[58] which underlie important aspects of language listening. However, with training, the animals regain normal temporal resolution.[58] Similarly, some aspects of disordered central auditory processing, associated with recurrent MEE in infancy, such as binaural masking level difference, recover spontaneously in teenagers, once MEE has resolved.[59]

The long-term effects of fluctuating hearing impairment, associated with middle ear effusion, during the early period of the development of language are not clear.[60] The result of prospective studies on this topic are difficult to interpret, as there are no standard inclusion and outcome criteria and many of the studies are poorly designed.[54]

Moreover, retrospective studies are difficult to evaluate, as the data are often not precise. The history of OME for example is subjectively elicited from the parents, rather than objectively based on otoscopy, tympanometry and audiometry. However, there is sufficient data to establish that there is an effect of OME on auditory perception,[61] speech, language development, cognition and behaviour.[62]

Balance

Children who present with chronic middle ear effusion can experience symptoms of dizziness and imbalance.[63–64] However, the symptoms frequently reported by parents are clumsiness and frequent falls.[65] A number of authors found, using a balance platform system, that children with chronic OME demonstrated greater sway than a control group.[66–68] It has also been demonstrated that resolution of the middle ear effusion led to improvement of the associated balance dysfunction.[63,69,70,71] Three mechanisms to explain vestibular involvement in OME have been proposed. One school of thought states that negative middle ear pressure changes are transmitted through the labyrinthine windows and cause secondary movement of the inner ear fluids.[65,69,67,72,73] The second school of thought proposes that the symptoms are caused by serous labyrinthitis, as a result of superadded infection of the middle ear effusion.[69,67,72,74] It had been found that bacteria can be cultured from 20% to 77% of chronic middle ear effusions.[75,76] A third mechanism has been suggested by Jones,[68] who has postulated a transfer of ions through the semi-permeable round window membrane, leading to a change in the chemical composition of the endolymph via the perilymph. This in turn, would lead to changes in the ionic channels of the kinocilia and stereocilia leading to a disturbance of balance.

Children with balance problems, as a result of chronic middle ear effusion, especially those with additional problems (such as speech and language delay, or behaviour problems) may not recover spontaneously and, therefore, should be referred for early surgical intervention.[77,78]

Other possible structural sequelae to chronic OME are tympanic membrane perforation, chronic suppurative otitis media, formation of cholesteatoma, retraction pockets of the tympanic membrane (Figure 23.8), patches of tympanosclerosis, mastoiditis, labyrinthitis, or facial paralysis. Many of these require surgical intervention (see Chapter 36).[79]

Management

Treatment of AOM and OME falls into three categories:

TREATMENT OF AOM AND OME

- Medical and preventative.
- Surgical.
- Rehabilitative.

Medical treatment of AOM

The first line of management of AOM is with an antibiotic agent sensitive to the most common pathogens, causing middle ear infection, such as Streptococcus pneumoniae, Haemophilus influenzae and Moraxella catarrhalis. The recommended drug

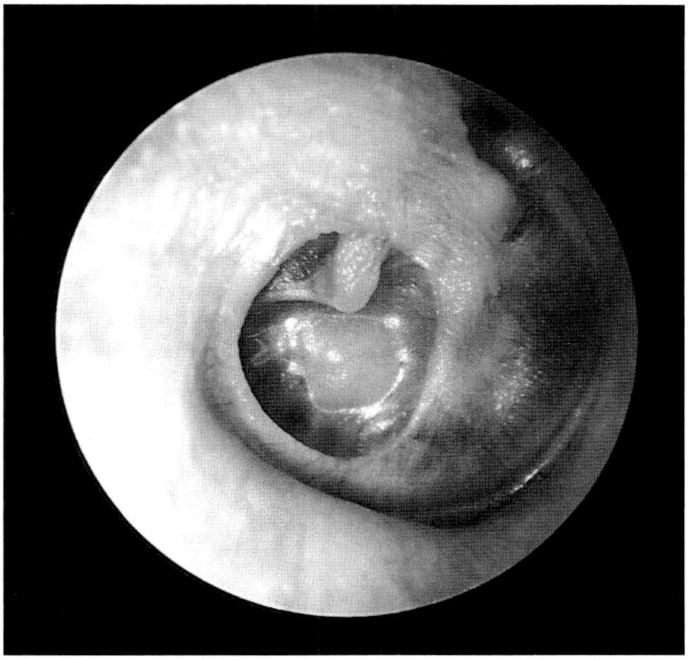

Figure 23.8 Retraction pockets.[20] The sequelaed negative middle ear pressure due to Eustachian tube dysfunction. (From Hawke and McCombe. *Diseases of the Ear Pocket Atlas.* Austin TX: Manticore Communications Inc, 1995.[20])

of choice is amoxycillin, which is effective, safe and inexpensive. A combination of amoxycillin and clavulanate is recommended as the second line treatment in North America, if amoxycillin alone is ineffective. A 10–14 day course is recommended.[80, 81] If the infection continues a change of antibiotics is advised, e.g. erythromycin or trimethoprim, together with a detailed examination to identify other foci of infection and tympanocentesis (incision and drainage of middle ear abscess). Culture and sensitivity of the causative pathogen, obtained from the middle ear fluid, will allow the use of the appropriate most sensitive antibiotic.

In parallel to antibiotic therapy, AOM could be treated symptomatically with analgesic, antipyretics, antihistamines and decongestants, although their efficacy has not been proven. Severe recurrent attacks of AOM should be investigated to exclude underlying conditions, such as an allergy or an immunological defect, which should be treated appropriately.[82] Environmental factors, predisposing to recurrent infection, should be excluded, such as passive smoking,[83] while attendance at the day nursery should be raised with the parents as a relevant predisposing factor.

Children with a history of recurrent otitis media (more than 6 attacks per year) and impaired immune responses, should be offered 7 valent type of conjugate pneumococcal vaccine[84] or influenza virus vaccine, or indeed long-term antimicrobial prophylaxis with amoxycillin or sulphonamide.[85]

If, despite prophylaxic treatment, the child continues to have episodes of otitis media, other options of treatment should be considered, such as the insertion of grommets (ventilation tube) alone, or in combination with adenoidectomy, if indicated by the symptoms of hypertrophied adenoids, obstructing the ostium of the Eustachian tube.

AOM may be followed by persistent OME, which should be kept under observation ('watchful waiting' before surgery), together with placement of the child on a provisional surgical waiting list. From this position, repeated assessments allow the child to be transferred for surgery as soon as required.[85, 86] However, if the OME resolves, this approach allows removal from the surgical list, with effective and economic management of healthcare resources.

Medical treatment of OME

Chronic OME has been treated with a variety of agents, such as systemic and intranasal decongestants and, antihistamine/-decongestant combinations, but clinical trials have not proven their efficacy.[80] Systemic corticosteroids have been used, but with uncertain effectiveness, and potential side effects, particularly in children, reduce their usefulness in the management of OME.[87]

Other methods, such as mucolytics and otovent autoinflation of the middle ear[88] have also proven of little benefit. In the case of usage of the otovent, there is the practical problem of poor compliance in children, and the theoretical risk of forcing infecting nasopharyngeal secretions into the middle ear.

An alternative approach has been the use of xylitol sugar chewing gum, which has been shown in a study of five-year-old children in day care to prevent AOM. Some success has been registered, as compared with children using sucrose gum.[89] Xylitol can be produced from birch tree, and is also found in raspberries and plums. It inhibits the growth of Streptococcus mutans, and is therefore, widely used in toothpaste to prevent dental caries. However, it has been shown, in vitro, to inhibit the growth of Streptococcus pneumoniae,[90] and these initial observations deserve further investigation.

Surgical management

Several different modalities of surgical intervention are of value in the management of OME (see Chapter 36).

SURGICAL MANAGEMENT

- Insertion of a ventilation tube (**grommet**) (Figure 23.9)[20] which maintains ambient pressure within the middle ear cleft and provides adequate draining through the grommet and Eustachian tube into the nasopharynx.
- **Adenoidectomy** (= the removal of hypertrophied lymphoid tissue from the ostium of the Eustachian tube and nasopharynx).

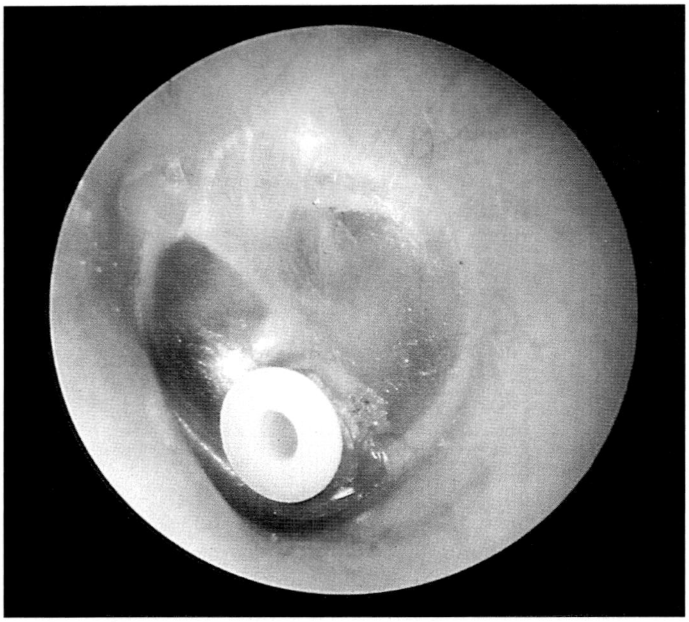

Figure 23.9 Ventilation tube (grommet). The tube is inserted in the anteriorinferior quadrant of the tympanic membrane, which allows the aeration of the middle ear bypassing the dysfunctional Eustachian tube. (From Hawke and McCombe. *Diseases of the Ear Pocket Atlas*. Austin TX: Manticore Communications Inc, 1995.[20])

- A combination of insertion of a **grommet and adenoidectomy.**
- **Adenotonsillectomy.**

The indications for surgical management are:

a) Chronic middle ear effusion of longer than 3 months' duration and occurring in both ears, leading to secondary sequelae such as:
   - Conductive hearing impairment of 20dB or more.
   - Speech and language delay associated with hearing impairment
   - Communication, behaviour difficulties
   - Balance problems, clumsiness, frequent falling.
   - Pathology of tympanic membrane such as the presence of retraction pockets (Figure 23.8).[20]
   - Middle ear changes arising from long term effects of negative middle ear pressure such as adhesions, ossicular involvement.

b) Recurrent episodes of AOM, superimposed on chronic otitis media.

c) Recurrent episodes of AOM without effusion between attacks, in which the medical treatment with antibiotics for each episode and prophylactic antibiotics have failed.[80]

The aim of treatment of OME is four-fold:

- To relieve the symptoms caused by middle ear conditions
- To resolve the underlying pathological abnormalities
- To prevent the development of sequelae
- To treat coexistent infections of the nose, sinuses and allergy.

The efficacy of the various modalities of surgical management of chronic OME has been widely studied.[91,92] The insertion of a grommet provides an immediate, however short term, hearing improvement up to 20dB. Longer term studies have shown the improvement only of 12dB or less per year post surgery.[88] The benefit of combined adenoidectomy with grommet insertion and tonsillectomy has been assessed by various authors.[93–95]

Maw reported a prospective controlled study of adenoidectomy and adenotonsillectomy on chronic OME in 322 children aged 2–11 years.[96, 97] He found that the children treated with the combination of adenoidectomy and insertion of grommet had the shortest duration of OME (Figures 23.10 and 23.11).[97]

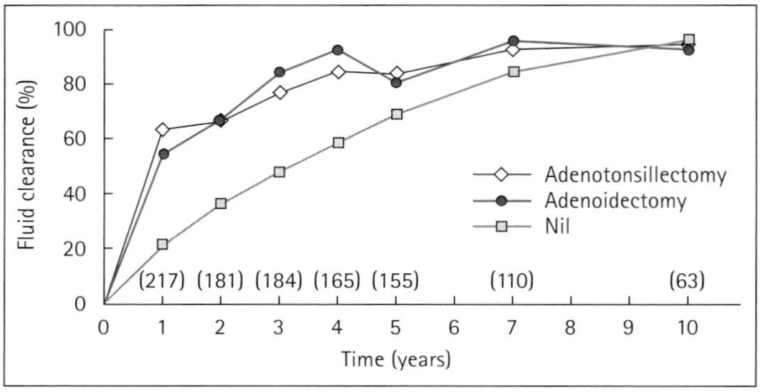

Figure 23.10 The rate of clearance of MEE after treatment by adenotonsillectomy, adenoidectomy, compared with the control (untreated) ears. (From Maw and Parker. *Acta Otolaryngol* 1988; 454 (suppl): 202–7.[96])

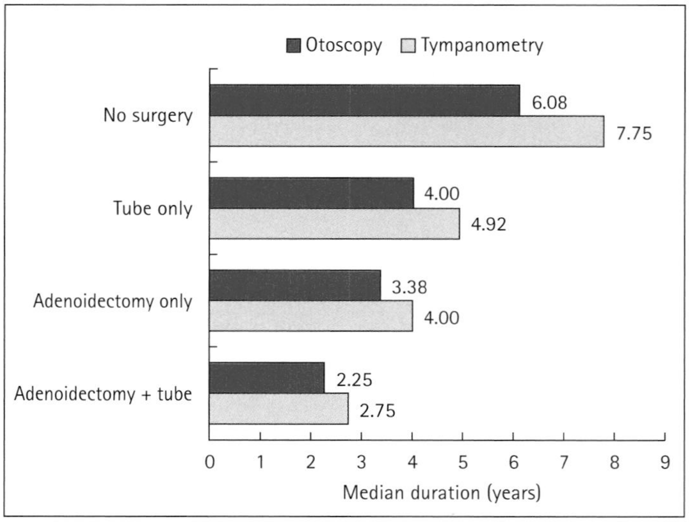

Figure 23.11 Median duration of chronic OME in ears treated with adenoidectomy and grommet, with adenoidectomy or, grommet (tube) insertion only, and in the ears without any treatment, as shown by otoscopy and tympanometry.[96]

There was no overall difference between the group with insertion of grommet or adenoidectomy only, but significant differences were shown when the two modalities of treatment were combined.

The recent UK Target (Trial of alternative regimes of glue ear treatment) multi-centre, randomized, controlled trial to determine the effectiveness of surgery in OME has established that in children with chronic OME, aged 3–7 years, the benefit of insertion of a grommet is only mildly successful, and up to 70% of such children would be better treated by a combination of grommet insertion and adenoidectomy.[98]

Rehabilitative management

OME is generally a self-limiting condition, the alternative to surgical management is temporary amplification. This should reduce the child's disability arising from hearing impairment associated with OME. The studies showed children's satisfaction with this type of management, and a reduction in disability.[99,100] However, this type of management requires very careful monitoring, such that the sequelae of OME leading to permanent damage of the middle ear do not occur.

Summary and conclusion

OME is one of the most common conditions in children, and may lead to fluctuating or stable conductive hearing impairment. The sequelae may not only affect the structure of the ME, but also lead to expressive more than receptive language, communication difficulties, disturbed behaviour and imbalance.

The treatment is in the first instance medical. However, chronic presentation of OME, with any sequelae, point to surgical management, which optimally is a combination of adenoidectomy and insertion of grommet.

References

1. Casselbrandt ML, Mandel EM, Rosenfeld RM, Bluestone CD, ed. Epidemiology. In: *Evidence Based Otitis Media.* Hamilton BC Decker Inc. 1999; 124.
2. Marchant CD, Shurin PA, Turozyk VA, Wasikowski DE, Tutihasi MA, Kinney SE. Course and outcome of otitis media in early infancy, a prospective study. *J Paediatr Child Health* 1984; **104**: 826–31.
3. Bartalozzi G, Sacchetti A, Scarane P & Becherucci P. Natural history of otitis media with effusion in children under six years of age. *Advances in Otolaryngology* 1992; **47**: 281–3.
4. Casselbrandt ML, Okeowo PA, Flaherty MR, Feldmann RH, Doyle WJ, Bluestone CD, Rogers KD & Hanley T. Prevalence and incidence of otitis media in a group of pre-school children in the United States. In: Lim DJ, Bluestone JO, Klein and Nelson JD, eds. *Recent Advances in Otitis Media with Effusion.* Philadelphia: Decker BL, 1984; 16–19.
5. Zielhuis GA, Straatman H, Rach GH and Van der Broek P. Analysis and presentation of data on the natural time course of otitis media with effusion in children. *Int J Epidemiol* 1990; **19**: 1037–44.
6. Zielhuis GA, Heuvelmans-Heinen EW, Rach GH & Van der Broek P. Environmental risk factors for otitis media with effusion in pre-school children. *Scand J Prim Health Care* 1987; **7**: 33–8.
7. Pelton SL, Shurin PA, Klein JO. Persistence of middle ear effusion after otitis media. *Paediatr Res* 1977; **11**: 504.
8. Casselbrant ML, Brostoff LH, Cantekin EI, Flaherty MR, Doyle WJ, Bluestone CD & Fria TJ. Otitis media with effusion in pre-school children. *Laryngoscope* 1985; **95**: 428–36.
9. Zielhuis GA, Roch GH, Van Der Bosch A, Van der Broek P. The prevalence of otitis media with effusion: a critical review of the literature. *Clin Otolaryngol.* 1990; **15**: 283–8.
10. Sadler-Kimes D, Siegel MJ, Todhunter JS. Age related morphological difference in the components of the eustachian tube/middle ear system. *Ann Otol Rhinol Laryngol* 1989; **98**: 854–8.
11. Proctor B. Embryology and anatomy of eustachian tube. *Arch Otolaryngol Head and Neck Surg* 1967; **86**: 503–26.
12. Giebink GS. Preventing otitis media. *Ann Otol Rhinol Laryngol Suppl* 1994; **163**: 20–3.
13. Kraemer MJ, Richardson MA, Weiss NS, Furukuwa CT, Shapiro GG, Pierson WE & Bierman W. Risk factors for persistent middle-ear effusions: otitis media, catarrh, cigarette smoke exposure and atopy. *JAMA* 1983; **249**: 1022–5.
14. Aniansson G, Alm B, Andersson B, Häkansson A, Larsson P, Nylen O, Peterson H, Rigner P, Svanborg, Sabharwal H & Svanborg C. A prospective cohort study on breast feeding and otitis media in Swedish children. *Pediatr Infect Dis J* 1994; **13**: 183–8.
15. Teele DW, Klein JO, Rosner B & Hue. Greater Boston Otitis Media Study Group. Epidemiology of otitis media during the first seven years of life in children in Greater Boston: A prospective cohort study. *J Infectious Diseases* 160: 83–94.
16. Owen MJ, Boldwin CD, Swank PR, Pannu AK, Johnson DL, Howie VM. Relation of infant feeding practice, cigarette smoke exposure and group child care to the onset and duration of otitis media with effusion in the first two years of life. *J Paediatr Child Health* 1993; **123**: 702–11.
17. Alho OP, Kilkku O, Oja H, Koivu H, & Sorri M. Control of the temporal aspect when considering risk factors for acute otitis media. *Arch Otolaryngol Head Neck Surg* 1993; **119**: 444–9.
18. Hardy AM, Fowler HG. Child care arrangements and repeated ear infections in young children. *Am J Public Health* 1993; **83**: 1321–5.
19. Klein JO, Naunton RF, Tos H, Ohyama M, Hussl B & Van Cauwenberge PB. Definitions and classification panel reports. *Ann Otol Rhinol Laryngol Suppl* 1989; **139**: 10.
20. Hawke M, McCombe A. *Diseases of the Ear Pocket Atlas.* Austin TX: Manticore communications Inc. 1995.
21. Bluestone CHD, Klein JO. Definitions, terminology and classifications. In: Ju Bluestone CHD, Klein JO, eds. *Otitis Media in Infants and Children.* 2nd Edition, Philadelphia: WB Saunders Co. 1995; 1–3.

22. Henderson FW, Roush J. Diagnosis of otitis media. *Otitis Media in Young Children*. In: Roberts JE, Wallace I F, Henderson FW, Paul H Brookes, eds. Baltimore: Baltimore Publishing Co., 1997; 43–60.
23. Jerger I, Jerger S, Mauldin L. Studies in impedance audiometry in middle ear disorders. *Arch Otolaryngol* 1974; **99**:165–71.
24. Browning GG, Acoustic impedance. In: Browning GG, ed. *Clinical Otology and Audiology* 2nd edition. Oxford: Butterworth-Heinemann, 1998: 185–90.
25. Medical Research Council Multi-Centre Target Report: The role of tympanometry in predicting associated hearing impairment in children with otitis media with effusion. *Clin Otolaryngol* 1998.
26. Politzer A. Uber die willkurlichen Bewegungen des Trommelfells. *Wiener Med Halle Nr*1862; **18**:103.
27. Bluestone CHD, Klein JO. Epidemiology. In: Bluestone CHD, Klein JO, eds. *Otitis Media in Infants and Children*, 3rd ed. Philadelphia: WB Saunders Co., 2001; 58–78.
28. Bluestone CD, Klein JO. Anatomy. In: Ju WB, ed. *Otitis Media in Infants and Children* 2nd ed. Philadelphia: Saunders Co. 1995; 5–15.
29. Bluestone CD, Berry QC, Andrew W. Mechanics of the eustachian tube as it influences susceptibility to and persistence of middle ear effusions in children *Ann Otol Rhinol Laryngol* 1974; **83**(11): 27–34.
30. Mills R Uttley A, McIntyre M. Relationship between acute suppurative otitis media and chronic suppurative otitis media: role of antibiotics. *J R Soc Med* 1984; **77**: 754–7.
31. Lewis ER. Otitis media and allergy. *Ann Otol Rhinol Laryngol* 1929; **38**: 185–8.
32. Jordan R. Chronic secretory otitis media *Laryngoscope* 1949; **59**: 1002–15.
33. Draper WL. Secretory otitis media in children: A study of 540 children. *Laryngoscope* 1967; **77**:636–53.
34. McMahan JT, Calenoft E, Croft J, Barenholtz L, Weber LD. Chronic otitis media with effusion and allergy. Modified RAST analysis of 119 cases. *Arch Otolaryngol Head Neck Surg* 1981; **89**:427–31.
35. Mogi G. Immunologic and allergic aspects of otitis media. In: Lim DJ, Bluestone CD Klein JO, Nelson JD, eds. *Recent Advances in Otitis Media with Effusion*. Burlington, Ontario; Decker Periodicals, 1993; 145–51.
36. Bluestone CD. Eustachian tube function and allergy in otitis media. *Paediatrics* 1978; **61**:753–60.
37. Bluestone CD. Eustachian tube function, physiology, pathophysiology and role of allergy in pathogenesis of otitis media. *J Allergy Clin Immunol* 1983; **72**:242–51
38. Scadding GK. The pathogenesis of otitis media with effusion-allergy revisited. *J Audiological Medicine* 1995; **4**(3):173–81.
39. Rynnel-Dagoo B, Freijd A. Immunodeficiency. In: Bernstein J, Ogra. P, eds. *Otitis Media in Immunology of the Ear*. New York: Raven Press, 1987; 363–80.
40. Sigurdardottir S, Otte W, Casselbrandt M, Fireman P. Abnormal immune responsiveness in older children with chronic otitis media with effusion. *Paediatric Res* 1991; **29**:163a.
41. Paradise JL, Bluestone CD, Felder H. The universality of otitis media in 50 infants with cleft palate. *Paediatrics* 1969; **44**: 35–42.
42. Paradise JL, Bluestone CD. Early treatment of the universal otitis media of infants with cleft palate. *Paediatrics* 1974; **53**:48–54.
43. White BL, Doyle WJ, Bluestone CD. Eustachian tube function in infants and children with Down's Syndrome. In: Lim DY, Bluestone CD, Klein JO, et al. (eds.) Recent Advances in Otitis Media with Effusion: Proceedings of the Third International Symposium. Philadelphia: BC Decker 1984; 62–6.
44. Diamant H, Diamant M. The mastoid air cells. In: McCabe BF, Sade J, Abramson M, eds. *Choleastatoma First International Conference* Birmingham: Aesculapius Publishing Co., 1977; 319–23.
45. Berry QC, Doyle WJ, Bluestone CD, Cantekin EI, Wiet RJ. Eustachian tube function in an American Indian population. *Otol Rhinol Laryngol* 1980; **89**:28–33.
46. Rasmussen F. Protracted secretory otitis media: The impact of familial factors and day-care centre attendance. *Int J of Paediatr Otorhinolaryngol* 1993; **26**:29–37.
47. Casselbrandt ML, Mandel EM, Kurs-Lasky H, Rockette HE, Bluestone CD. Otitis media in a population of black American and white American infants 0–2 years of age. *Int J Paediatr Otorhinolaryngol* 1995; **33**: 1–16.
48. Stenstrom R, Bernard PAM, Ben-Simon H. Exposure to environmental tobacco smoke as a risk factor for recurrent acute otitis media in children under the age of five years. *Int. J Paediatr Otorhinolaryngol* 1993; **27**:127–36.
49. Blakely JE. Smoking and middle ear diseases, are they related? A review article. *Otolaryngol Head Neck Surg* 1995; **112**: 441–6.
50. Zielhuis GA, Heuvelmans-Heinen EW, Rach GH, Broeck PVD. Environmental risk factors for otitis media with effusion in pre-school children. *Scand J Prim Health Care* 1989; **7**: 33–8.
51. Strachan DP, Jarvis MJ, Feyerabend C. Passive smoking, salivary cotinine concentrations and middle ear effusion in 7 year old children. *BMJ* 1989; **298**: 1549–52.
52. Etzel RA, Pattishall EN, Haley NJ, Fletcher RH, Henderson FW. Passive smoking and middle ear effusion among children in day care. *Paediatrics* 1992; **90**: 228–32.
53. Friel-Patti, Finitzo T. Language learning in a prospective study of otitis media with effusion in the first two yeaers of life. *J Speech Hearing Res* 1990; **33**: 188–94.
54. Roberts JE, Wallace JF. Language and Otitis Media. In: Roberts JE, Wallace JF, Hendersson FW, eds. *Otitis Media in Young Children. Medical Developmental and Educational Considerations*.. Baltimore: Paul Brookes Publishing Co., 1997: 133–61.
55. Maw AR. Presentation and diagnosis. In: Maw AR. *Glue Ear in Childhood, A Prospective Study of Otitis Media with Effusion*. London: Mackeith Press, 1995; 47–60.
56. Moore DR, Hogan SC, Kecelnik O, Parsons CH, Rose MM, Klug AJ. Auditory Learning as a cause and treatment of central dysfunction. *Audiol Neurootol* 2001; **6**(4): 216–20.
57. Hogan SC, Moore DR. Impaired binaural hearing in children produced by a threshold level of middle ear disease. *J Assoc Res Otolaryngol* 2002; Sept 23.
58. Moore DR, Hogan SC. Effects of OME on central auditory function. *The ESPO 2002 Book of Abstracts*. 8th International congress of paediatric otorhinolaryngology,Oxford, 2002; 11–14 Sept.

59. Hogan SC, Meyer SE, Moore DR. Binaural unmasking returns to normal in teenagers who had otitis media in infancy. *Audiol Neruootol* 1996; **1**(2): 104–11.
60. Bluestone CHD, Klein JO. Complication and sequelae: Intratemporal. In: Bluestone CHD, Klein JO. *Otitis Media in infants and children* 3rd edition. Philadelphia: WB Saunders Co. 2001; 299–309.
61. Mandell JR. Impact of otitis media on auditory function. In: Rosenfeld RM, Bluestone CHD. *Evidence-Based Otitis Media*. DC: Decker Hamilton, 1999; 337–51.
62. Vernon-Feagaus L. Impact of Otitis Media on speech, language, cognition & behaviour. In: Rosenfeld RM, Bluestone CHD. *Evidence Based Otitis Media*. DC: Decker, Hamilton, 1999; 353–73
63. Bower CM, Cotton RT. The spectrum of vertigo in children. *Arch Otolaryngol Head Neck Surg* 1995; **121**: 911–5.
64. Casselbrant ML, Furman JM, Rubenstein E, Mandel EM. Effect of otitis media on the vestibular system in children. *Ann Otol Rhinol Laryngol* 1995; **104**: 620–4
65. Busis SN. Dizziness in children. *Paediatr Ann.* 1988; **17**: 648–55.
66. Casselbrant ML, Black FO, Nashner L, Panion R. Vestibular function assessment in children with otitis media with effusion. *Ann Otol Rhinol Laryngol* 1983; **92** (Suppl 107): 46–7
67. Grace ARH, Pfleiderer AG. Dysequilibrium and otitis media with effusion: what is the association? *J Laryngol Otol* 1990; **104**: 682–4.
68. Jones NS, Radomski P, Prichard AJN, Snashall SE. Imbalance and chronic secretory otitis media in children: effect of myringotomy and insertion of ventilation tubes on body sway. *Ann Otol Rhinol Laryngol* 1990; **105**: 987–9.
69. Blayney AW, Colman BH. Dizziness in childhood. *Clin Otolaryngol* 1984; **9**: 77–85.
70. Fried MP. The evaluation of dizziness in children. *Laryngoscope* 1980; **9**: 1548–60.
71. Golz A, Westerman ST, Gilbert LM, Joachims HZ, Netzer A. Effect of middle ear effusion on the vestibular labyrinth. *J Laryngol Otol* 1991; **105**: 987–9.
72. Ben-David J, Podoshin L, Fradis M, Faraggi D,. Is the vestibular system affected by middle ear effusion? *Otolaryngol Head Neck Surg* 1993; **109**: 421–6.
73. Flisberg K. The effects of vacuum on the tympanic cavity. *Otolaryngol Clin North Am* 1970; **3**: 3–13.
74. Golz A, Netzer A, Angel-Yeger B, Westerman T, Gilbert LM, Joachims HZ. Effects of middle ear effusion on the vestibular system in children. *Otolaryngol Head Neck Surg* 1998; 695–9.
75. Calhoun KH, Norris WB, Hokanson JA, Stiernberg CM, Moore Quinn FB. Bacteriology of middle ear effusions. *South Med J* 1988; **81**: 332–6.
76. Post JC, Preston RA, Aul JJ, et al. Molecular analysis of bacterial pathogens in otitis media with effusion. *JAMA* 1995; **273**: 1598–604.
77. Cohen H, Friedman EM, Lai D, Pellicer M, Duncan N, Sulek M. Balance in Children with otitis media with effusion. *Int J Paediatr Oto Rhino Laryngol* 1997; **42**: 107–15.
78. Snashall S. Vestibular disorders. In: Kerr AG, Groves J, eds. *Scott-Brown's Otolaryngology*. 5th ed. London: Butterworths; 1987; 194–217.
79. Kenne MA, Diagnosis & management of acute otitis media & otitis media with effusion. In: Wetmore RF, Muntz HR, McGill TJ. *Paediatric Otolaryngology, Principles and Practice Pathways*. New York: Thieme, 2000; 263–79.
80. Bluestone CHD, Klein JO. Management. In: Bluestone CHD, Klein JO, eds. *Otitis Media in Infants and Children* 3rd ed. 2001; 180–298.
81. US Department of Health and Human Services. Otitis media in young children. In: *AHCPR Publication number 94–0622, (Clinical Practice Guidline; no12)*. 1994.
82. Bernstein JH. Role of allergy in eustachian tube blocleage and otitis media with effusion, a review. *Otolaryngol Head Neck Surg* 1996; **114**: 562–8.
83. Maw AR, Parker AJ, Lauce GN, Dilkes ME. The effect of parental smoking on outcomes after treatement for glue ear in children. *Clin Otolaryngol* 1992; **17**: 411–14.
84. Block S, Shinefield H, Fireman B et al. Efficacy of heptavolent pneumococcal conjugate vaccine in children. Northern California Kaiser permaeunte cavvince study group. *Paedr Infect Dis J* 2000; **19**: 187–95.
85. Berman S, Nuss R, Roark R, Huber-Navin C, Grose K, Herrera M. Effectiveness of continuous vs intermittent amoxycillin to prevent episodes of otitis media. *Paedtr Infect Dis J* 1992; **11**: 63–7.
86. Effective Health Care Bulletin. School of Public Health, University of Leeds, Centre for Health Economics, University of York; Research Unit, Royal College of Physicians. The treatment of persistent glue ear in children. 1992, 4.
87. Rosenfeld RM. What to expect from clinical treatment of otitis media. *Paedtre Inf Dis J* 1995; **14**: 731–37.
88. Maw AR. Treatment. In: Maw RD, ed. *Glue ear in Childhood – A Prospective study of otitis media with effusion*. Cambridge: Mac Keiten Press, 1995; 61–102.
89. Uhari M, Kontiokani T, Koskela M et al. Xylitol chewing gum in prevention of acute otitis media a double blind randomised trial.- *BMJ* 1996; **313**: 1180–4.
90. Kontiokari T, Uhari K, Koskela M. Effect of Xylitol on growth of nasopharyngeal bacteria in vitro. *Antimicide Agents Cheurother* 1995; **39**: 1820–3.
91. Maw AR, Bowden R. Spontaneous solution of severe chronic glue ear in children and the effect of adenoidectomy, tonsillectomy and insertion ventilation tubes. *BMJ* 1993; **306**: 256–60.
92. Todd DH, Stool SE. Surgical management of otitis media with effusion. In: Roberts JE, Wallace JF, Hendersson EW, eds. *Otitis media in young children*. Baltimore: Paul Brookes, 1997; 245–64.
93. ΩGates GA, Avery CA, Prihode TJ, Cooper JC. Effectiveness of adenoidectomy and tympanostomy tubes in the treatment of chronic media with effusion. *New Zealand J Med* 1987; **317**: 1444–51.
94. Paradise JC, Bluestone CD, Rogers KD, et al. Efficacy of adenoidectomy for recurrent otitis media in children previously treated with tympanostomy tube placement. Results of parallel randomised and non-randomised trials. *J Am Med Assoc* 1990; **263**: 2066–73.
95. Dempster JH, Browning CE, Gatehouse SG. A randomised study of the surgical management of children with persistent otitis

media with effusion associated with a hearing impairment. *J Laryngol Otolaryngol* 1993; **107**: 284–9.
96. Maw RD, Parker A. Surgery of the tonsils and adenoids in relation to secretory otitis media in children. *Acta Otolaryngol* 1988; **454** (suppl): 202–7.
97. Haggard M. The magnitude of developmental outcomes from surgery in OME. In: ESPO 2002, *Book of Abstracts 8th International Compass of Paediatrics*. Otorhinolaryngology, Sept 2002.
98. Flanagan PM, Knight LC, Thomas A, Browning S, August A & Clayton MJ. Hearing aids and glue ear. *Clin Otolaryngol* 1996; **21**: 297–300.
99. Jardine AH, Griffiths MV, Midgley E. The acceptance of hearing aids for children with otitis media with effusion. *The J Laryngol Otol* 1999; **113**: 314–17.
100. Bower CM, Cotton RT. The spectrum of vertigo in children. *Arch Otolaryngol Head Neck Surg* 1995; **121**: 911–15.

24 Disorders of the inner ear in children

Valerie Newton

Introduction

The reported prevalence of sensorineural hearing impairment in children has varied depending upon such factors as the country involved, the age of the children and the criteria for defining a hearing impairment. In the Trent region of the UK a prevalence of 1.2 per 1000 live births per annum was reported for children born between 1983 and 1988 and having a bilateral hearing impairment of at least 40 dB HL. Fifty per cent had a moderate hearing impairment (40–69 dB HL), 23% a severe impairment (70–94 dB HL), and 27% a profound hearing impairment (greater than 95 dB HL[1]. In developing countries, the prevalence of hearing impairment is greater. Mencher and Madriz Alfaro[2] found the prevalence in Costa Rica to be between 1.5 and 1.63 per 1000 live births, whereas Prasansuk[3] reported the prevalence to be between 3.5% and 5% in Thailand.

Conditions which affect the inner ear are the main causes of congenital hearing impairment in children and contribute significantly, but to a lesser degree, to hearing disability acquired during infancy and childhood. Studies indicate that in developed countries about half of the congenital causes are genetic in origin, whereas most of the acquired conditions are the result of infectious processes. In the developing economies of the south, infections cause a higher proportion of hearing impairment than in the countries of the north.

As sensorineural hearing impairment can have marked effects upon a child's emotional, social and educational development, it is of paramount importance that a hearing loss is detected as early as possible after the causative event and the child be habilitated or rehabilitated.

Genetic hearing impairment

It has been estimated that genetic hearing impairment is 70% autosomal recessive, 25% autosomal dominant and approximately 5% X-linked. Most genetic impairment is non-syndromal, and inheritance is mainly autosomal recessive.

Non-syndromic hearing impairment

Currently, more than 60 gene locations causing non-syndromic hearing impairment have been found. Several genes have been identified, and it has been shown that, in some instances, the same gene can cause both syndromal and non-syndromal hearing impairment. Lalwani and Castelein[4] described the general features of each type of hearing impairment. Non-syndromal autosomal recessive hearing impairment tends to be prelingual in onset, severe to profound in severity, and non-progressive, and involves all frequencies. Non-syndromal autosomal dominant hearing impairment is more variable, with a late onset, and progression, and is often in the high frequencies. In X-linked hearing loss, the onset is usually prelingual, but the clinical phenotype is too variable for generalization.

CAUSES OF HEARING IMPAIRMENT

- Genetic
  - Syndromal
  - Non-syndromal
- Genetic/sporadic
- Chromosomal
- Infections
- Congenital disorders/defects
- Perinatal factors
- Ototoxicity
- Unknown

Syndromal hearing impairment

Autosomal dominant conditions

Waardenburg syndromes (WS) (Figures 24.1 and 24.2)
The syndrome described by Waardenburg[5] was believed to occur in 1 in 42 000 of the population, or 1.43% of the congenitally deaf. Four types have subsequently been reported:

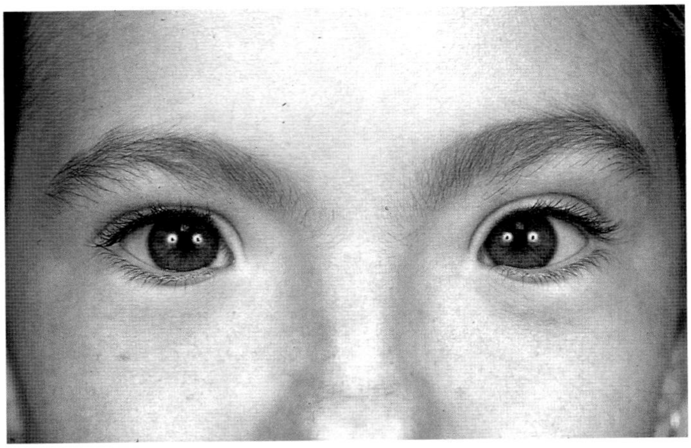

Figure 24.1 The typical eyelid appearance and lateral displacement of the inner canthi seen in Waardenburg syndrome type 1.

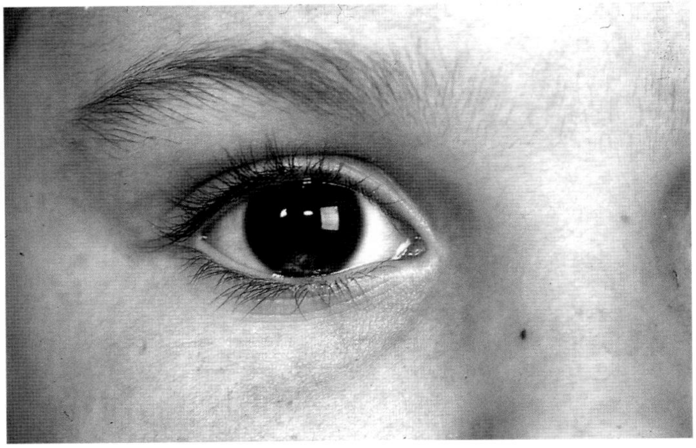

Figure 24.2 A sharply demarcated segment of the iris as found in the Waardenburg syndromes, mainly in type 2.

WS1–3 is autosomal dominantly inherited, whereas WS4 follows an autosomal recessive pattern.

Clinical features include: a white forelock, rarely one which is black or red; complete or partial iris heterochromia—the different-coloured segments are sharply demarcated and usually wedge-shaped; early greying of the hair, which may be poorer in texture; and the eyebrows bushy medially and confluent over the nose. An eyelid anomaly, with lateral displacement of the inner canthi (dystopia canthorum), is a feature of WS1 and WS3, and is associated with a high nasal root and nostrils with reduced flaring. Expressivity of the genes shows considerable inter- and intrafamilial variation.

EXAMPLES OF INHERITED CONDITIONS WITH HEARING IMPAIRMENT

- Autosomal dominant
  - Waardenburg syndrome
  - Marshall–Stickler syndrome
  - Branchio-oto-renal syndrome
  - Osteogenesis imperfecta
- Autosomal recessive
  - Usher syndrome
  - Pendred syndrome
  - Jervell and Lange–Neilsen syndrome
  - Mucopolysaccharidoses
  - Refsum syndrome
  - Cockayne syndrome
- X-Linked
  - Alport syndrome
  - Norrie's syndrome
  - Perilymphatic gusher
- Mitochondrial
  - Kearns–Sayre syndrome
  - MELAS

Balance disorders have been described occasionally.[6] There are radiological studies which indicate that whereas the commonest pathological defect is of the Scheibe or cochleosaccular type, more major defects affecting the vestibular apparatus may occasionally be found. Sprengel's shoulder, cleft palate and spina bifida have been described in association with the syndrome.

WS1 is caused by mutations in the *PAX3* gene on chromosome 2 which encodes a DNA-binding transcription factor. The effect of the mutations is to reduce the amount of protein produced. Expression of *PAX3* is switched on early in development and affects cells of the neural crest. Dystopia canthorum is the most prevalent feature of WS1 and is present in 99% of those affected. Whereas this may be evident clinically, in doubtful cases eye measurements can be used to calculate the W index.[7]

Hearing impairment is found in about 69% of those affected, and profound bilateral hearing impairment is the most common. Occasionally, an ascending audiogram or one depicting a mid-frequency hearing loss may be found, or a unilateral hearing impairment.[8] Pigmentation abnormalities are correlated with the degree of hearing loss, occuring more frequently in those with a severe or profound hearing impairment than in those with normal hearing.[9] Having more than one pigmentation defect increases the likelihood that an affected person will have a severe hearing impairment.

WS2 is a heterogeneous group, a proportion of which have been found to have mutations in the *MITF* gene on chromosome 3. The gene encodes a DNA-binding transcription factor which is believed to influence the pigmentary system. Hearing impairment is commoner in WS2, occuring in 87%, and there is a greater likelihood of asymmetrical hearing loss than in WS1. Partial heterochromia of the iris is more prevalent in WS2 than in WS1.[10]

WS3 is rare and is associated with upper-limb abnormalities in addition to features of WS1. It has been shown to be caused by mutations in *PAX3*, and the label WS3 is now largely redundant.

WS4, or Shah–Waardenburg syndrome, is an autosomal recessive condition consisting of Hirschsprung's disease associated with features of WS2, but is much less common. Patients with mutations in endothelin 3 or the gene for its receptor show this phenotype.

No relationships have been found between particular mutations in any of the genes identified and the phenotypes.

Stickler or Marshall syndrome

These syndromes overlap phenotypically and are often combined as the Marshall–Stickler syndrome. This is a connective tissue disorder with highly variable clinical manifestations.[10] Sensorineural or mixed hearing impairment is associated with various eye, skeletal and facial defects. Hearing impairment is not invariable but, when present, affects particularly the high frequencies and is progressive.

Myopia is the commonest eye defect, with retinal detachment being one of the associated risks. Whereas eye abnormalities are considered to be a main component of the syndrome, families without eye involvement have been reported.[11] Midfacial structures are undeveloped, giving rise to a flattened appearance. The nose is short and saddle-shaped, with anteverted nostrils. The philtrum may be extended. A cleft palate may be present, associated with underdevelopment of the lower jaw.

Arthropathy occurs with radiological signs. Mitral valve prolapse is found in 45% of affected individuals.[12] Genes identified are a type II procollagen gene (*COLIIA1*) on chromosome 12q and the collagen XI gene (*COLIIA2*) on chromosome 6.

Branchio-oto-renal syndrome

This syndrome involves the first and second branchial arches and the renal tract. Prevalence is estimated to be 1 in 40 000. Congenital hearing impairment is the feature found most frequently. In the study of Chen et al,[13] 93% had a hearing impairment. A mixed hearing impairment was the most common type (52%), with conductive (33%) and sensorineural (29%) hearing impairment also found. Different types of hearing impairment may be found in each ear. Hearing loss is usually severe, but can vary from mild to profound and may be either progressive or stable.

There is considerable inter-individual variation in physical signs.[14, 15] Pre-auricular pits are the commonest external feature. The pinna is frequently cup-shaped, and there may be stenosis or atresia of the external auditory canal. Approximately half of those affected have branchial fistulae, which may be unilateral or bilateral. Renal abnormalities vary in severity from mild defects to complete renal aplasia. Branchio-otic syndrome has a similar phenotype to branchio-oto-renal syndrome, but differs in that there is no renal dysplasia.[16]

Pathological defects include cochlear hypoplasia, dilated cochlear and vestibular aqueducts, and hypoplasia of the lateral semicircular canal.[13]

Mutations in *EYA1* are one cause of the syndrome, and a further gene has been localized to 1q31.

Osteogenesis imperfecta

This condition has been divided into four main categories on the basis of the mode of inheritance and the phenotypic appearance. The autosomal dominant type 1 is the most common type encountered.[17] The clinical features include bone fragility, blue sclerae, dentigenous imperfecta and a hearing impairment, and these vary in degree between affected individuals. The basic defect is in collagen type I, and causative genes have been found on chromosomes 7q and 17q.

The pathological defect is a softening of bone leading to ossicular fixation. Whereas initially a conductive hearing impairment is found, this progresses to a mixed hearing loss.

Autosomal recessive conditions

Usher syndromes

Three types have been described (Table 24.1). In type I, the hearing impairment is very severe or profound, and retinitis pigmentosa appears before adolescence. There is absent vestibular function, and children are late at sitting and walking.[18, 19] Six loci have been found, and four gene's—myosin VI1A USH1c or Harmonin, cadherin 23 and Proto cadherin 15.[20] Mutations in myosin VIIA cause USH1B. The protein encoded is present in the stereocilia, the cuticular plate and the synaptic region. It is believed that the protein has an important role in the morphogenesis of stereocilia and in their positional organization.[21]

In type 2, hearing impairment is moderate to severe, with an audiogram which slopes towards the higher frequencies (Figure 24.3). Vestibular function is normal. Retinitis pigmentosa generally appears after adolescence, but there is overlap between types 1 and 2 in this respect. At least two genes are involved in causing USH2,[22] and a gene has been found for USH2a on chromosome 1.[23]

Type 3 appears to be much less common than the other two types. It shows a progressive sensorineural hearing impairment with retinitis pigmentosa and either normal or subnormal vestibular function. The time of onset of retinitis pigmentosa is variable. USH3 in a Finnish family has been localized to chromosome 3q.[24]

An atypical form of Usher syndrome, which has features of USH3, has been found to be caused by a mutation in myosin VIIA.[25] In the 1990s, the genetic heterogeneity of Usher syndrome has begun to be unravelled[26] allowing clarification of phenotype expression.[27]

Table 24.1 Clinical features of the Usher syndromes

Type	Hearing loss	Vestibular function	RP Onset
USH1	Profound	Absent	1st decade
USH2	Moderate to severe	Normal	2nd–3rd decades
USH3	Progressive	Variable	1st or 2nd decade

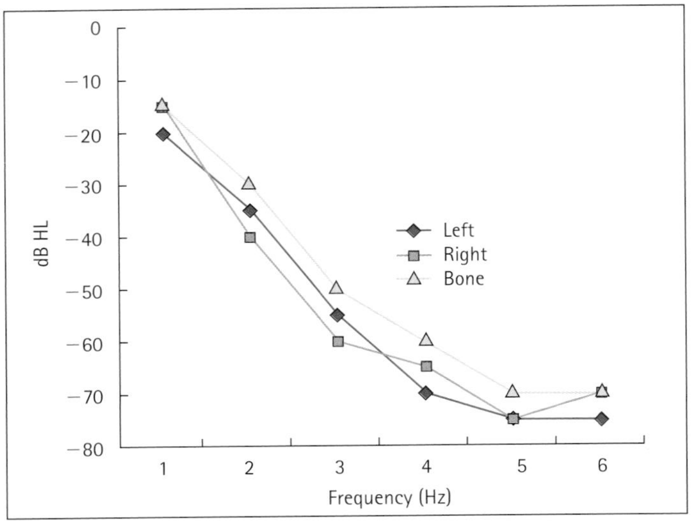

Figure 24.3 An audiometric configuration found frequently in Usher syndrome type 2.

Pendred syndrome

Congenital sensorineural hearing loss is associated with an organization defect of the thyroid gland. The defect is in the incorporation of iodide into the thyroxine molecule.

Hearing impairment is usually severe to profound, and vestibular function may be affected unilaterally or bilaterally. Patients are usually euthyroid, but may be hypothyroid. A goitre tends to appear after the age of 8 years but may be present in infancy. Thirty-six familial cases with linkage to the locus for the Pendred syndrome locus on chromosome 7q were investigated by Reardon et al,[28] and 73% had goitre. The perchlorate discharge test was negative in one instance. The perchlorate test is not always positive in Pendred's syndrome and is positive in other conditions, e.g. Hashimoto's disease.

Radiological abnormalities are found in 86% of affected individuals. Manifestations include Mondini cochleae and a dilated vestibular aqueduct.[29, 30] The latter is almost a constant feature.[29] Enlargement of the endolymphatic sac and duct in association with a dilated vestibular aqueduct was found in all 20 patients described by Phelps et al.[30]

A gene has been found on chromosome 7 which encodes a protein, pendrin, which is believed to be involved in ion transportation.

Jervell and Lange-Neilsen syndrome

In 1957, Jervell and Lange-Neilsen described a condition in which hearing impairment is associated with electrocardiographic changes. The prevalence of this condition is believed to be 1 in 100 000, and it involves congenital sensorineural hearing loss with a conduction defect of the heart. Typical electrocardiographic findings are a prolongation of the QT interval and inversion of the T wave.

Affected individuals have a bradycardia and this can be present in utero.[31] They are prone to develop arrhythmias in conditions of stress or exercise. There may be a history of syncopal attacks, usually lasting 3–5 min, or there may just be brief periods of altered consciousness. During these episodes, ventricular fibrillation or asystole may occur. These syncopal attacks may appear in infancy or later. Heterozygotes may also be prone to changes in heart rhythm.

It has been discovered that homozygous *KVLQT1* mutations cause the hearing impairment in this condition as a result of causing a truncated protein. The *KVLQT1* gene has been shown to be expressed in the stria vascularis in mice.[32] Autosomal dominant long-QT syndrome results from a mutation in *KVLQT1* in which affected individuals are heterozygous. *KVLQT1* protein joins with minK protein to form cardiac Iks potassium channels, and it is known that the gene encoding minK is expressed in the inner ear and that the protein affects the production of endolymph.[31]

Mucopolysaccharidoses (Figure 24.4)

These are a group of lysosomal storage diseases caused by an enzyme deficiency. The most common of these, Hurler's disease (MPS1), is due to an α-L-iduronidase deficiency. This results in an accumulation of glycosamines in the tissues and excretion of these in the urine. Hunter's disease (MPS 11) is the only one of these conditions which is X-linked, all others being inherited as autosomal recessive disorders.

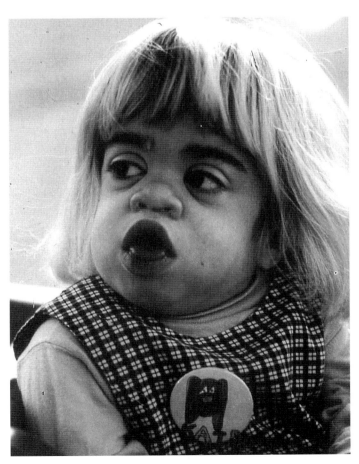

Figure 24.4 The typical facies of Hurler's syndrome.

Hearing impairment in the mucopolysaccharidoses is not invariable but, when it occurs, it is usually mixed.[33] There is evidence to indicate that bone marrow transplantation can result in stabilization of hearing or, in some instances, an improvement.[34, 35]

Refsum syndrome

This is a phytanic acid storage disease with peripheral neuropathy, cerebellar ataxia, retinitis pigmentosa, cardiac defects, and sensorineural hearing impairment.[36, 37] Treatment is with a diet low in phytol and phytanic acid.[38]

Cockayne syndrome

This premature ageing disorder is believed to be a form of leukodystrophy. The condition is characterized clinically by short stature, mental retardation, ataxia, retinal pigmentation and sensorineural hearing impairment. Hearing is normal initially and then deteriorates as the condition progresses. It has been suggested that the site of lesion is both peripheral and also involves the brainstem.[39]

X-linked conditions

Alport syndrome

Glomerulonephritis is associated with an acquired sensorineural hearing loss. About 85% of cases show an X-linked dominant inheritance, and about 10% autosomal recessive inheritance; a few cases of autosomal dominant transmission have also been described.[40] In the X-linked form, males are more severely affected than females; this is thought to be due to different patterns of X-chromosome inactivation in females.[41] In the autosomal recessive and autosomal dominant forms, males and females are equally affected.

In a study of 30 patients, Sirimanna and Stephens[42] found that 87% had a symmetrical hearing loss and 53% of the audiograms had a 'trough'configuration. Hearing loss was progressive, with the higher frequencies becoming involved after the middle frequencies. Hearing impairment was not necessarily correlated with severity of the renal involvement. Carriers have either a sensorineural hearing loss or dips in audiometric thresholds determined using the Audioscan method.[43]

Norrie's syndrome

Progressive sensorineural hearing loss is associated with optic atrophy and neurological deficits. The onset may be in childhood.

X-linked hearing impairment with perilymphatic gusher

This condition may become evident in the first years of life and is associated with progressive hearing impairment. Either a sensorineural or mixed hearing impairment may be found.[44] A CT scan may show a bulbous internal auditory meatus, deficient bone at the fundus of the internal auditory meatus, and a dilated facial canal.[45] The perilymphatic gusher becomes apparent if the stapes footplate is disturbed during surgery.

The condition has been found to be the result of mutations in *POU3F4*, which encodes a transcription factor. Fifty per cent of carrier females are reported to have abnormal audiograms, and affected males have vestibular abnormalities.[46]

Mitochondrial conditions

Mitochondrial mutations give rise to syndromal and non-syndromal sensorineural hearing impairment. Syndromal conditions include Kearns–Sayre syndrome, in which there is a progressive high-frequency sensorineural hearing loss, and MELAS (myoclonus, encephalopathy, lactic acidosis and stroke-like episodes), in which a high-frequency hearing loss may start in the second decade.

Mitochondrial mutations are believed to account for at least 2% of non-syndromal sensorineural hearing impairment of childhood origin.[47] One of the earliest mutations to be described was the A1555G mutation, which conveys a susceptibility to develop a sensorineural hearing impairment after the administration of aminoglycosides.[48] The hearing loss is non-syndromal and will develop eventually even if aminoglycosides are not given.

Hutchin et al[47] described mtDNA mutations—*A7445G*, *T7510*, and *A3243G*—in subjects with a family history of hearing impairment. The age of onset of the sensorineural hearing loss and severity varied widely in the families although the loss was always progressive. In a further article, Hutchin et al[49] described six families in which the heteroplasmic *7472insC* mutation in the *TRNA2*$^{ser(UCN)}$ gene was present. This mutation causes sensorineural hearing impairment associated with various neurological abnormalities, including ataxia and progressive myoclonic epilepsy.

Genetic/sporadic

Some conditions usually occur sporadically, but occasionally an inherited pattern is described.

Wildervanck syndrome

This syndrome is characterized by the Klippel–Feil anomalad, Duane retraction syndrome and congenital hearing impairment. Wildervanck specified sensorineural hearing impairment when defining the syndrome, but since then conductive and mixed hearing impairment has been described.[50, 51] The syndrome is found with a 10 to 1 female preponderance.

The Klippel–Feil anomalad consists of variable degrees of fusion of the spine occuring in the cervical, thoracic and sometimes the lumbar regions, associated with congenital hearing loss. The typical clinical appearance is of a short neck and a low posterior hairline. Associated features include Sprengel's shoulder. Hearing impairment may be mixed, sensorineural or conductive and unilateral as well as bilateral

EXAMPLES OF GENETIC/SPORADIC SYNDROMES AND ASSOCIATIONS

- Wildervanck syndrome
- Cornelia-de-Lange syndrome
- Noonan syndrome
- CHARGE association

hearing impairment has been described. Conductive hearing impairment is due to ossicular abnormalities.

Duane syndrome consists of lateral rectus palsy, with the globe of the affected eye being retracted on adduction. Sensorineural hearing impairment was found in 12 of 176 patients described by Kirkham.[52]

Radiological abnormalities of the inner ear in Wildervanck syndrome have shown a variety of abnormalitites, including Mondini deformities, absent modioli, and dilated vestibules.[53]

Cornelia de Lange syndrome (Figure 24.5)

The syndrome, also known as Brachmann de Lange syndrome, is characterized by multiple congenital malformations, otolaryngological abnormalities and intellectual disability. The otological abnormalities include external canal stenosis and cleft palate. Upper-limb abnormalities occur, and slight, moderate or severe sensorineural hearing impairment may be found.[54] The syndrome is often sporadic, but may be dominantly inherited.[55]

Noonan syndrome (Figure 24.6)

This syndrome was first described in 1963, and it is estimated that the prevalence is between 1 in 1000 and 1 in 2500 live births. Characteristic facies are found and cardiac defects, the most frequent of which is pulmonary valve stenosis due to a dysplastic or thickened valve. Aortic valve involvement can occur, and also dysplasia of other valves. Short stature, undescended testes, and intellectual disability may be present. Ocular manifestations include epicanthal folds, ptosis, hypertelorism, downward-slanting palpebral fissures and ocular proptosis. Hearing impairment may be progressive.

CHARGE association (Figure 24.7)

This represents a spectrum of defects, the name being an acronym for **C**oloboma, **H**eart, **A**tretic choanae, **R**etarded growth, **G**enital hypoplasia and **E**ar abnormalities. Additional

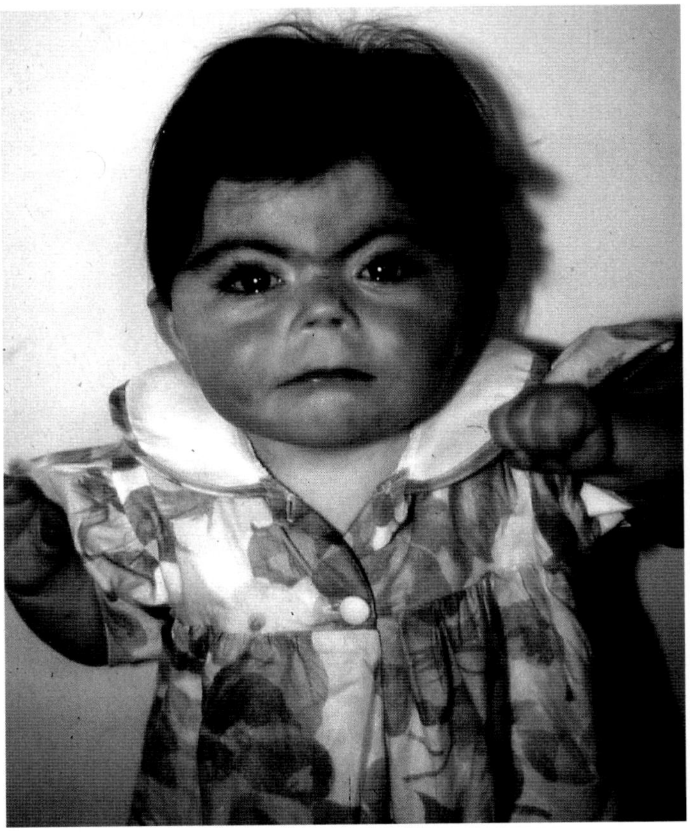

Figure 24.5 Cornelia-de-Lange syndrome, showing the typical facies and low hairline.

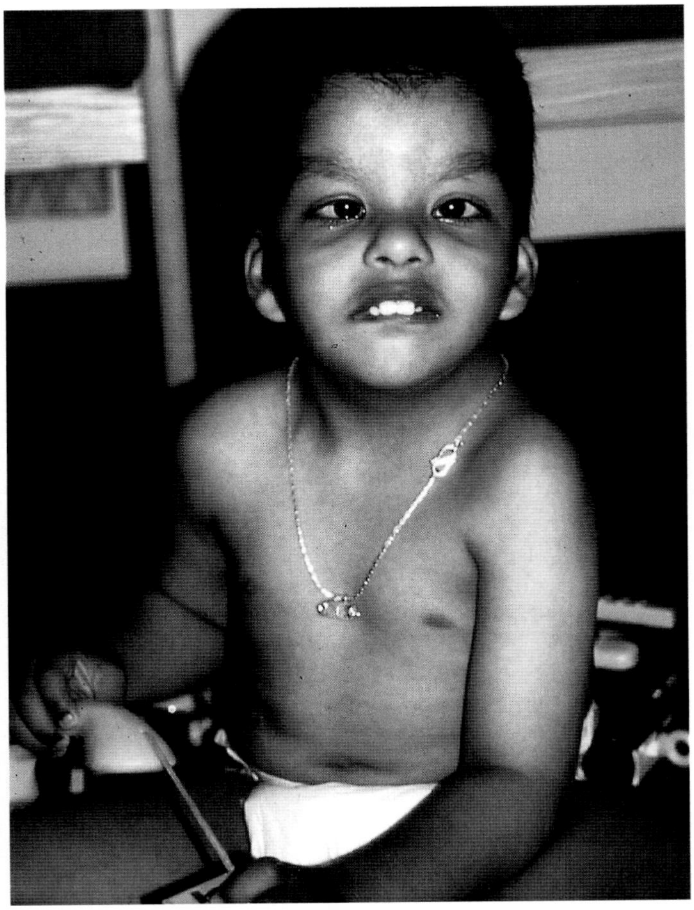

Figure 24.6 A child with Noonan's syndrome showing low-set ears.

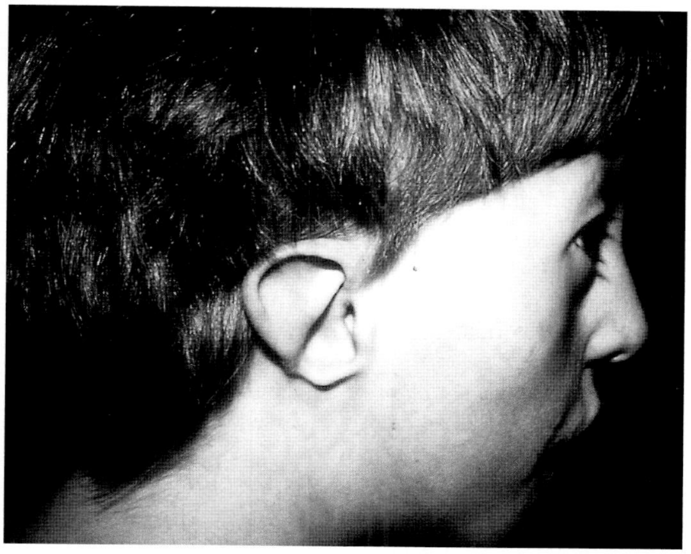

Figure 24.7 The cup-shaped pinna frequently found in CHARGE association.

abnormalities include facial weakness and orofacial clefting. The condition is usually sporadic but has been reported to be familial.[56]

The external ear is affected frequently, the ears being typically low set and cup-shaped. Hearing impairment is common and is usually severe. In a study described by Edwards et al,[57] 5 of 21 children had a sensorineural hearing impairment, four a bilateral mixed hearing impairment, and two a mixed hearing impairment in one ear and a conductive hearing loss in the other. Two of the children had cochlear dysplasias.

On the whole, a mixed hearing impairment is the most common type of hearing impairment, but sensorineural and conductive hearing impairment have been described. A characteristic radiological feature is absence of the semicircular canals.[58]

Chromosomal abnormalities

A number of chromosomal abnormalities are associated with sensorineural or mixed hearing impairment. Some of these are unique, e.g. as a result of rearrangements of chromosomes, deletions or extra chromosomal material. Examples of conditions associated with hearing loss of inner ear origin are as follows.

CHROMOSOMAL ABNORMALITIES WITH HEARING IMPAIRMENT

- Down's syndrome
- Turner's syndrome
- Trisomy 13
- Trisomy 18

Down's syndrome

Congenital sensorineural hearing impairment is found in about 5% of children born with Down's syndrome. Bilgin et al[59] found that those with Down's syndrome had a shorter cochlea than controls. A Mondini defect was identified in some, and a reduced number of spiral ganglion cells.

In a larger proportion, the hearing impairment is conductive, mainly as a result of otitis media with effusion, but also due to congenital ossicular abnormalities, usually affecting the stapes. Affected individuals may have pinna abnormalities and a narrow external auditory canal.

Turner's syndrome

The XO phenotype typically has low-set ears with rotation, a webbed neck, nuchal lymphoedema, short stature, shield-shaped chest, cubitus valgus, ovarian dysgenesis, congenital heart disease (coarctation of the aorta), and renal abnormalities, including horseshoe kidney. Various mosaics have been described.

There is a predisposition to otitis media. A history of otitis media was found in 21 of 24 patients, and sensorineural hearing impairment is progressive. Progression began in late childhood or early adulthood in 7 of 24 patients described by Sculerati et al.[60] Auricular abnormalitites and hearing loss due to otitis media are reported to occur more frequently in those with a total deletion of the p-arm of the chromosome rather than a partial deletion, possibly as a result of a loss of growth-regulating genes, e.g *SHOX*.[61]

Benazzo et al[62] examined 62 patients with Turner's syndrome aged 5–32 years, and found 13 to have a bilateral symmetrical sensorineural hearing loss; nine of these had a progressive high-frequency impairment, and the remaining four a dip in the mid-frequency range. In eight cases, the hearing loss was thought to be cochlear, and in five retrocochlear.

Radiological abnormalities have been found in the external ear and in the internal auditory meatus. An abnormal downward slope was seen in the external auditory canals, and the internal auditory meati were short, wide and sometimes asymmetrical.[62]

Trisomy 13

This is also known as Patau syndrome. Inner ear abnormalities are associated with middle ear and external ear malformations. Multiple abnormalities occur, including cardiac defects. Partial trisomies are more likely to survive into childhood. More than 50% of cases have a hearing impairment.

Trisomy 18

Edward's syndrome is found in about 0.3% of newborn babies. Multiple abnormalitites occur, including cardiac and renal defects. Ears may be low set, with deformed pinnae, and hearing impairment can be profound.

Infections

Infections are the cause of both congenital and acquired hearing impairment. The main infections giving rise to congenital hearing impairment are rubella, cytomegalovirus, toxoplasmosis and herpes simplex. Postnatal hearing impairment is mainly the result of organisms giving rise to meningitis or measles and mumps. In some countries in the northern hemisphere rubella, measles and mumps have been almost eliminated as a result of immunization programmes. The introduction of the HIB vaccine has also been effective in reducing this type of meningitis.

> **INFECTIONS**
>
> - Prenatal
>   - Rubella
>   - Cytomegalovirus
>   - Toxoplasmosis
>   - Syphilis
>   - Herpes simplex
> - Postnatal
>   - Meningitis
>   - Measles
>   - Mumps

Prenatal

Rubella

The risk of fetal infection is estimated as 75–90% after primary maternal infection in the first trimester, 25–39% in the second trimester, and 24–53% in the third trimester.[56]

There may be a history of contact, and the mother may develop a rash associated with cervical lymphadenopathy, or the infection could be subclinical.

Fetal infections in the first trimester usually result in eye, heart and ear defects, whereas sensorineural hearing impairment and pigmentary retinopathy are the only accompanying sequelae to infections in the middle or even the last trimester of pregnancy.[63] Hearing impairment is mainly sensorineural and bilateral, but unilateral hearing impairment may occur. Progression of hearing impairment is not infrequent.

Diabetes mellitus was found to be overt or latent in 20% of young adults with conigental rubella syndrome (CRS).[64]

Cytomegalovirus

Congenital infection of the fetus occurs mainly after a primary infection, but can occur after a secondary infection. The transmission rate is 20–50% after a primary maternal infection.[65] It is estimated that 1% of newborns are congenitally infected.[66] The majority of congenital infections are asymptomatic. Hearing impairment is more likely to follow a symptomatic rather than an asymptomatic infection. Periventricular radiolucencies or calcifications seen on a CT scan indicate an increased risk for hearing impairment.[67]

Fetal damage can occur in all three trimesters with apparently equal frequency.[66] Symptomatic infections are more likely to occur when infections occur in the first half of pregnancy. Hearing loss is more likely to follow a primary infection.[68] Hearing impairment is found in about 10% of those affected and is most commonly bilateral but can be unilateral. It is frequently progressive.

Deterioration has been documented up to the age of 4 years.[67] Other associated defects include language disorders and intellectual disability.

Toxoplasmosis

This is a protozoal infection, and primary infections occur with a frequency of 0.1–1%. Fetal infection occurs in 40% of cases.[69] Most infections are asymptomatic but, after a period, choroidoretinitis can develop, together with other neurological signs.[70] Hearing impairment is sensorineural, is usually bilateral, and may be mild, or more severe and profound. Toxoplasmosis has also been implicated in acquired hearing impairment.

Detection of infections is important, as treatment is possible. Early treatment and/or prolonged antimicrobial therapy were considered to be the possible reasons why none of the 30 children with congenital infections investigated by McGee et al[71] had a sensorineural hearing impairment.

Syphilis

Congenital syphilis is a cause of potentially reversible sensorineural hearing impairment. Ampicillin combined with steroids is effective in preventing hearing from becoming progressively worse.[72] Pathologically, endolymphatic hydrops occurs, together with degeneration of the organ of Corti and of the spiral ganglion.[73] Karmody and Schukneckt found that hearing impairment in childhood usually presented with a sudden onset of profound bilateral symmetrical hearing impairment without symptoms of vestibular disturbance.[73]

Herpes simplex

Sensorineural hearing impairment has been described after symptomatic neonatal herpes infection.

Postnatal

Meningitis

Meningitis is the main cause of acquired sensorineural hearing loss in children. It has been estimated that about 10% of children having a bacterial meningitis develop a hearing impairment. Bacterial meningitis is more likely than viral meningitis to result in hearing impairment. It is the most common single defect following meningitis, but may be associated with other neurological sequelae. Hearing loss is present early in the infection.[74] Given early in *Haemophilus influenzae* infections, dexamethasone may prevent a hearing impairment or cause a hearing impairment to be less severe than it might otherwise have been. In pneumococcal meningitis, dexamethasone was effective if given before or concomitantly with antibiotics.[75]

Streptococcus pneumoniae; *Neisseria meningitidis* and *Haemophilus influenzae* are the most common organisms involved. They are believed to cause a labyrinthitis which, if septic, may lead to a permanent hearing impairment. An aseptic labyrinthitis is thought to account for cases of temporary hearing loss.

Hearing loss is usually bilateral but may be unilateral. It is often profound. Occasionally, the high frequencies are preserved and a low-frequency ascending audiogram is obtained. Occasionally, there is progression of the hearing loss as a result of ossification of the lumen of the cochlea or fibrosis around blood vessels. Ossification of the lumen of the cochlea has important consequences for cochlear implantation (Figure 24.8). The time of onset is variable, and so children with a profound hearing impairment following meningitis should be referred early to cochlear implant programmes. Delay may result in full insertion of the implant device not being possible.

Loss of balance is usually associated with hearing loss as a result of meningitis, and may be present early in the course of the infection.

Measles

Hearing impairment after measles is usually bilateral and can be moderate or profound. A temporal bone study of hamster cochleae showed atrophy of the stria vascularis, loss of the organ of Cortia, 'rolled-up' tectorial membrane and cell infiltration into the scala media.[76]

Mumps

There is an acute onset of sensorineural hearing loss, usually unilateral but sometimes bilateral.[77] Hearing loss is usually profound and can be reversible. Disequilibrium can develop as a result of vestibular involvement.

Some children have developed a sensorineural hearing loss after mumps, measles and rubella vaccination (MMR), and this is thought to be related to the mumps component.[78]

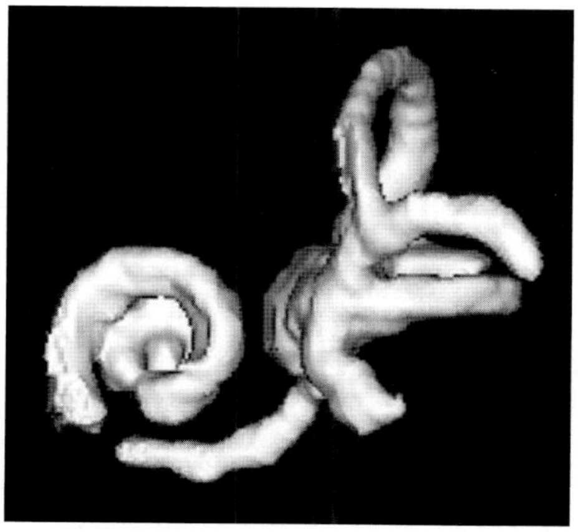

Figure 24.8 Surface shaded rendering MRI image of labyrinth with oclusive changes post meningitis.

Congenital disorders/defects

These account for a very small proportion of cases of hearing impairment.

Congenital hypothyroidism

The prevalence of primary congenital hypothyroidism is estimated as being between 1 in 3000 and 4000 live births. Unilateral or bilateral sensorineural hearing impairment may be found, mainly affecting the higher frequencies.[79] Mild impairment of auditory and vestibular function may be found in children, in spite of early treatment with thyroxine.[80] In this study, the severity of the abnormalities was related to the degree of hypothyroidism prior to treatment. In the study described by Rovet et al,[79] the age of onset of the hearing impairment was related to the presence of hearing impairment but not to disease severity or duration.

Perilymphatic fistula

This is an abnormal communication between the perilymphatic space and the middle ear. Perilymphatic fistulae may be congenital and associated with abnormalities of the inner ear, or they may be acquired, e.g. as a result of trauma. A retrospective study of 94 children (117 ears) by Weber et al[81] found that the majority had middle ear abnormalities but 16 (17%) children had inner ear abnormalities. Of the 25 ears with abnormalities of the inner ear, 14 had a dilated vestibular aqueduct, 7 had Mondini defects and 3 had 'Mondini-like' deformities.

Children present with a fluctuating progressive or sudden sensorineural hearing loss accompanied by tinnitus and with or without vertigo. Vertigo may be present with or without loss of hearing.[81, 82]

The degree of trauma needed to produce a fistula is not necessarily severe, and coughing, sneezing or straining may be sufficient.

Perinatal causes

There are several factors surrounding births which have the potential for causing a hearing impairment. Hypoxia may result from birth asphyxia or from recurrent episodes of apnoea and cause a sensorineural hearing impairment. Prolonged pre-peri- and postnatal hypoxia–ischaemia is a more important factor than pure hypoxia as a cause of both brain and ear damage during delivery.[83] Hearing impairment is found more frequently in children who have neurodevelopmental deficits after perinatal asphyxia than in those without such defects.[84]

PERINATAL FACTORS

- Low gestation/birthweight
- Hypoxia–ischaemia
- Hyperbilirubinaemia
- Sepsis
- Ototoxic drugs

Hyperbilirubinaemia may result in the deposition of bilirubin in the cochlear nuclei and cause a sensorineural hearing loss. The level of hyperbilirubinaemia which is potentially damaging depends upon the age of gestation of the baby. Those babies with sufficiently high levels to warrant exchange transfusion are considered to be at risk for developing sensorineural hearing impairment.

Low-gestation babies may be exposed to a number of potentially damaging factors. They have a greater vulnerability to the effects of hypoxia–ischaemia than full-term babies. They are more prone to hyperbilirubinaemia and more susceptible to its effects. In addition, they may develop sepsis around the time of birth, and this can potentiate the effects of hyperbilirubinaemia. Treatment of the infections with aminoglycosides presents an additional risk for sensorineural hearing impairment.

In spite of the occurrence of sensorineural hearing impairment after perinatal trauma, many babies emerge unscathed.[85, 86] It is, therefore, possible that babies who develop a hearing impairment may do so as a result of other causations, and the birth history may be a result of these conditions or be unrelated to the hearing impairment.

Ototoxicity

Children may be exposed to potentially ototoxic drugs in utero, in the perinatal period or postnatally, in particular, drugs for the treatment of severe sepsis, drugs which are used to control fluid and electrolyte balance and cytotoxic agents.

Aminoglycosides are bacteriocidal agents which are effective against Gram-negative infections. They are both ototoxic and nephrotoxic. Hypersensitivity to aminoglycosides occurs during the period of development of the inner ear. This is also a period when there is hypersensitivity to loop diuretics and especially to the combination of these with aminoglycosides.[87]

The aminoglycosides differ with regard to the degree to which they affect the cochlea or the vestibular apparatus. The mechanisms involved in causing ototoxicity are not fully understood, but it is believed that the ototoxic effects of gentamicin are caused by a metabolized form of the drug via an iron–gentamicin complex which produces free radicals.[88] Outer hair cells are destroyed preferentially in the basal turn and then extend towards the apex. Later, there is damage to the inner hair cells. Children with renal disease are at greater risk of ototoxic side-effects, as the drugs are excreted via the renal tract. Careful monitoring of the peak and trough levels is necessary to prevent potentially harmful serum levels.

Unknown

In spite of aetiological investigations, a definite cause for a hearing impairment may not be identified. In these instances, the cause is believed in most cases to be genetic. Lench et al[89] reported finding connexin 26 mutations in isolated cases of hearing impairment. With the rapid advances being made in molecular genetics, the 'unknown' causation group will, in time, increasingly diminish in numbers. Parker et al,[90] in a population-based investigation, found that 10% of those with a non-syndromal hearing loss had a connexin 26 35 delG mutation.

Conclusion

There are many potential causes of a sensorineural hearing impairment in childhood, and children found to be hearing impaired should have the causation of their hearing loss investigated as soon as possible after detection. Identification of the cause is becoming increasingly possible, and clinicians need to keep abreast of new developments, particularly in the field of medical genetics.

References

1. Davis A, Wood S, Healy R, Webb H, Rowe S. Risk factors for hearing disorders: epidemiological evidence of change over time in the UK. *J Am Acad Audiol* 1995; **6**: 365–70.
2. Mencher GT, Madriz Alfaro JJ. Prevalence of sensorineural hearing loss in children in Costa Rica. *Audiology* 2000; **39**: 278–83.
3. Prasansuk S. Incidence/prevalence of sensorineural hearing impairment in Thailand and Southeast Asia. **39**: 207–11.
4. Lalwani AK, Castelein CM. Cracking the genetic code: non-syndromic hereditary hearing impairment. *Am J Otol* 1999; **20**: 115–32.
5 Waardenburg PJ. A new syndrome combining developmental anomalies of the eyelids, eyebrows and nose root with pigmentary defects of the iris and head hair and with congenital deafness. *Am J Med Genet* 1951; **3**: 195–253.
6. Hageman M, Oosteveld WJ. Vestibular findings in 23 patients with Waardenburg syndrome. *Acta Otolaryngol* 1977; **103**: 648–52.
7. Read AP, Newton VE. Waardenburg syndrome. *J Med Genet* 1997; **34**: 656–65.

8. Newton VE. Hearing loss in Waardenburg syndrome. *J Laryngol Otol* 1990; **104**: 97–103.
9. Newton VE, Liu X, Read A. The association of sensorineural hearing loss and pigmentation abnormalities in Waardenburg syndrome. *J Audiol Med* 1994; **3**: 69–77.
10. Zlogotora J, Sagi M, Schuper A et al. Variability of Stickler syndrome. *Am J Med Genet* 1992; **42**: 337–9.
11. Sirko-Osadsa D, Murray MA, Scott JA et al. Stickler syndrome without eye involvement is caused by mutations in COL11A2, the gene encoding the a2 (X1) chain of type X1 collagen. *J Pediatrics* 1996; **132**: 368–71.
12. Liberfarb RM, Goldblatt A. Prevalence of mitral valve prolapse in the Stickler syndrome. *Am J Med Genet* 1986; **24**: 387–92.
13. Chen A, Francis M, Ni L et al. Phenotypic manifestations of branchio-oto-renal syndrome. *Am J Med Genet* 1995; **58**: 365–70.
14. Smith PG, Dyches T, Loomis RA. Clinical aspects of branchio-oto-renal syndrome. *Otolaryngol Head Neck Surg* 1984; **92**: 468–75.
15. Smith RJH, Kimberling WJ. Branchio-oto-renal syndrome. In: Martini A, Read A, Stephens D, eds. *Genetics and Hearing Impairment*. London: Whurr Publishers. 1996: 180–4.
16. Kumar S, Marres HA, Cremers CW et al. Autosomal-dominant branchio-otic (BO) syndrome is not allelic to the branchio-oto-renal (BOR) gene at 8q13. *Am J Med Genet* 1998; **76**: 395–401.
17. Beighton P. Auditory dysfunction in genetic disorders of the skeleton. In: Martini A, Read A, Stephens D, eds. *Genetics and Hearing Impairment*. London: Whurr Publishers, 1996: 130–40
18. Smith RJH, Peliaz MZ, Daiger S et al. Clinical variability and genetic heterogeneity within the Arcadian Usher Population. *Am J Med Genet* 1992; **43**: 964–9.
19. Smith RJH, Berlin CI, Hejtmancik JF et al. Clinical diagnosis of the Usher syndromes, Usher Syndrome Consortium. *Am J Med Genet* 1994; **50**: 32–8.
20. Astuto LM, Weston MD, Carney CA et al. Genetic heterogeneity of Usher syndrome: analysis of 151 families with Usher syndrome type 1. *Am J Hum Genet* 2002; **67**: 1569–74.
21. E1-Amraoui A, Petit C. Towards a molecular understanding of the pathophysiology of Usher syndrome. *J Audiol Med* 1997; **6**: 170–84.
22. Eudy JD, Weston MD, Yao S et al. Mutation of a gene encoding a protein with extracellular matrix motifs in Ushers Syndrome type IIa. *Science* 1998; **280**: 1753–7.
23. Leroy BP et al. Spectrum of mutations in USH2A in British patients with Usher syndrome type II. *Exp Eye Res* 2001; **72**: 503–9.
24. Pakarinen L, Karjalainen S, Smola KOJ et al. Usher's syndrome type 3 in Finland. *Laryngoscope* 1995; **105**: 613–17.
25. Liu XZ, Hope C, Walsh J et al. Mutations in the myosin VII A gene causing a wide phenotypic spectrum including atypical Usher syndrome. *Am J Med Genet* 1998; **63**: 909–12.
26. Petit C. Usher syndrome: from genetics to pathogenesis. *Annu Rev Genomics Hum Genet* 2001; **2**: 271–97.
27. Otterstedde et al. A new clinical classification for Usher's syndrome based on a new subtype of Usher's syndrome type 1. *Laryngoscope* 2001; **111**: 84–6.
28. Reardon W, Coffey R, Phelps PD et al. Pendred syndrome—100 years of underascertainment. *Q J Med* 1997; **90**: 443–7.
29. Cremers WR, Bolder C, Admiraal RJ et al. Progressive sensorineural hearing loss and a widened vestibular aqueduct in Pendred syndrome. *Arch Otolaryngol Head and Neck Surg* 1998; **124**: 501–5.
30. Phelps PD, Coffey RA, Trembath RC et al. Radiological manifestations of the ear in Pendred's syndrome. *Clin Radiol* 1998; **53**: 268–73.
31. Splawski I, Timothy KW, Vincent GM et al. Molecular basis of the long-QT syndrome associated with deafness. *N Engl J Med* 1997; **336**: 1562–7.
32. Neyroud N, Tesson F, Denjoy I et al. A novel mutation in the potassium channel gene causes the Jervell and Lange-Neilsen cardio-auditory syndrome. *Nature Genet* 1997; **15**: 186–9.
33. Briedenkamp JK, Smith ME, Dudley JP et al. Otolaryngologic manifestations of the mucopolysaccharidoses. *Ann Otol Rhinol Laryngol* 1992; **101**: 472–8.
34. Griffon N, Souillet G, Maire I et al. Follow up of nine patients with Hurler syndrome after bone marrow transplantation. *J Pediatrics* 1998; **133**: 119–25.
35. Papsin BC, Vellodi A, Bailey CM et al. Otologic and laryngologic manifestations of mucopolysaccharidoses after bone marrow transplantations. *Otolaryngol Head Neck Surg* 1998; **118**: 30–6.
36. Refsum S. Heredopathia atactica polyneuritiformis phytanic-acid storage disease, Refsum's disease: a biochemically well-defined disease with a specific dietary treatment. *Arch Neurol* 1981; **38**: 605–6.
37. Wierzbicki AS, Lloyd MD, Schofield CJ, Feher MD, Gibberd FB. Refsum's disease: a peroxisomal disorder affecting phytanic acid alpha-oxidation. *J Neurochem* 2002; **80**: 727–35.
38. Brown PJ, Mei G, Gibberd FB, Burston D, Mayne PD, McClinchy JE, Sidey M. Diet and Refsum's disease. The determination of phytanic acid and phytol in certain foods and the application of this knowledge to the choice of suitable convenience foods for patients with Refsum's disease. *J Hum Nut Diet* 1993; **6**: 295–305.
39. Iwisake S, Kaga K. Chronological changes of brainstem responses in Cockayne's syndrome. *Int J Pediatr Otorhinolaryngol* 1994; **30**: 211–21.
40. Brunner HG. Alport syndrome. In: Martini A, Read A, Stephens D, eds. *Genetics and Hearing Impairment*. London: Whurr Publishers, 1996: 166–71.
41. Vetrie D, Flinter F, Bobrow M, Harris A. X inactivation patterns in females with Alport syndrome: a means of selecting against a deleterious gene? *J Med Genet* 1992; **29**: 663–6.
42. Sirimanna T, Stephens D. Hearing loss in Alport's syndrome. *J Audiol Med* 1997; **6**: 71–8.
43. Sirimanna T, France L, Stephens D. Alport's syndrome: can the carriers be identified by audiometry? *Clin Otolaryngol* 1995; **20**: 158–63.
44. Nance WE. Genetic counselling for the hearing impaired. *Audiology* 1971; 222–3.
45. Reardon W, Bellman S, Phelps P, Pembrey M, Luxon L. Neuro-otological function in X-linked hearing loss: a multipedigree assessment and correlation with other clinical parameters. *Acta Otolaryngol* 1993; **113**: 706–14.

46. Brunner HG. X-linked hearing loss. In: Martini A, Read A, Stephens D, eds. *Genetics of Hearing Impairment*. London: Whurr Publishers, 1996: 231–5.
47. Hutchin TP, Thompson KR, Parker M, Newton V, Bitner-Glindzicx M, Mueller RF. Prevalence of mitochondrial DNA mutations in childhood/congenital onset non-syndromal sensorineural hearing impairment. *J Med Genet* 2000; **38:** 3–5.
48. Prezant TR, Agapian JV, Bohlmann MC et al. Mitochondrial ribosomal RNA mutation associated with both antibiotic-induced and non-syndromic deafness. *Nature Genet* **4**: 289–94.
49. Hutchin TP, Navarro-Coy NC, Van Camp G et al. Multiple origins of the mtDNA 7472insC mutation associated with hearing loss and neurological dysfunction. *Eur J Hum Genet* 2001; **9**: 385–7.
50. Wildervanke. The cervico-oculo-acousticus syndrome. In: Vinken PJ, Bruyn GW, Myranthopoulos NC, eds. *Handbook of Clinical Neurology*. Amsterdam: North-Holland, 1978: 123–30.
51. Cremers CWRJ, Hoogland GA, Kuypers W. Hearing loss in the cervico-oculoacoustic (Wildervanck) syndrome. *Arch Otolaryngol* 1984; **110**: 54–7.
52. Kirkham TH. Inheritance of Duane's syndrome. *Br J Opthalmol* 1970; **54**: 323–9.
53. West PDB, Gholkar A, Ramsden RT. Wildervanck's syndrome—unilateral Mondini dysplasia identified by computed tomography. *J Laryngol Otol* 1989; **103**: 408–11.
54. Marres HAM, Cremers CWRJ, Jongbloet PH. Hearing levels in the Cornelia de Lange syndrome. A report of seven cases. *Int J Pediatr Otorhinolaryngol* 1989; **18**: 31–7.
55. Robinson LK, Wolfsberg E, Lyons Jones K. Brachmann de Lange syndrome: evidence for autosomal dominant inheritance. *Am J Med Genet* 1985; **22**: 109–15.
56. Metlay LA, Smythe PS, Miller ME. Familial CHARGE syndrome: clinical report with autopsy findings. *Am J Med Genet* 1987; **26**: 577–81.
57. Edwards BM, van Riper LA, Kileny PR. Clinical manifestations of CHARGE Association. *Int J Pediatr Otorhinolaryngol* 1995; **33**: 23–42.
58. Morgan D, Bailey M, Phelps P et al. Ear nose–throat abnormalities in the CHARGE Association. *Arch Otolaryngol Head Neck Surg* 1993; **119**: 49–54.
59. Bilgin H, Kasemsuwan L, Schachern PA et al. Temporal bone study of Down's syndrome. *Arch Laryngol Head Neck Surg* 1996; **122**: 271–5.
60. Sculerati N, Oddoux C, Clayton CM et al. Hearing loss in Turner syndrome. *Laryngoscope* 1996; **106**: 992–7.
61. Barrenas M-L, Nylen O, Hansen C. The influence of karyotype on the auricle, otitis media and hearing in Turner syndrome. *Hear Res* 1999; **138**: 163–70.
62. Benazzo M, Lanza L, Cerniglia M et al. Otological and audiological aspects in Turner syndrome. *J Audiol Med* 1997; **6**: 147–59.
63. Griffiths KH. In: Kerr AG, Stephens D, eds. *Scott Brown's Otolaryngology*, Vol. 2, 6th edn. London: Butterworths, 1997: 7–12.
64. Wolinsky JS. Rubella. In: Fields BN, Knipe DM, Howley PM et al, eds. Field's *Virology*. Philadelphia: Lippincott-Raven Publishers, 1996: 899–921.
65. Marres HAM. Congenital abnormalities of the inner ear. In: Ludman H, Wright T, eds. *Diseases of the Ear*. London: Arnold, 288–9.
66. Nelson CT, Demmler GJ. Cytomegalovirus infection in the pregnant mother, foetus and newborn infant. *Clin Perinatol* 1997; **24**: 151–60.
67. Williamson WD, Demmler GJ, Percy AK et al. Progressive hearing loss in infants with asymptomatic congenital cytomegalovirus infection. *Pediatrics* 1992; **90**: 862–6.
68. Jones CA, Isaacs D. Predicting the outcome of symptomatic congenital cytomegalovirus infection. *J Paediatr Child Health* 1995; **31**: 70–1.
69. Stray-Pedersen B. Toxoplasmosis in pregnancy. *Clin Obstet Gynaecol* 1993; **7**: 107–37.
70. Stern H, Booth JC, Elek SD. Microbial causes of mental retardation. The role of prenatal infections with cytomegalovirus, rubella virus and toxoplasma. *Lancet* 1969; **2**: 443–8.
71. McGee T, Wolters C, Stein L et al. Absence of sensorineural hearing loss in treated infants and children with congenital toxoplasmosis. *Otolaryngol Head Neck Surg* 1992; **106**: 75–80.
72. Adams DA, Kerr AG, Smyth GD et al. Congenital syphilitic deafness. *J Laryngol Otol* 1983; **97**: 399–404.
73. Karmody CS, Schuknecht HF. Deafness in congenital syphilis. *Arch Otolaryngol* 1966; **83**: 18–27.
74. Richardson MP, Reid A, Tarlow MJ et al. Hearing loss during bacterial meningitis. *Arch Dis Child* 1997; **76**: 134–8.
75. McIntyre PB, Berkey CS, King SM et al. Dexamethasone as adjunctive therapy in bacterial meningitis. A meta-analysis of randomised clinical trials since 1988. *JAMA* 1997; **278**: 925–31.
76. Fukuda S, Ishikawa K, Inuyama Y. Acute measles infection in the hamster cochlea. *Acta Otolaryngol* 1994; **514**: 111–16.
77. Fuse T, Inamura H, Nakamura T et al. Bilateral hearing loss due to viral infection. *J Otorhinolaryngol Relat Specialties* 1996; **58**: 175–7.
78. Steward BJA, Prabhu PU. Reports of sensorineural deafness after measles, mumps and rubella immunisation. *Arch Dis Child* 1993; **69**: 153–4.
79. Rovet J, Walker W, Bliss B et al. Long term sequelae of hearing impairment in congenital hypothyroidism. *J Pediatrics* 1996; **128**: 776–83.
80. Bellman SC, Davies A, Fuggle PW et al. Mild impairment of neuro-otological function in early treated congenital hypothyroidism. *Arch Dis Child* 1996; **74**: 215–18.
81. Weber PC, Perez BA, Bluestone CD. Congenital perilymphatic fistula and associated middle ear abnormalities. *Laryngoscope* 1993; **103**: 160–4.
82. Pappas DG, Schneiderman TS. Perilymphatic fistula in pediatric patients with a pre-existing sensorineural loss. *Am J Otol* 1989; **10**: 499–501.
83. Borg E. Perinatal asphyxia, hypoxia, ischaemia and hearing loss. An overview. *Scan Audiol* 1999; **19**: 77–91.
84. Jiang ZD. Long term effect of perinatal and postnatal asphyxia on developing human auditory brainstem responses: peripheral hearing loss. *Int J Pediatr Otorhinolaryngol* 1995; **33**: 225–38.
85. Newton VE. Aetiology of bilateral sensorineural hearing loss in young children. *J Laryngol Otol* 1985; Suppl 10.

86. Das VK. Adverse perinatal factors in the causation of sensorineural hearing impairment in young children. *Int J Pediatr Otorhinolaryngol* 1991; **21**: 121–5.
87. Henley CM, Rybak. Developmental ototoxicity. *Otolaryngol Clin North Am* 1993; **26**: 857–71.
88. Song BB, Schacht JB. Variable efficacy of radical scavengers and iron chelators to attenuate gentamycin ototoxicity in guinea pigs in vivo. *Hear Res* 1996; **94**: 87–93.
89. Lench L, Houseman M, Newton V et al. Connexin-26 mutations in sporadic non-syndromal deafness. *Lancet* 351: 415.
90. Parker MJ, Fortnum HM, Young ID, Davis AC, Mueller RF. Population-based genetic study of childhood hearing impairment in the Trent Region of the United Kingdom. *Audiology* 2000; **39**: 226–31.

25 Management of the hearing-impaired child

Cliodna OMahoney

The detection of hearing loss, including via screening programmes, and the subsequent assessment and investigation of the nature (i.e. conductive or sensory, neural or central), degree and cause of the loss are addressed elsewhere (Chapters 20 and 22) and will only be briefly mentioned in this chapter, where appropriate.

The emphasis in this chapter is mainly on the management of permanent hearing impairment, including sensory (cochlear), neural, central and permanent conductive losses. Although common conductive hearing losses such as glue ear and ear infection are more common, they also often resolve spontaneously or are amenable to medical or surgical management. On the other hand, sensory/neural/central and long-term conductive problems usually demand more complex, long-term, multidisciplinary, rehabilitative rather than curative management strategies.

Table 25.1 Summary of the principles of management of bilateral permanent hearing loss

1. Reduce/abolish hearing impairment
2. Minimize the degree of handicap (habilitation/rehabilitation)
   - Amplification—various hearing aids available
   - Vibrotactile and electrotactile aids
   - Assistive listening devices
   - Environmental modifications
   - Speech/language/communication support
   - Educational support
   - Psychological/emotional issues
3. Identify the cause of hearing loss
4. Identify and manage associated vestibular pathology
5. Identify and manage associated pathology
6. Investigate other family members for similar auditory/associated pathology and refer for genetic advice as appropriate
7. Advise on hearing preservation measures
8. Practical information on grants/allowances/self-help organizations etc.

General principles of management

For a child with any form of hearing loss, addressing the broad areas outlined in Table 26.1 provides a useful framework on which to base a management plan for that particular child. In many instances, particularly in cases of temporary conductive hearing loss, some of these will not be problem areas for a given individual, and thus need only to be considered briefly.

Reduce/abolish the hearing impairment

> Curing hearing loss is more likely to be a feasible option in the case of conductive hearing losses or for the conductive component of a mixed loss.

Removal of a foreign body from the ear canal, antibiotics for outer or middle ear infection, and measures to combat allergic rhinitis (e.g. avoidance of dust mite, anti-allergic nasal sprays) in order to improve Eustachian tube function and so abolish 'glue ear' are relatively easy measures which may improve or normalize hearing. Insertion of grommets, reconstruction of ossicles in the case of trauma or congenital deformity, or stapedectomy for otosclerosis, are some of the surgical interventions which may be appropriate in order to restore hearing.

Sensorineural loss is rarely amenable to cure. However, there are some circumstances where the possibility of at least reducing the loss should be considered. For example, patients with hearing loss associated with widened vestibular aqueducts (e.g. Pendred syndrome) may have a fluctuating sensory hearing loss. In such children, there is evidence that head trauma or changes in pressure, such as during air travel or deep sea diving, can precipitate a deterioration in hearing. Advice about avoiding contact sports or other precipitating activities may be appropriate. Similarly, Menière's disease is associated with a fluctuating sensorineural loss which often responds to salt-reducing diet and diuretic therapy. However, Menière's disease, although common in adults, accounts for a very small proportion of hearing loss in children. Claims have also been made for the efficacy of steroids in reducing hearing loss in various conditions, e.g. autoimmune hearing loss, however, this remains to be proven conclusively.

Minimize the degree of handicap (habilitation/rehabilitation)

Where abolition of the hearing loss is not a possibility, or where it is likely to be delayed for a significant time, e.g. long waiting lists for grommet insertion, assessing the nature and degree of disabilities caused and how they affect, i.e. handicap, the individual child is necessary. The common, inter-related areas of life which are likely to be adversely affected include communication, education, social and emotional development, family relationships and, in the older child, vocational opportunities.

> (Re)habilitation of a child with hearing loss is an ongoing dynamic process, needing a coordinated team approach with input from a wide variety of professionals, including audiological physician, audiologist, speech and language therapist, social worker, ear, nose and throat (ENT) surgeon, psychologist and teachers.

One or more of the interventions below may be appropriate for a particular child.

Amplification

Air conduction hearing aids

The range of hearing aids currently available is vast. The most common type worn is the conventional behind-the-ear air conduction aid. These come in a variety of sizes to fit comfortably behind different-sized ears, colours to suit different hair/skin colours, and technical specifications to accommodate different degrees and shapes of hearing loss.

> Binaural fitting of aids is usually considered preferable to monaural (for bilateral loss, of course), as it gives rise to better localization skills, and the degree of amplification needed in each ear in order to achieve the same benefit is less in binaural than in monaural amplification.

Exceptions to binaural fitting include the following: where there is a 'dead ear' on one side, amplification on that side will be of no benefit, or when the degree of asymmetry of the hearing loss is such that each ear requires very different amplification. Binaural fitting in this latter case may give rise to different sound qualities and so confusion of the sound input, which is clearly undesirable. However, in most cases when an older child wears only one aid, it is most commonly the child's choice for cosmetic rather than acoustical reasons.

Other types of air conduction hearing aids include in-the-ear- and in-the-canal-type aids. At this point in time, the power and flexibility of these aids is limited relative to the conventional behind-the-ear aids. In-the-ear aids are most suitable for mild to moderate flat hearing losses, and in such situations are often the aid of choice of older children and adolescents, on account of their cosmetic acceptability. In addition, children with pinna deformities may be unable to retain a behind-the-ear aid in place, and an in-the-ear aid may be the most appropriate. In the young child, up until around the age of 12 or 13 years, the pinna and ear canal are changing shape and size. With a conventional behind-the-ear aid, this means that the moulds need to be changed frequently—three, four or even more times a year. As the mould encases the aid itself in the in-the-ear-type aid, a change of 'mould' means an entire change of casing, which is more expensive. Thus, in the current climate of budgetary constraints, many centres restrict the prescription of in-the-ear aids for cosmetic reasons to the over-12-year age group.

With the increasing range of powerful and yet very small behind-the-ear aids, the role of the body-worn hearing aid—apart from 'radio aids' (see below)—has become very much reduced. In the very young, profoundly deaf, child, acoustical feedback and whistling may be a problem with postaural aids, because of the small size of the ear canals and the difficulty in getting earmoulds to fit very accurately. In addition, the larger body-worn aid is less likely to get lost. Previously, body-worn aids had greater low-frequency amplification than postaural aids, and for the profoundly deaf this was an advantage, as it improved their chances of utilizing their minimal, residual, usually low-frequency, hearing. However, nowadays, many postaural aids have similar potential and tend to be the aid of choice.

Bone conduction hearing aids

Normally, sound is conducted to the inner ear through air-filled cavities, the outer and middle ears, and, when possible, air conduction is also the method of choice of delivery of amplified sound. However, there are circumstances under which this is not possible. For a child with recurrent ear infections giving rise to persistently discharging ears, having the mould of a hearing aid or a hearing aid itself occluding the ear canal may exacerbate the infections and, in addition, render the aid less effective if the canal is fluid/discharge filled. Also, external or middle ear anomalies such as atresia may give rise to a conductive hearing loss where a conventional air conduction aid cannot be fitted.

> **INDICATIONS FOR BONE CONDUCTION AID**
>
> - Persistently discharging ear
> - External ear anomalies
> - Middle ear anomalies

In such circumstances, bone conduction hearing aids provide the solution. Sound energy is converted to electrical energy and amplified in the usual way by a postaural aid fixed at one end of a headband. This electrical energy is conducted to an electromagnetic vibrator situated at the other end of the headband and held tightly against the opposite mastoid process. The vibrations are then conducted to the inner ear from the mastoid process across the skull bones and, to a lesser extent, the ossicles. This is obviously more cumbersome and less cosmetically appealing than a conventional postaural aid. Also, as the headband needs to fit tightly in order for the vibrator to make good contact with the mastoid area, some children find this uncomfortable and thus may limit the amount of time for which they will wear it. In addition, the presence of soft tissue and skin between the vibrator and the skull leads to loss of power and poorer quality of sound. However, for those children needing long-term bone conduction aiding, the advent of the bone-anchored hearing aid (BAHA) has greatly improved the situation. Briefly the bone BAHA consists of a small box, which contains a microphone, the circuitry to convert sound to electromagnetic vibration, and the vibrator itself or piston. The vibrator is coupled via a screw to a titanium implant surgically fixed into the underlying skull, usually placed behind the ear. This process of osseointegration means that vibrations are transferred more efficiently to the skull without the loss of power due to the interposition of skin and soft tissue, and clarity and sound quality are improved. It is also a more cosmetically acceptable (the box being almost completely hidden by hair) and comfortable option than the headband-type aid. The BAHA is a feasible option from the age of 5 years. If the child is younger than this, the skull bone is unlikely to be thick enough for the stable insertion of the osseointegrated screw.

Cochlear implants

Since the 1980s, when the first cochlear implants were inserted in children in the USA, France and UK, cochlear implantation has become well established in the repertoire of 'hearing aids' used in the management of childhood profound hearing loss, both congenital and acquired.

As this is the subject of a separate chapter, the various issues will only be mentioned here, and dealt with in greater detail in Chapter 26.

Several companies are now manufacturing cochlear implant systems with different specifications. Essentially, all devices consist of a receiving microphone connected to a signal processor, which in turn leads to a transmitter coil. This transmitter is bound magnetically to a receiver implanted under the skin postaurally. The signal passes from the receiver along the stimulating electrodes to the cochlea. The most commonly used devices nowadays are intracochlear and multichannel, i.e. multiple electrodes are implanted into the scala tympani along the length of the basilar membrane. In extracochlear devices, the single stimulating electrode (single channel) is placed at the round window.

The decision that a cochlear implant is a suitable form of amplification for a given child is a complex one based on many factors. Also, as local and worldwide experience grows, the indications for cochlear implantation change. However, the general rule is that cochlear implantation should be chosen when it is predicted that it will be more beneficial than conventional aids. Some of the various factors that need to be taken into account include: present age, age of onset of hearing loss, whether the loss is stable or progressive, aided thresholds with conventional aids, presence of an eighth nerve and whether the cochlear anatomy will permit the insertion of electrodes (e.g. dysplastic or ossified), presence of other disabilities which may limit the effectiveness of rehabilitation post-implantation (e.g. learning difficulties, primary speech/language problems), previous compliance with conventional hearing aids, medical fitness for surgery, social support and psychological factors. As successful habilitation requires a huge commitment from both the child and parent, realistic expectations of the likely outcome, cultural issues regarding whether the child will grow up in a hearing world or in a deaf culture, and the different ways in which cochlear implantation is often viewed by both communities, are also very important issues.

This is by no means an exhaustive list of the important issues, but highlights the importance of a team approach, mentioned above, to the management of children with profound hearing loss, in order to make the decision as to whether to implant or not. For those implanted, 'switching on' the implant, 'mapping' of the electrodes, and subsequent (re)habilitation are intensive, and also demand ongoing input from all members of the team.

Radio aids

Radio aid systems are systems where the transmitter and receiver are separated, the transmitter being close to or worn by the speaker, the receiver worn by the child and the two 'connected' via radio waves. Such a system improves the signal-to-noise ratio and is used when it is desirable that a child listen to speech from one source to the exclusion of other sounds (e.g. background noise). This situation arises most commonly in the classroom, where the aim is that the teacher's voice be amplified with as little interference as possible from background noise, e.g. from other children.

> The basic system consists of an FM radio transmitter worn by the teacher and a radio receiver and amplifier contained in a box worn by the child. The amplified signal is then conducted to the child's ears, and is nowadays usually routed directly into his or her postaural hearing aids, if the latter are suitable (i.e. have a socket into which the radio aid plugs).

While this kind of system improves the signal-to-noise ratio for the teacher's voice, the child can become isolated, unable to participate in group discussions. However, it operates over long distances and is suitable for outdoor use. The use of different frequencies of transmission in different classrooms overcomes the problem of interference from nearby classrooms.

Alternatives to this system of radio wave transmission (and so, strictly speaking, not radio aids) include the use of electromagnetic waves with a loop system—either where an electromagnetic loop is placed around the room, or the child wears an individual loop around his neck. The amplified output from the speaker induces an electromagnetic signal in the loop—either the room or the neck loop—which is then detected by the telecoil in the child's own hearing aid ('T' switch). Interference from electromagnetic transmission in nearby rooms can be a problem.

Other systems employ infrared waves for the transmission and detection of signals. Infrared has an advantage over electromagnetic transmission, in that infrared waves will not pass through walls, and this solves the problem of interference from adjacent classrooms seen with electromagnetic systems. However, it is not a suitable system for outdoor use, as sunlight interferes with the signal.

Vibrotactile and electrotactile aids

> These devices, which are usually worn on the wrist, convert acoustical signals to tactile signals, the tactile system being simulated either by small electrical stimuli (electrotactile) or vibration (vibrotactile).

The range of frequencies (below 1000 HZ) and intensities (above 55–60 dB), as well as the ability to detect timing and intensity differences, are much more limited in the tactile than in the auditory system. Thus, tactile aids have only been used in profoundly deaf children (and adults), often as an alternative to cochlear implants.

A very basic vibrotactile device was first introduced for profoundly deaf adults in 1924 by Gault.[1] Since then, many new devices have been developed, both single channel and multichannel. In multichannel systems, the speech signal is split into its component frequencies and the different frequencies routed to separate vibrators or electrical stimulators, e.g. on different fingers, using the principle of place coding for frequency as in the cochlea.[2] Thornton and Philips,[3] Philips et al[4] and Waldstein and Boothroyd[5] describe and compare some of the more well-known devices.

As 'hearing' through touch is a different skill from hearing through the auditory system, considerable training is necessary if the patient is to derive optimal benefit from these devices, in much the same way as intensive (re)habilitation is needed after cochlear implantation. If such training is provided, there is much evidence that tactile aids are effective, in terms of both the child's performance[6, 7] and electrophysiological measures.[8]

Although some workers have claimed that aspects of performance were similar when using an electrotactile aid as when using a cochlear implant,[9] and Brooks et al[10] reported a patient who had developed an extensive vocabulary using only a tactile aid, this has not been universally the case.[7] Generally, the use of vibrotactile and electrotactile aids tends to be limited to those patients who are unwilling or unable to have a cochlear implant, with the expectation that the chief benefit of tactile aids is improved lipreading skills[11] and awareness of environmental/alerting sounds.

Assistive listening devices

These are devices which are not worn by the hearing-impaired child, but help to make acoustical signals more accessible. They include doorbells with a ring that is louder or at a frequency which is easier for the individual to hear and doorbells which, when activated, cause the lights in the house to flash. Other devices include vibrating or flashing alarm clocks, flashing light smoke alarms, amplifiers for the telephone, or loop systems for the television, to mention just some of the devices available, often at no cost to the patient, through social services.

While such devices are routinely discussed with adult or adolescent patients, they are rarely mentioned to parents of young hearing-impaired children or infants, on the grounds that the infant/young child will not need to use the telephone or alarm clock, answer the door, etc. However, it is through watching others use these everyday objects that all children learn about the world around them. If the hearing-impaired child sees his parents/siblings run to pick up the telephone/answer the door randomly, as it seems to him, it makes no sense. But if he sees that every time the light flashes, the door or telephone is answered, he understands the association, and learns these important social skills, in the same way as a normally hearing child.

Assistive listening devices are discussed in greater detail in Chapter 30.

Environmental changes

> Identifying where a child experiences greatest handicap—often in school—and improving the acoustical environment in that place can be of great benefit.

Simple measures, such as moving the child's desk to the front of the class, or the side further away from outside traffic, playground noise, corridors etc., are simple but often very effective measures. Strategies which decrease reverberation can be more difficult to achieve, but very desirable, such as the use of soft furnishings, carpets and curtains.

Speech/language/communication

One of the main concerns of parents when their infant has been diagnosed as having a hearing loss is whether or not the child will learn to speak. Although it is not always easy to give the answer to this question, particularly in children with severe and profound loss, it may be appropriate that the issue be broadened into language and communication, rather than focusing solely on one form of communication, i.e. speech, and that the parents be made aware of other forms of communication, including the various signed languages. Access to a specialist speech and language therapist with particular expertise in problems associated with hearing loss, often in conjunction with a peripatetic teacher of the deaf, is an invaluable resource for parents. In the early months, advice to the parents/carers about how to stimulate and develop language skills in the hearing-impaired child is the main benefit, with more structured sessions with the therapist being appropriate later on.

> The decision about whether the child 'should sign or speak' is not made at one point in time, but gradually evolves over months and years.

Many factors need to be taken into account, including parental choice, the mode of communication within the family/community in which the child lives, and audiological factors. The most important concept to keep sight of while thinking about such problems is that communication, rather than any one particular form of language, is the key issue, and whatever method enhances the child's communication is probably the best method for that child at that particular point in time.

Educational support

The impact of hearing loss on a child's education is another of the major concerns of parents. Just as with speech, language and communication, the educational services should be informed and involved with a hearing-impaired child and his family as soon as possible after diagnosis. As mentioned above, the peripatetic teacher for the deaf is a useful resource for advice about promoting language development. This teacher will also be able to help parents come to a decision about what kind of school is right for their child, e.g. integrated in the local mainstream school, partially integrated into mainstream education with support from an attached unit for the hearing impaired or a special school for the deaf, day or boarding. In the case of a school for the deaf, the policies on communication differ in different schools; for example, some have a clear demarcation between aural/oral or signing traditions while others subscribe to a total communication policy, where both speech and signing are encouraged.

In the UK, the strengths and weaknesses of any child with a disability can be assessed and a statement of special educational needs drawn up, if appropriate; parents can have a large input into this. The kind of support needed, and which school can provide such support, can then be decided upon. The statement is subject to regular review, and the child's progress is monitored to ensure that he is achieving his potential.

Psychological/emotional issues in child and family

The news that their child has a permanent hearing loss is usually devastating for parents, and they need time to be able to grieve, express their fears and ask whatever questions they like. The issues mentioned above and below, such as communication, education, aetiology and the likelihood of recurrence, almost invariably arise sooner or later with every family. Parents find it easier to accept their child's hearing loss and get on with dealing with it and their lives in general if these issues can be tackled in a sensitive, well-informed and honest way as soon as they arise. Meeting other parents who have been in similar situations is also helpful for many families.

The psychological and emotional issues for the child vary greatly with age of the child and the age of onset of hearing loss. Inability to communicate effectively, feelings of being different, of never being part of 'normal life' and fears about the future, can be very frustrating and cause great sadness, even to the point of clinical depression in children/young adults—particularly in the teenage years. Counselling, psychological and psychiatric services specifically for the hearing impaired, or even voluntary social organizations where hearing-impaired children/adolescents can meet each other, can be of great benefit at such times.

Identify the cause of hearing loss

This area of the management of hearing loss is often neglected, as when the diagnosis of hearing loss is confirmed, attention often focuses on habilitation/rehabilitation, and aetiology is often presumed rather than proven. There are many reasons why the cause of hearing loss should always be sought. If the cause is not sought and identified, or at least certain causes excluded, parents may be given inaccurate information about recurrence risks or the existence of significant associated pathology, including vestibular pathology (see below). This may lead to mismanagement of the child. In addition, parents, especially mothers, often have their own ideas about the cause of the hearing loss, and quite often wrongly blame themselves, thinking that something they did during pregnancy has led to the hearing loss. If the issue of aetiology is not addressed, many of these parents harbour guilt feelings for many years which adversely affect their lives.

As the assessment of the hearing-impaired child is covered in Chapter 22, the details of investigation will not be discussed further here.

Identify and manage associated vestibular pathology

As there are close associaions, both anatomically and physiologically, between the auditory and vestibular systems at the level of the inner ear, eighth nerve and central connections, pathology which affects the auditory system may also give rise to vestibular dysfunction. Apart from academic interest, there are three important reasons why vestibular pathology should be sought in any child with sensorineural hearing loss, and perhaps also in patients with long-term conductive losses:

1. The presence or absence of vestibular involvement may be one of the distinguishing features in the diagnosis of a syndrome associated with hearing loss. For example, in making the distinction between Usher's type I and type II, the prognosis being very different for the two types, vestibular function is normal in type I but abnormal in type II.
2. Vestibular dysfunction, in particular congenital bilateral or insidious-onset bilateral symmetrical dysfunction, may, under most circumstances, be asymptomatic. However, the loss of vestibular function can become life-threatening in certain situations; for example, while swimming underwater, orientation relies largely on an intact vestibular system; when standing at the edge of a train platform, balance may be lost as a train flashes by and vision is thus compromised if the vestibular system is dysfunctional. Both these situations will be more dangerous for a child who, in addition to their orientation/ balance being compromised, also has a hearing loss and may not hear alerting sounds, e.g. the train approaching.
3. In the young child, vestibular dysfunction may present as delayed motor milestones. Particularly where there have been perinatal problems, it may be presumed that these problems have given rise on the one hand to hearing loss and on the other hand to global developmental delay, if it is not appreciated that vestibular pathology exists. Clearly, the management of a child with hearing loss and vestibular pathology is different to that of a child with hearing loss and developmental delay.

VALUE OF VESTIBULAR INVESTIGATION OF HEARING-IMPAIRED CHILD

- Facilitates aetiological diagnosis
- Defines vestibular failure and accompanying changes
- Allows appropriate management of condition

The management of vestibular dysfunction is dealt with in detail elsewhere, but interventions such as vestibular exercises—Cawthorne–Cooksey, Brandt–Daroff—and appropriate advice as regards safety need to be considered.

Identify and manage other associated pathology

In more than 30% of cases of childhood sensorineural hearing loss, the hearing problem is part of a syndrome. The actual figure is probably even higher, as in many cases children have not been investigated. In some cases, this is widely recognized and the hearing loss may be sought as a result of other features, e.g. Down's syndrome. However, the opposite is often the case, where the hearing loss is the first feature identified and no other abnormality is immediately obvious. Nevertheless, it behoves the physician to thoroughly investigate the cause of the hearing loss and refer to other specialties as appropriate, and in so doing to identify pathology elsewhere— such as in the eye (e.g. Usher's syndrome), thyroid gland (e.g. Pendred syndrome), kidneys (e.g. branchio-oto-renal syndrome), and heart (Jervell–Lange–Nielsen syndrome).

Failure to identify this pathology will lead to serious mismanagement of the child—with, for example, progressive renal failure or potentially fatal but treatable cardiac arrhythmias going undetected. In additon, the prognosis and genetic advice given will clearly be very different for a child with isolated hearing loss than where there is coexistent significant disease.

Investigate other family members for similar pathology

In all cases of childhood permanent hearing loss, first-degree relatives (siblings and parents), as well as any family member with a suspicious history, should have their hearing tested by whatever method is appropriate to their age. In addition, a history of associated pathology, including vestibular pathology, in the family members should be sought, whether or not the index case was found to have associated abnormalities. Two family members with the same condition may not necessarily have exactly the same manifestations or to the same degree.

Where parents have one child with a significant disability, almost invariably they are anxious to know what the chances are that a future child or grandchild will have the same condition and to what degree. Referral for genetic advice may be appropriate. In addition, informing parents of the availability of neonatal hearing screening (see Chapter 24) for the early detection of congenital loss is often very reassuring for parents, especially where a previous child's hearing loss has been diagnosed late.

Advice on hearing preservation measures

Whatever the cause of a child's hearing loss, even if, despite investigation, this remains unknown, part of the management strategy should include advice about preserving whatever hearing is left. Such advice should include information about the risks to hearing associated with leisure or occupational noise, and appropriate ways of protecting against such damage. In addition, as mentioned above, children with the abnormality of widened vestibular aqueduct seen on CT scan of the inner ear should be advised of the risks of hearing deteriorating further in association with head injuries, deep sea diving, etc.

Practical help and information

When a child has been diagnosed as having a permanent hearing impairment, as well as the medical, educational, psychological and emotional issues, practical problems arise within that family. These can include: financial problems, perhaps due to a parent needing time off work to attend appointments, arranging care for other siblings, etc.; logistical problems, such as getting the hearing-impaired child to a suitable school, which may be some distance away; finding social outlets for the child; meeting parents of other hearing-impaired children; getting advice about vocational opportunities for the older child; or just finding the extra time needed to support the child with a hearing disability. A social worker or a liaison worker with an interest in the problems surrounding hearing loss and a knowledge of the various allowances, organizations etc. is an invaluable resource for parents who often feel very isolated when they leave the hospital clinic and go back to their own communities.

Unilateral hearing loss

The prevelance of unilateral hearing loss among school-age children has been variously reported as being from 0.6 to 1.7 per 1000 live births.[12–14]

It is often thought that unilateral impairment causes only minor, irritating problems, e.g. with localization of sound, or use of the telephone, but no significant disability/handicap in the areas of speech/communication and learning. However, this is still an area of controversy, with many reports, particularly since the 1980s,[15–20] claiming that such children have language, educational and behavioural difficulties attributable to their hearing loss. On the other hand, Klee and Davis-Dansky[21] and Hallmo et al[22] found no such language or educational difficulties in their studies. Ito[23] also refuted the claim that unilateral hearing loss was a handicap to academic achievement, as he found a similar prevalence of unilateral hearing loss among the students in the very high-achieving University of Tokyo as in preschool and elementary schools.

The use of hearing aids for amplification of unilateral hearing loss is also somewhat controversial. Where there is residual hearing in the affected ear, the use of a postaural aid may be beneficial, assuming that the pinna and ear canals are suitable, e.g. not atretic. Many children find the difference in the quality of sound between the aided and non-aided ears confusing, however, and reject the aid. However, there is an argument, as yet unproven, that aiding the impaired side promotes auditory development, particularly in the young child, where there is a great deal of neural plasticity. The Contralateral routing of sound (CROS)-type aid, where sound is detected by a postaural microphone on the impaired side but routed to the good ear, is one option, especially where the loss is profound. However, nowadays few children will wear such an aid, their real benefit being in situations such as large meetings, where the listener has to be able to hear speakers from both sides, e.g. around a table. Generally, even in these circumstances, and certainly with children, strategies such as appropriate placement with respect to the speaker(s) are usually preferred.

Many or all of the management strategies discussed above, such as environmental modifications, educational support, and speech and language therapy, are appropriate to a greater or lesser extent in the child with a unilateral loss. The situation should be reassessed regularly, even if the hearing itself has not changed, as the effect of the loss will be different at different times in the child's life, and support which was not previously needed may become necessary as demands on hearing increase.

Central auditory dysfunction

The central auditory system denotes those pathways involved in auditory perception from the brainstem at the level of entry of the eighth nerve, up to and including the cerebral cortex.

Previously in this chapter, attention has been focused on the relatively well understood dysfunction of the peripheral auditory system. Functionally, the peripheral auditory system is comparatively simple, being involved in the detection, amplification and conversion of sound (acoustical energy) to neural impulses (electrical energy). Relatively little processing of the speech signal occurs at the peripheral level, although the nature of the response of the peripheral system to sound gives some information about basic frequency and intensity characteristics of the incoming signal. However, it is the function of the central auditory system to further analyse these complex signals at a more sophisticated level. The integration of different signals from each ear, the correct localization or temporal sequencing of sound, the ability to selectively attend to one signal over another (e.g. speech in background noise), and the attribution of meaning to perceived sounds, are just some of the complex functions of the central auditory system. This complexity of sound-processing function is reflected in the structure of the central auditory pathways, with each nerve fibre from the eighth nerve synapsing with several neurones in the brainstem, and the number of synapses further increasing between the brainstem and the auditory cortex.

It is only relatively recently that the nature and extent of disability associated with central auditory dysfunction has been recognized, and in the case of children, much of the impetus to understand and manage these conditions better has come from the educational rather than health fields.

TYPICAL INTER-RELATED PRESENTATIONS OF CENTRAL AUDITORY DYSFUNCTION

- difficulty in hearing in background noise, although hearing ability when in optimal conditions may be totally unimpaired.
- general complaints of bilateral hearing impairment despite normal standard audiometry
- poor school performance
- distractibility/poor attention—especially in situations of background noise, e.g. school
- poor behaviour—particularly in a crowded/noisy environment, e.g. school
- difficulty with multistep instructions
- poor music skills
- discrepancy between verbal and performance skills (verbal being lower) on psychological testing.

The details of the causes and assessment of central auditory function are beyond the remit of this chapter and are dealt with elsewhere (Chapter 29). Briefly, the assessment of a child suspected of having a central auditory processing disorder includes history (not forgetting an educational history/report), clinical examination, with particular emphasis on neurological examination to exclude a neurological deficit, standard audiological tests appropriate for the age of the child (which typically will show no abnormality), followed by specific tests of central auditory function.

As there is a great deal of redundancy in both normal speech and the central auditory system, in order to detect the often very subtle processing problems, most workers in this field suggest that several tests of central auditory function be applied to assess different aspects of central processing, i.e. a test battery.

These latter include:

- Behavioural tests of central auditory function. These may be monaural (stimulus presented to one ear only during any one test) or binaural, where different stimuli are presented to both ears either simultaneously (dichotic tests) or sequentially. In the monaural, the speech stimulus is modified (e.g. filtered or time compressed) in order to decrease the degree of redundancy and increase the difficulty of the task of understanding speech. Alternatively, the speech signal is presented in background noise. In binaural tests, where each ear only gets part of the test signal, the ability to fuse information (binaural integration) from each ear or to selectively attend (binaural separation) to one ear only is assessed.
- Objective tests, including electrophysiological tests (e.g. auditory evoked brainstem responses, middle latency response, mismatch negativity), ipsilateral and contralateral stapedial reflex threshold, and suppression of otoacoustical emissions via the poorly understood efferent auditory system.

As 'central auditory dysfunction' is an umbrella term for a wide range of pathologies—often unknown—which affect any parts of the central auditory pathways, and give rise to very variable symptoms and degrees of disability in different children, there can be no one management plan which will be appropriate for all affected children. In addition, high-quality, long-term research into the outcomes of different interventions is still relatively scarce. Therefore, many of the strategies used in these conditions remain empirical.

A multidisciplinary approach, including audiological physician, neurologist, speech and language therapist, psychologist, and specialist teacher, will be required to address the primary auditory problem as well as any secondary problems—educational, behavioural, emotional, psychological—which may have arisen as a result of perhaps long-standing, previously unrecognized, central auditory processing problems.

Strategies of management include:[24, 25]

1. full neurological assessment and appropriate neuroimaging to identify associated neurological disorders which may need specific intervention
2. alteration of the listening environment(s) in which the child is experiencing difficulty
3. auditory training
4. compensatory non-acoustical strategies to be developed in tandem with (2) and (3) above.

The most common situation in which children with central auditory dysfunction experience difficulty is in school. Apart from amplification, many of the general principles of management of the hearing-impaired child discussed above apply as much to children with central as with peripheral auditory problems. Awareness of the nature of the problem by sympathetic teachers, positioning near the teacher to improve attention, decreasing sound reverberation by the introduction of soft furnishings, (carpets, curtains, etc.), smaller group teaching, and use of a non-amplified FM system to cut down background noise, are some of the strategies which may improve the child's detection of speech.

An auditory training programme needs to be tailored to the requirements of the individual child, working on the specific skills where problems have been demonstrated.[25] For example, difficulty in extracting the signal from background noise means that the child is left having to guess missed words from the context. In such a case, improving the child's vocabulary may mean that he at least is not further disadvantaged by not understanding words which he *has* heard. For others, practising localization or sequencing skills may be the key to improved understanding. Much has been written about the plasticity of the central nervous system, and the effect of learning on stimulating new 'wiring' patterns in the central nervous system, including the central auditory system.[26–31] It is suggested that such auditory training operates by functionally altering the auditory pathways in this way.

There are many compensatory strategies which will limit the disability associated with central auditory dysfunction, although not directly addressing the pathology. Provision of written notes prior to teaching, note-takers during classes, and presentation of new material other than verbally, e.g. pictures, practical demonstrations, videos or computer programs, are just some of the non-auditory compensatory strategies that are commonly found to be beneficial.

Despite the fact that the management of central auditory dysfunction is still in its infancy, with few data as yet on efficacy, often the most therapeutic aspect for the child and his family is the objective demonstration of the problem in the first place. Many of these children will in retrospect have been experiencing problems and perhaps struggling in school years, being labelled as badly behaved, disruptive and/or of low intelligence. Being able to ascribe a diagnosis and draw up a management plan shifts the emphasis from a punitive, negative way of handling the problem to a positive, confidence-building approach.

Non-organic hearing loss

Non-organic hearing loss, also called functional hearing loss, pseudohypacusis or psychogenic hearing loss, describes a condition where a patient presents complaining of hearing loss but with objective evidence of normal hearing and where no organic pathology to account for a hearing deficit can be found. Its prevalence is thought to be underestimated, the condition often being misdiagnosed.[32]

In adults, this condition most commonly occurs where there is a compensation claim for injury pending and the hearing loss is consciously faked for financial gain.[33]

However, the situation is very different in children, where such malingering for financial gain is almost never the underlying motivation.[34]

> It is now generally accepted that non-organic hearing loss in children is a cry for help,[35, 36] a manifestation of an underlying psychological, emotional or educational[37] problem, although not invariably a serious or long-term problem.

Most studies have reported that non-organic hearing loss occurs more frequently in females than in males, in a ratio of 2 : 1 or 3 : 1, and it has been described from as young as 6 years of age, although it more typically presents between the ages of 10 and 14 years. Children with a wide range of IQ scores present, but with a preponderance in the low average to low range. Characteristically, affected children will have had a past history of transient hearing loss, e.g. due to glue ear, at which time the hearing loss may have given rise to secondary gain such as an excuse for poor school performance, or increased attention from parents or teachers.

The onset of the non-organic loss may be sudden and precipitated by some stress/conflict at home, school or elsewhere e.g. examinations, bereavement, or family problems, or may be insidious in onset with no obvious precipitating factors. The severity of impairment ranges from mild impairment to complete loss, and it has been suggested that the greater the degree of hearing loss, the more likely there is to be a significant underlying psychological/psychiatric problem.[36] Premorbid personalities of these children suggest a high level of anxiety and 'neuroticism', sometimes with evidence of other psychosomatic disorders, e.g. non-organic visual problems.

Non-organic hearing loss is a diagnosis of exclusion; that is, true hearing loss including central auditory problems must first be excluded. There are many strategies which can be used during behavioural testing which highlight the inconsistencies of responses and point to a non-organic cause. If there is still doubt, objective tests such as otoacoustic emissions and electrophysiological tests, including auditory brainstem evoked potentials and cortical evoked potentials, will help clinch the diagnosis.

When the diagnosis of non-organic hearing loss has been confirmed, nowadays most of the literature recommends a non-confrontational approach—i.e. not to confront the child or parents with the false nature of the abnormal hearing test. While this may force the child to retract the symptom of hearing loss, if there is a significant underlying problem, this may be further exacerbated by the parents' perception of their child's bad behaviour in pretending to have a hearing loss and/or it is likely that the child will somatize his problem in a different way e.g. develop recurrent abdominal pains or headaches. The recommended course of action is to accept that there is a hearing lass at present, but reassure all concerned that it is expected that it will be short-lived, will resolve spontaneously and will not need intervention in the form of amplification. This gives the child a 'face-saving' device, and some authors suggest that this is as far as management should go,[32] as to intervene further will only consolidate the loss.

However, others report that failure to address underlying problems leads to incomplete or only temporary resolution of the hearing problem, or, even if the hearing loss is 'cured', many of these patients go on to have persistent pyschological, psychiatric, learning and communication disorders, even into adulthood.[38]

Thus, although there is not as yet universal agreement, a pragmatic approach to management should probably comprise non-confrontation, reassurance vis-à-vis the prognosis for resolution of the hearing loss, and a screening assessment for underlying psychological, educational or communication problems. For those children in whom there is evidence of dysfunction in any of the above areas, appropriate medication, psychotherapy, counselling, speech and language therapy or remedial teaching should be instigated, while recognizing that not all children will require such input.

Finally, it is important to distinguish between non-organic hearing loss and spurious hearing loss. In the latter, an abnormal hearing test may be found, often in a school screening situation, but where, at least prior to this finding, there is no complaint of hearing problems. This is most commonly due to the inadequate acoustical environment in which many school tests are conducted, or, as Coles[39] pointed out, to poor attention on the child's behalf during testing giving rise to minor degrees of abnormality on the audiogram/hearing test.

References

1. Gault RH. Progress in experiments on tactual interpretation of oral speech. *J Abnorm Social Psychol* 1924; **19**: 294–9.
2. Mason JL, Frost BJ. Signal processing strategies for multichannel systems. In: Summers IR ed. *Tactile Aids for the Hearing Impaired.* London: Whurr, 1992: 128–45.
3. Thornton ARD, Philips AJ. A comparative trial of four vibrotactile aids. In: Summers IR, ed. *Tactile Aids for the Hearing Impaired.* London: Whurr, 1992: 231–52.
4. Philips AJ, Thornton ARD, Worsfold S, Downie A, Milligan J. Experience of using vibrotactile aids with the profoundly deafened. *Eur J Disord Commun* 1994; **29**(1): 17–26.

5. Waldstein RS, Boothroyd A. Comparison of two multichannel tactile devices as supplements to speechreading in a postlingually deafened adult. *Ear Hear* 1995; **16**(2): 198–208.
6. Kishon-Rabin L, Haras N, Berman M. Multisensory speech perception of young children with profound hearing loss. *J Speech Language Hear Res* 1997; **40**(5): 1135–50.
7. Sehgal ST, Kirk KI, Svirsky M, Ertmer DJ, Osberger MJ. Imitative consonant feature production by children with multichannel sensory aids. *Ear Hear* 1998; **19**(1): 72–84.
8. Suarez H, Cibils D, Caffa C, Silveira A, Basalo S, Svirsky M. Vibrotactile aid and brain cortical activity. *Acta Otolaryngol* 1997; **117**(2): 208–10.
9. Blamey PJ, Cowan RSC. The potential benefit and cost effectiveness of tactile devices in comparison to implants. In: Summers IR, ed. *Tactile Aids for the Hearing Impaired*. London: Whurr, 1992: 187–217.
10. Brooks PL, Frost BJ, Mason JL, Gibson DM. Continuing evaluation of the Queen's University tactile vocoder I: identification of open-set words. *J Rehabil Res Dev* 1986; **23**: 119–28.
11. Plant G. Training in the use of a tactile supplement to lipreading: a long-term case study. *Ear Hear* 1998; **19**(5): 394–406.
12. Kankkunen A. Pre-school children with impaired hearing. *Acta Otolaryngol (Stockh)* 1982; Suppl 391: 1–124.
13. Tarkkanen J, Aho J. Unilateral deafness in children. *Acta Otolaryngol (Stockh)* 1966; **61**: 270–8.
14. Vartianinen E, Karjalainen S. Prevalence and etiology of unilateral sensorineural hearing impairment in a Finnish childhood population. *Int J Pediatr Otorhinolaryngol* 1998; **43**: 253–9.
15. Bess FH. Children with unilateral hearing loss. *J Acad Rehabil Audiol* 1982; **15**: 131–44.
16. Bess FH, Tharpe SM, Gibler AM. Auditory performance of children with unilateral sensorineural hearing loss. *Ear Hear* 1986; **7**: 20–6.
17. Culbertson JL, Gilbert LE. Children with unilateral sensorineural hearing loss: cognitive, academic and social development. *Ear Hear* 1986; **7**: 38–42.
18. Brookhouser PE, Worthington DW, Kelly WJ. Unilateral hearing loss in children. *Laryngoscope* 1991; **101**: 1264–72.
19. Dancer J, Burl NT, Waters S. Effects of unilateral hearing loss on teacher responses to the SIFTER. *Am Ann Deaf* 1995; **140**(3): 291–4.
20. English K, Church G. Unilateral hearing loss in children: an update for the 1990's. *Language, Speech Hear Services Schools* 1999; **30**(1): 26–31.
21. Klee TM, Davis-Dansky E. A comparison of unilaterally hearing-impaired children and normal-hearing children on a battery of standardised language tests. *Ear Hear* 1986; **7**: 27–37.
22. Hallmo P, Moller P, Lind O, Tonning FM. Unilateral sensorineural hearing loss in children less than 15 years of age. *Scand Audiol* 1986; **15**: 131–7.
23. Ito K. Can unilateral hearing loss be a handicap in learning? *Arch Otolaryngol Head Neck Surg* 1998; **124**: 1389–90.
24. Chermak GD, Musiek FE. Managing central auditory processing disorders in children and youth. *Am J Audiol* 1992; **1**(3): 61–5.
25. Musiek FE, Chermak GD. Three commonly asked questions about central auditory processing disorders: management. *Am J Audiol* 1995; **4**: 15–18.
26. Hebb DO. *The Organization of Behaviour*. New York: Wiley, 1949.
27. Knudsen E, Knudsen P. Vision guides the adjustment of auditory localisation in young barn owls. *Science* 1985; **230**: 545–8.
28. Knudsden EJ. Early auditory experience shapes auditory localisation behavior in the spatial tuning of auditory units in the barn owl. In Raushecher J, and Marler P eds. *Imprinting and Cortical Plasticity* New York: John Wiley & Sons, 1987: 7–23.
29. Hall JW, Grose JH, Pillsbury HC. Predicting binaural hearing after stapedectomy from pre-surgery results. *Arch Otolaryngol Head Neck Surg* 1990; **116**: 946–50.
30. Hall JW, Grose JH. The effect of otitis media with effusion on the masking-level difference and the auditory brainstem response. *J Speech Hear Res* 1993; **36**: 210–17.
31. Irvine DRF, Rajan R, Wize LZ, Heil P. Reorganisation in auditory cortex of adult cats with unilateral restricted cochlear lesions. *Soc Neurosci* 1991; **17**: 1485.
32. Pracy JP, Bowdler DA. Pseudohypacusis in children *Clin Otolaryngol* 1996; **21**: 383–4.
33. Noble W. The conceptual problem of 'functional hearing loss'. *Br J Audiol* 1987; **21**: 1–3.
34. Brockman SJ, Hoversten GH. Pseudoneural hypacusis in children. *Laryngoscope* 1960; **70**: 825–39.
35. Northern JL, Downs MP. *Hearing in Children*. Baltimore: Williams and Wilkins, 1974: 158–9.
36. Aplin DY, Rowson VJ. Psychological characteristics of children with functional hearing loss. *Br J Audiol* 1990; **24**: 77–87.
37. Barr B. Psychogenic deafness in school children. *Int Audiol* 1963; **2**: 125–8.
38. Brooks DN, Geoghegan PM. Non-organic hearing loss in young persons: transient episode or indicator of deep-seated difficulty. *Br J Audiol* 1992; **26**: 347–50.
39. Coles RRA. Non-organic hearing loss. In: Gibb AG, Smith MFW, eds. *International Medical Reviews Otolaryngology: I Otology*. London: Butterworth Scientific, 1982: 150–76.

26 Cochlear implants for adults and children

Graeme M Clark

Introduction

Scope of chapter

Cochlear implants which use multiple-electrode speech-processing strategies are now an established clinical entity for children and adults, and, as a result, preoperative selection and (re)habilitation are key issues. It is now hard to realize that it was only in the 1960s and 1970s that many scientists and clinicians said that successful cochlear implants were not possible in the foreseeable future. The questions that had to be addressed by a multi-disciplinary research effort are discussed, and the solutions achieved from the University of Melbourne's perspective are presented. However, the main aim of this chapter is to focus on preoperative selection, and (re)habilitation, including the results obtained. These issues are discussed primarily with reference to data from the University of Melbourne's Cochlear Implant Clinic at the Royal Victorian Eye and Ear Hospital. As this is a book on audiological medicine, only an overview of surgical principles is presented. The surgical management of the patient is, of course, very important, so for more details the reader is referred elsewhere.[1–4] Cochlear implantation has also been the subject of quite intense ethical debate, particularly over its use for children. For this reason, a discussion of ethical issues is included. Finally, the chapter concludes with a vision of research in the new Millennium.

The need for cochlear implants

> The cochlear implant is of benefit to many severely-to-profoundly deaf people. These people cannot use powerful or speech-processing hearing aids to adequately communicate with normally hearing people.

Severely-to-profoundly deaf children also have more difficulty in learning written language than their normally hearing peers. For example, research at The University of Melbourne[5] has shown that severely-to-profoundly hearing-impaired schoolchildren do not reach as high a level of basic literacy as their normally hearing peers. For example, an 'average' normally hearing child at grade level 8 would have a reading level of grade 8; that is their reading is age-appropriate. An average deaf child at grade 8 would only be reading at a grade equivalent of 4.8, and the difference increases as the child gets older. At the age of 17, when normally hearing children are entering the workforce or university, an average deaf child has a reading age equivalent to a 12-year-old (a grade equivalent of 7.5). In addition, profound and total deafness prevents the development of normal speech and expressive language. The numbers of people likely to benefit from cochlear implants have not been clearly established. However, in Australia, 1 in every 2000 children born is severely or profoundly deaf.

Concept of the cochlear implant

The cochlear implant is an electronic device that replaces the inner ear when it does not function in severely-to-profoundly deaf people. It consists of a directional microphone which sends information to a small speech processor behind the ear or to a larger, more versatile, one attached to a belt (Figure 26.1). The speech processor extracts information of importance to speech understanding, produces a code for the signal, and transmits it by inductive coupling to the receiver–stimulator implanted in the mastoid bone. The receiver–stimulator decodes the signal and produces a pattern of electrical stimulus currents in an array of electrodes inserted around the basal turn of the cochlea.

Objections and solutions

When the idea of restoring hearing by electrical stimulation of the cochlear nerve was conceived, a number of objections were

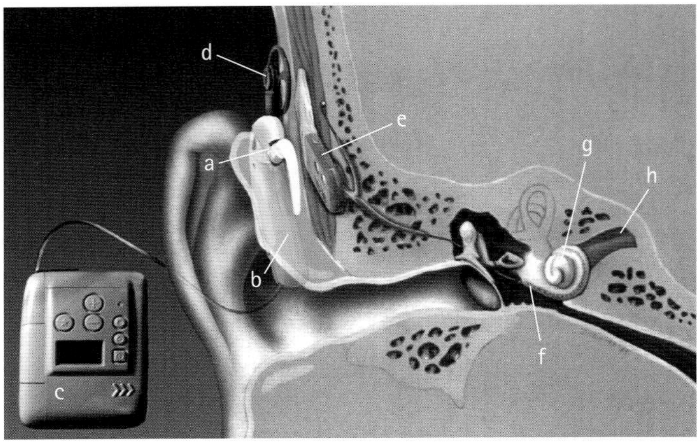

Figure 26.1 The Nucleus-24 multiple-channel cochlear prosthesis: (a) microphone; (b) behind-the-ear speech processor (ESPrit); (c) body-worn speech processor (SPrint); (d) transmitter coil; (e) receiver–stimulator; (f) electrode array; (g) cochlea; (h) cochlear nerve. This prosthesis was developed by Cochlear Limited in association with the Cooperative Research Centre for Cochlear Implant Speech and Hearing Reasearch.

raised by scientists and clinicians. These objections were reasonable in the light of the knowledge at the time. They had, however, to be answered before cochlear implants could be established as safe and effective.

First objection and solution

The first objection was: *a cochlear implant would destroy the very nerves it was hoped to stimulate*. This was overcome, first, by showing that the gentle insertion of electrodes, with the right biomechanical properties, would not lead to loss of ganglion cells. Second, it was found that biphasic, charge-balanced pulses did not cause long-term damage to the cochlea or auditory nerve. It was also necessary to keep the charge density below approximately 32 $\mu C/cm^2$ geom. per phase. The geometric (geom.) area is less than the 'real' area where electrochemical charge takes place.

Second objection and solution

In developing cochlear implants, another main objection was: *the cochlear hair cells and their nerve connections were too complex and numerous to be replaced by a small number of electrodes for the coding of sound.*[6] This was answered in part by research to see how well electrical stimulation could reproduce the coding of sound. Normally, the frequency of a sound is coded by the brain as both a timing and a place code. Furthermore, the coding of frequency correlates with pitch perception.

Reproduction of the temporal coding of frequency

The temporal coding of frequency is illustrated in Figure 26.2. On the left, it can be seen that brainstem action potentials occur in phase with the sound waves. The intervals between the action potentials can be plotted as a histogram, shown on the right. The intervals are multiples of the period of the sound wave. Up to 600 Hz, the first or predominant interval is the same as the period of the wave, but not at higher frequencies.

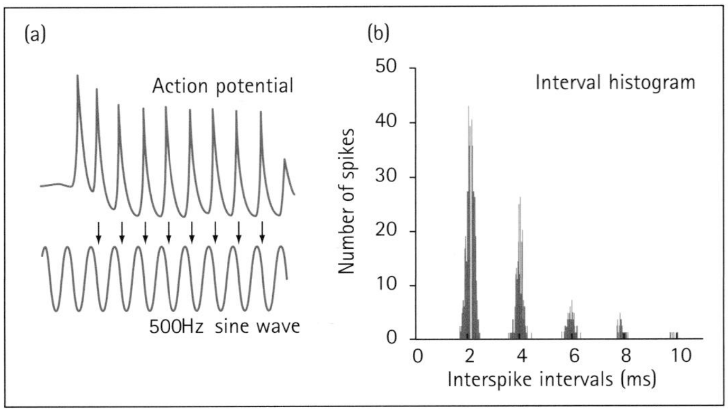

Figure 26.2 (a) The brainstem action potentials in response to a 500 Hz sine wave. (b) The interspike interval histogram of the responses to a 500 Hz tone. (Reprinted with permission from Clark. *J Clin Physiol Pharmacol Res* 1996; **23**: 766–76.[108])

The temporal coding of frequency with electrical stimulation was studied in the experimental animal by examining the suppression of brainstem field potentials, and by measuring the frequency discrimination for different rates of electrical stimulation. It was also studied in the human by measuring frequency discrimination and pitch perception. Figure 26.3 shows that field potentials in the brainstem of the cat were markedly suppressed at 100 pulses/s, presumably due to inhibition.[7]

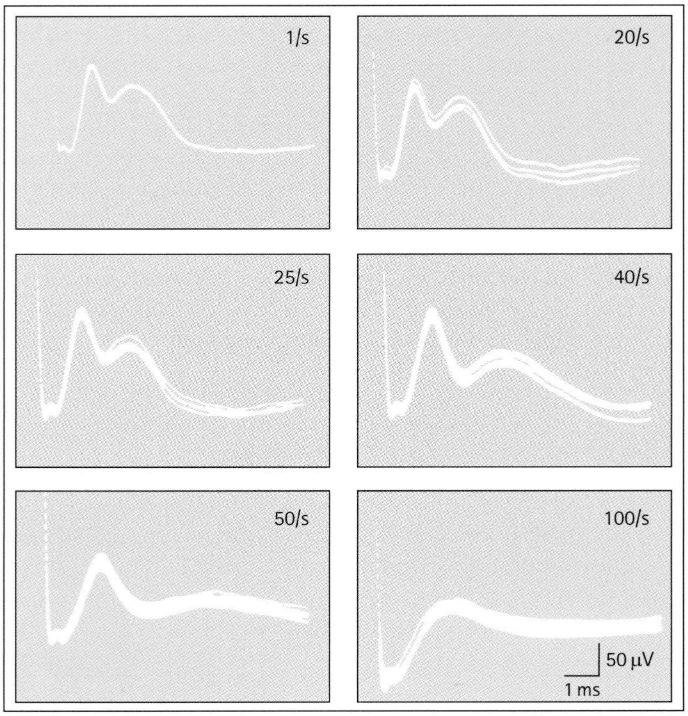

Figure 26.3 The brainstem field potentials in the cat in response to different rates of electrical stimulation. (From Clark. *Exp Neurol* 1969; **24**: 124–36.)[7]

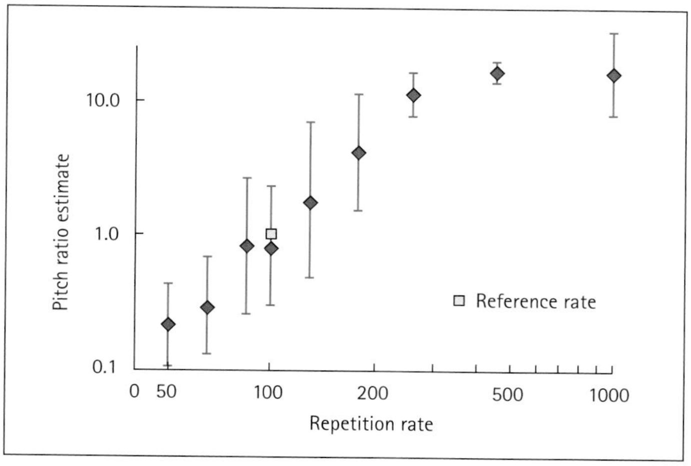

Figure 26.4 The pitch ratios for variations in rate of stimulation in the first multiple-channel cochlear implant patient in Melbourne. (From Tong et al. *J Acoust Soc Am* 1983; **74**: 73–80.[19])

Behavioural studies in the experimental animal demonstrated that rate difference limens were more comparable to those for sound at 100 and 200 pulses/s than at higher rates.[8, 9]

Furthermore, psychophysical research on temporal coding in the human showed that rate of electrical stimulation approximate normal frequency discrimination and pitch perception up to about 300 pulses/s, but not up to the 3000 pulses/s needed for speech understanding. Figure 26.4 shows that pitch ratios for test and reference rates in the human increased linearly up to 300 pulses/s and then reached a plateau.[10] Furthermore, as electrical stimulation separates the rate of stimulation from the place of stimulation, it has helped establish the importance of timing information in the coding of sound, at least for low frequencies.

The place coding of frequency

The place coding of frequency is illustrated in Figure 26.5. According to the place code, the pitch of a sound depends on the place of stimulation within the brain. This is illustrated by the fact that the cochlea, and the auditory pathways, are arranged tonotopically so that a frequency scale is preserved. Further evidence is that the cochlea also filters the sound, so that the responses from different places in the cochlea are sharply tuned.

Research to simulate place coding showed that electrical currents could be localized to discrete groups of nerve fibres within the cochlea.[11–13] In Figure 26.6, the neural threshold of units in the inferior colliculus is plotted against distance along the basilar membrane as determined for their bipolar and monopolar stimulation. It can be seen that there is much less spread for the bipolar pulses. These results were in the acute animal with fluid in the scalae. It has also been shown in the acute animal that if the electrodes are placed close to the neurones, localized stimulation may be achieved with monopolar stimulation.[14] Furthermore, in an implanted patient, where presumably fibrous tissue or bone had surrounded the array, monopolar stimuli with the banded array could give localized stimulation comparable to that for bipolar stimuli.[15] It was also established[16] that electrical currents should not be presented simultaneously to electrodes, as otherwise there would be an interaction of electrical fields, as shown in Figure 26.7. This interaction produced unpredictable variations in loudness.

Place coding studies on patients showed that, with localized electrical stimulation, they could rank the percepts for each electrode on the basis of timbre, but not true pitch. In the high-frequency areas of the cochlea, the percept was sharper (S), and on the lower-frequency side it was duller (D). The percept at each electrode was compared with the percepts at each of the

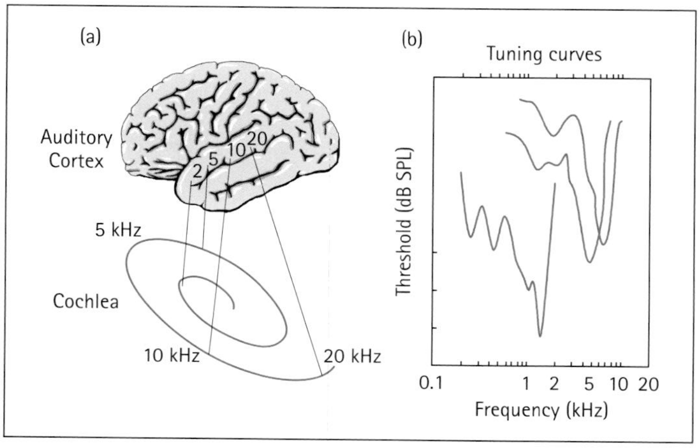

Figure 26.5 (a) The tonotopic organization from the cochlea to the auditory cortex in the human. (b) The turning curves for different frequencies stimulating the cochlea. (Reprinted with permission from Clark. *J Clin Physiol Pharmacol Res* 1996; **23**: 766–76.[108])

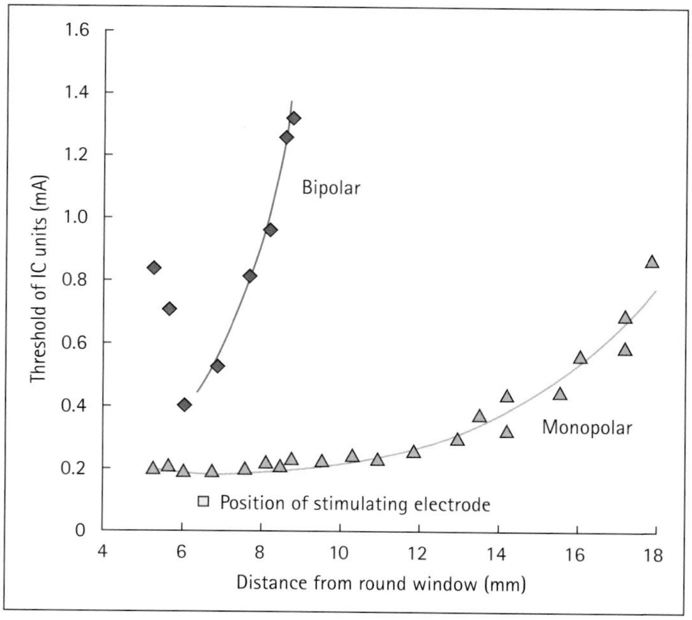

Figure 26.6 Inferior colliculus unit thresholds versus distance along the cochlea for bipolar and monpolar electrical stimulation in the acute cat experiments. (Reprinted with permission from Clark et al. Adv Otorhinolaryngol 1987; **38**: 1–181 (review).[110])

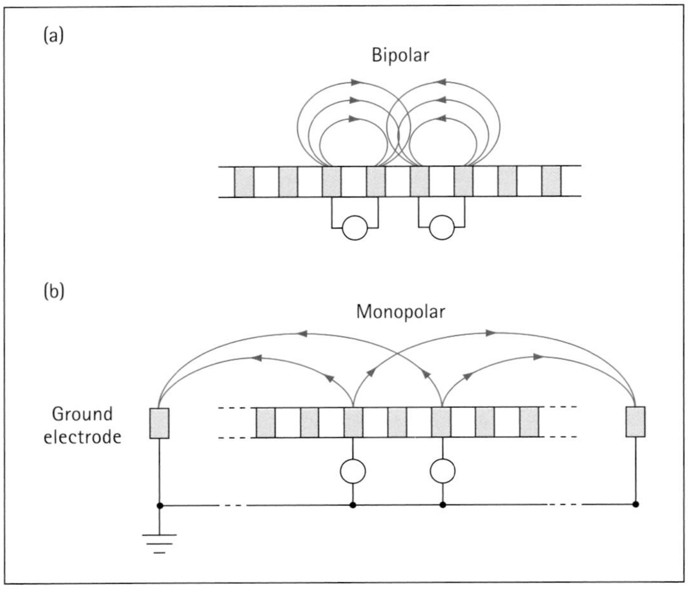

Figure 26.7 The electrical fields for (a) bipolar and (b) monopolar electrical stimulation, and the interaction of the fields with simultaneous stimulation.

other electrodes to produce a ranking of timbre or place pitch. Figure 26.8 shows the percept for the comparison electrode when compared with the standard or reference electrode.The electrodes are numbered from low to high, according to their placement in the lower- or higher-frequency areas of the cochlea. In general, the sharp and dull percepts lie on either side of the diagonal, indicating that there was good ranking of place pitch.

Standard stimulus (electrode no.): Low → High; Comparison stimulus: Low ↓ High; (Dull) above diagonal, (Sharp) below diagonal

Comparison stimulus \ Standard stimulus	1	2	3	4	6	7	8
1 (Low)	=	D	D	D	D	D	D
2	S	=	S	S	D	D	D
3	S	S	=	D	D	D	D
4	S	S	S	=	S	D	D
6	S	S	D	S	=	D	D
7	S	S	S	S	S	=	D
8 (High)	S	S	S	S	S	S	=

Figure 26.8 The ranking of timbre for different electrodes in the first Melbourne cochlear implant patient. (From Tong et al. *J Acoust Soc Am* 1982; **71**: 153–60.[10])

Reproduction of the intensity code

Variations in the amplitude of the speech signal also convey essential information. Initial research on patients in Melbourne using electrical stimulation,[17] illustrated in Figure 26.9 and confirming the findings of Simmons,[18] showed a steep linear function between the logarithm of current amplitude, plotted in decibels, versus loudness. The dynamic range for electrical stimulation was 5–10 dB, and is smaller than the 30–40-dB range for speech sounds or the more than 100-dB dynamic range for sound. However, the number of discriminable steps in loudness over the narrow dynamic range for electrical stimulation (5–10 dB) is greater than for sound over the same range. It can be calculated from the degree of overlap in the standard deviations and the d' values in the data shown in Figure 2 of Tong et al[19] that the just-discriminable steps in loudness for electrical stimulation were 0.3 dB. Therefore, the just-discriminable steps for electrical stimulation over a dynamic range of 5–10 dB are 15–30. For sound, the loudness difference limens vary with intensity from 0.7 dB at 40 dB to 0.3 dB at 80 dB.[20] Consequently, with an average difference limen of 0.5 dB, the number of discriminable steps for sound over the speech intensity range is approximately 60–80. The data thus indicated that if the amplitude variations of speech were also compressed into a narrower dynamic range, there would be enough loudness steps for electrical current to convey essential information.

Third objection and solution

The third objection was that *speech was too complex to be presented to the nervous system by electrical stimulation.*

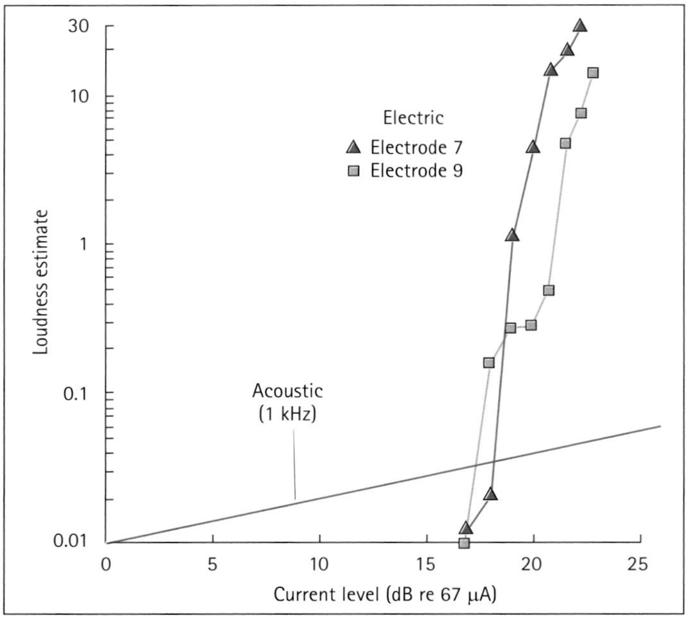

Figure 26.9 Loudness growth for electrical stimulation of the cochlea in our first patient on two representative electrodes stimulated at 200 pulses/s, compared to loudness growth for sound. (From Tong et al. *J Laryngol Otol* 1979; **93**: 679–95.[17])

Electroneural bottleneck

Although the experimental animal and human psychophysical data showed that the coding of the frequencies and intensities of speech sounds could be partially reproduced with electrical stimulation, there was still an 'electroneural bottleneck' between the world of sound and the central auditory nervous system for high-fidelity sound perception. The objection was resolved when it was found that the selection of important speech information and its appropriate presentation to the nervous system was required for optimal speech recognition. The selection of important speech information was necessary because of the 'electroneural bottleneck'. Then the most important questions became: what speech information should be selected, and how should the selected speech elements be transmitted by a multiple-channel cochlear implant system?

Selection of speech information

The answer to the question 'what speech information should be selected?' came when it was noted that the first Melbourne patient reported vowel sounds rather than simple sounds when each electrode was stimulated, and the vowels varied according to the site of stimulation. This is illustrated in Figure 26.10. It was realized that single formant vowels were perceived when similar locations in normally hearing people were excited.[21] In particular, /I/ and its longer-duration equivalent /i/ were perceived for a high-frequency area of the cochlea, /ʌ/ and /a/ at a mid- to low-frequency area, and /ʊ/ and /ɔ/ at a lower-frequency region induced by extra-cochlear current flow.

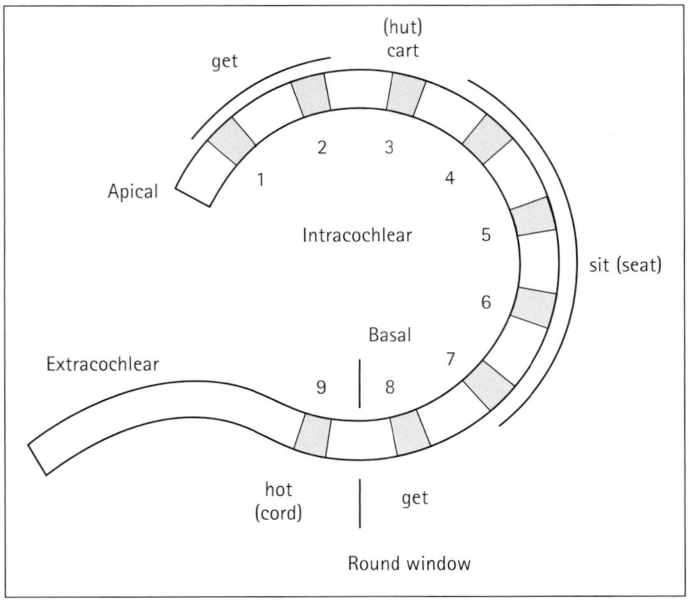

Figure 26.10 The vowels perceived when stimulating different sites within the cochlea in our first patient. (From Tong et al. *J Laryngol Otol* 1979; **93**: 679–95.[17])

As a result of these findings, it was decided to extract a single formant; however, it was considered that this should be the second formant frequency, as acoustically it carries the most information.[22] In addition, it was important to select the voicing frequency so that a distinction could be made, in particular, between the voiced and unvoiced speech sounds. Intensity was extracted, as it also carries important speech information.

Transmission of information to the auditory nervous system

Not only was it necessary to determine the key elements to be selected from speech, but it was also important to determine how to transmit the information through the 'electroneural bottleneck' to the central auditory pathways. As the second formant is high in frequency, it seemed appropriate to code it as place of stimulation, even though it was perceived as timbre. The amplitude of the second formant would be suitably coded as current level. On the other hand, the voicing frequency, which is a low frequency, was thought to be best coded as rate of stimulation, as the psychophysical studies had shown that only low rates could be discriminated.

Furthermore, speech is a complex and dynamic signal, and it was necessary to determine whether changes in place or rate of stimulation could be discriminated over durations of 25 ms, which are required for consonant recognition. A psychophysical study, to study the perception of time-varying place information, showed that the ability to discriminate a shift in the site of electrode stimulation was the same for durations of 25, 50 and 100 ms (Figure 26.11).[10] The first part of the test stimulus produced a shift in electrode stimulated from either electrode 4, 3, or 2 to electrode 1 over durations of 25, 50 and 100 ms. It then remained steady on electrode 1 for 100 ms. The

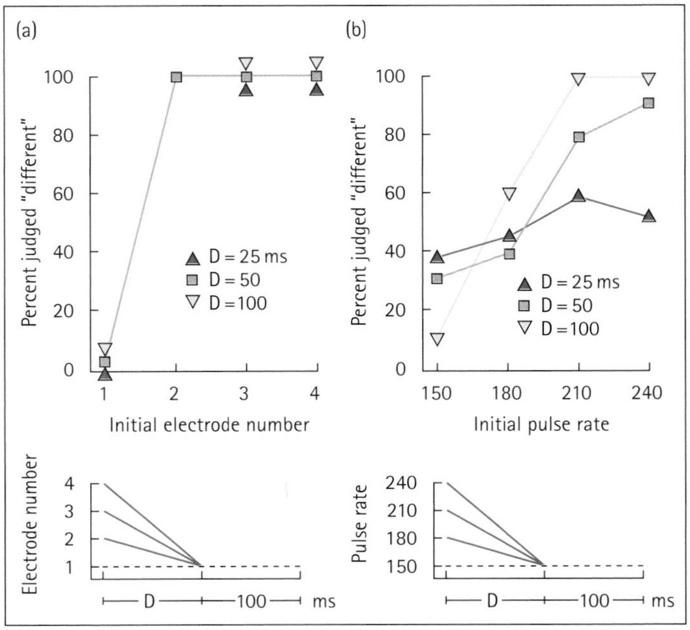

Figure 26.11 (a) Discrimination of changes in place of stimulation versus stimulus duration. (b) Discrimination of changes in rate of stimulation versus stimulus duration. (From Tong et al. *J Acoust Soc Am* 1982; **71**: 153–60.[10])

standard comparison stimulus remained steady on electrode 1. As can be seen, the percentage judgements called different reached 100%, whether the initial electrode was close (no. 2) or further away (no. 4) from the standard electrode (no. 1). There was also no difference in the discrimination ability, whether the duration was 25 ms as required for consonant recognition, or longer, at 100 ms.

These research findings were thus in support of a speech-processing strategy which used place of stimulation to code the rapid changes in formant frequencies of importance to speech. They also suggested that change in place of stimulation was a key coding mechanism for frequency-modulated signals.

A similar study to the above was undertaken using rate of stimulation. In Figure 26.11 the initial pulse rate at the beginning of a frequency ramp was plotted against percentage judgements called different. Note that for a duration of 25 ms, which is required for consonant identification, the performance was poor, but for the longer durations of 50 and 100 ms for vowels, the results were good.

Speech consists not only of segmental information represented by consonants, but suprasegmental or prosodic information conveyed by slow changes in the voicing frequency over time. The voicing frequency ranges on average from 120 Hz for men, to 225 Hz for women. It was essential to transmit this information as well as segmental information. Rate of stimulation was thus shown to be appropriate to code voicing.

The next question to be answered was, could rate not only be discriminated, but perceived as voicing or questions and statements? Furthermore, as place of stimulation would vary with the presentation of segmental speech frequencies, it was also desirable to see if rate changes would convey prosody not only on a particular electrode but also across electrodes. Selected data from one of these studies are illustrated in Figure 26.12.[19] The trajectories for rate are numbered from 1 to 6. The stimuli were categorized as questions if the subject thought that the trajectory was rising in pitch, or as a statement if it was falling. The results for a single electrode show a high success rate. This is also shown when the change in rate is shifted across electrode sites.

The results presented above thus supported the rationale of using rate of stimulation to convey voicing information with a cochlear implant speech-processing strategy. They also demonstrated that pitch from rate of stimulation is integrated into the one speech percept across different sites within the brain.

On the basis of the above psychophysical data and rationale, the inaugural speech-processing strategy extracted the second formant frequency, and stimulated an electrode on a frequency place coding basis. The current level was made proportional to the intensity of the formant frequency. The fundamental frequency or voicing was coded as rate of stimulation across electrodes. This strategy enabled patients to understand running speech when combined with lipreading, and some speech using electrical stimulation alone, as illustrated in Figure 26.13. It can also be seen, e.g. with electrical stimulation alone, that the scores improved over time.

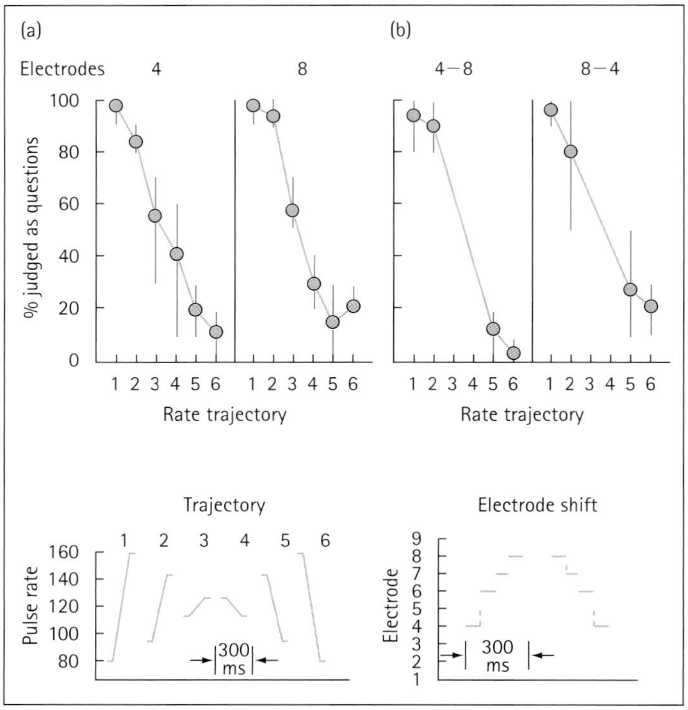

Figure 26.12 Percentage questions and statements for rising and falling pulse rates (a) on single electrodes and (b) across electrodes. (From Tong et al. *J Acoust Soc Am* 1983; **74**: 73–80.[19])

After establishing the concept of selecting maximal speech information and using the right coding strategy for the transmission of the second formant and voicing frequency through the 'electroneural bottleneck', further research was undertaken to expand the concept. This required examining whether improved speech recognition could be obtained by selecting the first and/or the third formants, as well as the second formant, and transmitting these on a place coding basis through the 'bottleneck'. For this reason, a psychophysical study was first undertaken to see if stimulating two sites within the cochlea for two formants would produce a percept with perceptual space that resulted from the two sites of stimulation. This in fact occurred, as shown in Figure 26.14, where it can be seen that, with multidimensional scaling, the result is best satisfied with two dimensions.[23] This result provided the psychophysical basis for more advanced speech-processing strategies which presented additional formant and other spectral information on a place coding basis.

Research then focused on which further speech elements to extract. It was first found that picking the energy in the first (F_1) as well as second formant (F_2) peaks, and presenting these on a place coding basis, gave improved results ($F_0/F_1/F_2$ strategy). It was then discovered that selecting energy in the high-frequency bands in the third formant region as well as the first and second formant gave even better results ('Multipeak' strategy). Most recently, it has been found that selecting 6–8 frequency bands with the greatest energy from a 16–20 bandpass filter bank, and presenting the information as a place code, results in a further

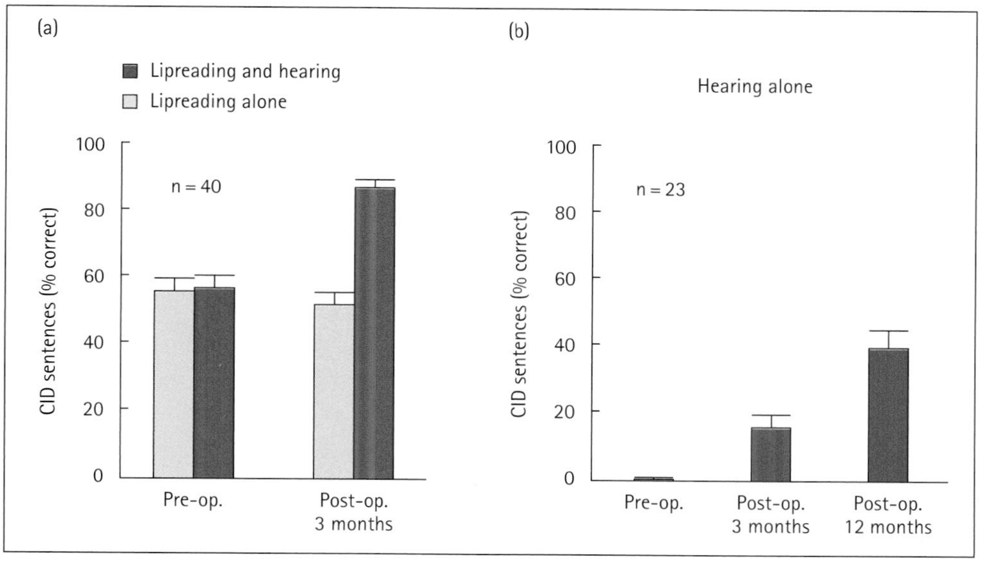

Figure 26.13 (a) The improvements in open-set Central Institute for the Deaf (CID) sentence scores 3 months postoperatively for the inaugural second formant/voicing speech processor for lipreading combined with electrical stimulation compared to lipreading alone. (b) The open-set CID sentence scores for electrical stimulation alone at 3 and 12 months postoperatively.

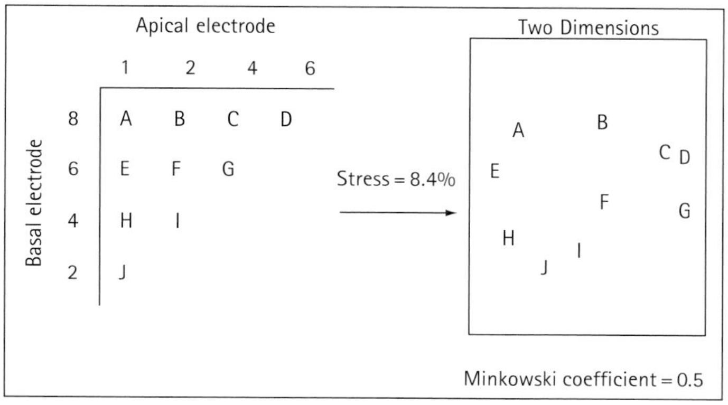

Figure 26.14 Multidimensional scaling of the percept from dual electrode stimulation. (Reprinted with permission from *Science* 1983; **219**: 993–4. © 1983 American Association for the Advancement of Science.[23])

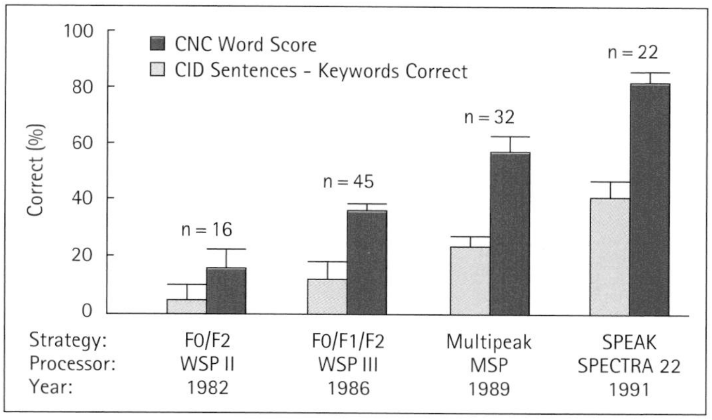

Figure 26.15 The average open-set word and sentence results for four speech-processing strategies which select progressively increasing spectral information for coding on a place basis. CNC, consonant–nucleus–consonant. (From Clark. *Cochl Implants Int* 2000; **1**: 1–17.[113])

improvement in speech recognition (SPEAK strategy). In this case, rate of stimulation is not used to convey voicing, but a constant rate of stimulation is produced, and voicing is conveyed through the amplitude variations in the signal. A constant rate of stimulation is used to avoid the interactions that take place in the electrical fields when neighbouring electrodes are excited. The improved results obtained by progressively increasing the amount of information presented on a place coding basis, as well as the way in which the information is extracted from speech, are shown in Figure 26.15.

Fourth objection and solution

The fourth objection was that *there would not be enough residual hearing nerves in the cochlea after die-back due to deafness for speech understanding*. This was partly answered in studies on experimental animals in which it was found that varying populations of spiral ganglion cells had no significant effect on discrimination of the rate of stimulation.[24] However, ultimately the question of nerve survival and speech understanding had to be resolved in patients. For this reason, speech recognition results have been compared for different aetiologies as they are thought to affect the auditory nerve and ganglion cell numbers.

Figure 26.16 shows the ranking of speech recognition versus aetiology for 808 subjects,[25] and the ranking of ganglion cell count versus aetiology for 66 subjects, based on the results of Nadol et al.[26] The ranking of speech recognition does not correspond with the ranking for ganglion cell counts, and this suggests that there is no significant relationship between spiral ganglion cell numbers and speech recognition for the present multiple-electrode system.

Fifth objection and solution

The fifth objection was: *children born deaf or deafened early in life would not develop the right neural connections for speech*

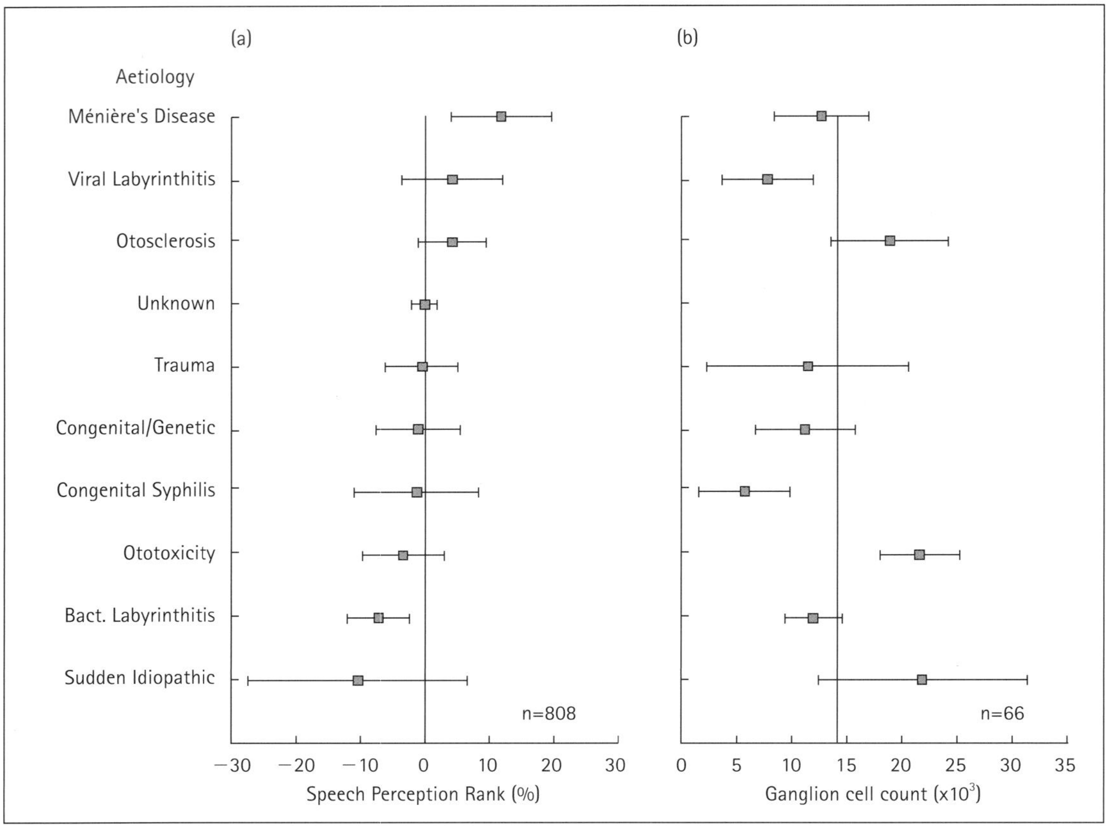

Figure 26.16 (a) Comparison between speech recognition scores and aetiology.[25] (b) Comparison between aetiology and ganglion cell numbers. (Reprinted with permission from Blamey et al. *Audiol Neurootol* 1996; **1**: 296–306[25] and Nadol et al. *Ann Otol Rhinol Laryngol* 1989; **98**: 411–16.[26])

understanding. This objection could not be answered until children who were born deaf or deafened early in life were implanted. In Melbourne, the first three children were implanted in 1985 and 1986 after establishing the benefits of the cochlear implant for adults. This was the start of an international trial for the US Food & Drug Administration (FDA).

The trial showed that 60% of children born deaf were able to understand some open-set speech, and the majority of the others had significant help in lipreading. Figure 26.17 shows the pre- and post- operative speech perception levels in children who were prelinguistically or postlinguistically deaf.[27] In both groups, closed-set and open-set speech perception was significantly better after the operation. The open-set score, however, was better for the postlinguistic group. Nevertheless, the results suggest that children born deaf (i.e. without exposure to sound) have or can develop the right neural connections for processing speech sounds presented through electrical stimulation.

The FDA approved the device as safe and effective for children 2 years of age and above in 1990. Furthermore, a subsequent analysis of our data on children has shown (Figure 26.18) that, although there is considerable variability in results, the younger the child, the better the speech perception, and, if extrapolated back, speech perception may be better if the child is younger than 2 years of age. These results indicate that age is a factor in children born deaf being able to develop the right neural connections for speech recognition.

To determine why speech recognition is better for younger children, the development of frequency discrimination and pitch perception with age, and their relationship to speech recognition, have been studied. Children's ability to discriminate electrode place of stimulation, in particular, has been investigated because of the importance of place coding in speech understanding. As shown in Figure 26.19, the younger the child, the better the discrimination of electrode place of stimulation. This suggests that there is a critical period of time over which the neural connectivity for place discrimination can occur.[28]

To help confirm the relationship between electrode place discrimination and speech perception, a comparison was made using a closed-set speech test. The findings in Figure 26.20 show that the smaller the separation between electrodes that could be detected, the better the speech perception. This supports the view that if the neural connections required for place coding are created during the critical period, then speech perception will be enhanced.[28]

On the other hand, when the ability of children to rank pitch tonotopically (i.e. whether it is higher or lower in pitch) rather than simply discriminate electrode place was compared with their speech perception scores, it can be seen, as shown in Figure 26.21, that not all children who could rank pitch had good speech recognition. For three-quarters of the 16 children in the study, a tonotopic ordering of pitch percepts was found. However, only 58% of these children with good ability to rank

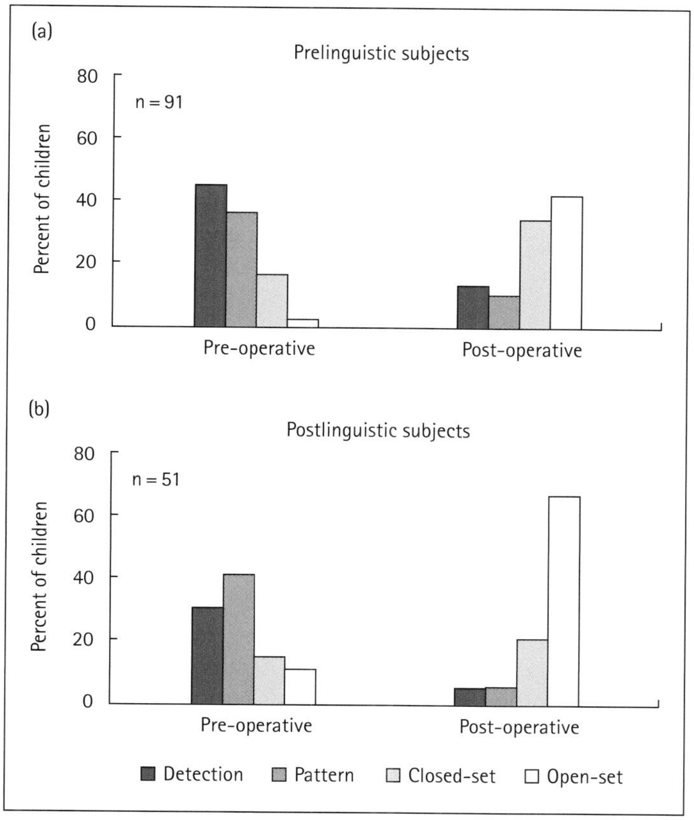

Figure 26.17 Pre- and postoperative highest communication categories achieved for children from 2 to 18 years of age using the Nucleus F_0/F_2 and $F_0/F_1/F_2$ speech processors 3 months postoperatively. The categories were sound detection, pattern recognition, closed-set word recognition, and open-set word recognition. The children were divided into (a) prelinguistic (deaf before speech developed) and (b) postlinguistic (deaf after speech developed) groups. The data were presented to the US FDA, and approval was given in 1990 for the use of the multiple-channel implant in children. The data for the construction of the graphs are from Staller et al. *Am J Otol* 1991; **12**: 126–36.[27]

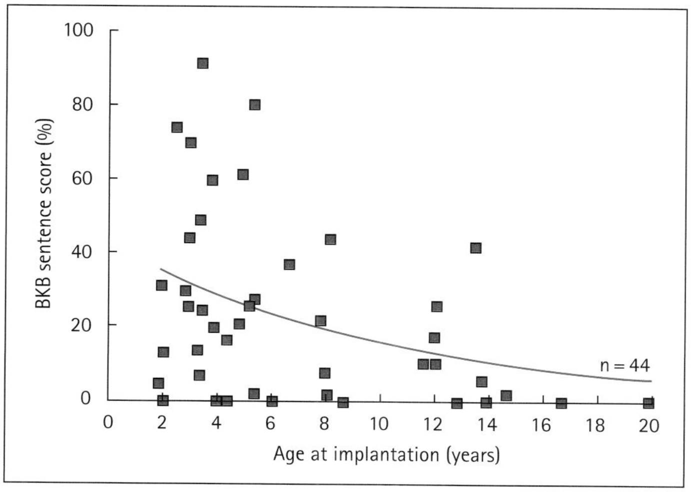

Figure 26.18 BKB open-set sentence scores for electrical stimulation alone versus age at implantation.

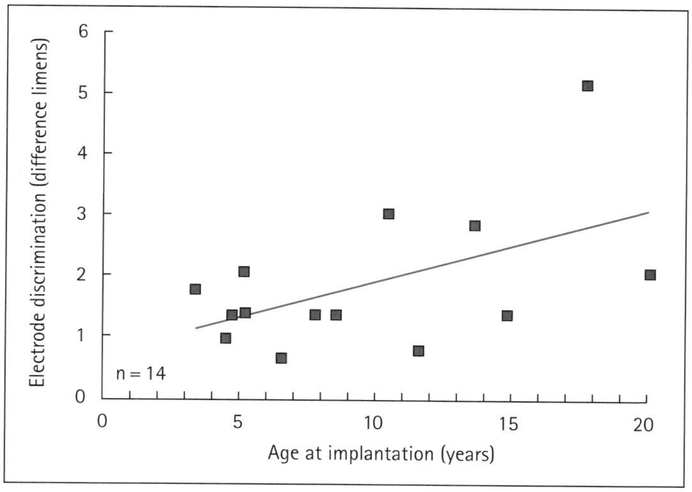

Figure 26.19 The discrimination of place of stimulation versus age at implantation in children. (Reproduced with permission from Clark. In: *Perpetual Learning*. Cambridge MA: MIT Press, 2002.[90])

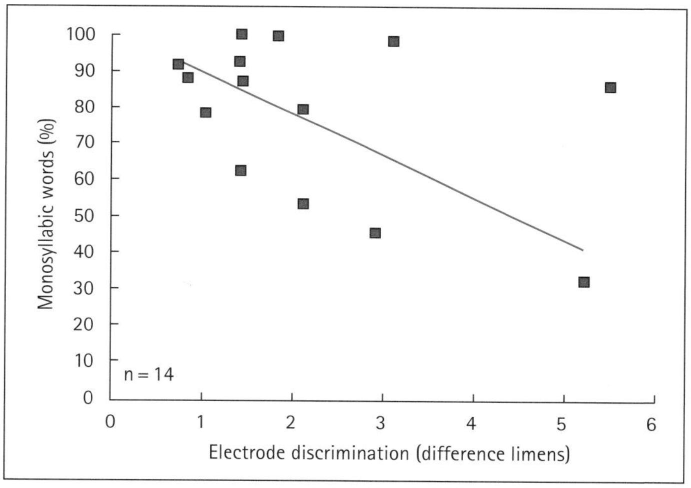

Figure 26.20 Monosyllable word scores versus electrode place discrimination recorded as difference limens. (Reproduced with permission from Clark. In: *Perpetual Learning*. Cambridge MA: MIT Press, 2002.[90])

pitch had satisfactory speech perception of 30% or more. Because the ability to rank pitch was not always associated with good speech perception, this suggests that a factor other than the neural connectivity associated with place discrimination is required for speech recognition.[28] Other studies have shown that this other factor is most probably language.[29]

Finally, as the data from the study on speech recognition versus age showed that extrapolation of results back to earlier than 2 years of age could lead to better results, operations on very young children were planned. However, before carrying out the operations, it was necessary to undertake and complete a series of biological studies to ensure that operating on a child of this age was safe. Young children have special problems. These are: first, the effects of head growth on the lead wire

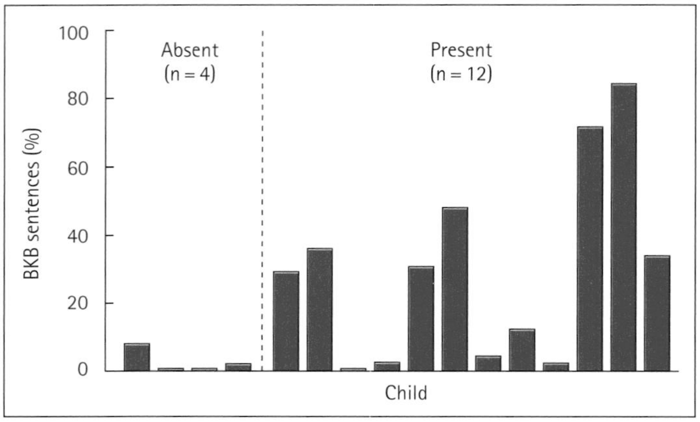

Figure 26.21 Open-set BKB sentence scores for children where tonotopic pitch-ordering ability is either absent or present. (Reproduced with permission from Clark. In: *Perpetual Learning*. Cambridge MA: MIT Press, 2002.[90])

assembly; second, any inner ear complications from otitis media leading to an extension of the infection around the electrode entry point; and third, the effects of electrical stimulation on the developing nervous system. This research was part of a special 5-year contract to the US National Institutes of Health[14] (Studies on Pediatric Auditory Prosthesis Implants, Contract NO-NS-7-2342/1987–1992). This research showed no cause for concern with regard to operations on young children.

Preoperative selection

The selection of a person for a cochlear implant requires a number of interviews, special tests, and counselling. This process must be undertaken by a number of professionals, and progress should be reviewed at appropriate stages by a clinical team headed by an audiological physician or otolaryngologist.

Medical

At the first consultation, a preliminary medical history should be taken, and an otological examination performed. The details of the hearing loss should be clarified, particularly its time and speed of onset, precipitating factors, severity, previous treatment, disability caused, and associated symptoms such as ear discharge, tinnitus, and disequilibrium. Any general medical and surgical issues that are relevant to the aetiology of the condition and its management need to be explored and corrected.

As otitis media and middle ear effusion are common in young children, they are frequently seen in many in this age group when being assessed for cochlear implantation. Previous animal experimental studies have shown that implantation with overt or incipient infection in the middle ear at the time of surgery is likely to produce suppurative labyrinthitis with marked loss of spiral ganglion cells.[30, 31] Therefore, preoperative selection and management should ensure that there is no active ear disease at the time of surgery. The otitis media should have completely resolved. On the other hand, middle ear effusions are usually sterile, and implantation can proceed more readily once the condition has been controlled with grommets and, when necessary, adenoidectomy.

The medical consultation will provide an opportunity to assess the expectations of the person, or the parents in the case of a young child. It is also desirable to discuss the communication options available for children, and find out whether the parents have adequately explored these.

Hearing, speech and language

In selecting children and adults for surgery, it is important to ensure that their hearing status is such that they would do better with an implant rather than a hearing aid.

Hearing status in adults

In the case of adults, it is necessary to carry out not only pure tone audiometry in unaided and aided conditions, but also extensive speech testing. As shown by the work of Flynn et al,[32] there is not always good agreement between audiometric thresholds and speech recognition results. Ultimately, the speech recognition scores are the most critical in determining suitability for an implant with an adult. As the mean CID sentence scores for electrical stimulation alone for the SPEAK strategy are now 80%, the University of Melbourne Cochlear Implant Clinic patients are considered for surgery when the hearing in the better ear is poorer than 40–50%. On particular occasions, patients may be considered with higher scores. The ability to communicate in noisy surroundings and the need for this skill is becoming an important issue in patient selection.

Hearing status in infants and young children

The hearing status in infants and young children needs to be accurately determined by both behavioural and objective tests. The tests should also elucidate the status of the central auditory pathways, and their ability to process information. There is still a long way to go to achieve this second goal.

Hearing loss in young children from 6 to 18 months of age, when this is considered as developmental age, can be assessed using visual reinforcement audiometry (or VRA). With normally hearing children, the test yields thresholds within 10 dB of thresholds obtained later with standard audiometry. A review of the literature shows that there are no satisfactory studies indicating how well it correlates for deaf children or the false-positive rates. Research is needed to clarify these questions, and the situation only serves to emphasize the need to use behavioural tests in conjunction with objective tests. Similarly, with play audiometry, which is applicable from 18 months and above, there are no comparisons of thresholds for deaf children with later results for standard audiometry.

An accurate objective threshold in infants and young children over the speech frequency range can be obtained using tone-burst evoked auditory brainstem responses (ABRs) with a 'notched-noise' masker. Stapells et al[33] showed that there was excellent correspondence between ABR with a 'notched-noise' masker and behavioural thresholds for the 500-Hz to 4-kHz range. However, the recording of steady-state evoked potentials (referred to as SSEPs)[34] is preferred for the objective assessment of children, as it is just as accurate as the ABR with 'notched-noise' for the severe-to-profound hearing losses, and has an automatic detection algorithm for judging when an ABR is present or absent.[35] With SSEPs, the auditory evoked potentials are recorded from the scalp in response to amplitude-modulated sound frequencies. A Fourier analysis of the evoked potentials is carried out to determine the amplitude and phase spectra of the waveform. The relationship between SSEPs and behavioural thresholds is shown in Figure 26.22.[36] Notice the particularly good correlation for the severe-to-profound losses.

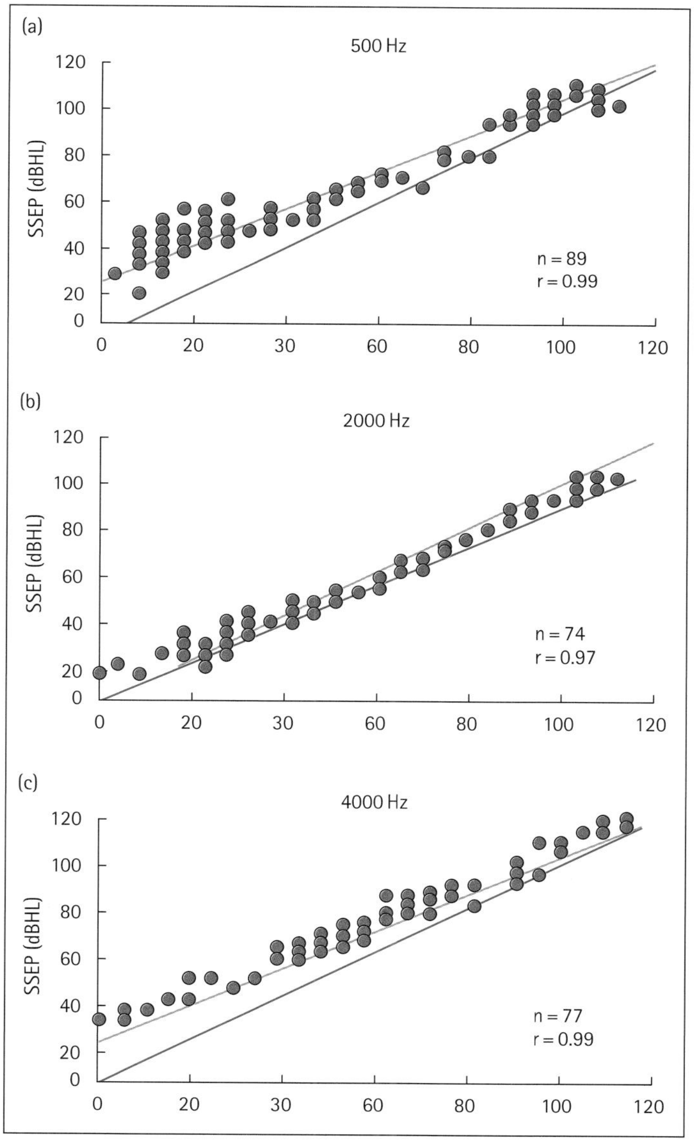

Figure 26.22 The relationship between steady-state evoked potentials (SSEPs) and behavioural thresholds for the frequencies (a) 500, (b) 2000 and (c) 4000 Hz. (From Rance et al. *Ear Hear* 1995; **16**: 499–507.[36])

Cochlear microphonics and summating potentials should also be recorded from children who are prospective cochlear implant recipients. Recent studies have shown that a small proportion of children with absent or elevated ABR or SSEP thresholds may have cochlear microphonics present. Some of these children may have normal hearing. On the other hand, those with a profound loss may do poorly with a cochlear implant. The cochlear microphonic can be recorded using click-evoked ABRs to rarefaction and condensation clicks, and a typical result is shown in Figure 26.23.

In Melbourne, 5199 children were screened with click ABRs, and 109 were found with raised thresholds. Thirty-seven had no ABRs. Of the 37 with no ABRs, there were 25 who also had no cochlear microphonics and they were severely-to-profoundly deaf. On the other hand, 12 had cochlear microphonics and hearing which ranged from normal to total loss. Those children with a severe loss were thought to have a neuropathy, and possibly should not be implanted. In this series, the majority had anoxia or kernicterus at birth.[37]

The recording of cochlear microphonics and slower potentials can also be done using transtympanic electrodes, and they may also play an important role in the preoperative assessment of children for a cochlear implant. It has been found that a small proportion of children with a severe-to-profound hearing loss have an abnormal positive potential, referred to as an APP[38]. The origin of this potential is not clear. It may reflect a retrocochlear as well as cochlear pathology. If a cochlear implant operation is carried out on children with abnormal potential, a proportion could have poor auditory perception postoperatively. These children would have little neural activity when electrically evoked potentials were recorded with their implants. The recording of otoacoustic emissions (OAEs) is not central to the assessment of hearing thresholds in the child, as it only correlates with thresholds up to 45 dB HL. However, as it is a measure of outer hair cell integrity, it should be used to study children where a neuropathy is suspected.

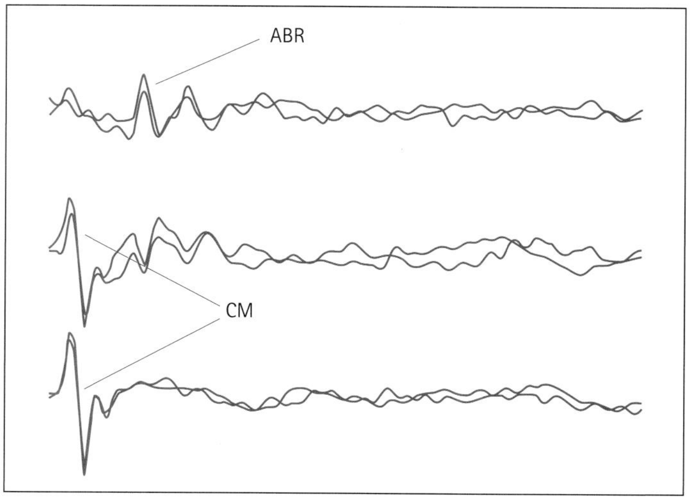

Figure 26.23 Click-evoked ABRs and cochlear microphonics (CM). (From Rance et al. *Ear Hear* 1995; **16**: 499–507.[36])

The relationship of the pure tone audiogram to expected speech perception with an implant

Hearing thresholds are very important in selecting infants and young children for implantation. The thresholds are required to determine whether the child has sufficient hearing to do better with a hearing aid rather than an implant. Hearing thresholds are important, as speech tests are not effective, due to their limited language. Multiple-channel implants can provide spectral information in the mid- to high-frequency range when this is not possible through amplification of sound with an aid. For this reason, pay particular attention to the thresholds for the frequencies above 1 kHz. As shown in Figure 26.24, if the unaided thresholds are greater than 90 dB for the frequencies 1.5, 2.0, 3.0 and 4.0 kHz, the child is a likely candidate. Furthermore, the aided thresholds for the above hearing losses when using a powerful hearing aid will just enter the speech spectrum for 70-dB speech presented at a distance of 1 m, as shown in Figure 26.25. Consequently, a child with an aided threshold at 2 kHz greater than 60 dB SPL is a likely recipient.

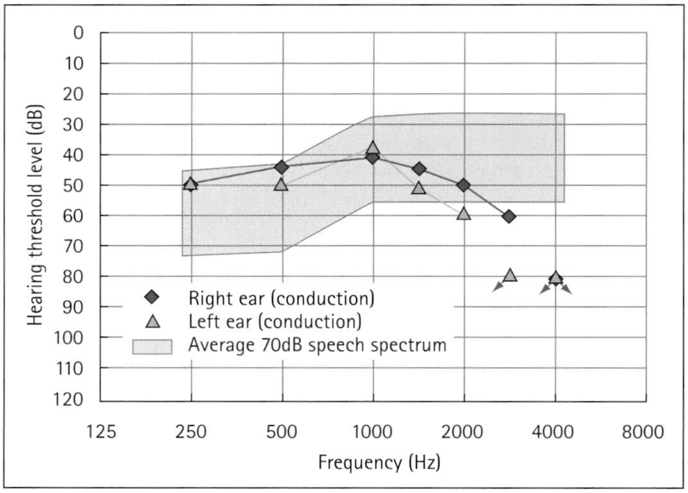

Figure 26.25 Aided audiogram showing the usual minimum threshold level required for selection for implantation

Family support and education

In addition to the medical as well as hearing, speech and language assessments, it is important to determine the level of family support and educational management of children. Family support is required for both adults and children. With adults, the family is needed, in particular, to help in the social adjustments required in adopting new modes of communication, such as answering the telephone. With children, parents play a crucial role in their child's education, especially at the preschool stage. The parents will need to understand how best to communicate with their child, be knowledgeable about the cochlear implant, and support their child socially and emotionally. If the child is at school level, the teacher's appraisal is essential. Before embarking on an implant, it it important to be sure that there will be optimal support for an auditory/oral education to achieve best results with the implant.

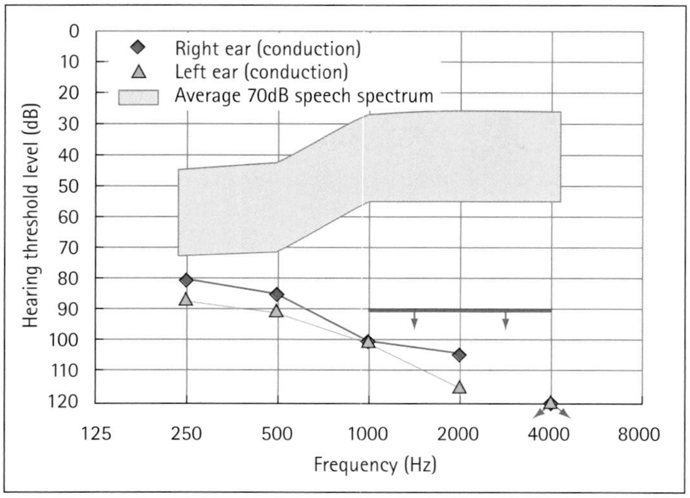

Figure 26.24 Unaided audiogram as a selection criterion for cochlear implantation. When thresholds are greater than the demarcated level, implantation can be considered.

Predictive factors

The factors that predict successful outcomes are important in helping to select patients for surgery. People, and in the case of children their parents, wish to know how well they are likely to perform after surgery. A better knowledge of the preoperative factors predicting outcomes will help answer their questions. Two studies on adults have shown that approximately 20% and 40% of the variance in the results can be accounted for by the predictive factors,[39, 40] and one study on children has shown that 50% of the variance can be accounted for this way.[41] Thus, it is still not possible to confidently tell a prospective patient or parent how well they or their child will perform, but in assessing the suitability of each person, the preoperative predictive factors are still quite important.

Preoperative predictive factors for adults and children

The preoperative predictive factors that are common to both the adult and child are: (1) aetiology; (2) age at implantation and duration of deafness; (3) progressive hearing loss; (4) length of insertion of the electrode array; (5) electrical stimulation of the promontory results; and (6) speech processing strategy.

With aetiology, Menière's disease correlates positively and meningitis negatively with results in the adult. In children, meningitis also correlates negatively with results. This may be due to a reduced number of electrodes which can be inserted because of labyrinthitis ossificans.[25]

Age at implantation and duration of deafness are both inter-related. In the adult, however, they can both be separated and both correlate negatively with results. With age, however, results are only poorer if the patient is over 60 years of age. In children, age at implantation and duration of deafness cannot be separated, as most children are congenitally deaf. Age at implantation probably has its effects because perceptual learning is more difficult the older the child or adult. On the other hand, with duration of deafness, it may have its effect because the longer the duration of the hearing loss, the greater the loss of the neurones and their connections.

The effect of a progressive hearing loss has not been determined, but it appears to correlate with good results in the clinic patients in Melbourne. This is probably due to the time required to learn how to process a degraded signal.

A positive relationship has been seen between the length of insertion or the number of electrodes in use and speech perception. Two studies have been carried out on adults and one on children,[39–41] and have shown that there is increasing benefit in having additional electrodes from 9 up to 21 (9 being the minimum number inserted in the patients in the study). These results highlight the importance of multiple-electrode stimulation, which is needed for the spectral information in speech.

There has been a positive correlation between preoperative tests of temporal processing via promontory stimulation of the auditory nerve and speech perception results. Discriminating gaps smaller than 50 ms for low rates of stimulation, and pitch changes for rates of 100 and 200 pulses/s, suggest a good result. The ability to detect changes in rate of stimulation and gaps between stimuli appears to be a more central function, and is important for segmenting speech and processing the slow frequency changes occuring in voicing.

The speech-processing strategy affects results in both children and adults. Improvements have primarily been seen by presenting additional frequency information on a place coding basis.[42]

Preoperative predictive factors relevant to children

There are additional preoperative predictive factors that are especially relevant to children. These factors are: (1) prelinguistic versus postlinguistic hearing loss; (2) language development; (3) communication strategy and mode of education; and (4) delayed cognitive and motor milestones.

The effects of prelingual (born deaf or lost hearing before learning language) versus postlingual hearing loss (lost hearing after learning language) on results were assessed for the F_0/F_2 and $F_0/F_1/F_2$ speech-processing strategies. This was done by analysing data from the international trial for the US FDA to determine whether the multiple-electrode cochlear implant would benefit both prelinguistic and postlinguistically deaf children. As discussed above, the trial showed that 60% of the children were able to understand some open-set speech, and the majority of the others had significant help in lipreading. The results were broken down into the pre- and postoperative highest speech perception categories achieved in children who were prelinguistically or postlinguistically deaf, and are shown in Figure 26.17.[27] In both groups, closed-set and open-set speech recognition was markedly better after operation. The open-set score, however, was better for the postlinguistic group.

In studying the relation between speech recognition and language, results have been analysed for 57 children with a bilateral severe or profound hearing loss.[29] Of these children, 33 were hearing aid users and 24 implant users. They attended deaf/oral schools or preschools, and the data are from a 4-year longitudinal study. The speech recognition results were comparable for the aided and implanted children. For the hearing aid children, the mean loss was 81 dB (averaged over 0.5, 1.0 and 2.0 kHz). For the implanted children, the mean preoperative loss in the better ear was greater than 100 dB HL. This indicates that the implanted children with thresholds of 100 dB HL were performing at a comparable level to children who had thresholds of 81 dB HL, and used a powerful hearing aid. As an 81 dB HL threshold at the frequencies of 0.5, 1.0 and 2.0 kHz equates with a hearing loss at 2.0 kHz of 90 dB HL, these data help confirm one of the University of Melbourne's criteria for selection of children. This criterion is that they are suitable for implantation if their thresholds are greater than 90 dB HL for frequencies above 1.0 kHz.

The receptive language for the aided and implanted group of children was also compared with their speech perception scores. The Peabody Picture Vocabulary Test (PPVT)[43] and Clinical Evaluation of Language Fundamentals (CELF)[44] tests were used. The PPVT is for children from 2 years and above, and the CELF is designed for children over 6 years. The receptive language results were slightly better for the aided children, but this was probably due to the fact they were older on average. When speech recognition (Figure 26.26) and receptive language (Figure 26.27) scores were both plotted against chronological age, there was a gradual increase in performance, but the increase did not keep up with that seen with normally hearing children.[29]

On the other hand, when speech recognition (word and sentence scores) was compared with receptive language (PPVT or CELF equivalent ages), there was a very close relationship between the two. For example, the auditory/visual word score

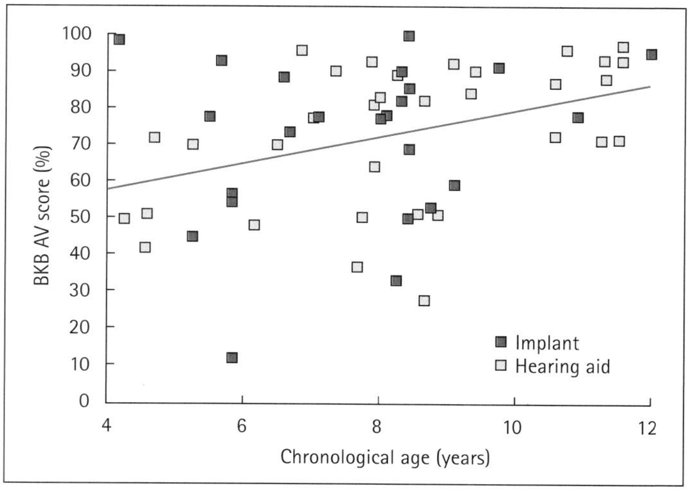

Figure 26.26 Speech recognition results in linear regression for hearing-aided and implanted children using the BKB sentences with audition and lipreading versus chronological age.

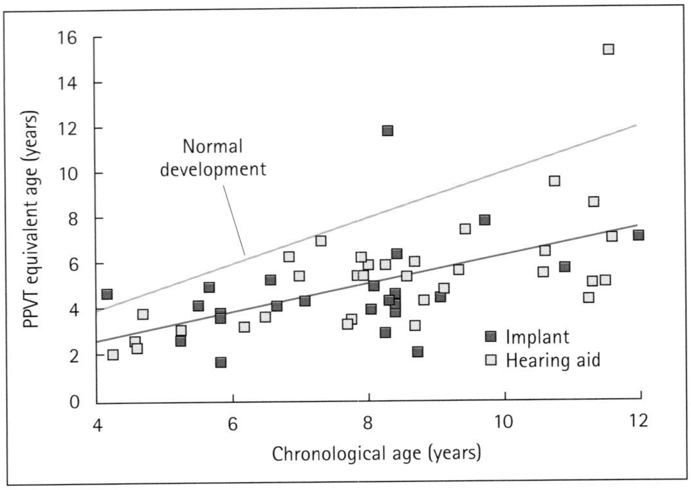

Figure 26.27 Receptive language results and linear regression for hearing-aided and implanted children using the PPVT as age-appropriate test versus chronological age. (From Blamey et al. *Ann Otol Rhinol Laryngol* 1992; **107**: 342–8.[39])

reached 100% at a PPVT or CELF age of 8–10 years (Figure 26.28). However, for audition alone, the slope was less steep, and a 100% score was reached later at 10–11 years. These results demonstrate the important relationship between speech recognition and language.

The communication strategy adopted before surgery influences results, and children do better if they have had an auditory–oral education.[41] The mode of education after surgery is important, and an auditory–oral education is required for best results. However, it has been said that the results for mode of education are subject to selection; that is, children who have poor speech perception may require total communication, or children who have the potential to do better are being selected for the auditory–oral programme. It is relevant, however, that the data from Melbourne, although there is a wide spread of

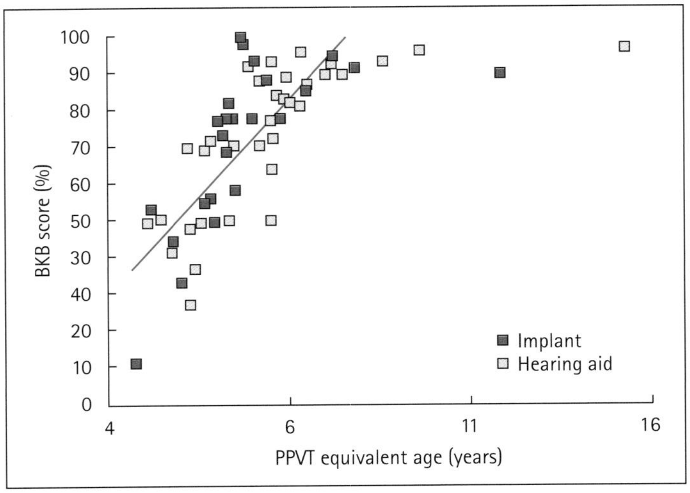

Figure 26.28 Auditory/visual speech recognition (BKB sentences) versus receptive language (PPVT). (From Blamey et al. *Ann Otol Rhinol Laryngol* 1992; **107**: 342–8.[39])

performance for both groups, show that children with open-set scores of 50% or more are only seen in the auditory–oral group.

To see if delayed motor and cognitive milestones affect the cochlear implant results, the perfomances for children with and without these disabilities have been compared. As some aetiologies (rubella, cytomegalovirus, meningitis, anoxia, prematurity, kernicterus, and certain syndromes) are likely to affect the central nervous system and so cause delayed motor and cognitive milestones, the study also compared performance across these aetiologies.[45] The results showed that the occurrence of motor and cognitive delays was fairly evenly spread across aetiologies, with the exception of cytomegalovirus, which had a higher than average prevalence in the delayed group. However, aetiology did not have a significant effect on speech recognition. On the other hand, children with delayed cognitive and motor milestones did significantly worse on both an analysis of variance and general linear model, as they had poorer speech recognition.

The percentages of normal and delayed children reaching five different speech recognition categories over time are shown in Figure 26.29. The categories are maximum performance levels of: 1—sound identification; 2—syllabic pattern recognition; 3—vowel identification; 4—consonant identification; and 5—varying degrees of open-set recognition. The data show that it takes much longer for children with developmental delays to reach targets, and this applies in particular for open-set recognition. Although the benefits are not as good in children with developmental delays, they may receive a greater relative benefit because of their handicap. A child has to have a very severe disability and not be able to follow instructions before the Melbourne clinic will advise against surgery. If the child's habilitation is slow, the staff of the clinic sometimes recommend that they have complementary signing help.

Technological features of selected multiple-channel cochlear implant systems

The findings discussed in this chapter apply to multiple-channel implants in general. However, the performance of an implant system not only depends on the underlying concept, but is inextricably linked to the engineering of the device. For this reason, it is important to understand how the variations in the technological features for the most commonly used products impact on present and future results. The technological details referred to are for the Cochlear Limited (Nucleus-24), Med-El (Combi-40), and Advanced Bionics (Clarion-S) devices (Table 26.1). The details are those available from the manufacturer's manuals, websites, patents and scientific papers. However, the rationale for the features is not in every case substantiated. The features to be discussed in particular are for the devices in regular clinical use in early 1999.

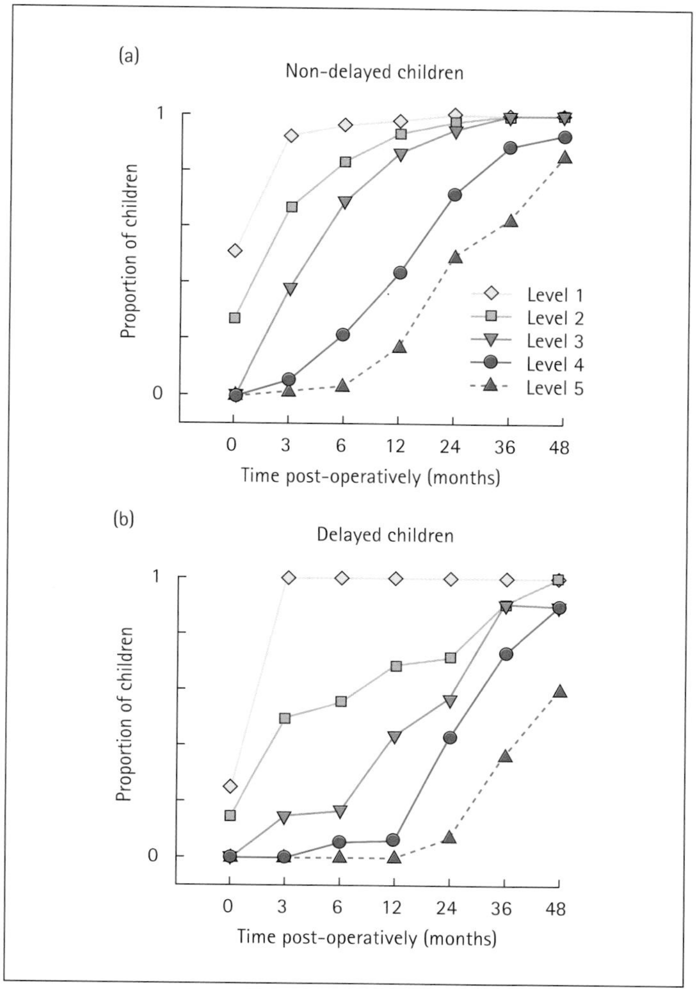

Figure 26.29 Speech recognition categories for children with (a) normal and (b) delayed motor and cognitive milestones. The categories are maximum performance levels of: 1—sound identification; 2—syllabic pattern recognition; 3—vowel identification; 4—consonant identification; and 5—varying degrees of open-set recognition. (Reprinted with permission from Pyman et al. *Am J Otol* 2000; **21**: 57–61.[45])

Standard speech-processing strategy

SPEAK

The SPEAK (Spectral Maxima Sound Processor) strategy used by the Nucleus system selects the 6–8 spectral maxima from the outputs of 16–20 bandpass filters, and presents the voltage outputs non-simultaneously on a place coding basis. A constant rate of stimulation is used to reduce channel interactions (250 Hz, and voicing is conveyed by variations in the amplitude of the signal. Variations of this strategy have been tested in pilot studies at the Cooperative Research Centre for Cochlear Implant Speech and Hearing Research in Melbourne. These include order of presentation of the stimuli, and the use of fundamental frequency or random rate instead of a constant rate. The present device allows for these and other variations to be used.

SAS

The SAS (Simultaneous Analogue Stimulation) strategy used by Clarion is a derivative of the strategy developed by both the Salt Lake City[46, 47] group and implemented as the Symbion or InnerAid device, and the University of San Francisco group,[48] and implemented as the Storz or MiniMed device. The InnerAid device presented the outputs of four fixed filters to the auditory nerve by simultaneous monopolar stimulation, and the Storz device used bipolar stimulation.This analog scheme was subsequently used with eight filters in the Clarion[49] processor.

Simultaneous stimulation was shown early in cochlear implant research to produce unpredictable variations in loudness, due to interactions in current flow.[16] To control loudness, an algorithm is needed to predict the voltage fields from two or more electrodes at all intensity levels. This has not been achieved. The only way to avoid the problem of channel interaction is to separate the stimulus channels so that the voltage fields do not overlap. An adequate separation of stimulus channels may be achieved if a curved electrode array is placed close to the spiral ganglion cells so that either monopolar or bipolar stimulation can produce localized neural excitation.

Analogue stimulation of the nervous system was evaluated by the pioneering neurophysiologists in the 1940s and 1950s, and found to be less suitable than pulsatile stimulation. The neurone integrates current to produce an action potential, whether the stimulus is analogue or pulsatile. With a pulse, the current can be more precisely controlled. However, a preliminary study by Clark[7] was undertaken to compare analogue and pulsatile stimuli and their effects on synchrony of firing, but with inconclusive results. A more detailed neurophysiological evaluation of the effects of both biphasic current pulses and sinusoidal current waveforms showed no significant differences in the temporal properties of the responses.[50, 51] There are, however, differences in synchrony of response, depending on pulse width and frequency.

The Symbion/InnerAid four fixed filter system, which used analogue waveforms, was compared with the Nucleus Multipeak-MSP system. The Multipeak-MSP was an earlier version of Nucleus systems extracting two formant peaks, and the energy in three high-frequency bands.[52] The well-controlled study[53] showed that there were better mean speech scores for the Multipeak-MSP system (75%) compared with the Symbion/InnerAid system (42%).

CIS

The CIS (Continuous Interleaved Sampler) strategy, like SPEAK, stimulates multiple channels non-simultaneously to reduce channel interactions, but does so at a higher rate. The outputs of six or more filters are sampled, and used to stimulate corresponding numbers of electrodes on a place coding basis. Various studies have been done to optimize the number of filters and stimulus rate.[54, 55] A constant stimulus rate between 833 and 1111 pulses/s per channel has been recommended.[49]

A comparison of the SPEAK and CIS strategies was first possible from data for comparable groups of patients using the

Table 26.1 Comparative Technology, March 1999—Nucleus-24, Combi-40, Clarion-S implant systems.

	Nucleus-24	Combi-40	Clarion-S
Standard speech-processing strategies	SPEAK CIS	CIS	CIS SAS
Maximum pulse rates: non-simultaneous stimulation	14 493	12 120	6500
Maximum sample rates simultaneous stimulation	Not applicable	Not applicable	104 000 samples/s
Maximum number of stimulus channels	22	8	8 (CIS) 7 (SAS)
Mode of stimulation	Monopolar Common ground Bipolar	Monopolar	Monopolar (CIS) Bipolar (SAS)
Speech strategies under investigation or proposed	ACE, ADRO, TESM	CIS+, Jitter–CIS	SPS, HAP, PPS,
Behind-the-ear speech processor	In regular use	In regular use	In regular use
Telemetry	CAP Impedance Compliance	Impedance	Impedance
Implant casing	Titanium	Ceramic	Ceramic
Reliability	99.6% adults at 1 year 98.7% chldren at 1 year	N/A	N/A
Number of years contributing to observed reliability	>3000	N/A	N/A

N/A, not available.

six-channel (electrode) SPEAK and six-channel CIS strategies in 1995 and 1996. SPEAK presented essentially six maxima, but this could be up to 9 or 10. The open-set CID sentence scores for electrical stimulation alone for the CIS-Clarion system (on 64 patients 6 months postoperatively)[56] and the SPEAK-Spectra-22 system (on 51 unselected patients tested from 2 weeks to 6 months after the start-up time) (data presented to the FDA, January 1996) were compared. The results showed that the performance for SPEAK was at least as good or possibly better.[57]

For more details of these strategies and their comparative results, see Clark.[57]

Maximum rates: non-simultaneous pulsatile stimulation

The manufacturers offer the CIS stategies at rates even higher than 800 pulses/s. Communication engineers can sample speech much more rapidly than can be processed through each nerve fibre. For example, an audio CD samples the sound wave at 44 100 samples/s. However, the cochlear nerve fibres have an absolute refractory period of approximately 0.5 ms, and a relative refractory period of approximately 2 ms. This refractoriness affects the ability of nerve fibres to respond to each pulse, and has been studied by Paolini & Clark.[58] Figure 26.30 shows the number of intervals between action potentials from cells in the cochlear nucleus for stimuli at 200, 800, 1200 and 1800 pulses/s. The duration of the relative refractory period is marked. At 200 pulses/s, the firing interval between action potentials is the same as the period of the stimulus, which is 5 ms. The firing is also very precise in time (deterministic). At the higher rate of 800 pulses/s, there are multiple firing intervals as occurs with sound; these are the first, second and third multiples of the period. The firing is less precise in time (stochastic), which is also seen with sound. This pattern in the intervals at 800 pulses/s is more similar to sound due to reduced responsiveness of the stimuli as they occur within the relative refractory period. At an even higher rate of 1200 pulses/s, the separateness of the interval peaks is markedly reduced. This suggests that at this frequency and above there

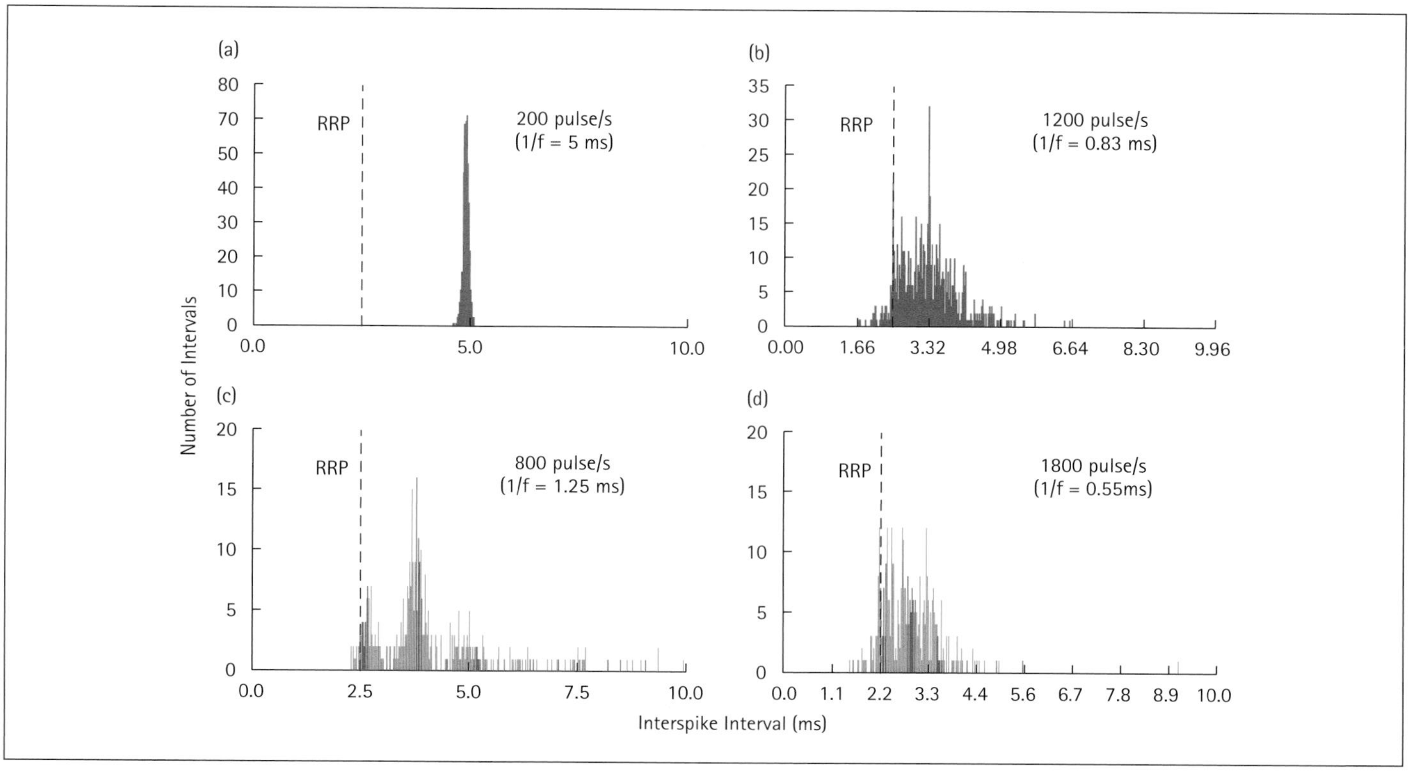

Figure 26.30 The intervals between the action potentials from the globular bushy cochlear nucleus neurones in the cat for stimulus rates of (a) 200, (b) 800, (c) 1200 and (d) 1800 pulses/s. The stimulus period and relative refractory period (RRP) are indicated.

is a progressive loss in the transmission of temporal information as the intervals between the electrical stimuli become less than the relative refractory period and enter the absolute refractory period.

Temporal information can also be conveyed by amplitude variations at high rates of stimulation through altering the population of nerves excited. Psychophysical studies, however, show that only low rates of modulation (100–200 Hz) can be adequately detected.[59–61]

While high stimulus rates used within clinically acceptable intensity levels are usually safe,[62] the high rate itself, especially at current levels and charge densities above those normally used clinically, may damage auditory neurones.[63, 64] Furthermore, the devices must be engineered so that charge recovery occurs between each pulse at the electrode–tissue interface. If this does not happen, a DC current will build up, and this too can, at certain levels (>2 μA), damage nervous and cochlear tissue.[65]

All the past neurobiological studies on safety emphasize the importance of evaluating in animal experimental studies the effects of any significantly altered rate of stimulation. The electronics to be used in patients to deliver the high pulse rates must also be included in the experimental trials. This safety information is important for patient management. With the Nucleus system, all significant changes in stimulus parameters and electrode geometry have been accompanied by experimental animal studies. There are very few detailed studies on the effects on safety of the use of increasingly higher rates of stimulation with the other systems.

A second reason for experimental animal safety studies with each device is that the charge density at the electrode–tissue interface may exceed acceptable levels. Studies[66–69] have demonstrated that stimuli with charge densities below 32 μC/cm^2 geom. per phase are safe. The upper limit for safety has not been established. The Nucleus banded-array has a large surface area for each electrode band (0.44–0.66 mm^2), and hence low charge density. The pulse width normally used in patients is 25 μs, but 50 μs may be needed. For the maximum current level that can be delivered (1.75 mA), the maximum charge density for the largest band on the Nucleus array is 19.9 μC/cm^2 per phase. The surface area of the Nucleus electrode is up to five times greater than the electrode areas of the Med El and Clarion devices, which are approximately 0.14 mm^2 for both (Med-El Combi-40 Manual; Clarion Device Description, Advanced Bionics Corporation). The Med El Combi-40 can deliver a maximum current of 2 mA for pulse widths varying from 40 μs to 640 μs, and so the maximum charge density could vary from 80 μC to 914 μC/cm^2 per phase. The Advanced Bionics Clarion system can produce a maximum current of 2.5 mA, and at its minimum pulse width of 77 μs, the charge density would be 137.5 μs/cm^2 per phase. The pulse width can be increased, and the charge density would become greater. The maximum charge densities possible with the Combi-40 and

Clarion-S devices are well in excess of the level that is known to be safe (32 μC/cm^2 geom. per phase). It is important to establish the upper safe levels for charge density, and in particular for the operating range of Combi-40 and Clarion-S.

Although the benefits of high rates of stimulation have not been established, companies emphasize the importance of the maximum rates that their devices can achieve. Clarion-S is reported to produce 104 000 samples/s, but this is only for one electrode (Clarion Device Description: Advanced Bionics Corporation). The term sample rate is ambiguous, and is not the same as biphasic pulse rate. They are the voltages used to represent simultaneous analogue/stimulation alone. Furthermore, seven and not eight electrodes are used for the bipolar stimulation required for SAS. Radial stimulation cannot always reach the dynamic ranges required on eight electrode pairs, so seven are placed longitudinally. Consequently, 91 000 samples/s are available to stimulate all seven electrodes. Furthermore, for simultaneous pulsatile stimulation (SPS), two output samples are required to produce one biphasic pulse, so that 45 500 pulses/s are available for distribution to stimulate the nerves. The sample rate is also confusing, as all the seven electrodes can only be updated every 77 μs, whether this be individual voltages or biphasic pulses. In other words, all seven electrodes can be stimulated at 12 987 samples or pulses/s. This will only produce quasi-stochastic responses conveying amplitude envelope information, as it is an impossibly fast rate to stimulate the nerves. For non-simultaneous stimulation, the Clarion-S device is subject to similar limitations in information transfer as the Nucleus-24 and Combi-40/40+ systems. In this case, only one electrode is stimulated at a time. As stated for the Clarion-S, the data update interval is 77 μs. This means a maximum rate of 12 987 samples or 6494 pulses/s for distribution across eight electrodes (i.e. approximately 812 pulses/s for each electrode) (Patent # 5,522,865).[70]

The Combi-40 stimulates non-simultaneously at up to 12 120 pulses/s and a newer version, the Combi-40+, at 18 180 pulses/s (I. Hochmair, personal communication). The Combi-40+, when using 12 electrodes, can stimulate at up to 1515 pulses/s on each electrode. With Nucleus-24 there is 25 μs for each phase of the pulse, an interphase gap of 7 μs for more efficient stimulation, and a shorting period of 12 μs between pulses to ensure no DC build-up and biological safety. The maximum rate of 14 400 pulses/s resulting can be applied to one electrode or divided across electrodes. There could be 1440 pulses/s on each of 10 electrodes, or 720 pulses/s on each of 20 electrodes.

Maximum number of stimulus channels

The number of stimulus channels (electrodes) is another important issue in speech processing for cochlear implants. The place coding of frequency achieved with multiple-electrode implants is the main reason why results with multiple-electrode systems are superior to those of single-electrode systems. The optimal number of channels for stimulation with the Nucleus-24, Combi-40 and Clarion-S systems has not been fully established. Our studies[39] have shown, however, that for the Nucleus system and the $F_0/F_1/F_2$ speech-processing strategy, the results are progressively better for electrode numbers greater than nine, the minimum number in the study being nine. An additional advantage for the Nucleus system in having 22 electrodes is that there are more electrodes available for stimulating areas of the cochlea where place of stimulation is more effective. This could be due to pathology causing variations in the density of the auditory neurones.

The mode of stimulation and the electrode geometry are relevant to channel separation and the number of channels to be used. Initial research[11–13,71] showed that bipolar and common ground stimulation would localize current to discrete groups of neurones, without it short-circuiting along the fluid compartments of the cochlea. With bipolar stimulation, the current passes between neighbouring electrodes, and with common ground stimulation, between an active electrode and the others on the cochlear array connected together electronically. It has subsequently been shown[72] that if the electrodes are placed close to neurones, then monopolar stimulation between an active and distant electrode may also allow localized stimulation. There is thus an interaction between stimulus mode, electrode geometry and cochlear anatomy for the optimal place coding of speech frequencies. Furthermore, if the electrodes are small, and not adjacent to the spiral ganglion cells, high current levels will be required with bipolar stimulation to cover the dynamic range. In this case, the implant may not be able to deliver the current required. The electrode separation for the biopolar stimulation will need to be increased, and this in turn will reduce channel separation.

Placement of electrodes close to spiral ganglion cells should reduce channel interaction, and permit more stimulus channels to be used. There has been debate[73] about the merit of using a moulded array to achieve placement close to the ganglion cells (e.g. the array developed at San Francisco).[74] This array was designed in particular to produce radial bipolar stimulation of the peripheral processes of the spiral ganglion cells, and because effective stimulation is not tolerant to small variations in electrode placement.[75] A comparison of the histological effects of a free fitting versus a moulded array was undertaken by Sutton et al,[76] and showed significantly more trauma for the moulded array. A number of studies[31, 77, 78] have established that this trauma can lead to the loss of spiral ganglion cells. As illustrated in Figure 26.31, a Teflon strip cutting the basilar membrane can lead to a marked loss of spiral ganglion cells in the hearing animal. Fractures of the osseous spiral lamina have also been shown to produce loss of the spiral ganglion cells in the deafened animal.[79] With electrodes now being inserted to lie close to spiral ganglion cells for improved information transfer, it is even more imperative that trauma be kept to a minimum to preserve adequate spiral ganglion cell numbers.

Recently, the safety of using a Teflon 'former' to push a Nucleus free-fitting banded array close to the modiolus after it has been inserted has been studied in the human temporal bone.[80] Furthermore, a wire former has been attached to the tip

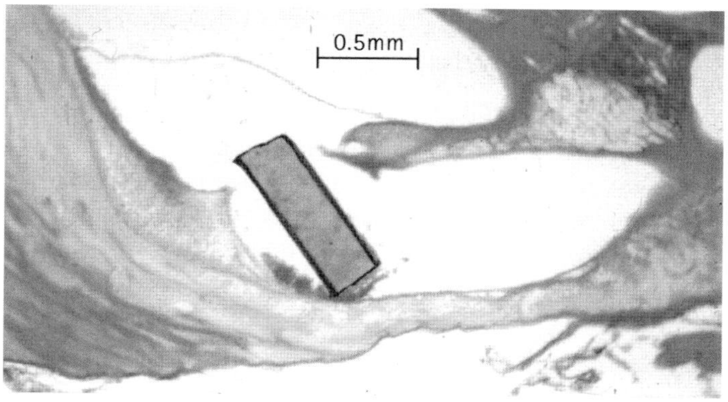

Figure 26.31 A photomicrograph of the cat cochlea after tearing of the basilar membrane with a Teflon strip, showing the marked loss of spiral ganglion cells. (Reprinted with permission from Clark and Lawrence. *Aust J Otolaryngol* 2000; 3(5): 516–22.[114])

of the Combi-40+ array to force it close to the inner spiral. A silicone plug attached to the Clarion-S array is also being trialed. All these formers are likely to produce significant trauma, as was seen in the earlier study of Sutton et al.[76]

The Nucleus array with a Teflon 'former' has been compared with a pre-curved array without 'former' in a number of human temporal bones subsequently sectioned to evaluate damage.[80] This 'former' was shown in a significant proportion of insertions to buckle, and to tear the basilar membrane, and enter the scala vestibuli, as illustrated in Figure 26.32. For this reason, an electrode with 'former' will not be used for advanced Nucleus systems. Sections of the human temporal bone have shown that a pre-curved array held straight before insertion is much less traumatic than an array with 'former'.[80]

Speech-processing strategies under investigation

Each manufacturer offers a number of variations of their standard speech-processing strategies. These variations are all at different stages of evaluation.

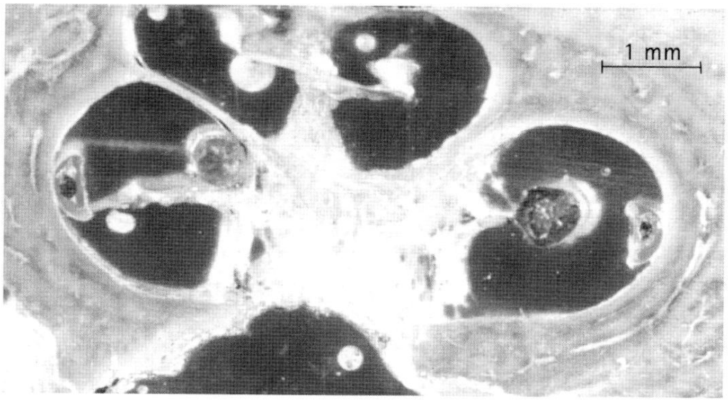

Figure 26.32 A photomicrograph of the human cochlea after the insertion of free-fitting electrode and Teflon 'former', showing them penetrating into the scala vestibuli. (Reprinted with permission from Clark and Lawrence. *Aust J Otolaryngol* 2000; 3(5): 516–22.[114])

Nucleus-24 system

The ACE strategy is being trialed with the Nucleus-24 system. ACE is a modification of SPEAK, with stimuli presented at high rates and/or with more channels of stimulation. This gives the clinician the opportunity to optimize the speech processor to obtain maximum benefit for individual subjects. The effect of a higher rate of stimulation (in particular 800 pulses/s) with Advanced Combination Encoder (ACE) has been compared with the SPEAK strategy, which uses a rate of 250 pulses/s. The study on a small group of subjects[81] showed that the average results did not improve for rates higher than 250 pulses/s. There was, however, patient variability, and so rate of stimulation could be varied to suit performance. A second strategy being trialed with SPEAK is one which optimizes the dynamic range for each frequency band by an adaptive dynamic range optimization mechanism (ADRO). Initial results indicate that it can give improved speech perception at low signal levels.[82] A third strategy emphasizes the transient information in speech of importance for intelligibility (TESM),[83] and may lead to advances in speech perception.

Combi-40 system

It has been proposed that the Combi-40 system use a high-rate CIS, CIS+, jitter CIS, variable-rate CIS, and '*n* of *m*'. The CIS+ strategy uses the Hilbert transform for envelope extraction. The Hilbert transform (a 90° phase shifter) is an efficient technique for detecting the speech wave envelope from each filter. The transform was first described by Hilbert early in the 20th century, and has been in regular use in communications engineering since the 1970s.[84] Jitter CIS means the addition of a random rather than a constant-rate stimulus. This is also available with the SPEAK strategy, and for some subjects it can make the sound more natural. '*n* of *m*' means the selection of *n* stimulus channels from *m* filter outputs. This is essentially the principle underlying all the Nucleus speech-processing strategies (F_0/F_2), ($F_0/F_1/F_2$), MULTIPEAK, and SPEAK. Studies undertaken at Melbourne University, including those under an NIH contract (Speech Processors for Auditory Prostheses: Contract NO1-DC-9-2400), have shown that SPEAK is the optimum '*n* of *m*' strategy.

Clarion system

Clarion offers the possibility of simultaneous analogue as well as pulsatile stimuli through SPS. The issues relating to simultaneous stimulation are discussed above. Partial simultaneous strategies that have been proposed are HAP (hybrid analogue pulsatile processor), QPS (quadruple pulsatile sampler), and PPS (paired pulsatile sampler).

HAP would use simultaneous analogue stimulation for the lower frequencies, and non-simultaneous pulsatile stimulation in the higher frequencies. This may lead to speech-processing improvements. This type of strategy was initially described by von Wallenberg et al.[85] They compared the results for a four-channel system in which a broadband analogue signal was presented on the most apical electrode, and the second formant as pulsatile stimuli to one of the three more basal electrodes. Vowel identification was significantly better for the hybrid than for the single-channel system. Furthermore, a hybrid speech processor has been developed in the Human Communication Research Centre, Melbourne (AMA 'Hear-Say', Australian Provisional Patent PN 3133, 18 May 1995). This strategy encoded voicing information on a separate apical electrode, and constant-rate spectral maxima information on the other electrodes. It was compared with a standard spectral maxima processor. The study[86] showed no difference in the scores for the hybrid scheme presenting suprasegmental information on a separate electrode. Another version of the hybrid strategy has been developed at the Cooperative Research Centre for Cochlear Implant Speech and Hearing Research in Melbourne. This uses single-channel stimulation on an apical electrode to provide temporal information for excitation of residual low-frequency hearing electrophonically, and electrical stimulation of the auditory nerves for high-frequency spectral information (Cochlear implant system for residual hearing stimulation, Australian Provisional Patent 8016, March 1993).

The PPS and QPS are systems for stimulating either two or four electrodes simultaneously with a CIS strategy. The electrodes are selected so that they are at a distance from each other to reduce interactions from overlapping electrical fields. At present this is an untested variation.

Behind-the-ear speech processor

A behind-the-ear speech processor is very desirable for a number of patients, particularly children older than about 4 years as well as adults. They find that it is more convenient to dispense with the leads passing from the microphone to the body-worn device, and it is more aesthetic, especially for teenagers. Keeping it small requires high-powered zinc–air batteries, and a low power consumption. This is easier to achieve for strategies that stimulate at low rates. SPEAK has been used with the Nucleus behind-the-ear speech processor, ESPrit, since 1997. It now uses ACE and CIS as well as SPEAK. It also has a whisper setting (ADRO) which improves understanding in quiet, and an integral telecoil for loop systems and the telephone. The zinc air batteries last for up to 3 days. A behind-the-ear speech processor was used with the Med-El device (Tempo+) in 1999. It provides the CIS coding strategy and uses zinc air batteries. Advanced Bionics commenced using one in 2001. It provides CIS and SAS strategies, but the rechargeable lithium ion batteries require a recharge every 4–8 hours of usage. There is also no on/off switch.

Telemetry

Telemetry transmits information from the implant to the external programming system, such as the voltages from electrodes on the array in response to a stimulus pulse. The transmitted voltages can be used to determine the tissue impedance around the array, and so assess pathological changes. The Nucleus system can also measure the very small voltages from the auditory nerve, referred to as the compound action potential (CAP). The CAP can help determine stimulus thresholds and dynamic ranges. Like all objective audiological procedures, it should be accompanied by behavioural measures. The CAP has advantages over the electrically evoked brainstem response (EABR) procedure, which is done using surface electrodes, as it can be made rapidly, and a child does not require an anaesthetic. The Nucleus 24 system also has an additional feature which can determine whether the stimulus has exceeded the voltage compliance, and hence whether a programming change is required.

Reliability

Reliability is an important issue for the surgeon when deciding how to best advise a prospective patient. It is essential to know the overall reliability of the different products, as well as the reliability of the most recent models. It takes time to accumulate meaningful statistics, and short-term estimates for recent models can be very misleading. The past history is important, as reliability depends on accumulated manufacturing experience. Specific information is also needed on the incidence of package failures, sealing leaks, cracks to the case, fractures of the electrodes or transmitting coil, and electronic failures. For children, in particular, it is important that the implant is resistant to blows to the head. Implant design should evolve to the point where all sporting activities are not contraindicated. Reliability data have been reported in the literature by Cochlear Limited, but at this point in time not to a similar extent by the other manufacturers. Uniform procedures and meaningful reporting are essential for the clinician.

Surgery

Surgery for cochlear implants is primarily carried out in the following stages.

Incision

Skin preparation for the incision requires shaving the hair so that there is sufficient room between the incision and the edge of the hair to prevent wound infection. The incision should be placed 45 mm behind the external osseous auditory meatus so that it does not overlie the implanted device. The direction of the incision for the Nucleus CI-24 receiver–stimulator device is different from that for the CI-22 system. As shown in Figure 26.33, it still remains within the postauricular sulcus, but then extends more vertically, as the Nucleus CI-24 can be placed at a greater angle to the horizontal (Frankfurt's plane).

Exposure of the middle ear and round window

The deep fascia and periosteum should be elevated to make an anteriorly based flap, so that the incision does not directly overlie the device or lead-wire assembly. This reduces the risk of the device being exposed to the exterior if there is wound infection

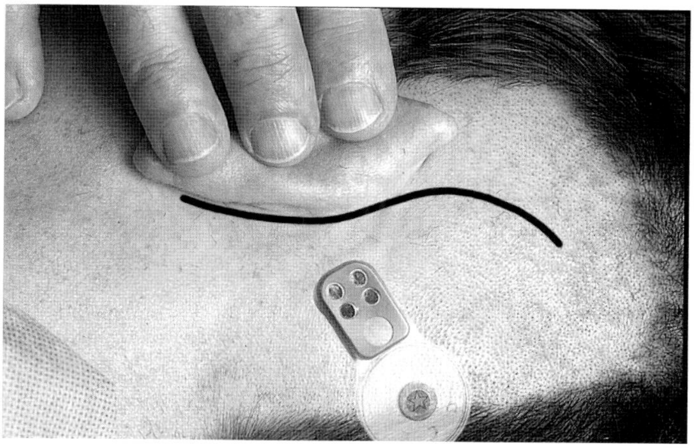

Figure 26.33 The incision for the implantation of the Nucleus CI-24 system.

or breakdown. A mastoid air cell exenteration is performed. This does not need to be complete, but sufficient to safely allow the completion of the posterior tympanotomy. The posterior tympanotomy is carried out with care, to avoid damaging the vertical section of the facial nerve. Once the middle ear is entered, the round window niche is identified.

Creation of bed for the receiver–stimulator

After the middle ear has been exposed and the round window identified, a bed is created in the mastoid bone to take the small flat stimulator section of the implant device. This may need to be drilled down to the underlying dura so that it fits comfortably in the skull. As stated above, it is important to ensure that the anterior margin of the receiver–stimulator lies sufficiently far behind the postauricular sulcus to ensure that the behind-the-ear speech processor does not rub any elevated skin over the anterior edge of the package.

Insertion of the electrode array and placement of the receiver–stimulator

After restraining ties for the lead wire are placed (platinum wires around the floor of the mastoid antrum), the opening into the cochlea is made for the insertion of the electrode bundle. The cochleostomy opening is sited approximately 1–2 mm antero-inferior to the round window niche. The package is opened, and the array inserted gently around the basal turn of the cochlea with the aid of a claw,[2, 87] until minimal resistance is felt. If an adequate depth of insertion is not achieved, this may be facilitated by withdrawing the electrode a little, and rotating it 90° clockwise in the case of the left cochlea, and anticlockwise for the right cochlea. It is then reintroduced. After insertion, the ties are tightened around the lead wire, which is protected by a Silastic sleeve. The package is placed in its bed and two sutures are inserted into the fascia surrounding the receiver–stimulator, and tied over it to prevent it from moving forward. Fascia is placed around the electrode entry to minimize the ingress of any infection at a later stage and to help establish a seal. After final haemostasis, the wound is closed in layers.

Postoperative management

Postoperatively, the wound needs to be inspected for pain, bleeding or discharge. Otherwise, in the usual uneventful recovery, the patient can be discharged from hospital after 3–4 days. The postoperative complications are minimal, the most common one being wound infection. This is usually treated conservatively with antibiotics. A haematoma requires needle aspiration. Sometimes, air is forced up the Eustachian tube and creates a pneumatocoele under the flap. This responds to a pressure dressing for a few days. More details of the surgery and the management of any complications can be found in Clark et al,[2] Webb et al.[3] Clark et al.[73] Cohen et al[88] and Clark et al.[89]

(Re)habilitation

It is important to know not only when to select adults and children for cochlear implantation, but how best to (re)habilitate them. (Re)habilitating a child, in particular, with a cochlear implant will depend in part on the plasticity of the central auditory nervous system, and how responsive it is to new information. (Re)habilitation will also depend on the cognitive processes required for speech perception, speech production, and the acquisition of language.

Mapping

After surgery, the device is switched on 2 or 3 weeks postoperatively, subject to the healing of the incision. (Re)habilitation requires establishing the intensity of the stimuli for the loudness thresholds, maximum comfortable levels, and dynamic ranges for each electrode. These levels are mapped into the person's speech processor so that the electrical representation of the acoustical signals remains within the operating range. The stimulus parameter responsible for neural excitation is electrical charge. This can be controlled by varying either the pulse amplitude or width.

The thresholds (T level) can be obtained by averaging a number of responses to an ascending and descending procedure. When ascending from no signal to the electrically induced percept, the threshold will be higher than when descending in amplitude. A more stable threshold can be obtained by also averaging the results for the two procedures. The maximum comfortable level (MC level) is the highest stimulus intensity that can be used without causing discomfort. The level is lower for an initial rather than a continuous presentation, as habituation occurs. As speech is a dynamic signal, often with short bursts to individual electrodes, the lower or more conservative value should be adopted to ensure that there are no unpleasant side-effects. Setting the MC level correctly is also important, as the greater part of the speech signal is mapped to the top 20% of the dynamic range. If the T levels and MC levels are high for bipolar stimulation, they can be brought more into the current output range of the receiver–stimulator by stimulating a greater area of the cochlea or number of neurones. This is achieved by stimulating between more widely separated electrodes.

Once the T and MC levels are set, it is important to determine whether the loudness percepts are comparable across electrodes at these intensities. This is done by sweeping the stimuli across the electrodes to see if the loudness is balanced. It is also necessary to evaluate the loudness growth function for increases in intensity at each electrode, as this may vary, and lead to unpleasant or non-optimal speech perception if it is not taken into consideration. The shape of the function can be roughly assessed by sweeping across electrodes at an intensity 50% between the T and MC levels. If an electrode sounds softer at this level, this may be because the loudness growth function is flat near threshold, so that the 50% level is too low on the normal steep section of the curve. Owing to changing pathology in the inner ear following implantation, especially during the early postoperative phase, repeated measurements of thresholds and comfortable levels are required.

In (re)habilitating children in the use of the cochlear implant, special care must be taken in establishing thresholds and maximum comfortable levels. If a stimulus is unpleasant and too loud, it will delay the child's confidence and learning. The procedure is carried out by the audiologist observing the behavioural responses to the stimuli, particularly an aversive or withdrawal reaction.[90] Assessment will also be improved with receiver–stimulators such as the Nucleus CI-24 system, which have telemetry. They can signal externally by radio waves the voltages in the auditory nerve, and these can be correlated with thresholds and comfortable levels.[90]

Speech recognition over time in adults

In (re)habilitating children and adults, it is necessary to know not only what changes in speech perception can occur, but also the time-course of these changes and the factors affecting this time-course. The degree of learning over 12 months for adults who have previously had hearing before going deaf and who used the inaugural F_0/F_2 strategy is shown in Figure 26.34. As can be seen, the mean open-set CID sentence score for electrical stimulation alone increased by 145% from 3 to 12 months postoperatively. The learning rate for speech perception with the SPEAK strategy on postlingually deaf adults is also shown in Figure 26.34. From this it can be seen that the scores arise to a plateau much more quickly. This suggests that the signal contains more information that is similar to natural speech, and less rehabilitation is required.

Speech recognition over time in children

The rate of learning over time has been examined for three groups of implanted children: those implanted under 3 years, from 3 to 5 years, and over 5 years. The results are shown in Figure 26.35. As can be seen with these preliminary data, the rate of learning for all three groups increases at the same rate for 2 years postoperatively, and only then starts to plateau for the over 5 age group (Dowell, personal communication). Why this occurs is not clear.

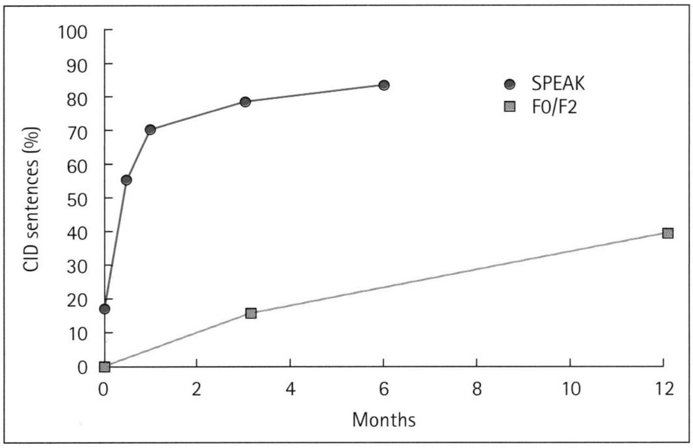

Figure 26.34 The open-set speech scores for electrical stimulation alone for adults using the inaugural F_0/F_2 and the recent 'SPEAK' cochlear implant strategies. (From *Clark*. In: Fahle and Poggio, eds. *Perceptual Learning*. Cambridge Mass: MIT Press, 2002: 147–60.[90])

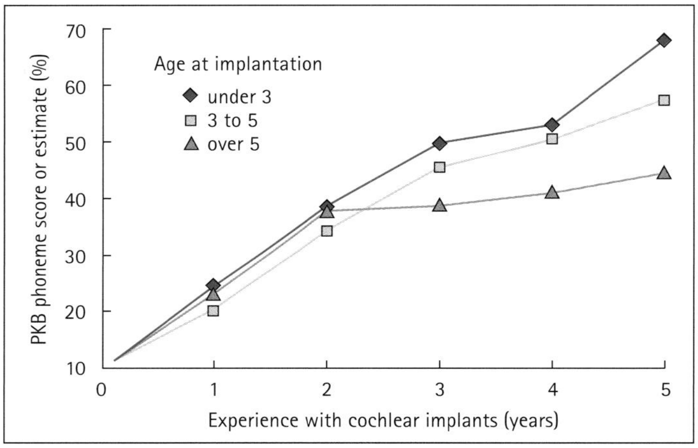

Figure 26.35 The phonetically balanced kindergarten (PBK) phoneme score or estimate plotted over time in children implanted under 3, 3–5 and over 5 years of age. (From *Clark*. In: Fahle and Poggio, eds. *Perceptual Learning*. Cambridge Mass: MIT Press, 2002: 147–60.[90])

Speech production over time in children

In (re)habilitating children, it is important to know their rate of learning not only for speech perception but also for speech production. The two are inter-related, and any particular delays may be correctable. To help in monitoring speech production in particular, a computer-aided speech and language assessment procedure (CASALA) has been developed.[91] The conversation is transcribed by a clinician into the appropriate written symbols, and the computer transcribes the written word into the correct phonetic representation of what was spoken. The program then analyses the data and produces an inventory of the vowels and consonants being used, the percentage of correctly identified phonemes, and the abnormal phonological processes being used by the child.

This information can then be used to monitor the progress of (re)habilitation, and identify where special help is needed. Progress in speech production versus receptive language has been plotted in a number of children. Its use in four children is demonstrated in Figure 26.36. This shows a plot over time of the percentage of phonemes produced correctly, and a measure of receptive language, PPVT, in equivalent age. The two children with auditory/oral skills (children 1 and 9) show the two curves parallel to each other. On the other hand, for the meningitic child (child 7), there is a loss of speech production before this catches up with language.

Changes in speech perceptual space in adults post-implantation

(Re)habilitation with electrical stimulation requires plasticity and adaptability of the neural pathways and perceptual processes. Evidence for adaptability in speech perception has been seen in a pilot study in an adult postlingually deaf cochlear implant patient. In this patient, the vowel spaces were mapped at two short intervals after implantation. With the normal two-formant vowel space, there is a limited range or grouping of frequencies required for the perception of each vowel. The study was undertaken by presenting 64 two-formant synthesized sounds to the subject via appropriately place-coded electrodes. He was then asked to identify which vowels he heard. If, for example, he heard vowels that had a higher second-formant frequency than the frequency of the stimulated electrode, the vowel centre was shown as moved upwards in frequency (Blamey and Dooley, personal communication). With electrical stimulation, it was found that at the end of the second week there was a wider range of electrodes contributing to the perception of each vowel. However, after the subject had learned to use the implant for a further week, the range of electrodes contributing to the perception of the vowels became more restricted, and the vowel spaces came to more closely resemble those for normal hearing. This result suggests that perceptual changes for vowel formant identification can occur quickly, but, as referred to above, the higher-level 'top-down' changes required for speech perception take longer.

Changes in speech recognition in children with 'bottom-up' or perceptual training

In (re)habilitating children, it is necessary not only to understand plasticity and perceptual learning with electrical stimulation, but to train them in using 'bottom-up' and 'top-down' information. The central processing for speech recognition is both 'bottom-up' and 'top-down', and both may be trained to improve speech recognition. With regard to 'bottom-up' processing, specific training in vowel formant discrimination has been undertaken in a group of five children with poor speech recognition.[92] In these children, vowel formant discrimination was worse than their ability to discriminate electrodes.

With speech-processing strategies, the formants are represented by place of electrode stimulation, and an index for assessing the spatial separation of electrodes representing the formants in vowel pairs was developed. This index is calculated

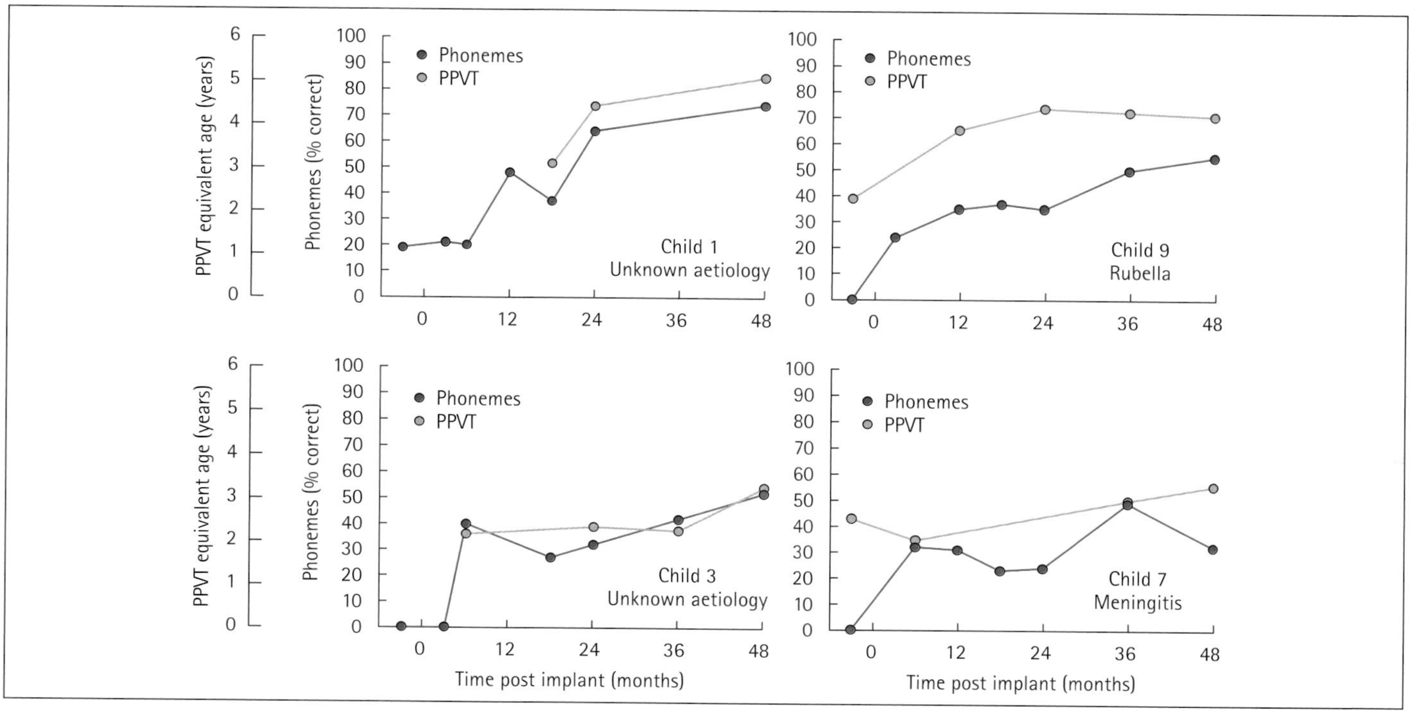

Figure 26.36 Plot of speech production over time with CASALA (Blamey, personal communication).

as the lengths of vectors in a Euclidean space. The distance between a pair of vowels is the square root of the sum of squares of the first and second formant electrode separations. The indices for some selected vowel pairs are shown in Figure 26.37. With four of the five children in the group, the perceptual space for the vowel formants that they could discriminate was much greater than their ability to discriminate electrode place. After training, two children (3 and 4) showed significant improvements in speech recognition which were more consistent with their electrode difference limens. This is illustrated for child 3 in Figure 26.38. Child 3 could discriminate 1.8 electrodes apart, which was sufficient for vowel discrimination down to a separation index of 2.8. As can be seen, the discrimination of head/hood, had/hod, had/hud and hud/hod could not be made pre-training. The training was carried out first to achieve discrimination of the vowel pairs where the formants were most widely separated. It was argued that this would result in the changes required for learning to discriminate more closely separated vowel pairs.

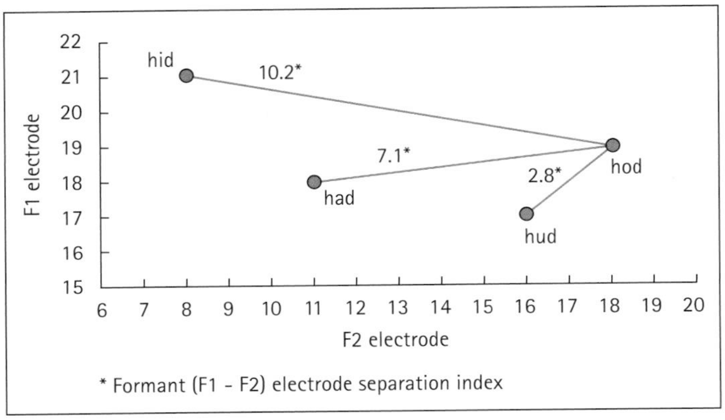

Figure 26.37 Formant separation indices for selected vowels. (From Clark. *Am J Otol* 1999; **20**: 4–8.[109])

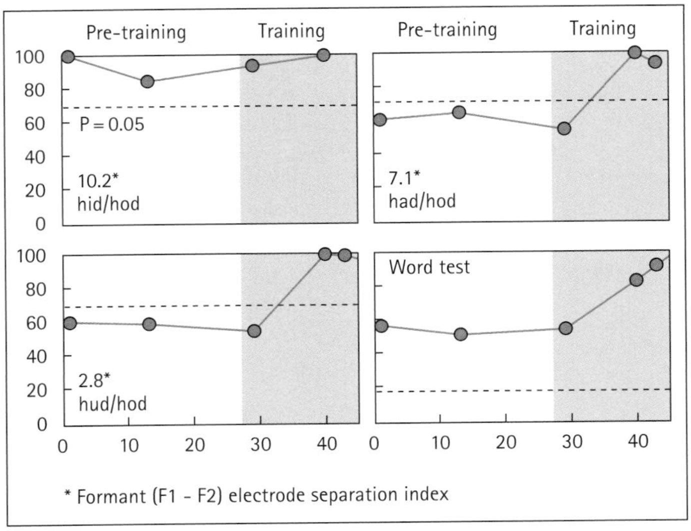

Figure 26.38 Specific training of vowels in child 3. (From Clark. *Am J Otol* 1999; **20**: 4–8.[109])

Child 3, and a second one, child 4, improved in their abilities to distinguish vowel pairs. In the child shown, gains in minimal vowel pair recognition carried over to improved speech recognition. In child 3, the gains in vowel perception generalized to consonants, as demonstrated by improvements in a monosyllable word test. In child 5, the overall speech perception was poorer than that of the other children pre- and post-training, and this was consistent with her wider apical electrode difference limens, which were 5.5–5.8. This child had deafness of genetic origin and was not implanted until 13 years of age. These results suggest that training to distinguish vowels with widely separated formant frequencies, and then carrying this over to more closely separated formants, can be effective, with the benefits being retained and extended to the perception of speech.

Changes in speech recognition in children with 'top-down' or language training

With regard to 'top-down' processing, the effects of language training on speech perception have been investigated in three implanted children.[93] They were trained in the use of tense and other grammatical concepts. The data showed a significant training effect. In another study, the children were educated in the meaning of words that they did not understand and then tested to find the effects of understanding on speech perception. The mean results showed that there was a very significant improvement for the unknown words compared with the known words when meaning was provided.

Ethics

Introduction

Medical ethics is generally considered in terms of beneficence, non-maleficence, and autonomy. Beneficence is defined as the duty to do the best for the individual patient,[94] non-maleficence is the duty to do no harm, and autonomy is the right of individuals to make decisions on their own behalf. The cochlear implant should be used clinically in accord with these guiding principles.

It is also ethically correct for cochlear implant research to be carried out in accordance with the principles laid down by the Helsinki Declaration on Biomedical Research adopted by the 18th World Medical Assembly, Finland 1969, and revised by the 29th World Medical Assembly in Tokyo in 1975. Research on children should also be in accordance with the convention of the Rights of the Child adopted by the General Assembly of the United Nations on 20 November 1989.

Beneficence

The need for beneficence is implied in the Helsinki declaration, where it states that: 'biomedical research involving human subjects cannot legitimately be carried out unless the importance of the object is in proportion to the inherent risk to a subject.'

Cochlear implantation complies with this requirement, as it has now been clearly shown that severely and profoundly deaf adults and children receive significant help with a cochlear implant, and this is better than they would get with the most powerful optimally fitted hearing aid or a tactile vocoder. The beneficial results have been reported in a number of studies.[95–97] The US National Institutes of Health Consensus statement concluded that: 'using tests commonly applied to children and adults with hearing impairments the perceptual performance with an implant increases with each succeeding year post-operatively. Furthermore, the performance may improve to match that of children who have residual hearing and are highly successful hearing aid users.[97] The outcomes, complications and cost-effectiveness of cochlear implants in the UK from 1990 to 1994 have also been documented by Summerfield et al[98] from the MRC Institute of Hearing Research University of Nottingham.

Non-maleficence

Non-maleficence is implied by the Helsinki Declaration that: 'every biomedical research project involving human subjects should be preceded by careful assessment of predictable risks in comparison with foreseeable benefits to the subject or to others. Concern for the interest of the subject must always prevail over the interests of science and society.'

The principle of doing no harm has always been central to the research conducted by the University of Melbourne and the Bionic Ear Institute. In Melbourne, a significant number of studies have been undertaken over the last two decades to ensure in the first instance that cochlear implants in adults and children from 2 to 18 years of age were safe as well as effective. These involved studies to determine the placement of the electrode array at an appropriate location in the cochlea so that the cochlear nerve would not be damaged, and there would be no adverse pathological changes in the cochlea.[31, 69, 99, 100] The studies also helped establish the electrical stimulus parameters that were required for continuous long-term stimulation without loss of neural elements.[101–103] The research undertaken by the Deparment of Otolaryngology at the University of Melbourne was crucial in the acceptance of the first multiple-channel cochlear implant to be approved by the US FDA in August 1985. Furthermore, as there was evidence to indicate that operating on children under 2 years of age is important, the University of Melbourne and the University of San Francisco were both awarded in 1987 US National Institutes of Health (NIH) contracts to study the safety of auditory prosthesis implants for paediatric patients.

As a result of the studies at the University of Melbourne, it was clearly shown that head growth had no effect on the electrode lead-wire assembly and that the implantation itself had no effect on head growth. Infection entering the inner ear from otitis media, common in young children, was investigated and was shown to be no greater a risk than if there was no implantation. These studies were undertaken in particular at the University of Melbourne under a 5-year contract.[14] The effect of electrical stimulation on the maturing nervous system was also investigated, and shown to be no different to that of an adult. In summary, the NIH studies demonstrated that cochlear implantation of children under 2 years of age was safe.

Autonomy

As far as autonomy is concerned, this is embodied in the statement of the Helsinki Declaration that:

> In any research on human beings, each potential subject must be adequately informed of the aims, methods, anticipated benefits and potential hazards of the study and the discomfort it may entail. He or she should be informed that he or she is at liberty to abstain from participation in the study and that he or she is free to withdraw his or her consent to paricipation at any time. The physician should then obtain the subject's freely-given informed consent, preferably in writing.

The advantages and disadvantages of a cochlear implant operation are always raised and discussed with prospective adult patients or parents of a young child at the University of Melbourne's Clinic at the Royal Victorian Eye & Ear Hospital. It is also the policy of the Cochlear Implant Clinic to make sure that children who are of an age when they can clearly understand the implications of the procedure and its benefits and risks are involved in the decision-making process concerning the operation.

Autonomy is also embodied in the statements of the convention of the Rights of the Child adopted by the General Assembly of the United Nations on 20 November 1989. Relevant ones are:

> Article 5
> State Parties shall respect the responsibilities, rights and duties of parents or, where applicable, the members of the extended family or community as provided for by local custom, legal guardians or other persons legally responsible for the child, to provide, in a manner consistent with the evolving capacities of the child, appropriate direction and guidance in the exercise by the child of the rights recognised in the present Convention.
>
> Article 12.1
> States Parties shall assure to the child who is capable of forming his or her own views the right to express those views freely in all matters affecting the child, the views of the child being given due weight in accordance with the age and maturity of the child.

It is important to recognize not only that parents have the right to decide the care needed for their child on the basis of the future needs of the child to fit into society, but also the communication needed at home. Parents with hearing will usually prefer their children to be able to communicate with them in an auditory–oral mode. Approximately 85–90% of deaf children are in families with normally hearing parents. On the other hand, if two deaf parents have a deaf or hearing child, there may be a need for the child to learn to sign. In both cases, the two educational modes should not be initially exclusive, provided that the cochlear implant is carried out at an early age during the child's critical period for speech and language development.[104]

Highest standard of clinical and scientific practice

The clinical use of cochlear implants as well as research studies should also only be considered ethical if the clinical, scientific and industrial management is carried out in accordance with the highest standards of practice. These are laid down by the Helsinki Declaration and its amendments, and the guidelines adopted by recognized bodies such as the US NIH and the National Health and Medical Research Council of Australia.

Summary

The ethical issues of importance for cochlear implantation are presented in more detail by Clark et al.[104]

The question of cochlear implantation in children needs to be presented sensitively, with due consideration for other communication options, in particular sign language of the deaf. It is important that people do not gain the impression that sign language leads to lives that are not worthwhile or fulfilled. It is ethical to only present the facts regarding the benefits and risks of a cochlear implant providing different levels of hearing.

Research directions

There are a number of challenges for the cochlear implant of the future with regard to further improvements in its performance. The first challenge is to provide a better reproduction of the coding of sound. Already, research is contributing answers to these questions. Research to improve the place coding of frequency is being undertaken by developing an array which will lie closer to the neural elements in the cochlea.[105] The present array lies peripherally, and needs to be placed close to the central axis of the cochlear spiral where the ganglion cells are located. To do this, an electrode array has been developed which is pre-curved and held straight before insertion and then released once inside the cochlea.[106] This array comes to lie close to the spiral ganglion cells in the central axis, as shown in the X-ray in Figure 26.39.

An initial group of patients have been implanted with this pre-curved array, and a masking study has been undertaken to evaluate the spread of current to the cochlear nerve fibres to see if better place coding could be achieved.[105] In these patients,

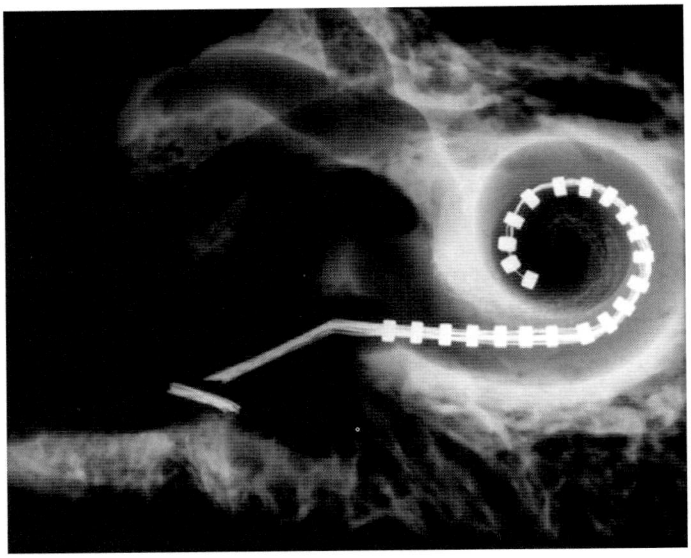

Figure 26.39 X-ray of the cochlea and pre-curved electrode.

the array was closer to the central axis at some points, and further away at other points. This enabled a comparison of current spread with distance from the central axis to be made in the one subject. In the study, a masking stimulus on a certain electrode was followed by probe stimuli on different electrodes. The intensity of the probes required for masking enabled a masking curve to be plotted, and this determined the spread of current around the masker electrode.

An example of the results is shown in Figure 26.40 for patient 1. For the basal electrode 10, which was at some distance from the inner wall, the masking curve is broad. On the other hand, where the apical electrode 18 lies very close to the inner wall, the masking curve is much narrower, indicating a discrete area of neural stimulation. The results from this preliminary study showed that, for the pre-curved array, electrode discrimination was better and neural excitation sharper with the electrodes close to the spiral ganglion cells.

Research into better reproduction of the temporal coding of frequency has first compared the pattern of interspike intervals from brainstem cells for acoustical and electrical stimulation in the experimental animal with frequency discrimination in both the experimental animal and human subject. Figure 26.41 shows the interspike interval histograms for units in the cochlear nucleus for acoustical and electrical stimulation at 400 Hz and 800 Hz. The patterns of these intervals are important in encoding frequency, but how the brain decodes this temporal information is not known.

For acoustical stimuli, the action potentials are phase-locked to the sound at both low and high frequencies, and there is some jitter in the phase locking referred to as stochastic firing. On the other hand, with electrical stimulation there is little jitter at low stimulus rates, and this is referred to as deterministic firing. At higher rates of 800 Hz and above, electrical stimulation produces stochastic firing similar to that of

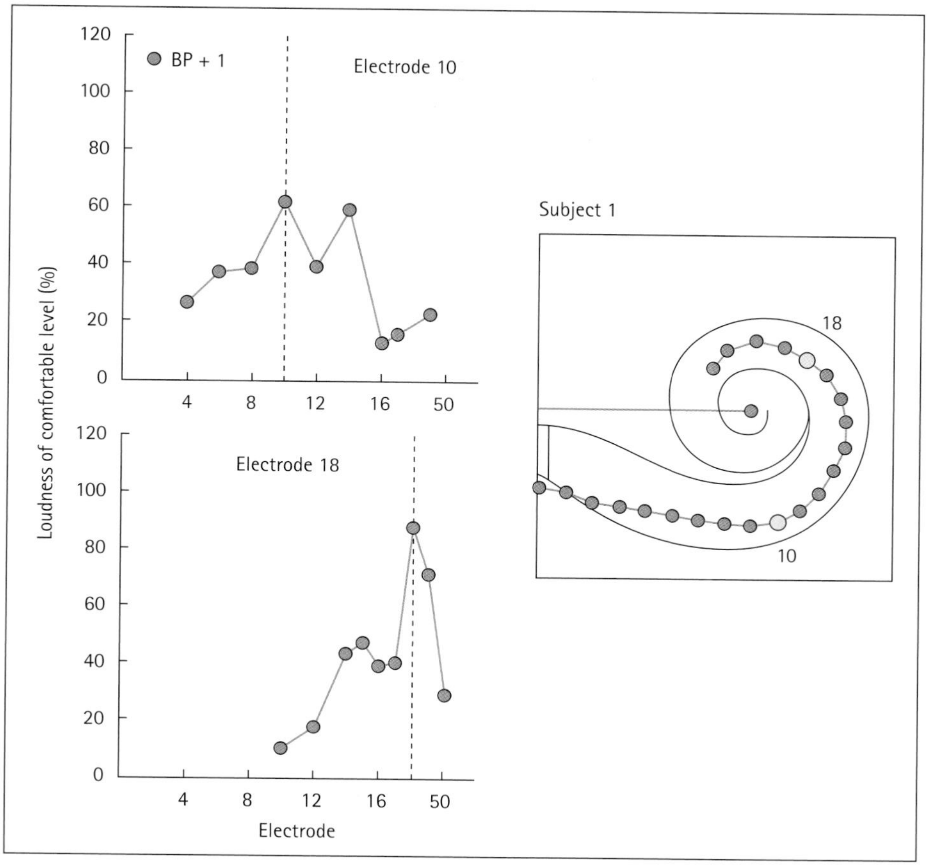

Figure 26.40 Masking of current spread using the pre-curved array; patient 1. Stimulation was bipolar with one intervening electrode. (Reprinted with permission from Shepherd et al. In: Clark, ed. *Cochlear Implants*. Bologna: Monduzzi Editore, 1997: 205–9.[115])

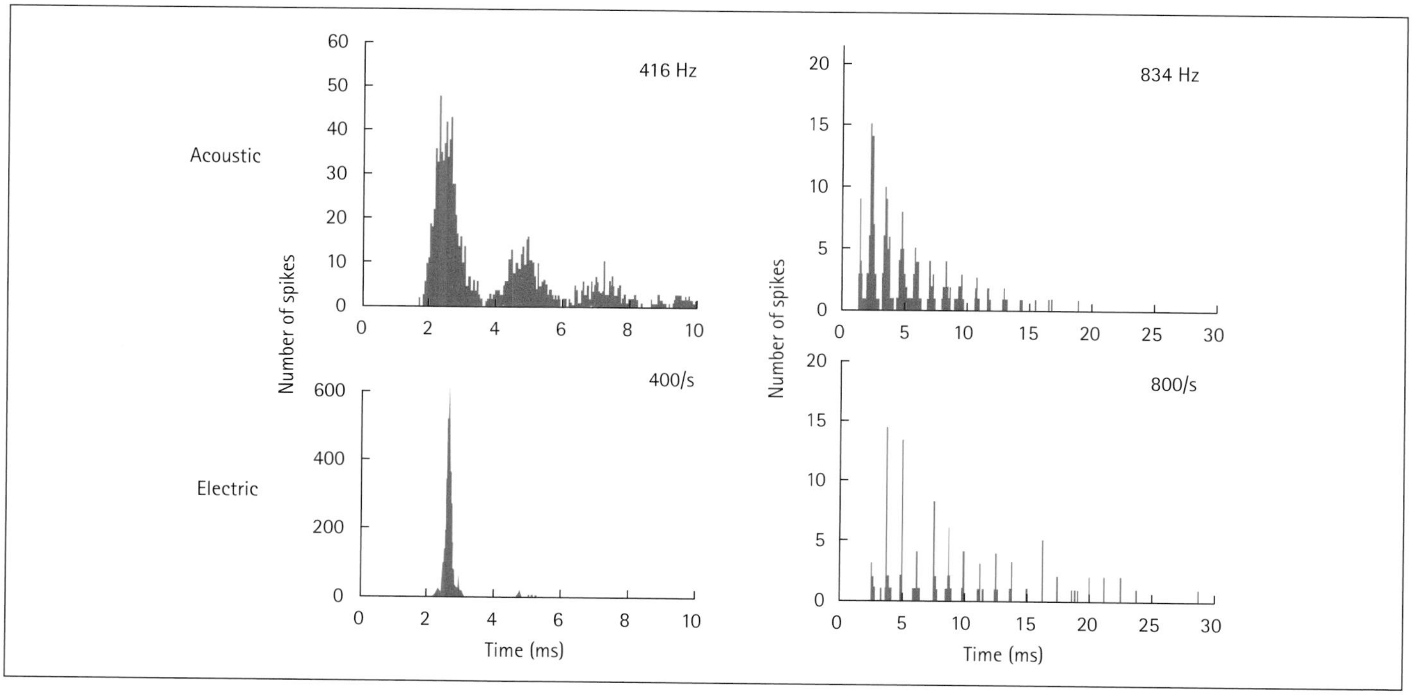

Figure 26.41 The interval histograms from cochlear nucleus cells in the cat for (a) acoustical and (b) electrical stimulation at low and high pulse rates. (From Clark. In: Greenberg and Ainsworth, eds. *Springer Handbook of Auditory Research: Speech Processing in the Auditory System*. Berkeley MA: Springer Verlag.[57])

sound. For acoustical stimulation, there are also a number of intervals, which are multiples of the period of the sound wave. For electrical stimulation at low rates, there is usually only one interval, which is the same as the period of the stimulus. At high rates there are a number of intervals, as seen with sound.

In summary, the pattern of interspike intervals for low rates of electrical stimulation is different from that of sound. It is, however, similar at high stimulus rates. On the other hand, frequency discrimination for low rates of electrical stimulation is similar to that for sound, but the discrimination of high stimulus rates is poor. If this discrepancy between the physiology and the psychophysics can be better understood, it may be possible to better reproduce frequency information with advanced cochlear implants.

The discrepancy may result from the fact that coding is not due primarily to the pattern of spikes in individual fibres in an ensemble, but to timing differences across the fibres due to the fact that sound induces a travelling wave along the basilar membrane, as illustrated in Figure 26.42. Temporal information across fibres could also be produced for acoustical stimuli through the rapid phase changes occurring in the area of maximum vibration, which are shown in Figure 26.43. To achieve this fine temporal and spatial pattern of responses for temporal coding, a new electrode array will be required, with many more electrodes to stimulate small groups of auditory nerve fibres, as illustrated in Figure 26.44. This array should also improve place coding.

The second important area of research for the future is to make the cochlear implant invisible. Teenagers, for example, are very sensitive about their deafness, and may not use their device in company. A total implant means implanting the speech processor as well as the microphone inside the body. There are a number of approaches to the problem (Figure 26.45). Sound vibrations may be detected with a piezoelectric microphone under the skin of the ear canal, and the electrical signal sent to the implanted electronics unit. Alternatively, the vibrations of the middle ear bones may be sensed by an inertia mass transducer or accelerometer, reflected light waves, and a cantilever. The electronics unit would be powered by an implanted rechargeable battery.

The inertia mass transducer responds to acceleration, and, as shown in Figure 26.46, movement is converted into electrical signals through the bending of a piezoelectric beam.

Another important area of research for the future is the use of nerve growth factors or neurotrophins to protect the cochlear nerve from die-back after deafness. This research may lead to better results with the cochlear implant, with more nerves to stimulate, and ultimately the pharmacological cure of a sensorineural hearing loss. Nerve growth factors can prevent nerve die-back and cause regeneration by activating the appropriate gene in the spiral ganglion cell. Nerve growth factors released into the inner ear are either actively transported back to the nucleus, or stimulate a signalling cascade of proteins. The acti-

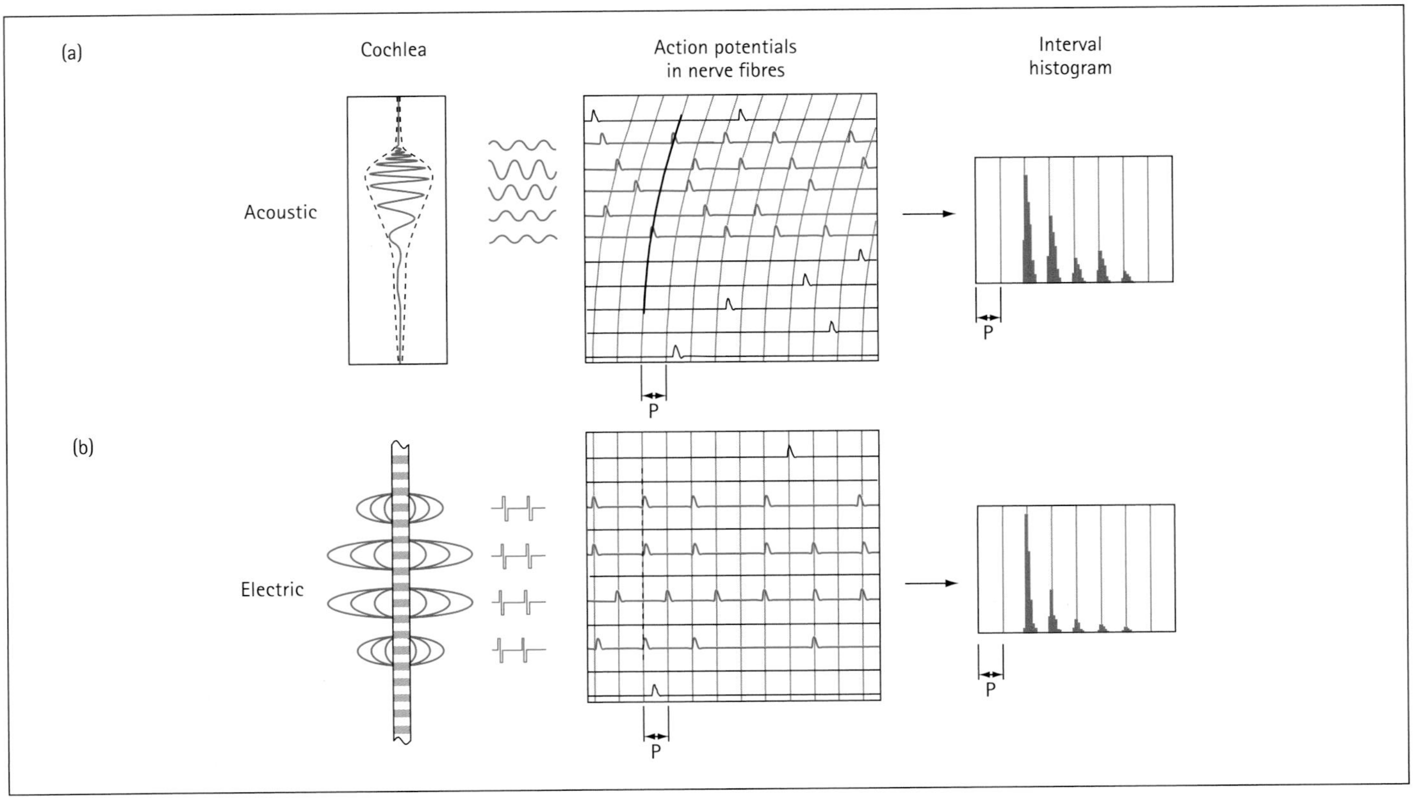

Figure 26.42 Temporal firing in an ensemble of fibres for (a) acoustical and (b) electrical stimulation and interspike interval histograms. P = period of stimulus. (From Clark. *Cochl Implants Int* 2000; **2**: 75–97.[116])

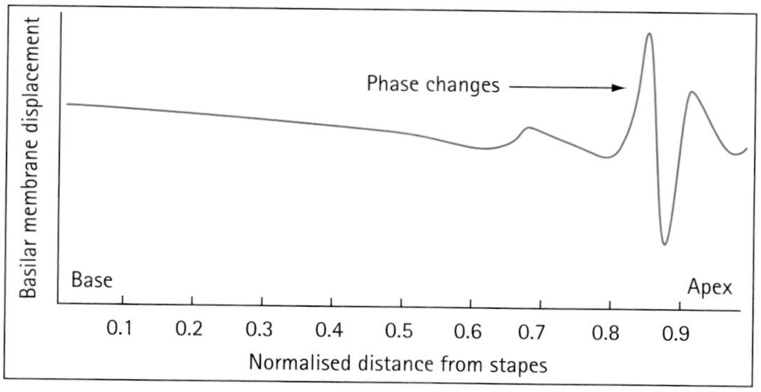

Figure 26.43 The basilar membrane phase changes at the maximum. (From Clark. *Am J Otol* 1999; **20**: 4–8.[109])

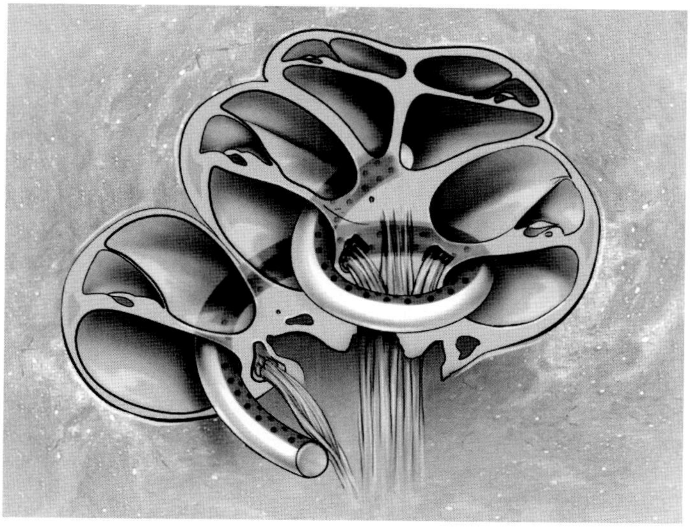

Figure 26.44 Advanced electrode array lying close to the spiral ganglion cells with increased number and density of electrode pads. (From Clark. *Am J Otol* 1999; **20**: 4–8.[109])

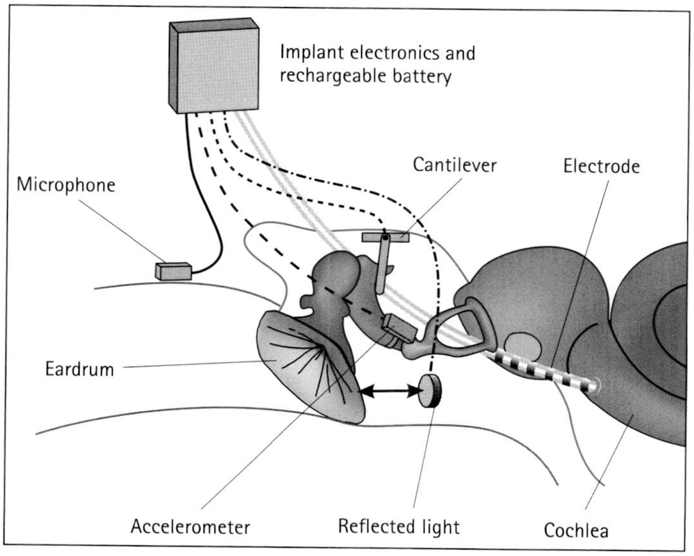

Figure 26.45 Implanted microphone, and vibration sensors for a totally implantable cochlear implant.

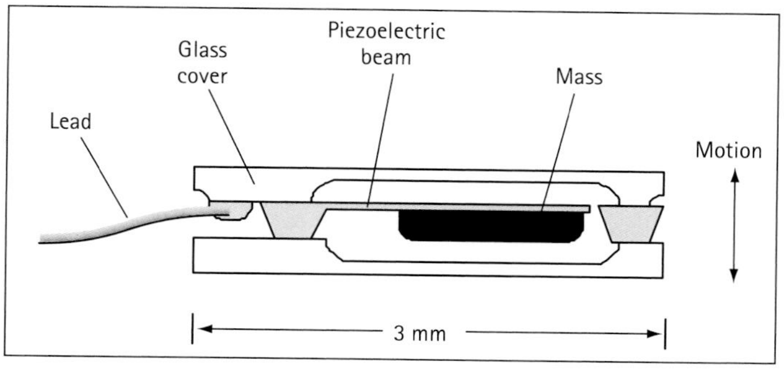

Figure 26.46 Inertia mass transducer (accelerometer): piezoelectric beam.[112]

vated gene then expresses the proteins required for neuronal health and regeneration (Figure 26.47).

Research has commenced to determine the best combinations of nerve growth factors to use. Results of studies by Marzella et al[107] on cultures of rat spiral ganglion cells are shown in Figure 26.48. This figure shows the ganglion cell counts for a constant dose of neurotrophin NT-3 with increasing concentrations of neuronal cytokine transforming growth factor TGF-β3. There is considerable facilitation in survival when the two drugs are used in combination. Possible ways of delivering the neutrophin to the site of action include a micropump, slow release from polymers, and viral vectors.

Finally, another application for neurotrophins will be the restoration of auditory plasticity in older children in whom the critical period has passed. Neurotrophins could facilitate a return of the plasticity required to develop the neural connections for coding speech frequencies. The release of neurotrophins into the inner ear of deaf children could not only improve nerve survival, but also facilitate synaptic transmission, as well as neuronal sprouting and connectivity. This could lead to improved cochlear implant results (Figure 26.49).

In summary, improved cochlear implant results are likely in the future, with a better understanding of how the brain codes sound as an electrical network, and an increased knowledge of molecular biology and how neurones respond to sound.

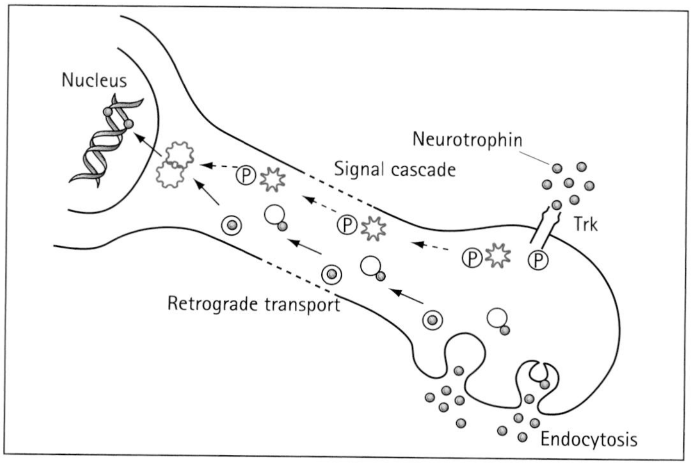

Figure 26.47 Neurotrophin transport along the axon to the nucleus and excitation of the appropriate gene.

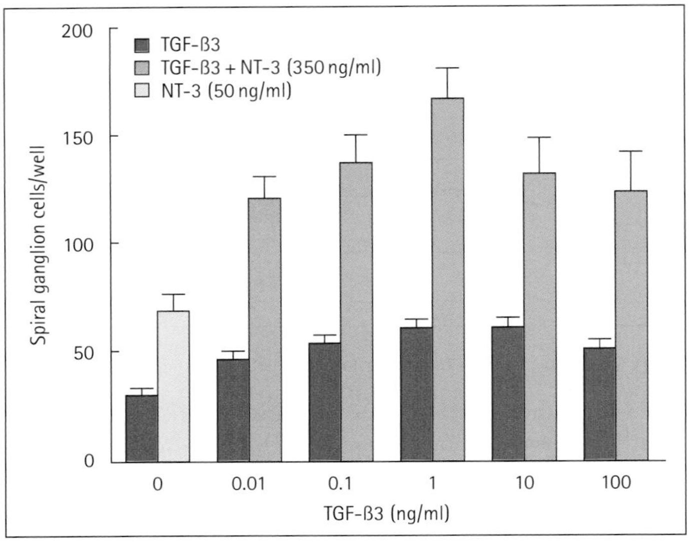

Figure 26.48 Combinations of neurotrophins to maximize the preservation of cultures of spiral ganglion cells. TGF, transforming growth factor; NT, neurotrophin. (Reprinted from Marzella et al. *Neuro Sci Letter* 1998; **240**: 77–80 with permission frm Elsevier Science.[107])

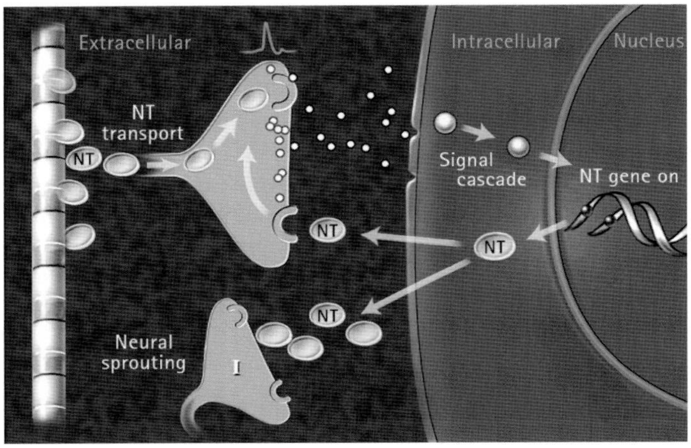

Figure 26.49 Action of neurotrophins on the higher auditory pathways, showing release from a cochlear implant electrode, anterograde and retrograde transport to the presynaptic region of the neurone, facilitation of transmitter release, excitation of the neurotrophin gene with protein production and release, and further facilitation of transmitter release and neural sprouting. (From Clark. *Am J Otol* 1999; **20**: 4–8.[109])

Acknowledgements

I would especially like to acknowledge Mrs Sue Davine, Dr David Lawrence, Mrs Helen Ried for their considerable help in the preparation of this chapter and also the many colleagues from the Department of Otolaryngology and The Bionic Ear Institute who have contributed to the research work over the last 30 years, as well as the bio-engineering achievements of Cochlear Limited. I would also like to thank Mr J.F. Patrick for reading the technology chapter section on comparative technology and for his helpful comments.

References

1. Clark GM, Pyman BC, Bailey QR. The surgery for multiple-electrode cochlear implantations. *J Laryngol Otol* 1979; **93**: 215–23.
2. Clark GM, Pyman BC, Webb RL, Bailey QR, Shepherd RK. Surgery for an improved multiple-channel cochlear implant. *Ann Otol Rhinol Laryngol* 1984; **93**: 204–7.
3. Webb RL, Pyman BC, Franz BK-HG, Clark GM. The surgery of cochlear prostheses. In: Clark GM, Tong YC, Patrick JF, eds. *Cochlear Prostheses*. London: Churchill Livingstone, 1990: 153–80.
4. Clark GM, Pyman BC, Webb RL. Surgery. In: Clark GM, Cowan RSC, Dowell RC, eds. *Cochlear Implantation for Infants and Children—Advances*. San Diego: Singular Publishing, 1997: 111–24.
5. Walker L, Rickards F. Reading comprehension levels of profoundly, prelingually deaf students in Victoria. *The Australian Teacher of the Deaf* 1993; **32**: 32–47.
6. Lawrence M. Direct stimulation of auditory nerve fibres. *J Arch Otolaryngol* 1964; **80:** 367–8.
7. Clark GM. Responses of cells in the superior olivary complex of the cat to electrical stimulation of the auditory nerve. *Exp Neurol* 1969; **24**: 124–36.
8. Clark GM, Nathar JM, Kranz HG, Maritz JS. A behavioral study on electrical stimulation of the cochlea and central auditory pathways of the cat. *Exp Neurol* 1972; **36**(2): 350–61.
9. Clark GM, Kranz HG, Minas H. Behavioral thresholds in the cat to frequency modulated sound and electrical stimulation of the auditory nerve. *Exp Neurol* 1973; **41**: 190–200.
10. Tong YC, Clark GM, Blamey PJ et al. Psychophysical studies for two multiple-channel cochlear implant patients. *J Acoust Soc Am* 1982; **71**: 153–60.
11. Merzenich MM. Studies on electrical stimulation of the auditory nerve in animals and man: cochlear implants. In: *The Nervous System, 3, Human Communication and its Disorders*. New York: Raven Press, 1974: 537–48.
12. Black RC, Clark GM. Electrical network properties and distribution of potentials in the cat cochlea. *Proc Aust Physiol Pharmacol Soc* 1978; **9**: 71.
13. Black RC, Clark GM. Differential electrical excitation of the auditory nerve. *J Acoust Soc Am* 1980; **67**: 868–74.
14. Studies on Pediatric Auditory Prosthesis Implants. NIH Contract NO1-NS-7-2342/1987–1992.
15. Cohen LT, Busby PA, Clark GM, Cochlear implant place psychophysics 2. Comparison of forward masking and pitch estimation data. *Audiol Neurootal* 1996; **1**: 278–92.
16. Laird RK. The bioengineering development of a sound encoder for an implantable hearing prosthesis for the profoundly deaf. MEng Sc Thesis, University of Melbourne, 1979.
17. Tong YC, Black RC, Clark GM et al. A preliminary report on a multiple-channel cochlear implant operation. *J Laryngol Otol* 1979; **93**: 679–95.
18. Simmons FB. Electrical stimulation of the auditory nerve in man. *Arch Otolaryngol* 1966; **84**: 2–54.

19. Tong YC, Blamey PJ, Dowell RC, Clark GM, Psychophysical studies evaluating the feasibility of a speech processing strategy for a multiple-channel cochlear implant. *J Acoust Soc Am* 1983; **74**: 73–80.
20. Riesz RR. Differential intensity sensitivity of the ear for pure tones. *Phys Rev* 1928; **31** series 2: 867–75.
21. Delattre P, Liberman AM, Cooper FS. An experimental study of the acoustic determinants of vowel color observations on one and two formant vowels synthesised from spectrographic patterns. *Word* 1952; **8**(3): 195–210.
22. Fant G. On the predictability of formant levels and spectrum envelopes from formant frequencies. In: Halle H, Lurnt M, Maclean H, eds. *For Roman Jakobson* The Hague: Mounton, 1956: 109–120.
23. Tong YC, Dowell RC, Blamey PJ, Clark GM. Two-component hearing sensations produced by two-electrode stimulation in the cochlea of a deaf patient. *Science* 1983; **219**: 993–4.
24. Black RC, Steel AC, Clark GM. Amplitude and pulse rate difference limens for electrical stimulation of the cochlea following graded degeneration of the auditory nerve. *Acta Otolaryngol* 1983; **95**: 27–33.
25. Blamey P, Arndt P, Bergeron S et al. Factors affecting auditory performance of postlinguistically deaf adults using cochlear implants. *Audiol Neurootol* 1996; **1**: 293–306.
26. Nadol JB, Young Y, Glynn RJ. Survival of spiral ganglion cells in profound sensory neural hearing loss: implications for cochlear implantation. *Ann Otol Rhinol Laryngol* 1989; **98**: 411–16.
27. Staller SJ, Beiter AL, Brimacombe JA, Arndt P. Paediatric performance with the nucleus 22-channel cochlear implant system. *Am J Otol* 1991; **12**: 126–36.
28. Busby PA, Clark GM. Pitch estimation by early deafened subject using a multiple electrode cochlear implant. *J Acoust Soc Am* 2000; **107**: 547–58.
29. Blamey PJ, Sarant JZ, Serry TA et al. Speech perception and spoken language in children with impaired hearing. In *Proceedings of the 5th International Conference on Spoken Language Processing*, Sydney, 30 November–4 December 1998; **1**: 288.
30. Clark GM, Knight LJ, Stanley GV. Auditory evoked potentials and auditory sequential memory. *Proc Aust Physiol Pharmacol Soc* 1974; 5(2): 185.
31. Clark GM. An evaluation of per-scalar cochlear electrode implantation techniques. A histopathogical study in cats. *J Laryngol Otol* 1977; **91**: 185–99.
32. Flynn MC, Dowell RC, Clark GM. Speech perception of hearing aid users versus cochlear implantees. In: Clark GM, ed. *Cochlear Implants*. Bologna: Monduzzi Editore, 1997: 261–5.
33. Stapells DR, Gravel JS, Martin BA. Thresholds for auditory brainstem responses to tones in notched noise from infants and young children with normal hearing or sensorineural hearing loss. *Ear Hear* 1995; **16**: 361–71.
34. Rickards FW, Clark GM. Steady-state evoked potentials to amplitude-modulated tones. In: Nodar RH, Barber C, eds. *Evoked Potentials II*. Boston: Butterworths, 1984: 163–8.
35. Cohen LT, Rickards FW, Clark GM. A comparison of steady-state evoked potentials to modulated tones in awake and sleeping humans. *J Acoust Soc Am* 1991; **90**: 2467–79.
36. Rance G, Rickards FW, Cohen LT, De Vidi S, Clark GM. The automated prediction of hearing thresholds in sleeping subjects using auditory steady-state evoked potentials. *Ear Hear* 1995; **16**: 499–507.
37. Rance G, Beer De, Cone-Wesson BK, Shepherd RK, Dowell RC, King A, Rickards FW, Clark GM. Clinical findings for a group of infants and young children with auditory neuropathy. *Ear Hear* 1999; **20**: 238–52.
38. O'Leary SJ, Mitchell TE, Gibson WP, Sanli H. Abnormal positive potentials in transtympanic electrocochleography. *Am J Otol* 2000; **21**: 813–18.
39. Blamey PJ, Pyman BC, Gordon M et al. Factors predicting postoperative sentence scores in postlinguistically deaf adult cochlear implant patients. *Ann Otol Rhinol Laryngol* 1992; **101**: 342–8.
40. Blamey PJ. Factors affecting auditory performance of postlinguistically deaf adults using cochlear implants: etiology, age, and duration of deafness. In: *100th NIH Consensus Development Conference on Cochlear Implants in Adults and Children*, Bethesda, Maryland, 1995, 1996: 15–20.
41. Dowell RC, Blamey PJ, Clark GM. Rehabilitation strategies for adult cochlear implant users. In: Clark GM ed. *Cochlear Implants*. Bologna: Monduzzi Editore, 1997: 35–40.
42. Clark GM. Cochlear implant research directions. In: Clark GM, ed. *Cochlear Implants*. Bologna: Monduzzi Editore, 1997: 55–60.
43. Dunn LM, Dunn LM. *PPVT-III Peabody Picture Vocabulary Test*, 3rd edn. Circle Pines, Minnesota: American Guidance Service, 1997.
44. Semel E, Wiig EH, Secord WA. *CELF 3—Clinical Evaluation of Language Fundamentals*, 3rd edn. San Antonio: Harcourt Brace, 1995.
45. Pyman BC, Blamey PJ, Clark GM. Development of speech perception in children using cochlear implants: effects of etiology and delayed milestones. *Am J Otol* 2000; **21**: 57–61.
46. Eddington DK. Speech discrimination in deaf subjects with cochlear implants. *J Acoust Soc Am* 1980; **68**: 886–91.
47. Eddington DK. Speech recognition in deaf subjects with multichannel intracochlear electrodes. *Ann NY Acad Sci* 1983; **405**: 241–58.
48. Merzenich M, Byers C, White M. Scala tympani electrode arrays. *Fifth Q Prog Rep*. NIH Contract NO1-59-2353 USCF San Francisco. 1984: 1–11.
49. Battmer R-D, Gnadeberg D, Allum-Mecklenburg DJ, Lenarz T. Matched-pair comparisons for adults using the Clarion or Nucleus devices. *Ann Otol Rhinol Laryngol* 1994; **104**(suppl 166): 251–4.
50. Hartmann R, Topp G, Klinke R. Discharge patterns of cat primary auditory fibers with electrical stimulation of the cochlea. *Hear Res* 1984; **13**: 47–62.
51. Hartmann R, Topp G, Klinke R. Electrical stimulation of the cat cochlea—discharge pattern of single auditory fibres. *Adv Audiol* 1984; **1**: 18–29.
52. Dowell RC, Whitford LA, Seligman PM, Franz BK-HG, Clark GM. Preliminary results with a miniature speech processor for the 22-electrode/cochlear hearing prosthesis. In: Sacristan T, ed.

Otorhinolaryngology, Head and Neck Surgery (XIV World Congress of Otorhinolaryngology Head and Neck Surgery, Madrid, 1990). Amsterdam: Kugler & Ghedini, 1990: 1167–73.

53. Cohen NL, Waltzman SB, Fisher SG. A prospective, randomised study of cochlear implants. *N Engl J Med* 1993; **328**: 233–82.
54. Wilson BS, Lawson DT, Zerbi M, Finley CC. Twelfth Quarterly Progress Report—Speech Processors for Auditory Prostheses, April 1992. NIH contract N01-DC-9-2401. Research Triangle Institute, North Carolina, 1992.
55. Wilson BS, Lawson DT, Zerbi M, Finley CC. Fifth Quarterly Progress Report—Speech processors for Auditory Prostheses, October 1993. NIH contract N01-DC-2-2401. Research Triangle Institute, North Carolina, 1993.
56. Kessler DK, Loeb GE, Barker MJ. Distribution of speech recognition results with the Clarion cochlear prosthesis. *Ann Otol Rhinol Laryngol* 1995; **104**(suppl 166): 283–5.
57. Clark GM. Speech processing for cochlear implants. In: Greenberg S, Ainsworth W, eds. *Springer Handbook of Auditory Research: Speech Processing in the Auditory System*. Berkeley, MA: Springer Verlag, in press.
58. Paolini AG, Clark GM. The effect of pulsatile intracochlear electrical stimulation on intracellularly recorded cochlear nucleus neurons. In: Clark GM, ed. *Cochlear Implants*. Bologna: Monduzzi Editore, 1997: 119–24.
59. Viemeister NF. Temporal modulation transfer functions based upon modulation thresholds. *J Acoust Soc Am* 1979; **66**(5): 1364–80.
60. Shannon RV. Temporal modulation transfer functions in patients with cochlear implants. *J Acoust Soc Am* 1992; **91**: 2156–64.
61. Busby PA, Tong YC, Clark GM. The perception of temporal modulations by cochlear implant patients. *J Acoust Soc Am* 1993; **97**: 124–31.
62. Xu J, Shepherd RK, Millard RE, Clark GM. Chronic electrical stimulation of the auditory nerve at high stimulus rates: a physiological and histological study. *Hear Res* 1997; **105**: 1–29.
63. Huang CQ, Shepherd RK, Seligman PM, Clark GM. Reduction in excitability of the auditory nerve in guinea pigs following acute high rate electrical stimulation. *Proc 16th Annu Meeting Aust Neurosci Soc* 1996; **7**: 227.
64. Huang CQ, Shepherd RK, Seligman PM, Clark GM. Reduction in excitability of the auditory nerve following electrical stimulation at high stimulus rates: III Capacitive versus non-capacitive coupling of the stimulating electrodes. *Hear Res* 1998; **116**: 55–64.
65. Tykocinski M, Shepherd RK, Clark GM. Reduction in excitability of the auditory nerve following electrical stimulation at high stimulus rates. II. Comparison of fixed amplitude with amplitude modulated stimuli. *Hear Res* 1997; **112**: 147–57.
66. Brummer SB, Turner MJ. Electrical stimulation with Pt electrodes. I—A method for determination of 'real' electrode areas. *IEEE Trans Biomed Engng* 1977; **24**(5): 436–9.
67. Brummer SB, Turner MJ. Electrical stimulation with Pt electrodes: II—estimation of maximum surface redox (theoretical non-gassing) limits. *IEEE Trans Biomed Engng* 1977; **24**(5): 440–3.
68. Brummer SB, Turner MJ. Electrochemical considerations for safe electrical stimulation of the nervous system with platinum electrodes. *IEEE Trans Biomed Engng* 1977; **24**(1): 59–63.
69. Shepherd RK, Clark GM, Black RC. Chronic electrical stimulation of the auditory nerve in cats, physiological and histopathological results. Acta Otolaryngol 1983(suppl 399): 19–31.
70. Schulman JH, Gord JC, Strojnik P, Whitmoyer DI, Wolfe JH. Voltage/current control system for a human tissue stimulator, 1996. US Patent 5,522,865.
71. Black RC, Clark GM. Electrical transmission line properties in the cat cochlea. *Proc Aust Physiol Pharmacol Soc* 1977; **8**: 137.
72. Leake PA, Snyder RL, Hradek GT. Spatial organization of inner hair cell synapses and cochlear spiral ganglion neurons. *J Comp Neurol* 1993; **333**: 257–70.
73. Clark GM, Blamey PJH, Busby PA et al. A multiple-electrode intracochlear implant for children. *Arch Otolaryngol* 1987; **113**: 825–8.
74. Michelson RP, Schindler RA. Multichannel cochlear implant preliminary results in man. *Laryngoscope* 1981; **91**: 38–42.
75. Clark GM, Busby PA, Roberts SA et al. Preliminary results for the Cochlear Corporation Multi-Electrode intracochlear implants on six prelingually deaf patients. *Am J Otol* 1987; **8**(3): 234–9.
76. Sutton D, Miller JM, Pfingst BE. Comparison of cochlear histopathology following two implant designs for use in scala tympani. *Ann Otol Rhinol Laryngol* 1980; **89**: 11.
77. Simmons FB, Glattke TJ. Comparison of electrical and acoustical stimulation of the cat ear. *Ann Otol Rhinol Laryngol* 1970; **81**: 731–8.
78. Schindler RA, Kessler DK, Barker MA. Clarion patient performance: an update on the clinical trials. *Ann Otol Rhinol Laryngol* 1995; **104**(suppl 166): 269–72.
79. Shepherd RK, Matsushima J, Martin RL, Clark GM. Cochlear pathology following chronic electrical stimulation of the auditory nerve: II Deafened kittens. *Hear Res* 1994; **81**: 150–66.
80. Tykocinski M, Cohen LT, Pyman BC et al. Comparison of electrode position in the human cochlea using various peri-modiolar electrode arrays. *Am J Otol* 2000; **21**: 205–11.
81. Vandali AE, Whitford LA, Plant KL, Clark GM. Speech perception as a function of electrical stimulation rate using the Nucleus 24 cochlear implant system. *Ear Hear* 2000; **21**: 608–24.
82. Blamey PJ, Sarant JZ, Serry TA et al. Speech perception and spoken language in children with impaired hearing. *Proc 5th Int Conf Spoken Language Processing* 1998 6: 2615–18.
83. Vandali A, Harrison JM, Huigen J, Plant K, Clark GM. Multichannel cochlear implant speech processing: further variations of the Spectral Maxima sound processor strategy. *Ann Otol Rhinol Laryngol* 1995; **104**(suppl 166): 378–81.
84. Stark H, Tuteur FB. In: *Modern Electrical Communications: theory and systems*. Englewood Cliffs, NJ: Prentice Hall, 1979.
85. Von Wallenberg EL, Hochmair ES, Hochmari-Desoyer IJ. Initial results with simultaneous analog and pulsatile stimulation of the cochlea. *Acta Otolaryngol* 1990; **469**: 140–9.
86. Jones OA, McDermott HJ, Seligman PM, Millar JB. Coding of voice source information in the Nucleus cochlear implant system. *Ann Otol Rhinol Laryngol* 1995; **104**(suppl 166): 363–5.
87. Clark GM, Patrick JF, Bailey QR. A cochlear implant round window electrode array. *J Laryngol Otol* 1979; **93**: 107–9.

88. Cohen NL, Hoffman RA, Stroschein M. Medical or surgical complications related to the Nucleus multichannel cochlear implant. *Ann Otol Rhinol Laryngol* 1988; **97**(suppl 135): 8–13.
89. Clark GM, Cohen LT, Shepherd RK. Surgical and safety considerations of multi-channel cochlear implants in children. *Ear Hear* 1991; **12**(suppl): 15–24.
90. Clark GM. Learning to understand speech with the cochlear implant. In: Fahle M, Poggio T, eds. *Perceptual Learning*. Cambridge, Mass: MIT Press, 2002: 147–60.
91. Serry TA, Blamey PJ, Spain P, James C. CASALA: Computer aided speech and language analysis. *Aust Commun Q* 1997; Spring: 27–8.
92. Dawson PW, Clark GM. Changes in synthetic and natural vowel perception after specific training for congenitally deafened patients using a multichannel cochlear implant. *Ear Hear* 1997; **18**: 488–501.
93. Sarant JZ, Blamey PJ, Cowan RS, Clark GM. The effect of language knowledge on speech perception: what are we really assessing? *Am J Otol* 1997; **18**: S135–7.
94. Breen KJ, Plueckhahn VD, Cordner SM. *Ethics, Law and Medical Practice*. St Leonards NSW: Allen & Unwin, 1997.
95. Skinner MW, Clark GM, Whitford L et al. Evaluation of a new Spectral Peak coding strategy for the Nucleus 22 channels cochlear implant system. *Am J Otol* 1994; **15**(suppl 2): 15–27.
96. Geers AE, Moog JS. Effectiveness of cochlear implants and tactile aids for deaf children. *Volta Rev* 1994; **96**(5): 1–198.
97. US National Institutes of Health. Cochlear implants in children. NIH Consensus statement, Bethesda, Maryland, 1995; **13**(2): 1–30.
98. Summerfield AQ, Marshall DH, Davis AC. Cochlear implantation: demand, costs, and utility. *Ann Otol Rhinol Laryngol* 1994; **104**: 245–8.
99. Clark GM. A hearing prosthesis for severe perceptive deafness—experimental studies. *J Laryngol Otol* 1973; **87**: 929–45.
100. Clark GM, Kranz HG, Minas H, Nather JM. Histopathological findings in cochlear implants in cats. *J Laryngol Otol* 1975; **8**: 495–504.
101. Agnew, WF, Yuen TGH, Pudenz RH, Bullara LA. Neuropathological effects of intracerebral platinum salt injections. *J Neuropathol Exp Neurol* 1977; **36**: 533–46.
102. Black RC, Hannakeer P. Dissolution of smooth platinum electrodes in biological fluids. *Appl Neurophysiol* 1979; **42**: 366–74.
103. Shepherd RK, Murray MT, Houghton ME, Clark GM. Scanning electron microscopy of chronically stimulated platinum intracochlear electrodes. *Biomaterials* 1985; **6**: 237–42.
104. Clark GM, Cowan RSC, Dowell RC. Ethical issues. In: Clark GM, Cowan RSC, Dowell RC, eds. *Cochlear Implantation for Infants and Children*. San Diego: Singular Publishing Group, 1997: 241–9.
105. Cohen LT, Saunders E, Clark GM. Psychophysics of a prototype peri-modiolar cochlear implant electrode array. *Hear Res* 2001; **155**: 63–81.
106. Treaba C, Xu J, Xu SA, Clark GM. Precurved electrode array and insertion tool. *Ann Otol Rhinol Laryngol* 1995; **104**(suppl 166): 438–41.
107. Marzella PL, Clark GM, Shepherd RK, Bartlett PF, Kilpatrick TJ. Synergy between TGF-B3 and NT-3 to promote the survival of spiral ganglia neurones in vitro. *Neurosci Lett* 1998; **240**: 77–80.
108. Clark GM. Electrical stimulation of the auditory nerve: the coding of frequency, the perception of pitch, and the development of cochlear implant speech processing strategies for profoundly deaf people. *J Clin Physiol Pharmacol Res* 1996; **23**: 766–76.
109. Clark GM. Cochlear implants in the third millenium. *Am J Otol* 1999; **20**: 4–8.
110. Clark GM, Blamey PJ, Brown AM et al. The University of Melbourne—Nucleus multi-electrode cochlear implant. *Adv Otorhinolaryngol* 1987; **38**: 1–181 (review).
111. Clark GM. Auditory central nervous system plasticity: application to cochlear implantation. In: Clark GM, ed. *Cochlear Implants*. Bologna: Monduzzi Editore, 1997: 19–23.
112. Roylance LM, Angell JB. A batch fabricated silicon accelerometer. *IEEE Trans Electron Devices* 1979; **ED-26**(12): 1911–17.
113. Clark GM. The cochlear implant: A search for answers. *Cochl Implants Int* 2000; **1**: 1–17.
114. Clark GM, Lawrence D. Technical features of the Nucleus, med-El and Clarion cochlear implants. *Aust J Otolaryngol* 2000; **3(5)**: 516–22.
115. Shepherd R, Treaba C, Cohen L, Pyman B, Huigen J, Xu J, Clark GM. Peri-modiolar electrode arrays: A comparison of electrode position in the human temporal lobe, In: Clark GM, ed. *Cochlear Implants*. Bologna: Monduzzi Editore, 1997: 205–9.
116. Clark GM. The cochlear implants: Climbing new mountains. *Cochl Implants Int* 2000; **2**: 75–97.

27 Disorders of the inner ear in adults

Alessandro Martini, Silvano Prosser

This chapter deals with inner ear disorders in adults. Rather than an extensive disease listing, we have attempted to provide a review oriented towards possible aetiological and pathogenetic mechanisms.

Epidemiological studies have pointed out that the percentages of the general population having a hearing loss exceeding 45 dB HL and 65 dB HL are around 1.3% and 0.3% respectively between ages 30 and 50, and 2.3% and 7.4% between ages 60 and 70.[1]

The auditory cells have a life cycle which is different from that of the cells of other sensory organs. Gustatory cells survive for 14–21 days, and olfactory cells survive for 30–90 days. Auditory cells have a lifespan of 70–100 years, but their number is less than 20 000, instead of 137 000 000 retina cells.

Loss of hearing has long been considered a permanent and untreatable consequence of ototoxicity, trauma, ageing, etc. Moreover, the biochemical mechanisms by which the hair cells are lost are partially known, and different pathways have been discovered.

Advances in molecular biology and molecular genetics have made a major contribution to the understanding of inner ear disease states.

This applies not only to congenital profound hearing losses: note the roles of connexin 26,[2–4] myosin VII,[5,6] pendrin[7] and usherin;[8] but also to late-onset/progressive hearing impairments: note the roles of *COL4A* genes in the basilar membrane in Alport syndrome,[9] the *Mpv17* glomerulosclerosis gene, deficiency of which leads to significant abnormalities of the inner ear structures,[10] and the *COCH* gene (in patients with mutation in the *COCH* gene, inner ear deposition of acidophilic ground substance, which can cause degeneration of cochlear and vestibular sensory axons and dendrites, probably due to strangulation, has been reported).[11]

Anatomical structures within the cochlea are relatively inaccessible to fluid and tissue sampling, and this has limited our understanding of many pathological states of the cochlea, which are frequently described not in terms of the actual causative abnormality but rather in terms of audiometric findings, i.e. threshold asymmetries, recruitment, threshold profile, hearing loss changes over time (sudden, progressive, fluctuating), or concomitant symptoms, e.g. vertigo or tinnitus. Certainly, some forms of cochlear hearing loss which show common symptoms and audiometric changes have different causative agents. The prototype of this is the hearing impairment found in Menière's syndrome, in which essentially all pathogenic mechanisms have been postulated to play a role, with the possible exception of neoplastic processes. In fact, the clinical definition of Menière's syndrome is still problematic.[12]

The rapid advances in the understanding of physiological and biochemical peculiarities of the cochlea rendered it a complex procedure for the association of deafness with any specific causative agents, i.e. the nosological classification of cochleopathies. The integrity of the structures contained in the cochlear duct largely depends on a locally controlled delicate homeostatic equilibrium.[13] The metabolism of hair cells, which are an extremely specialized form of neuroepithelium, depends on endolymph composition and on biochemical information exchanges with supporting cells. In turn, endolymph secretion and maintenance depend on the stria vascularis, itself a structure highly specialized in dealing with high metabolic cycling rates. Toxic substances can gain access to the cochlea through the bloodstream and cause abnormalities of either the neuroephithelial apparatus responsible for electromechanical transduction or of the vascular structure responsible for endolymph homeostasis. Moreover, the inner ear is capable of immune responses to invading viral or bacterial antigens, and can itself be the target of autoimmune diseases.

Given these assumptions, acquired disorders developing inside the cochlea can be classified on the basis of current knowledge as local effects of numerous factors which can be vascular, dysmetabolic, toxic, inflammatory or immune-mediated. Genetic as well as traumatic or neoplastic causes may also be involved. The effects of normal ageing are discussed in Chapter 3.

Cochleopathies of genetic origin

Although many kindreds with autosomal dominant (AD) progressive hereditary hearing impairment have been reported in the literature, no epidemiological information exists on the prevalence of genetic hearing impairment in the adult population.[14] The majority of these adult-onset forms are due to the interaction of environmental and genetic factors.[15] Animal studies have given valuable information on the degenerative processes developing in the auditory system as a function of age,[16] and a number of syndromes are recognized both in humans and mice in which hearing loss presents with a late onset.[17] In the 'neuroepithelial defects' group, the primary defect lies in the neuroepithelia of the inner ear: the auditory cells ultimately degenerate, but some developmental defects can be detected long before the onset of degeneration.[18] Cosgrove et al,[9] have reported that in a gene-knockout mouse model for Alport syndrome, mutagenesis of the *COL4A3* gene produces changes throughout the basement membranes of the cochlea and thickening of the basement membranes surrounding the vessels of the stria vascularis.

Genetically determined hearing impairments may develop at any age throughout life, either as the sole manifestation of the mutant gene, as part of an inherited syndrome, or as a result of the interaction with exogenous factors;[14] in fact, it is possible that mutations in some genes render the ear more susceptible to environmental factors causing inner ear damage (i.e. noise exposure, infection, injury and ototoxic drugs).[19]

> A genetically determined hearing loss, independently from onset-age and temporal progression, may develop as a result of:
>
> - occasional gene mutation
> - inherited gene alteration
> - interaction between gene alteration and exogenous factors

Even if many (and usually the most severe) forms of genetic sensorineural hearing losses (SNHLs) are congenital, a number of hearing impairments appear during or after the first decade of life and are progressive. The majority of postlingual non-syndromic sensorineural hearing impairments (NS-SNHIs) are AD.[20] Typical is the DFNA1 form ('Monge' hearing loss), in which low frequencies are involved during the early years, progressing to hearing impairment involving high frequencies in later years. Older individuals with this condition exhibit a loss involving all frequencies.[21,22] This is also true for some other non-syndromic hearing disorders which may initially have different audiometric patterns (e.g. involving medium or high frequencies) that become superimposable during adulthood, e.g. severe pantonal hypoacusis with possible high-frequency decapitation, (Figure 27.1, Table 27.1).[23,24]

The progression of the hearing impairment is typical of AD forms, as stressed by Van Egmond:[25] 'Dominant inner-ear deafness is rarely congenital. It develops in middle age, has a strong progression with frequent lengthy pauses, and loss of hearing for all frequencies'. A 'progressive hearing impairment' is an impairment of PTA ≥15 dB in a 10-year period, as defined by the European Work Group on Genetic Hearing Impairment.[26] Subjects over the age of 50 have to be analysed according to other criteria to allow for the possible overlapping of normal ageing effects[27,28] (Figure 27.2).

Even though a genetic cause is recognized, the underlying pathogenetic mechanism might be quite different (the most well-recognized example being represented by congenital abnormalities such as the hearing impairment associated with connexin 26). Various pathogenetic mechanisms are suggested by the different histopathological findings (see Figure 4.4). In some instances, a marked loss of ganglion cells, atrophy of stria vascularis, and degeneration of the organ of Corti (Paparella et al,[29] in AD mid-frequency SNHL) have been described; in AD progressive SNHL, Khetarpal et al[11] reported acidophilic deposits in the spiral ligament, spiral limbus and spiral lamina of all three turns of the cochlea.

Table 27.1 Genetic hearing loss with no associated abnormalities.

Autosomal dominant inheritance
AD congenital severe SNHL
AD congenital low-frequency SNHL
AD progressive low-frequency SNHL with childhood onset (Monge type)
AD mid-frequency SNHL
AD progressive low-frequency SNHL
AD progressive low-frequency mixed HL
AD unilateral SNHL
AD progressive vestibulocochlear dysfunction and SNHL
Autosomal recessive inheritance
AR congenital severe-to-profound SNHL
AR congenital retrocochlear HL
AR congenital moderate SNHL
AR early-onset progressive SNHL
AR progressive high-frequency SNHL
X-linked inheritance
X-linked congenital SNHL
X-linked early-onset SNHL
X-linked moderate SNHL
X-linked high-frequency SNHL
X-linked progressive mixed HL with perilymphatic gusher
Other forms of HL
Hereditary Menière syndrome

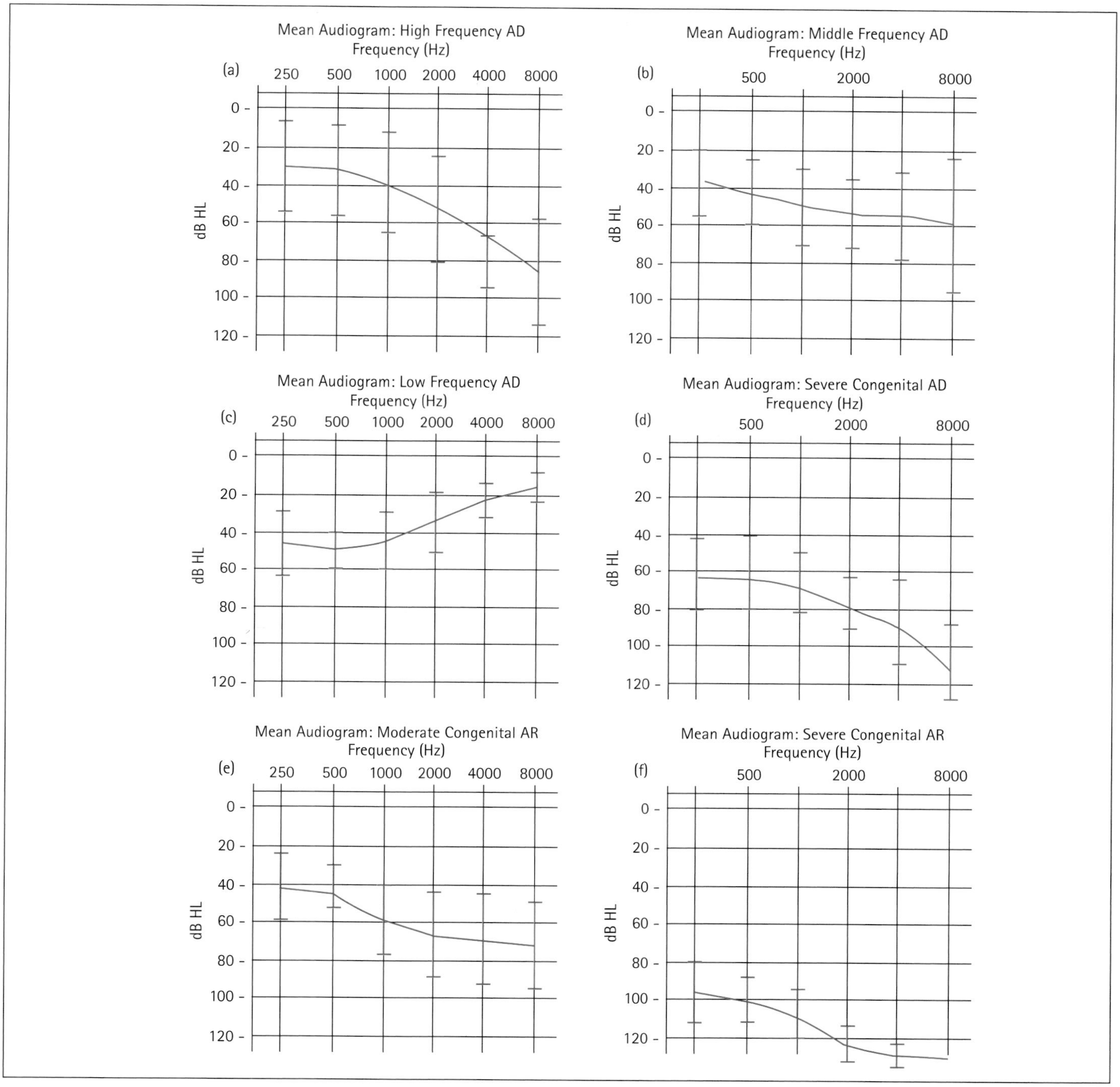

Figure 27.1 The most common audiogram shapes in hereditary non-syndromal sensorineural hearing impairments (From Martini et al. *Audiology* 1997; **36**: 228–36.[142]). AD, autosomal dominant; AR, autosomal recessive.

Syndromic hearing impairments

Evidence of hearing impairment progression was found in the CHARGE association[30] (Figure 27.3) and in several forms associated with eye disorders, apart from Usher syndrome. Namely, hearing loss is progressive in Alström, Refsum and Norrie syndromes (Figure 27.4), ocular albinism, some types of otic atrophy and 'cataracts and progressive SNHL'. In the latter hereditary condition, histopathological findings of severe cochleosaccular degeneration have been reported.[31]

Also, in Stickler syndrome (or hereditary arthro-ophthalmopathy), progressive sensorineural high-tone hearing loss has been reported in 80% of cases.[32]

Typically progressive is the hearing impairment in Alport syndrome (nephritis and SNHL), Epstein syndrome (macrothrombocytopenia, nephritis and SNHL), Lemieux–Neemeh syndrome (nephritis, motor and sensory neuropathy and SNHL), and Muckle-Wells syndrome (nephritis, urticaria, amyloidosis and SNHL); generally, hearing loss severity and its rate of progression is unrelated to the degree of the associated renal involvement.[33]

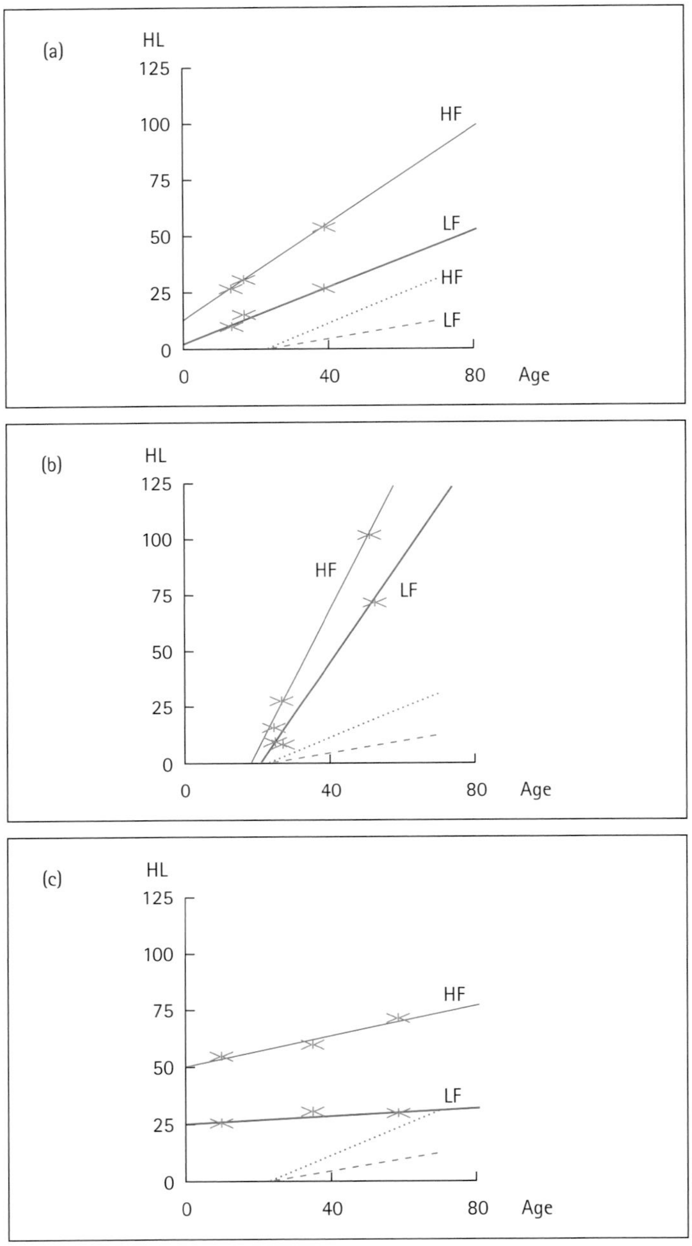

Figure 27.2 Three main possible patterns of evolution of a hereditary hearing impairment can be defined: (a) the hearing level may be relatively stable throughout adult life, and hence resistant to the typical age-dependent deterioration; (b) the hearing level may deteriorate progressively with an age-dependent rate parallel to that of a normally hearing population, hence showing a simple additional effect of hereditary hearing loss and age-related hearing loss; (c) the hearing level deteriorates from an early age, at a faster rate than that of the normally hearing population, hence showing an interaction between age-related hearing loss and hereditary hearing loss. (After Martini et al. *J Audiol Med* 1996; **6**: 141–56.[27]). HF, high frequency; LF low frequency.

In Alport s. the human temporal bone studies have reported a wide range of features, including collapse of the Reissner's membrane, severe degeneration of the Organ of Corti, loss of cochlear neurons and defects in the stria vascularis.[34,35]

The majority of genetic hearing abnormalities associated with nervous system disorders are progressive.[36] This is the case

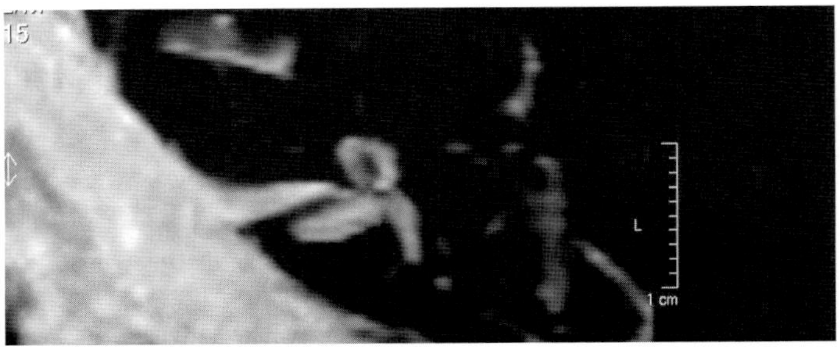

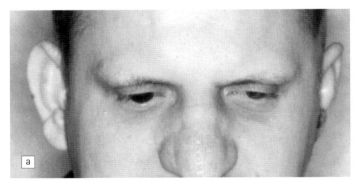

Figure 27.3 MR of the left temporal bone of a patient with a CHARGE association: the semicircular canals are severely malformed: lateral is absent, the superior and posterior are hypoplastic.

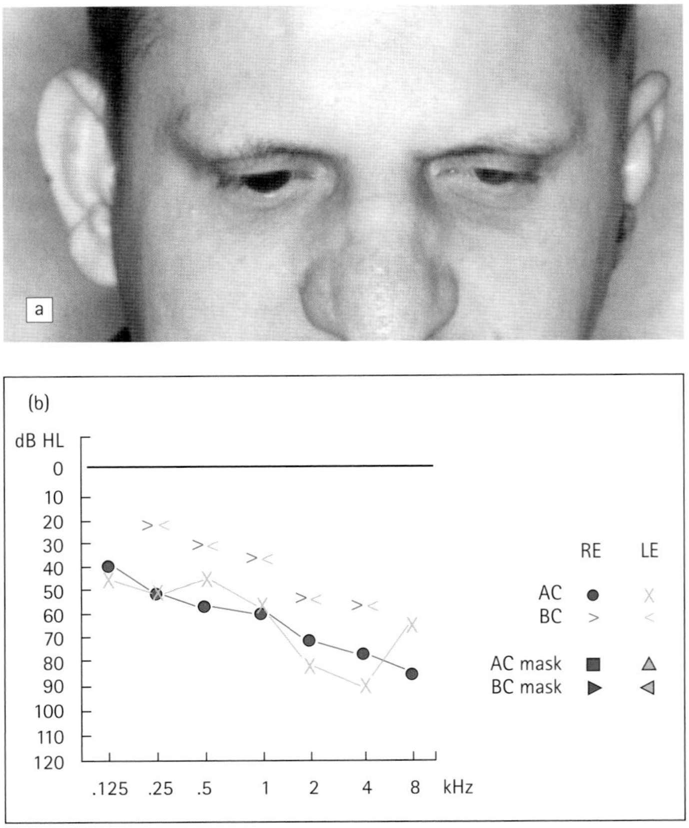

Figure 27.4 Norrie syndrome (oculoacousticocerebral dysplasia). (a) Eyes are deep-set and phthisic; the corneas are hazy. (b) Audiogram of the patient, 35 years old, showing moderate-to-severe bilateral mixed hearing loss. RE, right ear; LE, left ear; AC, air conduction; BC, bone conduction.

for syndromes associated with ataxia (Cockayne syndrome, Klippel-Durante syndrome, Hallgren syndrome, Richards–Rundle syndrome, etc.) (Figure 27.5), with neuromuscular disorders (Brown–Vialetto–Van Laere syndrome, AD Charcot–Marie–Tooth syndrome, Hagemoser syndrome, Pauli syndrome, etc.), and with sensory and autonomic neuropathies (Hicks syndrome, etc.), or mitochondrial syndromes such as Kearns–Sayre syndrome (ophthalmoplegia plus), MELAS (mitochondrial encephalomyopathy, lactic acidosis, stroke-like episodes and SNHL), or other forms such as Wells–Jankovic syndrome (spastic paraplegia, hypogonadism and SNHL). Few inner ear histopathological abnormalities have been reported: atrophy of the neuroepithelium, hair cell degeneration, prominent vessels with haemorrhage,[37] severe cochleosaccular degeneration and almost complete degeneration of spiral lamina nerve fibres,[38] gliosis of ventral cochlear nuclei, and degeneration of cochleovestibular nerves.[36]

SNHL especially involving high frequencies is a common finding in early adulthood in metabolic disorders such as alpha-D-mannosidosis,[39] Fabry disease,[40] Krabbe disease,[39] and adrenoleukodystrophy.[41] Mucopolysaccharidoses (MPS) are a group of metabolic disorders which involve heteroglycan metabolism, and each has a specific enzymatic deficiency. MPS are mainly paediatric diseases. MPS II (Hunter disease) mild form is compatible with survival to adulthood, and some degree of hearing loss develops in the majority of affected persons; the hearing impairment is usually mixed and results from a combination of middle ear infection and glycosaminoglycan infiltration of the otic ganglion.[42,43] MPS IV (Morquio syndrome) presents progressive sensorineural or mixed hearing loss which develops in late childhood.[44]

Also in the DIDMOAD syndrome (diabetes insipidus, diabetes mellitus, otic atrophy, sensorineural deafness or Wolfran syndrome), SNHL involving initially high frequencies progressively extends to lower frequencies and is probably related to atrophy of the stria vascularis.[45,46]

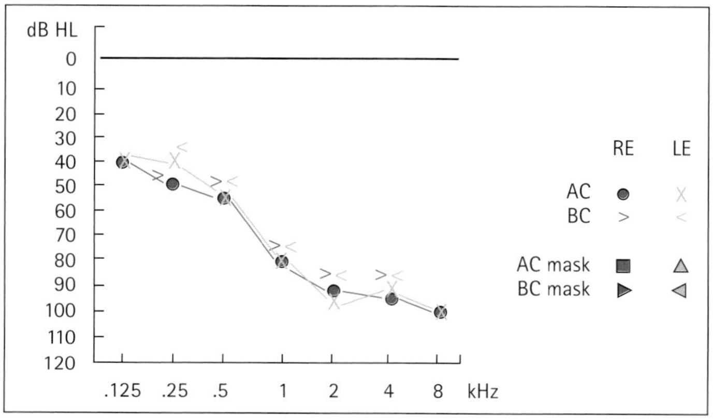

Figure 27.5 Audiogram of a 24-year-old woman with a Klippel–Durante syndrome (ataxia and SNHL); stapedial reflexes (SN) present only at 0.5 kHz; DPOAE absent; no auditory evolved brainstem response (ABR); normal saccades; smooth pursuit showed a reduced gain and optokinetic nystagmus (OKN) was dysrhythmic.

The majority of genetic hearing loss forms associated with integumentary or with oral–dental disorders are congenital and profound, but some present with progressive hearing loss, such as type II Waardenburg syndromes[47] 'multiple pigmented naevi and SNHL'[48] (Figure 27.6), Crandall syndrome,[49] otodental syndrome,[50] and, in some cases, ichthyosis[51] (Figure 27.7).

Auditory impairment in genetic disorders of the skeleton is dealt with later in the chapter.

The majority of X-linked hearing impairments are due to mutations in the *POU3F4* gene which cause either progressive mixed hearing loss or severe congenital SNHL.[52–54]

The SNHL associated with aminoglycoside therapy initially reported by Horiguchi in Japan in 1957[55] and later well characterized by Hu in 1991[56] is a peculiar situation and is dealt with later in the chapter.

Vascular factors

Sudden hearing loss and presbyacusis are generally considered to be due to vascular events. In fact, microthrombi, red cell slugging or spontaneous haemorrhages may cause rapid local perfusion defects which result in sudden hearing impairment. Such situations may typically occur in atherosclerotic disease, but also in haematological disorders such as leukaemia, macroglobulinaemia, polycythaemia, sickle cell disease, and systemic immune disorders with antiendothelial cell antibodies.[57] Even infectious processes such as syphilis may cause local bloodflow defects secondary to arteritis obliterans concomitantly with endolymph reabsorption defects.[58] Vasospasms have been postulated as being the cause of sudden deafness occurring in patients suffering from headaches.[59] The arteries involved in cochlear ischaemic phenomena are the anterior inferior cerebellar artery (AICA), the internal auditory artery, the main cochlear artery (common cochlear artery) with its vestibulocochlear branch, and the network of spiral and radial arteries which follow the conformation of the cochlea (Figure 27.8). Different degrees and types of hearing losses may occur, depending on the level of obstruction, e.g. low- and high-frequency deafness, and may be associated with other signs and symptoms due to ischaemia of contiguous structures, e.g. vertigo or facial palsy. Cochlear anoxia accounts for changes of microphonic potential and VIIIth nerve action potential that ensue over a few minutes.[60] If anoxia persists, permanent damage to hair cells occurs and the hearing deficit becomes irreversible. A slowly progressive vasculopathy has been associated with varying degrees of atrophy of the stria vascularis leading to degenerative processes of the organ or Corti. These events, occurring mostly in the elderly, define a 'vascular' form of presbyacusis that is identifiable pathologically.[61]

Anoxia consequent to vascular diseases affecting the inner ear blood supply leads to a damage of the hair cells. The resulting hearing loss may often be permanent, due to the cochlear vessel distribution, which is mostly terminal

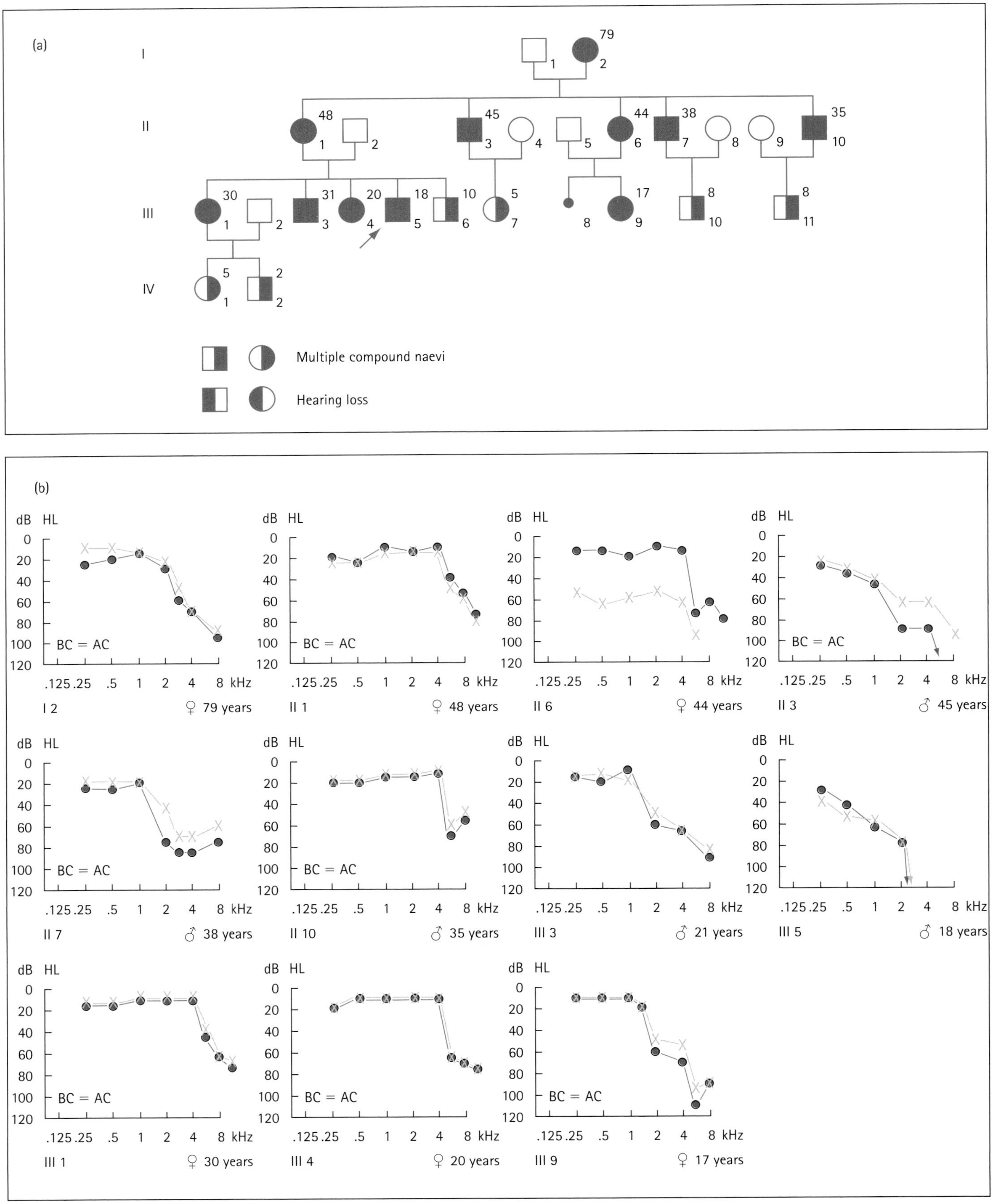

Figure 27.6 Multiple pigmented naevi and SNHL syndrome: (a) pedigree of family with multiple pigmented naevi and SNHL; (b) audiograms of patients;

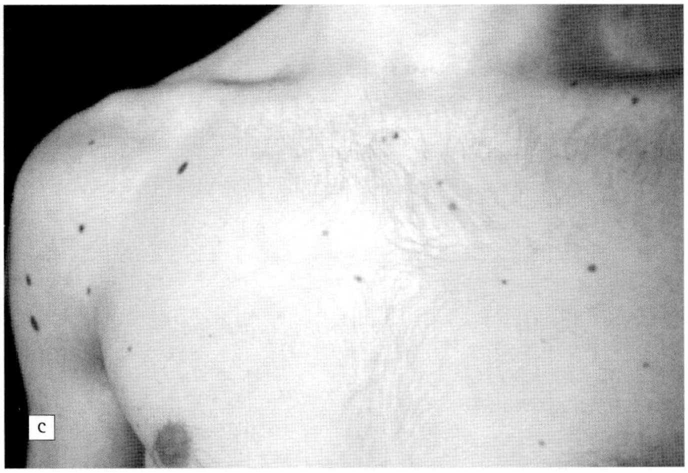

Figure 27.6 cont. Multiple pigmented naevi and SNHL syndrome: (c) photograph of the proband showing numerous pigmented naevi. (From Peserico et al. *Int J Pediatr Otorhinolaryngol* 1981; 3: 269–72.[48])

Immune and inflammatory factors

Inflammatory disorders

Middle ear or meningeal inflammatory processes may extend to the cochlea (Table 27.2), the former through the fenestra vestibuli or fenestra cochlea or via fistular tracts, so-called 'otogenous labyrinthitis' (Figures 27.9 and 27.10), and the latter by continuity through the cochlear aqueduct,[54] or via the internal auditory meatus, so-called 'meningogenic labyrinthitis'. The inflammatory response of the cochlea can be classified clinically as serous or purulent. The serous form, characterized by endolymphatic hydrops and increased protein concentration in the perilymph, is believed to be due to bacterial, viral or toxin antigens. It manifests itself as rapid-onset hearing loss, frequently associated with tinnitus and vertigo, and is generally reversible unless there has been permanent damage to cochlear membranous structures. The purulent form, due to pyogenic organisms gaining access to the labyrinth, is characterized by massive neutrophil infiltration of the perilymphatic spaces and,

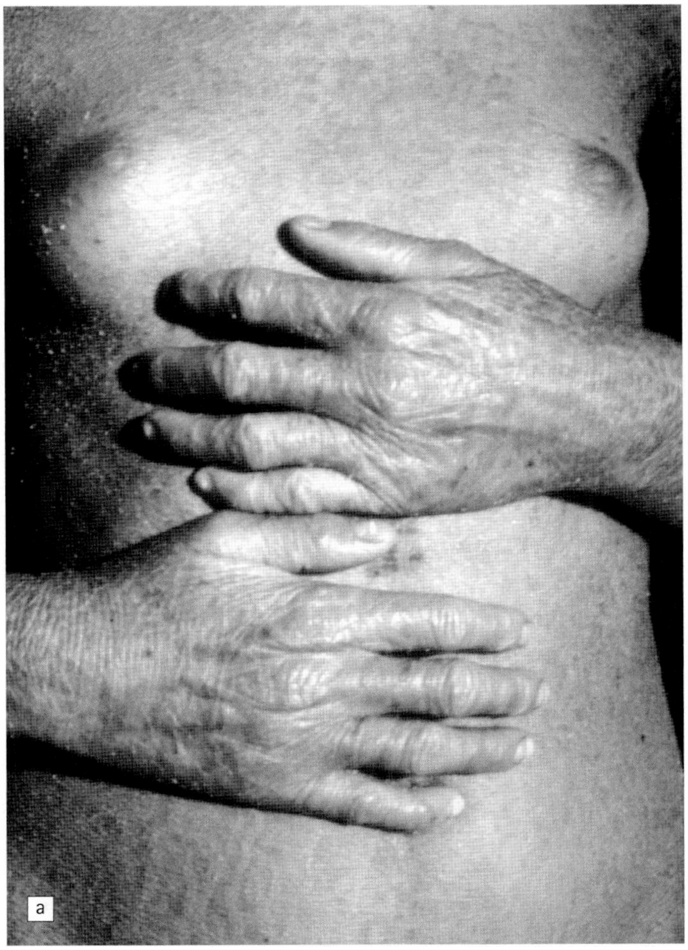

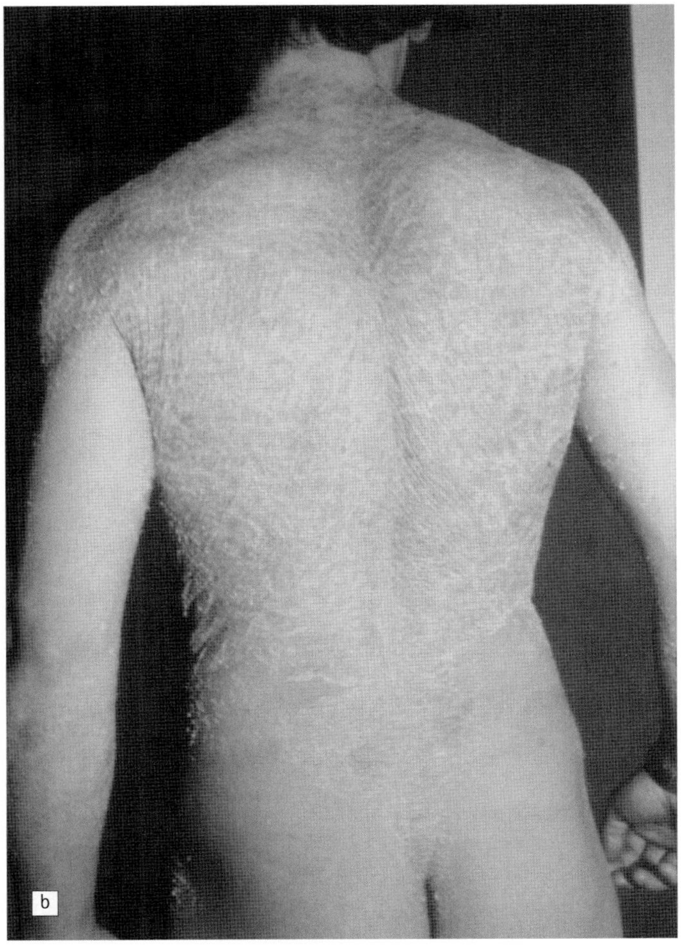

Figure 27.7 Extensive ichthyosiform dermatosis in a young female (a).Extensive ichthyosiform dermatosis in a young male (b), unrelated to the female in (a), presenting moderate SNHL. (Courtesy of Professor Andrea Peserico.)

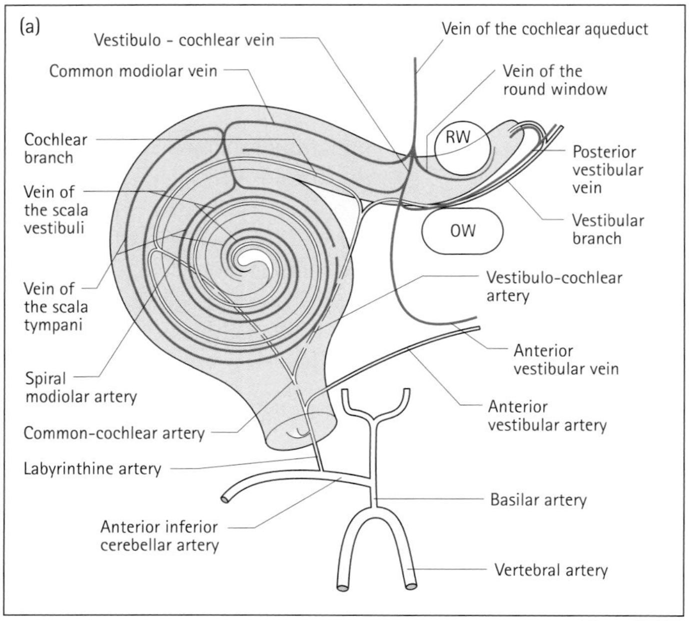

(b)

Main vascular diseases involved in sudden hearing loss

1. Atherosclerotic disease
2. Haematological disorders (leukaemia, macroglobulinaemia, polycythaemia, sickle cell disease)
3. Systemic immune disorders (autoimmune vasculitis)
4. Otosyphilis (vasculitis)

(c)

Local vascular mechanisms in sudden hearing loss

1. Occlusion
2. Haemorrhage
3. Vasospasm

Figure 27.8 (a) Cochlear blood supply. (b) Main vascular diseases involved in sudden hearing loss. (c) Local vascular mechanisms in hearing loss. (Part (a) is reproduced from *Audiologists' Desk Reference Volume 1. Diagnostic Audiology Principles, Procedures and Protocols.* 1st edition by Hall. © 1997. Reprinted with permission of Delmar Learning, a division of Thomson Learning: www.thomsonrights.com. Fax 800 730-2215.)

Table 27.2 Bacterial and viral agents most commonly associated with internal ear infections (see Figures 27.11 and 27.12).

Bacterial agents primarily acting in the middle ear
Streptococcus pneumoniae
Haemophilus influenzae
Staphylococcus aureus
Moraxella catarrhalis
Group A haemolytic streptococcus (*Streptococcus pyogenes*)
Bacterial agents primarily acting in the meningeal spaces
Haemophilus influenzae
Streptococcus pneumoniae
Neisseria meningitidis
Listeria monocytogenes
Bacterial agent acting through late endoarteritis
Treponema pallidum
Viral agents
Influenzae viruses
Measles virus
Rubella virus
Mumps virus
Cytomegalovirus
Varicella-zoster virus

subsequently, of the membranous portion, which undergoes proteolytic necrotic changes followed by ossification. In this situation, auditory function is permanently suppressed. The above-described events are due to an internal ear immune response,[63] made possible by the presence of antibodies in the perilymph and of immunocompetent cells in the endolymphatic sac. The former, probably deriving from blood or cerebrospinal fluid (CSF), participate in neutralization, opsonization and complement fixation. The latter may oppose bacterial or viral antigens directly or by eliminating infected cells, and by subsequently giving rise to local antibody production. The endolymphatic sac, which is considered to be crucial in internal ear immune function,[64] is capable of the production of cytokines such as interleukin-2 (IL-2), the early release of which may induce rapid immunocompetent cell recruitment from the bloodstream. Local neutrophil migration occurs initially, followed by T and B lymphocytes, while in situ antibody production occurs later. Concomitantly with the appearance of these immunocompetent cell populations, a dense extracellular matrix is formed which is tightly adherent to bone and provides a support for ossification.[65] The osteoblasts necessary for ossification processes may differentiate from mesenchymal cells dispersed in the extensive microvascular mesh of the cochlea.[66]

The severe hearing losses resulting from such situations are a consequence of degenerative processes involving the whole organ of Corti, the stria vascularis, and the spiral ganglion, at the completion of the inflammatory reaction.

The inner ear is the site of immune-mediated responses. They can be secondary to local inflammation (middle ear, temporal bone), or can be part of a more generalised immunity disorder. The consequences on the cochlea include vasculitis, Corti's organ atrophy, otospongiosis, ossification, hydrops, spireal ganglion degeneration. Hearing impairment may be either sudden or progressive, from a slight high frequency loss, to anacusis.

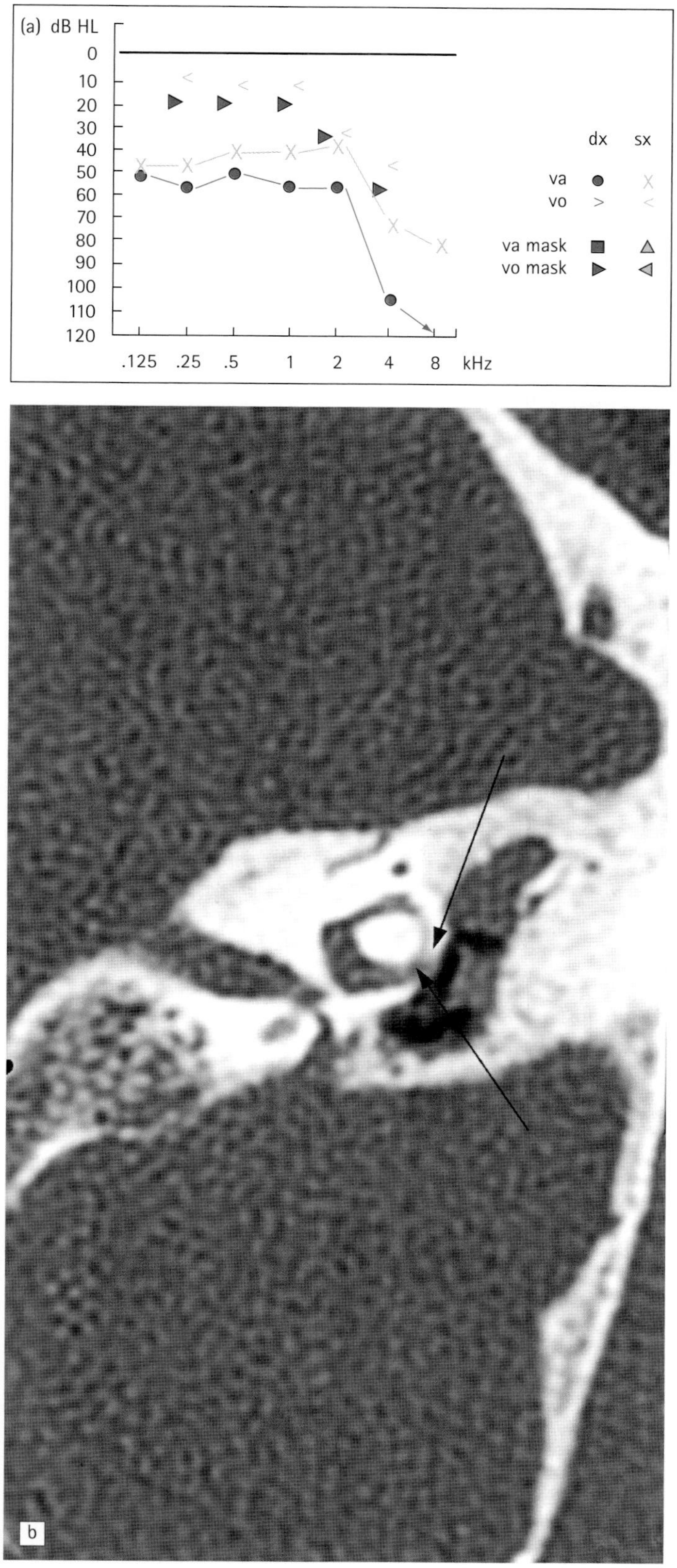

Figure 27.9 Male, 49 years old, complaining of moderate conductive right-ear hearing loss (a), with no dizziness, and presenting a fistula of the lateral semicircular canal (CT scan) (b) due to cholesteatoma.

Immune-mediated internal ear disorders

These are due to an 'uncontrolled' immune response, which in autoimmune disease is directed towards self-antigens. The internal ear may not be the primary target, but may rather be involved as an 'innocent bystander' by immunocomplex deposition[59] or by other mechanisms, whereas the inner ear is involved as part of a systemic autoimmune disease, e.g. relapsing polychondritis (Figure 27.13), systemic lupus erythematosus, rheumatoid arthritis, systemic vasculitis, Wegener syndrome (Figure 27.14), myasthenia gravis, systemic sclerosis, or Cogan's syndrome (Figure 27.15).

Immune-mediated cochlear disorders have variable clinical pictures. Most commonly, there is progressive bilateral hearing loss ensuing over a few months, but a Menière-type picture, as well as sudden uni- or bilateral deafness[67] or otosclerosis, can also occur. This clinical variability may be related to the different immune mechanisms underlying these disorders.[68] Cochlear pathological changes include cochlear vasculitis,[69] atrophy of the organ of Corti, otospongiosis of the otic capsule, endolymphatic hydrops, and spiral ganglion degeneration. Establishing a diagnosis can be difficult, since laboratory test results are not generally specific enough. The response to steroids or immunosuppressive drugs may contribute to the confirmation of a diagnostic suspicion.

Even though the autoimmune mechanisms acting in the cochlea are still unclear, autoimmunity directed towards type II collagen has been reported in patients with relapsing polychondritis, and antibodies specifically reacting with type II collagen have also been detected in patients with otosclerosis and Menière's syndrome.[70] This type of collagen is present in the membranous structures of the cochlea, the enchondral bushel, the interosseus corpuscles of the otic capsule, the spiral ligament, the limbus, and Rosenthal's channel. Laboratory evaluations may or may not be specific. The potentially diagnostic tests most commonly employed for initial screening[71] are: erythrocyte sedimentation rate (ESR), autoantibody screening (i.e. rheumatoid factor, antinuclear and antithyroglobulin antibodies), IgG, IgM, IgA, and complement (CH50, C3, C4, C1q). Other tests, the diagnostic applicability of which is incompletely defined, are: lymphocyte transformation and migration inhibition assays, indirect immunofluorescence, and Western blot analysis for cochlear antigens.[72]

Menière's disease

Menière's disease is defined as the idiopatic syndrome of endolymphatic hydrops. The condition of a hydropic distension of the endolymphatic system is thought to be responsible of the the clinical signs the disease more often displays: bounds of rotational vertigo, unilateral hearing loss with tinnitus and fullness. However, the clinical picture may be multiform, both in the consistency of the main symptoms, and in their temporal evolution. Clinical terms like 'cochlear Menière' or 'vestibular Menière' might express two extreme forms of the disease, with

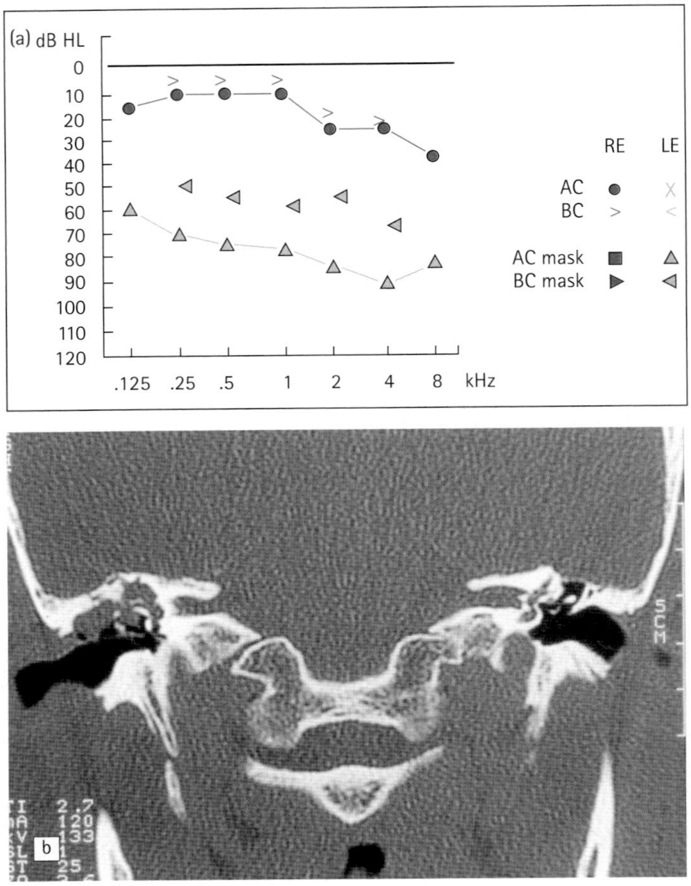

Figure 27.10 Male, 52 years old, complaining of severe mixed right-ear hearing loss (a) due to intralabyrinthic chronic cholesteatomatous otitis media (CT scan) (b).

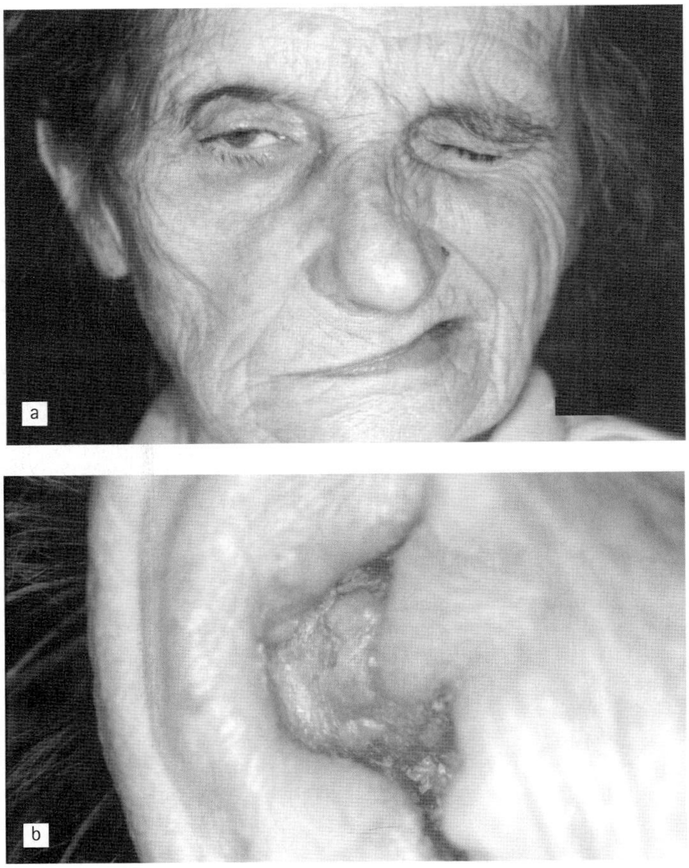

Figure 27.12 A woman, 72 years old, complaining of sudden severe SNHL and vertigo, and right facial palsy (a), and presenting the typical vesicles involving the pinna (b).

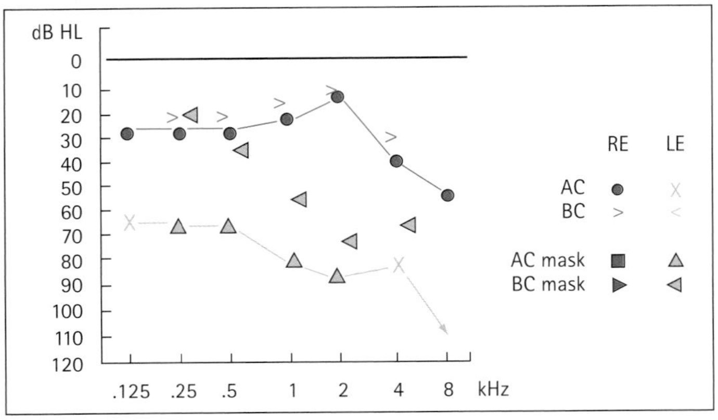

Figure 27.11 A woman, 76 years old, admitted to the hospital for sudden left hearing loss (see audiogram) and vertigo due to acute haemorrhagic otitis media.

only auditory or vestibular sympthoms respectively. A diagnostic scale for Menière disease has been proposed[73] providing useful criteria to help the clinician in staging the disease from 'possible' to 'probable', 'definite' to 'certain'.

According to the classical theory, the typical recurrencies of Menière disease are due to the increase of endolymph volume, distension of the whole endolymphatic system, and final ruptures in the membranes which separate the endo-perilymphatic compartments. A consequent concentration of potassium in perilymph space would inhibit the bio-electric activity of the labyrinthine receptors. It has been recognized that Menière disease has not a single causative factor. Rather, many pathological conditions could trigger the endolymphatic hydrop, even though such conditions are quite differing and uncorrelated to each other (endocrine disorders, unbalance of autonomic nervous system, allergy, infections, vascular disorders, autoimmune disorders). Recently, theories pointing to immunomediated events primarly taking place within the endolymphatic have been proposed. Results from several laboratories suggest that specific HLA antigen haplotypes could be associated to increased risk of developing inner-ear disorders as Menière.[74] Infectious diseases sustained by ototropic viruses (the more frequent could be CMV[75] could enter the endolymph, harbouring in a latent state within the endolymphatic sac. The consequent immune-mediated response could explain the temporal course of the disease, at least in a major proportion of cases.

The diagnostic key of Menière disease remains so far based on clinical observation. Instrumental (audiometry, ABR,

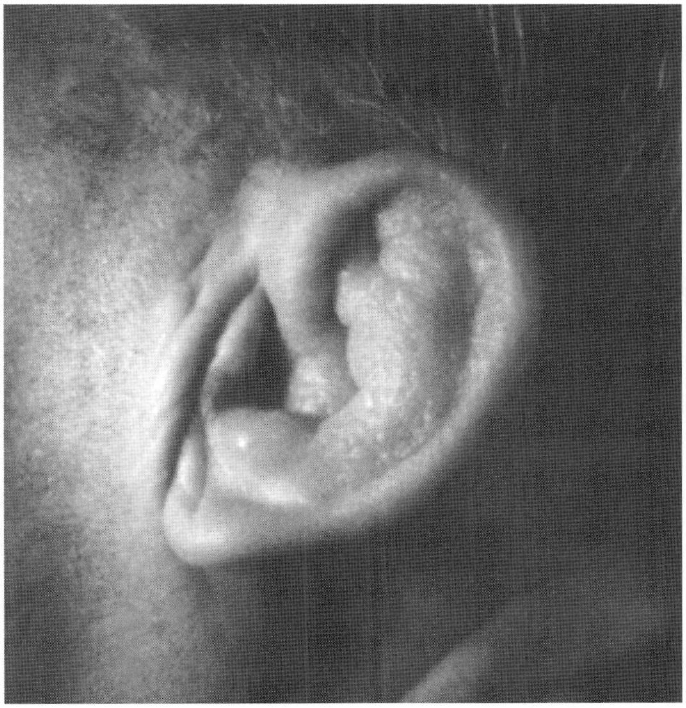

Figure 27.13 Relapsing polychondritis involving the auricle in a 58-year-old man.

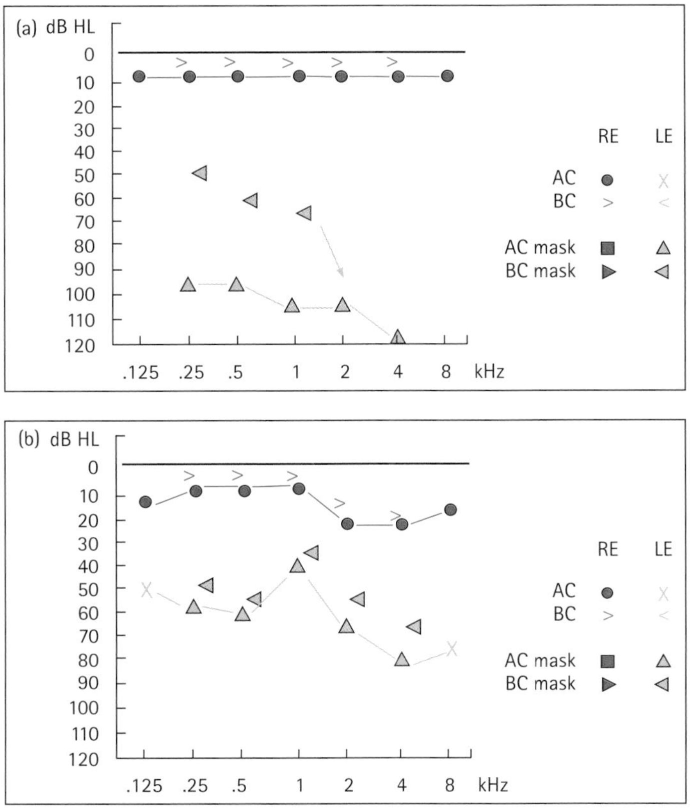

Figure 27.14 A man, 41 years old, who presented as first localization of Wegener left otitis; audiogram (a) before and (b) after cortisone treatment.

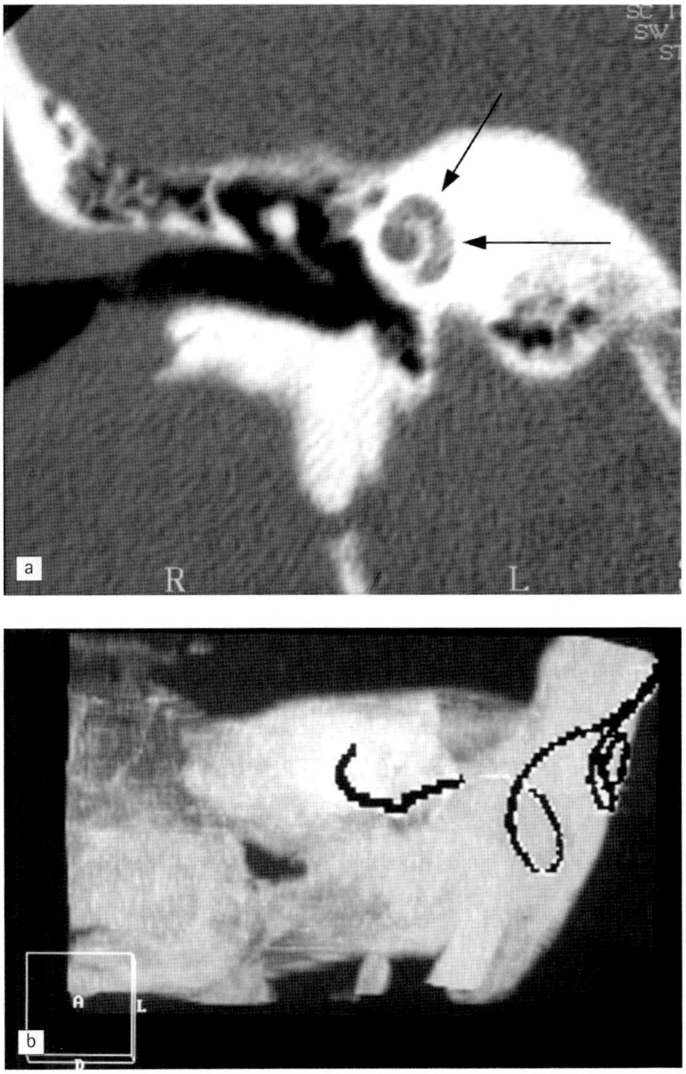

Figure 27.15 (a), Temporal bone CT scan of a 48-year-old woman who presented a rapidly bilateral progressive profound SNHL, due to Cogan's syndrome: the cochlear duct is partially occluded by fibrotic and bone tissue. The patient underwent cochlear implant surgery (postsurgery CT scan) (b).

electrocochleography, vestibular investigation) and imaging results (CT, MRI) serve to confirm a peripheral origin of the sympthoms, by excluding any kind of retrocochlear involvement. Clinical investigations concerning with endocrine, metabolic, cardiovascular, renal conditions are aimed to find out whether other factors may contribute to precipitate the disease.

For the medical treatment of Menière disease acute attack antihistamines are used for their anti-hemetic and vestibular sedative effect, or diazepam for its tranquilizing effect. Neuroleptic drugs are valid vestibular suppressor although they may have anticholinergic and extrapyramidal side-effects. For the long term treatment of Menière's disease a great number of medical and surgical remedies have been proposed, according to the belief of its pathogenesis. The medical therapy includes other than a dietary salt restriction (intake < 1 g/day), betahistine, diuretics (glycerol, hydrochlorothiazyde), vaso-active drugs (trimetazidine), cynarizine), steroids and amynoglycosides (streptomycin, gentamicin). These two latter classes of drugs can be administred via intratympanic injection.[76,77] While aminoglycosides may effectively control vertigo because of their destructive action on sensory vestibular cells, they may also be active on cochlear hair cells with a consequent severe-profound hearing loss. Among the surgical treatments the efficacy of endolymphatic sac surgery is controversial, while vestibular neurectomy can be an ultimate option for a little proportion of otherwise untreatable cases.[78]

Metabolic factors

Oxidative metabolism supplies the necessary energy to hair cells for neuroelectric transduction. High ATP concentrations favour those active ionic transport mechanisms performed by the stria vascularis on which endocochlear electrical potentials are dependent. Any metabolic derangement capable of interfering with such processes can result in hearing loss, e.g. diabetes mellitus, renal insufficiency, or hypothyroidism. The hearing defect is generally bilateral, initially involves high-pitch frequencies and later extends to middle–low frequencies. However, since metabolic diseases have generalized effects, this type of hearing problem may also depend on extracochlear lesions involving the VIIIth nerve or the central auditory pathways.

> The cochlear homeostasis is highly sensitive to disorders of general metabolism, which are mainly directed to the cochlear vascular supply and stria vascularis. As a consequence, hair cells and spiral ganglion degenerate with the functional result of a progressive bilateral hearing loss.

Acquired hypothyroidism occurs most frequently as a consequence of Hashimoto's thyroiditis. Even though the relationship between thyroid hormone levels and hearing loss is unclear, it has been postulated that a deficiency of these hormones may impair the oxidative phosphorylation leading to ATP synthesis and result in cellular dysfunction. This would in turn lead to atrophy of the stria vascularis, and hair cell and spiral ganglion degeneration.[79] Moderate hearing loss has been observed in 25–50% of patients with severe hypothyroidism. This finding, however, was not confirmed by studies in which advanced age was taken into consideration as an independent cofactor potentially accounting for hearing deficits.[80] Whether thyroid hormone replacement is able to restore hearing is also unclear.[81,82]

Type II and IV hyperlipidaemias may be responsible for some forms of hearing impairment[83] which frequently have a tendency to fluctuate. High blood lipids would result in hyperviscosity with the potential for partial or complete obstruction of the vascular network and hence for temporary or permanent cochlear function impairment. The reduction of blood lipid levels, and an appropriate diet, especially in younger patients, may improve hearing threshold.[84] This may be less likely to occur in the elderly, in whom other factors concomitant with dyslipidaemia, such as hypertension and excessive noise exposure, may have a synergistic effect and contribute to more permanent cochlear damage. However, studies have failed to show a straightforward relationship between hearing threshold and blood levels of serum lipids.[85,86]

Microangiopathies and polyneuropathies are typical of diabetes mellitus. The hearing loss frequently observed in patients with diabetes mellitus has been attributed to lesions of the cochlear vascular supply[87] consisting of endothelial proliferation and lipid deposition, or to degeneration of VIIIth nerve neural elements (Figures 27.16 and 27.17). However, it is still unclear whether the vascular cochlear lesions are specific to

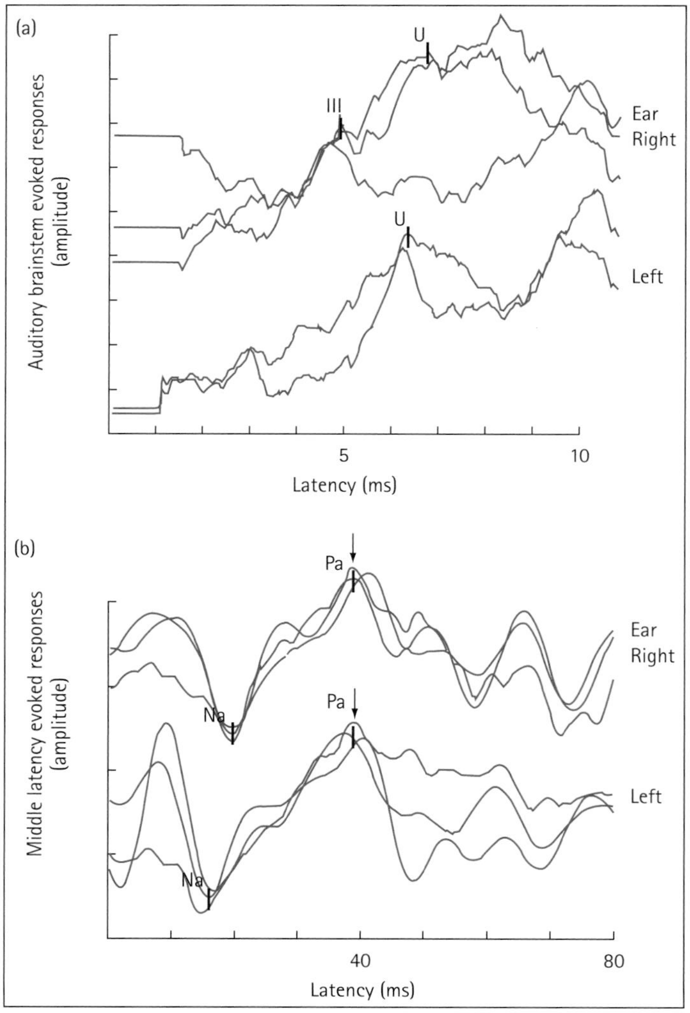

Figure 27.16 Diabetic patient with normal pure tone audiogram and with (a) a pathological ABR and (b) a normal MLR pattern.

diabetes mellitus[88] or rather a consequence of its associated complications, i.e. atherosclerosis, hypertension,[89] renal failure, and dyslipidaemia.

The association of renal failure and hearing loss has been frequently observed. This may be related to the many ionic transport function similarities between nephron and cochlea.

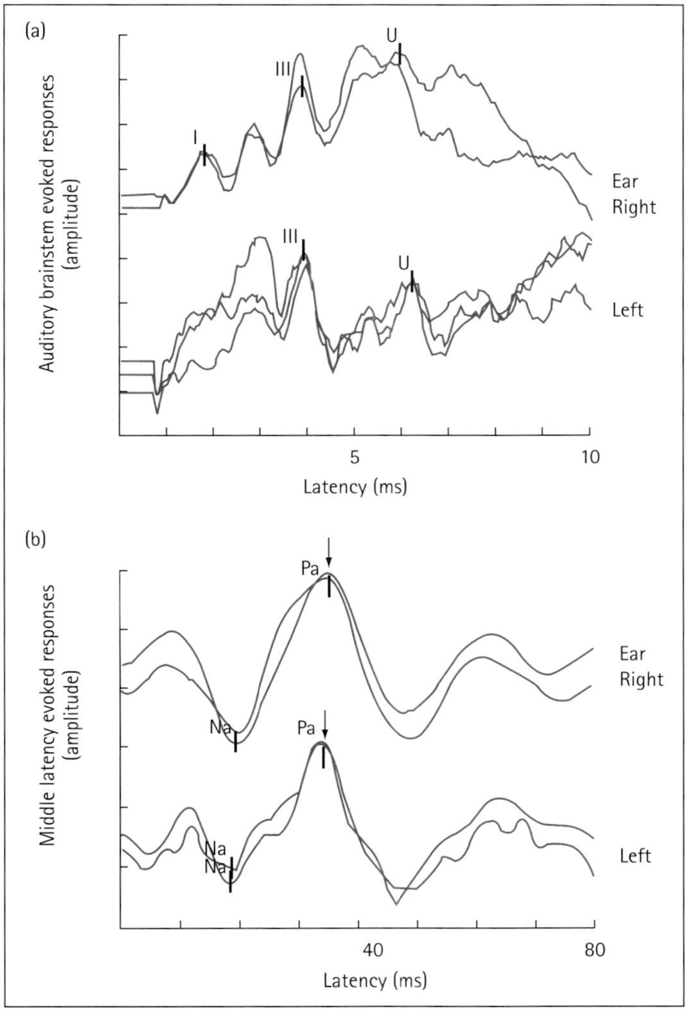

Figure 27.17 Diabetic patient with a normal audiogram showing a pathological ABR (a) and MLR pattern (b).

In addition, some drugs have been shown to be toxic to both organs. Cochlear lesions characterized by basophilic depositions in the stria vascularis and by varying degrees of hair cell degeneration have been reported.[90] It is still controversial, however, whether cochlear lesions are due to the same causative agents responsible for renal failure or whether they are the consequence of electrolyte disturbances, drug administration (e.g. aminoglycoside antibiotics, loop diuretics), haemodialysis, or concurrent hypertension.[91]

Ototoxic factors

A number of drugs have been recognized to potentially damage the inner ear,[92] and can be classified into four groups: aminoglycoside antibiotics, chemotherapeutic agents, anti-inflammatory drugs and quinine, and loop diuretics (Table 27.3). A continuous high-pitch tinnitus is frequently the initial complaint, and this may be related to basal turn hair cells being affected first. Threshold elevation is generally bilateral and begins for high frequencies. The severity of hearing loss depends on the offending drug plasma levels, renal function, and general clinical conditions. Hearing problems may ensue from a few minutes to several days after drug administration; however, late and slowly progressive hearing loss occurring several years later is possible, through synergistic effects between drugs and other noxious agents.[93]

Ototoxic agents, such as aminoglycosides and platinum compounds, exert their adverse effect on the hair cells, by interfering with membrane permeability, and mitochondrial, DNA, RNA systems. The resulting hearing loss is dose-dependent and permanent.

Aminoglycoside antibiotics

These bactericidal drugs act by inhibiting protein synthesis at the bacterial ribosome level. They are excreted unaltered in the urinary tract and tend to be tissue bound. Streptomycin,

Table 27.3 Common ototoxic drugs.

Antibiotics	Chemotherapics	Diuretics	Anti-inflammatory	Anti-malarial
Streptomycin	Cis-platinum	Ethacrynic acid	Salicylates	Quinine
Kanamicin	Dichloromethothrexate	Furosemide	Naproxen(?)	Chloroquine
Amikacin	Nitrogen mustard	Bumetanide		
Gentamicin				
Tobramycin				
Netilmicin				
Neomycin				

gentamicin, kanamycin, amikacin, and tobramycin have a two-stage toxicity for hair cells.[94] Initially, after the antibiotic has penetrated the endolymph, there is a reversible blockade of ionic channels. In the second stage, the drug becomes more strongly bound to cellular phospholipids and proteins, and cell permeability increases, causing a depletion of magnesium ions, which are present in particularly high amounts in the mitochondrial apparatus. This results in blockage of many enzymatic reactions, especially oxidative phosphorylation, leading to cell death.[95] Some studies suggest that the cytotoxicity of these antibiotics may be mediated by iron–antibiotic complexes with free radical production.[96] Other mechanisms possibly involving cellular DNA and RNA have been postulated in order to account for the different aspects relating to the degree of hearing loss and to its time-course. The incidence of aminoglycoside-related hearing loss occurring with therapeutic doses has been estimated to be from 2.5% to 14%.[97]

Several reports suggest a genetic component influencing the susceptibility to normal doses of aminoglycosides with variable penetrance, with a typically maternal inheritance pattern in most kindres.[56,98,99] Mitochondrial DNA mutations have been implicated in both syndromal and nonsyndromal sensorineural hearing loss;[100] the np 1555 mutation clearly interacts with aminoglycosides in causing SNHI in humans.[99] However, in other cases a need for co-operation between nuclear and mitochondrial DNA in the expression of the pathological phenotype has also been inferred.[101,102]

Chemotherapeutic agents

Platinum compounds (cisplatin and carboplatin), nitrogen mustards, amino-nicotinamide and dichloromethotrexate are well known to be ototoxic. Among these, cisplatin is the one most toxic to the cochlea, being associated with dose-dependent extensive and permanent damage (Figure 27.18). Functional and structural alterations are similar to those induced by aminoglycosides,[103–105] and may be related to cellular calcium channel blockage,[106] and to damage of the stria vascularis[107] resulting from inhibition of an important enzyme function, i.e. adenylate cyclase. Hearing loss may initially be for high frequencies, and occasionally a limited defect from frequencies above 8 kHz has been observed. The incidence of cisplatin-associated hearing problems has been estimated to be in the range of 17% with variations relating to both single dose levels and cumulative drug exposure,[108–110] or to additive toxicity with other drugs. In paediatric patients treated for brain tumours,[111] moderate-to-severe hearing loss may occur in up to half of the cases, most likely because of concomitant radiotherapy.

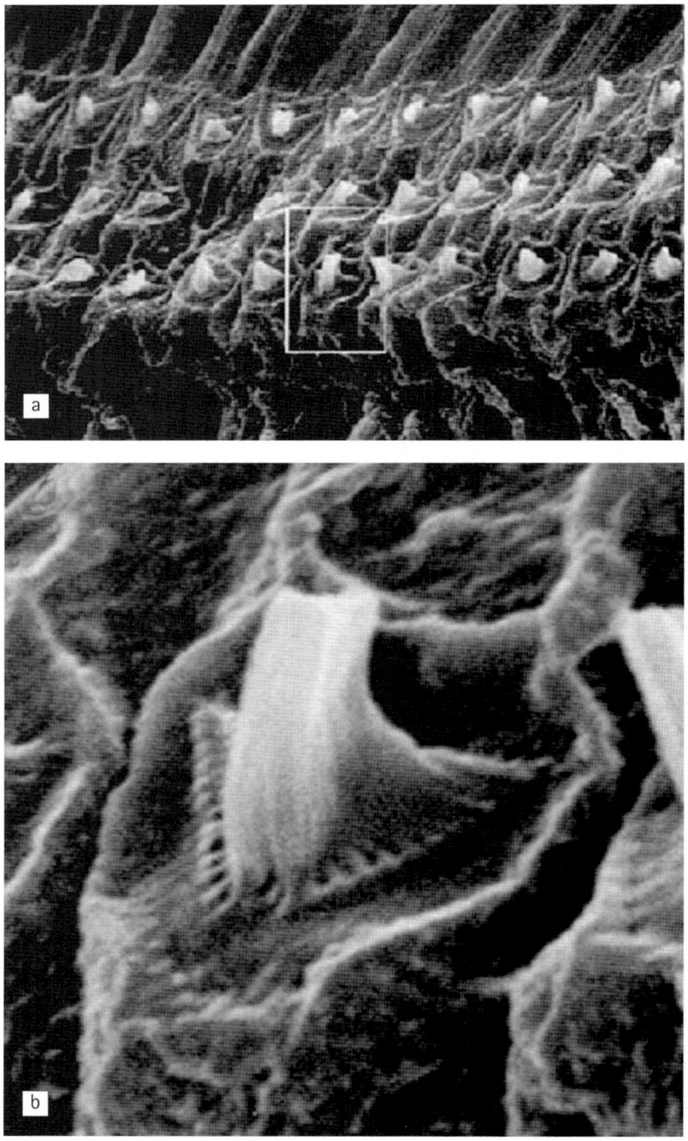

Figure 27.18 (a) Outer hair cell damage in a rat treated with cis-platinum (SEM); (b) magnification showing fusion of the cilia. (From Hatzopovlos et al. *Audiology* 2001; **40**: 253–64.[143])

Diuretics

The most commonly employed loop diuretics are furosemide and bumetanide. Ethacrynic acid is used less frequently. They act by inhibition of chloride and hence sodium reabsorption in the loop of Henle. These drugs cause a generally reversible hearing loss. This toxicity is most frequently of rapid onset, and resolution occurs when furosemide is discontinued, while ethacrynic acid ototoxicity is associated with a slower course and delayed recovery. Permanent hearing loss has been reported in patients with renal insufficiency treated with both loop diuretics and aminoglycoside antibiotics, which may have synergistic ototoxicity. Cochlear damage is most frequently at the level of the stria vascularis, with oedema of the marginal portion and endothelial rupture, followed by damage to the outer hair cell stereocilia, mostly of the basal turn of the cochlea. Adenylate cyclase enzyme complex abnormalities may be responsible for damage to the stria vascularis.[112] The latter results in ionic imbalance of endocochlear fluids and hair cell electromechanical transduction impairment.[113] More recently, studies of molecular biology applied to the electroneutral Na–K–2Cl cotransporter system within the cochlea revealed that this system is inhibited by loop diuretics, accounting for the different sensitivity of diuretic potency and ototoxicity often reported in clinical and experimental studies.[114]

Salicylates, NSAIDs and quinine

At high doses (4–5 g/day for acetylsalicylic acid), both salicylates and some of the non-steroidal anti-inflammatory drugs (NSAIDs) may cause moderate hearing loss which is generally reversible.[115] The ototoxicity mechanism may involve the outer hair cells; however, a reduced blood supply to the cochlea has also been postulated. Increased prostaglandin and decreased leukotriene synthesis and their effect on inflammatory processes may also be related to ototoxicity.

Quinine has been substituted by newer and less toxic antimalarial drugs. Its cochlear toxicity is similar to that of salicylates, i.e. dose dependent and generally reversible, while its labyrinth toxicity is more severe and permanent.[116] Even though quinine effects are less well understood than the effects of salicylates, they seem to be related to vasoconstrictive phenomena and to abnormalities of potassium-dependent channels of the stria vascularis and of the surface of the outer hair cells.

Trauma

A trauma can produce hearing (and vestibular) impairment in different ways: (1) ossicular chain injuries (Figure 27.19), (2) perilymphatic fistulae, (3) labyrinthine concussion, (4) barotrauma, (5) temporal bone fractures and (6) penetrating wounds (Figure 27.20). We will discuss here hearing impairments due only to labyrinthine concussion, barotrauma and temporal bone fractures. Noise trauma is discussed in Chapter 17.

Labyrinthine concussion

Balance and hearing loss may follow a blow to the head, even in the absence of radiologically evident labyrinth fractures.[117] Even if brain and brainstem haemorrhages have been reported, the principal mechanism involved is a concussion injury to inner ear structures.[118]

According to Schuknecht,[117] two possible mechanisms are involved: a pressure wave transmitted through bone to the cochlea, or a sudden movement of the stapes footplate due to the inertia of the tympanic membrane and ossicles when a sudden acceleration or deceleration is applied.

Regarding the severity of the head trauma, this usually must be enough to produce loss of consciousness; less severe trauma, however, can cause permanent SNHL.[117] The most frequent vestibular consequence is benign paroxysmal positional vertigo or cupulolithiasis.[119]

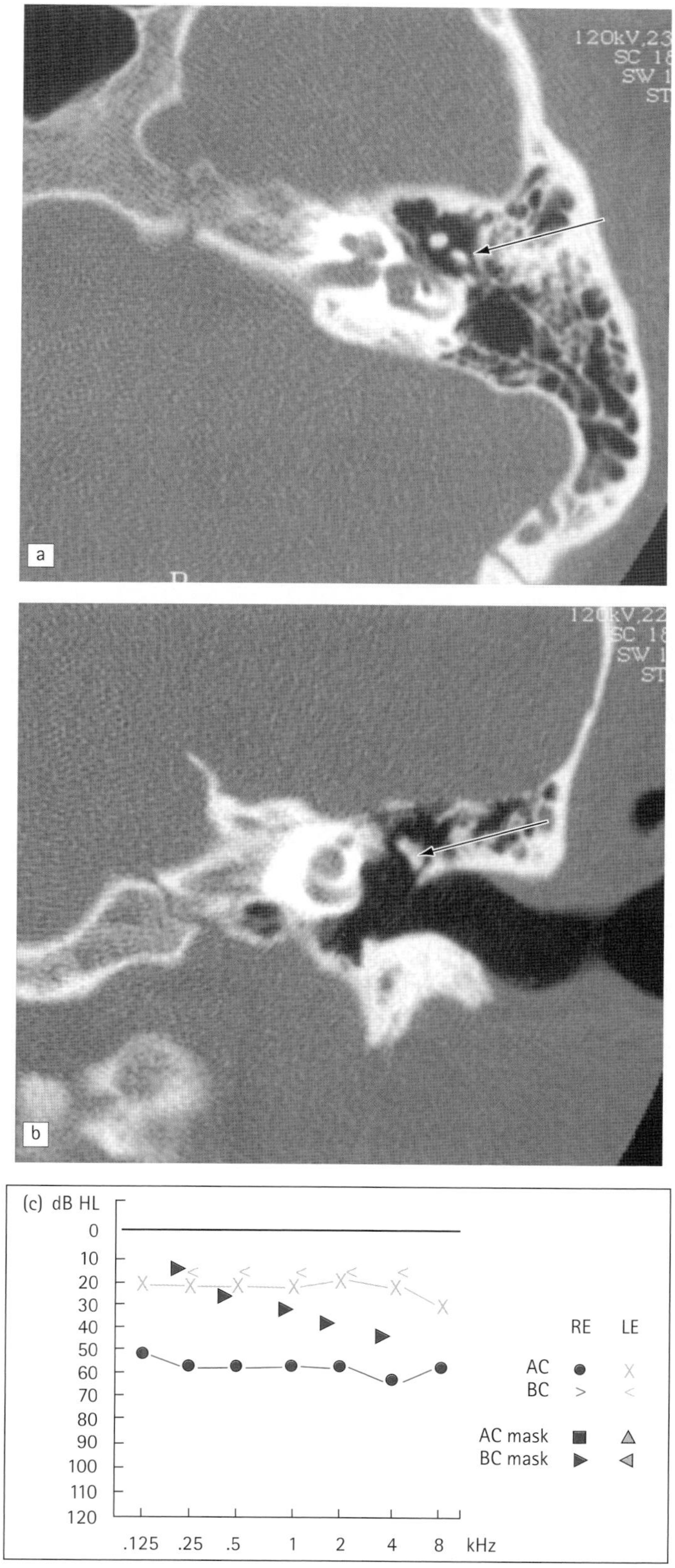

Figure 27.19 Temporal bone CT scan of a 34-year-old man, showing ossicular chain injuries with rotation of the incus ((a) b1 coronal and (b) b2 axial views) and (c) audiogram.

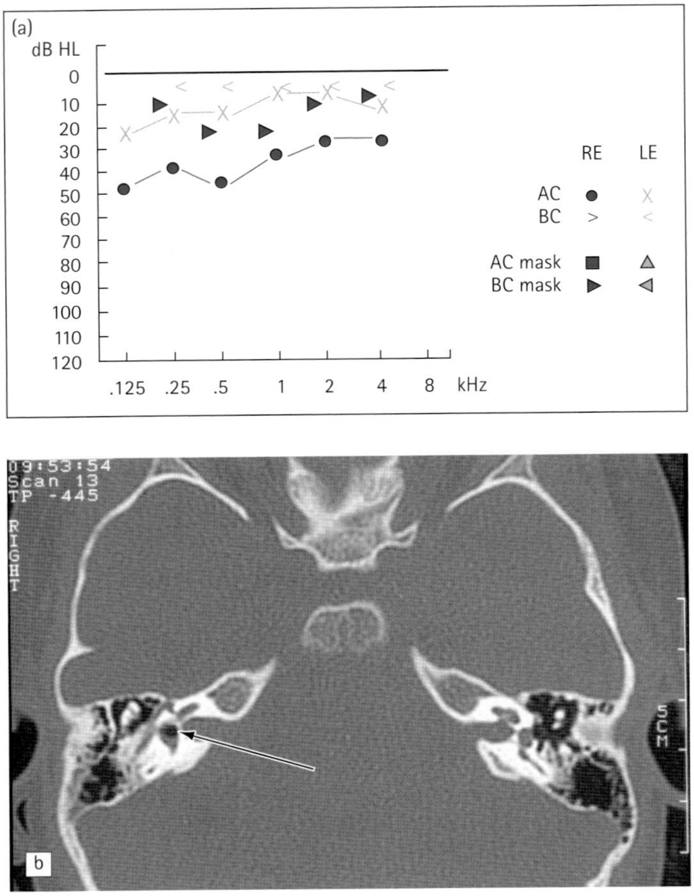

Figure 27.20 Audiogram of a patient demonstrating a small posterosuperior tympanic membrane perforation and left-beating spontaneous nystagmus after a toothpick trauma, presenting a right mixed hearing loss (a), and a bubble of blood inside the vestibule ((b), CT scan).

Toglia et al[120] reported that after whiplash injuries, vestibular abnormalities are present in 50% of patients, stressing the importance of electronystagmography.

Barotrauma

Aural barotrauma is caused by damage to the ear due to a sudden and significant change of air pressure at the level of the drum, as may occur in flying and diving, forced sniffing or a slap involving the ear. The acute change of pressure in the middle ear which is not equalized by the Eustachian tube may result in rupture of the oval or round window membranes with perilymphatic fistula and/or breaks of the cochlear membranes (in particular, Reissner's membrane). The symptoms of inner ear barotrauma include SNHL, tinnitus and persistent vertigo. In cases of persistent symptoms or worsening of inner ear functions, an exploratory tympanotomy may be warranted (Figure 27.21).

Temporal bone fractures

Temporal bone fractures have been classified as:

- longitudinal (i.e. linear breaks through the floor of the middle cranial fossa passing parallel and adjacent to the anterior margin of the petrous pyramid)
- transverse (i.e. perpendicular to the long axis of the petrous pyramid)
- mixed.[121,122]

A longitudinal temporal bone fracture usually results in SNHL limited to high frequencies and most severe at 4 kHz, similar to an acoustical trauma.[123]

A transverse fracture usually results in a complete loss of cochlear and vestibular function as it passes through the vestibule of the inner ear, causing extensive destruction of the membranous labyrinth[117] (Figures 27.22 and 27.23).

Possible complications of a temporal bone fracture are: endolymphatic hydrops,[124,125] perilymph fistula of the opposite ear,[117] delayed meningitis,[126] cholesteatoma,[127] and facial nerve palsy.

Disorders of bone

Many disorders of the temporal bone may produce impairment of audiovestibular function. Otosclerosis is the most common of these disorders, but osteogenesis imperfecta, Paget's disease and fibrous dysplasia can also be observed in clinical practice.

> Bone diseases involving the temporal bone, some of them having a genetic origin, as well as traumatic discontinuities of the otic capsule may damage the inner ear membranous structures. Hearing impairment strictly depends on the extent of the local lesion. Otosclerosis represents a bone disease limited to otic capsule. Although it becomes auditorily evident with a conductive loss due to the stape fixation, its long term effects may progressively involve the inner ear.

Otosclerosis

Otosclerosis is a disorder of the bony labyrinth which becomes clinically evident when the stapes footplate is involved by the disease. The aetiology of otosclerosis is not clear, and although the presence of siblings with otosclerosis in certain families has been described, the genetics remain poorly understood.[128] The majority of most recent studies indicate an AD mode of inheritance with incomplete penetrance. Multifactorial inheritance is likely to play a role in the expressivity or penetrance of otosclerosis. Recently, linkage studies of a family with otosclerosis have led to the localization of a gene for otosclerosis to chromosome 15q25–q26.[129]

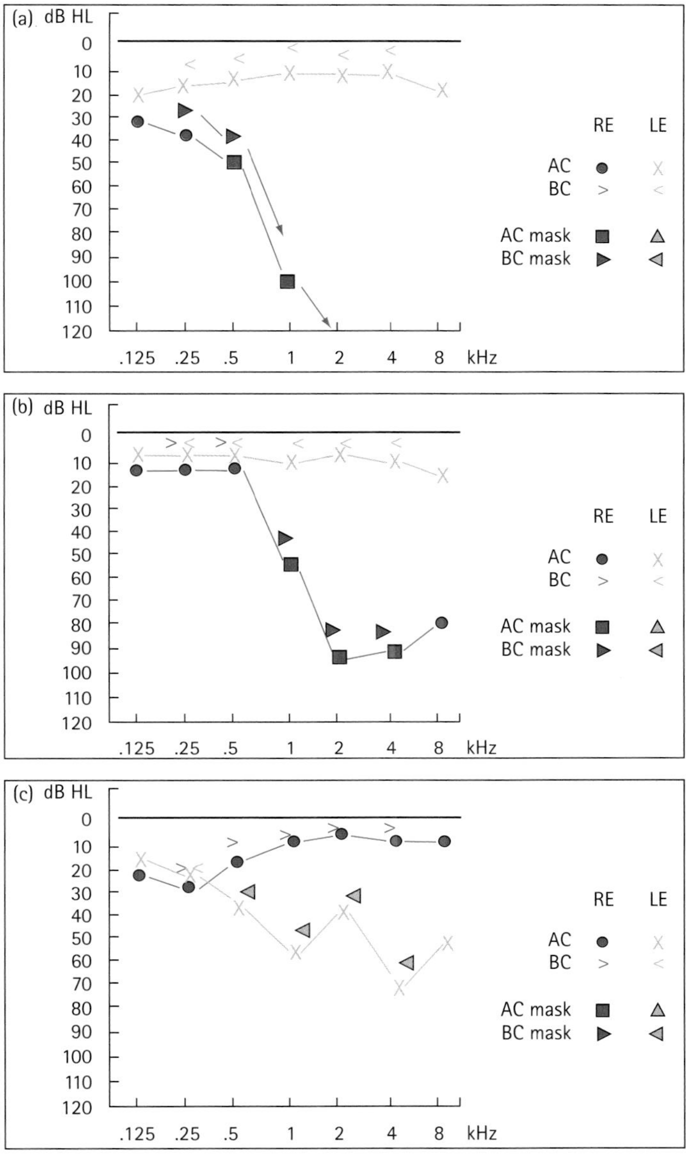

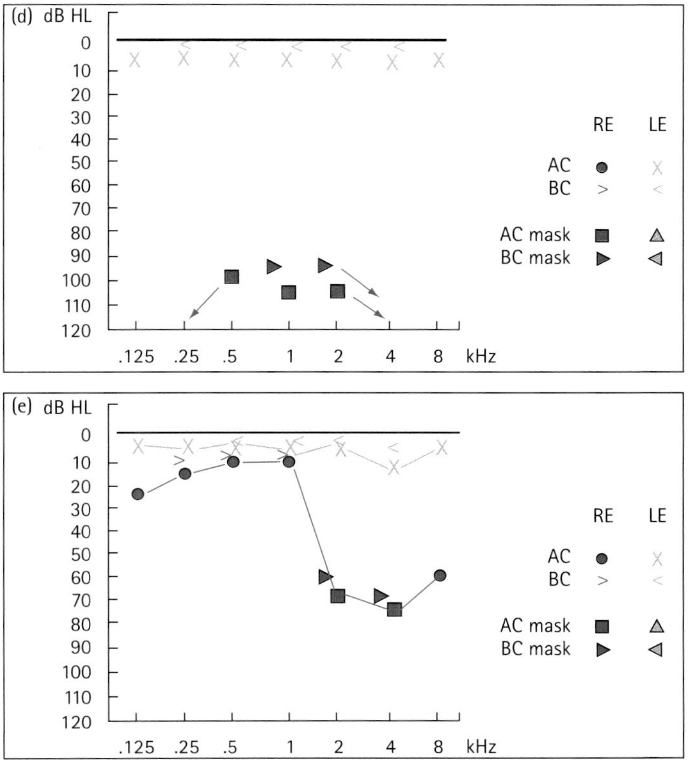

Figure 27.21 Audiograms of patients who presented with various degrees of SNHL due to barotrauma: MA, female aged 37, referred with a sudden hearing loss during diving: (a) before explorative tympanotomy; (b) some days after the closure of a round window fistula. (c) PA, male aged 22, referred sudden left hearing loss after diving; explorative tympanotomy showed a rupture of the round window membrane. (d) BL, male aged 31, referred a right sudden hearing loss after diving; an explorative tympanotomy was performed 10 days later for persisting severe dizziness and showed a fracture of the right footplate; patient referred after the closure of the fistula immediate improvement of the dizziness but the hearing did not improve. (e) NA, female aged 40, presented a sudden SNHL after a basketball ear trauma. Audiogram.

Otosclerosis can involve the inner ear and produce progressive SNHL.[130]

It is a common clinical practice observation that otosclerosis tends to progress with time to neurosensory involvement and that the operated ear worsens less than the contralateral nonoperated ear. (Figures 27.24 and 27.25).

There is no agreement as to the relationship between otosclerotic foci and hearing impairment. Keleman and Linthicum[131] showed a positive correlation between the magnitude of SNHL and the severity of atrophic change in the spiral ligament, while Schuknecht and Barber[132] found no significant correlation between the extent of endosteal involvement and the bone conduction threshold abnormality. The concept of cochlear otosclerosis itself has been questioned.[133,134]

Sclerosing bone dysplasias

The sclerosing bone dysplasias are a group of genetic disorders characterized by overgrowth and increased radiological density of the skeleton.[135] Severe auditory impairment is a consistent feature of many conditions in this group; it is progressive and mainly the result of the entrapment of the acoustical nerves by the bone overgrowth in the cranial foramina[136] (Figure 27.26).

In craniometaphyseal dysplasia, there are a number of progressive changes that impact on communicative impairment. The hearing loss, both conductive and sensorineural, becomes progressive in the second decade of life. However, the natural history also involves a progressive change in speech resonance, and the compression of the cranial nerves usually produces facial paresis and may impair articulation and oral resonance.[137]

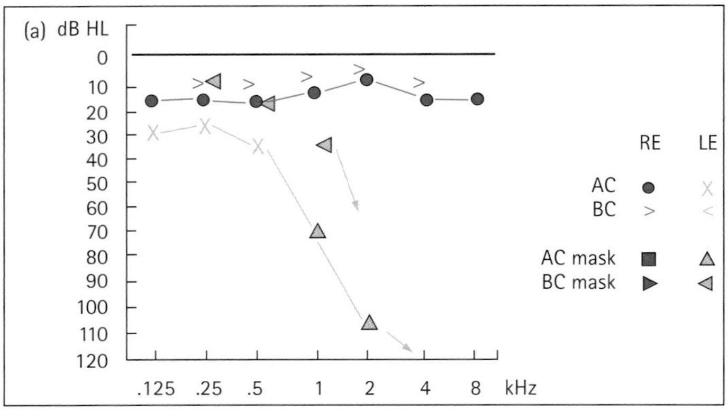

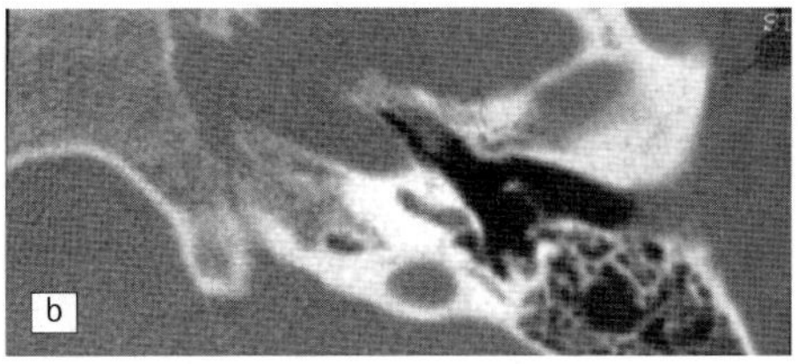

Figure 27.22 Male, 33 years old, complaining of a left SNHL (a) after a car accident with no evidence of a temporal bone fracture (CT scan, (b))

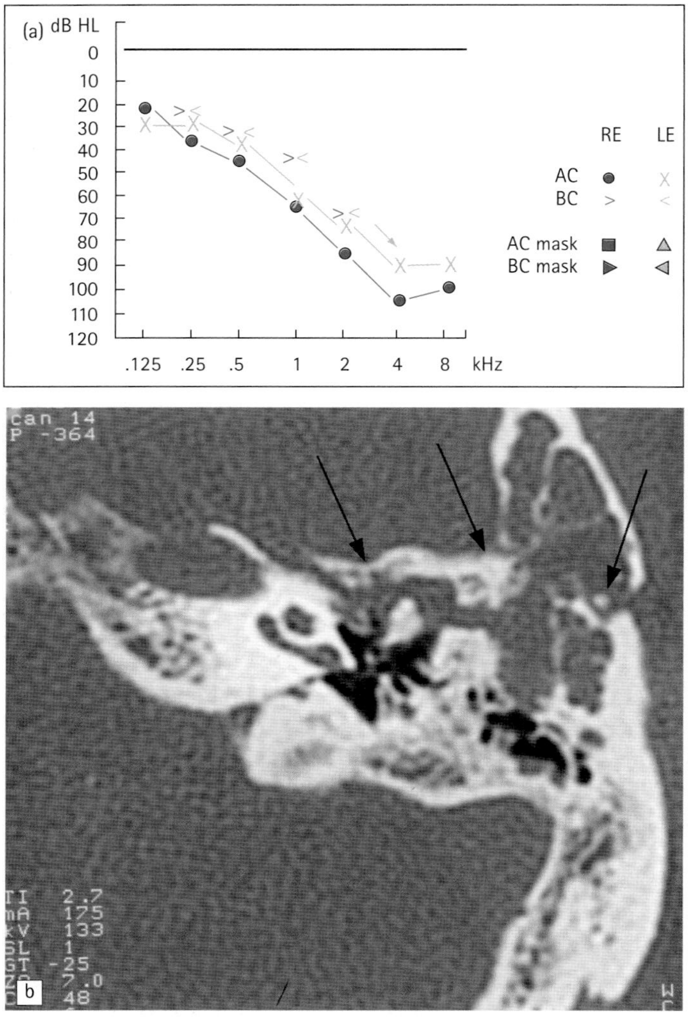

Figure 27.23 Male, 55 years old, complaining of a bilateral SNHL (a) after a car accident with severe left temporal bone fracture (CT scan, (b)).

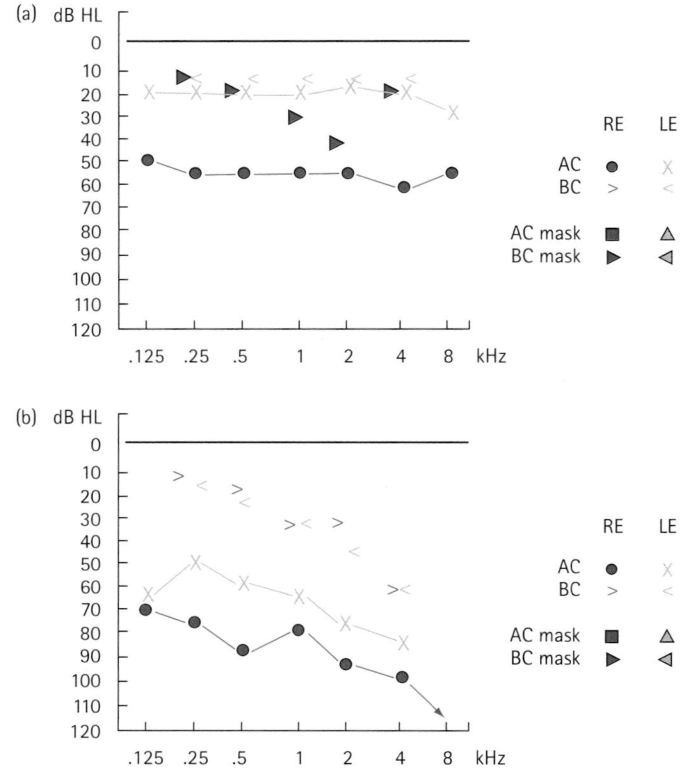

Figure 27.24 (a) and (b) Different degrees of hearing loss in otosclerotic subjects.

Paget's disease

This disorder, also known as osteitis deformans, may involve the skull, sacrum, pelvis, femur, and tibia. The neurocranium is commonly involved in this disease of unknown origin (autosomal dominant? due to viral infection?), and when the temporal bone is involved, it results in a thickening of the petrous pyramid with important structural deformity (i.e. displacement of the internal carotid artery, mastoid enlargement with cellular obliteration, narrowing of the internal auditory canal, fixation of the stapes, obliteration of the round window and cochlear duct, etc.) (Figure 27.27). The hearing loss is usually mixed conductive and sensorineural,[138] the latter generally being more sensorial than neuronal.[139] According to Khetarpal and Schuknecht,[140] the hearing loss is caused by changes in bone density, mass and shape that dampen the motion mechanics of the middle and inner ear.

Osteogenesis imperfecta (van de Hoeve's syndrome)

In this syndrome, hearing impairment (usually of the mixed type) is associated with blue sclerae and fragile bones. Type I is AD, and types II and III are AR; type IV may have both dominant and recessive inheritance. The main characteristic

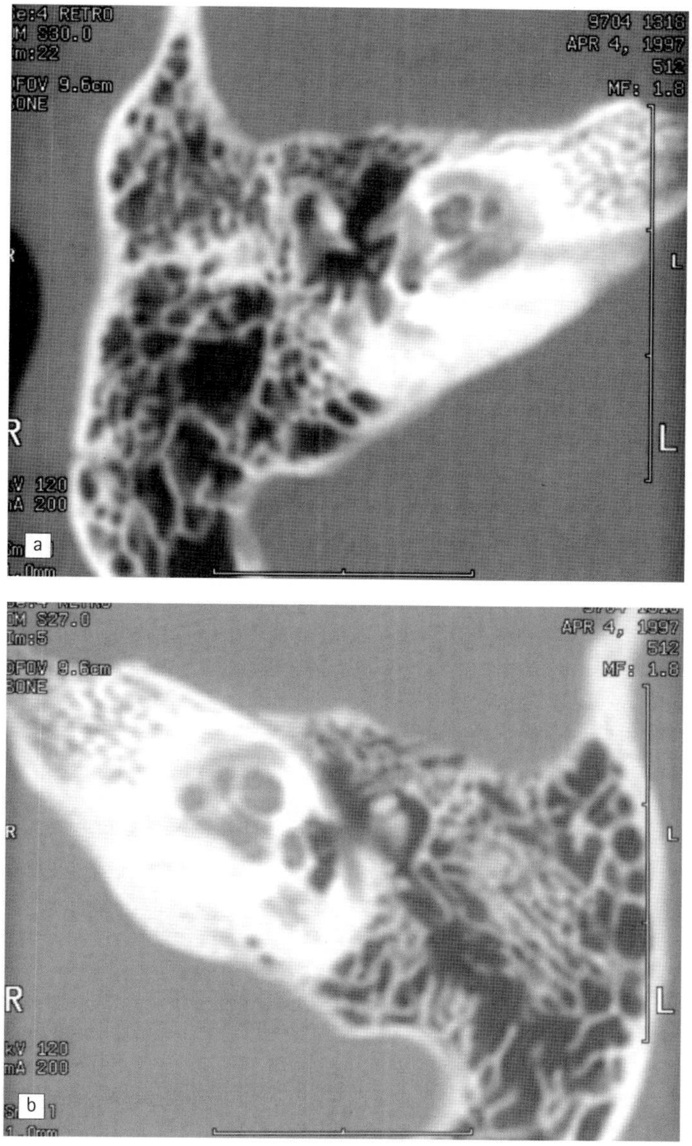

Figure 27.25 Temporal bone CT scan in a case of otosclerosis with cochlear involvement: in both the right (a) and left (b) axial images, the high degree of bone demineralization is evident.

histopathological findings are large remnants of cartilage in the enchondral bone, enchondral layer ossification delay, and periosteal bone formation.[117] Even if stapedectomy/stapedotomy can improve the conductive component of the hearing loss, the obliteration of the oval and round windows and the sensorineural component may eventually compromise the success of surgery[141] (Figure 27.28).

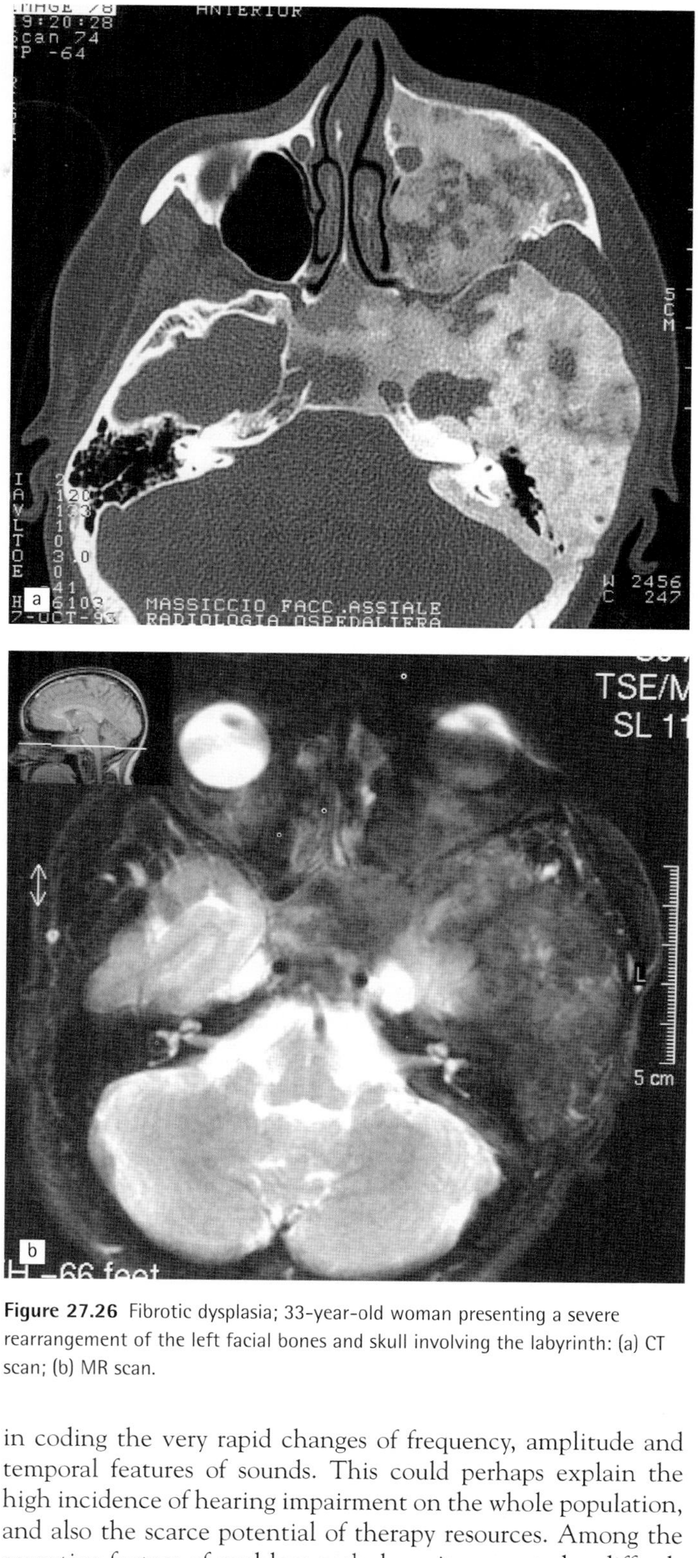

Figure 27.26 Fibrotic dysplasia; 33-year-old woman presenting a severe rearrangement of the left facial bones and skull involving the labyrinth: (a) CT scan; (b) MR scan.

Conclusions

The inner ear is extremely complicated in its functioning mechanisms. In fact it has to ensure an astonishing sensitivity in coding the very rapid changes of frequency, amplitude and temporal features of sounds. This could perhaps explain the high incidence of hearing impairment on the whole population, and also the scarce potential of therapy resources. Among the causative factors of cochlear pathology, it seems today difficult to propose a nosographic classification. A rather broad distinction could be done between pathologies which result from the action of environmental factors (trauma, noise ototoxic substances) and others from internal factors (inflammatory,

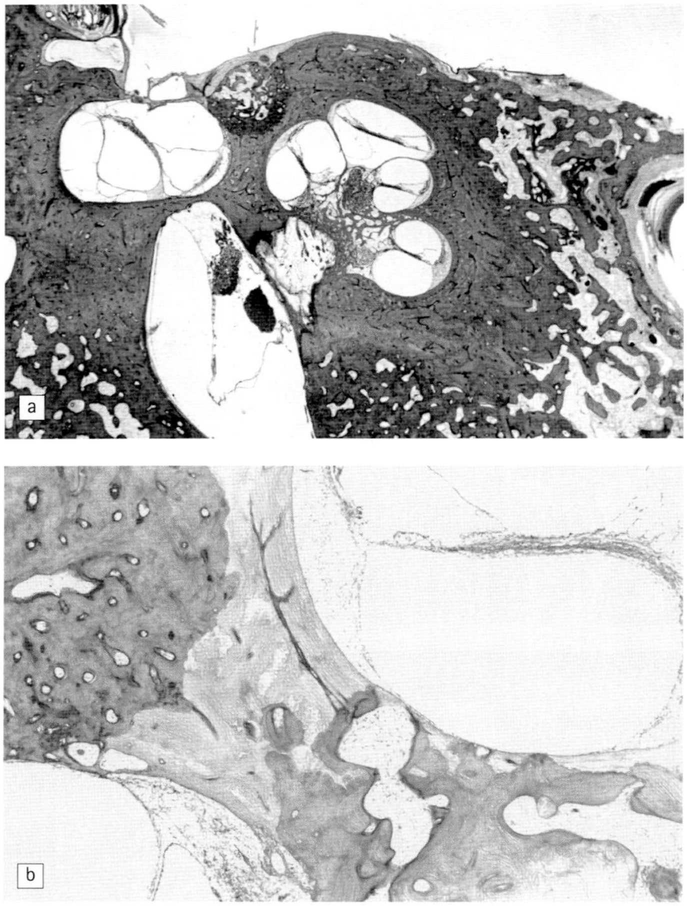

Figure 27.27 Paget's disease of bone (osteitis deformans). (a) Photomicrograph of the cochlear duct of a patient with Paget's disease. The labyrinthine capsule is extensively replaced by Paget bone, and the footplate is blocked in the oval window; (b) detail shows the Paget bone close to the stria vascularis. (Courtesy of Professor George Keleman.)

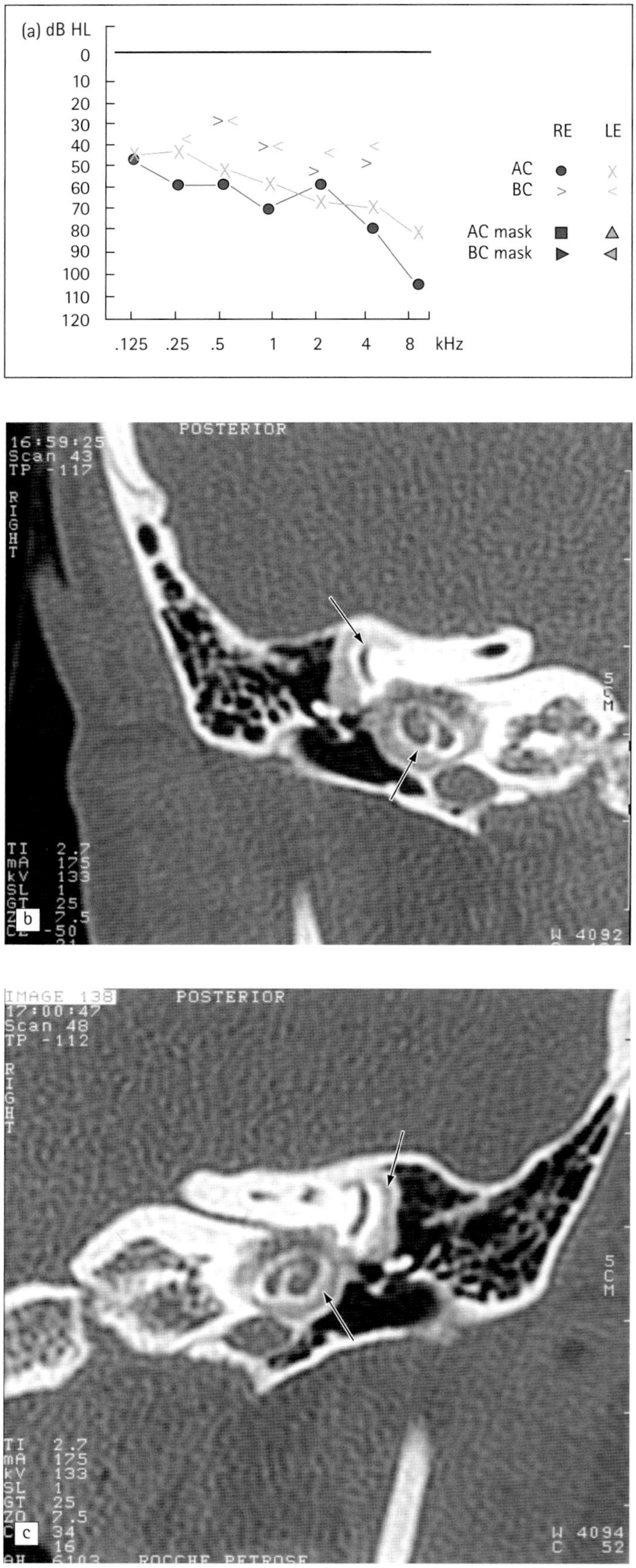

metabolic, vascular, genetic.) However, as molecular biology and genetics advance, it's clear that the majority of hearing impairments have a genetic basis. Even the susceptibility to noise or ototoxic effects may be to some extent genetically determined. As more is learned, this is likely to be also applied to the immune response the inner ear may develop against any factor which sets out of balance its homeostatis. The construction of cDNA libraries of the inner ear components will be a major step in the diagnosis of cochlear diseases. The identification of proteins unique to these structures will contribute to the knowledge of intimate molecular events underlying audition, and the modalities by which they could also be altered in the case of disease affecting other organs and systems. New therapies will soon be available for inner ear diseases, mainly acting on the defective genes responsible for the disorder. With such a perspective the ability of the clinician in correctly classifying the possible causative factor of a patient's sensorineural hearing loss will be more crucial than in the past.

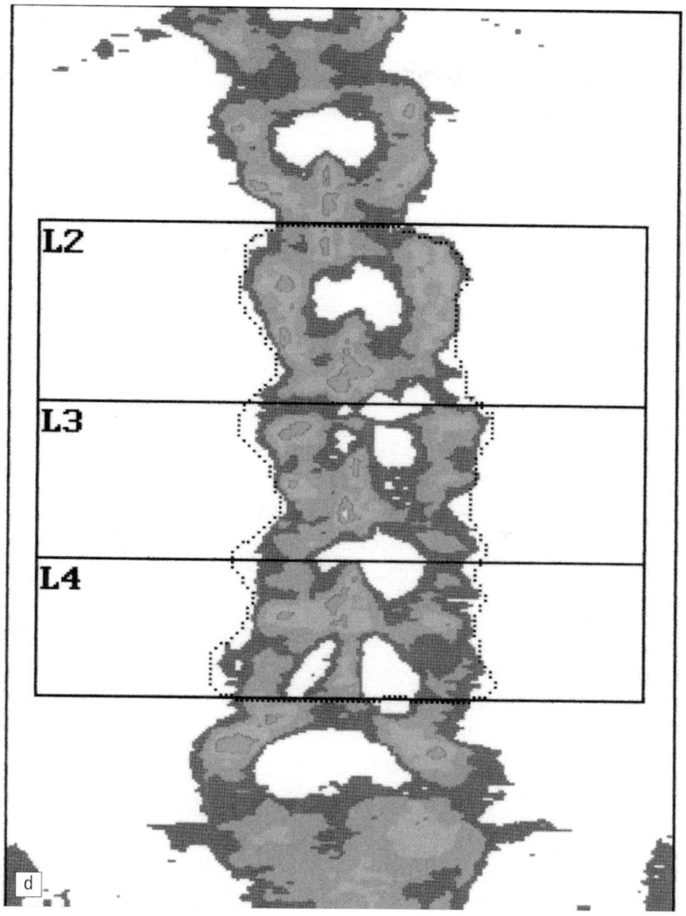

Figure 27.28 Mixed hearing loss: findings in a 21-year-old woman with osteogenesis imperfecta (van der Hoewe syndrome): (a) pure tone audiogram—mixed hearing loss; (b) CT scan, right coronal, and (c) left coronal views, which show diffuse demineralization of the bony labyrinth with a fluffy 'cotton wool' appearance, both at chochlear and vestibular level; (d) bone densitometry of lumbar vertebral tract, showing severe demineralization.

References

1. Davis A. The prevalence of hearing impairment and reported hearing disability among adults in Great Britain. *Int J Epidemiol* 1989; **18**: 911–17.
2. Kikuchi T, Kimura RS, Raul DL, Adams JC. Gap junctions in the rate cochlea: immunohistochemical and ultrastructural analysis. *Anat Embryol* 1995; **191**: 101–18.
3. Kelsell DP, Dunlop J, Stevens HP et al. Connexin 26 mutation in hereditary non-syndromic sensorineural deafness. *Nature* 1997; **387**: 80–3.
4. Steel KP. A new ear in the genetics of deafness. *N Engl J Med* 1998; **339**: 1545–7.
5. Gibson F, Walsh J, Mburu P et al. A type VII myosin encoded by the mouse deafness gene shaker-1. *Nature* 1995; **374**: 62–4.
6. Weil D, Blanchard S, Kaplan J. Defective myosin VIIa gene responsible for Usher syndrome type IB. *Nature* 1995; **374**: 60–1.
7. Everett LA, Glaser B, Beck JK *et al.* Pendred syndrome is caused by mutation in a putative sulphate transporter gene (PDS). *Nat Genet* 1997; **17**: 411–22.
8. Eudy JD, Weston MD, Yao S *et al.* Mutation of a gene encoding a protein with extarcellular matrix motifs in Usher syndrome type lia. *Science* 1998; **12**: 1753–7.
9. Cosgrove D, Samuelson G, Meehan DT et al. Ultrastructural, physiological, and molecular defects in the inner ear of a gene-knockout mouse for autosomal Alport syndrome. *Hear Res* 1998; **121**: 84–98.
10. Meyer zum Gottesberge AM, Eschen B, Reuter A, Kintrup L, Weiher H. Mpv17-glomerulosclerosis gene is essential for inner ear function. In: Stephens D, Read A, Martini A, eds. *Developments in Genetic Hearing Impairment.* London: Whurr, 1998: 148–55.
11. Khetarpal U, Schuknecht HF, Gacek RR, Holmes LB. Autosomal dominant sensorineural hearing loss. Pedigrees, audiological findings, and temporal bone findings in two kindreds. *Arch Otolaryngol Head Neck Surg* 1991; **117**: 1032–41.
12. Committee on Hearing and Equilibrium. Meniere's disease: criteria for diagnosis and evaluation of therapy for reporting. *Bull Am Acad Otorhinolaryngol Head Neck Surg* 1985; **4**: 6–7.
13. Wangemann P, Schacht J. Homeostatic mechanisms in the cochlea: In: Dallos P, Popper A, Fay RR, eds. *The Cochlea.* Springer-Verlag, 1996: 30–85.
14. Parving A. Epidemiology of genetic hearing impairment. In: Martini A, Read A, Stephens D, eds. *Genetics and Hearing Impairment.* London: Whurr, 1996: 73–81.
15. Sill AM, Stick MJ, Prenger VL, Phillips SL, Boughman JA, Arnos KS Genetic epidemiologic study of hearing impairment. *Am J Hum Genet* 1994; **54**: 149–53.
16. Steel KP. Similarities between mice and humans with hereditary deafness. *Ann NY Acad Sci* 1991; **630**: 68–79.
17. Brown SDM, Steel KP. Mouse models for human hearing impairment. In: Martini A, Read A, Stephens D, eds. *Genetics and Hearing Impairment.* London: Whurr, 1996: 53–63.
18. Steel KP, Palmer A. Basic mechanisms of hearing impairment. In: Martini A, Read A, Stephens D, eds. *Genetics and Hearing Impairment.* London: Whurr, 1996: 73–81.
19. van Camp G, Coucke P, Willems PJ. Autosomal dominant non-syndromal hearing loss. In: Martini A, Read A, Stephens D, eds. *Genetics and Hearing Impairment.* London: Whurr, 1996: 213–20.
20. Gorlin RJ. Genetic hearing loss with no associated abnormalities. In: Gorlin RJ, Toriello HV, Cohen MM, eds. *Hereditary Hearing Loss and its Syndromes.* Oxford: Oxford University Press, 1995: 42–61.
21. Konigsmark BW, Mengel M, Berlin CI. Familial low frequency hearing loss. *Laryngoscope* 1971; **81**: 759–71.
22. Leon PE, Bonilla JA, Sanchez JR et al. Low frequency hereditary deafness in man with childhood onset. *Am J Hum Genet* 1981; **33**: 209–14.
23. Liu X, Xu L, Newton V. Audiometric configuration in non-syndromal genetic hearing loss. *J Audiol Med* 1994; **3**: 99–106.
24. Martini A, Prosser S. Audiometric patterns of genetic hearing loss. In: Martini A, Read A, Stephens D, eds. *Genetics and Hearing Impairment.* London: Whurr, 1996: 92–9.

25. Van Egmond AAJ. Congenital deafness. *J. Laryng. Otol.* 1954; **68**: 429–43.
26. Martini A, Mazzoli M, Read A, Stephens D. *Definitions and Guidelines in Genetic Hearing Impairment*. London: Whurr, 2001.
27. Martini A, Prosser S, Mazzoli M, Rosignoli M. Contribution of age-related factors to the progression of non-syndromic hereditary hearing impairment. *J Audiol Med* 1996; **6**: 141–56.
28. Martini A. Ipoacusie progressive di tipo genetico. *Acta Otorhinolaryngol Ital Suppl* 1998; **59**: 21–7.
29. Paparella MM et al. Familial progressive sensorineural deafness. *Arch Otolaryngol* 1969; **90**: 44–51.
30. Thelin JW, Mitchell JA, Hefner MA, Davenport SL. CHARGE syndrome. Part II, hearing loss. *Int J Pediatr Otorhinolaryngol* 1986; **12**: 145–63.
31. Nadol JB, Burgess B. Cochleosaccular degeneration of the inner ear and progressive cataracts inherited as a dominant trait. *Laryngoscope* 1982; **92**: 1028–31.
32. Gorlin RJ. Genetic hearing loss associated with eye disorders. In: Gorlin RJ, Toriello HV, Cohen MM, eds. *Hereditary Hearing Loss and its Syndromes*. Oxford: Oxford University Press, 1995: 105–40.
33. Gorlin RJ, Wester DC, Carey JC. Genetic hearing loss associated with renal disorders. In: Gorlin RJ, Toriello HV, Cohen MM, eds. *Hereditary Hearing Loss and its Syndromes*. Oxford: Oxford University Press, 1995: 234–56.
34. Arnold W. Inner ear and renal diseases. *Ann Otol Rhinol Laryngol* 1984; **112**: 119–24.
35. Smith RJH, Steel KP, Barkway C, Soucek S, Michaels L. A histologic study of nonmorphogenetic forms of hereditary hearing impairment. *Arch Otolaryngol Head Neck Surg* 1992; **118**: 1085–94.
36. Dobyns WB. Genetic hearing loss associated with nervous system disorders. In: Gorlin RJ, Toriello HV, Cohen MM, eds. *Hereditary Hearing Loss and its Syndromes*. Oxford: Oxford University Press, 1995: 257–317.
37. Sylvester PE. Spino-cerebellar degeneration, hormonal disorder, hypogonadism, deaf mutism and mental deficiency. *J Ment Defic Res* 1972; **16**: 203–14.
38. Lyndsay JR, Hinojosa R. Histopathologic features of the inner ear associated with Kearns–Sayre syndrome. *Arch Otolaryngol* 1976; **102**: 747–52.
39. Gorlin RJ. Genetic hearing loss associated with endocrine and metabolic disorders. In: Gorlin RJ, Toriello HV, Cohen MM, eds. *Hereditary Hearing Loss and its Syndromes*. Oxford: Oxford University Press, 1995: 318–54.
40. Morgon SH et al. The neurological complications of Anderson–Fabry disease (alfa-galactosidase A deficiency)—investigation of symptomatic and presymptomatic patients. *Q J Med* 1990; **75**: 491–504.
41. Cotrufo R, Melone MA, Monsurro MR et al. Phenotype heterogeneity among hemizygotes in a family biochemically screened for adrenoleukodystrophy. *Am J Med Genet* 1987; **26**: 833–8.
42. Shapiro J, Stome M, Crocker A. Airway obstruction and sleep apnea in Hurler and Hunter syndrome. *Ann Otol Rhinol Laryngol* 1985; **94**: 458–61.
43. Zecner G, Moser M. Otosclerosis and mucopolysaccharidosis. *Acta Otolaryngol* 1987; **103**: 384–6.
44. Sataloff RT, Schiebel BR, Spiegel JR. Morquio's syndrome. *Am J Otolaryngol* 1987; **8**: 443–9.
45. Wolfram DJ, Wagener HP. Diabetes mellitus and simple optic atrophy among siblings: report of four cases. *Proc Mayo Clin* 1938; **13**: 715–18.
46. Cremers CWRJ, Wijdenveld PG, Pinkers AJ. Juvenile diabetes mellitus, optic atrophy, hearing loss, diabetes insipidus, atonia of the urinary tract and bladder, and other abnormalities (Wolfran syndrome). A review of 88 cases from the literature and personal observation on 3 patients. *Acta Paediatr Scand Suppl* 1977; **264**: 3–16.
47. Hildesheimer M, Maayan Z, Muchnik C. Auditory and vestibular findings in Waardenburg syndrome type II. *J Laryngol Otol* 1989; **103**: 1130–33.
48. Peserico A, Martini A, Tenconi R. Familial multiple pigmented naevi and sensorineural deafness. A new autosomal dominant syndrome? *Int J Pediatr Otorhinolaryngol* 1981; **3**: 269–72.
49. Crandall B, Samec L, Sparkes RS, Wright SW. A familial syndrome of deafness, alopecia, and hypogonadism. *J Pediatr* 1973; **82**: 461–5.
50. Cook RA, Cox JR, Jorgensen, RJ. Otodental dysplasia: a five year study. *Ear Hear* 1981; **2**: 90–4.
51. Torriello HV. Genetic hearing loss associated with integumentary disorders. In: Gorlin RJ, Toriello HV, Cohen MM, eds. *Hereditary Hearing Loss and its Syndromes*. Oxford: Oxford University Press, 1995: 355–412.
52. Brunner HG. X-linked hearing loss. In: Martini A, Read A, Stephens D, eds. *Genetics and Hearing Impairment*. London: Whurr, 1996: 231–5.
53. Cremers CWRJ. The X-linked recessive progressive mixed hearing loss syndrome with perilymphatic gusher during stapes surgery (DFN3). In: Martini A, Read A, Stephens D, eds. *Genetics and Hearing Impairment*. London: Whurr, 1996: 236–43.
54. de Kok YJM, van der Maarel SM, Bitner-Glindewiez M et al. Association between X-linked mixed deafness and mutations in the POU domain gene POU3F4. *Science* 1995; **267**: 685–8.
55. Horiguchi I. Familial streptomycin-induced hearing loss. *Jap J Otorhinolaryngol* 1957; **29**: 1396.
56. Hu DN, Oui WO, Wu BT et al. Genetic aspects of antibiotic induced deafness: mitochondrial inheritance. *J Med Genet* 1991; **28**: 79–83.
57. Ottaviani F, Cadoni G, Marinelli L et al. Anti-endothelial autoantibodies in patients with sudden hearing loss. *Laryngoscope* 1999; **109**: 1084–7.
58. Linthicum FH, El-Rahman AGA. Hydrops due to syphilitic endolymphatic duct obliteration. *Laryngoscope* 1987; **97**: 568–74.
59. Viirre ES, Baloh RW. Migraine as a cause of sudden hearing loss. *Headache* 1996; **36**: 24–8.
60. Mattox D, Simmons FB. Natural history of sensorineural hearing loss. *Ann Otol Rhinol Laryngol* 1977; **86**: 463–80.
61. Schucknecht HF, Gacek CW. Cochlear pathology in presbycusis. *Ann Otol Rhinol Laryngol Suppl* 1993; **102** (158): 1–16.
62. Schucknecht HF, Montandon P. Pathology of the ear in pneumococcal meningitis. *Arch Klin Exp Ohr Nas Kehlkheilk* 1970; **195**: 207–25.

63. Harris JP, Heydt J, Keithley EM, Chen MC. Immunopathology of the inner ear: an update. *Ann NY Acad Sci* 1997; **830**: 166–78.
64. Tomiyama S, Harris JP. The role of endolymphatic sac in inner ear immunity. *Acta Otolaryngol* 1987; **103**: 182–8.
65. Chen MC, Harris JP, Keithley EM. Immunohistochemical analysis of proliferating cells in a sterile labyrinthitis animal model. *Laryngoscope* 1998; **108**: 651–6.
66. Paparella MM, Sugiura S. The pathology of suppurative labyrinthitis. *Ann Otol Rhinol Laryngol* 1967; **76**: 554–86.
67. Dereby MJ, Rao VS, Siglok TJ, Linthicum FH, Nelson RA. Meniere's disease: an immune mediated illness? *Laryngoscope* 1991; **103**: 1027–34.
68. Garcia Berrocal JR, Vargas JA, Ramirez Camacho RA et al. Deficiency of naive T cells in patients with sudden deafness. *Arch Otolaryngol Head Neck Surg* 1997; **123**: 712–17.
69. Dornhoffer JL, Arenberg JG, Arenberg IK, Shambaugh Jr GE. Pathophysiological mechanisms in immune inner ear disease. *Acta Otolaryngol Suppl* 1997; **526**: 30–6.
70. Yoo TJ, Tomoda K, Stuart JM, Kang AH, Townes AS. Type II collagen autoimmunity in otosclerosis and Meniere's disease. *Science* 1982; **17**: 1153–5.
71. Hughes GB, Barna BP, Kinney SE, Calabrese LH, Nalepa NL. Predictive value of laboratory tests in 'autoimmune' inner ear disease: preliminary report. *Laryngoscope* 1986; **96**: 502–5.
72. Harris JP, Sharp P. Inner ear autoantibodies in patients with rapid progressive sensorineural hearing loss. *Laryngoscope* 1990; **97**: 63–76.
73. Commitee on hearing and equilibrium of the American Academy of Otolaryngology—Head and Neck Surgery. Commitee on hearing and equilibrium gidelines for the diagnosis and evaluation of therapy in Menière's disease. *Otolaryngol Head Neck Surg* 1995; **113**: 181–5.
74. Melchiorri L, Martini A, Rizzo R, Berto A, Adinolfi E, Baricordi OR. HLA-A,B,C, DR antigens and soluble HSA-class I serum level in Menière's disease. *Acta Otolaryngol* 2002 (accepted).
75. Arenberg IK, Lemke C, Shambaugh GE Jr. Viral theory for Meniere's disease and endolymphatic hydrops: overview and new therapeutic options for viral labyrinthitis. *Ann NY Acad Sci* 1997; **830**: 306–13.
76. Schuknecht H. Ablation therapy in the management of Menière's disease. *Acta Otolaryngol Suppl* 1957; **132**: 1–41.
77. Blakley BW. Update on intratympanic gentamicin for Meniere's disease. *Laryngoscope* 2000; **110**: 236–40.
78. van de Heyning PA, Verlooy J, Schatteman I et al. Selective vestibual neurectomy in Menière's disease: A review. *Acta Otolaryngol Suppl* 1997; **526**: 58–66.
79. Kohonen A, Jauhiainen T, Liewendahl K, Tarkkanen J, Kaimio M. Deafness in experimental hypo- and hyperthyroidism. *Laryngoscope* 1971; **81**: 947–56.
80. Parving A. Hearing sensitivity in elderly patients with mixoedema. *Adv Audiol* 1985; **3**: 147–51.
81. Ritter FN. The effects of hypothyroidism upon the ear, nose and throat. *Laryngoscope* 1967; **77**: 1427–79.
82. Post JT. Hypothyroid deafness. *Laryngoscope* 1964; **74**: 221–32.
83. Spencer JT. Hyperlipoproteinemias in the etiology of inner ear disease. *Laryngoscope* 1973; **83**: 639–78.
84. Strome M, Toff P, Vernick DM. Hyperlipidemia in association with childhood sensorineural hearing loss. *Laryngoscope* 1988; **98**: 165–9.
85. Lee FS, Matthews LJ, Mills JH, Dubno JR, Adkins WY. Analysis of blood chemistry and hearing levels in a sample of older persons. *Ear Hear* 1998; **19**: 180–90.
86. Jones NS, Davis A. A prospective case-controlled study of patients presenting with idiopathic sensorineural hearing loss to examine the relationship between hyperlipidaemia and sensorineural hearing loss. *Clin Otolaryngol* 1999; **24**: 531–6.
87. Jorgensen MB. The inner ear in diabetes mellitus. *Arch Otolaryngol* 1961; **74**: 31–9.
88. Harner SG. Hearing in adult-onset diabetes mellitus. *Otolaryngol Head Neck Surg* 1981; **89**: 322–7.
89. Duck SW, Prazma J, Bennett PS, Pillsbury HC. Interaction between hypertension and diabetes mellitus in the pathogenesis of sensorineural hearing loss. *Laryngoscope* 1997; **107**: 1596–605.
90. Oda M, Preciado MC, Quick CA, Paparella MM. Labyrinthine pathology of chronic renal failure patients treated with hemodialysis and kidney transplantation. *Laryngoscope* 1974; **84**: 1489–506.
91. Bergstrom LV, Thompson P, Sando I et al. Renal disease: its pathology, treatment, and effects on the ear. *Arch Otolaryngol* 1980; **106**: 567–72.
92. Aran JM. Current perspective on inner ear toxicity. *Otolaryngol Head Neck Surg* 1995; **112**: 133–44.
93. Aran JM, Hiel H, Hayashida T et al. Noise, aminoglycosides and diuretics. In: Dancer A, Henderson D, Salvi RJ, Hamenrik RP, eds. *Noise Induced Hearing Loss*. Philadephia: BC Decker, 1991: 188–95.
94. Lim DJ. Effect of noise and ototoxic drugs at the cellular level in the cochlea: a review. *Am J Otol* 1986; **7**: 73–98.
95. Schacht J. Biochemical basis of aminoglycoside ototoxicity. *Otolaryngol Clin North Am* 1993; **26**: 845–856.
96. Priuska EM, Shacht J. Formation of free radicals by gentamicin and iron and evidence for an iron/gentamicin complex. *Biochem Pharmacol* 1995; **50**: 1749–52.
97. Kahlmeter G, Dalager J. Aminoglycoside toxicity and review of medical studies published between 1975 and 1982. *J Antimicrob Chemother* 1984; **13**: 9–22.
98. Higashi K. Unique inheritance of streptomycin-induced deafness. *Clin Genet* 1989; **35**: 433–36.
99. Prezant TR, Agapian JV, Bohlman MC, Bu X, Otzas S, Qui W-Q, Amos KS, Cortopassi GA, Jaber L, Rotter JI, Shohat M, Fischel-Ghodsian N. Mitochondrial ribosomal RNA mutation associated with both antibiotic-induced and non-syndromic deafness. *Nature and Genetics* 1993; **4**: 289–94.
100. Jacobs HT, Shah ZH, Migliosi V, Lehtinen SK, Rovio A, O'Dell K. Nuclear canditates genes for 'mitochondrial deafness'. In Stephens D, Read A, Martini A, eds. *Developments in Genetic Hearing Impairments*, London: Whurr, 1998; 104–15.
101. Braverman I, Jaber L, Levi H et al. Audiovestibular findings in patients with deafness caused by a mitochondrial susceptibility

mutation and precipitated by an inherited nuclear mutation or aminoglycosides. *Arch Otolaryngol–Head and Neck Surgery* 1996; **122**: 1001–4.

102. Jacobs HT. Phenotype/genotype correlation of hearing impairment associated with mitochondrial DNA mutations. In Martini A, Mazzoli M, Read A, Stephens D, eds. *Definitions, Protocols and Guidelines in Genetic Hearing Impairment*, London: Whurr, 2001: 152–6.
103. Chapman P. Rapid onset hearing loss after cysplatia therapy: case report and literature review. *J Laryngol Otol* 1982; **96**: 159–62.
104. Evans WE, Yee GC, Crom WR et al. Clinical pharmacology of bleomycin and cisplatin. *Otolaryngol Head Neck Surg* 1981; **4**: 98–110.
105. Helson L, Okonkwo E, Anton L et al. Cisplatinum ototoxicity. *Clin Toxicol* 1978; **13**: 469–78.
106. Saito T, Moataz R, Dulon D. Cisplatin blocks depolarization induced calcium entry in isolated cochlear outer hair cells. *Hear Res* 1991; **56**: 143–7.
107. MacAlpine D, Johnstone BM. The ototoxic mechanisms of cisplatin. *Hear Res* 1990; **47**: 191–204.
108. Kopelman F. Ototoxicity of high dose cisplatin by bolus administration in patients with advanced cancers and normal hearing. *Laryngoscope* 1988; **98**: 858–63.
109. Pollera C. Very high dose of cisplatin-induced ototoxicity: Preliminary report on early and long term effects. *Cancer Chemother Pharmacol* 1988; **21**: 61–4.
110. Waters RA, Ahmad M, Katsarkas A et al. Ototoxicity due to cis-diaminedichloroplatinum in the treatment of ovarian cancer: influence of dosage and schedule of administration. *Ear Hear* 1991; **12**: 91–102.
111. Pasic TR, Dobie RA. Cis-platinum ototoxicity in children. *Laryngoscope* 1991; **101**: 985–91.
112. Paloheimo S, Thalmann R. Influence of 'loop' diuretics upon Na+ K+-ATPase and adenlate cyclase of the stria vascularis. *Arch Otorhinolaryngol* 1977; **17**: 347–59.
113. Bosher SK. The nature of otoxic actions of ethacrynic acid upon the mammalian endolymph system. I. Functional aspects. *Acta Otolaryngol* 1980; **89**: 407–18.
114. Ikeda K, Oshima T, Hidaka H, Takasaka T. Molecular and clinical implications of loop diuretic ototoxicity. *Hear Res* 1997; **7**: 1–8.
115. Jung TTK, Rhee CK, Lee CS, Park YS, Choi DC. Otoxicity of salicylate, nonsteroidal antiinflammatory drugs and quinine. *Otolaryngol Clin North Am* 1993; **26**: 791–809.
116. Claessen FA, vanBoxtel CJ, Perenboom RM, Tange RA, Wetsteijn JC, Kager PA. Quinine pharmacokinetics: ototoxic and cardiotoxic effects in healthy Caucasian subjects and in patients with falciparum malaria. *Trop Med Int Health* 1998; **3**(6): 482–9.
117. Schuknecht HF. *Pathology of the Ear*, 2nd edn. Phildelphia: Lea and Febiger, 1993.
118. Schuknecht HF. Mechanisms of inner ear injury from blows to the head. *Ann Otol Rhinol Laryngol* 1969; **78**: 253–62.
119. Schuknecht HF. Cupulolithiasis. *Arch Otolaryngol* 1969; **90**: 765–78.
120. Toglia JU, Rosenberg PE, Ronis ML. Posttraumatic dizziness. Vestibular, audiologic, and medicolegal aspects. *Arch Otolaryngol* 1970; **92**: 485–92.
121. McHugh HE. The surgical treatment of facial paralysis and traumatic conductive deafness in fractures of the temporal bone. *Ann Otol Rhinol Laryngol* 1959; **68**: 855–89.
122. Khan AA, Marion M, Hinojosa R. Temporal bone fractures: a histopathologic study. *Otolaryngol Head Neck Surg* 1985; **93**: 177–86.
123. Schuknecht HF, Davison RC. Deafness and vertigo from head injury. *Arch Otolaryngol* 1956; **63**: 513–28.
124. Pulec JL. Symposium on Meniere's disease. I. Meniere's disease: results of a two and one-half-year study of etiology, natural history and results of treatment. *Laryngoscope* 1972; **82**: 1703–15.
125. Clark SK, Rees TS. Posttraumatic endolymphatic hydrops. *Arch Otolaryngol* 1977; **103**: 725–6.
126. Applebaum E. Meningitis following trauma to the head and face. *JAMA* 1960; **173**: 1818–22.
127. Freeman J. Temporal bone fractures and cholesteatoma. *Ann Otol Rhinol Laryngol* 1983; **92**: 558–60.
128. Mazzoli M, Rosignoli M, Martini A. Otosclerosis: are familial and isolated cases different disorders? *J Audio Med* 2001; **10**: 49–59.
129. Tomek MS, Brown MR, Sabitha RM et al. Localization of a gene for otosclerosis to chromosome 15q25-q26. *Hum Mol Genet* 1998; **7**: 285–90.
130. Linthicum FH, Neely JG. Unrelated sensorineural hearing loss in patients with otosclerosis. A report of three cases. *Laryngoscope* 1977; **87**: 1746–52.
131. Kelemen G, Linthicum FH Jr. Labyrinthine otosclerosis. *Acta Otolaryngol Suppl* 1969; **253**: 1–68.
132. Schuknecht HF, Barber W. Histologic variants in otosclerosis. *Laryngoscope* 1985; **95**: 1307–17.
133. Shambaugh GE Jr. Clinical diagnosis of cochlear (labyrinthine) otosclerosis. *Laryngoscope* 1965; **75**: 1558–62.
134. Schuknecht HF. Cochlear otosclerosis. An intractable absurdity. *J Laryngol Otol Suppl* 1983; **8**: 81–3.
135. Beighton P, Cremin B. *Sclerosing Bone Dysplasias*. Berlin: Springer Verlag, 1980.
136. Beighton P. Auditory dysfunction in genetic disorders of the skeleton. In: Martini A, Read A, Stephens D, eds. *Genetics and Hearing Impairment*. London: Whurr, 1996: 130–40.
137. Shprintzen RJ. *Genetics, Syndromes, and Communication Disorders*. San Diego: Singular Publishing Group, 1997.
138. Lindsay JR, Suga F. Paget's disease and sensori-neural deafness: temporal bone histopathology of Paget's disease. *Laryngoscope* 1976; **86**: 1029–42.
139. Clemis JD, Boyles J, Harford ER, Petasnick JP. The clinical diagnosis of Paget's disease of the temporal bone. *Ann Otol Rhinol Laryngol* 1967; **76**: 611–23.
140. Khetarpal U, Schuknecht HF. In search of pathologic correlates for hearing loss and vertigo in Paget's disease. A clinical and histopathologic study of 26 temporal bones. *Ann Otol Rhinol Laryngol Suppl* 1990; **145**(99): 1–16.

141. Garretsen TJTM, Cremers CWRJ. Stapes surgery in osteogenesis imperfecta: analysis of postoperative hearing loss. *Ann Otol Rhinol Laryngol* 1991; **100**: 120–30.
142. Martini A, Milani M, Rosignoli M, Mazzoli M, Prosser S. Audiometric patterns of genetic non-syndromal sensorineural hearing loss. *Audiology* 1997; **36**: 228–36.
143. Hatzopoulos S, Di Stefano M, Campbell KCM, Falgione D, Ricci D, Rosignoli M, Finesso M, Albertin A, Previati M, Captani S, Martini A. Cisplatin ototoxicity in the Sprague Dawley rat evaluated by distortion product otoacoustic emissions. *Audiology* 2001; **40**: 253–64.

28 Noise-induced hearing loss

Ilmari Pyykkö, Jukka Starck, Esko Toppila, Mats Ulfendahl

Introduction

Although the severity of hearing loss has decreased in the last decades in industrialized countries, the total number of cases of noise-induced hearing loss (NIHL) has declined only slightly.[1,2] In population studies, risk analysis for NIHL is well established.[3,4] In individual cases, confounding factors make exact risk prediction for NIHL difficult.[5–7] The shortage of well evaluated databases containing information on individual exposure, the use of hearing protective devices (HPDs), social noise exposure and various biological confounding factors may explain the inaccuracy in risk evaluation.[8] Problems arise also from sampling techniques, and the selection and duration of samples.[9] A common database including all the confounding factors and exposure-linked variables could provide a base of knowledge from which individual noise susceptibility could be determined. Further, a database is important in the identification of adverse phases of work and in monitoring the hearing of workers.

In the present chapter, we will focus on the vulnerability of the inner ear to noise, the evaluation of hazardous limits for environmental noise, and on prevention of NIHL by using database-based programs.

Current databases used in the risk assessment of NIHL

CURRENT DATABASES USED IN DIFFERENT NORMS

- Kryter (1967)[10]
- Baughn (1973)[12]
- Burns and Robinson(1970)[13]
- Passchier-Vermeer (1974)[17]
- Johnson (1973)[19]

Kryter[10] proposed one of the first databases used in risk estimation. The damage risk criteria were presented as a group of curves based on laboratory experiments on temporary threshold shift (TTS). Also, some data collected in 1955–56 on permanent threshold shifts (PTS) in workers exposed to industrial noise were included. The Committee on Hearing, Bioacoustics and Biomechanics (CHABA)[10] used these data in establishing the first norm for noise damage assessment. Recently, Melnick[11] has criticized this approach.

Baughn[12] published the first epidemiological database. He studied a large (6835) population working in stable locations and with known noise exposure.[12] The exposure durations extended up to 45 years, with average noise exposure levels of 78, 86 and 92 dB. Baughn recommended that the hearing loss of subjects exposed to the 78 dB (A) noise would be considered as representative of typical non-noise-exposed males.

Burns and Robinson established their database by studying 759 otologically normal workers. Based on the noise exposure, 422 males were classified into four exposure groups, ranging from 87 dB(A) to 97 dB(A).[13] The maximum length of exposure was 49 years. As controls, 97 subjects not exposed to noise were used. The authors developed a mathematical model for the prediction of hearing loss.[14,15] The model introduced the equal-energy principle, which enabled the combination of different sound levels.[16] The hearing loss was divided into two parts: age-dependent hearing loss (presbyacusis) and NIHL. After correcting for age and gender, the distribution of NIHL was calculated by using the specified formulae. The separation of presbyacusis and NIHL resulted in a smaller NIHL component than in other models.

Passchier-Vermeer[17] collected a database including 19 studies, each consisting of a limited number of cases; 12 studies had 50 cases or less. The data agreed well with the data of Robinson[4] at most frequencies, but large differences were found at some frequencies. One reason was in the definition of the audiometer zero level used in some of the studies.[18]

STANDARDS AND NORMS BASED ON DATABASES:

- CHABA 1966[131]
- EPA 1974[132]
- NIOSH 1974[20]
- ISO 1975[21]
- ISO 1990[22]

Johnson[19] collected a database for the US Environmental Protection Agency (EPA), to be used to predict noise-induced permanent theshold shift (NIPTS) for exposure to continuous noise. The report was based on the data of Burns and Robinson[13] and Passchier-Vermeer.[17] The data of Baughn[12] were also used in the evaluation of the hearing loss of the non-exposed population. For this reason, the hearing loss of the non-exposed population is somewhat less than that of Burns and Robinson[13] and Passhier-Vermeer.[17]

The National Institute for Occupational Safety and Health (NIOSH) collected a database from industrial workers exposed to noise levels of 85, 90 and 95 dB(A) and control subjects exposed to noise at levels less than 80 dB(A).[20] The study consisted of 792 otologically screened noise exposed subjects and 380 controls. The NIHL was determined as a function of exposure level and duration.

The International Organization for Standardization (ISO) published in 1975 a standard for assessing occupational noise exposure for hearing conservation.[21] The database on which this standard was based is not evident, but according to Suter,[22] the norm is based on the data of Baughn.[12] The standard adopted the equal-energy principle for the calculation of different sound exposures from the Robinson model. According to ISO tables, 50% of non-noise-exposed people will have a hearing loss, whereas the respective figure in Robinson and Sutton's model[23] was 10% and that in the US public health services study[24,25] was 20%. A mathematical form for the hearing loss was given in order to produce the present standard model.[3]

System approach for hearing protection programmes

KEY AREAS IN HEARING CONSERVATION PROGRAMME

- Usage rate of HPD
- Identification of noise source
- Free-time noise exposure
- Combination of different types of noise

The approach to protecting workers against noise (described in the directive 86/188/EC) is based on the identification of the

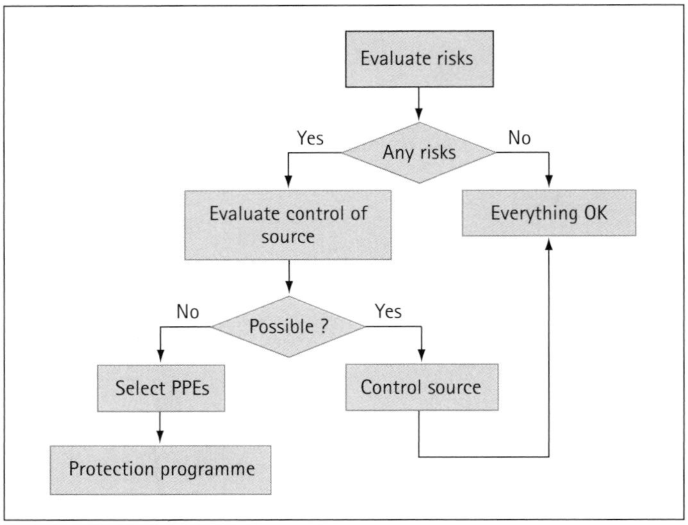

Figure 28.1 The general approach to the hearing conservation programme. PPE, personal protective equipment.

risks in the workplace (Figure 28.1). If there is a risk for NIHL, the employer must establish a hearing conservation programme (HCP). Qualified personnel should carry out the risk assessment. The first task is to evaluate the sources of noise and the possibilities of reducing the levels of noise by technical means. If reduction of the noise source is not possible, the workers should be provided with HPDs and should be informed about the risks and the correct use of the selected HPDs in an appropriate manner.

These guidelines alone, however, may not be sufficient to ensure an effective HCP in practice. The following problems must be solved:

1. How to guarantee that the hearing protection devices (HPDs) are used properly.
2. How to identify risky workplaces or tasks.
3. How to address all aspects of protection against noise emission, especially if the greatest exposure occurs in leisure time.
4. How to collect and combine various exposures with different physical characteristics.

By solving these questions, the minimal legal requirements of an HCP will be achieved. A good HCP contains additional elements, which are included to increase the power of the HCP.

The contents of a good HCP will be discussed in the following section.

Risk assessment of NIHL based on ISO 1999–1990

The ISO model[3] uses three input parameters in the evaluation of NIHL: age, exposure to noise, and gender. Exposure to noise is evaluated using the equal-energy principle. Age is corrected in a dichotomized way. Different correction factors for gender

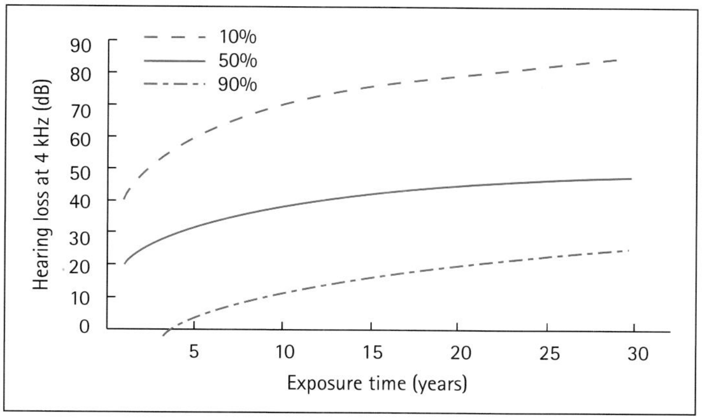

Figure 28.2 The mean hearing loss with 10% and 90% confidence limits of a male worker exposed to 100-dB(A) noise as a function of time.

are given. Based on these parameters, the distribution of NIHL can be calculated. The variation is large; the difference between the 10% and 90% percentiles is 60 dB when subjects are exposed to a noise of 100 dB(A) after 30 years (for males see Figure 28.2).

According to the standard ISO 1999–1990, PTS is due to a combination of ageing and noise effects. It is used for the estimation of the hearing impairment due to noise in a population free from hearing loss due to other causes. The standard may also be used for estimating the permanent effects of noise on the perception of everyday acoustical signals. The appreciation of music or the effect of one specific frequency on hearing is not addressed by the standard. Although the standard is intended for population studies and should not be applied to individuals, it has been used to evaluate the probability of NIHL in individual subjects, particularly in medico-legal cases.

Factors to be controlled in establishing a database for NIHL

The factors influencing the degree of hearing loss in noise-exposed subjects are shown in Figure 28.3. To increase the efficiency of an HCP, it would be very profitable to be able to predict NIHL more accurately than shown in Figure 28.2.

The first section identifies exposure variables important in the aetiology of NIHL from the exposure point of view. The first element shows work noise variables and protection provided by individual HPDs. The second element consists of leisure time and military service noise. The third element controls the exposure to ototoxic solvents and drugs. The harmful effects of noise on hearing depend on the energy content of the noise transmitted to the ear. The energy content of noise—comprising the level of noise exposure, the frequency of noise, and the duration of exposure—is determined by means of the A-weighted equivalent sound pressure level. This principle is well suited for determining risk in the case of steady-state constant noise, but it underestimates risk in the case of impulsive noise.

The second section shows confounding factors used to explain individual susceptibility to noise. These factors include cholesterol level, blood pressure and smoking, and may explain the large variation in the individual development of NIHL.

The third section shows the results of otological examination and describes the effects on the inner ear that are measured or considered.

Impulse noise

Impulse noise differs from steady-state noise in time-domain properties. Impulse noise contains rapid pressure transients,

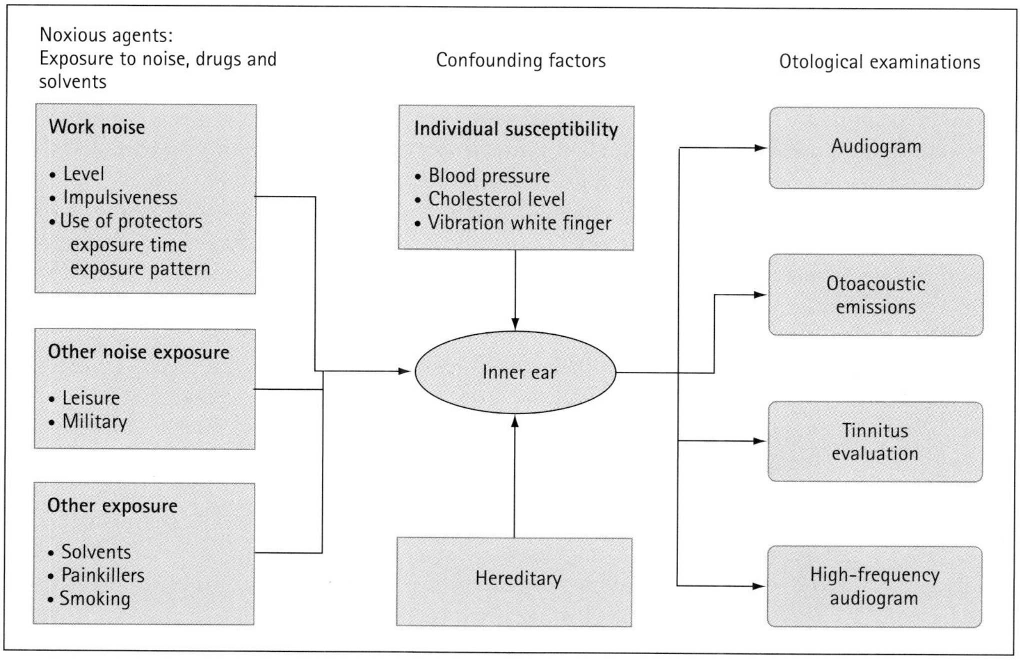

Figure 28.3 Factors known or suspected to contribute to the development of hearing loss.

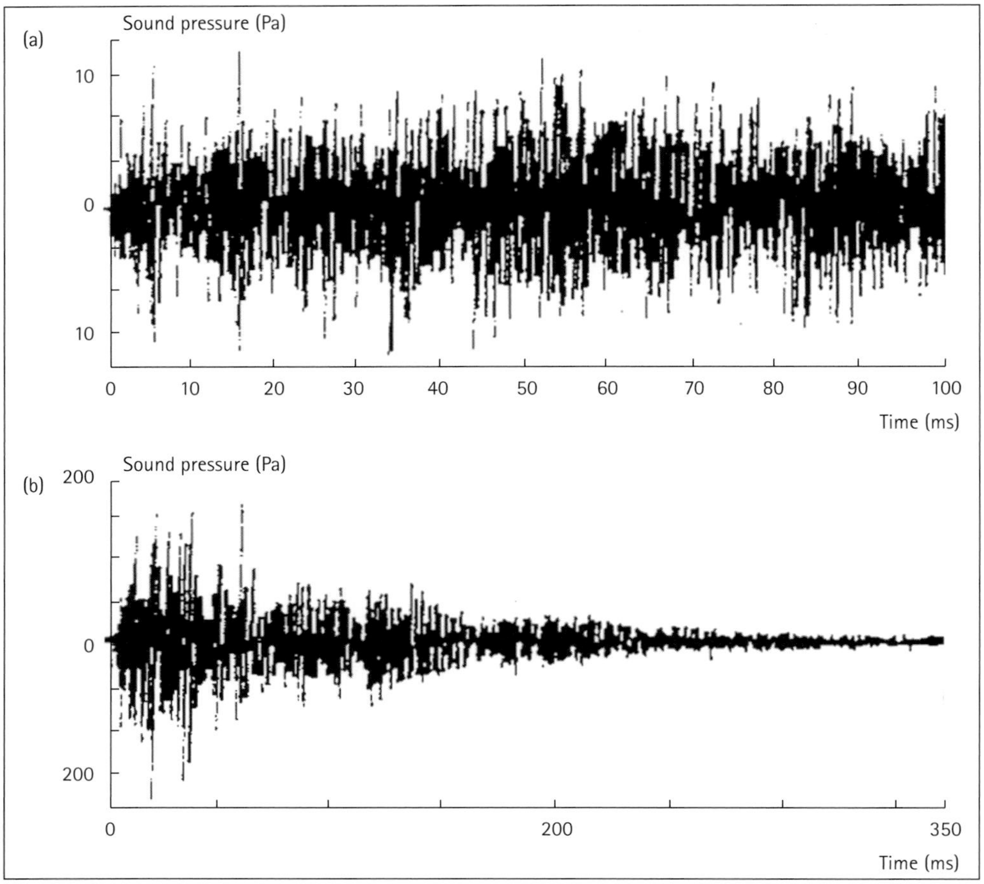

Figure 28.4 Impulses from (a) chisel hammer and (b) hammer blow.

which do not always give a fully audible response but can reach the sensory hair cells located in the inner ear (Figure 28.4). The criteria presented for impulse noise are based on the repetition rate of peaks of sound pressures. Impulse noise has also been defined as noise consisting of single bursts with duration of less than 1 s and with peak levels 15 dB higher than background noise. Several parameters can be measured and displayed to describe the impulse properties in time domain: peak level, rise time, decay time, repetition rate and frequency content.

In industrial workplaces, impulses are seldom identical (even repetitive) and are not produced regularly. Several machines producing impulses may be used at the same time, and the workers often move around at different distances from noise sources. Generally, workers' exposure to noise consists of impulses spaced randomly in time and mixed with steady-state noise. Thus, the acoustical evaluation will require statistical analyses for impulse noise parameters. Recently, a statistical distribution for crest factor has been proposed to determine the impulsiveness of industrial impulse noise.[26]

Impulse noise and hearing

Properties of impulse noise can be described by the instantaneous time function. The parameters generally used are the peak level, rise time and duration of the impulse. In peak level measurements, the time constant of the measuring device has to be less than 50 μs, preferably 20 μs. The duration of an impulse can be determined in at least four different way: the effective impulse duration, or the A- , B- or C-duration.[27,28] Physically, the effective duration is uniformly defined, as it is the length of a rectangular impulse with the same energy as the actual impulse. Duration A is determined for an idealized gunshot, in which the duration is defined as the time of the first positive transient. B- and C- duration are idealized hammer blows on a piece of metal. These noise peaks can be very intensive but extremely short, and therefore do not contribute significantly to the measuring result of L_{eq} or the total noise dose.

The risk of NIHL is higher in occupations where workers are exposed to impulse noise. In many occupations, the impulses are so brief that they contribute only a small increase to the energy content of noise. Comparative studies showed that, for example, shipyard workers who are exposed to impulse noise had 10 dB greater hearing loss than was predicted by the ISO 1999 model. In forest workers who are exposed to steady-state noise, the observed and predicted hearing threshold levels were consistent.[26,29] Target shooting and hunting constitute a risk for hearing loss.[30] Forest workers exposed to shooting noise demonstrate an approximately 10-dB greater NIHL than those with only occupational exposure to chainsaw noise.[31] The NIHL appears at a younger age in military personnel than in other groups of workers exposed to noise.[30] Soldiers exposed to large-calibre weapons have a higher risk of NIHL, as HPDs are less effective in this situation, due to the non-linear attenuation against very high peak levels and the low-frequency components of large-calibre weapons.[26,32–35]

It is therefore important that any database on NIHL contains information on impulsiveness of noise. As the method of quantification of impulsiveness is not yet standardized, the impulsiveness should be indicated with no/yes questions.

Hearing protectors

HPDs used in a noisy working environment must meet the specified minimum requirements for attenuation. The test method is standardized by ISO[36,37] and CEN.[38,39] The attenuation of an HPD will be measured as a difference between hearing thresholds without and with hearing protector using 16 test persons. The mean value (M_f) and standard deviation (S_f) will be calculated. The assumed protection value ($APV_{f,x}$) can then be calculated by the formula

$$APV_{f,x} = M_f - \alpha S_f \text{ (dB)}$$

where the subscript x is the percentage of users who will obtain at least the attenuation $APV_{f,x}$. The percentage x depends on the factor α. In the CEN standard, x is 84% and the respective α value is 1.

Minimum attenuation in accordance with the $APV_{f,84}$ values should not be less than those given in Table 34.1 The testing house has to identify the parameters presented above. Moreover, the indices denoted H, M, L (used in HML methods) and SNR are defined and used for selection purposes. H is the HPD attenuation against high-frequency noise, M against medium-frequency noise, and L against low frequency noise. SNR is overall attenuation against typical industrial noise.

Effect of the usage rate

Figure 28.5 shows the importance of usage rate when hearing protectors are worn. If a 30-dB hearing protector is used for only 4 h out of 8 h a day, the effectiveness of HPDs is not more than 3 dB.

The best HPD is one with a usage rate of 100%. This emphasizes the importance of comfort of HPDs. Relatively low minimum requirements for attenuation may allow for the manufacturers to develop more lightweight and, especially, more comfortable devices according to the new standards.[38,40]

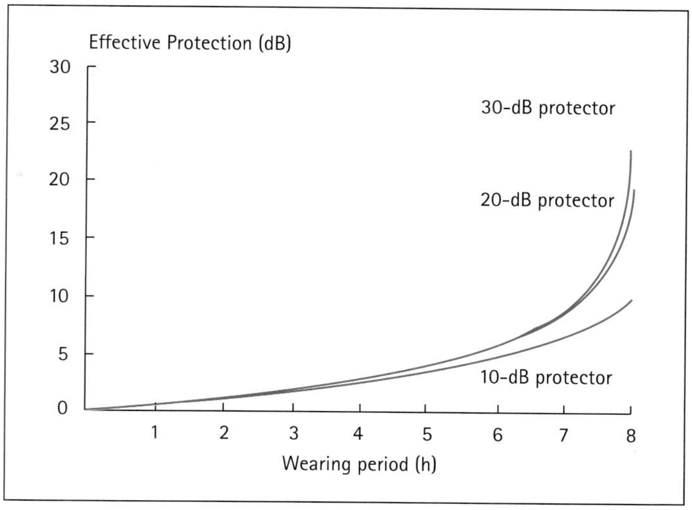

Figure 28.5 Reduction of effectiveness of hearing protectors with decreased usage rate.

User education and training for the development of HCPs

The use of HPDs has a significant impact on protection against environmental noise.[34,41] In a database, attenuation of an HPD is retrieved from the result of the type tests. However, even with the most sophisticated protectors, the average noise attenuation in practice may not be more than 17 dB when measured with the miniature microphone method.[42,43] In 10% of the workers examined, the attenuation of HPDs was less than 5 dB.[44] The same studies indicated that HPDs attenuate industrial impulse noise even more effectively than steady-state noise. This is due to the high-frequency content of the impulses, which are attenuated effectively by earmuffs. The efficiency of the attenuation also depends on environmental factors. Thus in a cold environment, as in forest work in Nordic countries, the stiffening of the cushion rings causes a slight but systematic worsening in the attenuation.[45] The deterioration of the cushions and the reduction in their spring force also affects attenuation. In the winter, northern forest workers use helmet liners, which in some cases nullify the attenuation of the hearing protectors.[33] All of these factors tend to reduce the protection efficiency of HPDs. Thus, the values provided for the HPDs are frequently overestimations of the attenuation in actual working conditions and reduce the efficacy of HCPs.

Table 28.1 Attenuation requirements (APV_f) for hearing protectors at octave bands

Frequency (Hz)	125	250	500	1000	2000	4000	8000
APV_{f84}(dB)	5	8	10	12	12	12	12

ATTENUATION OF HPDs (MEAN 17 dB)

- Education
- Usage rate
- Condition of cushion rings
- Shape of the skull

The reduction of noise exposure by HPDs is most effective in motivated users. Low motivation to wear HPDs is seen as low usage rate and respectively as low attenuation values.[46] Motivation to use HPDs can be obtained via appropriate education and training. Users need training on maintenance, installation and use of HPDs. The attenuation of protectors remains good only if they are well maintained.[40] Good maintenance consists of cleaning, changing of replaceable parts like cushions, and overall monitoring of the state of the HPD. Usage must be established before entering the noisy area.[40] If earplugs are used, special attention to the proper installation technique must be paid.[46,47] According to recommendations, the users must be informed about the effects of noise and the risks in their workplace (89/188/EC). The most informative approach is to use personal audiometric data.[48]

Other noise exposure

Military service and noise exposure

Exposure to assault rifle noise and bazookas often damages the hearing of conscripts. It is noteworthy that a single shot at a noise level exceeding 140 dB can have a measurable effect on hearing.[49] Even a few shots with bazookas or artillery, when the immission noise level exceeds 170 dB (for heavy bazookas, 184 dB), may be detrimental to hearing.[32] The military noise exposure of conscripts, especially during the handling of heavy weapons, causes an average of 5-dB hearing loss at 4000 Hz.[31] Thus exposure to military noise in humans may cause a significant threshold shift in hearing that is commonly disregarded when occupational NIHL is evaluated. At present, military noise causes hearing loss in 10% of conscripts. This is mainly due to shooting with blanks in forest rehearsals, when HPDs are not worn.

Exposure to leisure time noise

The most frequent leisure time hazard is exposure to music. The highest music exposure rates are from rock music. The noise level in a concert or a disco exceeds, in general, 100 dB(A). Thus only one attendance in a week causes an exposure that exceeds the occupational action limit. Similar levels are reported in the users of portable cassette recorders (for review see Clarck[50]). With classical music the levels are lower, but the musicians still have a risk of hearing loss. Among musicians, the use of HPDs is low, but is increasing, notably during rehearsals.[41] The role of music in NIHL is not well understood. In many studies conducted among young people, no changes in the audiogram have been found.[51] It has been suggested that the effect of music exposure would show up later. This is in accordance with a study in which people attending discotheques were three times more likely to complain of tinnitus than those who seldom visited discotheques. The severity of tinnitus was shown to correlate with hearing loss.[51]

Other exposures

Smoking

Tobacco smoking has been linked to hearing loss in population studies.[52] Thus, it could be expected that smoking acts as a risk factor for NIHL. Smoking in combination with noise exposure or other risk factors has been shown to significantly aggravate NIHL.[53] However, some authors[54–56] were not able to demonstrate that smoking was a risk factor for NIHL. This may be due to the fact that the effect of smoking may be confounded by other risk factors, e.g. ageing, elevated blood pressure and vibration-induced white finger disease (VWF), and therefore remains silent in the statistical analysis.[56]

Analgesics

The effect of indomethacin-type pain-alleviating drugs on hearing loss, as regards acute, toxic effects, is well documented in the literature, but little is known about long-term effects. The same is true for salicylates. After high doses of salicylates, very few morphological changes occur in the inner ear.[57] Hawkins[58] was one of the first workers to demonstrate that salicylates reduce cochlear bloodflow by causing capillary narrowing. The narrowing of vessels appears to be caused by swollen endothelial cells and possibly pericyte contraction.[59] In humans, the critical ototoxic salicylate level is high,[60] corresponding to the ingestion of 10–15 g salicylic acid a day.[61] The acute effect on hearing is characterized by a sudden onset, but is reversed within 1–10 days.[57]

Acute exposure to noise seems to increase the hearing loss induced by salicylates. Eddy et al.[62] demonstrated in acute experiments on chinchillas that a TTS produced by combined noise (85 dB) and salicylates (20–40 mg/100 mg) was significantly greater (55 dB) than that produced by noise (35 dB) or salicylates (30 dB) alone. So far, it is not known whether salicylates in combination with environmental noise would increase the likelihood of a permanent NIHL. Miller et al.[63] showed that salicylates, in very low doses, may act as free oxygen scavengers and protect hearing from noise damage. The exclusion of salicylate consumers from the rest of the forest workers in one study improved the average hearing level by 0.9 dB.[64] Such an increase may be substantial, though not statistically significant, and supports the theory that even moderate use of salicylates in conjunction with environmental noise may be hazardous to cochlear function.

Organic solvents

Exposure to organic solvents and noise has a synergistic damaging effect on hearing. In a paper mill, workers in the chemical section (exposed to organic solvents) showed a pronounced NIHL in spite of lower noise levels (80–90 dB) that was in contrast to the workers in a non-chemical section, who had higher noise levels of 95–100 dB.[65] According to Morata et al,[66] exposure to toluene and noise increased the relative risk of hearing loss by 11 times among rotogravure printing workers. Exposure to noise or toluene increased the risk of NIHL by four and by five times, respectively.[66] The effect of solvents seems to depend on the solvent concentration. In the glass-fibre reinforced plastic industry in the Netherlands, Muijser et al.[67] found that with higher levels of styrene there was a significant change in hearing threshold at high frequencies. In animal experiments, noise combined with a high level of styrene (600 ppm/m^2) caused a threshold shift in hearing of 25 dB.[68] When the animals were exposed to noise or styrene alone, the respective hearing losses were 3 and 5 dB, respectively. Such a high level of styrene is seldom encountered in industry, and the solvent-linked NIHL must be less than 25 dB in humans.

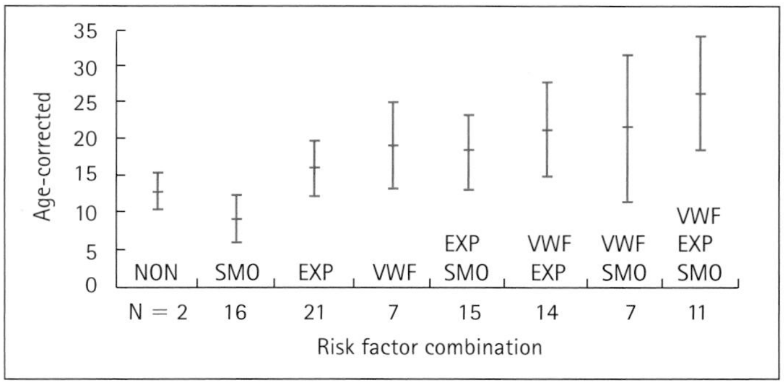

Figure 28.6 Age-corrected hearing level among forest workers due to various risk factors separately and in combination. NON, no risk factors; SMO, smoking; EXP, exposure; VWF, vibration white finger.

Individual risk factors

Individual susceptibility to NIHL seems also to depend on biological factors (for a review see Ward[69]). The findings of Rosen et al.[70] and Rosen and Olin[71] suggested that major cardiovascular risk factors, such as elevated total cholesterol, promote hearing loss. The factors discussed most commonly are cholesterol level, blood pressure, and presence of VWF.[72] Any database should contain information on these factors. The cholesterol level is correlated with hearing loss, and when combined with noise exposure and hypertension, produces more prominent hearing loss than each factor alone.[72] We have calculated that an elevated cholesterol level alone explains about 2–4 dB of hearing loss at a frequency of 4 kHz.[64] This cholesterol-linked hearing loss is age-dependent and is observed in subjects aged 40 years or over. The effect of total cholesterol on hearing may be mediated as a 'small vessel disease', as indicated by Pillsbury,[73] but may also be a direct effect on outer hair cells in the cochlea. Oghalai et al[74] demonstrated cholesterol in the lateral wall of the outer hair cells, and Nguyen and Brownell[75] observed that elevated total cholesterol reduces the stiffness of the outer hair cells leading to deterioration of hearing.

Hypertension significantly reduces hearing,[76,77] especially at 4 kHz. The effect of hypertension on hearing is still under discussion as some researchers find that noise is the reason for hypertension, and these factors jointly cause the adverse effects on hearing.[78] The other possibility is that noise and hypertension independently or in combination cause hearing loss. Animal studies have indicated that hypertension accelerates age-related hearing loss.[76,79] In epidemiological studies, the antihypertensive medication may partly mask the effect of elevated blood pressure on NIHL, as antihypertensive subjects under medication have normal or near normal blood pressure.[64]

Smoking together with hypertension increases NIHL.[7] The connection between smoking and hearing level may be confounded by cessation of smoking.[80] Smoking together with hypertension heightens the role of smoking in causing NIHL.[80] At present, there is not sufficient evidence to show whether the effects of noise and hypertension are additive or synergistic.

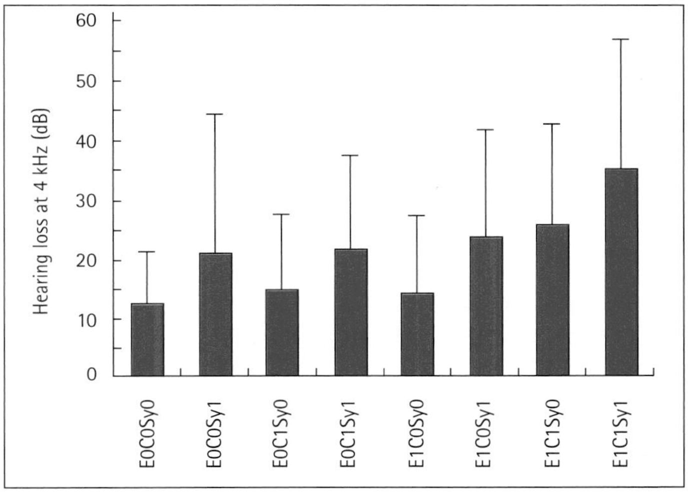

Figure 28.7 Effect of exposure to cholesterol and systolic blood pressure on hearing. E, exposure; C, cholesterol; Sy, systolic blood pressure; 0, below median; 1, above median.

VWF syndrome is a risk factor that causes about 10 dB greater hearing loss than if this syndrome were not present.[7,55,80] The effect of VWF and noise seems to be synergistic (Figure 28.6). Also the effects of cholesterol and hypertension are synergistic when the exposure to noise is long duration (Figure 28.7).

Genetic factors

Genetically induced hearing loss may occur in a hereditary or sporadic form.[81] In syndromic form it is relatively easy to detect, but in non-syndromic form it is often difficult to separate from NIHL. It is often age-dependent and increases with ageing. In the extension of the Framingham study, a good correlation was found with early onset of hearing loss and extent of presbyacusis within the family.[82] In men, the relationship was not as evident as in females, possibly because environmental noise was a confounding factor.[82] The genetic background of non-syndromic hearing loss is heterogeneous, and to date 33 different gene loci for non-syndromic hearing loss have been defined

(13 autosomal recessive hearing loss, 13 autosomal dominant hearing loss, 5 X-linked HL and two mitochondrial mutations).[2] Of these gene mutations, the connexin 26 (Cx26) mutation is most frequent and can be observed in 3% of the population.[83] In recessive form, the Cx26 mutation is observed in 50% of the population.[83]

There are insufficient data available on the relationship between NIHL and genetic background. One study indicated that analgesics and military noise exposure aggravated the hearing loss but the connection is not evident in occupational noise exposure.[84] Such data are urgently needed, as they could explain the great variability in noise vulnerability in population studies. The results of the Framingham study indicate that genetic factors play a significant role in the development of age-dependent hearing loss and consequently in NIHL. In future, subjects with indications of genetically induced hearing loss might be tested for a possible defect in the Cx26 gene and possibly also for some mitochondrial defects. The number of new known gene mutations is constantly increasing, and the readers are advised to look at the home page for genetic hearing loss.[2]

Hearing measurements

TO CONTROL IN AUDIOLOGICAL EVALUATION:

- Type of audiometry
- Annual calibration of audiometry
- Sound isolation of booth

Audiometry

Such technical factors as measurements of hearing threshold level with clinical, automatic or screening audiometer may cause considerable differences in HCP between various work plants. Melnick[11] proposed that in clinical audiometry a 10-dB hearing level (HL) shift at any frequency is significant but in screening audiometry, a 15-dB HL shift should be considered significant. The automatic audiometer using 1-dB HL steps may be more accurate than the clinical audiometer, which uses 5-dB HL steps,[85] since greater variability was found in clinical audiometry than in automatic audiometers. They consequently proposed the use of automatic audiometry in screening hearing in industry. Nevertheless, the automatic audiometer, using 1-dB steps, is not inherently more accurate than clinical audiometry, provided that in routine use the standardized procedure is strictly followed.[86]

The background noise of a soundproof room is seldom measured, and in many cases hearing is measured in non-isolated but quiet rooms. These do not allow the measurement of hearing threshold levels down to 0 dB. Automatic audiometers may introduce another error in the measurement if the test environment does not fulfil the requirements for ambient noise. At frequencies where thresholds exceed the screening level, they are measured with essentially the same accuracy and reliability as in a clinical procedure. Moreover, Royster and Royster[87] pointed out that audiometer calibration should be adequately carried out, as otherwise the audiometry results may be biased. In addition to relevant calibration, these authors proposed that normal controls with normal hearing be mixed with the noise-exposed population. Finally, the quality of audiometric data is dependent on training, education and attention, of both subject and tester. A shortage of information on the purpose of the test, and careless recording of threshold values and control of background noise, may severely reduce the value of the audiometric data.

Any database should include data on the type and calibration of the audiometer and the quality of the soundproof room where the tests took place.

HEARING MEASUREMENT:

Audiometry
- Clinical audiometry
- Screening audiometry
- Automatic audiometry

Otoacoustic emissions
- Spontaneous
- Transient
- Distortion product
- Contralateral inhibition

High-frequency audiometry

Otoacoustic emission

The term otoacoustic emission (OAE) refers to sounds emitted by the ear.[88] The emitted sounds originate from the outer hair cells and may be helpful in the early identification of sensorineural hearing loss (SNHL) caused by occupational noise exposure. Three OAE forms exist, all of which are evoked by particular stimuli. In the normal ear, spontaneous otoacoustic emissions (SOAEs) are present in the absence of acoustical stimulation among 70% of the subjects. After even subtle lesion, the SPOAEs seem to disappear.[89] Transient evoked otoacoustic emissions (TEOAEs) are elicited by brief stimuli, such as clicks or tone pips. Distortion-product otoacoustic emissions (DPOAEs) are elicited by the non-linear interaction of two simultaneous, long-lasting pure tones.[90] The evoking tones are referred to as the f1 and f2 primaries in humans, the largest DPOAE occurs at the frequency equivalent to 2f1–f2.

Contralateral inhibition of distortion product (DPI) is recognized by the reduction in the amplitude of evoked OAE upon stimulation of the opposite ear. The OAE is vulnerable to noxious stimuli, such as ototoxic drugs, intense noise and hypoxia, which are all known to affect the cochlea. They are absent with cochlear hearing loss greater than 35 dB. The type of OAE most commonly used for clinical purposes is TEOAE. TEOAEs are attractive for use as a screening procedure, as the test procedure is short and no cooperation of the subject is needed. DPOAEs may be more sensitive than TEOAEs in discriminating subjects with NIHL.[91] However, an analysis of the efficacy of OAEs in assessing NIHL is not yet available. So far, few databases exist with data on OAE.

High-frequency audiometry

High-frequency audiometry refers to threshold testing at frequencies from 8 kHz to 20 kHz. It is assumed that high-frequency audiometry assists in the early detection of NIHL, revealing hearing impairment before it is detectable at the frequencies normally measured. In NIHL, improvement in hearing may be seen at 10 kHz, 12 kHz and 14 kHz. In age-related hearing loss, this may not be observed.[41]

In high-frequency audiometry, thresholds tend to deteriorate after the age of 18–24 years.[92] High-frequency audiometry seems to be of value among young subjects with normal hearing before any noise-induced alteration in hearing. The use of high-frequency audiometry is limited by the reliability and repeatability of such audiometers,[93] and, so far, few databases exist with data on high-frequency audiometry.

Construction of a database

Interface

The interface between the computer program and the user must satisfy several demands: it must be user-friendly, i.e. the content of the questions and input data must be easy to comprehend, and it must be self-controlling for input errors. It must be self-explanatory and, when needed, provide help for inputting or using the interface. Recently, the graphical display has surpassed the traditional string commands. The advantage of the graphical display is that the item can be selected easily by one hand, and interest can be focused constantly on the item on the screen. The objects on the screen can be self-explanatory and, accordingly, easy to understand.

An example of the interface for entering data or evaluating data on the expert program 'NoiseScan' is provided in Figure 28.8. In the program, several buttons are provided on the computer screen. However, only those that are relevant for the current tasks are activated, and, when selected, the explanatory text is displayed in red at the bottom of the screen.

Work noise

An unlimited number of exposure periods can be entered, with data on the possible impulsiveness, usage of HPDs and frequency content of noise (Figure 28.9). The program calculates the total occupational exposure to noise, considering the protection efficiency of HPDs and the usage rate. In the case of missing exposure data, the program helps to make an estimate from the results in the register of employment measurements. The attenuation of HPDs is evaluated using the HML-check method of the standard EN 458.[40]

Other exposure

Information regarding smoking, the use of analgesics and exposure to solvents is entered with respect to time periods. Smokers are divided into non-smokers, smokers and heavy smokers. A similar division is made for the use of analgesics. Exposure to solvents is indicated with a yes/no answer.

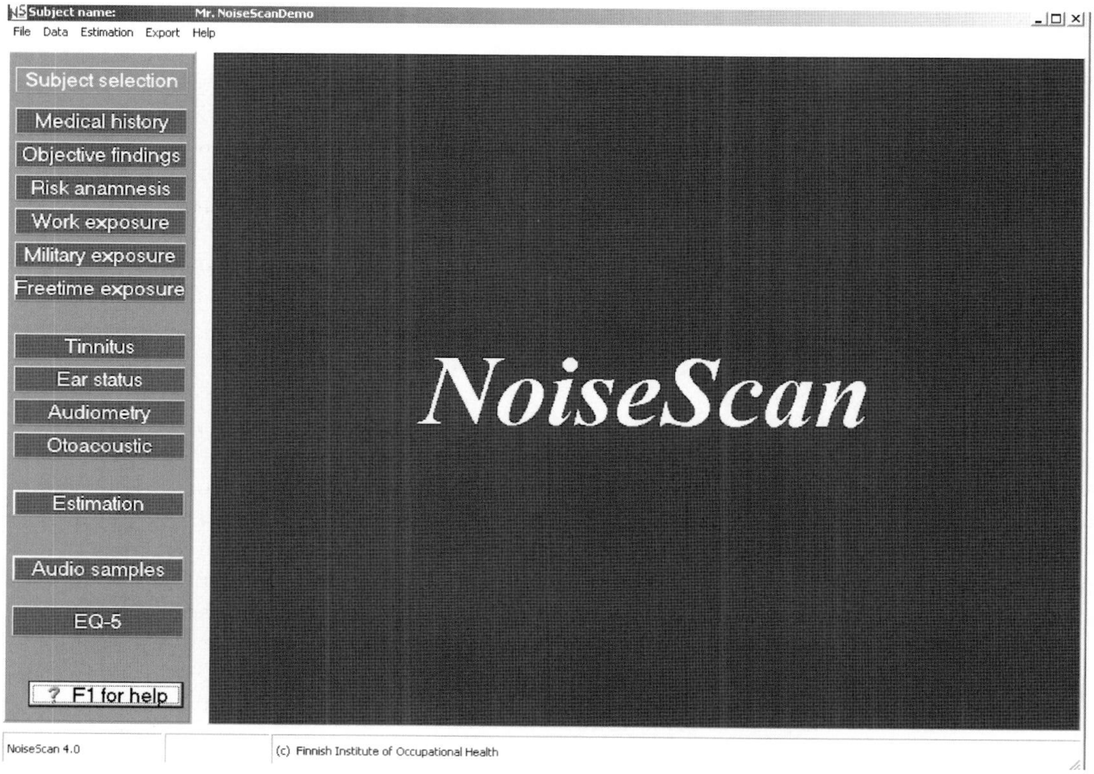

Figure 28.8 Main screen of the database for the expert programme 'NoiseScan'.

Other noise exposure

The recorded non-occupational noise exposures include music, shooting, use of power tools and exposure during military service. All these exposures are collected in periods. The form used for the collection of military service exposure is also used to collect exposure data for professional soldiers.

Music exposure is considered in detail. Rock playing, classical playing, use of portable stereos and visits to discos are identified separately. For each activity, evaluations of the loudness and the use of HPDs are sought (Figure 28.10). On the same form, there are questions about the use of power tools, public noise events and shooting. Some questions are also added about leisure time exposure to solvents.

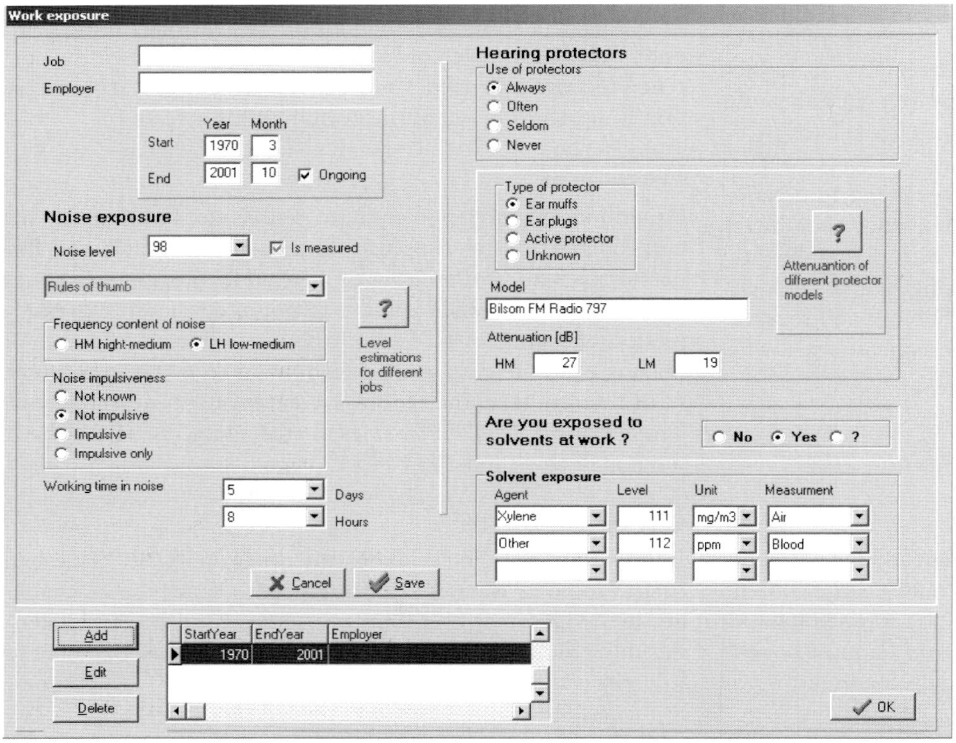

Figure 28.9 Data sheet for work noise.

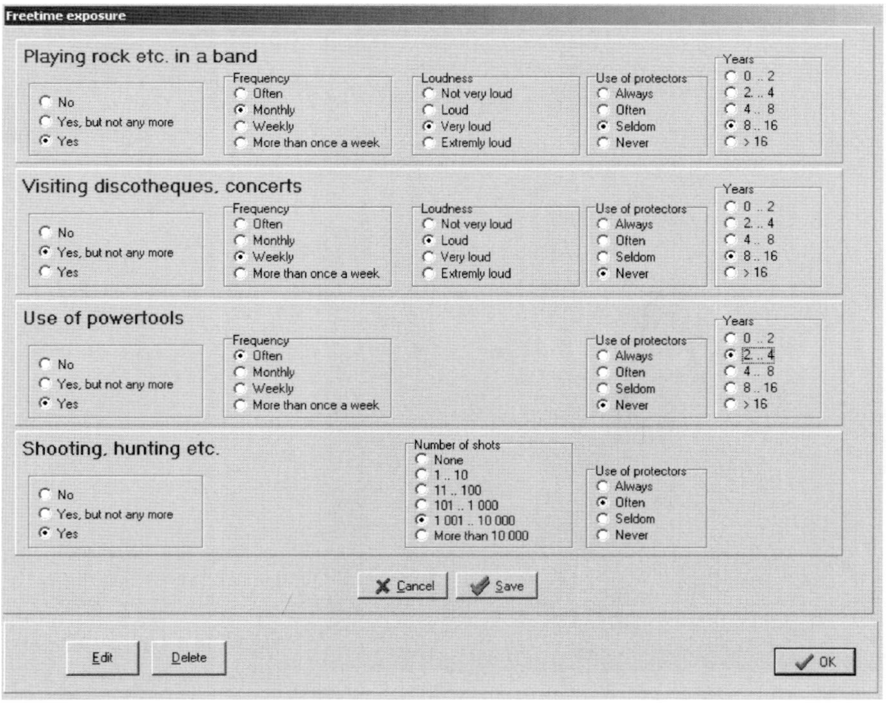

Figure 28.10 Questionnaire screen for free time exposure.

Control parameters

Hereditary factors are identified on a separate sheet for those people having an early hearing loss or relatives with early hearing loss. Skin sensitivity to sun is also identified, as subjects sensitive to sunburn are reported to develop greater NIHL.[94,95]

The individual susceptibility factors consist of blood pressure readings and cholesterol level. These factors are collected during each study occasion for each employee.

In addition to the above factors, other health-related symptoms or factors which may explain hearing loss are collected. Such factors include ear infections, ear surgery, skull and head trauma, vertigo, ototoxic drugs, central nervous system disorders, migraine and possible central nervous system infections.

Prediction of hearing level

NoiseScan provides two models for hearing level prediction, the ISO 1999–1990 model and the NoiseScan model.

The ISO 1999 model takes as input the work noise level outside the HPD.[3] Based on this figure, the ISO 1999 model gives the distribution of hearing losses. NoiseScan provides the prediction based on population A (screened population) of ISO 1999.[21] NoiseScan prints the latest audiogram on top of these statistical curves. In addition, NoiseScan evaluates on the same screen the possible other sources of exposure, i.e. free-time noise and military noise.

Unlike the ISO 1999 model, the NoiseScan model tries to predict the NIHL at an individual level. For this purpose the NoiseScan model utilizes as input the individual risk factors (Figure 28.11). In distinction to the ISO 1999 model, the NoiseScan models use the total noise exposure to the ear as the input parameter.[96]

Finally, NoiseScan calculates a prediction of the likely progression of the NIHL based on the assumption that the present exposure with the present use of HPDs continues. For simulation purposes, NoiseScan provides the possibility of predicting the effect of full-time use of protectors.

Mechanism for cellular vulnerability to noise

So far, no database has collected systematic information on possible preventive agents of NIHL, such as dietary antioxidants, dietary supplements competing with calcium homeostasis or drugs effective in blocking the *N*-methyl-D-aspartate (NMDA) receptors.

In the Israeli army, Attias et al.[97] have successfully given Mg^{2+} ions as a dietary supplement to prevent the accumulation of Ca^{2+} in hair cells and reduce NIHL. Small doses of acetylsalicylic acid may rescue hair cells from noise damage.[98] Other drugs that may be used to rescue hair cells are melatonin,[99] iron chelators,[100] dietary glutathione,[100] and NMDA antagonists.[98] Therefore, various drugs and dietary supplements are constitute relevant information to include in a database.

In the following, a short summary of the postulated mechanisms leading to NIHL is given. Most research has focused on the structural results of noise exposure and has correlated damaged stereocilia bundles or missing hair cells with hearing dysfunction. However, information on the cellular and subcellular

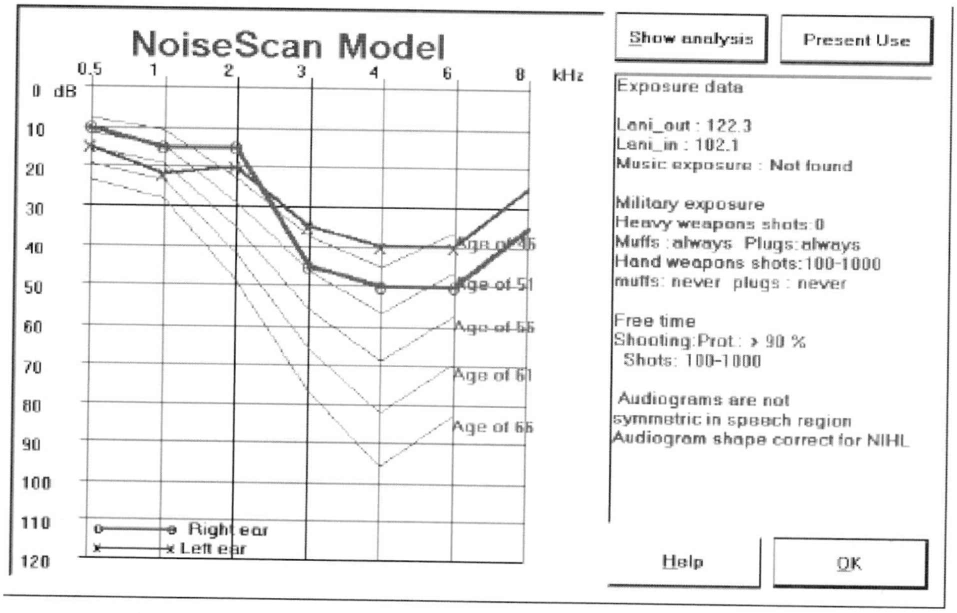

Figure 28.11 NoiseScan model. NoiseScan displays the latest audiogram for right and left ears and predicts the development of NIHL in 5-year intervals. Exposure data are summarized and the comparison of the configuration forms of audiograms is made.

processes involved is sparse. In addition, as the importance of the 'cochlear amplifier' for auditory performance is now generally accepted, injury processes related to the outer hair cell body must be recognized as being as significant as those of the sensory hair bundles.

Normal auditory stimulation elicits pressure differences across the cochlear partition, causing a number of mechanical events within the organ of Corti: vibrations, shearing motion, and stereocilia deflection (for a review see Ulfendahl[101]). The end-result is excitation of the outer and inner hair cells, and, following release of transmitter substances, increased activity in the auditory nerve. Obviously, noise or excessive auditory stimulation will elicit similar events but at much larger amplitudes. There are two fundamentally different ways in which overstimulation may lead to cochlear injury: mechanical or metabolic.[102] Large-amplitude motion may mechanically alter or disrupt cochlear structures. Cellular distortion, disorganization of stereocilia and possible ruptures of cell membranes disable the cochlear fluid barriers and cause immediate reduction of auditory sensitivity.[103–110]

On the other hand, sound-induced overstimulation and overactivity of the cochlea can result in disturbed cochlear homeostasis and subsequent functional impairment, in the absence of direct and immediate mechanical damage. Experimental evidence suggests a critical level around 125 dB SPL,[111] at which the cause of damage changes from predominantly metabolic to mechanical. Thus, at moderate sound pressure levels, damage would mainly be caused by metabolic mechanisms, while at higher levels, mechanical mechanisms would dominate. As changes in homeostasis will occur also after mechanical trauma, and the effects of metabolic stress are also likely to be expressed as mechanical damage, it is not meaningful to make a strict separation between metabolic and mechanical causes of NIHL.

There are several steps leading from acoustical overstimulation to cellular damage (Figure 28.12). Some of the mechanisms are mainly related to metabolic changes, e.g. oxidative stress, synaptic hyperactivity and altered cochlear bloodflow, while others are predominantly mechanical. It is likely, however, that the resulting damage to the auditory system is partly mediated by similar mechanisms, irrespective of the cause. Although definite evidence of a 'common final pathway' is missing, experimental data suggest that free radicals and other highly reactive endogenous substances play a significant role in NIHL.

PROTECTION AGAINST NOISE:

- Antioxidants
- Ca^{2+} antagonists
- NMDA receptor blockers
- Growth factors

It is well known from other biological systems that reactive oxygen metabolites (ROMs) are important mediators of cell injury. ROMs are free radicals or other molecules which have a chemical structure that makes them extremely reactive. As they react very easily with cellular components such as lipids, proteins and DNA, they are potentially cytotoxic. ROMs are produced continuously as part of normally occurring reactions, e.g. in the mitochondria. However, protection is offered by several endogenous antioxidants. These are either enzymes

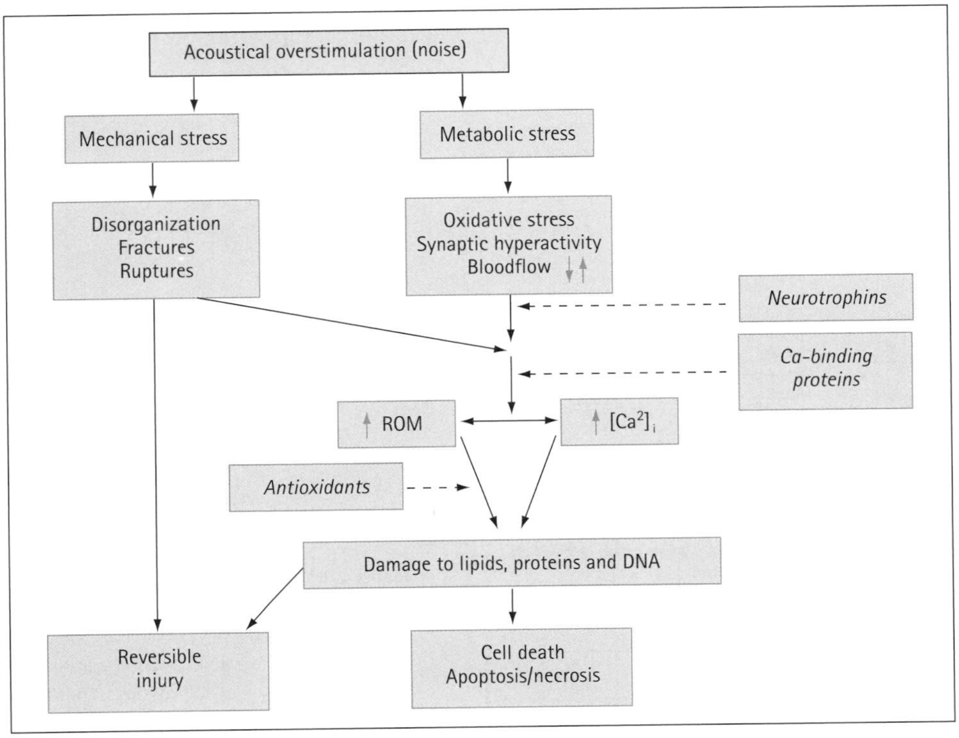

Figure 28.12 Pathways for noise-induced injury to the peripheral auditory system. ROM, reactive oxygen metabolites; Ca, calcium. (Modified after J.M. Miller, personal communication.)

catalysing reactions neutralizing the ROMs, or scavengers binding them. When there is an imbalance between the production of ROMs and the endogenous protective mechanisms, the tissue is under oxidative stress. Increased ROM production can cause cell death, whereas overactive protective mechanisms may lead to tumour growth. In the auditory system there are several reports demonstrating elevated levels of either ROMs or antioxidants following noise exposure,[8,112,113] and reduced hearing loss after treatments increasing antioxidant levels.[100,114,115]

During intense sound exposure, the inner hair cells are overstimulated, resulting in synaptic hyperactivity and an excessive release of transmitter substance. The afferent neurotransmitter is most likely glutamate, which, like other excitatory amino acids, has toxic effects when released in large amounts. The resulting overstimulation of the glutamate receptors elicits inflow of calcium ions, which in combination with other ions bring about the entry of water and subsequent swelling of the nerve endings. The result may be a total disruption of the synapses between the inner hair cells and the afferent nerve fibres in the auditory nerve.[116]

POSSIBLE ROM SCAVENGERS:

- Glutathione
- *N*-acetylcysteine
- Ascorbic acid
- Salicylic acid
- Melatonin
- α-Tocopherol
- Iron chelator (desferrioxamine)
- Mannitol

Changes in cochlear bloodflow have generally been suggested to contribute to NIHL.[63,117–119] Recent findings have clearly demonstrated noise-induced alterations in cochlear microcirculation causing local ischaemia.[120,121] The effect varies with intensity and duration of the exposure, but when vascular insufficiency is manifest, the reduced oxygen and energy supply to the cochlea, and the accumulation of metabolites, will be accompanied by severe functional alterations. It has been shown experimentally that applying drugs blocking vasoconstriction prevents noise-induced microcirculatory ischaemia, and maintains normal hearing thresholds.[122] However, the exact role of local bloodflow alterations is unclear, and it should be noted that it has been observed that hearing loss and cochlear hypoxia may actually precede changes in cochlear bloodflow.[120]

In addition to the accumulation of ROMs seen following metabolic and/or mechanical stress, it has been demonstrated that acoustical overstimulation leads to a significant rise in intracellular calcium levels in the outer hair cells.[123,124] A sustained increase in the intracellular calcium concentration is known to elicit severe cell injuries, such us cytoskeletal breakdown, membrane defects and DNA damage.[125,126] One probable consequence of the increased calcium concentration in the outer hair cells is the loss of cell body stiffness observed after intense acoustical stimulation.[127] Moreover, a structural reorganization of the organ of Corti has recently been demonstrated following acoustical overstimulation.[103] The noise-induced changes in cellular stiffness and structure of the hearing organ seem to be at least partly reversible, and the results may thus contribute to knowledge about mechanisms underlying reversible injuries.

When the metabolic and/or mechanical stress is too large, the cells die and a permanent hearing loss is manifest. Cell death is a result of either apoptosis or necrosis. Apoptosis is a strictly controlled process to eliminate dysfunctional cells without affecting surrounding tissue. It can be viewed as a counterbalance to cell division, and a disturbance may, for example, result in degenerative disorders or tumour growth. Necrosis, on the other hand, is a more passive type of cell death, involving a rapid and disorganized breakdown of a cell, often as a consequence of acute trauma (toxic substances, ischaemia, etc.). As the cell contents are released directly into the surrounding tissue, an inflammatory reaction usually follows. Thus, for the organism, apoptosis is the preferred method when it is necessary to eliminate cells. In the auditory system there is no conclusive evidence that apoptosis plays a significant role. Structural observations of DNA fragmentation may suggest the involvement of either apoptotic[128] or necrotic mechanisms[129] during peri- and postnatal development of the inner ear. One study on autopsy material from subjects with no history of acoustical trauma suggests that apoptosis does not contribute significantly to the regulation of the cell population in the normal adult inner ear.[130] Nevertheless, apoptosis may be involved during noise-induced trauma, although there is, to date, no such evidence.

Increased knowledge of the processes leading to cell injuries is of fundamental importance in order to develop clinical means for protection and repair. Many recent reports on the protection against noise-induced hearing loss offered by drugs like antioxidants and neurotrophins are promising for the future.

Diagnosis of noise-induced hearing loss

DIAGNOSIS OF NOISE-INDUCED HEARING LOSS SHOULD BE BASED ON:

- Relevant exposure data
- Shape of the audiogram (high-frequency hearing loss)
- Symmetry of audiograms between both ears (mean of speech frequencies not exceeding 10 dB between the ears).

According to ISO 1999–1990, noise vulnerability is linked to A-weighted sound energy entering the ear. No changes are to be expected at speech frequencies in the audiogram if the A-weighted equivalent noise level is less than 80 dB. However, in most countries, if compensation is to be awarded a higher level of 85 or 90 dB(A) is required. The criteria for NIHL are country-dependent, and may include other criteria than those related to the audiogram, such as speech intelligibility. In scientific papers, the criterion for acceptance of evidence of NIHL is a mean hearing loss of 25 dB across the speech frequencies. Usually, the NIHL starts in the 3–6-kHz area, where a typical notch in the audiogram can be observed. When the noise damage increases, the notch becomes wider and deeper, and later the audiogram starts to flatten, indicating damage at speech frequencies. With prolonged and very severe noise exposure, the NIHL levels out across the high frequencies at 60–80 dB HL but the low frequencies are less affected than the high frequencies. Usually both ears are involved to the same extent, and if the difference at speech frequencies exceeds 10 dB HL, the inner ear damage should be assumed to be complicated by other factors than noise. These criteria are helpful for diagnosing NHL and facilitating differentiation from other high-tone SNHL.

PROBLEMS IN AUDIOMETRIC EVALUATION

1. No baseline audiogram for an employer. Underlining ear disorders may confound NIHL.
2. Inadequate instructions in measurement. Variable hearing test results.
3. Ears not inspected (wax, foreign body). Hearing results variable.
4. A 16-h noise free period not honoured, allowing TTS to bias movement.
5. Noisy background in the hearing test room. Difficult to evaluate correct hearing level.
6. Background noise during testing not exceeding 40 dB(A). Difficult to evaluate correct hearing level.

The primary goal of an industrial HCP must be the prevention (or, at least, limitation) of NIHL associated with exposure to industrial noise.[85] Other goals may be formulated in addition to this primary goal, such as reduction of employee stress and absenteeism, and reduction of workplace accidents. An HCP is costly and demands resources and personnel. Often, due to these factors, only selected personnel are tested audiologically. Newly employed persons are not always tested. If a hearing test is not carried out before a person starts work, it may be difficult later to show that the hearing loss is of pre-employment origin. It is strongly recommended that all persons entering jobs with a risk of development of NIHL should be tested.

Often, the people who carry out industrial audiometry have little experience and education in the field. Earwax may not be removed, and the ears may not have been inspected. We often observe workers with blocked ear canals or with noise protection cotton in the ear canal, and such situations may cause unexpected hearing threshold shifts in audiometry. On certain occasions, the subject may not understand the instructions and may provide inaccurate responses and an unreliable audiogram. Instructions should be simple and given verbally before the test. Importantly, the noise-free period should be 16 h to allow hearing threshold measurement that is free from TTS caused by environmental or occupational noise. Therefore, the test should be done first thing in the morning and the subject should not have been exposed to noise the previous evening. Attention should be paid to the background noise of the audiometry booth, and this noise should be measured, as even at low frequencies it may mask the tone pips in the audiometric frequencies such that 0-dB threshold values cannot be measured. As a rule, the background should not exceed 30 dB(A) in the booth, to allow 0-dB threshold values to be measured. In industry, screening audiometry is performed for 25-dB hearing level at any frequency. For this purpose, background noise should not exceed 40 dB(A) in the booth.

Who then should be referred to an otologist? A worker with a 10-dB hearing change at two frequencies between the last two audiograms should be referred, as the change may indicate NIHL or an ear disorder. Also, if the threshold shift is greater than 25 dB at any frequency, the worker should be referred to an otologist. The American Academy of Otolaryngology—Head and Neck Surgery has provided proposals for the referral (AAO-HNS 1983).

In addition, to complete the exposure history and audiograms, the case history must have documented other factors that may cause SNHL. These include the possible use of ototoxic drugs such as streptomycin and cis-platinum. Heavy use of anti-inflammatory agents such as salicylates and indomethacin-type antiphlogistics may cause reversible or non-reversible hearing loss and aggravate the NIHL.[96] Some inner ear diseases, such as idiopathic tinnitus, Menière's disease, otosclerosis, and sudden deafness, may begin with a pure inner ear component affecting only hearing or masking the hearing, as tinnitus may do. Infectious ear diseases, such as chronic otitis media or tympanosclerosis, cause hearing loss. Hereditary hearing losses, either symptomatic or asymptomatic, may be difficult to detect, as these occur in about half of the cases. So far, it is not known whether genetic (hereditary) hearing loss is more susceptible to NIHL. However, general opinion favours the idea of increased vulnerability or predisposition. Therefore, for subjects with a family history of deafness, the use of ear protection is a must, and sometimes changes of work or working tasks are advisable. Furthermore, it is worth mentioning that the most common genetic disorder is connexin 26 (*DNFB3*). It is present in 3% of the population.

Summary

The aim of developing an industrial database for hearing conservation is four-fold. It includes: (1) screening of workers who may be at risk of developing NIHL in selected work tasks or sites; (2) warning against excessive noise pollution in selected work tasks or sites; (3) allowing the comparative assessment of success among various Hips, and finally (4) calling attention to individual susceptibility. To fulfil these demands, the database must include all known factors that affect hearing loss. Such factors are audiometric testing methods, the testing environment, efficiency of the HPDs, and exposure to military and leisure time noise. It must provide accurate data from lifetime noise exposure in various jobs or work tasks. The database must also have adequate information on the type and use of HPDs. Finally, confounding factors must be controlled, such as elevated blood pressure, the presence of VWF syndrome, elevated serum cholesterol level, and use of various ototoxic drugs. Such factors can explain a significant variation in the extent of hearing loss in individual cases. In the present database, we have attempted to include such factors, known to be relevant for the HCP.

References

1. Koton S, Ifrah A, Lerman Y et al. Worker's health in Israel. *Public Health Rev* 1998; **26**: 189–203.
2. Van Camp G, Smith RJH. Hereditary Hearing Loss Homepage. http://dnalab-www.uia.ac.be/dnalab/hhh.html
3. International Organization for Standardization. *Acoustics—Determination of Occupational Noise Exposure and Estimation of Noise-induced Hearing Impairment*, ISO1999–1990. Geneva: ISO 1990.
4. Robinson DW. Estimating the risk of hearing loss due to continuous noise. In: Robinson DW, ed. *Occupational Hearing Loss*. London: Academic Press, 1971.
5. Borg A, Canlon B, Engström B. Individual variability of noise-induced hearing loss. In: Dancer AL, Henderson D, Salvi RJ et al., eds. *Noise-Induced Hearing Loss*. St Louis: Mosby Year Book, 1992: 467–75.
6. Humes LE. Noise induced hearing loss as influenced by other agents and by some physical characteristics of the individual. *J Acoust Soc Am* 1984; **76**: 1318–29.
7. Pyykkö I, Pekkarinen J, Starck J. Sensory-neural hearing loss in forest workers. An analysis of risk factor. *Int Arch Occup Environ Health* 1986; **59**: 439–54.
8. Yamane H, Nakai Y, Takayama M et al. The emergence of free radicals after acoustic trauma and strial blood flow. *Acta Otolaryngol (Stockh) Suppl* 1995; **519**: 87–92.
9. International Organization for Standardization. *Acoustics—Guidelines for the Measurements and Assessment of Exposure to Noise in Working Environment*. ISO 9612.2. Geneva: ISO, 1997.
10. Kryter KD. Damage risk criterion and contours based on permanent and temporary hearing loss data. *J Am Ind Hyg Assoc* 1965; **26**: 34–44.
11. Melnick W. Evaluation of industrial hearing conservation programs: a review and analysis. *Am Ind Hyg Assoc J* 1984; **45**: 459–67.
12. Baughn WL. *Relation Between Daily Exposure and Hearing Loss Based on Evaluation of 6835 Industrial Noise Exposure Cases*. Dayton: Wright-Patterson Air Force Base, Report AMRL-TR-7353. US Air Force, 1973.
13. Burns W, Robinson DW. *Hearing and Noise in Industry*. Her Majesty's Stationery Office, 1960.
14. Robinson DB, Shipton MS. *Tables for the Estimation of Noise-induced Hearing Loss*. NPL Acoustics Report Ac. 61, 2nd edn. British ARC, 1977.
15. Robinson DW. *The Relationship between Hearing Loss and Noise Exposure*. NPL Aero Report Ac. 32. British ARC, 1968.
16. Burns W. Permanents effects of noise on hearing. In: Burns W, *Noise and Man* 2nd edn., London: John Murray, 1973.
17. Passchier-Vermeer W. Hearing loss due to continuous exposure to steady-state broad-band noise. *J Acoust Soc Am* 1974: **46**(5): 1585–93.
18. Glorig A, Nixon J. Distribution of hearing loss in various populations. *Ann Otol Rhinol Laryngol* 1980; **69**(2): 497–516.
19. Johnson D. *Prediction of NIPTS due to Continuous Noise Exposure*. Report No. AMRL-TR-73-91. US Air Force, 1973.
20. National Institute for Occupational Safety and Health (NIOSH). Occupational noise and hearing 1968–72. NIOSH Pub. No 74-116, 1974.
21. International Organization for Standardization. *Acoustics—Assessment of Occupational Noise Exposure for Hearing Conservation Purposes*. ISO 1999. Geneva: ISO, 1975.
22. Suter AH. The development of federal standard and damage risk criteria. In: Libscomb DM, ed. *Hearing Conservation in Industry, Schools, and the Military*. San Diego: Singular Publishing Group, 1994: 45–66.
23. Robinson DW, Sutton GJ. Age effects in hearing—a comparative analysis of published threshold data. *Audiology* 1979; **18**: 320–34.
24. Glorig A, Roberts J. *Hearing Levels of Adults by Age and Sex: United States 1960–1962*. Report PHS-PUB-100-SER-11-11. Nat Cent Health Serv Res and Dev, 1965.
25. Rowland M. *Basic Data on Hearing Levels of Adults 25–74 years*. DHEW Publication no. (PHS) 80-1663, series 11, no. 215. US Department of Health, Education and Welfare, 1980; 49p.
26. Starck J, Pekkarinen J. Industrial impulse noise: crest factor as an additional parameter in exposure measurements. *Appl Acoust* 1987; **20**: 263–74.
27. Pfander F. *Das Knalltrauma*. Berlin, Heidelberg, New York: Springer Verlag, 1975.
28. Ward D. Auditory effects of noise. In: Berger EH, Ward WD, Morrill JC, Royster LH, eds. *Noise and Hearing Conservation Manual*. AIHA, 1986.
29. Starck J, Pekkarinen J, Pyykkö I. Impulse noise and hand–arm vibration in relation to sensory neural hearing loss. *Scand J Work Environ Health* 1988: **14**: 265–71.
30. Ylikoski M, Ylikoski J. Hearing loss and handicap of professional soldiers exposed to gunfire noise. *Scand J Work Environ Health* 1994; **20**: 93–100.
31. Pekkarinen J, Iki M, Starck J et al. Hearing loss risk from exposure to shooting impulses in workers exposed to occupational noise. *Br J Audiol* 1993; **27**: 175–82.
32. Pekkarinen J, Starck J, Ylikoski J. Hearing protection against high level shooting impulses in relation to hearing damage. *J Acoust Soc Am* 1992; **91**: 196–202.
33. Starck J, Pekkarinen J, Aatola S. Attenuation of earmuffs against low frequency noise. *J Low Frequency Noise Vibration* 1987; **6**(4): 167–74.

34. Toppila E, Starck J, Pihlström A et al. The evaluation of protection efficiency of hearing protectors for hearing conservation programs. *Adv Noise Res* 1998; **2**: 167–76.
35. Ylikoski J, Pekkarinen J, Starck J. The efficiency of earmuffs against impulse noise from firearms. *Scand Audiol* 1987; **16**: 85–8.
36. International Organization for Standardization. *Acoustics–Hearing Protectors. Subjective Method for the Measurement of Sound Attenuation*. ISO-4869-1. Geneva: ISO, 1990.
37. International Organization for Standardization. *Acoustics—Hearing Protectors. Estimation of Effective A-weighted Pressure Levels When Hearing Protectors are Worn*. ISO-4869-2.2. Geneva: ISO, 1992.
38. EN 352 *Hearing Protectors—Safety Requirements and Testing*—parts 1–3, 1993.
39. prEN 13819–2 *Hearing Protectors—Testing—part 2: Acoustic Test Methods*, 2000.
40. EN 458 *Hearing Protectors—Recommendations for Selection, Use, Care and Maintenance*, 1993.
41. Sataloff RT, Sataloff J. Hearing loss in musicians, In: Sataloff RT, Sataloff J, eds. *Occupational Hearing Loss*, New York: Marcel Dekker, 1993.
42. Liu Chang-Chun, Pekkarinen J, Starck J. Application of the probe microphone method to measure attenuation of hearing protectors against high impulse sound levels. *Appl Acoust* 1989; **27**: 13–25.
43. Starck J, Pekkarinen J. Objective measurements of hearing protector attenuation for weapons noise exposure. In: *Proceedings 1992; Hearing Conservation Conference*, 1992: 89–92.
44. Pekkarinen J. Industrial noise, crest factor and the effect of earmuffs. *Am Ind Hyg Assoc J* 1987; **48**: 861–6.
45. Toppila E, Starck J, Pekkarinen J. Hearing protection efficiency in forestry. In: Blombäck P, Heikkonen J, Jokiluoma H et al, eds. *Proceedings of the Seminar on Clothing and Safety Equipment in Forestry*. Kuopio: University Printing Office, 1994: 183–7.
46. Foreshaw S, Cruchley J. Hearing protector problems in military operations. In: Alberti P, ed. *Personal Hearing Protection in Industry*. New York: Raven Press, 1982.
47. Berger EH. Using the NRR to estimate the real world performance of hearing protectors. *Sound Vibration* 1983; **17**(1): 12–18.
48. Lipscomp DM. The employee education program In: Lipscomb DM, ed. *Hearing Conservation in Industry, Schools and the Military*. San Diego: Singular Publishing Group, 1994: 81–230.
49. Price G. Relative hazard of weapons impulses. *J Acoust Soc Am* 1983; **73**: 556.
50. Clarck WW. Noise exposure from leisure activities: a review. *J Acoust Soc Am* 1991; **90**: 175–81.
51. Smith P, Davis A, Ferguson M et al. The prevalence and type of social noise exposure in young adults. *Noise and Health* 2000; **6**: 41–56.
52. Cruickshanks KJ, Klein R, Klein BE, Wiley TL, Nondahl DM, Tweeeds TS. Cigarette smoking and hearing loss: the epidemiology of hearing loss. *JAMA* 1998; **279**: 1715–59.
53. Starck J, Toppila E, Pyykkö I. Management of a sophisticated hearing conservation program. *Am J Ind Med* 1999, **1** (Suppl): 47–50.
54. Drettner B, Hedstrand H, Klockhoff I et al. Cardiovascular risk factors and hearing loss. *Acta Otolaryngol* 1975; **79**: 366–71.
55. Friedman GD, Siegelan AB, Seltzer CC. Cigarette smoking and exposure to occupational hazards. *Am J Epidemiol* 1969; **98**: 175–83.
56. Pyykkö I, Koskimies K, Starck J et al. Evaluation of factors affecting sensory neural hearing loss. *Acta Otolaryngol (Stockh) Suppl* 1988; **449**: 155–60.
57. Myers EN, Bernstein JM. Salicylate ototoxicity. *Arch Otolaryngol* 1965; **82**: 483–93.
58. Hawkins JE. Vascular patterns of the membranous labyrinth. In: Graybiel A, ed. *Third Symposium on the Role of the Vestibular Organs in Space Exploration*. Washington: NASA, 1967: 241–58.
59. Smith I, Lawrence M, Hawkins JE. Effects of noise and quinine on the vessels of the stria vascularis: an image analysis. *Am J Otolaryngol* 1985; 5.
60. Graham JDP, Parker WA. The toxic manifestation of sodium salicylate therapy. *Q J Med* 1948; **17**: 153–63.
61. Crifo S. Aspirin ototoxicity in the guinea pig. *ORL J Otorhinolaryngol Relat Spec* 1975; **37**: 27–34.
62. Eddy LB, Morgan RF, Carney HC. Hearing loss due to combined effects of noise and sodium salicylate. *ISA Trans* 1976; **15**: 103–8.
63. Miller JM, Ren TY, Dengerink HA et al. Cochlear blood flow changes with short sound stimulation. In: Axelsson A, Borchgrevink H, Hamernik RP, Hellstrom P, Henderson D, Salvi RJ, eds. *Scientific Basis of Noise-Induced Hearing Loss*, New York: Theime Medical Publishers, 1996: 95–109.
64. Pyykkö I, Koskimies K, Starck J et al. Risk factors in the genesis of sensory neural hearing loss in Finnish forestry workers. *Br J Ind Med* 1989; **46**: 439–46.
65. Bergström B, Nyström B. Development of hearing loss during long-term exposure to occupational noise. *Scand Audiol* 1986; **15**: 227–34.
66. Morata TC, Dunn DE, Kretchmer LW, et al. Effects of occupational exposure to organic solvents and noise on hearing. *Scand J Work Environ Health* 1993; **19**: 245–54.
67. Muijser H, Hoogendijk EM, Hooisma J. The effects of occupational exposure to styrene on high-frequency hearing threshold. *Toxicology* 1988; **49**: 331–40.
68. Mäkitie A. The ototoxic effect of styrene and its interactions with an experimental study in rats. Academic Dissertation, University of Helsinki, Helsinki University Hospital, 1997.
69. Ward WD. Endogenous factors related to susceptibility to damage from noise. *Occup Med* 1995; **10**: 561–75.
70. Rosen S, Pleater D, El-Mofty A et al. Relation of hearing loss to cardiovascular disease. *Trans Am Acad Ophthalmol Otolaryngol* 1964; **68**: 433–44.
71. Rosen S, Olin P. Hearing loss and coronary heart disease. *Arch Otolaryngol* 1965; **82**: 236–43.
72. Pyykkö I, Toppila E, Starck J et al. Database for a hearing conservation program. *Scand Audiol* 2000; **29**: 52–8.
73. Pillsbury HC. Hypertension, hyperlipoproteinemia, chronic noise exposure: is there synergism in cochlear pathology? *Laryngoscope* 1986; **96**: 1112–38.
74. Oghalai JS, Nakagawa T, Patell AA et al. Cholesterol partitioning within the outer hair cell lateral wall. *Otolaryngol Head Neck Surg* 1997; **117**: 91.

75. Nguyen T-V, Brownell WE . Contribution of membrane cholesterol to outer hair cell lateral wall stiffness. *Otolaryngol Head Neck Surg* 1998; **119**: 14–20.
76. Borg E. Noise-induced hearing loss in normotensive and spontaneously hypertensive rats. *Hear Res* 1982; **8**: 117–30.
77. Johnsson A, Hansson L. Prolonged exposure to a stressful stimulus (noise) as a cause of raised blood pressure in man. *Lancet* 1977; **I**: 86–7.
78. Talbot EO, Findlay RC, Kuller LH et al. Noise-induced hearing loss: a possible marker for high blood pressure in older noise-exposed populations. *J Occup Med* 1990; **32**: 890–7.
79. McCormic G, Harris DT, Hartley CB et al. Spontaneous genetic hypertension in the rat and its relationship to reduce cochlear potentials: implications for preservation of human hearing. *Proc Natl Acad Sci USA* 1982; **79**: 2668.
80. Starck J, Toppila E, Pyykkö I. Smoking as risk factor in sensory neural hearing loss among workers exposed to occupational noise. *Acta Otolaryngol* 1999; **119**: 302–5.
81. Morton NE. Genetic epidemiology of hearing impairment. *Ann NY Acad Sci* 1991; **630**: 16–31.
82. Gates GA, Couropmitree NN, Meyers RH. Genetic associations in age-related hearing thresholds. *Arch Otol Head Neck Surg* 1999; **125**: 654–9.
83. Green CE, Scott DA, McDonald JM et al. Carrier rates in the mid western United States for GJB2 mutations causing inherited deafness. *JAMA* **281**: 2211–16.
84. Kaksonen R, Pyykkö I, Kere J et al. Hereditary hearing loss—the role of environmental factors. *Acta Otolaryngol (Stockh)* 2001; **30**: 85–7.
85. Royster LH, Lilley LT, Thomas WG. Recommended criteria for evaluating effectiveness of hearing conservation program. *Am Ind Hyg Assoc* 1980; **41**: 40–8.
86. International Organization for Standardization. *Acoustics. Audiometric Test Methods.* Part 1: *Basic Pure Tone Air and Bone Conduction Threshold Audiometry.* ISO 8253-1:1. Geneva: ISO, 1989.
87. Royster JD, Royster LH.Using audiometric data base analysis. *J Occup Med* 1986; 28: 1055–68.
88. Kemp DT. Stimulated acoustic emissions from within the human auditory system. *J Acoust Soc Am* 1978; **64**: 1386–91.
89. Furst M, Reshef I, Attias J. Manifestation of intense noise stimulation on spontaneous otoacoustic emission and threshold microstructure: experiment and model. *J Acoust Soc Am* 1992; **91**: 1003–14.
90. Avan P, Bonfils P. Frequency specificity of human distortion product otoacoustic emissions. *Audiology* 1993; **32**: 12–26.
91. Oeken J. Topodiagnostic assessment of occupational noise-induced hearing loss using distortion-product otoacoustic emissions compared to the short increment sensitivity index test. *Eur Arch Otorhinolaryngol* 1999; **256**: 115–21.
92. Hallmo P, Borchgevink HM, Mair IW. Extended high-frequency thresholds in noise-induced hearing loss. *Scand Audiol* 1995; **24**: 47–52.
93. Chery-Croze S, Truy E, Morgon A. Contralateral suppression of transiently evoked otoacoustic emissions and tinnitus. *Br J Audiol* 1994; **28**(4–5): 255–66.
94. Barrenäs M-L. The influence of melanin-binding drug on temporary threshold shift in humans. *Scand Audiol* 1994; **23**: 93–8.
95. Barrenäs M-L, Hellström PA. The effect of low-level acoustic stimulation on susceptibility to noise in blue- and brown-eyed young human subjects. *Ear & Hear* 1996; **7**: 63–8.
96. Pyykkö I, Kaksonen R, Toppila E et al. Development of a sophisticated hearing conservation programme. In: Prasher D, Luxon L, Pyykkö I, eds. *Advances in Noise Research*, Vol 2. *Protection Against Noise*. London: Whurr Publishers, 1998: 219–23.
97. Attias J, Weisdz G, Almog A et al. Oral magnesium intake reduces permanent hearing loss induced by noise exposure. *Am J Otolaryngol* 1994; **15**: 26–32.
98. Sha SH, Schacht J. Salicylate attenuates gentamicin-induced ototoxicity. *Lab Invest* 1999; **79**: 807–13.
99. Lopez-Gonzales MA, Guerrero JM, Rojas F et al. Melatonin and other antioxidants prolong the postmortem activity of the outer hair cells of the organ of Corti: its relation to the type of death. *J Pineal Res* 1999; **27**: 73–7.
100. Yamasoba T, Schacht J, Shoji F et al. Attenuation of cochlear damage from noise trauma by an iron chelator, a free radical scavenger and glial cell line-derived neurotrophic factor in vivo. *Brain Res* 1999; **815**: 317–25.
101. Ulfendahl M. Mechanical responses of the mammalian cochlea. *Prog Neurobiol* 1997; **53**: 331–80.
102. Lim DJ, Melnick W. Acoustic damage of the cochlea. A scanning and transmission electron microscopic observation. *Arch Otolaryngol* 1971; **94**: 294–305.
103. Borg E, Canlon B, Engstrom B. Noise-induced hearing loss. Literature review and experiments in rabbits. Morphological and electrophysiological features, exposure parameters and temporal factors, variability and interactions. *Scand Audiol Suppl* 1995; **40**: 1–147.
104. Dew LA, Owen RG Jr, Mulroy MJ. Changes in size and shape of auditory hair cells in vivo during noise-induced temporary threshold shift. *Hear Res* 1993; **66**: 99–107.
105. Flock Å, Flock B, Fridberger A et al. Supporting cells contribute to control of hearing sensitivity. *J Neurosci* 1999; **19**: 4498–507.
106. Lyons GD, Dodson, Casey DA et al. Round window rupture secondary to acoustic trauma. *South Med J* 1978; **71**: 71–3.
107. McNeil PL, Steinhardt RA. Loss, restoration and maintenance of plasma membrane integrity. *J Cell Biol* 1997; **137**: 1–4.
108. Saunders JC, Dear SP, Schneider ME. The anatomical consequences of acoustic injury: a review and tutorial. *J Acoust Soc Am* 1985; **78**: 833–60.
109. Slepecky N. Overview of mechanical damage to the inner ear: noise as a tool to probe cochlear function. *Hear Res* 1986; **22**: 307–21.
110. Ulfendahl M, Khanna SM, Löfstrand P. Changes in the mechanical tuning characteristics of the hearing organ following acoustic overstimulation. *Eur J Neurosci* 1993; **5**: 713–23.
111. Luz GA, Hodge DC. Recovery from impulse-noise induced TTS in monkeys and men: a descriptive model. *J Acoust Soc Am* 1971; **49**: 1770–7.
112. Ohlemiller KK, Wright JS, Dugan LL. Early elevation of cochlear reactive oxygen species following noise exposure. *Audiol Neurootol* 1999; **4**: 229–36.

113. Yamasoba T, Harris C, Shoji F et al. Influence of intense sound exposure on glutathione synthesis in the cochlea. *Brain Res* 1998; **804**: 72–8.
114. Hu BH, Zheng XY, McFadden SL et al. R-phenylisopropyladenosine attenuates noise-induced hearing loss in the chinchilla. *Hear Res* 1997; **113**: 198–206.
115. Seidman MD, Bhagylakshmi G, Shivapuja G et al. The protective effects of allopurinol and superoxide dismutase on noise-induced cochlear damage. *Otolaryngol Head Neck Surg* 1993; **109**: 1052–6.
116. Puel JL, Ruel J, Gervais d'Aldin C et al. Excitotoxicity and repair of cochlear synapses after noise-trauma induced hearing loss. *Neuroreport* 1998; **9**: 2109–14.
117. Axelsson A, Denjerink H. The effects of noise on histological measures of cochlear vasculature and red blood cells: a review. *Hear Res* 1987; **31**: 183–92.
118. Hawkins JE. The role of vasoconstriction in noise-induced hearing loss. *Ann Otol Rhinol Laryngol* 1971; **80**: 903–14.
119. Scheibe F, Haupt H, Ludwig C. Intensity-related changes in cochlear blood flow in the guinea pig during and following acoustic exposure. *Eur Arch Otol Rhinol Laryngol* 1993; **250**: 281–5.
120. Lamm K, Arnold W. Noise-induced cochlear hypoxia is intensity dependent, correlates with hearing loss and precedes reduction of cochlear blood flow, 1996.
121. Quirk WS, Seidman MD. Cochlear vascular changes in response to loud noise. *Am J Otol* 1995; **16**: 322–5.
122. Goldwin B, Khan MJ, Shivapuja B. Sarthran preserves cochlear microcirculation and reduces temporary threshold shifts after noise exposure. *Otolaryngol Head Neck Surg* 1998; **118**: 576–83.
123. Fridberger A, Flock Å, Ulfendahl M et al. Acoustic overstimulation increases outer hair cell Ca^{2+} concentrations and causes dynamic contractions of the hearing organ. *Proc Natl Acad Sci USA* 1998; **95**: 7127–32.
124. Fridberger A, Ulfendahl M. Acute mechanical overstimulation of isolated outer hair cells causes changes in intracellular calcium levels without shape changes. *Acta Otolaryngol (Stockh)* 1996; **116**: 17–24.
125. Orrenius S, McCabe MJ, Nicotera P. Ca^{2+}-dependent mechanisms of cytotoxicity and programmed cell death. *Toxicol Lett* 1992; **64/65**: 357–64.
126. Trump BF, Berezesky IK. Calcium-mediated cell injury and cell death. *FASEB J.* 1995; **9**: 219–28.
127. Chan E, Suneson A, Ulfendahl M. Acoustic trauma causes reversible stiffness changes in auditory sensory cells. *Neuroscience* 1998; **83**: 961–8.
128. Nishikori T, Hatta T, Kawauchi H et al. Apoptosis during inner ear development in human and mouse embryos: an analysis by computer-assisted three-dimensional reconstruction. *Anat Embryol (Berl)* 1999; **200**: 19–26.
129. Orita Y, Nishizaki K, Sasaki J et al. Does TUNEL staining during peri- and post-natal development of the mouse inner ear indicate apoptosis? *Acta Otolaryngol (Stockh) Suppl* 1999; **540**: 22–6.
130. Jokay I, Soos G, Repassy G et al. Aptoptosis in the human inner ear. Detection by in situ end-labeling of fragmented DNA and correlation with other markers. *Hear Res* 1998; **117**: 131–9.
131. CHABA. Proposed damage-risk criterion for impulse noise (gunfire). Report of working group 57, National Academy of Sciences Research Council. Washington DC: Committee of Hearing, Bioaccoustics and Biomechanics, 1968.
132. Johnson DL. Prediction of NIPTS due to continuous noise exposure. EPA-550/9-73-001-BO.

29 Central auditory disorders

Jane A Baran, Frank E Musiek

Introduction

The central auditory nervous system (CANS) is a complex and intricate network of neural pathways extending from the cochlear nucleus complex through the primary auditory reception areas of the temporal lobes and beyond. As sensory information travels within the CANS, the processing of the signal undergoes several levels of processing. This processing occurs not only in a hierarchical or serial order as the signal travels up the CANS, but also in a parallel manner. The result of this combined serial and parallel processing of information is a highly efficient, but redundant, system (see Chapter 11).

One of the benefits of such a redundant neural system is that compromise of the CANS seldom leads to complete loss of auditory function. It is much more common for the effects of lesions within the CANS to be subtle, and frequently these effects can be identified only when sophisticated test procedures are used to tease out the deficits. Because of the intrinsic complexity of the CANS and the unique processing that occurs at various levels of the system, the auditory deficits that are observed in individuals with compromise of the CANS are frequently quite diverse. Therefore, it must be recognized that central auditory processing disorders (CAPD) represent a heterogeneous group of disorders with a variety of etiological bases, including both developmental and pathological conditions, as well as behavioral manifestations.[1] It is for this reason that no one test will identify all disorders affecting the CANS. Assessment procedures must include a number of tests that tap specific auditory processes and levels of processing (e.g. brainstem versus cortical). Likewise, management procedures need to be tailored to the specific deficits and needs of each individual patient.

History

Assessment of central auditory function can be traced back to the mid-1950s, when two Italian physicians utilized a sensitized speech test (low-pass filtered speech) in an effort to tease out the auditory difficulties which were being reported by patients with temporal lobe lesions.[2,3] Their findings indicated that, while routine peripheral hearing tests failed to identify the auditory difficulties being experienced by these patients, use of a modified speech test did result in abnormal performance in the ear contralateral to the affected hemisphere. Since the time of these early investigations, the interest in central auditory assessment has grown steadily, and currently there are numerous tests available for use in the assessment of CANS function. These early efforts to use monaural low-redundancy speech tests were quickly followed by utilization of binaural integration tests,[4,5] dichotic speech tests,[6,7] temporal patterning tests,[8–10] and electrophysiological procedures[11–14] in a variety of clinical research investigations. Although many of these early clinical research instruments and test protocols did not become common assessment tools, they laid the foundation for the development of many of the tests that are used today in the assessment of patients considered to be at risk for CAPDs.[15,16]

Definition

Along with efforts to develop tests sensitive to dysfunction along the CANS came several attempts to define CAPD. What emerged was a number of definitions which were embraced by some professionals, but not universally by all professionals. Many professionals argued that CAPD did not represent a unique clinical entity, but rather that any auditory deficits noted were simply manifestations of other disorders, such as language-processing disorders or attention deficits. Recognizing the need to achieve some consensus on several issues surrounding CAPD, the American Speech–Language–Hearing Association convened a task force in 1993. One of the outcomes of the deliberations of this task force was the development of the following definitions for central auditory processes and CAPD.

> **Central auditory processes** are the auditory system mechanisms and processes responsible for the following behavioral phenomena: sound localization and lateralization,

> auditory discrimination, auditory pattern recognition, temporal aspects of audition including temporal resolution, temporal masking, temporal integration, and temporal ordering, and auditory performance with degraded acoustic signals.[17] (p. 41)
>
> A **central auditory processing disorder** is an observed deficiency in one or more of the above listed behaviors. For some persons, CAPD is presumed to result from the dysfunction of processes and mechanisms dedicated to audition; for others, CAPD may stem from some more general dysfunction, such as an attention deficit or neural timing deficit, that affects performance across modalities. It is also possible for CAPD to reflect co-existing dysfunction of both types.[17] (p. 41)

Of significance in this definition of CAPD is the recognition that the disorder can result from dysfunction of the mechanisms dedicated to audition, as well as from more global deficits such as language, memory or attention deficits, as long as these deficits impact negatively upon the processing of auditory information.

More recently, participants in a consensus conference held in April 2000 on the Diagnosis of Auditory Processing Disorders in School-Aged Children recommended a change in terminology and offered the following definition of an auditory processing disorder (APD).

> An APD may be broadly defined as a deficit in the processing of information that is specific to the auditory modality. The problem may be exacerbated in unfavorable acoustic environments. It may be associated with difficulties in listening, speech understanding, language development, and learning. In its pure form, however, it is conceptualized as a deficit in the processing of auditory input.[18] (p. 468)

This change in terminology was recommended by the expert panel of 14 senior-level researchers and clinicians in an effort to maintain an operational definition for the auditory deficits experienced by many school-aged children who presented with normal auditory thresholds, while avoiding the imputation of anatomical loci, and underscoring the potential for interactions between disorders originating at both peripheral and central sites. Although the consensus conference focused specifically on problems in diagnosing school-aged children with auditory processing deficits, the proposed definition of APD would appear to have applications for both younger and older individuals who may experience similar auditory deficits. Since APD is a new term that is not yet widely recognized by hearing healthcare professionals, and since most of the investigations reviewed in this chapter used CAPD to refer to the auditory disorders being studied, both abbreviations will be used in the remainder of this chapter.

> Many neurocognitive mechanisms and processes are involved in the recognition and discrimination of auditory stimuli. Some of these mechanisms are dedicated to the processing of acoustic signals, whereas others, such as attentional mechanisms and long-term language representation, are not. In the latter case, the term *central auditory processing* is used to refer to the deployment of these non-dedicated processes and mechanisms in the processing of acoustic information.

Prevalence

There is little information available on the prevalence of APD/CAPD. This is due in large part to the heterogeneous nature of the disorder, the lack of an agreed upon definition of APD/CAPD, the high comorbidity of APD/CAPD with other medical, developmental and psychoeducational disorders or disabilities, and the lack of well-designed epidemiological studies. Chermak and Musiek[16] have estimated the prevalence of APD/CAPD in children to be between 2% and 3%. These authors based this estimate upon data provided in published clinical reports, a review of prevalence data for other comorbid conditions, and their own personal clinical experience. Estimates of the prevalence of the disorder in the aging population are considerably higher and range from a low of 17% to a high of 90%.[16,19] The large disparity in these estimates is believed to be due to a number of factors, including the age of the population studied in the various investigations reviewed, the central tests administered as part of the research protocols, and the inclusion/exclusion of subjects with peripheral hearing loss or cognitive deficits in the experimental groups. Unfortunately, many of these studies did not control for peripheral hearing loss and/or cognitive status. Therefore, it is difficult to determine the prevalence of APD/CAPD in the elderly population at this time. However, given the fact that age-related changes are known to occur in the brainstem and cortical structures, as well as the auditory periphery,[20–24] it is anticipated that a significant number of elderly patients will experience an APD/CAPD related to normal degenerative processes occurring within the CANS. Additional information on central auditory function in the elderly, as well as a discussion of the potential effects of peripheral and cognitive factors on performance, can be found in Chapter 17, as well as in other sources.[25–28]

Etiological bases

Research on children and adults with APD/CAPD has revealed a number of etiological bases for the auditory deficits that these patients experience. In many individuals, the deficits can be linked to frank neurological lesions or disease processes that affect the integrity of the CANS. Frank neurological bases for APD/CAPD include trauma, neoplasms, degenerative disorders, metabolic dysfunction, neurotoxicity, viral infections, and surgical lesions.[1] In other individuals, the deficits are related to benign CANS dysfunction. These etiological bases include delays in the neuromaturational development of the CANS,[29] cerebromorphological abnormalities,[30] and age-related changes.[15]

> APD/CAPD can have a number of etiological bases. These can include benign cerebromorphological abnormalities, delays in the neuromaturational development of the central nervous system, and normal aging processes occurring within the CANS, as well as frank neurological involvement.

Comorbid conditions

Although APD/CAPD may exist in isolation, it much more frequently coexists in an individual with other developmental and/or acquired disorders. Common comorbid conditions include speech and language disorders, learning disabilities, attention deficit disorders with or without hyperactivity, psychological and emotional disorders, and social and behavioral problems. Although there have been many attempts to establish cause-and-effect relationships between these various disorders, the relationships remain elusive at this time, and more than likely not unidirectional. More critical to the management of the individual with comorbid disorders than the establishment of these cause-and-effect relationships is the identification of the various disorders or disabilities which coexist within the individual, so that an effective program can be developed in an effort to address each area of deficit or disability. Since assessment and management may cut across professional boundaries, it is critical that professionals from a variety of disciplines provide input into the development of an assessment and management program whenever comorbid conditions may exist.

> Since many individuals with APD/CAPD are likely to have other comorbid conditions, an interdisciplinary model for assessment is recommended, whenever feasible.

Clinical presentation

The CANS is a complicated and extensive neural network, with lesions potentially occurring at a number of distinct sites along its pathways. Since different types of processing occur at various sites along the CANS, the symptoms which patients experience are likely to vary with the site of lesion. Moreover, many of the auditory symptoms related to CANS dysfunction may be subtle and unusual. This is related to the fact that processing of an incoming acoustic signal occurs in an overlapping or parallel fashion, as well as in a serial fashion. It is therefore important that background information be solicited carefully from each patient at risk for APD/CAPD. If not, some symptoms may be missed, as many are qualitative in nature.

Some of the more commonly reported symptoms include: (1) difficulty hearing in noise or highly reverberant rooms; (2) subjective tinnitus, typically localized to the mid-line of the head; (3) auditory hallucinations or unusual auditory sensations; (4) difficulty following complex auditory directions; (5) poor utilization of prosodic information; (6) auditory inattentiveness and high distractibility; (7) difficulty localizing sound sources; (8) auditory memory deficits; and (9) marked decrease in the appreciation of music. In addition to these complaints, there are a number of other behavioral or academic issues which may be heralding an APD/CAPD. Many individuals with APD/CAPD experience concomitant spelling, reading, writing and organizational skill deficits. Several behavioral checklists have been developed for use in determining which children should be considered at risk for APD/CAPD.[31–34] These can be used to provide valuable insights into the nature of the difficulties which the individual presenting for assessment may be experiencing. Finally, it should be mentioned that although all of the checklists referenced above have been developed for use with children, many can easily be modified for use with adults.

Assessment protocols

There have been numerous classification systems developed in an effort to categorize the various central auditory tests which can be used to assess CANS function. For the purposes of the present discussion, a five-category classification system will be used. The categories include binaural interaction tests, dichotic speech tests, monaural low-redundancy speech tests, temporal patterning tests, and electrophysiological procedures. Space limitations preclude an exhaustive discussion of each of these five categories and the many tests that fall within each of these categories. However, a brief discussion of a representative test within each of the categories is presented. Additional information on these and other CANS tests can be found in Table 29.1 and in a number of other sources.[1,15,16,19]

Table 29.1 Behavioral tests frequently employed in the assessment of central auditory nervous system function[a]

Test	Category	Stimulus	Mode	Onset	Result
Masking level difference[35]	Binaural interaction	Spondees in noise/pulsed pure tones in noise	Binaural/ diotic	Simultaneous	dB difference
Rapidly alternating speech perception[36]	Binaural interaction	Sentences	Binaural	Alternating segments (300 ms)	Percentage correct
Binaural fusion[36]	Binaural interaction	Spondees[b]	Binaural	Simultaneous	Percentage correct
Dichotic digits[37]	Dichotic speech/divided attention	Digits (1–10, not 7)	Dichotic	Simultaneous	Percentage correct
Dichotic CVs[38]	Dichotic speech/divided attention	CVs (pa, ta, ka, ba, da, ga)	Dichotic	Simultaneous or delayed	Percentage correct
Staggered spondaic words[39]	Dichotic speech/divided attention	Spondees	Dichotic	Staggered, overlapping	Percentage correct
Synthetic sentence identification with contralateral competition[40]	Dichotic speech/directed attention	Third-order sentence approximations with a story as competition	Dichotic	Not applicable	Percentage correct
Dichotic sentences[41]	Dichotic speech/divided attention	Third-order sentence approximations	Dichotic	Simultaneous	Percentage correct
Competing sentences[36]	Dichotic speech/directed attention	Sentences	Dichotic	Simultaneous	Percentage correct
Compressed speech[42]	Monaural low-redundancy speech	Monosyllabic words[c]	Monaural	Not applicable	Percentage correct
Low-pass filtered speech[36]	Monaural low-redundancy speech	Monosyllabic words[d]	Monaural	Not applicable	Percentage correct
Synthetic sentence identification with ipsilateral competition[40]	Monaural low-redundancy speech	Third-order sentence approximations with a story as competition	Monaural	Not applicable	Percentage correct
Frequency patterns[43]	Temporal patterning	Sequences of three tonal stimuli[e]	Monaural[g]	Not applicable	Percentage correct
Duration patterns[44]	Temporal patterning	Sequences of three tonal stimuli[f]	Monaural[g]	Not applicable	Percentage correct

From Baran and Musiek.[45] Adapted with permission from Butterworth-Heinemann Medical Publishers.

[a] The descriptions provided represent test parameters which are in common clinical use. There are several alternatives for many of these tests. Therefore, it is important to determine the parameters used by the tester when reviewing test data as different parameters may affect normative data.

[b] The stimuli are passed through a low-bandpass filter (500–700 Hz) and a high-bandpass filter (1900–2100 Hz). The low-bandpass filtered information is presented to one ear, and the high-bandpass filtered information to the other ear. The order of presentation may then be reversed.

[c] The stimuli are subjected to 60% time compression, with the end-result being that the compressed stimuli are only 40% of their original durations.

[d] The stimuli are passed through a low-bandpass filter with a 500 Hz cut-off frequency and an 18 dB per octave rejection rate.

[e] The stimuli consist of high (1122 Hz) and low (880 Hz) pure tones of a constant duration (150 ms with a 10-ms rise–fall time) in the following six sequences: HHL, HLL, HLH, LLH, LHH, and LHL. The ISI between consecutive tones within each sequence is 200 ms.

[f] The stimuli consist of long (500 ms) and short (250 ms) pure tones of a constant frequency (1000 Hz) in the following six sequences: LLS, LSS, LSL, SSL, SLL, and SLS. Rise–fall times are 10 ms and the ISI between consecutive tones within each sequence is 300 ms.

[g] The stimuli may be presented diotically or in the sound field.

Binaural interaction tests

Binaural interaction tests, or binaural integration tests, encompass those tests that require the interaction of both ears in order to effect integration of information that is separated by time, intensity, or frequency factors to the two ears. The tests in this category are designed to assess the ability of the CANS to take disparate information presented to the two ears and to unify this information into one perceptual event. This unification of auditory information from the two ears is presumed to occur in the brainstem. For this reason, tests that fall into this category are believed to be sensitive to brainstem pathology. They can, however, also be affected by cerebral lesions (Table 29.2).

One of the more sensitive of the tests in this category is the masking level difference test. The test paradigm involves the presentation of a stimulus (either spondee words or pulsed pure tones) to both ears at the same time that a broadband masking noise is delivered to the two ears.[46] The patient is tested under two conditions, a homophasic condition and an antiphasic condition. In the homophasic condition, the stimulus and the noise are presented in phase to both ears (S_0N_0), whereas in the antiphasic condition, one of the two signals is presented 180° out of phase while the other signal is maintained in phase between the two ears (Figure 29.1). For example, in the $S_{\pi}N_0$ antiphasic condition, the noise is maintained in phase between the two ears, and the signal is presented 180° out of phase. Subtracting the threshold established in the homophasic condition from that found in either of the antiphasic conditions results in a difference score referred to as the masking level difference. In individuals with normal brainstem function, the threshold noted in the antiphasic condition is noticeably better than the threshold obtained in the homophasic condition. This is considered to represent a 'release from masking', which is considered to originate at the level of the CANS where information from the two ears is first integrated.

Dichotic speech tests

Dichotic speech tests involve speech tests in which different speech materials are presented to the two ears in a simultaneous or overlapping manner. Test stimuli can involve any type of speech stimulus, ranging from consonant–vowel combinations (CVs), through monosyllabic words to sentences. In addition, patients can be asked to divide their attention (i.e. to repeat all stimuli heard in both ears) or to direct their attention (i.e. repeat only the stimuli perceived in the right ear or the left ear). Research findings suggest that when the CANS is stimulated with dichotic speech materials, the weaker ipsilateral pathways tend to be suppressed, and the neural impulses travel up the preeminent contralateral pathways to reach the auditory reception areas of the cerebrum.[6,7] Dichotic speech tests are particularly sensitive to lesions of the auditory cortex and interhemispheric fibers, and to a lesser degree to auditory brainstem lesions (Table 29.2). Most typically contralateral ear effects are noted with lesions of the auditory cortex, whereas left-ear deficits are commonly noted in patients with lesions involving the interhemispheric pathways. In cases of brainstem pathology, ipsilateral ear deficits are more common in patients with extra-axial lesions (i.e. lesions originating from the periphery of the brainstem), whereas bilateral, contralateral or ipsilateral ear effects may be observed with intra-axial lesions (i.e. lesions originating from within the brainstem).

One of the more commonly used tests in this category is the dichotic digits test. In this test, two digit pairs (i.e. four digits) are presented to the patient at 50 dB SL (re: SRT) and the patient is asked to repeat all digits perceived (Figure 29.2). The digits used include the numbers from 1 to 10 (except 7) and are carefully aligned in terms of their stimulus onsets. Patients are encouraged to guess, and informed that it is not necessary to repeat the digits in any particular order. A percentage correct score is derived for each ear and compared to age-appropriate norms.

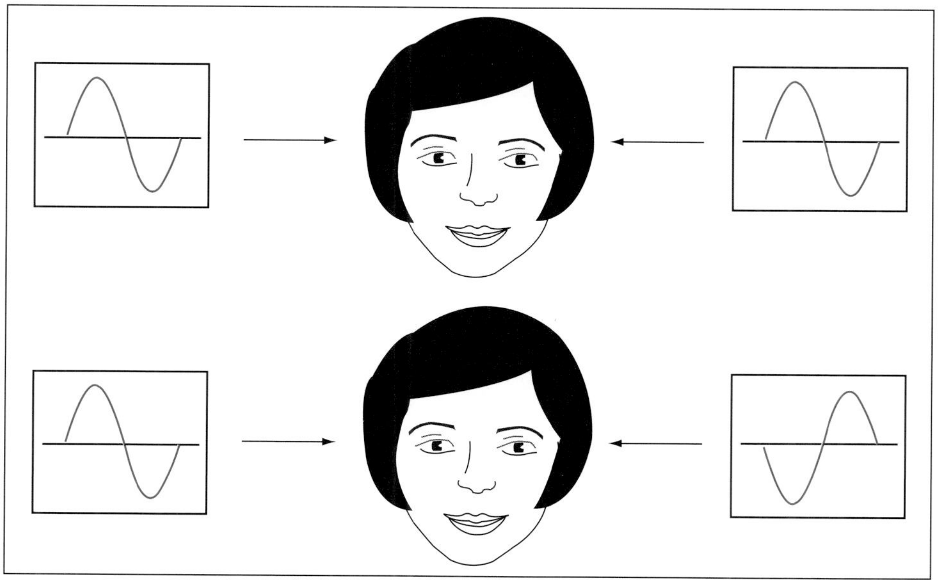

Figure 29.1 Example of the procedure used to derive a masking level difference (MLD). The upper panel shows a pure tone test stimulus being presented in phase to the two ears (i.e. homophasic condition), whereas the lower panel depicts the presentation of the pure tone stimuli 180° out of phase between the two ears (i.e. the antiphasic condition). In each condition, a noise stimulus (not shown) is presented in phase between the two ears, and a pure tone detection threshold is derived. The difference between these two thresholds represents the MLD.

Table 29.2 Patterns of central test results that may be observed in patients with lesions at various sites along the CANS.

Test category	Low brainstem	High brainstem	Auditory cortex	Interhemispheric pathways
Binaural interaction	Binaural deficit[a] (2)	Little or no deficit (3)	Little or no deficit (3)	Little or no deficit (3)
Dichotic speech	Ipsilateral ear deficit (2)	Contralateral ear deficit (2) Bilateral deficits (2) Ipsilateral ear deficit (2)	Contralateral ear deficit (3) Bilateral deficits (1)	Contralateral ear deficit (3)
Monaural low-redundancy speech	Ipsilateral ear deficit (2)	Contralateral ear deficit (2) Bilateral deficits (2) Ipsilateral ear deficit (1)	Contralateral ear deficit (3)	No deficit (3)
Temporal patterning	Ipsilateral ear deficit (1)	Contralateral ear deficit (1) Bilateral deficits (1) Ipsilateral ear deficit (1)	Bilateral deficits[b] (3)	Bilateral deficits[b] (3)
Auditory brainstem response[c]	Ipsilateral abnormality (3) Bilateral abnormalities (1) Contralateral abnormality (1)	Contralateral abnormality (2) Bilateral abnormality (1) Ipsilateral abnormality (1)	No deficit (3)	No deficit (3)
Middle latency response[c]	Ipsilateral ear effect (1)	Contralateral ear effect (2) Bilateral effects (1) Ipsilateral effect (1)	Abnormality at electrode nearest pathology (2) Contralateral ear effect (2)	Little or no deficit (3)
Late response (N1 and P2)[c]	Ipsilateral ear effect (1)	Contralateral ear effect (1) Bilateral ear effects (1) Ipsilateral ear effect (1)	Abnormality at electrode nearest lesion (2) Contralateral ear effect (2)	Little or no deficit (3)
Auditory cognitive (P3 or P300)[c]	Same as late response	Same as late response	Non-localizing abnormality (2)	Little or no deficit (3)

From Baran and Musiek. In: Wall, ed. Hearing for the Speech-Language Pathologist and Healthcare Professional.[45]

Adapted with permission from Butterworth-Heinemann Medical Publishers.

Key: (3) high probability of occurrence; (2) moderate probability of occurrence; (1) low probability of occurrence.

[a] Binaural is used in this context, since both ears are receiving segments of the stimulus and only one score is derived.

[b] Specified deficits would be predicted if the patient was asked to verbally describe the patterns perceived.

[c] Abnormal results may be noted for one or more of the indices derived during the electrophysiological procedure (see Chapter 16). The use of the singular form in this context indicates that any abnormalities that exist are limited to one ear.

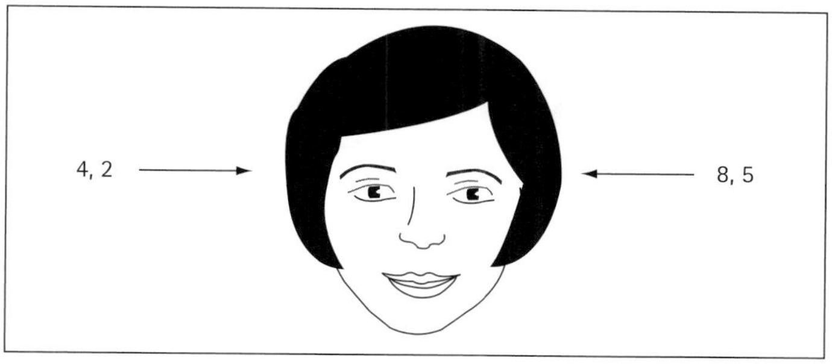

Figure 29.2 Example of a test stimulus from the dichotic digits test. The digit, 4, is presented to the right ear at the same time that 8 is presented to the left ear; this is followed by 2 to the right ear and 5 to the left ear.

Monaural low-redundancy speech tests

Monaural low-redundancy speech tests include tests in which the stimuli have been degraded by modifying the frequency, temporal or intensity characteristics of the undistorted signal. Common to all these tests is the monaural presentation of a speech signal that has undergone some type of signal degradation. Clinical research has demonstrated that these types of tests tap auditory closure abilities and are moderately sensitive to cortical lesions—in which case, contralateral ear deficits are most commonly noted (Table 29.2). In individuals with left-hemisphere compromise, bilateral deficits may also be noted. In these cases, it is likely that the auditory areas subserving speech recognition have been compromised. Monaural low-redundancy tests are less sensitive to brainstem lesions, and, as was the case for the dichotic speech tests, the laterality effects noted are likely to differ with the specific location of the lesion. Finally, test performance on monaural low-redundancy speech tests is unlikely to be affected in patients with interhemispheric pathway compromise.

An example of a monaural low-redundancy speech test is the compressed speech test. Some of the more commonly used versions of this test utilize monosyllabic words that have been compressed using time compression ratios of 60% or 65%. This is achieved by removing brief segments of the original signal until either 60% or 65% of the original speech signal has been removed. The remaining segments are then abutted to achieve a new speech signal that contains only 40% or 35% of the original signal. These compressed stimuli are presented to each ear individually at 40 dB SL (re: SRT), and percentage correct scores are derived for each ear. These scores are compared to age-appropriate norms.

Temporal patterning tests

Temporal patterning tests involve feature detection, frequency or duration discrimination, and acoustic contour recognition. In addition, if the patient is asked to label the patterns perceived, then linguistic processing is also tapped. These tests have been shown to be sensitive to compromise of the auditory cortex in the right hemisphere, which is responsible for the processing of the acoustic contour of the patterns. In addition, if a verbal response is required, the test is sensitive to lesions in the left hemisphere (responsible for verbally labeling the patterns perceived) and/or the interhemispheric pathways. Deficits are less common in patients with brainstem lesions (Table 29.2).

The frequency pattern sequences test is one of the more popular tests within this category. It is composed of test sequences consisting of three tone bursts. In each of the sequences, two tone bursts are of the same frequency while the third is of a different frequency (Figure 29.3). The two tone bursts used on commercially available tests include a low-frequency tone (880 Hz) and a high-frequency tone (1122 Hz). All tone bursts have a 10-ms rise–fall time and a total duration of 150 ms, and there is a 200-ms interstimulus interval between successive tones in each sequence. Given these parameters, a total of six different sequences are possible: high-high-low, high-low-high, high-low-low, low-low-high, low-high-low, and low-high-high. It is normal practice to have the patients describe the sequences perceived using the words 'high' and 'low'. Thirty sequences are presented at 50 dB SL (re: SRT) to each ear individually, and a percentage correct score is derived for each ear. However, experience has shown that ear differences are uncommon on this test. Therefore, it is possible to derive a single score either diotically under headphones or in the sound field. In addition, if a patient is unable to describe the sequences, he or she may be asked to hum the sequences. If this is done, the test assesses primarily right-hemisphere function. In either instance, test scores are compared to age-appropriate norms for the specific test procedure administered.

Electrophysiological procedures

Several of the auditory evoked potentials discussed in other chapters of this text are of value in assessing CANS integrity and can serve as a valuable adjunct to the behavioral tests discussed thus far. Electrophysiological procedures can be used to evaluate function of the auditory pathways, beginning with the cochlear nerve and progressing through the cortical levels of the CANS.

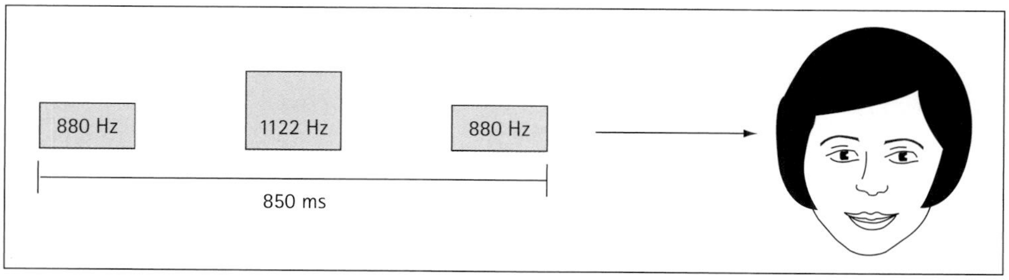

Figure 29.3 Example of a test stimulus from the frequency pattern sequences test, showing the acoustic stimulus consisting of a series of three tone bursts, with two tone bursts of the same frequency and a third tone burst of a different frequency.

The auditory brainstem response (ABR) is an early latency response which is frequently abnormal in patients with lesions of the cochlear nerve and/or caudal brainstem, whereas lesions in the thalamic regions and above are likely to result in normal ABR findings. The middle latency response (MLR) is sensitive to lesions located more rostrally within the CANS (thalamus and primary auditory projections), and the late auditory evoked response (LAER) and P300 assess cortical functions (Table 29.2). Recently, interest has grown in the use of the mismatch negativity responses to assess a patient's ability to discriminate or selectively attend to certain stimuli. Physiological tests offer an advantage over behavioral tests, due to their objectivity, and, in general, absence of a need for a cooperative patient. The reader interested in additional information on these test protocols is referred to Chapter 16 as well as to other sources.[47,48]

Range of severity

As mentioned previously, the deficits noted in many individuals with APD/CAPD are often subtle and may not be detected during routine audiological testing. On the other end of the continuum are individuals who present with dramatic auditory deficits, including 'deafness' of a central origin, whose deficits are quite striking and are obvious even during routine pure tone testing. In fact, if testing were limited to routine peripheral assessment procedures, the 'deafness' noted in these patients might well be misdiagnosed as peripheral in origin. In the past, a number of terms have been used to refer to the auditory disorders that these individuals experience. Among these terms are central deafness, cortical deafness, auditory agnosia, verbal auditory agnosia, and word deafness.

The term central deafness has been used to refer to the disorder experienced by individuals with bilateral hemispheric involvement of the auditory areas of the brain. These individuals often show no subjective experience of 'hearing' and will frequently present with a profound hearing loss during routine pure tone assessments. However, if electroacoustic and electrophysiological testing of the auditory periphery is conducted in these cases (e.g. otoacoustic emissions and ABR), they will typically reveal normal peripheral auditory function. Abnormal central auditory function is implicated in these individuals by the observation of abnormal test results for the latter auditory potentials (MLRs and LAERs). Although the term central deafness has been used to refer to bilateral hemispheric lesions, it must be recognized that the auditory deficits noted in this particular disorder can be caused by extensive bilateral lesions of the auditory tracts located within the cortex, subcortex, and/or brainstem.[1]

The term cortical deafness has been used to refer to a condition where the damage in the central nervous system is limited to the primary auditory areas of the cortex. Concerns have been raised that this use of terminology may not accurately reflect the site of lesion in many of these patients, as it is quite uncommon for damage to be confined to the primary auditory areas. In fact, it has been suggested that regions of the subcortex are additionally involved in most cases of cortical deafness.[49]

Auditory agnosia refers to the inability to identify environmental sounds in the presence of normal hearing sensitivity and is frequently accompanied by amusia (i.e. the inability to recognize music), whereas the terms verbal auditory agnosia and word deafness are used to refer to the inability to decode phonology in the presence of normal hearing sensitivity.[50] It has been argued that patients with the latter condition will usually experience difficulty in recognizing any sound stimulus (verbal or non-verbal) that requires a high degree of temporal resolution. Therefore, most of the individuals who experience verbal auditory agnosia or word deafness will also experience difficulty in processing non-verbal signals (i.e. auditory agnosia).[51]

It is important to note that central deafness, cortical deafness, auditory agnosia and word deafness are not distinct entities. In most cases, there is considerable overlap in the deficits noted.[1] Moreover, not all patients with central deafness experience significant losses of threshold sensitivity, and, in many cases, the auditory deficits noted are not stable over time. With changes in hearing sensitivity, there are likely to be concomitant changes in the type and extent of the central auditory problem(s) noted. It is therefore essential that extensive psychoacoustic and electrophysiological testing be done on these patients in order to document the nature, extent and variability of the deficits experienced by these individuals.

Effects of peripheral hearing loss

A major consideration in the use of any central auditory processing test is the presence of a peripheral hearing impairment in the patient to be assessed. It is not unusual to find significant cochlear distortion effects in an individual with a peripheral hearing loss. If depressed scores are noted on routine speech audiometric procedures, then depressed scores would be anticipated for any test that requires the processing of speech stimuli. For many years, it was common practice for the audiologist to avoid the administration of any of the central auditory tests if a peripheral hearing loss was present. Although such a practice avoided the need to account for the potential contribution of the peripheral hearing loss to the central test results, it often failed to meet the needs of the patient as a central hearing disorder may coexist with a peripheral hearing impairment and its identification may have important implications for management of the individual with hearing loss.[27,52,53]

To date, there have been a number of investigations which have studied the effects of peripheral hearing loss on central auditory test results. These investigations have shown that the presence of a peripheral hearing loss can have a negative effect on the results of a number of central auditory tests.[35,41,54–63] However, in spite of the finding that virtually all central auditory tests can be affected by peripheral hearing loss, some of these studies have shown that certain tests may be less affected by peripheral hearing loss than others. Both the dichotic digits test[59,63] and the dichotic sentence identification test[41] appear to be less affected by the presence of mild-to-moderate hearing losses than most of the other speech recognition tests. In addition, the frequency pattern sequences and the auditory duration patterns tests have been shown to be relatively resistant to the potential confounding effect of mild-to-moderate peripheral hearing loss.[43,44] Given these findings, these tests should be given serious consideration for administration whenever a central auditory assessment is being conducted on a patient with a peripheral hearing loss.

Despite the potential confounding effects of peripheral hearing loss and the limited number of tests that appear to be somewhat resistant to the confounding effects of peripheral hearing loss, the assessment of central auditory function in individuals with mild-to-moderately severe peripheral hearing impairment should not be abandoned. The presence of normal or abnormal central auditory function can be implicated in a number of situations, and this can lead to more effective management of the individual with hearing loss. These situations include the following: (1) if hearing loss is present and central test results fall within the normal range for both ears, then the presence of CANS compromise or an APD/CAPD can be ruled out; (2) if a bilaterally symmetrical hearing loss is present and the central test results are more depressed in one ear than in the other, then the presence of CANS compromise or an APD/CAPD is implicated; (3) if a hearing loss is present but it is asymmetrical or unilateral and the 'better ear' shows the poorer performance, then CANS compromise or an APD/CAPD is implicated; (4) if a symmetrical hearing loss is present and abnormal middle and/or late potentials are noted from electrodes over one hemisphere versus the other (i.e. a significant electrode effect), CANS involvement should be suspected; and (5) if a symmetrical hearing loss is present and an 'ear effect' is noted during electrophysiological testing, then the possibility of CANS involvement should be entertained.[27] In these cases, a determination as to the status of the central auditory system can be made with a certain degree of confidence. For those individuals who do not fall into one of these categories, determination of the status of the CANS is difficult, if not impossible to make. However, one may still be able to manage the deficits identified in such a way as to improve the quality of life for the patient with these auditory difficulties, even though the etiological basis for the deficits cannot be determined.

A significant confounding variable in the assessment of APD/CAPD is the presence of a peripheral hearing loss. However, the presence of a peripheral impairment need not pre-empt assessment of central auditory processing skills. Knowledge of the effects of peripheral loss on test performance, along with the careful selection of tests that are most resistant to cochlear confounds, can result in a test battery that is interpretable.

Need for a test battery

As mentioned above, the CANS is a complex neural system that is responsible for the processing of acoustic information at various sites along its pathways. The nature of the processing is complex, and different types of processing occur at different levels. Therefore, it is unlikely that any one test, or even a small group of tests, will be appropriate for each individual presenting with a potential CANS lesion. For this reason, reliance on one test is not advisable. If compromise of one level of the auditory system is suspected based upon case history information, then tests shown to be sensitive to lesions at that level of the system should be targeted for use. For instance, if a cerebral lesion is suspected, administration of a dichotic speech test along with a temporal patterning test would probably provide more information than use of a single dichotic speech test, two dichotic speech tests that are essentially testing the same processes, or even a binaural interaction test and a dichotic speech test. On the other hand, if a brainstem lesion is suspected, then an electrophysiological test (i.e. ABR) and the MLD may be utilized, with less reliance on tests for cortical and/or interhemispheric pathway function.

The CANS is a complex, but highly redundant, neural system. For this reason, the deficits that accompany disorders affecting the CANS are often subtle and may vary with the site of lesion. Therefore, it is essential that a battery of tests be used to assess auditory function in the patient considered to be at risk for an APD/CAPD. The test battery should include tests that assess the various auditory processes that underlie normal auditory function, as well as functioning at various levels within the CANS.

Management protocols

Non-medical management of the individual with an APD/CAPD has essentially taken one or more of three approaches. These include: (1) improving the quality of the signal; (2) enhancing the individual's auditory perceptual skills; and (3) enhancing the individual's linguistic and cognitive skills. The specific approach or approaches employed with any given individual will depend on a number of factors, including the age and cognitive abilities of the individual, and the exact nature of the APD/CAPD. Typically, the younger the patient, the greater the likelihood that management will focus on efforts to improve the patient's auditory perceptual skills, whereas with older patients efforts are more likely to focus on strategy instruction.

Auditory plasticity

The foundation for many of the direct intervention strategies used in the remediation of APD/CAPD is the concept of brain plasticity. Research efforts in this area have provided a substantial body of evidence that demonstrates that auditory stimulation can result in the development or a reorganization of the auditory neural substrate.[64] The evidence, however, does implicate age as a factor in terms of brain plasticity; that is, young brains are highly plastic and change more rapidly with appropriate stimulation than more mature brains.[65]

> Auditory plasticity serves as the foundation for many of the direct intervention strategies that will be used in the remediation of APD/CAPD. The term is used to refer to the alteration of nerve cells to better conform to immediate environmental influences. This type of alteration of nerve cells is facilitated by repetitive auditory stimulation and is typically associated with behavioral change.

Enhancing the quality of the speech signal

Clear speech

Clear speech is the process where the speaker attempts to produce every word in an utterance in a precise, accurate and clearly articulated manner. As a result of these efforts, speech tends to become slower and louder, intonation tends to become more varied, and stress on certain words or phrases becomes more prominent, thereby increasing the perceptual saliency of these words or phrases. In addition, the speech stream tends to become more clearly segmented through the insertion of pauses between phrases and sentences, and individual speech sounds or phonemes are less likely to be omitted or reduced. These techniques have been employed with individuals with peripheral hearing impairment, and the results have demonstrated that improvements in speech intelligibility are realized when the speaker makes such conscious efforts to speak clearly.[66–68] Given the difficulty that individuals with APD/CAPD have in processing rapidly changing brief acoustic information, it is logical to assume that such efforts would enhance the ability of the individual with APD/CAPD to process auditory information.

Classroom acoustics

One of the most common problems encountered by individuals with APD/CAPD is increased difficulty in listening in noisy or reverberant backgrounds. Efforts can be made to improve these adverse listening environments. These include the application of acoustic ceiling tiles, window treatments, carpeting, and other architectural changes which serve to absorb sound in the room and minimize the amount of reverberation in the listening environment.[16,69]

FM systems

Another method of attempting to improve the individual's ability to follow conversation is the provision of an assistive listening device (i.e. FM system) to improve the signal-to-noise ratio. The FM system includes a microphone which picks up the voice of the speaker and transmits it to a receiver, where the signal is amplified and then transduced back to an acoustic signal. These types of systems include both personal and classroom types of systems. Both have been shown to be effective in assisting individuals with APD/CAPD to overcome many of the difficulties experienced when having to listen under adverse listening conditions.[16,69,70]

Enhancing the individual's auditory perceptual skills

Auditory training

Auditory training programs for the individual with APD/CAPD are similar to those designed for individuals with peripheral hearing impairments. Training often initially focuses on tasks such as frequency, temporal and intensity discrimination and then progresses through activities focused on pattern recognition, to discrimination and recognition of syllables, words, phrases, sentences, and connected speech. The intervention program can be tailored to each individual's abilities and modified as appropriate.[16,69] For example, if a given individual has good frequency, temporal and intensity discrimination abilities, then activities focusing on the development of these skills can be bypassed with initial intervention activities focused on discrimination and recognition of speech materials.

Enhancing the individual's linguistic cognitive skills

The management procedures that follow include procedures which can be incorporated into a comprehensive management plan in an effort to assist the individual with APD/CAPD to overcome the potentially devastating effects of these deficits. This is achieved by providing the individual with access to alternative knowledge bases and/or strategies which can be utilized to derive meaning from an auditory event which would otherwise be a challenging, if not impossible, listening activity. It should be noted, however, that although these efforts are directed at improving linguistic or cognitive skills, it is not uncommon to see some improvements in auditory perceptual skills as a byproduct of many of these intervention strategies or procedures.[71,72]

Phonological awareness

Phonological awareness refers to the ability to recognize and manipulate the various sound units characteristic of the language (i.e. phonemes, syllables, and words). Individuals with deficits in this area have difficulty in perceiving, decoding, storing and retrieving verbal information. Phonemic awareness, a component of phonological processing, is the ability to recognize and manipulate the individual sounds in words (e.g.

phonemes). Phonological processing difficulties are quite common in individuals with APD/CAPD, since the efficient processing of speech is based upon the ability to process brief acoustic events which are changing rapidly in their temporal, spectral and intensity characteristics. It is quite likely that management of the individual with APD/CAPD, especially if the individual is a child, will involve some type of phonemic awareness or phonological processing training.

Skill areas typically targeted during phonemic awareness training include: auditory discrimination, sound blending, sound segmentation, phoneme identification, recognition of sound and sound position in word, and rhyming. Two commercial programs[73,74] released within the past few years have prompted a great deal of interest in this particular management strategy. Although there has been considerable interest generated in the use of these two programs to remediate poor phonemic awareness skills, it should be noted there are a number of other workbooks and therapy materials which are commercially available, and management materials in this area can be easily developed.[75,76] Efficacy data for this type of intervention are beginning to emerge, and the available evidence appears to support the continued use of this type of treatment for individuals with phonological processing disorders.[72,77]

Morphology

Morphological markers are frequently not processed efficiently by individuals with APD/CAPD, due, in large part, to their unstressed and weak acoustic representation within the speech stream. Individuals with APD/CAPD who must deduce the existence of these markers solely on the basis of their auditory experiences with spoken language are likely to demonstrate significant delays in the acquisition of these linguistic markers. Therefore, efforts should be directed at remediating any delays in the individual's expressive or receptive use of these markers.

Vocabulary

The acquisition of new lexical items is often challenging for the individual with an APD/CAPD. This is due in large part to the difficulty that the individual has in processing the brief and rapidly changing acoustic stream that represents the new lexical item, deducing the underlying phonological representation of the new word, storing the phonological representation in his or her mental lexicon, and then retrieving this phonological representation from the mental lexicon for future use. Efforts to foster the development of new vocabulary items can take a number of forms. One procedure which has proven to be particularly advantageous for the child with APD/CAPD is vocabulary previewing or pretutoring. In this procedure, challenging vocabulary items that are to be introduced in the class the following day are provided to a parent or aid the day before so that the adult can introduce the novel vocabulary items in a less stressful environment. To obtain maximum benefits from this approach, it is desirable to have the activities conducted in a quiet environment free from auditory and visual distractions. The adult should provide the child with an auditory stimulus supported by visual aids (i.e. the word in print along with a pictorial representation, if possible) and then the child should be asked to repeat the word. Additional activities could include a review of the definition of the new vocabulary item and use of the new item in a sentence. The benefit of this type of approach is that it allows the child to use a variety of sensory input modalities (sight, hearing, and kinesthetic) to assist in the processing, acquisition and storage of new information. This integration of sensory information helps to facilitate the individual's ability to recognize, recall and retrieve the information when the word or words are introduced in the classroom.[15,78]

Prosody

Prosody or intonation is an important linguistic marker that can often change the meaning of an utterance. A declarative sentence spoken with a rising as opposed to a falling intonation takes on a different meaning and requires a different type of response from the communicative partner. Differences in prosody can also form the basis for humor. Simply putting the stress on a different syllable within a sentence can significantly alter the meaning of the sentence. Many individuals with APD/CAPD experience difficulty in processing the acoustic envelope of an ongoing acoustic stream. As a result, they are often unaware of subtle differences in intonation patterns which signal alternative linguistic meanings or intentions. Hence, this is an area which frequently requires intervention. Training should focus on contrasting intonation patterns, to foster recognition of the alternative semantic interpretations of sentences which may have otherwise identical phonological, syntactic and semantic structures.

Metacognition

Metacognition refers to the processes through which an individual: (1) reflects on the demands inherent in an activity or situation; (2) recognizes the skills that he or she brings to the activity or situation; (3) identifies the variables that can affect performance; and (4) uses this information and knowledge to plan, monitor and regulate behaviors such as attention, memory, listening, comprehension, and the use of language. For many individuals, metacognitive processes are automatic and relatively effortless. They are derived or activated with little conscious effort.[79,80] For other individuals, however, these processes require conscious focus on the cognitive demands associated with the context or behavior, a recognition of the individual's goals with respect to the context or behavior, and the mental processes needed to meet both the demands and goals.[81]

The latter situation is one that is frequently encountered by individuals with APD/CAPD. For these individuals, formalized strategy instruction is warranted. Most of the procedures that have been advocated to date involve a number of steps, which include activities such as: (1) pretesting and commitment to strategy development and use; (2) description of the strategy; (3) modeling of the strategy; (4) verbal rehearsal of the strategy; (5) controlled practice and feedback; (6) post-testing; and (7) generalization.[82–91] In addition, since it is unlikely that one strategy will meet the needs of the individual in all contexts and environments, the ability to identify and use additional strategies needs to be fostered.[89] In other words, the individual must be trained to become strategic. To do so, the individual must be capable of recognizing the underlying similarities in new problems which may parallel patterns noted in previously solved problems.[89] The professional can help facilitate the individual's move toward strategic actions by providing hints, discussion and reflection, and allowing the individual to teach or demonstrate strategic actions.[90]

Space limitations preclude a detailed discussion of the various strategies that can be used with individuals with APD/CAPD. A few selected procedures are provided to illustrate the various types of procedure available. The reader interested in additional strategies and strategy instruction is referred to other sources.[16,74,91–94]

Contextual derivation

Context can often be used to derive word meaning and enhance message comprehension when an individual encounters an unfamiliar lexical item or phrase.[95] Unfortunately, many individuals with APD/CAPD focus their efforts on bottom-up types of processing (i.e. they attempt to process the sounds heard or orthographic symbols seen to achieve word recognition), rather than shifting to a more top-down type of processing when unfamiliar words or phrases are encountered. As a result, comprehension often breaks down. By using linguistic context which is represented within the utterance or written statement, the efficient listener or reader can frequently achieve grammatical closure and message understanding despite the fact that they have no knowledge of, or experience with, one or more of the lexical items within the utterance. In context-derived comprehension instruction, the individual is encouraged to use their world and linguistic knowledge to deduce word meaning and achieve message comprehension. For example, in the sentence 'The thief absconded with the jewels and the money' the meaning of the word 'absconded' can be deduced from the semantic information contained in the rest of the utterance.

Discourse cohesion devices and schema induction

Discourse cohesion devices are linguistic conventions that connect propositions into complex messages.[96] These devices allow communicative partners to formulate and comprehend complex messages in an efficient manner by establishing distinct relationships between words (for example, the words 'and', 'therefore', 'before', 'although' and 'instead of', signal additive, causal, temporal, adversative and disjunctive relationships, respectively). Schema is a psychological construct used to account for knowledge organization which is invoked when discrete cognitive tasks are undertaken.[97] A schema is an organized assemblage of related concepts, a set of expectations, abstract and generic knowledge stored in long-term memory which preserves the relationships among the constituent concepts, and generalized knowledge about an event, object, or message. It provides the individual with a conceptual framework that can guide interpretation, as it represents a multidimensional map which connects inter-related ideas and concepts. Formal schemata are linguistic conventions that serve to organize, integrate and predict relationships among propositions.[98] The discourse cohesion devices discussed above represent formal schemata, as they can be used to organize, integrate and predict relationships among propositions. Other linguistic conventions include linguistic markers that would signal parallelism or correlative status (e.g. not only ... but also, neither ... nor), causation or speculation (e.g. if ... then), temporal relationships (first, finally), and so forth.

It has been established that many individuals with language-processing disorders have difficulty in formulating these types of schemata.[99,100] Management efforts for these individuals should be directed at developing the ability to first recognize the presence of these types of discourse elements within utterances and then to discern the unique relationships between the propositions being signaled by these discourse elements. This should assist the individual with an APD/CAPD in processing complex spoken information, as utilization of these skills and abilities during listening and/or reading activities should trigger certain expectations about the message, narrow the possible alternatives for interpretation, and provide the individual with direction in processing the information.[16]

Cognitive style and reasoning

Individuals differ along a number of different cognitive style continua (flexibility/inflexibility, field independent/field dependent, convergent/divergent, and impulsive/reflective). Some of these cognitive styles will serve to facilitate one's ability to adjust to various listening and learning situations, whereas others will impede such adjustments. It is essential to the success of the management program that the individual be encouraged to assume or develop a more facilitative cognitive style (e.g. flexible, reflective), if needed. This can be accomplished by various behavioral modification techniques.

> Several approaches have been advocated for the management of the auditory difficulties experienced by individuals with APD/CAPD. These include: (1) improving the quality of the acoustic signal; (2) enhancing the individual's auditory perceptual skills; and (3) enhancing the individual's cognitive and listening skills. In developing a comprehensive management plan, consideration should be given to all three approaches. However, the extent to which each of the three approaches will be incorporated into a given patient's management plan will probably depend on a number of factors (e.g. the specific nature of the patient's deficits, the age and cognitive abilities of the patient, the availability of technology resources, and the presence/absence of any comorbid conditions).

Case presentation

History

A left-handed male was 10 years old when he was evaluated at our medical facility. He had been delivered by emergency Cesarean section following a motor vehicle accident at 34 weeks of gestation. His neonatal history was complicated by hyaline membrane disease, jaundice, respiratory distress syndrome, and hepatitis of unknown etiology. As a result of these complications, he remained in the NICU for 6 weeks postpartem and was then discharged to home.

At the age of 5 months, concerns were raised regarding his increasing head circumference and a CT scan was ordered. The scan revealed markedly dilated lateral ventricles, with the left ventricle being more involved than the right. At that time, a ventricular peritoneal shunt was inserted on the left. A revision procedure was conducted when the child was 6 years of age. At the age of 4 years, this child began to experience complex partial seizures, which were managed with 100 mg of Dilantin daily.

ABR testing was performed at the age of 4½ months. The results suggested borderline normal hearing in the low frequencies and a mild loss of hearing in the high frequencies for the right ear, and a severe-to-profound loss in the left ear. Results of periodic audiological testing over a 2-year period following this initial assessment were consistent with these early findings. However, subsequent audiological evaluations revealed hearing thresholds which were within normal limits bilaterally.

Developmental assessment conducted in kindergarten reportedly indicated that this child's development was delayed by 6 months. At the present time, he is reported to be functioning 1–2 years behind the grade level in most academic areas, and receives remedial services in school for speech and language, reading, writing, and spelling.

Audiological findings

Results of pure tone testing revealed hearing thresholds which fell within normal limits bilaterally (Figure 29.4). Speech recognition scores were excellent in both ears.

Results of behavioral central testing (Figure 29.5) revealed depressed scores for the right ear on two dichotic speech tests (dichotic digits and competing sentences), and for both ears on a monaural low-redundancy speech test (low-pass filtered speech) and two temporal patterning tests (frequency pattern sequences and auditory duration patterns). When the patient was asked to hum the frequency pattern sequences instead of verbally describing the sequences, performance rose to within normal limits for both ears.

Results of ABR/MLR testing conducted with insert receivers revealed a well-defined ABR wave V for both ears and normal MLR responses (Na and Pa) for all recording montages with right-ear stimulation (Figure 29.6). With left-ear stimulation, the MLR responses did not replicate well. A questionable Pa was noted on the left ear recordings. However, if this is a Pa response, it is delayed in latency and reduced in amplitude when compared to the right-ear response (i.e. an ear effect).

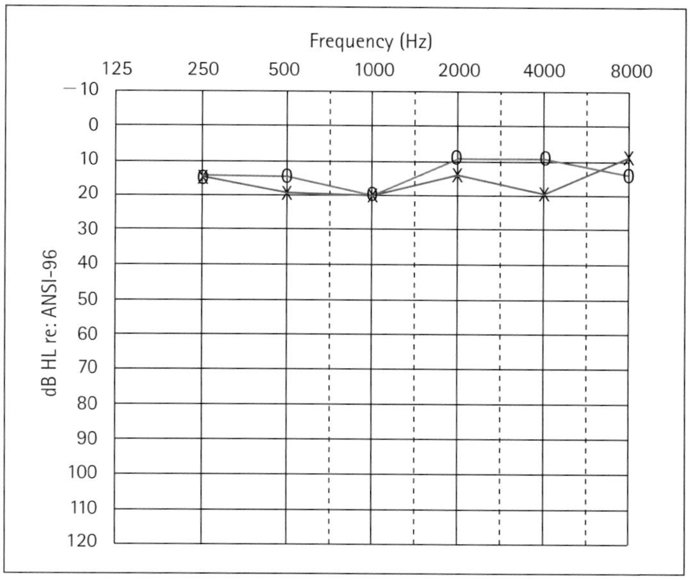

Figure 29.4 Audiogram (right ear O; left ear X) of a 10-year-old male diagnosed with asymmetrical hydrocephalus of the lateral ventricles.

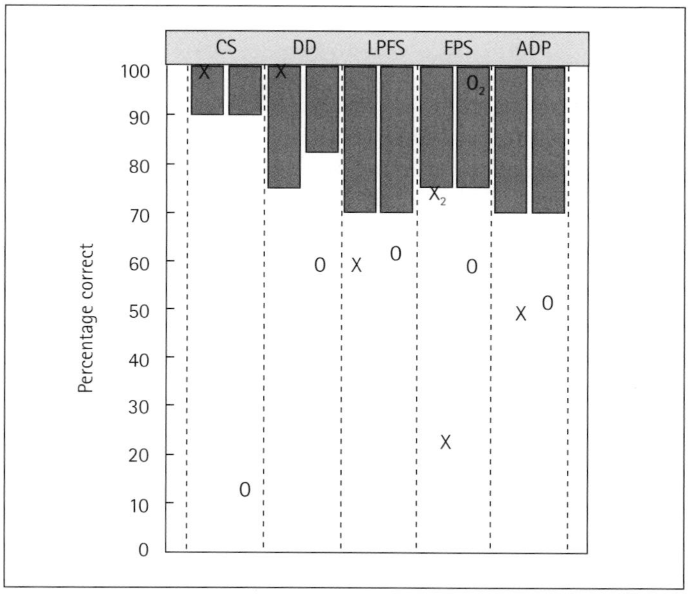

Figure 29.5 Central auditory test results for the patient described in Figure 29.4. Data are presented for two dichotic speech tests (CS, competing sentences; DD, dichotic digits), a monaural low-redundancy speech test (LPFS, low-pass filtered speech), and two temporal patterning tests (FPS, frequency pattern sequences; ADP, auditory duration patterns) for the right (O) and left (X) ears. For the FPS test, results are provided for both verbal (O and X) and hummed (O_2 and X_2) responses. The shaded areas represent the range of normal performance for each test.

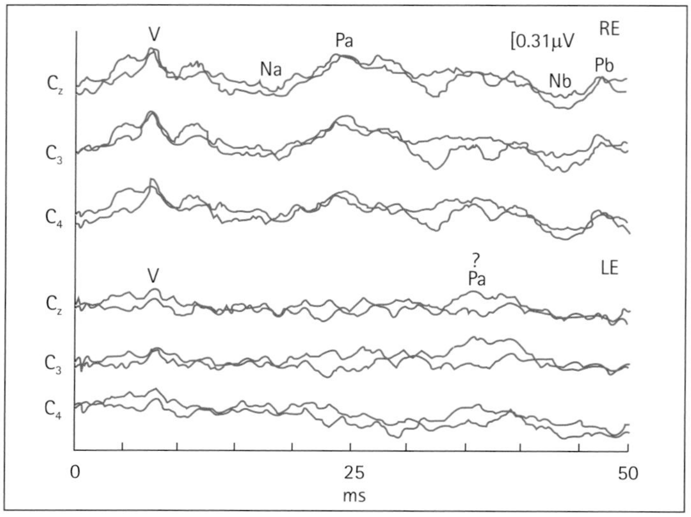

Figure 29.6 Combined ABR and MLR recordings for the right and left ears for the patient described in Figure 29.4.

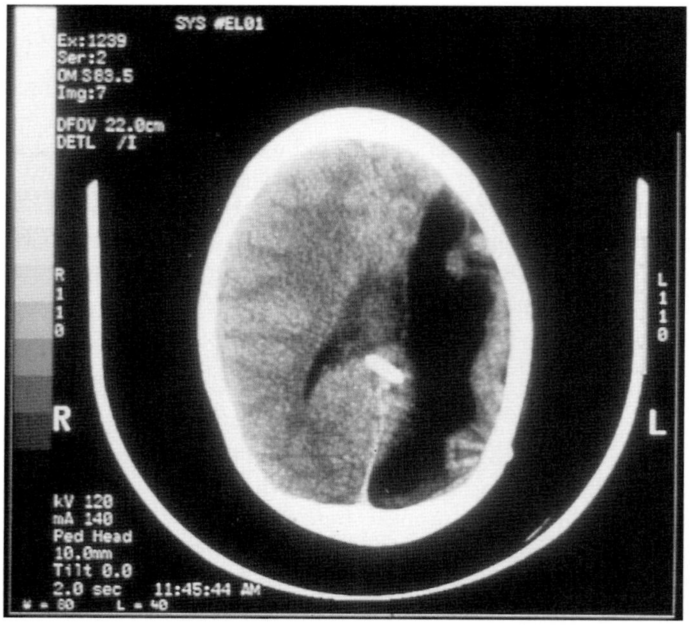

Figure 29.7 CT scan for the patient described in Figure 29.4, showing marked dilatation of the left lateral ventricle and less marked, but significant, dilatation of the right lateral ventricle.

Radiological findings

A CT scan conducted at 5 months of age revealed marked dilatation of the left lateral ventricle and less marked, but significant, dilatation of the right lateral ventricle. In addition, the third ventricle was dilated. A diagnosis of asymmetrical hydrocephalus was made (Figure 29.7).

Management

This child continues to receive speech and language and academic services in his school, with remedial activities focused on many of the linguistic interventions suggested earlier in this chapter. Since he is receiving appropriate services within his school district and the family lives at some distance from our center, we are not providing ongoing management services at this time. We met with the child's mother and a number of school professionals (speech–language pathologist, classroom teacher, special education teacher, and educational plan coordinator) following our evaluation, to review the child's current management plan and identify a number of strategies which can be used at home and in school to help the child overcome the auditory processing difficulties he is experiencing as a result of his CANS lesion.

Comments

This case demonstrates the utilization of central tests in cases of central nervous system lesions and the importance of a 'team approach' to management. The behavioral results showed large right-ear deficits with normal left-ear performance for the dichotic tests. These deficits represent the 'classic' contralateral ear deficit (see Table 29.2) often noted with a lesion of the auditory cortex (likely to be secondary to the lateral ventricle hydrocephalus). In addition, the pattern of results on the temporal patterning tests implicates a significant left-sided lesion, since verbal labeling of the frequency pattern sequences resulted in depressed scores bilaterally, while mimicking (or humming) the patterns resulted in normal performance for both ears. The bilateral deficits noted on the monaural low-redundancy test, with the more prominent depression observed for the right ear, may be accurately reflecting the asymmetric structural lesion noted during radiological assessment; that is, both hemispheres were affected, but the extent of the lesion was much greater for the left side. Finally, the MLR tracings revealed an ispilateral ear effect which may reflect some compromise in the thalamic region. Given the extent of the dilatation of the left lateral ventricle and the question of third ventricle involvement in this case, it is possible that both auditory cortex and high brainstem function were affected by the hydrocephalus.

Concluding comments

There have been a number of significant developments in the field of central auditory processing assessment since the first attempts to assess CANS function in patients with neurological lesions. Our understanding of the neuroanatomy and neurophysiology of the CANS has grown tremendously since the time of these early attempts. Many new tests have been introduced in an effort to tease out the various deficits observed in individuals with APD/CAPD, and there are a number of innovative assessment protocols which are being investigated in research laboratories at the present time. It is anticipated that many of these tests will find their way into the assessment arena and will serve to increase the sensitivity of current assessment protocols as well as to provide the opportunity for more comprehensive assessment of the auditory deficits experienced by individuals with CANS lesions. In addition, the past decade has seen an increase in the attention paid to the development of effective management strategies for use with individuals with APD/CAPDs. It is anticipated that management programs will be refined as technology is used to a greater extent and the efficacies of the various approaches currently being used are established. The end-result of all these endeavors should be an improved quality of life for those individuals who present with an APD/CAPD.

References

1. Musiek FE, Baran JA, Pinheiro ML. *Neuroaudiology: Case Studies*. San Diego: Singular Publishing Group, 1994.
2. Bocca E, Calearo C, Cassinari V. A new method for testing hearing in temporal lobe tumors. *Acta Otolaryngol* 1954; **44**: 219–21.
3. Bocca E, Calearo C, Cassinari V, Migliavacca F. Testing 'cortical' hearing in temporal lobe tumors. *Acta Otolaryngol* 1955; **45**: 289–304.
4. Sanchez-Longo LP, Forster FM. Clinical significance of impairment of sound localization. *Neurology* 1958; **8**: 1191–225.
5. Sanchez-Longo LP, Forster FM, Auth TL. A new clinical test for sound localization and its applications. *Neurology* 1957; **7**: 653–5.
6. Kimura D. Cerebral dominance and the perception of verbal stimuli. *Can J Psychol* 1961; **15**: 166–71.
7. Kimura D. Some effects of temporal lobe damage on auditory perception. *Can J Psychol* 1961; **15**: 157–65.
8. Milner B. Laterality effects in audition. In: Montcastle VB ed. *Interhemispheric Relations and Cerebral Dominance*. Baltimore: John Hopkins Press, 1962: 117–95.
9. Milner B, Kimura D, Taylor LB. Nonverbal auditory learning after frontal or temporal lobectomy in man. Paper presented at a meeting of the Eastern Psychological Association, Boston, April 1968.
10. Shankweiler D. Effects of temporal damage on perception of dichotically presented melodies. *J Comparative Physiol Psychol* 1966; **62**: 115–19.
11. Jerger JF, Weikers NJ, Sharbrough FW, Jerger S. Bilateral lesions of the temporal lobe: a case study. *Acta Otolaryngol* 1969; **258**: 5–51.
12. Starr A, Achor LJ. Auditory brainstem responses in neurological disease. *Arch Neurol* 1975; **32**: 761–8.
13. Stockard JJ, Rossiter VS. Clinical and pathologic correlates of brain stem auditory response abnormalities. *Neurology* 1977; **27**: 316–25.
14. Robinson K, Rudge P. Abnormalities of the auditory evoked potentials in patients with multiple sclerosis. *Brain* 1977; **100**: 19–40.
15. Baran JA, Musiek FE. Behavioral assessment of the central auditory nervous system. In: Musiek FE, Rintelmann WF, eds. *Contemporary Perspectives in Hearing Assessment*. Boston: Allyn & Bacon, 1999: 375–413.
16. Chermak GD, Musiek FE. *Central Auditory Processing Disorders: New Perspectives*. San Diego: Singular Publishing Group, 1997.
17. American Speech–Language–Hearing Association. Central auditory processing: current status and implications for clinical practice. *Am J Audiol* 1996; **5**: 41–54.
18. Jerger J, Musiek F. Report of the consensus conference on the diagnosis of auditory processing disorders in school-aged children. *J Am Acad Audiol* 2000; **11**: 467–74.
19. Baran JA. Speech perception test materials for central auditory processing assessment. In: Mendel LL, Danhauer JL, eds. *Audiologic Evaluation and Management and Speech Perception Assessment*. San Diego: Singular Publishing Group, 1997: 147–68.
20. Brody H. Organization of cerebral cortex: III. A study of aging in human cerebral cortex. *J Comparative Neurol* 1955; **102**: 511–36.
21. Kirikae I, Sato T, Shitara T. A study of hearing in advanced age. *Laryngoscope* 1964; **74**: 205–20.
22. Smith BH, Sethi PH. Aging and the nervous system. *Geriatrics* 1975; **30**: 109–15.
23. Schnuknecht HF. Further observations on the pathology of presbycusis. *Arch Otolaryngol* 1964; **80**: 369–82.
24. Schnuknecht HF. *Pathology of the Ear*. Cambridge, MA: Harvard University Press, 1974.
25. Humes LE, Christopherson L, Cokely C. Central auditory processing disorders in the elderly: fact or fiction? In: Katz J, Stecker N, Henderson D, eds. *Central Auditory Processing: A Transdisciplinary View*. St Louis: Mosby Year Book, 1992: 141–50.
26. Kricos PB, Lesner SA. *Hearing Care for the Older Adult: Audiologic Rehabilitation*. Boston: Butterworth-Heinemann, 1995.
27. Musiek FE, Baran JA. Amplification and the central auditory nervous system. In: Valente M, ed. *Hearing Aids: Standards, Options, and Limitations*. New York: Thieme Medical Publishers, 1996: 407–38.
28. Weinstein BE. Presbycusis. In: Katz J, ed. *Handbook of Clinical Audiology*, 4th edn. Baltimore: Williams & Wilkins, 1994: 553–67.
29. Musiek FE, Gollegly KM, Baran JA. Myelination of the corpus callosum in learning disabled children: theoretical and clinical correlates. *Semin Hear* 1984; **5**: 231–42.
30. Musiek FE, Gollegly KM, Ross MK. Profiles of types of central auditory processing disorders in children with learning disabilities. *J Child Commun Disord* 1985; **9**: 43–61.
31. Fisher LI. *Fisher's Auditory Problems Checklist*. Bemidji, MN: Life Products, 1976.
32. Kelly DA. *Central Auditory Processing Disorders: Strategies for Use with Children and Adolescents*. San Antonio, TX: Communication Skill Builders, 1995.
33. Smoski WJ, Brunt MA, Tannahill JC. Listening characteristics of children with central auditory processing disorders. *Language Speech Hear Services Schools* 1992; **23**: 145–52.
34. Willeford JA, Burleigh JM. *Handbook of Central Auditory Processing Disorders in Children*. Orlando, FL: Grune and Stratton, 1985.
35. Olsen WO, Noffsinger D, Carhart R. Masking level differences encountered in clinical populations. *Audiology* 1976; **15**: 287–301.
36. Willeford J. Differential diagnosis of central auditory dysfunction. In: Bradford L, ed. *Audiology: An Audio Journal for Continuing Education*, Vol. 2. New York: Grune & Stratton, 1976.

37. Musiek FE. Assessment of central auditory dysfunction: the dichotic digit test revisited. *Ear Hear* 1983; **4**: 79–83.
38. Berlin CI, Lowe-Bell SS, Jannetta PJ, Kline DG. Central auditory deficits after temporal lobectomy. *Arch Otolaryngol* 1972; **96**: 4–10.
39. Katz J. The use of staggered spondaic words for assessing the integrity of the central auditory system. *J Auditory Res* 1962; **2**: 327–37.
40. Jerger JF, Jerger SW. Auditory findings in brainstem disorders. *Arch Otolaryngol* 1974; **99**: 342–9.
41. Fifer RC, Jerger JF, Berlin CI, Tobey E, Campbell J. Development of a dichotic sentence identification test for hearing impaired adults. *Ear Hear* 1983; **4**: 300–5.
42. Beasley DS, Schwimmer S, Rintelmann WF. Intelligibility of time-compressed CNC monosyllables. *J Speech Hear Res* 1972; **15**: 340–50.
43. Musiek FE, Pinheiro ML. Frequency pattern in cochlear, brainstem, and cerebral lesions. *Audiology* 1987; **26**: 79–88.
44. Musiek FE, Baran JA, Pinheiro ML. Duration pattern recognition in normal subjects and patients with cerebral and cochlear lesions. *Audiology* 1990; **29**: 304–13.
45. Baran JA, Musiek FE. Central auditory processing disorders in children and adults. In: Wall LG, ed. *Hearing for the Speech–Language Pathologist and Health Care Professional*. Boston: Butterworth-Heinemann, 1995: 415–40.
46. Licklider JCR. The influence of interaural phase relations upon the masking of speech by white noise. *J Acoust Soc Am* 1948; **20**: 150–9.
47. Hall JW. *Handbook of Auditory Evoked Responses*. Boston: Allyn and Bacon, 1992.
48. Musiek FE, Lee WW. Auditory middle and late potentials. In: Musiek FE, Rintelmann WF, eds. *Contemporary Perspectives in Hearing Assessment*. Boston: Allyn and Bacon, 1999: 243–72.
49. Tanaka Y, Kamo T, Yoshida M, Yamadori A. So called cortical deafness: clinical, neurophysiological and radiological observations. *Brain* 1991; **114**: 2385–401.
50. Rapin I. Cortical deafness, auditory agnosia, and word deafness: how distinct are they? *Human Commun* 1985; **5**: 29–37.
51. Phillips D, Farmer M. Acquired word deafness and the temporal grain of sound representation in the primary auditory cortex. *Behav Brain Res* 1990; **40**: 85–94.
52. Stach BA. Hearing aid amplification and central processing disorders. In: Sandlin RE, ed. *Handbook of Hearing Aid Amplification*. Vol. II: *Clinical Considerations and Fitting Practices*. Boston: College-Hill Press, 1990: 87–111.
53. Stach BA, Spretnjak ML, Jerger JF. The prevalence of central presbycusis in a clinical population. *J Am Acad Audiol* 1990; **1**: 109–15.
54. Divenyi PL, Haupt RM. Audiological correlates of speech understading in elderly listeners with mild-to-moderate hearing loss. I: Age and lateral asymmetry effects. *Ear Hear* 1997; **18**: 42–61.
55. Divenyi PL, Haupt RM. Audiological correlates of speech understanding in elderly listeners with mild-to-moderate hearing loss. III: Factor representation. *Ear Hear* 1997; **18**: 189–201.
56. Grimes AM, Mueller HG, Williams DL. Clinical considerations in the use of time-compressed speech. *Ear Hear* 1984; **5**: 114–17.
57. Kurdziel S, Noffsinger D, Olsen W. Performance by cortical lesion patients on 40 and 60% time-compressed materials. *J Acoust Soc Am* 1976; **2**: 3–7.
58. Miltenberger G, Dawson G, Raica A. Central testing with peripheral hearing loss. *Arch Otolaryngol* 1978; **104**: 11–15.
59. Musiek FE, Gollegly KM, Kibbe K, Verkest-Lenz S. Proposed screening test for central auditory disorders: follow-up on the dichotic digits test. *Am J Otolaryngol* 1991; **12**: 109–13.
60. Noffsinger D. Clinical applications of selected binaural effects. *Scand Audiol* 1982; **15**: 156–62.
61. Orchik DJ, Burgess T. Synthetic sentence identification as a function of the age of the listener. *J Am Acoust Soc* 1977; **3**: 42–6.
62. Roeser R, Johns D, Price L. Dichotic listening in adults with sensorineural hearing loss. *J Am Auditory Soc* 1976; **2**: 19–25.
63. Speaks C, Niccum N, Van Tasell D. Effects of stimulus material on the dichotic listening performance of patients with sensorineural hearing loss. *J Speech Hear Res* 1985; **28**: 16–25.
64. Musiek FE, Berge BE. A neuroscience view of auditory training/stimulation and central auditory processing disorders. In: Masters MG, Stecker NA, Katz J, eds. *Central Auditory Processing Disorders: Mostly Management*. Boston: Allyn and Bacon, 1998: 15–32.
65. Hassmannova J, Myslivecek J, Novakova V. Effects of early auditory stimulation on cortical centers. In: Syka J, Aitkin L, eds. *Neural Mechanisms of Hearing*. New York: Plenum, 1981: 355–9.
66. Picheny MA, Durlach NI, Braida LD. Speaking clearly for the hard of hearing I: Intelligibility differences between clear and conversational speech. *J Speech Hear Res* 1985; **28**: 96–103.
67. Picheny MA, Durlach NI, Braida LD. Speaking clearly for the hard of hearing II: Acoustic characteristics of clear and conversational speech. *J Speech Hear Res* 1986; **29**: 434–46.
68. Picheny MA, Durlach NI, Braida LD. Speaking clearly for the hard of hearing III: Attempts to determine the contribution of speaking rate to differences in intelligibility between clear and conversational speech. *J Speech Hear Res* 1989; **32**: 600–3.
69. Bellis TJ. *Assessment and Management of Central Auditory Processing Disorders in the Educational Setting: From Science to Practice*. San Diego: Singular Publishing Group, 1996.
70. Stein RL. Application of FM technology to the management of central auditory processing disorders. In: Masters MG, Stecker NA, Katz J, eds. *Central Auditory Processing Disorders: Mostly Management*. Boston: Allyn and Bacon, 1998: 89–102.
71. Merzenich MM, Jenkins WM, Johnston P, Schreiner C, Miller SL, Tallal P. Temporal processing deficits of language-learning impaired children ameliorated by training. *Science* 1996; **271**: 77–81.
72. Tallal P, Miller SL, Bedi G et al. Language comprehension in language-learning impaired children improved with acoustically modified speech. *Science* 1996; **271**: 81–4.
73. *Earobics*. Evanston, IL: Cognitive Concepts, Inc., 1997.
74. *FastForWord*. Berkely, CA: Scientific Learning Corporation, 1997.
75. Masters MG, Stecker NA, Katz J, eds. *Central Auditory Processing Disorders: Mostly Management*. Boston: Allyn and Bacon, 1998.
76. Sloan C. *Treating Auditory Processing Difficulties in Children*. San Diego: College-Hill Press, 1986.
77. Edelen-Smith PJ. How now brown cow: phoneme awareness activities for collaborative classrooms. *Intervent School Clinic* 1997; **33**: 103–11.

78. Baran JA. Management of adolescents and adults with central auditory processing disorders. In: Masters MG, Stecker NA, Katz J, eds. *Central Auditory Processing Disorders: Mostly Management*. Boston: Allyn and Bacon, 1998: 195–214.
79. Flavell JH. *Cognitive Development*, 2nd edn. Englewood Cliffs, NJ: Prentice Hall, 1985.
80. Siegler R, Shipley C. Variation, selection, and cognitive change. In: Simon T, ed. *Developing Cognitive Competence*. Hillsdale, NJ: Lawrence Erlbaum Associates, 1995: 31–76.
81. Siegler R, Shrager J. Strategy choices in addition and subtraction: how do children know what to do? In: Sophian C, ed. *Origin of Cognitive Skills*. Hillsdale, NJ: Lawrence Erlbaum Associates, 1984: 229–93.
82. Deshler DD, Schumaker JB, Lenz BK, Ellis ES. Academic and cognitive interventions for LD adolescents: Part II. *J Learn Disabil* 1981; **17**: 170–87.
83. Deshler DD, Alley GR, Warner MM, Schumaker JB. Instructional practices for promoting skill acquisition and generalization in severely learning disabled adolescents. *Learn Disabil Q* 1981; **4**: 415–21.
84. Harris KR, Graham S, Pressley M. Cognitive-behavioral approaches in reading and writing language: developing self-regulated learners. In: Singh NN, Beale IL, eds. *Learning Disabilities: Nature, Theory, and Treatment*. New York: Springer-Verlag, 1991: 415–51.
85. Meichenbaum D, Goodman J. Training impulsive children to talk to themselves: a means of developing self-control. *J Abnorm Psychol* 1971; **77**: 115–26.
86. Palinscar AS, Brown DA. Interactive teaching to promote independent learning from text. *Reading Teacher* 1987; **39**: 771–7.
87. Pressley M, Borkowski JG, O'Sullivan JT. Memory strategy instruction is made of this: metamemory and durable strategy use. *Educational Psychologist* 1984; **19**: 94–107.
88. Wilson CC, Lanza JR, Barton JS. Developing higher level thinking skills through questioning techniques in the speech and language setting. *Language Speech Hear Services Schools* 1988; **19**: 428–31.
89. Wynn-Darcy ML, Gillam RB. Accessing long-term memory: metacognitive strategies and strategic action in adolescents. *Topics Language Disord* 1997; **18**: 32–44.
90. Crisafi M, Brown A. Analog transfer in very young children: combining two separately learned solutions to reach goal. *Child Dev* 1986; **57**: 953–68.
91. Bender WA. *Learning Disabilities: Characteristics, Identification, and Teaching Strategies*, 2nd edn. Boston: Allyn and Bacon, 1995.
92. Chermak GA. Metacognitive approaches to managing central auditory processing disorders. In: Masters MG, Stecker NA, Katz J, eds. *Central Auditory Processing Disorders: Mostly Management*. Boston: Allyn and Bacon, 1998: 49–62.
93. Gillam RB, ed. *Memory and Language Impairments in Children and Adults: New Perspectives*. Gaithersburg, MD: Aspen Publishers, 1998.
94. Hallahan DP, Kauffman JM, Lloyd JW. *Introduction to Learning Disabilities*. Boston: Allyn and Bacon, 1996.
95. Miller GA, Gildea PM. How children learn words. *Sci Am* 1987; **257**: 94–9.
96. Halliday MAK, Hasan R. *Cohesion in English*. London: Longman, 1976.
97. Kintsch W. The role of knowledge in discourse comprehension: a construction–integration model. *Psychol Rev* 1988; **95**: 165–85.
98. Dillon GL. *Constructing Texts*. Bloomington: Indiana University Press, 1981.
99. Liles BZ. Cohesion in the narratives of normal and language-disordered children. *J Speech Hear Res* 1985; **28**: 123–33.
100. Liles BZ. Episode organization and cohesive conjunctions in narratives of children with and without language disorders. *J Speech Hear Res* 1987; **30**: 185–96.

30 Audiological rehabilitation

Dafydd Stephens

Introduction and definition

Audiological rehabilitation has been given many definitions by various authors.[1–3] The working definition used in this chapter is 'a problem-solving process aiming to minimize the disablements experienced by individuals with hearing disorders and to maximize their quality of life'. In terms of the International Classification of Functioning, Disability and Health of the World Health Organization (ICF),[4] it entails the minimization of activity limitation (disability) and participation restriction (handicap). I propose here to make no distinction between audiological rehabilitation, aural rehabilitation, auditory rehabilitation and hearing rehabilitation, which can be regarded as different terms for the same process. I shall indicate that we are dealing with patient (client)-orientated processes driven by the difficulties encountered by the individual and those around him in their actual environment. It relates essentially to concepts of ecological audiology developed by Noble and others.[5–7]

Within this chapter, I shall start by discussing the final draft of the World Health Organization Classification of Functioning Disability and Health (ICF), which provides a useful framework, albeit with weaknesses, within which the difficulties experienced by the patient can be considered. This leads on to an updated 'management model' derived from that of Goldstein and Stephens,[8] and which provides a coherent structure for the evaluation and appropriate management of the individual concerned. Finally, I shall consider ways in which the process can be best evaluated, both from the standpoint of the individual patient and also in a broader context in order to assess the cost-effectiveness of the system.

Disablements

In 2001, the World Health Organization published, as ICF,[4] a revision of their earlier classification of Impairments, Disabilities and Handicaps,[9] taking into account further studies and criticisms of the earlier version, published in 1980. This new document changed aspects of the terminology from the two previous versions and referred to the umbrella concept of disability covering the impairments and their consequences for the individual. This new structure is shown in Figure 30.1. This shows that the underlying disease or developmental defect can give rise to an impairment of function or structure which in turn may affect the individual's activity or activities and consequently cause some restriction of participation in aspects of society within which the individual might be expected to participate. It may be noted that there is not a straightforward right-to-left progression from impairment to participation restriction, but that this is a two-way process which can be modified by interventions or changes in environmental and personal factors.

Such modifiers, both external and internal, can act at different stages in the process. Some ways in which this can occur, and perhaps even be measured, have been discussed by Borg[7] in his concept of ecological audiology. The work of Noble and Hétu[6] concentrates in more detail on the influences of environmental factors.

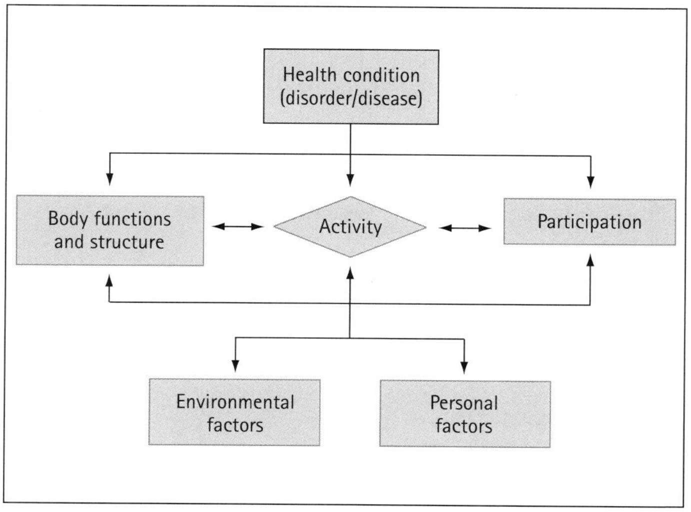

Figure 30.1 Outline of the ICF framework.

Structure and function

The WHO concept of impairments is divided into two, functional and structural impairments. Elsewhere, we have argued that, apart from gross abnormalities of the external ear, the concept of structural impairments is of little practical relevance in the field of audiological rehabilitation,[10] and further discussion will concentrate on functional impairments.

Functional impairments entail abnormal psychological or physiological function which can be measured in a standardized way, using psychophysical or physiological measures.

This is usually defined in terms of the auditory threshold, which is a reflection of the auditory sensitivity of the individual but may be a measure of a variety of other auditory functions, including intolerance of noise or even tinnitus, as shown in Table 30.1. In this table, it may also be seen that there are various auditory impairments in addition to impaired threshold sensitivity, derived particularly from damage to the transducer mechanism of the inner ear. These are discussed in Chapter 12.

The inclusion of tinnitus here is somewhat debatable, as it is more analogous to pain, and possibly both should be considered as discomforts separate from the general concept of impairments. The same is possibly true of intolerance of noise when considered in isolation and not related to an abnormal growth of loudness in a damaged ear (recruitment).

Activity limitation

This is broadly analogous to the former concept of 'disability', which concerns the hearing or listening activities which are affected in the individual's life. It will depend not only on the impairments affecting the individual, but also on the demands placed on the auditory system. It is defined as 'difficulties an individual may have in executing activities'. Activity limitation may be assessed by asking the individual about their specific difficulties, but also by the use of a variety of questionnaires. These may be constrained or open-ended. It may also be assessed by testing the individual using situation-specific tests, e.g. recording the noise from the workplace and assessing the individual's ability to recognize relevant speech in that context.

Table 30.1 Classification of hearing and related functions.

b2300	Sound detection
b2301	Sound discrimination
b2302	Localization of sound source
b2303	Lateralization of sound
b2304	Speech discrimination
b2400	Ringing in ears or tinnitus
b2404	Irritation in the ear
b2405	Aural pressure
b2408	Phonophobia or hyperacusis

A classification of activities, based on ICF is shown in Tables 30.2 and 30.3. This has significant weaknesses in that, communication aside, there is only one subsidiary category (a115—Listening) which covers almost all other auditory activity limitations. We would argue that the approach adopted in the intermediate (β1) classification[11] is more appropriate, and this is what has been adopted here in a modified version.

Different individuals with the same functional impairment, such as a bilateral high-frequency sensorineural hearing impairment, may experience very different activity limitations. Examples of such different problems experienced by different individuals could be steelworkers who may not be aware of any activity limitation, particularly as friends and colleagues probably have a similar hearing loss; secretaries who may be aware of problems only when in an open-plan office; and teachers whose work situation may become impossible because of the problem as they cannot hear their pupils.

Participation restriction

It may be seen that these problems of activity limitation lead on easily into participation restriction, the effects of impairment and/or activity limitation on the individual's lifestyle. It may be more easily defined as 'the non-auditory consequences of hearing impairment', and is influenced by a variety of psychosocial and

Table 30.2 Communication activities.

d310	Receiving spoken messages
d315	Receiving nonverbal messages
d320	Receiving formal sign language messages
d325	Receiving written messages
d350	Conversation
d360	Using communication devices and techniques

Table 30.3 Potential classification of listening activity.

1. Ability to receive loud auditory signals (in noise or quiet)
2. Hearing when there is background noise
3. Hearing when sounds come from different directions
4. Ability to hear moderately loud noises (in noise or quiet)
5. Ability to hear soft sounds (in noise or quiet)
6. Recognizing
7. Recognizing distance, e.g. footsteps, traffic, birds
8. Recognizing direction, e.g. warning signals, traffic, birds
9. Ability relating to noise tolerance
10. Environmental awareness

environmental factors. ICF defines it as the 'problems an individual may experience in involvement in life situations'. The activity construct addresses the question as to whether the individual 'can' do the activity, whereas the participation construct addresses the question as to whether the individual 'does' do the task.

Participation restriction is determined particularly by the activity limitations experienced, but may occur in the presence of hearing impairment without any experienced activity limitation. It is generally assessed by interview or questionnaires, but may also be assessed by indirect measures such as numbers of days of work lost, or related medical consultations. As participation restriction extends broadly across the consequences of a variety of impairment types such as visual or locomotor impairments, approaches using quality of life measures may be relevant here.

Furthermore, participation restriction, more than other elements of disablement, is the factor most likely to determine whether or not the individual seeks help for their hearing loss.[12]

The domains of participation are shown in Table 30.4, which mirrors the domains of activity. It may be seen from this that these cover a wide range of areas which can also be influenced by other (non-auditory) impairments. Among these, the most important and commonly related areas are those of reduced participation in social interaction at a variety of levels, ranging from with partners and family members through to with strangers. Communication domains at a participation level cover the individual's exclusion from a conversation or telephone call, rather than their perceived difficulties in hearing in these circumstances. Restriction in work and educational environments may even create particular problems for the individuals in their 80s seeking to improve their knowledge.

Contextual factors

The contextual factors or modifiers which may influence the individual's degree of activity limitation and participation restriction may be considered in the two broad categories of environmental factors — external to the person concerned and personal, relating to the personality, experiences and the coping strategies which the individual adopts to deal with a range of experienced problems.

The environmental factors cover a range of areas, both human and inanimate, and even include societal attitudes towards hearing impairment and approaches to its management. Another area is devices, which may be used to alleviate the individual's problems, including both hearing aids and environmental aids (assistive listening devices). This area in particular highlights the way in which activity limitation and participation restriction constitute a dynamic, continually changing process which may be altered by changes in environmental factors.

Thus use of an appropriate hearing aid system may reduce activity limitation and consequently increase some aspects of participation. However, stigmatizing societal reactions to the wearing of a hearing aid may subsequently result in the individual using it only at home, so increasing his activity limitation or participation restriction with regard to involvements outside the home. The contextual factors are shown in Table 30.5 and 30.6.

A management model

The model development by Goldstein and Stephens in 1981[8] aimed to be sufficiently broad to cover all types of hearing

Table 30.4 Domains of activity and participation.

1.	Learning and applying knowledge
2.	General tasks and demands
3.	Communication
4.	Movement
5.	Self-care
6.	Domestic life
7.	Interpersonal interactions and relationships
8.	Major life areas
9.	Community, social and civic life

Table 30.5 Environmental factors.

1.	Products and technology
2.	National environment and human-made changes to the environment
3.	Support and relationships
4.	Attitudes
5.	Services, systems and policies

Table 30.6 Proposed classification of personal factors.

1.	Personal and demographic characteristics – age, race, gender
2.	Education profession
3.	Past and current experience
4.	Overall behaviour pattern and character style
5.	Individual psychological assets
6.	Other health conditions, fitness
7.	Lifestyle, habits, upbringing
8.	Coping styles
9.	Social background

problems and to be relevant on an individual basis to each person with such problems. It should be applicable within all sociomedical systems. We argued that it was important to consider all relevant factors, if only to dismiss many immediately as being irrelevant. The model was based on the principle of integrating instrumental and non-instrumental aspects of rehabilitation, so facilitating intervention which was appropriate to the individual's needs.

The model was updated in detail in 1997,[13,14] while retaining the fundamental principles of the original concept. The main ideas gave increased emphasis to the problems (activity limitations and participation restrictions) reported by the individual concerned, and also increased emphasis on the role of significant others. Within the following account, further minor amendments are incorporated, aimed at integrating some of the other aspects of ICF.

The overall model is shown in Figure 30.2. The main changes from the 1997 version are the renaming of the first section as Activity and Participation, and the third section as Contextual Factors, bringing in here the individual's physical environment in addition to the psychosocial factors which have predominated in previous versions of the model. The fourth section is now called Related Functions and Activities. Finally, an element of environmental modification has been incorporated, with the final section previously known as 'Communication Training' being renamed 'Continuing remediation', as it includes factors other than communication skills.

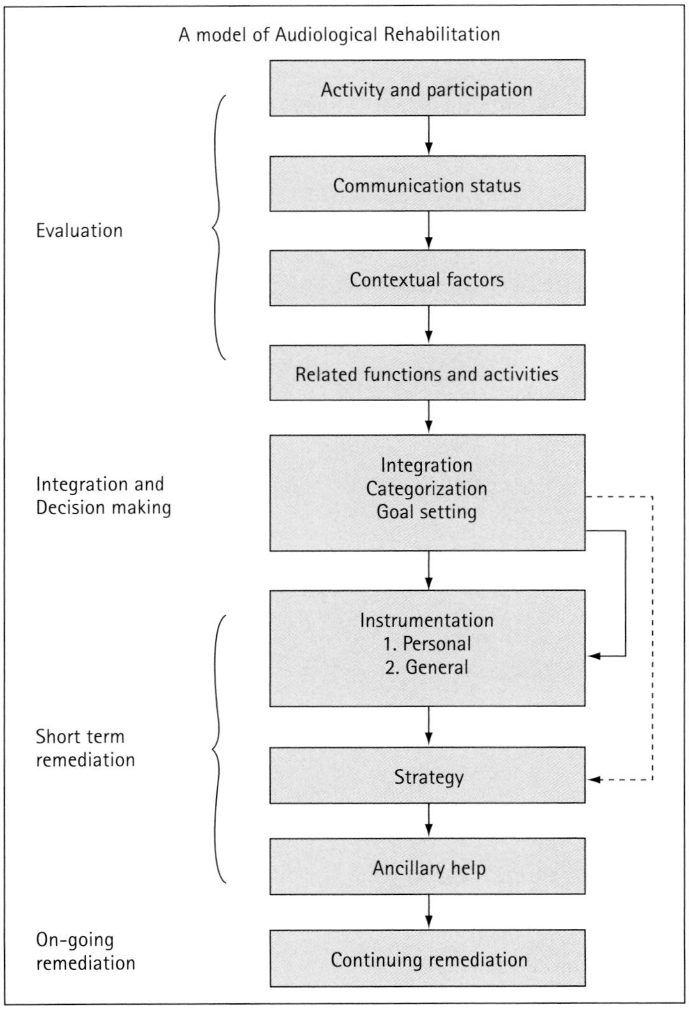

Figure 30.2 Management model for rehabilitation.

This management model will be used to provide the framework for the remainder of this chapter. Overall, it will be seen that it comprises four basic sections:

1. Evaluation — determining the problems and the 'raw materials' with which the professional has to work.
2. Integration and decision making — drawing together this basic information and making appropriate initial decisions.
3. Short-term remediation — immediate actions and procedures implemented over a short period of time.
4. Ongoing remediation — the continuing process of remediation.

Evaluation

As mentioned earlier, this is the stage in which it is important to consider all possibly relevant factors, if only to dismiss some immediately. A range of evaluative techniques may be used, extending from brief observation to detailed testing, and have been discussed in some detail elsewhere.[1,14] The approach chosen will depend on the individual, their set of problems, and also what is relevant to the interventions which might be considered. There is little point in wasting time collecting detailed information which will not have any bearing on the choice or details of interventions.

Activity and participation

This is the key point, as it determines the specific problems which the patient is encountering and which they would like addressed. They are usually tapped by a combination of techniques, including direct questioning, and open-set and closed-set questionnaires. Other, more objective, approaches are available but rarely used. These could include testing the individual's recognition of a relevant sample of speech in background noise recorded where they have problems, surveying communicative interactions, or examining their help-seeking behaviours in different contexts.

Determination of the individual's specific problems may be performed using the Problem Questionnaire,[15] which asks simply 'Please make a list of the difficulties you have with your hearing. List them in order of importance, starting with the biggest. Write down as many as you can think of.' This has the advantage of tapping into what the patient sees as relevant and does tend to be effective at defining relevant activity limitations, such as general conversation, hearing the television, hearing the doorbell, speech in noise and telephone conversations. It is, however, less effective at tapping into participation restriction.[16,17] In this context, we have recently adopted a new questionnaire, 'Please make a list of the effects of hearing loss on your life. Write down as many as you can think of.' About half of the responses to this are still activity limitations, but about a quarter are now participation restrictions, with a further 20% being personal contextual factors/effects.[17]

This open-set approach may be used in a quantitative way to assess changes in specific problems as a result of intervention, such as on repeated occasions after a cochlear implant (Figure 30.3).[18] A widely adopted use of this approach is also found in Dillon's COSI (Client Orientated Scale of Improvement)[19,20] and in a section of Gatehouse's Glasgow Hearing Aid Benefit Profile.[21]

A variety of questionnaires tapping different aspects of activity limitation and participation restriction have appeared since the introduction of the Hearing Handicap Scale[22] in 1964, which, in fact, measured predominantly speech hearing activity limitations. A number of the most recent of these measures are listed in Table 30.7, and they have been recently reviewed in the context of self-report outcome measures in audiological rehabilitation.[23] Unfortunately, many are rather confused in terms of the ICF dimensions, and relatively few set out to specifically assess participation restriction, which, as mentioned earlier, is not well delineated by open-set questionnaires. It is in this domain that such measures[17] could continue to have a useful role in the assessment of the needs of the specific individual. Their use as outcome measures is probably restricted to the assessment of specific interventions in particular groups of subjects, and this is discussed further later in this chapter.

Communication status

The components of this section, which covers, broadly speaking, the raw materials of communication, are shown in Table 30.8.

Auditory

This represents essentially the impairments of function which are relevant to the rehabilitative process. The first, and generally most crucial, is a measure of sensitivity, usually a pure tone audiogram. The type and details will be relevant to the rehabilitative approach and, in individuals with an audiometric configuration which changes rapidly across the frequency range, a sweep frequency measure like Békésy or Audioscan audiometry may be more relevant (see Chapter 11).

Most sophisticated techniques of non-linear processing in hearing aids emphasize the need for measures of the dynamic range. While most measures of most comfortable loudness levels (MCLLs) show considerable intra-subject variability, the uncomfortable loudness level (ULL) measures are more consistent, and MCLLs may be extrapolated from these.[24]

Speech recognition scores are important in deciding which ear to aid and which instrumental approach may be most appropriate. However, they should not be the only factor in such decisions, as some individuals with poor speech recognition in one ear may still wish to use that ear to provide a three-dimensional approach and to enable them to hear and locate relevant environmental sounds.

With the advent of digital hearing aids including binaural systems, a range of other psychophysical measures of binaural and monaural signal processing are becoming relevant, depending on the system being considered. As elsewhere, the procedures to be adopted will depend on them being relevant to the rehabilitative approach considered suitable for the individual concerned.

Visual

While whether or not the individual uses spectacles, and how often they use them, may have some bearing on the broad type

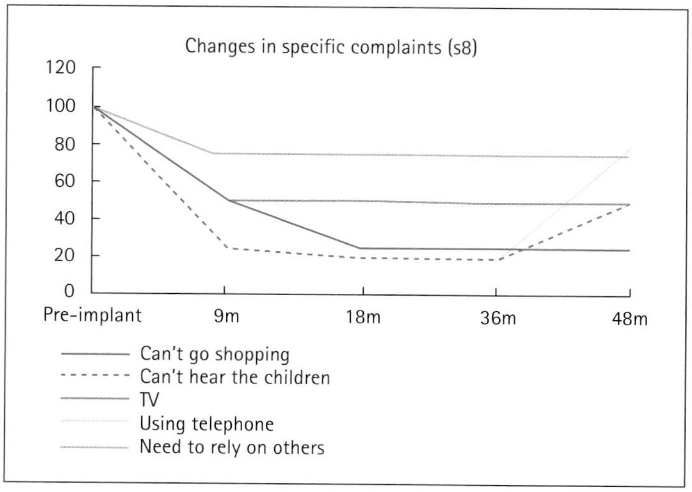

Figure 30.3 Changes in ratings of disablements by a patient with a cochlear implant, before and up to 4 years post-implant.

Table 30.7 Some recent scales of activity limitation and participation restriction

- Amsterdam Inventory for Auditory Disability & Handicap – Kramer *et al.*[58]
- Communication Scale for Older Adults – Kaplan *et al.*[59]
- Gothenburg Profile – Ringdahl *et al.*[60]
- Hearing Disability & Handicap Scale – Hétu *et al.*[61]

Table 30.8 Communication status

- Auditory
- Visual
- Speech Production
- Manual
- Non-verbal Skills
- Previous Rehabilitation
- Overall

of hearing aid to be selected, the use of smaller-in-the-ear and behind-the-ear aids, together with the disappearance of spectacle aids, has made this of less relevance than formerly.

Visual acuity, aided where relevant, is of more importance in deciding on the emphasis to be given to binaural hearing aid fittings, and is also something to check and correct in order to improve the individual's speech-reading (lipreading) ability. Such ability may be assessed in a variety of ways, although in recent years the emphasis has been on testing the recognition of individual phonemes and sentences and on connected discourse tracking (CDT).[25] These are illustrated in Table 30.9.

The approach to be adopted will depend on the aim of the assessment. Sentence lists (e.g. BKB lists,[26] CID lists[27]) may be used to obtain a broad overall picture of the individual's abilities relative to this. They can also be used to compare auditory, visual and audiovisual recognition of speech by the same person.

CDT, in which the number of words per minute of a text read by the tester or correctly repeated is scored, is a valuable measure of change in performance over time and following intervention. It can be chosen from a text compatible with the individual's needs and lexicon. Video-recorded versions have been used, but most testing uses live presentations.

Tests of recognition of individual phonemes or phoneme groups — usually consonants in the form aka/asa/ada, or vowels in the form hid/had/hod or bid/bad/bod — are used for defining specific problems which the individual experiences and the effectiveness of the particular therapeutic approach in reducing them. The pattern of errors found can help focus the training on particular sources of errors made by the individual patient.

Speech and language production

Speech and language production effects may also be considered in the context of the individual within their social and environmental situation and with regard to their more specific problems. Thus, in the first context, it is important to be aware of the individual's dominant language and, where relevant, the dialect of that language. In addition, the rehabilitative training programme may be structured differently according to the individual's lexicon and lexical needs, according to, for example, whether the person concerned is a farmer or a computer programmer.

Hearing impairments of most types will influence the phonological elements of the individual's speech production, that is to say how they pronounce different components of speech, and this needs to be defined. Thus high-frequency hearing losses will mainly affect the fricatives for which the individual receives no acoustical feedback. The pragmatic elements of speech, influenced predominantly by intonation patterns, on the other hand, will be influenced more by the low-frequency hearing level. Inability to hear this can, for example, affect the individual's ability to differentiate between a question and a statement, or the stress on particular parts of a sentence.

While these are relevant to all types of hearing loss, congenital and acquired, semantic and syntactic aspects of speech production are abnormal generally only in those with congenital hearing impairments who have not learned the rules for these in the spoken language, which may be very different from those in the dominant sign language culture of the country concerned. This must be understood before an in-depth rehabilitation programme is planned.

Sign language

Sign language (or manual communication) may be classified into three types (Table 30.10). First, there are sign languages, usually associated with the local deaf culture, which have their own syntax and vocabulary and can be regarded as languages in their own right. While these have a high status in certain societies, such as parts of the USA, in other countries such as the UK, they tend to be eschewed by the education system. In such countries, there is more emphasis on sign systems which use the syntax of the dominant aural/oral culture, such as 'Signs Supporting English' or the Paget Gorman System. In any case, it is important for the individual planning the rehabilitation service to be aware of these differences and evaluate the patient's fluency in production/reception of the relevant sign system.

Other systems are concerned with signs which support or complement speech reading. The two main systems in this context are the American Cued Speech (Cornett)[28] and the Danish Mouth–hand System.[29] The latter is one which purely complements speech reading, just providing cues on voicing, nasality and place, whereas cued speech is a more complex system, giving information on most aspects of speech. In addition, elements of finger spelling may be used to complement speech reading by signing elements of speech such as voicing/nasality which are not usually lipreadable. Thus, in the differentiation

Table 30.9 Speechreading tests

- Consonant confusions; e.g. /aba/, /ada/
- Vowel confusions; e.g. /hid/, /had/
- Word recognition; e.g. Boothroyd
- Sentence recognition; e.g. BKB sentences
- Connected discourse tracking

Table 30.10 Types of manual communication

- Support to speechreading; e.g. Cued speech, mouth–hand system, (finger spelling)
- Systems based in the spoken language of the society; e.g. Paget Gorman, signed English
- Autonomous sign languages; e.g. British sign language, American sign language

of 'Pan', 'Ban' and 'Man', the first letter of the word may be signed to clarify which is being said.

Non-verbal communication

Non-verbal communication, the use of gestures and expressions in communication, will be well established in most individuals who lose their hearing in later life, and is unlikely to be impaired. However, many individuals with a congenital hearing impairment may never have acquired these skills, which may need to be taught to enhance the person's communication skills. The other group in whom this is important comprises immigrants from another society in which the code of non-verbal communication is different. It will be helpful for them, if hearing impaired, to learn the non-verbal symbolism of their adopted society in order to improve their overall communication skills.

Previous rehabilitation

It is important, as well, to be aware of what rehabilitative help the individual has received previously, to build on the positive aspects and work to overcome the negative experiences. Thus, the context will be set by the individual's attitude to what has been done for them previously, whether positive or negative, and this will need to be known before approaching the specific details. These details will cover instrumental help, hearing aids and environmental aids, and any speech-reading training or other skill-building techniques, including sign language training. For example, if an inappropriate hearing aid system has been fitted previously, the professional's approach will be very different in overcoming the individual's problems, convincing them that a more appropriate aid may be helpful, than if they have an appropriate aid which merely needs updating or to be complemented with other approaches.

Overall

Finally within this section, it is important to remember that the individual's overall communication ability will not necessarily be the same as the total of the separate elements of their communication which have been assessed — it may be less or it may be more. It is thus important to assess their communication ability in the favoured mode of communication, whether it is audiovisual, signing plus speech reading, etc.

Contextual factors

These are the components which will influence the professional's overall approach to the rehabilitation of the individual concerned. Formerly, we have restricted this to the individual's human environment, but it is important to consider their physical environment as well. Thus a person living in an isolated detached bungalow will have a very different set of needs and approaches from one living in a block of flats in a city.

The two contextual components of environmental and personal factors can be regarded as referring to the external and internal environments in which the individual operates. The latter will cover predominantly the psychological components and experiences of the individual together with their motivation and approaches to coping.

The main grouping of these factors is shown in Tables 30.5 and 30.6, derived from ICF.[4]

Environmental factors

The first section, 'Products and technology', will be defined by the nature of the society in which the person lives on both the macro- and microlevels and will generally change with time. The two main areas of relevance here are 'Products for personal use in daily living' and 'Products for communication'. The former includes both general devices such as computers, and also the availability of assistive technology (environmental aids), which includes alarm and alerting technologies.

Likewise, 'Products for communication' covers both general communication devices and the modified versions of these, which may be used to promote access for hearing-impaired people. It is interesting that expansion of the available technology in this field is paralleling the change in Western society from production-based employment to communicative employment.[30]

Within the context of 'Natural environment and human changes to this', the area of the noise in the environment in which the person lives and works is the most relevant, although illumination will have an important second-order effect.

'Support and relationships' covers the main sociological factors of the previous version of the model. Here we are concerned about those significant others playing an important role in the individual's life, from family through friends to work colleagues and carers, and their attitudes towards the individual and their problems.

This overlaps with the grouping 'Attitudes, values and beliefs' which influences these relationships. Such attitudes will be those held by the significant others of the hearing-impaired person, but also those of society as a whole. The broad societal attitudes, values and beliefs may well be reflected in the group around the individual, or alternatively some or all of the group may have very different attitudes to the prevailing pattern within the particular society. This can have a major knock-on effect on aspects of the stigma experienced by the patient.[31]

The needs of and provisions for the patient will be influenced by the social, health, educational and employment services available locally, which may vary in different parts of any one country, as well as between countries, in terms of the availability of free or subsidised provision of environmental aids or FM radio systems.

This again comes within the broader concept of the general systems and policies of the country concerned; these will determine access to different provisions, which may be paid for from central taxation, insurance; or from the pocket of the individual concerned.

Personal factors

These cover basically the attitudes, values and beliefs of the individual with a hearing impairment together with their personality and approaches to coping. These will all have a key role in the approaches to be adopted in the rehabilitative process in terms of what will be acceptable, what needs to be encouraged, and what problems need to be overcome. They will cover the attitudes towards having rehabilitative help at all, and also towards different parts of the process—e.g. hearing aids, speechreading. It will further determine whether the individual can see the positive as well as the negative dimensions of their disability and adopt a positive attitude towards the problems being faced.

Such an approach will also influence the effects of the hearing impairment on the individual's psychological state, which could lead to the individual becoming more isolated, suffering form increased depression, or becoming more anxious as a result of concerns about not hearing intruders in their homes.

Related functions and activities

Whereas the contextual factors influence the broad-based approach to the rehabilitative process, this is an area of the assessment of the individual which impacts on detailed aspects of the process, such as determining specific types of instrumentation to be used, the balance between hearing aids and environmental aids, and which ear(s) to fit hearing aids to. It also governs the approach to presenting these to the patient and instructing them.

The factors which influence this are shown in Table 30.11, which again broadly follow the earlier approach of 'Related conditions'. The area of 'Mental functions' is new, and covers broadly the intellectual, attention and memory functions of the patient. Such an individual may range from an alert, vigorous person living in their own home to a cognitively compromised individual with Alzheimer's disease or Down's syndrome in an institution. Their acceptance of the intervention may be positive but the means by which it is presented will need to be tied to the individual's ability to understand and remember any instructions. Generally, significant others will play a greater role.

Sensations associated with hearing and vestibular function cover three particularly relevant areas, 'Ringing in the ears or tinnitus', 'Irritation in the ear', and 'Aural pressure'. In addition, the vestibular section could be assumed to include the Tullio phenomenon, in which loud sounds may induce vertigo. This would be a contraindication to having too high a maximum output of a hearing aid which would induce dizziness.

Table 30.11 Related functions and activities

- Mental functions
- Sensations associated with hearing and vestibular function
- Touch function
- Manipulative activities
- Walking activities

The presence of tinnitus will usually be a positive indication to fitting a hearing aid to the affected ear or ears, which will generally result in some relief from tinnitus.[32] It is important, however, to use as open an earmould as possible, as occlusion of the meatus can increase the level of the tinnitus. In addition, a small proportion of patients, even fitted with non-occlusive earmoulds, may report an increase in the level of the tinnitus, so such a fitting should be avoided in these cases.

Irritation and related discharge from an ear can be aggravated by a hearing aid fitting and, indeed, in such an infected ear, a fitting may precipitate a severe infection.

The sensation of blockage in the ear, while in many people's minds associated with otitis media with effusion, is a common occurrence in cochlear disease, particularly endolymphatic hydrops. In patients complaining of this symptom, an occlusive earmould should be avoided, and as open a mould as possible should be used. Even in severe hearing losses, the use of a vent with a sintered filter may relieve the occlusion without resulting in feedback.

'Touch function', particularly in the fingers, can influence the difficulty individuals have in fitting hearing aid systems to the ear and in controlling settings of the hearing aids. This will need to be taken into account in the detailed selection of the hearing aid systems, to ensure that fitting and controlling the hearing aid and the earmould are within the tactile capabilities of the individual concerned.

This links closely to the activity of 'Fine hand use' (manipulating), limitations of which tend to run in parallel with loss of sensation, particularly in elderly people.

The final section here comprises 'Walking activities', which defines the mobility of the individual and, by extension, his or her likelihood of encountering different environments. For individuals whose mobility is so limited that they are bedbound or housebound, it may be more reasonable to concentrate on pertinent environmental aids rather than hearing aids, unless the individual has difficulties in face-to-face conversations.

Integration and decision-making

The stage has now arrived for all the information acquired in the evaluative stage of the rehabilitative process to be pulled together and relevant management decisions made with and for the patient. This will include any relevant information obtained from significant others. In particular, elements of the individual's 'attitude' towards their hearing loss and its management will need to be taken into account and, if inappropriate, some effort made to modify it. Their 'understanding' of what has happened to them and what can be done to help can also influence the process, as can their 'expectations' of the outcome of the process. These again can sometimes be manipulated to ensure that not too high an expectation exists which, if it is not achieved, can result in disillusionment and rejection of the entire process. Further, if expectations are too low, the individual may not persist with the rehabilitation. The skilled clinician must aim at achieving a happy medium of realistic expectations.

We have argued that the next stage is one of categorization of the individual. The four-way classification[8] proposed in 1981 seems to have withstood the passage of time and is summarized in Table 30.12.

Basically those classified as type 1 are strongly motivated to have help for their problems and are prepared, within reason, to accept any appropriate intervention. They have no complicating factors obvious either to themselves or to the audiological professional and may expect to pass quickly through the system. They will probably be fitted with a hearing aid system, be reviewed to ensure that they are coping well, and receive further advice and adjustments of their hearing aid, and advice on environmental aids and hearing tactics, and then generally be discharged on the understanding that they will return should there be any significant problems.

Type 2 patients will similarly be positively motivated but have some complicating factors. They may have severe tinnitus or otorrhoea, have manipulative problems, tremor etc. or may have either a very severe or very mild hearing impairment. All these will be broadly apparent to the patient. The professional may also see that they have an audiometric configuration that will be difficult to fit, e.g. a low-frequency sensorineural hearing loss or a ski-slope high-frequency loss. They may also have somewhat unrealistic expectations or concerns. These patients will need more time with audiological professionals and require extensive counselling and training, together with repeated adjustments of their hearing aids, before they are optimally helped. While for many of these patients this may take only three or four sessions, in others, particularly those with a profound hearing loss, the rehabilitation may continue over months or years.

Type 3 patients are seeking help, but are very negative about certain approaches which would, in principle, be helpful for them. Most commonly, this aversion concerns hearing aids. Others may be convinced that a hearing aid system will solve all their problems with relationships and are reluctant to accept the concepts of hearing tactics, counselling or psychological help. In both cases, the professional needs to be devious, using an indirect approach. An immediate straightforward hearing aid fitting would be inappropriate in both cases, being rejected immediately in the first case, and being rejected when the patient sees that it does not achieve the perceived goal in the second case.

Table 30.12 Category types

- 1. Positively motivated and straightforward
- 2. Positively motivated with complicating factors
- 3. Want help, but problems with elements of the rehabilitation process
- 4. Deny problems

The use of group sessions with a mixture of individuals can be helpful in these cases, with the idea of hearing aids introduced by hearing-impaired peers, in a way which the patient feels to be less threatening than when the idea comes from a professional. Groups will also include some elements of counselling, which can lead on to individual counselling sessions to meet the specific needs of the particular individual.

Type 4 patients are negative about any helpseeking, either not being conscious of any disablement or refusing to admit to one. They will attend the clinic as a result of pressure from significant others and may or may not openly articulate their problems. It is important that, in part of the evaluative session at least, they should be assessed separately from any significant others so that their true feelings can be determined.

Intervention in these cases is counterproductive. If the individual denies any disablement, their opinion must be respected and the patient discharged with the clear option of returning should they feel they have any problems at a later date. At the same time, wherever possible, the significant others should be contacted by the hearing therapist (or other relevant professional), who can discuss the importance of the patient's views on this matter, no matter how loud their television, and also give advice on communication tactics and environmental aids, which the patient may accept as being nothing directly to do with their disablement.

Following this initial categorization of the individual from the professional's standpoint, the professional should work with the individual and also with any relevant significant other to define some initial goals which are both important for the patient and realistically achievable. While in most type 1 and 2 patients this will entail some instrumental provision/fitting, in a small number of individuals with mild hearing impairment or with King Kopetzky syndrome, the professional may proceed directly to the strategy stage of the remediation process, depending on the specific goals. These goals are important in assessing the ultimate efficacy of the rehabilitative process and are incorporated in the use of COSI[20] as an outcome measure.

Instrumentation

This section covers all aspects of instrumental help which may be provided for a patient. The particular instrumentation falls into two groups — personal (hearing aids, tactile aids and cochlear implants), which are tailored to the specific individual, and environmental (assistive listening devices — ALDs) which may be appropriate for and used by a wide range of people. All need to be accompanied by appropriate training.

Personal instruments

Most aspects of hearing aids, cochlear implants and their selection are dealt with elsewhere in this book (Chapters 27 and 34). Here it is important to consider just a few general principles, mainly non-acoustical. Examples of how the information obtained in the evaluation process can be applied in the selection of both the hearing aid and the earmould as well as the cochlear implant or tactile aid have been discussed elsewhere.

While the particular signal processing strategy to be used in the aid continues to develop and become more sophisticated, the individual, generally elderly, person using it, does not. Thus there are two main factors which come into play here and which often work in opposite directions. The first is the stigma of having to use a hearing aid adding to the stigma already experienced of having a hearing impairment.[31] This will make the individual seek an aid which, ideally for them, is invisible — essentially an all-in-the-canal instrument. The problems which then arise are those of manipulating the controls, fitting the aid to the ear, and changing the battery. While the first can be overcome by an infrared remote control system, the second and third remain problematic without increasing dependence on a sympathetic significant other who may themselves have similar tactile and manipulative problems as the patient. In addition, such an 'invisible' aid is not going to have the effect on a communication partner of alerting them to the fact that the individual is hearing impaired and that they may need to adjust their speech appropriately.

Manufacturers of hearing aids have traditionally paid little attention to ergonomically friendly hearing aids, despite the need within the elderly community; such aids can be easily designed (e.g. Figure 30.4 which shows such a device produced as an undergraduate engineering project[33]), but need to be accepted. Many patients need to be fitted first with an aid of a size acceptable to them and acoustically appropriate. By this means, they will realize the sound benefits which they are obtaining and further realize the impossibility of handling it, and then be more enthusiastic about trying a larger, more manageable aid.

The culture is now beginning to change with the development of coloured and bejewelled aids which, together with more attractive earmoulds, are beginning to make hearing aids more acceptable, particularly to younger people.

Such cosmetic considerations also apply to a lesser extent to cochlear implants, for which there was also much patient pressure for the development of head-worn systems and, ultimately, 'invisible' systems. Again, however, they will never completely 'normalize' the individual's hearing, and the need to signal to the communication partner to make more effort with their speech will still be there.

Environmental aids

Within the ICF, these come within the context of 'Products and technology' of 'environmental factors'. There they come into two areas, 'Products for personal use in daily living' and 'Products for communication'. This approach is in line with earlier audiological approaches, in which the former have sometimes been defined as alerting and warning systems, and the latter as communication devices. In both cases, a variety of approaches have been adopted to improve access for the hearing-impaired individual to the particular system concerned.

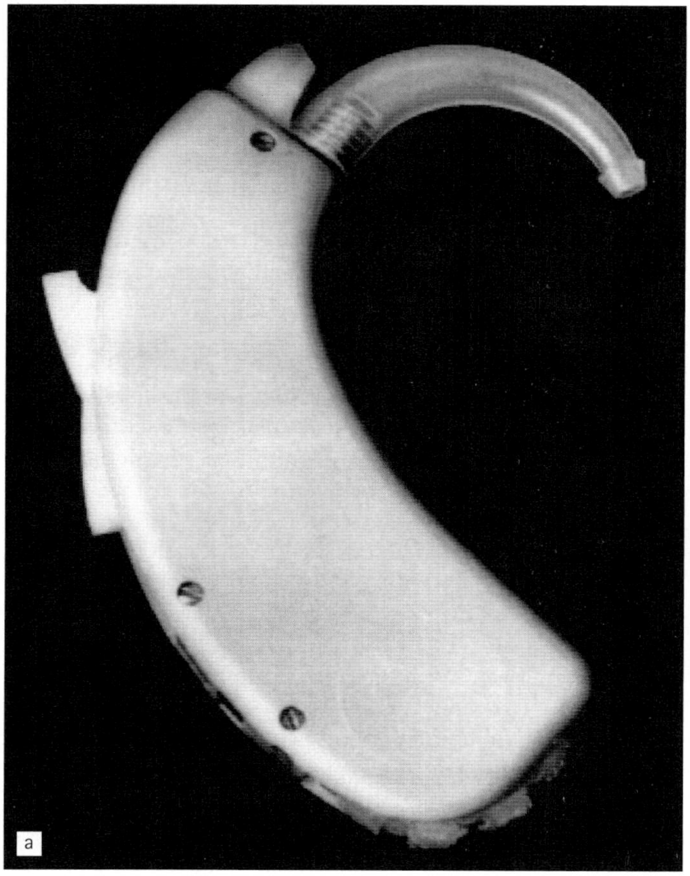

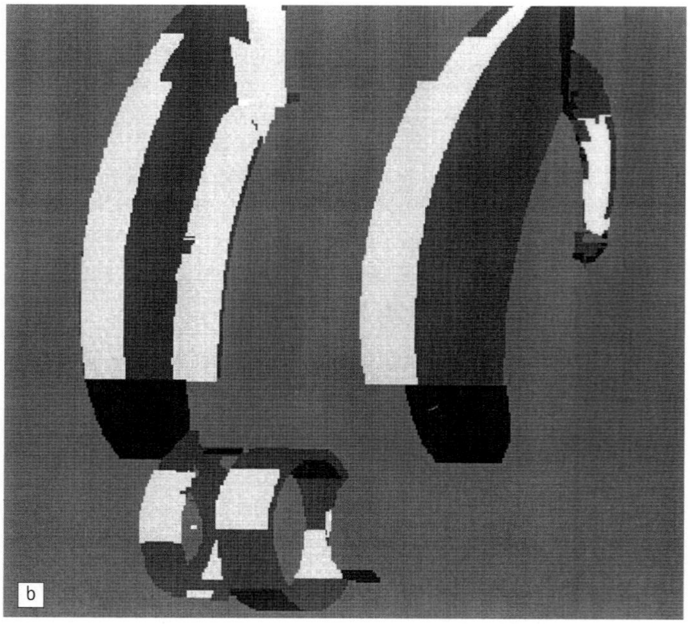

Figure 30.4 Ergonomic hearing aid, showing simple on–off switch (a) and the volume control incorporating the battery compartment (b). (After Roberts. *An ergonomic investigation into the design of a behind the ear (BTE) hearing aid to overcome handling difficulties experienced by elderly users.* Undergraduate dissertation, University of Glamorgan, 1992.[33])

Products for use in daily living Table 30.13 shows the types of aids which are available in the 'use in daily living' category and the approaches to making them accessible to hearing-impaired people. It may be seen that approaches range from increasing sound amplitude and the signal/noise ratio through to various types of sensory substitution. The most recent developments include multipurpose portable devices providing a tactile, visual or auditory warning with different variants on the stimulus presented, according to whether the doorbell is being rung, the telephone bell is ringing or a smoke alarm has been triggered.

In many respects, the simplest are the most effective, with an extension to the doorbell being located in the room where the individual watches the television. Even if no extension is used for the doorbell, replacing a sophisticated high-frequency bell with a cheap low-frequency buzzer may be the best solution for an individual with a high-frequency hearing loss living in a small house or flat. As in all elements of the rehabilitative programme, the approach must be tailored to the needs of the particular hearing-impaired individual within their normal environment.

Problems with the telephone bell not being heard in certain parts of the house are being reduced by the increasing use of mobile telephones and cordless phones which the individual can keep with them. In addition, there may be different extension telephones located in different strategic points of a large house. Where these present problems, or the individual is profoundly impaired and uses a text telephone, a visual alerting system, either built into the telephone or hard-wired into the house lighting system, may be used, which flashes the lights with the rings of the phone. This can also be linked to a portable vibrator system.

Related assistive technology for communication While current changes in employment from manufacturing to communication-based skills present a difficulty for those with hearing impairment,[30] the concomitant developments in technology provide better access in many ways for those with such problems.

Modes of communication that can be helped by technological developments include telephone communication, television/videos, public address systems, radios, teaching environments, banks and ticket offices, cinema/theatre, churches and within public transport, including aeroplanes. In most cases, this entails improving the signal/noise ratio, but some provide visual substitution. The range of facilities is summarized in Table 30.14.

Most progress is currently being made in telephone systems, which are also being replaced in certain contexts by increasing use of the Internet, with which people with hearing problems can communicate equally easily with others with hearing problems and with the normally hearing world. Among telephone devices themselves, the simplest is an additional earpiece, which can be used by a hearing partner of the hearing-impaired individual, who can then lipspeak or sign what is being said to the patient. Other long-standing approaches entail the incorporation of an additional amplifier into the handset and also the use of a built-in loop system. With normal telephones, these roles can be fulfilled by clip-on devices which can be fixed to the handset by an elastic band, and either amplify the acoustical signal or convert it to an electromagnetic field, which can be picked up by a hearing aid on the telecoil system.

More recent developments include the video-phone system, which enables the individual to obtain speech-reading cues or signs from the individual with whom they are communicating. It is, however, likely to be a few years before this is widely available, although the World Wide Web is having a major impact in this respect. More currently readily available are text telephones (e.g. Minicom and several mobile telephone systems), although these usually need to pass through the intermediary of a human interpreter when the hearing-impaired

Table 30.13 Types of aids for daily living.

	Doorbell	Phone bell	Alarm clock	Smoke alarm	Burglar alarm
Auditory					
Low-frequency	+	±	+	+	+
Loud	+	+	+	+	+
Extensions	+	+			
Mobile with patient	+	+	(watch)		
Visual					
Built-in light	+	+	+		
Link to lighting system	+	+			
Separate strobe system	+		+	+	+
Tactile					
Mobile vibrator	+	+	+	+	
Fan alarm			+		

Table 30.14 Types of aids for communication.

		Acoustical				
	Additional speaker	Additional amplifier	Loop	Infrared	FM	Text supplement
Telephone	+	+	+			
TV/Video	+	+	+	+	±	+
PA systems			+			
Lectures/classrooms, theatres	+	+	+	+	+	+
Places of worship	+	+	+			
Cinemas/theatres		+	+	+	+	
Banks/ticket offices	+	+	+			
Buses/trains	+					+
Aircraft				+		+

person is communicating with a hearing individual. These are likely to be replaced by automatic speech recognition and production systems as technology improves.

Mobile telephones, particularly digital systems, at the present time present more of a problem for hearing aid users with pickup of electronic noise. Some of this problem may be reduced by distancing the speaker from the hearing aid and the use of a neckloop system in digital signal-processing hearing aids.

Many loudspeakers in television sets are of poor quality, and the clarity of the output sound signal can be improved by the use of an external speaker or headphone or by taking the output via a high-fidelity system. This can be combined with an additional amplifier fed directly from a television output, or by having a microphone attached close to the television speaker, leading to an amplifier and either a headset or a loop system. Such a loop system may range from a silhouette or neckloop system through to one creating an electromagnetic field in the whole room. The quality of the field produced by such loop systems is sometimes poor, and better quality can be obtained by transmitting the sound to the individual using either an infrared or FM radio system. These have the additional difficulty of needing to be linked to the patient with the receiver connected to the hearing aid either indirectly via a neck loop or directly via an audio input.

Many television films and other programmes now have a subtitling or captioning facility which is being increasingly used and which is made easier by new digital technology. The replacement of video cassettes by DVDs, which generally have the option of subtitling one or more languages, can be helpful in this context. In addition, various television systems, particularly news and sport, may have information fully available in written form, although this role has gradually been taken over by the World Wide Web/Internet.

Finally some programmes of particular relevance, e.g. news bulletins, may have the announcer 'shadowed' by a signer to make the information more accessible to the deaf community. This is more widely available in some countries than in others.

The acoustical systems discussed above are also available for the use of people listening to the radio or recorded music.

Public address systems, particularly in stations and airports, present a considerable problem for most hearing-impaired people. The background noise is high, as is the reverberation. Sometimes information is presented by a loop system in certain demarcated areas. More commonly, there is a visual presentation of the information via television monitors or specifically designed information boards.

With all instrumental approaches, ranging from wearable hearing aids through cochlear implants to text telephones, appropriate instruction and training will be necessary to ensure that the patient is deriving optimal benefit from the device. In particular, this entails monitoring their progress after it has been fitted or provided.

Strategy

This section is concerned with the development of behavioural strategies to help the individual cope with their hearing problems in a real-life environment. Much of the need for such an approach is based on the premise that no hearing aid or implant system can restore their hearing to its pristine state. However, such strategies are also relevant for normally hearing people in difficult listening circumstances and also for those individuals with King Kopetzky syndrome (obscure auditory dysfunction (OAD): auditory disability with normal hearing (ADN)) who have normal octave-band audiometric thresholds but difficulty in hearing in the presence of any background noise. Hearing aids will not help such individuals.

The approach of teaching 'Hearing tactics' was developed particularly in Denmark in the 1970s[34,35] and entails manipulating one's environment, both animate and inanimate, to facilitate hearing—usually conversation. However, before such appropriate techniques may be taught or developed, it is important to define the specific auditory goals which the individual is trying to achieve and the broad gamut of approaches which would be acceptable to the particular individual.

The process of developing an appropriate strategy passes through various stages as outlined in Table 30.15.

Goal setting
This must be an interactive approach involving the patient, the professional and, usually, one or more significant others. However, such significant others must not be allowed to dominate the preferences of the hearing-impaired individuals.

The starting point returns to a consideration of the particular activity limitations and participation restrictions experienced by the patient and which they find as having the most important impact on their life. The Problem Questionnaire[15] may be used as a starting point, but the problems listed there are often very general — such as 'hearing conversation', which may be refined by discussing the circumstances, the types of conversation, and the particular individuals with which the person may have most difficulty. The patient also needs to be prompted for participation restrictions that they encounter, which tend to be under-represented in the Problem Questionnaire. Significant others may be helpful in highlighting areas in this respect, but only after probing first with the patient themselves.

Philosophy/personality
This concerns the approach of the individual to different circumstances as well as their overall approach to life. While one individual may be very shy or very outgoing in all circumstances, others may have different views according to their self-confidence or experience in dealing with particular groups of people.

Thus someone who is an expert in archaeology may have a very different approach at a meeting dealing with archaeological topics, being very dominant and controlling the meeting, than if he attends a political meeting to raise a particular local issue, where he may be very reserved. In developing appropriate tactics for the individual, the professional needs to take into account what he sees as the individual's own very particular needs and devise, in conjunction with him, the set of tactics for such particular circumstances.

Table 30.15 Strategy

- Goal definition
- Personality
- Significant others
- Hearing tactics
  - Manipulating social interaction
  - Manipulating physical environment
  - Observation

Hearing tactics
This term was coined by Von der Lieth[34] in Denmark to define the behavioural approaches that could be used by an individual to optimize their communication. In this early work, it generally entailed adopting a rather assertive approach, which is reflected in the publication *Hearing Tactics.*[35] Subsequently, Field and Haggard[36] published a broader classification of hearing tactics (Table 30.16), opening the way for a consideration of more passive behaviours as well as assertive behaviours. They subdivided tactics into 'Manipulating social interaction', 'Manipulating the physical environment' and 'Observations' but did not include 'withdrawal' from a communicative situation among their valid tactics. This has even been regarded by some as a maladaptive behavioural response.[37]

Elsewhere we have argued that withdrawal is an appropriate response in certain circumstances,[38] in terms of saving face and maintaining a self-image. Further, we have found that social withdrawal is one of the commonest tactics adopted by hearing-impaired people, being reported as frequently as asking others to repeat what they said and more frequently than passive positioning of themselves, interrupting and pretending to have heard.[39] Their use of these tactics is shown in Figure 30.5.

Pichora-Fuller et al[40] have highlighted the differences between 'transactional' aspects of communication aimed at achieving a specific, if limited, aim, and 'interactional' aspects aimed at maintaining or building relationships. They have found that someone with high social skills may maintain the

Table 30.16 Hearing tactics (after Field & Haggard[36])

- Manipulating social intervention; e.g. asking talker to face you, asking speaker to specify topic
- Manipulating physical environment; e.g. reducing background noise, soft furnishings to reduce reverberation
- Observation; e.g. watching face of speaker, noting non-verbal communication

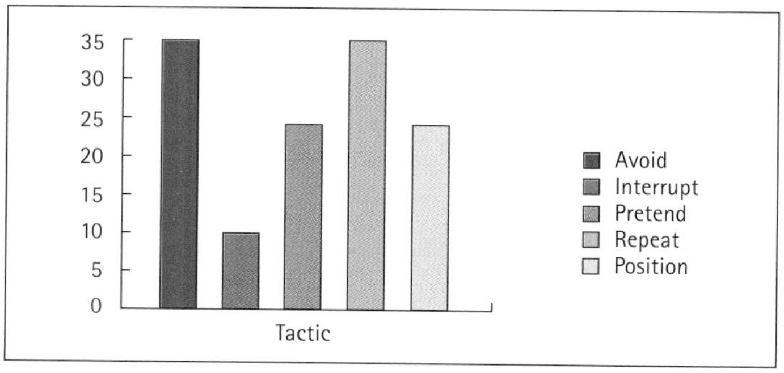

Figure 30.5 Percentage reported use of different hearing tactics—always or often. (After Stephens et al. *Br J Audiol* 1999; **33**: 17–27.[39])

latter without their communicative ability being put into question, as it might if they were noticed to make major mistakes in the former. This is an area of communication tactics which merits and indeed needs further study.

Ancillary help (services)

This is the stage at which it is important to consider other support services which will complement the rehabilitative support given to the hearing-impaired individual. This covers areas related to that provided in the normal rehabilitative services but which cannot be covered to the same degree or in the same respects.

Within ICF, these come within the realms of 'Environmental factors—services', which can have an impact on the disablements encountered by the hearing-impaired individual, in particular participation restriction. Referrals to such agencies complement the rehabilitative service, but should be considered in parallel with what is being done in related aspects of rehabilitation. The components of this section are summarized in Table 30.17, following the ICF classification of services.

Social services

These have a different role in different countries, and the needs for their intervention will depend on social problems highlighted by the evaluation process of the patient. These may range through housing and support for self-care through to aspects of possible abuse. Within the UK, in addition, under the terms of the Chronically Sick and Disabled Persons Act 1970 the social services have a responsibility for the provision of environmental aids (ALDs) although the degree and conditions in which such a provision is made vary throughout the UK.

Health services

These will play a different role according to the structure of the rehabilitative service in the particular centre concerned. In many centres in Europe, the rehabilitative service is based on medical departments, and related aural conditions such as otorrhoea, wax and vertigo can be dealt with as part of the service. In other countries, particularly the USA and Canada, they may be based on non-medical departments, so such aural conditions will call for referral to other appropriate services. In all cases, the management of the patient may highlight other important untreated health conditions, e.g. tremors affecting the rehabilitative management of the patient which may call for appropriate referral either to the patient's primary physician or to a relevant specialist.

The other aspect of health service referral pertinent to the rehabilitative process is for psychological or psychiatric help. This may be necessary in the individual severely emotionally affected by their hearing impairment, or in cases where inadequately treated underlying psychological/psychiatric conditions interfere with the individual's ability to participate adequately in the rehabilitative process.

Education and training services

While close liaison with such services is a traditional part of paediatric audiology, often including teachers within the rehabilitative team, it is frequently not implemented as well as it could be. Good relationships between the rehabilitative and educational services are essential from the age of diagnosis, with both services providing valuable inputs for the hearing-impaired child. The rehabilitative service can provide advice on the latest aspects of amplification and environmental aids and provide speech therapy support, but must take care to avoid clashes with the domains covered by the teachers.

Such liaison with education services does not finish when the individual reaches 16 or 18 years of age. Further and higher education now continues through colleges, universities and other training establishments for much of the individual's life, and links to ensure appropriate support, environmental help, note-takers, interpreters and sophisticated communication systems should continue for most of the individual's life. Indeed, many people well into their 80s attend evening and other part-time classes or television-based university studies, and liaison with appropriate support individuals in these contexts will be important.

Labour and employment services

The role of disability employment advisors in this respect has been highlighted in many Western countries by the passing of disability discrimination legislation. The support of such individuals in facilitating the retraining or support of hearing-impaired individuals in their chosen domain of work can be vital. They also have an important role in liaison with appropriate employers, alerting them to the needs of employees with hearing impairments, and what can be done to facilitate their participation in the workplace in the context of the acoustical environment and environmental aids.

Voluntary organizations

Many individuals with hearing impairment feel isolated within society and unable to find non-professionals with whom they can discuss their problems. The various voluntary organizations for deaf children, deaf adults, hard-of-hearing adults and those with profound acquired hearing impairment have an important role in meeting these needs. This is particularly important for parents of deaf children, but many adults with acquired hearing

Table 30.17 Ancillary help (services)

- Social services
- Health services
  - Other medical, psychological, etc.
- Education and training services
- Labour and employment services
- Voluntary organizations

impairment also find that support from hard-of-hearing peers can be helpful, particularly in the early stages of adjustment to their hearing impairment. Obviously, such organizations have other campaigning and support roles, but the source of contact is the main element of immediate relevance to the newly treated hearing-impaired individual. Information about voluntary organizations should be made available within the rehabilitative departments but not forced on the individuals concerned.

Continuing remediation

This differs from other aspects of the remediation process, in that it may continue over a period of weeks, months or even years, while the bulk of the other components are achieved in two or three sessions immediately following the evaluation and decision-making stages. While in some rehabilitative programmes this is a fixed-duration process which all patients pass through, we would argue that it is a process which should be tailored to the needs of the specific individual concerned. Thus, while for some category 1 patients it may comprise merely a short part of one session, in other cases, such as some patients with profound acquired hearing loss or severe auditory distortions stemming from brainstem injuries, it may extend over a considerable period of time.

However, in all cases it is important to consider each of the stages shown in Table 30.18 to determine what, if anything, needs to be done to alleviate the individual's disablements.

Table 30.18 Continuing remediation

- Information provision
- Skill-building
- Instrument modification
- Counselling
- Changes to the physical and cultural environment

Information provision

This may cover a wide range of matters, from the structure of the ear and what has happened to it in the individual's case, through to the basic signal processing used in the latest digital hearing aid. It is a very patient-centred process and must be organized to meet the needs of the particular person. Some may be obsessed with the cause, mechanism and prognosis of their otosclerosis, whereas others will only be concerned about the long-term prognosis for their hearing. Some patients will want to know all about the processing strategies and capabilities of a cochlear implant, whereas others will prefer to treat it as a black box. The level of sophistication of the information provision will depend on the background and understanding of the individual concerned, but, in all cases, the information must be presented in an easily comprehensible manner. For many patients, such an understanding of what is affecting their hearing and what any of the treatment options can be expected to achieve, and how, is a precondition for their acceptance of their condition and any further intervention.

Skill-building

This area is one in which many aspects of the rehabilitative process are elaborated. It can range from training the elderly tremulous patient to fit an earmould and hearing aid into their ear, to learning how to supplement their visual input from a tactile stimulator or frequency transposition hearing aid.

All these aspects are important in order to help the individual to minimize the difficulties which they have as a result of their hearing impairment and improve their participation in their chosen lifestyle. They thus range from using their instrumentation optimally through practising and refining appropriate tactics to improving their audiovisual communication skills.

From an instrumental standpoint, the biggest initial problem experienced by most patients, particularly the elderly, is fitting their hearing aid system to their ears. Without this, they will derive inadequate benefit from their aid and may reject the whole process. The skill-building here is to help the patient achieve this fitting successfully and effortlessly. This may entail cutting down the earmould as well as working with the patient to develop a technique to fit their aid to the most difficult-shaped ears.

In order to obtain optimal benefit from their hearing aid, tactile aid or cochlear implant, the patient must learn to obtain optimal benefit from it in the difficult listening situations which they normally encounter. This will entail auditory training, i.e. learning to utilize and understand distorted or altered inputs such as from a frequency transposition or tactile aid, and to integrate this with their visual input. This can be achieved by training with different but relevant practice materials, and computerized video-based techniques can be helpful in this respect.[41]

Such auditory and audiovisual training techniques can also be important in patients with essentially normal hearing sensitivity but distorted recognition of speech, such as those with central auditory dysfunction (see Chapter 29). Related to this is training in speechreading (lipreading), although there is little evidence to suggest that general lipreading classes can help the overall lipreading performance of an individual, except by improving their self-confidence.

In many, if not all, cases this approach is not sufficient to meet all the needs of the patient, and the role of hearing tactics must be considered here. While the short-term aspects of the remedial process may cover a presentation and discussion of the different tactics which can be used, some individuals lack the confidence or understanding to implement them and require training to cope with specific difficult situations, such as meetings around a table, or group discussions. The training in these circumstances is often optimal with a group of patients being supported by one or more therapists.

Instrument modification

This covers two broad areas, that of the support for the long-term adaptation to a particular hearing aid system, and the selection of appropriate environmental aids after hearing aid fitting.

Barfod,[42] in a theoretical discussion, highlighted the fact that an aid which acoustically may be appropriate for an individual's hearing impairment may be unacceptable, as the individual has become used to a distorted input (e.g. reduced high frequencies). This may lead to a biasing in the individual's recognition mechanism towards the type of acoustical input to which they are accustomed. Adding more high frequencies will result in what, to the patient, is a distorted input, and they will reject the aid. Barfod suggested that patients need to be weaned onto the ideal hearing aid characteristics by increasing the high-frequency amplification gradually over time in steps acceptable to the individual until they are able to both appreciate the sound of the aid and benefit from the appropriate frequency configuration.

Gatehouse[43] and others have extensively studied this adaptation process and have shown that it may occur over a period of 3–6 months, particularly when sophisticated signal-processing strategies are used. The audiologist must ensure that the fitting is acceptable to the patient so that they continue to use the hearing aid and are moving in a direction which should result in optimal performance.

Some environmental aids, such as systems for hearing the doorbell or the alarm clock, where the patient will be receiving the sound in the presence of background noise, is unaffected by the hearing aid, or is not using their aid(s), can be selected at an early stage of the rehabilitative process. In other cases, such as watching the television in the company of a normally hearing partner, the hearing aid may reduce or minimize all their problems. In these cases it is important to see which problems remain after the hearing aid fitting and which environmental aids will then be appropriate to resolve these. The same may also be true of a variety of other communication and alerting systems, where the hearing aid system may alleviate many of the difficulties.

In addition to the adaptation to the hearing aids, the particular hearing aid system selected may not meet the specific needs of the patient in their chosen environments and may need to be modified or changed according to the expressed problems. It must be remembered that the best hearing aid prescription formulae provide only a guide to the optimal hearing aid settings for a given hearing loss and cannot allow for the particular environments in which the individual may need to use their aid. Thus, fine-tuning may be necessary over a period of time. However, the professional must be alert for the individual who is always complaining and requesting further adjustments to the hearing aid fitting, when really he is trying to tell the professional that he is rejecting the hearing aid system altogether.

Counselling

This is a key part of any continuing remediation, supporting the patient in their continuing needs and difficulties. There are many counselling techniques[44] aimed mainly at improving the patient's adjustment to their disablements, and the professional must adopt an approach in harmony with their philosophy and orientation.

The counselling may, in some individuals, entail practical discussions of how to cope with a specific situation which has arisen. In others, it may entail attempting to change their approach to the whole rehabilitative process and could involve endeavouring to convert patients in the type 3 category into those more amenable to intervention.

In the context of particular sets of problems, it is also important to involve significant others in the counselling process, if the patient is amenable to such an approach. The behavioural modifications may well involve these significant others and they can support the patient in various ways.

Changes to the physical and cultural environment

These may be specific to the environment of the patient or they may have an influence in the society as a whole, or at least in the local situation.

What these will entail is an attempt to change the acoustical, visual and stress-related problems confronting the patient through involvement of the patient, his family, employers, educators and others in a position to influence the environment. All this, obviously, must be done only with the full agreement of the patient.

In a broader context, the professional has a responsibility to attempt to change the attitudes and approaches of the society in which the patient lives, in order to facilitate the individual's full participation within this environment. This may entail liaising with media professionals to, for example, cut down on the use of any background noise or music during spoken broadcasts. This can have knock-on effects to benefit other hearing-impaired individuals, and not just the particular target person. The need for such actions may be highlighted by the complaints of one particular individual, who can then act as a trigger for something which may be of broad general benefit.

The professionals can also, by use of the media, attempt to reduce the stigmatizing attitudes of society towards hearing impairment in general and hearing aids in particular. This can be achieved only slowly, but steps can be made by broad public health education approaches and by seeking role models capable of influencing the views of the public at large.

Outcome measures

In the context of any rehabilitative programme, it is important to use appropriate outcome measures which can enable those working in the programme to assess the effectiveness of what they are doing for the particular individual. They have other applications, as are discussed below.

Performance-based measures

These are usually orientated towards a particular technology such as hearing aids or cochlear implants and may entail four different approaches (e.g. Table 30.19). The first three are broadly self-explanatory and are covered elsewhere in this book, in the context of hearing aids (Chapter 31).

The quality and quantity of spontaneous communication may apply to the linguistic and interactive elements of the speech of children receiving implants, hearing aids or sign language programmes. It may also apply to an assessment of individuals in retirement homes, with regard to their various types of communicative interactions with staff and other residents before and after rehabilitative interventions.

Satisfaction measures

Various ad hoc approaches have been used in this context for satisfaction with the approach, process or particular interventions received. These may be tailored towards the particular approach under study. Cox and Alexander[45] published their well-researched 'Satisfaction with Amplification in Daily Life Scale' (SADL), which has subscales of 'Positive effects', 'Service and cost', 'Negative features' and 'Personal image'. This is capable of modification for other circumstances.

Improvement in activity and participation (reduction in disability and handicap)

A great variety of such scales have been described, dating back to the Hearing Handicap Scale of High, Fairbanks and Glorig,[22] which was a measure of speech communication activity limitation. Many of these have been discussed by Noble[46] and by Bentler and Kramer.[23] They all largely come under the category of 'standardized scales'—see Table 30.7.

In addition, there are patient-generated scales, of which the most promising would appear to be the 'Cliented Orientated Scale of Improvement' (COSI).[20] In this the patient is required to specify the major problem areas during the assessment process. At the end of the rehabilitation, they then rate the improvement and residual problems in each of these areas.

The 'Glasgow Hearing Aid Benefit Profile' (GHABP)[21] can be regarded as a hybrid of these two, with fixed standardized components as in the first group, and patient-generated complaints as in the second. The main problem here is obtaining the relevant balance between the two sections, which should, arguably, be scored separately.

Simple ratings have been used elsewhere,[18] in which the patients lists their problems as in COSI and in the second part of the GHABP and then rate the magnitude of these problems on a visual analogue-type scale, rating them again at the end of the rehabilitative process.

Table 30.19 Performance-based measures

1. Speech in noise recognition
2. Threshold improvement
3. Quantity and quality of spontaneous communication
4. Hearing aid use, etc.

Improvement in quality of life

These are usually performed using standardized scales such as the SF36[47] or Health Utilities Index,[48] all of which have some limitations from an audiological standpoint. Alternatively, the patient may be asked to rate their quality of life or the effects of their hearing on their quality of life, before and after intervention, as used in the Euroquol thermometer.[49]

A global assessment of any programme should use a combination of these approaches, depending on what is being assessed, and for what purpose. The groupings of uses of these, particularly the questionnaire-based measures, have been discussed by Cox et al.[50] They list four goals for these measures, as follows.

Assessment of the rehabilitative outcomes for an individual hearing-impaired person

This is a key function in all patient-centred rehabilitative processes.

A key tool to use in such an assessment is COSI,[26] which measures improvement and residual problems in a range of dimensions specified by the patient at their initial assessment. It is important also at the initial assessment to probe for participation restrictions (handicaps), which tend to be listed less than activity limitations (disabilities). It is also important in the formulation of this to seek views of significant others, if present, as to what major problems may be. A useful starting point for both the individual and the significant others is the Problem Questionnaire,[15] which can be sent to the patient with their clinic appointment. This can also be used with significant others, who can complete their version while the patient is being tested.[51]

This measure may be supplemented by one or more questions as to the patient's satisfaction with the rehabilitative process, ranging from a simple question such as 'Overall, how satisfied are you with the rehabilitation service?' through to more extensive measures, primarily hearing aid orientated, such as SADL.[45]

The assessment of the effectiveness of the service(es) provided by a particular clinical unit or agency

This enables purchasers to decide between a variety of competing service providers.

In this context, as well, COSI is a useful tool, which has been found in Australia to provide a valuable outcome measure, and which relates well to a pool of other measures.[20] Again, it should be supplemented with a satisfaction measure, and in this context, the two following questions would appear to be useful:

1. 'How satisfied were you with the approach of the professionals you saw about hearing problems?'
2. 'How satisfied are you with the extent to which your hearing problems have been reduced?'

Finally, the individuals should be asked to list the benefits and shortcomings of the service which they had received, as used by Stephens and Meredith[52] in a hearing aid study, and subsequently in other studies.[53]

The assessment of the effectiveness of new instrumental technologies

These may include different hearing aid systems, cochlear implants or environmental aids.

In this context, performance-based measures will come into their own in order to best define the differences between two broadly similar approaches. They also have the advantage that they are more resistant to biasing from patient and experimenter preferences (the Hawthorn effect). There have been very few double-blind comparisons of different hearing aid systems. The most widely used tests in this context are speech-in-noise tests (e.g. FAAF)[54] and triplet tests (e.g. letter–digit–letter), which enable the tester to determine the speech threshold in a certain level of background noise. Tests such as the BKB test[26] may also be used to determine the optimal speech recognition score in such noise.

Other surrogate performance scores may include assessments of device use, either self-report, or using some measuring system. In addition, a variety of rating scales of sound quality have been used.

In terms of specific hearing aid benefits, SHAPIE (Shortened Hearing Aid Performance Inventory for the Elderly)[55,56] has been rigorously evaluated, and can be recommended. This asks questions as to the benefit which the individual derives from the hearing aid in a range of situations. However, other tools may be more relevant under other circumstances, depending on the aims of the particular new technology.

The evaluation of the effect of hearing rehabilitation services on the quality of life

This last is important from a public health standpoint, when considering resources which should be provided to audiological services against, for example, services treating varicose veins.

Health-related quality of life measures are the key tools in this respect. All have many limitations in the weighting which they attach to hearing and communication problems in relation to more physical or life-threatening conditions. The two most relevant, and widely used in this context are the SF36[47] and the Health Utilities Index.[48] The latter is probably the most useful in this field, and has achieved acceptance in the domain of cochlear implants.[57]

References

1. Stephens D. Audiological rehabilitation. In: Stephens D. (ed.) *Scott Brown's Otolaryngology*, 5th edn. London: Butterworth, 1987: 446–80.
2. Tye-Murray N. *Foundations of Aural Rehabilitation*. San Diego: Singular.
3. Alpiner JG, McCarthy PA (eds). *Rehabilitative Audiology: Children and Adults*, 2nd edn. Baltimore: Williams and Wilkins, 1993.
4. World Health Organization. *ICF: International Classification of Functioning, Disability and Health*. Geneva: WHO, 2001.
5. Noble W. Hearing, hearing impairment and the audible world: a theoretical essay. *Audiology* 1983; **22**: 325–38.
6. Noble W, Hétu R. An ecological approach to disability and handicap in relation to impaired hearing. *Audiology* 1994; **33**: 117–26.
7. Borg E. Audiology in an ecological perspective — development of a conceptual framework. *Scand Audiol* 1998; **27**(suppl 49): 132–9.
8. Goldstein DP, Stephens SDG. Audiological rehabilitation: management model: I. *Audiology* 1981; **20**: 432–52.
9. World Health Organization. *The International Classification of Impairments, Disabilities, and Handicaps — a Manual Relating to the Consequences of a Disease*. Geneva: WHO, 1980.
10. Stephens D, Kerr P. Auditory disablements: an update. *Audiology* 2000; **39**: 322–32.
11. World Health Organization. *International Classification of Impairments, Activities and Participation* — ICIDH-2. (Beta-1 draft). Geneva: WHO, 1997.
12. Stephens SDG, Meredith R, Callaghan DE, Hogan S, Rayment A. Early intervention and rehabilitation: factors influencing outcome. *Acta Ololaryngol Suppl* 1991; **476**: 221–5.
13. Stephens SDG. Hearing rehabilitation in a psychosocial framework. *Scand Audiol* 1996; **25**(suppl 43): 57–66.
14. Stephens D. Audiological rehabilitation. In: Stephens D, ed. *Scott Brown's Otolaryngology*, 6th edn. Oxford: Butterworth Heinemann, 1997: 2/13/1–36.
15. Barcham LJ, Stephens SDG. The use of an open ended problem questionnaire in auditory rehabilitation. *Br J Audiol* 1980; **14**: 49–54.
16. Stephens SDG. People's complaints of hearing difficulties. In: Kyle JG, ed. *Adjustment to Acquired Hearing Loss*, Bristol: Centre for Deaf Studies, 1987: 37–47.
17. Stephens D, Gianopoulos I, Kerr P. Determination and classification of the problems experienced by hearing-impaired elderly people. *Audiol* 2001; **40**: 294–300.
18. Stephens D, Jaworski A, Kerr P, Zhao F. Use of patient-specific estimates in patient evaluation and rehabilitation. *Scand Audiol* 1998; **27**(suppl 49): 61–8.
19. Dillon H, Birtles G, Lovegrove R. Measuring the outcomes of a national rehabilitation program: normative data for the Client Oriented Scale of Improvement (COSI) and the Hearing Aid User's Questionnaire (HAUQ). *J Am Acad Audiol* 1999; **10**: 67–79.
20. Dillon H, James A, Ginis JA. The Client Oriented Scale of Improvement (COSI) and its relationship to several other measures of benefit and satisfaction provided by hearing aids. *J Am Acad Audiol* 1997; **8**: 27–43.

21. Gatehouse S. Glasgow hearing aid benefit profile: derivation and validity of a client-centred outcome measure for hearing aid services. *J Am Acad Audiol* 1999; **10**: 80–93.
22. High WS, Fairbanks G, Glorig A. Scale for the self assessment of hearing handicap. *J Speech Hear Disord* 1964; **19**: 215–30.
23. Bentler RA, Kramer SE. Guidelines for choosing a self-report outcome measure. *Ear Hear* 2000; **21**: 37S–49S.
24. Stephens SDG. Auditory rehabilitation. *Br Med Bull* 1987; **43**: 999–1026.
25. De Filippo CL, Scott BL. A method for training and evaluating the reception of ongoing speech. *J Acoust Soc Am* 1978; **63**: 1186–92.
26. Bench J, Bamford J. (eds). *Speech-Hearing Tests and the Spoken Language of Hearing-Impaired Children*. London: Academic Press, 1979.
27. Hirsh IJ, Davis H, Silverman SR, Reynolds EG, Eldert E, Benson RW. Development of materials for speech audiometry. *J Sp Hear Dis* 1952; **17**: 321–37.
28. Cornett RD, Beadles R, Wilson B. Automatic cued speech. In: Pickett JM, ed. *Papers from the Research Conference on Speech-Processing Aids for the Deaf* Washington, DC: Gallaudet College, 1982: 224–39.
29. Forchammer G. *Om nodvendigheden af sikre meddelelsesmidler i Dovestumm eundervisningen*. København: Frimodt, 1903.
30. Ruben RJ. Redefining the survival of the fittest: communication disorders in the 21st century. *Laryngoscope* 2000; **110**: 241–5.
31. Hétu R. The stigma attached to hearing impairment. *Scand Audiol* 1994; **25**(suppl 43): 12–24.
32. Vernon JA, Meikle MB. In: Tyler RS, ed. *Tinnitus Masking in Tinnitus Handbook*, Vol. 14. 2000; **14**: 313–55.
33. Roberts P. *An ergonomic investigation into the design of a behind the ear (BTE) hearing aid to overcome handling difficulties experienced by elderly users*. Undergraduate dissertation, University of Glamorgan, 1992.
34. Von der Lieth L. Hearing Tactics I & II. *Scand Audiol* 1972; **1**: 155–60.
35. Vognsen S (ed.). *Hearing Tactics*. Copenhagen: Oticon, 1976.
36. Field DL, Haggard MP. Knowledge of hearing tactics 1: assessment by questionnaire and inventory. *Br J Audiol* 1989; **23**: 349–54.
37. Demorest ME, Erdman SA. Development of the communication profile for the hearing impaired. *J Speech Hear Disord* 1987; **52**: 129–43.
38. Jaworski A, Stephens D. Self-reports on silence as a face-saving strategy by people with hearing impairment. *Int J Appl Linguistics* 1998; **8**(1): 61–80.
39. Stephens SDG, Jaworski A, Lewis P, Aslan S. An analysis of the communication tactics used by hearing-impaired adults. *Br J Audiol* 1999; **33**: 17–27.
40. Pichora-Fuller MK, Johnson CJ, Roodenburg KEJ. The discrepancy between hearing impairment and handicap in the elderly: balancing transaction and interaction in conversation. *J Appl Commun Res* 1998; **26**: 99–119.
41. Tye-Murray N, Tyler RS, Bong B, Nares T. Computerised laser videodisc programs for training speechreading and assertive communication behaviours. *J Acad Rehabil Audiol* 1988; **21**: 143–52.
42. Barfod J. Speech perception processes and fitting of hearing aids. *Audiology* 1979; **18**: 430–41.
43. Gatehouse S. Report of the First Eriksholm Consensus Conference on Auditory Deprivation and Acclimatization. *Ear Hear* 1996; **17**.
44. Erdman SA. Counselling hearing-impaired adults. In: Alpiner JG, McCarthy PA, eds. *Rehabilitative Audiology: Children and Adults*, 2nd edn. Baltimore: Williams & Wilkins, 1993: 374–413.
45. Cox RM, Alexander GC. Measuring Satisfaction with Amplification in Daily Life: the SADL Scale. *Ear Hear* 1999; **20**: 306–20.
46. Noble W. *Self Assessment of Hearing and Related Functions*. London: Whurr, 1998.
47. Brazier JT, Usherwood, Harper R, Thomas K. Deriving a preference-based single index from the UK SF-36 Health Survey. *J Clin Epidemiol* 1998; **51**: 1115–28.
48. Torrance GW. Measurement of health state utilities for economic appraisal — a review. *J Health Economics* 1986; **5**: 1–30.
49. Euroquol Group. A new faculty for the measurement of health related quality of life. *Health Policy* 1990; **16**: 199–208.
50. Cox R, Hyde M, Gatehouse S et al. Optimal outcome measures, research priorities and international cooperation. *Ear Hear* 2000; **21**: 106S–15S.
51. Stephens SDG, France L, Lormore K. Effects of hearing impairment on the patient's family and friends. *Acta Otolaryngol* 1995; **115**: 115–17.
52. Stephens SDG, Meredith R. Qualitative reports of hearing aid benefit. *Clin Rehabil* 1991; **5**: 225–9.
53. Stephens D, Board T, Hobson J, Cooper H. Reported benefits and problems experienced with bone-anchored hearing aids. *Br J Audiol* 1996; **30**: 215–20.
54. Foster JS, Haggard M. The four alternative auditory feature test (FAAF)—linguistic and psychometiric properties of the material with normative data in noise. *Br J Audiol* 1987; **21**: 165–74.
55. Dillon H. Shortened Hearing Aid Performance Inventory for the Elderly (SHAPIE): a statistical approach. *Aust J Audiol* 1997; **16**: 37–48.
56. Walden BE, Demores ME, Hepler EL. Self-report approach to assessing benefit derived from amplification. *J Speech Hear Res* 1984; **27**(1): 49–56.
57. Summerfield AQ, Marshall DH. *Report by the MRC Institute of Hearing Research on the Evaluation of the National Cochlear Implant Programme. Main Report. Cochlear Implantation in the UK, 1990–1994.*
58. Kramer SE, Kapteyn TS, Festen JM, Tobi H. Factors in subjective hearing disability. *Audiology* 1995; **34**: 167–99.
59. Kaplan H, Bally S, Brandt, Busacco D, Pray J. Communication Scale for Older Adults (CSOA). *J Am Acad Audiol* 1997; **8**: 203–17.
60. Ringdahl A, Eriksson-Mangold M, Andersson G. Psychometric evaluation of the Gothenburg Profile for measurement of experienced hearing disability and handicap: applications with new hearing aid candidates and experienced hearing aid users. *Br J Audiol* 1998; **32**: 375–85.
61. Hétu R, Getty L, Philbert L, Desilets F, Noble W, Stephens D. Mise au point d'un outil clinique pour la mesure d'incapacités et de handicaps. *J Speech Language Pathol Audiol* 1994; **18**: 83–95.

31 Auditory amplification in adults

Stuart Gatehouse

Fitting of a hearing aid or hearing aids remains the only viable management option for the vast majority of listeners with sensorineural hearing impairment, and a smaller though still significant number of people with conductive impairment for whom surgery has either been refused, is not appropriate, or perhaps has been unsuccessful. However, as an opening statement, this sentence is in itself incomplete, as it tends to view a hearing aid fitting in isolation. The realistic object of intervention at present is not to provide a 'cure' for sensorineural hearing impairment (however laudable and desirable such an aim might be) but, rather, to provide a process which attempts to overcome the disabilities and handicaps of hearing-impaired listeners and their families and others with whom they interact. Thus, while this chapter restricts itself to considerations of amplification per se, it would be unwise to read and interpret the information contained herein in isolation from the other contributions in this book, which address the overall components of a rehabilitation service for hearing-impaired individuals.

The content of this chapter is aimed at physicians and surgeons who have the overarching responsibility for the management of hearing-impaired listeners, and who might have the responsibility for the organization and delivery of a hearing rehabilitation service containing at its core the provision of amplification. As such, it is not aimed at technical specialists in audiology in the detail it provides. A search of the scientific and clinical literature will identify an extensive collection of information addressing hearing aids and their fitting—indeed, this author's own collection of published papers in this field (which is by no means extensive or complete) runs to some 3500 items, and the reader will readily identify any number of specialist texts relating to signal processing for hearing aids, the fitting of hearing aids, and the verification and evaluation of their performance. No single chapter could possibly hope to provide a comprehensive description of this knowledge base, and, therefore, certain strategies and decisions have been taken in configuring the content. This chapter aims to identify the major decision-points and the dimensions of those options which a clinician might face in the management of individual hearing-impaired listeners or the organization of a service. It attempts to summarize current knowledge and to provide an accessible synopsis. It does contain a relatively extensive bibliography (though not 3500 strong!) to direct the reader to the evidence base from which the conclusions are drawn. Where the line of argument becomes more extensive, a short-form conclusion is provided and highlighted. Given that in the UK the great majority of hearing aid fittings are undertaken by the National Health Service (NHS), much of the information provided makes reference to current and potential future practice within the NHS. However, to address only NHS concerns would be overly restrictive, particularly in view of the currently narrow range of technological options open to the NHS and rehabilitative contexts within which those technological options are delivered. This is particularly apposite given the initiatives at the time of writing to upgrade the status, organization and content of hearing aid services offered by the NHS. Therefore, this chapter does indeed consider technologies which are currently not available through the NHS, but which might well become part of a clinician's armoury in years to come.

As has been mentioned, the fitting of a hearing aid is, at all of its stages, inextricably linked to the overall rehabilitation programme that the service delivers. The detailed descriptions of rehabilitative options are available elsewhere in this book but, for the purposes of configuring this chapter, the overly simplified schematic shown in Figure 31.1 is used as an artifice to

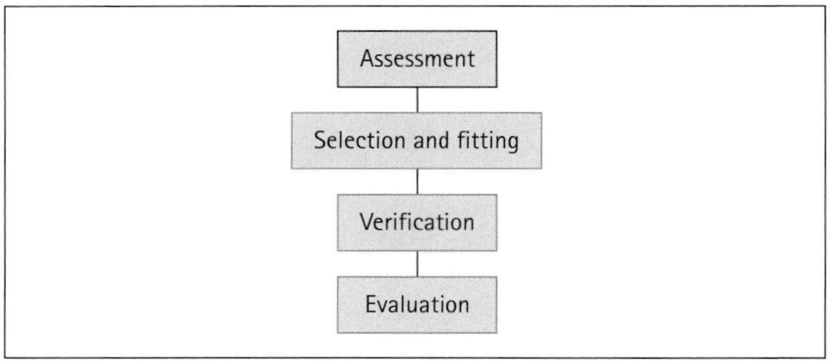

Figure 31.1 Schematic representation of the hearing aid fitting and rehabilitation process.

delineate some of the major stages, and identifies four main components comprising assessment, selection and fitting, verification and evaluation.

This chapter enters the process at the point where the clinician has taken the decision that the management of disability and handicap should contain an element of amplification—that is, a hearing aid or aids are to be fitted. There are, of course, a whole host of elements which enter into that decision, of which only a minority are audiological in nature. Clearly, for a hearing aid to be appropriate, it is helpful if the patient has a hearing impairment so that the device has the opportunity to make audible sounds that were previously inaudible (although, as will be mentioned later, there are potential roles for processing features such as directional microphones which improve the signal-to-noise ratio even for listeners with very minor auditory impairments). At the other end of the impairment spectrum, for profound losses the role of acoustical amplification gives way to management via electrical stimulation (cochlear implants) and tactile devices. It is unwise to try to generate, at either end of the severity distribution, levels or configurations of hearing impairment which delineate people whose hearing is regarded as 'too good' to be helped by amplification from those who are hearing aid candidates, and from those whose hearing is regarded as 'too impaired' to benefit from acoustical amplification. Certainly, current practice in adult cochlear implantation is to manage as well as possible using hearing aids, and then the restricted benefits derived from those devices itself form candidature criteria for implantation. Similarly, listeners who complain of hearing disability and wish to try amplification should not be discouraged because of an arbitrary limit in the impairment domain. Indeed, it is more likely that the clinician will need to persuade an unwilling candidate that amplification offers a viable option. Candidature criteria in the impairment domain are useful for epidemiological and service planning purposes,[1] but should not be used to restrict access on an individual basis.

When a clinician makes a recommendation to a hearing-impaired individual concerning the likely benefits of amplification, he will of course address a number of non-audiological issues, including lifestyle demands, motivations, physical and cognitive function and manipulation abilities, both in the initial decision regarding management and in the choice of hearing aid management.

Selection and fitting of hearing aid features

Following the decision to include a hearing aid fitting as part of an individual's management, there is a host of options concerning the features of that hearing aid fitting which are available to the clinician. Some of these features concern the various signal-processing options within hearing aids, while others are more general 'features' which include the different physical options for hearing aids and the ways in which they are coupled to the impaired auditory system. All of these different styles of feature are relevant to the hearing aid fitting process, and are addressed here in turn.

Hearing aid style

Under this heading we consider some of the physical aspects of a hearing aid,[2] in terms of its size, and some of the electronic and electroacoustical elements of the way in which a hearing aid functions. Early electronic aids to hearing consisted of a battery-pack and electronics worn on the belt or body which were coupled via cables to a transducer at the patient's ear. Such 'body-worn' devices are now rarely used, except in rare cases where feedback issues become paramount (discussed below) or where the physical ability to manipulate controls is severely compromised. The vast majority of modern hearing aids are of the 'at-the-ear' type. The two broad divisions are shown in Figures 31.2 and 31.3. Figure 31.2 shows two postaural units (behind-the-ear (BTE)) of differing physical size. With the advances in battery technology, transducer technology and electronic circuitry, it has proved possible to manufacture BTE devices that are much less cumbersome than those available hitherto. The requirement for large postaural casings has largely been removed. Since the relatively early days of integrated circuit technology, the hearing aid industry has striven to reduce the size of devices, and to fit them in the ear canal itself with the primary objective of making the hearing aid 'invisible' (a central point of much hearing aid advertising). Figure 31.3 shows instances of devices which are conventionally labelled as 'in-the-ear' (ITE), 'in-the-canal' (ITC) and 'completely in-the-canal' (CIC), with progressive degrees of miniaturization. The primary drive for this miniaturization is cosmetic, and might at first consideration appear to be a purely technical issue. However, there is here an interaction with the overall rehabilitation concept which is worthy of mention. When most hearing-impaired listeners are first seeking help and being fitted with hearing aids, they express a strong desire for their hearing aids

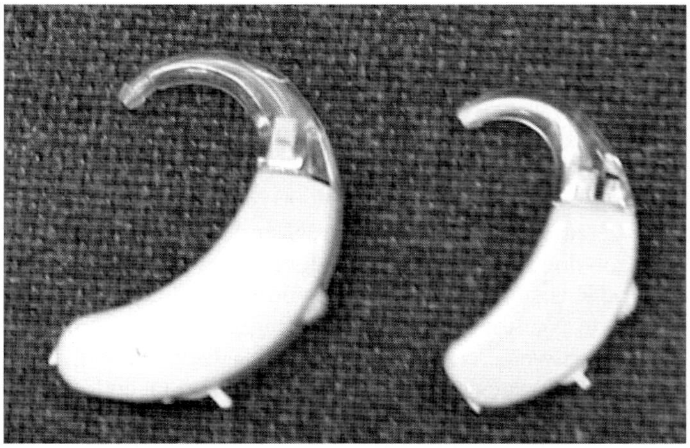

Figure 31.2 Styles of behind-the-ear (BTE) hearing aids.

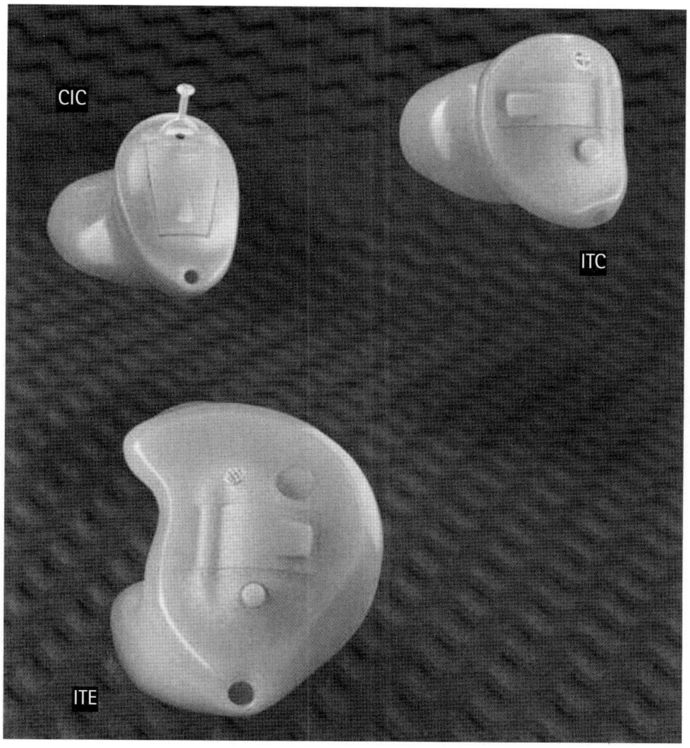

Figure 31.3 Styles of in-the-ear (ITE) hearing aids. CIC, completely in the canal; ITC, in the canal.

to be as invisible as possible so that it is not apparent to others that the impaired person has a hearing problem. The whole issue of stigma associated with both hearing impairment and with hearing aids, and the implications that this has for hearing aids themselves, and the design and delivery of rehabilitation services, contains many elements. Perhaps one of the most important is that the cosmetic drive towards miniaturization can be part of an unwanted and unhelpful avoidance on the part of the hearing-impaired person of the existence of problems and the impact this has both on their own lives and those of their companions. It is instructive to contrast this approach with reports from experienced users of hearing aids who positively suggest that they wish their hearing aid to signal to other people that they do have a hearing problem, and that appropriate communication strategies should be adopted. The tension between the desire of hearing aid manufacturers and hearing-impaired people to have invisible devices, and the comprehensive approach to the rehabilitation of disability and handicaps, remains unresolved.

Although the primary motivation for miniaturization remains cosmetic, there are a number of acoustical advantages in devices which are fitted in rather than behind the ear. A BTE hearing aid delivers its sound to the tympanic membrane via a tube and earmould (Figure 31.4). The tube and earmould has an acoustical effect which is often undesirable. If the output of a hearing aid is delivered closer to the tympanic membrane, there are advantages in terms of the power that is needed to drive the device, and the fidelity of the sound that is produced (provided

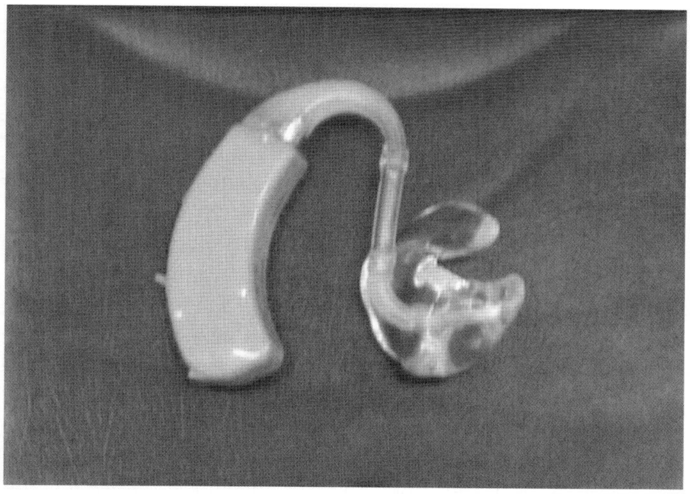

Figure 31.4 A post-aural (BTE) hearing aid and earmould coupling.

that undue engineering compromises are not required in the miniaturization process itself). A further set of potential benefits arise from the fact that in ITE devices the hearing aid microphone is located in a more 'natural' position and serves to better preserve some of the cues which underpin sound localization and aspects of binaural hearing.

There are, however, significant disadvantages associated with progressively smaller devices. As the separation between the microphone and the hearing aid output decreases, the likelihood of feed back increases. The smaller the device and its associated controls, the greater will be the difficulties experienced in physically fitting and adjusting the device by (predominantly elderly) people whose manipulation abilities are compromised. In addition, ITE devices are naturally more prone to blockage and damage by wax than are postaural units. Cleaning or replacing an earmould is easier and more convenient than replacing a hearing aid. Nevertheless, ITE as opposed to BTE fittings are desired by hearing-impaired people and play an increasing role in provision. A discussion of the issues surrounding the benefits and problems of ITE and BTE devices can be found in the literature.[3–11]

A simplified representation of the functional elements of a hearing aid is shown in Figure 31.5. Sound in the environment

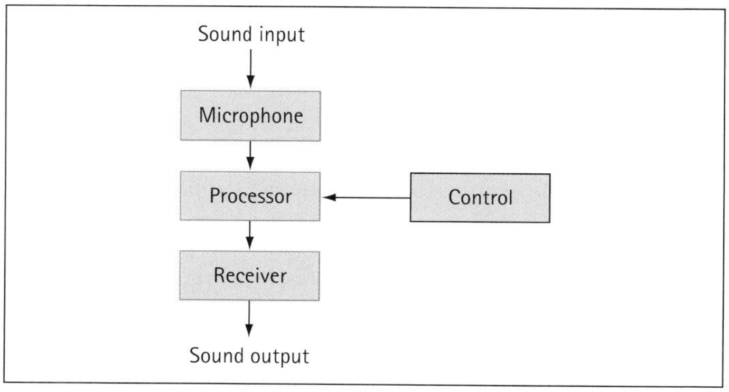

Figure 31.5 Basic elements of a hearing aid.

is converted by the microphone into an electrical signal. This electrical signal is then processed (e.g. amplified) and reconverted via the hearing aid receiver (output transducer) into sound to be delivered into the ear canal. There is usually some form of control (at the disposal of the hearing-impaired listeners or of the dispensing audiologist) over the characteristics of the processor (at its simplest level, this might be a volume control). The three broad classifications of the electronic means by which the hearing aid achieves its processing are analog, digitally programmable and fully digital. At one stage, all hearing aids were analog in nature, whether they were based upon valve technology, transistor technology or integrated circuits, and whatever control was available was achieved by external mechanical elements accessed by either switches, volume wheels or internal screwdriver potentiometers.[12] A subsequent development was the emergence of electronic circuits whose characteristics could be controlled by a computer or other external programming devices.[13] The fundamental processing of the signal was still analog in nature,[14] but increased range and flexibility of control elements were available, not least because of the relaxation of the requirement for physical external controls. Recent years have seen the development of fully digital devices,[15] whose first processing stage is to convert the analog signal from the microphone into a discrete digitized signal which is then processed (by the equivalent of a miniature computer) and reconverted to an analog signal for presentation at the receiver. (Technical developments make this description overly simplistic, but this chapter is not the place for a more detailed consideration of those issues.) One of the prime developments in recent years has been the explosion of claims for the benefit of 'digital' hearing aids over analog counterparts and pressure upon health services to deliver such devices. One further development comprises remote control facilities. Here the user has a small hand-held unit which communicates with the hearing aid via infrared or wireless technology to control some functions of the hearing aid.

Because of the sheer pace of technological developments, any contribution which attempts to survey the details of processing options and their deliverable benefits will, of necessity, be out of date. At the time of writing, numerous studies have been published concerning the benefit provided by digital signal processing.[16–34] Most studies have demonstrated that digital signal processing does not provide better speech recognition in noise than hearing aids with analog signal processing. However, most studies have demonstrated a subjective preference for digital signal processing, and improvements in sound quality, ease of listening etc., using a wide range of measures. Many of these subjective tools include questions related to preferences, benefits and/or satisfaction in recognizing speech-in-noise. It is unknown whether the subjective reported benefits for digital signal processing are simply a result of the ways in which all elements of society automatically recognize 'digital' as superior. In any event, this chapter adopts the standpoint that the particular engineering implantation of a hearing aid feature is largely unimportant. It is almost certainly the case that all new hearing aids will be digital in nature, because that is the direction that hearing aid manufacturers are pursuing in their research and development divisions. It is also undoubtedly true that some features can only be realized by digital signal processing (or perhaps realized much more easily, effectively and cost-effectively) and, despite the marketing pressures, what a clinician needs to try and determine are the ways in which various features of a hearing aid and its fitting might deliver benefits to hearing-impaired listeners.[35–38] Also, at the time of writing, there is an initiative by the NHS to run comprehensive trials of the effectiveness of digital hearing aids within the mass-provision service whose outcome is presently unknown.

In-the-ear fittings are desired by listeners primarily for cosmetic reasons. They do confer acoustical benefits and benefits in spatial hearing. Drawbacks include susceptibility to feedback, problems with manipulation and susceptibility to blockage with wax.

Unilateral versus bilateral fittings

Most listeners have two ears and normal hearing listeners use the signals arriving at their two ears to advantage in a number of domains. Figure 31.6 shows a representation of a sound source which is located on the right side of a listener. The path length between the sound source and the right ear is shorter than that between the source and left ear. Hence, the sound will arrive at the right ear before it arrives at the left. Thus, for any part of the waveform, there is an interaural time difference (ITD) between the two ears.[39] This ITD provides an important cue for the location of the sound source in the horizontal plane. A further effect is that the head casts an acoustical shadow so that the sound arriving at the left ear is attenuated relative to that arriving at the right ear.[40] The resultant interaural intensity difference (IID) is a second important cue for sound localization. The combination of the (predominantly low-frequency) ITD and the (predominantly high-frequency) IID provides the auditory system with sufficient information to determine the

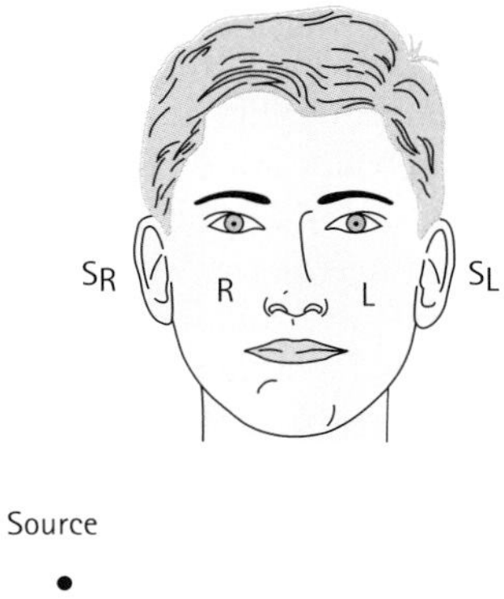

Figure 31.6 Schematic representation of a single off-axis sound source.

location of sound sources in the environment in the horizontal plane.[41–46] There are further complex head and pinna effects which, in combination with head movements, allow the listener to determine location in elevation and to resolve confusions between sound sources located in the frontal plane and those behind the listener. While listeners with sensorineural hearing impairment can and do suffer from deficits in the ability to process these localization cues, if the sounds are made audible at the two ears then at least partial use can be made of both the ITD and IID cues.[47]

Now consider the arrangement in Figure 31.7, where a speech source is located in front of the listener on the mid-line and some interfering noise source is located on the right-hand side (notice that this is a listening circumstance of some ecological relevance, as we usually orientate conversations so that speaker and listener are facing each other). In this circumstance, the speech sound arriving at the two ears is identical (as the speech is on the mid-line), while the interfering noise differs in the ways described in Figure 31.6. Thus, the noise arriving at the left ear is 'shadowed' relative to the noise arriving at the right ear. Hence, the signal-to-noise ratio (the level of the speech relative to the level of the noise) at the left ear will be more advantageous than that arriving at the right ear. Thus, in this circumstance, the listener can 'choose' to listen through their left ear—the ear with the more advantageous signal-to-noise ratio. The listener now finds himself in the environment represented in Figure 31.8 where the interfering noise source occurs on the left side. Now the more favourable signal-to-noise ratio occurs at the right ear. Thus, a listener with two functioning ears gains an advantage over the equivalent 'one-eared' person in always having the option of listening at either the left ear or the right ear, depending upon which has the more advantageous signal-to-noise ratio.

Another advantage can occur in the situation represented in Figure 31.9 where the speech and noise are both located on the mid-line and, hence, the signals arriving at the two ears are identical. This circumstance is referred to as diotic listening, and the normal auditory system uses the identical information arriving at the two ears to advantage by a process referred to as 'binaural redundancy'.

In addition to head-shadow advantages and diotic advantages, the binaural auditory system uses and combines the information arriving at the right ear (less advantageous signal-to-noise ratio) with that arriving at the left ear (more advantageous signal-to-noise ratio) in Figure 31.7 to improve performance yet further by a process referred to as 'binaural squelch'.

For normal hearing listeners, depending on the spectrum and content of the speech material and the location of the speech and noise sources, the advantages from head shadow effects can be around 10 dB of signal-to-noise improvement, the advantages of binaural squelch around some 3 dB in terms of signal-to-noise ratio improvements, and those of diotic advantage approximately 2 dB of signal-to-noise ratio improvement.[48] It will be apparent that the advantages from head shadow

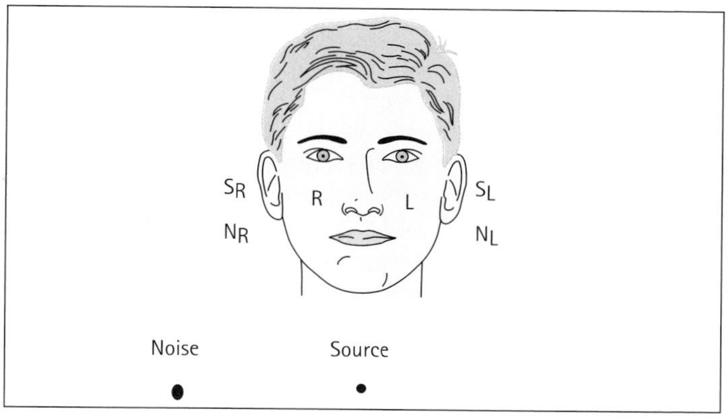

Figure 31.7 Schematic representation of spatially separated speech and interfering noise sources.

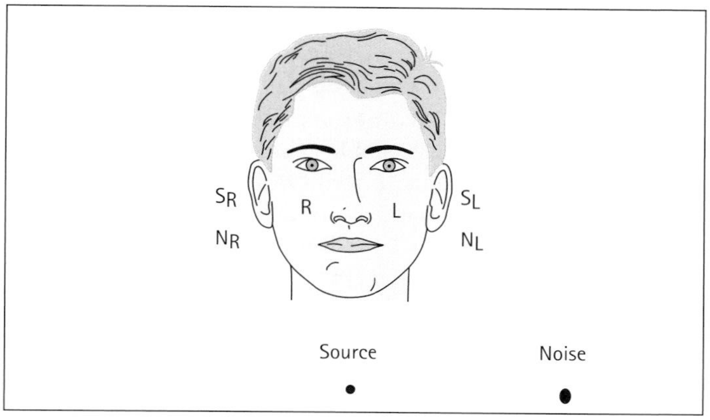

Figure 31.8 Schematic representation of spatially separated speech and noise sources with the noise located to the other ear.

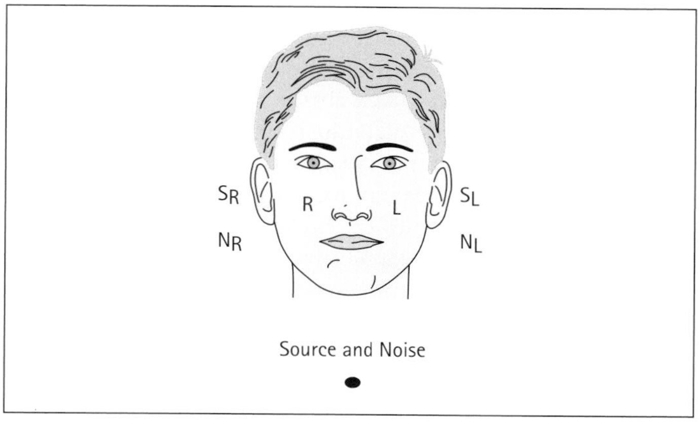

Figure 31.9 A diotic listening situation where the signals arriving at the two ears are identical.

(which result from simple physical acoustics independent of sensorineural hearing impairment) will also be delivered to listeners with sensorineural hearing impairment. Although there is some evidence of diminished advantages in binaural squelch and diotic summation, those advantages still do occur in listeners with sensorineural hearing loss. Thus, there are advantages to the gain in making signals audible to the two ears of such a listener with sensorineural hearing loss.

At this point, some clarification of terminology is required. The term 'binaural listening' is used to represent the situation where a signal is available at both ears. The term 'binaural aiding' or 'binaural hearing aids' is not used. Rather, the term 'bilateral fitting of hearing aids' is advocated. The reason for this is that fitting two hearing aids does not necessarily imply that the desired signals are audible at both ears and, similarly, fitting of a single hearing aid does not imply that the desired signals are only available at the fitted ear. Therefore, binaural listening and bilateral or unilateral fitting of hearing aids can be, to some extent, independent.

There is a substantial body of literature suggesting that listeners with sensorineural impairment can and do gain benefit from bilateral fitting of hearing aids in a number of domains for different listening circumstances.[41–45, 49–54] These benefits are largely independent of asymmetries in hearing, provided that listeners have two ears that are impaired and two ears whose impairment is acoustically aidable. The determining factors are the range of environments in terms of location of desired and unwanted signals and magnitude of desired and unwanted signals in the environments that listeners experience, and the importance of those environments to everyday listening. Thus, it would appear that the great majority of hearing-impaired listeners are realistic candidates for the bilateral fitting of hearing aids. Contrast this with standard practice in the UK NHS, where the great majority of fittings are unilateral. It has to be stated that the main reason that underpins this policy is economic rather than audiological. There are, however, potential disadvantages to bilateral fittings which have to be taken into consideration. It has already been mentioned that there is a degree of stigma associated with hearing impairment and hearing aids, and a common reaction from hearing impaired listeners, when offered bilateral hearing aids, is 'I'm not that deaf, doctor'. Part of the reason for this is associated with current practice, in that it is only individuals with severe and profound hearing impairments who are routinely offered and fitted with bilateral amplification, thus reinforcing the stereotype. Other disadvantages associated with bilateral fitting occur when patients with material manipulative and cognitive deficits find the burden of coping with two prosthetic devices unacceptable. A very small number of patients suffer from a phenomenon referred to as 'binaural interference' in which the sound at the second ear actively disrupts their ability to perceive and process that at the first.[55] However, there is also evidence that long-term listening through a unilateral fitting leads to a process of auditory deprivation in the unaided ear.[56–59]

Overall, the evidence in favour of bilateral fittings is sufficiently substantial to recommend that a sensible default position (independent of economic considerations) should be to offer bilateral fittings to all candidates rather than the current practice of recommending unilateral fittings in all but special cases.

> Most patients are candidates for bilateral fitting of hearing aids. Most patients will benefit from bilateral fittings. Bilateral fittings should be the default norm.

Frequency shaping for linear fittings

The simplest form of hearing aid is one which provides linear amplification—that is, an input signal is amplified by the same amount, independent of its level. Figure 31.10 shows a representation of the input/output function for such an amplifier at any particular given frequency. As the input level is increased by any given amount, the output level also increases by the same degree. Such a representation shows what happens at any particular frequency. It is well recognized that most listeners with sensorineural hearing loss have thresholds which are poorer at high frequencies by amounts greater than at low frequencies. Clearly, then, the audibility of high-frequency sounds will be compromised to a greater extent than the audibility of low-frequency sounds. A very natural response to this is to attempt to amplify high-frequency sounds by greater amounts than low-frequency sounds, leading to a gain characteristic which is a function of frequency. Such a characteristic is shown in Figure 31.11, and is fairly typical of a current postaural fitting employed by the UK NHS. When confronted with a hearing-impaired listener who is to be fitted with a hearing aid, the clinician needs to decide what is the most appropriate frequency gain characteristic to use. Unfortunately, at this point, the clinician encounters a wide variation in the audiological literature. Many prescription regimens exist which attempt to predict, from the hearing thresholds as a function of frequency, the gain that is likely to be required at each frequency to optimally compensate for the hearing loss.[37, 60–73] These prescription regimens have different conceptual origins and, indeed, can lead to different frequency gain characteristics. Perhaps the most commonly used prescription regimen originates from the National Acoustic Laboratories (NAL) in Australia. The NAL regimen

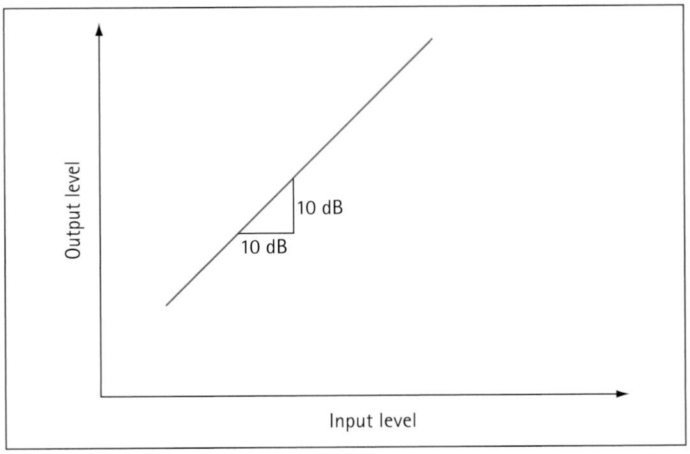

Figure 31.10 The input–output function for a simple linear hearing aid.

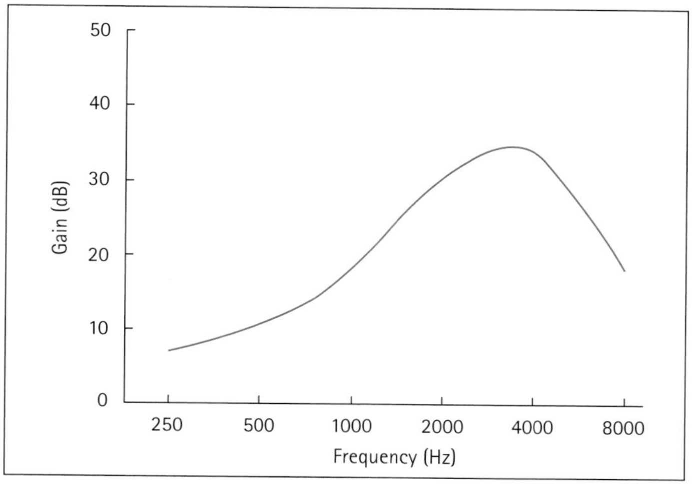

Figure 31.11 An example of a frequency–gain characteristic.

also happens to be the procedure which has received the greatest experimental verification and one which has as its theoretical basis a well-thought-out set of assumptions and implementations. Although this chapter is not the place for an in-depth discussion of the origins, merits and demerits of the various alternatives, it is perhaps worth stating that the NAL prescription regimen aims to make different frequency bands of speech equally loud to hearing-impaired listeners, so that no one frequency region of the speech spectrum dominates the perception of the loudness of the speech signal. With the flexibility of modern technology, there is every opportunity to realize a particular target gain for the frequencies which are important for speech understanding. A reasonable issue that clinicians might raise is the question of whether matching a target actually matters, in terms of the benefits delivered to hearing-impaired listeners. Certainly, the verification work which underpins the various prescription regimens would suggest that this is an issue of potential importance. Indeed, within the context of the very limited technological options hitherto available to the UK NHS, there is also a body of evidence suggesting that user preferences for and benefits from hearing aid prescriptions which more closely match a clinically achievable and soundly based prescription regimen do indeed result in increased benefits.[74, 75]

> Clinicians should select the frequency gain characteristic of a hearing aid on the basis of a rationale with a verifiable evidence base.

Output limiting

Any hearing aid has a limit to the amount of output that can be produced, and, indeed, there are levels for both normal hearing listeners and listeners with sensorineural hearing impairment above which sound becomes uncomfortably loud. For a linear hearing aid, the output will increase by 10 dB for each 10-dB increase in the input until the hearing aid limit is reached and the hearing aid is driven into saturation. When considering the maximum output that a hearing aid can deliver, the gain characteristic shown in Figure 31.11 is not the most appropriate representation and the output characteristic shown in Figure 31.12 is preferable. This displays the output of the hearing aid in dB SPL as a function of frequency. When the maximum output of the hearing aid is reached, then an increase in the input level will not result in an increase in the output level. The corresponding input/output function is shown in Figure 31.13. Here, above a certain level, the hearing aid saturates. For a simple linear hearing aid, as the device is driven into saturation, there are some undesired effects of this saturation on the input signal.[76–78] These are illustrated in Figure 31.14, which shows the increase in the input signal as the input increases, and the 'clipping' of the output signal as the input increases beyond the saturation point. This is perceived by the listener as distortion of the signal, and can lead to further problems in the intelligibility of

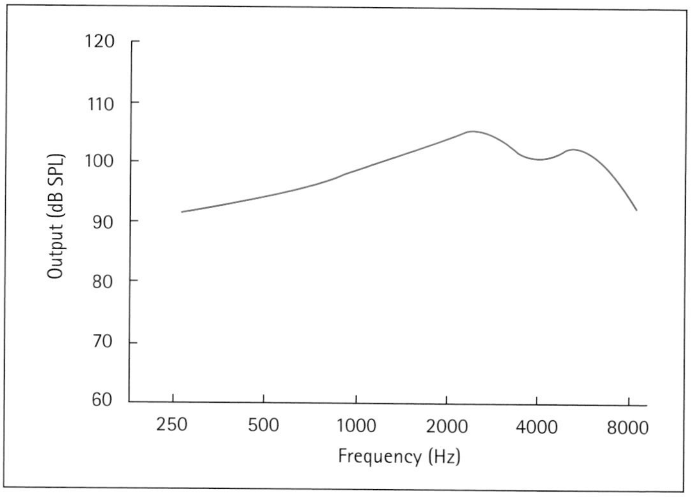

Figure 31.12 An example of a hearing aid output characteristic.

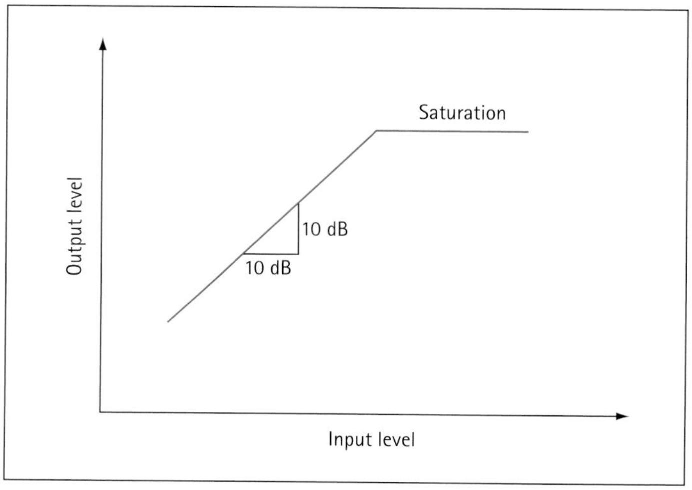

Figure 31.13 A hearing aid input–output function demonstrating saturation.

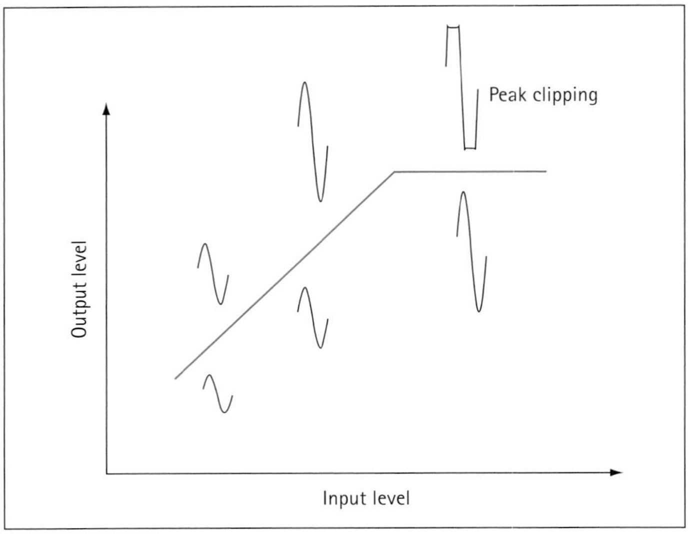

Figure 31.14 The input–output function of a peak clipping hearing aid.

speech. Given that the aim of any amplification device is to present the signal with minimal loss of fidelity, such a process is clearly undesirable. Many linear hearing aids still achieve limitation on their output via this process of peak-clipping, though for many years alternatives have been available. The primary alternative has been output compression limiting, shown in Figure 31.15. Here, above a certain threshold (the compression threshold), increases in input level result in much smaller increases in output level, with minimal distortion of the signal. Experimental studies have shown that the great majority of hearing-impaired listeners both prefer and perform better with output compression-limiting devices than those which are limited via peak-clipping. The exception would appear to be some listeners with severe and profound hearing losses who express preferences for peak-clipping devices. It is unclear whether this preference is simply a result of an engineering limitation of output compression devices, whereby the maximum gain and output that can be delivered is reduced over the equivalent peak-clipping circuitry, or whether it is a genuine perceptual link to and preference for the peak-clipped signal (which might appear unlikely). Despite this extensive body of evidence, at the time of writing, output limiting by peak-clipping in NHS hearing aids is still the norm rather than the exception.

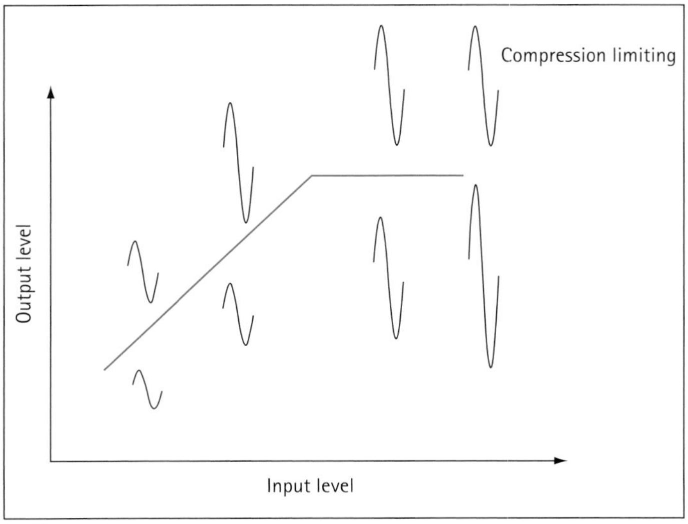

Figure 31.15 The input–output function of a compression limiting hearing aid.

Most hearing aids, whether of the output compression or the peak-clipping type, contain the ability to adjust the level at which the hearing aid is driven into saturation. This is usually adjusted so that the loudest sounds that the hearing aid can produce do not exceed the threshold of uncomfortable loudness for a hearing-impaired listener. As companions to prescription regimens for the frequency gain characteristic, there are predictions from auditory threshold of average settings for thresholds of uncomfortable listening and, hence, maximum power output from hearing aids.[69, 79–82] It might appear more direct to measure the threshold of uncomfortable listening and adjust the hearing aid accordingly, although there are a number of complicated intervening factors, such as the calibration differences between audiometric measures on sinusoids and hearing aid characteristics in couplers and the extent to which broadband sounds exhibit differing loudness relationships to narrow-band sinewaves. If the maximum power output (MPO) is set too low, then signals in the environment will regularly drive the device into saturation, and the listener is likely to complain that louder sounds are often distorted. An MPO set too high is likely to result in complaints that a hearing aid is 'too loud' even if the frequency gain characteristic is appropriate for the listener's hearing thresholds.

> Inappropriate output limiting can compromise hearing aid acceptance and benefit. Clinicians should, as a routine, adjust the maximum power output of a device in the light of patient characteristics.

Earmoulds

It has already been mentioned that for postaural hearing aids the sound is conducted from the hearing aid to the ear canal via tubing[83] and earmoulds. These earmoulds have acoustical effects, and are themselves the subject of an extensive literature. Of more practical importance is the extent to which an earmould in a listener's ear leads to the occlusion effect.[84, 85] The occlusion effect can manifest itself as a feeling of blockage, but it also has an important acoustical element in the way that sounds are presented and perceived. Perhaps the easiest way to demonstrate this is for a normal hearing listener to place a finger into their own ear canal, and then to speak and observe the effect on the listener's own voice. Although effects on signals are not limited to one's own voice, they are perhaps most obvious for that signal. A normal hearing listener will clearly perceive the differences in timbre and loudness that occlusion of the ear canal produces. Many earmoulds are designed to not completely occlude the ear canal, but to allow a degree of venting to address both the overall 'blockage' perception and to counteract, at least in part, some of the acoustical problems of occlusion and to allow entry of low-frequency sounds from outside unprocessed by the hearing aid. The particular styles and characteristics of earmoulds are varied, and perhaps the easiest summary is to recommend that an earmould with the largest degree of venting and the least degree of occlusion that is compatible with the patient's hearing loss and amplification characteristics without encountering feedback problems is the desired choice. There is some evidence that the deep canal fittings which accompany completely in-the-canal hearing aids lead to decreased problems with the acoustical aspects of occlusion.

One of the advantages of ITE hearing aids is that the unwanted acoustical effects of tubing and earmoulds (independent and not associated with occlusion) can be relatively easily overcome, leading to better high-frequency responses and output than from postaural devices. Although they find little favour and application in world markets, it is possible to use ITE devices of a modular type (Figure 31.16) which contain a basic unit to which is attached a custom shell. Modular devices have the advantage of not requiring total custom shells, so that in the event of a malfunction in a hearing aid, the standard unit can be replaced immediately, and the listener does not have to forego amplification while a repair is undertaken.

> Earmould selection should be based on a compromise between minimization of the occlusion effect and prevention of feedback.

Compression and multichannel processing

Above we considered linear processing, which amplifies a signal by an amount which is independent of its input level. Hearing-impaired listeners exhibit elevated hearing thresholds, but also have thresholds of uncomfortable listening which are similar to or only mildly elevated above those exhibited by listeners with normal hearing. Thus, listeners with sensorineural hearing impairment exhibit a reduced dynamic range between the threshold of hearing and the threshold of uncomfortable listening. Furthermore, as most sensorineural hearing losses slope from low frequencies to high frequencies, such listeners also exhibit reduced dynamic range at high frequencies compared to that at low frequencies. Thus, a hearing aid is faced with the task of mapping signals in the auditory environment into an available range of hearing which is less than that enjoyed by normal hearing listeners, and is more compromised at high frequencies than it is at low frequencies. One clear approach to this is to configure the amplification so that it amplifies low-level sounds by a greater amount than higher-level sounds. The input/output function of such a scheme is shown in Figure 31.17. Here, once the input level reaches a certain point (the compression knee-point) the increase in the output level is less than the increase in the input level. For a compression ratio of 2 : 1, for each 10-dB increase in the input level, the output level increases by 5 dB. Numerous experiments on amplitude compression systems have been conducted over the years, and it is now normally accepted that compression ratios of greater than around 3 : 1 are undesirable because of deleterious effects on speech intelligibility.

Given that, for a hearing-impaired listener, the reduction in dynamic range at high frequencies is greater than at low frequencies, there is the natural consequence that the desirable compression characteristics for high-frequency signals will differ from those for low-frequency signals. This introduces the concept of multi-band processing, where the hearing aid has different characteristics as a function of frequency, not only in terms of the gain that is delivered but in the ways in which gain varies as a function of input level. A reasonable question is then 'How many channels do we need?' If one looks at the commercial hearing aid market, then multi-channel devices are available with anything from 2 to 20 channels, although there is some potential confusion between the concepts of a 'frequency band' and a 'compression channel'. Modern devices have a number of frequency bands which allow the matching of a particular target with a degree of precision, and this can be different

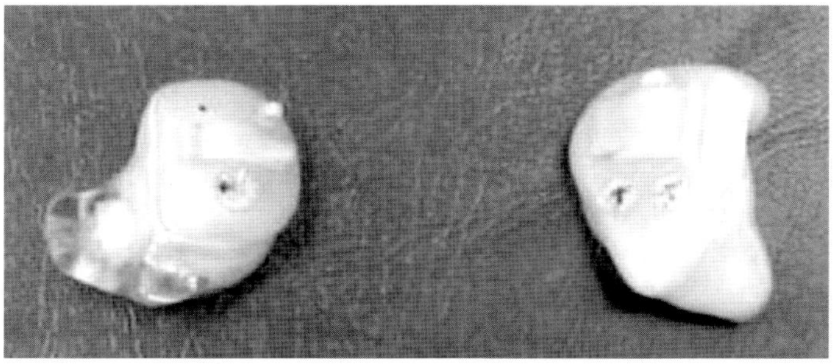

Figure 31.16 Example of modular and custom in-the-ear (ITE) hearing aids.

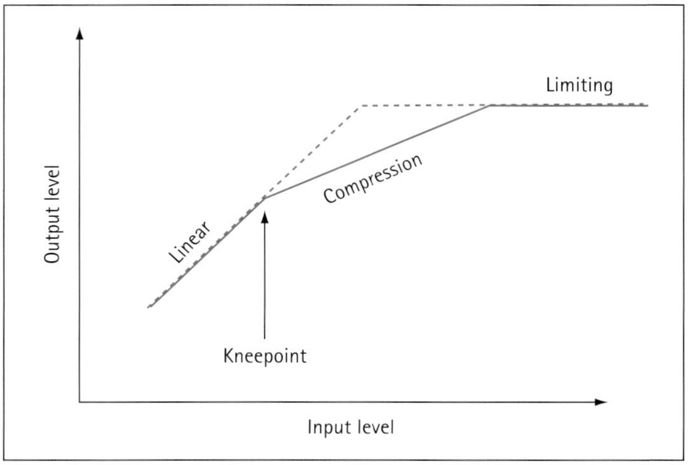

Figure 31.17 Schematic representation of the input–output function for one frequency in a simple compression hearing aid.

from the number of independent compression channels within which it is possible to implement different dynamic relationships in terms of the input/output function. Although there is an absence of evidence from robust clinical trials, there is a reasonable supposition that somewhere between four and eight independent frequency bands might be required to properly compensate for a particular audiometric configuration, whereas somewhere between two and four independent dynamic compression channels might be useful.

One aspect of compression that has not yet been considered is that of time constants. When considering output compression limiting, it is reasonable to assume that the compression system should act as rapidly as possible in order to protect the listener from loud transient sounds in the environment, such as a door slamming. The issue is not necessarily as clear-cut when considering compression to compensate for restrictions in dynamic range (and the distortions in frequency and temporal processing which are almost an inevitable accompaniment to sensorineural hearing loss). Here there are broadly two approaches, referred to as 'slow-acting automatic volume control' (AVC), and fast-acting wide dynamic range compression (WDRC). Slow-acting AVC attempts to compensate for the changes that occur in the acoustical environment as the background that the listener experiences or the desired signals within that environment themselves change. Examples of this might be the differing requirements placed on hearing aids when one exits from a quiet house into a busy street, or the differing requirements when conversing with one's 'quietly-spoken Scottish or Welsh grandmother', compared with the stentorian tones of a 'gruff English uncle'. Here the hearing aid processing attempts to alter its characteristics as the acoustical environment in which it functions alters. The environment changes relatively slowly, and time constants of hundreds of milliseconds, or even seconds, are appropriate.

In contrast, WDRC attempts to compensate more directly for some of the characteristics of a sensorineural hearing loss. The objectives of WDRC processing can be illustrated by consideration of the utterance 'asa'. This consists of a relatively intense, relatively low-frequency vowel 'a' followed by a relatively less intense, relatively high-frequency, consonant 's', followed by another incidence of the vowel 'a'. A device employing fast-acting WDRC will provide greater amplification and greater high-frequency amplification during the consonant 's' than in the preceding and successful vowels 'a' in an attempt to make available on a moment-to-moment basis as much of the acoustical information contained within the speech waveform as is feasible. Clearly, processing which reconfigures its characteristics across syllables and phonemes has to act more rapidly than processing which attempts to compensate for environmental changes, and here time constants of milliseconds and tens of milliseconds are appropriate.

Although there are almost as many implementations of compression systems as there are manufacturers, and, indeed, many modern devices contain elements of both AVC and fast-acting WDRC, either within or between frequency bands, the differing overall objectives of the two approaches remain in force.

There is an extensive and contradictory literature on the implementation, benefits and limitations of a variety of compression systems, both in the laboratory and in wearable hearing aids.[83, 86–104] Perhaps a reasonable summary would suggest that there are unlikely to be benefits of any compression system when compared to linear amplification which has been adjusted and optimized for any particular listening environment, be that in quiet or in noise. However, compression systems do allow listeners to function in a wider range of acoustical environments and to process a wider range of input signal characteristics than is the case for more constrained linear amplification, and that the benefits can reside in aspects of improved sound quality and ease of listening as well as measures of speech identification performance.

There is some preliminary evidence[105] that the diversity and importance of the acoustical environments that listeners experience and are required to function in can be an important factor in determining candidature for linear as opposed to nonlinear processing.

> Current compression rationales do not improve speech identification in noise relative to optimized linear processing. They do permit improved functioning in a wider range of auditory environments than linear fittings.

Multi-memory fittings

The previous section on amplitude compression systems considered the ways in which hearing aid processing can be configured to obtain optimal function in a variety of acoustical environments. This makes the assumption that there is a simple mapping between aspects of the environment (e.g. overall signal level) and the processing that is required and, furthermore, it makes the assumption that the desirable properties of processing for a particular environment will not change over time. There is reasonable evidence that the characteristics of a hearing aid that are optimum for speech intelligibility are not necessarily those that are optimum for sound quality or listening comfort, and may differ yet again from those that are optimum for spatial hearing and localization. It may be that within any given environment at different times, the hearing-impaired listener has differing goals and requirements and, therefore, a hearing aid that is configured with one particular predominant goal in mind may not be suitable for different environments in different circumstances. An alternative to the automatic approach is to configure a number of different control programmes in the hearing aid, and then allow the listener to select the different programmes, depending upon the environments that they find themselves in, and their particular wishes and priorities when in those environments. Such an approach gives the user more control over the desirable properties of the processing for any given listening experience. This philosophy can be extended to give the hearing aid user some input to or control over the basic types of processing built into devices.[106] The physical and electrical characteristics of hearing aids were discussed above, and one of the available options is to control the characteristics of the hearing aid remotely, rather than having to constantly adjust switches on the device, with the consequent problems that occur with feedback and small control elements. A convenient remote control device which communicates with the hearing aid, using infra red or wireless technology, can be used to select one of a number of programmes (usually between two and four), with different inherent characteristics according to the environment and wishes of the listener. Such an approach places the listener in a position of greater control over the signals that they are receiving. Although detailed field trials of such devices are in their relative infancy, information is becoming available regarding the configuration of and candidature for such multi-memory devices.[107, 108]

Multi-memory devices are beneficial to listeners who require to function in a wide range of auditory environments with a diverse set of listening demands.

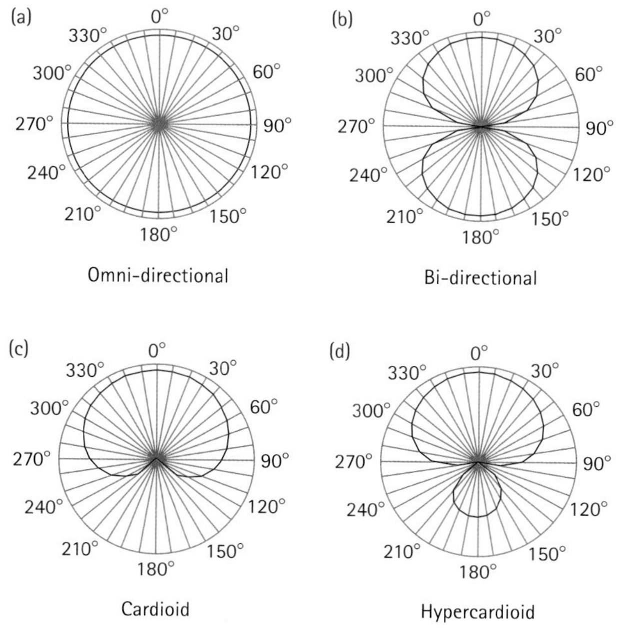

Figure 31.18 Directivity patterns for some hearing aid microphone systems.

Directional microphones

Most microphones have (in the free field) a characteristic which is referred to as omni-directional. This is illustrated in Figure 31.18a. Here, the sensitivity of the microphone (indexed by the distance from the centre of the circle) is independent of the origin of the sound source. Microphones can be configured to have particular directional characteristics, and directional microphones have been available for many years. They had been relatively unsuccessful in hearing aid applications until the advent of switchable directional microphones. Conventional directional microphones achieve their directionality by having dual inlet ports in the microphone so that sound from some particular location is 'cancelled out' while sound from other locations is not. The technological development was to replace the single dual-port directional microphone with a pair of omnidirectional microphones. The signals from those two microphones can then be processed in a variety of ways (usually by subtraction with varying time delays) to achieve directivity patterns with a variety of different characteristics. Some of these are shown in Figure 31.18 b, c, d. The bi-directional microphone is equally sensitive towards the front and the rear, but is insensitive to sounds arising from the left-hand and right-hand sides. The cardioid microphone has no sensitivity from the back but still has reasonable sensitivity to the sides, while the hyper-cardioid characteristic attempts to minimize the influence from the left- and right-hand sides, while retaining some suppression from the rear. This can be seen from the characteristics in Figure 31.18 (which, it must be stressed, are schematic illustrations—the actual directivity patterns of real microphones in real hearing aids worn on real heads and in real ears are somewhat more complex). The polar patterns can locate the nulls and maxima in the directivity response in a variety of locations.

One of the reasons why directional microphones only began to find substantial applications in hearing aids when they became switchable is that there are listening circumstances whereby a directivity pattern which, for example, suppressed sound from the sides might be definitely disadvantageous. If I am travelling in a car, either as the passenger or the driver, and wish to converse with my companion, the last thing (particularly if I am the driver) that I wish to do is to have to turn towards my companion to be able to hear what they are saying. Similar factors can come into play, for example, around a dinner table, or in music environments. The opportunity to be able to switch between omnidirectional and directional characteristics allows the listener to access different components of the environments which match their listening needs. Depending upon the configuration of the sound sources in the environment, the benefits of directional microphones are established and unequivocal and, indeed, are an example of one of the few types of processing which does physically improve the signal-to-noise ratios of signals delivered to hearing-impaired listeners.[36, 109–124] Indeed, one might argue that listeners with marginal hearing losses (marginal in the sense of gaining benefit from amplification, that is) can gain benefits from the improvements in signal-to-noise ratio that accompany low-gain hearing aid fittings with directionality available. When coupled with the availability of multi-programme devices as described in the previous section, it is possible to combine the advantages of selectable directional microphones with other aspects of a hearing aid processing strategy so that optimized parameters, e.g. directed at listening in noisy environments, can be derived and selected using remote control facilities.

Directional microphones are the single hearing aid feature with an evidence base to improve speech identification ability in noise.

Feedback management

Feedback is one of the commonest causes of complaint from hearing aid users, and a significant bar to achieving hearing aid use and benefit. The concept of feedback is illustrated in Figure 31.19. When a hearing aid amplifies the sound input to produce a sound output, a certain amount of the energy produced has the opportunity to return to the microphone via a feedback leakage path. One of the reasons for earmoulds, and the importance of properly fitting ITE devices, is to reduce this feedback path to manageable proportions, but with vented earmoulds and increasingly small ITE devices where the microphone input and receiver input are brought closer and closer together, the opportunities for feedback become ever greater. When the amplification provided by the hearing aid processor exceeds the attenuation that is present in the feedback path, then oscillatory feedback takes place and the hearing aid is driven into saturation. The whistling hearing aid is a phenomenon with which all clinicians will be all too familiar. The first approach to feedback management is to reduce the feedback leakage path, either by improvements in the earmould or ITE fitting, or by the reduction of venting availabilities. However, such measures are not always successful, particularly when hearing aids

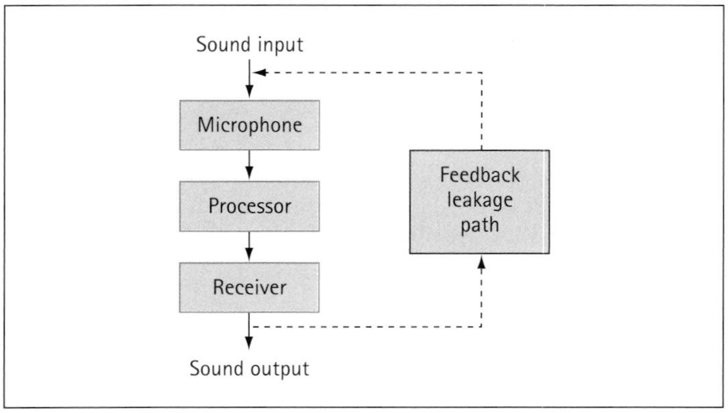

Figure 31.19 Schematic representation of the feedback process in a hearing aid system.

with high gain are required. The problem can also be exacerbated in amplitude compression systems where high gains are applied to low-level signals. There are two further approaches to feedback management. The first of these is to try and identify when feedback might be occurring or about to occur, and to reduce the gain of the device for those signals which are likely to lead to feedback. With the advent of digital signal processing, and the ability to adjust the frequency gain characteristics of hearing aid processing in narrow-frequency bands, it is possible to not eliminate, but reduce, the occurrence of feedback without altering the overall gain characteristic to a material extent and, hence, without compromising access to many components of the input signal. The extent to which hearing aids can dynamically configure their frequency gain characteristics, depending upon the occurrence or likely occurrence of feedback, is a factor of hearing aid processing that is developing rapidly with the advent of digital signal-processing techniques. At present, feedback management techniques are becoming an integral component of many digital hearing aids, though with varying degrees of sophistication and effectiveness. A further approach to feedback management is to detect the feedback path that is occurring, and then to introduce an artificial signal into the hearing aid processing which attempts to cancel the feedback and, hence, allow use of greater gain without driving the system into oscillatory feedback. Such devices are in their relative infancy, but are becoming available to increase the headroom that is available to hearing-impaired listeners. A discussion of the various approaches to feedback management can be found in the literature.[125–130]

Modern digital signal-processing options are a material addition to the traditional procedures in management of feedback.

Noise reduction systems

The primary complaint of all listeners with sensorineural hearing loss, and the prime limitation of all hearing aids, is the ability to understand speech in noisy or other adverse environments. The 'Holy Grail' of hearing aid processing is to amplify those signals to which the listener wants access while suppressing those which are undesired. Such a goal is distant, but currently available digital signal-processing techniques are beginning to make advances.

The first element is the extent to which the hearing-impaired listener might be aware of the internal noise of the hearing aid itself, particularly in quiet environments where amplitude compression systems will configure high gain. In such a situation, the hearing aid processing can detect the aspects of the environment (e.g. the input level), can detect whether or not there is a 'interesting' signal present, and, if a decision is made that such a signal is not present, can suppress the hearing aid output and, hence, the internal noise of the hearing aid amplifier.

A more ambitious approach is to try and identify the nature of the input signal. This is usually done on a frequency-by-frequency band basis. Within any particular frequency band, a variety of statistics from the input signal are derived (often aspects of the modulation spectrum and the coherence of inter-band envelopes) to determine whether the input signal is likely to be classified as speech, or as a non-speech input. Those frequency regions where the input is classified as predominantly speech can then be selectively amplified with respect to those frequency regions where the input is classified as a non-speech signal. Such techniques are a natural development of previous regimens to introduce reductions in low-frequency amplification when an extraneous noise signal has been detected,[131] but do so on a much more sophisticated basis. Clearly, it would be unreasonable to suppress all signals which were classified as non-speech, as the listener would then have no access to environmental sounds in occurrences where a speech signal was not present. Such an implementation would be clearly dangerous. Of all the topics within this chapter, this element concerning noise reduction is likely to be the one that becomes most rapidly dated, given the increasing access to sophisticated processing techniques in digital signal processing.

Bone conduction fittings

Bone conduction hearing aids have been part of the armoury of amplification for many years. They usually find application where acoustical coupling of the hearing aid to the middle ear is not possible, because of a disease process, traumatic injury or congenital malformations. In these cases, coupling has been achieved by placing a mechanical vibrator on the bony mastoid process and stimulating the cochlea via bone conduction. Such devices have poor sound quality, are uncomfortable, and have limited gain characteristics. In recent years, bone conduction coupling, using either transcutaneous electro-magnetic coupling,[132] or percutaneous direct coupling,[133–139] has been developed. Such devices still find application in the relatively small number of listeners for whom acoustical coupling is not appropriate. There are instances of application of such devices to middle ear problems such as otosclerosis as options for acoustical amplification.[140] It must be pointed out, however, that at present, the controlled trials comparing such devices with appropriate acoustical amplification (and many of the trials have not used appropriate acoustical amplification) have yet to be conducted.

Implantable hearing aids

As a potential alternative to acoustical coupling to the middle ear, it is possible to implant electromagnetic or piezoelectric transducers directly on the ossicular chain.[141–143] Such devices can be the internal component driven by an external device or can form part of a totally implantable unit. It is suggested that such devices might be suitable for listeners for whom wearing of an earmould is impossible (e.g. congenital abnormalities) or where the listener refuses to countenance an earmould (because of, for example, extensive problems with occlusion). In addition, the relatively low forces that are required to stimulate the ossicular chain might make such devices appropriate for individuals with severe or profound hearing impairment who are not suitable for cochlear implants and for whom acoustical devices deliver insufficient gain and, hence, benefit, although this latter possibility is not yet realized because of output limitations of the experimental units. It is doubtful whether such devices will find widespread application in the routine management of sensorineural hearing impairment, because of the requirements for surgery and the high cost of devices and the associated health-economic issues.

Personal communicators

There are some situations where the wearing of a hearing aid can be unacceptable and inappropriate. In such circumstances, a portable personal communicator which allows the speaker to present amplified sound to a hearing-impaired listener can be a useful aid to communication (Figure 31.20). Such devices tend to find application in long-stay healthcare facilities for elderly patients with multiple deficits.

Verification

In the light of the needs of the hearing-impaired listener and the availability of the various technological options and other features of a hearing aid fitting discussed above, the clinician will select and fit a hearing aid or hearing aids. Depending upon the decisions that have been taken, this will be achieved via a variety of means. A simple linear fitting might, for example, be implemented via a prescribed target gain, while the fitting of a more complex multi-channel amplitude compression device might be implemented via one of the published regimens to achieve equal loudness or normalized loudness. Perhaps more likely will be the increasing use of manufacturer-specific fitting tools associated with particular products. No matter what the details of the implementation, the regimen is always based upon the ways in which a relatively large number of hearing-impaired listeners perform with any given device and its fitting. Inevitably, an individual hearing-impaired listener can and will differ from the prescribed average, both in terms of the acoustical characteristics of their auditory system and the ways in

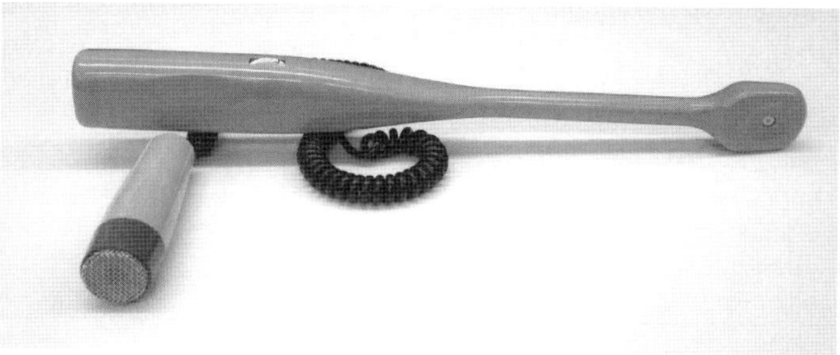

Figure 31.20 Example of a portable communicator.

which their impaired hearing mechanism processes the sound signals. It is, therefore, imperative that clinicians do not rely on the assumption that the individual hearing-impaired listener under their care will conform to the 'average client' but that an individual process by which the hearing aid fitting is verified and fine-tuned is undertaken as a matter of routine.[144]

Acoustical verification

The ways in which hearing aids perform in standard couplers is different from the ways in which they perform in real ears.[145–147] It is possible to assess the performance of a hearing aid in a coupler which represents the average of a set of human ears,[148, 149] but the acoustical characteristics of ears to be fitted can and do vary. This is true for simple linear amplification, but becomes more of an issue when more complex signal processing is employed in the hearing aid fitting.

Although at present only a small component of clinical practice in the UK NHS, it is argued here that real-ear measurement of the acoustical characteristics of a hearing aid fitting should become part and parcel of routine clinical practice.

This chapter is not the place to discuss the technical details of real-ear measurement systems and procedures,[149–154] and a brief description only is given. All systems consist of a flexible probe tube which can be placed in close proximity to the listener's tympanic membrane and, hence, can measure the sound pressure level delivered into the ear canal. The measurement is performed without a hearing aid to assess the acoustical characteristics of the listener's ear prior to fitting. The measurement is then repeated with the hearing aid in place and adjusted according to the particular prescription regimen. The difference between the two measures is the effect of fitting the hearing aid which can then be compared with the particular prescription target. There is a relatively diverse set of terminologies used in real-ear measures. For the purposes of this chapter, we use only three concepts, whose definitions are given in Table 31.1. The real-ear unaided response (REUR) represents the acoustical characteristics of the unaided ear, the real-ear aided response (REAR) represents the acoustical performance of the hearing aid in the listener's ear, while the difference between the two, the real-ear insertion response (REIR), represents the ways in which the hearing aid processes the sound.

For a simple linear fitting, a plot of the real-ear insertion as a function of frequency (see Figure 31.11 for an illustrative example) can be compared to the target prescription, and a similar process can be repeated for the maximum power output of the hearing aid (in that case, the hearing aid gain is set to maximum and a loud input signal is used). Such a fitting is relatively simple and constrained, and the particular characteristics of the signal that are used to assess the REIR are largely immaterial, as, for the linear system, the gain is independent of input level and the spectral characteristics of the signal.

For more complex hearing aid fitting, this no longer holds. Instead of producing a single target as in Figure 31.11, which needs to be verified, there will be a whole family of targets for signals with different input levels, e.g. when fitting a WDRC device. Furthermore, the device will perform differently depending upon the spectral characteristics of the input signal. Current practice, therefore, uses a broadband input signal with spectral characteristics similar to those of conversational speech.[155] This, however, is not necessarily the end of the story. For an amplitude compression device, the performance of the hearing aid fitting depends not only on the signal that is currently being presented, but also on signals that have previously been presented, and this becomes a particular problem in hearing aids with long time constants whose characteristics vary only slowly. At the time of writing, the hearing aid industry and the audiological community have not converged upon a set of agreed standards for the specification of more complex hearing aids. One of the challenges that faces both researchers and clinicians is the development of verification procedures which can more realistically characterize the ways in which hearing aids perform for realistic signals when worn by hearing-impaired listeners.

As a matter of routine, hearing aid fittings should be acoustically verified by a measure of real-ear performance.

Table 31.1 Terminology used in real-ear measures for acoustical verification.

Real-ear unaided response (REUR)	Real-ear aided response (REAR)	Real-ear insertion response (REIR)
A plot of the sound-pressure level arriving in the ear canal as a function of frequency for a given input signal presented at a given level from a given orientation measured in the listener's open ear.	A plot of the sound-pressure level arriving in the ear canal as a function of frequency for a given input signal presented at a given level from a given orientation in the listener's open ear measured with the hearing aid adjusted and in situ.	The REUR subtracted from the REAR to provide a representation of the effect of the hearing aid on a given input signal.

Table 31.2 Examples of environments which might be employed in a fine-tuning process.

Soft speech presented in-quiet
Soft speech presented in-noise
Conversational speech presented in-quiet
Conversational speech presented in-noise
Loud speech presented in-quiet
Loud speech presented in-noise
Listener's own voice
Traffic noise

Fine-tuning

As has been mentioned previously, a particular fitting rationale locates a set of hearing aid characteristics that are thought to be appropriate for the average of hearing-impaired listeners, with, for example, audiometric thresholds, thresholds of uncomfortable listening, and loudness growth relationships, depending on the input to the rationale. Any given hearing-impaired listener is likely to differ from the overall average in ways that are not necessarily connected with the detailed acoustics of their ear (as appropriate to the verification process) but associated with their perceptions of different sound of different spectrum and intensity. It is, therefore, necessary to conduct a process of fine-tuning so that the listener's perception of a range of different sounds is appropriate for the hearing aid fitting. Table 31.2 contains a possible list of the sorts of sound situations which might be presented to a listener and their responses elicited. These attempt to encompass the range of listening environments likely to occur in everyday life and that are, therefore, appropriate to the hearing aid fitting. They include listening to speech in quiet and noise in a variety of presentation levels in addition to loud extraneous sound represented by traffic noise and the important perception of the listener's own voice. It is clear that some of these can be conducted informally between the fitter and hearing-impaired listener, though increasingly practitioners will access calibrated systems of pre-recorded material so that listeners can be assessed and questioned in more controlled environments. The sorts of responses that will be informative to the fitter will include 'too quiet', 'too loud', 'too boomy', and 'too tinny', and depending upon the controls available, adjustment of the hearing aid devices and their fitting packages provide fine-tuning guides which couple to the hardware and software controls on the hearing aid in an interactive manner. Indeed, researchers are developing fitting rationales of an adaptive nature whereby the listener's perceptions of different sound signals feed back in an interactive manner to the characteristics of the hearing aid fitting itself.

> Systematic fine-tuning of a hearing aid fitting, considered over a range of auditory environments, should become part of practice as technological flexibility increases.

Evaluation

Even when a clinician has fully assessed the needs and characteristics of a hearing-impaired listener, and properly verified and fine-tuned the fitting to achieve a good technological match and acceptance by the user, the process is by no means ended. There is abundant evidence that ongoing care is required to maximize the benefit that listeners derive from hearing aid fittings and that continued information and support is required to minimize residual disabilities and handicaps.[156–163] Therefore, all hearing aid programmes should contain elements whereby listeners are followed up to assess the success or otherwise of a hearing aid fitting and the extent to which further intervention might be required.

If it is accepted that the objective of intervention is to minimize the disabilities and handicaps experienced by hearing-impaired listeners, then it naturally follows that the success or otherwise of a hearing aid fitting should be assessed by measures of those very entities. Almost independent of the mode of healthcare delivery (but increasingly important in systems such as the UK NHS) is an evaluation culture whereby services are required to document the quality standards that they employ and to strive for continuously improved performance. The funding agencies for services wish to know the extent to which the facilities they provide are clinically effective and cost-effective, and as the range of technological options and rehabilitative contexts available to practitioners increases, then targeting those options to hearing-impaired listeners will require routine information regarding the performance of a service and its various components.

This background implies that a routine component of hearing aid fitting should be an evaluation of the extent to which the fitting has alleviated the disabilities and handicaps experienced by hearing-impaired listeners as a means of making sensible decisions about the future management of individual hearing-impaired listeners, and also providing information concerning the performance of the healthcare system. The requirements placed upon an outcome measure become quite severe when the intention to provide system information regarding the extent to which a practice, clinic or service is meeting its objectives is coupled with the need to provide clinically useful information regarding management of hearing-impaired listeners. Any practical outcome measure must have high face validity for both the hearing-impaired listener and the audiologist (that is, it must be clear to both parties that the information that is being gathered is relative and appropriate). If the outcome measure is used in the optimization and development of services, it must be sensitive to changes in both the technological content (the hearing aids themselves and their fittings) and the rehabilitative context. A useful outcome measure should have the discriminatory power to reliably identify appropriate changes in the effectiveness and cost-effectiveness. Furthermore, outcome measures which have a clinical utility in the management process (that is, they actually help clinicians with the task of patient management) are more likely to find widespread acceptance than instances which serve only as some form of quality control. Thus, an outcome measure aims to fulfil both the system evaluation requirement and the requirement to guide management of individual patients. A myriad of hearing disability and handicap scales have been used to assess the effectiveness of hearing aid fittings in the past, and there is a substantive body of literature documenting the psychometric evaluation and the properties of such scales.[119, 164–173] Although naturally partisan because of this author's own activity, a little space is devoted here to one particular outcome measure (The Glasgow Hearing Aid Benefit Profile—GHABP), which is finding increasing relevance in the UK NHS context.[174–176] This is given as an example of the sort of measure and application that is envisaged.

In considering the desirable properties of an outcome measure, it is suggested that in addition to the required psychometric abilities, an outcome measure should recognize and appropriately access the different dimensions of disability and benefit. It should retain the ability to address the relevant concerns of individual hearing-impaired listeners while providing outputs which are analytically tractable and psychometrically viable. It is argued that good audiological practice will require, in addition to some measure of auditory impairment prior to hearing aid fitting, an assessment of recognition of the disability experienced by the client, and the extent to which that disability impacts upon the client's life (hearing handicap). Where an audiologist wishes to ascertain the extent to which intervention has been successful, it will be required to have some indication of the extent to which the client makes use of the hearing aid, the extent to which the hearing aid fitting has delivered benefit to the client, the extent to which the client has residual problems which may or may not require further intervention, and the extent to which the client is satisfied with the overall delivery of service. The GHABP attempts to access these dimensions while allowing the client to participate in the problem-setting and -solving exercise by determining the goals of the intervention. Space in this chapter does not permit a full description of the steps and principles that have entered into the generation or validation of the GHABP, and the details are available elsewhere. A tool such as the GHABP can be appropriate for the evaluation of the system, and is sensitive to changes in the technological content of a service, the hearing aids and the rehabilitative context within which those devices are prescribed. Although a different clinical setting might lead to a different choice of particular outcome measure, it is argued that routine evaluation of the extent to which a hearing aid fitting has achieved its required objectives should be an essential component of modern clinical practice.

> Routine evaluation of the extent to which hearing aid fittings alleviate disability and handicap should accompany hearing aid fittings as a matter of routine to guide individual management decisions and as part of system quality standards.

Future developments

Any contribution which attempts to survey hearing aids and their fitting in a time of rapid technological change will, of necessity, date rapidly. The particular devices that are available and the processing that they employ have changed enormously over the last 2–3 years, and the only safe prediction that one can make is that this pace of change will increase rather than decrease. The flexibility of devices that are available to clinical practitioners will increase, although the extent to which a state-funded health care system such as the UK NHS will have access to that technology remains unclear. Consequences of this rapid technological change are that the clinical trial information that is required to validate particular processing and its fitting to hearing-impaired listeners will almost inevitably lag behind the availability of the devices, and that as hearing aids employ more complex processing specific to individual manufacturers (incorporated, among other motives, for sales and marketing reasons), particular fitting rationales and regimens are likely to be manufacture-specific rather then generic. Clinical practitioners will have to exercise care to understand the particular motivation and content of different hearing aid processing and fitting, and themselves garner information concerning the extent to which different devices and rationales are providing benefits to their patients and clients. Given the wide range of technological possibilities and the different and sometimes conflicting rationales which underpin them, it would appear likely that there are different groups of hearing-impaired listeners who will gain benefit from different rationales and approaches. One of the prime challenges for future researchers and clinicians is to determine sets of principles which match the technological features of hearing aids and their fittings to the characteristics and needs of hearing-impaired listeners to maximize the benefit that they receive, and to package such procedures into forms which can be applied clinically with all of the constraints on time and resources that that requirement imposes.

References

1. Haggard MP, Gatehouse S. Candidate for hearing aids: justification for the concept and two-part criterion. *Br J Audiol*. 1993; **27**: 271–6.
2. Olsen W. Physical characteristics of hearing aids. In: Hodgson W, ed. *Hearing Aid Assessment ands Use in Audiologic Habilitation*. Baltimore: Williams and Wilkins, 1986; 13–37.
3. Clasen T, Vesterager V. In-the-ear hearing aids: a comparative investigation of the use of custom-made versus modular type aids. *Scand Audiol* 1987; **16**(4) 195–200.
4. Henrichsen J, Noring E. In-the-ear hearing aids. The use and benefit in the elderly hearing-impaired. *Scand Audiol* 1988; **17**: 209–12.
5. Henrichsen J, Noring E. The use and benefit of in-the-ear hearing aids: a four-year follow-up examination. *Scand Audiol* 1991; **20**(1): 55–9.

6. Jerivall L, Almqvist B. Clinical trial of in-the-ear hearing aids. *Scand Audiol* 1983; **12**: 63–70.
7. Meredith R, Stephens D. In-the-ear and behind-the-ear hearing aids in the elderly. *Scand Audiol* 1993; **2**: 211–16.
8. Parving A, Boisen G. In-the-canal hearing aids. *Scand Audiol* 1990; **19**: 25–30.
9. Pumford J, Seewald R, Scollie S, Jenstad L. Speech recognition with in-the-ear and behind-the-ear dual-microphone hearing instruments. *J Am Acad Audiol* 2000; **11**(1): 23–35.
10. Stuart A, Allen R. The effects of venting on in-the-ear canal, and completely-in-the-ear-canal hearing aid shell frequency responses: real-ear measures. *J Speech Language Hear Res* 1999; **42**: 804–13.
11. Turk R. A clinical comparison between behind-the-ear and in-the-ear hearing aids. *Audiol Acoust* 1986; **25**: 76–86.
12. Agnew J. Hearing aid adjustment through potentiometers and switch options. In: Valente M, ed. *Hearing Aids: Standards, Options and Limitations*. New York: Thieme Medical Publishers, 1996; 210–51.
13. DeJonge R. Microcomputer applications for hearing aid selection and fitting. *Trends Ampl* 1996; **1**(3): 114.
14. Fortune T. Amplifiers and circuit algorithms of contemporary hearing aids. In: Valente M, ed. *Hearing Aids: Standards, Options and Limitations*. New York: Thieme Medical Publishers, 1996; 152–209.
15. Agnew J. Digital hearing aid terminology made simple: a handy glossary. *Hear J* 2000; **53**(3): 37, 40–44.
16. Arlinger S, Billermark E. One-year follow-up of users of a digital hearing aid. *Br J Audiol* 1999; **33**: 223–32.
17. Arlinger S, Billermark E, Oberg M, Lunner T, Hellgren J. Clinical trial of the Oticon Digifocus hearing aid. *Scand Audiol* 1998; **27**: 51–61.
18. Berminger E, Karslsson KK. Clinical study of Widex Senso on first-time hearing aid users. *Scand Audiol* 1999; **28**: 117–25.
19. Bille M, Jensen A, Kjarbol E, Vesterager V, Sibelle P, Nielsen H. Clinical study of a digital versus an analogue hearing aid. *Scand Audiol* 1999; **28**: 127–35.
20. Boymans M, Dreschler W, Schoneveld P, Verschure H. Clinical evaluation of a full-digital in-the-ear hearing instrument. *Audiology* 1999; **38**: 99–108.
21. Bray V, Nilsson M, Ghent R, Johnson J. Results from a clinical evaluation of a new DSP hearing aid using an optimized platform. Poster presentation at the 11th meeting of the American Academy of Audiology, Miami Beach, FL, 1999.
22. Knebel S, Bentler R. Comparison of two digital hearing aids. *Ear Hear* 1998; **19**(4): 280–9.
23. Lunner T, Hellgren J, Arlinger S, Elberling C. A digital filterbank hearing aid: three digital signal processing algorithms—user preference and performance. *Ear Hear* 1997; **18**(5): 373–87.
24. Lunner T, Arlinger S, Hellgren J. 8-channel digital filter feedbank for hearing aid use: preliminary results in monaural, diotic and dichotic modes. *Scand Audiol* 1993; **38**(suppl): 75–81.
25. Lunner T, Hellgren J, Arlinger S, Elberling C. A digital filterbank hearing aid: improving a prescriptive fitting with subjective adjustments. *Scand Audiol* 1997; **26**: 169–76.
26. Lunner T, Hellgren J, Arlinger S, Elberling C. A digital filterbank hearing aid: predicting user preference and performance for two signal processing algorithms. *Ear Hear* 1997; **18**(5): 12–25.
27. Lunner T, Hellgren J, Arlinger S, Elberling C. Non-linear signal processing in digital hearing aids. *Scand Audiol* 1998; 27(suppl 49): 40–9.
28. Murray D, Hanson J. Application of digital signal processing to hearing aids: a critical survey. *J Am Acad Audiol* 1992; **3**: 145–52.
29. Newman C, Sandridge S. (1998). Benefit from, satisfaction with, and cost effectiveness of three different hearing aid technologies. *Am J Audiol* 7(2):115–28.
30. Ringdahl A, Magnusson L, Edberg P, Thelin L. Clinical evaluation of a digital power hearing instrument. *Hear Rev* 2000; **7**(3): 59–62, 64.
31. Roeser R, Taylor K. Audiometric and field trials with a digital hearing instrument. *Hear Instr* 1988; **39**(4): 14–6, 18, 20, 22.
32. Sweetow R. Selection and fitting of programmable and digital hearing aids. In: Valente M, Roeser R, Hosford-Dunn H, eds. *Audiology: Treatment Strategies*, New York: Thieme Medical Publishers, 1999.
33. Valente M, Fabry D, Potts L, Sandlin R. Comparing the performance of the Widex Senso digital hearing aids with analog hearing aids. *J Am Acad Audiol* 1998; **9**: 342–60.
34. Valente M, Sweetow R, Potts L, Bingea B. Digital versus analog signal processing: effect of directional microphone. *J Am Acad Audiol* 1999; **10**: 133–50.
35. Byrne D. Key issue in hearing aid selection and evaluation. *J Am Acad Audiol* 1992; **3**: 67–80.
36. Byrne D. Hearing selection for the 1990s: Where to? *J Am Acad Audiol* 1996; **7**: 377–95.
37. Hawkins D. Selection of hearing aid characteristics. In: Hodgson W, ed. *Hearing Aid Assessment and Use in Audiologic Habilitation*. Baltimore: Williams and Wilkins, 1986; 128–51.
38. Walden BE. Toward a model clinical-trials protocol for substantiating hearing aid user-benefit claims. *Am J Audiol* 1997; **6**(2): 13–24.
39. Kuhn G F. Model for the interaural time differences in the azimuthal plane. *J Acoust Soc Am* 1997; **62**: 157–67.
40. Shaw E A G. Transformation of sound pressure level from the free field to the eardrum in the horizontal plane. *J Acoust Soc Am* 1975; **56** : 1848–61.
41. Byrne D, Noble W. Effects of hearing aids on localization of sounds by people with sensorineural and conductive/mixed hearing loss. *Aus J Audiol* 1995; **17**(2): 79–86.
42. Byrne D, Noble W. Effects of earmold type on ability to locate sounds when wearing hearing aids. *Ear Hear* 1996; **17**: 3.
43. Byrne D, Noble W. Optimising sound localization with hearing aids. *Trends Ampl* 1998; **3**: 49–73.
44. Byrne D, Sinclair S. Open earmold fittings for improving aided auditory localization for sensorineural hearing losses with good high-frequency hearing. *Ear Hear* 1998; **19**: 62–71.
45. Lorenzi C, Gatehouse S, Lever C. Sound localization in noise in normal-hearing listeners. *J Acoust Soc Am* 1999; **105**(3): 1810–20.
46. Noble W, Byrne D. Auditory localization under conditions of unilateral fitting of different hearing aid systems. *Br J Audiol* 1991; **15**: 237–50.

47. Lorenzi C, Gatehouse S, Lever C. Sound localization in noise in hearing-impaired listeners. *J Acoust Soc Am* 1999; **105**(6): 3454–63.
48. Zurek PM. Binaural advantages and directional effects in speech intelligibility. *Acoustical Factors Affecting Hearing Aid Performance*. 2nd edn. Studebaker GA and Hockberg I, eds. Boston, Allyn-Bacon, 1980: 255–76.
49. Byrne D. Clinical issues and options in binaural hearing aid fitting. *Ear Hear* 1987; **2**(5): 187–93.
50. Colburn HS, Zurek PM. Binaural directional hearing-impairments and aids. *Directional Hearing*. Yost WA and Gourevitch G. New York, Springer-Verlag, 1987: 261–78.
51. Day GA, Browning GG, Gatehouse S. Benefit from binaural hearing aids in individuals with severe hearing impairment. *Br J Audiol* 1988; **22**: 273–7.
52. Gatehouse S, Haggard M P. The influence of hearing asymmetries on benefits from binaural amplification. *Hear J* 1986; **22**(1): 15–20.
53. Hawkins DB, Yacullo WS. Signal-to-noise ratio advantage of binaural hearing aids and directional microphones under different levels of reverberation. *J Speech Hear Dis* 1984; **49**: 278–86.
54. Jerger J, Carhart R, Dirks D. Binaural hearing aids and speech intelligibility. *J Speech Hear Res* 1961; **4**(2): 137–48.
55. Chmiel R, Jerger J. Unsuccessful use of binaural amplification by an elderly person. *J Am Acad Audiol* 1997; **8**: 1–10.
56. Emmer M. Review of late-onset auditory deprivation and clinical implications. *Hear J* 1999; **52**(11): 26, 28–30, 32.
57. Hurley R. Recovery from the unaided ear effect. *Hear J* 1999; **52**(11): 35–6, 38 ,40. *Hear Rev* **5**(9): 40–2, 71.
58. Palmer C. Deprivation and acclimatization in the human auditory system: do they happen? Do they matter? *Hear J* 1999; **52**(11): 2323–4.
59. Silman S, Gelfand SS. Late-onset auditory deprivation: effects of monaural versus binaural hearing aids. *J Acoust Soc Am* 1984; **76**(5): 1357–62.
60. Byrne D. Implications of the National Acoustic Laboratories (NAL) research for hearing gain and frequency response selection strategies. In: *Acoustical Factors Affecting Hearing Aid Performance*. Studebaker GA, Hochberg I, Boston: Allyn-Bacon, 1980: **8**: 119–31.
61. Byrne D, Dillon H. The National Acoustic Laboratories (NAL) new procedure for selecting gain and frequency response of a hearing aid. *Ear Hear*, 1986; **7**: 257–65.
62. Byrne D, Parkinson A, Newall P. Hearing aid gain and frequency response requirements for the severely/profound hearing impaired. *Ear Hear* 1990; 11: 40–9.
63. Humes LE. An evaluation of several rationales for selecting hearing aid gain. *J Speech Hear Dis 1986;* **51**: 272–81.
64. Humes LE, Halling D. Overview, rationale and comparison of suprathreshold-based prescriptive methods. In: Valente M, ed. *Strategies for Selecting and Verifying Hearing Aid Fittings*, New York: Thieme Medical Publishers, 1994; 19–37.
65. Leijon A, Lindkvist A, Ringdahl A, Israelsson B. Sound quality and speech reception for prescribed hearing aid frequency responses. *Ear Hear* 1991; **12**(4): 251–60.
66. Libby R. The 1/3–2/3 insertion gain hearing aid selection guide. *Hear Instr* 1986; **37**: 27–8.
67. McCandless G. Hearing aid formulae and their application. In: Sandlin R, ed. *Handbook of Hearing Aid Amplification*, Vol. 1. Boston: Little Brown and Company, 1988; 221–38.
68. McCandless G. Overview and rationale of threshold-based hearing aid selection procedures. In: Valente M, ed. *Strategies for Selecting and Verifying Hearing Aid Fittings*. New York: Thieme Medical Publishers, 1994; 1–18.
69. McCandless G, Lyregaard P. Prescription of gain/output (POGO) for hearing aids. *Hear Instrum 1983;* **34**: 16–21.
70. Macrae JH, Dillon H. Gain, frequency response and maximum output requirements for hearing aids. *J Rehab Res Dev* 1996; **33**(4): 363–76.
71. Moore BCJ, Glasberg B R. Use of a loudness model for hearing-aid fitting. 1. Linear hearing aids. *Br J Audiol* 1998; **32**: 317–35.
72. Palmer C, Lindley G, Mormer E. Selection and fitting of conventional hearing aids. In: Valente M, Roeser R, Hosford-Dunn H, eds. *Audiology: Treatment Strategies*. New York: Thieme Medical Publishers 1999.
73. Valente M, Bentler R, Seewald R, Trine T, Van Vliet D. Guidelines for hearing aid fitting for adults. *Am J Audiol* 1998; **7**: 5–13.
74. Harrowven R. Insertion gain versus median ear corrected coupler gain: a comparison of two fitting methods in new NHS hearing aid users. *Br J Audiol* 1998; **32**: 153–65.
75. Swan I R C, Gatehouse S. The value of routine in-the-ear measurement of hearing aid gain. *Br J Audiol* 1995; **29**: 271–7.
76. Fortune TW, Preves DA. Hearing aid saturation and aided loudness discomfort. *J Speech Hear Res* 1992, **35**: 175–85.
77. Gabrielsson A, Sjogren H. Perceived sound quality of hearing aids. *Scand Audiol* 1979; **8**: 159–69.
78. Stelmachowicz P, Lewis D, Hoover B, Keefe D. Subjective effects of peak clipping and compression limiting in normal and hearing-impaired children. *J Acoust Soc Am* 1999; **105**: 412–22.
79. Dillon H, Storey L. The National Acoustic Laboratories' procedure for selecting the saturation sound pressure level of hearing aids: theoretical derivation. *Ear Hear* 1998; **19**: 255–66.
80. Mueller, HG, Bright, KE. Selection and verification of maximum output. In: Valente M, ed. *Strategies for Selecting and Verifying Hearing Aid Fittings*. New York: Thieme Medical Publishers, 1994; 38–63.
81. Pascoe DP. Clinical measurement of the auditory dynamic range and their relation to the formulas for hearing aid gain. In: Jensen JH, ed. *Hearing Aid Fitting: Theoretical and Practical Views*. 13th Danavox Symposium. Copenhagen: Stougaard Jensen, 1988; 129–52.
82. Storey L, Dillon H. The national acoustic laboratories procedure for selecting the saturation sound pressure level of hearing aids: experimental validation. *Ear Hear* 1998; **19**: 267–79.
83. Moore B. Benefits of linear amplification and multichannel compression for speech comprehension in backgrounds with spectral and temporal dips. *J Acoust Soc Am* 1999; **105**: 400–11.
84. Dempsey JJ. The occlusion effect created by custom canal hearing aids. *Am J Otol* 1990; **11**(1): 44–6.
85. Mueller HG, Northern BK. Studies of the hearing aid occlusion effect. *Semin Hear* 1996; **17**(1): 21–32.

86. Barker C, Dillon H. Client preferences for compression threshold in single-channel wide dynamic range compression hearing aids. *Ear Hear* 1999; **20**: 127–39.
87. Chouard C, Ouayoun M, Meyer B et al. Auditory performances of a 3–4–7 programmable numeric filter hearing aid. *Audiology* 1997; **36**: 339–53.
88. Cornelisse L, Seewald R, Jamieson D. Wide dynamic range compression hearing aids: the DSL[i/o] approach. *Hear J* 1995; **47**(10): 23–4, 26, 28–9.
89. Cox RM. (1995). Using loudness data for hearing aid selection: the IHAFF approach. *Hear J* 1995; **48**(2): 10, 39–44.
90. Dillon H. Compression in hearing aids. In: Sandlin R, ed. *Handbook of Hearing Aid Amplification*, Vol. 1. Boston: Little Brown and Company, 1988; 121–46.
91. Dillon H, Byrne D, Brewer S, Katsch R, Ching T, Keidser G. NAL non-Linear (NAL-NL1). (Version 1.01 User Manual). Chatswood, 1998.
92. Hickson L, Thyer N, Bates D. Acoustic analysis of speech through a hearing aid: consonant–vowel ratio effects with a two-channel compression amplification. *J Am Acad Audiol* 1999; 10: 549–56.
93. Jenstad L, Pumford J, Seewald R, Cornelisse L. Comparison of linear gain and wide dynamic range compression hearing aid circuits II: aided loudness measures. *Ear Hear 2000;* **21**: 32–44.
94. Jenstad L, Seewald R, Cornelisse L, Shantz J. Comparison of linear gain and wide dynamic range compression hearing aid circuits: aided speech perception measures. *Ear Hear* 1999; **20**: 117–26.
95. Kam A, Wong L. Comparison of performance with wide range compression and linear amplification. *J Am Acad Audiol* 1999; **10**: 445–57.
96. Keidser G, Dillon H, Brewer S. Using the NAL-NL1 prescriptive procedure with advanced hearing instruments. *Hear Rev* 1999; **6**(11): 8, 10, 12, 16, 18.
97. Kochkin S. Customer satisfaction and subjective benefit with high performance hearing aids. *Hear Rev* 1996; **3**(12): 16–26.
98. Kuk F. Rationale and requirements for a slow-acting compression hearing aid. *Hear J* 1998; **51**(6): 45–53, 79.
99. Lindley G, Palmer C. Fitting wide dynamic range compression hearing aids: DSL [i/o], the IHAFF protocol, and FIG6. *Am J Audiol* 1997; **6**: 19–28.
100. Moore BCJ, Glasberg BR. A comparison of four methods of implementing automatic gain control (AGC) in hearing aids. *Br J Audiol* 1988; **22**: 93–104.
101. Moore BCJ, Glasberg BR. Optimization of a slow-acting automatic gain control system for use in hearing aids. *Br J Audiol* 1991; 25: 171–82.
102. Moore BCJ, Glasbert BR. Use of a loudness model for hearing aid fitting: III A general method for deriving initial fittings for hearing aids with multi-channel compression. *Br J Audiol* 1999; **33**: 241–58.
103. Stelmachowicz P, Dalzell S, Peterson D, Kopun J, Lewis D, Hoover B. A comparison of threshold based fitting strategies for nonlinear hearing aids. *Ear Hear* 1998; **19**: 131–8.
104. Stone MA, Moore BCJ. Comparison of different forms of compression using wearable digital hearing aids. *J Acoust Soc Am* 1999; **106**(6): 3603–19.
105. Gatehouse S, Elberling CE, Naylor G. Aspects of auditory ecology and psychoacoustic function as determinants of benefits from and candidature for non-linear processing in hearing aids. In: Rasmussen AN ed. *Auditory Models and Non-linear Hearing Instruments*, 18th Danavox Symposium Holmens Trykkeri, 1999; 221–34.
106. Elberling CE, Hansen KV. Hearing instruments—interaction with user preference. In Rasmussen AN ed. *Auditory Models and Non-linear Hearing Instruments*, 18th Danavox Symposium, Holmens. Trykkeri, 1999, 341–8.
107. Keidser G. The relationship between listening conditions and alternative amplification schemes for multiple memory hearing aids. *Ear Hear* 1995; **16**(6): 575–86.
108. Keidser G, Dillon H, Byrne D. Guidelines for fitting multiple memory hearing aids. *J Am Acad Audiol* 1996; **7**: 406–18.
109. Cox RM, Gilmore C. Development of the profile of hearing aid performance (PHAP). *J Speech Hear Res* 1990; **33**: 343–57.
110. Frank T, Gooden RG. The effect of hearing aid microphone types on speech scores in a background of multi-talker noise. *Maico Audiol Library Series* 1973; **11**(5): 1–4.
111. Hoffman M, Stewart R. Simulation of multi-microphone hearing aids in multiple interference environments. *Br J Audiol* 1996; **30**: 249–60.
112. Leeuw AR, Dreschler WA. Advantage of directional hearing aid microphones related to room acoustics. *Audiology* 1991; **3**: 330–44.
113. Lentz WE. Speech discrimination in the presence of background noise using a hearing aid with a directionally-sensitive microphone. *Maico Audiol Library Series* 1972; **10**(9): 1–4.
114. Lurquin P, Rafhay S. Intelligibility in noise using multi-microphone hearing aids. *Acta Otorhinlarynol (Belg)* 1996; **50**: 103–9.
115. Madison TK, Hawkins DB. The signal-to-noise ratio advantage of directional microphones. *Hear Instr* 1983; **34**(2): 18, 49.
116. Nielson HB. A comparison between hearing aids with a directional microphone and hearing aids with a conventional microphone. *Scand Audiol* 1973; **2**: 45–8.
117. Nielson HB, Ludvigsen C. Effects of hearing aids with directional microphones in different acoustic environments. *Scand Audiol* 1978; **7**: 217–24.
118. Ricketts T, Dhar S. Comparing performance across three directional hearing aids. *J Am Acad Audiol* 1999; **10**: 180–9.
119. Ricketts T. Directivity quantification in hearing aids: fitting and measurement effects. *Ear Hear* 2000; **21**: 45–58.
120. Ricketts T, Mueller G. Making sense of directional microphone hearing aids. *Am J Audiol* 1999; **8**(2): 117–27.
121. Sung GS, Sung RJ, Angelelli RM. Directional microphone in hearing aids. *Arch Otol* 1975; **101**: 316–19.
122. Upfold LLP. Directional advantage with lower gain directional hearing aids. *Aust J Audiol* 1996; **18**(1): 35–45.
123. Valente M, Fabry D, Potts L. Recognition of speech in noise with hearing aids using dual microphones. *J Am Acad Audiol* 1995; **6**: 440–9.
124. Voss T. Clinical evaluation of multi-microphone hearing instruments. *Hear Rev* 1997; **4**(9): 36, 45–6, 74.

125. Dyrlund O, Bisgaard N. Acoustic feedback margin improvements in hearing instruments with a prototype DFS (digital feedback suppression system). *Scand Audiol* 1991; **20**: 49–53.
126. Dyrlund O, Henningsen L. Bisgaard N, Jensen J. Digital feedback suppression (DFS). Characteristics of feedback-margin improvement in a DFS hearing instrument. *Scand Audiol* 1994; **23**: 135–8.
127. Dyrlund O, Ludvigsen C. Hearing aid measurements with speech and noise signals. *Scand Audiol* 1994; **33**(3): 153–7.
128. Engebretson M, French-St M, O'Connell G, O'Connell MP. Adaptive feedback stabilization of hearing aids. *Scand Audiol* 1993; **38**: 56–64.
129. Hellgren J, Lunner T, Arlinger S. System identification of feedback in hearing aids. *J Acoust Soc Am* 1999; **105** (6): 3481–96.
130. St George MF, Wood DJ. Behavioural assessment of adaptive feedback equalization in a digital hearing aid. *J Rehab Res Dev* 1993; **30**(1): 17–25.
131. Van Tasell DJ, Crain TR. Noise reduction hearing aids: release from masking and release from distortion. *Ear Hear* 1992; **13**(2): 114–21.
132. Browning GG. The British experience of an implantable, subcutaneous bone conduction hearing aid (Xomed Audiant). *J Laryngol Otol* 1990; **104**: 534–8.
133. Carlsson P, Hakansson B. A speech-to-noise ratio test with the bone-anchored hearing aid: a comparative study. *Otol Head Neck Surg*, 1986; **94**: 421–6.
134. Cooper HR, Burrell SP. The Birmingham bone anchored hearing aid programme: referrals, selection, rehabilitation, philosophy and adult. *J Laryngol Otol* 1996; BAHA Suppl: 13–20.
135. Hakansson B, Tjellstrom A. The bone-anchored hearing aid. *Acta Otol (Stockh)* 1985; **100**: 229–39.
136. Mylanus EAM, Snik AFM. Audiological results for the bone-anchored hearing aid HC220. *Ear Hear* 1994; **15**: 187–92.
137. Mylanus EAM, Snik AFM. Patients' opinions of bone-anchored vs conventional hearing aids. *Arch Otol Head Neck Surg* 1995; **121**: 421–5.
138. Ringdahl A, Eriksson-Mangold M. Perceived sound quality of three bone-anchored hearing aid models. *Br J Audiol* 1995; **29**: 309–14.
139. Ringdahl A, Israelsson B. Paired comparisons between the classic 300 bone-anchored and conventional bone-conduction hearing aids in terms of sound quality and speech intelligibility. *Br J Audiol* 1995; **29**: 290–307.
140. Burrell SP, Cooper HC. The bone anchored hearing aid. The third option for otosclerosis. *J Laryngol Otol 1996;* BAHA Suppl: 31–7.
141. Gyo K, Saiki T, Yanaghihara N. Implantable hearing aid using a piezoelectric ossicular vibrator: a speech audiometry study. *Audiology* 1996; **35**: 271–6.
142. Yanagihara N, Aritoma H, Yamanaka E, Gyo K. Implantable hearing aids. *Arch Otol Head Neck Surg* 1987; **113**: 869–72.
143. Yanagihara N, Hinohira Y. Surgical rehabilitation of deafness with partially implantable hearing aid using piezoelectric ceramic bimorphiossicular vibrator. *Auris Nasus Larynx* 1997; **24**: 91–8.
144. Bentler R. Future trends in verification strategies. In: Valente M, ed. *Strategies for Selecting and Verifying Hearing Aid Fittings*. New York: Thieme Medical Publishers, 1994: 343–62.
145. Fikret-Para S, Revit LJ. Individualised correction factors in the pre-selection of hearing aids. *J Speech Hear Res* 1992; **35**: 384–400.
146. Munro K, Hatton N. Customized acoustic transform functions and their accuracy in predicting real-ear hearing aid performance. *Ear Hear* 2000; **21**: 59–69.
147. Mueller HG, Hawkins D, Northern J. *Probe Microphone Measurements. Hearing Aid Selection and Assessment*. San Diego: Singular Press, 1992.
148. American National Standards Institute. *Specification of Hearing Aid Characteristics* ANSI S3.22-1987. New York: Acoustical Society of America, 1987.
149. American National Standards Institute. *American National Standard for Specification of Hearing Aid Characteristics*. ANSI S3.22-1996. New York: ANSI, 1996.
150. Cole W, Sinclair S, Block M, Baer J, Groth J, Majest B. Equipment to assess the performance of nonlinear hearing aids. *Trends Ampl* 1998; **3**(4): 122–71.
151. DeJonge R. Real-ear measures: individual variations and measurement error. In: Valente M, ed. *Hearing Aids: Standards, Options and Limitations*. New York: Thieme Medical Publishers, 1996: 72–125.
152. Preves D, Curran J. Hearing aid instrumentation and procedures for electroacoustic testing. In: Valente M, Roeser R, Hosford-Dunn H, eds. *Audiology: Treatment Strategies*, New York: Thieme Medical Publishers 1999.
153. Revit L. Real-ear measures. In: Valente M, Roeser R, Hosford-Dunn H, eds. *Audiology: Treatment Strategies*. New York: Thieme Medical Publishers 1999.
154. Tecca J. Use of real-ear measures to verify hearing aid fitting. In: Valente M, ed. *Strategies for Selecting and Verifying Hearing Aid Fittings*. New York:Thieme Medical Publishers, 1994: 88–107.
155. American National Standards Institute. *American National Standard for Testing Hearing Aids with a Broad-band Noise Signal*. ANSI S3.42-1992. New York: ANSI, 1992.
156. Brooks D N. Counselling and its effect on hearing aid use. *Scand Audiol* 1979; **9**: 101–7.
157. Brooks D N. The time course of adaption to hearing aid use. *Br J Audiol* 1996; **30**: 55–62.
158. Gatehouse S. The time course and magnitude of perceptual acclimatization to frequency responses: evidence from monaural fitting of hearing aids. *J Acoust Am* 1992; **92**: 1258–68.
159. Gatehouse S. Role of perceptual acclimatization in the selection of frequency responses for hearing aids. *J Am Acad Audiol* 1993; **4**: 296–306.
160. Lindley G. Adaptation to loudness: implications for hearing aid fittings. *Hear J* 1999; **52**(11): 50, 52, 56–7.
161. Sweetow RW. Counselling: it's the key to successful hearing aid fitting. *Hear J* 1999; **52**(3): 10–17.
162. Ward PR. Effectiveness of aftercare for older people prescribed a hearing aid for the first time. *Scand Audiol* 1981; **10**: 99–106.

163. Ward PR, Gowers JI. Fitting hearing aids: the effects of method of instruction. *Br J Audiol* 1980; **14**: 15–18.
164. Cox RM, Alexander GC. The abbreviated profile of hearing aid benefit. *Ear Hear* 1995; **16**: 176–86.
165. Dillon H. Shortened hearing aid performance inventory for the elderly (SHAPIE): a statistical approach. *Aust J Audiol* 1994; **16**(1): 37–48.
166. Dillon H, James A, Ginis J. Client-oriented scale of improvement (COSI) and its relationship to several other measures of benefit and satisfaction provided by hearing aids. *J Am Acad Audiol* 1997; **8** :27–43.
167. Erdman S, Demorest M. *CPHI Manual: A Guide for Clinical Use*. Simpsonville, MD: CPHI Services, 1990.
168. Malinoff RL, Weinstein B E. Measurement of hearing aid benefit in the elderly. *Ear Hear* 1989; **10**(6): 354–6.
169. Mason D, Popelka. Comparison of hearing aid gain using functional, coupler, and probe-tube measurements. *J Speech Hear Res* 1986; **29**: 218–26.
170. Newman CW, Weinstein BE. The hearing handicap inventory for the elderly as a measure of hearing aid benefit. *Ear Hear* 1988; **9**(2): 81–5.
171. Newman C, Weinstein B, Jacobson G, Hug G. The hearing handicap inventory for adults: psychometric adequacy and audiometric correlates. *Ear Hear* 1990; **11**: 430–3.
172. Noble W. *Self-assessment of Hearing and Related Functions*. London: Whurr, 1998.
173. Noble W, Atherley G. The hearing measure scale: a questionnaire for the assessment of auditory disability. *J Aud Res* 1970; **10**: 229–50.
174. Gatehouse S. The Glasgow Hearing Aid Benefit Profile: derivation and validation of a client-centred outcome measure for hearing aid services. *J Am Acad Audiol* 1999; **10**: 80–103.
175. Gatehouse S. A self-report outcome measure for the evaluation of hearing aid fittings and services. *Health Bulletin* 1999; **57**(6): 424–36.
176. Gatehouse S. The Glasgow hearing aid benefit profile. *Hear J* 2000; **53**(3): 10, 12, 14, 16, 18.

32 The pathophysiology and assessment of tinnitus

Kajsa-Mia Holgers, Marie-Louise Barrenäs

Tinnitus aetiology and pathophysiology

Definition

Tinnitus can be defined as a sound sensation in the absence of an external sound or electrical stimulation. Tinnitus may also be generated by internal body sounds, i.e. sounds from blood vessels. This is called objective tinnitus, since a sound generator is present and because the sound may be heard by others. This presentation will mainly focus upon subjective tinnitus which cannot be explained by the presence of external or internal sound sources.

Epidemiology

Tinnitus is a common symptom, occurring in 10–15% of the general population. In 1–2% of sufferers, tinnitus affects daily life severely.[1, 2] Tinnitus is often related to an auditory dysfunction, and approximately two-thirds of the sufferers have hearing loss.[1, 3–5] More men than women seek help for tinnitus. They are also younger and have worse hearing loss than women.[5–8] In women, the tinnitus frequency is lower and the characterization is more complex than in men.[6]

The knowledge of tinnitus in children is limited. The incidence of tinnitus in children has been reported to vary between 6% and 36%.[9–12] In children with hearing loss, the incidence is reported to be much higher, up to 76%.[9–12] The reported incidence of tinnitus varies between studies, and the variability is greater in children than in adults. This might reflect the difficulties faced when interviewing children. To increase the reliability of the answers given in the tinnitus interview, Stouffer and co-workers included only children who, at the beginning of the interview, had given reliable answers to practical questions which did not concern tinnitus. In their study of 120 children, 13% with normal hearing had experienced tinnitus. Similar results (12%) were found in a study of 961 7-year-old school children.[13,14] Among the schoolchildren with and without hearing loss, 9% and 13% respectively had experienced tinnitus to a varying extent.[13,14]

> Tinnitus can be defined as a sound sensation in the absence of a sound generator or electrical stimulation.
>
> 10–15% of the general adult population perceive tinnitus and 10–20% of these cases have tinnitus severe enough to affect daily life. The occurrence of tinnitus in children is less well known, but is presumably 12–13%.

Tinnitus aetiology

Tinnitus is a multifactorial symptom which can be induced by a number of conditions (Figure 32.1). Lesions at different locations in the auditory system, somatic disorders, psychiatric conditions and drug effects are all associated with tinnitus.[15–20] Moreover, psychological factors play an important role[21–23] in the intrusiveness of tinnitus. Usually, tinnitus aetiology is classified by type and underlying disorders[24] (Figure 32.2). However, tinnitus is not regarded as an organic disease but more as a functional system or disorder of the auditory system, including the interpretation of auditory activity by the auditory cortex.

> Tinnitus is not regarded as an organic disease but more as a functional system or a disorder of the auditory system, including the interpretation of auditory activity by the auditory cortex.

The mechanisms of tinnitus sensation have been discussed, and several reviews on the different theoretical hypotheses of the neural origin of subjective tinnitus have been presented.[25–27] The value of these models is limited, because no single model can explain the fact that, although damage to the auditory system may induce tinnitus, patients with hearing loss will not necessarily perceive tinnitus. Nonetheless, the models have increased the understanding of different mechanisms by which tinnitus may be induced and maintained. Models focusing upon the mechanisms underlying the severity of tinnitus have also been proposed.[8, 28]

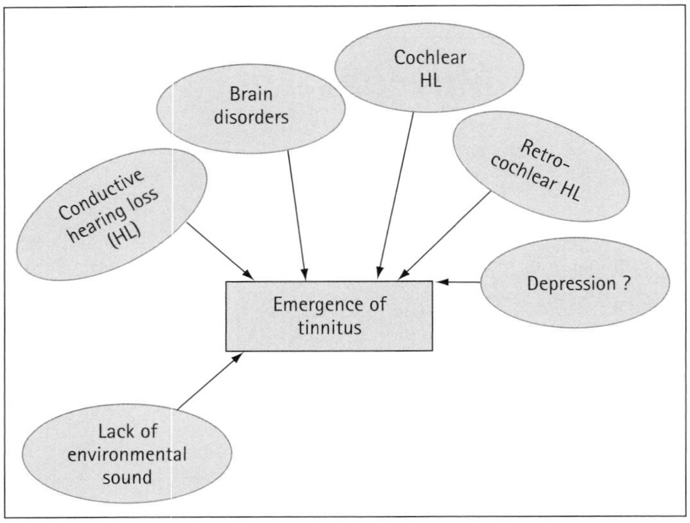

Figure 32.1 Different aetiological factors for the emergence of tinnitus. Used with permission of Holgers In: Hazell, ed. *Sixth International Tinnitus Seminar*, Cambridge. Kings Lynn: Biddles Short Run Books, 1999: 218–19.[13]

Tinnitus is a common phenomenon but not everyone who is aware of tinnitus 'suffers' from the symptom. Therefore, it is very important to distinguish tinnitus awareness from tinnitus complaint. Some hypotheses provide explanations as to why some patients suffer more than others and provide great help to the clinician when explaining possible mechanisms of the generation of the symptom to the patient. It has been suggested that noise damage but also other initial insults may induce plastic changes in the central auditory structures and, after some time, these changes could be consolidated as neural patterns that represent tinnitus. This consolidation may be facilitated by different causes. A new model based on the aetiology of tinnitus suffering has been introduced which divides tinnitus complaint into three categories: somatic tinnitus, depression–anxiety-related tinnitus complaint, and audiological tinnitus suffering.[8] Somatic tinnitus is when abnormalities in the musculoskeletal apparatus influence suffering from tinnitus by possible interactions between the auditory and somatosensory systems. Anxiety- and depression-related tinnitus suffering is connected with anxiety and depressive disorders. Audiological tinnitus is present when the patient has significant limitations in life due to the combination of severe hearing loss and persistent tinnitus. The severity of tinnitus will be further discussed later in this chapter.

It is beyond the scope of this chapter to describe all the theoretical models that have been described in the literature to explain the aetiology of tinnitus. Instead, emphasis has been placed on those models which we have found to be illustrative and useful when describing tinnitus mechanisms to patients and students.

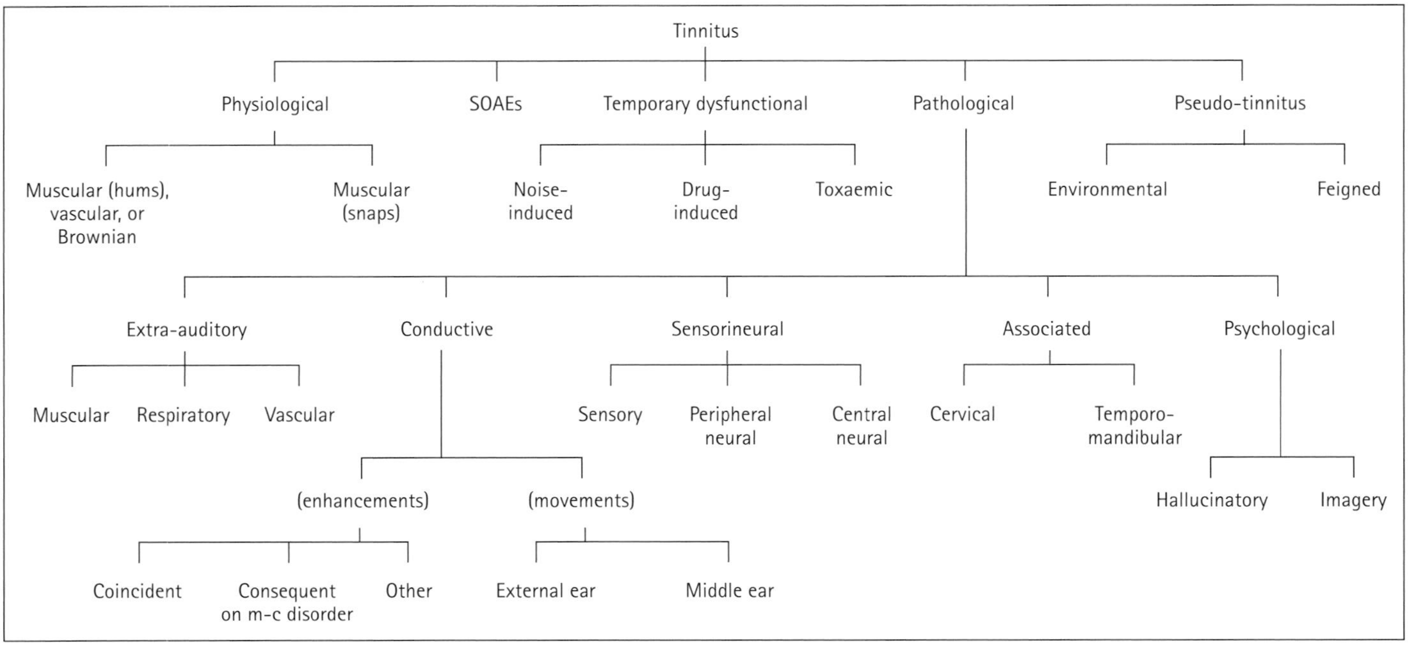

Figure 32.2 Aetiology of tinnitus based on underlying disorders. SOAE, spontaneous otoacoustic emissions. (From Coles. *Proc 5th Int Tinnitus Sem*, Portland, OR, USA. Reprinted with permission from the American Tinnitus Association, www.ata.org: 1995, 25–9.[24])

Experimental animal models

In experimental settings, tinnitus is often induced by drugs or noise. A prerequisite for animal research is to induce tinnitus and to interpret and evaluate behavioural changes due to tinnitus in the animal, which is difficult. Therefore, current experimental models are only valid to a limited extent in modelling the psychophysical and clinical features of tinnitus. Owing to these circumstances, conclusions based on results from animal models are open to debate. However, animal research offers a good opportunity to study changes of calcium homeostasis, cochlear bloodflow, distortion otoacoustic emission (DPOAE), tinnitus-related neuronal signals and potential central mechanisms related to tinnitus, including the investigation of spontaneous neural and metabolic activity, neurotransmitters and plastic changes in the central nervous system.[29–32]

General tinnitus hypotheses

The following general hypotheses are linked to the models which we will describe later in this chapter:

1. Tinnitus is regarded as a perceptual consequence of altered spontaneous activity within the auditory system.
2. The induction of tinnitus usually involves some kind of damage to the peripheral auditory structures that results in altered spontaneous inputs to the central auditory system.
3. The generation, maintenance and intrusiveness of tinnitus involves central auditory structures which are not necessarily impaired, e.g. the limbic system and the autonomic nervous system.

The most important characteristics of tinnitus

- Tinnitus persists even after destruction of the cochlea or the VIIIth nerve.
- Tinnitus can be masked both ipsi- and contralaterally, but its masking behaviour differs from that of an external sound.
- Tinnitus can show residual inhibition by masking by external sound.
- Tinnitus can be transiently masked by intravenous administration of lidocaine.
- Tinnitus may sometimes change through manipulations of the musculoskelatal system.

Neuropathophysiological tinnitus models

A major task of the auditory cortex is to determine whether a particular activity pattern in afferent auditory neurons is caused by an external sound stimulus, or represents spontaneous 'nonsense' activity. Under non-pathological silent conditions, the spontaneous activity from the afferent auditory neurones is completely irregular and almost non-existent (Figure 32.3a). Normally, this stochastic spontaneous discharge pattern is not perceived by the central auditory system as a sound. An external sound stimulus will increase the action potential rate and modulate the temporal action potential pattern from irregular to regular. These changes will be recognized by the auditory cortex as 'sound' (Figure 32.3b) (note that the action potentials are synchronized when induced by an external sound).

In the case of tinnitus, it is believed that the rate and/or the stochastic temporal pattern of the spontaneous neural activity is altered by the pathological process from irregular (non-sound pattern) to synchronized (sound pattern). Accordingly, the pathology will produce neural activity, which simulates the presence of an acoustical signal, although there is no true acoustical input. It is believed that tinnitus is mainly a consequence of an abnormal synchronized action potential pattern of the spontaneous activity within the central auditory pathways. An altered firing rate seems to be less important; both increased and decreased firing rates have been reported in association with tinnitus (increased by salicylate and decreased by Co^{2+} or Mn^{2+}).

The pathologically synchronized spontaneous activity from the auditory nerve is processed by the same central auditory structures and physiological mechanisms as external sounds. Therefore, the afferent system will interpret the pathologically synchronized spontaneous activity as a non-pathological sound. Accordingly, the auditory cortex will interpret a non-sound as an acoustical 'signal', and the patient will perceive tinnitus.

Model 1—The synaptic synchronization of the hair cell by Ca^{2+} influx

In the absence of mechanical stimulation, the normal hair cell is partially depolarized as a result of a leakage of K^+ flowing through the transduction channels at the top of the hair cells. This steady depolarization opens the Ca^{2+} channels, allowing Ca^{2+} to enter into the cell, as Ca^{2+} ions only enter when the hair cell is depolarized. The entry of Ca^{2+} ions into the hair cell results in spontaneous transmitter release of glutamate in the synapse between the inner hair cell and the afferent auditory neurone. For example, ion channel dysfunction of the inner hair cells (IHCs) located at the maximum locus of the hearing loss can become a source of leakage currents, which in turn continuously generate a depolarization and transmitter depletion of the synapse.[33]

Another possible mechanism is damage to the hair cell cilia, a common finding due to noise trauma, resulting in a constant influx of K^+ ions, causing Ca^{2+} entry. In both conditions, the Ca^{2+} influx might alter the spontaneous input from the IHCs to the auditory nerve from being non-synchronized to synchronized. Then the central auditory system will interpret the regular spontaneous activity as an external sound, instead of silence, and the patient will perceive tinnitus.

The benefit of this model is that it can explain why tinnitus is induced by noise trauma or ototoxic drugs. A shortcoming is

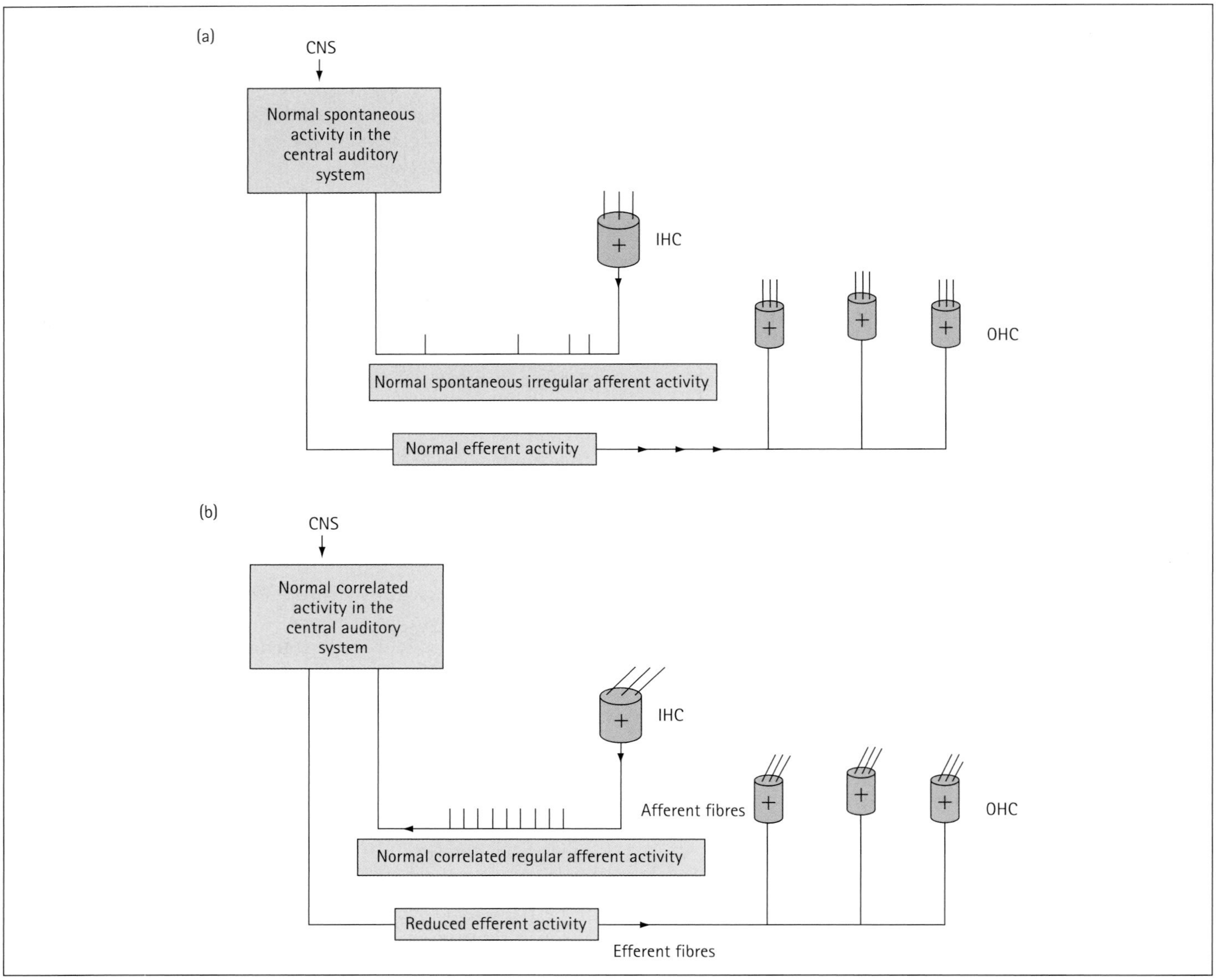

Figure 32.3 (a) Normal nervous activity in a silence condition (undamaged cochlea). (b) Normal nervous activity in a noisy condition (undamaged cochlea).

that it does not explain why not all patients with sensorineural hearing loss (SNHL) due to hair cell damage perceive tinnitus.

Model 2—Induction of tinnitus by outer hair cell damage, including the influence of the efferent system

In most tinnitus patients, an SNHL is found.[1–5] Usually, the SNHL is caused by outer hair cell (OHC) damage. The OHCs may be damaged by a variety of different underlying mechanisms, such as presbyacusis, noise, ototoxic drugs, and Menière's disease. The activity of the OHCs is modulated by the efferent system, which originates from the superior olivary complex. The efferent nerve fibres are mainly arranged in the crossed olivocochlear bundle, which terminates predominantly on the OHCs. The uncrossed bundle terminates on the IHCs. The efferent system, the OHCs, the IHCs, the VIIIth nerve and the superior olivary complex are linked together, forming a feedback system. The function of this feedback system is to regulate the micromechanics of the cochlea, which, in turn, are controlled by the central nervous system. The efferent system modulates the OHC activity to provide an optimum operation point for the amplification of the travelling wave, in order to increase the afferent input from the IHCs. Thus the IHCs are rendered more sensitive.

In a silent environment, the afferent auditory input is small or non-existent. It is hypothesized that this will also be the case if the OHCs are damaged or lacking (Figure 32.3c). In order to increase the afferent auditory input, the efferent system will

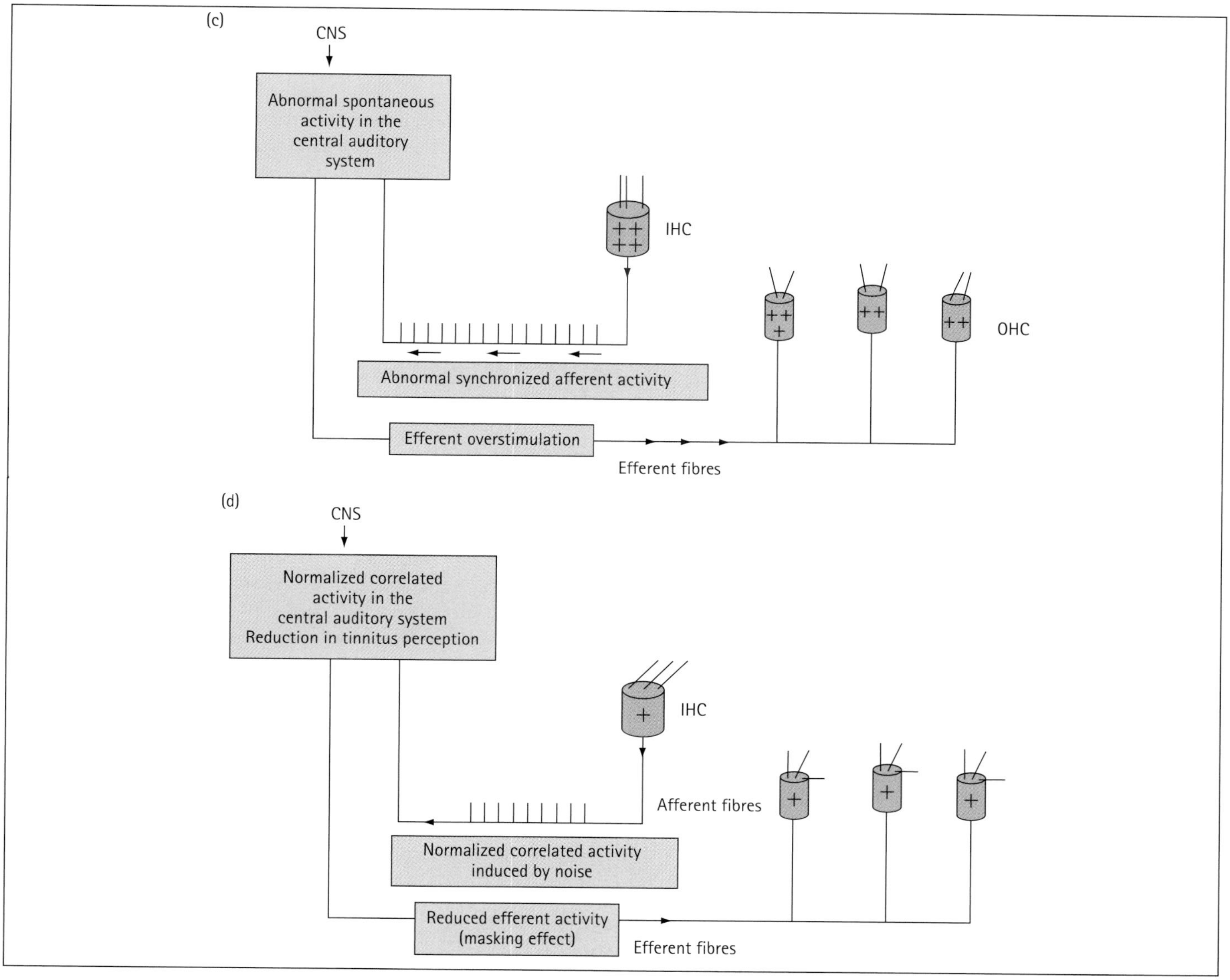

Figure 32.3 (c) Abnormal nervous activity (damaged outer hair cells). (d) Masking of tinnitus by noise. Normalized nervous activity in a noisy condition (damaged outer hair cells). (Opposite situation compared to (c).) CNS, central nervous system; IHC, inner hair cell; OHC, outer hair cell.

activate the remaining OHCs at the edge of the hair cell loss by stimulating the IHCs. Consequently, the few intact OHCs will become 'hyperactive'. This, in turn, will increase the firing rate from the IHCs. If the spontaneous activity in the auditory nerve becomes synchronized, then a 'cochlear tinnitus' is induced. When people with normal hearing and no tinnitus are placed in a noisy environment, the afferent input is increased by the acoustical stimulation. In turn, the activity in the efferent system will be reduced. It is suggested that this is also the case for patients with tinnitus, explaining why tinnitus is often reduced by noise, i.e. the masking effect (Figure 32.3d).

The benefit of this model is that it offers an interpretation for the masking phenomenon, but it does not explain why not all patients with hearing loss perceive tinnitus.

Model 3—The 'gate control' theory

Tonndorf[34] focused upon the similarities between chronic tinnitus and chronic pain, when presenting the 'gate control hypothesis for tinnitus' in analogy with that for pain. Both conditions are wholly subjective and continuous sensations. However, with time, they may change in both quality and character. In selected cases, both sensations can be alleviated, masked or even totally suppressed by suitable inputs, e.g. different stimulations of the somatosensory system. In both tinnitus and pain, the alleviation of the pathological sensation may outlast the cessation of the alleviating stimulus (residual inhibition). Finally, anaesthetic agents can suppress both sensations.

The 'gate control' theory implies the joint action of two different fibre systems, which together with relay neurones in the brainstem form a 'gate control system'. The 'gate' regulates the input of information from the peripheral to the central auditory system. If the input is increased as a result of damaged hair cells, then the gate will stay open for a longer period of time as a result of adaptation.

A benefit of this model is that it opens up options for treatment programmes like physiotherapy or treatment of temporomandibular dysfunctions. A shortcoming is that this theory is very theoretical and has still not been verified for tinnitus.

Model 4—The neural model of ephaptic transmission for tinnitus

The neural model of ephaptic interaction between nerve fibres seems to be valid in cases of tinnitus caused by auditory nerve damage (e.g. acoustical neurinoma, demyelinating diseases).[25,26] If the myelin sheaths of the nerve fibres are damaged and the electrical isolation between the fibres is lost, this might lead to ephaptic transmission across or 'cross-talk' between fibres. This will alter the normally stochastic spontaneous activity in the auditory nerve, because the neural activity between fibres will be pathologically synchronized and interpreted as 'sound' by the central auditory system. This model is also valid for tinnitus caused by surgery on the VIIIth nerve. A benefit of this model is that it is supported by both clinical and experimental studies. In humans, a gaze-evoked tinnitus may occur after deafferentation that can be turned on and off by eye movements.[35]

The mechanisms and neuroanatomical sites of this phenomenon are not known. According to the neural sprouting hypothesis, gaze-evoked tinnitus is caused by a regeneration of neurones and new synapse formation between the para-abducens nucleus and the cochlear nucleus or between the auditory pathways and the neural integrator for eye movements. Owing to reactive synaptogenesis, intact axons will grow and replace those lost by injury. This possibility is supported by experimental studies on animals in which both degenerative and regenerative changes are found in the peripheral and central auditory pathways, after complete unilateral deafferentation of the auditory periphery (cochlea and/or auditory nerve). Changes in gaze can also act as powerful triggers and/or suppressors of a variety of phantom sensory and motor events. These findings are in accordance with the suggestion that synchronous neural activity from the ocular motor system can be transmitted to the auditory system and the central auditory system will interpret this activity as 'sound'.

The benefit of this model is that it is supported by experimental studies. A shortcoming is that only a few patients suffer from this particular phenomenon.

> It is crucial to distinguish between the aetiology of the onset of tinnitus and the aetiology of the development of tinnitus suffering.

Neurophysiological models of tinnitus suffering

It is of great importance to be aware of all aspects of possible mechanisms leading to suffering associated with tinnitus. In each case, a careful audiological and neuro-otological approach requires evaluation to investigate the aetiology of the onset of tinnitus, but also factors relevant to why the patient suffers from tinnitus. To differentiate between the aetiology of tinnitus and the aetiology of tinnitus suffering is crucial. It is not uncommon for patients who have had tinnitus many times or have had it for many years to suddenly develop persistent tinnitus and/or tinnitus that becomes a troublesome problem.

The neurophysiological model

As we have pointed out earlier, one has to separate the induction of tinnitus from the maintenance of tinnitus leading to suffering complaint. Jastreboff and Hazell[28] suggest why some patients suffer more from the symptoms of tinnitus than others. The model focuses on the network of neural activity in the parasympathetic and sympathetic autonomic nervous systems, the auditory system and the limbic system (including the cortical structures (the olfactory cortex, hippocampal formation, cingulate gyrus, subcallosal gyrus) and subcortical areas, including the amygdala, septum, hypothalamus, epithalamus, anterior thalamic nuclei and parts of the basal ganglia). The auditory periphery is described as the source of tinnitus. All levels of the auditory pathways, from the cochlea, auditory subcortical centres to the auditory cortex, are necessary in creating the perception of tinnitus. The pathological spontaneous activity which results from cochlear damage is processed by subcortical auditory centres and by the limbic system, before the action potentials reach the auditory cortex. In non-sufferers, it is suggested that the tinnitus-related neural activity remains constrained within the auditory pathways. Therefore, the person is not bothered by tinnitus. However, in tinnitus sufferers, activation of the limbic and autonomic nervous systems plays a crucial role by establishing strong negative emotions related to the tinnitus sensation and also, simultaneously, various defence responses of the body. These researchers point out the importance of focusing upon such reactions in the management of tinnitus patients. Tinnitus retraining therapy (TRT) is based on this theory.[36,37]

The model is highly relevant clinically, because it is well understood by patients. The benefit of this model is that involvement of the limbic system in tinnitus perception was demonstrated by PET-scan studies demonstrating increased bloodflow in the limbic system and in the auditory cortex when tinnitus was turned on and off by orofacial movements.[38] However, the theory that tinnitus is generated in the cochlea is not supported by PET-scan studies.

In non-sufferers, it is suggested that the tinnitus-related neural activity remains constrained within the auditory pathways. In tinnitus sufferers, activation of the limbic and autonomic nervous systems plays a crucial role by establishing strong negative emotions related to the tinnitus sensation and also, simultaneously, various defence responses of the body.

Somatic modulation of tinnitus

The interpretation of the 'tinnitus signal' is also considered to be related to the activity of the central nervous system other than the auditory system, the limbic system and the autonomic nervous system. Activity in the somatosensory systems may influence the tinnitus sensation, and is called 'somatic modulation of tinnitus'. By stimulating the median nerve, tinnitus loudness was altered,[39] suggesting a connection between the auditory and somatosensory systems. It is also well known that the annoyance of tinnitus is increased if the patient has pain, i.e. in the neck or head, or suffers from temporomandibular dysfunction (TMD).[39–42] TMD is a collective term for a number of clinical problems that involve the masticatory muscles, the temporomandibular joint and associated structures. Tinnitus is one of the otological symptoms frequently reported by patients with TMD; additionally, Rubinstein[41] reported that 30% of tinnitus patients could change their tinnitus with jaw movements. Moreover, extremity and head or neck manipulations modulate tinnitus, and head or neck manoeuvres are twice as likely to alter the tinnitus signal as extremity manipulations.[42] Somatic–auditory interactions are hypothesized to take place at the level of the dorsal cochlear nucleus, which receives ipsilateral auditory and somatic inputs. One hypothesis is that the interaction between these signals determines whether or not the patients will be aware of the tinnitus signals. Accordingly, a somatic modulation of tinnitus has been suggested.

Neurophysiological model of the aetiology and treatment of tinnitus suffering

Another more recent description also distinguishes between the mechanisms of the awareness of tinnitus and those involved in the suffering. This model is based on research focusing on the severity of tinnitus.[13, 14, 20, 40, 43] High scores on all dimensions of the NHP (Nottingham Health Profile), such as 'Emotional disturbances', 'Sleep disturbances', 'Pain', 'Physical mobility', 'Social isolation' and 'Energy', were found in patients with tinnitus who had tinnitus that severely influenced their working capacity.[20] They also had high scores on several items of the Tinnitus Severity Questionnaire. The strongest predictors for the development of such severe tinnitus were the depression factors and the physical immobility factor in the NHP. However, the pure tone averages of hearing thresholds at the low and middle frequencies were moderate predictors only. It has also been found that the occurrence of depression and anxiety disorder according to DSM-IIIR was 75% in consecutive tinnitus patients seeking help at an audiological department.[20, 43] Preliminary results have shown that the occurrence of depression and anxiety disorders is even higher in patients with a high risk of developing incapacitating tinnitus. Based on these findings, which are in accordance with those of other researchers, it is possible to categorize the suffering of tinnitus into:

- somatic tinnitus
- depression–anxiety-related tinnitus
- audiological tinnitus.

A schematic model has been proposed to describe the development of severe tinnitus suffering starting from the occurrence of tinnitus (Figure 32.4). By identifying the aetiology or aetiologies of the patients suffering, the rehabilitation may thereafter be chosen based on these aetiology/aetiologies found in each individual case. This approach is presented in Figure 32.5 and is aimed at stopping or reducing the negative development of persistent severe tinnitus, following the onset of tinnitus.

The onset of tinnitus is suggested to be a consequence of different types of damage which have resulted in hearing impairment. Mainly, the suffering of tinnitus can be due to somatic disorders, audiological disorders or depressive and anxiety disorders, or a monoaminergic vulnerability.

Monoaminergic-vulnerability model of tinnitus

As already described, the majority of consecutive tinnitus patients who seek help at an audiological clinic have anxiety and depressive disorders.[43]

This common comorbitidy of psychiatric symptoms and tinnitus raises questions about the possibility of common neurochemical dysfunctions.[44] The neurotransmitter serotonin is a likely candidate, because of its involvement in the modulation of the sensory processing in the primary auditory cortex,[45, 46] and the serotonin transporter is reported to be involved in unipolar as well as bipolar depression.[47] Antidepressant drugs which modulate serotonergic functions in the brain have been used in a clinical trial by Dobie et al,[48] and they reported on the positive effect of nortriptyline in the treatment of patients with tinnitus and depressive symptoms. Their results showed a reduction in depression parameters, functional disability, and the audiometrically measured tinnitus loudness and frequency.

Salvi and collegues suggested that the plastic changes in the auditory pathways after noise trauma created a hyperexcitability which could create the tinnitus sensation.[49] The plastic changes in the auditory cortex consisting of the generation of new synaptic contacts are likely to be random in nature.

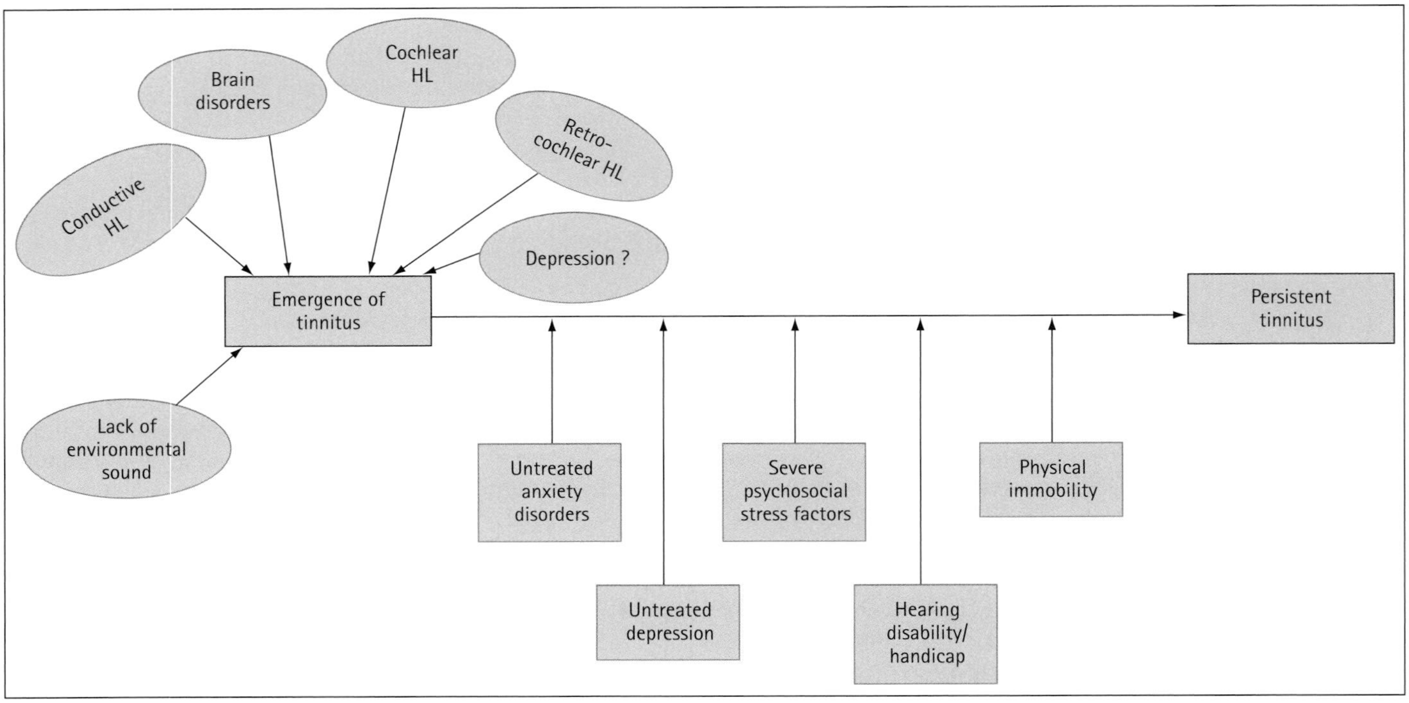

Figure 32.4 Different aetiological factors for the development of persistent tinnitus. HL, hearing loss. (Translated from Holgers,[14] used by permission.)

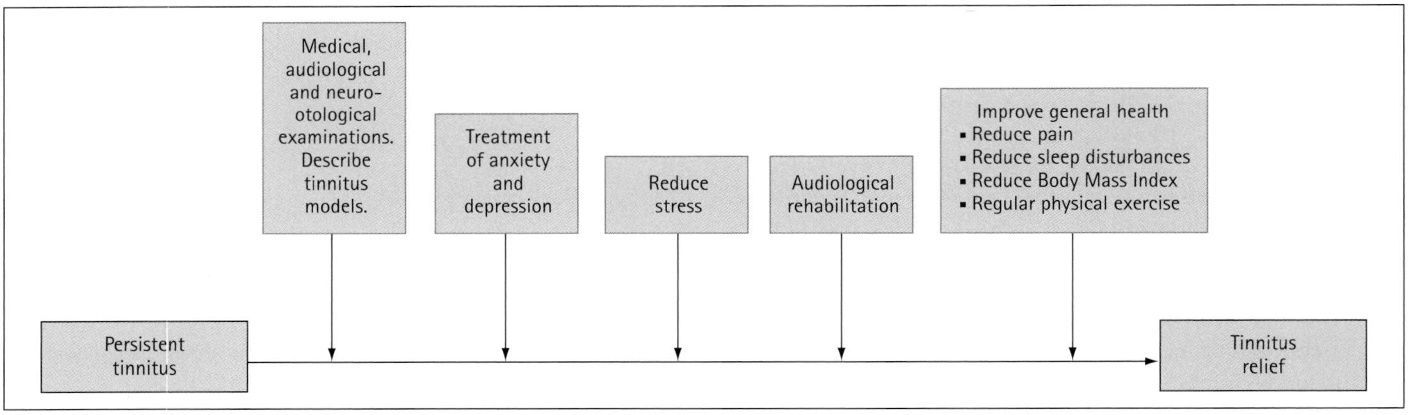

Figure 32.5 Aetiologically based tinnitus therapy, a model for management of tinnitus. (Translated from Holgers. Tinnitus vårdprogram 2000 Stockholm: National Board of Health and Welfare, 1999.[14] Used by permission.)

In some individuals, these changes may include contact between neurones that represents tinnitus, while in others the neurological changes could be insignificant.

It has been suggested that it is possible that there is a vulnerability in the monoaminergic system, presumably in the serotonergic system, in patients who perceive severe tinnitus.[43,44] Serotonergic nerve endings are present in the auditory nuclei, such as the superior olivary complex, the lateral leminiscus, the inferior colliculus and the cochlear nucleus, as well as in the primary auditory cortex.[50–52] It is possible that changes in the neurotransmission, changes in the monoaminergic receptors or changes of the transporters are present, due to a vulnerability in these neurochemical systems. This vulnerability may lead to the development of severe tinnitus.

The neurochemical-vulnerability model, according to Holgers and Zöger,[44] suggests that it is possible that a vulnerable monoaminergic system is present in patients who develop severe tinnitus, as it is in patients developing depression. It is also possible that the mechanisms behind these changes may lead to tinnitus in some patients, to depression in others, and to both depression and tinnitus in others.

The neurochemical-vulnerability model suggests that it is possible that a vulnerable monoaminergic system is present in patients who develop severe tinnitus, as it is in patients developing depression.

Clinical tinnitus assessment

In the authors' clinical experience, the majority of tinnitus patients only visit the clinic once or twice, during an 18-month period. However, more persistent tinnitus generates more suffering. This makes a patient seek more frequent help in order to try to reduce the symptoms. If tinnitus treatment is to be successful, it is of great importance to use instruments and methods by which patients who are at a high risk of severe persistent tinnitus can be identified. It is also important to identify the predictive factors which have a strong impact on the daily life and wellbeing of the tinnitus patient.

In the clinical management of tinnitus patients, it is essential to have reliable tools to examine the tinnitus symptoms and predictors and to be able to analyse the effect of different tinnitus therapies. Usually, tinnitus is assessed by clinical gradings, psychometrically and/or psychoacoustically.

Clinical gradings

The degree of tinnitus can be described by using clinical gradings based on judgements of tinnitus severity, such as grading into different categories (not always present (I) /always present (II) and always disturbing (III)).[53] Based on epidemiological data from the MRC Institute of Hearing Research, Coles categorized tinnitus annoyance into none, slight, moderate and severe, and also by the degree of tinnitus effect on life—none, slight, moderate, severe.[3] Some authors have categorized patients into help-seeking or not help-seeking and complainers or non-complainers.[54, 55] A rather robust method is to determine whether or not tinnitus affects the working capacity.[8]

Patients are also often asked to describe both the quality of their tinnitus sounds and the localization of their tinnitus. The subjective description of tinnitus (ringing, buzzing, whistling, pulsatile) has been reported not to correlate with tinnitus aetiology.[56] It is reported that 'tonal tinnitus' and tinnitus of high pitch are the most common descriptions, and bilateral tinnitus is more common than unilateral.[57, 58]

The degree of tinnitus can be described in different ways:

- how often tinnitus occurs
- how intrusive tinnitus is perceived to be
- how tinnitus causes limitations in daily life
- how tinnitus affects the patient mentally
- the effect on working capacity
- how tinnitus affects general health and life quality.

However, one major problem in the assessment of tinnitus is the lack of objective measurements. The character of tinnitus symptoms is multi-dimensional and very complex. Therefore, it is important to use instruments that assess a variety of faces of tinnitus suffering, such as concentration, sleep problems, hearing difficulties, anxiety, depression disorders, and different psychosomatic problems. Owing to the subjectivity of tinnitus symptoms, a variety of questionnaires for measuring different aspects and perceptions of tinnitus severity have been used.[5, 8, 21–23, 54, 55, 59–68]

> The character of tinnitus symptoms is multi-dimensional and very complex. Therefore, it is important to use instruments that assess a variety of facets of tinnitus suffering.

In Table 32.1, examples of well-known instruments and measurements are outlined, including the number of items, levels, dimension of the instruments and reliability. In Table 32.2, correlations between these instruments/measurements and other parameters such as hearing parameters, psychological measurements and aspects of general health are summarized. When investigating the outcome of an intervention, instruments should be chosen that assess the aspects of tinnitus focused upon by the intervention.

Psychoacoustical measurements

Psychoacoustical measurements include matching of tinnitus quality, pitch, loudness and masking levels.[69–78]

Tinnitus pitch is often a high-frequency sound in patients with noise-induced hearing loss,[79] but it is not possible to use pitch measurements as indicators of noise-induced hearing loss. Tinnitus loudness often appears to be close to the hearing thresholds at the poorest audiometric frequency.[79, 80] The individual tinnitus sensation level, i.e. the difference between the tinnitus audiometric level and hearing threshold, is approximately 5 dB HL.[79, 80]

The maskeability of tinnitus can be regarded as a possible method to describe the intrusiveness of tinnitus by analysing the sound level needed to mask tinnitus. Both narrow- and broadband noise have been used.[81–85] When performing measurements of the maskeability of tinnitus, the localization of the masking noise generator (left or right ear) did not seem to matter.[81] This implies that central components of tinnitus awareness are important. The value of these assessments is in dispute as, often, only weak correlations have been reported between perceived tinnitus severity and psychoacoustical tinnitus measurements.

Questionnaires

Many different questionnaires are used in the management of tinnitus. There are two main types, namely non-diagnosis-specific and tinnitus-specific questionnaires.

Usually, questionnaires are self-assessed and distributed to the patient by mail or in the clinic. The questionnaires may also be used as tools when conducting face-to-face interviews. When using different questionnaires, it is of great importance to have information about the quality of each specific instrument, e.g. the reliability, i.e. test–rest reliability, or the internal

Table 32.1 Examples of instruments and measurements, number of items, levels and dimension.

Instruments and/or clinical instruments	Number of items and levels	Reliability/consistency	Dimensions
TSQ Coles et al,[59] Baskill et al,[60] Erlandsson et al,[23] Holgers and Barrenäs,[5] Erlandsson and Holgers[40]	10 items 5 levels	Test-retest 0.62–0.72 High internal consistency	I General tinnitus severity II Life quality III Psychological aspects
THI Newman et al,[63] Newman et al,[62] Newman et al[61]	25 items 3 levels	Cronbach $\alpha = 0.93$ THI versus THQ $r = 0.78$	I Functional II Emotional III Catastrophic
THQ Kuk et al,[64] Newman et al,[63] Newman et al,[62] Newman et al,[61] Meric et al[7]	27 items scale of 0–100	Cronbach $\alpha = 0.93$ THI versus THQ $r = 0.78$ Test-retest $r = 0.89$	I Effects of tinnitus on social emotional and physical behaviours II Hearing ability III Patient's view of tinnitus
TRQ Meric et al,[7] Wilson et al[65]	26 items 5 levels	Test-retest 0.88 Cronbach $\alpha = 0.96$	I General distress II Interference with work and leasure activities III Severe signs of distress IV Avoidance of activities
STSS and clinical ratings (1–3) Halford et al[66]	16 items 2 levels	Clinical validity versus STSS $r = 0.73$ $r = 0.76$	I Distress intrusion II Cognitive focus III Irritant IV Constancy focus V Distraction
THSS Erlandsson et al[23]	28 items 5 levels		I Perceived attitudes II Social support NS III Disability handicap–0.66
TQ Hallam,[67] Goebel and Hiller[68]	40 items 3 levels	Test-retest 0.94 Cronbach $\alpha = 0.94$	I Emotional and cognitive distress II Intrusiveness III Hearing difficulties IV Sleep disturbances V Somatic complaints
Help-seeking (H) Non Help-seeking (NH) Attias et al,[54] Hallberg and Erlandsson[55]	2 levels		Help-seeking/non help-seeking related to tinnitus
AWT ± Holgers et al[8]	2 levels		Sick leave related to tinnitus

TSQ, Tinnitus Severity Questionnaire; THI, Tinnitus Handicap Inventory; THQ, Tinnitus Handicap Questionnaire; TRQ, Tinnitus Reaction Questionnaire; STSS, Subjective Tinnitus Severity Scale; H, Help-seeking; NH, Non-Help-seeking; AWT, Absence from Work; NHP, Nottingham Health Profile; BDI, Beck Depression Inventory; MMPI, Minnesota Multiphasic Personality Inventory; BMI, body mass index; PTA, pure tone average; SRSL, Symptom Rating Scale List; NS, not significant.

Table 32.2 Correlations between the instruments/measurements and psychoacoustical, psychological measurements and aspects of general health are presented.

Instruments and/or clinical gradings	Correlation with audiometry	Correlation with psychology	Correlation with general health
TSQ Coles et al,[59] Baskill et al,[60] Erlandsson et al,[23] Holgers and Barrenäs,[5] Erlandsson and Holgers[40]	TSQ versus hearing parameters NS TSQ versus PTA 3; 4; 6 kHz moderate	TSQ versus perceived attitudes (THSS) low TSQ versus disability/handicap (THSS) moderate TSQ versus emotional disturbances (NHP) high	Frequent headache low Dizziness/vertigo low Oversensitivity to sounds low TSQ versus pain and sleep/NHP moderate
THI Newman et al,[63] Newman et al,[62] Newman et al[61]	THI versus pitch and loudness low	THI versus BDI week versus SRSL high	THI versus MSPQ week THQ versus general health moderate
THQ Kuk et al,[64] Newman et al,[63] Newman et al,[62] Newman et al,[61] Meric et al[7] Loudness match–NS Mean hearing thresholds–moderate	THQ versus loudness match NS PTA NS–moderate	THQ versus MMPI low versus perceived loudness moderate versus depression moderate versus life satisfaction moderate	THQ versus general health moderate
TRQ Meric et al,[7] Wilson et al[65]		TRQ versus MMPI low	
STSS and clinical ratings (1–3) Halford et al[66]	STSS versus loudness match at 1 kHz moderate	Clinical ratings versus STSS high	
THSS Erlandsson et al[23]			
Help-seeking (H) Non Help-seeking (NH) Attias et al,[54] Hallberg and Erlandsson[33,55]	Pure tone thresholds lower in H than NH	More concentration difficulties, irritability and psychiatric symptomatology in the H group	
AWT ± Holgers et al[8]	AWT versus hearing thresholds moderate Speech recognition test NS	ANT versus emotional reactions, social isolation (NHP) high	NHP; physical immobility, sleep, pain Energy (NHP) moderate–high BMT; physical exercise

TSQ, Tinnitus Severity Questionnaire; THI, Tinnitus Handicap Inventory; THQ, Tinnitus Handicap Questionnaire; TRQ, Tinnitus Reaction Questionnaire; STSS, Subjective Tinnitus Severity Scale; H, Help-seeking; NH, Non-Help-seeking; AWT, Absence from Work; THSS, Tinnitus Handicap and Support Scale; NHP, Nottingham Health Profile; BDI, Beck Depression Inventory; MMPI, Minnesota Multiphasic Personality Inventory; MSPQ, Modified Somatic Perception Questionnaire; PLU, Personal Loudness Units; NS, not significant.

consistency (Cronbach's α), but also the validity, i.e. correlations with other measurements.

The review presented in Table 32.2 focuses upon tinnitus-specific questionnaires, and how they correlate with psychoacoustical audiometric variables and with different dimensions of non-diagnosis-specific questionnaires and different clinical gradings. As can be observed upon review, when analysing tinnitus severity in relation to inner ear damage, non-significant or weak correlations have often been reported between perceived tinnitus severity and psychoacoustically measured tinnitus and hearing function. Nonetheless, some reports have presented moderate correlations between tinnitus severity and audiometric parameters, such as pure tone averages and tinnitus loudness match. However, the relationship between audiometry and tinnitus severity is reported to be weaker than the correlation between tinnitus severity and psychological factors, e.g. depression, concentration problems and irritability. Other important aetiological factors influencing tinnitus severity are poor general health, poor sleep patterns, and pain. The suffering of tinnitus is also correlated with frequent headaches, dizziness and oversensitivity to sound, as can be seen in Table 32.2. It is important to be aware of those symptoms that may be considered by the patient to be related to tinnitus suffering but that may also be due to a depressive disorder. It is of great importance to identify and treat depressive disorders early.

> The relationship between audiometry and tinnitus severity is reported to be weaker than the correlation between tinnitus severity and psychological factors. Symptoms related to tinnitus may also be symptoms of a current depressive disorder.

Other techniques for measuring tinnitus

Auditory brainstem responses (ABRs)

Several studies have evaluated the ABR responses in tinnitus patients, aiming to localize tinnitus and assess central auditory dysfunction.[86–92] In some reports, the test stimuli during ABR recording can mask tinnitus and, therefore, it can be difficult to use ABR in these patients.[86]

Four main types of observation have been reported:

- changes in morphology of the ABR waveform
- fluctuation in amplitude of waves III and V
- prolonged brainstem transmission time
- lidocaine effect on the morphology of the waveform.

Rosenhall and Axelsson[89] reported on prolonged responses of wave I accompanied by a prolongation of waves III and V in tinnitus patients compared to normal controls. A lengthening of the III–V interpeak latencies was also reported. These findings indicate both peripheral dysfunction and dysfunction in the brainstem. Lemaire and Beutter[90] reported that the ABR findings in tinnitus patients differed by gender. However, tinnitus was always associated with a significant lengthening of 0–I and I–V latencies on the tinnitus-affected side. However, when comparing ABR responses from tinnitus patients and normal controls, the changes have not always been conclusive.[91, 92]

Compression of the intracranial portion of the cochlear nerve has been suggested to cause severe tinnitus. In patients with severe tinnitus, a prolonged interpeak latency of peaks I–III (0.2 ms or more) or a prolonged interpeak latency of III–V (0.2 ms or more) has been used as an inclusion criterion for microvascular decompression surgery of the cochlear nerve.[93, 94] However, there is a high incidence of asymptomatic individuals who have compression of the nerve without having any symptoms,[94] so this treatment should be used very carefully. This treatment should not be performed without investigating the psychological/psychiatrical status of the patients.[8]

Auditory evoked magnetic field (AEF)

Hoke et al.[95,96] and Pantev et al.[97] reported that the amplitude ratio of the two major waves of the auditory evoked magnetic field (AEF), M200/M100, could be used as an objective measurement allowing discrimination between individuals suffering from tinnitus (ratio less than 0.5) and individuals without tinnitus (ratio greater than 0.5). However, Jacobson et al.[98] could not verify these findings. This inconsistency could be due to the selection of subjects tested. Hoke et al.[99] also reported on the age effect on these responses. In normally-hearing individuals, the average amplitude ratio decreases linearly with age.

Functional magnetic resonance imaging

By using functional magnetic resonance imaging (fMRI), it seems possible to investigate tinnitus-related abnormalities in brain function in patients with lateralization of tinnitus. The method is, however, based on masking noise stimulus which is used to change tinnitus loudness and examining the corresponding changes in activity of the inferior colliculus (IC). For lateralized tinnitus subjects, the sound-evoked activation showed an asymmetric IC, but in the control group, the right versus left IC did not differ significantly.

Positron emission tomography

The bloodflow in the brain can be measured using positron emission tomography. Increased activity in the primary auditory cortex in tinnitus patients compared to normal controls was reported in a study by Arnold et al.[100] This study was supported by other researchers,[38] who also found indices for the involvement of the hippocampus. In Denmark, Mirz et al.[101] reported that the increased neuronal activity caused by tinnitus occurred predominantly in the right hemisphere, with significant foci in the middle frontal and middle temporal gyri, in addition to lateral and mesial posterior sites. These results are consistent with the hypothesis that the sensation of tinnitus is associated with activity in cortical areas functionally linked to functions such as attention, emotion and memory, and supports the neurophysiological models earlier presented.

Conclusion

Different models focus on the results of damage to the sensory cells in the cochlea as the aetiology of tinnitus. However, these models do not explain why tinnitus causes suffering in some persons. Since not all patients with hearing loss suffer from tinnitus, additional explanations are necessary. The depression factor had a very strong impact on working ability for tinnitus patients, so a procedure for identifying depressive and anxiety disorders in tinnitus patients should be included in the early contact with tinnitus patients. Tinnitus comorbidity with depressive and anxiety disorders is high, and a monoaminergic-vulnerability model has been suggested to be a predisposing factor to induce the development of severe tinnitus. It is of great importance to be aware of all aspects of possible mechanisms beyond the symptom of tinnitus. A careful audiological, somatic and neuro-otological approach must be carried out in each patient, to investigate the aetiology of the debut of tinnitus and to find out the reason why the patient suffers from tinnitus.

Acknowledgement

We are grateful to the Regional Health Authority in West Sweden and the National Board of Health and Welfare for financial grants. We would also like to acknowledge Professor Linda Luxon and Dr Derek N. Eder for valuable comments.

References

1. Axelsson A, Ringdahl A. Tinnitus—a study of its prevalence and characteristics. *Br J Audiol* 1989; **23**: 53–62.
2. Davies AC. *Hearing in Adults*. London: Whurr, 1995.
3. Coles RRA, David AC, Haggard MP. Epidemiology of tinnitus. In: Evered D, Lauresson G, (eds.), London: *Tinnitus CIBA Foundation Symposium* 85. Pitman 1981.
4. Davies AC. The prevalence of hearing impairment and reported hearing disability among adults in Great Britain. *Int J Epidemiol* 1989; **18**: 911–17.
5. Holgers KM, Barrenäs ML. The correlation between speech recognition scores in noise in patients with no, mild or severe tinnitus. In: XXIII *International Congress Of Audiology*, Bari, 1996.
6. Meikle MB, Griest SE. Gender based differences in characteristics of tinnitus. *Hear J* 1989; **42**: 68–76.
7. Meric C, Gartner M, Collet L, Chéry-Croze S. Psychopathological profile of tinnitus sufferers: evidence concerning the relationship between tinnitus features and impact on life. *Audiol Neurootol* 1998; **3**: 240–52.
8. Holgers K-M, Erlandsson SI, Barrenäs M-L, Predictive factors for the severity of tinnitus. *Audiology* 2000; **39**: 284–91.
9. Nodar RH. Tinnitus aurium in school age children: a survey. *J Audiol Res* 1972; **12**: 133–5.
10. Mills RP. Tinnitus in childhood. *Clin Otolaryngol* 1986; **11**: 431–4.
11. Graham J. Tinnitus in hearing-impaired children. *Tinnitus*. 1987; **7**: 137–43.
12. Stouffer JL, Tyler RS, Booth JC Buckrell B. Tinnitus in normal-hearing and hearing-impaired children. In: Aran JM, ed. *Proceedings of the Fourth International Tints Seminar*. New York: Kugler, 1991: 255–8.
13. Holgers KM. Tinnitus in children. In: Hazell J, ed. *Sixth International Tinnitus Seminar*, Cambridge. King's Lynn: Biddles Short Run Books Ltd, 1999: 218–19.
14. Holgers KM. *Tinnitus vårdprogram '2000* Stockholm: National Board of Health and Welfare, 1999.
15. Chole RA, Parker WS. Tinnitus and vertigo in patients with temporomandibular disorders. *Arch Otolaryngol Head Neck Surg* 1992; **118**: 817–21.
16. Vernon J, Griest S, Press L. Attributes of tinnitus that may predict temporomandibular joint dysfunction. *J Craniomand Pract* 1992; **10**: 282–7.
17. Rubinstein B, Erlandsson S. A stomatognatic analysis of patients with disabling tinnitus and craniomandibular disorder. *Br J Audiol* 1991; **25**: 77–83.
18. Seligmann H, Podoshin L, Ben-David J, Fradis M, Goldsher M. Drug-induced tinnitus and other hearing disorders. *Drug Safety* 1996; **14**(3): 198–212.
19. Iwarsson S, Andersson D, Gretzer-Quick I. et al. (eds). *FASS 2000*. Stockholm: LINFO AB, 2000.
20. Holgers KM, Zöger S, Svedlund J, Erlandsson SI. Psychiatrical profiles of tinnitus patients seeking help at an audiological clinic. In: Hazell JW ed. *Sixth International Tinnitus Seminar*. King's Lynn: Biddles Short Run Books Ltd, 1999: 283–5.
21. Gerber KE, Nehemikis AM, Chawter RA, Jones HC. Is tinnitus a psychological disorder? *Int J Psychiatry* 1985/86; **15**: 81–7.
22. Collet L, Moussu MF, Disant F, Ahami T, Morgan A. Minnesota Multiphasic Personality inventory in tinnitus disorders. *Audiology* 1990; **28**: 101–6.
23. Erlandsson S, Hallberg L, Axelsson A. Psychological and audiological correlates of perceived tinnitus severity. *Audiology* 1992; **31**: 168–79.
24. Coles R. In: Reich GE, Vernon JA, eds. *Proceedings of the Fifth International Tinnitus Seminar*, Portland, Oregon, USA. American Tinnitus Association, 1995: 25–9.
25. Eggermont JJ. On the pathophysiology of tinnitus; a review and a peripheral model. *Hear Res* 1990; **48**: 111–24.
26. Moller AR. Pathophysiology of tinnitus. *Ann Otol Rhinol Laryngol* 1984; **93**(1 Pt 1): 39–44.
27. Lenarz T, Schreiner C, Snyder RL, Ernst A. Neural mechanisms of tinnitus. *Eur Arch Otorhinolaryngol* 1993; **249**(8): 441–6.
28. Jastreboff PJ, Hazell JWP. A neurophysiological approach to tinnitus: clinical implications. *Br J of Audiol* 1993; **27**: 7–17.
29. Eggermont JJ, Kenmochi M. Salicylate and quinine selectively increase spontaneous firing rates in secondary auditory cortex. *Hear Res* 1998; **117**(1–2): 149–60.
30. Jastreboff PJ, Brennan JF, Sasaki CT. Animal models of tinnitus. *Laryngoscope* 1988; **98**: 280–286.
31. Kellerhals B, Zogg R. Tinnitus-induced weight loss in rats. An

animal model for tinnitus research. *ORL J Otorhinolaryngol Relat Spec* 1991; **53**(6): 331–4.
32. Jastreboff P, Sakai CT. Salicylate-induced changes in the spontaneous activity of single units in the inferior colliculus of the guinea pig. *J Acoust Soc Am* 1986; **80**: 1384–91.
33. Zenner HP, Ernst A. Cochlear-motor, transduction and signal-transfer tinnitus: models for three types of cochlear tinnitus. *Eur Arch Otorhinolaryngol* 1993; **249**(8): 447–54.
34. Tonndorf J. The analogy between tinnitus and pain: a suggestion for a physiological basis of chronic tinnitus. *Hear Res* 1987; **28**(2–3): 271–5.
35. Cacace A, Lovely T, Parnes S, Winter D, McFarland D, Gaze-evoked tinnitus following unilateral peripheral auditory deafferentation: a case for anomalous crossmodal plasticity. In: Salvi RJ, ed. *Auditory System Plasticity and Regeneration*. New York: Thieme Medical Publishers Inc., 1996: 354–8.
36. Jastreboff P, Jastreboff M, How TRT derives from the neurophysiological model. In: *Proceedings of the VIth International Tinnitus Seminar* 1999.
37. Hazell JWP. The TRT method in practice. In: *Proceedings of the VIth International Tinnitus Seminar* 1999.
38. Lockwood AH, Salvi RJ, Coad ML, Towsley ML, Wack DS, Murphy BW. The functional neuroanatomy of tinnitus: evidence for limbic system links and neural plasticity. *Neurology* 1998; **50**(1): 114–20.
39. Moller AR, Moller MB, Yokota M. Some forms of tinnitus may involve the extralemniscal auditory pathway. *Laryngoscope* 1992; **102**: 1165–71.
40. Erlandsson SI Holgers KM. The relationship between perceived tinnitus severity and health-related quality of life with aspects of gender. *Noise Health*.
41. Rubinstein B. Tinnitus and craniomandibular disorders. Is there a link? Doctoral thesis, University of Göteborg, 1993.
42. Levine RA. Somatic modulation appears to be a fundamental attribute of tinnitus. In: Hazell JW, ed. *Sixth International Tinnitus Seminar*. Biddles Short Run Books, King's Lynn: 1999; 193–7.
43. Zöger S, Svedlund J, Holgers KM. Psychiatric disorders in tinnitus patients without severe hearing impairment: 24 month follow-up of patients at an audiologic clinic. *Audiology* 2001; **40**: 133–40.
44. Holgers KM, Zöger S. *1st Etiologically Based Tinnitus Therapy Course*, Thorskog, Sweden, 1999.
45. Hegerl U, Juckel G. Intensity dependence of auditory evoked potentials as indicators of central serotonergic neurotransmission —new hypothesis. *Biol Psychiatry* 1993; **33**: 173–87.
46. Juckel G, Monar M, Hegerl U, Csèpe V, Karmos G. Auditory evoked potentials as indicator of brain serotonergic activity—first evidence in behaving cats. *Biol Psychiatry* 1997; **41**: 1181–95.
47. Ressler KJ and Nemeroff CB. Role of serotonergic and noradrenergic systems in the pathophysiology of depression and anxiety disorders. *Depression and Anxiety* 2000; **12**: 2–19.
48. Dobie R, Sakai CS, Sullivan MD, Katon WJ, Russo J. 'Antidepressant treatment of tinnitus patients: report of a randomized clinical trial and clinical prediction of benefit.' *Am J Otol* 1993; **14**(1): 18–23.
49. Salvi R, Wang J Powers N. Rapid functional reorganization in the inferior colliculus and cochlear nucleus after acute cochlear damage. In: Salvi R, Henderson D, Fiorino F, Colletti V eds. Auditory System Plasticity and Regeneration. New York: Thieme Medical Publishers Inc., 1996: 275–96.
50. Woods CI, Azeredo WJ. Noradrenergic and serotonergic projections to the superior olive: potential for modulation of olivocochlear neurons. *Brain Res* 1999; **836**: 9–18.
51. Thompson GC, Thompson AM, Garrett KM, Britton BH. Serotonin and serotonin receptors in the central auditory system. *Otolaryngol Head Neck Surg* 1994; **110**: 93–103.
52. Andorn AC, Vittorio JA, Bellflower J. ^{3}H-spiroperidol binding in human temporal cortex (Brodmann areas 41–42) occurs at multiple high affinity state with serotonergic selectivity. *Psychopharmacology* 1989; **99**: 520–5.
53. Klockhoff I, Lindblom U. Meniere's disease and hydrochlorothiazide (Dichlotride)—a critical analysis of symptoms and therapeutic effects. *Acta Otolaryngol (Stockh)* 1967; **63**: 347–65.
54. Attias J, Shemesh A, Bleich A et al. Psychological profile of help-seeking and non-help-seeking tinnitus patients. *Scand Audiol* 1995; **24**: 13–18.
55. Hallberg L, Erlandsson S. Tinnitus characteristics in tinnitus complainers and noncomplainers. *Br J Audiol* 1993; **27**: 19–27.
56. Alberti PW. Tinnitus in occupational hearing loss: nosological aspects. *J Otolaryngol* 1987; **16**: 34–5
57. Stouffer JL, Tyler RS. Characterization of tinnitus by tinnitus patients. *J Speech Hear Res* 1990; **55**: 439–53.
58. Meikle MB, Taylor-Walsh E. Characteristics of tinnitus and related observations in over 1800 tinnitus clinic patients. *J Laryngol Otol* 1984; **9**: 17–21.
59. Coles RRA, Lutman ME, Axelsson A, Hazell JWP. Tinnitus severity gradings; cross sectional studies. In: Aran JM, Dauman R, eds. *Tinnitus 91 Fourth International Tinnitus Seminar*. Bordeaux: Kugler, 1991; 453–5.
60. Baskill JL, Coles RRA, Lutman ME, Axelsson A. Tinnitus severity grading: longitudinal studies. In: Aran JM, Dauman R, eds. *Proceedings of the Fourth International Tinnitus Seminar*. Bordeaux: Kugler, 1991; 457–60.
61. Newman CW, Sandridge SA, Jacobson GP. Psychometric adequacy of the tinnitus handicap inventory (THI) for evaluating treatment outcome. *J Am Acad Audiol* 1998; **9**: 153–160.
62. Newman CW, Jacobson GP, Spitzer JB. Development of the tinnitus handicap inventory. *Arch Otolaryngol Head Neck Surg* 1996; **122**: 143–8.
63. Newman CW, Wharton JA, Shivapuja BG, Jacobson GP. Relationships among psychoacoustic judgements, speech understanding ability and self-perceived handicap in tinnitus subject. *Audiology* 1994; **33**: 47–60.
64. Kuk F, Tyler RS, Russell D, Jordan H. The psychometric properties of a tinnitus handicap questionnaire. *Ear Hear* 1990; **11**: 434–45.
65. Wilson PH, Henry J, Bowen M, Haralambous G. Tinnitus reaction questionnaire: psychometric properties of a measure of distress associated with tinnitus. *J Speech Hear Res* 1991; **34**: 197–201.
66. Halford JBS, Stewart D, Andersson M. Tinnitus severity measured by a subjective scale, audiometry and clinical judgement. *J Laryngol Otol* 1991; **105**: 89–93.

67. Hallam RS. *Manual of the Tinnitus Questionnaire (TQ)*. London: Psychological Corporation, 1996.
68. Goebel G, Hiller W. *Tinnitus-Fragebogen (TF) Ein instrument zur Erfassung von Belastung und Scheregrad bei Tinnitus (Mannual)* Göttingen: Hogrefe Verlag, 1998.
69. Coles RRA, Baskill JL, Sheldrake J. Measurement and management of tinnitus. *J Laryngol Otol* 1984; **98**: 1171–6.
70. Josephson EM. A method of measurement of tinnitus. *Arch Otolaryngol* 1931; **14**: 282–3.
71. Wegel RL. A study of tinnitus. *Arch Otolaryngol* 1931; **14**: 158–65.
72. Tyler RS, Stouffer JL. A review of tinnitus loudness. *Hear J* 1989; **42**: 52–7.
73. Tyler RS, Conrad-Armes D. Tinnitus pitch: a comparison of three measurement methods. *Br J Audiol* 1983; **17**: 101–7.
74. Burns EM. A comparison of variability among measurements of subjective tinnitus and objective stimuli. *Audiology* 1984; **23**: 426–40.
75. Penner MJ.Variability in matches to subjective tinnitus. *J Speech Hear Res* 1983; **26**: 263–7.
76. Fowler EP. The 'illusion of loudness' of tinnitus—its etiology and treatment. *Laryngoscope* 1942; **52**: 275–85.
77. Hinchcliffe R, Chambers C. Loudness of tinnitus: an approach to measurement. *Adv Otorhinolaryngol* 1983; **29**: 163–73.
78. Tyler RS, Conrad-Armes D. Masking of tinnitus compared to masking of pure tones. *J Speech Hear Res* 1984; **27**: 106–11.
79. Axelsson A, Sandh A. Tinnitus in noise-induced hearing loss. *Br J Audiol* 1985; **9**: 271–6.
80. Man A, Naggan L. Characteristics of tinnitus in acoustic trauma. *Audiology* 1981; **20**: 70–8.
81. Tyler RS. Tinnitus maskers and hearing aids for tinnitus. *Semin Hear* 1987; **8**: 49–61.
82. Feldmann H. Homolateral and contralateral masking of tinnitus by noise-bands and pure tones. *Audiology* 1971; **10**: 138–44.
83. Penner MJ. Masking of tinnitus and central masking. *J Speech Hear Res* 1987; **30**: 147–52.
84. Shailer MJ, Tyler RS, Coles RRA. Critical masking bands for sensorineural tinnitus. *Scand Audiol* 1981; **10**: 157–62.
85. Smith PA, Parr VM, Lutman ME, Coles RRA. Comparative study of four noise spectra as potential tinnitus maskers. *Br J Audiol* 1991; **25**: 25–34.
86. Shulman A, ABR and tinnitus—an overview. *J Laryngol Otol* 1984; **9**: 170–7.
87. Ikner CL, Hassen AH. The effect of tinnitus on ABR latencies. *Ear Hear* 1990; **11**(1): 16–20.
88. Maurizi M, Ottaviani F, Paludetti G, Almadori G, Tassoni A. Contribution to the differentiation of peripheral versus central tinnitus via auditory brain stem response evaluation. *Audiology*. 1985; **24**(3): 207–16.
89. Rosenhall U, Axelsson A. Auditory brainstem response latencies in patients with tinnitus. *Scand Audiol* 1995; **24**(2): 97–100.
90. Lemaire MC, Beutter P. Brainstem auditory evoked responses in patients with tinnitus. *Audiology* 1995; **34**(6): 287–300.
91. Attias J, Urbach D, Gold S, Shemesh Z. Auditory event related potentials in chronic tinnitus patients with noise induced hearing loss. *Hear Res* 1993; **71**(1–2): 106–13.
92. Barnea G, Attias J, Gold S, Shahar A. Tinnitus with normal hearing sensitivity: extended high-frequency audiometry and auditory-nerve brain-stem-evoked responses. *Audiology* 1990; **29**(1): 36–45.
93. Moller MB, Moller AR, Janetta PJ. Vascular decompression surgery for severe tinnitus: selection criteria and results. *Laryngoscope* 1993; **17**: 421–7.
94. Vasama JP, Moller MB, Moller AR. Microvascular decompression of the cochlear nerve in patients with severe tinnitus. Preoperative findings and operative outcome in 22 patients. *Neurol Res* 1998; **20**: 242–8.
95. Hoke M, Feldmann H, Pantev C, Lutkenhoner B, Lehnertz K. Objective evidence of tinnitus in auditory evoked magnetic fields. *Hear Res* 1989; **37**(3): 281–6.
96. Hoke M. Objective evidence for tinnitus in auditory-evoked magnetic fields. *Acta Otolaryngol Suppl* 1990; **476**: 189–94.
97. Pantev C, Hoke M, Lutkenhoner B, Lehnertz K, Kumpf W. Tinnitus remission objectified by neuromagnetic measurements. *Hear Res* 1989; **40**(3): 261–4.
98. Jacobson GP, Ahmad BK, Moran J, Newman CW, Tepley N, Wharton J. Auditory evoked cortical magnetic field (M100–M200) measurements in tinnitus and normal groups. *Hear Res* 1991; **56**(1–2): 44–52.
99. Hoke M. Objective evidence for tinnitus in auditory-evolved magnetic fields. *Acta Otolaryngol* 1990; **479**: 189–94.
100. Arnold W, Bartenstein P, Oestreicher E, Romer W, Schwaiger M. Focal metabolic activation in the predominant left auditory cortex in patients suffering from tinnitus: a PET study with [18F]deoxyglucose. *ORL J Otorhinolaryngol Relat Spec* 1996; **58**(4): 195–9.
101. Mirz F, Pedersen B, Ishizu K et al. Positron emission tomography of cortical centers of tinnitus. *Hear Res* 1999; **134**(1–2): 133–44.

33 Management of the tinnitus patient

Richard S Tyler, Soly Erlandsson

Introduction

This chapter provides a general outline for the management of the tinnitus patient. It does not review the entire subject of tinnitus (see other reviews: Tyler and Babin,[1] Coles[2]), and nor does it provide details about specific treatments. Instead, this chapter focuses on overall strategies for the 'everyday clinical management' of typical and distressed patients with sensorineural tinnitus.

This approach is founded on three levels of tinnitus severity, based on our clinical experiences (Table 33.1). Most patients require only simple information and reassurance. We refer to these as level 1 patients. However, some patients require more detailed explanations regarding tinnitus and its treatments. Once they have a better understanding of causes and treatments, they are satisfied with this knowledge. These patients are at level 2. Finally, a few patients with a severe reaction to tinnitus require specific formal treatments. These patients are referred to as level 3.

Typically, we assume that patients are at level 1. As the counseling session progresses, it usually becomes apparent if they require level 2 assistance. We prefer to let patients go home (with a handout) and consider what they have learned. Usually, a second appointment is scheduled if they are at level 3.

We realise that this is an oversimplification. Some patients may move from one level to another, and some patients may require level 3 therapy immediately. Nonetheless, this a useful, overall plan.

Table 33.1 Outline of approach in three levels of treatment.

Level	Overall goal	Focus areas
1	Basic information	▪ Listen to the patient ▪ Provide hearing aid if necessary ▪ Provide general information about the background and treatment of tinnitus ▪ Determine if there is a need for further treatment
2	Preliminary counseling	▪ Listen to the patient ▪ More detail about tinnitus ▪ More detail about treatments ▪ Assess individual needs ▪ Provide plan for self-treatment ▪ Determine if further treatment needed
3	Tinnitus assessment and treatment	▪ Listen to the patient ▪ Assess tinnitus handicap ▪ Measure tinnitus ▪ Assess psychological wellbeing ▪ Provide information about treatments ▪ Assess treatment plan options and decide on treatment(s)

Level 1—Basic information

Listen to the patient

It is always important to let the patient share what is bothering them about their tinnitus. This provides some insight into what direction the counseling should take and how much depth is required. It is also therapeutic for the patient.

Many people with tinnitus are not handicapped by it. Normally, the initial onset results in some concern and distress. There is a period of adjustment, and patients eventually become less attentive to the tinnitus, and focus on other aspects of their life; tinnitus then becomes less important. Although patients are occasionally aware of their tinnitus, they are able to move forward without a tinnitus handicap.

Other patients, however, are not as fortunate. Tinnitus becomes a major focus of their life.[3] Their reaction to the tinnitus becomes worse, they cannot or are unable to ignore their tinnitus, and there is an increased alertness to the symptoms.

Patients with tinnitus almost always have a hearing loss. Therefore, most patients will improve their communication with a hearing aid. In some patients, the hearing aid will also help the tinnitus. If the patient requires a wearable noise generator (see below), then the provision of a noise generator and a hearing aid in a 'combination unit' should be considered. Before providing the hearing aid, it would be desirable to introduce the concept of noise generators and allow the person to listen to a low-level broadband noise (from the audiometer or from an in-stock noise generator).

Hearing aids can help tinnitus because they:

- improve communication and reduce stress
- amplify low-level background noise, which can be useful for masking, habituation, and distraction
- produce noise, when can be useful for masking, habituation, and distraction.

It may be desirable to adjust the frequency response of the hearing aids to:

- extend the low- or high-frequency range of amplification to activate a broader frequency range of the auditory system
- amplify more low frequencies to enhance environmental sounds.

Provide general information about background and treatment

Table 33.2 describes the general information that can be provided at an initial session. Most patients are surprised and comforted to know what causes tinnitus and how common it is. It will help some to understand that tinnitus is often a 'natural' part of the aging process. The fact that different external agents (e.g. noise exposure) cause tinnitus often reassures them that it is not something just 'in their head'.

Patients need to know that there is no 'magic pill' to cure tinnitus. However, they should also be told at the same time that there are lots of things people can do to help themselves. It is the clinician's responsibility to provide the patients with the guidance and resources so that they can help themselves. Sufficient information should be provided so that the patient is aware of the help that is available, and the different professionals providing this help. This knowledge can be helpful to patients in case they decide to return for more help in the future.

Approximately 1 in 10 people has tinnitus, and about 1 in 200 has a very bothersome tinnitus that interferes with their ability to lead a normal life. In about 75% of patients, tinnitus remains the same throughout life. In about 10% of patients, the tinnitus gets worse, and in about 15% it improves over time.[4] Most patients learn to adjust to it.

Assess need for further treatment

Most patients are satisfied with this general information. They now have reliable information about tinnitus, are aware of the treatments available, and know where to receive treatment. They can contact their therapist in the future if they require further help. However, other patients remain anxious, depressed, or just unclear, and require additional counseling.

Table 33.2 General information about tinnitus to be provided at initial contact.

Information area	Content
Prevalence	▪ About 1 in every 10 people experiences some tinnitus ▪ About 1 in every 200 people is severely bothered by tinnitus
Causes	▪ Stress ▪ Noise-induced hearing loss ▪ Aging ▪ Medications ▪ Head injury ▪ Almost anything that causes hearing loss
Treatments	▪ No magic pill ▪ Strategies to help yourself ▪ Hearing aids, counseling, relaxation, psychological therapies, maskers, habituation

Level 2—Preliminary counseling

Patients should be considered for the preliminary counseling level if they:

- are not satisfied with the discussion at the initial contact
- express an interest in further treatment
- are depressed or anxious.

Listen to the patient

At this level, it can be useful to ask more probing questions about what troubles the patient. They now have some accurate information about tinnitus. It is useful if they have had time to consider this information. If possible, provide them with an informational handout, which they can review at home before the appointment.

A few questions that are helpful include the following:

- What troubles you most about your tinnitus?
- What would you like to happen next?
- What can I do to help you the most?

More details about tinnitus

Review the material presented in Table 33.2 regarding causes, prevalence, and treatments. In some patients, providing more details can be helpful. In others, simply restating what has already been said is sufficient. The level and detail of information provided must match the level of interest and sophistication of the patient.

Additional information can be discussed relating the mechanisms of tinnitus and regarding the patient's reaction to tinnitus (Table 33.3). Although the specific mechanisms of tinnitus are unknown, discussing possible mechanisms in a concrete fashion makes the tinnitus more tangible. It is a real physiological mechanism that is reinforced by emotional reactions. It is not something they are imagining.

Separating the tinnitus and the patient's reaction to tinnitus is the basis for cognitive behavior modification.[5,6] For most patients, it is useful to distinguish 'hearing' the tinnitus and the patient's reaction to the tinnitus. Patients often benefit from seeing how they can have some control over their reaction.

Normally, nerve fibers throughout the auditory system have some level of activity, even in the absence of sound. This spontaneous activity is normal and is not perceived as sound. When a sound is presented, action potentials are produced and this pattern of activity is interpreted by the brain as sound. Some places in the auditory system have inhibitory neural circuits, such that the presentation of sounds can actually decrease spontaneous activity.

Because the presence of sound is coded by action potentials, the obvious correlate of tinnitus would be high rates of spontaneous activity. However, when animal physiologists have examined nerve fibres in animals exposed to a noise-induced hearing loss, for example, the spontaneous discharge rate has actually decreased. Furthermore, understanding the mechanisms of tinnitus is difficult, because it is not possible to ask animals if they have tinnitus. Thus, theories are speculative.

There are many different theories regarding how tinnitus is coded in the auditory system. These theories can broadly be categorized in the following areas:

- increased spontaneous rate
- bursts of increased spontaneous firing
- decreased spontaneous rate
- the edge between normal and decreased spontaneous rate
- coordinated activity across nerve fibers
- brain reorganization resulting in a greater than normal representation of one frequency region.

Table 33.3 Additional areas to discuss for patients at level 2.

Information area	Content
Mechanisms	■ Spontaneous activity in the nervous system ■ Probably an increase in spontaneous activity ■ Probably involves entire auditory pathway from cochlea to brain
Separate tinnitus from reaction to tinnitus	■ Tinnitus can be loud or soft, low- or high-pitched, composed of one or many sounds ■ Sound of tinnitus is different from reaction to tinnitus, people can learn new reactions

More details about treatments

At this point, the patient could have learned about treatment options from various sources:

- from you at an earlier counseling session
- from other health care professionals
- from friends or acquaintances with tinnitus
- from the media or internet.

Determine what treatments the patient is particularly interested in. At this point, the patient is ready for more detailed information regarding what treatments are available. The information needs to be sufficiently detailed to allow the patient to decide if she/he wants to pursue a treatment and, if so, which one. Table 33.4 provides a broad outline of some different treatments.

Provide plan for self-treatment

It can be very useful to provide some general guidelines that give the patient a clear plan and something to do for their tinnitus. It should give them a feeling of control. Table 33.5 has some suggestions that are helpful for most patients.

Table 33.4 General treatments available for tinnitus.

Treatments	Information
Refocus	■ Attention on tinnitus or attention on engaging activity ■ Develop plan for when reaction to tinnitus is bad
Hearing aids	■ Improving communication and therefore reduce stress ■ Amplify low-level background noise, which can be useful for masking, habituation, and distraction ■ Produce noise which can be useful for masking, habituation, and distraction
Sound therapy	■ Mask or cover up sound ■ Reduce the loudness of tinnitus ■ Distract (divert) attention from tinnitus ■ Facilitate habituation
Medications for coping	■ Not a cure ■ Help sleeping ■ Help relax ■ Help anxiety, depression

Table 33.5 General plan appropriate for most patients.

Areas to address	Relevant questions
Awareness of problems	What problems are perceived to be related to tinnitus?
Awareness of environmental factors	In what situations is tinnitus worse?
Possible solutions	When is patient least disturbed by tinnitus?
Potential use of solutions	What activities can be used to reduce tinnitus?
Plan to implement solutions	What will patient do in specific situation when reaction to tinnitus is worse?

Patients can describe the problems that they think are related to their tinnitus. They can keep a diary, identifying daily situations where they perceive their tinnitus to be the most problematic. They can also list times during the day when their tinnitus is not bothersome, and things that they do successfully to cope with their tinnitus.

Based on these observations, the patient may produce their own strategy for coping with tinnitus by:

- reducing time spent in situations where tinnitus is problematic.
- increasing time in situations where tinnitus is not a problem
- having plans to perform activities that render tinnitus less problematic when tinnitus is bothersome.

Although this can be easier said than done, it can empower some patients.

Determine if further treatment is needed

The patient should now have a more thorough understanding of treatment options. The patient can then decide if additional treatment is desired. Sometimes it is helpful to give the patient a handout to go home with, allowing time to consider the options and schedule a follow-up appointment if desired.

Most patients benefit from joining the American Tinnitus Association for support and information (PO Box 5, Portland, OR, 97207-0005: 1-800-634-8978, E-mail: tinnitus@ata.org, web page: http://www.ata.org), and other similar organizations worldwide.

Level 3—Tinnitus assessment and treatment

At this level of intervention, a more direct therapy is probably going to be selected. Therefore, more time is spent measuring tinnitus and related difficulties to be able to later quantify the benefits of treatment.

Assess tinnitus handicap

We use three approaches to quantify the disability and handicap (Table 33.6). We have patients assigned a value to the severity of their tinnitus on a scale from 0–100, 0 being the least severe tinnitus they can imagine and 100 being the most severe. They are then given the open-ended Tinnitus Problems Questionnaire.[7] Patients are asked to list the problems that they believe have been 'caused' by their tinnitus. This is helpful, because it allows the patient to consider what is important to them. A closed set of questions might not ask the right question. The most common complaints involve sleep difficulties, speech understanding, anxiety and depression.

It is often useful to quantify the handicapping nature of tinnitus on standardized questionnaires. There are several well-studied questionnaires available.[8] These include the Tinnitus Reaction Questionnaire,[9] the Tinnitus Handicaps Questionnaire,[10] and the Tinnitus Handicap Inventory.[11] With the Tinnitus Handicap Questionnaire, the severity of a patient's handicap can be compared directly with other patients who have completed the questionnaire to determine their handicap related to others. This provides a more concrete assessment of the severity of their handicap.

Measure tinnitus

Measuring the psychoacoustical aspects of tinnitus can be helpful for many reasons, including:

- confirmation to the patient that their tinnitus is real
- to monitor changes of the magnitude of the tinnitus
- to provide some insights into the mechanism
- to aid in the fitting of a device (for example, it can be helpful to know if the tinnitus can be masked and at what level, or to know if the tinnitus can be masked in the contralateral ear)
- to determine reliability in legal cases

Table 33.6 Handicap assessment tools.

General tool	
Category scale severity rating	0–100
Problems important to patient	Open-ended questionnaire
Formal questionnaire of tinnitus handicap or disability	■ Tinnitus Reaction Questionnaire ■ Tinnitus Handicap Inventory ■ Tinnitus Handicap Questionnaire

Table 33.7 Audiological measurement of tinnitus.

Measurement	Details
Description	▪ Ringing ▪ Roaring ▪ Pulsing ▪ Humming
Localization	▪ Left ear ▪ Right ear ▪ Bilateral ▪ In the head ▪ Outside of the head
Pitch	At least 5 replications reporting each match
Loudness	At least 3 replications reporting each match
Broadband noise masking	▪ Ipsilateral ear ▪ Contralateral ear
Uncomfortable loudness levels (for hyperacusis)	Ascending method, caution needed in some patients

These measurements should only be made when there is a clear purpose in mind, such as those listed above.

Table 33.7 makes some general suggestions about measuring tinnitus. Tinnitus pitch can be measured by adjusting the frequency of a pure tone to have the same pitch as the most prominent pitch of the tinnitus. Similarly, the intensity of a tone can be adjusted to have the same loudness as the tinnitus, The level of a broadband noise can be adjusted so that it just masks the tinnitus in the ipsilateral and/or contralateral ear. Details regarding procedures can be found in the literature.[12, 13]

Loudness and minimal masking can be useful to quantify the magnitude of the tinnitus. Comparing ipsilateral and contralateral can suggest ipsilateral and contralateral involvement.

Assess psychological wellbeing

The patient must be understood and treated in the context of their environment and their psychological self. Table 33.8 highlights a few areas that should be addressed. The role of gender for the experience of tinnitus suffering should also be taken into consideration, as the life situation and the gender roles of women are different from those of men.[3] Gender differences in the perceived health-related quality of life among tinnitus patients have been reported.[20]

What expectations does the patient have about the therapy? Do they expect to be cured? Are they simply looking for reassurance? What previous therapies have they tried? Is this their first attempt to treat their tinnitus? Have they traveled around the country to several clinics?

Tinnitus affects interpersonal relationships.[3] It is difficult for others to understand the devastating nature of tinnitus.

Table 33.8 Background and psychological areas of assessment.

Area to evaluate
Expectations from tinnitus therapy
Previous tinnitus treatments tried and results
Interpersonal relationships/support system in place
Sleep difficulties
Anxiety
Depression
Suicide

Problems occur with spouses, children, and co-workers. Are there any critical external circumstances that could be relevant? Has the patient changed jobs, experienced changes in marriage, or had a death in the family? Are there any events that could have triggered the tinnitus or made it worse? Is the tinnitus only one symptom of many difficulties faced by the patient? What kind of support system does the patient have? Does the patient live alone? Were they accompanied to the clinic with a sympathetic partner?

Sleep problems are often reported with tinnitus. Referrals to a 'sleep clinic' can be necessary. Some basic suggestions include:

- getting to sleep at the same time each evening
- reserving the bed as a place to sleep, not read or think
- not drinking or eating before bedtime.

What is the personality of the patient? Some patients may be anxious, whereas others can be depressed. Consultation or referrals to psychologists or psychiatrists may be helpful. What is the overall wellbeing of the patient? Are they happy with their life? Do they enjoy their work? Do they have hobbies? Do they have a general positive outlook?

Finally, one should not overlook the fact that some tinnitus patients consider and commit suicide. If the patient mentions or hints at suicide, a referral to a psychiatrist is essential.

Assess treatment plan options

After carefully assessing the patient, a clear and complete description of therapies and options should be discussed.

Provide specific treatment

Table 33.9 reviews a number of specific treatment options that are available.

Counseling

General counseling can be helpful to assist the patient to develop successful coping strategies, to reduce distress and modify maladaptive behavior. The specific problem that compels the patient to seek help might be an overwhelming anxiety; not over a feared physical disease, but over the risk of suffering a

Table 33.9 Treatments available.

Treatment	References
Counseling	Tyler et al[17] Wilson and Henry[6]
Relaxation	Erlandsson[3]
Cognitive behavior modification	Sweetow[5] Wilson and Henry[6]
Masking	Vernon[18] Tyler and Bentler[19]
Habituation	Jastreboff and Hazell[15]
Sound therapy	See text
Refocus therapy	See text

mental breakdown.[21] When effective, counseling can help to open up new possibilities, increased awareness, empowerment and enhanced quality of life.[22]

Relaxation

Relaxation is aimed at gaining control over tension and being able to relax when necessary. These techniques can be used routinely, or particularly when tinnitus appears worse. This has the additional benefit that it increases confidence. There are many techniques that help patients relax when they are particularly bothered by their tinnitus. Examples include videotapes, using recorded soft music, or biofeedback. As with most things, results are typically better when relaxation therapy is provided by someone trained in the procedure.

Cognitive behavior modification

Cognitive therapy involves separating the tinnitus from a patient's reaction to the tinnitus. It evaluates the way in which patients talk and think about their tinnitus. The intent is to have them think about their tinnitus in a realistic fashion, to adjust their thoughts about tinnitus, and to design therapies to change their reaction to tinnitus.

Masking

Tinnitus masking can involve covering up tinnitus so that the tinnitus is inaudible, or partially masking it so that the tinnitus loudness is decreased. Wearable noise generator devices, maskers, portable tape players, combination hearing aids and maskers, or non-wearable devices can be used to produce noise. Environmental noise can be used to produce masking. These devices can also be used to help the patient get to sleep.

Habituation or retraining therapy

The brain naturally habituates to sounds that are unimportant.[14] For example, within seconds of entering a room, our brain ignores a noisy refrigerator. Retraining therapy combines counselling (Table 33.10) and habituation (Table 33.11) to reduce the fear of tinnitus and structure the environment to ensure that the patient is frequently in the presence of low levels of background noise.[15] Both wearable and non-wearable noise generators and environmental noise can be used. The noise level is adjusted to where the tinnitus begins to break up, the 'mixing point'.

Table 33.10 Counseling specific to tinnitus retraining therapy.

The link between the tinnitus, the brain and emotions
The general principles of the habituation process
The specific mechanisms by which tinnitus can be habituated
Retraining of thinking—altering the beliefs and thoughts about tinnitus so they do not fear tinnitus, and do not feel threatened or in danger
The importance of maintaining audibility of the tinnitus
The importance of continued use of the noise generators
Inform the patients that we expect them to benefit from the treatment because others with similar tinnitus have benefited from this treatment in the past

Table 33.11 General principles of habituation.

Treat hyperacusis first if it is present
Use hearing aids if there is a communication handicap
Use hearing aid/noise generator combination units if background sound amplified by hearing aids is insufficient to reduce tinnitus. The tinnitus must be audible
If tinnitus is exacerbated by noise, start sound level below mixing point and gradually increase over weeks
Routine daily exposure to low-level background sound is advised (minimally about 8 h per day)
Wearable binaural noise generators are most desirable, although habituation through environmental sounds with or without hearing aids is possible
Avoid silence during all waking hours
Do not focus on the tinnitus
Provide follow-up contact to ensure compliance with mixing point and noise exposure

Sound therapy

Most patients report that the presence of background noise or music is helpful. These sounds can:

- mask (cover up) the tinnitus
- reduce its loudness (while still hearing the tinnitus)
- distract the patient from attending to the tinnitus.

The types of sound used in sound therapy include:

- Broadband noise—many patients report that it is easier to listen to the noise than it is to listen to their tinnitus.

- Music—usually soft, light, background music (e.g. classical baroque, simple piano music).
- Sound produced particularly for relaxation or distraction (e.g. waves lapping against the shore, raindrops falling on leaves—sometimes these are combined with light music).

There are several different devices that produce these sounds:

- Wearable devices that resemble hearing aids. These sound generators can be worn inside the ear canal or behind the ear.
- Wearable devices with earphones or insert earphones (portable cassette or CD players).
- Non-wearable devices that include radios, tape players, compact disk players or sound generators specifically produced for relaxation or tinnitus. Some are meant to be used at the bedside with timers and different sound types.

Sound therapy does not have to be used all the time.

Refocus therapy

Many patients focus their attention on their tinnitus. They think about their tinnitus much of the day. The more they think about their tinnitus, the worse it gets, and the worse it gets, the more they think about it. Tinnitus becomes a critical part of their life. They spend much of their time trying to 'fix' their tinnitus, learn more about it, and trying numerous 'popular' cures.

We have found that many patients need to redirect their attention away from their tinnitus and onto other aspects of their life. Tinnitus is real, and it is probably not going to go away. However, most people in life have some intrusion they have to manage. They may have some other serious illness, or be responsible for the care of someone who does. Few of us escape the challenges of life.

We have also found that some patients benefit from a frank conversation about the importance of the other activities in their life that they enjoy. Many of the patients have people who love and care about them. Many get great satisfaction from their work. Others have interesting and captivating hobbies. Patients can also be encouraged to develop new interests. We call this strategy 'refocus therapy'. The clinician's role is to help them put the handicap resulting from their tinnitus in perspective, and to help them to focus on other activities in their life. It is important for all of us to focus our attention on things in life that we enjoy.

Table 33.12 Influencing patient expectations to facilitate therapy.

Attributes	Details
Be perceived as a knowledgeable professional	■ Act professional ■ Impact useful knowledge ■ Be organized and clear
Be sympathetic towards the patient	■ Listen ■ Acknowlegde problems
Demonstrate that you understand tinnitus	■ Discuss ■ Problems ■ Causes ■ Treatments
Provide a clear therapy plan	
Show that you sincerely care	■ Be sincere ■ Provide follow-up

Influencing patient expectations

The manner in which we interact with the patient can have an enormous impact on the success of our therapy. Table 33.12 provides an outline of some of the critical factors involved in nurturing patient expectations.[16] Patient expectations influence the success of many treatments. Many of these critical factors that influence patient expectations can and should be utilized to influence therapy.

The patient will feel more confident if they perceive the therapist as competent, sympathetic, and having a good knowledge of tinnitus. This can be complicated, because although there are some common aspects of tinnitus, there are also individual aspects that are unique to each patient. The therapy plan, whatever it is, should be clear and understood by the patient. The therapy should produce feelings of hope and mastery in the patient. The patient should be empowered to engage in therapy and turn their hopes into concrete expectations.

Summary

Tinnitus can be treated, but not all patients require the same approach. We have organized treatment levels depending on the needs of the patient. These approaches are helpful to most patients encountered.

Most patients with sensorineural tinnitus entering an audiology/otology clinic require only a simple explanation about tinnitus (level 1). They benefit from having someone listen to their difficulty, but do not need detailed counseling or treatment. The initial contact section is sufficient, and they can be welcomed back should they have problems in the future.

Other patients need a more detailed explanation about the causes and treatments of tinnitus (level 2). They have more serious questions, but are satisfied when they have a deeper understanding of what options are available to them. Many will benefit from a simple plan to monitor their tinnitus for a few weeks and strategies for using background sound.

Finally, some patients require participation in a specific therapy (level 3). For these patients, we measure tinnitus and the handicap resulting from it. Following a thorough understanding of the patient's environments and needs, a detailed description of treatment options can be provided and the patient directed to appropriate professionals.

References

1. Tyler RS, Babin RW. Tinnitus. In: Cummings CW, Fredrickson JM, Harker L, Krause CJ, Schuller DE, eds. *Otolaryngology—Head and Neck Surgery*. St Louis: CV Mosby Co., 1993: 3031–53.
2. Coles RRA. Tinnitus and its management. In: Stephens SDG, Kerr AG, eds. *Scott-Brown's Otolaryngology*. Guildford: Butterworth, 1989: 368–414.
3. Erlandsson S. Psychologic profiles. In: Tyler RS, eds. *Handbook on Tinnitus* San Diego, CA: Singular Publishing Group, 2000: 25–57.
4. Stouffer JL, Tyler RS. Characterization of tinnitus by tinnitus patients. *J Speech Hear Disord* 1990; **55**: 439–53.
5. Sweetow RW. Cognitive aspects of tinnitus patient management. *Ear Hear* **7**: 390–6.
6. Wilson PH, Henry JL. Psychological management. In: Tyler RS, ed. *Handbook of Tinnitus*. San Diego, CA: Singular Publishing Group, 2000: 263–79.
7. Tyler RS, Baker LJ. Difficulties experiences by tinnitus sufferers. *J Speech Hear Disord* 1983; **48**: 150–4.
8. Tyler RS. Tinnitus disability and Handicap Questionnaires. *Semin Hear* 1993; **14**: 377–84.
9. Wilson PH, Henry J, Bowen M, Haralambous G. Tinnitus Reaction Questionnaire: Psychometric properties of a measure of distress associated with tinnitus. *J Speech Hear Res* 1991; **34**: 197–201.
10. Kuk F, Tyler RS, Russell D, Jordan H. The psychometric properties of a tinnitus handicap questionnaire. *Ear Hear* 1990; **11(6)**: 434–42.
11. Newman CW, Jacobson GP, Spitzer JB. Development of the Tinnitus Handicap Inventory. *Arch Otolaryngol Head Neck Surg* 1996; **122**: 143–8.
12. Tyler RS. Psychoacoustical measurement. In: Tyler RS ed. *Handbook on Tinnitus*. San Diego, CA: Singular Publishing Group, 2000.
13. Henry JA, Flick CL, Gilbert A, Ellingson RM, Fausti SA. Reliability of tinnitus loudness matches under procedural variation. *J Am Acad Audiol* 1999; **10**: 502–20.
14. Hallam RS, Jakes SC, Hinchcliffe R. Cognitive variables in tinnitus annoyance. *Br J Clin Psychol* 1988; **27**: 213–22.
15. Jastreboff PJ, Hazell JWP. A neurophysiological approach to tinnitus: clinical implications. *Br J Audiol* 1993; **27**: 7–17.
16. Tyler RS. The use of science to find successful tinnitus treatments. In: Hazell J, eds. *Proceedings of the Sixth International Tinnitus Seminar*. London: The Tinnitus and Hyperacusis Centre, 1999: 3–9.
17. Tyler RS, Stouffer JL, Schum R. Audiological rehabilitation of the tinnitus patient. *J Acad Rehabil Audiol* **22**: 30–42.
18. Vernon JA. *Tinnitus: Treatment and Relief*. Needham Heights, MA: Allyn & Bacon, 1998.
19. Tyler RS, Bentler RA. Tinnitus maskers and hearing aids for tinnitus. *Semin Hear* 1987; **8(1)**: 49–61.
20. Erlandsson SI, Holgers KM. The impact of perceived tinnitus severity on health-related quality of life with aspects of gender. *Noise Health* 2001 **10**: 39–52.
21. Erlandsson SI. Psychological counselling in the medical setting—some clinical examples given by patients with tinnitus and Menières disease. *Int J Adv Counsel* 1998; **20**: 265–76.
22. Robertson SE, Brown RI (eds). *Rehabilitation Counselling*. Approaches in the Field of Disability. Suffolk, UK: Chapman & Hall, 1992

34 Aspects of the paracuses

Ronald Hinchcliffe

Introduction

The subject of this chapter will be the paracuses other than diminutions of hearing sensitivity. These encompass a variety of disturbances of auditory perception which patients, unless they are musicians, infrequently admit to, let alone complain about. Many of the terms are inappropriate and are used differently, or not at all, by different writers (see Glossary). Many patients are also unable to recognize, or confuse, these various disturbances, so that they are brought to light only by a clinical examination.[1] Nevertheless, this is a topic of increasing interest.

Classifications of various aspects and disturbances of auditory perception are shown in Figures 34.1 and 34.2.

Intensity-related phenomena

Loudness is the subjective magnitude of the physical magnitude (intensity, pressure) of sound. Like any other sensory magnitude, it bears a particular mathematical relationship (power function) to the physical magnitude of the sensory stimulus, the power law of the psychophysical function.[2,3] An international standard[4] prescribes two methods[5–7] for calculating the loudness of environmental noises. Just as one can calculate the loudness of a sound in sones so one can calculate the noisiness of a sound in noys.[8,9] There are individual differences in loudness functions (the rate at which loudness grows with increase in sound level).[10]

Noise caused by traffic and industrial or recreational activities is one of the main environmental problems in the world and the source of an increasing number of complaints. Different acoustical features are responsible for annoyance at different sound levels: 'at low levels, the feature of tonality is dominant above absolute level. However at higher noise levels, the feature of absolute level is more dominant than tonality.'[11] Moreover, 'the wide variety of descriptions of the characteristics of the noise stimuli highlighted the large number of subjective descriptors for the perceived character of a noise resulting from a physical feature. It appears that a noise can be judged by different features by different listeners.'[12]

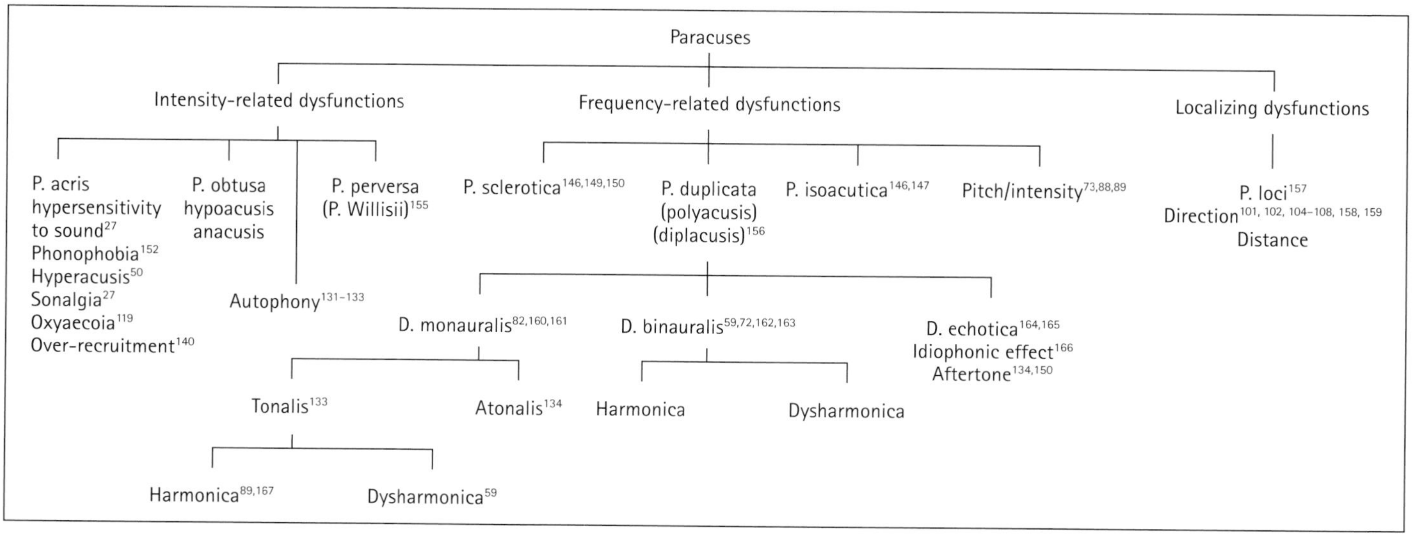

Figure 34.1 Aspects of the paracuses. The meanings of the various terms are given in the Glossary.

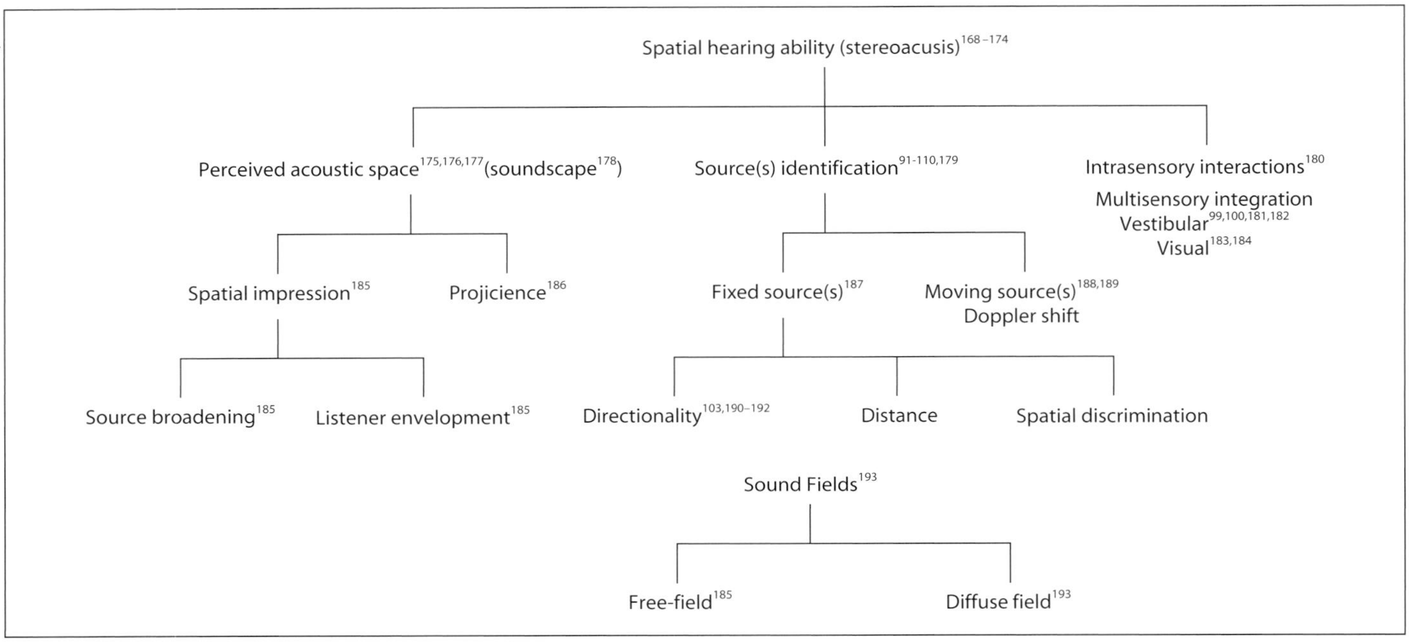

Figure 34.2 Aspects of stereoacusis (spatial hearing ability). The meanings of the various terms are given in the Glossary.

'Physically identical sound may become noise to one person and music to another, depending on whether one likes Mozart or rock and roll . . . The noise of the neighbor's lawnmover (*sic*) may be annoying if (s)he mowed the lawn two days ago, but a pleasant relief if (s)he just returned from a six weeks vacation to clean up an overgrown front yard.'[13] Indeed the non-acoustical properties of noises, e.g. controllability, fears, or beliefs about maleficent effects, are more important determinants of individual annoyance than are the acoustical properties of the noises.[14]

Reductions in the annoyance properties of noises can be approached not only by altering the perceptions of the listeners but also by modifing the nature and quality of the noise. Yehudi Menuhin made the plea that ambulances need not shriek and police cars need not wail—they should make harmonious sounds (alternating thirds), pleasing to the human ear, as they do in France.[15] Even helicopter noise can be aestheticized. In the composition *Choppers and strings*, Stockhausen merged the sounds of helicopters with those of musical instruments.[16]

Hyperacusis

This is an unfortunate term, since it implies that an affected individual would have better hearing than a normally hearing person. In that sense it would be equated with oxyaecoia. Such is rarely the case. The alternative description of hypersensitivity is no better, since many describe the hearing threshold level as a measure of auditory sensitivity.

The Hyperacusic Network[17] defines hyperacusis as 'a collapsed tolerance to normal environmental sounds. It is a rare hearing disorder where the individual becomes highly sensitive to noise.' As with other conditions, any prevalence figure will be determined by the criteria adopted for its diagnosis. For example, if hyperacusis is defined 'by the onset of symptoms of loudness discomfort from everyday sounds that previously had not bothered the patient and/or uncomfortable loudness levels for pure tones in the 500–4000 Hz range of less than 70 dB HL',[18] then a higher prevalence would obtain than if one noted how many patients actually complained of an intolerance to loud sounds. Judging from other auditory percepts, it could make a difference in prevalence of 50 to 1. Deciding on the normal range for thresholds of uncomfortable loudness is a similar problem to that of deciding on the normal range for thresholds of hearing. It has been proposed that the phrase 'clinical limits' be used to refer to the 2½ and 97½ percentage points to the distribution of healthy persons.[19] It is not stated to what centile a threshold of uncomfortable loudness (TUL) of 70 dB HL corresponds. Moreover, there is also the question of to what extent a low TUL is of central origin[20] and results from anxiety.[21] Different diagnostic criteria could well account for the difference between 'In our Tinnitus Clinic, where more than 4000 patients have been seen, hyperacusis has been seen only 4 times,'[22] and 'about 40% [of tinnitus patients] exhibited hyperacusis in varying degrees.'[23] However, the American Tinnitus Association rates the prevalence of hyperacusis among tinnitus patients as of the order of 2%.[24] Preferred loudness levels do, however, appear to be lower in patients with tinnitus. The mean most comfortable loudness level for tinnitus patients is 17 dB lower than that for a normal control group.[25]

An individual's hypersensitivity to sound may be associated with hypersensitivity to other sensory stimuli,[26, 27] e.g. light and touch, with headaches and migraine,[27, 28] with sound distortion,[27] and with tinnitus,[23] where it may be more troublesome than the tinnitus.[18]

Hypersensitivity to sound is characteristic of acute noise damage to hearing.[29, 30] but not of chronic occupational noise damage to hearing,[31–34] with the exception of those occupations where the exposure is to music.[27] 'In persons regularly exposed to industrial noise the limit of discomfort is generally found to be shifted to considerably higher sound levels . . . the higher sound tolerance of workers accustomed to noise is due only to a process of central adaptation'.[35]

Hypersensitivity to sound is observed in Bell's palsy,[36] where its presence is a poor prognostic sign,[37] and in Ramsay Hunt syndrome.[38] It is reported to be a symptom of VIIIth nerve vascular compression syndrome,[39] and is a feature of GM1 gangliosidosis type 2,[40] Tay-Sachs disease[41] and Williams syndrome.[42] It is also observed in autistic children.[17]

Intolerable hypersensitivity to sound is an adverse effect of trifluoromethane.[43] Along with photophobia, it is a feature of the benzodiazepine withdrawal syndrome.[44]

It has been suggested that 'central hyperacusis' is a symptom of 5-hydroxytryptamine (5-HT; serotonin) dysfunction.[20] 5-HT has a role in the control of anxiety.[45]

SOUND INTOLERANCE: INVESTIGATION
Anamnesis
Clinical otological, neurological and psychological examination.
Audiometry [preferably Békésy type]
- Threshold measurements
- MCLL
- TUL
- Individual loudness functions
- Speech audiometry
  - in quiet
  - in noise
- Acoustical stapedius reflexes (?)

The investigation of patients with hypersensitivity to sound includes not only a detailed history and a clinical otological, neurological and psychological examination, but also audiometric tests. These should include measurements of hearing threshold levels, most comfortable loudness levels and TULS. Békésy audiometry is eminently suitable for these purposes.[46, 47] The same technique can be used to construct individual loudness functions.[25] The determination of TULs for specific sounds, as well as speech audiometry in the quiet and in a noisy background, may also be indicated.[27] The patient may or may not tolerate acoustical stapedius reflex studies.

Schemes for grading[48, 49] and classifying[20, 27, 49, 50] patients with hypersensitivity to sound have been published. However, the classifications are mainly intuitive and not based on taxonometric methods.[51]

SOUND INTOLERANCE: MANAGEMENT
Passive attenuator
Desensitization
Electronic loudness supression devices
Cochlear labyrinthectomy (unilateral cases, rarely)

Management includes psychological methods, including desensitization. For example, a good response of hyperacusis in tinnitus patients is reported to treatment with low-level wideband noise to the affected ear for 6 h per day for several months.[26] Most if not all hyperacusic patients wear some form of passive attenuator. Indeed, this behavior can be considered to be the pathognomonic sign of the condition. Subjects fitted binaurally with electronic loudness suppression devices reported that they benefited from the devices in at least some listening conditions.[24] These devices supply low-level amplification followed by an extreme form of amplitude compression. Very rarely, hyperacusis may be sufficiently bad as to justify surgical destruction of the affected ear.[52]

Paracusis Willisii

This is perhaps the best known of the paracusias. It is a feature not only of otosclerosis but of conductive hearing impairments in general. It has been attributed to a speaker unconsciously raising his voice to communicate with a hearing-impaired individual. It is named after Thomas Willis, who described the phenomenon in 1672, although William Holder had described it 3 years earlier.[53]

Frequency-related phenomena

There are a multiplicity of disorders of auditory perception that have been described as a result of damage to the sound-analyzing organ of the internal ear,[54] although these paracuses can arise, if but rarely, from central lesions also.[55, 56]

Diplacusis

Diplacusis is a feature of Menière's disease,[57] where it is the first sign to disappear in response to treatment.[58] Its presence has been reported as indicative of cochlear otosclerosis[59] and it has been reported after both stapedectomy and fenestration operations.[60] It has been reported as an adverse effect of potassium iodide medication[61] and chloroform inhalation.[62] Binaural diplacusis was experienced by a non-factory worker following exposure to factory noise.[63] In respect of ONIHL, the UK Health and Safety Commission (HSC) stated 'auditory symptoms other than impairment of hearing which result from noise damage to hearing [the clinical source of this section is not stated]: Tinnitus ('ringing in the ears') can become permanent. Many people find this as distressing as the hearing loss [but this picture is not that which has emerged from direct examinations over the years of workers in Britain exposed to hazardous occupational noise levels,[31, 64–66] and tinnitus occurs early, if at all, in the course of hazardous occupational noise exposure and is not a prominent feature of such exposure]. Diplacusis (double hearing) in which a sound will have a different tone in each ear, or will sound rough. This will contribute to lowered intelligibility of speech which cannot be improved by a hearing aid.'[67] Nevertheless, it is clear that people in both Canada[68] and the UK[69] with noise-damaged hearing can obtain substantial benefit from hearing aids.

Reports of diplacusis associated with the central nervous system are rare, but a lesion of the posterior thalamus resulted in diplacusis binauralis.[56]

The investigation of diplacusis includes not only a detailed history and a clinical otological, neurological and psychological examination, but also hearing tests of a more sophisticated kind than are usually employed. Diplacusimetry,[70] an adaptation of Békésy audiometry, provides measures of binaural diplacusis. There is not normally a difference of more than 4% for a pair of tones that are matched to give the same pitch perception to the two ears. In Menière's disease, the difference may amount to 37% (maximum at 250 Hz) and, in high frequency hearing losses, 17% (maximum at 4000 Hz). There is an upward shift in perceived pitch on the affected side.[71] The maxima for binaural frequency differences correspond to the maxima in hearing threshold differences for the two ears.[72]

More sophisticated psychoacoustical testing would include the determination of psychophysical tuning curves, pitch–intensity functions, masking patterns, and frequency just-noticeable differences (jnds) as well as diplacusis measures.[73] Temporal acuity, normally about 2 ms,[74] would also be of interest.

However, many of these functions, e.g. frequency selectivity and frequency discrimination, and speech discrimination (in the quiet or in noise) are highly correlated with one another and so may reflect the same basic process(es).[75, 76] It is not possible to establish a primary relationship between, say, impaired frequency resolution, pure tone threshold and speech intelligibility.[77] Nevertheless, in noise-induced threshold shifts, impaired binaural pitch matching[78] and frequency resolution changes[79] may be demonstrated in regions where the threshold of hearing is normal.

Moreover, neither impaired frequency selectivity nor impaired temporal resolution is specific to any one type of internal ear disorder.[80]

Diplacusis cannot be demonstrated in all subjects with sensorineural hearing loss, and nor is it absent in subjects with otherwise normal hearing.[81]

Otoacoustical emissions should also be studied in individuals with diplacusis. The consumption of aspirin by one subject with monaural diplacusis reduced the spontaneous otoacoustical emissions (SOAEs) into the noise floor and eliminated the monaural diplacusis.[82]

Pitch–intensity aberrations

Pitch is primarily a function of the frequency of a tone.[83] However, it is secondarily a function of the intensity of the tone.[84–88] Even in normally hearing subjects, a given tone seems lower in pitch as it becomes more intense and higher as it grows weaker.[84]

Accentuation of the pitch–intensity relationship is associated with diplacusis.[89] Pitch–intensity function aberrations are best investigated with psychophysical tuning curves, masking patterns, frequency jnd's and diplacusis measurements.[73]

Patients who are neither musicians nor psychoacousticians will not usually be complaining of diplacusis, pitch–intensity aberrations or other related paracuses. All these aberrations are subsumed under the term 'distortion', and they will consider this to affect their ability to enjoy life to a greater degree than does any tinnitus.[90] This serves to emphasize the greater attention that needs to be paid to these paracuses.

Sound Localization

There are a number of component abilities that govern sound localization, e.g. direction perception, distance perception and spatial resolution.[91] Studies of what have been said to be 'sound localization' have almost exclusively been concerned with sound directionalization.

Both intensity[92] and phase[93] differences are important for sound directionalization.[94, 95] Time differences, which are reflected in phase differences at the two ears, are of considerable importance.[96] The role of the auricles in all this is paramount. Each gives rise to time delays and stimulus redundancy, which provide a unique temporal pattern for every locus in space.[97]

Stereoacusis is dependent on normal vestibular function.[98] Elevation (vertical plane) directionalization requires the ability to move the head.[99, 100]

There are no differences in localization acuity between sides, but there are significant differences between front and back regions. Azimuth (horizontal plane) and elevation error are well matched and low in the front. However, azimuth error increases in the regions behind the head, particularly for azimuth positions 120° to 160°. Larger increases are found for positions in the upper elevations of this region. Elevation error also increases in the upper elevations behind the head. A comparison of auditory and visual data indicates that this pattern of error is not due to motor factors. These findings relate to the structural characteristics of the auricles and the modifications that they impose on incoming sound energy.[101]

Dysstereoacusis

Thirty-three of the forty-two patients with supratentorial neurological disease had defects in azimuth (horizontal) directionalization on the side opposite to the involved hemisphere; in three cases the directionalization defect was bilateral. None of the patients with neurological disease which was not supratentorial showed directionalization defects.[102] Disturbed directional hearing is common among patients with sensory aphasia.[103]

A sophisticated study of '140 subjects, including 69 with different types of hearing impairments, 32 with neurological diseases, and 39 with normal hearing,' concluded 'There exist characteristic impairments of sound localization in different types of hearing impairments tested. On a general level, the results are consistent with the concept that the localization of sound relies on a decision made by the central auditory system based on a number of cues present in the acoustic signal at the two ears. The cues tested in our study are: 1) the interaural time difference, 2) the interaural intensity difference, and 3) the spectrum of the received signal at each ear. At a more specific level, the sound localization impairments found in conductive hearing losses are interpreted as bone-conduction effects, the results found in sensorineural hearing losses are interpreted as consequences of impaired or preserved spectral processing, the results in neurinomas are interpreted as impaired signal transmission in the auditory nerves, and the results of subjects with central involvements suggest that separate processors exist at some level in the central auditory system for the different localization cues.'[104] Although the study referred to 'sound localization', it was concerned with the purely directional aspects of stereoacusis (as the authors conceded).

Different mechanisms are involved for the two planes. Vertical plane directionalization requires the possession of normal high-frequency auditory acuity. For example, normal horizontal plane directionalization, but impaired vertical plane directionalization, has been observed in a patient with a bilateral abrupt high-tone loss above 4 kHz (90 dB HL at 6 kHz; 75 dB at 8 kHz); the converse ability was observed in a patient with a total unilateral hearing loss.[105] Vertical plane directionalization thus depends on the ability to correlate head movement with high-frequency acoustical clues. Neurological cases may similarly show different behavior in the two planes. For example, a man with a parietal glioblastoma showed normal (or near normal) vertical plane directionalization, but impaired horizontal plane localization. The converse behavior is sometimes associated with brainstem lesions.[106]

Hearing-impaired children behave significantly poorer on horizontal sound directionalization tasks than do their normally hearing counterparts; individual differences among the hearing impaired can be attributed to age and hearing threshold differences.[107] None of 44 children with a severe unilateral hearing loss directionalized a 500-Hz pure tone as well as normally hearing controls, although nine were able to directionalize a high-pass noise as accurately as those with normal hearing. This was attributed to better use of auricular information by these nine children.[108] The contribution of the auricles to stereoacusis also explains the ability of many individuals with a unilateral hearing loss to localize sounds accurately,[109–111] although in surveys of the general population, sound localization ability (assessed by a questionnaire) was highly correlated with measures of hearing impairment in the worse ear.[112]

DYSSTEREOACUSIS: INVESTIGATION

Clinical otological and neurological
Auditory function measurements
- Pure tone threshold for air (and bone) conduction
- Phase audiometry
- Minimal audible angles (right–left; front–back)

Vestibular examination
Neuro-imaging

Impaired sound localization may be the presenting symptom for patients with a vestibulocochlear schwannoma. There are also individuals with impaired sound localization as the presenting symptom who are found to have normal manual pure tone and speech audiograms, no unusual findings on routine neurological examination, normal interaural time and intensity jnds, and normal minimal audible angle for right–left distinctions but abnormal minimal audible angle for front–back distinctions. This condition might be referred to as idiopathic dysstereoacusis. One of two affected individuals had a history of recurrent embolic disease of unknown origin.[104]

Dysstereoacusis must be distinguished from auditory inattention.[113, 114] The latter applies to conditions in which the subject reacts as though acoustical stimuli (whether unilateral or bilateral) were coming from one side only. The condition occurs in certain hemisphere lesions. In parietal lesions, there is no response to contralateral stimuli, and in frontal lesions, no response to ipsilateral stimuli.

For clinical purposes, directional hearing can be measured using phase audiometry.[115] An interaural phase lag produces a sensation of lateralization of the sound inside the head towards the side of the ear which has the lead in phase. However, if appropriate equipment is available, the minimal audible angle for both front–back and right–left distinctions should also be determined, since one or other may be abnormal when interaural time and intensity jnds are normal. Moreover, sound directionalization in the vertical plane should be tested as well as that in the horizontal plane, because this function may be impaired when that in the horizontal plane is normal, and vice versa.

Conclusions

Disorders of the ears and of the central nervous system may produce a number of aberrations of auditory sensations other than shifts in the absolute threshold of hearing. These paracuses may betoken disease of which clinicians need to be aware and so must be adequately investigated. Moreover, these paracuses may be compensable under the English common law.[116] Medical examinations of hearing will therefore need to be more extensive than they have been hitherto.

References

1. Hinchcliffe R. Clinical tests of auditory function in the adult and in the schoolchild. In: Beagley HA, ed. *Audiology and Audiological Medicine* Vol. 1. Oxford: Oxford University Press, 1981: 320–64.
2. Stevens SS. The measurement of loudness. *J Acoust Soc Am* 1955; **27**: 815–29
3. Scharf B, Stevens JC. The form of the loudness function near threshold. In: Cremer L ed. *Proceedings of the 3rd International Congress on Acoustics*, Stuttgart. Amsterdam: Elsevier, 1959.
4. International Organization for Standadization. ISO 532: 1975. *Acoustics—Method for Calculating Loudness Level*. Geneva: ISO, 1975.
5. Stevens SS. Calculation of the loudness of complex noise. *J Acoust Soc Am* 1956; **28**: 807–32.
6. Zwicker E. Ein Verfahren zur Berechnung der Lautstarke. *Acustica* 1960; **10**: 304–8.
7. Zwicker E. Subdivision of the audible frequency range into critical bands (*Frequenzgruppen*). *J Acoust Soc Am* 1961; **33**: 248.
8. Kryter KD. Scaling human reactions to the sound from aircraft. *J Acoust Soc Am* 1959; **31**: 1415–29.
9. Kryter KD, Pearsons KS. Modification of noy tables. *J Acoust Soc Am* 1964; **36**: 394–7.
10. Barbenza CM de, Bryan ME, McRobert H, Tempest W. Individual loudness susceptibility. *Sound* 1970; **4**: 75–9.
11. Berry BF, Porter ND. The evaluation of acoustic features in industrial noise. In: *Proceedings of Inter-noise 94*, Yokohama, 1994: 803–8.
12. Porter ND. *The Assessment of Industrial Noise—Subjective Listening Tests and Objective Assessment Procedures*. NPL Report RSA(EXT) 0057A. Teddington: National Physical Laboratory, 1995.
13. Berglund B, Lindvall T (eds). *Community Noise*. Archives of the Center for Sensory Research Vol 2, Issue 1. Document prepared for the World Health Organization. Stockholm: Stockholm University and Karolinska Institute, 1995.
14. Borsky PN. Review of community response to noise. In: Tobias JV, Jansen G, Ward WD, eds. *Proceedings of the Third International Congress on Noise as a Public Health Problem*, Freiburg 1978. ASHA Report 10. Rockville, Maryland: American Speech-Language-Hearing Association, 1980: 453–74.
15. Lister D. Tuneful sirens, please. *Independent*; 12 November 1998: 9.
16. http://www.u.arizona.edu/~jkandell/music /stock/stock_prem.html (1997).
17. http://www.hyperacusis.net/
18. Coles RRA. Tinnitus. In: Stephens D, ed. *Scott-Brown's Otolaryngology* 6th edn, Vol. 2, *Adult Audiology*. London: Butterworth-Heinemann, 1997: 2/18/1–34.
19. Elvebach LR, Guillier CL, Keating Jr FR. Health, normality and the ghost of Gauss. *J Am Assoc* 1970; **211**: 69–75.
20. Marriage J, Barnes NM. Is central hyperacusis a symptom of 5-hydroxytryptamine (5-HT) dysfunction? *J Laryngol Otol* 1995; **109**: 915–21.
21. Stephens SDG, Anderson CMB. Experimental studies on the uncomfortable loudness level. *J Speech Hear Res* 1971; **14**: 262–70.
22. Vernon JA. Pathophysiology of tinnitus: a special case—hyperacusis and a proposed treatment. *Am J Otol* 1987; **8**: 201–2.
23. Jastreboff PJ, Gray WC, Gold SL. Neurophysiological approach to tinnitus patients. *Am J Otol* 1996; **17**: 236–40.
24. Sammeth CA, Preves DA, Brandy WT. Hyperacusis: case studies and evaluation of electronic suppression devices as a treatment approach. *Scand Audiol* 2000; **29**: 28–36.
25. Hinchcliffe R, Chambers C. Loudness of tinnitus: an approach to measurement. *Adv Otorhinolaryngol* 1983; **29**: 163–73.
26. Hazell JWP, Sheldrake JB. Hyperacusis and tinnitus. In: Aran J-M, Dauman R eds. *Tinnitus 91: Proceedings of the Fourth International Tinnitus Seminar*, Bordeaux 1991. Amsterdam: Kugler, 1992: 245–8.
27. Anari M, Axelsson A, Eliasson A, Magnusson L. Hypersensitivity to sound. *Scand Audiol* 1999; **28**: 219–30.
28. Woodhouse A, Drummond PD. Mechanism of increased sensitivity to noise and light in migraine headache. *Cephalalgia* 1993; **13**: 417–21.
29. Elonka DR. Acute acoustic trauma after acoustic reflex testing. *Am J Otol* 1986; **7**: 164–5.
30. Axelsson A, Hamernik RP. Acute acoustic trauma. *Acta Otolaryngol* 1987; **104**: 225–33.
31. Barr T. Enquiry into the effects of loud sounds upon the hearing of boilermakers and others who work among noisy surroundings. *Proc Glasgow Phil Soc* 1886; **17**: 223–39.
32. Larsen B. Investigations of professional deafness in shipyard and machine factory labourers. *Acta Otolaryngol (Stockh)* 1939; Suppl 36: 3–255.
33. Committee on the Problem of Noise. *Noise: Final Report*. Cmnd. 2056. London: HMSO, 1963.
34. Alberti PW. Noise and the ear. In: Stephens D, ed. *Scott-Brown's Otolaryngology, 6th edn*, Vol. 2, *Adult Audiology*. London: Butterworth-Heinemann, 1997: 2/11/1–34.
35. Niemeyer W. Relations between the discomfort level and the reflex threshold of the middle ear muscles. *Audiology* 1971; **10**: 172–6.
36. Lucae A. Ueber Gehörstörungen bei Facialislähmung. *Verhandlung Berl Med Gesellschaft* 1866; **1**: 134.
37. Kar N, Banerjee SK. Prediction of recovery of Bell's palsy from clinical manifestations. *J Ind Med Assoc* 1992; **90**: 267–9.
38. Adour KK. Otological complications of herpes zoster. *Ann Neurol* 1994; **35** (Suppl): S62–4.
39. Brandt T, Dieterich M. VIIIth nerve vascular compression syndrome: vestibular paroxysmia. *Baillière's Clin Neurol* 1994; **3**: 565–75.
40. Gascon GG, Ozand PT, Erwin RE. GM1 gangliosidosis type 2 in two siblings. *J Child Neurol* 1992; **7** (Suppl): S41–50.
41. Arisoy AE, Ozden S, Ciliv G, Ozalp I. Tay–Sachs disease: a case report. *Turkish J Pediatr* 1995; **37**: 51–6.
42. Nigam A, Samuel PR. Hyperacusis and Williams syndrome. *J Laryngol Otol* 1994; **108**: 494–6.
43. Fagan SC, Rahill AA, Balakrishnan G, Ewing JR, Branch CA, Brown GG. Neurobehavioral and physiologic effects of trifluoromethane in humans. *J Toxicol Environ Health* 1995; **45**: 221–9.

44. Lader M. Anxiolytic drugs: dependence, addiction and abuse. *Eur Neuropsychopharmacol* 1994; **4**: 85–91.
45. Marsden CA. 5–hydroxytryptamine receptor subtypes and new anxiolytic drugs: an appraisal. In: *Psychopharmacology of Anxiety* Tyrer P, ed. Oxford: Oxford University Press, 1989: 3–27.
46. Hinchcliffe R. Audiology. In Maran AGD, Stell PM, eds. *Clinical Otolaryngology*. Oxford: Blackwell, 1979.
47. Hinchcliffe R. Hearing: symptoms, examination, disorders. In: Oosterveld WJ, ed. *Otoneurology*. Chichester: John Wiley, 1984: 221–66.
48. Axelsson A, Anari M. Hyperacusis. *Z Lärmbekämpf* 1995; **42**: 18–20.
49. Goldstein B, Shulman A. Tinnitus—Hyperacusis and the loudness discomfort level test—a preliminary report. *Int Tinnitus J* 1996; **2**: 83–9.
50. Brandy W, Lynn J. Audiologic findings in hyperacusic and nonhyperacusic subjects. *Am J Audiol* 1995; **4**: 46–51.
51. Sokal RR, Sneath PHA. *Principles of Numerical Taxonomy*. San Francisco: Freeman, 1963.
52. Cherry JR, Brown MJ. Relief of severe hyperacusis and diplacusis in a deafened ear by cochlear labyrinthectomy. *J Laryngol Otol* 1996; **110**: 57–8.
53. Weir N. *Otolaryngology: An Illustrated History*. London: Butterworths, 1990.
54. Stephens SDG. The input for a damaged cochlea. *Br J Audiol* 1976; **10**: 97–101.
55. Auerbach SH. Central razzle: a central auditory pain syndrome. *Arch Neurol* 1981; **38**: 671.
56. Ghosh P. Central diplacusis. *Eur Arch Otorhinolaryngol* 1990; **247**: 48–50.
57. Lee J-S. http://madang.ajou.ac.kr/~ajouorl/meniere.htm
58. Williams HL. *Menière's Disease* Springfield, IL: Charles Thomas, 1952: 109.
59. Shambaugh GE Jr. Diplacusis: a localising symptom of disease of the organ of Corti. *Arch Otolaryngol* 1940; **31**: 160–4.
60. Rossberg G. Beobachtungen von Diplacusis binauralis nach Fensterungsoperation bei Otosklerose. *Z Ohrenkeilkunde* 1954; **33**: 236–42.
61. Moos S. Doppelhören in Folge einer Jodkaliumcur. *Z Ohrenkeilkunde* 1882; **11**: 52–3.
62. Moos S. *Klinik der Ohrenkrankheiten: ein Handbuch fur Studirende und Aerzte*. Vienna: Wilhelm Braumüller, 1866.
63. Spalding FA. Diplacusis binauralis. Eine Selbstbeobachtung. *Z Ohrenkeilkunde* 1881; **10**: 143–6.
64. McKelvie WB. The effect of noise on hearing. *The Medical Press and Circular* 1937; **195**: 401–2.
65. Johnston CA. A field study of occupational deafness. *British Journal of Industrial Medicine* 1953; **10**: 41–50.
66. Atherley GRC, Nobel WG. Clinical picture of occupational hearing loss obtained with the hearing measurment scale. In *Occupational Hearing Loss*. DW Robinson (ed) London: *Academic Press* 1971, pp 193–216.
67. Health and Safety Commission. *Prevention of Damage to Hearing from Noise at Work: Draft Proposals for Regulations and Guidance*. Consultative document. London: HMSO, 1987.
68. Alberti PW. In: Salvi RJ, Henderson D, Hamernik RP, eds. *Basic and Applied Aspects of Noise-Induced Hearing Loss*. New York: Plenum Press, 1986.
69. Harrowven RGC, Greener JDF, Stephens SDG. A double blind cross-over study of high-frequency emphasis hearing aids in individuals with noise-induced hearing loss. *Br J Audiol* 1987; **21**: 209–19.
70. Albers GD. Diplacusimetry. In: *Proceedings of VIII International Congress of Otolaryngology*, Tokyo, 1965. Amsterdam: Excerpta Medica, 1966: 401.
71. Jones RO, Pracy R. An investigation of pitch discrimination in the normal and abnormal hearing adult. *J Laryngol Otol* 1971; **85**: 795–802.
72. van den Brink G. Diplacusis and threshold audiogram. *Int Audiol* 1966; **5**: 439–41.
73. Burns EM, Turner C. Pure-tone pitch anomalies. II. Pitch–intensity effects and diplacusis in impaired ears. *J Acoust Soc Am* 1986; **79**: 1530–40.
74. Forrest TG, Green DM. Detection of partially filled gaps in noise and the temporal modulation transfer function. *J Acoust Soc Am* 1987; **82**: 1933–43.
75. Scharf B. Comparison of normal and impaired hearing. *Scand Audiol 1978;* Suppl 6: 49–54.
76. Bonding P. *On Auditory Frequency Selectivity and Loudness of Noise Bands—Normative and Clinical Data*. Copenhagen: FADL's Forlag, 1981.
77. Tyler RS, Wood EJD, Fernandes M. Frequency resolution and hearing loss. *Br J Audiol* 1982; **16**: 45–63
78. Brandt JF. Frequency discrimination following exposure to noise. *J Acoust Soc Am* 1967; **41**: 448–57.
79. Tyler RS, Fernandes M, Wood EJ. Masking, temporal integration and speech intelligibility in individuals with noise-induced hearing loss. In: Taylor IG, Markides A, eds. *Disorders of Auditory Function III*. London: Academic Press, 1980.
80. Schorn K, Zwicker E. Frequency selectivity and temporal resolution in patients with various inner ear disorders. *Audiol* 1990; **29**: 8–20.
81. Robinson DO. Diplacusis associated with bilateral high frequency hearing loss. *J Speech Hear Res* 1975; **18**: 5–16.
82. Long G. Perceptual consequences of the interactions between spontaneous otoacoustic emissions and external tones. I. Monaural diplacusis and aftertones. *Hear Res* 1998; **119**: 49–60.
83. Boring EG. *Sensation and Perception in the History of Experimental Psychology*. New York: Appleton-Century, 1942.
84. Urbantschitsch V. Zur Lehre von der Schallempfindung. *Arch gesamte Physiol* 1881; **24**: 574–95.
85. Zurmühl G. Abhängigkeit der Tonhöhenempfindung von der Lautstärke und ihre Beziehung zus Helmholtzschen Resonanztheorie des Hörens. *Z Sinnesphysiol* 1930; **61**: 40–86.
86. Stevens SS. The relation of pitch to intensity. *J Acoust Soc Am* 1935; **6**: 150–4.
87. Morgan CT, Garner WR. Further measurements of the relation of pitch to intensity. *Am Psychologist* 1947; **2**: 433.
88. Burns EM. Pure-tone anomalies. I. Pitch–intensity effects and diplacusis in normal ears. *J Acoust Soc Am* 1982; **72**: 1394–402.
89. Gradenigo G. Ueber Diplacusis monauralis. *Z Ohrenkeilkunde* 1892; **23**: 251–3.

90. Hinchcliffe R, Gordon A. Subjective magnitude of symptoms and handicaps related to hearing impairment. In: Tobias JV, Jansen G, Ward WD, eds. *Proceedings of the Third International Congress on Noise as a Public Health Problem*, Freiburg 1978. ASHA Report 10. Rockville, MD: American Speech-Language-Hearing Association, 1980.
91. Blauert J. *Räumliches Hören*. Stuttgart: Hirzel, 1974.
92. Kries J von, Auerbach F. Die Zeitdauer einfachster psychicher Vorgänge. *Arch Anat Physiol* 1877; **1**: 297–378.
93. Thompson SP. Phenomena of binaural audition. *Philosophical Magazine* 1878; **6**: 383–91.
94. Stevens SS, Newman EB. The localization of pure tones. *Proc Acad Sci, Washington* 1934; **22**: 668–72.
95. Stevens SS, Newman EB. The localization of actual sources of sound. *Am J Psychol* 1936; **48**: 297–306.
96. Hornbostel EM von, Wertheimer M. Ueber die Wahrnehmung der Schallrichtung. *Akademisch Wissenschaft Wien* 1920; **15**: 388–96.
97. Batteau DW. The role of the pinna in human localization. *Proc R Soc Series B* 1967; **168**: 158–80.
98. Laborde J-V. Essai d'une détermination expérimentale et morphologique du rôle fonctionnel des canaux semi-circulaires. *Bull Soc Anthropol, Paris* 1881; **4**: 797–840.
99. Young PT. The role of head movements in auditory localization. *J Exp Psychol* 1931; **14**: 95–124.
100. Wallach H. The role of head movements and vestibular and visual cues in sound localization. *J Exp Psychol* 1940; **27**: 339–68.
101. Oldfield SR, Parker SP. Acuity of sound localisation: a topography of auditory space. I. Normal hearing conditions. *Perception* 1984; **13**: 581–600.
102. Klingon GH, Bontecou DC. Localisation in auditory space. *Neurology* 1966; **16**: 879–86.
103. Rosenhall U, Norrsell U, Ramsing S, Blomstrand C. Directional hearing and aphasia. *J Audiol Med* 1998; **7**: 200–8.
104. Haüsler R, Colburn S, Marr E. Sound localization in subjects with impaired hearing. *Acta Otolaryngol Suppl* 1983; **400**.
105. Butler RA. The effect of hearing impairment on locating sound in the vertical plane. *Int Audiol* 1970; **9**: 117–26.
106. Walsh EG. An investigation of sound localization in patients with neurological abnormalities. *Brain* 1957; **80**: 222–50.
107. Humes LE, Allen SK, Bess FH. Horizontal sound localization skills of unilaterally hearing-impaired children. *Audiology* 1980; **19**: 508–18.
108. Newton VE. Sound localisation in children with a severe unilateral hearing loss. *Audiology* 1983; **22**: 189–98.
109. Jongkees LBW, van der Veer RA. On directional sound localization in unilateral deafness and its explanation. *Acta Otolaryngol* 1958; **49**: 119–31.
110. Bauer RW, Matuzsa JL, Blackmer RF, Glucksberg S. Noise localization after unilateral attenuation. *J Acoust Soc Am* 1966; **40**: 441–4.
111. Freedman SJ, Fisher SG. The role of the pinna in auditory localization. In: Freedman SJ, ed. *The Neuropsychology of Spatially Oriented Behaviour*. Homewood, IL: Dorsey, 1968.
112. Lutman ME, Brown EJ, Coles RRA. Self-reported disability and handicap in the population in relation to pure-tone threshold, age, sex and type of hearing loss. *Audiology* 1987; **21**: 45–58.
113. Heilman KM, Pandya DN, Karol EA, Geschwind N. Auditory inattention. *Arch Neurol Chicago* 1971; **24**: 323–5.
114. Soroker N, Calamaro N, Glicksohn J, Myslobodsky MS. Auditory inattention in right hemisphere-damaged patients with and without visual neglect. *Neuropsychologia* 1997; **35**: 249–56.
115. Nilsson R, Lidén G. Sound localization with phase audiometry. *Acta Otolaryngol* 1976; **81**: 291–9.
116. Clement-Evans C. New developments in noise-induced hearing loss. *ENT News* 1998; **7**: 28–9.
117. Laird DA. Acuity of hearing. *Science* 1935; **82**: 152–3.
118. Dickson EDD, Ewing AWG, Littler TS. The effects of aeroplane noise on the auditory acuity of aviators: some preliminary remarks. *J Laryngol Otol* 1939; **54**: 531–48.
119. Jepsen O. *Studies on the Acoustic Stapedius Reflex in Man*. Aarhus: Aarhus University, 1953.
120. Lawton RW, Robinson DW. *A Concise Vocabulary of Audiology and Allied Topics*. Southampton: University of Southampton's Institute of Sound and Vibration Research, 1999.
121. McBride P. *A Guide to the Study of Ear Disease*. Edinburgh: Johnston, 1884: 156.
122. Bergman PS. Unilateral auditory hallucinations. *Trans Am Neurol Assoc* 1965; **90**: 226–7.
123. Currie S, Heathfield KWG, Henson RA, Scott DF. Clinical course and prognosis of temporal epilepsy: a survey of 666 patients. *Brain* 1971; **60**: 13–21.
124. Ross ED, Jossman PB, Bell B, Sabin T, Geschwind N. Musical hallucinations in deafness. *JAMA* 1975; **231**: 620–2.
125. Goodwin PE. Tinnitus and auditory imagery. *Am J Otol* 1980; **2**: 5–9.
126. Berrios GE. Musical hallucinations: a historical and clinical study. *Br J Psychiatry* 1990; **156**: 188–94.
127. Nayani TH, David AS. The auditory hallucination: a phenomenological survey. *Psychol Med* 1996; **26**: 177–89.
128. Ishigaki T, Tanno Y. The signal detection ability of patients with auditory hallucination: analysis using the continuous performance test. *Psychiatry Clin Neurosci* 1999; **53**: 471–6.
129. Formby C, Gjerdingen DB. Pure-tone masking of tinnitus. *Audiology* 1980; **19**: 519–35.
130. Gulick WL, Gescheider GA, Frisina RD. *Hearing: Physiological Acoustics, Neural Coding, and Psychoacoustics*. Oxford: Oxford University Press, 1989.
131. Brunner G. The etiology and symptomatology of autophony. *Arch Otol* 1883; **12**: 238–44.
132. Knapp H. A personal experience of an acute attack of autophony. *Arch Otol* 1900; **29**: 325–8.
133. O'Connor AF, Shea JJ. Autophony and the patulous eustachian tube. *Laryngoscope* 1981; **91**: 1427–35.
134. Ward W. Tonal monaural diplacusis. *J Acoust Soc of Am* 1955; **27**: 365–72.
135. Hyde ML, Stephens SDG. Psychoacoustical experimentation. In: Beagley HA, ed. *Auditory Investigation*. Oxford: Oxford University Press, 1979.

136. Hood JD, Poole JP. Tolerable limits of loudness: its clinical and physiological significance. *J Acoust Soc Am* 1966; **40**: 47–53.
137. Simmons FB, Dixon RF. Clinical implications of loudness balancing. *Arch Otolaryngol* 1966; **83**: 449–54.
138. Fowler EP. Some attributes of loudness recruitment. *Trans Am Acad Ophthalmol Otol* 1965; **53**: 78–84.
139. Davis H, Goodman AC. Subtractive hearing loss, loudness recruitment, and decruitment. *Ann Otol Rhinol Laryngol* 1966; **75**: 87–94.
140. Morrison AW. Menière's disease. In: Dix MR, Hood JD, eds. *Vertigo*. Chichester: John Wiley, 1984: 133–52.
141. Dix MR, Hallpike CS, Hood JD. Observations upon the loudness recruitment phenomenon, with a special reference to the differential diagnosis of disorders of the internal ear and eighth nerve. *Proc R Soc Med* 1948; **41**: 516–26.
142. Dix MR. Observations upon the nerve fibre deafness of multiple sclerosis, with particular reference to the phenomenon of loudness recruitment. *J Laryngol Otol* 1965; **79**: 695–706.
143. Davis H, Silverman SR. *Hearing and Deafness*. New York: Holt, Rinehart and Winston, 1978.
144. Ward WD. Effects of noise exposure on auditory sensitivity. In: Lee DHK, ed. *Handbook of Physiology*. Vol. 9: *Reaction to Environmental Agents*. Bethesda: American Physiological Society, 1977: 1–15.
145. Kemp DT. Evidence of mechanical nonlinearity and frequency selective wave amplification in the cochlea. *Arch Otolaryngol* 1979; **224**: 37–45.
146. Daae H. Ueber Doppelhören. *Z Ohrenkeilkunde* 1894; **25**: 251–68.
147. Bunch CC. Hearing aids. *Trans Am Acad Ophthalmol Otol* 1942; **46**: 163–78.
148. Evans EF. The sharpening of cochlear frequency selectivity in the normal and abnormal cochlea. *Audiology* 1975; **14**: 419–42.
149. Itard JMG. *Traité des maladies de l'oreille et de l'audition*. Paris: Méquignon-Marvis, 1821: 42.
150. Bacon SP, Viemeister NF. A case study of monaural diplacusis. *Hear Res* 1985; **19**: 49–56.
151. Hallam R, Jakes SC, Chambers C, Hinchcliffe R. A comparison of different methods for assessing the 'intensity' of tinnitus. *Acta Otolaryngol (Stockh)* 1985; **99**: 501–8.
152. Tschiassny K. Stapedioparalytic phonophobia ('hyperacusis') in a dead ear; case reports including studies on analysis of the phenomenon and suggestions for applications of phonophobia test. *Laryngoscope* 1949; **59**: 886–903.
153. Small AM. Pure-tone masking. *J Acoust Soc Am* 1959; **31**: 1619–25.
154. Leschowitz B, Lindstrom R, Zurek P. Psychophysical tuning curves in normal and hearing impaired ears. *J Acoust Soc Am* 1975; **58**: S71.
155. Gibson WPR. The physical and functional examination of the ear. In: Ballantyne J, Groves J, eds. *Scott-Brown's Diseases of the Ear, Nose and Throat*. Vol. 2 *The Ear*. London: Butterworths, 1984.
156. Lempp O. Ueber Diplakusis und musikalisches Falschhören. *Hals-, Nasen-, Ohrenartz* 1938; **46**: 193–255.
157. Politzer A. Studien über die Paracusis loci. *Arch Ohrenheilkunde* 1876; **11**: 231–6.
158. Oldfield SR, Parker SP. Acuity of sound localisation: a topography of auditory space. II. Pinna cues absent. *Perception* 1984; **13**: 601–17.
159. Oldfield SR, Parker SP. Acuity of sound localisation: a topography of auditory space. III. Monaural hearing conditions. *Perception* 1986; **15**: 67–81.
160. Berthold E. Ueber diplacusis monauralis. *Arch Ohrenkeilkunde* 1902; **55**: 17–25.
161. Formby C, Gjerdingen DB. Some systematic observations on monaural diplacusis. *Audiology* 1981; **20**: 219–33.
162. Moos S. Ein einfaches Verfahren zur Diagnose einseitig simulierter Taubheit. *Arch Augenheilkunde* 1869; **1**: 240–4.
163. Shambaugh GE Jr. Syndrome of diplacusis and nerve deafness for low tones. *Arch Otolaryngol* 1935; **21**: 694–702.
164. Gruber J. *Lehrbuch der Ohrenheilkunde*. Vienna: Carl Gerold's Sohn, 1888.
165. Treitel L. Ueber Diplacusis binauralis. *Arch Ohrenkeilkunde* 1891; **32**: 215–24.
166. Flottorp G. Pure-tone tinnitus evoked by acoustic stimulation: the idiophonic effect. *Acta laryngologica* 1953; **43**: 396–415.
167. Steinbrügge H. Ein Fall von Diplacusis. *Z Ohrenkeilkunde* 1882; **11**: 53–5.
168. Medical Research Council. *The Localisation of Sound*. Report of the Committee on the Physiology of Hearing III. MRC Special Report Series No. 207. London: Medical Research Council, 1936.
169. Blauert J. *The Psychophysics of Human Sound Localisation*. Cambridge, MA: MIT Press, 1997.
170. Gilkey RH, Anderson TR (Eds) *Binaural and Spatial Hearing in Real and Virtual Environments*. New York: Erlbaum, 1997.
171. Bernstein LR. Auditory processing of interaural timing information: new insights. *J Neurosci Res* 2001; **66**: 1035–46.
172. Mrsic-Flogel TD, King AJ, Jenison RL, Schnupp JW. Listening through different ears alters spatial response in ferret primary cortex. *J Neurophysiol* 2001; **86**: 1043–46.
173. Euston DR, Takahashi TT. From spectrum to space: the contribution of level difference cues to spatial receptive fields in the barn owl inferior colliculus. *J Neurosci* 2002; **22**: 284–93.
174. Lewald J, Foltys H, Topper R. Role of the posterior parietal cortex in spatial hearing. *J Neurosci* 2002; **22**: RC207.
175. Tohyama M, Suzuki H, Ando Y. *The Nature and Technology of Acoustic Space*. New York: Academic Press, 1995.
176. Recanzone GH, Guard DC, Phan ML, Su TK. Correlation between the activity of single auditory neurons and sound-localization behavior in the macaque monkey. *J Neurophysiol* 2000; **83**: 723–39
177. http://www.sfu.ca/sonic-studio/handbook/Acoustic_Space.html (accessed 28 May 2002).
178. http://www.sfu.ca/sonic-studio/handbook/Soundscape.html (accessed 28 May 2002)
179. Koch U, Grothe B. Interdependence of spatial and temporal coding in the auditory midbrain. *J Neurophysiol* 2000; **83**: 2300–14
180. Pratt H, Bleich N, Mittelman N. Echo suppression in the human cortex is affected by the spatial and temporal proximity of the primary sound and echo. *J Basic & Clinical Physiol & Pharmacol* 2001; **12**: 109–23.

181. Lewald J, Karnath HO. Vestibular influence on human auditory space perception. *J Neurophysiol* 2000; **84**: 1107–11.
182. DiZio P, Held R, Lackner JR *et al.* Gravitoinertial force magnitude and direction influence head-centric auditory localization. *J Neurophysiol* 2001; **85**; 2445–60
183. Frassinetti F, Pavani F, Ladavas E. Acoustical vision of neglected stimuli: interaction among spatially converging audiovisual inputs in neglect patients. *J Cogn Neurosci* 2002; **14**: 62–9.
184. Pavani F, Ladavas E, Driver J. Selective deficit of auditory localisation in patients with visuospatial neglect. *Neuropsychologia* 2002; **40**: 291–301.
185. Morfey CL. *Dictionary of Acoustics*. New York: Academic Press, 2001.
186. http://www.sfu.ca/sonic-studio/handbook/Projicience.html (accessed 28 May 2002)
187. Mickey BJ, Middlebrooks JC. Responses of auditory cortical neurons to pairs of sounds: correlates of fusion and localization. *J Neurophysiol* 2001; **86**: 1333–50.
188. Ingham NJ, Hart HC, McAlpine D. Spatial receptive fields of inferior colliculus neurons to auditory apparent motion in free field. *J Neurophysiol* 2001; **85**: 23–33
189. Xiang J, Chuang S, Wilson D et al. Sound motion evoked magnetic fields. *Clin Neurophysiol* 2002; **113**: 1–9.
190. Reale RA, Brugge JF. Directional sensitivity of neurons in the primary auditory (AI) cortex of the cat to successive sounds ordered in time and space. *J Neurophysiol* 2000; **84**: 435–50.
191. Su TI, Recanzone GH. Differential effect of near-threshold stimulus intensities on sound localization performance in azimuth and elevation in normal human subjects. *Jaro* 2001; **2**: 246–56.
192. Tollinn DJ, Yin TC. The coding of spatial location by single units in the lateral superior olive of the cat. II. The determinants of spatial receptive fields in azimuth. *J Neurosci* 2002; **22**: 1468–79.
193. Yost WA. *Fundamentals of Hearing*, Fourth edition. San Diego: Academic Press, 2000.

Glossary

Acoustic space–The perceived volume encompassed by a *soundscape*, either an actual environment, or an imagined one such as produced with a tape recording and several loudspeakers.

Agnosia, auditory–Inability to recognize music, words or other organized sounds because of a defect of the hearing part of the brain.

Anacusis–Complete elevation of the hearing threshold level, i.e. total loss of hearing.

Anechoic room (chamber)–A room or chamber that attempts to obtain *free-field* conditions; this is achieved by lining the room surfaces with sound-absorbing material, usually in the form of wedges.

Auditory acuity–A term to denote sharpness of hearing; used to refer to the hearing threshold level[117–119] or, more broadly, to also cover other auditory functions, e.g. frequency and intensity discriminations.[120]

Auditory hallucinations–Hearing organized sounds (in contrast to tinnitus), e.g. voices or music, which are not audible to others and where there is no corresponding external stimulus.[121–128]

Auditory sensitivity–A term to denote hearing sensitivity without any commitment as to whether or not the hearing is within the range of normality or outside it, and, if the latter, whether it is better or poorer, and, if the latter, whether it amounts to an impairment (material or otherwise) or a hearing loss and whether or not it results in one or more inabilities, disabilities or handicaps.[129,130]

Autophony–Increased resonance of one's own voice, breath or other body sounds which is perceived in association with upper respiratory tract and middle ear cleft disorders,[131,132] including patulous auditory tube.[133]

Combination tone–A tone which may be heard when an acoustical stimulus is delivered to the ear but is not present physically in that stimulus; it must therefore have arisen from non-linear distortion in the auditory system; the case which is usually being considered is when the acoustical stimulus comprises two pure tones of different frequencies.

Critical band–The range of frequencies that are centered on some specified frequency and whose width is a measure of the frequency resolution (selectivity) of the ear at that frequency.

Diffuse field–Where reflecting surfaces are such that the sound intensity is uniform.

Diplacusis–An abnormal perception of sound in respect of time or pitch in which one sound is heard as two (or more) sounds; strictly speaking, the phenomenon should be referred to as 'polyacusis'.[134]

Diplacusis, binaural–A given sound is perceived as two different sounds in the two ears.

Diplacusis echoica–A sound heard in the affected ear is perceived as being repeated.

Diplacusis, monaural–A sound heard in the affected ear is perceived as two sounds; more precisely, the phenomenon is said to exist when an acoustical stimulus consisting of a single sinusoid and presented monaurally is judged to be plural.[134]

Diplacusis, monaural, atonal–The perceived sound is buzzing, noisy or rough.

Diplacusis, monaural, tonal–The perceived sound is of two or more pure tones.

Directionalization, sound–A term to denote an individual's ability to determine the direction from which a sound is coming.[135]

Discrimination, frequency–The ability to distinguish two successively presented tones.

Doppler shift–Shift in perceived sound frequency as a sound source moves towards (increase in frequency) or away from (decrease in frequency) an observer.

Dysacusis–A term that has been applied to any impairment of auditory perception that is not primarily a loss of auditory sensitivity, so that it has been used to cover the diplacuses, dysstereoacusis, hyperacusis, speech discrimination loss, auditory agnosia, auditory inattention, and King–Kopetzky syndrome.

Dysstereoacusis–Impaired ability to localize sound in space (syn. paracusis loci).
Echoic (reverberation) room (chamber)–A room or chamber that attempts to obtain *diffuse-field* conditions; used to investigate reverberation times; these increase when sound absorption decreases and the volume of the sound spaces increases.
EOAE–Evoked otoacoustic emissions (Kemp 'echoes').
Free field–An environment free of sound scattering or reflecting boundaries so that outgoing sound waves never return towards their source origin. In a truly free field change in sound intensity conforms to the *inverse square law*.
Hallucinations, auditory–Hearing organized sounds (in contrast to tinnitus), e.g. voices or music, which are not audible to others and where there is no corresponding external stimulus.
Health and Safety Commission–The official body in the UK which is responsible for the care of factory workers.
Hearing loss–An impairment of hearing that exceeds a criterial level; no units, but may be qualified, in terms of severity, as 'mild', 'severe' etc. Neither the term 'hearing loss' nor the term 'hearing gain' should be used to describe hearing which is, respectively, greater than, or less than, the average hearing threshold level, just as the terms 'height loss' or 'height gain' would not be used to describe the height of someone who was less than, or greater than, average height, unless it had been shown that a loss or a gain in height had occurred, e.g. by serial measurements.
Hearing status–A description of the degree to which the hearing of an individual functions normally with respect to accepted criteria (analogous to health status).
Hearing threshold level (HTL)–For a particular ear, and a given frequency and test system, it is an individual's threshold of hearing (i.e. the quietest sound that he can hear) as determined in a stated manner and expressed by the system's indicated 'hearing level' value. Expressed in decibels, i.e. as dB HTL.
HSC–Health and Safety Commission.
HSS–Hypersensitivity to sound.[27]
5-HT–Abbreviation for 5-hydroxytryptamine.
HTL–Abbreviation for hearing threshold level.
5-Hydroxytryptamine–Synonym for serotonin.
Hyperacusis–Abnormal sensitivity to one or other sound; also defined more strictly as a condition in which the patient, with or without hearing loss, experiences severe loudness discomfort from everyday environmental sound levels;[50] 'It is incorrect to use the term as a general designation, as it only rarely signifies an increased auditory acuity, but more frequently a hypersensitiveness to loud sounds.'[119]
Hyperacusis, threshold–Hyperacusis associated with abnormally low auditory thresholds (≥10 dB better than the age-related norm)[50]
Hyperacusis, suprathreshold–Discomfort from sounds less than about 65 dB SPL when hearing is normal.[50]
Hypoacusis–Partial impairment of hearing as indicated by an elevated hearing threshold level.
Inverse square law–In an acoustic *free-field* the sound intensity is inversely proportional to the distance from the sound squared. Thus doubling the distance produces a fall in the sound intensity by a factor of four, i.e. 6 dB (10 log 4). Since the sound pressure is proportional to the square root of the intensity, doubling the distance produces a fall in the sound pressure by a factor of two. This still represents a 6 dB change (20 log 2).
jnd–Just-noticeable difference.
LDL–Loudness discomfort level[136] (but since there are many loudness discomfort levels, it is preferable to refer to the threshold of uncomfortable loudness (TUL), which the LDL test purports to determine).
Listener envelopment–The sense of being surrounded by sound, especially in a concert hall. Listener envelopment is a component of *spatial impression*; it is considered to be related to the later reverberant sound received by the listener and to increase with sound level.
Localization, sound–Encompasses both directionalization and distance perception.
Loudness–The subjective dimension of the objective (physical) dimension of sound (intensity, pressure); unit is the sone; as a rule of thumb, a 1-dB increase in the SPL of a noise gives a 10% increase in loudness, and a 10-dB increase produces a doubling of the loudness.
Loudness adaptation–Decrease in the loudness of a steady tone over time.
Loudness decrement–Synonym loudness derecruitment.[137]
Loudness derecruitment–The converse of loudness recruitment, i.e. the presence of an abnormally slow growth in loudness.[138, 139]
Loudness level–The loudness level, in phons, of a sound is numerically equal to the sound pressure level in decibels (relative to a pressure of 20 μPa) of a simple tone of frequency 1 kHz which is judged by the median listener to be equivalent in loudness.[4]
Loudness over-recruitment–A condition in which the growth of loudness results not only in normal loudness for a given sound pressure but continues to rise so that a greater loudness than would otherwise be the case is reached; this phenomenon may be associated with abnormal sensitivity to sound.[140]
Loudness recruitment–The growth of the sensation of loudness more rapidly than is normally the case.[141]
Loudness reversal–Synonym for loudness derecruitment.[142]
MAA–Minimum audible angle; a measure of spatial discrimination for sound sources.[104]
MCLL–Most comfortable loudness level.
mel–The unit of pitch; 1000 mels is the pitch of a 1000-Hz tone at a sensation level of 40 dB.
Most comfortable loudness level–The level at which an individual registers what he considers to be the most comfortable loudness for a sound (tone, speech units) that is presented to him (usually from an audiometer); provides a measure of loudness tolerance and an index of loudness recruitment.
Neurotransmitter: a specific body chemical that transmits the information contained in a nervous impulse from one nerve cell to the next.

Noise–Unwanted sound, but 'physically identical sound may become noise to one person and music to another, depending on whether one likes Mozart or rock and roll . . . The noise of the neighbor's lawnmover [*sic*] may be annoying if (s)he mowed the lawn two days ago, but a pleasant relief if (s)he just returned from a six weeks vacation to clean up an overgrown front yard.'[13]

Noise pollution level–An index of noise annoyance which takes into account not only the level of noise but also the fluctuation in that level (abbreviation NPL; symbol L_{NP})

Normal threshold of hearing–'A term which should be avoided because of its medical and medicolegal implications.'[143] There is no single normal threshold of hearing; there are indeed a number of normal thresholds of normal hearing.

Nosoacusis–Hearing loss due to all factors other than aging, and industrial and non-industrial noise exposure.[144]

noy–The unit (subjective) of noisiness, i.e. parallels the sone for loudness; thus a sound of 4 noys is four times as noisy as a sound of one noy.

OAE–Otoacoustical emissions (may be SOAE or EOAE).

ONIHL–Occupational noise induced hearing loss

Otoacoustic emissions–Sound energy which is emitted by the internal ear (more specifically, the outer hair cells of the cochlea), either spontaneously or evoked.[145]

Oxyacoa–Synonym for oxyaecoia.

Oxyacoia–Synonym for oxyaecoia.

Oxyaecoia–Enhanced sensitivity to sounds due to having a threshold of hearing that is lower than that of the average person.

para-–A prefix that denotes a departure from the normal.

Paracusis–A term applied to one or other of the various disorders of auditory perception which may have a peripheral or central origin.

Paracusis acris–Synonym for hyperacusis.

Paracusis duplicata–Synonym for diplacusis.

Paracusis isoacutica–A condition in which all frequencies in a particular frequency band are perceived as being of the same pitch;[146, 147] the pathophysiological basis could be the loss of 'tips' of the tuning curves of cochlear neural elements with degradation to a very broad tuning.[148]

Paracusis loci–Impaired, including absent, ability to determine the location of a sound source.

Paracusis obtusa–Impaired, including absent, hearing, so covering hypoacusis and anacusis.

Paracusis perversa–Synonym for parcusis Willisii.

Paracusis sclerotica–If this form of paracusis is present, the patient will say that the sound is distorted, harder (hence the term, paracusis sclerotica), harsher, rougher or out of tune on one or other side;[7, 146, 149, 150] this percept can be considered as a variant of paracusis duplicata in the sense that it can be looked upon as atonal polyacusis.

Paracusis Willisii–The symptom of hearing a speaker better in noisy environments than in quiet ones; synonym for false paracusis.

Personal loudness unit–The unit of a scale of loudness that has been determined for a specific individual.[25] Only audiometric matches of the tinnitus 'intensity' in terms of PLUs are significantly correlated with reported loudness; unlike other measures of tinnitus 'intensity', PLU transformations of tinnitus 'intensity' produce tinnitus 'intensity' values that are generally independent of other audiometric measures.[151]

phon–The unit of loudness level; 40 phons is the loudness level of a 40 dB SPL 1-kHz tone.

Phonophobia–A morbid fear of one or other sound, including one's own voice, although term also used as a synonym for hyperacusis.[152]

Pitch–The subjective magnitude of frequency; unit is the mel.

PLU–Personal loudness unit

Post-traumatic stress disorder–A psychiatric disorder (F43.1 of ICD-10) that arises as a delayed or protracted response to a stressful event or situation (of either brief or long duration) of an exceptionally threatening or catastrophic nature, which is likely to cause pervasive distress in almost anyone. Predisposing factors, such as personality traits or previous history of neurotic illness, may lower the threshold for the development of the syndrome or aggravate its course, but they are neither necessary nor sufficient to explain its occurrence. Typical features include episodes of repeated reliving of the trauma in intrusive memories ('flashbacks'), dreams or nightmares, occurring against the persisting background of a sense of 'numbness' and emotional blunting, detachment from other people, unresponsiveness to other people, unresponsiveness to surroundings, anhedonia, and avoidance of activities and situations reminiscent of the trauma.

Projicience–The sense of depth of a sound in *acoustic space* (http://www.sfu.ca/sonicstudio/handbook/Projicience.html (accessed 28 May 2002)).

Psychophysical function–The mathematical expression that relates the subjective magnitude of a stimulus to its physical magnitude; until the 1950s, this was considered to be a logarithmic function; the scientific evidence accumulated over the past half-century indicates it to be a power function.

Psychophysical tuning curve–A measure of the frequency selectivity of the ear.[153, 154]

Psychophysics–The science that studies the relationship between physical stimuli and the resulting sensations.

PTC–Psychophysical tuning curve.

Range–The difference between the minimum and maximum values for a measurement.

Range of normal hearing–The scatter of actual determinations of hearing sensitivity of normally hearing persons with respect to age and gender. Sometimes, the limit is taken arbitrarily as two standard deviations from the mean, sometimes as the 95th percentile.

Selectivity, frequency–The ability to detect one frequency in the presence of others.

Semeion–Any untoward phenomenon, or departure from the normal in structure, function or sensation, which is experienced by an individual, or noted by another person, but which is

elicited only by direct questioning and is not spontaneously reported; such a person is termed a respondent (not a patient).
Serotonin–A neurotransmitter (physiological chemical), 5-hydroxytryptamine, that influences the calibre of blood vessels, body secretions and psychological states.
SOAE–Spontaneous otoacoustical emissions.
Sonalgia–Pain experienced by sound exposure.[27]
sone–The unit of loudness; one sone is the loudness of a sound whose loudness level P is 40 phons; loudness S in sones is related to loudness level in phons by the relation:[4]

$$S = 2^{(P-40)/10}$$

Sound field–Any environment that contains sound.
Soundscape–A sound environment, with emphasis on the way it is perceived and understood by the individual, or by a society. It thus depends on the relationship between the individual and any such environment. The term may refer to actual environments, or to abstract constructions such as musical compositions and tape montages, particularly when considered as an artificial environment.
Source broadening–The sense that a sound source, especially the orchestra or players in a concert hall, occupies a larger region than its physical extent. It is one component of *spatial impression*.
Spatial impression–The sense, due to sound heard by the ears, of being in three-dimensional space. Spatial impression in concert halls is currently thought to consist of two separate components, i.e. *source broadening* and *listener envelopment*.
Stereoacusis–Spatial hearing ability.
Symptom–Any untoward phenomenon, or departure from the normal in structure, function or sensation, which is experienced by a patient, or noted by another person, and spontaneously reported to the doctor when medical advice is sought.
TUL–Threshold of uncomfortable loudness (as determined by audiometric testing, usually for pure tones).
ULL–Uncomfortable loudness level (but since there are many uncomfortable loudness levels, it is preferable to refer to the threshold of uncomfortable loudness (TUL), which the ULL test purports to determine).

35 Psychological aspects of hearing impairment and tinnitus

Laurence McKenna, Gerhard Andersson

Introduction

The application of clinical psychology within the fields of audiological medicine and otolaryngology is relatively new. Most of the clinical psychology research in this field has taken place since the early 1980s in a few centres around the world, particularly in the UK, Sweden and Australia. The amount of psychological research done in this area has not matched that seen in other areas of health care such as pain management, primarily because the number of psychologists involved in audiology is still relatively few. In spite of this, psychologists have made important contributions to our understanding of the nature and management of distressing audiological symptoms. The body of psychological work has been reviewed in a number of places[1, 2] and this chapter seeks to highlight the more salient aspects of the psychological literature on tinnitus and acquired hearing loss and to update the earlier reviews.

Tinnitus

> To view tinnitus as a complaint about a noise in the ears or head that varies only in its psychophysical parameters is inadequate. People's complaints about tinnitus are complex and usually multidimensional.

There are a number of descriptions of the negative consequences of tinnitus.[3–7] These accounts indicate that tinnitus complaint includes references to factors such as sleep disturbance and emotional distress as well as auditory perceptual disorders. It is important to note that there are large individual differences in the extent to which people experience these problems. It is also the case that different treatments may be expected to affect different aspects of tinnitus complaint. Recent work[8] suggests that children's experiences of tinnitus are parallel to those of adults.

Tinnitus and emotional distress

The link between tinnitus and emotional distress has been investigated in several studies.[9–16] Most studies on the emotional consequences of tinnitus have been conducted on highly selective samples of patients with severe tinnitus distress[17] and the conclusions drawn may not apply to all tinnitus patients. Some studies have found relatively low (but significant) correlations between tinnitus distress and psychological complaints.[10, 18]

> 45% of those whose main complaint was tinnitus showed signs of significant psychological disturbance,[13] while 63% of tinnitus sufferers could be classified as psychiatrically disturbed and 46% had mood disorder as assessed by the Structured Interview for the DSM-III-R (SCID).

Russo et al.[19] used the DSM-IV to estimate the prevalence of psychiatric disorder among tinnitus patients. A number of studies have used the Beck Depression Inventory (BDI)[20] in the assessment of tinnitus patients. Kirsch et al.[12] reported that the mean BDI score for a group of tinnitus patients was within the normal range, but other researchers[21] and unpublished data from a Swedish population (Andersson, unpublished data), using larger samples, revealed mean scores within the range of mild mood disturbance. Erlandsson[22] theorized that there are two psychological reactions to tinnitus, one characterized by anxiety and one by depression, but these thoughts have not yet been validated empirically. In a review by Hinchcliffe and

King[23] depression was found to be the principal distinguishing feature between tinnitus complainers and non-complainers. However McKenna,[24, 25] reported that anxiety, and in particular trait rather than state anxiety,[26] is a characteristic of tinnitus patients. Subsequent, unpublished data from the same author[27] indicated BDI scores within the normal range for a group of tinnitus patients. As with hearing impairment, psychoacoustical measures (e.g. matching of tinnitus loudness) have not been found to be good predictors of tinnitus discomfort.[28]

A number of self-report scales for the assessment of tinnitus-related distress have been developed.[7, 21, 29] Most of these scales have good psychometric properties, and the Tinnitus Effects Questionnaire[7] has been applied both in Germany[30] and in Sweden.[31] It is recognized that much of the severity of tinnitus relates to the individual's psychological response to the stimulus, and it has been recommended that these self-report scales form part of the assessment of tinnitus severity in both clinical and medico-legal contexts.[32] Daily measures of tinnitus distress and loudness on Visual Analogue Scales have been used in clinical and research settings,[33, 34] even though the use of repeated measures designs is relatively rare. Self-report measures like the BDI,[20] the Beck Anxiety Inventory,[35] and other measures of psychological problems, such as personality and coping, may well be used in audiological populations, given some consideration of the group being assessed. Self-report is becoming an important tool in audiological research and rehabilitation. It has a potential value for research on rehabilitation effectiveness and for the treatment itself. A structured interview has been developed in Uppsala, Sweden, with which all patients referred to the psychologist for tinnitus treatment are assessed. The interview is structured along cognitive behavioural principles. In addition to descriptions of the tinnitus, detailed information is sought about its antecedent variables (affecting changes in it) and consequences, and its severity is graded on a three-point scale.[36] The information gathered then guides the psychological treatment offered.

Psychological model of tinnitus

Among the earliest and most significant of contributions from psychologists within the field was Hallam, Hinchcliffe and Rachman's[4] psychological model of tinnitus. The authors suggested that the natural history of tinnitus is characterized by the process of habituation. They conceived of patients' complaints of distress associated with tinnitus as a failure of habituation. They suggested that habituation to tinnitus follows the same rules as habituation to any other constant stimulus. They pointed out that habituation is slowed by factors such as a high level of tonic arousal and by the stimulus acquiring an emotive significance.

This original model has been challenged.[37] Dishabituation may be another way of describing the process of developing tinnitus-related distress, in that the emotional colouring of the tinnitus sound is interpreted as a warning signal that short-circuits the habituation.[38] However, relatively little research has been done to support these other approaches, and the above model[4] remains the main inspiration for clinical work, suggesting that psychological treatment should focus on reducing patients' arousal and changing the emotional significance of the tinnitus, i.e. a cognitive behaviour therapy (CBT) approach to tinnitus management.

Cognitive behavioural therapy

A CBT approach to tinnitus management has been suggested by others.[39] Other psychological treatment styles, besides a strict CBT approach, have also been suggested, but most, like CBT, are aimed at decreasing the psychological distress associated with tinnitus, rather than lessening the sound itself. Andersson et al.[40] reviewed psychological outcome studies employing hypnosis, biofeedback, relaxation, and CBT with or without applied relaxation. They concluded that CBT approaches received the most empirical support. The clearest benefits observed were in terms of reduced tinnitus annoyance, with weaker improvements in negative affect and sleep disturbance. Improvements were reported in tinnitus loudness immediately following treatment.

Perhaps the most challenging aspect of the psychological model is its reference to cognitive therapy. Implicit within this approach to treatment is the idea that tinnitus per se is less important than the patients' beliefs about it. Many patients do not find this an intuitively appealing idea, and a certain amount of convincing or 'socializing' of patients to this model is often needed.

Cognitive therapy is a form of psychotherapy that focuses on discovering people's thought processes and changing these when they are unrealistically negative or unhelpful.

It is based on the cognitive model of Aaron Beck,[41] and forms the basis for the practice of many clinical psychologists in the UK and elsewhere. The model proposes that people's thoughts influence their emotional state, and that negative thoughts are not only a feature of emotional disturbance, but maintain the disorder. Negative beliefs relate to the person, the world and the future. They are maintained by cognitive distortions such as 'all or nothing thinking' or the selective acceptance of information that confirms the person's ideas and rejection of information that contradicts them. Cognitive distortions are, in turn, thought to occur as a consequence of the poor emotional state. Cognitive therapy is pragmatic in style and is usually brief, ranging from as few as six to about twenty sessions, over a course of months rather than years. Part of the therapeutic effort is to elucidate the person's thoughts about his or her circumstances. People are often unaware of the content of their thoughts until they pay specific attention to them, and they are commonly much more aware of the emotions than the thoughts produced. Thoughts often have an automatic quality and take the form of a 'running commentary' or 'dialogue' and are frequently in a shorthand form. Automatic thoughts are not necessarily the result of reasoning or reflection on a situation, but instead often arise spontaneously. They tend to be specific and can be plausible in-spite of evidence that contradicts them. They do not necessarily arise as a result of external events but can be provoked by ruminations or memories. Techniques such as questioning and diary-keeping help to reveal the content of automatic thoughts. Another part of the therapy involves assessing the accuracy of automatic thoughts through the use of techniques such as questioning (rather than persuasion) or behavioural experiments. The discovery of negative distortions in one's automatic thoughts leads to the thoughts being reformulated and a consequent improvement in the associated emotion. In addition to day-to-day thoughts, the person can be helped to become aware of deeper 'core' beliefs that are formed through early learning experiences. These are more difficult to articulate and may take some effort to access. These core beliefs are generalized in nature and ultimately have a determining influence on how the person thinks about all events. Most people maintain relatively positive core beliefs, most of the time, but at times of emotional distress negative beliefs can emerge and become dominant. When they have a negative content, core beliefs are commonly concerned with the idea that the person is 'not good enough' in terms of being either inadequate or unloveable in some way. Intermediary beliefs in the form of attitudes, rules and assumptions lie between the core beliefs and the day-to-day automatic thoughts. Intermediate beliefs help the person to cope with painful ideas inherent in the core beliefs. Initially, therapy usually focuses on identifying and changing automatic thoughts in order to produce symptom relief. Subsequently, intermediate and core beliefs, which are common to many situations, become the focus of the treatment.

Neurophysiological model of tinnitus

There are striking parallels between Hallam's[4] model and the more recent neurophysiological model of tinnitus suggested by Jastreboff and Hazell.[42] Although different language is used, both emphasize the role of central rather than peripheral factors in tinnitus perception, both point to the importance of autonomic nervous system arousal, and both highlight the importance of the emotional significance of the tinnitus.

> The neurophysiological model, however, extends the psychological one by suggesting that the use of sound enrichment serves to disrupt neuronal networks that process tinnitus information.

Tinnitus retraining therapy (TRT), the treatment that derives from this model, involves a combination of counselling and sound enrichment. This model further extends the psychological one by suggesting that TRT leads not only to habituation of reaction to tinnitus but in some cases also to habituation of perception of tinnitus.

The similarities and differences between the neurophysiological and psychological models and the relative merits of both have been a focus of debate. A particular confusion has been between the counselling element of TRT, known as directive counselling, and CBT. Early papers on the neurophysiological model seem to use the terms 'directive counselling' and 'cognitive therapy' interchangeably, and the intention of the directive counselling process is to change patients' beliefs about their tinnitus. Psychologists,[43] however, have suggested that directive counselling does not equate to cognitive therapy, as it does not meet the rigorous standards and protocols of that therapy. Jastreboff[44] also sought to highlight differences between TRT and cognitive therapy. However, the descriptions of the directive counselling provided are again reminiscent of those associated with cognitive therapy. She has suggested that psychological therapy will not lead to lasting improvements in tinnitus complaints. It is suggested that, while both psychological therapy and TRT seek to modify the emotional significance of tinnitus, TRT extends this by addressing patients' subconscious non-verbal processing of tinnitus information, presumably through the use of sound enrichment. The contention[44] is that only by influencing both conscious and subconscious processes can enduring improvements be achieved. The evidence, to date, does not support this contention. A number of methodological difficulties with TRT studies have been highlighted by Wilson et al.[43] and it is not yet clear that the benefits of TRT extend beyond those that might be offered by directive counselling. One of the most recent psychological therapy outcome studies[45] reported results that were as favourable, or more so, than the suggested standards for TRT.[46]

Cognitive measures in tinnitus sufferers

The focus on central factors in tinnitus perception has led to studies on measures such as evoked potentials,[47] regional cerebral blood flow,[48] and auditory brain stem responses.[49] It has also led to a small series of studies on the cognitive functioning or information-processing abilities of tinnitus patients.[24, 25, 27] This work has focused on a hitherto neglected aspect of tinnitus complaint, i.e. concentration problems. The findings suggest that tinnitus patients do experience some inefficiency in cognitive processing that cannot be accounted for simply in terms of emotional disturbance. A clearer understanding of the exact nature of the difficulties is still awaited, but it may be that tinnitus occupies part of the capacity of the working memory system, a series of cognitive structures that hold information on its arrival in the system until it can be processed further. Research on tinnitus and cognitive performance has led to a modified psychological theory of tinnitus in which it is regarded as a 'changing-state' stimulus (i.e. it comes and goes because of masking environmental sound or it is a variable stimulus in itself).[50] This reasoning is influenced by cognitive psychology and the finding that an auditory stimulus that changes in pitch has the capacity to negatively affect cognitive processing to an equal degree as irrelevant speech.[51] Given that tinnitus can be regarded as a 'changing-state' stimulus it is not surprising to find that tinnitus patients often complain of concentration problems and that many people do not manage to habituate to tinnitus. The psychology of tinnitus continues to develop.

Hearing loss

Hearing-impaired people are commonly regarded as suffering from psychological disturbances such as depression or paranoia,[52] although this observation has only partly been investigated in the empirical literature.[53] It has also been observed that people who use hearing aids are regarded less favourably by others than people without a hearing aid.[54] There are certainly good reasons to suppose that hearing loss might influence the onset of psychological disturbance. Acquired hearing impairment involves losses of one kind or another. Depression may come about when a person experiences a sense of loss and/or helplessness, i.e. a sense that one's actions do not influence events. Anxiety may arise when a person anticipates loss, or believes that things will go wrong in some way.

> There are many descriptions of the negative emotional consequences of hearing loss. For example, McKenna et al.[13] reported that 27% of people attending a neuro-otology clinic with a main complaint of hearing loss were suffering from significant psychological disturbance. This is considerably higher than the prevalence of psychological disturbance among the general population (approximately 5% have significant psychopathology). It is, however, lower than the prevalence rates reported to be associated with other audiological symptoms such as tinnitus and vertigo.[13, 55, 56]

A different approach to the question has been to examine the extent of hearing loss among populations of known psychiatric patients, but the results are far from clear. However, there is the potential for a hearing loss to lead to mis-classification in psychiatric cases, and it is important for this to be taken into account in the diagnostic process.[57] When other health problems have been taken into consideration, the correlations between hearing loss and anxiety and depression are weaker. The experience of multiple symptoms leads to a greater likelihood of a person suffering from significant psychological distress. The high comorbidity between hearing loss and tinnitus is particularly relevant in this respect; many hearing-impaired people may experience significant psychological distress as a consequence of the combined effects of that loss and tinnitus.

It is clear that the relationship between hearing loss and psychological wellbeing is a complex one. This point is highlighted by the fact that many people, particularly older people, do not complain about their hearing loss. It is often the case that older people tolerate a greater degree of impairment before taking action than do younger people, and they regard a hearing aid as of little use to them. It has been noted that some people deny that they have a hearing problem even when confronted with audiometric evidence of a hearing loss.[58] It is also the case that the link between audiological measures and psychological disturbance is unclear. If hearing loss is associated with psychological disturbance then it might be expected that there would be a relationship between the extent of the hearing loss and the extent of the psychological problems. Many studies,[58–61] however, have found that this is not the case. One study,[60] however, suggested that while there was no clear relationship between degree of hearing loss and psychological disturbance for most of the population assessed, there was a higher degree of disturbance among a subgroup of people with particularly severe hearing loss and poor speech discrimination, and who received little benefit from hearing aids.

Therefore, at first sight, the evidence on the relationship between hearing loss and psychological well-being seems mixed. In part, this may be because of an overly simple approach to assessing psychological status. Many studies[59, 60, 62–64] have used an approach that classifies people as either psychiatrically disturbed or not. This runs the risk of neglecting those people who experience emotional distress but who fall short of a classification as dysfunctional. For example, it seems reasonable to suppose that because it involves loss, acquired hearing impairment might lead to a grief reaction. Clearly, not everyone experiencing grief about hearing loss will react in ways that would allow them to be classified as psychiatrically dysfunctional. One recent study used a different approach to the study of hearing loss. The researchers[61] used a questionnaire method and factor analysis to discover the subjective experiences of people with acquired hearing loss. They emphasized the multidimensional nature of the experience and described the effects of hearing loss in terms of six factors.

SUBJECTIVE EXPERIENCE OF ACQUIRED HEARING LOSS

- Communication problems
- Social restrictions
- Poor interaction with others
- Psychological dimension
  - distress
  - social isolation
- Sense of loss/bereavement
- Positive experiences
  - social support
  - philosophical resources

Only one of these factors referred to the communication problems that one might expect to be associated with hearing loss. One factor was concerned with social restrictions such as employment difficulties and strained family relationships. Another factor referred to poor interactions on the part of others, that is, deafened people perceive others as using strategies that undermine the hearing-impaired person. The other factors emphasized the psychological dimensions of the experience. One factor was concerned with the distress associated with interactions and a sense of social isolation. Another factor highlighted a sense of loss and bereavement and a sense that hearing people do not understand what it is like to be deafened. The last factor was concerned with positive experiences associated with hearing loss, such as social support and greater inner philosophical resources. In common with other studies, Kerr and Cowie[61] found that audiological factors did not allow one to say how much impact a hearing loss would have on a person's life.

The finding that hearing loss might be associated with some positive consequences may seem surprising. However, there are other sources of evidence that the effects of hearing loss are not always those that one might intuitively think of. For example, it is worth noting that not all cochlear implant users report a positive psychological outcome, even when the implant provides obvious acoustical benefit. It is sometimes the case that the 'restoration of hearing' provided by the implant does not lead to the changes in life that the person hoped for and, just as with hearing aids, a proportion of implant recipients do not use their devices.[65]

The World Health Organization model applied to hearing loss

The complexity of the relationship between hearing loss and emotional wellbeing can be accounted for by the fact that hearing loss does not occur in a vacuum but rather within the 'rich tapestry of life'. To restate the point: two people with the same level of hearing loss may have quite different life experiences. The World Health Organization (WHO) 1980[66] classification of impairment, disability and handicap has been appealed to when seeking to explain the lack of a clear relationship between the extent of hearing loss and the level of psychological disturbance.

WHO (1980) Classification	
Impairment	The defective function that may be measured using psychoacoustical techniques.
Disability	The auditory problem experienced, and complained of, by the individual.
Handicap	The non-auditory problems that result from hearing impairment and disability.

Stephens and Hétu[67] provided definitions of impairment, disability and handicap within an audiological context. They defined impairment as the defective function that may be measured using psychoacoustical techniques and suggested that it is independent of psychosocial factors. Stephens and Hétu[67] defined disability as the auditory problem experienced, and complained of, by the individual. They refer to handicap as the non-auditory problems that result from hearing impairment and disability and suggested that this is determined by the social and cultural context within which the hearing impairment occurs. As handicap refers to the disadvantage that the individual experiences, there is not a direct relationship between impairment, disability and handicap.

The WHO 1980[66] model has been challenged in other areas of health-care.[68] Johnston[68] summarized a number of difficulties with the traditional model as applied to physical disorders and suggested amendments to it. The WHO 1980 model[66] assumes that different health professionals would rate a person's behaviour in a similar way. Johnston[68] reported that, in fact, nurses consistently rated patients as more disabled than physiotherapists and occupational therapists did and sought to explain this observation in terms of social circumstances influencing the level of disability observed. Some psychological models used in the study of people with chronic disease postulate that people cope with their mental representations of the problem rather than with the problem per se. Studies have also indicated that patients' perceptions of the control they have over recovery and level of disability influence the outcome of rehabilitation, even allowing for original level of disability.

The theory of planned behaviour: a psychological model

It can not be assumed that all disabled people have an equal and full intention to perform everyday tasks. For example, past failures to perform tasks may lead a person to give up even when there has been a recovery from impairment. Johnston[68] argued that levels of disability are influenced by a combination of an intention to behave in a certain way and perceived control over being able to do so. Johnston cited the Theory of Planned Behaviour[69] in this context. This theory suggests that a person's intention to perform a task is determined by a combination of a change in attitudes to the behaviour, the subjective norm for the behaviour, and the person's perception of control over the behaviour. In a hearing rehabilitation context, the behaviour in question might be speaking with others. A change in attitude associated with this might be 'when I speak to people I mishear and feel embarrassed and I dislike embarrassment'. The subjective norm might be 'my spouse wishes to do the talking for me and I am happy to go along with this' and an example of perceived control over the behaviour could be 'I am not confident that I can hear what people say'. Applying the Theory of Planned Behaviour to the WHO 1980 model,[66] Johnston[68] proposed that physical impairment influences mental representations, which, in turn, determine behavioural intentions and disabled behaviour. In summary, the suggestion is that disability, like handicap, refers to behaviour that is subject to manipulation in the same way as any other behaviour. The ideas of famous behavioural psychologist B. F. Skinner add to this view of hearing.[70] Hearing can be viewed as an operant, i.e. as a behaviour classified on the basis of its effects and also that is under the influence of contingencies of reinforcement. During his later years, Skinner extended his theories into the field of ageing and hearing loss.[71] He advocated an assertive approach while acknowledging that when it is impossible to hear: 'You do best to stop trying to hear things when you are having trouble. You are probably not enjoying what is said in a television program if you are straining to hear it'[71] (p. 44). The point that social factors influence the level of disability was recognized by Stephens and Hétu.[67] While the social model of disability[72,73] emphasizes social barriers as the determinants of disability, (for example a wheel-chair user is disabled because there are steps rather than a ramp), Johnston's[68] argument goes beyond this by highlighting not only social determinants of disability but also cognitive or mental ones. The relative contributions of social and psychological factors and their place in the models of disability are discussed by Arnold.[74]

While the notion that hearing-impaired people face social barriers is now considered self-evident, from a clinical point of view it is also apparent that they encounter psychological obstacles through factors such as anxiety or reduced motivation. The evidence suggests that the effects of acquired hearing loss go beyond communication problems, and there are strands of support for the idea that psychological factors influence hearing disability directly. One piece of research from the field of cochlear implants[75] adds to this picture. An assessment was carried out of a group of implant users' retrospective perceptions of changes in their psychological status. The assessment indicated that almost all of the group studied believed that their lives were close to ideal prior to the onset of hearing loss, and that this was radically changed by hearing loss. It seems implausible that so many in any group would have had near-perfect lives before losing their hearing. It seems unlikely that this perception is the consequence of only social factors. It seems likely that this represents a cognitive manoeuvre or a change in people's mental maps of their psychological space. The effect is to increase the perception of the loss experienced, and this in turn is likely to be a determinant of the subsequent disability behaviour.

A new WHO model

A new classification of impairments, disability and handicap has been developed by the WHO.[76] The proposed new classification again refers to three levels of disablement: losses or abnormalities of bodily function and structure (previously referred to as impairments), limitations of activities (previously disabilities), and restriction in participation (previously handicaps).

NEW WHO (2001) CLASSIFICATION OF FUNCTIONING, DISABILITY AND HEALTH

- Loss or abnormalities of bodily function and structure
- Limitations of activities
- Restriction in participation

The proposed new classification is set within the context of the social model of disability. It suggests that disablement occurs within and by means of contextual factors. Two sorts of contextual factors are identified: social and environmental factors, and personal factors. Social and environmental factors include physical conditions such as climate and terrain as well as aspects of the social environment such as social attitudes, laws, policies and social and political institutions. Personal factors include gender, age, other health conditions, coping styles, social background, education, profession, past and current experience, overall behaviour pattern, character style and other factors that influence how disability is experienced by the individual. This new classification is broad enough to incorporate the ideas put forward within the psychological model.[68] However, Johnston's[68] model delineates more clearly the role of psychological factors.

Treatment perspectives regarding hearing loss

From a psychological point of view, much of the emphasis within a clinical setting has been on providing a psychotherapeutic or counselling response to the emotional consequences of hearing loss. Clinically, an emphasis is often placed on working through a grief process or changing a person's beliefs about the implications of the loss through the use of cognitive therapy.[41] There is therefore an overlap with the psychological therapy approaches to tinnitus. A behavioural perspective to the management of people with hearing loss has also been suggested. Within a behavioural approach emphasis is placed on considering each patient as unique and requiring a tailor-made set of rehabilitation strategies.[2] The behaviours that need changing are identified, together with the factors that control them. It needs to be remembered that the patient experiences hearing loss in his or her own environment. Identifying the controlling factors involves observing those circumstances in which the relevant behaviour takes place and also observing the consequences of the behaviour.

McKenna[77] described a behavioural approach to audiological rehabilitation based on goal-planning principles. This system involves the use of clear behavioural language in the description of the patient's needs and the things that each person involved in the rehabilitation will do. Abstract concepts are avoided, and goals are described in terms of what the person says or does. For example, rather than having a vague objective for a patient, such as 'better communication', specific goals may be stated, such as 'he needs to wear his hearing aids for six hours a day' or 'he needs to tell people how to talk to him'. These goals are then broken down into achievable steps, and each person's role in achieving the steps is described. An emphasis is placed on abilities rather than disabilities and positive language is used, e.g. 'the patient needs to practise relaxation techniques' rather than 'he cannot relax'. Goal-planning does not impose any theoretical framework or dictate what therapies should be used in the rehabilitation. Rather, it is a framework for organizing the rehabilitation process. It is a means of stating what should be achieved but does not dictate the method of intervention.

A cognitive behavioural approach to the management of hearing loss in elderly people has been described in a series of studies by Andersson et al.[78–81] These have focused on the use of hearing tactics, i.e. the methods used by hearing impaired people to solve the everyday problems resulting from the hearing loss. The treatment involves setting individualized treatment goals and achieving these through the use of behavioural tasks and communication strategies. It includes the rehearsal of tactics and teaching relaxation and coping skills. Overall, the results indicate that subjects treated in this way were better able to cope with their hearing loss, and evidence of some long-term benefit was also found. Andersson et al. concluded that disability resulting from hearing impairment could be regarded as a behavioural problem and that this behaviour can be the central focus of rehabilitation. They suggested that cognitive, and especially motivational, factors are of the utmost importance in how hearing disability is viewed.

Conclusions

> Whether or not hearing loss or tinnitus are problematic is dependent as much, if not more, on psychological factors as on physical ones.

People's responses to tinnitus and to hearing loss are not always easily predictable. They depend on cognitive, behavioural and social influences as well as the changes in acoustical ability.

> An approach to auditory rehabilitation that focuses only on an attempt to alter acoustical input runs the risk of ignoring fundamental aspects of the experience and therefore faces the prospect of only limited success.

This is evidenced in the large variation in people's acceptance and use of devices such as hearing aids or tinnitus instruments. The management of acquired hearing loss needs to go beyond the provision of hearing aids to the manipulation of many factors, including psychological ones. This was recognized over 20 years ago when Goldstein and Stephens[82] recommended that aural rehabilitation should address psychological factors. Our understanding of the issues involved has improved since then, and the argument for the involvement of clinical psychologists in rehabilitation of hearing-impaired people has become all the more persuasive. It now seems likely that not only is the handicap associated with a hearing loss psychologically determined but that the level of disability is also the product of psychological factors. The future direction of psychology within the field of hearing loss may be in manipulating the determinants of disability as much as moderating handicap. Psychological treatment of tinnitus is now well established in major centres. However, there is a need for these treatments to be refined so that they become efficacious across a wider spectrum of tinnitus complaint. For example, the efficacy of psychological treatments on tinnitus-related insomnia is limited,[83] and not well studied.[84] To date, the treatment strategies have not specifically addressed sleep disturbance, and it seems likely that psychological treatments that specifically tackle insomnia may lead to greater success. Given the limited success that psychological treatments have had on auditory perceptual aspects of tinnitus complaint,[40] it may be that this is another area in which a refinement of treatment approaches would lead to greater success. The greater understanding of tinnitus complaint that psychologists have developed in recent years, including of the difficulties in concentration associated with tinnitus, may lead to a more sophisticated and more useful cognitive model of tinnitus. The main impediment to these developments is the continuing paucity of psychologists working in audiology.

References

1. Jakes S. Otological symptoms and emotion. A review of the literature. *Adv Behav Res Ther*, 1988; **10**: 53–103.
2. McKenna L, Andersson G. Hearing disabilities. In: Bellack A, Hersen M. eds. *Comprehensive Clinical Psychology*, Vol. 9: *Diverse Populations*. Oxford: Pergamon Press, 1998: 69–83.
3. Fowler E. The emotional factor in tinnitus aurium. *Laryngoscope*. 1948; **58**: 145–54.
4. Hallam RS, Rachman S, Hinchcliffe R. Psychological aspects of tinnitus. In: Rachman S, ed. *Contributions to Medical Psychology*. Oxford: Pergamon Press, Vol 3. 1984: 31–53.
5. Tyler R, Baker L. Difficulties experienced by tinnitus sufferers. *J Speech Hear Disord*, 1983; **48**: 150–4.
6. Hallam R. *Living with Tinnitus: Dealing with the Ringing in Your Ears*. Wellingborough: Thorsons, 1989.
7. Hallam R, Jakes S, Hinchcliffe R. Cognitive variables in tinnitus annoyance. *Br J Clin Psychol*, 1988; **27**: 213–22.

8. Kentish RC, Crocker SR, McKenna L. Children's experiences of tinnitus: a preliminary survey of children presenting to a psychology department. *Br J Audiol* 2000; **34**: 335–40.
9. Zöger S, Holgers K-M, Svedlund J. Psychiatric disorders in tinnitus patients without severe hearing impairment: 24 month follow-up of patients at an audiological clinic. *Audiology* 2001; **40**: 133–40.
10. Halford J. Anderson S. Anxiety and depression in tinnitus sufferers. *J Psychosom Res*,1991; **35**: 383–90.
11. Harrop-Griffiths J, Katon W, Dobie R, Sakai C, Russo J. Chronic tinnitus: association with psychiatric diagnoses. *J Psychosom Res*. 1987; **31**: 613–21.
12. Kirsch C, Blanchard E, Parnes S. Psychological characteristics of individuals high and low in their ability to cope with tinnitus. *Psychosom Med* 1989; **51**: 209–17.
13. McKenna L, Hallam RS, Hinchcliffe R. The prevalence of psychological disturbance in neuro-otology outpatients. *Clin Otolaryngol*. 1991; **16**: 452–6.
14. Simpson RB, Nedzelski JM, Barber HO, Thomas MR. Psychiatric diagnoses in patients with psychogenic dizziness or severe tinnitus. *J Otolaryngol* 1988; **17**: 325–30.
15. Stephens S, Hallam R. The Crown Crisp experiential index in patients complaining of tinnitus. *Br J Audiol* 1985; **19**: 151–8.
16. Wood K, Webb W, Orchik D, Shea J. Intractable tinnitus: psychiatric aspects of treatment. *Psychosomatics* 1983; **24**: 559–65.
17. Briner W, Risey J, Guth P, Noris C. Use of the million clinical multiaxail inventory in evaluating patients with severe tinnitus. *Am J Otolaryngol* 1990; **11**: 334–7.
18. Hiller W, Goebel G, Rief W. Reliability of self rated tinnitus distress and association with psychological symptom patterns. *Br J Psychol* 1994; **33**: 231–9.
19. Russo J, Katon W, Sullivan M, Clark M, Buchwald D. Severity of somatisation and its relationship to psychiatric disorders and personality. *Psychosomatics* 1994; **35**: 546–56.
20. Beck A, Ward C, Mendelson M, Mock J, Erbaugh J. An inventory for measuring depression. *Arch Gen Psychiatry* 1961; **4**: 561–71.
21. Wilson P, Henry J, Bowen M, Haralambous G. Tinnitus reaction questionnaire: psychometric properties of a measure of distress associated with tinnitus. *J Speech Hear Res* 1991; **34**: 197–201.
22. Erlandsson S. Tinnitus: tolerance or threat? Psychological and psychophysiological perspectives. Doctoral Thesis, University of Goteborg, 1990.
23. Hinchcliffe R, King P. Medicolegal aspects of tinnitus. 1: Medicolegal position and current state of knowledge. *J Audiol Med* 1992; **1**: 38–58.
24. McKenna L, Hallam RS, Shurlock L. Cognitive functioning in tinnitus patients. In: Reich GE, Vernon JA. ed. *Proceedings of the Fifth International Tinnitus Seminar*, 1995/1996. Portland: American Tinnitus Association, 1996: 589–95.
25. McKenna L., Hallam R. A neuropsychological study of concentration problems in tinnitus patients. In: Hazell J, ed. *Proceedings of the Sixth International Tinnitus Seminar*, Cambridge, UK: The Tinnitus and Hyperacusis Centre; 1999: 108–113.
26. Speilberger C, Gousuch A, Lushene A. *Test Manual of the State-Trait Anxiety Inventory*. Palo Alto: Consulting Psychology Press; 1970.
27. McKenna L. Audiological disorders: psychological state and cognitive functioning. Unpublished doctoral thesis, The City University, London, 1997.
28. Dobie RA. A review of randomized clinical trials in tinnitus. *Laryngoscope* 1999; **109**: 1202–11
29. Kuk F, Tyler R, Russell D, Jordan H. The psychometric properties of a tinnitus handicap questionnaire. *Ear Hear* 1990; **11**: 434–45.
30. Hiller W, Goebel G. A psychometric study of complaints in chronic tinnitus. *J Psychosom Res* 1992; **36**: 337–48.
31. Andersson G. The role of optimism in patients with tinnitus and in patients with hearing impairment. *Psychol Health* 1996; **11**: 697–707.
32. McCombe A, Baguley D, Coles R, McKenna L, McKinney C, Windle Taylor P. Guidelines for the grading of tinnitus severity: the results of a working group commissioned by the British Association of Otolaryngologists, Head and Neck Surgeons. *Clin Otolaryngol* 2001; **26**: 388–93.
33. Andersson G, Hägnebo C. Dysphoria, optimism, confidence in activities and daily symptoms of Menière's disease. *J Audiol Med* 1996; **5**: 83–91.
34. Lindberg P, Scott B, Melin L, Lyttkens L. The psychological treatment of tinnitus: an experimental evaluation. *Behav Res Ther* 1989; **27**: 593–603.
35. Beck A, Epstein N, Brown G, Steer R. An inventory for measuring clinical anxiety. Psychometric properties. *J Consult Clin Psychol* 1988; **56**: 893–7.
36. Andersson G, Lyttkens L, Larsen HC. Distinguishing levels of tinnitus distress. *Clin Otolaryngol* 1999; **24**: 404–410.
37. Carlsson S, Erlandsson S. Habituation and tinnitus: an experimental study. *J Psychosom Res* 1991; **35**: 509–14.
38. Baltissen R, Boucsein W. Effects of a warning signal on reactions to aversive white noise stimulation: does warning 'short-circuit' habituation? *Psychophysiology* 1986; **23**: 224–31.
39. Scott B, Lindberg P, Melin L, Lyttkens L. Psychological treatment of tinnitus. An experimental group study. *Scand Audiol* 1985; **14**: 223–30.
40. Andersson G, Melin L, Hägnebo C, Scott B, Lindberg P. A review of psychological treatment approaches for patients suffering from tinnitus. *Ann Behav Med*. 1995; **17**: 357–66.
41. Beck A. *Cognitive Therapy and the Emotional Disorders*. Madison, CT: International Universities Press, 1976.
42. Jastreboff P, Hazell J. A neurophysiological approach to tinnitus: clinical implications. *Br J Audiol* 1993; **27**: 7–17.
43. Wilson P, Henry J, Lindberg P, Andersson G, Hallam R. A critical analysis of directive counselling as a component of tinnitus retraining therapy. *Br J Audiol* 1998; **32**: 273–86.
44. Jastreboff MM. Controversies between cognitive therapies and TRT counselling. In: Hazell J, ed. *Proceedings of the Sixth International Tinnitus Seminar*, Cambridge, UK: The Tinnitus and Hyperacusis Centre; 1999: 288–291.
45. Henry J, Wilson P. Cognitive behavioural therapy for tinnitus related distress: an experimental evaluation of initial treatment and relapse prevention. In: Hazell J, ed. *Proceedings of the Sixth International Tinnitus Seminar*, Cambridge, UK: The Tinnitus and Hyperacusis Centre; 1999: 118–124.

46. McKinney C, Hazell J, Graham R. An evaluation of the TRT method. In: Hazell J, ed. *Proceedings of the Sixth International Tinnitus Seminar*. Cambridge, UK: The Tinnitus and Hyperacusis Centre; 1999: 99–105.
47. Attias J, Urbach D, Gold S, Sheemesh Z. Auditory event related potentials in chronic tinnitus patients with noise induced hearing loss. *Hear Res* 1993; **71**: 106–13.
48. Andersson G, Lyttkens L, Hirvelä C, Furmark T, Tillfors M, Fredrikson M. Regional cerebral blood flow during tinnitus: a PET case-study with lidocaine and auditory stimulation. *Acta Otolaryngol* 2000; **120**: 967–972.
49. Rosenhall U, Axelsson A. Auditory brainstem response latencies in patients with tinnitus. *Scand Audiol* 1995; **24**: 97–100.
50. Andersson G, Khakpoor A, Lyttkens L. Masking of tinnitus and mental activity. *Clin Otolaryngol* 2002; **27**: 270–4.
51. Jones D, Macken W. Irrelevant tones produce an irrelevant speech effect. *J Exp Psychol Learning Memory Cognition* 1993; **19**: 369–81.
52. Jones E, White AJ. Mental health and acquired hearing impairment. A review. *Br J Audiol* 1990; **24**: 3–9.
53. Andersson G. Hearing as behaviour. Psychological aspects of acquired hearing impairment in the elderly. Doctoral dissertation, Acta Universitas Upsaliensis, 1995.
54. Danhauer J, Johnson CE, Kasten R, Brimacombe J. The hearing aid effect. Summary, conclusions & recommendations. *Hear J* 1985; **38**: 12–14.
55. Asmundson GJG, Larsen DK, Stein MB. Panic disorder and vestibular disturbance: an overview of empirical findings and clinical implications. *J Psychosom Res* 1998; **44**: 107–20.
56. Meric C, Gartner M, Collet L, Chéry-Croze S. Psychopathological profile of tinnitus sufferers: evidence concerning the relationship between tinnitus features and impact on life. *Audiol Neurootol* 1998; **3**: 240–52.
57. Kreeger JL, Raulin ML, Grace J, Priest BL. Effect of hearing enhancement on mental status ratings in geriatric psychiatric patients. *Am J Psychiatry* 1995; **152**: 629–31.
58. Gilhome Herbst K, Humphrey C. Hearing impairment and mental state in the elderly living at home. *BMJ* 1980; **281**: 903–5.
59. Mahapatra S. Deafness and mental health: psychiatric and psychosomatic illness in the deaf. *Acta Psychiatr Scand* 1974; **50**: 596–611.
60. Thomas A, Gilhome Herbst K. Social and psychological implications of acquired deafness for adults of employment age. *Br J Audiol* 1980; **14**: 76–85.
61. Kerr P, Cowie R. Acquired deafness: a multidimensional experience. *Br J Audiol*; 1997; **31**: 177–88.
62. Knapp P. Emotional aspects of hearing loss. *Psychosom Med* 1948; **10**: 203–22.
63. Ingalls G. Some psychiatric observations on patients with hearing deficit. *Occup Ther Rehabil* 1946; **25**: 62–6.
64. Singerman B, Reidner E, Folstein M. Emotional disturbance in hearing clinic patients. *Br J Psychiatry* 1980; **137**: 58–62.
65. McKenna L. The psychological assessment of cochlear implant patients. *Br J Audiol* 1986; **20**: 29–34.
66. World Health Organization. *International Classification of Impairments, Disabilities and Handicaps*. Geneva: WHO, 1980.
67. Stephens SDG, Hétu R. Impairment, disability and handicap in audiology: towards a consensus. *Audiology* 1991; **30**: 185–200.
68. Johnston M. Models of disability. *Psychologist* 1996; May: 205–10.
69. Azjen I. *Attitudes, Personality and Behaviour*. Milton Keynes: Open University Press, 1988.
70. Skinner B F. *Verbal Behavior*. New York: Appleton-Century-Crofts, 1957.
71. Skinner BF, Vaughan ME. *Enjoy Old Age. A Program for Self-management*. London: Hutchinson. 1983.
72. Finkelstein V. *Attitudes and Disabled People*. New York: World Rehabilitation Fund, 1980.
73. Finkelstein V. 'We' are not disabled, 'you' are. In: Gregory S, Hartley G, eds. *Constructing Deafness*. London: Pinter/Milton Keynes: Open University Press, 1990: 265–71.
74. Arnold P. Is there still a consensus on impairment, disability and handicap in audiology? *Br J Audiol* 1998; **32**: 265–71.
75. McKenna L, Denman C. Repertory grid technique in the assessment of cochlear implant patients. *J Audiol Med* 1993; **2**: 75–84.
76. WHO. International Classification of Functioning, Disability and Health. 2001; Geneva: World Health Organization.
77. McKenna L. Goal planning in audiological rehabilitation. *Br J Audiol* 1987; **21**: 5–11.
78. Andersson G, Melin L, Scott B, Lindberg P. Behavioural counselling for subjects with acquired hearing loss. A new approach to hearing tactics. *Scand Audiol* 1994; **23**: 249–56.
79. Andersson G, Melin L, Scott B, Lindberg P. An evaluation of a behavioural treatment approach to hearing impairment. *Behav Res Ther* 1995; **33**(3): 283–92.
80. Andersson G, Melin L, Scott B, Lindberg P. A two-year follow-up examination of a behavioural treatment approach to hearing tactics. *Br J Audiol* 1995; **29**: 347–54.
81. Andersson G, Green M, Melin L. Behavioural hearing tactics: a controlled trial of a short treatment programme. *Behav Res Ther* 1997; **35**: 523–30.
82. Goldstein DP, Stephens SDG. Audiological rehabilitation: Management model I. *Audiol* 1981; **20**: 432–52.
83. McKenna L. Tinnitus and insomnia. In: Tyler RS, ed. *Tinnitus Handbook*. San Diego: Singular Publishing; 2000: 59–84.
84. Andersson G, Lyttkens L. A meta-analytic review of psychological treatments for tinnitus. *Br J Audiol* 1999; **33**: 201–10.

36 Surgical management of hearing impairment in audiological medicine

Paul Van de Heyning, Jos Claes, Jan Brokx, Frank Declau, An Boudewyns, Evert Hamans, Erwin Koekelkoren, Dirk De Ridder

Introduction

For many decades, ear surgery has endeavoured to improve hearing impairment. Initially, ear surgery was aimed at eradicating infectious middle ear pathology, but with better public health and the advent of antibiotics, tumour surgery, especially acoustical neuroma surgery, and the surgical treatment of incapacitating vertigo developed. Progressively, the aim of hearing improvement became more and more important, and a branch of ear surgery evolved aimed at purely functional hearing restoration. This has been named cophosurgery or functional ear surgery. International societies focusing on otosurgery (e.g. Politzer Society) have developed, and many international conferences and workshops, together with dedicated industrial technology, have contributed immensely to the broad application of functional ear surgery.

The main indication for hearing improvement with functional ear surgery was, and still is, conductive hearing loss. This is achieved by direct action on the structures of the outer ear canal, tympanic membrane, ossicles or middle ear structures. A specific place is taken by bone-anchored hearing aids (BAHAs), which bypass the outer and middle ear amplifier.

The last 30 years have been characterized by the progressive development of cochlear implantation, making it possible to restore hearing in severe or profound bilaterally hearing-impaired patients to a level comparable with moderate to moderate–severe hearing loss. As well as adults, children have benefited from this technology, insofar as it has radically changed the approach towards the failing organ of Corti. Moreover, recently, the field of surgically implanted hearing aids for sensorineural hearing loss has been established, especially as totally implantable systems are becoming a reality.

Last, the otoneurosurgical approach to the distressing audiological symptom of tinnitus is discussed as an adjunct to the neurocognitive approaches to tinnitus, such as tinnitus retraining therapy, tinnitus coping therapy and noise generators.

Outcome research in functional ear surgery

Outcome analysis of functional ear surgery comprises many aspects, mainly related to the desired improvement of hearing level, but also linked to the initial pathology treated, the contralateral hearing level, the environment, the subjective self-evaluation of the patient concerning his or her quality of life, and the adverse effects of the sound quality (e.g. distortion and hyperacusis) or surgery, such as pain, discomfort, changes of taste and dizziness.[1] Indeed, important aspects of outcome may remain unnoticed if only objective measures are used.[2,3]

Applied to hearing disablements, WHO guidelines recommend three domains of evaluation: functional impairment, disability or the ability to perform daily activities, and handicap for the degree of participation in socio-economic aspects of life.

The only guidelines existing on functional outcome in conductive hearing loss were issued in 1995 by the Committee on Hearing and Equilibrium of the American Academy of Otolaryngology and Head and Neck Surgery (AAO-HNS).[4] The Committee recommended that the average air–bone gap at 0.5, 1, 2 and 3 kHz calculated from postoperative bone and hearing thresholds be reported. The Committee also encouraged the reporting of raw data. Simple visual representations of these raw data have been proposed.[5] The air–bone gap evaluates, in particular, the result of the technical surgical intervention. These data have to be complemented by data on the comparison of pre- and postoperative bone conduction thresholds, to detect overclosure or iatrogenic cochlear damage.

In many countries outside the USA, the 4 kHz is more frequently measured than the 3 kHz, and thus, in these instances, the 3 kHz should be calculated as the mean of 2 and 4 kHz. In the majority of publications, when dealing with the results of conductive hearing loss, auditory threshold values are the basis of reporting the level of success. A frequently used technique is to report the percentage of achieved air–bone closure to within 10 or 20 decibels. It should be noted that the frequencies used to calculate this mean air–bone gap often comprise the combination of 0.5, 1 and 2 kHz.[6–8] In many publications, postoperative air thresholds are also compared with preoperative bone thresholds. Investigations have shown that the use of the mean of 0.5, 1 and 2 kHz, as well as the combination of preoperative bone thresholds with postoperative air thresholds, appear better than is actually the case. Using the gain of the speech reception thresholds (SRTs) as an external criterion, the best correlations of hearing gain were achieved with the combination of 0.5, 1, 2 and 3 or 4 kHz, supporting the guidelines of the AAO-HNS.[9,10] The inclusion of the 4-kHz thresholds gives a better indication for speech in noise. Indeed, the all-or-none inclusion of 4 kHz in defining hearing impairment has an important effect on the prevalence figures of hearing impairment in general[11] and success rates in particular.[10]

It has to be emphasized that the determination of exact thresholds in bilateral mixed hearing loss, as is often found in chronic otitis media and otosclerosis, is compromised by the difficulty of masking. Also, the preoperative influence of the Carhart effect[12] renders the preoperative estimation of the true cochlear function problematic. This can be partially overcome by the use of insert phones, although the use of these phones has not become a standard procedure, and nor has it been included in the guidelines or recommendations. Indeed, with deep insertion of insert phones, interaural attenuation is considerably larger, leading to more robust masking procedures. The postoperative air–bone gap is not necessarily representative of the benefit perceived by the patient in terms of satisfactory social hearing following surgery.[13]

Evaluation of activities and participation is typically assessed with validated questionnaires. These include generic questionnaires, such as the SF 36,[14] or disease-specific questionnaires. These latter questionnaires can focus on auditory capacities (e.g. the Hearing Handicap Inventory for Adults[15]) and different listening conditions and tasks, such as speech recognition in noise and in quiet, the discrimination of sounds and sound quality or directional hearing,[16] or can be complemented by different patient-specific items, as evaluated in the Client Oriented Scale of Improvement (COSI).

In order to assess the benefit of an operation for the patient based on air conduction thresholds, the Belfast rule of thumb (success is achieved when postoperative airconduction is equal or better than 30 dB or the interaural difference is 15 dB or less[17]) was introduced, and afterwards elaborated by the Glasgow Benefit Plot.[18] Based on this approach, the benefit from bilateral stapedectomy[19] or from BAHA was demonstrated, and others subsequently simplified this method for defining patient success.[20] Outcome instruments for evaluating the treatment of specific hearing disorders were also developed, mainly for research purposes (e.g. cochlear implants,[21] and for conductive hearing loss[22]).

To date, none of these disability-oriented methods has gained universal application in the evaluation of the correction of conductive hearing loss, partially due to the lack of good validated studies and partially due to the initial aim of the surgeon of focusing on the surgical result itself. Nevertheless, a multidimensional outcome approach is becoming almost compulsory, in terms of both evidence-based medicine and finance—the latter dictated by the healthcare insurers. This approach has been able to analyse the preference of patients for functional ear surgery in comparison to hearing aids.[3,23] However, to date, only a few studies have complied with the principles of evidence-based medicine and good clinical practice.[24]

The method of reporting results of conductive hearing loss contrasts with the more broadly applied methodology to assess hearing improvement, whether using hearing aids (e.g. abbreviated profile of hearing aid benefit[25]) or evaluating or treating sensorineural hearing loss.[26] Functional results are reported in terms of hearing gain or achieved hearing level based on air conduction threshold values, most often based on the mean of 0.5, 1, 2 and 3 or 4 kHz, on speech recognition tests in quiet and in noise, and on disease-specific questionnaires. The use of phonetically balanced monosyllables has gained wide acceptance as a measure of assessing cochlear performance. Sentence tests, on the other hand, tend to evaluate speech comprehension and, hence, are essentially monitoring the process of acclimatization. The results after cochlear implantation in pre-lingually deaf children include educational, receptive and expressive speech and language developmental measures as well.

Comparing hearing improvement outcomes by surgery or by fitting auditory prostheses

Elements and essential considerations involved in the decision-making process

Decisions about the best approach for solving auditory problems by surgery or the provision of auditory prostheses may not be

OUTCOME MEASURES IN THE SURGICAL TREATMENT OF HEARING LOSS

- the use of the mean for four frequencies (0.5, 1, 2 and 3 or 4 kHz) derived from the same postoperative audiogram
- postoperative air–bone gap in case of conductive hearing loss
- air conduction hearing gain in case of sensorineural hearing loss
- comparison of pre- and postoperative bone conduction
- speech recognition of monosyllables
- assess the disability and handicap with validated disease-specific questionnaires

based on the evaluation of auditory impairments alone. Also, the consequences of the impairments in daily life in terms of disablements and handicaps also need to be evaluated separately. A good overview of these individual components, together with knowledge of the advantages and disadvantages of each approach, ensure that the elements for a good decision-making process are available.

In most countries, the estimation of hearing disability is based on a pure-tone average of auditory thresholds. Analysis ($N = 274$) of the 'Inventory for Auditory Disability and Handicap' from Kramer showed that more factors are involved than the detection of sounds alone. Discrimination and recognition of sounds, localization, speech intelligibility in silence and speech intelligibility in noise are independent dimensions.[27–30] Also, intolerance to noise is an important dimension for many patients. Analysis of the data has shown that not all of these factors are of equal importance. Poor speech perception in noise appears to be the most important factor for most hard-of-hearing individuals.

Handicap is much more than the sum of the disabilities of disordered auditory functions, and describes the individual negative consequences in daily life functioning. Of interest is the distinction that Kramer makes between primary and secondary handicaps. Primary handicaps are the disadvantages experienced in daily life, while secondary handicap elements reflect the mental effort and concentration problems caused by the hearing loss.

Kramer's approach was developed for the validation of a hearing loss. In fact, the same elements are relevant when distinguishing between a surgical intervention and a technical solution using hearing aids.

Other factors that have to be taken into account are the advantages and disadvantages of the use of hearing devices. For different patient groups, such as the multisensory and the mentally disabled these factors or the impact of these factors may be different.

Some disadvantages of hearing devices could be as follows:

- Intolerance of materials used for earmoulds or devices.
- Problems in handling by the client or by the management.
- Directional hearing or environmental orientation. This is an important factor when dealing with the multisensory handicapped. In many cases, environmental orientation is more relevant than optimal speech understanding.
- For some multisensory handicapped or mentally disabled patients, the non-linear behaviour and the environmental adaptive properties of modern digital hearing devices may cause disorientation.

A different approach using the COSI method

Another way of obtaining information about the added value of a certain approach is the COSI. This is a client-oriented review system developed by the Australian Hearing Services (NAL).[31]

In a comparative study on result measurements in hearing aid fitting, the Hearing Aid User's Questionnaire (HAUQ), the Hearing Difficulties Inventory (HDI), the Global Satisfaction Scale (GSA), the Profile of Hearing Benefit (PHAB), the Shortened Hearing Aid Performance Inventory (SHAPIE) and the COSI were compared. In this study, the SHAPIE was the best, but proved to be impractical because of the 25-item questionnaire. In terms of the ease of testing, COSI was the second best and scored only the items which were of relevance for each individual client. With the COSI system, specific needs, expectations and their relevance for the client can be assessed in an easy way. This information relates to the total intervention and also facilitates the measurement of results.

The setup is very simple. First, the specific needs and expectations of a client are listed. Second, the needs are ranked in an interview with the client, such that any proposed intervention will focus on the items with the highest priorities. After the intervention, the list can be evaluated and improvements can be estimated on a five-point scale: worse, no difference, a little better, better and much better. If the items with the highest rank order do not improve satisfactorily, a new intervention is appropriate, followed by a repeat evaluation.

This easy and practical system was developed for the hearing aid fitting process, but can be applied to almost all interventions. Moreover, a similar application can be adapted for use with the independent disability and handicap elements of the Kramer approach. The specific needs can be listed and ranked, and the advantages and disadvantages of a certain intervention can be evaluated.

For the client, personal problems can be considered and expectations become more realistic. Above all, personal involvement is obtained. For the surgeon, the COSI gives a patient's point of view, and to date there are no generally accepted alternatives. Further, COSI gives a structure for the client needs in the decision-making process, leads to other interventions or fine-tuning and, finally, measures the level of a client's satisfaction.

For research purposes, a modified COSI can be proposed. This is illustrated in an unpublished study considering the preference for analogue or digital hearing aids among a specific group of clients with Usher's syndrome type II.[32] These clients have an average hearing loss (across 0.5, 1, 2 and 4 kHz) of about 70 dB HL and retinitis pigmentosa.

From an inventory, it became clear that these clients, because of their combined auditory and visual disabilities, had different degrees of handicap in respect of certain situations: communication at home, communication at work, orientation/mobility at home, and orientation/mobility outside.[32] For each of these situations, a separate COSI was undertaken. The responses after the intervention, i.e. the fitting of a digital hearing aid, could be evaluated on a seven point scale. For analysis purposes, the responses were weighted as follows: much worse, −3; worse, −2; a little worse, −1; no difference, 0; a little better, +1; better, +2; much better, +3. For each of the four situations, the client could identify his three most important needs. Then, the responses for the items with the highest priority were multiplied by 3, the responses for the item of second priority by 2, and the responses for the item with the lowest priority by 1. In this way, per situational COSI, a maximum of 18 points could be obtained when a maximal improvement was scored for all three levels of need.

The results of this experiment showed a significant improvement of speech perception in all listening situations and also better orientation/mobility at home. However, orientation/mobility outside was disturbed by the ongoing adaptations to the varying listening situations of the digital hearing aids. For a number of these clients, the integrity of the perceived environmental sounds was of such importance that they preferred an analogue hearing aid, despite the poorer speech perception in nearly all listening situations.

This example illustrates the potential power of the client-oriented approach. When surgery or fitting hearing devices are alternatives, a COSI might help in the decision-making process. The elements of the disorder and the handicap can be considered, and the client may be able to rank his or her needs and expectations. The feedback from the COSI gives the surgeon quantified information about the decisions that were made together with the client. In some cases, a modified COSI can be helpful, especially when there is interference by impairments.

ESSENTIAL ELEMENTS IN THE DECISION-MAKING PROCESS

- auditory thresholds
- discrimination and recognition of sounds
- localizing sounds
- speech perception in silence and in noise
- intolerance of noises
- problems in handling
- mental effort and concentration problems

Client Oriented Scale of Improvement (COSI)
Easy-to-use system for assessing specific needs, expectations and their relevance for the client. Developed for hearing aid fitting but applicable in most interventions.

Surgery in conductive hearing loss being a part of a congenital or hereditary syndrome

Congenital middle ear abnormalities can be divided into major and minor anomalies: the major malformations represent the congenital atresias of the external auditory canal, the minor relate to the congenital defects of the ossicular chain.

The prevalence of major anomalies can be estimated as 1 in 10 000 births; there are no proper data on the prevalence or incidence of minor anomalies. The latter are syndromal in 25% of cases.

These congenital anomalies cause moderate-to-severe hearing loss and require early detection after birth, within 3 months, of the hearing level by evoked potentials. Also, genetic counselling is required, not only to establish the hereditary pattern, but also to rule out associated anomalies in other organ systems. In bilateral anomalies, amplification by air or bone conduction hearing aids, within 6 months after birth, is essential to avoid delays in speech or language development. During early childhood, it is important to check both ears regularly for the presence of otitis media. In unilateral atresia cases, it is especially important to check the normal ear regularly to exclude otitis media with effusion. If secretory otitis media is present, prompt medical and/or surgical therapy is needed. Also, the atretic ear may be involved and exhibit signs of acute otitis media. If this diagnosis is suspected in the atretic ear, prompt antibiotic treatment should be commenced to minimize the risk of complications such as coalescent mastoiditis or subdural abscess.

The classification of the minor middle ear anomalies, is modified after Teunissen and Cremers[33] (Table 36.1), has been approved by the HEAR consensus group of the European Workgroup on Genetics of Hearing Impairment. This classification is based on the peroperative findings and has direct impact on the reconstruction technique applied.

This classification is not based on the degree of abnormality, but depends on the degree of fixation of the stapedial footplate or on the presence or absence of accompanying anomalies of the other ossicles. With the exception of severe dysplasia or aplasia of the oval and/or round window (group IV), a postoperative air–bone gap of $\leq$20 dB was found in 72% of the operated cases. Preoperative inclusion criteria are: (1) older than 10 years; (2) no intermittent periods of secretory otitis media; (3) tonal and speech audiogram as well as tympanometry with contralateral stapedial reflexes performed; and (4) high-resolution CT scan performed.

Table 36.1 HEAR classification for ossicular malformations.

I	Isolated congenital stapes ankylosis
	A. Footplate fixation
	B. Stapes suprastructure fixation
II	Idem + another ossicular chain anomaly
	A. Discontinuity of the chain
	B. Epitympanic fixation
	C. Tympanic fixation
III	Congenital anomaly of the ossicular chain but a mobile stapes footplate
	A. Discontinuity of the chain
	B. Epitympanic fixation
	C. Tympanic fixation
IV	Congenital aplasia or severe dysplasia of the oval or round window: aplasia or dysplasia; crossing nerve VII; persistent stapedial artery

Table 36.2 HEAR classification for congenital atresia of the external ear canal

Type I:	mild–tympanic membrane is hypoplastic; various kinds of ossicular malformations
Type II:	moderate–atretic plate; tympanic cavity is within normal limits
IIa:	tympanic bone is hypoplastic; course of the facial nerve usually normal
IIb:	tympanic bone is absent; abnormal course of the facial nerve
Type III:	severe–atretic plate with a severely hypoplastic tympanic cavity

Further rehabilitation of atresia patients is performed either with a surgical correction or with a BAHA. Atresia repair surgery should only be performed in carefully selected patients after a thorough investigation of all parameters involved. A proper selection based on stringent audiological and radiological criteria is obligatory. Preoperatively, a complete audiometric survey is performed, as well as a high-resolution CT scan of the temporal bones.

The atresias are classified, according to a modification of the classification of Altmann[34] (Table 36.2). This classification is based on the degree of malformation present. Type II is further classified into types IIa and IIb according to the tympanic bone and the course of the facial nerve[35,36] (Figure 36.1) or depending on the thickness of the atretic plate.[37]

As radiological criteria, the scoring system defined by Jahrsdoerfer et al[38] is recommended.

A meta-analysis of the surgical results published in the last 30 years[39] demonstrated a mean hearing gain of 20–25 dB in atresia type II and 30–35 dB in atresia type I. Surgical correction is only recommended if postoperative hearing better than 25–30 dB can be realized. The long-term results remain almost unchanged.[37] Most frequently, the anterior approach is used to open the atretic plate. This type of surgery can be performed from the ages of 5 to 6 years. In the literature, no agreement can be found on surgery for unilateral cases: some surgeons will not operate on these cases, while others wait until the age of 18, so that the patient can decide. Patients who do not meet the criteria for surgical intervention should be helped by BAHAs. The results of the BAHA show not only a hearing gain in 89%, but also better comfort when compared to classical bone conduction hearing aids.[40] Also, the speech discrimination and intelligibility scores are also much better.[41,42] The age limit for implantation has been set around 5 years in most centres. In children, it is performed under general anaesthesia using a two-stage procedure: in the first stage, the titanium fixtures (usually two) are placed in the bone at the mastoid and 2 months later, after osseointegration has taken place, the fixtures are liberated and the external hearing aid attached to the bone-anchored implant.

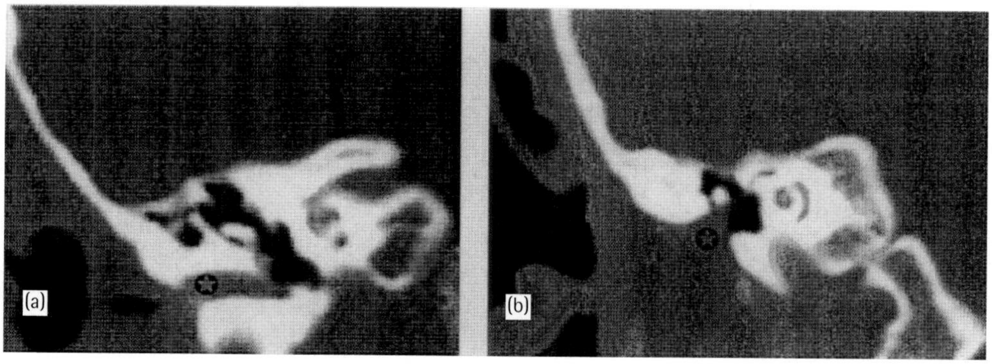

Figure 36.1 Classification of atresia type II according to Marquet. (a) Atresia type IIa. Coronal view through the external auditory canal; incomplete bony closure by atretic plate (*) formed by squamosal bone and malformed tympanic bone. Abnormal ossicular chain. Normal course of facial nerve in its mastoid segment. (b) Atresia type IIb. Absence of tympanic bone; incomplete bony closure by atretic plate formed by squamosal and petrous bone (*). Superficial hypotympanum and dysplastic ossicular chain. Abnormal anterior course of the facial nerve in its mastoid segment.

In surgery for minor middle ear anomalies, a postoperative air–bone gap of ≤20 dB may usually be expected in most cases.
In surgery for congenital ear atresia, a mean hearing gain of 20–25 dB in atresia type II and 30–35 dB in atresia type I may be expected.
BAHA is a good alternative in patients who do not meet the criteria for surgical intervention.

Otosclerosis

Definition

Otosclerosis is a hereditary disease of the otic capsule, characterized by deposits of abnormal bone. About half of the cases are assumed to be caused by specific gene defects, with variable penetrance and expression. The sites of predilection for otosclerotic foci are the fissura ante fenestram, and the round and oval windows. Otosclerotic foci near the oval window may be asymptomatic, but often result in ankylosis of the stapes footplate, causing a conductive hearing loss. Otosclerosis in the cochlear turns or vestibulum may result in sensorineural hearing loss and vertigo. The clinical expression is most often a mixed hearing loss.

Otosclerosis is a relatively frequent cause of hearing loss. Declau et al examined a large series of non-selected temporal bones and found histological features of otosclerosis in 2.5% of 236 temporal bones studied.[43] This provides an extrapolated clinical prevalence of 0.30–0.38% The pathogenesis is most likely multifactorial: hormonal influences, fluoride deficiency, viral infection (measles) and genetic deficits are recognized as contributing factors.[44]

Audiometric findings

The characteristic of otosclerotic hearing loss is a progressive, bilateral conductive hearing loss, which is often more pronounced in one ear, this difference being maintained over the years. An additional sensorineural hearing loss may develop later on (due to cochlear involvement, ageing or noise exposure) or may be the only manifestation (Figure 36.2).

The hearing loss in otosclerosis can be explained by a reduction in the effectiveness of sound transmission at the lower frequencies and increased resonance frequency. In the earlier stages of the disease, audiometry shows a progressive low-frequency hearing loss, which is often not noticed by the patient until it reaches a threshold of about 25 dB. As the growth of otosclerotic foci progresses and the footplate becomes completely fixed, a stabilization of low-frequency thresholds is found, accompanied by a progressive increase of high-frequency thresholds and a progressive widening of the air–bone gap. In the absence of cochlear involvement, complete fixation of the stapes footplate results in a maximum conductive hearing loss of 60–65 dB.

However, in many cases the cochlea becomes involved in the disease process, and a mixed hearing loss becomes apparent.

Fixation of the stapes footplate results in an impaired bone conduction response. The audiometric hallmark of otosclerosis is the Carhart notch, characterized by elevation of bone conduction thresholds of approximately 5 dB at 500 Hz, 10 dB at 1000 Hz, 15 dB at 2000 Hz and 5 dB at 4000 Hz.[12] Importantly, the Carhart notch is a mechanical artefact and does not represent the true cochlear reserve; it disappears with closure of the air–bone gap after successful surgery, a phenomenon known as 'overclosure' of the air–bone gap. (Figure 36.4).

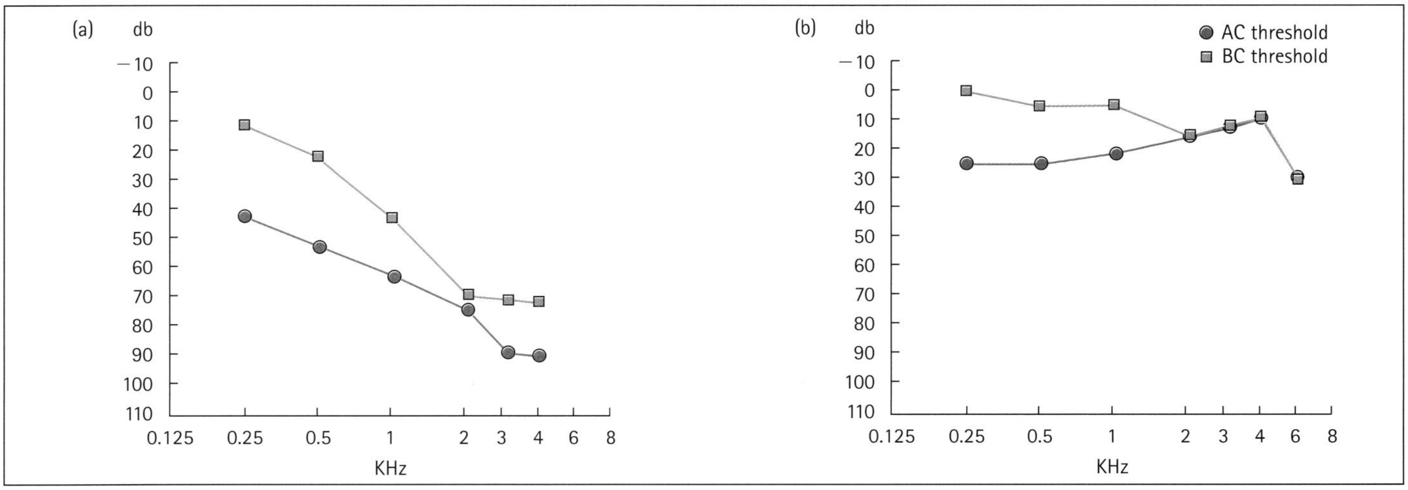

Figure 36.2 Pure tone audiometry of otosclerosis of a mainly conductive hearing loss (a) and of a mainly sensorineural hearing loss (b)

Speech audiometry in cases with a pure conductive hearing loss demonstrates a speech reception threshold in agreement with a three-frequency (500–1000–2000 Hz) pure tone average (±6 dB), and word identification accuracy at suprathreshold levels is 90–100%. Abnormalities (on/off phenomenon) or absence of acoustical reflexes in the affected ear on ipsi- and contralateral stimulation become evident fairly early in the disease process.[45]

It is important to differentiate preoperatively between fixation of the malleus and stapes fixation. Causse and Causse report that malleus fixation occurs in as many as 10.6% of cases of primary stapedectomies.[46] Malleus fixation may occur as a primary disorder or in association with otosclerosis. A conductive hearing loss of 10–15 dB is more often found with isolated malleus fixation, and the air–bone gap is seldom more than 30 dB.[47] The presence of a Carhart notch is of no value for differential diagnosis, because it may also be seen with malleus fixation due to ossicular chain pathology.

Surgical technique

The aim of surgical intervention for otosclerosis is to restore sound transmission at the level of the oval window and to improve speech understanding. Rosen in 1952 and Shea in 1958 laid the cornerstones for modern stapes surgery.[48]

Stapes surgery is based on three major anatomical and physiological principles (Figure 36.3):[49]

- At least a small part of the stapes footplate should be removed.
- By using a prosthesis, a solid connection should be established between the long process of the incus and the cochlear fluids beneath the opening, with no adhesion to the edges of the oval window niche.
- A watertight seal of the labyrinth at the opening should be created in order to avoid fistulization or possible infection.

There has been tremendous variation in surgical techniques for stapes surgery over recent years, with variations in the type of prosthesis used (Teflon, Teflon–steel), the diameter of the prosthesis, and the amount of stapes footplate removed (total removal, partial removal or small-hole stapedotomy). The advantages and disadvantages of cutting the stapedial tendon, the use of grafted material to seal the oval window and the employment of laser surgery have all been debated. An in-depth discussion of these issues is beyond the scope of this chapter and the reader is referred to surgical textbooks for a more detailed description.[49]

The major surgical techniques are 'stapedectomy' and 'stapedotomy'. The first steps are similar for both procedures. An endaural approach with the creation of a tympanomeatal flap is advocated. The tympanomeatal flap is elevated until the fibrous annulus can be identified. Subsequently, the tympanic membrane is lifted out of the sulcus so that the posterior half can be folded forwards over the handle of the malleus. The chorda tympani is then identified and gently displaced forwards. This is followed by the identification of the inducostapedial joint and the stapes footplate, which may necessitate a partial removal of the bony canal wall. Thereafter, one must carefully verify the presence of stapes fixation and normal mobility of the malleus. A calibration rod is now employed to measure the length of the prosthesis which is to be used subsequently. The incudostapedial joint is then disconnected, followed by fragmentation of the posterior and anterior crus of the stapes and removal of the stapes superstructure. Some authors advocate preservation of the stapes tendon, but this is not universally accepted.

During stapedectomy, the previous steps are followed by fracturing of the stapes footplate and gentle removal of the footplate fragments. In order to prevent fistulization, the oval window may be covered or filled with a soft tissue graft prepared from a compressed vein or earlobe fat. A calibrated Teflon or steel prosthesis is then placed between the centre of the graft and the long process of the incus. The loop of the prosthesis is secured around the incus.

With stapedotomy, removal of the crura is followed by fenestration of the footplate (small hole technique).[50] This is achieved by drilling a calibrated hole through the footplate by means of micro-instruments,[50] a microdrill[48,51] or laser.[52] The hole should be 0.1 mm larger than the prosthesis. The prosthesis is placed in such a way that it enters the hole and encircles the long crus of the incus, where it is tightened to avoid dislocation.

At the end of the procedure, the tympanomeatal flap is turned back and the outer ear canal filled with an earpack.

Difficult or unusual cases may require a specialized approach, adopted by the surgeon during the procedure.[53]

Results of stapes surgery

The results of stapes surgery are considered to be highly successful. In the hands of very experienced surgeons, over 90% of patients achieve a closure of the air–bone gap to less than 10 dB.[6, 54–56] Cremers et al compared differences in hearing gain 1 year after stapedotomy, partial platinectomy, or total stapedectomy for otosclerosis at different frequencies and concluded that hearing gain for air conduction was significantly better by an average of 7.4 dB for all frequencies combined, after either stapedotomy or partial platinectomy compared to total stapedectomy.[56]

Indications for surgery in otosclerosis

The risk of surgery should be weighed against the expected benefit. Therefore, the air–bone gap should be at least 15 dB and there should be a speech discrimination score of 60% or more to obtain a good hearing improvement. Surgery might also be considered in patients with a severe hearing loss of 90–100 dB and without measurable cochlear reserve on speech discrimination. In those cases, the aim of surgery is to improve hearing to a level where a hearing aid may be of help.

Formal contraindications for stapes surgery are:

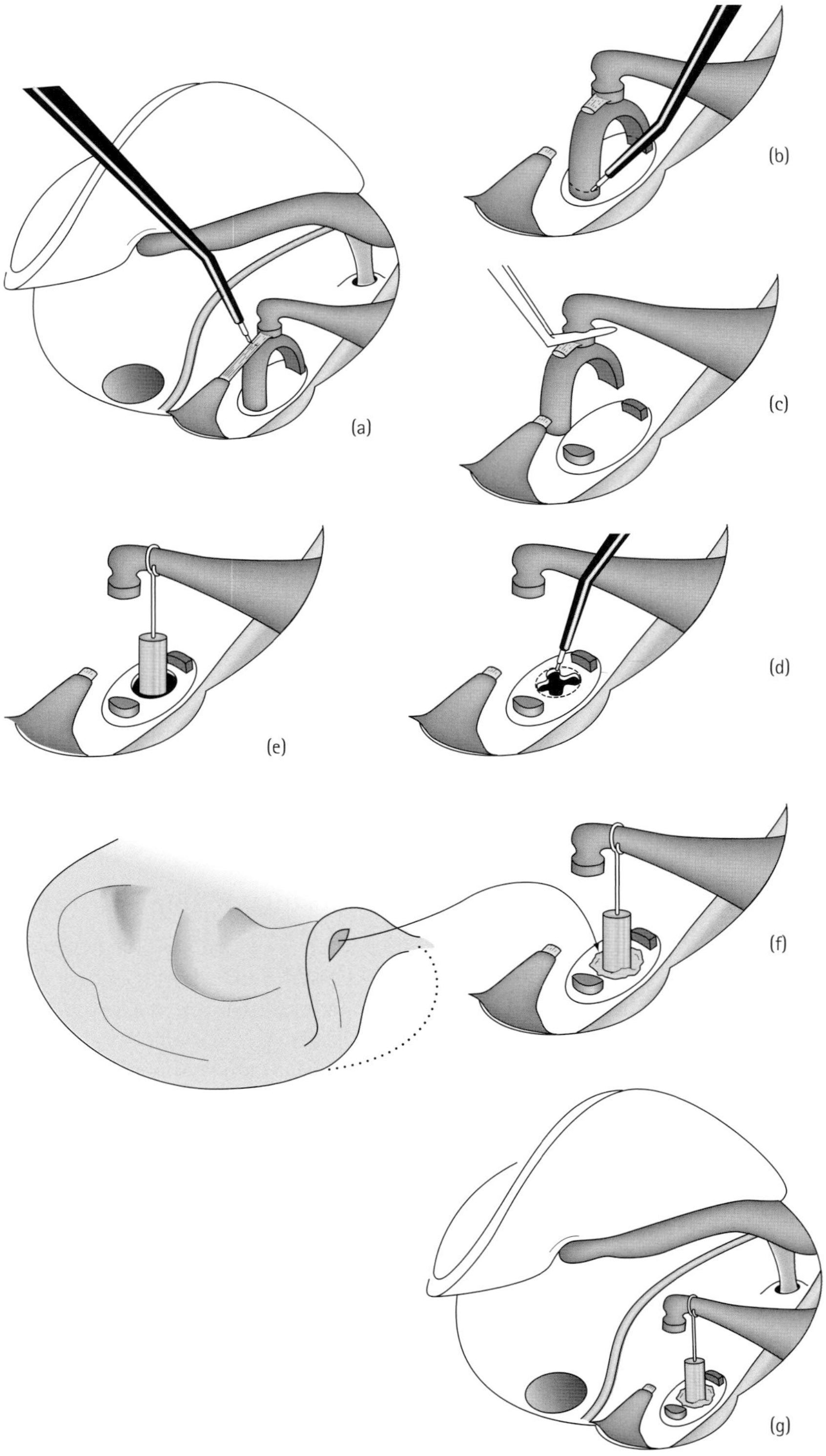

Figure 36.3 Schematic surgical technique illustrated with the use of a laserprobe. For details see text. (From Häusler. *Laryngorhinootologie* 2000; **79**(S2): 59–139.[53] Georg Thieme Verlag)

- a patient unfit for surgery due to the presence of general medical disease, especially patients with bleeding disorders or an excessively unstable autonomic system
- the presence of an infection in the ear to be operated on
- a tympanic membrane perforation
- chronic otitis media
- tympanosclerosis (because of the likelihood of concomitant malleus fixation).

Relative contraindications are:

- a patient with only one hearing ear
- the presence of vertigo and clinical evidence of endolymphatic hydrops or labyrinthine fistula
- congenital malformations of the middle or inner ear, because these are associated with an increased risk for pre- or postoperative perilymph leakage and sensorineural hearing loss.

When treatment counselling is provided to a patient with otosclerosis, the possibilities of surgery or hearing aids should be discussed. It must be explained that even after an initially successful surgical procedure, a progressive worsening of bone conduction thresholds may develop as time passes postoperatively. Long-term worsening of hearing acuity is mainly sensorineural and can be attributed to presbyacusis or cochlear otosclerosis. Whereas many patients will eventually need a hearing aid in the long term, it has been demonstrated that stapes surgery can postpone the need for a hearing aid for more than 20 years. In addition, some authors have found bone conduction thresholds to be maintained better in operated as opposed to unoperated ears.[57]

Risks of stapes surgery

The major surgical risks of stapes surgery are perilymph fistula and sensorineural hearing loss. A perilymph fistula gives rise to dysequilibrium and hearing loss, and is associated with an increased risk for meningitis. A fistula may develop years after the initial procedure.

Postoperative or late sensorineural hearing loss occurred in 23 of 2521 ears (0.91%) of patients undergoing stapes surgery by Marquet.[8] Causes of sensorineural hearing loss after stapes surgery are perilymph fistula, surgical trauma, noise from surgical drilling or viral infection. Facial palsy is a rare complication, with a reported incidence of 0.1%.[7] It is considered to be an idiopathic form of facial palsy without direct trauma to the nerve.

Future perspectives

Although small innovations in surgical technique are still possible, major innovations in the management of patients with otosclerosis are likely to be found in the field of molecular biology and genetics. Up to now, two genes involved in the development of otosclerosis have been discovered and their mode of inheritance unravelled.[58,59]

> **OTOSCLEROSIS**
> Otosclerosis is characterized by a mixed or sensorineural hearing loss due to deposition of otosclerotic foci in the middle ear and cochlea. Surgery consists of the interposition of a calibrated piston between the oval window and the long process of the incus in order to restore sound transmission at the level of the stapes footplate. Both stapedotomy and stapedectomy are highly successful in most cases, provided that a proper preoperative assessment of the patient and his audiometric and radiological data has been performed. Patients considered not to be surgical candidates can be fitted with a hearing aid.

Chronic otitis media and its surgical management

Definition and approach

Chronic otitis media (COM) is a collective noun for different forms of chronic middle ear disease. Middle ear atelectasis, adhesive otitis media and chronic otitis media with or without cholesteatoma are all part of a chronic (non)-infectious state of the middle ear.

The prevalence of COM has decreased over the last 20 years, due to antibiotic treatment and the use of ventilation tubes. The prevalence is estimated to be between 1.5% and 2.6%.[32]

COM can lead to infectious complications, including acute and chronic mastoiditis, petrositis and intracranial infections. The non-infectious sequelae, including chronic perforation of the tympanic membrane, ossicular erosion, labyrinthine erosion and tympanosclerosis, are major causes of hearing loss.

The decision regarding surgical management of COM requires a complete assessment of the patient's problem. Aural discharge and hearing loss are the principal symptoms. Sometimes, there may be hardly any hearing loss, because the cholesteatoma is itself transmitting sound. Otalgia is uncommon. The development of headache, vertigo, fever or facial palsy is evidence of complications. Early diagnosis of intracranial complications is a prerequisite for a favourable outcome.

Otoscopic examination of the ear will reveal the nature of the disease. The extent of the disease has to be examined with audiological assessment and radiological imaging.

A pure tone audiogram, including air and bone conduction with full masking, is essential to evaluate the degree of hearing loss and to determine the air–bone gap. In cases in which an attempt to improve hearing is being considered, a speech audiogram and self-assessment are valuable.

Hearing thresholds vary considerably in cases of COM, ranging from normal hearing to a dead ear. The characteristics of the hearing loss will significantly influence the possibility of surgical hearing improvement and therefore will influence the decision-making.

Most patients with COM will present with a conductive hearing loss due to tympanic membrane perforation, ossicular fixation or destruction and tympanosclerosis.

In addition to the conductive hearing loss, many patients have a degree of sensorineural hearing loss.[60] Cochlear damage has been attributed to the diffusion of toxic products of inflammation through the scala tympani via the round window membrane.

The anatomy of the temporal bone is well demonstrated by CT scanning. Extension of the disease may be observed in a case of cholesteatoma, erosion of the ossicular chain is sometimes visible, a labyrinth fistula can be predicted, and intracranial complications can be demonstrated. Chronic inflammatory tissue or exudate presents as clouding in the tympanic space or mastoid. The specificity of this clouding is very low. CT scan and MRI are no adequate substitute for a 'second look' operation in the assessment of cases which have undergone canal wall surgery for cholesteatoma.[3]

Pathophysiology

Middle ear atelectasis is thought to result mainly from longstanding Eustachian tube dysfunction. One of the main functions of the Eustachian tube is ventilation. Opening of the Eustachian tube allows the exchange of gases and equalization between the environment and middle ear. The middle ear gases also are exchanged via the middle ear mucosa. Bilateral diffusion between the middle ear cavity and the blood may also be an important factor in the development of atelectasis, because the gas composition of the middle ear basically resembles that of venous blood and differs from that of air.[61]

Aural cholesteatomas are epidermal inclusion cysts of the middle ear or mastoid. They contain the desquamated debris (keratin) from their keratinizing, squamous epithelial lining.

It is generally accepted that cholesteatomas may be congenital or acquired. Congenital cholesteatomas, by definition, originate from areas of keratinizing epithelium within the middle ear cleft. The pathogenesis of acquired cholesteatomas has been debated for more than a century. There are four basic theories: (1) invagination of the tympanic membrane (retraction pocket); (2) basal cell hyperplasia; (3) epithelial ingrowth through a perforation (migration); and (4) squamous metaplasia of middle ear epithelium.

Chronic otomastoiditis without cholesteatoma is marked by the presence of irreversible inflammatory changes within the middle ear and mastoid. Very frequently, there is a tympanic membrane perforation, but the factors that allow acute infections within the middle ear and mastoid to develop into chronic infections are not clear. Chronic obstruction of the attic and antrum with infection may lead to this chronic status.

Tympanosclerosis is thought to be a consequence of resolved otitis media or trauma, in which acellular hyaline and calcified deposits accumulate within the tympanic membrane and the submucosa middle ear. Osteoneogenesis can occur in these lesions, and bone deposition leads to ossicular fixation, mainly involving the malleus and incus.

In most patients, these plaques are clinically insignificant and cause no or little hearing impairment. Ossicular chain fixation leads to conductive hearing loss, but results of surgical treatment are often unpredictable. This significantly influences the decision-making concerning surgery.

Secretory otitis media (SOM) is the accumulation of fluid in the middle ear cavity behind an intact tympanic membrane without symptoms of acute infection. Eustachian tube dysfunction, failure of ciliary clearance and bacterial invasion in the middle ear are responsible factors.

Surgical management

The most important surgical aim in COM is to eradicate the pathology that causes the patient's symptoms of aural discharge and hearing loss. This aspect needs a complete and convincing explanation to the patient to prevent the development of unrealistic expectations, especially concerning hearing improvement. If the pathology is not or incompletely eradicated, recurrent or residual pathology will result in complications or unsatisfactory hearing improvement in the short and long term.

Decision-making regarding surgery includes many aspects of both medical and non-medical importance, and should be evidence-based. There are few evidence-based arguments in the literature regarding hearing improvement after surgery for COM. Critical appraisal of evidence-based medicine in the general literature shows little sign that the approach is effective and indicates that further rigorous evaluation is a priority.[62]

In evaluating an ear, the following questions should be asked. What is the nature of the disease? What is the extent of the disease? Are the ossicles involved? What is the status of hearing in the contralateral ear? Do voice and tuning fork tests confirm audiometric tests? What is the status of the middle ear mucosa? What is the condition of the external ear canal? Is a semicircular canal fistula present? What is the status of Eustachian tube function?

Prognostic factors influencing the functional outcome of tympanoplasty are dry status of the mucosal lining, availability of the malleus handle, mastoidectomy, tympanic membrane perforation, preoperative air–bone gap, contralateral absence of pathology, and younger age.[63,64]

The primary pathology is the most important determining factor in decision-making. If the pathology is aggressive or complications are present or expected in the future (in the case of cholesteatoma), surgery is necessary. If the pathology is chronic, but no further evolution is expected, other factors will help in decision-making. Frequent episodes of aural discharge, aural pain or hearing loss can be very annoying for the patient and can justify surgery. If hearing loss is the one and only problem from a medical point of view, hearing aids can be a very effective alternative to surgery.

Tympanic membrane perforations often cause few symptoms. The decision of whether to operate or not is therefore based on the potential benefits to the patients: (1) prevention of recurrent discharge; (2) hearing improvement; and (3) ability to swim.

Frequent episodes of discharge provoke inflammatory changes in the middle ear and tympanosclerosis. Postponing surgery, e.g. in children, will possibly result in less hearing improvement because of these changes, while functional results of tympanoplasty are good in the childhood population.[65] In 88% of cases, the surgery resulted in a closed tympanic membrane and a median hearing gain of 10 dB.

In cases of middle ear atelectasis, the tympanic membrane becomes retracted onto the promontory and the ossicles, and otitis media with effusion is usually coexistent. In atelectatic ears, the middle ear space is partially or completely obliterated. This results in changes in the mucosa of the middle ear and may lead to erosion of the long process of the incus and the stapes superstructure.

Middle ear atelectasis may be reversible with ventilation tubes. The tympanic membrane can revert to its normal position and hearing will improve. Hearing improvement is explained by the evacuation of the effusion and by the restoration of the normal vibrating function of the tympanic membrane.

Cholesteatomas can only be eradicated by surgical resection. There is, however, a small group of elderly and medically unfit patients who are best managed by regular suction clearance in the outpatient clinic.

In the early days of chronic ear surgery, radical mastoidectomy, with removal of the incus, malleus and tympanic membrane, was the operation of choice. This proved to be effective as a means of eradicating the disease, but was associated with poor hearing and a high incidence of chronic discharge. The modified radical operation, with preservation of the malleus handle and a remnant of drum tissue, was devised to overcome these disadvantages. Intact canal wall surgery was introduced by Jansen in the late 1950s.[66] With this 'closed technique', an open cavity with its inherent problems could be avoided, functional reconstruction was facilitated, and the ability to fit a hearing aid in a dry ear with a suitable external auditory meatus was improved.

The purpose of surgery is eradication of disease and management of complications, and, secondarily, reconstruction of the middle ear to improve hearing.

Restoration of hearing can be achieved by reconstruction of the tympanic membrane and the ossicular chain. The long-term audiometric results of this surgery are generally disappointing.

After 10 years of follow-up, gain of the air conduction between 1 and 10 dB was reported.[49,67]

Ossicular destruction leads to hearing loss. To improve hearing, reconstruction of the sound-transmitting chain is needed. Whether this reconstruction should resemble the original anatomical structures can be debated. In the early 1960s, tympano-ossicular allografts were introduced in the field of middle ear reconstruction. The alleged advantage was the perfect anatomical reconstruction ability. This technique was successful in improving hearing when an intact stapes superstructure

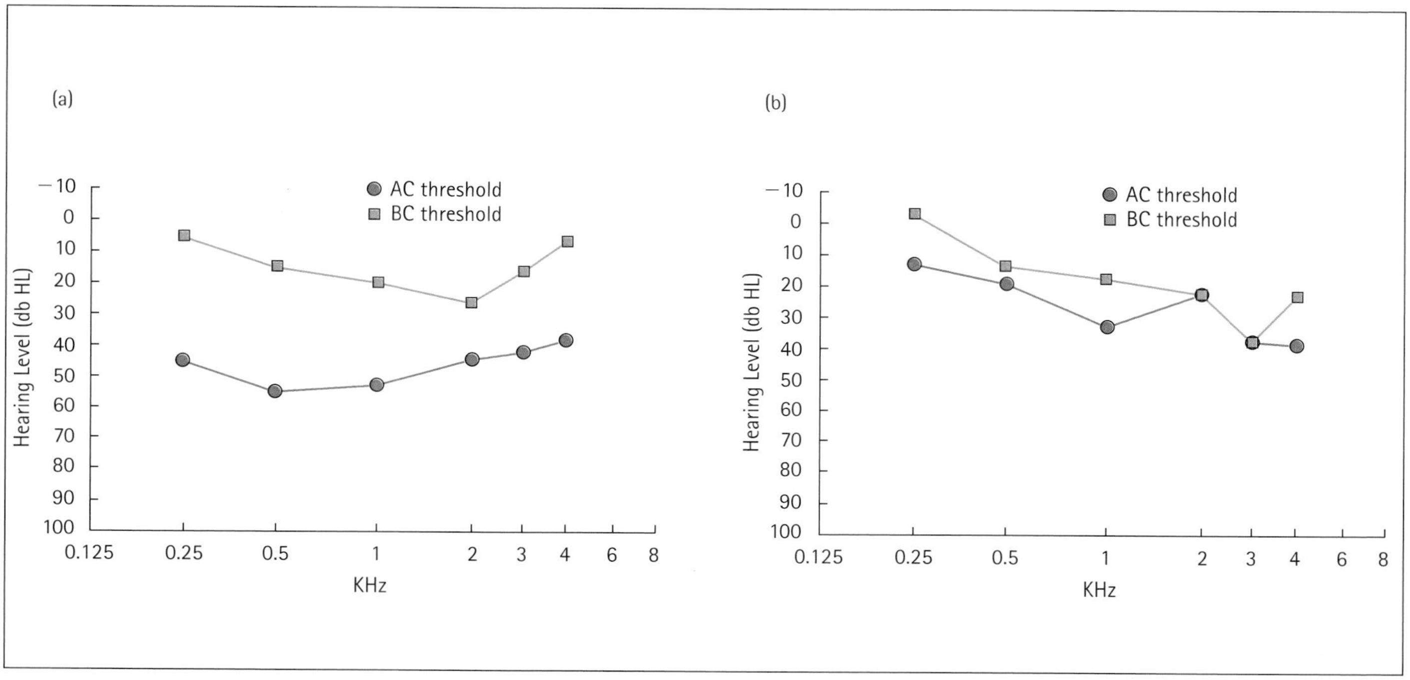

Figure 36.4 Pre- (a) and postoperative (b) audiogram of a patient with otosclerosis of the right ear. Note the presence of a Carhart notch at 2000 Hz on the preoperative audiogram and an improvement of both air and bone conduction postoperatively (overclosure).

was present. It was less successful in those ears in which only a mobile stapes footplate remained.[68]

In recent years, collaborative efforts between biomaterial scientists and surgeons have led to the manufacture of metals, solid and porous polymer materials and a range of ceramic materials, specifically designed for implantation. These materials are biotolerant or biocompatible in order not to provoke inflammatory reactions or extrusion of the implant.

Audiological results of ossicular reconstruction are very variable in the literature, depending mostly on the primary pathology, which led to ossicular destruction. An inflammatory mucosa, tympanosclerosis, bad Eustachian tube function, absence of the malleus and revision surgery were all bad prognostic factors influencing the audiological outcome.[31]

Malleus-to-footplate prostheses seem to provide good results compared with other techniques. A high degree of biocompatibility and stability and therefore optimal sound transfer is responsible for this.[21,69]

Reconstruction of an eroded incus with a malleus handle present and an intact stapes results in a postoperative air–bone gap within 20 dB in 85% of cases.[70]

Malleus ankylosis is an unusual pathology but should be systematically assessed during surgery and preferably after separation of the incudostapedial joint. A preoperative diagnosis is difficult to ascertain. A postoperative air–bone gap smaller than 10 dB is obtained in 77% of cases in the short term.[33]

Tympanosclerosis within the middle ear is histologically similar to that occurring within the tympanic membrane, but it often leads to conductive hearing loss caused by ossicular fixation. Ossicular reconstruction can be performed in ears with tympanosclerosis, but the risk of cochlear damage appears to be greater than in other middle ear diseases because of the extensive dissection that is required in tympanosclerotic ears.

Surgical mobilization of the ossicular chain results in better hearing in the short term. In the long term, tympanosclerosis has a tendency to relapse. On the one hand, it is the nature of the disease that causes the relapse, but on the other hand, every surgical act in the middle ear evokes scar tissue and will enhance the process of tympanosclerosis. Therefore, the patient should be well informed about the limitations of surgery. The surgeon should be conservative in his decision-making, and hearing aids should be considered.

SOM or otitis media with effusion are two terms used for the chronic condition in which there is an accumulation of non-purulent fluid in the middle ear for more than 12 weeks.[9] SOM has its highest prevalence in the first 2 years of life and decreases thereafter. It is preceded by acute otitis media in most cases. Risk factors for SOM are male gender, bottle feeding, contact with other daycare children, allergy, socio-economic status, smoking by the mother and viral upper airway infections.[71]

The fluid-containing middle ear results in a conductive hearing loss of about 35–40 dB. In rare cases of acute otitis media with purulent bulging of the drum, there may be a sensorineural hearing loss, caused by toxic inflammatory agents. The adverse effects of this hearing loss on the development of cognitive, linguistic, auditive and communication skills have long been debated.

The otologic sequelae of SOM are perforation of the tympanic membrane, COM, tympanosclerosis, adhesive otitis media and retraction pockets of the tympanic membrane.

The diagnosis of SOM is made by otoscopy and tympanometry. The hearing loss is assessed by audiometry and otoacoustical emissions.

Management of SOM can be medical and surgical. Antibiotic treatment is used in the USA, but this is much debated, since the effusion in the middle ear is not proven to be due to bacterial infection. Surgical treatment is often recommended for prompt remediation of the hearing loss and avoidance of long-term sequelae. In children younger than 3 years of age, who have persistent otitis media, prompt insertion of tympanostomy tubes does not measurably improve developmental outcomes at the age of 3 years.[44]

Insertion of ventilation tubes is the treatment of choice. The decision regarding surgical treatment should be postponed for several weeks, because the effusion has a tendency to resolve by itself. Thus, a balance must be reached between the probability of spontaneous resolution versus the sequelae of prolonged morbidity and the risk of intercurrent infection. Surgery is recommended more often in the autumn, because of the high likelihood of exacerbation of the condition during winter.

Other, more urgent, indications for surgical intervention, regardless of the time of year, relate to structural abnormalities of the tympanic membrane that may lead to ossicular erosion and cholesteatoma, namely retraction pockets.

The rationale for using tympanostomy tubes is prolonged ventilation of the tympanic cavity. The mucosal hyperplasia will revert to a more normal condition with aeration.

The efficacy of adenoidectomy for SOM is debated. Children with a history of upper airway infections, especially purulent rhinitis, are considered good candidates for adenoidectomy. Indeed, adenoidectomy is considered by many authors to be disease-modifying.

> The first aim of surgery in chronic otits media is cure of the diseased middle ear and eradication of the pathology.
> The perceived hearing improvement will be dependent on factors other than the air–bone gap alone.
> A correct assessment of the preoperative status, a sound judgement of the influencing risk factors and an operative plan are essential for the medical and functional outcome.
> Many factors in COM surgery are uncontrolled, e.g. Eustachian tube function, mucosal function, scar tissue and tympanosclerosis formation during the healing process.

Bone-anchored hearing aids (BAHAs)

Principle

The basic principle of treatment with BAHAs is simple: sound vibrations are directly transmitted to the skull bone via a skin-penetrating titanium implant and then are further transmitted to the cochlea, bypassing the middle ear.[40]

Bone conduction stimulation of the cochlea results from:

- sound radiation in the external ear canal (predominantly the high frequencies)
- the inertial response of the middle ear ossicles and the inner ear fluids (predominant contribution at the low frequencies)
- the compression response of the inner ear spaces (predominant response at the middle frequencies).[72]

For BAHAs, the latter two responses are the most important, and the end result will depend on the sensorineural functional level of the cochlea. However, sound radiation in the ear canal is still possible with the use of the BAHA, which does not occlude the external ear canal, and this is one of the major benefits of this form of amplification.

For patients with chronic middle and external ear diseases and atresias, the use of a conventional bone-conducting hearing aid, fixed on the arms of spectacles or on a headset, usually results in poor auditory rehabilitation, for several reasons, e.g.

- low pressure of the sound transducer or movements on the mastoid
- damping properties of the skin and the subcutaneous tissues, with inconsistency in sound quality
- discomfort from the continuous pressure.[73]

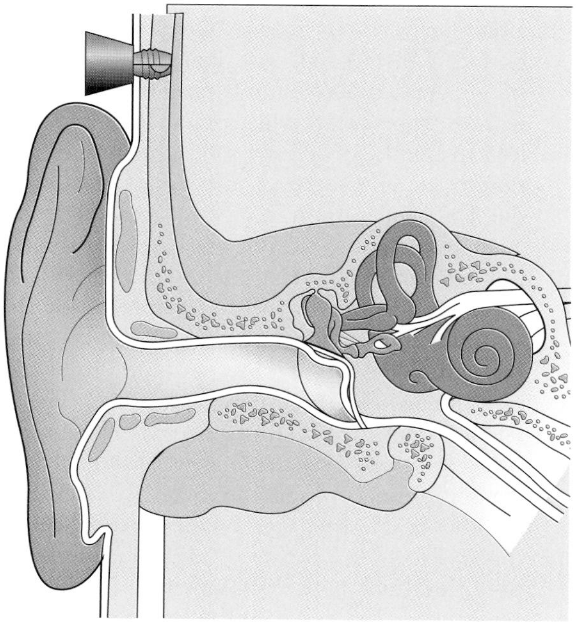

Figure 36.5 Schematic view of the BAHA in place.

By using a percutaneous osseointegrated stable titanium implant as the fixing point, a BAHA will overcome these disadvantages and stimulate the cochlea ipsilaterally and even contralaterally by bone conduction. The reported results are very good, especially in cases with a pure conductive hearing loss in which problems of recruitment, distortion or phonemic redundancy are not present.[40,60,72] Problems of acoustical feedback are not mentioned, but Snik[74] demonstrated that a percutaneous device gives better results than a transcutaneous device.

Disadvantages include the higher costs in comparison to a classic air conduction hearing aid, the surgical procedure necessary to implant the titanium fixing screw, and the limited power transferred by the bone conductor implant into the skull bone. In this way, good results (>90% of the cases successfully treated) for hearing losses up to 45 dB pure tone bone conduction average (0.5–3 kHz) can be obtained with the classic or compact sound processor.

For higher hearing losses from 45 to approximately 60 dB pure tone bone conduction average (0.5–3 kHz), satisfactory functional results can be achieved by using a powerful body-worn sound processor connected to the transducer on the implant.

Indications

The current criteria for the application of a bone conductor as hearing aid include:

1. Sensorineural hearing loss in which the use of a conventional air conduction hearing aid is not possible for reasons of recurrent infections associated with the occlusion of the external ear canal by the prosthesis, or skin reactions in the external ear canal, e.g. contact allergy or eczema reaction, making the use of a conventional hearing aid impossible.
2. Congenital malformation with agenesis or atresia of the external and/or middle ear structures or acquired stenosis of the external meatus. Most of these patients have a major conductive or mixed hearing loss with preservation of the inner ear function resulting in good bone conduction thresholds. In children, the limiting factor is the thickness of the dense cortical bone in the temporo-occipital region of the skull. High-resolution multiplanar CT scanning and the use of three-dimensional image reconstruction for pre-operative examination together with the use of computer-guided navigation during surgery will highly benefit the success rate of osseointegration of the implant. In this way, early implantation (even before the age of 2 years) will make it possible to minimize the delay in speech and language development in children with bilateral congenital agenesis or atresia of the ear.[75] In these cases, the combined application of a BAHA and an auricular prosthesis fixed onto an osseointegrated implant will not only result in a functional benefit but also offer the possibility of a very good aesthetic rehabilitation with major psychoemotional

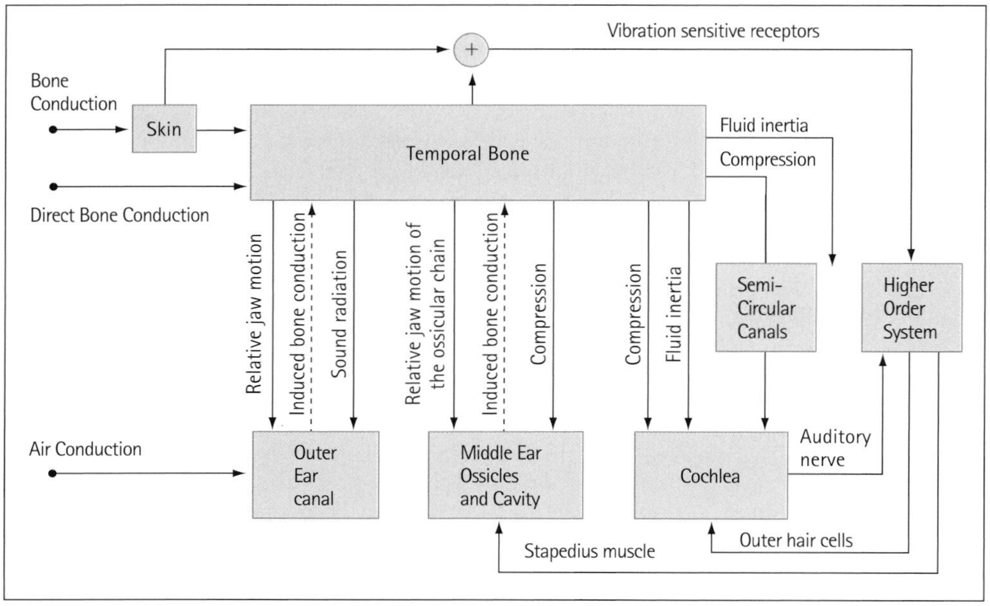

Figure 36.6 The acoustical pathways to the cochlea, when stimulated by air conduction (ac), bone conduction (bc), and direct bone conduction (dbc). Note the bypass of external and middle ear achieved by bone conduction hearing devices. (From Huttenbrink. *Otolaryngol Clin North Am* 2001; **34**: 315–35.[66])

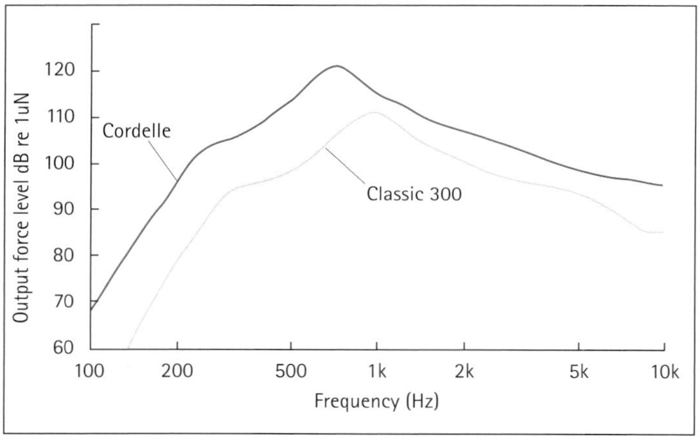

Figure 36.7 The maximum output level of the BAHA Classic 300 and the BAHA Cordelle. μN micro Newtons. (From Huttenbrink. *Otolaryngol Clin North Am* 2001; **34**: 315–35.[66])

benefits. Moreover, for the patients using eyeglasses, a stable support can be offered.[76] It should be emphasized that for cases of ear malformation, a BAHA can be a temporary solution that neither damages the inner ear nor excludes the possibility of functional tympano-ossicular surgery when the child is older, provided that the anatomical conditions are favourable.[61]

3. Otosclerosis or chronic middle ear pathology (e.g. cholesteatoma) in a unilateral hearing patient, in whom the risk of failure of surgical intervention, e.g. a stapedotomy operation, is complete deafness.[77] When the sensorineural hearing threshold of the inner ear is preserved and the conductive hearing loss becomes too high, the use of a bone conductor will give better functional results and resolve the discomfort of the classical hearing aid, e.g. the distortion and the tendency to provoke acoustical feedback or Larsson effect.
4. Major radical mastoidectomy cavities, with which the use of the conventional hearing aid is not possible for a number of reasons: the acoustical features of the cavity (uncontrollable feedback when using an air conduction aid); humidity resulting in recurrent foul-smelling ear discharge and responsible for recurrent technical problems of a standard AC aid.

Newer recent indications for BAHA are :

- Congenital or acquired unilateral deafness as, for example, after resection of an acoustical neuroma, where the application of a BAHA will contribute to the restoration of the stereophonic aspects of hearing. The audiological results of such an application remain premature and too limited to lead to definite conclusions, but the initial subjective reactions of patients suggest significant satisfaction, especially if the delay between onset of the unilateral deafness and the commencement of the use of a BAHA is short.
- Bilateral use of a BAHA in cases of bilateral moderate and severe conductive or mixed hearing loss with symmetric sensorineural thresholds after, for example, chronic middle ear pathology with persistent intermittent ear discharge even after several surgical interventions.[78] The advantage of bilateral application has been found in better localization of sound in space, resulting in stereophonic hearing. In quiet, the speech recognition threshold was 3–6 dB better for a binaural BAHA than for a monaural application. In noise, the results show a significant difference in speech recognition threshold between monaural and binaural BAHA application, depending on the localization of the noise and the side of initial fitting.[79–81]

Surgery

The use of a pure titanium implant screw as the fixing point is best suited to guarantee a sure osseointegration. The placement is performed following a standard method of controlling the forces exerted with maximum cooling during drilling, tapping the screwthread and inserting the titanium implant device, in order to keep the heat production as low as possible to prevent osseolysis at the site of implantation and allow the process of osseointegration. The location of the implant site is determined by use of a BAHA dummy and, if possible, by using a peroperative image-guiding navigation system.

This latter technique offers a special benefit in cases of congenital malformation, in which the skull bone is often very irregular and thin in some places. During the implantation procedure, contamination of the titanium surface of the implant device by contact with metal material other than titanium has to be avoided. Therefore, one part of the surgical equipment is manufactured out of pure titanium and will be separated from the other tools during the entire surgical intervention. On the other hand, a low-speed drilling motor, with controlled force, is absolutely necessary.

The surgical intervention can be performed under general or local anaesthesia, during a short stay in hospital (±2 days).

To fit the hearing aid to the implant screw, a percutaneous device, the so-called 'abutment', has been developed and produced in pure titanium. This abutment has a special design, initially adapted for a so-called 'bayonet'-connection. Currently, however, a completely different, so-called 'snap'-connection, is used to guarantee stable and fixed positioning of the hearing aid with guaranteed holding forces, but safe loosening capacities in response to accidental forces on the hearing aid, and also allowing safe removal.

During surgical implantation, a skin modification with reduction of the subcutaneous tissue at the implant site has to be performed to get an area of hair-free skin with close adherence to the periosteum in order to diminish the skin mobility around the abutment. In this way, reduced accumulation of skin debris will prevent the intrusion of an infection around the implant, which could be responsible for the extrusion and loss of the implant screw.

In most cases, the implantation of the screw and the adaptation of the skin is actually performed in one stage. In cases where the osseointegration could be at risk (e.g. in very young children or patients with a congenital atresia or radiated skull bone area), a two-stage procedure may be used. In the former two situations, a longer delay (usually at least 6 months) before loading the implant is necessary.

Loading of the implant can be performed safely after completed osseointegration, which takes 3–4 months, although in practice a tendency exists to perform loading at an earlier stage.

To guarantee the best chance of good osseointegration and stable fixation of the implant in the long term, implant location in dense cortical skull bone is necessary. This will not only result in stable positioning of the hearing aid, but also give better functional results. In order to achieve this, the use of high-resolution multiplanar CT scanning, with three-dimensional imaging and preoperative planning, together with the use of intraoperative computer-guided navigation, can be helpful.

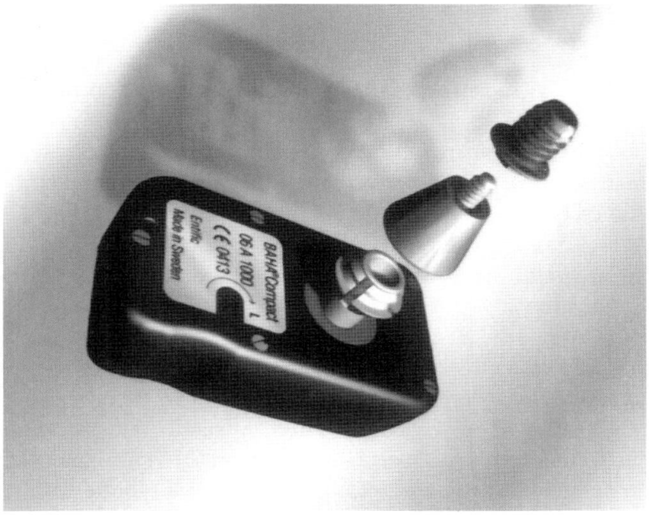

Figure 36.8 The BAHA Compact with snap coupling and the percutaneous abutment and fixture screw.

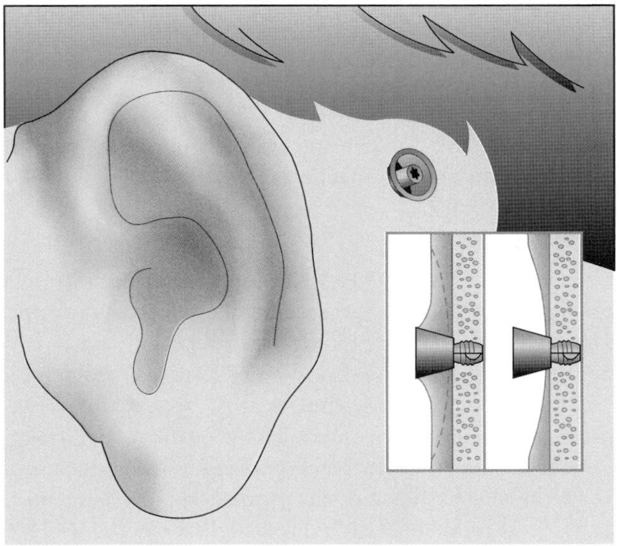

Figure 36.9 Schematic view of the abutment for snap coupling and the skin adaptation.

Contraindications

The following limitations mitigate against an optimal result:

- pure tone average bone conduction thresholds (0.5–3 kHz) worse than 60 dB HL
- age less than 2 years.

Results

The surgical procedure is minor, well established and almost risk-free.[40] A success rate of 97% for osseointegration has been reported.[60]

Skin-penetrating abutments cause only a few cases of adverse skin reactions, which are mostly temporary and can be resolved easily.[40,60]

If necessary, the removal of the skin-penetrating coupling can be performed without anaesthesia and without future complications.

The subjects' positive opinions about the BAHA were confirmed by results obtained from both patients' questionnaires and audiological tests.[40,60,72,79]

Mylanus et al[82] demonstrated a small but significant improvement in the speech recognition in noise test. This improvement was related to the size of the air–bone gap: the greater the air–bone gap, the poorer the results with conventional air conduction hearing aids.

The contribution to improvement in quality of life of BAHAs, compared with conventional hearing aids, for hearing-impaired patients with chronically draining ears, malformed ears, or otosclerosis or tympanosclerosis can be characterized by:

- improvement of the quality of sound
- improved comfort
- better appearance
- diminished risk for ear infections, improving healing of ongoing chronic ear infection.

Conclusions

Currently, the use of a BAHA can fulfil the criteria for a valuable surgical treatment for specifically selected problems of hearing rehabilitation, not only for adults but also for children.[75,83,84] Although some shortcomings, such as problems with the telephone, wind noise and hearing speech in noise, are reported, there are many practical, acoustical, psychological and medical benefits reported by patients.[85] A significant quality of life benefit has been demonstrated by Arunachalam, who measured the result of the BAHA surgical intervention using the Glasgow Benefit Inventory. The maximum benefit was noted in patients with congenital atresias followed by discharging mastoid cavities. The general benefit score was comparable to that with middle ear surgery, but just below the benefit from cochlear implant.[86]

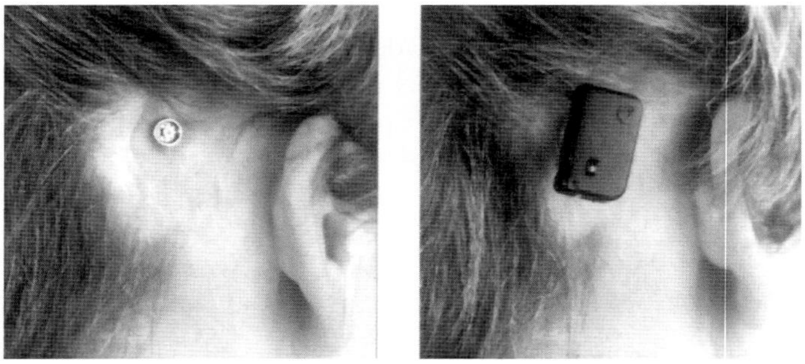

Figure 36.10 The abutment for snap coupling on the left, the Compact BAHA in place on the right photograph.

Actual experiences based on long-term follow-up in many patients are leading to the introduction of new indications for BAHA application which seem to offer satisfactory results.

Some of them, e.g. the use of BAHAs in pure sensorineural hearing impairment[87] or in unilateral conductive or mixed hearing loss,[88] are only pilot studies.

More and more ENT doctors and patients are becoming familiar with this specialized hearing aid. Possible developments for the future are miniaturization and semi-implantable bone-conducting devices, percutaneous electrical coupling, and a BAHA for tinnitus suppression.[75]

> Bone-anchored hearing aids use bone conduction stimulation of the cochlea. The end result will depend on the sensorineural functional level of the cochlea.
> The application of the BAHA needs a surgical procedure, which is minor, well established and almost risk-free. The high success rate is based on the process of osseointegration of a titanium fixture screw and the use of a titanium skin-penetrating abutment.
> Bypassing the external and middle ear structures, the classical indications for application of the BAHA are the cases with a pure conductive hearing loss, e.g. in congenital agenesis of the external and middle ear structures, otosclerosis or chronic middle ear pathology (e.g. cholesteatoma) in a unilateral hearing patient.
> However, all cases, even those with a sensorineural hearing loss, in which the use of a conventional air conduction hearing aid is not possible are potential indications for the use of a BAHA.
> Based on the good functional results and the high patient satisfaction, newer indications are found in: congenital or acquired unilateral deafness (e.g. after resection of an acoustical neuroma) and in the bilateral application for patients with bilateral moderate and severe conductive or mixed hearing loss with symmetrical sensorineural thresholds (e.g. chronic middle ear pathology with persistent intermittent ear discharge even after several surgical interventions).

Cochlear implantation

The concept

Cochlear implantation is a method designed to improve the communication abilities of severely hearing-impaired people with bilateral cochlear dysfunction, who derive little or no benefit from amplified sound through traditional hearing aids.

CIs have evolved into an accepted standard of care for severely to profoundly hearing-impaired adults and children.[89]

A CI is a partially implantable neurostimulator of the cochlear nerve, replacing the organ of Corti and hence bypassing the outer, middle and inner ear. It comprises an internal surgically implantable part—the implant—and an external part consisting of a microphone system, a speech processor, a battery compartment empowering the CI and an emitting coil (Figure 36.11).

For nearly a decade, the intracochlear multichannel CI has become the widely accepted auditory prosthesis for both adults and children with a severely dysfunctional or failing organ of Corti.[90,91] The vast majority of these patients derive substantial benefit, especially when used in conjunction with (cued) speech reading according to the NIH Consensus Statement.[92] It has to be stressed that access to optimal educational and rehabilitation services is important to adults and critical to children in order to maximize the benefits available from cochlear implantation.

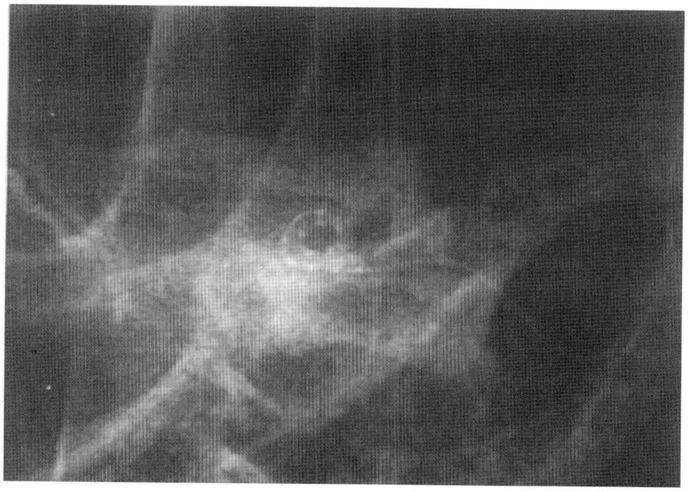

Figure 36.11 Postoperative X-ray Medel Combi 40+ electrode array in place in the cochlea.

Therefore, the CI is not just a device or a surgical intervention, but has evolved over 30 years into a whole concept of care for the person with a failing organ of Corti.

Owing to the driving force of technical improvement and the reliability of many implants, the concept of cochlear implantation and holistic rehabilitation has dramatically changed the approach to the severe to profoundly hearing impaired person and has led to an enormous amount of scientific research concerning every aspect of ear, hearing, hearing impairment, deafness, rehabilitation and technical innovations.[89,93] Indeed, every progress in this field can eventually be implemented in the CI care programme, leading to improved communication skills.

The importance of technological innovation is demonstrated by the substantial improvement of auditory capacities of CI users. Moreover, the success of CIs is evidenced by the very low rate of non-users.[94]

An overview of working principles, candidate selection and results in terms of expressive and receptive speech outcomes is given.

Schematic functioning and place of CI surgery

CIs replace the inner and outer hair cell function, by transforming sound and speech to meaningful electrical stimulation of the dendrites and the ganglion cells of the spiral ganglion. Table 36.3 summarizes the addresses of the major CI companies. Figure 36.11 represents a schema of a CI.

First, the sound is captured by a microphone, which sends the signal to the speech processor. At this level, initial processing, designated as pre-processing, occurs. A novel example of processing development is the two-microphone noise reduction system,[95] as enhancing the signal-to-noise ratio by 10 dB. The microphone is most often fitted behind the ear, but may be remote, using a microphone coupled with an FM system.

The speech processor converts the microphone signal to a digital code of instructions for the implanted neurostimulator. The operating program of the speech processor executes the speech-coding strategy, i.e. the way in which sound is converted

Table 36.3 General Information on Cochlear Implant Companies

	Medel	Cochlear	Advanced Bionics	M.X.M.
Name of implant	Combi 40+	CI 24R	CLARION CII Bionic Ear system	Digisonic DX10
Origin	Austria	Australia	USA	France
Company	Medel Fürstenweg 77a 6020 Innsbruck Austria Tel: 43/512/288889 Fax: 43/512/293381	Cochlear A.G. Margarethenstrasse 47 4053 Basel Switzerland Tel: 41/61/050404 Fax: 41/61/050405	Advanced Bionic Corp., 12740 San Fernando Road, Sylmar, CA 91342, USA Tel: 1/818/3627588 Fax: 1/818/3625069 E-mail: info@advancedbionics.com europe@advancedbionics.com	Laboratoires M.X.M. Les Mimosas Quartier Croix Rouge 06600 Antibes France Tel: 33/93331413 Fax: 33/93335376

into electrical signals for the brain to interpret. The speech coding has to deliver a combination of temporal and spectral information that is optimal for the CI user. Although physiological data of a normally hearing ear are fundamental, they are not necessarily optimal[96] or even exploitable[97] for the affected auditory system and, moreover, may not even be similar for all patients.[98]

All the speech-processing systems pass the signal through a filter bank, mimicking the simultaneous tonotopy of passive filtering of the cochlea. The active cochlear amplifier and the stochastic stimulation of the nerve fibres which occur in normal cochlear nerves, however, are more difficult to replicate. Adaptations, e.g. amplitude enhancement, jitter-like stimulation, background noise injection[64] and signal interaction cancelling (G. F. Smoorenburg, personal communication), are possible future refinements currently under investigation.

Physically, the speech processor, together with the battery compartment, is built into a body-worn device, or a behind-the-ear (BTE) processor. In the latter case, the microphone system is also included in the BTE. Progress is to be expected in battery technology, allowing further miniaturization of the BTE. The use of BTE speech processors has improved both the comfort of and acceptance by the patient.[99]

Via an RF link between the external emitting coil and the receiving internal coil, the information and the power are transmitted to the internal part of the device, which is the surgically implanted part of the CI. To improve the information transfer, resolutions are developed enhancing the artificial intelligence of the implant and allowing more transfer capacity for the fluctuation of the captured sound. The implanted part of the device itself has no battery. The electronic and neurostimulator part is embedded in a recess drilled in the skull in the retroauricular region. Owing to smaller receiving coils in the implant, minimal invasive approaches can be used with smaller retroauricular incisions of 3–4 cm.[100] This makes it feasible to perform this surgery with only an overnight hospital stay, or as a day case depending on the facilities in the hospital.

The electrode array carries 12–24 independent electrodes. The electrode array is brought into the scala vestibuli of the cochlea, each electrode corresponding to a certain tonotopically (frequency-to-place relationship) defined frequency region. High tones correspond with electrodes located at the basal part of the array, and low tones with those at the apical part. The approach to the scala tympani is through a mastoidectomy and a posterior tympanotomy (Figure 36.12). There is also experience with a retroauricular, transcanal approach or a supralabyrinthine approach. The electrodes are sequentially activated using pulsatile electric signals, or they are activated simultaneously with analog electrical signals. The most common technique is the former, but a significant part of the fine structure information is lost in this way. The latter has the disadvantage of channel interaction of the instantaneous electrical fields.[62]

The stimulation mode may be hybrid, in which case the lower tones are stimulated in an analog way, while the higher frequencies are stimulated in a digital way.

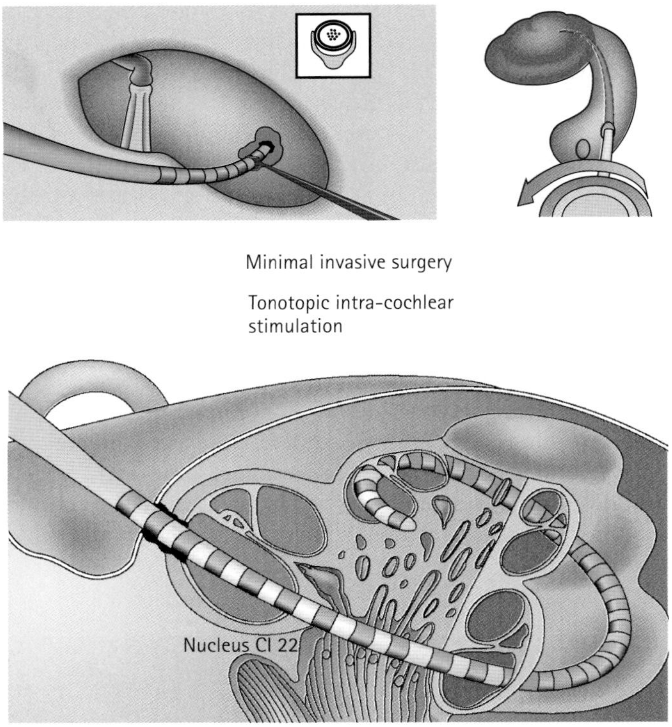

Figure 36.12 Intracochlear position of an electrode array.

An increase in efficacy of conveying the electrical current to the remaining nerve fibres in the spiral ganglion is achieved by the application of so-called 'modiolar hugging' electrodes facing the cochlear neural compartment. This is achieved by the intrinsic shape characteristics of the electrode, or by the addition of an electrode-positioning system (Figure 36.13). Lower stimulation thresholds and less across-patient variability have been reported.[101]

The CI can not only stimulate the nerve, but can also collect information about the functionality of the system by back telemetry. For instance, electrode impedances and CI characteristics can be analysed. Using the CI, the electrically evoked compound action potentials can be recorded from activated spiral ganglion cells stimulated by the same CI. A customized algorithm (Neural Response Telemetry, NRT) has been implemented in the CI24 for clinical and research use.[102,103] This allows for peroperative checking of the integrity of the implant, the intracochlear neural system and the correct functioning of the device. Experiments have demonstrated that the use of NRT will be helpful for the fitting procedures (G. F. Smoorenburg, personal communication).[104,105]

The fitting procedure itself commences about 4 weeks after cochlear implantation and is integrated into the auditory rehabilitation. Threshold levels (T-levels) and maximal comfortable levels (C-levels) are defined in several fitting sessions, and the pitch and loudness perception eventually adjusted.

Complications of CIs, including device failure, occur in 0.9–10% over a 10-year period. Especially for parents of small

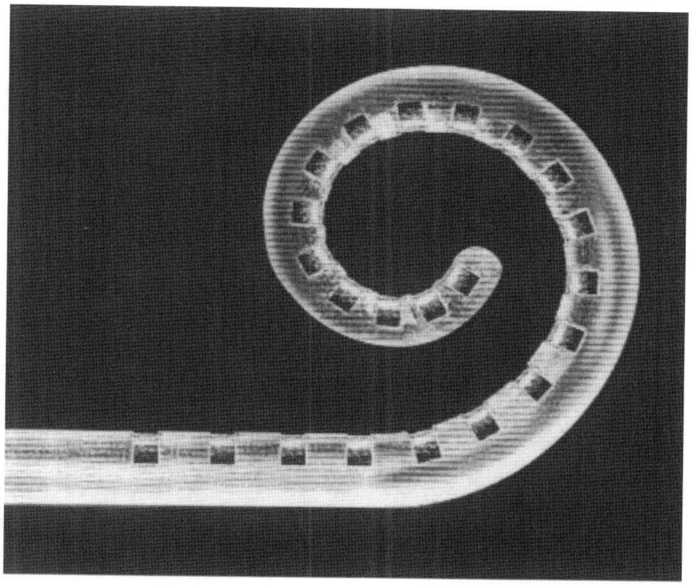

Figure 36.13 Radiological image of a perimodiolar Contour electrode array.

children, reimplantation is an emotionally loaded event, and has to be anticipated when discussing CIs.

Cochlear implant candidacy

The general condition for candidacy for cochlear implantation is the presence of bilateral severe-to-profound hearing impairment not obtaining sufficient benefit from optimal conventional hearing aids. There should also be no formal medical or (neuro)anatomopathological contraindications, evidence that oral communication will be used, and the presence of favourable mental and social conditions to participate in an active rehabilitation programme. These include realistic expectations. When considering CIs, an elaborate and comprehensive multidisciplinary evaluation is set up.

It is argued that non-aided auditory thresholds cannot represent the only auditory criterion. Aided speech recognition tests after following a rehabilitation programme have to be included.[106,107] As a general guideline for adults, the mean thresholds at 500, 1 and 2 kHz of the better-hearing ear should be worse than 85 dB HL, and maximal aided speech recognition for spondee lists should be 40% or less.

If the hearing is better than these criteria, the domain of experimental exploration of the limits of CI is entered and, occasionally, a conventional hearing aid might be better or at least as good.

In prelingual children, conventional hearing aids are nearly always fitted first and an intensive course of auditory training is initiated. If it becomes clear after at least 3 months that the child has no benefit, a CI can be considered. Specific tools to monitor the progress of sound production, auditory capabilities and communication development are instrumental for this assessment.[108–110]

The actual minimal age for cochlear implantation according to FDA regulations is 18 months. Many children younger that 18 months and even 12 months, however, have been implanted. As claimed by studies with hearing aids, it is expected that cochlear implantation in these very young children may produce a better result than later implantation. As results become available, it will be clear whether the warnings of some groups of educators are well founded.[111]

From a theoretical viewpoint, the hearing loss should be due primarily to outer and inner hair cell failure. Although a good neural reserve seems to predict better outcome, the link between ganglion population counts and speech intelligibility is weak. Moreover, the majority of severely to profoundly hearing-impaired patients still have enough neural reserve in order to benefit from cochlear implantation. Even in specific conditions, e.g. congenital malformations[112] or auditory neuropathy,[113] cochlear implantation provided substantial benefit. In the absence of any auditory nerve, such as in neurofibromatosis, direct electrical stimulation of the cochlear nuclei with auditory brainstem implants (ABIs) can result in improved communication.

An important element in candidacy is the evidence that the patient will comply with the fitting procedure, will use oral communication with the implant and, especially for children, will follow an intensive rehabilitation programme.

A number of conditions deserve special attention, and may influence the decision of the multidisciplinary implant team on whether or not to implant the patient.

The first one is severe to profound hearing impairment due to bacterial meningitis. A considerable risk exists of endocochlear bone formation (labyrinthitis ossificans). This condition is also characterized by a more extensive loss of ganglion cells. Once this process is observed on high-resolution CT scan, cochlear implantation is an emergency. In the case of a blocked scala vestibuli due to labyrinthitis ossificans, specific drill-outs to embed the electrode arrays and implants with split electrode carriers may overcome the problem.[68,114,115]

On average, the results will be significantly inferior than with cochlear implantation in normal patent cochleae.

The second situation is bilinguism at home and/or at school. At least a sufficient amount of auditory training and stimulation has to be provided in order to obtain benefit from cochlear implantation.[110] Some studies have shown better auditory skills with pure auditory–verbal training. On the other hand, mixed education, including the acquisition of sign language, has advantages from the total relational viewpoint, and studies have not shown inferior speech development.[116] This approach allows children to belong to both worlds, the hearing world and the deaf community. The third situation is the case of a second implant, creating a bilateral CI. Preliminary results show increased patient satisfaction and increased speech recognition in noise. It is not clear, and certainly not in all patients, whether this increased speech understanding is the result of head shadow effects, or whether there is a true dichotic or squelch effect. In conventional hearing aids, bilateral use has been shown to result in improved speech understanding in difficult listening conditions.

Results

The outcomes in prelingually deaf children and postlingually deaf adults are fundamentally different. Both situations have to be discussed separately.

Among postlingual adults, the majority of CI patients demonstrate clearly increased open-set speech recognition as early as 3 months post-fitting.[117,118] Further improvement in performance may extend over a time course of 3–4 years. Many series show mean open-set speech understanding for sentences of >80%, with ceiling effects occurring in the test material. For this reason, more difficult listening tests have been developed, in particular speech-in-noise. Preoperative prognostic factors predicting auditory capacity outcome are mainly duration of deafness and hearing level.[119] Old age is not a contraindication, but the potential for rehabilitation and relearning may be diminished. There are no studies showing whether intensive speech therapy improves the result in comparison with fitting sessions and aural communication.

Speech tests best predicting the CI speech recognition outcome are the monosyllable tests. In properly selected postlingual candidates, scores range from 10% to 70%, with a mean of 40–50%.[107,118]

Progress and evolution in congenital and prelingually implanted children are followed up by evaluating auditory function (speech reception),[109] and expressive capabilities (speech production). In comparison with conventional hearing aids, both aspects of speech improve significantly after cochlear implantation, as shown in many studies.[110,120]

If no other handicaps exist or develop, severely and profoundly hearing-impaired children implanted before the age of 2 years can follow mainstream education at the age of 5 years. The majority of children implanted before the age of 5 years with oral language as their sole means of communication will develop significant and usable open-set speech perception.[121] Implantation at a young age and oral communication were the most important determinants of later speech perception in one study.[110]

Regular testing for developmental retardation is mandatory, as in some series up to 50% of the severely or profoundly hearing-impaired children eventually develop a selective or more general developmental deficit. When children with congenital or prelingual profound hearing impairment are implanted at an older age, the results become less favourable. When prelingually profoundly hearing-impaired children have reached the age of 10 years, patients may exceptionally be allowed onto the CI programme after very extensive counselling. This does not apply to the congenitally hearing-impaired patients who have substantial benefit from conventional hearing aids but who suffered, at a later age, further deterioration of their hearing. They appear to have fairly good outcomes.

> Cochlear implantation bypasses the inner ear.
> Candidate selection is not merely based on non-aided auditory thresholds, but aided speech recognition tests in quiet and in noise after a rehabilitation period may be decisive.
> The vast majority of severely or profoundly hearing-impaired persons can benefit from cochlear implantation.
> Cochlear implantation restores hearing in 80% of postlingually deaf adults to a level allowing normal conversation, using the telephone and even understanding in a limited amount of background noise.
> Congenitally severely or profoundly hearing-impaired children implanted before the age of 2 years will outperform patients operated on at a later age.
> Cochlear implantation is not just a technique, but the driving force behind an elaborate care programme for the severely hearing-impaired patient.

Implantable electronic devices for sensorineural hearing loss

Description

Conventional hearing aids continue to have important limitations, even when vigorous patient selection and device adaptation is used. Many patients with sensorineural hearing loss (SNHL) paradoxically avoid the use of a hearing aid. Apart from psychological factors, distortion of the sounds amplified by the device is often cited as a major reason for this attitude. The presence of a hearing aid in the external ear canal is described as uncomfortable, cosmetically unacceptable and stigmatizing. Occlusion may cause external otitis or wax accumulation. Acoustical transmission of amplified sound has several limitations. Acoustical feedback phenomena occur at high frequencies and high intensities. A small receiver has large distortions at low frequencies. These problems degrade speech understanding and limit the gain that can be achieved with conventional hearing aids.

The design of a hearing aid that does not use acoustical transmission of sound and is preferably totally implantable would probably meet the needs of a large population of patients with SNHL.

Advantages over conventional hearing aids and principles of functioning

Implantable electronic devices transmit acoustical sound to the cochlea as a mechanical vibration, in most cases applied to the ossicular chain; they are therefore often referred to as 'direct drive' transducers. A piezoelectric element, electromagnetic force or even hydrostatic force can generate the mechanical vibration.

Obviously, these systems make occlusion of the external ear canal and the use of sound speakers unnecessary, and therefore appear user-friendlier and promise better quality of amplified hearing.

The coupling of the driving element of these devices to the ossicular chain is a critical issue.

Our knowledge of the micromechanics of the normal ossicular chain as a sound transducer is evidently incomplete. These notions nevertheless are equally or even more important than considerations of technical and surgical feasibility when a coupling system is designed. The mass load effect of a device, the direction of force transmission to the ossicular chain and the condition of the interface between implant and ossicle in the long term are issues still under evaluation today.[66]

Types of implants currently available for clinical implantation

Four types of implants are currently available for clinical use under FDA and/or CE approval.

The Vibrant Soundbridge (Symphonix Devices, San Jose, California, USA) is a semi-implantable device consisting of an electromagnetically driven transducer (also called 'floating mass transducer'), which is attached to the long process of the incus. The internal receiver of the device is implanted in a recessed seat in the temporal fossa, similar to a CI. A wire links the internal receiver to the floating mass transducer. A mastoidectomy with posterior tympanotomy is necessary for exposition of the long process of the incus, to which the floating mass transducer is attached. The audio processor is worn externally like the external coil of a CI, and is coupled to the internal receiver by telemetry (Figure 36.14).

The Totally Implantable Communication Assistance device (TICA, Implex AG, Munchen, Germany) picks up sounds transcutaneously in the external ear canal and transforms them into microvibrations that are delivered to the ossicular chain. The microphone is a membrane sensor implanted in the posterior bony external ear canal, underlying the canal skin. The transducer is a piezoelectric element, which allows minimal power consumption, and is implanted in a mastoidectomy cavity. The processor module and battery are implanted subcutaneously in the postauricular skin. It is plug-connected to the transducer and microphone and can be replaced separately. The battery lifetime is 3–5 years and expected to become longer with technical progress. The battery is an accumulator cell that has to be transcutaneously recharged by induction. The transducer has a titanium rod that can be coupled to the long incus process with a clip or directly to the body of the incus. Coupling to a piston prosthesis, the stapes head or perilymph directly is under development. A titanium micromanipulator is integrated into the transducer, and allows safe manipulation and application of the titanium rod to the ossicular chain (Figure 36.15).

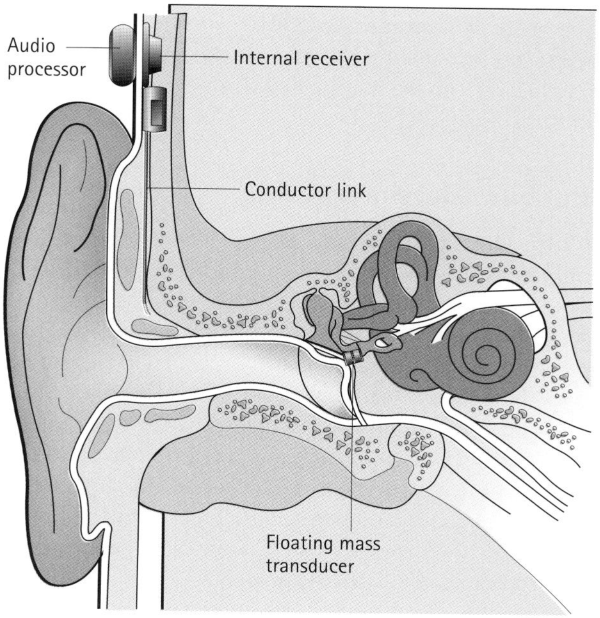

Figure 36.14 The Vibrant Soundbridge system.

The Otologics Middle Ear Transducer (MET, Otologics, Boulder, Colorado, USA) consists of an external audio processor which is worn on the skin overlying the temporal fossa, and an internal receiver–transducer that drives an aluminium oxide probe that is coupled to the incus body. The electromagnetic transducer is mounted into a atticomastoidectomy cavity. A hole is made in the body of the incus with a laser, and a micrometer screw is used to position the probe in this hole. The receiver capsule with electronics is embedded in a temporal fossa seat, much like is done in cochlear implant surgery (Figure 36.16).

The Soundtec Direct Hearing System (Soundtec Inc., Oklahoma City, Oklahoma, USA) consists of an external and an internal portion. The external part carries a microphone and a sound processor connected to an electromagnetic coil; it can be worn in the ear canal or behind the ear with a custom ear canal mould in which

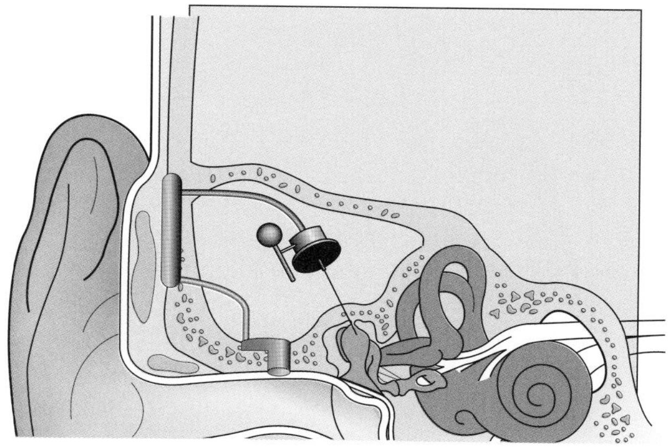

Figure 36.15 The TICA system.

the coil is incorporated. The internal part is a magnet that is attached to the incudostapedial joint (Figure 36.17). It can be implanted through a transmeatal tympanotomy.

Patient selection criteria

Only adult patients are selected for Vibrant Soundbridge implantation today. There should be an SNHL loss, which is not of retrocochlear origin. Middle ear anatomy must be normal, and there should be no air–bone gap greater than 10 dB at two or more frequencies at 0.5, 1, 2 and 4 kHz. The hearing loss must be stable in time. The use of a conventional hearing aid must be contraindicated for medical reasons or rejected by the patient after optimal fitting and a reasonable period of use. The pure tone unaided hearing levels of the fitted ear must lie within the boundaries given in Figure 36.18. Speech understanding should be at least 50% in open-set word tests at the most comfortable listening level.

For the TICA device, selection criteria include the lack of benefit from conventional hearing aids, a normal volume of the mastoid as evaluated with Schuller's radiograph, and SNHL levels within the boundaries shown in Figure 36.19.

Speech intelligibility test scores are not included in the criteria. Although only patients with pure SNHL have been implanted until today, coexistent conductive hearing loss will probably not remain an exclusion criterion, since the company is developing coupling devices to stapes head, piston prosthesis or perilymph.

The selection criteria for the MET implant include adult patients with SNHL, no signs of conductive or retrocochlear hearing loss, and no history of recurrent otitis media. The hearing loss must be stable, of postlingual onset and lie within the limits given in Figure 36.20.

Patients should have realistic expectations of their device's benefit.

The Soundtec aims at patients of 18 years or older, with normal middle ear anatomy and function (bone thresholds within 10 dB of air thresholds), who have an SNHL within the limits of what is defined in Figure 36.21. The SNHL should be stable over the last 2 years, and there is also a speech discrimination score criterion.

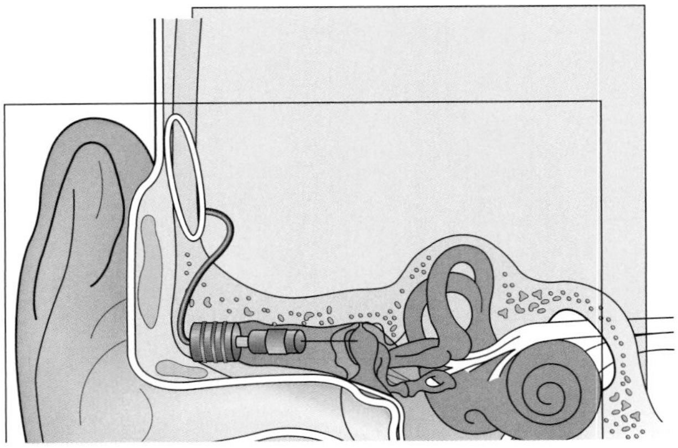

Figure 36.16 The MET system.

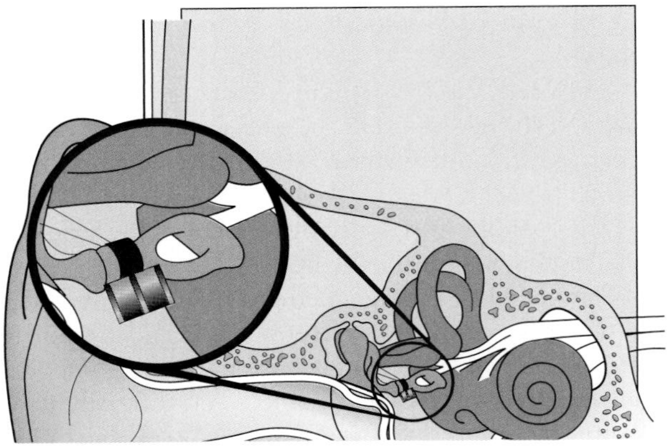

Figure 36.17 The Soundtec Direct Hearing system.

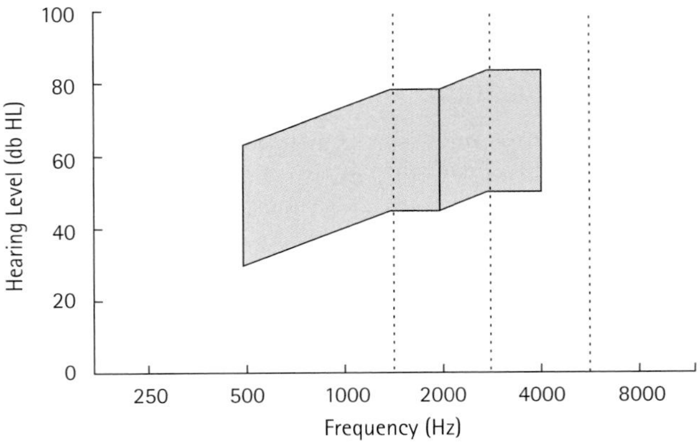

Figure 36.18 Audiological selection criteria for Vibrant Soundbridge.

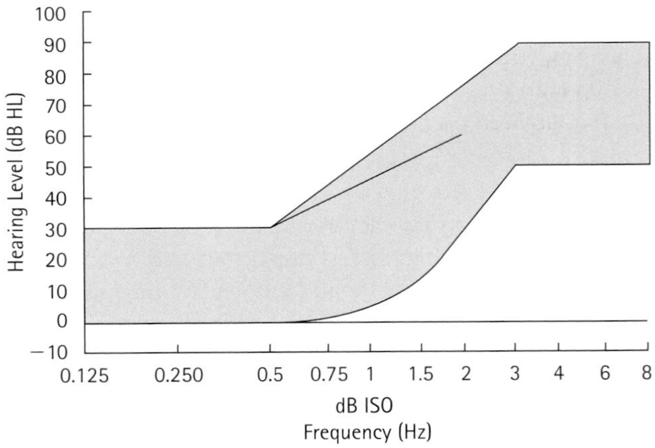

Figure 36.19 Audiological criteria for TICA: a maximum hearing loss of 30 dB at 0.5 kHz and 90 dB at 3 kHz and higher, with a slope of 30 dB or more between 0.5 and 2 kHz.

Results

There are several reports by different European centres on results after implantation of the Vibrant Soundbridge system.[71,122–124] All of these reports concern rather small series of patients, the largest being a series of 34.[124] A multicentre audiometric results report (on a total number of 63 patients) has been published.[125] In this report, an overall conclusion states that most of the patients clearly benefited from the Vibrant Soundbridge, with, however, a subgroup of patients experiencing a low gain (at threshold or at conversational sound level) that could not be explained by their preoperative degree of hearing impairment. Speech recognition scores after implantation are comparable to results obtained with conventional hearing aids, with, however, a large spread of results. Unsatisfactory results in some of the patients are attributed to problems with positioning and fixation of the floating mass transducer, as well as to suboptimal programming of the audio processor. With regard to the subjective evaluation of sound quality after implantation, patients report undistorted hearing resulting in a better speech understanding even in situations with loud background noise.[124]

Since the TICA device has only been implanted clinically in one centre until now,[126] reports are only available from that centre. The most recent summary of their results on 20 implanted patients mentions a statistically significant increase of monosyllabic word recognition score as well as in sentence recognition in quiet and in the presence of noise, when the system is compared with the unaided preoperative status.[127]

The MET implant system has only recently entered the phase of multicentre clinical study. The phase I FDA clinical trial results indicate good tolerance of the implant with superior sound quality, but a need for higher amplification. The output of the implant now in phase II study has therefore been increased.[16]

There are three studies available, performed by two different centres, which report on the results of clinical implantation of the Soundtec system.[70,128,129] Results of, respectively, 10, 5 and 23 implanted subjects suggest a considerable gain over traditional hearing aids, especially in the high-frequency range. The subjective evaluation of the acoustical performance of the device was clearly in favour of the device.

In none of the clinical studies were local or general adverse effects or significant hearing loss caused by the implantation reported. There is long-term experience of at least 10 years in a large series of Japanese patients with an investigative piezoelectric device. Deterioration of bone conduction caused by use of the device was not noted in any of the patients.[130]

Conclusion

After a long period of experimental studies and research, the implantable electronic hearing devices for SNHL are now on the verge of broad clinical application. The first clinical results are very promising, and the currently used devices are safe and functional. They will probably become a good alternative for those patients who are dissatisfied with their conventional hearing aid. It is also clear that some changes in the technical aspects of implantation—especially in the design of the ideal coupling between transducer and ossicular chain—are needed before these hearing aids will become widely accepted.

> Implantable electronic devices for sensorineural hearing loss have a number of theoretical advantages that make them a valuable solution for patients who do not tolerate a conventional hearing aid. The technical progress made over the last 30 years has made these devices possible today. The early clinical experience seems to support the predicted advantages. Some issues—specifically on the coupling of the device to the human auditory system—are still open to improvement.

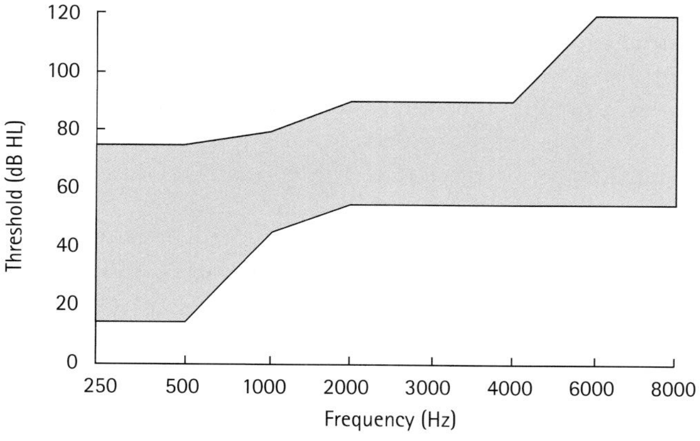

Figure 36.20 Audiological criteria for MET.

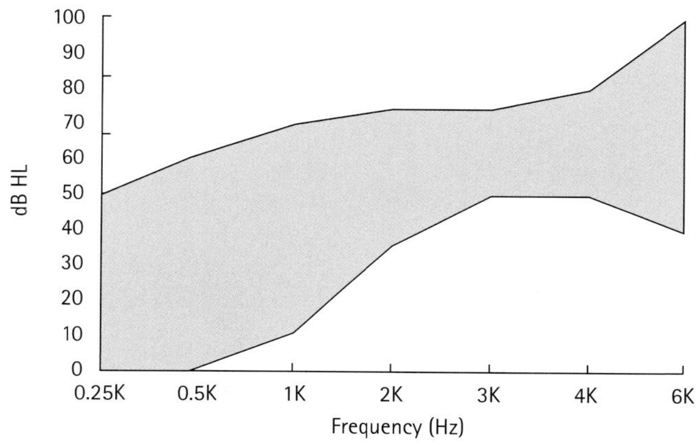

Figure 36.21 Audiological criteria for Soundtec.

Otoneurosurgical treatment of tinnitus

Introduction

Tinnitus is a distressing symptom affecting 15% of the population. It leads to depression or insomnia in half of the patients and causes an important decrease in the quality of life in 20% of tinnitus sufferers.[131]

Tinnitus can be subdivided into two completely different entities, pulsatile and non-pulsatile tinnitus. Pulsatile tinnitus is the result of a normally functioning auditory system in which vascular anomalies create a resonance effect in the petrous bone, and can be subdivided into an arterial pulse-synchronized tinnitus and a venous hum. The venous hum originates either from primary venous disease or from conditions producing increased intracranial pressure.[132] Non-pulsatile tinnitus, on the contrary, is caused by an abnormally functioning auditory system and can be considered an auditory phantom phenomenon,[133–136] similar to phantom pain. It is caused by a reorganization of the auditory tract and auditory cortex and it probably develops in two phases. An initial reversible phase tends to turn into an irreversible tinnitus after 2–3 years.[137,138] This might warrant surgical treatment of non-pulsatile tinnitus to be considered as relatively urgent.[137,139]

Surgical treatment of pulsatile tinnitus

Almost all causes of pulsatile tinnitus can be diagnosed by MRI and magnetic resonance angiography, except for the most frequent cause of pulsatile tinnitus, benign intracranial hypertension.

Table 36.4 Surgically treatable causes of tinnitus.

Pulsatile tinnitus	Non-pulsatile tinnitus
Venous	Vestibular schwannoma (acoustical neuroma)
Benign intracranial hypertension	Other cerebellopontine angle lesions
Chiari malformation	Arachnoid cyst
High jugular bulb	Menière's disease
	Otosclerosis
Arterial	Brain tumour
Carotid stenosis	Chiari malformation
Glomus tumour	Microvascular compression
Vascular lesions of petrous bone/skull base	
Arteriovenous malformation	
Aneurysm	
Microvascular compression	

Venous hum

Benign intracranial hypertension is a clinical entity usually affecting obese women who suffer from a venous hum, headache and blurry vision. Importantly, the venous hum, even unilaterally, can be the only presenting symptom.[132] Clinically, it can be diagnosed by compressing the ipsilateral jugular vein, causing the venous hum to disappear. Except for the rarely diagnosed condition of sinus thrombosis,[140] magnetic resonance angiography and MRI are usually negative, and the diagnosis is confirmed by lumbar puncture (pressure >20 cm water). Treatment consists of weight loss, diuretics or ventriculoperitoneal or lumboperitoneal shunting.

The Chiari malformation is a clinical entity in which there is a tonsillar herniation into the foramen magnum (Figure 36.22). Of these patients, 7–10%[141] suffer from tinnitus, and it can be both non-pulsatile and pulsatile.[142] The pulsatile tinnitus consists of a venous hum caused by raised intracranial pressure and worsens on bending over, but disappears on ipsilateral jugular vein compression, which also results in an improvement of the hearing (masking). No brainstem auditory evoked potential changes are noted in this kind of tinnitus. After the surgical decompression, this form of tinnitus disappears.[142]

Non-pulsatile tinnitus, on the other hand, is usually intermittent and the cause is not known. It is due either to stretching of the cochlear nerve, e.g. by microvascular compression, or to brainstem traction.[143] Brainstem auditory evoked potential changes are noted in 75% of the patients, and consist of an IPL III–V prolongation in 100% of the patients (brainstem traction and/or contralateral microvascular compression?) and of IPL I-III prolongation in 30%[143] (ipsilateral microvascular compression?). Posterior fossa decompression, which consists of opening the foramen magnum and widening the dura mater, results in abolishing the non-pulsatile tinnitus if tinnitus is of recent origin.

The high jugular bulb can generate a venous hum, as a result of intimate direct contact with the cochlea. This venous hum disappears on compressing the ipsilateral jugular vein and can be diagnosed by CT imaging. Surgically ligating or lowering the jugular bulb and interposing Teflon or bonewax can abolish or diminish this form of tinnitus.[144,145]

Arterial pulse-synchronous tinnitus

Carotid stenosis is the most frequent cause of arterial pulsatile tinnitus. The pulsatile tinnitus disappears on compressing the ipsilateral, internal carotid artery. Diagnosis can be confirmed by angiography. Treatment of the extracranial carotid artery stenosis consists of dilatation and stenting or carotid endarterectomy. As for the rarer intracranial carotid artery stenosis (Figure 36.23a) two approaches can be followed. An initial balloon occlusion test under transcranial doppler and EEG monitoring can verify whether the ipsilateral carotid artery can be sacrificed. If so, one option is to ligate the symptomatic carotid artery. The other option is to dilate and stent (Figure 36.23b) the intracranial portion of the carotid artery, resulting in a disappearance of the arterial pulsatile tinnitus.[146]

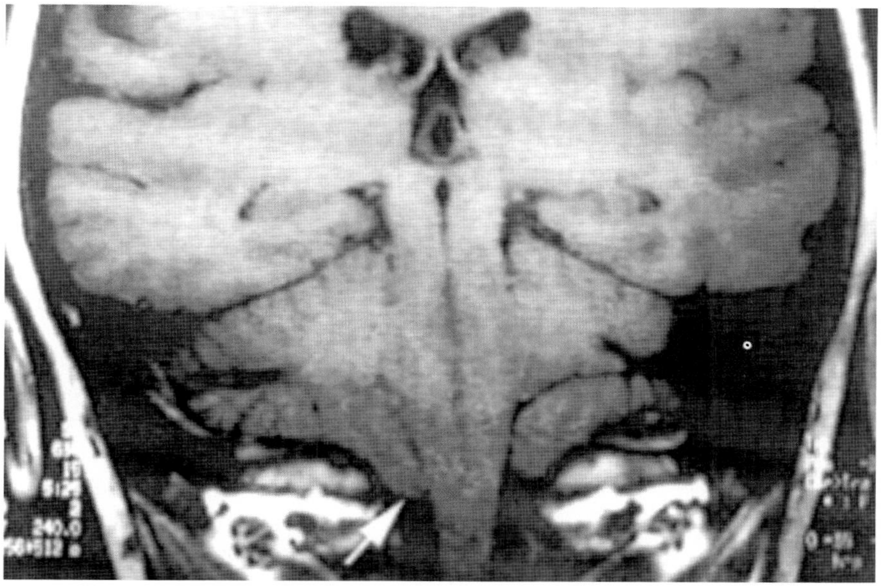

Figure 36.22 Tonsilar herniation (white arrow) leading to ipsilateral venous hum or non-pulsatile tinnitus. Arnold-Chiari malformation. This very discrete unilateral herniation resulted in ipsilateral non-pulsatile tinnitus, disappearing after surgery.

A major problem still faced today is that stents tend to occlude, and thus this elegant technique still remains experimental until the coagulation problems are better controlled.[146]

Glomus tumours, or paraganglioma, are found in women presenting with unilateral hearing loss and pulsatile tinnitus. As they are benign lesions growing to less than 2 cm in 5 years, treatment options are a 'wait and see' policy or embolization and surgery.[147]

Other vascular lesions of the petrous bone or skull base, such as haemangiopericytoma,[148] plasmacytoma[148] and giant cell tumours,[149] among others, are also known to generate a treatable pulsatile tinnitus.

Dural arteriovenous malformations (AVM) result from chronic mastoiditis or other causes leading to occlusion of the sigmoid transverse sinus. Vascular bypasses develop around the occlusion, resulting in a dural AVM (Figure 36.24a). If the dural AVM is symptomatic or if it is asymptomatic with leptomeningeal drainage, these lesions should be embolized (Figure 36.24b), usually in multiple sessions. If intractable with endovascular treatment, surgical excision of the AVM and dura can be proposed.[150]

Microvascular compressions of the cochlear nerve can cause incapacitating low-pitch pulsatile or high-pitch non-pulsatile tinnitus.[139] This difficult diagnosis is based on the clinical picture and confirmed by auditory brainstem evoked potentials and MRI (Figure 36.25).[137,139,151,152] Results of microsurgical vascular decompression are related to the surgical delay, the preoperative hearing status, MRI imaging and gender. In general, we can state that if the tinnitus has been present for less than 3 years,[137] if there is serviceable or normal hearing,[139] and if the MRI demonstrates vascular compression[139,151,152] in women[137]—the results can be good. Vascular compressions of the vestibulocochlear nerve are found in many asymptomatic patients[153,154] (21.5% and 12.5% respectively), but this discrepancy is also found in trigeminal neuralgia (14%),[155] and even in herniated lumbar disks (36%),[156] where this is not considered an argument against the pathophysiological importance of the neural compression in generating symptoms.

Non-pulsatile tinnitus

Any lesion along the auditory tract altering its normal function can cause non-pulsatile tinnitus. Menière's disease, vestibular schwannoma, cerebellopontine angle lesions, arachnoid cysts, microvascular compressions, Chiari malformation and brain tumours are causes of non-pulsatile tinnitus that can be treated surgically.

In vestibular schwannoma, the high-pitch tinnitus (ringing or steam from a kettle) is present in 60–85% of patients. Recently, vestibular schwannomas have often been treated by radiosurgery. This seems to have almost no effect on the tinnitus,[157] whereas with microscopic surgery 40–50% of the tinnitus disappears.[158] Unfortunately, microsurgery also creates tinnitus in many patients.[159]

Other cerebellopontine angle lesions (CPAs),[160] such as meningiomas, epidermoid tumours, lipomas, choroid plexus papillomas, epithelial cysts, teratomas, cavernomas, and haemangiomas, can present with non-pulsatile tinnitus, usually with associated symptoms, depending on the location of the lesion and the degree of brainstem, cerebellar or cranial nerve compression.

Arachnoid cyst is a rare cause of non-pulsatile tinnitus (Figure 36.26). It is a congenital or post-traumatic/postinflammatory disorder[161–164] leading to vague symptoms. Arachnoid cysts producing tinnitus can occur in the cerebellopontine angle, but can also be retroclival and retrocerebellar. Usually,

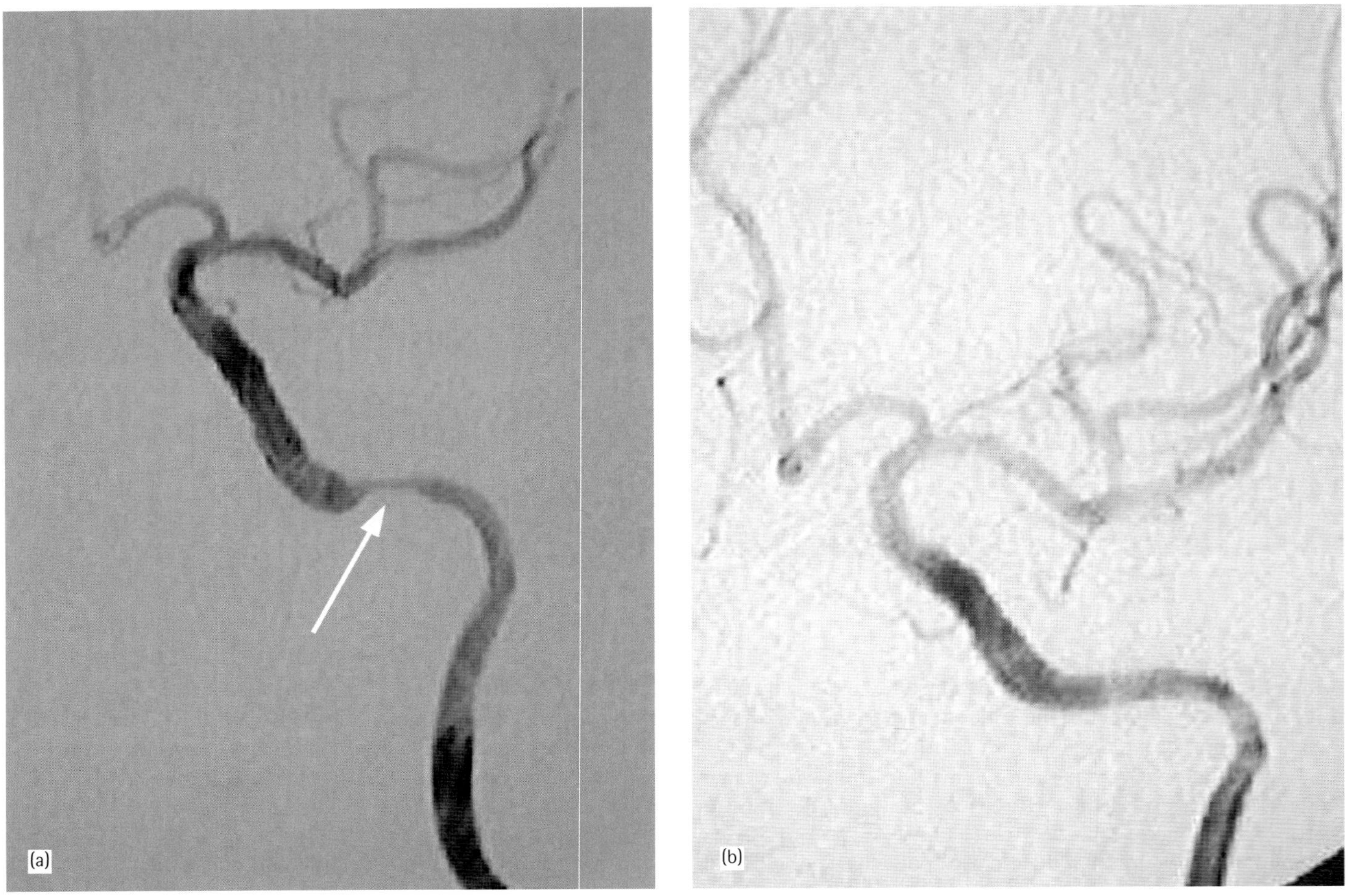

Figure 36.23 (a) Intracranial petrous carotid artery stenosis (arrow) causing arterial pulsatile tinnitus; (b) postdilation and stenting of petrous carotid artery stenosis resulting in abolishing pulsatile tinnitus.

symptoms of intracranial hypertension are associated with non-pulsatile tinnitus.[65,165] Surgical treatment consists of marsupialization or excision of the cyst.[65,165]

In Menière's disease no kind of surgery, whether vestibular nerve section, cochlear nerve section, endolymphatic sac surgery[131] or gentamicin injections,[166] seems to produce greater than 50% tinnitus control—a marginal improvement upon the 30% spontaneous disappearance in its natural history.[167]

In otosclerosis, relief of the non-pulsatile tinnitus by successful stapedectomy can be expected in about 40–64% of cases.[168,169]

A brain tumour compressing the auditory cortex (Figure 36.27) can cause a low-pitch (cortical tonotopy), non-pulsatile tinnitus as the sole symptom, probably due to a direct influence on normal cortical sound processing. Removal of the lesion results in abolishing the tinnitus.[170] Tumours elsewhere along the auditory tract, e.g. the brainstem, usually give rise to additional symptoms related to the closeness of other neural structures.

For intractable non-pulsatile tinnitus, auditory brainstem implants[171] and auditory cortex stimulations can be expected to give some relief in intractable non-pulsatile tinnitus, in a similar manner to dorsal column stimulation and motor cortex stimulation, used for intractable phantom pain. The advantage of both approaches in comparison to electrical stimulation via CI is that both techniques could be used to preserve hearing.

Conclusion

Tinnitus actually consists of two entirely different entities with different pathophysiologies, different clinical symptoms and different treatment. For pulsatile tinnitus, whether of arterial or venous origin, a cause can usually be found, and thus surgical treatment can be proposed.

However, the cause of non-pulsatile tinnitus, especially in unilateral non-pulsatile tinnitus, producing abnormal function

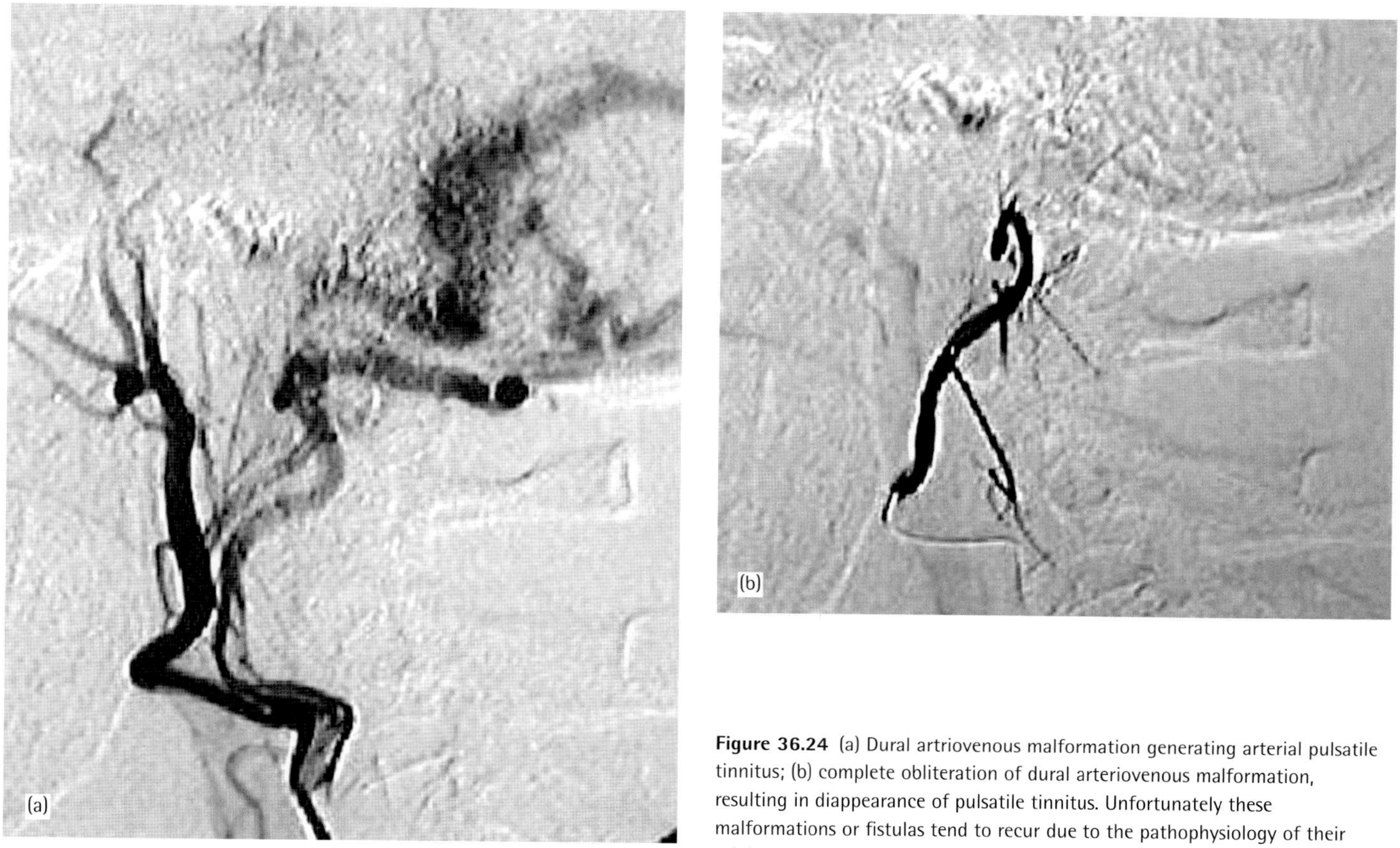

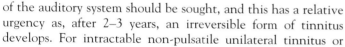

Figure 36.24 (a) Dural artriovenous malformation generating arterial pulsatile tinnitus; (b) complete obliteration of dural arteriovenous malformation, resulting in diappearance of pulsatile tinnitus. Unfortunately these malformations or fistulas tend to recur due to the pathophysiology of their origin.

of the auditory system should be sought, and this has a relative urgency as, after 2–3 years, an irreversible form of tinnitus develops. For intractable non-pulsatile unilateral tinnitus or bilateral tinnitus future developments consisting of auditory brainstem implants and auditory cortex stimulation might provide help and benefit.

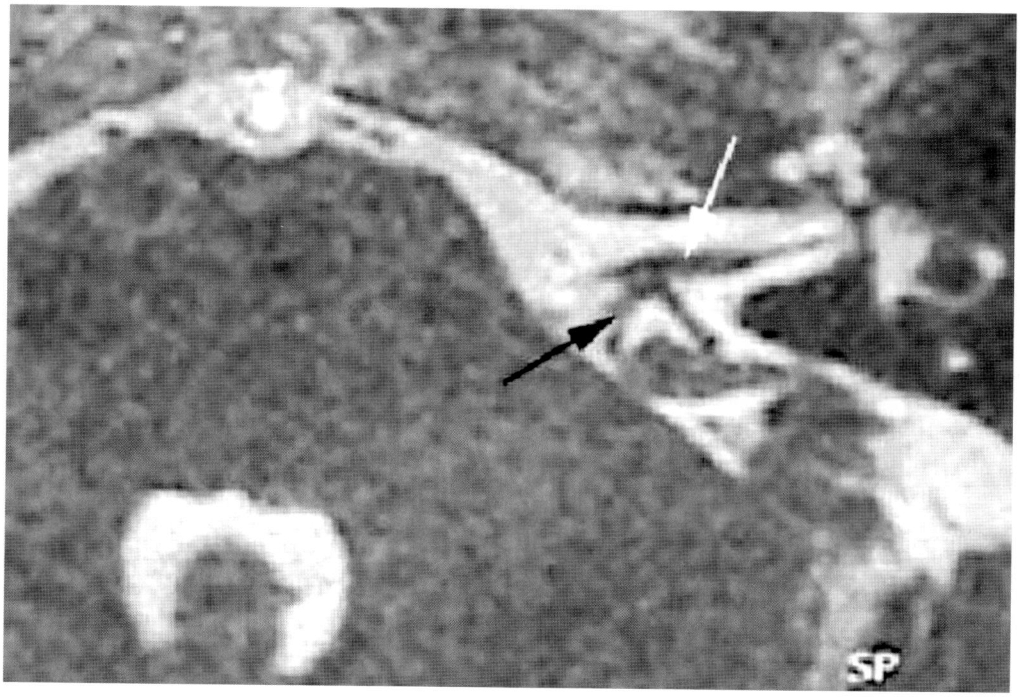

Figure 36.25 Microvascular (black arrow) compression of vestibulocochlear nerve (white arrow) generating high non-pulsatile or low pitch pulsatile tinnitus

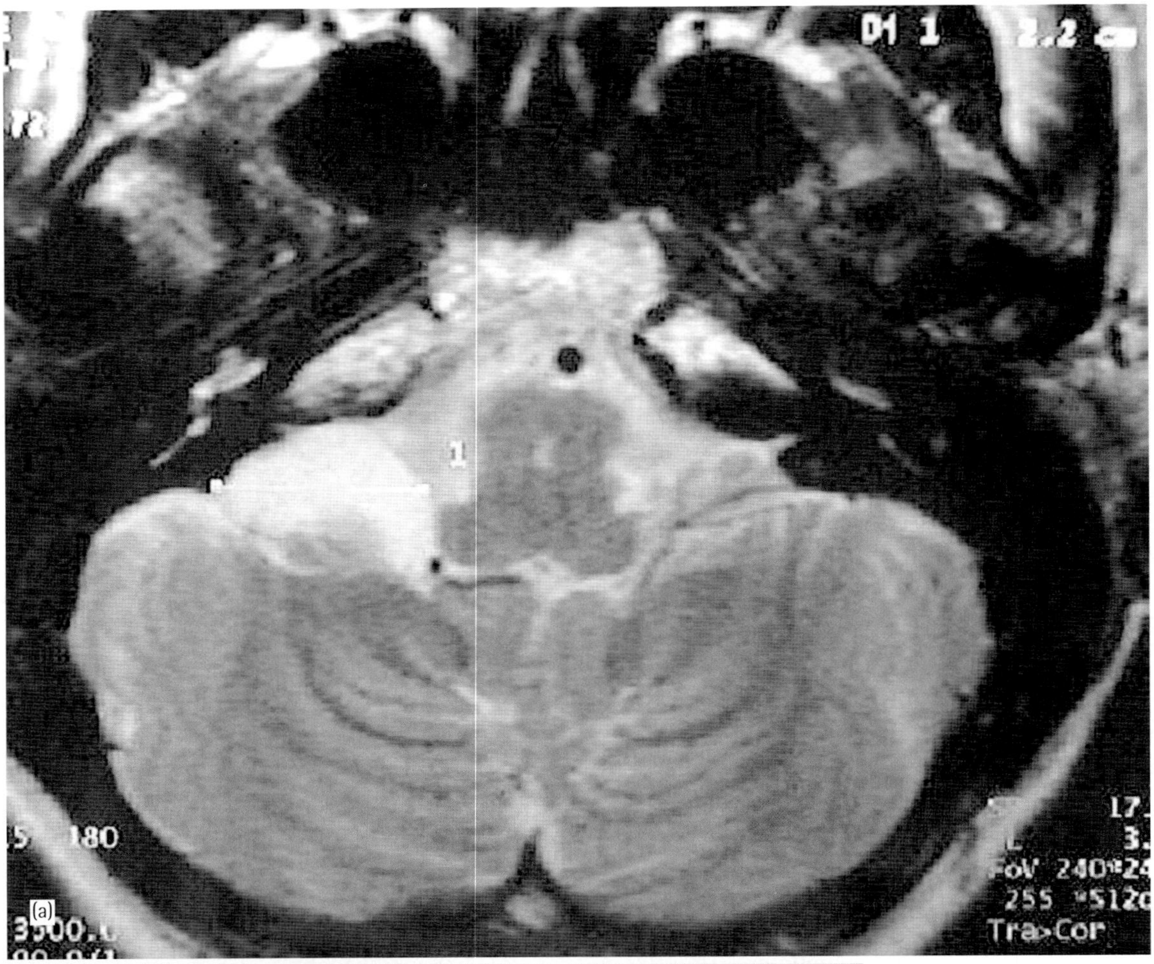

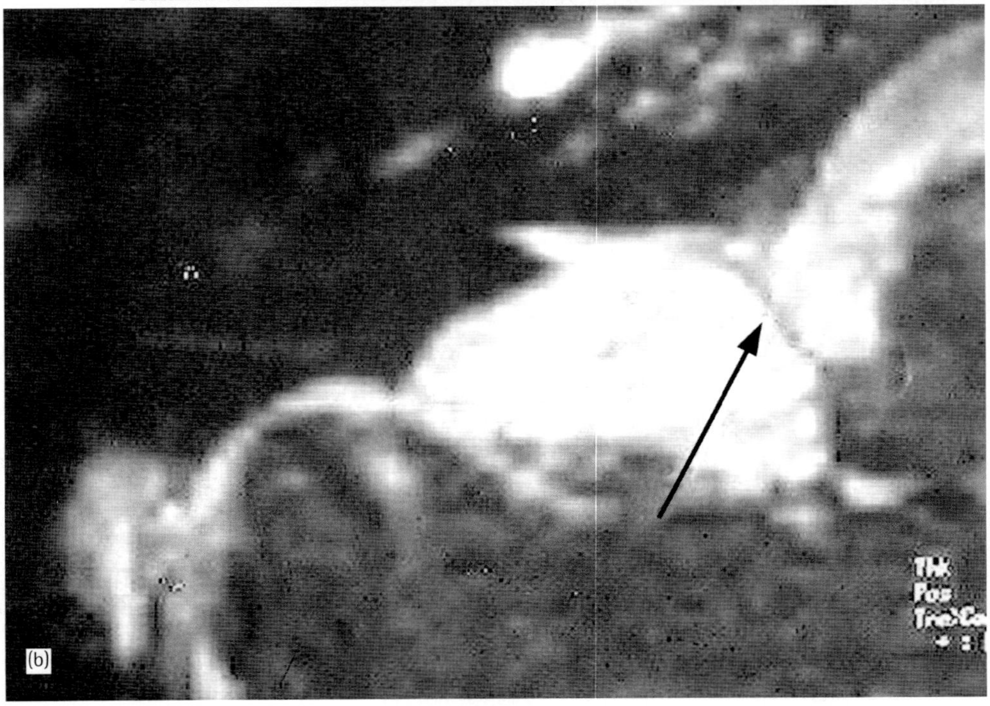

Figure 36.26 (a) Arachnoid cyst at cerebellopontine angle causing non-pulsatile tinnitus; (b) detail of arachnoid cyst stretching the vestibulocochlear nerve (black arrow)

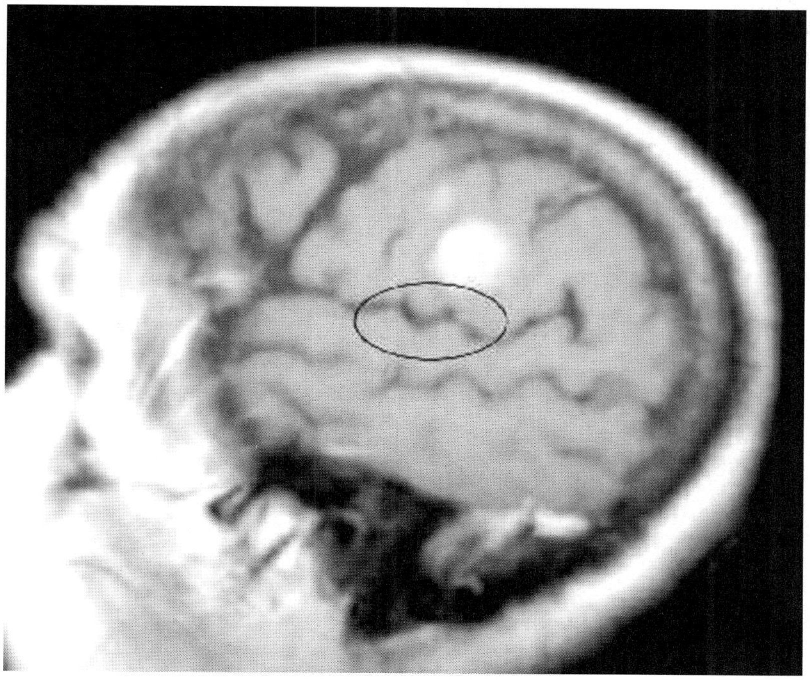

Figure 36.27 Meningioma of auditory cortex area (ovoid) causing low pitch (tonotopy) non-pulsatile tinnitus that disappeared after surgical removal

Highlights
Tinnitus = pulsatile or non-pulsatile tinnitus
Pulsatile tinnitus = normal function of auditory system, resonance effect in petrous bone
Pulsatile tinnitus = arterial pulse-synchronous or venous hum
Venous hum = venous disease or raised intracranial pressure
Non-pulsatile tinnitus = pathological auditory system = auditory phantom phenomenon
Pulsatile tinnitus can be cured
Non-pulsatile tinnitus is to be treated relatively urgently

Final remarks

Functional ear surgery has an important place in the treatment of hearing impairment. When considering surgery, not only the otological criteria have to be taken into account, but also general aspects and contraindications regarding operability, pregnancy, drug abuse, mental and emotional status and a correct understanding by the patient of the intervention. Realistic expectations are a cornerstone of patient satisfaction with respect to the offered health intervention. For this reason, assessment must include not only the hearing capability itself, but also the impact on the quality of life of the patient.

The option of the use of a combination of methods, i.e. surgery and hearing aids, has to be considered. In cases of advanced mixed hearing loss, neither surgery nor a hearing aid can provide enough improvement to provide a socially serviceable hearing level. However, surgery can reduce conductive hearing loss to a level within reach of conventional hearing aids. A specific situation consists of open cavities in which the posterior bony ear canal is rebuilt to render a more favourable acoustical situation for hearing aids. A second situation is that of a mixed hearing loss, in which the sensorineural component is more than 70 dB, such that the precise bone conduction hearing level cannot be determined. Stapedectomy in advanced otosclerosis creates a situation in which conventional hearing aids yield good speech understanding and cochlear implantation can be avoided.

An emerging field is the implantation of drug delivery systems (e.g. round window microcatheter or Otowick) to the inner ear to treat sensorineural hearing loss. These systems are currently being evaluated in the treatment of vertigo. It is to be expected that trials with corticosteroids, and also with neurotransmitters and neurotrophic factors, will find an indication in the treatment of hearing impairment and tinnitus.

Acknowledgements

The authors especially thank Professor Linda Luxon for her important support, and Miss S. Beckers and the late D. De Saegher for their technical assistance.

References

1. Ramsay H, Karkkainen J, Palva T. Success in surgery for otosclerosis: hearing improvement and other indicators. *Am J Otolaryngol* 1997; **18**: 23–8.

2. Sperling NM, Patel N. A patient-benefit evaluation of unilateral congenital conductive hearing loss presenting in adulthood: should it be repaired? *Laryngoscope* 1999; **109**: 1386–91.
3. Stewart MG, Coker NJ, Jenkins HA et al. Outcomes and quality of life in conductive hearing loss. *OtolaryngolHeadNeckSurg* 2000; **123**: 527–32.
4. Monsell EM, Balkany TA, Gates GA. Committee on Hearing and Equilibrium guidelines for the evaluation of results of treatment of conductive hearing loss. *Otolaryngol Head Neck Surg* 1995; **113**: 186–7.
5. De Bruijn AJG, Tange RA, Dreschler WA. Efficacy of evaluation of audiometric results after stapes surgery in otosclerosis. II. A method for reporting results from individual cases. *Otolaryngol-HeadNeckSurg* 2001; **124**: 84–9.
6. Shea JJ. Stapedectomy technique and results. *Am J Otol* 1985; **6**: 61–2.
7. Shea JJ. Thirty years of stapes surgery. *J Laryngol Otol* 1988; **102**: 14–19.
8. Somers T, Govaerts P, Marquet T et al. Statistical analysis of otosclerosis surgery performed by Jean Marquet. *Ann Otol Rhinol Laryngol* 1994; 945–51.
9. Berliner KI, Doyle KJ, Goldenberg RA. Reporting operative hearing results in stapes surgery: does choice of outcome measure make a difference? *Am J Otolaryngol* 2001; **17**: 521–8.
10. De Bruijn AJG, Tange RA, Dreschler WA. Efficacy of evaluation of audiometric results after stapes surgery in otosclerosis. I. The effects of using different audiological parameters and criteria on success rates. *OtolaryngolHeadNeckSurg* 2001; **124**: 76–83.
11. Duijvestijn JA, Anteunis LJC, Hendriks JJ et al. Definition of hearing impairment and its effect on prevalence figures: a survey among senior citizens. *Acta Otolaryngol (Stockh)* 1999; **119**: 420–3.
12. Carhart R. Effects of stapes fixation on bone conduction responses. In: Schuknecht H, ed. *International Symposium on Otosclerosis*. Boston: Little-Brown, 1962: 175.
13. Lundman L, Mendel L, Bagger-Sjoback D et al. Hearing in patients operated unilaterally for otosclerosis: self assessment of hearing and audiometric results. *Acta Otolaryngol (Stockh)* 1999; **119**: 453–8.
14. Ware JE, Snow KK, Kosinski M et al. *SF-36 Health Survey. Manual and Interpretation Guide*. Boston: Nimrod Press, 1993.
15. Newman CW, Weinstein BE, Jacobson GP et al. The hearing handicap inventory for adults: psychometric adequacy and audiometric correlates. *Ear Hear* 1990; **11**: 430–3.
16. Kapteyn TS, Kramer SE. Validiteitsbeoordeling op grond van vragenlijst en testbatterij. In: Dreschler WA, ed. *Validiteit van het gehoor*. 1999: 91–123.
17. Smythe GDL, Patterson CC. Results of middle ear reconstruction. Do patients and surgeons agree? *Am J Otol* 1985; **6**: 276–9.
18. Browning GG, Gatehouse S, Swan IRC. The Glasgow benefit plot: a new method for reporting benefits from middle ear surgery. *Laryngoscope* 1991; **101**: 180–5.
19. Porter MJ, Zeitoun H, Brookes GB. The Glasgow benefit plot used to assess the effect of bilateral stapedectomy. *Clin Otolaryngol* 1995; 20: 68–71.
20. Bulman CH. Audit of stapedectomy in the north west of England for 1996: an analysis of the criteria used to describe success. *Clin Otolaryngol* 2000; **25**: 542–6.
21. Hinderink JB, Krabbe PF, Van den Broek P. Development and application of a health-related quality-of-life instrument for adults with cochlear implants: the Nijmegen cochlear implant questionnaire. *Otolaryngol Head Neck Surg* 2000; **123**: 756–65.
22. Stewart MG, Jenkins HA, Coker NJ et al. Development of new outcomes instrument for conductive hearing loss. *Am J Otol* 1997; **18**: 413–20.
23. Eriksson-Mangold M, Erlandsson SI, Jansson G. The subjective meaning of illness in severe otosclerosis: a descriptive study in three steps based on focus group interviews and written questionnaire. *Scand Audiol* 1996; **43**(S): 34–44.
24. Robinson K. Evidence-based medicine and its implications for audiological science. *Br J Audiol* 1999; **33**: 9–16.
25. Cox R, Alexander GC. The abbreviated profile of hearing aid benefit. *Ear Hear* 1995; **16**: 176–86.
26. Chiossoine-Kerdel JA, Baguley D, Stoddart RL, Moffat DA. An investigation of the audiologic handicap associated with unilateral sudden sensorineural hearing loss. *Am J Otol* 2000; **21**: 645–51.
27. Kramer SE, Kapteyn TS, Festen JM et al. Factors in subjective hearing disability. *Audiology* 1995; **34**: 311–20.
28. Kramer SE, Kapteyn TS, Festen JM et al. The relationship between self-reported hearing disability and measures of auditory disability. *Audiology* 1996; **35**: 277–87.
29. Kramer SE, Kapteyn TS, Festen JM et al. Assessing aspects of hearing handicap by means of pupil dilatation. *Audiology* 1997; **36**: 155–64.
30. Kramer SE, Kapteyn TS, Festen JM. The self-reported handicapping effect of hearing disabilities. *Audiology* 1998; **37**: 301–12.
31. Dillon H, James A, Ginis J. Client Oriented Scale of Improvement (COSI) and its relationship to several other measures of benefit and satisfaction provided by hearing aids. *J Am Acad Audiol* 1997; **8**: 27–43.
32. Brokx J, Pepers A. Betekenis van digitale hoortoestellen voor mensen met gecombineerde auditieve en visuele problemen. Unpublished report, Instituut voor Doven, The Netherlands 1999.
33. Teunissen E, Cremers CW. Classification of congenital middle ear anomalies. Report on 144 ears. *Ann Otol Rhinol Laryngol* 1993; **102**: 606–12.
34. Altmann F. Congenital aural atresia of the ear in man and animals. *Ann Otol Rhinol Laryngol* 1955; **64**: 824–58.
35. Marquet J. Allografts and congenital aural atresia. *Adv Otorhinolaryngol* 1988; **40**: 15–23.
36. Declau F, Offeciers F, Van de Heyning P. Classification of the non-syndromal type of meatal atresia. In: Devranoglu I, ed. In: *Proceedings of the XVth World Congress of ORL and Head and Neck Surgery: panel discussions*. 1997: 135–7.
37. Cremers CW, Oudenhoven J, Marres EH. Congenital aural atresia. A new subclassification and surgical management. *Clin Otolaryngol* 1984; **9**: 119–27.
38. Jahrsdoerfer RA, Yeakley JW, Aguilar EA et al. Grading system for the selection of patients with congenital aural atresia. *Am J Otol* 1992; **13**: 6–12.

39. Declau F, Cremers C, Van de Heyning P. Diagnosis and management strategies in congenital atresia of the external ear canal. *Br J Audiol* 1999; **33**: 313–27.
40. Håkansson B, Liden G, Tjellström A et al. Ten years of experience with the Swedish bone-anchored hearing system. *Ann Otol Rhinol Laryngol* 1990; **99** (suppl 151): 1–16.
41. Powell RH, Burrell SP, Cooper HR et al. The Birmingham bone anchored hearing aid programme: paediatric experience and results. *J Laryngol Otol* 1996; Suppl 21: 21–9.
42. Snik AF, Mylanus EA, Cremers CW. The bone-anchored hearing aid compared with conventional hearing aids. Audiological results and the patients' opinions. *Otolaryngol Clin North Am* 1995; **28**: 73–83.
43. Declau F, Van Spaendonck M, Timmermans P et al. Prevalence of otosclerosis in an unselected series of temporal bones. *Otol Neurol* 2001; **22**: 596–602.
44. Niedermeyer HP, Arnold W, Schuster M et al. Persistent measles virus infection and otosclerosis. *Ann Otol Rhinol Laryngol* 2001; **110**: 897–903.
45. Causse JR, Causse JB. Otospongiosis as a genetic disease. *Am J Otol* 1984; **5**: 211–23.
46. Causse JR, Causse JB. Eighteen-year report on stapedectomy. I: problems of stapedial fixation. *Clin Otolaryngol* 1980; **5**: 49–59.
47. Powers WH, Sheehy JL, House HP. The fixed malleus head. A report of 35 cases. *Arch Otolaryngol* 1967; **85**: 77–181.
48. Shea JJ. Fenestration of the oval window. *Ann Otol Rhinol Laryngol* 1958; **67**: 932–51.
49. Portmann M, Portman D. The surgery of deafness (operations for function). In: Portman M, Portman D, ed. *Otologic Surgery: Manual of Oto-surgical Techniques*. London: Singular Publishing Group, 1998: 16.
50. Marquet J, Creten WL, Van Camp KJ. Considerations about the surgical approach in stapedectomy. *Acta Otolaryngol* 1972; **74**: 406–10.
51. House J. Stapedectomy technique. *Otolaryngol Clin North Am* 1993; **26**: 389–3.
52. Häusler R, Messerli A, Romano V et al. Experimental and clinical results of fiberoptic argon laser stapedotomy. *Eur Arch Otolaryngol* 1996; **253**: 193–200.
53. Häusler R. Fortschritte in der Stapeschirurgie. *Laryngorhinootologie* 2000; **79**(S2): S95–139.
54. Fisch U. Stapedotomy versus stapedectomy. *Am J Otol* 1982; **4**: 112–17.
55. Causse JB, Causse JR, Parahy C. Stapedectomy technique and results. *Am J Otol* 1985; **6**: 68–75.
56. Cremers CWRJ, Bensen JMS, Huygen PLM. Hearing gain after stapedotomy, partial platinectomy or total stapedectomy for otosclerosis. *Ann Otol Rhinol Laryngol* 1991; **100**: 959–61.
57. Smyth GDL, Hassard TH. Eighteen years experience in stapedectomy. The case for the small fenestra operation. *Ann Otol Rhinol Laryngol* 1978; **2**(suppl 49): 1–36.
58. Van den Bogaert K, Govaerts PJ, Schatteman I et al. A second gene for otosclerosis (OTSC2) maps to chromosome 7q34–36. *Am J Hum Genet* 2001; **68**: 495–500.
59. Tomek MS, Brown MR, Mani SR et al. Localization of a gene for otosclerosis to chromosome 15q25–q26. *Hum Mol Genet* 1998; **7**: 285–90.
60. Mylanus E. The bone anchored hearing aid. Clinical and audiological aspects. Thesis, Nijmegen, 1994.
61. Portmann D, Boudard P, Vdovytsya O. Bone-anchored hearing aids BAHA: 10 years' experience. *Ren Stomatol Chir Maxillofac* 2001; **102**: 274–7.
62. Pelizzone M. Auditory speech reception, signal processing and strategies for representing speech. In: Babighian G, ed. *Consensus on Auditory Implants: first European Conference on Cochlear and Brainstem Implants and State of the Art Symposium on Implantable Hearing Aids*. Padova: Azienda Ospidaliera Padova, 2001: 8–9.
63. Albu S, Babighian G, Trabalzini F. Prognostic factors in tympanoplasty. *Am J Otol* 1998; **19**: 136–40.
64. Chatterjee M, Robert ME. Noise enhances modulation sensitivity in cochlear implant listeners: stochastic resonance in a prosthetic sensory system? *JARO* 2001; **2**: 159–71.
65. Haberkamp T, Mansell M, House W et al. Diagnosis and treatment of arachnoid cysts of the posterior fossa. *Otolaryngol Head Neck Surg* 1990; **103**: 610–14.
66. Huttenbrink KB. Middle ear mechanics and their interface with respect to implantable electronic otologic devices. *Otolaryngol Clin North Am* 2001; **34**: 315–35.
67. Paradise J, Feldman H, Campbell T et al. Effect of early or delayed insertion of tympanostomy tubes for persistent otitis media on developmental outcomes at the age of three years. *N Engl J Med* 2001; **344**: 1179–87.
68. Lenarz T, Battmer RD, Lesinski A et al. Nucleus double array: a new approach for ossified cochleae. *Am J Otol* 1997; **18**: 39–41.
69. Choi J, Kim D. Pathogenesis of arachnoid cyst: congenital or traumatic? *Pediatr Neurosurg* 1998; **29**: 260–6.
70. Hough J, Dyer R, Matthews P et al. Early clinical results: SOUNDTEC implantable hearing device phase II study. *Laryngoscope* 2001; **111**: 1–8.
71. Snik AF, Cremers CW. First audiometric results with the Vibrant soundbridge, a semi-implantable hearing device for sensorineural hearing loss. *Audiology* 1999; **38**: 335–8.
72. Van der Pouw C. Bone anchored hearing. Short and long term results. Thesis, Nijmegen, The Netherlands, 1998.
73. Snik AF, Mylanus EA, Cremers CW. Speech recognition with the bone-anchored hearing aid determined objectively and subjectively. *Ear Nose Throat J* 1994; 73.
74. Snik AF, Dreschler WA, Tange RA et al. Short- and long-term results with implantable transcutaneous and percutaneous bone-conduction devices. *Arch Otolaryngol Head Neck Surg* 1998; **124**: 265–8.
75. Tjellstrom A, Hakansson B, Granstrom G. Bone-anchored hearing aids: current status in adults and children. *Otolaryngol Clin North Am* 2001; **34**: 337–64.
76. Proops DW. The Birmingham bone anchored hearing aid programme: surgical methods and complications. *J Laryngol Otol Suppl* 1996; **21**: 7.
77. Burrell SP, Cooper HC, Proops DW. The bone anchored hearing aid—the third option for otosclerosis. *J Laryngol Otol Suppl* 1996; **21**: 31–7.

78. Hamann C, Manach Y, Roulleau P. Bone anchored hearing aid. Results of bilateral applications. *Rev Laryngol Otol Rhinol (Bord)* 1991;112:297–300
79. Snik AF, Mylanus EA, Cremers CW. Binaural application of the bone-anchored hearing aid. *Ann Otol Rhinol Laryngol* 1998; **107**: 187–93.
80. Van der Pouw KT, Snik AF, Cremers CW. Audiometric results of bilateral bone anchored hearing aid application in patients with bilateral congenital aural atresia. *Laryngoscope* 1998; **108**: 548–53.
81. Bosman AJ, Snik AF, van der Pouw CT et al. Audiometric evaluation of bilateral fitted bone anchored hearing-aids. *Audiology* 2001; **40**: 158–67.
82. Mylanus EA, van der Pouw KC, Snik AF, Cremers CW. Intraindividual comparison of the bone-anchored hearing aid and the air-conduction hearing aids. *Arch Otolaryngol Head Neck Surg* 1998; **124**: 271–6.
83. Papsin BC, Sirimanna TK, Albert DM et al. Surgical experience with bone anchored hearing aids in children. *Laryngoscope* 1997; **107**: 801–6.
84. Lustig LR, Arts HA, Brackmann DE et al. Hearing rehabilitation using the BAHA bone-anchored hearing aid: results in 40 patients. *Otol Neurotol* 2001; **22**: 328–34.
85. Stephens D, Board T, Hobson J et al. Reported benefits and problems experienced with bone-anchored hearing aids. *Br J Audiol* 1996; **30**: 215–20.
86. Arunachalam PS, Kilby D, Meikle D et al. Bone-anchored hearing aid quality of life assessed by Glasgow Benefit Inventory. *Laryngoscope* 2001; **111**: 1260–3.
87. Stenfelt S, Hakansson B, Jonsson R et al. A bone-anchored hearing aid for patients with pure sensorineural hearing impairment: a pilot study. *Scand Audiol* 2000; **29**: 175–85.
88. Wazen JJ, Spitzer J, Ghossaini SN et al. Results of the bone-anchored hearing aid in unilateral hearing loss. *Laryngoscope* 2001; **111**: 955–8.
89. Waltzman SB, Cohen NL. *Cochlear Implants*. New York: Thieme, 2000.
90. Cohen NL, Waltzman SB, Fisher SG. A prospective, randomized study of cochlear implants. *N Engl J Med* 1993; **328**: 233–7.
91. Miyamoto RT, Osberger MJ, Cunningham L. Single to multichannel conversions in pediatric cochlear recipients. *Am J Otol* 1994; **15**: 40–6.
92. National Institutes of Health. *Cochlear Implants in Adults and Children*. Consensus statement no. 100. NIH, 1995: **13**: 1–30.
93. Babighian G. *Consensus on Auditory Implants: first European Conference on Cochlear and Brainstem Implants and State of the Art Symposium on Implantable Hearing Aids*. Padova: Azienda Ospedaliera Padova, 2001: 220–9.
94. Archbold S, O'Donoghue G, Nikolopoulos T. Cochlear implants in children: an analysis of use over a three-year period. *Am J Otol* 1998; **19**: 328–31.
95. Wouters J, Vanden Berghe J. Speech recognition in noise for cochlear implantees with a two-microphone monaural adaptive noise reduction system. *Ear Hear* 2001; **22**: 420–30.
96. Loizou PC, Poroy O. Minimal spectral contrast needed for vowel identification by normal hearing and cochlear implant listeners. *J Acoust Soc Am* 2001; 110: 1619–27.
97. Friesen LM, Shannon RV, Baskent D et al. Speech recognition in noise as a function of the number of spectral channels: comparison of acoustic hearing and cochlear implants. *J Acoust Soc Am* 2001; **110**: 1150–63.
98. Giraud AL, Truy E, Frackowiak RSJ et al. Differential recruitment of the speech processing system in healthy subjects and rehabilitated cochlear implant patients. *Brain* 2000; **123**: 1391–402.
99. Baumgartner W, Van de Heyning PH, Probst R et al. *Subjective Evaluation of the Tempo1+ Speechprocessor in Comparison to the Cispro1+ processor in Children and Adults*. Los Angeles: House Ear Institute, 2001: 78.
100. O'Donoghue GM. Minimal access surgery for cochlear implantation. In: Babighian G, ed. *Consensus on Auditory Implants: first European Conference on Cochlear and Brainstem Implants and State of the Art Symposium on Implantable Hearing Aids*. Padova: Azienda Ospidaliera Padova, 2001: 88.
101. Donaldson GS, Peters MD, Ellis MR et al. Effects of the clarion electrode positioning system on auditory thresholds and comfortable loudness levels in pediatric patients with cochlear implants. *Arch Otolaryngol Head Neck Surg* 2001: **127**: 956–60.
102. Abbas P, Brown C, Shallop J et al. Summary of results using the Nucleus CI24 implant to record the electrically evoked compound action potential. *Ear Hear* 1999; **20**: 45–59.
103. Dillier N, Lai WK, Almquist B et al. Measurement of the electrically evoked compound action potential (ECAP) via a neural response telemetry (NRT) system. *Ann Otol Rhinol Laryngol* 2002; **111**: 407–14.
104. Brown CJ, Hughes M L, Luk B et al. The relationship between EAP and EABR thresholds and levels used to program the Nucleus 24 Speech Processor: data from adults. *Ear Hear* 2000; **21**: 151–63.
105. Van de Heyning PH, Craddock L, Cooper H et al. Comparison between NRT based MAPS and behaviourally measured MAPS a different stimulation rates: a multi center investigation. In: Babighana, ed. *Consensus on Auditory Implants: First European Conference on Cochlear and Brainstem Implants and State of the Art Symposium on Implantable Hearing Aids*. Padova: Azienda Ospidalieva Padova, 2001.
106. Flynn MC, Dowell RC, Clark GM. Aided speech recognition abilities of adults with a severe or severe-to-profound hearing loss. *J Speech Language Hear Res* 1998; **41**: 285–99.
107. Hamzavi J, Franz P, Baumgartner WD et al. Hearing performance in noise of cochlear implant patients versus severely-profound hearing-impaired patients with hearing aids. *Audiology* 2001; **40**: 26–31.
108. Archbold S, Lutman ME, Marshall DH. Categories of auditory performance. *Ann Otol Rhinol Laryngol* 1995; **104**(suppl 166): 312–14.
109. Nikolopoulos T, Archbold S, O'Donoghue G. The development of auditory perception in children following cochlear implantation. *Int J Pediatr Otorhinolaryngol* 1999; **49**(suppl 1): 189–91.
110. O'Donoghue G, Nikolopoulos T, Archibold SM. Determinants of speech perception in children after cochlear implantation. *Lancet* 2000; **356**: 466–8.

111. Gregory S. Ethical aspects and counselling. In: Babighian G, ed. Consensus on auditory implants: first European Conference on Cochlear and Brainstem Implants and state of the art symposium on implantable hearing aids. Padova: Azienda Ospedale Padova, 2001: 10–11.
112. Weber BP, Dillo W, Dietrich B et al. Pediatric cochlear implantation in cochlear malformations. *Am J Otol* 1998; **19**: 747–53.
113. Shallop JK, Peterson A, Facer GW et al. Cochlear implants in five cases of auditory neuropathy: postoperative findings and progress. *Laryngoscope* 2001; **111**: 555–62.
114. Bredberg G, Lindström B, Löppönen H et al. Electrodes for ossified cochleas. *Am J Otol* 1997; **18**: S42–3.
115. Balkany T, Bird PA, Hodges AV et al. Surgical technique for implantation of the totally ossified cochlea. *Laryngoscope* 1998; **108**: 988–92.
116. Connor CM, Hieber S, Aerts HA et al. Speech, vocabulary, and the education of children using cochlear implants: oral or total communication? *J Speech Language Hear Res* 2000; **43**: 1185–204.
117. Aschendorff A, Marangos N, Laszig R. Early and long-term results of rehabilitation of cochlear implant patients. *Laryngorhinootologie* 1997; **76**: 275–7.
118. Helms J, Müller J, Schön F et al. Evaluation of performance with the COMBI 40 Cochlear Implant in adults: a multicentric clinical study. *ORL* 1997; **59**: 23–35.
119. Tyler RS, Summerfield AQ. Cochlear implantation: relationships with research on auditory deprivation and acclimatization. *Ear Hear* 1996; **17**: 38S–50S.
120. Vermeulen AM, Beijk CM, Brokx JPL et al. Development of speech perception abilities of profound deaf children: a comparison between children with cochlear implants and those with conventional hearing aids. *Ann Otol Rhinol Laryngol* 1995; **104**: 215–17.
121. Waltzman SB, Cohen NL, Gomolin RH et al. Open-set speech perception in congenitally deaf children using cochlear implants. *Am J Otol* 1997; **18**: 342–9.
122. Lenarz T, Weber BP, Mack KF et al. The Vibrant Soundbridge System: a new kind of hearing aid for sensorineural hearing loss. 1: Function and initial clinical experiences. *Laryngorhinootologie* 1998; **77**: 247–55.
123. Dazert S, Shehata-Dieler WE, Dieler R et al. 'Vibrant Soundbridge' middle ear implant for auditory rehabilitation in sensory hearing loss. I. Clinical aspects, indications and initial results. *Laryngorhinootologie* 2000; **79**: 459–64.
124. Lenarz T, Weber BP, Issing PR et al. Vibrant Sound Bridge System. A new kind of hearing prosthesis for patients with sensorineural hearing loss. 2. Audiological results. *Laryngorhinootologie* 2001; **80**: 370–80.
125. Snik AF, Mylanus EA, Cremers CW et al. Multicenter audiometric results with the Vibrant Soundbridge, a semi-implantable hearing device for sensorineural hearing impairment. *Otolaryngol Clin North Am* 2001; **34**: 373–88.
126. Zenner HP, Leysieffer H, Maassen M et al. Human studies of a piezoelectric transducer and a microphone for a totally implantable electronic hearing device. *Am J Otol* 2000; **21**: 196–204.
127. Zenner HP, Leysieffer H. Total implantation of the Implex TICA hearing amplifier implant for high frequency sensorineural hearing loss: the Tubingen University experience. *Otolaryngol Clin North Am* 2001; **34**: 417–46.128.
128. Hough J, Dyer R, Matthews P et al. Early Semi-implantable electromagnetic middle ear hearing device for moderate to severe sensorineural hearing loss. *Otolaryngol Clin North Am* 2001; **34**: 401–16
129. Roland PS, Shoup AG, Shea MC et al. Verification of improved patient outcomes with a partially implantable hearing aid, the SOUNDTEC Direct Hearing System. *Laryngoscope*, 2001; **111**: 1682–90.
130. Yanagihara N, Sato H, Hinohira Y et al. Long-term results using a piezoelectric semi-implantable middle ear hearing device: the Rion device E-type. *Otolaryngol Clin North Am* 2001; **34**: 389–400.
131. Meyershoff W, Ridemour B. Tinnitus. In: Meyershoff, Ria, eds. *Otolarangology Head and Neck Surgery*, Philadelphia, PA: WB Saunders, 1992: 435–46.
132. Sismanis A. Pulsatile tinnitus, a 15 year experience. *Am J Otol* 1998; **19**: 472–7.
133. Moller A. Similarities between severe tinnitus and chronic pain. *J Am Acad Audiol* 2000; **11**: 115–24.
134. Mühlmichel W, Elbert T, Taub E et al. Reorganization of auditory cortex in tinnitus. *Proc Natl Acad Sci USA* 1998; **95**: 10340–3.
135. Pantev C, Lütkenhöner B. Magnetoencephalographic studies of functional organization and plasticity of the human auditory cortex. *J Clin Neurophysiol* 2000; **17**: 130–2.
136. Torndorf J. The analogy between tinnitus and pain: a suggestion for a physiological basis of chronic tinnitus. *Hear Res* 1987; **28**: 271–5.
137. Moller M, Moller A, Jannetta P et al. Vascular decompression surgery for severe tinnitus: selection criteria and results. *Laryngoscope* 1993; **103**: 421–7.
138. Wiech K, Preissl H, Lutzenberges W et al. Cortical reorganisation after digit to hand replantation. *J Neurosurg* 2000; **93**: 876–83.
139. Ryu H, Yamamoto S, Sugiyama K et al. Neurovascular compression syndrome of the eighth cranial nerve. What are the most reliable diagnostic signs? *Acta Neurochir (Wien)* 1998; 140: 1279–86.
140. Donaldson J. Pathogenesis of pseudotumor cerebri syndromes. *Neurology* 1981; **31**: 877–80.
141. Paul K, Lye R, Strang F et al. Arnold–Chiari malformation; review of 71 cases. *J Neurosurg* 1983; **58**: 183–7.
142. Wiggs W, Sismanis A, Laine F. Pulsatile tinnitus associated with congenital central nervous system malformations. *Am J Otol* 1996; **17**: 241–4.
143. Ahmmed A, Mackenzie I, Das V et al. Audio-vestibular manifestations of Chiari malformation and outcome of surgical decompression: case report. *J Laryngol Otol* 1996; **110**: 1060–4.
144. Couloignier V, Grayeli A, Bouccara D et al. Surgical treatment of the high jugular bulb in patients with Menière's disease and pulsatile tinnitus. *Eur Arch Otorhinolaryngol* 1999; **256**: 224–9.
145. Golueke P, Panetta T, Sclafani S, Varughese G. Tinnitus originating from an abnormal jugular bulb: treatment by jugular vein ligation. *J Vasc Surg* 1987; **6**: 248–51.

146. De Ridder D, Fransen H, Cammaert T et al. Intracranial stenting for pulsatile tinnitus. Poster presentation at Tinnitus Seminar, Fremantle Australia, 2001; 3: 5–7.
147. Jackson C, Harris P, Glasscock M et al. Diagnosis and management of paragangliomas of the skull base. *Am J Surg* 1990; **159**: 389–93.
148. Megerian C, McKenna M, Nadol J. Non-paraganglioma jugular foramen lesions masquerading as glomus jugulare tumors. *Am J Otol* 1995; **16**: 94–8.
149. Rosenbloom J, Storper I, Aviv J et al. Giant cell tumors of the jugular foramen. *Am J Otolaryngol* 1999; 20: 176–179.
150. Awad I, Barrow D, eds. *Dural Arteriovenous Malformations*. Park Ridge, IL: American Association of Neurological Surgeons, 1993.
151. Brookes G. Vascular decompression surgery for severe tinnitus. *Am J Otol* 1996; **17**: 569–76.
152. Ko Y, Park C. Microvascular decompression for tinnitus. *Stereotact Funct Neurosurg* 1997; **68**: 266–9.
153. Makins A, Nikolopoulos T, Ludman C et al. Is there a correlation between vascular loops and unilateral auditory symptoms? *Laryngoscope* 1998; **108**: 1739–42.
154. Reisser C, Schuknecht H. The anterior inferior cerebellar artery in the internal auditory canal. *Laryngoscope* 1991; **101**: 761–6.
155. Hamlyn P. Neurovascular relationships in the posterior cranial fossa, with special reference to trigeminal neuralgia. 2. Neurovascular compression of the trigeminal nerve in cadaveric controls and patients with trigeminal neuralgia: quantification and influence of method. *Clin Anat* 1997; **10**: 380–8.
156. Boden S, Davis D, Dina T et al. Magnetic resonance scans of the lumbar spine in asymptomatic patients. *J Bone Joint Surg* 1990; **72A**: 403–8.
157. Noren G. Long-term complications following gamma knife radiosurgery of vestibular schwannoma. *Stereotact Funct Neurosurg* 1998; **70**(suppl 10): 65–73.
158. Dandy WE. Surgical treatment of Menière's disease. *Surg Gynaecol Obstet* 1941; **72**: 421–5.
159. Berliner K, Shelton C, Hitselburger W et al. Acoustic tumours: effect of surgical removal on tinnitus. *Am J Otol* 1992; **13**: 13–17.
160. Lalwani A. Meningiomas, epidermoids, and other non acoustic tumors of the cerebellopontine angle. *Otolaryngol Clin North Am* 1992; **25**: 707–28.
161. Bengochea F, Blanco F. Arachnoid cysts of the cerebellopontine angle. *J Neurosurg* 1954; **12**: 66–71.
162. Lesoin F, Dhellemes P, Rousseoux M et al. Arachnoid cysts and head injury. *Acta Neurochir* 1983; **69**: 43–51.
163. Pappas D, Brackmann D. Arachnoid cysts of the posterior fossa. *Otolaryngol Head Neck Surg* 1981; 89: 328–32.
164. Yanaka K, Enomoto T, Nose T et al. Post-inflammatory arachnoid cyst of the quadrigeminal cistern. Observation of development of the cyst. *Childs Nerv Syst* 1988; **4**: 302–5.
165. Daspit C. Neurotologic aspects of posterior fossa arachnoid cysts. In: Jackler RK, Brackmann DE, eds. *Neurotology*. St Louis: Mosby–Year Book, 1994: 939–44.
166. Kaasinen S, Pyykko I, Ishizak H et al. Effect of intratympanic administered gentamycin on hearing and tinnitus in Meniere's disease. *Acta Otolarygol Suppl* 1995; **52**: 184–5.
167. Vernon J, Johnson R, Schleuning A. The characteristics and natural history of tinnitus in Menière's disease. *Otolaryngol Clin North Am* 1980; **13**: 611–19.
168. Gersdorff M, Nouwen J, Gilain C et al. Tinnitus and otosclerosis. *Eur Arch Otolaryngol* 2000; **257**: 314–16.
169. Glasgold A, Thedinger B, Cueva R. The effect of stapes surgery on tinnitus in otosclerosis. *Laryngoscope* 1966; **76**: 1524–32.
170. De Ridder D, Krahel N, De Waele L et al. Auditory cortex meningeoma causing low pitch non-pulsatile tinnitus. Poster presentation at Tinnitus Seminar, Fremantle Australia, 2002; **3**: 5–7.
171. Soussi T, Otto S. Effects of electrical brainstem stimulation on tinnitus. *Acta Otolaryngol* 1994; **114**: 135–40.

Further Reading

Bluestone C. Current concepts of pathogenesis of otitis media with effusion. *Pediatr Ann* 1984; **13**: 417–21.

Browning G, Gatehouse S. The prevalence of middle ear disease in the adult British population. *Clin Otolaryngol* 1992; **17**: 317–21.

Claes J, Van de Heyning PH, Creten W et al. Allograft tympanoplasty: predictive value of preoperative status. *Laryngoscope* 1990; **100**: 1313–18.

Colletti V, Fiorino F. Malleus-to-footplate prosthetic interposition: experience with 265 patients. *Otolaryngol Head Neck Surg* 1999; **120**: 437–44.

Dornhoffer J, Gardner E. Prognostic factors in ossiculoplasty: a statistical staging system. *Otol Neurotol* 2001; **22**: 299–304.

Hamans E, Govaerts P, Somers T et al. Allograft tympanoplasty type 1 in the childhood population. *Ann Otol Rhinol Laryngol* 1996; 871–6.

Hough J, Dyer R, Matthews P et al. Semi-implantable electromagnetic middle ear hearing device for moderate to severe sensorineural hearing loss. *Otolaryngol Clin North Am* 2001; **34**: 401–16.

Huttenbrink K. The mechanics and function of the middle ear. Part 1: The ossicular chain and middle ear muscles. *Laryngorhinootologie* 1992; **71**: 545–51.

Iurato S, Marioni G, Onofri M. Hearing results of ossiculoplasty in Austin–Kartush group A patients. *Otol Neurotol* 2001; **22**: 140–4.

Jansen C. The combined approach for tympanoplasty (report on 10 years experience). *J Laryngol Otol* 1968; **82**: 779–93.

Janssens S, Govaerts PJ, Casselman J et al. The LAURA multichannel cochlear implant in a true Mondini dysplasia. *Eur Arch Otorhinolaryngol* 1996; **253**: 301–4.

Kasic JF, Fredrickson JM. The Otologics MET ossicular stimulator. *Otolaryngol Clin North Am* 2001; **34**: 501–13.

Marquet J. Twelve years experience with homograft tympanoplasty. *Otolaryngol Clin North Am* 1977; **3**: 581–93.

Paparella M, Brady D, Hoel R. Sensorineural hearing loss in chronic otitis media and mastoiditis. *Trans Am Acad Ophthalmol Otolaryngol* 1970; **741**: 108–15.

Pepers-van Lith G, Brokx J, Vriens R. Enquete over auditieve mogelijkheden met hoorapparatuur bij cliënten met het syndroom van Usher type II. Unpublished report, Instituut voor Doven, The Netherlands, 1996.

Quaranta N, Fernandez-Vega Feijoo S, Piazza F et al. Closed tympanoplasty in cholesteatoma surgery: long-term (10 years) hearing results using cartilage ossiculoplasty. *Eur Arch Otorhinolaryngol* 2001; **258**: 20–4.

Ryu H, Yamamoto S, Sugiyama K et al. Neurovascular decompression of the eighth cranial nerve in patients with hemifacial spasm and incidental tinnitus: an alternative way to study tinnitus. *J Neurosurg* 1998; **88**: 232–6.

Sadé J, Luntz M, Levy D. Middle ear gas composition and middle ear aeration. *Ann Otol Rhinol Laryngol* 1995; **104**: 369–73.

Schatteman I, Somers T, Govaerts P et al. Long-term results of allograft tympanoplasty in adult cholesteatoma. In: *6th International Conference on Cholesteatoma and Ear Surgery, Abstract book*, FP 75, P11, 2000.

Teele D, Klein J, Rosner B. Epidemiology of otitis media during the first seven years of life in children in greater Boston: a prospective cohort study. *J Infect Dis* 1989; **160**: 83–94.

Vanden Abeele D, Coen E, Parizel P et al. Can MRI replace a second look operation in cholesteatoma surgery? *Acta Otolaryngol* 1999; **119**: 555–61.

Vincent R, Lopez A, Sperling N. Malleus ankylosis: a clinical, audiometric, histologic and surgical study of 123 cases. *Am J Otol* 1999; **20**: 717–25.

Section IV
Vestibular science

37 The pathology of the vestibular system

Francesco Scaravilli

Anatomy

Labyrinth, vestibular nerve and nuclei

The inner ear includes the vestibular component of the cochleovestibular system. It consists of three semicircular ducts, the utricle and the saccule, all involved in maintaining the equilibrium, orientation in space, gaze and muscle tone.

The ducts, each with a terminal dilatation (ampulla), are arranged at right angles to each other (Figure 37.1). The ampulla contains a transversely orientated ridge (crista ampullaris) covered by the cupula; its columnar epithelium consists of neuroepithelial hair cells (the receptor). Following the displacement by angular acceleration of the endolymphatic fluid within the ducts, a movement of the cupula follows, which results in stimulation of the hair cells. The utricle and the saccule form the otolith organ; their sensory epithelium (macula) possesses hair cells in contact with gelatinous material containing concretions (otoliths). Whereas the utricle is sensitive to gravitational forces, the saccule responds to linear acceleration in the ventro-dorsal axis of the body.

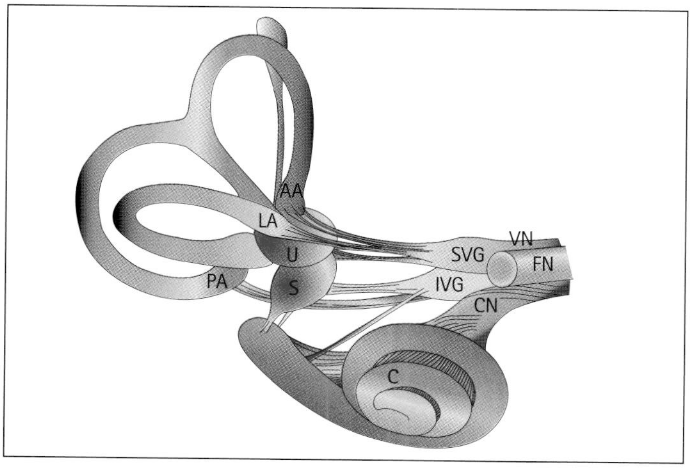

Figure 37.1 Anatomy of vestibular structures within the inner ear: AA, LA, PA = anterior, lateral and posterior ampulla; C: cochlea; CN: cochlear nerve; FN: facial nerve; IVG and SVG: inferior and superior vestibular ganglion; S: saccule; U: utricule; VN: vestibular nerve.

The vestibular ganglion (of Scarpa) is located in the internal auditory meatus and consists of superior and inferior parts, joined by a thin bridge (Figure 37.1). Vestibular nuclei are located predominantly in the floor of the fourth ventricle, spanning craniocaudally from slightly beyond the level of the VIth cranial nerve nucleus to a level rostral to the nucleus of the hypoglossus. The four components of the vestibular nucleus are arranged in two longitudinal columns, the lateral including the superior, lateral and inferior nuclei, and the medial consisting exclusively of the medial nucleus, the largest (Figure 37.2).

Primary vestibular pathways

The vast majority of fibres entering the brainstem with the vestibular nerve bifurcate into ascending and descending branches and terminate in the four nuclei. Cells of the superior vestibular ganglion (from the utricular macula) project to the ventrolateral nucleus and those of the inferior ganglion (saccular macula) to the dorsolateral parts of the inferior vestibular

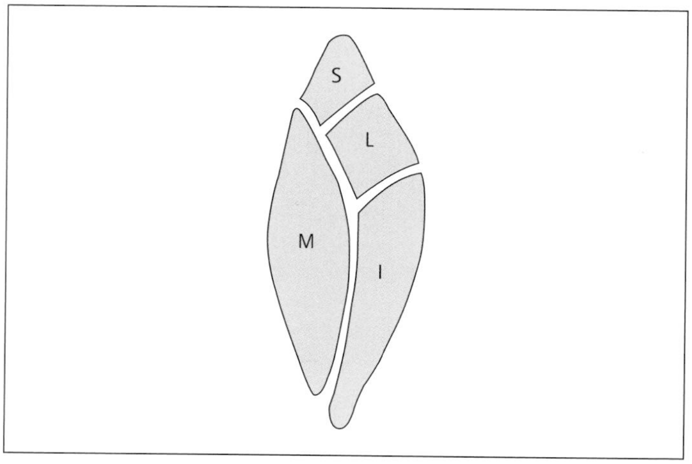

Figure 37.2 Components of the vestibular nucleus: M: medial; S: superior; L: lateral; I: inferior cell groups.

nucleus. Fibres from the cristae of the semicircular ducts terminate in the superior vestibular and rostral parts of the medial vestibular nucleus. A small contingent of primary vestibular fibres traverse the lateral and superior vestibular nuclei and proceed, as primary vestibulocerebellar fibres, directly to the ipsilateral nodulus and uvula of the cerebellum.[1]

Afferent projections to the vestibular nuclei

The vestibular nuclei receive afferent fibres from the cerebellum (the most numerous).[2] They arise from the ipsilateral flocculus, nodulus and ventral uvula, and are directed to the superior and medial nuclei, from the ipsilateral anterior vermis to the dorsal part of the lateral vestibular and dorsorostral part of the inferior vestibular nuclei. The spinal projection connects the forelimb region of the anterior lobe with the forelimb region of the lateral vestibular nucleus. No fibres from the cerebral cortex, striatum or superior colliculi reach the vestibular nuclei. On the other hand, the medial vestibular nucleus is reached by fibres from the interstitial nucleus of Cajal, via the medial longitudinal fasciculus. Fibres from ganglion cells innervating the cristae of the semicircular ducts and reaching the contralateral superior and medial vestibular nuclei, via commissural projections, have inhibitory effects; contralateral fibres from the maculae of the otoliths are, on the other hand, excitatory.

Secondary vestibular fibres

From the vestibular nuclei fibres project:

1. To the cerebellum — from the inferior and medial vestibular nuclei to the ipsilateral nodulus, uvula and flocculus through the juxtarestiform body.
2. To the nuclei of the three oculomotor nerves (III, IV, VI) — crossed and uncrossed fibres via the medial longitudinal fasciculus (MLF). They pass medially in the region of the nucleus of the VI nerve to form the fasciculus. The function of these fibres is to provide a simultaneous contraction of the lateral rectus on one side and of the medial rectus muscle on the opposite side, in order to achieve the conjugate lateral gaze. Those which terminate on motor neurones exert inhibitory influence on these cells.[3] The MLF contains, in addition, non-vestibular fibres from: (a) interstitial nucleus of Cajal (interstitiospinal tract); (b) superior colliculus (tectobulbar and tectospinal tract); (c) pontine reticular formation (reticulospinal tract) and fibres from rostral brainstem nuclei directed to the inferior olive.
3. To the most caudal regions of the spinal cord via the anterior and lateral funiculi (vestibulospinal tract, ipsilateral). These fibres are somatotopically arranged. The lateral vestibular nucleus, which receives impulses from the vestibular nerve and a number of cerebellar areas, mediates the muscular responses in the trunk and extremities, which are aimed at facilitating the tone of extensor muscles.

Pathology of the vestibular system

The whole vestibular system can be affected by primary and secondary lesions (Table 37.1).

Malformations

These include underdevelopment or malformation of the vestibule, absence, thinning or malformation of the oval window, and calcification of its annular ligament. The vestibular aqueduct may be underdeveloped or displaced, and the utricle and saccule absent, underdeveloped or malformed. Maculae may be abnormal. The endolymphatic duct and sac may be underdeveloped, short or wide and the utriculoendolymphatic valve abnormal.

The internal auditory meatus may be absent or underdeveloped; its vestibular component can also be displaced. There may be abnormality of the blood vessels.

With regard to the aetiology of the malformations, it is unknown for some (congenital absence of the round window), and known for others. Some are genetically transmitted: the cardio-auditory syndrome (Jervell Lange–Nielsen syndrome (JLNS) is a recessive disorder with congenital deafness and long QT (LQTS1) on the EEG. Mutations in the potassium channel gene KVLQT1 have been identified in JLNS and in the autosomal dominant LQT syndrome.[4] Waardenburg syndrome is an autosomal dominant disorder characterized by sensorineural hearing loss, pigmentary disturbances and other developmental defects,[5] and is caused by defective function of the embryonic neural crest.[6] Depending on additional symptoms, it is further classified into four subtypes (WS1, 2, 3 and 4).[7] Mutations in the microphthalmia-associated transcription factor (MITF) and PAX3 are responsible for WS2 and WS1/3, respectively,[7] bearing in mind that WS3 is an extreme form of WS1. Usher syndrome is an autosomal recessive disorder characterized by sensorineural hearing loss and visual impairment secondary to retinitis pigmentosa. The disorder is clinically and genetically heterogeneous; several subtypes of Usher type 1 have been described, the most frequent being USH1B, located on chromosome 11q13.5.[8]

Pendred syndrome is an autosomal recessive disorder with a defective organic binding of iodine leading to goitre, hypoplasia of the cochlea and widened vestibular aqueduct.[9] The gene

Table 37.1 Pathology of the vestibular system.

Malformations
Positional vertigo
Bone lesions
Ageing and degenerative diseases
Ototoxicity
Infectious and inflammatory diseases
Vascular lesions
Neoplasms

responsible for the disorder has been mapped to chromosome 7q31.[10]

The genetics related to acoustical neuroma will be dealt with later in this chapter. Chiari malformation was first described in 1891, and includes three subtypes.[11]

Type 1 presents with conical elongation of the cerebellar tonsils and adjacent cerebellar tissue into the vertebral canal. Spina bifida is not a feature, whereas adult patients can develop hydrocephalus. After studying 32 patients, Shady et al[12] concluded that tonsillar herniation is the consequence of bony occipital dysplasia.

Type 2 is found most commonly in infants together with myelomeningocele and hydrocephalus. Pathological changes consist of elongation of the inferior vermis and brainstem, which are displaced in the cervical spinal canal. The disorder is associated with abnormalities of the bone and dura and, in 50% of the patients, the lower medulla bends to form an S-shaped curve over the cervical cord.[13] In addition, patients have macroscopic polygyria.[14] The pathogenesis of the disorder is controversial, although a skeletal defect appears the most likely possibility.[13]

Type 3 is very rare. Pathological changes include occipitocervical or high cervical bone defects leading to cerebellar herniation. Associated changes are breaking of the tectum, elongation and folding of the brainstem, and lumbar spina bifida.

Vestibular symptoms in Chiari malformation are reported.[15–17]

Positional vertigo

This is a clinical symptom with no definite pathological counterpart, as pathological lesions outside the vestibular system, in particular in the cerebellum, can be responsible for it.[18] In a study by Lindsay and Hemenway[19] atrophy of the superior division of the vestibular nerve, utricle and crista of the lateral semicircular canal were described. Dix and Hallpike[20] and Cawthorne and Hallpike[21] showed degeneration of the macula of the utricle and of the cristae of the lateral and superior semicircular canals and of the superior vestibular nerve. Schuknecht[22] described, in two cases of positional vertigo, basophilic deposits adhering to the posterior surface of the cupula of the left posterior semicircular canal. The author suggested that the abnormal material could derive from otoconia in a degenerated utricular macula. This type of abnormality is called cupulolithiasis as opposed to canalithiasis which is due to free-floating debris in the long arm of the posterior canal.[23]

In a study of 363 patients presenting with vertigo,[24] 32% were found to have migraine. Common migraine can be defined as a unilateral, pulsating headache, lasting one to several days, which may be associated with nausea and vomiting.[25] Migraine, as well as oral contraceptives, is a common risk factor for cerebral infarction in young women.[26] Organic lesions associated with migraine include meningocortical calcifying angiomatosis,[27] mitochondrial cytopathy,[28–30] CADASIL,[31–35] hereditary endotheliopathy with retinopathy, nephropathy and stroke (HERNS), a disorder distinct from CADASIL,[36] moyamoya disease,[37] and giant cell arteritis.[38]

Bone lesions

Presentation and discussion of the disorders due to bone pathology go beyond the scope of this chapter, and the reader is invited to consult specialized books on this topic.[39,40] Here, only inherited hyperostoses will be mentioned.

Camurati–Englemann (or Englemann) disease, an uncommon condition inherited as an autosomal dominant trait,[41] is characterized radiologically by symmetric diaphyseal sclerosis involving the tubular bones, and clinically by limb pain, muscle weakness, waddling gait and sometimes deafness.[42] Hearing impairment is reported in 18% of the patients.[43] Hanson and Parnes[44] reported compression of the vestibular nerve, and Wilhelm et al[45] described vestibular disturbances and facial paralysis, in addition to damage to the optic nerves. The pathogenesis of the disorder consists of the narrowing of the internal auditory canal.[43]

Paget's disease of the bone, or 'osteitis deformans', is a disorder characterized by rapid remodelling resulting in abnormal bone formation. It affects 3–5% of people over 40 years. Genetic linkage analysis of families with this disease shows linkage to a region of chromosome 18q, near the polymorphic locus D18S42.[46]

Vestibular dysfunction has been reported by Proops et al,[47] who also described the pathological features of the disorder.

Ageing and degenerative diseases

Elderly people may present with disturbances of balance (presbyastasis) resulting in dysequilibrium, vertigo, light-headedness and falls. The disorder can be permanent or episodic.[48] Vestibular changes include degeneration of the saccular and, to a lesser extent, the utricular macula and loss of otoconia.[49] Rosenhall[50] described epithelial cysts in the sensory epithelium of the posterior and superior ampullary cristae, whereas reduction in the number of vestibular ganglion cells has not been confirmed.

With regard to neurodegenerative diseases, the lateral vestibular nucleus was found to harbour numerous neurofibrillary tangles in patients with Alzheimer's disease, albeit without nerve cell loss.[51] Neuronal loss, gliosis and neurofibrillary tangles in vestibular nuclei were described in progressive supranuclear palsy[52] (Figure 37.3a) and in a patient with thalamic degeneration of 20 years' duration.[53] Multisystem atrophy includes a group of disorders which were formerly described separately as olivopontocerebellar atrophy, Shy–Drager syndrome and striatonigral degeneration. These disorders are characterized by nerve cell loss in various regions and by the presence of characteristic glial inclusions.[54] Vestibular nuclei (Figure 37.3b), together with the primary motor and premotor cortex, putamen, globus pallidus, subthalamic nucleus, pretectal area, pontine nuclei, motor nuclei of the V, VII and XII cranial

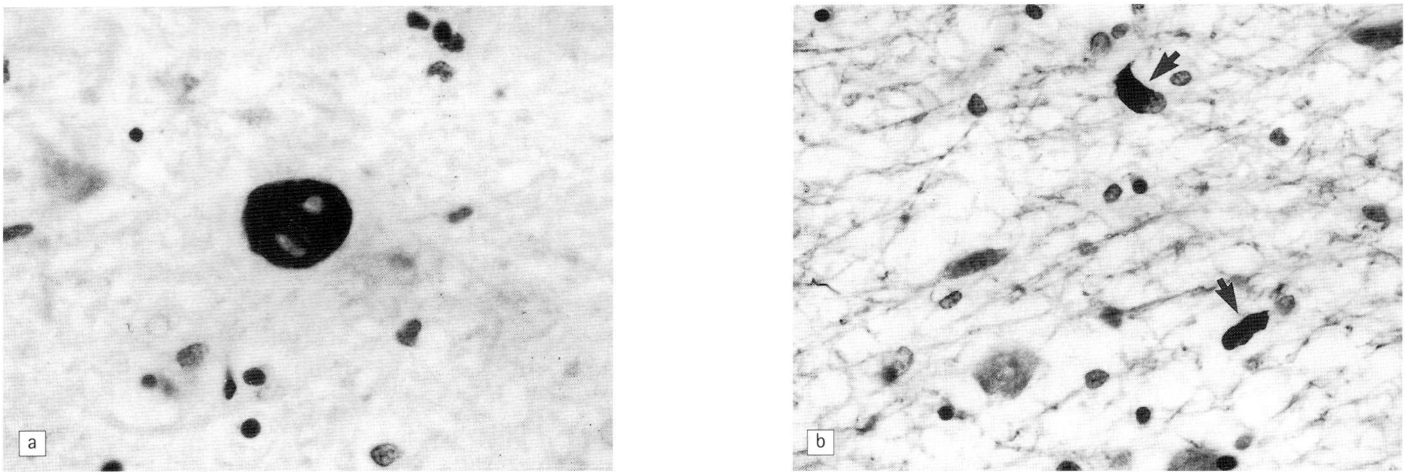

Figure 37.3 Neurone of the vestibular nucleus containing a *tau*-positive neurofibrillary tangle in a patient with progressive supranuclear palsy (a). Similar changes can be found in a number of neurodegenerative disorders, including Alzheimer's disease. (b) In MSA (multisystem atrophy), a number of glial cells (oligodendrocytes) contain typical cytoplasmic inclusions (arrows), best visualized by the Gallyas metod. X360.

nerves, pontomedullary reticular centres and intermediolateral column of the spinal cord are among the areas with the highest density of these inclusions.

A growing number of neurodegenerative disorders are presently known to be caused by an expanded CAG trinucleotide repeat that encodes polyglutamine in the disease protein.[55] To date, these disorders include Huntington's disease, spinal and bulbar muscular atrophy, dentatorubropallidoluysian atrophy and eight spinocerebellar ataxias (SCA1, 2, 3, 6, 7, 10, 12 and 17). The characteristic pathological feature common to all of them is the presence of ubiquitin-positive intranuclear inclusions within neurones. Involvement of the vestibular nuclei has not been reported in SCA1 and 2,[56] whereas it has been described in many patients with SCA3[57–59] (Figure 37.4). Moreover, vestibular nuclei are also abnormal in dentatorubropallidoluysian atrophy (all three cases in Iizuka et al;[60] case 4 in Hayashi et al[61]).

Gerstmann–Sträussler–Scheinker disease is a familial form of prion disease known to have mutations, first found at codons 102, 105 and 117 and subsequently also at codons 145, 198 and 217. Pathological changes include amyloid, kuru-like plaques, spongiform changes of variable severity, nerve cell degeneration and reactive gliosis. Among the various regions of the brain involved, Kuzuhara et al[62] found cell loss also in the vestibular nuclei.

Ototoxicity

Damage to the inner ear has been described following administration of a number of drugs. Five classes are considered by Michaels.[40]

1. Aminoglycoside antibiotics (streptomycin, kanamycin, gentamicin, tobramycin, viomycin and aminokacin). As these drugs also induce damage to the kidney, any delay in clearing the drug from the circulation would increase ototoxicity. This is the direct result of action by the drug on sensory cells and is further enhanced in patients with elevated serum iron.[63] The effect of tobramycin on the human ear has been documented by Sone et al[64] in six patients. Four of their temporal bones showed loss of hair cells and degeneration of ganglion cells. Moreover, six bones revealed degeneration of the spiral ganglion. In aminoglycoside[65] and gentamicin[66] toxicity, hair cell loss in the cochlea takes place via apoptosis.
2. Ethacrynic acid, a loop diuretic, has been involved in ototoxicity. It damages the hair cells of the cochlea and vestibule.[67] Vestibular changes are described as cyst formation in the sensory epithelium of the posterior semicircular canal and the saccular macula.[40] It should be mentioned that ethacrynic acid enhances ototoxicity induced by streptomycin, by addition (not potentiation) of the effects.[68]
3. The effect of salicylates on the vestibular system has been interpreted by Pickrell et al[69] as being due to potentiation of the action of ototoxins, probably by increasing the levels of these toxins in the endolymphatic fluid. No pathological changes have been reported in experimental studies, and there are no human temporal bone studies.
4. Quinine and **5.** cytotoxic drugs are not known to induce changes of the vestibular structures.

Infectious and inflammatory diseases

Agents of inflammatory diseases include bacteria, protozoa, fungi, metazoa and viruses. Involvement of the vestibular system follows various routes and takes place at different levels.

Bacterial infections

Invasion of the labyrinth may occur either from an otitis media, by far the most frequent occurrence, or via the meninges. In the first instance, infection enters via the oval or round windows,

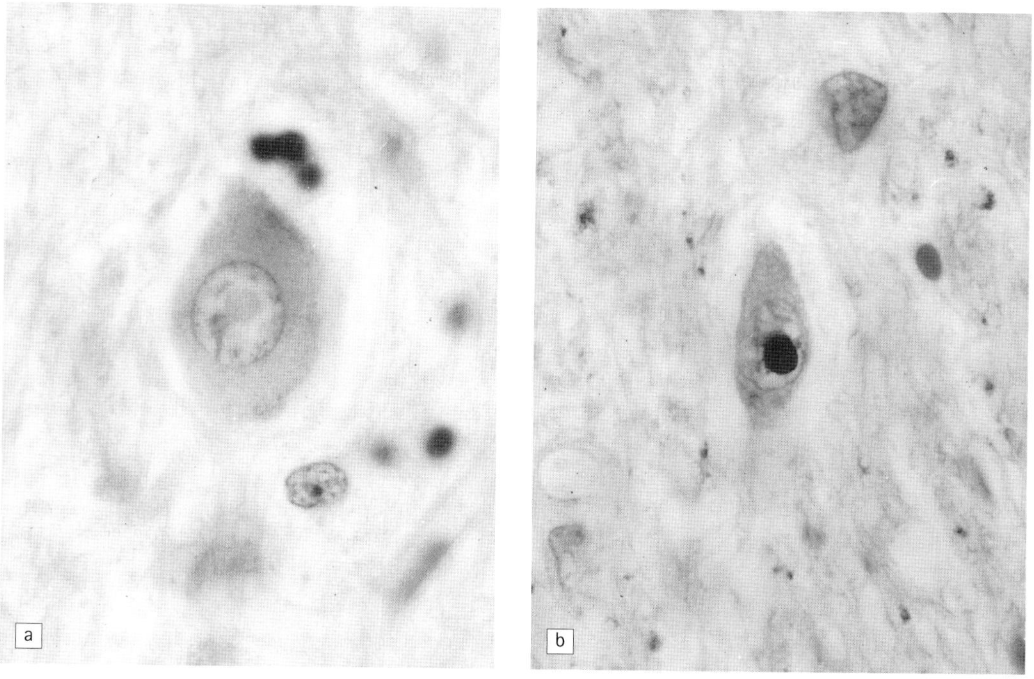

Figure 37.4 Photomicrographs of intranuclear inclusions in the vestibular nuclei of a patient suffering from SCA3/MJD. In H&E-stained sections, the pale inclusion is seen adjacent to a small nucleolus (a). Inclusions are strongly ubiquitin-and 1C2-positive. (b) ×900.

producing bone damage resulting in a fistula between the middle ear and labyrinth which may extend to the leptomeninges.[70] As for the meningeal route, involvement occurs via the internal auditory meatus and the cochlear aqueduct. In a study of 41 patients with bacterial meningitis,[71] suppurative labyrinthitis occurred in 20 of them.

The role of meningitis in producing bilateral vestibular failure (BVF) was evaluated by Brandt[72] and confirmed by Rinne et al.[73] The latter authors found that BVF was secondary to meningitis in 11% of 53 patients. The long-lasting effects of meningitis were followed up by Hugosson et al,[74] who detected subclinical vestibular pathology in 6 of 9 adults who had suffered from meningitis in childhood.

With regard to the aetiology of meningitides, damage to the vestibular system was revealed in patients who had survived meningococcal group B meningitis.[75,76] In *Haemophilus influenzae* meningitis, the loss of vestibular functions was attributed to ampicillin,[77] whereas tetracyclines, used in the treatment of *Chlamydia*, *Mycoplasma pneumoniae*, rickettsial and gonococcal infections, may also cause vestibular damage.[78] Vestibular areflexia was reported as a sequel in 13 of 111 patients with previous pneumococcal meningitis.[79] One case of vestibular nerve damage was reported by Heininger et al[80] in a boy with borreliosis, whereas McNeil and Gordon[81] report lack of labyrinthine function as a sequel of *Streptococcus suis* type II meningitis.

Tuberculous meningitis may occasionally affect the middle ear. The incidence of this infection is now increasing again, particularly among destitute people. The vestibular nerve and pathways may appear as a tuberculoma which, when localized to the cerebellopontine angle, may mimic the symptoms of the schwannoma of the VIII nerve.

The histological appearances of the process are similar to those seen elsewhere and include a granulomatous reaction with epithelioid and multinucleated giant cells of Langhans' type as well as lymphocytes (Figure 37.5). Caseous necrosis occurs with a meningeal localization, but is considered rare in the bone.[39] The diagnosis is confirmed by histochemical visualization of acid-fast organisms with light microscopy (Zeehl–Neelsen method), fluorescence (auramine–rhodamine) or culture.

Because of the many morphological similarities with tuberculosis, it is appropriate to describe sarcoidosis at this point. This systemic disease of unknown aetiology is found predominately among women, and appears morphologically as non-caseating granulomas consisting of closely packed epithelioid cells which often include Langhans' or foreign body multinucleated giant cells (Figure 37.6). Necrosis is usually absent and never has a caseating appearance. In chronic cases, a ring of fibrous or hyaline tissue may surround the granuloma. Laminated calcified concretions (Schaumann bodies) and asteroid bodies may be seen within giant cells. Neither type of body is pathognomonic.

Sarcoidosis has a predilection for the meninges at the base and therefore affects cranial nerves. The VIII nerve has been found to be involved in 5% of patients,[82] making it the fourth most commonly involved cranial nerve,[83] the facial nerve being the most affected.[84] Hooper and Holden[85] described both acoustical and vestibular signs. In their patient 2, functional tests suggested a non-labyrinthine lesion, possibly located in the brainstem.

In congenital syphilis, the infection may appear as gummae involving the bone marrow and periosteum and as diffuse petrositis.[40] Deafness is present in over a third of patients with congenital syphilis,[86] and indeed it is one of the components of the Hutchinson's triad (together with interstitial keratitis and deformed incisor teeth).

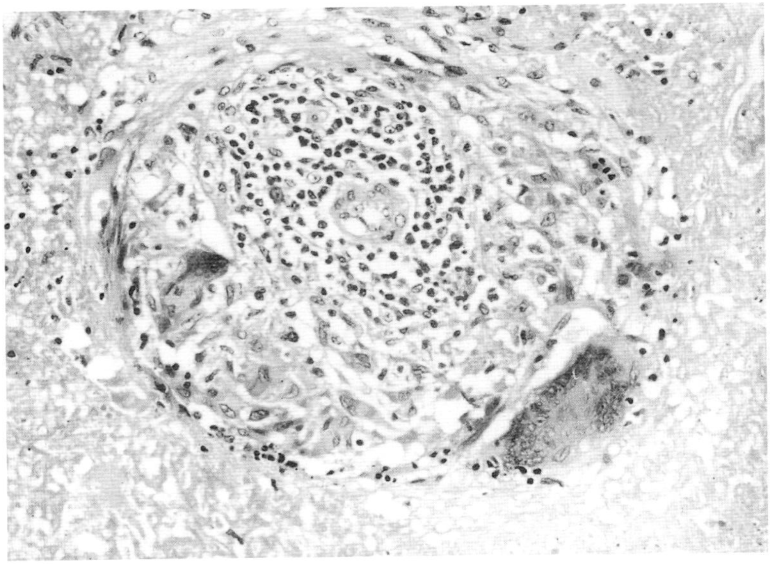

Figure 37.5 Tuberculous granulomas consist of epithelioid cells, lymphocytes and Langhans' multinucleated giant cells and are associated with caseous necrosis, which is seen in this picture surrounding the granuloma. H&E, ×220.

In the acquired infection, the central nervous system (CNS) is regularly involved in early syphilis, and sensorineural hearing loss is the commonest symptom. In association with HIV infection, tertiary syphilis may appear at an earlier stage than in the penicillin era (within 2 years of onset of *Treponema* infection). Musher et al[87] reported 40 such patients with asymptomatic neurosyphilis, meningitis or cranial nerve abnormalities. Cranial nerves involved included the optic and VIII nerves.

Protozoa

The four main groups of protozoa which produce infections of the nervous system in humans (amoebae, including free living amoebae, *Plasmodium*, *Toxoplasma* and *Trypanosoma*) do not appear to affect the vestibular system, except as part of a more generalized involvement of the nervous system.

Fungi

Although the incidence of mycoses has been increasing in the last three decades because of the growing number of immunosuppressed patients, infections of the inner ear and peripheral vestibular system remain rare. In most cases they take place via the bloodstream, although on occasion (see mucormycosis below) they spread by contiguity through the bone.

Infection of the inner ear by *Candida* has been reported.[88] In an experimental study by Ashman et al[89] systemic infection by *Candida albicans* in ageing inbred mice produced lesions of the utricle, adjacent parts of the semicircular canals, and also of the saccule and scala vestibuli. In another study,[90] involvement of the vestibule seemed to proceed from the brain and pachymeningitis that eroded the petrous bone.

A granulomatous meningitis due to *Coccidioides immitis*, a fungus endemic in South America (particularly Argentina and

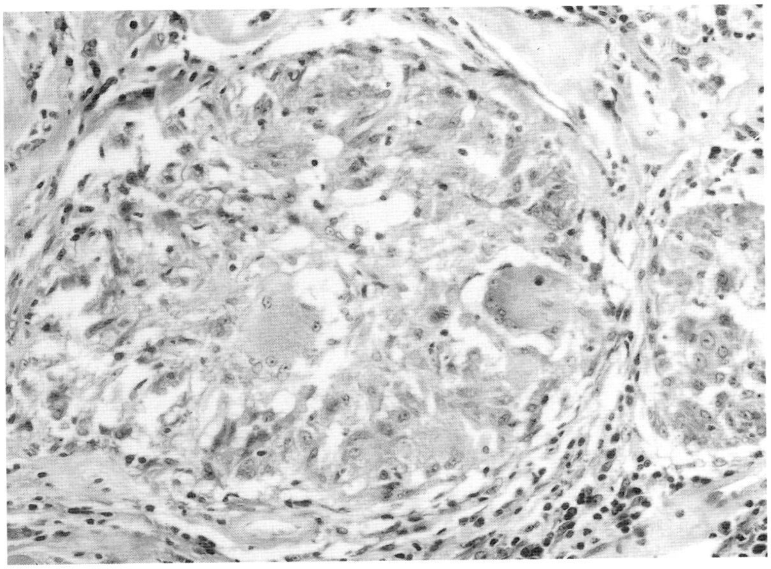

Figure 37.6 In sarcoidosis, granulomas are similar to those described in tuberculosis, but typically lack the necrosis. H&E, ×220.

Paraguay), Mexico, and also southern California,[91] affecting the vestibular nerve, was reported in a dog.[92]

Destruction of the VIII nerve and end organs was described in a 19-year-old woman with cryptococcal meningitis,[93] and Teuscher et al[94] reported a vestibular syndrome associated with *Cryptococcus neoformans* in a horse. Meningitis is different in immunocompetent and immunocompromised patients. In the former it shows a cellular component consisting of small inflammatory cells, including multinucleated giant cells. In the latter it includes almost exclusively organisms extensively infiltrating the central and peripheral nervous system (Figure 37.7).

As a number of members of the orders Mucorales and Entomorphthorales affect the head and neck, including bone and soft tissues, they can spread to the vestibular system. Meyerhoff et al[88] reported on a mildly diabetic patient in whom mucor infection had reached the middle ear, producing multiple cranial nerve (including the VIII) involvement. The infection had started as a focus in the pharynx and had spread to the base of the skull by contiguity.

Metazoa

Involvement of the vestibular system in metazoal infections depends on the localization of the parasite.

In cysticercosis, caused by the pig tapeworm *Taenia solium*, cysts tend to be multiple and localized within the brain parenchyma, in the meninges, in the ventricles, and sometimes in the spinal cord. Meningeal cysts often have a basal localization and can affect the vestibular nerve; as parenchymal cysts, they can involve the central vestibular pathways. In one patient reported by Ronge et al[95] cysts, localized in the cerebellopontine angle, produced a deficit of the cochleovestibular nerve.

Hydatid disease, the infection due to *Echinococcus granulosus*, is a worldwide problem. Whereas in humans the most involved organ is the liver (55%), the brain is affected in less than 1% of patients. Cyst formation in the brain is usually solitary, spherical and unilocular. Cysts are almost always found in the cerebral hemispheres. A patient with a cyst involving the cerebellar vermis and right cerebellar hemisphere was described by Palomico-Nicas and Pachon-Diaz.[96]

Viral infections

These can involve the central and peripheral vestibular pathways. With regard to the former, a viral aetiology is still a controversial issue in most cases. Although Menière's disease is widely regarded as being more probably due to endolymphatic hydrops, Adour et al[97] concluded that it results from a ganglionitis caused by herpes simplex virus (HSV). Indeed, intense vertiginous spells of sudden onset were observed by Mangabeira-Albernaz and Gananca[98] in patients with previous viral infections. Neuro-otological examination revealed central vestibular involvement. Furuta et al[99] examined at postmortem 26 vestibular ganglia. Using PCR, in situ hybridization and immunohistochemistry, they detected HSV DNA in 6 of 10 ganglia. However, as the latency-associated transcript (LAT) of HSV-1 was negative in all 16 ganglia examined, they concluded that ganglia are latently infected and that LAT is transcribed weakly or not at all. In another study by Shimizu et al[100] various viruses were investigated (HSV and *Herpes zoster* virus (HZV), cytomegalovirus, Epstein–Barr virus (EB), adenovirus, influenza type A and B, parainfluenza 3, mumps, rubella and measles virus) in 57 patients with vestibular neuronitis. HSV-1 IgM was found in only one case. In a study of 232 patients with acute peripheral vestibulopathy, usually attributed to viral inflammation or ischaemia of the extra-axial vestibular portion of the VIII nerve, 45 showed electrophysiological signs of pontine involvement. Possible causes included vertebrobasilar ischaemia (22 patients) or multiple sclerosis (8 patients).[101] The pathology is poorly documented. In an ultrastructural study of the ganglion of Scarpa and vestibular nerve, Friedmann and

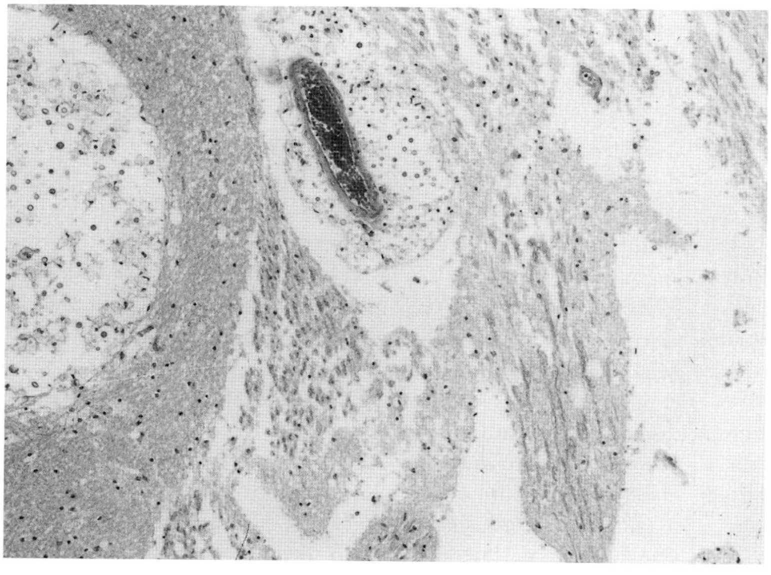

Figure 37.7 Cryptococcus meningoencephalitis involving the medulla and the cochleovestibular nerve in an immunocompromised patient. Note that in these patients the organisms, appearing as spherical structures in a pale and mucoid background, are not accompanied by inflammatory cells. H&E, ×90.

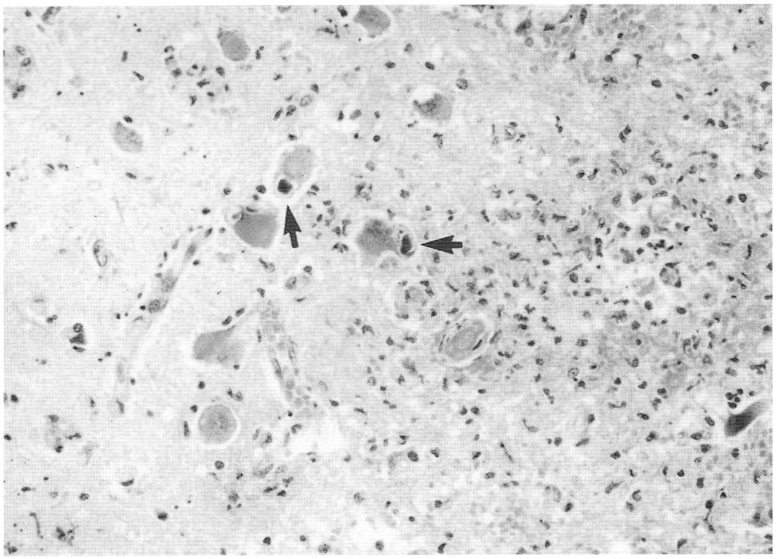

Figure 37.8 The inflammatory process, shown here to involve the vestibular nuclei in CMV encephalitis, includes a spotty area of necrosis, microglial hyperplasia and two large astrocytes with an intranuclear inclusion (arrows). H&E, ×220.

House[102] described degenerative neuronal changes and axonal lesions, both non-specific.

Although involvement of the central vestibular pathways in viral diseases does take place, signs and symptoms are not so frequently reported, as they are probably overshadowed by more severe ones elicited by the diffuse involvement of the brain.

HSV encephalitis has, in most cases, a hyperacute course, with haemorrhagic and necrotic lesions located predominantly in areas of the brain forming the limbic system. However, in cases with a subacute course, it shows the features of micronodular encephalitis. Localization to the brainstem shows these appearances. Kaji et al[103] analysed data from 27 patients: although limbic encephalitis was by far the commonest occurrence, two patients were found to also have a brainstem localization. Using in situ hybridization, Schmidbauer et al[104] revealed HSV DNA in 16 of 34 patients (43%) with brainstem (microglial nodule) encephalitis, thus confirming HSV as the cause of nodular encephalitis; the authors do not mention the cochleovestibular nuclei among those involved by the process.

The brainstem may be involved in HZV encephalitis;[105] a brainstem localization of cytomegalovirus (CMV) with truncal ataxia was reported by Fuller et al[106] in a patient suffering from AIDS (Figure 37.8).

The pathology depends on the causative agent; however, pathognomonic features (intranuclear inclusion bodies in many encephalitides) may be absent. Common abnormalities include perivascular cuffings, usually by lymphocytes and occasionally plasma cells, hypertrophy and proliferation of microglial cells, reactive gliosis, occasional foci of necrosis and neuronal changes (chromatolysis and neuronophagia).[105] In progressive multifocal leukoencephalopathy, localization to the brainstem occurs, albeit not frequently. The main pathological changes are severe myelin loss, scanty perivascular lymphocytic cuffs, macrophages and transformation of a number of surviving oligodendrocytes into large cells, many of which contain intranuclear inclusions of papovavirus.

The reader is referred to texts of neuropathology for more detailed descriptions regarding bacterial, fungal, protozoal, metazoal and viral diseases.[91,105,107]

Inflammatory diseases

These include disorders with an inflammatory pattern, but whose aetiology is either not known or definitely not infectious. The central vestibular pathways may be involved if the disorder has a brainstem localization. They can be grouped as follows:

1. multiple sclerosis
2. autoimmune encephalitis
3. vasculitides
4. paraneoplastic encephalomyelitis.

Multiple sclerosis (MS)

This is the most frequent and frequently identified disorder in this group and affects the central myelin. It is characterized by relapses and remissions of neurological disturbances with progressive deterioration. This can take place in a steadily progressive way from the onset (primary progressive MS) or through progression after an incomplete remission (secondary progressive MS). It affects individuals from 15 to 50 years at onset, and there is a 1.5 : 1 female predominance. The course spans from a few months to many decades, with an average life-expectancy of 25 years. In Europe its incidence increases with increasing latitude, and in the UK it varies between 175/100 000 and 99/100 000 between Scotland and the south of England. Genetic factors, in addition to environment, also play a role: MS has a low incidence among Orientals, and shows a 30% concordance among identical twins. In most populations, the disease is associated with HLA-DR15.

MS can present as an acute, subacute or chronic illness affecting the white matter of any region of the CNS. One of its most characteristic features is its lack of respect for any anatomical boundary. Therefore, with regard to the vestibular, as indeed any other, system, the whole or part of it may be involved, together with adjacent regions (Figure 37.9). Other characteristic pathological features of the typical lesions (plaques) are their multiplicity, the sharp demarcation from the surrounding normal white matter, the predominantly subependymal or subpial location, and their different age. Moreover, plaques are accompanied by perivenous lymphocytic cuffing. Areas of remyelination may also be present (shadow plaques). As white matter is ubiquitous in the CNS, including within the cortical grey matter, so are plaques.

The cellular composition of the plaques varies according to their stage of evolution. Inactive chronic plaques are hypocellular, contain predominantly astrocytes, no oil red O-positive material (indicative of a rather acute process), sparse oligodendrocytes, thickened veins with inflammatory cells, and normal or beaded axons. In active chronic stages, myelin breakdown is in progress at the edges of the plaque, there is oil red O- or myelin basic protein-positive material in macrophages, and oligodendrocytes may be either increased or decreased in number, whereas astrocytes do not take an active part. Remyelinating (shadow) plaques contain palely stained myelinated fibres. They may either persist indefinitely or further demyelinate. In acute plaques, myelin breakdown is associated with the presence of microglia and macrophages. The vessels are initially normal, and astrocytes and lymphocytes are fewer in number. The fate of oligodendrocytes varies, whereas axons are beaded. Two to three months later, enlarged astrocytes become obvious, myelin-laden macrophages disappear progressively, and lymphocytes increase in number.

As for the aetiology of MS, a viral hypothesis is supported by: (1) abnormal immune responses to a number of viral agents shown by patients; (2) long latencies and recurrences shared with some viral diseases; and (3) destruction of oligodendrocytes, as seen in some viral diseases. However, in MS, demyelination cannot be seen as a bystander of inflammation, as the latter appears late. In favour of an autoimmune process are the following data: (1) induction of spontaneously relapsing/remitting disorders following injection of myelin components; (2) MS-like lesions induced in humans after injection of nervous tissue; and (3) similarities between myelin destruction in MS and experimental allergic encephalomyelitis (EAE). However, there are morphological differences between MS and EAE, and autoreactive T cells or anti-myelin and anti-oligodendrocyte antibodies, similar to those seen in MS, are detected in other inflammatory diseases of the CNS.

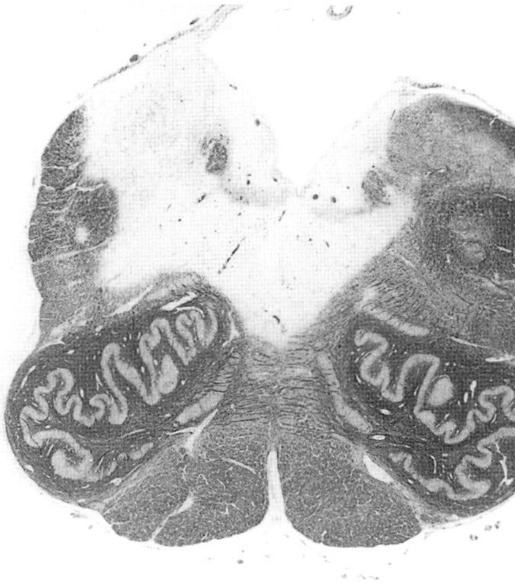

Figure 37.9 A plaque of multiple sclerosis in the medulla is shown to involve the vestibular nuclei. The plaque is sharply demarcated from the surrounding normal myelin and bears no relationship to any boundaries or systems. Luxol fast blue/cresyl violet.

Autoimmune encephalitides include: (1) perivenous encephalomyelitis in its post-infectious and post-vaccinal forms; and (2) acute haemorrhagic leukoencephalomyelitis. The latter (Hurst's disease), usually fatal, is characterized by abrupt onset, preceded in 50% of the cases by a febrile illness. It affects individuals between 2 and 36 years and can be considered as a hyperacute form of perivenous encephalomyelitis affecting the white matter. Pathological features include small vessel necrosis with fibrinoid degeneration, petechial haemorrhages and neutrophil infiltration. With regard to the aetiology of these lesions, a direct viral hypothesis appears to have been ruled out on the basis of: (1) failure to recover a virus from the brain or to demonstrate either viral antigens or nucleic acid in the nervous system in patients with perivenous encephalomyelitis;[108,109] and (2) pathological features that are quite different from those of any known viral encephalitis. On the other hand, the possibility that autoimmunity plays a role is supported by the following observations: (1) the stereotyped pattern of the reaction; (2) the delay between contact of the agent with the subject and development of the disorder; (3) pathological similarities with changes seen in EAE induced by whole white matter or myelin;[110] and (4) detection of lymphocytes reactive to myelin basic protein in peripheral blood and cerebrospinal fluid (CSF) in patients who develop perivenous encephalomyelitis following various viral infections.[111,112]

Brainstem involvement has been documented in acute haemorrhagic leukoencephalitis in humans[113,114] and in a dog.[115] No reports have been published on similar involvement in perivenous encephalomyelitis.

Vasculitis

This includes primary forms and those which are a manifestation of systemic diseases. Among the former are: (1) Takayasu's arteritis; (2) giant cell (temporal) arteritis; and (3) primary angiitis of the CNS. The latter include: (1) systemic lupus erythematosus (SLE); (2) polyarteritis nodosa; (3) Wegener's granulomatosis; (4) Churg–Strauss syndrome; (5) Sjögren syndrome; and (6) Behçet syndrome. Pathological features of these disorders are described in detail by Kalimo et al.[116]

Brainstem involvement, and hence possible vestibular complications, have been reported in SLE,[117,118] Sjögren syndrome[119] and Behçet disease.[120,121]

Vasculitis may also occur in individuals taking phenylpropanolamine or amphetamine, methamphetamine and ephedrine, the latter being sympathomimetics with chemical structures similar to that of phenylpropanolamine.[122] Vascular damage usually results in brain haemorrhage.

Paraneoplastic disorders

Paraneoplastic syndromes (PNS) include a number of uncommon disorders associated with systemic non-invasive malignancies. The incidence of paraneoplastic disorders varies depending on the criteria applied to their definition.[123] Moreover, the correlation between type of neoplasm and appearance of the changes in the central and peripheral nervous systems is not absolute or is even absent. These syndromes may become clinically evident before, after or at the time of the discovery of the neoplasm.

The detection, in patients with PNS, of antibodies reacting both with neuronal antigens and tumours supports an autoimmune pathogenesis. Various antibodies are known, whose description and properties go beyond the scope of this chapter.[124]

PNS are chronic encephalomyelitides or ganglionitis which share the following morphological features:[125]

1. predominant involvement of the grey matter, ganglia and nerves
2. presence of inflammatory changes, including perivascular lymphocytic cuffing and microglia hyperplasia and formation of neuronophagic nodules
3. absence of vasculitic changes
4. non-specific astrocytic hypertrophy
5. white matter changes secondary to neuronal loss.

The central and peripheral nervous systems can be involved separately or together, and the following clinico-pathological subtypes are described:

1. limbic encephalitis
2. brainstem encephalitis
3. myelitis
4. ganglioradiculoneuritis and autonomic neuropathy.

Particularly relevant for neuro-otologists is subtype (2). It poses differential diagnostic problems with vascular disorders, motor neurone disease, MS, infections and inflammatory disorders and intrinsic tumours, mainly before the tumour has become manifest. The inflammatory process may involve any of the nuclei of the brainstem, and Gulya[126] has reported cochleovestibular dysfunction in personal cases (Figure 37.10).

Vascular lesions

The CNS is highly dependent on the continuous flux of oxygen and nutrients through the blood vessels, and adequate blood supply can be affected by abnormalities of these vessels. The main vascular lesions responsible for an impaired circulation are the following:

1. atherosclerosis
2. hypertensive angiopathy
3. inflammatory
4. aneurysms
5. vascular malformations
6. miscellaneous disorders.

Atherosclerosis

This is the commonest vascular disorder, and many risk factors are considered. They include dyslipidaemia, hypertension, diabetes mellitus and smoking. Its incidence among ethnic groups varies, reflecting also differences in socio-economic conditions. Various hypotheses have been put forward regarding its pathogenesis: (1) the lipid hypothesis; (2) the response to injury; and (3) a unifying theory. Atherosclerotic lesions undergo stages, beginning with intimal changes, which lead ultimately to the degeneration of part of the wall, with either dilatation or severe reduction of the lumen.

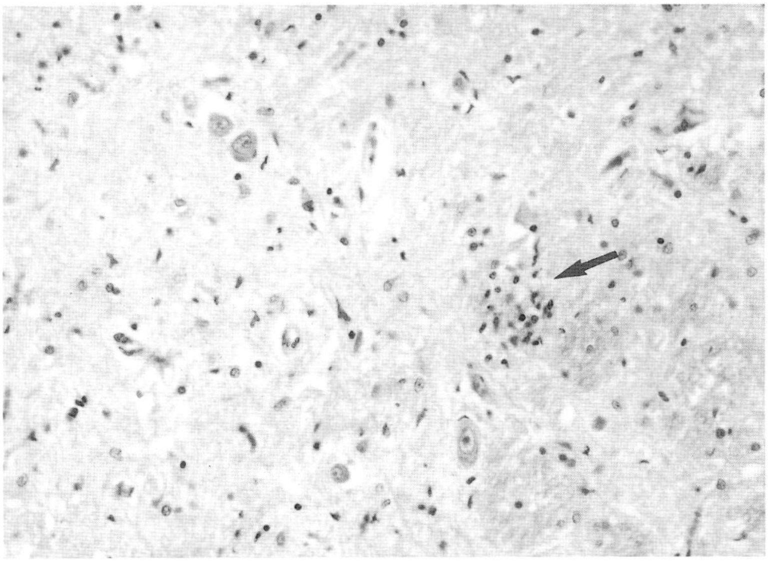

Figure 37.10 Photomicrograph of the vestibular nuclei in a patient with the bulbar localization of paraneoplastic encephalomyelitis. Note the small microglial nodule (arrow) in the place of an absent nerve cell. H&E, ×220.

The vertebrobasilar sector of the cerebral vessels is frequently affected. According to Stebhens[127] the extracranial segment of the vertebral arteries escapes atherosclerosis, except at its origin. On the other hand, Fisher et al[128] state that the carotid and vertebral arteries suffer equally in their intra- and extracranial portions. Meyer and Beck[129] described segmental involvement of the vertebral arteries in their cervical course, plaques tending to affect wider or ectatic segments between the foramina of the transverse processes. The brainstem can suffer from cerebrovascular accidents. With regard to the vestibular system, the size and location of its nuclei and pathways within the brainstem are such that vascular changes in this area involve more than one cranial nerve, in addition to long ascending and descending tracts. On the other hand, the distribution of the various branches is so stereotyped and the chances of collateral circulation so small that well-defined neurological sequelae can follow damage to the small branches of the vertebrobasilar system.

Wallenberg's syndrome results from occlusion either of the posterior inferior cerebellar artery or of the bulbar branches of the vertebral artery, producing a well-circumscribed area of infarct (Figure 37.11). Although the commonest cause is atherosclerosis, syphilitic arteritis has also been blamed. The syndrome may develop gradually or suddenly, and is characterized clinically by: (1) ipsilateral analgesia of the face with loss of the corneal reflex; (2) miosis, enophthalmos and ptosis and sometimes anhydrosis; (3) ipsilateral coarse ataxia; (4) contralateral insensitivity to pain and temperature of the trunk and extremities; (5) ipsilateral paralysis of the soft palate, pharynx and larynx; (6) variable involvement of the VI, VII and VIII cranial nerves; and (7) rare contralateral hemiparesis.

Hypertensive angiopathy

Chronic hypertension damages the nervous system in two ways: it worsens changes due to atherosclerosis in both extra- and intracranial arteries and induces damage to the small arteries. The latter is considered to be specific to hypertension.

Pathological changes are seen in small arteries and arterioles located within the brain tissue. They show thickened walls, due, initially, to proliferating smooth muscle fibres. Subsequently, they become homogeneously eosinophilic and contain fewer cells (Figure 37.12). The eosinophilic appearance may consist of fibrinoid change in the early stages and hyaline tissue late in the process.

Another change traditionally associated with hypertension is the so-called micro-aneurysm of Charcot and Bouchard,[130] a microscopic saccular formation in vessels ranging in diameter from 25 to 250 μm.[131,132] Its existence is controversial,[132,133] and it is possible that racial differences may account for this discrepancy between the authors. Localization of these aneurysms includes particularly the thalamus, but they are found also in the pons, cerebral cortex, claustrum, cerebellum and cerebellar peduncles.

Within the group of vascular disorders associated with hypertension, Binswanger's disease[134] is a subtype usually associated with dementia. It has the typical CT scan appearances of periventricular low densities and is found predominantly among hypertensive patients. Sufferers are usually between 50 and 70 years, and there is no sex predominance.

Microscopic examination shows myelin pallor throughout the whole hemispheric white matter. In some areas there may be necrosis, and axons are constantly severely damaged and/or reduced in number. There is also a variable amount of astrocytic hyperplasia. Arterioles in affected areas resemble those seen in hypertensive patients.

Pathological changes have been seen to extend to the brainstem,[135] with potential involvement of the vestibular nuclei and pathways.

The disorder is probably related to deficient blood supply due to vessel damage produced by hypertension. The damaged blood–brain barrier results in leakage of blood proteins. Repeated bursts of oedema, known to spread more easily through the white than the grey matter, induce white matter damage.[116]

In the past, a number of patients with pathological changes resembling those of Binswanger's disease did not appear to be hypertensive. In these cases, the disease presented in families

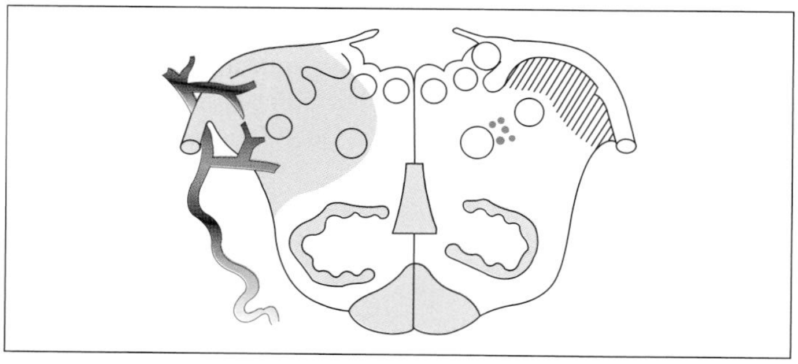

Figure 37.11 Drawing of the medulla showing (shaded area) the distribution of the softening responsible for Wallenberg's syndrome; the artery parallel to the left edge of the medulla is the inferior cerebellar artery.

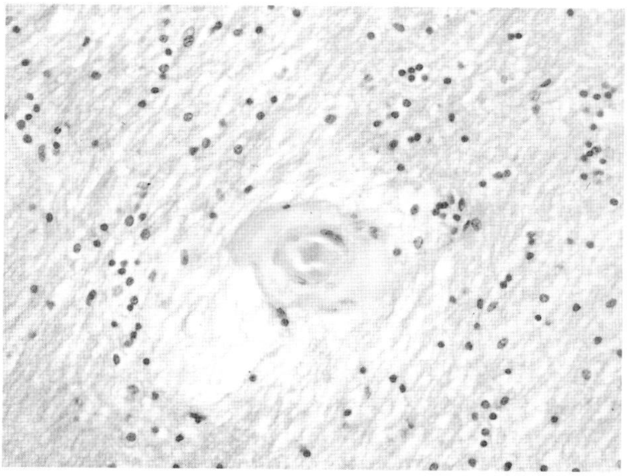

Figure 37.12 In the late stages of hypertensive angiopathy, small-calibre intraparenchymal blood vessels show a thick wall consisting of fibrous tissue. Their lumina are reduced in diameter. H&E, ×220.

with an autosomal dominant mode. It was first described by Sourander and Wålinder in 1977[136] and in 1993 Tournier-Lasserve et al[137] established it as a genetic disorder due to a defective chromosome 19q12. The disease was given the name CADASIL, an acronym for cerebral autosomal dominant arteriopathy with subcortical infarcts and leukoencephalopathy.

Morphologically, the vessels show non-arteriosclerotic, non-amyloid arteriopathy affecting the meninges, vessels penetrating the white matter as well as those in nerves, muscles and skin. Changes consist of concentric fibrohyaline thickening of the arterial walls, involving both the media and adventitia.[138] The former, which shows degenerative changes of muscle fibres, is PAS (periodic acid Schiff)-positive and contains, in addition, PAS-positive and basophilic granules. Mayer et al[139] described involvement of the brainstem in two members of a German family affected by the disorder.

Inflammatory diseases

Inflammatory diseases involving intracerebral vessels have been dealt with above.

Aneurysms

These include saccular, fusiform, infectious aneurysms as well as the Charcot–Bouchard type, which has been dealt with above.

Fusiform aneurysms are usually seen in patients with severe forms of atherosclerosis (see above).

Infectious aneurysms are produced by septic emboli and are seen in about 3% of patients with infective endocarditis. They can rupture with consequent intracerebral haemorrhage, the risk being 3–7% in patients with infective endocarditis.[140] The middle cerebral artery is the most frequently affected, the superior cerebellar artery having been involved in only one patient. The organisms most commonly involved are *Streptococcus viridans* and *Staphylococcus aureus*. Mycotic aneurysms can also be seen, the genus *Aspergillus* being the commonest culprit.

Morphologically, the segment of the arterial wall adherent to the embolus is oedematous, necrotic and infiltrated predominantly by polymorphs.

Saccular (berry) aneurysms appear as dilatations of part of the wall of large intracranial arteries. Their incidence is 2–5%, depending on the accuracy with which they are investigated.[141] Rare in children, they increase in frequency with age, 60% of them being found in patients between 40 and 60 years, predominantly women (female/male ratio 3:2) and they may appear in families.[142,143] About 40–70% rupture before death.

Virtually all saccular aneurysms originate in close proximity to, or at, the bifurcation of the main intracranial arteries. These, unlike their extracranial counterparts, are characterized by a rather thin muscle wall and absence of the external elastic lamina.

About 85–90% of them arise in the carotid arteries or their main branches, 5–10% in the vertebrobasilar arteries (Figure 37.13), and 5% in their minor branches, this distribution being reversed in children, in whom 40–45% have a posterior location.

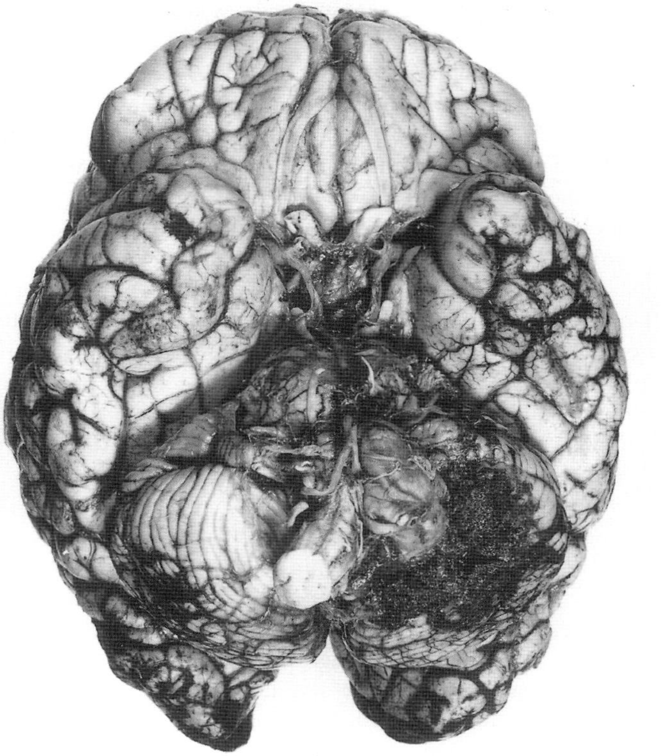

Figure 37.13 A large saccular aneurysm originating from the posterior inferior cerebellar artery (PICA) appears to compress the (left) lateral side of the medulla. The stretched VII and VIII nerves are seen on its anterior aspect.

Aneurysms vary in size, some reaching 'gigantic' proportions (over 2.5 cm). Their wall varies in colour from grey to yellow or dark red, depending on the presence and age of the blood component.

Histologically, their walls consist exclusively of endothelium (whenever present) and fibrous tissue. A blood clot may occupy a variable part of the sac, and the fibrous tissue may contain blood, haemosiderin, areas of necrosis or inflammatory cells.

Vascular malformations

These differ from each other with regard to localization within the meninges or the nervous system and the type of their component vessels (arteries, veins or a mixture of both). They are considered congenital, although irradiation of the brain and occlusion of the dural sinuses can induce lesions similar to the congenital ones.

Vascular malformations have been classified by Kalimo et al[116] as shown in Table 37.2. This classification is adapted from Challa et al.[144]

Arteriovenous malformations (AVMs)

These consist of irregular aggregates of arteries, veins and connecting vessels and can become clinically evident at any age, but particularly during the second, third and fourth decades.

Table 37.2 Intracranial vascular malformations.

Congenital malformations within the brain parenchyma
Arteriovenous malformations
Variant: malformation of the vein of Galen
Venous angioma and varicose vein
Cavernous angiomas
Capillary telangiectasia
Mixed:
Cavernous and venous
Cavernous and capillary
Other: haemangioma calcificans
Congenital malformations within the meninges
Arteriovenous malformations
Venous angioma and varicose vein
Cavernous haemangioma
Malformations as part of CNS or generalized syndromes
Phakomatoses
Hereditary haemorrhagic teleangiectasia
Others
Acquired vascular lesions simulating vascular malformations
Radiation-induced lesions of the white matter
Lesions secondary to venous sinus obstruction

They are localized predominantly in the supratentorial regions and at the surface of the brain or in the deep grey nuclei, but are also found in the dura.

The walls of these vessels are irregular in thickness, and a number of veins may appear arterialized, as shown by the presence of the internal elastic lamina. An important morphological feature of AVMs is the presence of brain tissue separating the vessels, which shows reactive gliosis and haemosiderin-laden macrophages (Figure 37.14).

The so-called aneurysm of the vein of Galen is an arteriovenous fistula, the vein undergoing aneurysmal dilatation. The feeding vessels are either one or both posterior cerebral arteries, and less frequently small posterior branches of the middle cerebral artery or carotid or basilar arteries.

Venous angiomas

These consist exclusively of aggregates of veins. They are often asymptomatic, but can give rise to epilepsy or haemorrhage.

Cavernous malformations (or cavernous angiomas)

These are aggregates of thin-walled vessels located both in brain and leptomeninges, including the brainstem. They usually become clinically manifest during the second or third decades, with seizures, headache and, less frequently, haemorrhages.

They appear as sharply demarcated nodules of variable size. Their thin vessels consist of endothelium and a surrounding ring of collagen of variable thickness. Angiomas in the brain can be associated with similar lesions in kidney, liver, lung and skin.

Capillary teleangiectasias

These consist of dilated capillaries separated by quasi-normal brain tissue. They are rarely symptomatic and are found predominantly in the pons. In addition, vascular malformations are known which combine the features of several lesions mentioned above.

Miscellaneous disorders

Cerebral amyloid angiopathy (CAA) results from extracellular deposition of protein fibrils (amyloid) in the walls of blood vessels of brain and meninges. The fibrils consist of β-pleated sheet secondary structures and are typically Congo red-positive. β-amyloid angiopathies are the commonest forms of amyloid deposition. The protein is encoded on chromosome 21. Presence of apolipoprotein Eε4 (ApoEε4) is a risk factor for CAA.

In sporadic cases, CAA is responsible for 5–12% of primary haemorrhages; however, the brainstem is not primarily involved by CAA.

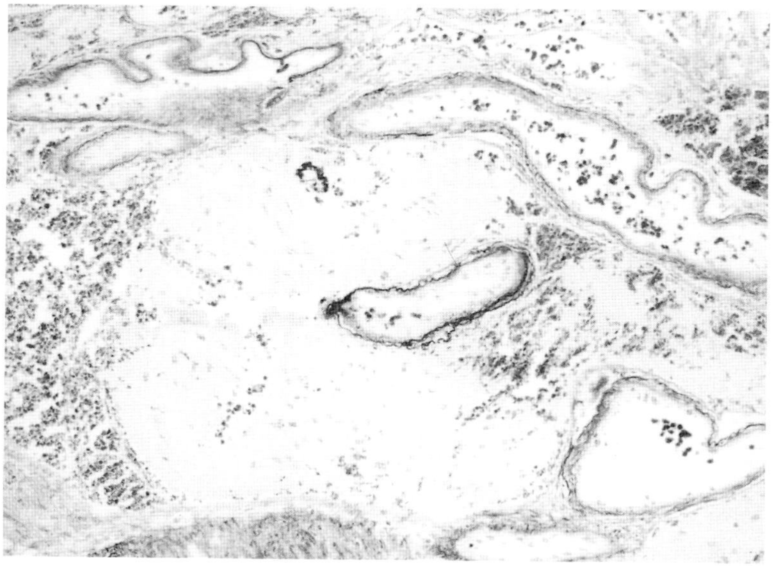

Figure 37.14 Photomicrograph of an arteriovenous malformation appearing as a tuft of vessels surrounded by brain tissue. The vessels have thin walls, some of which possess a complete or incomplete elastic lamina, appearing as a black thin line just beneath the endothelial lining. Elastin-van Gieson, ×90.

In fibromuscular dysplasia arteries are affected by a non-inflammatory thickening of the vessel wall. It occurs at any age, particularly in adults, is more common in women, and involves predominantly the mid-portion of the cervical internal carotid artery, mostly bilaterally. The extradural portion of the vertebral arteries is less frequently affected and involvement of the intracranial arteries is rare. However, Saygi et al[145] reported changes in the basilar artery and found five cases in the literature.

Any layer of the arterial wall may be affected, but it is the media that shows the most severe changes. These consist of fibrosis with segmental narrowing of the lumen which alternates with dilated portions of the vessel.

Haemosiderosis of the nervous system is the result of recurrent or persistent haemorrhages within the subarachnoid spaces, leading to deposition of large quantities of iron pigment in the subpial, subependymal tissue of the brain and spinal cord and leptomeninges. It was seen following hemispherectomy.[146] Koeppen and Wood[147] studied five cases and discussed the following causes: a small arteriovenous malformation of the inferior medullary velum, ependymoma of the cauda equina, undiagnosed chronic subdural haematoma and recurrent glioma. In the fifth case, a spinal arteriovenous malformation was suspected. Morita et al[148] reported haemosiderosis in a family with caeruloplasmin deficiency.

The lesion is quite uncommon; in advanced cases, patients present the typical triad of symptoms of progressive cerebellar ataxia, hearing loss and myelopathy. Both CT scan and MRI can help in the clinical diagnosis by confirming the presence of iron.[147]

Macroscopic examination reveals fibrous thickening and brown discoloration of the leptomeninges over the cerebral and cerebellar hemispheres; the VIII cranial nerve is involved, whereas the adjacent VII is free of pigment. The ependymal lining is also abnormal.

Histological examination shows reactive gliosis and presence of iron within astrocytes, macrophages and perivascular cells (Figure 37.15), as well as free in the tissue.

With regard to the pathogenesis of the lesion, two findings deserve attention: the particular vulnerability of the content of the posterior fossa, and that of the VIII nerve compared with the others. An important role in the process is played by ferritin, which is instrumental in sequestration and detoxification of iron,[149] and whose biosynthesis is stimulated by free iron molecules.[150,151] The biosynthesis of ferritin takes place in microglia, whereas the Bergmann glia is the source of iron- and haeme-responsive ferritin-repressor protein (FRP). Most of the haemosiderin formation (from haemoglobin, via haeme, iron and ferritin) occurs in microglia and macrophages, and the vulnerability of the cerebellar molecular layer probably depends on the large number of microglia and presence of Bergmann glia.[152] The severe damage of the VIII nerve is related to the fact that, in the subarachnoid space, its myelin is of the central type (and hence includes microglia), as the transition from CNS to peripheral nervous system is located quite distally, in proximity to the internal acoustical meatus, rather than near the exit from the brainstem, as occurs in the other cranial nerves from the III to the XII.[153,154]

Tumours

The brainstem can be the site of any primary and secondary tumours. However, some neoplasms are more common than others, while others, such as the schwannoma of the VIII nerve, are characteristic features of this region.

Peripheral nerve tumours

These include those consisting exclusively or partly of: (1) Schwann cells (schwannomas); (2) sheath fibroblasts; and (3) perineurial cells.

Schwannomas are the commonest type accounting for 7–8% of all primary intracranial tumours. Those arising from the VIII nerve represent 80–90% and, although they derive from its vestibular branch, the whole nerve (as well the facial) is affected. This neoplasm is found predominantly during the

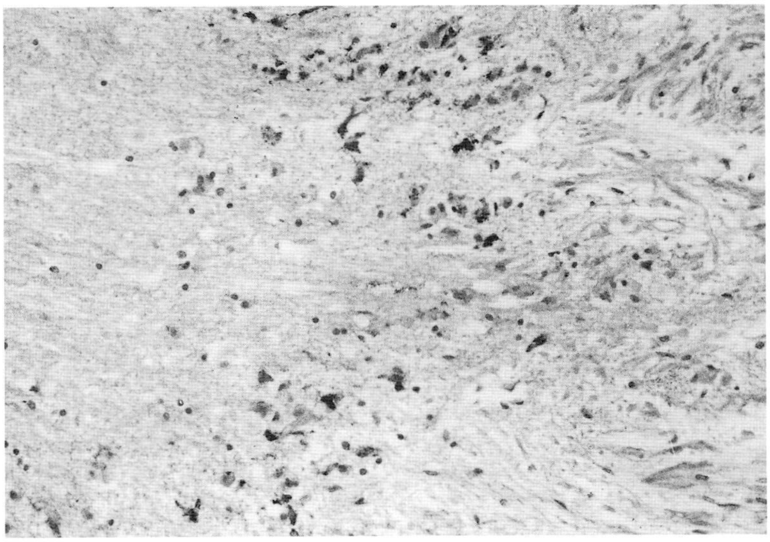

Figure 37.15 The vestibular nerve in a brain with haemosiderosis. Note the cluster of iron-containing cells at the transition between central (left) and peripheral (right) myelin. Perls, ×220.

5th decade and among women (female/male ratio 1.5 : 2/1)[155,156] and is unusual in children. About 95% are solitary; 5% are bilateral and part of the neurofibromatosis type 2 (NF2, see below) syndrome.

Other less frequent localizations are the trigeminal nerve roots and the ganglion. The tumour is found predominantly in sensory nerves, but motor ones (facial, hypoglossal, abducens and trochlear nerves) can also be affected, particularly in a setting of neurofibromatosis. Schwannomas of the nerve roots account for 16–30% of all spinal tumours, are particularly frequent in the lumbosacral region and cauda equina, and are found predominantly in males.

Intraparenchymal schwannomas also exist with both intracranial and spinal localizations. In the cerebral hemispheres they are periventricular, but they can be seen also in the brainstem and 4th ventricle. The absence of Schwann cells in both regions suggests that their origin is either from Schwann cells of nerves within vessels, from nerves running in the dura, or from ectopic neural crest cells.

Schwannomas are well-encapsulated formations, whose shape depends on the size and the compression they receive from adjacent structures (bone, brain, vessels). The VIII nerve of origin and the facial nerve may be stretched on the surface and appear as thin whitish filaments (Figure 37.16). On cut sections, the neoplasm is grey with yellow areas, but may contain areas of recent or old haemorrhage. Cystic areas may also be included.

Histologically, schwannomas reveals two main patterns irregularly intermingled and called Antoni type A and B. The former consists of interweaving fascicles of elongated cells, whose cytoplasm has ill-defined borders and whose nuclei are hyperchromatic and elongated. The arrangement of the latter in palisades may be seen (Figure 37.17a). The Antoni B (Figure 37.17b) pattern is characterized by spindle or stellate cells in a loose myxoid and microcystic background.

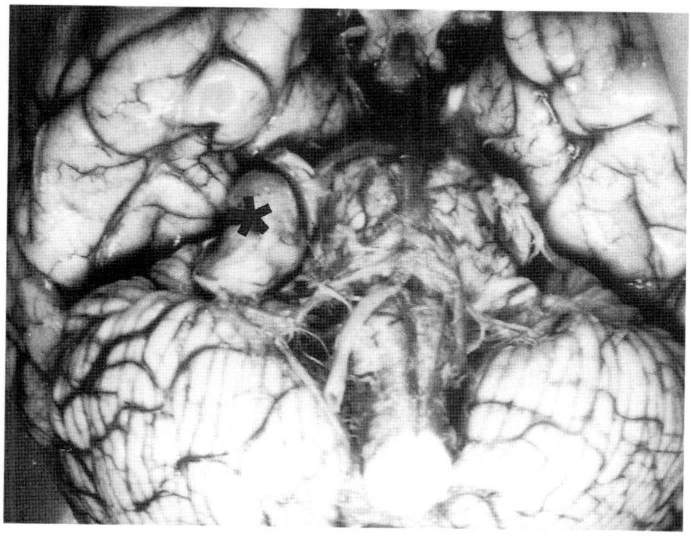

Figure 37.16 A cerebellopontine angle tumour (asterix) exerting compression in the region of the VII and VIII nerves.

Schwannomas also include hyalinized vessels, areas of fresh haemorrhage or foci of haemosiderin-laden macrophages, moderate nuclear pleomorphism, and, at least in tumours of the VIII nerve, total absence of mitoses.

Schwannomas are S-100 (Figure 37.17c) and vimentin positive. GFAP (glial fibrillary acidic protein) has also been demonstrated.[157,158]

Histological variants include cellular and melanotic schwannomas.

The former are unusual tumours found in younger individuals, predominantly females. Half of the cases in the series by Carney[159] were part of the Carney complex. In these instances, there was no sex predominance and the average age was 22.5 years. Font and Truong[160] reviewed the literature: the most frequent locations were the spinal nerve roots and adjacent structures (12 patients), the soft tissue (5), and heart, oesophageal wall, acoustic nerve and mandible (1 each). Further reports of this tumour localized to the acoustic nerve are those by Miller et al[161] and Earls et al,[162] the latter authors describing a malignant one.

NF2 is an autosomal dominant disorder with 95% penetrance; it affects 1/40 000–50 000 individuals and is associated with a gene abnormality on chromosome 22q12,[163] which acts as a tumour suppressor gene. The gene was cloned;[164,165] its product is merlin (or schwannomin). In addition to schwannomas, meningiomas or meningiomatosis, gliomas, particularly in the cord and microhamartomas are described.

NF1 is also an autosomal dominant disorder with 100% penetrance; approximately 1/3000 individuals are affected, and 2–29% of them progress to have malignant tumours. The gene responsible for the disorder has been located on chromosome 17q, and the protein it encodes is called neurofibromin. Affected patients present multiple, including paraspinal, neurofibromas, plexiform neurofibromas, optic nerve gliomas, and rarely paraspinal and pilocytic or high-grade astrocytomas.

Tumours of the meninges

These include meningiomas, mesenchymal tumours, primary melanocytic lesions and tumours of uncertain origin.

Meningiomas represent 13–19% of intracranial tumours; those with spinal localization represent 12%. Most of them appear between 45 and 55 years, have a female/male ratio of 1.8 : 1) and are rare during the first and second decades, when, however, they tend to be more aggressive. Meningiomas localized to the lower spinal regions are found exclusively in women.

They can develop anywhere, including inside the ventricles, predominantly in the lateral ones, only 15% and 5% being found in the 3rd and 4th, respectively. Extracranial meningiomas can also be seen. Multiple meningiomas, which are of the same histological type as single ones, are most commonly associated with NF2.

Although meningiomas are, on the whole, benign tumours, between 13%[166] and 29%[167] of all patients show recurrences, incomplete resection representing the main cause.

Meningiomas are of variable size (Figure 37.18), and their appearances depend on their location. In the majority of cases,

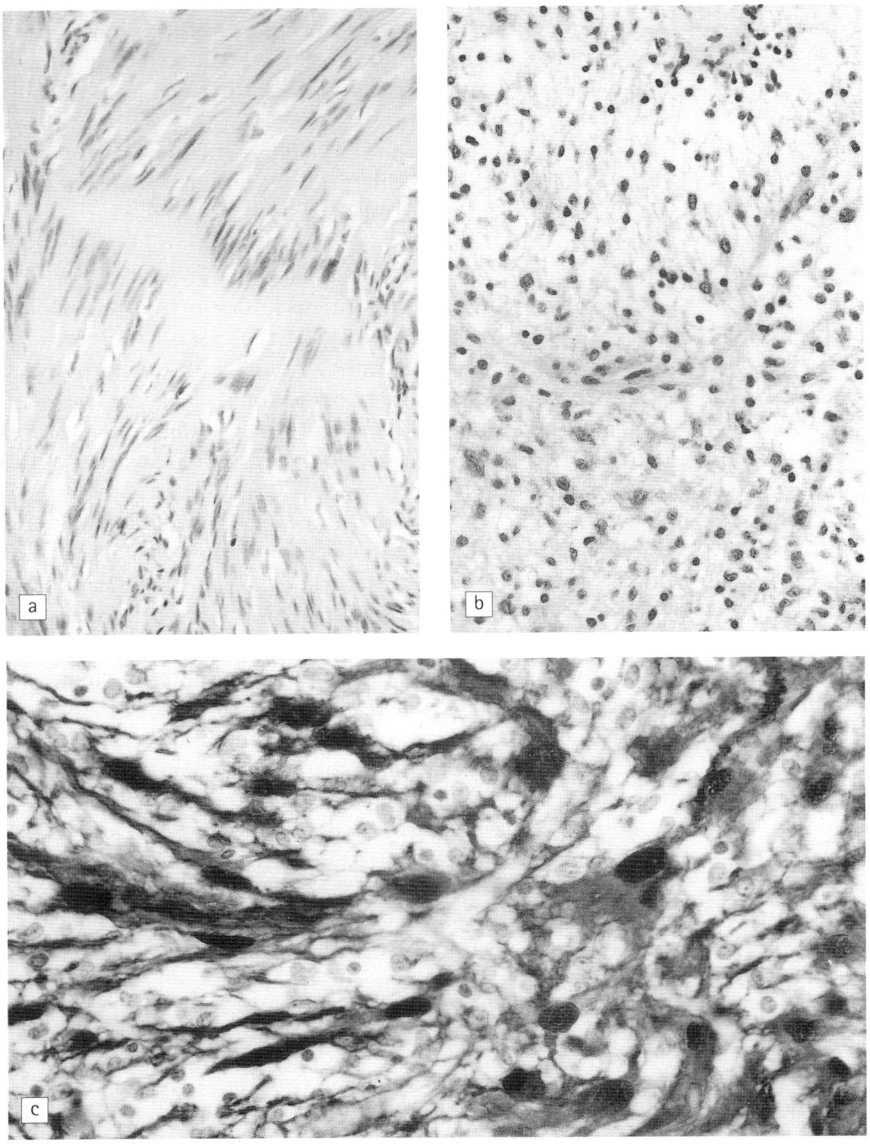

Figure 37.17 Schwannomas of the VIII nerve can present with two main histological appearances. In Antoni type A (a), cells are bipolar and their nuclei are often arranged to palisades. In Antoni type B (b), cell nuclei are seen in a loose microcystic background. Tumour cells are strongly S-100-positive; immunostaining involves both nuclei and cytoplasm of Schwann cells (c). (a, b): H&E, ×220; (c): S-100 immunostaining, ×600.

they are firmly adherent to the dura and their consistency varies from soft to firm and fibrotic. The so-called meningiomas *en plaque* grow by expanding widely instead of forming nodular structures; they are found predominantly at the base, on the sphenoid wing. Some tumours extend through the dura and may infiltrate the bone and even extend to the adjacent muscle. This behaviour is not considered, in the absence of other features, a criterion for malignancy.

The following histological subtypes have been described: (1) meningothelial (Figure 37.19a); (2) fibrous; (3) transitional; (4) psammomatous (Figure 37.19b); (5) angiomatous; (6) microcystic; (7) secretory; (8) clear cell (Figure 37.19c); (9) chordoid; (10) lymphoplasmacytic; and (11) metaplastic. On immunohistochemistry, all meningiomas are EMA (epithelial membrane antigen)-positive (Figure 37.19d).

The reader is referred to texts of neuropathology for more detailed descriptions of these subtypes.[168]

All the varieties mentioned above are classified as WHO grade 1. More aggressive tumours (grade 2) have the following features: increased mitotic activity and cellularity, high nuclear/cytoplasmic ratio, prominent nucleoli, patternless growth, necrosis and high Ki67 labelling index.

Anaplastic meningiomas have a poorly differentiated appearance, a high mitotic rate, areas of necrosis and brain invasion. They predominate during the 6th and 7th decades, with female predominance and a 100% tendency to recur.

The papillary variant of meningioma (Figure 37.20), is characterized by a perivascular pattern, reminiscent of ependymomas, and lacks any features of typical meningiomas. It develops at younger ages (50% in children), is invasive and tends to recur and metastasize. It is classified as grade 2–3.

Mesenchymal tumours of the meninges include: (1) haemangiopericytoma; (2) meningeal sarcomas; (3) fibrosarcomas; (4) chondrosarcomas; (5) rhabdomyosarcomas; (6)

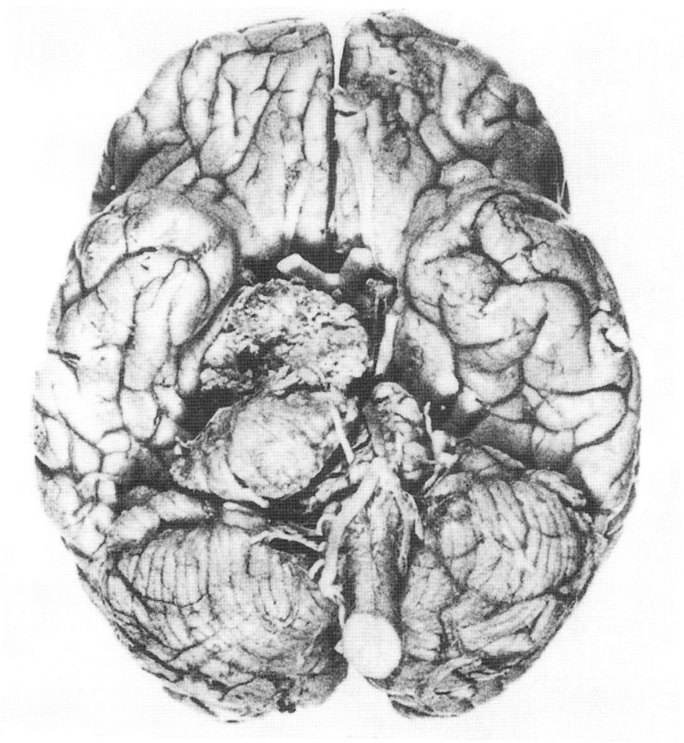

Figure 37.18 The meningioma shown in this photograph was located in the posterior fossa compressing the brainstem, including the VIII nerve.

meningeal sarcomatosis; and (7) solitary fibrous tumours of the meninges.

Haemangiopericytomas have an incidence of 2.5–7% of meningeal tumours and affect individuals in the 4th to 6th decades, with no sex predominance. Their common presentation in the tentorium and posterior fossa may affect the VIII nerve. Spinal and multiple tumours are also reported. Their cells are uniform in shape and size, with oval and hyperchromatic nuclei, and ill-defined borders, and surround thin capillaries (Figure 37.21). Reticulin is seen surrounding small clusters of cells. The tumour may include areas of necrosis, variable mitotic activity and obvious signs of anaplasia. Haemangiopericytomas are vimentin, CD34, desmin, actin and laminin positive, and EMA, GFAP and S-100 negative.

Haemangiopericytomas, particularly those originating from the posterior fossa and tentorium, should be regarded as malignant tumours with a high rate of recurrence and a tendency to invade.

Primary melanocytic lesions include diffuse melanosis, melanocytomas and malignant melanomas. As melanomas spread easily along nerve roots, whenever they develop within the posterior fossa they can involve multiple cranial nerves, including the VIII.

Chordomas are rare tumours (0.2% of brain tumours)[168] which occur at any age, although intracranial localizations are more frequent at a younger age than spinal ones. They are found predominantly in males (2 : 1).[169] Localization to the clivus accounts for 36%[169] and may produce vestibular symptoms.[170]

Chordomas vary in size from small and asymptomatic to large, soft and gelatinous masses. They consist of cells with small, round and hyperchromatic nuclei and abundant cytoplasm which may contain vacuoles (hence the name physaliphorous cells). Cells form clusters or elongated, branching aggregates which are located within a mucinous, alcian blue-positive matrix. Tumour cells are S-100 and cytokeratin positive, unlike the morphologically similar chondrosarcoma, which is only S-100 positive.

Among the tumours of uncertain origin, haemangioblastomas deserve a mention, as they are localized predominantly in the posterior fossa (93%); the next commonest site, the spinal cord, contributes with 3.8%, whereas supratentorial tumours represent only 2.9% of the cases. Their incidence is 1–2% of intracranial tumours and they may be seen at any age (peak at 35–45 years), with a male/female ratio of 2 : 1. Their association with von Hippel–Lindau disease is well known.

Haemangioblastomas are well encapsulated and vary in size from one to several centimetres. Their colour betokens their high levels in blood. Cystic cavities of variable size are not uncommon.

Histological examination shows a rich meshwork of capillaries surrounded by 'stromal' cells. These are relatively large, and have small hyperchromatic nuclei and cytoplasm that may appear homogeneously eosinophilic or finely vacuolated (Figure 37.22a). The content of the vacuoles consists of lipids. Mitotic activity is ususally not a feature. The reticulin component is rich and surrounds single cells or small clusters (Figure 37.22b).

Neuroepithelial tumours

These include the following subgroups:

1. astrocytomas
2. oligodendrogliomas
3. ependymomas
4. mixed gliomas
5. choroid plexus papillomas and carcinomas
6. neuroepithelial tumours of uncertain origin
7. neuronal and neuronal–glial tumours
8. pinealomas/pineoblastomas
9. embryonal tumours.

All these subgroups can involve, either directly or indirectly, the posterior fossa and the brainstem, and damage the cochleovestibular pathways. Some of them, however, are more common at this site and are briefly described.

Pilocytic astrocytomas

These are slow-growing tumours representing 6% of intracranial neoplasms and are the most frequent tumours in children: indeed 75% are found in patients below 20 years of age, with a peak between 8 and 13; there is no sex predominance. Preferred sites are the midline structures such as the optic nerve and chiasma, brainstem, spinal cord and cerebellum. The temporal lobe is the most frequent cerebral localization.

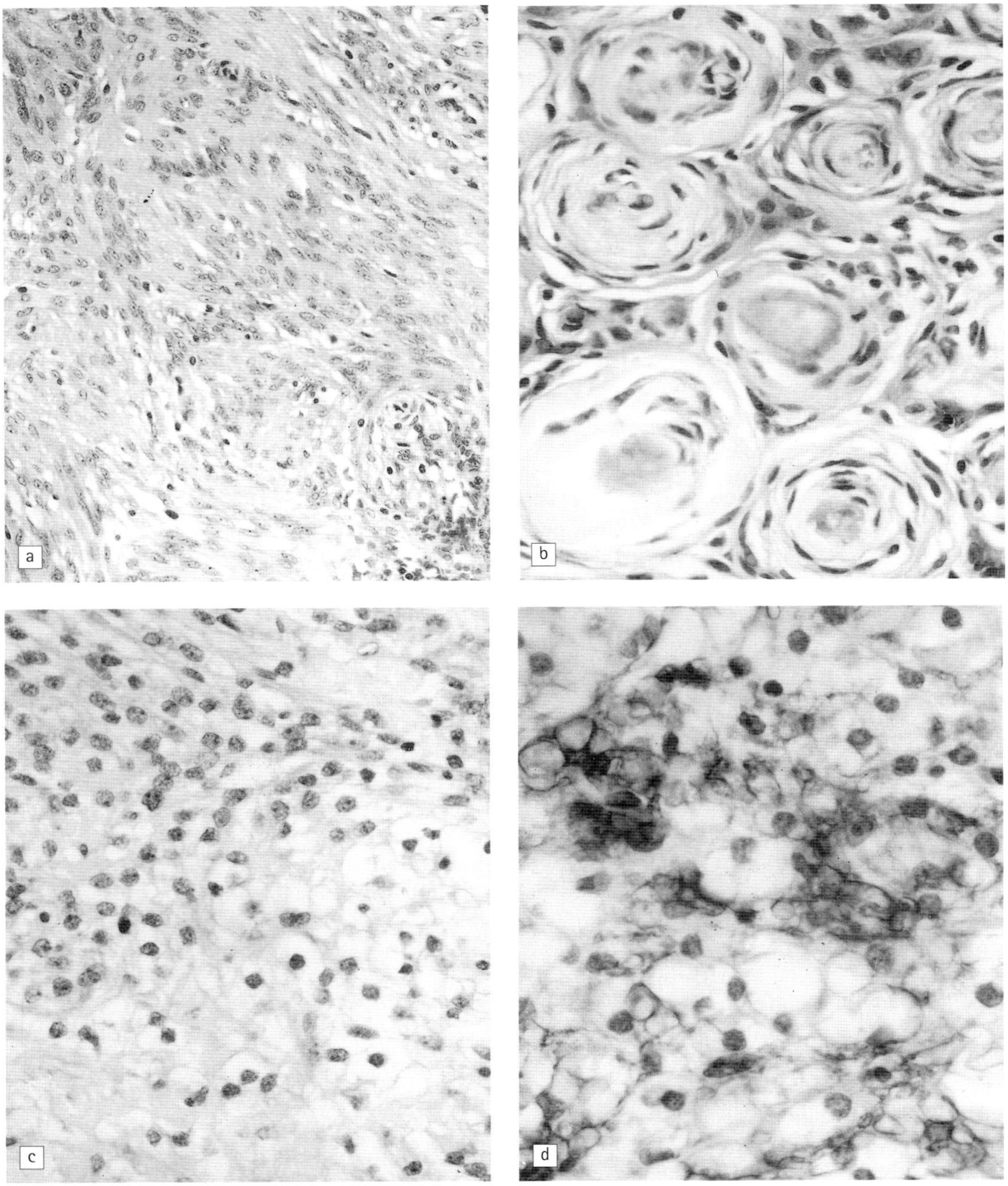

Figure 37.19
Photomicrographs of meningothelial (a), psammomatous (b) and clear cell (c) meningiomas. Immunohistochemically, all meningiomas are characterized by positive anti-EMA staining (d). (a, b, c): H&E; (a, c): ×220; (b, d): ×600.

Macroscopically they are generally well demarcated, except when they involve the optic nerves, and expand rather than infiltrate, with frequent cyst formation. Microscopically, they show a biphasic pattern consisting of pilocytic and microcystic areas; nuclei may have a considerable degree of pleomorphism, and blood vessels may show endothelial proliferation. Characteristic features of this neoplasm are the granular bodies and Rosenthal fibres. The reticulin component may be conspicuous, and the tumour can be seen invading the leptomeninges. Pilocytic astrocytomas are regarded as grade 1 tumours.

Diffuse astrocytomas are ubiquitous, but predominate in the cerebral hemispheres. They are characteristic of adulthood, infiltrate adjacent structures and tend to progress towards malignancy. They are classified as WHO grade 2–4. They may involve the brainstem, thus producing symptoms localized to one or more cranial nerves, including the VIII.

Mentioned by the WHO among the neuroepithelial tumours of uncertain origin, gliomatosis cerebri is a rare tumour involving the cerebral hemispheres and posterior fossa, and extending even to the spinal cord. Affected brains show global enlargement.

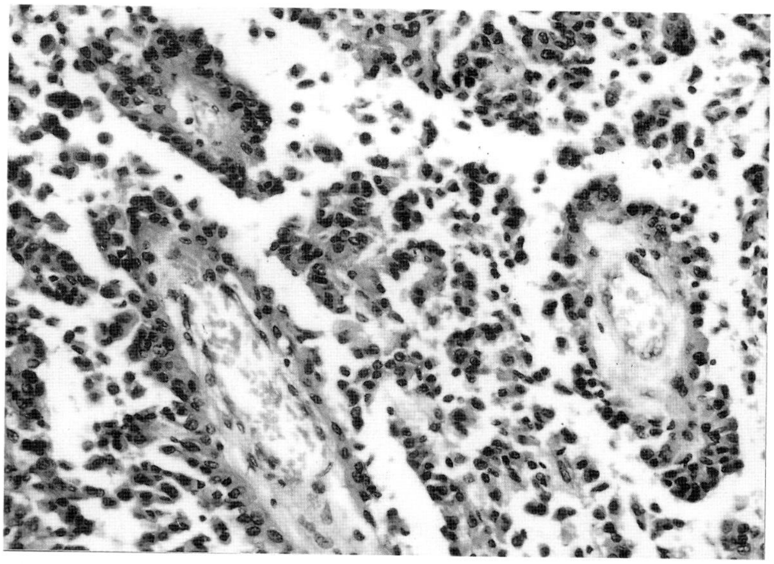

Figure 37.20 In the papillary variant of meningioma, cells are arranged in a pattern that is suggestive of ependymomas. H&E, ×220.

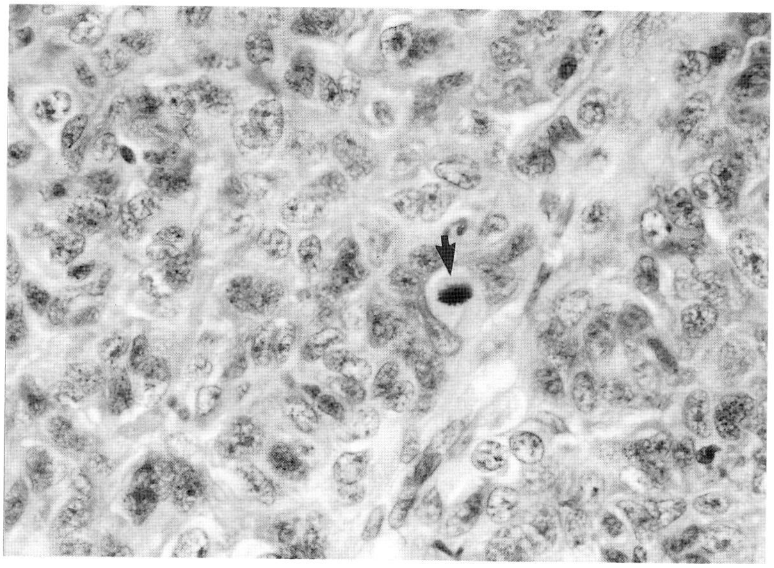

Figure 37.21 Photomicrographs of a haemangiopericytoma, showing closely packed cells surrounding thin-walled capillaries. Cells show some degree of pleomorphism and have nucleolated nuclei. Mitoses are usually seen (arrow). H&E, ×360.

Histological examination reveals oval or fusiform glial cells, with hyperchromatic and slightly pleomorphic nuclei, infiltrating the brain tissue without inflicting excessive distortion on its structures. GFAP positivity is variable. Their diagnosis can be made only at postmortem.

Because of their frequent localization to the 4th ventricle, ependymomas may produce vestibular symptoms. Their incidence varies between 1% and 6% of intracranial tumours, and they are most frequent from childhood to adulthood in both sexes. After the 4th ventricle, which represents the commonest site, the lateral and 3rd ventricles follow. In the spinal cord (cervicothoracic level), ependymomas are the most frequent neoplasm and may also occur outside the nervous system.

The following histological subtypes are described: cellular, papillary (rare), clear cell and tanycytic (reminiscent of astrocytomas).

The typical ependymoma is graded 2, and its proliferative index, as established by Ki67, is 2.6 ± 2.5%. It has a 44% tendency to recur, and a better prognosis in adults than in children and when localized to the spinal cord. Spinal seeding is now considered a rarer event than previously thought. Recurrences may be local or extradural.

A number of ependymomas, varying from 5% to 7%, are considered anaplastic and rated as WHO grade 3. About 27% of these can occur in the posterior fossa. Their diagnostic criteria are loss of ependymal differentiation, pleomorphism, necrosis, high mitotic rate and local invasion.

Mixed neuronal and neuronal–glial tumours

This group includes gangliogliomas with their anaplastic and desmoplastic infantile variants, the desmoplastic cerebral astrocytoma of infancy, ganglioneuromas and desmoplastic neuroepithelial tumours.

Gangliogliomas represent 0.4–6% of primary brain tumours, but amount to 20% of the epilepsy-related lesions. They develop at all ages, but are found predominantly around

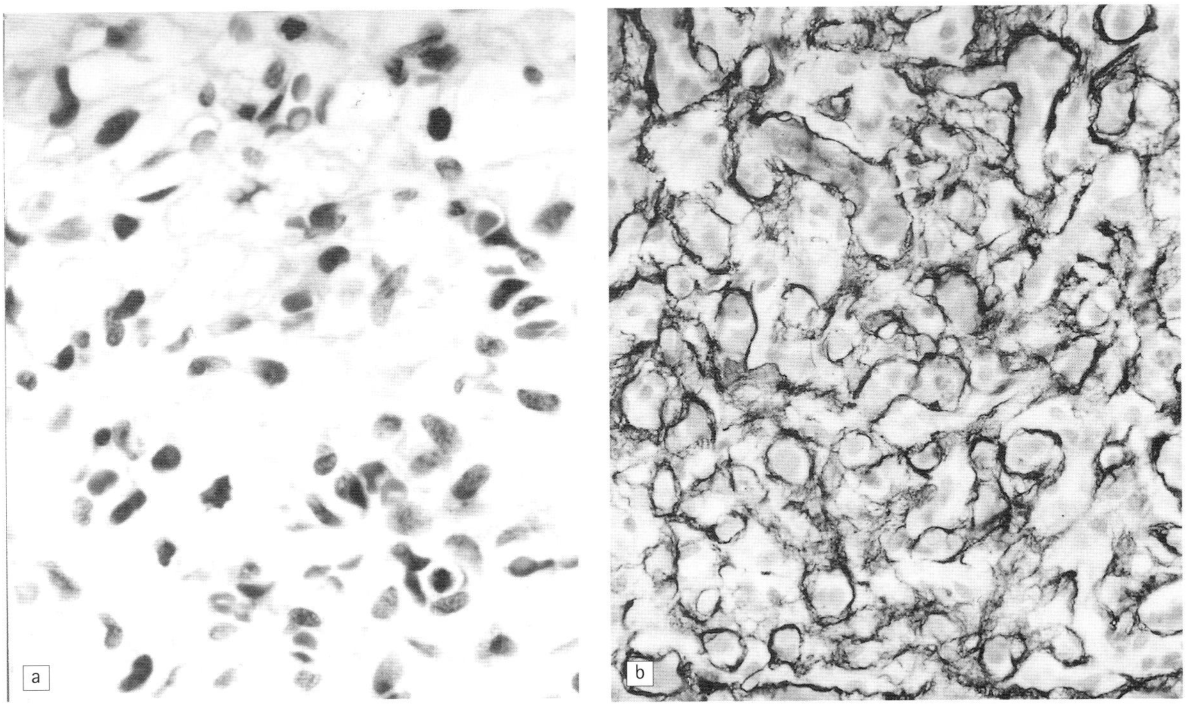

Figure 37.22
The histological appearances of haemangioblastomas include the presence of large cells with dark nuclei and pale, in places finely vacuolated, cytoplasm (a). Single or small clusters of cells are surrounded by a fine meshwork of reticulin fibrils (b). (a) H&E, ×360; (b) silver impregnation for reticulin, ×360.

20 years (14 years in the brainstem location) and have a male/female ratio of 1.3 : 1. They can be found in all the cerebral lobes, cerebellum, brainstem, sella, optic nerve and chiasma and spinal cord. There is no association with phakomatoses, but they are associated with neuronal migration disorders, Down's syndrome, agenesis of the corpus callosum, cerebral micropolygyria, cortical glioneuronal hamartias and vascular malformations.

Their histological features include the presence of neoplastic ganglion cells and neoplastic glia, some areas appearing exclusively glial, a variable stromal component and the presence of focal perivascular lymphocytic infiltrates.

When gangliogliomas progress towards malignancy, this takes place in the glial component, which may become indistinguishable from glioblastoma multiforme.

References

1. Brodal A. Anatomy of the vestibular nuclei and their connections. In: *Handbook of Sensory Physiology: Vestibular System*, Vol. 6. Kornhuber HH, ed. Berlin: Springer-Verlag, 1974; 239–352.
2. Brodal A, Hoivik B. Site and mode of termination of primary vestibulo-cerebellar fibres in the cat. *Arch Ital Biol* 1964; **102**: 1–21.
3. Wilson VJ, Yoshida M. Monosynaptic inhibition of neck motoneurons by the medial vestibular nucleus. *Exp Brain Res* 1969; **9**: 365–80.
4. Schulze-Bahr E, Haverkamp W, Wedekind H et al. Autosomal recessive long QT syndrome (Jarvell Lange–Nielsen syndrome) is genetically heterogeneous. *Hum Genet* 1997; **100**: 573–6.
5. Attaie A, Kim E, Wilcox ER, Lalwani AK. A splice-site mutation affecting the paired box of PAX3 in a three generation family with Waardenburg syndrome type 1 (WS1). *Mol Cell Probes* 1997; **11**: 233–6.
6. Pingault V, Bondurand N, Kuhlbrodt K et al. SOX10 mutations in patients with Waardenburg–Hirschprung disease. *Nat Genet* 1998; **18**: 171–3.
7. Watanabe A, Takeda K, Ploplis B, Tachibana M. Epistatic relationship between Waardenburg syndrome genes MITF and PAX3. *Nature Genet* 1998; **18**: 283–6.
8. Espinos C, Najera C, Millan JM et al. Linkage analysis in Usher syndrome type 1 (UST1) families from Spain. *J Med Genet* 1998; **35**:391–8.
9. Cremers WR, Bolder C, Admiraal RJ et al. Progressive sensorineural hearing loss and a widened vestibular aqueduct in Pendred syndrome. *Arch Otolaryngol Head Neck Surg* 1998; **124**: 501–5.
10. Mustapha M, Azar ST, Moglabey YB et al. Further refinement of Pendred syndrome locus by homozygosity analysis to a 0.8 cM interval flanked by D7s496 and D7s2425. *J Med Genet* 1998; **35**: 202–4.
11. Chiari H. Über die Veränderungen des Kleinhirns, des Pons, und des Medulla oblongata infolge von congenitaler Hydrocephalie des Grosshirns. *Dtsch Med Wochenschr* 1891; **27**: 1172–5.
12. Shady W, Metcalfe RA, Butler P. The incidence of craniocervical bony anomalies in the adult Chiari malformation. *J Neurol Sci* 1987; **82**: 193–203.
13. Harding BN, Copp AJ. Malformations. In: Graham DI, Lantos PL, eds. *Greenfield's Neuropathology*, Vol. 1. London: Arnold, 1997: 397–533.
14. McLendon RE, Crain BJ, Oakes WJ, Burger PC. Cerebral polygyria in the Chiari type II (Arnold–Chiari) malformation. *Clin Neuropathol* 1985; **4**: 200–5.

15. Hain TC, Zee DS, Maria BL. Tilt suppression of vestibulo-ocular reflex in patients with cerebellar lesions. *Acta Otolaryngol (Stockh)* 1988; **105**: 13–20.
16. Perez-Garrigues H, Yaya R, Lopez-Arlandis J et al. Oculographic findings in the Arnold–Chiari malformation type 1. *An Otorinolaringol Ibero-Am* 1991; **18**: 479–90.
17. Bronstein AM, Miller DH, Rudge P, Kendall BE. Down beating nystagmus: magnetic resonance imaging and neuro-otological findings. *J Neurol Sci* 1987; **81**: 173–84.
18. Rudge P. *Clinical Neuro-otology*. Edinburgh: Churchill Livingstone, 1984.
19. Lindsay JR, Hemenway WG. Postural vertigo due to unilateral sudden partial loss of vestibular function. *Ann Otol* 1956; **65**: 692–706.
20. Dix MR, Hallpike CS. The pathology, symptomatology and diagnosis of certain common disorders of the vestibular system. *Ann Otol Rhinol Laryngol* 1952; **61**: 987–1016.
21. Cawthorne TE, Hallpike CS. A study of the clinical features and pathological changes within the temporal bones, brainstem and cerebellum of an early case of positional nystagmus of the so-called benign paroxysmal type. *Acta Otolaryngol (Stockh)* 1957; **48**: 89–105.
22. Schuknecht HF. Cupolithiasis. *Arch Otolaryngol* 1969; **90**: 765–78.
23. Herdman SJ, Tusa RJ, Zee DS et al. Single treatment approaches to benign paroxysmal positional vertigo. *Arch Otolaryngol Head Neck Surg* 1993; **119**: 450–4.
24. Savundra PA, Carroll JD, Davies RA, Luxon LM. Migraine-associated vertigo. *Cephalalgia* 1997; **17**: 505–10.
25. Szirmai A. Vestibular disorders in patients with migraine. *Eur Arch Otorhinolaryngol Suppl* 1997; **1**: S55–7.
26. Barinagarrementeria F, Gonzalez-Duarte A, Miranda L, Cantu C. Cerebral infarction in young women: analysis of 130 cases. *Eur Neurol* 1998; **40**: 228–33.
27. La Mantia L, Pollo B, Savoiardo M et al. Meningo-cortical calcifying angiomatosis and celiac disease. *Clin Neurol Neurosurg* 1998; **100**: 209–15.
28. Prayson RA, Wang N. Mitochondrial myopathy, lactic acidosis and stroke-like episodes (MELAS) syndrome: an autopsy report. *Arch Pathol Lab Med* 1998; **122**: 978–81.
29. Ohno K, Isotani E, Hirakawa K. MELAS presenting as migraine complicated by stroke: case report. *Neuroradiology* 1997; **39**: 781–4.
30. Sano M, Ozawa M, Shiota S et al. The T-C 8356; mitochondrial DNA mutation in a Japanese family. *J Neurol* 1996; **243**: 441–4.
31. Desmond DW, Moroney JT, Lynch T et al. CADASIL in a North American family: clinical, pathologic and radiologic findings. *Neurology* 1998; **51**: 844–9.
32. Mellies JK, Baumer T, Muller JA et al. SPECT study of a German CADASIL family: a phenotype with migraine and progressive dementia only. *Neurology* 1998; **50**: 1715–21.
33. Taillia H, Chabriat H, Kurtz A et al. Cognitive alterations in non-demented CADASIL patients. *Cerebrovasc Dis* 1998; **8**: 97–101.
34. Chabriat H, Joutel A, Vahedi K, et al. CADASIL: Cerebral Autosomal Dominant Arteriopathy with Subcortical Infarcts and Leukoencephalopathy. *Rev Neurol (Paris)* 1997; **153**: 376–85.
35. Rubio A, Rifkin D, Powers JM et al. Phenotypic variability of CADASIL and novel morphologic findings. *Acta Neuropathol* 1997; **94**: 247–54.
36. Jen J, Cohen AH, Yue Q et al. Hereditary endotheliopathy with retinopathy, nephropathy and stroke (HERNS). *Neurology* 1997; **49**: 1322–30.
37. Battistella PA, Carollo C. Clinical and neuroradiological findings of moyamoya disease in Italy. *Clin Neurol Neurosurg* 1997; **99** Suppl 2: S54–7.
38. Gurwood AS, Brilliant R, Malloy KA. The enigma of giant cell arteritis: multidisciplinary management of two cases. *J Am Optom Assoc* 1998; **69**: 501–9.
39. Friedman I. *Pathology of the Ear*. Oxford: Blackwell Scientific Publications, 1974: 119–26.
40. Michaels L. *Ear, Nose and Throat Histopathology*. London: Springer-Verlag, 1987.
41. Naveh Y, Kaftori JK, Alon U et al. Progressive diaphyseal dysplasia: genetics, clinical and radiologic manifestations. *Pediatrics* 1984; **74**: 399–405.
42. Heymans O, Gebhart M, Alexiou J, Sokolow Y. Camurati–Englemann disease: effects of corticosteroids. *Acta Clin Belg* 1998; **53**: 189–92.
43. Higashi K, Matsuki C. Hearing impairment in Englemann disease. *Am J Otol* 1996; **17**: 26–9.
44. Hanson W, Parnes LS. Vestibular nerve compression in Camurati–Engelmann disease. *Ann Otol Rhinol Laryngol* 1995; **104**: 823–5.
45. Wilhelm KR, Lenarz T, Weise D et al. Value of various radiological study results in the follow-up of Camurati–Engelmann disease. *ROFO Fortschr Geb Rontgenstr Nuklearmed* 1987; **147**: 278–82.
46. Nellissery MJ, Padalecki SS, Brkanac Z et al. Evidence for a novel osteosarcoma tumor-suppressor gene in the chromosome 18 region genetically linked with Paget disease of the bone. *Am J Hum Genet* 1998; **63**: 817–24.
47. Proops D, Bayley D, Hawke M. Paget's disease and the temporal bone. A clinical and histopathological review of six temporal bones. *J Otolaryngol* 1985; **14**: 20–9.
48. Belal A, Glorig A. Dysequilibrium of ageing (presbyastasis) *J Laryngol Otol* 1986; **100**: 1037–41.
49. Johnsson LG, Hawkins JE. Pathologic changes in idiopathic labyrinthine hydrops. *Acta Otolaryngol (Stockh)* 1972; **73**: 402–12.
50. Rosenhall U. Epithelial cysts in the human vestibular apparatus. *J Laryngol Otol* 1974; **88**: 105–12.
51. Ransmayr G, Benesch H, Nowakowski C et al. Neurofibrillary tangles without cell loss in the lateral vestibular nucleus of patients with Alzheimer's disease. *Neurosci Lett* 1994; **177**: 11–14.
52. Jankovic J. Progressive supranuclear palsy. Clinical and pharmacologic update. *Neurol Clin* 1984; **2**: 473–86.
53. Pilz P, Erhart P. Thalamic degeneration. *Acta Neuropathol Suppl* 1981; **7**: 362–4.
54. Papp MI, Kahn JE, Lantos PL. Glial cytoplasmic inclusions in the CNS of patients with multiple system atrophy (striatonigral degeneration, olivoponto-cerebellar atrophy and Shy–Drager syndrome). *J Neurol Sci* 1989; **94**: 1–3.

55. Bates G. Expanded glutamines and neurodegeneration — a gain of insight. *Bioassays* 1996; **18**: 175–8.
56. Robitaille Y, Lopes-Cendes I, Becher M et al. The neuropathology of CAG repeat diseases: review and update of genetic and molecular features. *Brain Pathol* 1997; **7**: 901–26.
57. Woods BT, Schaumburg HH. Nigrospinodentatal degeneration with nuclear ophthalmoplegia. A unique and partially treatable clinicopathological entity. *J Neurol Sci* 1972; **17**: 149–66.
58. Romanul FCA, Fowler HL, Radvany J et al. Azorean disease of the nervous system. *N Engl J Med* 1977; **296**: 1505–8.
59. Coutinho P, Guimarães A, Scaravilli F. The pathology of machadoJoseph disease. Report of a possible homozygous case. *Acta Neuropathol* 1982; **58**: 48–54.
60. Iizuka R, Hirayama K, Maehara K. Dentato-rubro-pallido-luysian atrophy: a clinico-pathological study. *J Neurol Neurosurg Psychiatry* 1984; **47**: 1288–98.
61. Hayashi Y, Kakita A, Yamada M et al. Hereditary dentatorubral–pallidoluysian atrophy: detection of widespread ubiquitinated neuronal and glial intranuclear inclusions in the brain. *Acta Neuropathol* 1998; **96**: 547–52.
62. Kuzuhara S, Kanazawa I, Sasaki H et al. Gerstmann–Sträussler–Scheinker's disease. *Ann Neurol* 1983; **14**: 216–25.
63. Conlon BJ, Smith DW. Supplemental iron exacerbates aminoglycoside ototoxicity *in vivo*. *Hear Res* 1998; **115**: 1–5.
64. Sone M, Schachern PA, Paparella MM. Loss of spiral ganglion cells as primary manifestation of aminoglycoside ototoxicity. *Hear Res* 1998; **115**: 217–23.
65. Nakagawa T, Yamane H, Takayama M et al. Apoptosis of guinea pig cochlear hair cells following chronic aminoglycoside. *Eur Arch Otorhinolaryngol* 1998; **255**: 127–31.
66. Nakagawa T, Yamane H, Shibata S, Nakai Y. Gentamycin ototoxicity induced apoptosis of the vestibular hair cells of guinea pig. *Eur Arch Otorhinolaryngol* 1997; **254**: 9–14.
67. Matz GJ. The ototoxic effects of ethacrynic acid in man and animals. *Laryngoscope* 1976; **86**: 1065–86.
68. Mathog RH, Capps MJ. Ototoxic interactions of ethacrynic acid and streptomycin. *Ann Otol Rhinol Laryngol* 1977; **86**: 158–63.
69. Pickrell JA, Oehme FW, Cash WC. Ototoxicity in dogs and cats. *Semin Vet Med Surg Small Anim* 1993; **8**: 42–9.
70. Kangsanarak J, Navacharoen N, Fooanant S, Ruckphpaopunt K. Intracranial complications of suppurative otitis media: 13 years' experience. *Am J Otol* 1995; **16**: 104–9.
71. Merchant SN, Gopen Q. A human temporal lobe study of acute bacterial meningogenic labyrinthitis. *Am J Otol* 1996; **17**: 375–85.
72. Brandt T. Bilateral vestibulopathy revisited. *Eur J Med Res* 1996; **1**: 361–8.
73. Rinne T, Bronstein AM, Rudge P et al. Bilateral loss of vestibular function: clinical findings in 53 patients. *J Neurol* 1998; **245**: 314–21.
74. Hugosson S, Carlsson E, Borg E et al. Audiovestibular and neuropsychological outcome of adults who had recovered from childhood bacterial meningitis. *Int J Pediatr Otolaryngol* 1997; **42**: 149–67.
75. Moss PD. Outcome of meningococcal group B meningitis. *Arch Dis Child* 1982; **57**: 616–21.
76. Naess A, Halstensen A, Nyland H et al. Sequelae one year after meningococcal disease. *Acta Neurol Scand* 1994; **89**: 139–42.
77. Koskiniemi M, Pettay O, Raivio M, Sarna S. *Haemophilus influenzae* meningitis. A comparison between chloramphenicol and ampicillin therapy with special reference to impaired hearing. *Acta Paediatr Scand* 1978; **67**: 17–24.
78. Wilson WR, Cockerill FR. Tetracyclines, chloramphenicol, erythromycin and clindamycin. *Mayo Clin Proc* 1987; **62**: 906–15.
79. Rasmussen N, Johnsen NJ, Bohr VA. Otologic sequelae after pneumococcal meningitis: a survey of 164 consecutive cases with follow-up of 94 survivors. *Laryngoscope* 1991; **101**: 876–82.
80. Heininger U, Ries M, Christ P, Harms D. Simultaneous palsy of facial and vestibular nerve in a child with Lyme borreliosis. *Eur J Pediatr* 1990; **149**: 781–2.
81. McNeil NI, Gordon T. Meningitis caused by Streptococcus suis type II. *Postgrad Med J* 1986; **62**: 743–4.
82. Delaney P. Neurologic manifestations in sarcoidosis: review of the literature, with a report of 23 cases. *Ann Intern Med* 1977; **87**: 336–45.
83. Jahrsdoerfer RA, Thompson EG, Johns MM, Cantrell RW. Sarcoidosis and fluctuating hearing loss. *Ann Otol Rhinol Laryngol* 1981; **90**: 161–3.
84. Briner VA, Muller A, Gebbers JO. Neuro Sarcoidosis *Schweiz Med Wochenschr* 1998; **128**: 799–810.
85. Hooper R, Holden H. Acoustic and vestibular problems in sarcoidosis. *Arch Otolaryngol* 1970; **92**: 386–91.
86. Karmody CS, Schuknecht HF. Deafness in congenital syphilis. *Arch Otolaryngol* 1966; **83**: 18–27.
87. Musher DM, Hamill RJ, Baughn RE. Effect of human immunodeficiency virus (HIV) infection on the course of syphilis and on the response to treatment. *Ann Intern Med* 1990; **113**: 872–81.
88. Meyerhoff WL, Paparella MM, Oda M, Shea D. Mycotic infections of the inner ear. *Laryngoscope* 1979; **89**: 1725–34.
89. Ashman RB, Papadimitriou JM, Fulurija A. Acute labyrinthitis associated with systemic *Candida albicans* infection in ageing mice. *J Laryngol Otol* 1996; **110**: 13–18.
90. Papadimitriou JM, Ashman RB. The pathogenesis of acute systemic candidiasis in a susceptible inbred mouse strain. *J Pathol* 1986; **150**: 257–65.
91. Scaravilli F, Cook GC. Parasitic and fungal infections. In: Graham DI, Lantos PL, eds. *Greenfield's Neuropathology*, 6th edn, Vol. 2. London: Arnold, 1997: 65–111.
92. Burtch M. Granulomatous meningitis caused by Coccidioides immitis in a dog. *J Am Vet Med Assoc* 1998; **212**: 827–9.
93. Igarashi M, Weber SC, Alford BR et al. Temporal bone findings in cryptococcal meningitis. *Arch Otolaryngol* 1975; **101**: 577–83.
94. Teuscher E, Vrins A, Lemaire T. A vestibular syndrome associated with Cryptococcus neoformans in a horse. *Zentralbl Veterinarmed A* 1984; **31**: 132–9.
95. Ronge J, Aidoo GA, Kruger G. Cysticercosis of the brain. *Fortschr Neurol Psychiat Grenzgeb* 1978; **46**: 269–86.
96. Palomico-Nicas ME, Pachon-Diaz J. Hydatidosis of the posterior fossa. *An Med Interna* 1989; **6**: 257–9.
97. Adour KK, Byl FM, Hilsinger RL, Wilcox RD. Menière disease as a form of cranial polyganglionitis. *Laryngoscope* 1980; **90**: 392–8.

98. Mangabeira-Albernaz PL, Gananca MM. Sudden vertigo of central origin. *Acta Otolaryngol* 1988; **105**: 564–9.
99. Furuta Y, Takasu T, Fukuda S et al. Latent Herpes simplex type 1 in human vestibular ganglia. *Acta Otolaryngol Suppl* 1993; **503**: 85–9.
100. Shimizu T, Sekitani T, Hirata T, Hara H. Serum viral antibody titer in vestibular neuronitis. *Acta Otolaryngol Suppl* 1993; **503**: 74–8.
101. Thömke F, Hopf HC. Pontine lesions mimicking acute peripheral vestibulopathy. *J Neurol Neurosurg Psychiatry* 1999; **66**: 340–9.
102. Friedman I, House W. Vestibular neuronitis. Electron microscopy of Scarpa's ganglion. *J Laryngol Otol* 1980; **94**: 877–83.
103. Kaji M, Kusuhara T, Ayabe M et al. Survey of Herpes simplex virus infections of the central nervous system, including acute disseminated encephalomyelitis in the Kyushu and Okinawa regions of Japan. *Mult Scler* 1996; **2**: 83–7.
104. Schmidbauer M, Budka H, Ambros P. Herpes simplex virus (HSV) DNA in microglial nodular brainstem encephalitis. *J Neuropathol Exp Neurol* 1989; **48**: 645–52.
105. Esiri MM, Kennedy PGE. Viral diseases. In: Graham DI, Lantos PL eds. *Greenfield's Neuropathology*, 6th edn, Vol. 2. London: Arnold, 1997: 3–63.
106. Fuller GN, Guiloff RJ, Scaravilli F, Harcourt-Webster JN. Combined HIV–CMV encephalitis presenting with brainstem signs. *J Neurol Neurosurg Psychiatry* 1989; **52**: 975–9.
107. Gray F, Nordmann P. Bacterial infections. In: Graham DI, Lantos PL, eds. *Greenfield's Neuropathology*, Vol. 2. London: Arnold, 1997: 113–52.
108. Moench TR, Griffin DE, Obriecht CR et al. Acute measles in patients with or without neurological involvement: distribution of measles virus antigen and RNA. *J Infect Dis* 1988; **158:** 433–42.
109. Gendelman HE, Wolinsky JS, Johnson RT et al. Measles encephalomyelitis: lack of evidence of viral invasion of the central nervous system and quantitative study of the nature of demyelination. *Ann Neurol* 1984; **15**: 353–60.
110. Levine S. Relationship of experimental allergic encephalomyelitis to human disease. In: Rowland LP, ed. *Immunological Disorders of the Nervous System*, Vol. 49. Baltimore: Research Publications, Association for Research in Nervous and Mental Diseases, Williams and Wilkins, 1971: 33–49.
111. Behan PO, Geschwind N, Lamarche JB et al. Delayed hypersensitivity to encephalitogenic protein in disseminated encephalomyelitis. *Lancet*, 1968; **2**: 1009–12.
112. Johnson RT, Griffin DE, Hirsch RL et al. Measles encephalomyelitis: clinical and immunologic studies. *N Engl J Med* 1984; **310**: 137–41.
113. Posey K, Alpert JN, Langford LA, Yeakley JW. Acute hemorrhagic leukoencephalitis: a cause of acute brainstem dysfunction. *South Med J* 1994; **87**: 851–4.
114. Graham DI, Behan PO, More IA. Brain damage complicating septic shock: acute haemorrhagic leukoencephalitis as a complication of the generalized Schwartzman reaction. *J Neurol Neurosurg Psychiatry* 1979; **42**: 19–28.
115. Sawashima Y, Sawashima K, Taura Y et al. Clinical and pathological findings of a Yorkshire terrier affected with necrotizing encephalitis. *J Vet Med Sci* 1996; **58**: 659–61.
116. Kalimo H, Kaste M, Haltia M. Vascular diseases. In: Graham DI, Lantos PL, eds. *Greenfield's Neuropathology*, Vol. 1. London: Arnold, 1997: 315–96.
117. Keane JR. Eye movement abnormalities in systemic lupus erythematosus. *Arch Neurol* 1995; **52:** 1145–9.
118. Smith RW, Ellison DW, Jenkins EA et al. Cerebellum and brain stem vasculopathy in systemic lupus erythematosus. *Ann Rheum Dis* 1994; **53**: 327–30.
119. Bromberg MB, Junck L, Gebarski SS, McLean MJ, Gilman S. The Marinesco–Sjögren syndrome examined by computed tomography, magnetic resonance and 18F-2–fluoro-2–deoxy-D-glucose and positron emission tomography. *Arch Neurol* 1990; **47**: 1239–42.
120. Fukuyama H, Kameyama M, Nabatame H et al. Magnetic resonance images of neuro-Behçet syndrome show precise brain stem lesions. Report of a case. *Acta Neurol Scand* 1987; **75**: 70–3.
121. Iwasaki Y, Kinoshita M, Ikeda K et al. Central nervous system magnetic resonance imaging findings in neuro-Behçet syndrome. *Comput Med Imaging Graph* 1990; **14**: 85–7.
122. Forman HP, Levin S, Stewart B et al. Cerebral vasculitis and hemorrhage in an adolescent taking diet pills containing phenylpropanolamine: case report and review of the literature. *Pediatrics* 1989; **83**: 737–41.
123. Henson RA, Urich H. *Cancer and the Nervous System*. Oxford: Blackwell Scientific Publications, 1982.
124. Giometto B, Scaravilli F, eds. Symposium on paraneoplastic disorders. *Brain Pathol* 1999; **9**: 220–3.
125. Scaravilli F, An SF, Groves M, Thom M. The neuropathology of paraneoplastic syndromes. *Brain Pathol* 1999; **9**: 251–60.
126. Gulya AJ. Neurologic paraneoplastic syndromes with neurootologic manifestations. *Laryngoscope* 1993; **103**: 754–61.
127. Stebhens WE. *Pathology of the Cerebral Blood Vessels*. St Louis: Mosby, 1972: 98–130.
128. Fisher CM, Gore I, Okabe N, White PD. Atherosclerosis of the carotid and vertebral arteries — extracranial and intracranial. *J Neuropathol Exp Neurol* 1965; **24**: 455–76.
129. Meyer WW, Beck H. Das röntgenanatomische und feingewebliche Bild der Arteriosklerose im intrakranielle Abschitt der A. Carotis interna. *Virch Arch* 1955; **326**: 700.
130. Charcot J-M, Bouchard C. Nouvelles recherches sur la pathogénie de l'hémorrhagie cérébrale. *Arch Physiol (Paris)* 1869; **1**: 110, 643, 725.
131. Fisher CM. Cerebral miliary aneurysms in hypertension. *Am J Pathol* 1972; **66**: 313–30.
132. Wakai S, Nagai M. Histological verification of microaneurysms as a cause of cerebral haemorrhage in surgical specimens. *J Neurol Neurosurg Psychiatry* 1989; **52**: 595–9.
133. Challa VR, Moody DM, Bell MA. The Charcot–Bouchard aneurysms controversy: impact of a new histologic technique. *J Neuropathol Exp Neurol* 1992; **51**: 264–71.
134. Binswanger O. Die Abgrenzung des allgemeinen progressiven Paralysie. *Klin Wochenschr* 1894; **31**: 1103–5, 1137–9, 1180–6.

135. Janota I. Dementia, deep white matter damage and hypertension: 'Binswanger's disease'. *Psychol Med* 1981; **11**: 39–48.
136. Sourander P, Wålinder J. Hereditary multi-infarct dementia. *Acta Neuropathol* 1977; **39**: 247–54.
137. Tournier-Lasserve E, Joutel A, Melki J et al. Cerebral autosomal dominant arteriopathy with subcortical infarcts and leukoencephalopathy maps to chromosome 19q12. *Nature Genet* 1993; **3**: 256–9.
138. Lammie GA, Rakshi J, Rossor MN et al. Cerebral autosomal dominant arteriopathy with subcortical infarcts and leukoencephalopathy (CADASIL) — confirmation by cerebral biopsy in 2 cases. *Clin Neuropathol* 1995; **14**: 201–6.
139. Mayer M, Dichgans M, Gasser T et al. Hereditary CADASIL cerebral arteriopathy. Report of a family. *Nervenharzt* 1995; **66**: 927–32.
140. Masuda J, Yutani C, Waki R et al. Histopathological analysis of the mechanisms of intracranial hemorrhage complicating infective endocarditis. *Stroke* 1992; **23**: 843–50.
141. Weir B. *Aneurysms Affecting the Nervous System*. Baltimore: Williams and Wilkins, 1987.
142. Norrgård O, Ängquist K-A, Fodstad H et al. Intracranial aneurysms and heredity. *Neurosurgery* 1987; **20**: 236–9.
143. Ronkainen A, Hernesniemi J, Ryynänen M. Familial subarachnoid hemorrhage in East Finland 1977–90. *Neurosurgery* 1993; **33**: 787–97.
144. Challa VR, Moody DM, Brown WR. Vascular malformations of the central nervous system. *J Neuropathol Exp Neurol* 1995; **54**: 609–21.
145. Saygi S, Bolay H, Tekkok IH et al. Fibromuscular dysplasia of the basilar artery: a case with brain stem stroke. *Angiology* 1990; **41**: 658–61.
146. Oppenheimer DR, Griffith HB. Persistent intracranial bleeding as a complication of hemispherectomy. *J Neurol Neurosurg Psychiatry* 1966; **29**: 229–40.
147. Koeppen AH, Wood GW. Superficial siderosis of the central nervous system. In *Proceedings of the 10th International Congress of Neuropathology*, Stockholm, Gotab, 1986: 206.
148. Morita H, Ikeda S, Yamamoto K et al. Hereditary ceruloplasmin deficiency with hemosiderosis: a clinico-pathological study of a Japanese family. *Ann Neurol* 1995; **37**: 646–56.
149. Iancu T. Iron overload. In: Baum J, Gerlely J, Fanburg BL, eds. *Molecular Aspects of Medicine*, Vol. 6. Oxford: Pergamon Press, 1982: 1–100.
150. Chu LLH, Feinberg RA. On the mechanism of iron-induced synthesis of apoferritin in Hela cells. *J Biol Chem* 1969; **244**: 3847–54.
151. Zähringer J, Baliga BS, Munro HN. Novel mechanism for translational control in regulation of ferritin synthesis by iron. *Proc Natl Acad Sci USA* 1976; **73**: 857–61.
152. Koeppen AH, Dickson AC, Chu RC, Thach RE. The pathogenesis of superficial siderosis of the central nervous system. *Ann Neurol* 1993; **34**: 646–53.
153. Skinner HA. The origin of the acoustic nerve tumours. *Br J Surg* 1928; **16**: 440–63.
154. Rasmussen AT. Studies of the 8th cranial nerve in man. *Laryngoscope* 1940; **50**: 67–83.
155. Barker DJP, Weller RO, Garfield JS. Epidemiology of primary tumours of the brain and spinal cord: a regional survey in southern England. *J Neurol Neurosurg Psychiatry* 1976; **39**: 290–6.
156. Curley JW, Ramsden RT, Howell A et al. Oestrogen and progesterone receptors in acoustic neuroma. *J Laryngol Otol* 1990; **104**: 865–7.
157. Gould VE, Moll I, Lee I et al. The intermediate filament complement of the spectrum of nerve sheath neoplasms. *Lab Invest* 1986; **55**: 463–4.
158. Gray MH, Rosenberg AE, Dickersin GR, Bhan AK. Glial fibrillary acidic protein and keratin expression by benign and malignant nerve sheath tumors. *Hum Pathol* 1989; **20**: 1089–96.
159. Carney JA. Psammomatous melanotic schwannoma. A distinctive heritable tumor with special association, including cardiac myxoma and the Cushing syndrome. *Am J Surg Pathol* 1990; **14**: 206–22.
160. Font RL, Truong LD. Melanotic schwannoma of the soft tissues. Electron microscopic observations and review of the literature. *Am J Surg Pathol* 1984; **8**: 129–38.
161. Miller RT, Sarikaya H, Sos A. Melanotic schwannoma of the acoustic nerve. *Arch Pathol Lab Med* 1986; **110**: 153–4.
162. Earls JP, Robles HA, McAdams HP, Rao KC. General case of the day. Malignant melanotic schwannoma of the eighth cranial nerve. *Radiographics* 1994; **14**: 1425–7.
163. Rouleau GA, Wertelecki W, Haines JL et al. Genetic linkage of bilateral acoustic neurofibromatosis to a DNA marker in chromosome 22. *Nature* 1987; **329**: 246–8.
164. Rouleau GA, Merel P, Lutchman M et al. Alteration in a new gene encoding a putative membrane-organizing protein causes neurofibromatosis type 2. *Nature* 1993; **363**: 515–21.
165. Trofatter JA, MacCollin MM, Rutter JL et al. A novel moesin-, ezrin-, radixin-like gene is a candidate for the neurofibromatosis 2 tumor suppressor. *Cell* 1993; **72**: 791–800.
166. Malamed Sh, Sahar A, Beller AJ. The recurrence of intracranial meningiomas. *Neurochirurgia* 1979; **22**: 47–51.
167. Baird M, Gallagher PJ. Recurrent intracranial and spinal meningiomas: clinical and histological features. *Clin Neuropathol* 1989; **8**: 41–4.
168. Lantos PL, Vandenberg SR, Kleihues P. Tumours of the nervous system. In: Graham DI, Lantos PL, eds. *Greenfield's Neuropathology*, London: Arnold, 1997: 583–879.
169. Heffelfinger MJ, Dahlin DC, MacCarthy CS, Beabout JW. Chordomas and cartilagineous tumours at the skull base. *Cancer* 1973; **32**: 410–20.
170. Charachon R. Signal symptoms in tumours of the petrous bone. *Ann Otolaryngol Chir Cervicofac* 1981; **98**: 181–8.

38 Function and dysfunction of the vestibular system

Herman Kingma

The vestibular system contributes to three major tasks: spatial orientation, gaze stabilization and balance control, including head stabilization. However, these tasks can only be fulfilled in combination with input from many other sensory systems (Figure 38.1). Reflexes associated with vestibular function are the vestibulo-ocular reflex, the vestibulo-spinal reflex and the vestibulo-collic reflex. The clinical implication of the fact that vestibular function is associated with spatial orientation, gaze stabilization and balance control is that a dysfunction of the system may result in a variety of complaints and is not restricted to the classical rotatory vertigo, nausea or balance disorders. Moreover, problems with sensorimotor control (eye–head–hand coordination) or visual inspection of moving targets (quality control of objects on an assembly line) and fear or anxiety in conditions where self-motion and motion of the environment may be difficult to distinguish (e.g. busy supermarkets) from vestibular disorder. In addition, vestibular dysfunction may force patients to direct selective attention to otherwise subconscious reflexes and lead to faster fatigue.

Figure 38.2 shows the basic pathways that relate the vestibular, visual and proprioceptive systems with these tasks. To facilitate a basic understanding of vestibular function, a short introduction to these pathways is given. The labyrinths detect head orientation relative to gravity and head movements. This information is transmitted to the vestibular nuclei (VN) and the cerebellum (CER). The labyrinths detect head movements through accelerations only, which makes the system insensitive for movements with constant velocities. Information about the actual acceleration is therefore stored via the vestibular nuclei in the nucleus prepositus hypoglossi

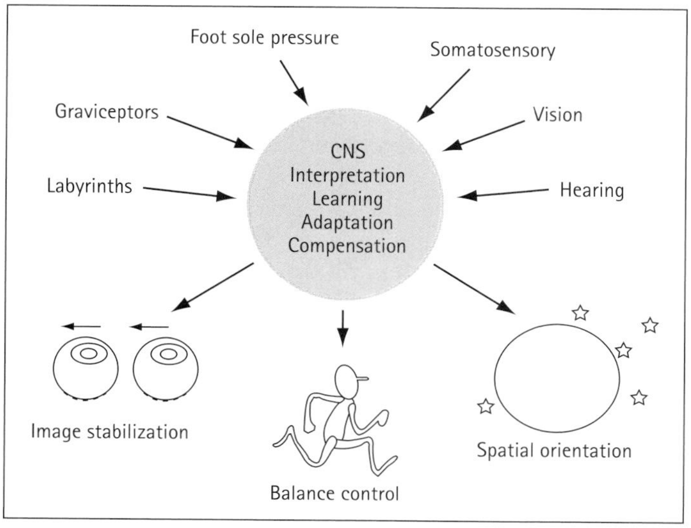

Figure 38.1 Schematic representation of the multi-sensory control of image stabilization, balance control and spatial orientation. CNS: central nervous system.

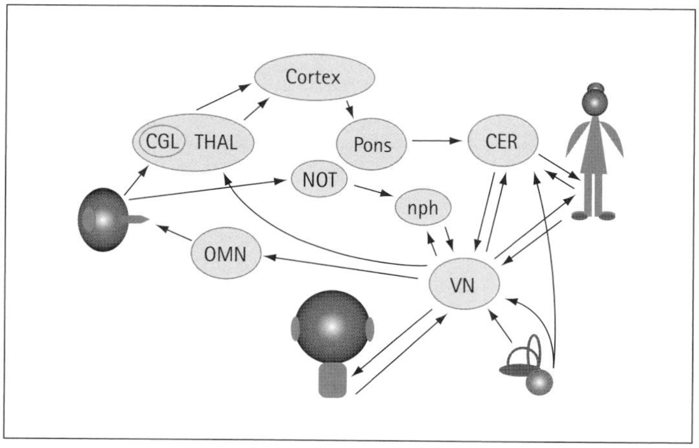

Figure 38.2 Simplified schematic overview of the major pathways involved in image stabilization, balance control and spatial orientation. VN: vestibular nuclei. OMN: oculo-motor nuclei. THAL: thalamus. CGL: corpus geniculatum laterale. NOT: nucleus of the optic tract. Pons: parapontine reticular formation. CER: cerebellum. nph: nucleus prepositus hypoglossi.

(NPH) to expand the perception of movements in time by a factor of three (velocity storage mechanism). Perception of self-movement and spatial orientation are major cortical functions of the vestibular system. The labyrinths project via the VN and the thalamus (THAL) to the vestibular cortex. The vestibular cortex function seems to be distributed among several multisensory areas in the parietal and temporal cortices and is integrated in a larger network for spatial attention and sensorimotor control. The parietoinsular vestibular cortex has been postulated to be the core region within the vestibular cortical system. Representation is bilateral, with a right-hemispheric dominance.[1]

Spatial orientation

Spatial orientation is a crucial ability for any animal: it is a prerequisite for postural control, locomotion and interaction with the environment. Optimal spatial orientation requires input from all senses (Figure 38.1). A fast and reliable interpretation of the multisensory input requires learning and preknowledge about what can be expected and may prevent erroneous interpretation of exactly what is happening. Nevertheless, spatial orientation is difficult even under rather simple, frequently occurring conditions, despite the multisensorial input and our intelligence. For example, assume that you are sitting in a train, which is expected to leave soon. Through the window you look at the train standing beside yours. When that train starts to move, most people will have the sensation that their train is moving in the opposite direction (Figure 38.3b). A fraction of a second later, we will realize that our train did not move at all. The explanation of this phenomenon is relatively simple when we apply our current insights into spatial orientation. Our labyrinths sense head accelerations (canals and maculae) and the absolute orientation of the head relative to the gravitation vector (maculae). Proprioceptors and other graviceptors in the body, in concert with the internal body scheme, inform the brain about the orientation of the body (and body segments) relative to the contact surface of the body with the environment (feet on the ground, hands on the table, etc.). Cervical proprioception allows integration of detected spatial orientations of head and body. Hearing allows orientation of the head relative to external sound sources (this modality is highly developed in bats). However, spatial orientation is far from optimal without vision. When we walk with eyes closed, we lose the absolute sense of direction and distance within seconds. All other senses are apparently unable to provide the brain with accurate information about our absolute position in space. Labyrinthine input is especially inaccurate in this respect. As noted above, the labyrinths only sense acceleration, and the brain therefore has to integrate this input twice to calculate position; a slight offset in the signal or small error in integration will then result in a major error in position. Also, as the labyrinths do not sense constant velocity, substantial displacement can occur without detection by the vestibular system. All these features point to the necessity to reorient us from time to time and to correct for the errors made in absolute position.

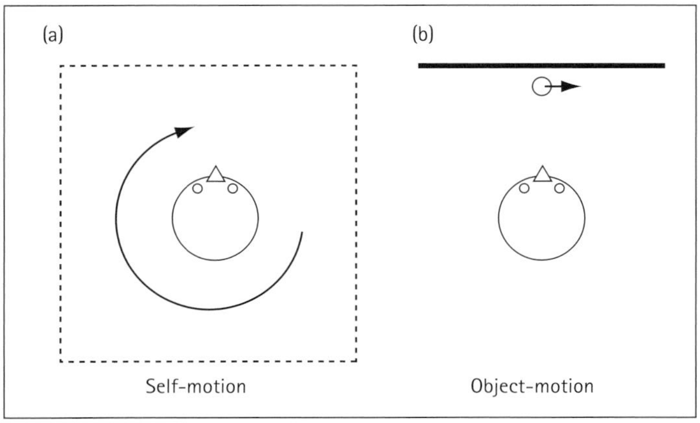

Figure 38.3 (a) Self-motion; (b) object-motion

A similar problem is encountered with navigation of airplanes: for detection of absolute position, external references are required (radar or satellites). We use vision as a source of external reference: frequent visual inspection of our orientation relative to the environment helps us to determine absolute position. Through experience, we learn to rely on visual orientation. When we start walking in infancy, we learn that the whole visual scene is moving over the retina during self-motion. As a consequence, we interpret such a visual stimulation as indicative of self-motion (Figure 38.3a). This also happened in the example of the train: the optokinetic stimulation of the retina with the moving neighboring train suggests self-motion. A fraction of a second later, we will realize that we were fooled by the visual input. The labyrinths will tell us that no acceleration occurred, no pressure of the seat or vibrations from the motors were sensed by proprioception, and we did not hear the noise that fits with the acceleration of our train. This example indicates how difficult spatial orientation is, despite the multisensorial input and learning. It also stresses that every sensory system contributing to spatial orientation plays a specific role and is highly relevant. Loss of any sensory system will therefore reduce performance, despite some overlap in function. Labyrinthine input is especially important as, in contrast to the other senses, it is very sensitive for fast, high-frequency head movements (1–10 Hz) and is characterized by short latencies (see below). These features allow fast detection and perception of motion in space and enable fast and adequate responses. Labyrinthine dysfunction, however, leads to impaired spatial orientation during fast head movements, which cannot be compensated by input from other senses.

As indicated above, even a healthy labyrinth shows deficiencies related to sensing motion due to specific limitations of the sensor. These drawbacks do not only relate to the semicircular canals. Spatial orientation based upon vestibular input is also difficult, because the statolith system is unable to distinguish linear accelerations from tilts or rolls (Figure 38.4). For example, a forward acceleration and a retroflexion of the head

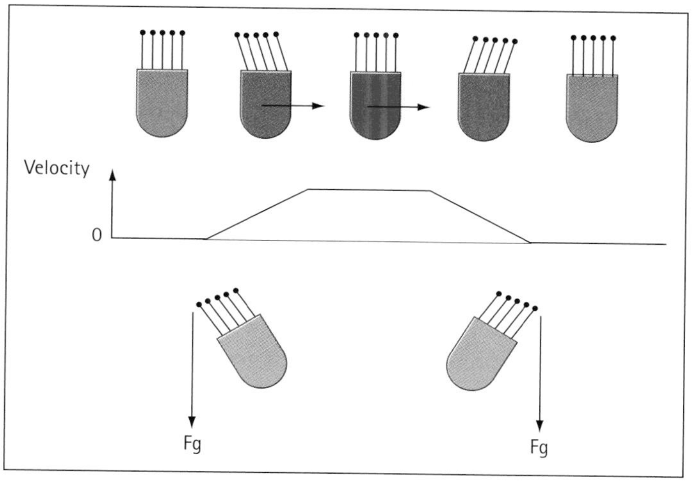

Figure 38.4 Schematic representation of the statolith hair cell response to linear translation (two upper trace) and to head tilts (lower trace). Fg: gravitational force.

result in similar deflection patterns of the cilia in the maculae. Perception is also confusing: a pilot in a quickly accelerating plane senses both acceleration and upward tilt instead of pure acceleration. This, combined with constant accelerations sensed by the labyrinth, easily leads to spatial disorientation. Spatial disorientation at least partly accounts for motion sickness. The example given below is a simplification of the actual problems, but nevertheless nicely demonstrates how spatial orientation can fail and lead to kinetosis (Figure 38.5).

First, we need to introduce the concept of the so-called efference copy.

> An efference copy is a learned sensorimotor pattern that is stored in the brain and that reflects the sensory input and motor output signals that fit with a specific stimulus condition.

For example, in a stationary condition, standing on a stable floor, the corresponding efference copy contains relatively stationary input signals (minor movements) and output signals (minor corrections). Any movement made will be detected by the senses involved. The input signals will be compared with the efference copy, resulting in a fast interpretation of movement and spatial orientation and generation of adequate, almost automatic, motor signals. As soon as we stand on a slowly moving ship, still using the efference copy applicable for a stationary environment, errors will occur in the motor commands that have to adjust posture and gate. We all know that it is not easy to keep balance while walking on a ship. We will therefore need to switch our selective attention to the most reliable sensory input for knowing how we move relative to gravity and how we move relative to the ship, features that are no longer correlated. The labyrinths are not reliable sensors, as

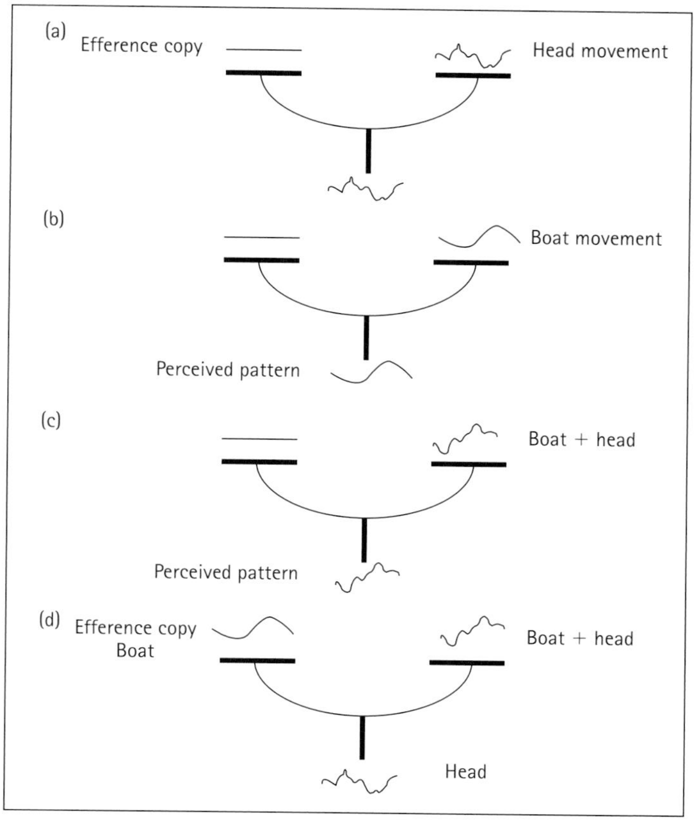

Figure 38.5 Motion sickness and spatial orientation: basic framework of thinking. (a) head motion in a stationary environment; (b) head fixed on a sailing boat; (c) head motion on a sailing boat; (d) head motion on a sailing boat after adaptation to the boat movement.

they detect the sum of boat and head motions, and are incapable of distinguishing between linear accelerations and roll (see below). Therefore, we tend to rely on the relatively slow visual input. Looking at the horizon and the ship, we can detect self-motion and boat motion. In contrast, visual orientation below deck is worse and easily induces motion sickness. Despite this, most people will become disoriented when boat movement is complex, and we will be warned by vegetative symptoms that we are at risk of falling. As long as we stay on the boat, we will be able to try to learn the relatively regular movements of the boat and build up a new, specific efference copy. As soon as we have made such a copy, we will be able to compare the sensory input during stance and locomotion with the 'known' boat movement, will experience normal spatial orientation again, and will be able to generate the required muscle activity. Now, we will experience a problem when we get off the boat: still using the 'moving' efference copy, we will experience motion (sea legs) despite the fact that the sensory input is nil during stance. This phenomenon is called 'mal de debarquement' and decays in time and disappears completely as soon as we activate the correct 'stationary' efference copy again.

Although spatial orientation is hardly tested in the clinic, it relies, to a major extent, on vestibular function.

Gaze stabilization

Information about head acceleration passes from the VN via the oculomotor nuclei (OMN) to the extraocular muscles to generate compensatory eye movements. The velocities of these eye movements need to match the velocity of the head movements within 3°/s accuracy. The image of the visual scene will then move over the retina (retinal slip) with a velocity of less than 3°/s. This is slow enough to allow the visual system to perceive all the necessary details of the image. It also allows us to guide gaze accurately to any desired visual target during head movements. It must therefore be stressed that the VOR is a velocity-controlled system. The latency of this vestibulo-ocular reflex (VOR) is only 7–10 ms.

CHARACTERISTICS OF VOR

- Velocity-controlled system
- Optimal frequency responses between 1 and 10 Hz
- Latency of VOR 7–10 msec
- Easy adaptation

The VOR is kept optimal by visual feedback: persistent poor gaze stabilization is detected on the retina and perceived in the visual cortex, and a correction signal is generated for both eyes in the horizontal gaze center in the pons, and transferred to the cerebellum; this decreases or increases the inhibition of the VN and thus the VOR. The VOR can be easily adapted. Adaptation of the VOR by visual feedback can occur within minutes. Melvil Jones even showed that the VOR could be inverted within 3 days by wearing inverted prisms.[2] Proprioception seems to have an equivalent in the podokinetic adaptation reported by Melvil Jones and co-workers.[3] They reported that subjects who are adapted to walking in circles lose their sense of direction as they adapt to an asymmetric proprioceptive input.

Most functional tests of the VOR are performed in the dark (caloric test, rotatory tests) to prevent optokinetic reflexes or visual suppression. However, the VOR is meant to stabilize images and is therefore not functional physiologically in the dark. In the dark, the mental setting and preknowledge of the patient influence the VOR marked: when the patient is almost asleep, hardly any VOR can be elicited, whereas the VOR is close to maximum when the patient is anxious or mentally fixating an imaginary target in a stationary environment. One of the challenges of current vestibular testing is to overcome this problem.

The sensitivity of the vestibular apparatus depends on the stimulus frequency, similar to any other sensory system. Melvil Jones and Groen calculated the frequency dependence based upon a theoretical second-order model of the canals and the maculae.[4,5] According to their findings, the canals are optimally sensitive to angular velocities with frequencies between roughly 1 and 10 Hz. How should we interpret this frequency dependence? As mentioned already, the labyrinths detect accelerations only, which implies that a constant velocity (0 Hz!) is not sensed. However, a change of angular velocity implies substantial angular acceleration. The faster the fluctuations in velocity, the higher the accelerations and the better the canals will sense the modulation of velocity. The fact that the labyrinthine sensitivity is limited to about 20 Hz is associated with the mechanical properties of the canal system. In delicate experiments Collewijn and co-workers showed that the VOR induced by passive head-shaking is indeed close to optimal in the range 1–10 Hz.[6] Owing to several technical problems, most diagnostic tests evaluate the VOR below 1 Hz, and do not picture the relevant physiological working range of the canals.

Eye movements can also be induced by steadily moving visual targets. Such a movement is called smooth pursuit in the case of foveal fixation. A smooth pursuit movement needs to be very accurate, as the fovea has only 1° of arc, and the image on the fovea of the moving object may easily slip off this region with high spatial resolution. Therefore, in contrast to the VOR, the smooth pursuit needs to be a very accurate *position-*controlled system, and uses foveal visual input for eye position control. The cortical optokinetic reflex (OKR) is another visually guided eye movement and is a velocity-controlled system like the VOR, using visual input from the entire retina. This reflex is elicited, for example, when we look at a train that passes by. The image of the train moves over the retina, and the visual system calculates the velocity of the image in the visual cortex. Based upon this information, usual signals are processed in two ways. The cortical pathway is similar to that for the smooth pursuit system, and information passes via the corpus geniculatum laterale (CGL) in the thalamus (THAL), the visual cortex, the pons, the cerebellum, the VN and the OMN to the extraocular muscles to generate conjugated eye movements with a velocity that again matches the retinal image motion with an accuracy within 3°/s, to allow the visual system to perceive all the necessary details of the image. Parallel to the cortical OKR, humans demonstrate a second subcortical OKR. Vision is poorly developed during the very first months of life: there is no smooth pursuit, and only large, attention-attracting targets seem to be observed. In this period, infants stabilize moving visual scenes on the retina by the subcortical OKR. The velocity of the image is now calculated for each eye separately in both nuclei of the optic tract (NOT), which, via the velocity storage memory (located in the NPH), the VN, the OMN, leads to an activation of the extraocular muscles. This pathway is also active in adults when we gaze at moving targets subconsciously. The subcortical OKR needs time to build up; it needs to fill the velocity storage memory before eye movements can start. Also, the remaining activity stored in the memory accounts for the fact that eye movements (nystagmus) continue when the visual stimulus is suddenly switched off. This phenomenon is known as optokinetic after nystagmus (OKAN) and is frequently studied to investigate whether the velocity storage function is intact. Dysfunction of the velocity storage, or reduced input from the labyrinths (labyrinthine deficits), generally leads to a shortening of post-rotatory responses.

> Vestibular function loss leads to impaired gazed stabilization, especially during fast head movements.[1] Smooth pursuit and optokinetic reflexes are too slow to compensate for this functional loss above 2–3 Hz. Below 2–3 Hz, visually guided gaze stabilization can take over.

As a consequence, many patients try to cope with their impaired gaze stabilization by preventing fast head movements. In the case of a unilateral vestibular deafferentation, central compensation can restore the tonic balance at the level of the vestibular nuclei. However, each labyrinth has a preponderance for stimulation to the ipsilateral side (Ewald's law). In the case of a unilateral deafferentation, this direction preponderance remains, and is especially apparent at higher frequencies, where visually guided gaze stabilization cannot contribute. The diagnostic head-impulse test is based upon this principle: a fast head rotation to the affected side leads only to minimal gaze stabilization and necessitates compensatory corrective saccade(s) that can be easily observed.

Balance control

> Balance and postural control involves maintenance of the alignment of body posture, stability and bodily orientation in the environment and also serves as a mechanical support for action. We should be aware that postural control is a prerequisite for voluntary skills, because almost every movement that an individual makes is made of postural components that stabilize the body.[7]

Labyrinthine input, predominantly from the statolith system, is relayed via both the VN (fast reflexes) and the cerebellum (precision of movement, adaptation, learning) to the postural muscles and is used for balance control (Figure 38.2). This labyrinthine input regulates the tonic activity of the postural extensor muscles to control the joints of the limbs and the orientation of the head in space, and provide appropriate body rigidity. Postural tone not only depends on the tonic labyrinthine input, but is also modulated through the myotatic reflex loop, neck reflexes, lumbar reflexes and positive supporting reactions.

In humans, where the supporting surface is narrow, there is a direct regulation of the center of body mass by displacement of body segments. This is in contrast to the situation in cats: here the brain does not control the orientation of the center of body mass, but regulates the orientation of the limbs. After a fall, the limbs will be oriented vertically as fast as possible to ensure that the cat will land on its feet. The main substrate as the basis for body orientation is the so-called postural body schema, an internal representation of body posture, which includes a representation of body geometry, body kinetics, and the body orientation with respect to gravity (vertical). Information regarding orientation with respect to verticality comes from the labyrinths, vision and possibly body graviceptors.[7,8] Visual and vestibular cues allow detection of the orientation of the head in space, while somatosensory sensors are necessary to relate head orientation to body orientation. Balance control requires the detection of verticality and the orientation of the support phase. It seems unambiguous that the support-phase orientation can be detected with the somatosensory sensors alone, specially those in the soles of the feet. However, the absolute support-phase orientation in space can only be estimated by relating the sensed support-phase orientation to the perceived subjective vertical, i.e. the direction of the gravitation vector. The multiple sensory inputs are integrated and resolved by the postural system to provide a coherent interpretation of the body's orientation and dynamic equilibrium to preserve balance. This information is then thought to be compared to the above-mentioned internal model of the body. Any resulting error signals are used to generate motor commands in order to maintain and regain body equilibrium.

Many studies have tried to quantify the contributions of the various senses towards postural control. It was assumed that in the case of a vestibular deficit, subjects would rely more on the other intact senses. Although this might be true, motor strategies and sensory dependence vary too widely in healthy subjects to allow a simple discrimination between normal and abnormal dependence on any sensory input in cases of limited sensory deficits.

Postural control is not organized as a single unit. Independent control of the position or orientation of segments such as the head, trunk and forearm has been shown to exist. These segments serve as a reference frame for perception and action processes. The execution of destabilizing voluntary movements is preceded by activation of postural muscles, called anticipatory postural adjustments. These adjustments serve to compensate in advance for changes in equilibrium or posture caused by the movement. So, apart from feedback processes, the postural system is also able to anticipate center of body mass displacements and environmental conditions.[7]

As mentioned above, labyrinthine input is used to control postural tone and to control the orientation of the center of body mass relative to the supporting phase (the ground) to prevent falling. Balance control, particularly, is optimized by motor learning and varies widely between healthy subjects. A dysfunction of the labyrinth initially leads to a tendency to fall to the deafferented side but is normally centrally compensated within weeks to months. Then, due to the large inter-individual variability, balance control may even be better in a well-trained, centrally compensated patient with labyrinthine function loss than in an inactive healthy subject. Reduced motor abilities and multisensory deficit may be the primary cause of frequent falls in the elderly. The injuries associated with the falls, and the fear of falling, again reduce mobility and the quality of life considerably. The role of vestibular dysfunction in this situation is still unclear.

References

1. Brandt T. *Vertigo. Its Multisensory Syndromes*. London: Springer Verlag, 1999.
2. Jones GM, Davies P. Adaptation of cat vestibulo-ocular reflex to 200 days of optically reversed vision. *Brain Res* 1976; **103** (3): 551–4.
3. Weber KD, Fletcher WA, Gordon CR, Melvill-Jones G, Block EW. Motor learning in the 'podokinetic' system and its role in spatial orientation during locomotion. *Exp Brain Res* 1998; **120** (3): 377–85.
4. Wilson VJ, Melvill Jones G. *Mammalian Vestibular Physiology*. New York: Plenum Press, 1979.
5. Groen JJ, Lowenstein O, Vendrik AJH. The mechanical analysis of the responses from the end organs of the horizontal canal in the isolated elasmobranch labyrinth. *J Physiol (Lond)* 1952; **117**: 329–46.
6. Tabak S, Collewijn H. Evaluation of the human vestibulo-ocular reflex at high frequencies with a helmet, driven by reactive torque. *Acta Otolaryngol Suppl* 1995; **520** Pt 1: 4–8.
7. Massion J, Woollacott MH. Posture and equilibrium. In: Bronstein AM, Brandt T, Woollacott MH, eds. *Clinical Disorders of Balance, Posture and Gait*. London: Arnold Publishers, 1996: 1–19.
8. Mittelstaedt H. Interaction of eye-, head-, and trunk-bound information in spatial perception and control. *J Vestib Res* 1997; **7**: 283–302.

39 Effects of aging on control of stability

Brian E Maki, William E McIlroy

Introduction

> Postural instability and falling are among the most serious problems associated with aging.[1–3]

Age-related changes in the neural, sensory and musculoskeletal systems can lead to balance impairments that have a tremendous impact on the ability to move about safely, and the consequences of instability and falling, in terms of healthcare costs and quality of life, are extensive (Tables 39.1 and 39.2). Injuries due to falls, such as hip fractures, place an enormous burden on the healthcare system. For example, in the USA alone, there are 300 000 hip fractures each year (90% due to falls), with associated healthcare costs estimated at $7–10 billion.[4] Up to 40% of hip-fracture victims die within 6 months of sustaining the injury,[5] and those who survive seldom regain their former level of mobility. In addition to serious injury, instability and falling are often associated with fear of falling, which can lead to anxiety, social withdrawal and activity restriction and attendant loss of quality of life.[6–9] The net effect of fall-related injury or fear is often a loss of ability to live independently. In fact, over 40% of nursing-home admissions are related to falls.[2,10]

Table 39.1 Age-related changes affecting falling risk.

Sensory systems
Reduced visual acuity, contrast sensitivity, depth perception and dark adaptation
Reduced vestibular function
Reduced proprioception
Reduced cutaneous sensation
Musculoskeletal system
Reduced muscle strength
Slowing of muscle contraction
Increased muscle fatigue
Increased joint stiffness
Reduced range of motion
Nervous system
Slowing of nerve conduction
Slowing and impairment of information processing

Table 39.2 Medical risk factors for instability and falls.

Sensory disorders
Cataracts, macular degeneration, glaucoma
Labyrinthitis, vestibular neuritis, Ménière's disease, acoustical nerve tumor
Neurological disorders
Parkinson's disease, hemiplegia (stroke), normal-pressure hydocephalus, dementia, peripheral neuropathy (diabetes, pernicious anemia, nutritional)
Disorders causing transient disturbances
Cardiac arrhythmia, transient ischemic attack, ocular ischemia, orthostatic or postprandial hypotension
Other conditions
Foot abnormalities, musculoskeletal disorders
Acute illness, seizure, syncope, incontinence
Medications and drugs
Antidepressants, benzodiazepines, alcohol

Identifying specific causes of instability in older adults and developing improved methods to diagnose and treat individuals with compromised balance will provide a significant opportunity to reduce healthcare costs and improve independence and quality of life. The challenge in meeting this objective arises due to the multifactorial nature of falls, the complexity of the balance control mechanisms, and the variable effects of aging on the neural, sensory and musculoskeletal substrates of balance control. Age-related pathology, as well as medication use, can also have profound effects on balance control. Although distinctions betwen effects of aging and borderline pathology are not always clear-cut,[11,12] the focus of this chapter is on the effects of those age-related changes that do not appear to be associated with any specific disease or drug. Understanding the complex and interacting effects due to age-related changes in the neural, sensory and motor systems is likely to be one of the more challenging tasks facing the clinician who needs to manage instability in an older clientele.

Basic principles of balance control

To maintain upright stance in the presence of gravity, the central nervous system (CNS) must regulate the static and dynamic relationship between the center of mass (COM) of the body and the base of support (BOS).[13–16] The BOS is usually defined by the feet, but may include the arms when touching an object for support.[17–19] In the absence of arm support, static equilibrium requires the COM to be positioned over the feet, and the perimeter of this foot area can be considered to represent the static stability limits associated with the BOS. If we model the body as an inverted pendulum that rotates about the ankle joint, then it becomes apparent that it is necessary to generate stabilizing ankle torque in order to counter the effects of gravity or other forces acting on the body (Figure 39.1a). The ability to maintain static equilibrium is dependent on the characteristics of the BOS, because the dimensions of the BOS

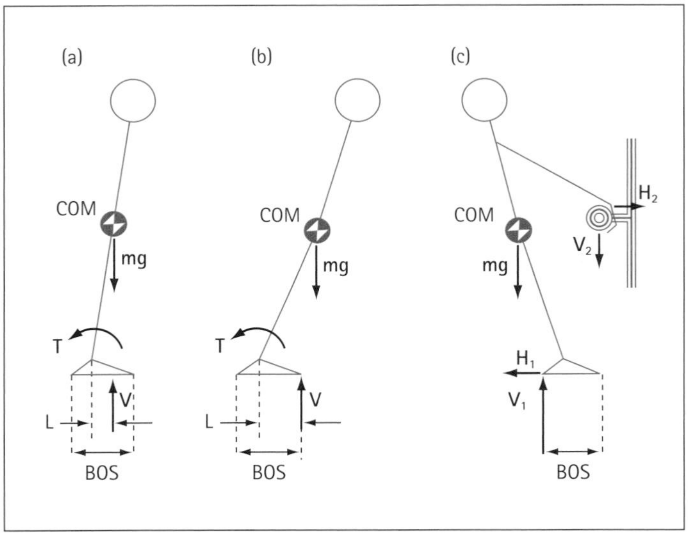

Figure 39.1 Biomechanical requirements for static equilibrium. In (a), the center of mass (COM) is situated within the anterior and posterior limits of the base of support (BOS). In (b), the COM is located at the anterior static stability limit. Note that the muscle-generated ankle torque (*T*), which is equal to the product of the vertical ground reaction force (*V* = mg; *m* = body mass; *g* = acceleration due to gravity) and the moment arm (*L*), is limited by the finite length of the BOS (maximum torque is generated in the case shown in (b)). (c) depicts a situation where grasping an object for support allows static equilibrium to be achieved even though the COM is outside the BOS limits. Although the examples shown depict stability requirements in the sagittal plane, analogous requirements apply in the frontal plane.

established by the feet limit the magnitude of stabilizing torque that can be generated (Figure 39.1b). By displacing the feet (Figure 39.2b) or using the arms to push against an object for support (Figure 39.2c), the stability limits of the BOS can be extended. Actual grasping of the object allows additional stabilizing forces to be generated and can extend the static stability limits beyond the perimeter of the BOS, provided that the grip is sufficiently strong to allow the necessary forces to be generated (Figure 39.1c).

> In order to maintain upright stability, the CNS must regulate the relationship between the COM of the body and the BOS, by controlling movement of the COM or by changing the BOS.

Dynamic equilibrium takes into account the additional requirement of controlling the momentum associated with movement of the COM.[20,21,198] If the COM is moving with sufficient horizontal velocity, it is possible for the body to be dynamically unstable, even when the COM is positioned over the BOS. Conversely, it is possible for the body to be dynamically stable even though the COM is located outside the static stability limits of the BOS, provided that the COM is moving toward the BOS with sufficient velocity that it can eventually be repositioned over the BOS. In a dynamic situation, horizontal shear force must be generated at the foot–ground interface in order to decelerate the COM (Figure 39.2a). The biomechanical capacity to generate this force is limited, again, by the dimensions of the BOS;[22] inadequate surface friction may, in some situations, place additional limits on the force that can be generated.

In situations where the COM cannot be stabilized with respect to the existing BOS, it may be possible to re-establish stability by altering the BOS, e.g. by taking a step or by using the upper limbs to push against or grasp an object for support (Figures 39.2b,c). Ultimately, failure to re-establish dynamic equilibrium within the time available will result in a fall, which is most commonly defined as an unintentional impact of the body with a lower surface (e.g. the ground, a bed, a chair).

> Given that the body is initially in a state of equilibrium, two things must happen in order for a fall to occur: (1) there must be a disturbance to postural equilibrium, i.e. a perturbation, that precipitates the loss of balance; and (2) there must be a failure of the balance control system to compensate adequately for the perturbation.

Precipitants of loss of balance

The perturbations that precipitate loss of balance are often inferred to involve mechanical effects, i.e. a change in the forces acting on the body. These *mechanical perturbations* act

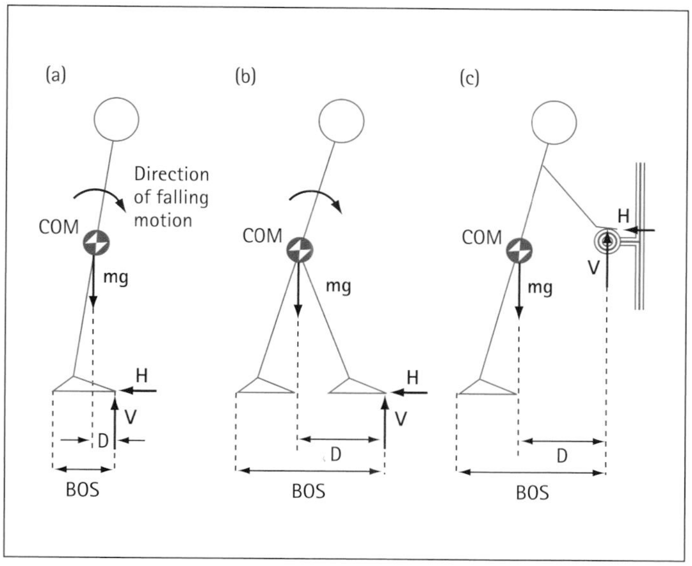

Figure 39.2 Recovery of dynamic equilibrium: comparison of fixed-support reactions (a) and change-in-support reactions (b, c). In the dynamic situation, the postural reaction must generate a horizontal ground-reaction shear force (*H*) in order to decelerate the horizontal motion of the body's COM. Note that the stepping reaction (b) and reach-and-grasp reaction (c) both have the potential to greatly amplify the moment arm (*D*) between the COM and the contact force (*V*), as well as the length of the BOS. This helps to decelerate the COM in two ways: (1) larger stabilizing shear force can be generated (this shear force is approximately proportional to the distance *D*);[22] and (2) there is more time available to decelerate the COM (the COM has to travel a larger distance to reach the limit of the BOS). Although the examples shown depict stability requirements in the sagittal plane, analogous requirements apply in the frontal plane.

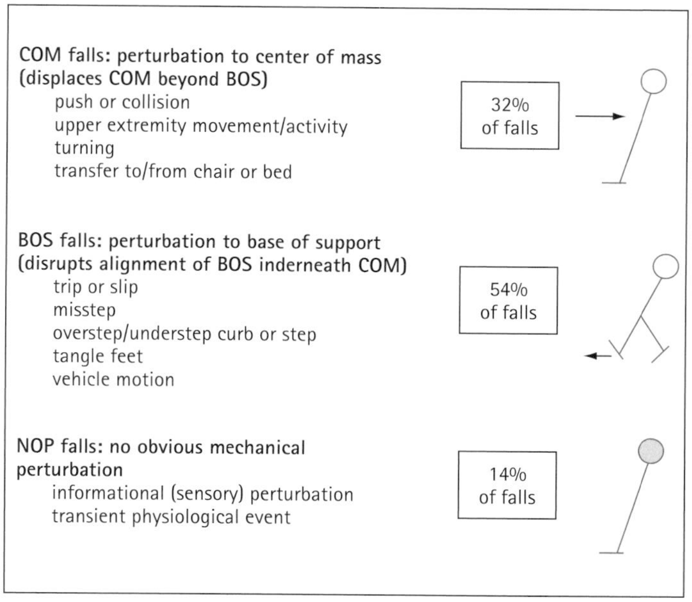

Figure 39.3 Precipitants of falls: mechanical (perturbations to COM and/or BOS) and non-mechanical (informational and physiological perturbations). The percentages of falls attributed to each category of perturbation were derived from interviews with 59 residents (age 62–96) of apartment-style self-care facilities who reported experiencing a total of 120 falls during a 1-year prospective monitoring period (18 of these falls could not be classified, due to insufficient information).[72,73]

either to displace the COM beyond the BOS (e.g. a push or collision) or to prevent the BOS from being appropriately aligned beneath the COM during ongoing movement (e.g. a slip, trip or misstep); see Figure 39.3. The destabilizing forces can be imposed by the environment (e.g. an impact from a swinging door or sliding door, a jostle from a crowd, standing in a moving vehicle) or may be self-induced, occurring during volitional movements such as walking, rising from a chair, bending over, reaching forward or pushing on a door. The destabilization associated with volitional movement can arise from the motion of the COM, but can also be related to the control of the BOS. During gait, for example, the control of stability is highly dependent on the placement of the swingfoot;[23] see Figure 39.4. It is also important to recognize that the upright body is inherently unstable due to the force of gravity; hence, even a quiet unperturbed stance requires ongoing postural stabilization.

Perturbations may also involve transient changes in the nature of the orientational sensory information that is available to the CNS; we have termed such changes *informational perturbations*.[15] Such perturbations may create transient conflicts between the visual, vestibular and somatosensory inputs (e.g. moving visual fields that create an illusion of self-motion, or carpets that distort proprioceptive information from the foot

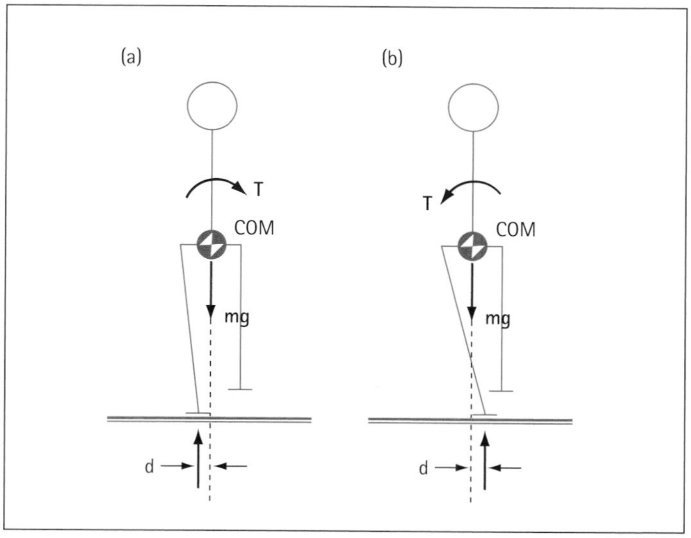

Figure 39.4 An example of perturbation arising due to errors in BOS control, i.e. foot placement, during gait. Lateral motion of the COM toward the unsupported side occurs during each step. During gait, this lateral falling motion is normally decelerated by controlling the foot to land laterally with respect to the mid-line, so that the body weight generates a stabilizing 'torque', $T = mg\ d$ (a). Errors in control of the foot placement affect the magnitude of the torque, and can even result in a situation (b) where the torque *T* acts to *increase* the lateral acceleration of the body.

and ankle), or may simply involve a transient change in the quality of the sensory input (e.g. dim lighting or glare which can interfere with visual inputs). In what appears to be a relatively small proportion of falls, an internal *physiological perturbation* may momentarily disrupt the operation of the balance control system itself,[15] by interfering with perfusion of postural centers in the brain or brainstem (e.g. transient ischemic attacks, postural or postprandial hypotension, cardiac arrhythmias) or by disrupting the sensorimotor systems (e.g. episodes of dizziness or vertigo).

Mechanisms for maintaining and recovering balance

The neural control of COM stability may be *predictive* (anticipatory) or *reactive*[24] (Figure 39.5). Predictive control is possible if the characteristics of the destabilization are known in advance, e.g. when compensating for the destabilizing effect of a planned voluntary movement. In general, however, sensory information about the body orientation and motion is also required, particularly when balance is disturbed unexpectedly. This sensory information is used to detect instability and to generate appropriate stabilizing reactions, either by triggering and scaling preprogrammed feedforward reactions or by continuously updating ongoing feedback corrections. Because reactive control is the only recourse in the event of unexpected perturbation (e.g. slips, trips, pushes, errors in volitional movement), it is likely to play a critical role in preventing falls.[15] In reviewing the literature on reactive control, it is important to note that many studies have used relatively predictable perturbations. This promotes the ability to preplan aspects of the response,[25–28] which may not be applicable to situations in daily life, where balance is threatened unexpectedly.

The role of specific sensory sources in controlling postural reactions is somewhat controversial. It has been suggested that the visual, vestibular and somatosensory inputs are weighted, in an 'adaptable hierarchy', in order to optimize the feedback for given task conditions.[29] This would be appropriate, since different sensory modalities are more sensitive to specific stimulus bandwidths.[30,31] Vision is generally thought to be limited to stabilizing balance at low frequencies;[32–34] however, there is evidence that vision may also modulate responses to rapid perturbations.[35–37] Although it has been suggested that the vestibular system serves primarily as a 'comparator' to resolve sensory conflicts,[29] others have assigned it a more extensive role in generating stabilizing responses.[38–40] Studies of somatosensory contributions have usually focused on ankle proprioception, an important role of muscle spindles. Many believe that such input is critical in initiating responses to perturbation.[29,40–42] Until recently, the contribution of cutaneous mechanoreceptors on

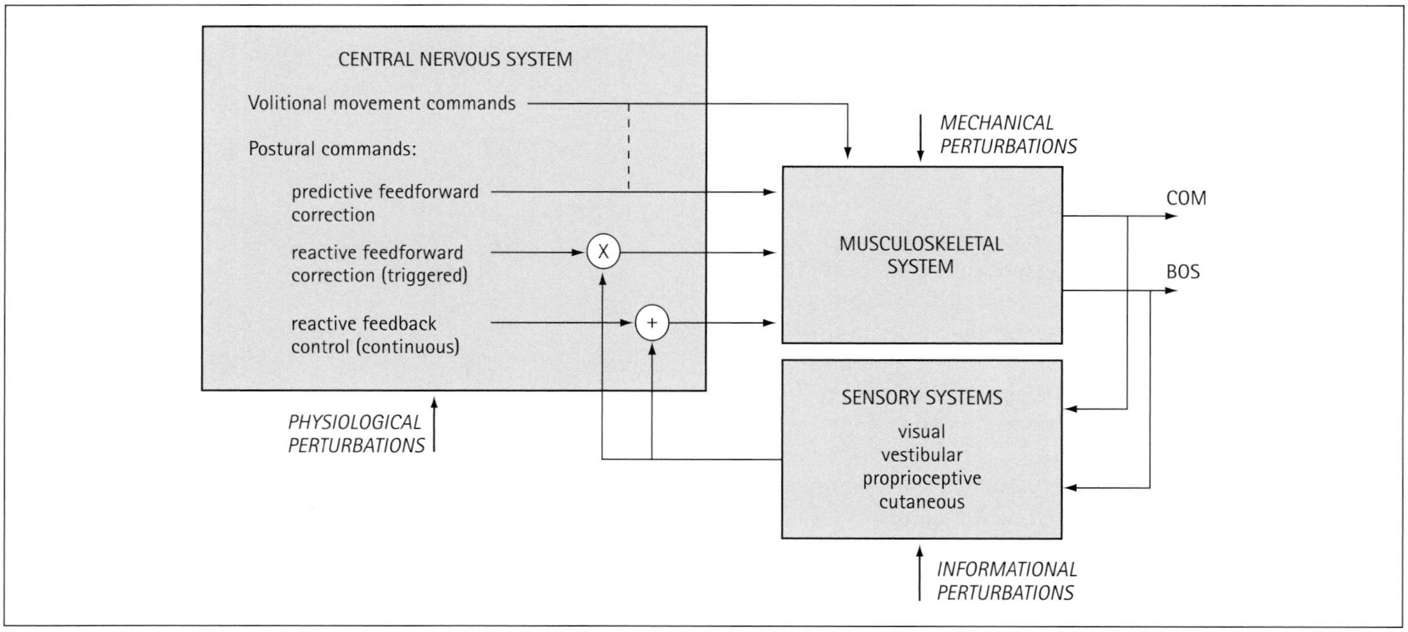

Figure 39.5 A conceptual model of the balance control system. The system acts to regulate the static and dynamic relationship between the body COM and the BOS established by the feet and/or arms, in the presence of: (1) mechanical perturbations (changes in forces acting on the body due to gravity, movement or interaction with the environment); (2) informational perturbations (transient changes in the nature of the orientational information available from the environment); or (3) physiological perturbations (transient internal events that disrupt the operation of the neural control system). Corrective changes to the COM are implemented via torque generation at the joints of the limbs and trunk; corrective changes to the BOS involve stepping or reach-and-grasp movements. In feedback control, sensory information is used to continuously update the corrections. In feedforward control, preprogrammed stabilizing reactions are released, either predictively (anticipatory postural adjustments) or in reaction to sensory information pertaining to the state of instability (triggered postural reactions). Anticipatory adjustments often precede volitional movements, and act to compensate for the destabilizing effects of the movement. (Adapted from Maki and McIlroy. *Clin Geriatr Med* 1996; **12**: 635–58.[15])

the plantar surface of the feet ('pressoceptors') to stabilization of posture has been largely discounted;[43] however, a number of studies support the view that these receptors can play an important role in controlling specific aspects of balance.[40,44–52] 'Haptic' cues arising during light touch of the hands with external objects can also have a pronounced effect on stabilization.[53]

It is important to recognize that functional balancing reactions are likely to involve multiple sensory inputs and highly adaptable triggered reactions, rather than stereotyped short-latency reflexive responses arising primarily from a single source of afferent drive (e.g. vestibulospinal reflex, myogenic stretch reflex). These sophisticated triggered reactions are believed to involve polysynaptic spinal and supraspinal neural pathways.[54] Furthermore, although balance control is often considered to be 'automated', a number of studies have demonstrated involvement of high-level cognitive and attentional systems. In dual-task experiments, performance on cognitive tasks has been shown to deteriorate as postural demands increase,[55–59,181] and reciprocal effects of cognitive task on control of balance have also been observed.[60–62,138,182–184] Furthermore, it appears that the different phases of postural reactions have differing attentional demands, and that rapid switching of attention is used to reallocate attentional resources as required.[185–186] The timing and scaling of the initial ankle-muscle activation evoked by a perturbation appear to be unaffected by the cognitive task; however, later phases of the stabilizing reaction may be altered.[185–188] It appears that reactions to perturbation are not as stereotyped as once believed, but are in fact highly adaptable to the functional demands of maintaining stability, i.e. regulating the relationship between COM and BOS.[13,14,63–65] Although some have speculated that critical afferent information for determining the state of the COM may arise from load receptors such as Golgi tendon organs,[65] it is important to recognize that maintaining stability also requires information about the state of the BOS and the direction of a gravitational (or gravito-inertial) reference vector (Figure 39.6). In contrast to the traditional view that the vestibular otoliths provide the reference vector, others have suggested a construct based on multiple sensory modalities.[66,67] Determination of the BOS state is also probably dependent on multiple sensory inputs, although it appears that the plantar cutaneous mechanoreceptors may play a particularly critical role in providing information pertaining to BOS stability limits and the state of contact between foot and ground.[50,52]

Traditionally, studies of reactive control have tended to focus on fixed-support reactions that involve maintaining the COM over an unchanging BOS, during unperturbed stance or in response to perturbations delivered (most commonly) using moveable platforms. These fixed-support reactions involve coordinated patterns of muscle activation which serve to generate the necessary stabilizing torques at the joints of the supporting limbs, trunk and neck. For stabilization in the anteroposterior direction, two fixed-support response 'strategies' have been identified: the 'ankle strategy', which relies primarily on ankle torque to stabilize the COM (see Figure 39.1), and the 'hip strategy', which involves the use of the hip flexors or extensors to generate shear forces at the feet in order to decelerate the COM.[68] The ankle strategy appears to predominate at small levels of perturbation, whereas increasing levels of hip activation are added as the postural challenge increases.[69] For stabilization in the mediolateral direction, the hip musculature appears to play a predominant role.[70,71] Although, historically, relatively little attention has been paid to lateral stability, it is particularly relevant to the falling problem, since a large proportion of falls involve lateral motion (42 of 95 falls in one

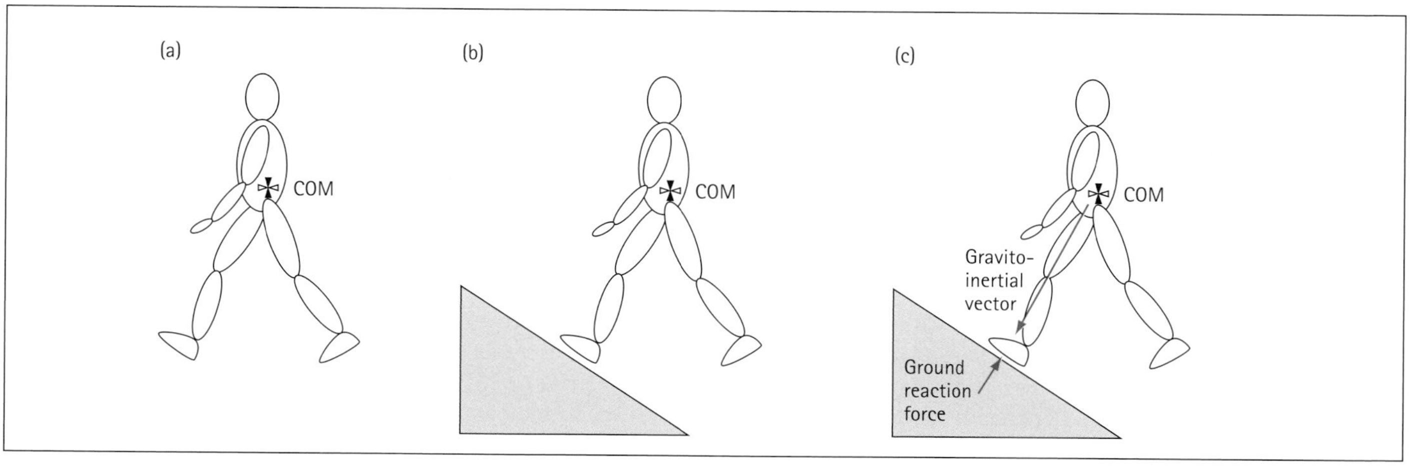

Figure 39.6 Sensory information required to maintain postural stability. The central nervous system (CNS) could, in theory, utilize a chain of proprioceptive information (from the joints and associated musculature of the different limb and axial body segments), in conjunction with stored information about the mass and COM of each segment, to estimate the position of the whole-body COM relative to the feet (a). However, in order to determine the state of stability, the CNS must also have access to information about the state of the BOS, i.e. which limbs are in contact with the environment and the nature of that contact (b). In addition, the CNS must have information about the direction of gravity (or the 'gravito-inertial' vector if the whole body is accelerating, e.g. when standing in a moving vehicle) (c). Assumptions that the ground surface was horizontal, in (a), or that the direction of gravity was vertical, in (b), would lead to erroneous conclusions about the actual state of stability depicted in (c).

study[72,73]), and debilitating hip-fracture injuries are most likely to occur as a result of lateral falls.[74]

The emphasis on fixed-support reactions that dominates the balance control literature has evolved largely on the basis of studies in which there are implicit or explicit constraints on limb movement; that is, there is no space to step or handholds to grasp and/or subjects are instructed not to move their feet or arms. However, when subjects are allowed to respond naturally, it becomes apparent that they will often step or move their arms so as to alter their BOS, even when the level of instability is relatively small.[16,75,76] These change-in-support reactions, i.e. compensatory stepping and grasping, ultimately have the potential to make a much greater contribution to stabilization, in comparison with fixed-support reactions, and are the only viable option in the event of large perturbation;[16,21,77] see Figure 39.2. In contrast to the view that the fixed-support 'hip strategy' plays an important role in responding to anteroposterior perturbation, it appears that individuals will normally elect to execute a change-in-support reaction, in preference to the hip strategy, when allowed to respond naturally.[16] Control of change-in-support reactions appears to differ, in some fundamental ways, from volitional limb-movement control. Compensatory stepping and grasping reactions are initiated and executed much more rapidly than reaction-time volitional movements (elicited, for example, by a visual cue).[16,75,78,79] In addition, rapid compensatory stepping reactions typically lack the large, functional anticipatory postural adjustments that invariably precede lifting of the swing limb during gait initiation or volitional leg movement[80–83] (the anticipatory adjustment acts to propel the COM toward the stance leg, prior to foot lift, in order to reduce the potential for the body to fall laterally toward the unsupported side after lifting the leg). It should be noted, however, that large anticipatory adjustments can be included, at very rapid latency, when task conditions demand a long interval of single-limb support, e.g. when withdrawing the foot from a noxious stimulus[189] or when execution of the compensatory stepping reaction requires clearance of an obstacle.[190]

Although the vast majority of studies have investigated balance control under conditions where the initial posture involves quiet stance, a number of investigators have studied reactions of young adults to perturbation during gait, applied most commonly via treadmill acceleration or motion of a platform or obstruction built into a walkway. These studies have revealed patterns of stabilizing muscle activation that are similar, in some respects, to the fixed-support reactions occurring during perturbation of quiet stance;[84] however, there are also distinct differences, e.g. phase-dependent modulation of reflex gain or pattern of muscle activation (according to the phase of the gait cycle)[85–87,199] and bilateral asymmetry in muscle activation.[88,89] Studies that have addressed the stability of gait have typically examined control of the COM without giving explicit consideration to the BOS control, i.e. foot placement, although it has been noted that foot-placement control actually appears to be the most important factor affecting stability;[23,90,91] see Figure 39.4.

Effects of aging on the substrates of balance control

The extent to which age-related balance impairment is due to sensory deficits, musculoskeletal factors or changes in CNS integrative mechanisms has not been well established. Although it appears that all of these factors are important,[15] some studies suggest that CNS factors are predominant.[92–94] Limitations due to CNS factors may manifest as an impaired ability to cope with heightened task demands. This is supported by studies showing that concurrent cognitive tasks have a greater effect on balance performance in older adults than in younger subjects.[60,95] In addition, two recent studies have shown that falling risk is associated with the tendency to 'stop walking when talking'[96] and to slow down when performing concurrent mobility and manual tasks.[97]

> Age-related changes in sensory systems, neural processing and musculoskeletal mechanics call all impact on the control of balancing reactions.

Sensory systems

Age-related changes, due primarily to loss of receptor cells and associated nerve cells or changes in receptor morphology, occur in all of the sensory systems that subserve balance control: visual, vestibular, proprioceptive and cutaneous.[98–102] These sensory impairments are often cited as an important contributor to age-related instability.[11,12,103,104] Sensory impairments could also lead to perceptual errors that increase the likelihood of experiencing perturbations, e.g. tripping on obstacles. Studies of associations between sensory function and falling risk in older adults have reported that individuals who experience falls are more likely to have decreased cutaneous sensation, proprioception, low-contrast visual acuity and contrast sensitivity.[105]

Musculoskeletal systems

Loss of muscle strength, associated primarily with loss and atrophy of muscle fibers, as well as loss of motoneurons, is one of the most well-documented changes associated with aging.[106] Slowing of muscle contraction and increased susceptibility to fatigue have also been well documented.[106] Whether these changes are a result of a biological aging process or are secondary to factors such as inactivity, impaired ability to generate muscle force is a fundamental biomechanical limitation that has the potential to affect the ability of the CNS to execute the stabilizing actions and reactions required to maintain upright stance. Relationships to falling risk have, in fact, been demonstrated. Severe compromise in the strength of the ankle dorsiflexors has been documented in nursing-home residents with a history of falling.[107] Other studies of less impaired individuals have also found evidence of associations between leg muscle weakness and increased falling risk.[105,108–111] In addition to problems in generating adequate muscle force, there may be age-related increases in intrinsic muscle stiffness which could potentially interfere with control of balance and movement.[112] Age-related decrease in flexibility and range of motion might also affect the ability to control volitional movement or compensatory postural responses. Although it appears that normal age-related loss of range of motion is actually rather small,[113] there is some evidence that individuals with a history of falling may have a smaller range of motion, in comparison to 'non-fallers'.[114]

Neural systems

Aging is associated with a number of changes to the CNS that could impact on balance control: loss of neurons, dendrite loss and reduced branching, impaired cerebral metabolism, reduced cerebral perfusion and altered transmitter metabolism.[115] It is likely that such changes disrupt the mobilization of complex postural responses, as well as reducing the ability to compensate for age-related impairments in sensory input. In addition, a general slowing of information processing,[92] in conjunction with an age-related decrease in nerve conduction velocity, may delay and further disrupt postural reactions. The functional significance of such changes is supported, indirectly, by observed associations between increased reaction time and falling risk.[105,111,116] To compound the problem, older adults appear to exhibit increased dependence on using high-level CNS resources for controlling balance,[59,60,182–184,200] as well as impaired ability to inhibit (and redirect) attention allocated to distracting tasks;[117,186] hence, they may experience particular difficulty in controlling balance in situations of daily life where attention is distracted from postural tasks. An impaired ability of the CNS to integrate sensory information is also thought to be an important contributor to increased risk of falling.[92–94] In support of this, older subjects experienced greater instability than young adults when somatosensory and/or visual cues were disrupted experimentally,[94,103,118,119] and subjects with a history of falling were less able to suppress inappropriate compensatory responses elicited by movement of the visual field, in comparison to 'non-fallers'.[120] In addition to effects on the balance recovery mechanisms, CNS impairments may contribute to an increased risk of sustaining a loss of balance, as a result of destabilization arising from errors in motor control or effects of impaired cognitive function (e.g. engaging in destabilizing motor behavior, failing to take account of environmental hazards).

Effects of aging on precipitants of falling

Sufficiently severe perturbations will result in falls, even in healthy young adults, and the ability to avoid falling, in any given situation, is entirely dependent on the extent to which the perturbation challenges the stabilizing capabilities of the individual's balance control system. Older adults are at risk for two reasons. First, because of age-related deterioration in the balance recovery mechanisms, the magnitude of perturbation that can be tolerated by older adults is reduced. Second, the problem is exacerbated by the fact that older adults may be more likely to experience perturbations, due to: (1) destabilization arising from impaired control of gait and volitional movement; (2) impairments of the anticipatory postural adjustments that normally act to mitigate such destabilization; and (3) cognitive or perceptual deficits that impair ability to identify and avoid environmental hazards, such as slippery surfaces and obstacles, during ongoing movement. The tendency to avoid more demanding activities, and to perform movements more slowly, may help to mitigate the risk of experiencing perturbations that exceed the individual's balancing capabilities. Nonetheless, the perturbations experienced by older adults may become problematic because of the decreased ability to compensate for what would, in many cases, represent only a relatively minor challenge for younger individuals.

Perturbation during gait

Perceptual errors could increase the likelihood of tripping over obstacles or slipping during gait. In addition, impaired control of toe clearance during the swing phase could increase the risk of tripping, and impaired control of foot velocity at heel contact could increase the risk of slipping. The latter problem is supported by reports of higher heel-contact 'skid velocity' in older, versus young, subjects;[121] however, at least one study has found no evidence of age-related differences in toe clearance during the swing phase, and in fact has shown that healthy older adults tend to exhibit less variability in the control of the toe clearance.[122] Errors in control of the foot placement during gait, i.e. missteps, may also perturb stability; reports that increased stride-to-stride variability in the control of stride length is associated with an elevated falling risk[123] could reflect such an effect. Conceivably, impaired ability to sense foot position and pressure on the sole of the foot could affect the ability to adapt the gait to accommodate changing ground conditions (e.g. surface irregularities, slipperiness, floor compliance), which could also increase the risk of misplacing the foot or slipping. In addition to problems associated with foot placement, impaired control of the COM during gait could also perturb stability. Such impairment (excessive lateral momentum) has been observed to occur in older adults who have vestibular hypofunction.[124]

Interestingly, it appears that older adults tend to modify their gait in a manner that actually acts to reduce many of these potential risk factors. Specifically, older adults tend to walk more slowly, with reduced stride length and increased duration of double-limb support,[122] and these stabilizing modifications tend to be more pronounced in individuals who have a fear of falling.[123] Additionally, in stepping over obstacles, older adults tend to exhibit greater toe clearance (thereby reducing risk of tripping) and tend to avoid forward motion of the foot at time of landing (thereby reducing risk of slipping), in comparison to young adults.[125] Age-related difficulty in stepping over or avoiding obstacles becomes apparent, however, when the individual must react suddenly to an obstacle that appears unpredictably;[126–128] these difficulties are exacerbated when subjects are distracted by a secondary cognitive task.[129]

Perturbation during volitional movement

In addition to problems in controlling gait, impairments in control of other volitional movements could act to increase the destabilizing effect of these movements. In general, however, it is difficult to dissect instability arising from errors in performing the movement from instability due to impaired ability to react to, and compensate for, the destabilizing effects of the movement. Nonetheless, it can be noted that studies have demonstrated age-related impairment in control of movements such as transferring from a chair.[130] In addition, some studies have shown that clinical balance assessments that involve rating performance on tasks such as rising from a chair, turning, bending and reaching can, to some degree, predict the risk of experiencing falls in older adults.[131,132] Furthermore, impaired performance on specific tasks—transfer, reaching and turning—was found to be predictive of increased risk of experiencing falls during the same types of activities in daily life.[72] Although errors in the control of these movements could be responsible for heightened destabilization, it should also be noted that older adults often tend to perform movements more slowly than younger individuals,[133] which may mitigate the destabilizing effect.

One potentially important aspect of this problem pertains to the control of the anticipatory postural adjustments that normally begin prior to the onset of the volitional movement. These anticipatory adjustments are widely believed to help compensate for the destabilizing effects of the volitional movement, although it should be noted that recent simulation studies have raised questions about the functional importance of the anticipatory adjustments that occur during certain types of movements.[134] Studies of the anticipatory activation of postural muscles that precedes movement of the arms have shown that older individuals are more likely to lack these anticipatory adjustments or to show changes in the relative timing of the postural and voluntary muscle activity.[135,136] Another study provided evidence that the magnitude of the anticipatory change in ground-reaction force, relative to the destabilizing effect of the arm movement, was actually larger in subjects who were at highest risk of falling, suggesting perhaps a disordered motor programming in these individuals.[137]

Effects of aging on control of stabilizing reactions

Control of balance with respect to a fixed base of support

Unperturbed stance

The majority of studies of balance and aging have focused on the control of quiet, unperturbed stance. The small movements that occur during unperturbed stance, as well as the postural activity that acts to control these movements, are often referred to as 'static' or 'spontaneous' postural sway. Spontaneous-sway measures are susceptible to confounding effects due to factors such as fear of falling and anxiety[7,138] and the extent to which the subject strives to minimize the sway;[139] therefore, one must be cautious in interpreting these measures. Nonetheless, spontaneous-sway tests are widely used, both clinically and experimentally, and it is commonly assumed that increases in the postural activity occurring during quiet stance are indicative of deterioration in the balance control system.

Numerous studies have documented age-related changes in measures related to the control of spontaneous postural sway,[11,94,98,118,140–147] and others have shown associations between these measures and risk of falling.[72,73,98,105,109,111,140,143,148–151] Most commonly, these measures are derived in terms of the displacement of the center of foot pressure (COP) (measured using force plates), which reflects the generation of stabilizing ankle torque (anteroposterior direction) and lateral 'weight shift' (mediolateral direction). Effects of aging are most pronounced in measures related to the rate at which the postural activity occurs,[15,73,143,145,152] whereas measures that characterize the amplitude of the corrective activity seem to be better indicators of the actual level of stability attained and the risk of experiencing falls.[73,143] Although, traditionally, relatively few studies of older adults have examined the control of lateral sway, one study in the early 1990s found the amplitude of mediolateral COP displacement, during blindfolded stance, to be the single best predictor of future falling risk, out of a wide range of static and dynamic balance measures.[73] Furthermore, the impairments in control of mediolateral sway observed in 'fallers' versus 'non-fallers' were disproportionately large relative to the impairments in control of anteroposterior sway;[153] see Figure 39.7a. More recent studies have since found further evidence to support a strong association between falling risk and lateral insta-

> Age-related difficulty in controlling lateral stability–evident during stance, during gait and during compensatory stepping–is of crucial importance because of the direct link between lateral falls and increased risk of sustaining a debilitating, and life-threatening, hip-fracture injury.

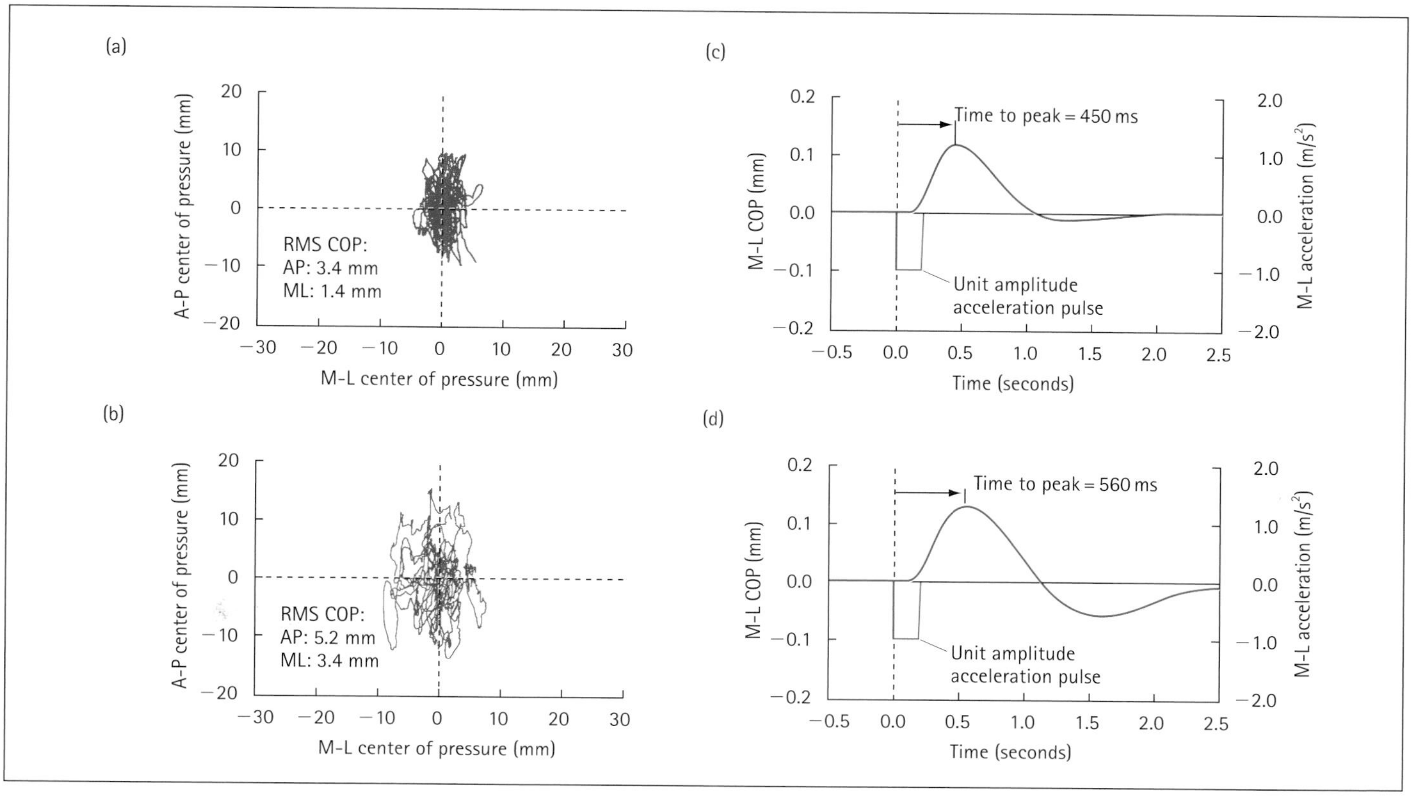

Figure 39.7 Changes in control of fixed-support reactions associated with risk of falling: spontaneous sway (a,b) and reactions to perturbation (c,d). Representative results are shown for elderly 'non-fallers' (a,c) and 'fallers' (b,d: falling status was based on 1 year of prospective fall monitoring). (a) and (b) show the anteroposterior (a–p) and mediolateral (m–l) displacement of the center of foot pressure (COP), relative to the mean location, recorded during 75 s of quiet standing (subjects blindfolded); the root-mean-square (RMS) COP displacement amplitudes are indicated on the graphs. Note that the COP displacement was larger in both directions in the 'faller'; however, the increase in the mediolateral direction was disproportionately large relative to the increase in the anteroposterior direction. (c) and (d) compare representative responses to mediolateral platform acceleration. The perturbation involved continuous pseudorandom platform motion (duration 96 s); a transfer function model fitted to the measured m–l acceleration and m–l COP data was used to predict the response to a sudden transient pulse of platform acceleration, as shown. Note the larger, and slower, response in the 'faller'.[73] (Adapted from Maki and McIroy. *Clin Geriatr Med* 1996; **12**: 635–58.[15])

bility during unperturbed stance, as well as other postural tasks.[196,201]

Efforts to model the control of spontaneous sway have suggested that older adults tend to exhibit longer intervals of unstable 'open-loop' (feedforward) control, coupled with more vigorous 'closed-loop' (feedback) corrections.[147] In addition, age-related reduction in the high-frequency content of the postural sway activity[152] has been interpreted to reflect loss of 'complexity' in the control mechanisms, which is thought to indicate a loss of adaptability.[115] To increase the level of challenge, the control of static stance is often characterized under altered BOS conditions: standing with feet together, heel to toe or on one leg.[154] Another approach is to instruct subjects to lean or reach as far as possible, in different directions, so as to characterize the 'functional BOS'.[155–157] Although such studies have demonstrated age-related differences and associations with falling risk, it is important to recognize that tests that require subjects to challenge their own balance are susceptible to confounding effects due to fear of falling. Thus, for example, in timing the maximum duration of one-leg stance, fearful subjects tend to 'bail out' early and hence perform poorly on the test; this poor performance may or may not be indicative of their physical ability to do the test.[7,73] Analogous effects, in which subjects underestimate their BOS stability limits, can occur during maximal lean/reach tests.[11]

Fixed-support reactions to perturbation

Whereas spontaneous-sway measures reflect reactions to the intrinsic instability of the upright body (due to gravity), these measures relate only indirectly, at best, to the ability to respond to overt perturbation. To study this ability directly, controlled perturbations are applied to the subject, most commonly by means of motion of the supporting (platform) surface. Studies of fixed-support reactions to perturbation have demonstrated that the sequence of muscle activation that is normally evoked by sudden transient anteroposterior platform translation is often disordered in older subjects, that there may be greater co-contraction of antagonistic muscles, and that the onset of the muscle activation and associated joint torque may be slightly delayed.[12,94,103,119,158] Studies of responses to toes-up and toes-down platform-tilt perturbations have also shown age-related increase in latency, as well as increased activation in certain muscles.[159] For the platform translation perturbations, small but consistent age-related increases in magnitude of body segment motion and joint torque have been noted, particularly in the upper body.[119,160,161] Older adults also tend to show less ability to control the head motion,[162] which may impact on the ability to stabilize the visual field and to use the vestibular system in controlling balancing responses. Observations of age-related increases in flexion–extension hip torque and hip rotation[119,160] appear to tie in with reports that older adults are more likely than the young to utilize the 'hip strategy';[12] however, it should be reiterated that the natural preference (in the absence of instructions to try not to step) is to take a step to recover balance, rather than executing a hip strategy.[16] Very few studies have examined whether falling risk is associated with an impaired control of fixed-support transient-perturbation reactions; the studies to date have indicated that there is little or no difference, between subjects with and without a prior history of falling, in terms of the latency, magnitude or pattern of the early 'automatic' muscle activation.[114,163]

Other studies have examined stabilizing reactions to continuous, rather than transient, perturbation. This approach facilitates the identification of control system models, which can provide insight into the nature of the control problem. Whereas responses to sudden transient perturbation are believed to involve the triggering (and scaling) of a preprogrammed response, the need to respond continuously to an ongoing, but unpredictable, perturbation demands a reliance on ongoing sensory feedback; hence, assessment of transient and continuous responses may provide complementary information about the integrity of the feedforward and feedback control processes, respectively. Older adults have been found to exhibit larger stabilizing responses to continuous pseudorandom platform motion, in comparison to young adults,[139,143] and delays in the responses to mediolateral perturbations (predicted by control models fitted to the data) were found to be highly associated with future risk of falling;[73] see Figure 39.7.

Causes of age-related changes in fixed-support control

Observed changes in fixed-support balance regulation and control may be due, in part, to age-related sensory loss. A number of studies have demonstrated small, but statistically significant, associations between sensory impairment and control of postural sway in older adults.[98,104,141,164,165] Generally, these studies have found that measures of lower-limb cutaneous sensation and proprioception tend to show the strongest correlations with the postural measures. In support of the importance of cutaneous sensation, it appears that facilitation of plantar cutaneous sensation (i.e. standing on an array of small skin indentors) has the potential to increase the speed of stabilizing responses to lateral perturbation in older adults with impaired plantar sensitivity.[15] In addition, correlations between plantar insensitivity and the degree of head motion resulting from transient antero-posterior platform perturbation have been reported.[166] With regard to other sensory modalities, at least one study of older adults has shown an association between visual acuity and postural sway,[150] and others have shown that visual acuity, contrast sensitivity and/or stereopsis become important when ankle and plantar sensation (as well as joint stiffness) are disrupted by standing on a compliant (foam rubber) surface.[104,146,197] In a study of community-dwelling females, the level of vestibular dysfunction was found to be associated with the amplitude of sway only when vision, as well as accurate ankle–foot somatosensation, were both deprived during the sway measurements.[146]

As outlined earlier, age-related neural changes may also play an important role, although most experimental evidence pertains to adaptability to task conditions. One study found that postural sway actually increased in older subjects when sensory inputs were suddenly augmented (i.e. during transitions from absence to presence of vision), whereas young adults were able to adapt rapidly and use the visual information to reduce their sway.[93] Analogous findings were reported for transitions between conditions where ankle proprioception was or was not disrupted (via tendon vibration).[167] In addition, it appears that older adults are less able to adapt to predictable task conditions. In response to repeated presentations of small perturbations, older subjects did not show the progressive reduction in sway observed in young adults.[168]

The contribution of impaired musculoskeletal function to the control of fixed-support reactions is somewhat controversial. Some studies have demonstrated small, but statistically significant, correlations between leg muscle strength and measures of postural sway;[104,146] however, other evidence raises some questions about the extent to which normal age-related loss of muscle strength directly affects the ability to execute fixed-support postural reactions. Studies of fixed-support reactions to antero-posterior postural perturbation have indicated that the muscle force required to generate these reactions, as well as the range of joint motion, is well within the capabilities of healthy older adults,[160] however, it appears that studies have not yet examined possible problems due to impaired speed of force generation.

Control of change-in-support reactions

To date, studies of age-related changes in change-in-support reactions have been largely limited to compensatory stepping. Studies of age-related changes in compensatory grasping, to date, have shown that older adults are more dependent on using arm reactions than younger subjects[173,175] yet the speed at which they can initiate and execute the grasping movements is delayed.[191] Increased dependence on arm reactions and slowing of these reactions are both predictive of increased risk of falling.[191]

> Older adults tend to be more reliant than young adults on using the arms to recover balance, yet their grasping reactions are slower.

Stepping behavior

A number of studies have demonstrated age-related difficulties in the ability to recover balance by stepping, and it has been reported that these difficulties appear to be more pronounced in individuals who have a history of falling.[169,170]

> Rapid compensatory stepping and grasping reactions play a critical role in preventing falls.

In apparent support of age-related control difficulty, several studies have shown that older subjects are more likely than young adults to take multiple steps, rather than a single step, in responding to anteroposterior perturbation.[169,171–173] It appears that these multiple-step responses may often emerge as a consequence of events arising *after* the initiation of the first step, rather than as a strategy planned in advance.[173] Impaired ability to control the tendency of the COM to fall laterally toward the unsupported side during step execution appears to be a particular problem. In one study,[173] over 30% of the initial forward- or backward-stepping reactions in the older adults were followed by steps that were directed so as to recover lateral stability, a tendency that was rarely seen in young adults (Figure 39.8a).

> Older adults often appear to experience difficulty in controlling lateral stability during the execution of stepping reactions, and there may be additional problems associated with the control of lateral leg movement (i.e. collisions with the stance limb) when stepping laterally.

Findings that older subjects with a history of falling tended to include lateral foot movement in the initial step of the reaction, when stepping in response to forward instability,[82,174,192] would also appear to indicate difficulty in controlling lateral stability during anteroposterior step execution. Attempts to compensate for lateral instability in this manner could represent a predictive strategy, which may have been facilitated by the more predictable perturbation conditions used in that study. It is also possible that such an adaptation is specific to subjects with a recent history of unsteadiness and falling. A prospective study found that the tendency to take multiple steps to recover balance, to follow an initial forward or backward step with a lateral step and to experience collision between the swing foot and stance limb were predictive of increased risk of falling.[191]

Studies of stepping reactions evoked by lateral perturbation have revealed further age-related difficulty in conrolling lateral stability. Older adults were more likely than the young to step in response to lateral platform perturbation, and were also more likely to take multiple steps or to use arm reactions to regain equilibrium.[175] Furthermore, there were age-related differences in the pattern of stepping. The predominant pattern of stabilizing response in young adults involved 'crossing over' with the leg that tended to be unloaded by the lateral COM motion induced by the perturbation.[176] This response required a long and relatively complex swing trajectory, and a prolonged swing duration, in order to move the foot across (either in front or behind) the body while circumventing the stance leg. Older subjects tended to avoid these demands by using instead a sequence of small 'side-steps' (Figure 39.8b). Nonetheless, older adults still experienced difficulty in avoiding collisions between the swing foot and stance limb. These difficulties were greatly exacerbated when the demands of controlling balance during gait were simulated by asking subjects to walk 'in place' on the platform prior to perturbation.

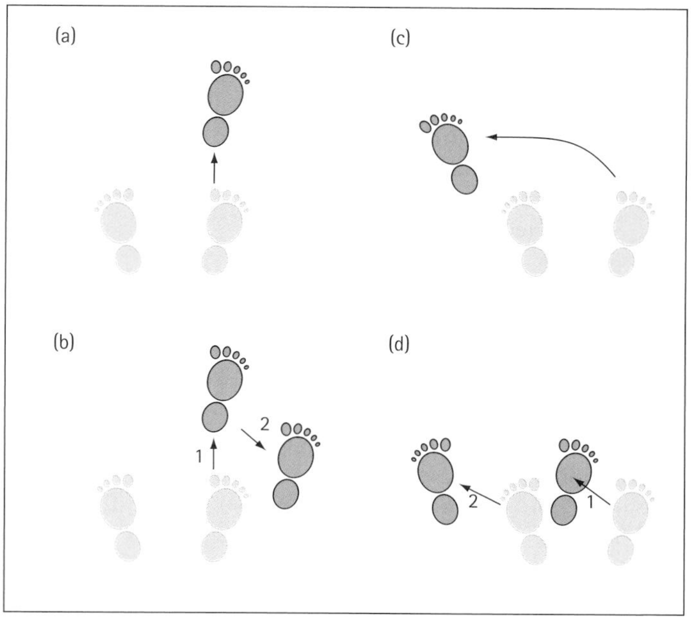

Figure 39.8 Age-related changes in patterns of compensatory stepping, in response to anteroposterior (a–p) perturbation (a, b) and mediolateral (m–l) perturbation (c, d) in young (a, c) and old (b, d). The feet outlines that are depicted with light shading represent the initial stance position. Although the examples shown only depict responses to instability in the forward (a–p) and leftward (m–l) directions, analogous behavior occurs for backward and rightward falls. Note that older adults are much more likely to take multiple steps in responding to anteroposterior instability (b), in contrast to the single-step response commonly exhibited by young adults (a). Although various patterns of multiple stepping can occur, the second step is often likely to include a lateral component, as shown here.[173] In responding to lateral perturbation, young adults tend to use a crossover step (c), which requires a long and relatively complex swing trajectory, and a prolonged duration of single-leg support, in order to move the foot across the body while circumventing the stance leg.[176] Even healthy and active older adults tend to avoid the demands associated with the crossover step, instead using a sequence of small side-steps (d); however, these older individuals are still more likely to require additional reactions (stepping or grasping) in order to recover equilibrium.[175] Moreover, older adults often appear to experience difficulty in controlling the swing-foot motion and are more likely to sustain collisions between the swing foot and stance limb.

Control of step initiation

With regard to control of compensatory step initiation, it has been observed that older adults are less likely to execute an anticipatory postural adjustment, prior to lifting the swing leg, when stepping in response to anteroposterior perturbation.[82,173] This, however, is unlikely to jeopardize safety. The anticipatory postural adjustments that occur during rapid compensatory stepping reactions are typically too small or brief to provide much functional benefit with regard to lateral stabilization.[83] In fact, the absence of the anticipatory phase is likely to be beneficial, because the delay in response associated with the inclusion of the anticipatory phase could actually jeopardize safety. In general, it appears that age-related differences in the timing of step initiation tend to be small,[173,177,193] suggesting instead that many of the difficulties are associated with control of the swing phase and/or landing. However, results to the contrary, i.e. earlier foot-lift in older subjects, have also been reported.[171,172] The reason for this discrepancy may lie in differences in instructions given to the subjects. It may be that younger subjects are, in fact, able to respond more rapidly when allowed to respond naturally or when given prior instructions to step, but may be more willing to delay step initiation (and risk instability) when told to try not to step.

Causes of age-related changes in stepping

The age-related changes in stepping behavior that have been observed could be a consequence of decrements in musculoskeletal capacity, sensory function and/or neural processing. Again, the contribution of impaired musculoskeletal function is controversial. The flexion–extension joint torques, as well as range of joint motion, required to initiate rapid backward compensatory steps appear to be well within the capabilities of healthy older adults.[171,172] However, it appears that the torque demands in certain muscles (e.g. hip abductors, hip flexors, knee extensors) during later phases of the stepping response can actually be very close to the strength limits measured in older adults,[77] and loss of strength is associated with the tendency to take multiple steps to recover balance.[194] This raises the possibility that age-related strength loss may, in some older individuals, contribute to difficulty in controlling stability during the swing phase and landing. Rate of muscle-force production may also be an important limiting factor. Although it appears that healthy older adults are well able to generate rapid anteroposterior stepping movements in responding to moderate levels of perturbation,[173,177] they seem to be unable to generate the faster movements that are required to deal with more severe postural challenge.[177]

Studies pertaining to the effect of neural impairments on the control of compensatory stepping have addressed pathological changes associated with stroke-induced hemiparesis[77,178] and Parkinson's disease.[179,195] With regard to effects of normal age-related changes in neural function, it has been shown that delay in volitional reaction time is associated with the tendency to take multiple steps to recover balance.[194] With regard to sensory function, it appears quite likely that age-related loss of cutaneous sensation, from the plantar surface of the foot, is an important factor contributing to impaired control of compensatory stepping. In support of this, facilitation of sensation from the boundaries of the plantar foot surface (using skin indentors) was found to decrease the frequency of multiple-step reactions, during forward 'falls', in older adults with moderate levels of cutaneous insensitivity.[52] This finding is complemented by the results of a study involving young adults, whereby attenuation of plantar sensation, via hypothermic anesthesia (cooling the foot sole in ice water), led to an increased frequency of multiple-step reactions in responding to forward instability.[50] Results from another study suggest that the level of cutaneous sensitivity, in older adults, may be associated, in a complex way, with the propensity for taking 'extra' steps or executing additional arm reactions; age-related changes in vestibular, visual and proprioceptive function did not correlate with the observed stepping behavior.[180,194] The observed effects of cutaneous facilitation/ attenuation on control of forward stepping appear to be related to the ability to sense and control heel contact and subsequent weight transfer during step termination.[77] Other observed contributions of the cutaneous receptors, in sensing the posterior stability limits and in maintaining stability during the prolonged swing phase of lateral crossover steps,[50,52] may tie in with other age-related changes in stepping behavior, i.e. increased tendency to step in response to backward instability and avoiding use of crossover steps.

> Loss of cutaneous sensation from the foot, impaired capacity to integrate multiple sensory inputs, slowing the reaction time, limits on strength and speed of muscle contraction, and impaired ability to rapidly switch attention to the balancing task appear to be amongst the most important contributors to age-related impairment in controlling various aspects of balance.

Summary

> Clinical assessment and treatment of balance impairments should include a focus on lateral stability and control of compensatory stepping and grasping. Efforts should be directed, during assessment, at simulating the heightened demands of controlling balance in daily life, i.e. effects of ongoing physical and cognitive activity, as well as environmental constraints on movement.

In order to maintain upright stability, the CNS must regulate the relationship between the COM of the body and the BOS established by the feet (and, in some situations, the arms). Thus, the perturbations that precipitate falls must ultimately affect the COM and/or the BOS, and the stabilizing responses to these perturbations must involve a movement of the COM and/or a change in the BOS.

To accomplish the task of maintaining stability, the CNS must rapidly integrate sensory information from visual, vestibular, proprioceptive and cutaneous sources, and use this information to generate complex motor responses that are appropriate, in terms of timing, direction and magnitude, to the characteristics of the balance disturbance, the current postural state (e.g. foot position, ongoing movement) and the constraints of the surrounding environment (e.g. friction of the support surface, unobstructed space to step, availability of handholds to grasp). Age-related changes in sensory systems, neural processing and musculoskeletal mechanics could all impact on this process.

It is possible that older adults may be more likely than the young to experience perturbations during certain activities and movements due to errors in motor control, impaired control of anticipatory postural adjustments and/or perceptual/cognitive deficits; however, it appears that age-related slowing of movement, and other adaptations, may help to limit the magnitude of the destabilizing effect in some situations. Nonetheless, the potential for increased frequency of experiencing perturbations is problematic because of the deterioration in the ability to compensate for balance disturbance.

Traditionally, researchers and clinicians have tended to focus on the control of the COM displacement over a fixed BOS, and numerous studies have documented age-related changes in the control of fixed-support balance regulation during quiet standing and fixed-support reactions to applied perturbation. There is, in general, a slowing and disordered control of fixed-support control in older adults, and difficulty in controlling lateral stability, in particular, appears to be a strong predictor of increased risk of falling. It is not yet clear to what extent these problems are due to sensory impairments versus problems in neural integration, although it is very likely that both factors are important. It does appear, however, that normal age-related reduction in muscle strength or range of motion is not typically a limiting factor in generating compensatory fixed-support reactions during stance; possible effects due to limits on speed of muscle contraction need to be explored further.

Over the last several years, increasing attention has been directed toward the control of changes in the BOS, i.e. compensatory limb movement, as an important element of the postural repertoire. By removing constraints on postural behavior, it becomes apparent that such limb movements are very often the predominant reaction to instability. Older adults appear to be more dependent than the young on using the arms to recover balance yet their grasping reactions are slower. There also appears to be a profound impairment in the control of compensatory stepping movements in older adults. Again, lateral instability appears to be a major problem, related to the challenge of controlling the COM during the movement and placement of the swing foot. Additional problems arise in attempting to control lateral movement of the swing foot, due to the challenge of avoiding collision with the stance limb. With regard to mechanisms, early findings implicate age-related loss of cutaneous sensation, from the plantar surface of the foot, as an important contributing factor. Limits on strength and speed of muscle contraction could also play a role.

Older adults exhibit an impaired ability to adapt rapidly to changing environmental conditions, and this may also contribute to increased falling risk. Studies also show a decreased ability to adapt to predictable testing conditions, but this is less likely to bear a relation to falls, which seem to occur most commonly when events happen unpredictably. Caution must be exercised in interpreting results derived from relatively predictable test conditions, since age-related differences recorded under such conditions could well be due to differences in adaptive capabilities, rather than other age-related factors. It also appears that older adults may attempt to compensate for deterioration in sensorimotor systems by relying, to a greater extent than the young, on high-level CNS resources in order to control their balance; this may lead to difficulties in situations where attention is distracted by ongoing cognitive or physical tasks.

In attempting to extrapolate from the results of laboratory or clinical balance tests (Table 39.3) so as to understand the

Table 39.3 Techniques for balance assessment.

Semiquantitative tests
Ability to adopt challenging postures (e.g. one-leg stance)
Ability to lean or reach
Activity-based performance assessment
Traditional 'posturography'
Spontaneous postural sway
Fixed-support reactions to external perturbation
Anticipatory postural adjustments (during volitional movement)
Newer approaches
Compensatory stepping reactions to external perturbation
Compensatory grasping reactions to external perturbation
Reactions to perturbations during ongoing movement

Table 39.4 Confounding effects due to fear of falling.

Clinical balance tests
Poor score on timed one-leg stance test
Poor scores on elements of activity-based performance assessments
Tendency to underestimate functional stability limits
Posturographic balance tests
Large anteroposterior center-of-pressure displacement during blindfolded stance
Tendency to lean forward
Tendency to adopt a wider base of support
Gait assessment
Small stride length
Slow walking speed
Greater proportion of gait cycle spent in double-support

problems faced by older adults in controlling stability in their daily lives, future work will likely benefit by: (1) mimicking, as much as possible, the varied and unpredictable nature of the events that often precipitate falls in daily life; (2) simulating the heightened demands of maintaining balance while performing concurrent cognitive or motor tasks; (3) removing constraints on postural behavior that may artificially promote specific control strategies (e.g. hip strategy) in preference to others (e.g. stepping); and (4) delineating effects that are associated with fear, rather than risk, of falling (Table 39.4). Control of lateral stability should be a major focus (Table 39.5) in choosing techniques to assess balance and falling risk and in developing interventions to help prevent falls (Tables 39.6 and 39.7). Addressing the difficulties that older adults appear to experience in controlling lateral stability may be of particular importance in reducing the risk of sustaining debilitating, and potentially life-threatening, hip-fracture injuries.

Table 39.5 Evidence of lateral instability in older adults.

Fixed-support balance control
Large mediolateral center-of-pressure displacement during quiet stance
Large, and slow, response to mediolateral perturbation
Stepping to recover balance
Anteroposterior perturbation
Extra steps in the lateral direction
The initial step may include a lateral component
Lateral perturbation
Avoidance of large crossover steps
Extra stepping or grasping reactions required to recover equilibrium
Collisions between the swing foot and stance limb
Control of balance during gait
Large stride width
Increase in lateral momentum

Table 39.6 Prevention of falls and their consequences.

Identify the high-risk individual
History of falling, unsteadiness or dizziness
If no obvious problems, perform balance/gait screening tests
Identify/treat medical factors
Diagnosis and treatment of specific disorders
Correct visual impairment
Review and adjust medications and dosages
Treatment to reduce osteoporosis
Interventions
Train balance during volitional movement (e.g. Tai Chi) and functional balance recovery (including compensatory stepping and grasping)
Train balance confidence (self-efficacy)
Train how to get up after a fall
Education with regard to risk factors and risk-taking behavior
Change footwear (low heels, moderate friction, minimal cushioning)
Prescribe walking aids, wheelchairs, hip padding
Use bed alarms, for high-risk patients in institutional settings
Environmental modifications ('fall-proof' the home or room)

Table 39.7 Environmental modifications to prevent falls and their consequences.

Floor coverings
Non-skid wax on floors; non-skid strips in bathtub
Avoid area rugs; tape down edges of rugs/carpets
Avoid transitions (carpet–tile) or tie to visual cues (e.g. doorways)
Avoid carpets/tiles with misleading visual cues
Eliminate trip hazards (even small edges), obstacles
Use thin carpets to provide 'padding'
Lighting/vision
Uniform and bright; no glare
Night-lights in bedroom
Wear properly prescribed lenses; avoid bifocals
Handrails and grab-bars
Highly visible, graspable, securely mounted
Install on all stairs (both sides) and in bathrooms
Vertical poles near chairs, bed, toilet, bath
Seating
Armrests on chairs, stable base
Avoid low chairs, overly compliant cushions
Toilets and bathtubs
Raise height of toilet base, add armrests
Install bathtubs with low walls and/or transfer aids
Stairways
No visual distractions; edges of treads well marked
Well lighted (always on, or switch at top and bottom)
No loose carpeting; no obstacles
New stairways: adequate tread size, no tread-to-tread variation in dimensions
Emergency response systems
Always accessible and operable

Acknowledgments

This work has been supported by Grants No. MT-10576 and MT-13355 from the Canadian Institutes of Health Research (CIHR; formerly, Medical Research Council) and Grants No. AG-06357 and AG-12165 from the National Institute on

Aging (USA). B. E. M. holds a CIHR Senior Scientist career award. The authors thank G. R. Fernie for comments and suggestions.

References

1. Baker SP, Harvey AH. Fall injuries in the elderly. *Clin Geriatr Med* 1985; **1**: 501–12.
2. Kennedy TE, Coppard LCE. The prevention of falls in later life (report of the Kellog International Work Group on the Prevention of Falls by the Elderly). *Danish Med Bull* 1987; **34**(suppl 4): 1–24.
3. Black SE, Maki BE, Fernie GR. Aging, imbalance and falls. In: Barber H, Sharpe J, eds. *Vestibulo-ocular Reflex, Nystagmus and Vertigo*. New York: Raven Press, 1993: 317–35.
4. Hayes WC, Myers ER, Robinovitch SN et al. Etiology and prevention of age-related hip fractures. *Bone* 1996; **18**: 77S–86S.
5. Grimley Evans J, Prudham D, Wandess I. A prospective study of fractured proximal femur: incidence and outcome. *Public Health* 1979; **93**: 235–41.
6. Murphy J, Isaacs B. The post-fall syndrome: a study of 36 elderly patients. *Gerontology* 1982; **28**: 265–70.
7. Maki BE, Holliday PJ, Topper AK. Fear of falling and postural performance in the elderly. *J Gerontol* 1991; **46**: M123–31.
8. Arfken CL, Lach HW, Birge SJ et al. The prevalence and correlates of fear of falling in elderly persons living in the community. *Am J Publ Health* 1994; **84**: 565–70.
9. Tinetti ME, Mendes de Leon CF, Doucette JT et al. Fear of falling and fall-related efficacy in relationship to functioning among community-living elderly persons. *J Gerontol* 1994; **49**: M140–7.
10. Tinetti ME, Williams CS. Falls, injuries due to falls, and the risk of admission to a nursing home. *New Engl J Med* 1997; **337**: 1279–84.
11. Horak FB, Shupert CL, Mirka A. Components of postural dyscontrol in the elderly: a review. *Neurobiol Aging* 1989; **10**: 727–38.
12. Manchester D, Woollacott M, Zederbauer-Hylton N et al. Visual, vestibular and somatosensory contributions to balance control in the older adult. *J Gerontol* 1989; **44**: M118–27.
13. Gollhofer A, Horstmann GA, Berger W et al. Compensation of translational and rotational perturbations in human posture: stabilization of the centre of gravity. *Neurosci Lett* 1989; **105**: 73–8.
14. Horstmann GA, Dietz V. A basic posture control mechanism: the stabilization of the centre of gravity. *Electroencephalogr Clin Neurophysiol* 1990; **76**: 165–76.
15. Maki BE, McIlroy WE. Postural control in the older adult. *Clin Geriatr Med* 1996; **12**: 635–58.
16. Maki BE, McIlroy WE. The role of limb movements in maintaining upright stance: the 'change-in-support' strategy. *Phys Ther* 1997; **77**: 488–507.
17. Marsden CD, Merton PA, Morton HB. Human postural responses. *Brain* 1981; **104**: 513–34.
18. Nashner LM. Adaptation of human movement to altered environments. *Trends Neurosci* 1982; **5**: 358–61.
19. Britton TC, Day BL, Brown P et al. Postural electromyographic responses in the arm and leg following galvanic vestibular stimulation in man. *Exp Brain Res* 1993; **94**: 143–51.
20. Pai YC, Patton J. Center of mass velocity–position predictions for balance control. *J Biomech* 1997; **30**: 347–54.
21. Maki BE, McIlroy WE. The control of foot placement during compensatory stepping reactions: does speed of response take precedence over stability? *IEEE Trans Rehabil Eng* 1999; **7**: 80–90.
22. Jian Y, Winter DA, Ishac MG et al. Trajectory of the body COG and COP during initiation and termination of gait. *Gait Posture* 1993; **1**: 9–22.
23. MacKinnon CD, Winter DA. Control of whole body balance in the frontal plane during human walking. *J Biomech* 1993; **26**: 633–44.
24. Frank JS, Earl M. Coordination of posture and movement. *Phys Ther* 1990; **70**: 855–63.
25. Horak FB, Diener HC, Nashner LM. Influence of central set on human postural responses. *J Neurophysiol* 1989; **62**: 841–53.
26. Beckley DJ, Bloem BR, Remler MP et al. Long latency postural responses are functionally modified by cognitive set. *Electroencephalogr Clin Neurophysiol* 1991; **81**: 353–8.
27. Maki BE, Whitelaw RS. Influence of expectation and arousal on centre-of-pressure responses to transient postural perturbations. *J Vestib Res* 1993; **3**: 25–39.
28. McIlroy WE, Maki BE. The 'deceleration response' to transient perturbation of upright stance. *Neurosci Lett* 1994; **175**: 13–16.
29. Nashner LM. Adaptation to altered support and visual conditions during stance patients with vestibular deficits. *J Neurosci* 1982; **2**: 536–44.
30. Nashner LM. Analysis of stance posture in humans. In: Towe AL, Luschei ES, eds. *Handbook of Behavioral Neurobiology*. New York: Plenum Press, 1981: 527–65.
31. Diener HC, Dichgans J. On the role of vestibular visual and somatosensory information for dynamic postural control in humans. *Prog Brain Res* 1988; **76**: 253–61.
32. Dichgans J, Mauritz KH, Allum JHJ et al. Postural sway in normals and ataxic patients analysis of the stabilizing and destabilizing effects of vision. *Agressologie* 1976; **17**: 15–24.
33. Lestienne F, Soechting J, Berthoz A. Postural readjustments induced by linear motion of visual scenes. *Exp Brain Res* 1977; **28**: 363–84.
34. Diener HC, Dichgans J, Bruzek W et al. Stabilization of human posture during induced oscillations of the body. *Exp Brain Res* 1982; **45**: 126–32.
35. Nashner LM, Berthoz A. Visual contribution to rapid motor responses during postural control. *Brain Res* 1978; **150**: 403–7.
36. Ledin T, Odkvist M. Visual influence on postural reactions to sudden antero-posterior support surface movements. *Acta Otolaryngol Stockh* 1991; **111**: 813–19.
37. Timmann D, Belting C, Schwarz M et al. Influence of visual and somatosensory input on leg EMG responses in dynamic posturography in normals. *Electroencephalogr Clin Neurophysiol* 1994; **93**: 7–14.
38. Allum JHJ, Pfaltz CR. Visual and vestibular contributions to pitch sway stabilization in the ankle muscles of normals and patients with bilateral peripheral vestibular deficits. *Exp Brain Res* 1985; **58**: 82–94.

39. Allum JHJ, Keshner EA, Honegger F et al. Organization of leg–trunk–head equilibrium movements in normals and patients with peripheral vestibular deficits. *Prog Brain Res* 1988; **76**: 34–45.
40. Horak FB, Nashner LM, Diener HC. Postural strategies associated with somatosensory and vestibular loss. *Exp Brain Res* 1990; **82**: 167–77.
41. Dietz V, Quintern J, Berger W. Afferent control of human stance and gait: evidence for blocking of group I afferents during gait. *Exp Brain Res* 1985; **61**: 153–63.
42. Inglis JT, Horak FB, Shupert CL et al. The importance of somatosensory information in triggering and scaling automatic postural responses in humans. *Exp Brain Res* 1994; **101**: 159–64.
43. Diener HC, Dichgans J, Guschlbauer B et al. The significance of proprioception on postural stabilization as assessed by ischemia. *Brain Res* 1984; **296**: 103–9.
44. Watanabe I, Okubo J. The role of the plantar mechanoreceptor in equilibrium control. *Ann NY Acad Sci* 1981; **374**: 855–64.
45. Magnusson M, Enbom H, Johansson R et al. Significance of pressor input from the human feet in anterior–posterior postural control. *Acta Otolaryngol Stockh* 1990; **110**: 182–8.
46. Do MC, Bussel B, Breniere Y. Influence of plantar cutaneous afferents on early compensatory reactions to forward fall. *Exp Brain Res* 1990; **79**: 319–24.
47. Do MC, Roby-Brami A. The influence of a reduced plantar support surface area on the compensatory reactions to a forward fall. *Exp Brain Res* 1991; **84**: 439–43.
48. Asai H, Fujiwara K, Tachino K. Limiting factor for movable range of the centre of foot pressure in backward direction. In: Taguchi K, Igarashi M, Mori S, eds. *Vestibular and Neural Front*. Tokyo: Elsevier, 1994: 525–8.
49. Wu G, Chiang JH. The significance of somatosensory stimulations to the human foot in the control of postural reflexes. *Exp Brain Res* 1997; **114**: 163–9.
50. Perry SD, McIlroy WE, Maki BE. The role of cutaneous mechanoreceptors in the control of compensatory stepping reactions evoked by unpredictable, multi-directional perturbation. *Brain Res* 2000; **877**: 401–6.
51. Thoumie P, Do MC. Changes in motor activity and biomechanics during balance recovery following cutaneous and muscular deafferentation. *Exp Brain Res* 1996; **110**: 289–97.
52. Maki BE, Perry SD, Norrie RG et al. Effect of facilitation of sensation from plantar foot–surface boundaries on postural stabilization in young and older adults. *J Gerontol* 1999; **54A**: M281–7.
53. Jeka JJ. Light touch contact as a balance aid. *Phys Ther* 1997; **77**: 476–87.
54. Dietz V. Human neuronal control of automatic functional movements: interaction between central programs and afferent input. *Physio Rev* 1992; **72**: 33–69.
55. Kerr B, Condon SM, McDonald LA. Cognitive spatial processing and the regulation of posture. *J Exp Psychol* 1985; **11**: 617–22.
56. Teasdale N, Bard C, LaRue J et al. On the cognitive penetrability of posture control. *Exp Aging Res* 1993; **19**: 1–13.
57. Lajoie Y, Teasdale N, Bard C et al. Attentional demands for static and dynamic equilibrium. *Exp Brain Res* 1993; **97**: 139–44.
58. Lassau-Wray ER, Parker AW. Neuromuscular responses of elderly women to tasks of increasing complexity imposed during walking. *Eur J Appl Physiol Occupat Physiol* 1993; **67**: 476–80.
59. Lajoie Y, Teasdale N, Bard C et al. Upright standing and gait: are there changes in attentional requirements related to normal aging? *Exp Aging Res* 1996; **22**: 185–98.
60. Stelmach GE, Zelaznik HN, Lowe D. The influence of aging and attentional demands on recovery from postural instability. *Aging* 1990; **2**: 155–61.
61. Geurts CH, Mulder TW, Ninhuis B et al. Dual-task assessment of reorganization of postural control in persons with lower limb amputation. *Arch Phys Med Rehabil* 1991; **72**: 1059–64.
62. Schlesinger A, Redfern MS, Dahl RE et al. Postural control, attention and sleep deprivation. *Neuroreport* 1998; **9**: 49–52.
63. Clement G, Gurfinkel VS, Lestienne F et al. Changes of posture during transient perturbations in microgravity. *Aviat Space Environ Med* 1985; **56**: 666–71.
64. Dietz V, Horstman GA, Trippel M et al. Human postural reflexes and gravity—an under water simulation. *Neurosci Lett* 1989; **106**: 350–5.
65. Dietz V, Gollhofer A, Klieber M et al. Regulation of bipedal stance: dependency on 'load' receptors. *Exp Brain Res* 1992; **89**: 229–31.
66. Stoffregen TA, Riccio GE. An ecological theory of orientation and the vestibular system. *Psychol Rev* 1988; **95**: 3–14.
67. Gurfinkel VS, Ivanenko YP, Levik YS et al. Kinesthetic reference for human orthograde posture. *Neuroscience* 1995; **68**: 229–43.
68. Horak FB, Nashner LM. Central programming of postural movements: adaptation to altered support-surface configurations. *J Neurophysiol* 1986; **55**: 1369–81.
69. Runge CF, Shupert CL, Horak FB et al. Ankle and hip postural strategies defined by joint torques. *Gait Posture* 1999; **10**: 161–70.
70. Winter DA, Prince F, Frank JS et al. Unified theory regarding a/p and m/l balance in quiet stance. *J Neurophysiol* 1996; **75**: 2334–43.
71. Henry SM, Fung J, Horak FB. Control of stance during lateral and anterior/posterior surface translations. *IEEE Trans Rehabil Eng* 1998; **6**: 32–42.
72. Topper AK, Maki BE, Holliday PJ. Are activity-based assessments of balance and gait in the elderly predictive of risk of falling and/or type of fall? *J Am Geriatr Soc* 1993; **41**: 479–87.
73. Maki BE, Holliday PJ, Topper AK. A prospective study of postural balance and risk of falling in an ambulatory and independent elderly population. *J Gerontol* 1994; **49**: M72–84.
74. Cummings SR, Nevitt MC. Non-skeletal determinants of fractures: the potential importance of the mechanics of falls. *Osteoporosis Int* 1994; **1**: S67–70.
75. McIlroy WE, Maki BE. Task constraints on foot movement and the incidence of compensatory stepping following perturbation of upright stance. *Brain Res* 1993; **616**: 30–8.
76. Rogers MW, Hain TC, Hanke TA et al. Stimulus parameters and inertial load: effects on the incidence of protective stepping responses in healthy human subjects. *Arch Phys Med Rehabil* 1996; **77**: 363–8.

77. Maki BE, McIlroy WE. Control of compensatory stepping reactions: age-related impairment and the potential for remedial intervention. *Physiother Theory Pract* 1999; **15**: 69–90.
78. Burleigh AL, Horak FB, Malouin F. Modification of postural responses and step initiation: evidence for goal-directed postural interactions. *J Neurophysiol* 1994; **72**: 2892–902.
79. McIlroy WE, Maki BE. Early activation of arm muscles follows external perturbations of upright stance. *Neurosci Lett* 1995; **184**: 177–80.
80. McIlroy WE, Maki BE. Do anticipatory postural adjustments precede compensatory stepping reactions evoked by perturbation? *Neurosci Lett* 1993; **164**: 199–204.
81. McIlroy WE, Maki BE. Adaptive changes to compensatory stepping responses. *Gait Posture* 1995; **3**: 43–50.
82. Rogers MW. Disorders of posture, balance and gait in Parkinson's disease. *Clin Geriatr Med* 1996; **12**: 825–45.
83. McIlroy WE, Maki BE. The control of lateral stability during rapid stepping reactions evoked by antero-posterior perturbation: does anticipatory control play a role? *Gait Posture* 1999; **9**: 190–8.
84. Nashner LM. Balance adjustments of humans perturbed while walking. *J Neurophysiol* 1980; **44**: 650–64.
85. Yang JF, Stein RB. Phase-dependent reflex reversal in human leg muscles during walking. *J Neurophysiol* 1990; **63**: 1109–17.
86. Duysens J, Tax AAM, Nawijn S et al. Gating of sensation and evoked potentials following foot stimulation during human gait. *Exp Brain Res* 1995; **105**: 423–31.
87. Sinkjaer T, Andersen JB, Larsen B. Soleus stretch reflex modulation during gait in humans. *J Neurophysiol* 1996; **76**: 1112–20.
88. Berger W, Dietz V, Quintern J. Corrective reactions to stumbling in man: neuronal co-ordination of bilateral leg muscle activity during gait. *J Physiol* 1984; **357**: 109–25.
89. Eng JJ, Winter DA, Patla AE. Strategies for recovery from a trip in early and late swing during human walking. *Exp Brain Res* 1994; **102**: 339–49.
90. Townsend MA. Biped gait stabilization via foot placement. *J Biomech* 1985; **18**: 21–38.
91. Redfern MS, Schumann T. A model of foot placement during gait. *J Biomech* 1994; **27**: 1339–46.
92. Stelmach GE, Worringham CJ. Sensorimotor deficits related to postural stability: implications for falling in the elderly. *Clin Geriatr Med* 1985; **1**: 679–4.
93. Teasdale N, Stelmach GE, Breunig A et al. Age differences in visual sensory integration. *Exp Brain Res* 1991; **85**: 691–6.
94. Wolfson L, Whipple R, Derby CA et al. A dynamic posturography study of balance in healthy elderly. *Neorology* 1992; **42**: 2069–75.
95. Maylor EA, Wing AM. Age differences in postural stability are increased by additional cognitive demands. *J Gerontol* 1996; **51**: P143–54.
96. Lundin-Olsson L, Nyberg L, Gustafson Y. 'Stops walking when talking' as a predictor of falls in elderly people. *Lancet* 1997; **349**: 617.
97. Lundin-Olsson L, Nyberg L, Gustafson Y. Attention, frailty, and falls: the effect of a manual task on basic mobility. *J Am Geriatr Soc* 1998; **46**: 758–61.
98. Brocklehurst J, Robertson D, James-Groom P. Clinical correlates of sway in old age—sensory modalities. *Age Ageing* 1982; **11**: 1–10.
99. Skinner HB, Barrack RL, Cook SD. Age-related declines in proprioception. *Clin Orthop Related Res* 1984; **184**: 208–11.
100. Verrillo RT, Verrillo V. Sensory and perceptual performance. In: Charnes N, ed. *Aging and Human Performance*. New York: John Wiley & Sons, 1985: 1–46.
101. Kenshalo DR. Somesthetic sensitivity in young and elderly humans. *J Gerontol* 1986; **41**: 732–42.
102. Paige GD. The aging vestibulo-ocular reflex (VOR) and adaptive plasticity. *Acta Otolaryngol Stockh* 1991; **481**(suppl): 297–300.
103. Woollacott M, Shumway-Cook A, Nashner LM. Aging and posture control: changes in sensory organization and muscular coordination. *Int J Aging Hum Dev* 1986; **23**: 97–114.
104. Lord SR, Clark RD, Webster IW. Postural stability and associated physiological factors in a population of aged persons. *J Gerontol* 1991; **46**: M69–76.
105. Lord SR, Ward JA, Williams P et al. Physiological factors associated with falls in older community-dwelling women. *J Am Geriatr Soc* 1994; **42**: 1110–17.
106. Vandervoort AA. Effects of ageing on human neuromuscular function: implications for exercise. *Can J Spt Sci* 1992; **17**: 178–84.
107. Whipple RH, Wolfson LI, Amerman RN. The relationship of knee and ankle weakness to falls in nursing home residents. *J Am Geriatr Soc* 1987; **35**: 13–20.
108. Tinetti ME, Williams TF, Mayewski R. Fall risk index for elderly patients based on number of chronic disabilities. *Am J Med* 1986; **80**: 429–34.
109. Campbell AJ, Borrie MJ, Spears GF. Risk factors for falls in a community-based prospective study of people 70 years and older. *J Gerontol* 1989; **44**: M112–17.
110. Robbins AS, Rubenstein LZ, Josephson KR et al. Predictors of falls among elderly people—results of two population-based studies. *Arch Intern Med* 1989; **149**: 1628–33.
111. Lord SR, Clark RD, Webster IW. Physiological factors associated with falls in an elderly population. *J Am Geriatr Soc* 1991; **39**: 1194–200.
112. Blanpied P, Smidt GL. The difference in stiffness of the active plantarflexors between young and elderly human females. *J Gerontol* 1993; **48**: M58–63.
113. Roach KE, Miles TP. Normal hip and knee active range of motion: the relationship to age. *Phys Ther* 1991; **71**: 656–65.
114. Studenski S, Duncan PW, Chandler J. Postural response and effector factors in persons with unexplained falls: results and methodologic issues. *J Am Geriatr Soc* 1991; **39**: 229–34.
115. Lipsitz LA, Goldberger AL. Loss of 'complexity' and aging. *JAMA* 1992; **267**: 1806–9.
116. Grabiner MD, Jahnigen DW. Modeling recovery from stumbles: preliminary data on variable selection and classification efficacy. *J Am Geriatr Soc* 1992; **40**: 910–13.
117. McDowd JM. Inhibition in attention and aging. *J Gerontol* 1997; **52**: P265–73.
118. Peterka RJ, Black FO. Age-related changes in human posture control: sensory organization tests. *J Vestib Res* 1990; **1**: 73–85.

119. Shepard N, Schultz A, Alexander NB et al. Postural control in young and elderly adults when stance is challenged: clinical versus laboratory measurements. *Ann Otol Rhinol Laryngol* 1993; **102**: 508–17.
120. Ring C, Nayak USL, Isaacs B. Balance function in elderly people who have and who have not fallen. *Arch Phys Med Rehabil* 1988; **69**: 261–4.
121. Winter DA. *The Biomechanics and Motor Control of Human Gait: Normal, Elderly and Pathological*, Vol. 2 Waterloo: University of Waterloo Press, 1991.
122. Winter D, Patla A, Frank J et al. Biomechanical walking pattern changes in the fit and healthy elderly. *Phys Ther* 1990; **70**: 340–7.
123. Maki BE. Gait changes in older adults: predictors of falls or indicators of fear? *J Am Geriatr Soc* 1997; **45**: 313–20.
124. Kaya BK, Krebs DE, Riley PO. Dynamic stability in elders: momentum control in locomotor ADL. *J Gerontol* 1998; **53**: M126–34.
125. Patla AE, Prentice SD, Gobbi LT. Visual control of obstacle avoidance during locomotion: strategies in young children, young and older adults. In: Ferrandez AM, Teasdale N, eds. *Changes in Sensory Motor Behavior in Aging*. Amsterdam: Elsevier, 1996: 257–77.
126. Chen HC, Ashton-Miller JA, Alexander NB et al. Effects of age and available response time on ability to step over an obstacle. *J Gerontol* 1994; **49**: M227–33.
127. Cao C, Ashton-Miller JA, Schultz AB et al. Abilities to turn suddenly while walking: effects of age, gender, and available response time. *J Gerontol* 1997; **52**: M88–93.
128. Cao C, Ashton-Miller JA, Schultz AB et al. Effects of age, available response time and gender on ability to stop suddenly when walking. *Gait Posture* 1998; **8**: 103–9.
129. Chen HC, Schultz AB, Ashton-Miller JA et al. Stepping over obstacles: dividing attention impairs performance of old more than young adults. *J Gerontol* 1996; **51**: M116–22.
130. Riley PO, Krebs DE, Popat RA. Biomechanical analysis of failed sit-to-stand. *IEEE Trans Rehabil Eng* 1997; **5**: 353–9.
131. Tinetti ME, Speechley M, Ginter SF. Risk factors for falls among elderly persons living in the community. *N Engl J Med* 1988; **319**: 1701–7.
132. Berg KO, Wood-Dauphinee SL, Williams JT et al. Measuring balance in the elderly: validation of an instrument. *Can J Publ Health* 1992; **42**: 75–9.
133. Bennett KMB, Castiello U. Reach to grasp: changes with age. *J Gerontol* 1994; **49**: P1–7.
134. Ramos CF, Stark LW. Simulation experiments can shed light on the functional aspects of postural adjustments related to voluntary movements. In: Winters JM, Woo SL-Y, eds. *Multiple Muscle Systems: Biomechanics and Movement Organization*. New York: Springer-Verlag, 1990: 507–17.
135. Inglis B, Woollacott M. Age-related changes in anticipatory postural adjustments associated with arm movements. *J Gerontol* 1988; **43**: M105–13.
136. Rogers MW, Kukulka CG, Soderberg GL. Age-related changes in postural responses preceding rapid self-paced and reaction time arm movements. *J Gerontol* 1992; **47**: M159–65.
137. Maki BE. A biomechanical approach to quantifying anticipatory postural adjustments in the elderly. *Med Biol Eng Comput* 1993; **31**: 355–62.
138. Maki BE, McIlroy WE. Influence of arousal and attention on the control of postural sway. *J Vestib Res* 1996; **6**: 53–9.
139. Maki BE, Holliday PJ, Fernie GR. A posture control model and balance test for the prediction of relative postural stability. *IEEE Trans Biomed Eng* 1987; **BME-34**: 797–810.
140. Overstall PW, Exton-Smith AN, Imms FJ et al. Falls in the elderly related to postural imbalance. *BMJ* 1977; **1**: 261–4.
141. Era P, Heikkinen E. Postural sway during standing and unexpected disturbance of balance in random samples of men of different ages. *J Gerontol* 1985; **40**: 287–95.
142. Hayes KC, Spencer JD, Lucy SD et al. Age-related changes in postural sway. In: Winter DA, Norman RW, Wells RP et al. eds. *Biomechanics IX-A*. Champaign, Illinois: Human Kinetics Publishers, 1985: 383–7.
143. Maki BE, Holliday PJ, Fernie GR. Aging and postural control: a comparison of spontaneous- and induced-sway balance tests. *J Am Geriatr Soc* 1990; **38**: 1–9.
144. Prieto TE, Myklebust JB, Myklebust BM. Characterization and modelling of postural steadiness in the elderly: a review. *IEEE Trans Rehabil Eng* 1993; **1**: 26–34.
145. Baloh RW, Fife TD, Zwerling L et al. Comparison of static and dynamic posturography in young and older normal people. *J Am Geriatr Soc* 1994; **42**: 405–12.
146. Lord SR, Ward JA. Age-associated differences in sensori-motor function and balance in community dwelling women. *Age Ageing* 1994; **23**: 452–60.
147. Collins JJ, DeLuca CJ, Lipsitz LA. Age-related changes in open-loop and closed-loop postural control mechanisms. *Exp Brain Res* 1995; **104**: 480–92.
148. Fernie GR, Gryfe CI, Holliday PJ et al. The relationship of postural sway in standing to the incidence of falls in geriatric subjects. *Age Ageing* 1982; **11**: 11–16.
149. Kirshen AJ, Cape RDT, Hayes HC et al. Postural sway and cardiovascular parameters associated with falls in the elderly. *J Clin Exp Gerontol* 1984; **6**: 291–307.
150. Lichtenstein MJ, Shields SL, Shiavi RG et al. Clinical determinants of biomechanics platform measures of balance in aged women. *J Am Geriatr Soc* 1988; **36**: 996–1002.
151. Thapa PB, Gideon P, Brockman KG et al. Clinical and biomechanical measures of balance as fall predictors in ambulatory nursing home residents. *J Gerontol* 1996; **51**: M239–46.
152. McClenaghan BA, Williams HG, Dickerson J et al. Spectral characteristics of ageing postural control. *Gait Posture* 1995; **3**: 123–31.
153. Maki BE. Direction- and vision-dependence of postural responses in elderly 'fallers' and 'non-fallers'. *Facts Res Gerontol (L'annee gerontologique)* 1995; **9**(suppl): 83–96.
154. Rossiter-Fornoff JE, Wolf SL, Wolfson LI et al. A cross-sectional validation study of the FICSIT common data base static balance measures. *J Gerontol* 1995; **50A**: M291–7.
155. Duncan PW, Weiner DK, Chandler J et al. Functional reach: a new clinical measure of balance. *J Gerontol* 1990; **45**: M192–7.

156. Blaszczyk JW, Lowe DL, Hansen PD. Ranges of postural stability and their changes in the elderly. *Gait Posture* 1994; **2**: 11–17.
157. King MB, Judge JO, Wolfson L. Functional base of support decreases with age. *J Gerontol* 1994; **49**: M258–63.
158. Stelmach GE, Phillips J, DiFabio RP et al. Age, functional postural reflexes, and voluntary sway. *J Gerontol* 1989; **44**: B100–6.
159. Nardone A, Siliotto R, Grasso M et al. Influence of aging on leg muscle reflex responses to stance perturbation. *Arch Phys Med Rehabil* 1995; **76**: 158–65.
160. Alexander NB, Shepard N, Gu MJ et al. Postural control in young and elderly adults when stance is perturbed: kinematics. *J Gerontol* 1992; **47**: M79–87.
161. Wu G. Age-related differences in body segmental movement during perturbed stance in humans. *Clin Biomech* 1998; **13**: 300–7.
162. Keshner EA, Chen KJ. Mechanisms controlling head stabilization in the elderly during random rotations in the vertical plane. *J Motor Behav* 1996; **28**: 324–36.
163. Smith BN, Segal RL, Wolf SL. Long latency ankle responses to dynamic perturbation in older fallers and non-fallers. *J Am Geriatr Soc* 1996; **44**: 1447–54.
164. Duncan G, Wilson JA, MacLennan WJ et al. Clinical correlates of sway in elderly people living at home. *Gerontology* 1992; **38**: 160–6.
165. Hughes MA, Duncan PW, Rose DK et al. The relationship of postural sway to sensorimotor function, functional performance, and disability in the elderly. *Arch Phys Med Rehabil* 1996; **77**: 567–72.
166. Wu G. The relation between age-related changes in neuromusculoskeletal system and dynamic postural responses to balance disturbance. *J Gerontol* 1998; **53A**: M320–6.
167. Hay L, Bard C, Fleury M et al. Availability of visual and proprioceptive afferent messages and postural control in elderly adults. *Exp Brain Res* 1996; **108**: 129–39.
168. Stelmach G, Teasdale N, DiFabio RP et al. Age related decline in postural control mechanisms. *Int J Aging Hum Dev* 1989; **29**: 205–23.
169. Wolfson LI, Whipple R, Amerman P et al. Stressing the postural response: a quantitative method for testing balance. *J Am Geriatr Soc* 1986; **34**: 845–50.
170. Chandler JM, Duncan PW, Studenski SA. Balance performance on the postural stress test: comparison of young adults, healthy elderly, and fallers. *Phys Ther* 1990; **70**: 410–15.
171. Luchies CW. Fall arrest biomechanics: sway and stepping responses in healthy young and old adults. Doctoral dissertation. Ann Arbor, Michigan: University of Michigan, 1991.
172. Luchies CW, Alexander NB, Schultz AB et al. Stepping responses of young and old adults to postural disturbances: kinematics. *J Am Geriatr Soc* 1994; **42**: 506–12.
173. McIlroy WE, Maki BE. Age-related changes in compensatory stepping in response to unpredictable perturbations. *J Gerontol* 1996; **51A**: M289–96.
174. Rogers MW, Cain TD, Hanke TA. Association of age and fall risk with changes in lateral stance control during induced forward stepping. In: McGill S, Gross M, Patia A, eds. *Proceedings of the Third North American Congress on Biomechanics*, Waterloo, Canada: University of Waterloo, 1998: 23–4.
175. Maki BE, Edmondstone MA, McIlroy WE. Age-related differences in laterally directed compensatory stepping behavior. *J Gerontol* 2000; **55A**: M270–7.
176. Maki BE, McIlroy WE, Perry SD. Influence of lateral destabilization on compensatory stepping responses. *J Biomech* 1996; **29**: 343–53.
177. Thelen DG, Wojcik LA, Schultz AB et al. Age differences in using a rapid step to regain balance during a forward fall. *J Gerontol* 1997; **52A**: M8–13.
178. Jiang N, McIlroy WE, Black WE et al. Control of compensatory limb movement in chronic hemiparesis. In: McGill S, Gross M, Patia A, eds. *Proceedings of the Third North American Congress on Biomechanics*, Waterloo, Canada: University of Waterloo, 1998: 263–4.
179. Burleigh-Jacobs A, Horak FB, Nutt JC et al. Step initiation in Parkinson's disease: influence of levodopa and external sensory triggers. *Movement Disord* 1997; **12**: 206–15.
180. Perry SD, Edmondstone MA, McIlroy WE et al. Sensory correlates of impaired compensatory stepping performance in healthy older adults. In: McGill S, Gross M, Patia A, eds. *Proceedings of the Third North American Congress on Biomechanics*, Waterloo, Canada: University of Waterloo, 1998: 285–6.
181. Yardley L, Gardner M, Bronstein A *et al.* Interference between postural control and mental task performance in patients with vestibular disorder and healthy controls. *J Neurology, Neurosurgery and Psychiatry* 2001; (in press).
182. Maylor EA, Wing AM. Age differences in postural stability are increased by additional cognitive demands. *J Gerontol* 1996; **51**: P143–54.
183. Shumway-Cook A, Woollacott M, Kerns KA *et al.* The effects of two types of cognitive tasks on postural stability in older adults with and without a history of falling. *J Gerontol* 1997; **52A**: M232–40.
184. Shumway-Cook A, Woollacott M. Attentional demands and postural control: the effect of sensory context. *J Gerontol* 2000; **55A**: M10–16.
185. McIlroy WE, Norrie RG, Brooke JD *et al.* Temporal properties of attention sharing consequent to disturbed balance. *NeuroReport* 1999; **10**: 2895–9.
186. Maki BE, Zecevic A, Bateni H *et al.* Cognitive demands of executing rapid postural reactions: does aging impede attentional switching? *NeuroReport* 2001; **12**: 3583–7.
187. Brown LA, Shumway-Cook A, Woollacott MH. Attentional demands and postural recovery: the effects of aging. *J Gerontol* 1999; **54A**: M165–71.
188. Rankin J, Woollacott MH, Shumway-Cook A *et al.* Cognitive influence on postural stability: a neuromuscular analysis in young and elders. *J Gerontol* 2000; **55A**: M112–19.
189. McIlroy WE, Bent LR, Potvin JR *et al.* Anticipatory balance control precedes withdrawal response to noxious stimulation. *Neurosci Lett* 1999; **267**: 197–200.
190. Zettel JL, Maki BE, McIlroy WE. Can features of triggered stepping reactions be modulated to meet environmental constraints? *Exp Brain Res* 2002; **145**: 397–308.

191. Maki BE, Edmondstone MA, Perry SD *et al.* Control of rapid limb movements for balance recovery: do age-related changes predict falling risk? In: Duysens J, Smits-Engelsman BCM, Kingma H (eds) *Control of Posture and Gait*. International Society for Posture and Gait Research, Maastricht, Netherlands, 2001: 126–9.
192. Rogers MW, Hedman LD, Johnson ME *et al.* Lateral stability during forward-induced stepping for dynamic balance recovery in young and older adults. *J Gerontol* 2001; **56**: M589–94.
193. Luchies CW, Wallace D, Pazdur R *et al.* Effects of age on balance assessment using voluntary and involuntary step tasks. *J Gerontol* 1999; **54**: M140–4.
194. Perry SD, McIlroy WE, Maki BE. Does neural, musculoskeletal or sensory impairment predict compensatory stepping behavior in the older adult? Submitted for publication.
195. Damiano NK, McIlroy WE, Maki BE *et al.* Compensatory stepping in Parkinson's Disease: Do PD patients use external cues to decrease postural instability? *Soc Neurosci Abstr* 2000; **26**: 164.
196. Lord SR, Rogers MW, Howland A *et al.* Lateral stability, sensorimotor function and falls in older people. *J Amer Geriat Soc* 1999; **47**: 1077–81.
197. Lord SR, Menz HB. Visual contributions to postural stability in older adults. *Gerontology* 2000; **46**: 306–10.
198. Pai YC, Maki BE, Iqbal K *et al.* Thresholds for step initiation induced by support-surface translation: a dynamic center-of-mass model provides much better prediction than a static model. *J Biomech* 2000; **33**: 387–92.
199. Tang PF, Woollacott MH. Phase-dependent modulation of poximal and distal postural responses to slips in young and older adults. *J Gerontol* 1999; **54**: M89–102.
200. Brauer SG, Woollacott M, Shumway-Cook A. The interacting effects of cognitive demand and recovery of postural stability in balance-impaired elderly persons. *J Gerontol* 2001; **56**: M489–96.
201. Brauer SG, Burns YR, Galley P. A prospective study of laboratory and clinical measures of postural stability to predict community-dwelling fallers. *J Gerontol* 2000; **55**: M469–76.

40 Vestibular influences on cardiovascular control during movement

Bill J Yates, Michael J Holmes, Brian J Jian, Ilan A Kerman

Introduction

Vestibular dysfunction and/or stimulation has long been known to evoke autonomic responses, including nausea and vomiting (see Yates et al[1] for a recent review). Because these autonomic responses appeared to be maladaptive responses to unusual conditions in which conflicting multiple sensory cues regarding body position in space were available, it was difficult to assign the responses a physiological role. More recently, however, evidence has accumulated to suggest that vestibular inputs, which signal body position in space and the direction and velocity of movements,[2] may be important in eliciting compensatory autonomic responses during movement. For example, standing in humans and nose-up rotations during climbing maneuvers in quadrupeds place the body's long axis parallel with the gravitoinertial vector, and can induce peripheral blood pooling if compensation does not occur quickly.[3] Since a particular pattern of vestibular inputs occurs during these postures, it would seem practical for vestibular signals to trigger compensatory cardiovascular responses that prevent orthostatic hypotension from occurring. A stereotyped pattern of vestibular inputs may also occur during locomotion and exercise, and thus labyrinthine signals could also potentially contribute to 'exercise pressor responses'.[4]

This chapter will review the evidence suggesting that vestibular signals comprise one of several sensory inputs that induce cardiovascular responses during movement and changes in posture. In particular, this chapter will highlight recent research indicating that: (1) a particular 'pattern' of changes in sympathetic nervous system activity is elicited by vestibular stimulation; (2) cardiovascular responses can be induced by vestibular stimulation in humans; (3) vestibular lesions impair the ability to correct blood pressure precisely during movement; and (4) the cerebellum may be an important component of the neural circuitry that mediates vestibulocardiovascular responses.

Although this chapter will concentrate on vestibular influences on cardiovascular control, both classical and recent studies have shown that additional autonomic responses are also affected by vestibular stimulation. The reader is referred to other reviews and manuscripts that discuss the role of the vestibular system in triggering changes in respiratory activity during movement,[5,6] influencing alertness and arousal through actions on brainstem monoaminergic neurons,[7–10] controlling background excitability of brainstem neurons that regulate sleep–waking cycles,[11] and eliciting nausea and vomiting during motion sickness.[1,12] Table 40.1 summarizes some of the facets of autonomic control that may be influenced by the vestibular system.

Table 40.1 Autonomic responses elicited by vestibular stimulation.

- Changes in blood pressure
- Changes in respiratory muscle activity
- Changes in alertness and arousal
- Changes in sleep–wake cycles
- Nausea and vomiting

Evidence suggesting that the vestibular system influences control of blood pressure

Two general types of experiment have been conducted to show that the vestibular system influences the control of blood pressure: those that observe cardiovascular responses to selective stimulation of vestibular afferents, and those that monitor orthostatic hypotension that occurs during whole-body movements following vestibular lesions. Some of the first experiments demonstrating a role of the vestibular system in cardiovascular control involved recording responses from sympathetic nerves during electrical stimulation of the vestibular nerve. Examples of these 'vestibulosympathetic reflexes' are illustrated in Figure 40.1. The sympathetic nerves that have been shown to respond to electrical vestibular stimulation are listed in Table 40.2. All of these nerves contain efferents that innervate structures involved in cardiovascular control, including the heart, blood vessels, and adrenal gland. Control experiments have indicated that these responses are the result of activation of vestibular afferents, and not non-target afferents outside of the vestibular nerve, as they are abolished by lesions of the medial and inferior vestibular nuclei.[13–15] Despite the fact that the activity of many sympathetic nerves is affected by vestibular stimulation, the relative sizes of responses in different nerves vary greatly. This issue is discussed below.

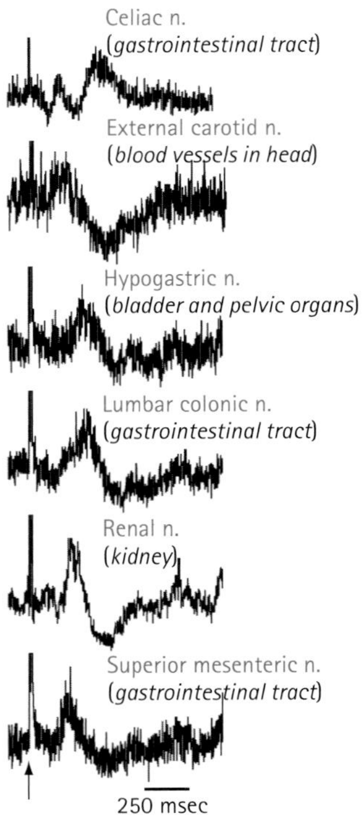

Figure 40.1 Examples of sympathetic nerve responses to electrical stimulation of vestibular afferents (5-shock train with a 3-ms interpulse interval delivered at the time of the arrow). Upward deflections represent an increase in nerve activity, whereas downward deflections represent an inhibition of activity. Traces are the average of over 100 sweeps. The stimulation intensity used was 350–500 μA. The onset latency of the responses was 100–140 ms, which is due to the slow conduction velocities of sympathetic efferents. All of the sympathetic nerves whose responses are illustrated innervate blood vessels, although some (celiac n., hypogastric n., lumbar colonic n., superior mesenteric n.) also innervate motility-regulating smooth muscle. (Adapted from Kerman and Yates. *Am J Physiol* 1998; **275**: R824–35.[13])

Table 40.2 Sympathetic nerves whose activity is altered by electrical vestibular stimulation.

Nerve	Reference
Adrenal	[13]
Celiac	[13]
Cervical sympathetic	[30]
External carotid	[13]
Hypogastric	[13]
Inferior cardiac	[64]
Lumbar colonic	[13]
Renal	[13, 65, 66]
Splanchnic	[14, 64, 67]
Superior mesenteric	[13]

Recently, cardiovascular responses elicited by selective natural vestibular stimulation have been reported. Vestibular stimulation was produced by rotation of the head on a fixed body following denervations to remove non-vestibular inputs that might be elicited by head movement. These denervations included transection of the IXth, Xth and sometimes the Vth cranial nerves and the upper cervical dorsal roots.[15–17] Nose-up rotations in this preparation elicited an increase in sympathetic nervous system activity[15] (Figure 40.2a), blood pressure[17] (Figure 40.2b), and blood catecholamine levels[18,19] (Figure 40.2c). However, changes in blood pressure and sympathetic nervous system activity are not elicited by ear-down rotations in quadrupeds, indicating that these responses have directional specificity.[15,17] Because nose-up vestibular stimulation signals the attainment of a posture that should result in an orthostatic challenge in a quadruped, vestibulosympathetic responses appear to be a practical adaptation to maintain stable blood pressure.

Other evidence that the vestibular system participates in adjusting blood pressure comes from experiments that record the effects of selective electrical or natural vestibular stimulation on the activity of brainstem neurons that control sympathetic nervous system activity. The neural circuitry necessary for the production of vestibulosympathetic reflexes, as indicated by anatomical, electrophysiological and lesion studies in animal preparations,[14,15,20–26] is shown in Figure 40.3. Over 70% of the putative cardiovascular-regulatory neurons in the major 'pressor' area of the cat brainstem, which is located in a confined region of the rostral ventrolateral medulla,[27–29] receive labyrinthine signals.[20,21] Lesions of this region abolish vestibulosympathetic reflexes,[22] indicating that the rostral ventrolateral

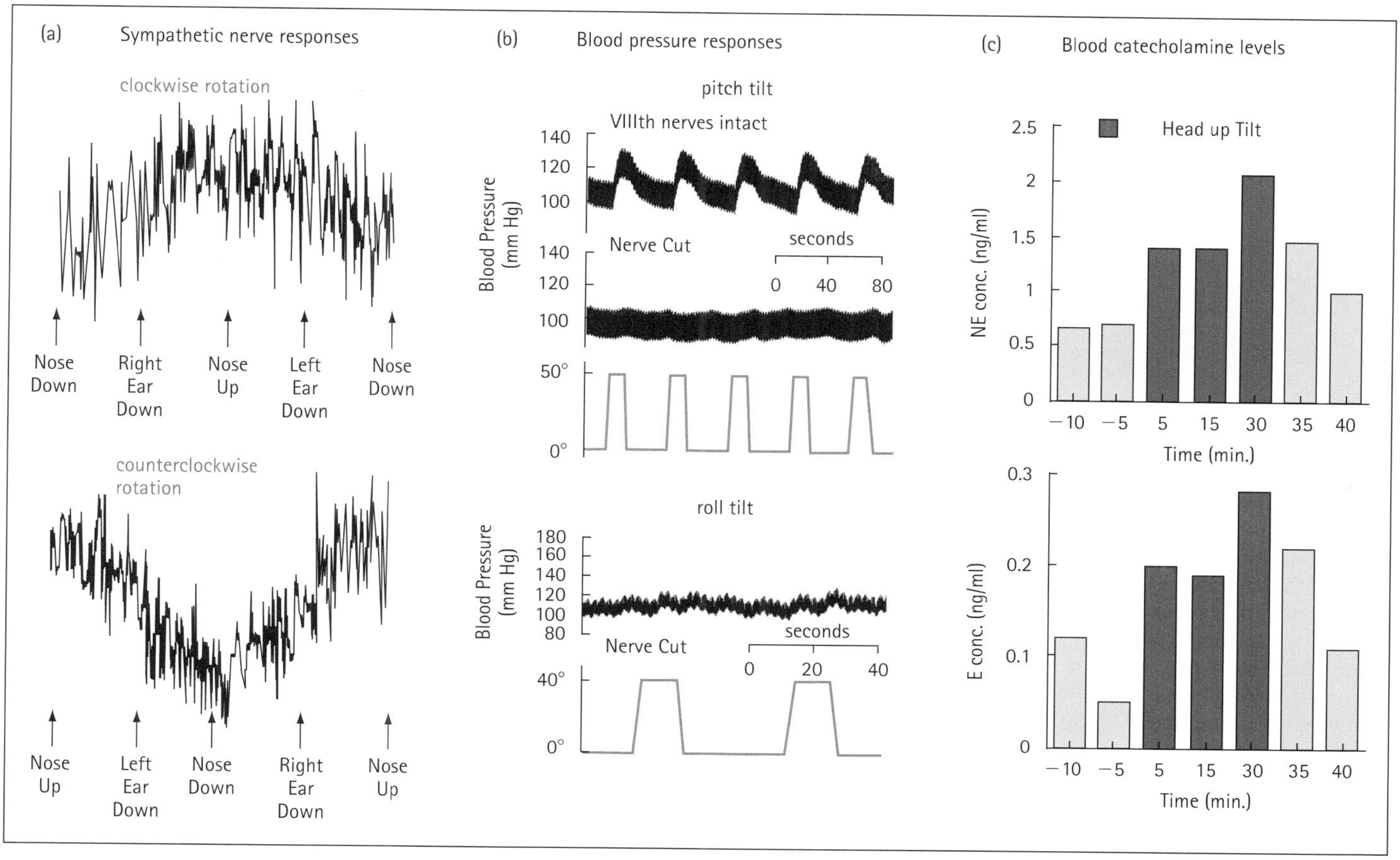

Figure 40.2 Cardiovascular responses to natural vestibular stimulation. (a) Averaged changes in activity of a sympathetic nerve (the splanchnic nerve) in response to 15° sinusoidal head rotations that incorporated roll and pitch. The responses were recorded from cats whose upper cervical dorsal roots were transected to remove inputs from the neck, and whose IXth and Xth cranial nerves were transected to remove autonomic inputs that might be elicited by head movement. In this preparation, head rotations presumably mainly stimulated vestibular afferents. Activity in this sympathetic nerve was dependent on head position, and was maximal during nose-up rotations and minimal during nose-down rotations. (From Yates and Miller.[15]) (b) Increases in blood pressure elicited by static head tilts in animals whose upper cervical dorsal roots and IXth and Xth cranial nerves were transected. Nose-up tilts elicited an increase in blood pressure of approximately 20 mmHg; these responses were abolished by transection of the VIIIth cranial nerves, indicating that they were due to stimulation of the vestibular system. In contrast, ear-down (roll) tilt had little effect on blood pressure. (From Woodring et al.[17]) (c) Blood norepinephrine (NE, top panel) and epinephrine (E, bottom panel) concentrations before, during and after 50° nose-up head tilt in the preparation described above. From 0 to 30 min the head was tilted nose-up by 50°, and blood was sampled at the indicated times. Nose-up head tilt produced over a two-fold increase in blood catecholamine levels. (From Yates and Kerman. *Brain Res Rev* 1998; **28**: 73–82.[19])

medulla is critical for transmitting vestibular signals to sympathetic 'output' neurons in the spinal cord. Lesions of the rostral ventrolateral medulla also abolish or greatly attenuate sympathetic nervous system responses to baroreceptor stimulation,[27–29] which suggests that baroreceptor and vestibular signals may converge on common neurons in this region. This hypothesis has been supported by recording studies, which demonstrated that rostral ventrolateral medulla neurons respond to electrical stimulation of both the carotid sinus nerve (which carries baroreceptor afferents) and the vestibular nerve.[20] However, not all neurons in the brainstem that are part of the baroreceptor reflex arc have activity that is modulated by labyrinthine signals. For example, neurons in the nucleus tractus solitarius that receive primary baroreceptor inputs, as well as inhibitory neurons in the baroreceptor reflex arc located in the caudal ventrolateral medulla, fail to respond to vestibular nerve stimulation.[23,24] The implications of this pattern of convergence of vestibular and baroreceptor inputs are not yet known. Vestibular signals also differ from many other inputs that affect blood pressure, in that they appear to affect mainly sympathetic outflow to the blood vessels, but not parasympathetic outflow to the heart. Tang and Gernandt[30] showed that electrical stimulation of the vestibular nerve produced robust changes in sympathetic nerve activity, but no change in vagus nerve activity other than in branches innervating upper airway muscles. Because all parasympathetic outflow to the heart is carried by the vagus nerve,[31] this experiment suggests that the parasympathetic and sympathetic systems are differentially affected by labyrinthine inputs. Cumulatively, these observations show that the vestibular system has influences on only some of the central nervous system circuitry responsible for the control of blood pressure. These selective influences may form the neural substrate of the 'patterning' of sympathetic nervous system activity elicited by vestibular stimulation (see next section).

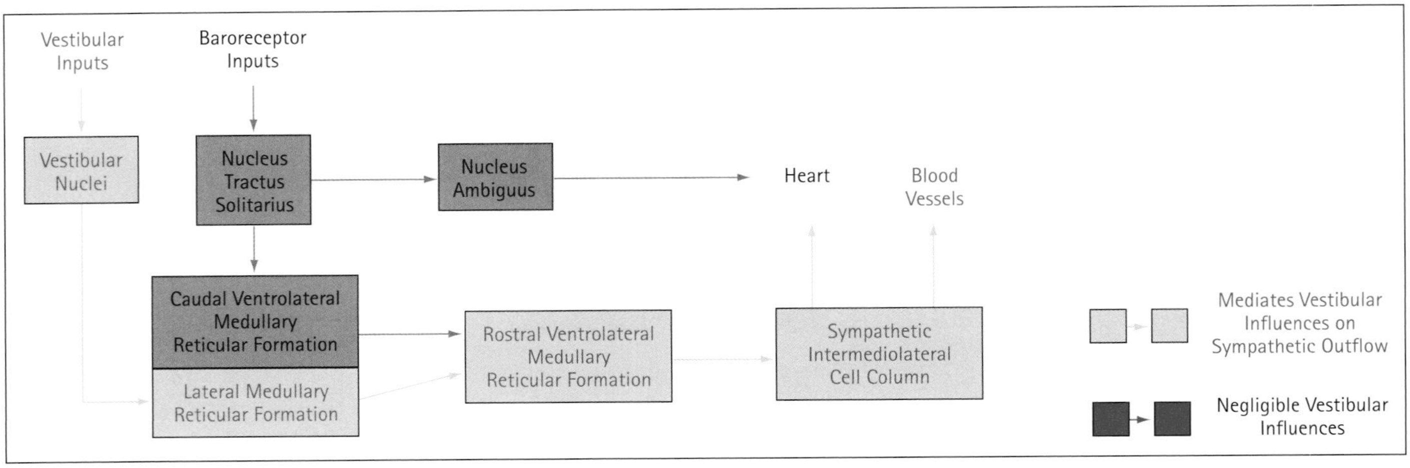

Figure 40.3 Schematic diagram of the brainstem and spinal cord pathways required for production of vestibulo-sympathetic and baroreceptor reflexes. Baroreceptor afferents terminate in the nucleus tractus solitarius. Baroreceptor effects on the sympathetic nervous system are mediated by inhibitory interneurons in the caudal ventrolateral medulla and pre-sympathetic neurons in the rostral ventrolateral medulla that directly innervate sympathetic preganglionic neurons in the spinal cord. In addition, baroreceptor-sensitive neurons in the nucleus tractus solitarius make direct connections with cardiac parasympathetic preganglionic neurons located in and near the nucleus ambiguus. Vestibular signals affect sympathetic outflow through a neural circuit including the vestibular nuclei, neurons in the lateral medullary reticular formation (but excluding cells with powerful baroreceptor inputs in the caudal ventrolateral medulla), and pre-sympathetic neurons in the rostral ventrolateral medulla. Thus, neurons in the rostral ventrolateral medulla represent the first site of convergence between baroreceptor and vestibular signals in pathways that control sympathetic outflow. The vestibular system appears to have negligible effects on parasympathetic outflow to the heart, which is mediated through parasympathetic preganglionic neurons located in and around the nucleus ambiguus. (Adapted from Yates and Kerman. *Brain Res Rev* 1998; **28**: 73–82.[19])

It should be noted, however, that the circuitry illustrated in Figure 40.3 probably does not reflect the entirety of connections involved in producing vestibular-induced or motion-induced cardiovascular responses in awake animals. For example, it is likely that the cerebellum is involved in modulating these responses (see below). Additionally, vestibular signals are integrated with many other inputs reflecting body position in space, including proprioceptive, visual and visceral signals, in order to produce precise cardiovascular adjustments during movement. For example, removal of neck inputs through transection of the upper cervical dorsal roots has been shown to potentiate greatly the effects of head rotation on sympathetic outflow.[32] This finding suggests that neck and vestibular inputs are integrated in a manner such that cardiovascular responses are elicited by whole-body movement (which only stimulates vestibular receptors), but not head movements on a stable body that elicit both neck and vestibular inputs. Furthermore, as discussed below, removal of vestibular inputs only produces a severe deficit in correcting blood pressure when other sensory signals regarding body orientation are also eliminated. Thus, vestibular influences on blood pressure should not be considered as isolated responses, but as a component of other highly integrative responses.

Patterns of sympathetic nerve responses to vestibular stimulation

The classical ideas regarding the function of the sympathetic nervous system were first proposed by Walter Cannon. Cannon[33,34] postulated that the sympathetic nervous system discharges in a unitary fashion so as to activate all of its outflows simultaneously in response to a variety of stimuli. Though the model proposed by Cannon is appealing and is still presented in many medical textbooks, more recent experimental evidence suggests that it is not entirely correct. There are numerous experimental examples that demonstrate that the sympathetic nervous system responds in a finely tuned and specific manner to various environmental challenges. Such responses are advantageous, as specific patterning of sympathetic outflow to address particular challenges is the most efficient way of maintaining homeostasis. For instance, during exposure to cold, one of the primary goals of the organism is to minimize heat loss. This is accomplished by increased piloerection and redistribution of blood away from the skin to the mesentery. Activity of cutaneous sympathetic nerves has been shown to increase during exposure to cold, while that of the splanchnic nerve (which innervates structures in the abdomen) simultaneously decreases; the opposite responses are observed during warming.[35,36] Many other examples of 'patterned' sympathetic nervous system responses to particular stimuli have also been observed.[31]

The idea that sympathetic efferents innervating different target tissues and organs are controlled individually is reflected by the fact that each type of sympathetic nerve efferent possesses an individual 'physiological signature', and only responds to a unique set of stimuli. For example, sympathetic nerves projecting to the gastrointestinal tract contain fibers that innervate blood vessels and those that innervate motility-regulating smooth muscle. However, these two classes of sympathetic efferents respond in different manners to different stimuli.

Vasoconstrictor efferents, which regulate blood flow to the gut, are silenced by increases in blood pressure and have discharges that are synchronized with the respiratory rhythm, but their excitability is unaffected by distension of the gut wall.[37,38] In contrast, motility-regulating fibers, which play no role in control of blood flow, are unresponsive to blood pressure alterations but are strongly excited by distension of the gut wall.[38,39] Clearly, these data demonstrate that the sympathetic nervous system is not controlled in an 'all-or-none' fashion such that each sympathetic efferent is excited or inhibited by the same stimuli.

The patterning of vestibulosympathetic reflexes has been investigated in anesthetized or decerebrate cats using electrical stimulation to activate vestibular afferents. As discussed above (see Table 40.2 and Figure 40.1), sympathetic nerves innervating many different target tissues and organs respond to vestibular stimulation. However, the sympathetic nerves whose activity is influenced by vestibular stimulation all contain vasoconstrictor efferents. Because excitability of vasoconstrictor efferents can be selectively inhibited by increasing blood pressure,[37–39] the role of these fibers in mediating vestibulosympathetic reflexes can be evaluated by comparing vestibular-elicited sympathetic nerve responses when blood pressure is normal versus when it is elevated. As illustrated in Figure 40.4, the magnitude of vestibulosympathetic reflexes is profoundly reduced when blood pressure is elevated.[13] Thus, it is likely that vestibulo-sympathetic reflexes are predominantly mediated by sympathetic fibers innervating blood vessels.

During postural changes, blood flow to the head and brain must remain adequate to prevent orthostatic hypotension. Because standing in humans and nose-up rotations in quadrupeds tend to pull blood towards the lower extremities, it would be expected that vasoconstriction in the lower body would be stronger than in the upper body during these movements. If vestibulosympathetic reflexes participate in orthostatic responses, it would be anticipated that the excitability of sympathetic efferents innervating the lower body would be more powerfully affected by vestibular inputs than sympathetic efferents innervating blood vessels of the upper body. To investigate this possibility, the relative amplitudes of vestibulo-sympathetic responses in two nerves known to be made up only of vasoconstrictor efferents, the renal[40] and external carotid[41] nerves, were compared. Renal nerve responses to vestibular stimulation (as a fraction of the maximal nerve response elicited by stimulation of the preganglionic part of the nerve) were much larger than those of the external carotid nerve.[13] This finding suggests that vasoconstrictor fibers located more caudally along the neuraxis may be preferentially influenced by vestibular inputs. However, this hypothesis must be explored in a more systematic manner in order to be verified.

The demonstration that a precise pattern of sympathetic outflow is induced by vestibular stimulation has specific functional implications. Clearly, vestibular signals are not simply 'non-specific inputs' that alter background excitability in the sympathetic nervous system. Instead, it appears that vestibulo-sympathetic reflexes are part of a carefully augmented autonomic response that serves to maintain homeostasis.

Human cardiovascular responses to vestibular stimulation

Far fewer data concerning vestibulo-cardiovascular effects are available from humans than from animals. This paucity of data is mainly a result of the difficulty in performing the appropriate

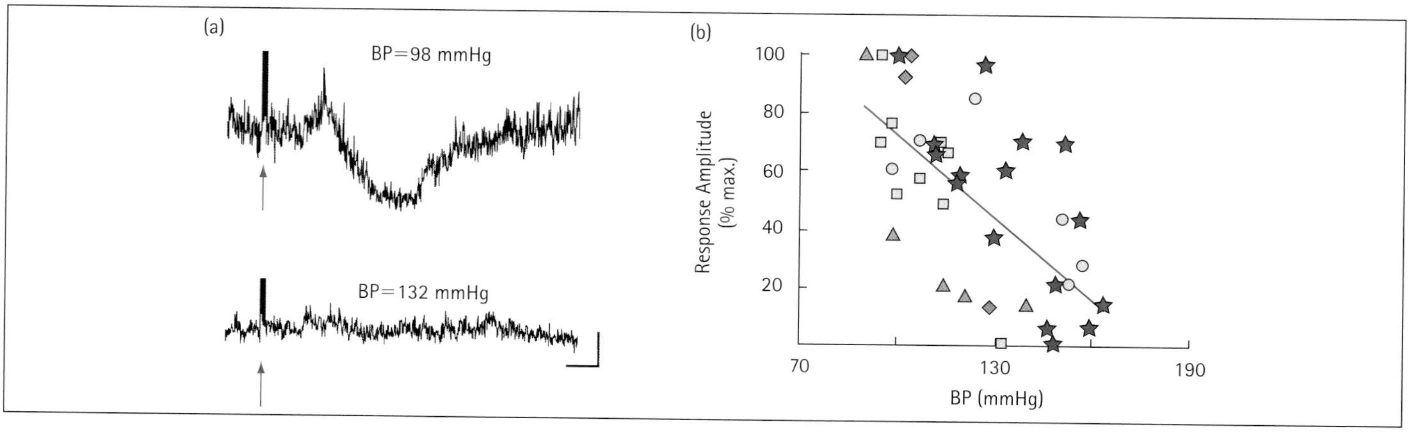

Figure 40.4 Effects of alterations in blood pressure (BP) on the magnitude of vestibulosympathetic reflexes. BP was increased using an intravenous infusion of the α-adrenergic agonist Aramine. (a) Effect of increasing mean BP on averaged vestibulosympathetic responses recorded from the superior mesenteric nerve. The five-shock stimulus to the vestibular nerve that elicited the responses was delivered at the latency indicated by the arrow. Note that when BP was high (132 mmHg), the magnitude of the vestibulo-sympathetic response was markedly less than when BP was near normal (98 mmHg). Vertical calibration, 1 μV; time scale, 100 ms. (b) Correlation between amplitude of the vestibulosympathetic reflex recorded from the superior mesenteric nerve and mean BP. Response amplitudes were expressed as a percentage of the maximal response recorded. Different symbols indicate measurements from different animals. The correlation between magnitude of responses and BP levels was examined using a linear regression analysis, and shown to be statistically significant ($p < 0.05$). (Adapted from Kerman and Yates. *Am J Physiol* 1998; **275**: R824–35.[13])

control experiments to prove that the apparent effects on the sympathetic nervous system are due to activation of labyrinthine receptors, and not visceral receptors or baroreceptors.[42] For example, a number of studies have shown that caloric vestibular stimulation can induce changes in blood pressure,[43] but this stimulus can also result in nausea and discomfort that might lead to psychologically induced cardiovascular effects. Hemmingway[44] showed that 150° swinging of human subjects has effects on both heart rate and blood pressure, but did not account for the possibility that activation of baroreceptors or other visceral receptors could have produced the responses. However, this scarcity of evidence from older experiments does not suggest that vestibular effects on the cardiovascular system are absent in humans, but only that these responses are difficult to study. Some anecdotal evidence does in fact suggest that vestibular actions on the sympathetic nervous system may be clinically relevant in humans. In one study, blood pressure was monitored in patients with peripheral vestibular disease after standing from a supine position, and it was noted that a significant fraction of these patients were more susceptible to orthostatic hypotension than normal subjects.[45]

Several recent studies have attempted to demonstrate that vestibulocardiovascular influences occur in humans. Shortt and Ray showed that static head-down neck flexion in prone subjects elicits marked increases in muscle sympathetic nerve activity and calf vascular resistance.[46] Similarly, Normand et al[47] showed that the same maneuver triggered decreases in both calf and forearm bloodflow. However, unlike most 'non-specific' stimuli that act on the sympathetic nervous system, head-down neck flexion does not produce changes in skin sympathetic outflow.[48] Alterations in sympathetic outflow do not occur during horizontal movements of the head or neck flexion in subjects lying on their side; these maneuvers activate receptors in the neck, but elicit a different pattern of vestibular inputs than is produced during head-down neck flexion in prone subjects. Thus, the prominent cardiovascular effects during head flexion in prone subjects are not due to stimulation of neck proprioceptors.[49,50] Unfortunately, however, these studies have not yet fully demonstrated that the responses to head-down neck flexion are due to labyrinthine stimulation. For example, they have not discounted the possibility that blood pooling in the head during static head-down tilt could have triggered the observed cardiovascular changes. Further control experiments will be necessary to verify that vestibular stimulation produced by head-down neck flexion in humans can affect the cardiovascular system.

Another approach that has been used to study potential vestibulocardiovascular responses in humans is to record blood pressure and heart rate changes during brief pulses of linear acceleration. As illustrated in Figure 40.5a, forward and backward linear acceleration of 0.2 g can induce changes in blood pressure of over 15 mmHg in some subjects.[51] Figure 40.5b shows that the interval between heartbeats becomes shorter just after acceleration onset (i.e. the heart rate increases), but then increases after the acceleration is complete. However, linear acceleration produces minimal cardiovascular effects in labyrinthine-defective subjects, indicating that the responses in labyrinth-intact individuals are due to activation of the vestibular system. The cardiovascular responses to linear acceleration do not adapt (become smaller) with repeated stimulus exposures, suggesting that they are not due to non-specific effects such as startle. Furthermore, there was no correlation between the magnitude of cardiovascular responses to linear acceleration and motion sickness susceptibility. These data thus support the hypothesis that vestibular influences on cardiovascular control in humans are not the result of motion discomfort, but instead occur as part of a reflex that acts to stabilize blood pressure during changes in posture.

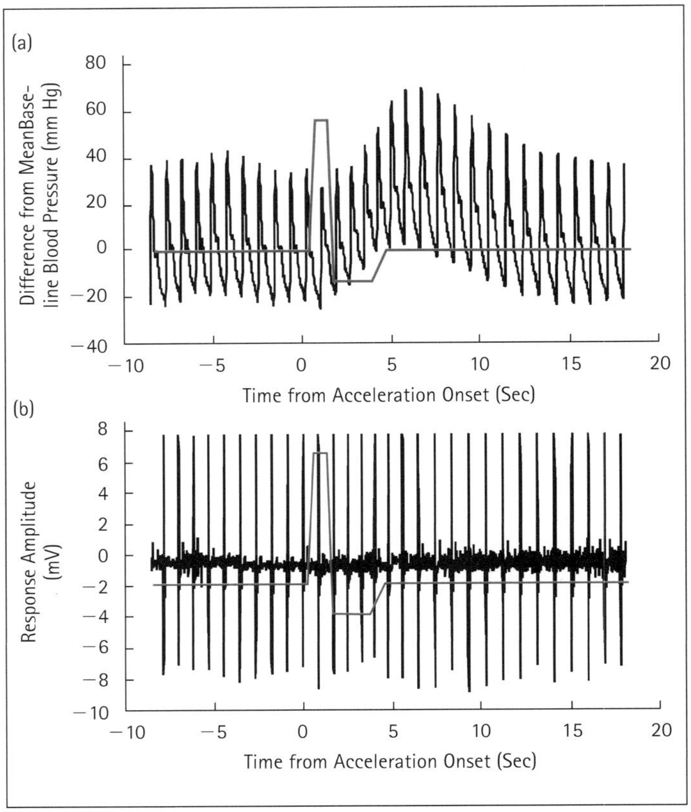

Figure 40.5 Cardiovascular responses to linear acceleration in a human subject. Cardiovascular responses were induced by a forward linear acceleration of 0.2 g, attaining a velocity of 2 m/s in 900 ms, and then deaccelerating for 3 s at approximately 0.07 g. The subject was seated facing the direction of acceleration with head restrained in the upright position. (a) Change in blood pressure induced by linear acceleration; note that blood pressure is plotted with respect to mean pressure before the onset of the stimulus. The acceleration profile (red trace) is superimposed on the blood pressure response (black trace). (b) ECG recording during linear acceleration; the acceleration profile (red trace) is superimposed on the recording (black trace). Note that the R–R interval (period between heartbeats) becomes shorter during the forward acceleration (i.e., the heart speeds up), and then becomes longer. (Adapted from Yates et al. *Exp Brain Res* 1999; **125**: 476–84.[51])

Effects of vestibular lesions on orthostatic tolerance

Some of the first evidence suggesting that the vestibular system plays an important role in cardiovascular control during movement came from lesion experiments. Doba and Reis[52] analyzed the effects of transecting the VIIIth cranial nerves on blood pressure stability during nose-up tilt in anesthetized, paralyzed cats. As shown in Figure 40.6, this experiment demonstrated that orthostatic tolerance was drastically reduced by removal of vestibular inputs. However, alert animals have more sensory inputs (proprioceptive, visual, etc.) available that indicate body position in space, and thus may not experience the same deficits following vestibular lesions. To examine this possibility, blood pressure was monitored during static nose-up rotations up to 60° in amplitude in alert cats that were trained to lie on a tilt table.[53] Changes in blood pressure during tilts were compared before and after the VIIIth cranial nerves were transected. As illustrated in Figure 40.7, these lesions impaired orthostatic tolerance significantly, particularly when the visual environment also rotated with the animal (thereby eliminating visual cues indicating body position in space). However, the deficit in adjusting blood pressure during tilt only persisted for about 1 week after removal of labyrinthine signals, perhaps because the animals learned to use other sensory inputs to determine body position in space. These findings are consistent with the hypothesis that vestibular inputs comprise one of several sensory cues used to trigger compensatory cardiovascular responses during movement.

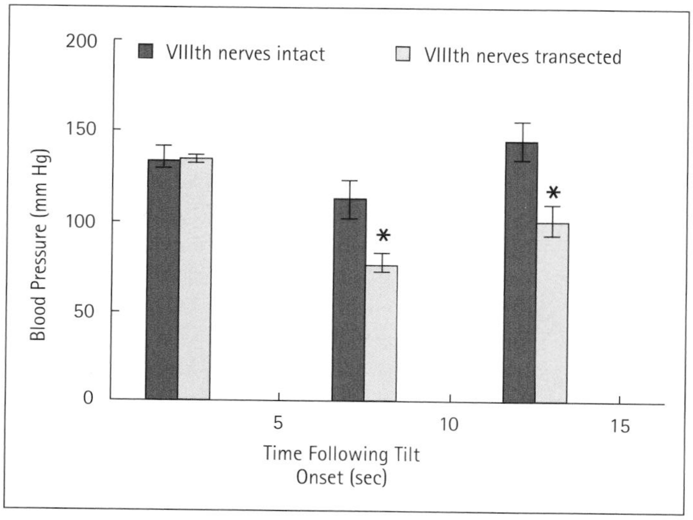

Figure 40.6 Effects of 60° nose-up tilt on blood pressure, in paralyzed and anesthetized animals before and after the VIIIth cranial nerves were transected. Solid bars represent the averaged results from eight animals, and error bars indicate one standard error of the mean. Elimination of vestibular inputs significantly ($p < 0.05$, paired Student's t-test) compromised the ability of the animals to adjust blood pressure during nose-up tilt. These significant differences are indicated by asterisks. (Adapted from Doba and Reis. *Circulation Res* 1974; **34**: 9–18.[52])

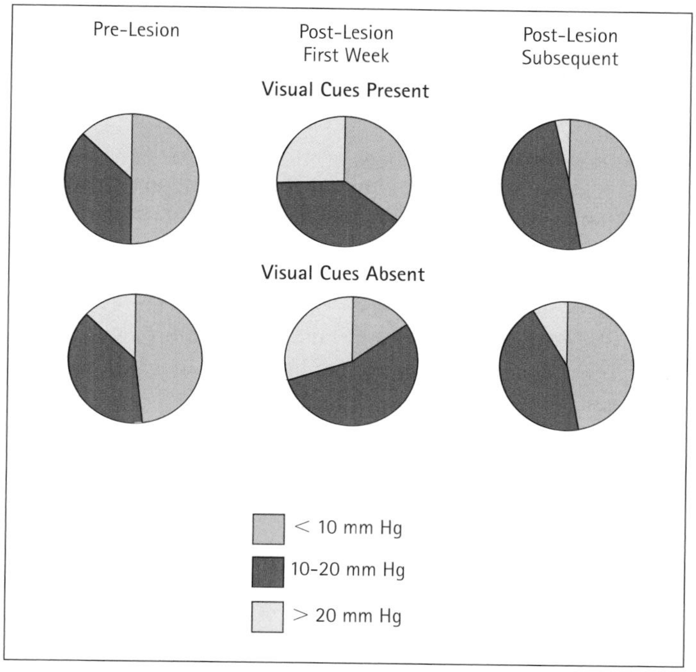

Figure 40.7 Percentage of experimental trials, before and after bilateral transection of the VIIIth cranial nerves, in which the maximal change in mean blood pressure during 60° nose-up tilt was small (< 10 mmHg; depicted by green areas), moderate (10–20 mmHg; depicted by purple areas), or large (> 20 mmHg; depicted by red areas). Responses recorded before the vestibular lesion, in the first week following the lesion, and at subsequent times are shown in different columns. Responses from trials in which visual cues concerning body position in space were present or eliminated are shown in separate rows. These graphs reflect the pooled data from five animals. Before the vestibular lesion, a change in blood pressure > 20 mmHg (red area in figures) occurred in only a small fraction of trials. However, after the vestibular lesion, blood pressure was unstable during tilt, particularly when animals were also deprived of visual cues regarding body position in space. This deficit in correcting blood pressure during body rotations persisted for only about 1 week. (Adapted from Jian et al. *J Appl Physiol* 1999; **86**: 1552–60.[53])

Cerebellar modulation of vestibulosympathetic reflexes

The results discussed above suggest that vestibular signals comprise one input to a brainstem 'integrator' that evaluates parameters of ongoing movements, determines the challenges to maintenance of homeostasis provided by those movements, and elicits appropriate compensatory autonomic responses. Furthermore, this integrator appears to exhibit a great deal of plasticity, as evidenced by the observation that recovery from the effects of vestibular lesions on cardiovascular control occurs over a period of days to weeks.[53] Although the neural circuitry involved in modulating vestibulo-cardiovascular responses is yet to be elucidated, there is considerable evidence to suggest that regions of the cerebellum form part of that circuitry. Some of this evidence comes from an analysis of the role of the cerebellum in modulating other vestibular-elicited reflexes.

Although the cerebellum is not required for the production of vestibulo-ocular and vestibulospinal reflexes, it is known to modulate the gain of these responses.[54] For example, adaptive plasticity in the vestibulo-ocular reflex is lost following ablations of the flocculonodular lobe of the cerebellum.[55] Further more, regions of the cerebellum that influence vestibulospinal and vestibulo-ocular reflexes integrate a variety of sensory inputs, including vestibular, visual and somatosensory signals, such that the reflex characteristics are more complex than can be attributed to processing vestibular inputs alone.[56] These observations suggest that cerebellar circuits may also have the proper characteristics to modify vestibulocardiovascular responses.

Several studies have shown that portions of the cerebellar vermis both receive visceral inputs and influence the activity of brainstem cardiovascular regulatory circuitry. Most of these studies have focused on the role of the caudal cerebellar vermis (including the uvula) in autonomic control, although there is some evidence that more rostral portions of the vermis and the fastigial nucleus may also participate in autonomic regulation (see Balaban[57] and Balaban and Yates[58] for reviews). In anesthetized and decerebrate rabbits, electrical stimulation of visceral afferents in the vagus nerve elicits evoked potentials in both the uvula and nodulus.[59] The same study also demonstrated that the nodulus and uvula receive blood pressure-related signals from aortic baroreceptors. Anatomical studies have suggested that the uvula has direct projections to the parabrachial nucleus, which is involved in autonomic control.[60] Stimulation of the uvula, and perhaps the nodulus, also evokes changes in heart rate and blood pressure.[61–63] Because the uvula and other regions of the cerebellar vermis receive powerful vestibular inputs and influence cardiovascular control, it is reasonable to speculate that these areas participate in modulating vestibulocardiovascular responses. Nonetheless, these is no direct evidence to demonstrate that the uvula or other regions of the cerebellum that integrate multiple sensory inputs and influence cardiovascular control are responsible for triggering autonomic adjustments during movement. Future studies will be required to elucidate the role of the cerebellum in cardiovascular regulation.

Summary and conclusions

Stimulation of vestibular receptors, and in particular otolith receptors, during nose-up tilt in quadrupeds (and presumably during standing in humans) induces a 'pattern' of activation of sympathetic efferents innervating vascular smooth muscle. Vestibular stimulation has an especially strong effect on the excitability of sympathetic fibers innervating blood vessels of the lower body. Because standing in human and nose-up tilt in quadrupeds tend to induce orthostatic hypotension, vestibulosympathetic reflexes appear to form part of a homeostatic mechanism to maintain stable blood pressure during changes in posture. In accordance with this hypothesis, animals and perhaps humans lacking vestibular inputs are more susceptible to orthostatic hypotension than normal subjects. However, vestibular inputs comprise only one of several sensory inputs that are integrated in order to trigger compensatory cardiovascular responses during movement. The cerebellum may play a role in controlling blood pressure during movement, as this structure receives the appropriate inputs, has the appropriate integrative circuitry, and possesses the pertinent outputs to accomplish this function.

Acknowledgements

The authors' research is supported by the National Institutes of Health of the United States, grants R01 DC00693, R01 DC03732, and P01 DC03417. M.J.H, B.J.J, I.A.K are supported by NASA's Graduate Student Researcher's Program.

References

1. Yates BJ, Miller AD, Lucot JB. Physiological basis and pharmacology of motion sickness: an update. *Brain Res Bull* 1998; **47**: 395–406.
2. Wilson VJ, Melvill Jones G. *Mammalian Vestibular Physiology*. New York: Plenum Press, 1979.
3. Yates BJ. Vestibular influences on cardiovascular control. In: Yates BJ, Miller AD, eds. *Vestibular Autonomic Regulation*. Boca Raton, FL: CRC Press, 1996: 97–111.
4. Kramer JM, Waldrop TG. Neural control of the cardiovascular system during exercise: an integrative role for the vestibular system. *J Vestib Res* 1998; **8**: 71–80.
5. Yates BJ, Miller AD. Physiological evidence that the vestibular system participates in autonomic and respiratory control. *J Vest Res* 1998; **8**: 17–25.
6. Yates BJ, Miller AD. Vestibular respiratory regulation. In: Miller AD, Bianchi AL, Bishop BP, eds. *Neural Control of the Respiratory Muscles*. Boca Raton, FL: CRC Press, 1996: 271–83.
7. Furman JM, Jacob RG, Redfern MS. Clinical evidence that the vestibular system participates in autonomic control. *J Vestib Res* 1998; **8**: 27–34.
8. Jacob RG, Furman JM, Perel JM. Panic, phobia and vestibular dysfunction. In: Yates BJ, Miller AD, eds. *Vestibular Autonomic Regulation*. Boca Raton, FL: CRC Press, 1996: 197–227.
9. Jacob RG, Furman JM, Durrant JD, Turner SM. Panic, agoraphobia, and vestibular dysfunction. *Am J Psychiatry* 1996; **153**: 503–12.
10. Furman JM, Jacob RG. Psychiatric dizziness. *Neurology* 1997; **48**: 1161–6.
11. Hobson JA, Stickgold R, Pace-Schott EF, Leslie KR. Sleep and vestibular adaptation: implications for function in microgravity. *J Vestib Res* 1998; **8**: 81–94.
12. Money KE, Lackner JR, Cheung RSK. The autonomic nervous system and motion sickness. In: Yates BJ, Miller AD, eds. *Vestibular Autonomic Regulation*. Boca Raton, FL: CRC Press, 1996: 147–73.

13. Kerman IA, Yates BJ. Regional and functional differences in the distribution of vestibulosympathetic reflexes. *Am J Physiol* 1998; **275**: R824–35.
14. Yates BJ, Jakus J, Miller AD. Vestibular effects on respiratory outflow in the decerebrate cat. *Brain Res* 1993; **629**: 209–17.
15. Yates BJ, Miller AD. Properties of sympathetic reflexes elicited by natural vestibular stimulation: implications for cardiovascular control. *J Neurophysiol* 1994; **71**: 2087–92.
16. Rossiter CD, Hayden NL, Stocker SD, Yates BJ. Changes in outflow to respiratory pump muscles produced by natural vestibular stimulation. *J Neurophysiol* 1996; **76**: 3274–84.
17. Woodring SF, Rossiter CD, Yates BJ. Pressor response elicited by nose-up vestibular stimulation in cats. *Exp Brain Res* 1997; **113**: 165–8.
18. Kerman IA, Yates BJ. Adrenal nerve responses to vestibular nerve stimulation in the cat. *Soc Neurosci Abst* 1996; **22**: 92.
19. Yates BJ, Kerman IA. Post-spaceflight orthostatic intolerance: possible relationship to microgravity-induced plasticity in the vestibular system. *Brain Res Rev* 1998; **28**: 73–82.
20. Yates BJ, Yamagata Y, Bolton PS. The ventrolateral medulla of the cat mediates vestibulosympathetic reflexes. *Brain Res* 1991; **552**: 265–72.
21. Yates BJ, Goto T, Bolton PS. Responses of neurons in the rostral ventrolateral medulla of the cat to natural vestibular stimulation. *Brain Res* 1993; **601**: 255–64.
22. Yates BJ, Siniaia MS, Miller AD. Descending pathways necessary for vestibular influences on sympathetic and inspiratory outflow. *Am J Physiol* 1995; **268**: R1381–5.
23. Yates BJ, Grélot L, Kerman IA, Balaban CD, Jakus J, Miller AD. Organization of vestibular inputs to nucleus tractus solitarius and adjacent structures in cat brain stem. *Am J Physiol* 1994; **267**: R974–83.
24. Steinbacher BC, Yates BJ. Processing of vestibular and other inputs by the caudal ventrolateral medullary reticular formation. *Am J Physiol* 1996; **271**: R1070–7.
25. Steinbacher BC, Yates BJ. Brainstem interneurons necessary for vestibular influences on sympathetic outflow. *Brain Research* 1996; **720**: 204–10.
26. Yates BJ, Balaban CD, Miller AD, Endo K, Yamaguchi Y. Vestibular inputs to the lateral tegmental field of the cat: potential role in autonomic control. *Brain Res* 1995; **689**: 197–206.
27. McAllen RM, Dampney RAL. The selectivity of descending vasomotor control by subretrofacial neurons. *Prog Brain Res* 1989; **81**: 233–42.
28. Dampney RAL, Goodchild AK, McAllen RM. Vasomotor control by subretrofacial neurons in the rostral ventrolateral medulla. *Can J Physiol Pharmacol* 1987; **65**: 1572–9.
29. Dampney RAL. The subretrofacial vasomotor nucleus—anatomical, chemical and pharmacological properties and role in cardiovascular regulation. *Prog Neurobiol* 1994; **42**: 197–227.
30. Tang PC, Gernandt BE. Autonomic responses to vestibular stimulation. *Exp Neurol* 1969; **24**: 558–78.
31. Loewy AD, Spyer KM. *Central Regulation of Autonomic Functions*. New York: Oxford University Press, 1990.
32. Bolton PS, Kerman IA, Woodring SF, Yates BJ. Influences of neck afferents on sympathetic and respiratory nerve activity. *Brain Res Bull* 1998; **47**: 413–19.
33. Cannon WB. *Bodily Changes in Pain, Hunger, Fear and Rage*. New York: Harper Torcbooks, 1929.
34. Cannon WB. *The Wisdom of the Body*. New York: W. W. Norton, 1963.
35. Iriki M, Simon E. Differential autonomic control of regional circulatory reflexes evoked by thermal stimulation and by hypoxia. *Aust J Exp Biol Med Sci* 1973; **51**: 283–93.
36. Walther O-E, Iriki M, Simon E. Antagonistic changes of blood flow and sympathetic activity in different vascular beds following central thermal stimulation. II. Cutaneous and visceral sympathetic activity during spinal cord heating and cooling in anesthetized rabbits and cats. *Pflügers Arch* 1970; **319**: 162–84.
37. Bahr R, Bartel B, Blumberg H, Jänig W. Functional characterization of preganglionic neurons projecting in the lumbar splanchnic nerves: vasoconstrictor neurons. *J Autonomic Nervous System* 1986; **15**: 131–40.
38. Jänig W. Spinal cord reflex organization of sympathetic systems. *Prog Brain Res* 1996; **107**: 43–77.
39. Bahr R, Bartel B, Blumberg H, Jänig W. Functional characterization of preganglionic neurons projecting in the lumbar splanchnic nerves: neurons regulating motility. *J Autonomic Nervous System* 1986; **15**: 109–30.
40. Dorward PK, Burke SL, Jänig W, Cassell J. Reflex responses to baroreceptor, chemoreceptor and nociceptor inputs in single renal sympathetic neurones in the rabbit and the effects of anaesthesia on them. *J Autonomic Nervous System* 1987; **18**: 39–54.
41. Weaver LC. Organization of sympathetic responses to distension of urinary bladder. *Am J Physiol* 1985; **248**: R236–40.
42. Mittelstaedt H. Somatic versus vestibular gravity reception in man. *Ann N Y Acad Sci* 1992; **656**: 124–39.
43. Preber L. Vegetative reactions in caloric and rotatory tests. *Acta Otolaryngol* 1958; Suppl 144: 1–119.
44. Hemmingway A. Cardiovascular changes in motion sickness. *J Aviation Med* 1945; **16**: 417–21.
45. Ohashi N, Imamura J, Nakagawa H, Mizukoshi K. Blood pressure abnormalities as background roles for vertigo, dizziness and disequilibrium. *Otorhinolaryngology* 1990; **52**: 355–9.
46. Shortt TL, Ray CA. Sympathetic and vascular responses to head-down neck flexion in humans. *Am J Physiol* 1997; **272**: H1780–4.
47. Normand H, Etard O, Denise P. Otolithic and tonic neck receptors control of limb blood flow in humans. *J Appl Physiol* 1997; **82**: 1734–8.
48. Ray CA, Hume KM, Shortt TL. Skin sympathetic outflow during head-down neck flexion in humans. *Am J Physiol* 1997; **273**: R1142–6.
49. Ray CA, Hume KM. Neck afferents and muscle sympathetic activity in humans: implications for the vestibulosympathetic reflex. *J Appl Physiol* 1998; **84**: 450–3.
50. Ray CA, Hume KM, Steele SL. Sympathetic nerve activity during natural stimulation of horizontal semicircular canals in humans. *Am J Physiol* 1998; **275**: R1274–8.

51. Yates BJ, Aoki M, Burchill P, Bronstein AM, Gresty MA. Cardiovascular responses elicited by linear acceleration in humans. *Exp Brain Res* 1999; **125**: 476–84.
52. Doba N, Reis DJ. Role of the cerebellum and vestibular apparatus in regulation of orthostatic reflexes in the cat. *Circulation Res* 1974; **34**: 9–18.
53. Jian BJ, Cotter LA, Emanuel BA, Cass SP, Yates BJ. Effects of bilateral vestibular lesions on orthostatic tolerance in awake cats. *J Appl Physiol* 1999; **86**: 1552–60.
54. MacKay WA, Murphy JT. Cerebellar modulation of reflex gain. *Prog Neurobiol* 1979; **13**: 361–417.
55. Robinson DA. Adaptive gain control of vestibuloocular reflex by the cerebellum. *J Neurophysiol* 1976; **39**: 954–69.
56. Ito M. *The Cerebellum and Neural Control*. New York: Raven Press, 1984.
57. Balaban CD. The role of the cerebellum in vestibular autonomic function. In: Yates BJ, Miller AD, eds. *Vestibular Autonomic Regulation*. Boca Raton, FL: CRC Press, 1996: 127–44.
58. Balaban CD, Yates BJ. Vestibulo-autonomic interactions: a teleologic perspective. In: Highstein SM, Fay RR, Popper AN, eds. *Anatomy and Physiology of the Central and Peripheral Vestibular System*. Heidelberg: Springer-Verlag, 2002: in press.
59. Nisimaru N, Katayama S. Projection of cardiovascular afferents to the lateral nodulus-uvula of the cerebellum in rabbits. *Neurosci Res* 1995; **21**: 343–50.
60. Paton JF, La Noce A, Sykes RM et al. Efferent connections of lobule IX of the posterior cerebellar cortex in the rabbit—some functional considerations. *J Autonomic Nervous System* 1991; **36**: 209–24.
61. Henry RT, Connor JD, Balaban CD. Nodulus-uvula depressor response: central GABA-mediated inhibition of alpha-adrenergic outflow. *Am J Physiol* 1989; **256**: H1601–8.
62. Bradley DJ, Ghelarducci B, Paton JFR, Spyer KM. The cardiovascular responses elicited from the posterior cerebellar cortex in the anesthetized and decerebrate rabbit. *J Physiol* 1987; **383**: 537–50.
63. Bradley DJ, Pascoe JP, Paton JFR, Spyer KM. Cardiovascular and respiratory responses evoked from the posterior cerebellar cortex and fastigial nucleus in the cat. *J Physiol* 1987; **393**: 107–21.
64 Cobbold AF, Megirian D, Sherrey JH. Vestibular evoked activity in autonomic motor outflows. *Arch Ital Biol* 1968; **106**: 113–23.
65 Ishikawa T, Miyazawa T. Sympathetic responses evoked by vestibular stimulation and their interactions with somatosympathetic reflexes. *J Autonomic Nervous System* 1980; **1**: 243–54.
66 Uchino Y, Kudo N, Tsuda K, Iwamura Y. Vestibular inhibition of sympathetic nerve activities. *Brain Res* 1970; **22**: 195–206.
67 Megirian D, Manning JW. Input-output relations in the vestibular system. *Arch Ital Biol* 1967; **105**: 15–30.

41 The physiology of the vestibulo-ocular reflex

Bernard Cohen, Martin Gizzi

Overview

Angular and linear accelerations are encountered with virtually every movement. The vestibular system senses these accelerations and uses the information to perform a number of clearly defined functions that maintain stability of the body, head and eyes in three-dimensional space. The vestibulo-ocular reflex (VOR) acts as a guidance system for the visual system. Utilizing both angular and linear components, the VOR stabilizes gaze by moving the eyes so that they compensate for head and body movement. This 'fixes' images on the retina, enabling clear sight. The VOR also 'orients' the eyes toward linear acceleration, which tends to maintain the position of the retina with regard to the spatial or gravitational vertical and aligns them with the linear acceleration generated during movement. The visual and somatosensory systems interact with the vestibular system and contribute to the perception of movement and to the production of compensatory eye movements. From the combined input of these sensory systems, the brain fashions a sense of spatial orientation. Vestibulospinal and vestibulocollic (neck) reflexes provide postural control during standing and help stabilize the body during walking and running. There are also important vestibular–autonomic functions. Heart and respiratory rates are altered to maintain blood pressure every time we stand erect. It is not surprising, therefore, that lesions of a system that has such protean functions can cause frightening or disabling symptoms or that physicians have been intrigued by the causes and treatment of vertigo for thousands of years. The purpose of this chapter is to provide an overview of the physiology of the VOR to provide a basis for understanding its functions and its disorders.

The vestibular labyrinth

The vestibular apparatus and the cochlea make up the inner ear, and are contained within the bony labyrinth in the petrous portion of the temporal bone (Figure 41.1). There are three principal portions of the labyrinth: the semicircular canals, the otolith organs and the cochlea. The central vestibule contains the otolith organs, the utricle and saccule. The membranous canals, which are filled with the viscous endolymph, lie in the bony canals surrounded by perilymph. At one end of each semicircular canal is a bulge known as the ampulla, which holds the sensory apparatus. At the base of the ampulla is the crista, which contains the neurons and the sensory epithelium. The sensory epithelium—made up of hair cells and supporting cells—is covered by a gelatinous mass, called the cupula, which extends across the diameter of the ampulla (Figure 41.2a). The cupula closes the canal, restricting the flow of endolymph. When the head is turned, the motion of the endolymph within the semicircular canals causes the cupula to move like a diaphragm, deflecting the hair cells embedded in the cupula (Figure 41.2b). This process underlies sensing angular movement of the head (Figure 41.2b, c).

The maculae of the otolith organs, the utricle and saccule, resemble inertial accelerometers. Each consists of hair cells, nerve fibers that innervate them, and an overlying gelatinous substance in which the otoliths are embedded (Figure 41.2d). The structure of the otolith organs differs significantly from the crista of the semicircular canals in that calcium carbonate $Ca(CO_3)_2$ crystals, which form the otoliths or otoconia, are embedded over the hair cells in the gelatinous mucopolysaccharide matrix. Initially during development, the calcium carbonate is laid down as calcite,[1] but in the adult it is converted to aragonite, a denser form of the mineral. A scanning electronmicrograph of the otoconia of a ground squirrel with polymorphic aragonite crystals is shown in Figure 41.3. Since the specific gravity of the crystals is greater than that of the endolymph, they are displaced in the direction of the gravity when the head is tilted, bending the hair cells (Figure 41.2e). Their inertia and the fluid in which they are embedded also cause them to lag and bend the hair cells away from the direction of linear acceleration when the head is translated (moved linearly) forward-and-back, side-to-side or up-and-down (Figure 41.2f). The utricular macula is oriented roughly horizontally, and the saccular macula is roughly vertical (Figure 41.4[2]), although both have substantial curvature.[3] Thus, the saccule is

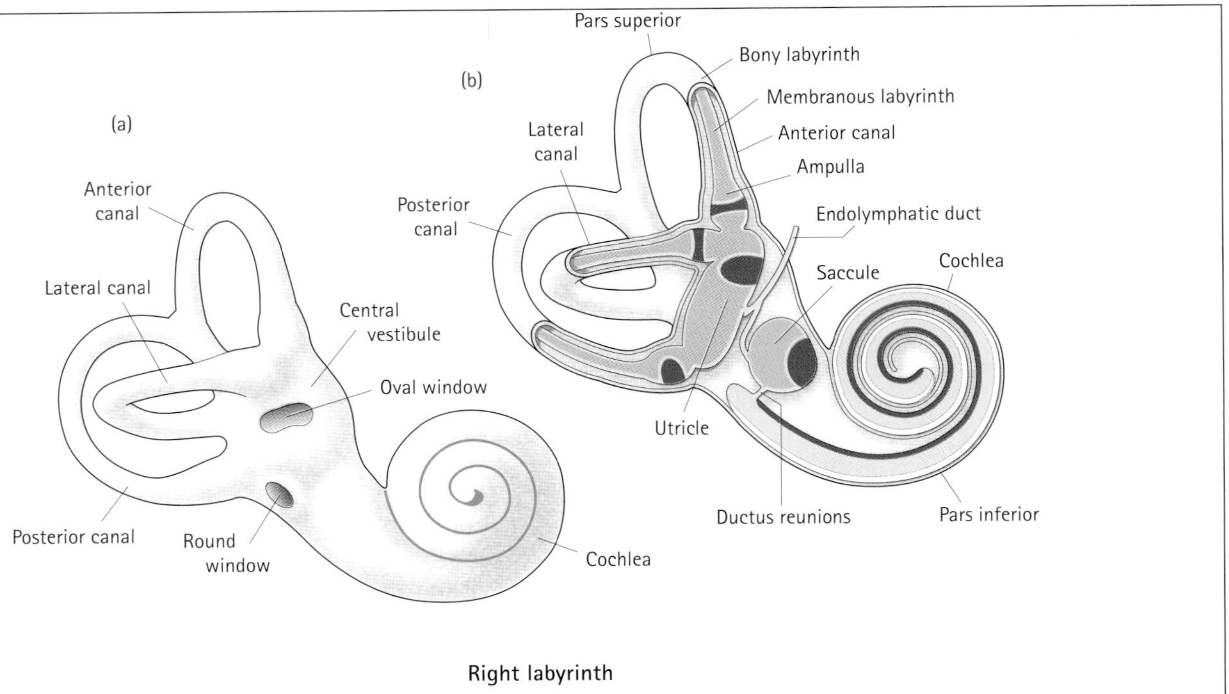

Figure 41.1 Bony structure of the right labyrinth (a), exploded in (b) to show membranous canals and the otolith organs, the saccule and utricle. (Adapted from Hudspeth. *Sci Am* 1983; **248**: 54–64.[89]).

well equipped to sense vertical head acceleration and the constant pull of gravity, whereas the utricles sense linear head motion in the horizontal plane. The utricles also play an important role in signaling the spatial upright when the head is tilted with regard to gravity.

Hair cells

There are two general classes of hair cells in both the canals and otolith organs. These are the goblet-shaped, type 1 hair cells, and the cylindrical, type 2 hair cells (Figure 41.5). Type 1 hair cells are surrounded by chalice-like nerve endings that ensure secure synaptic transmission.[4] Type 1 cells tend to be clustered at the top of the cristae of the canals or along the striola on the surface of the maculae of the utricle and saccule (Figure 41.6). Type 2 hair cells lie along the slopes of the crista and laterally on the maculae. Whether a stimulus raises or lowers the resting potential of a hair cell depends on the orientation of that cell with regard to the stimulus. Each hair cell has a cluster of stereocilia that are short on one end of the cell and gradually increase in length on the opposite end. The stereocilia create a surface that slopes upward and ends at the solitary kinocilium (Figure 41.5). Deflection of the stereocilia toward the kinocilium leads to depolarization and an increased firing rate in the eighth nerve; deflection away from the kinocilium leads to hyperpolarization and a decreased firing rate in the nerve; orthogonal deflections have no effect.[5–7] This principle of excitation holds for hair cells in both the cristae of the semicircular canals and maculae of the otolith organs. The hair cells of the semicircular canals have the same orientation on the crista so that they are all excited or inhibited by the flow of endolymph in the same direction (Figure 41.6a). This is in contrast to the hair cells on the maculae of the utricle and saccule, which have different orientations. The striola, the region where the excitatory direction of polarization of the hair cells is reversed (Figure 41.6b), forms a line across the middle of both of the otolith organs. Uchino et al[8] have shown that cells with opposite polarization vectors, which lie on opposite sides of the striola, are simultaneously excited or inhibited when the head is moved. An interposed neuron in the vestibular nuclei converts the inhibition from the hair cells on one side of the striola to excitation in the vestibular nuclei and feeds back the activity onto cells receiving input from the other side of the macula. Thus, the inputs from both sides of the striola are coordinated in the central vestibular system, and a common excitatory or inhibitory direction is produced from each macula.

An extensive network of nerve fibers connects the various types of hair cells in most parts of the crista as well as in the maculae (Figure 41.6)[9,10] This pattern of connectivity may account for some of the discharge characteristics of the hair cells.[11,12] The discharge of type 1 cells tends to be irregular, whereas type 2 cells exhibit a more regular discharge rate. This difference has been formalized using a coefficient of variation

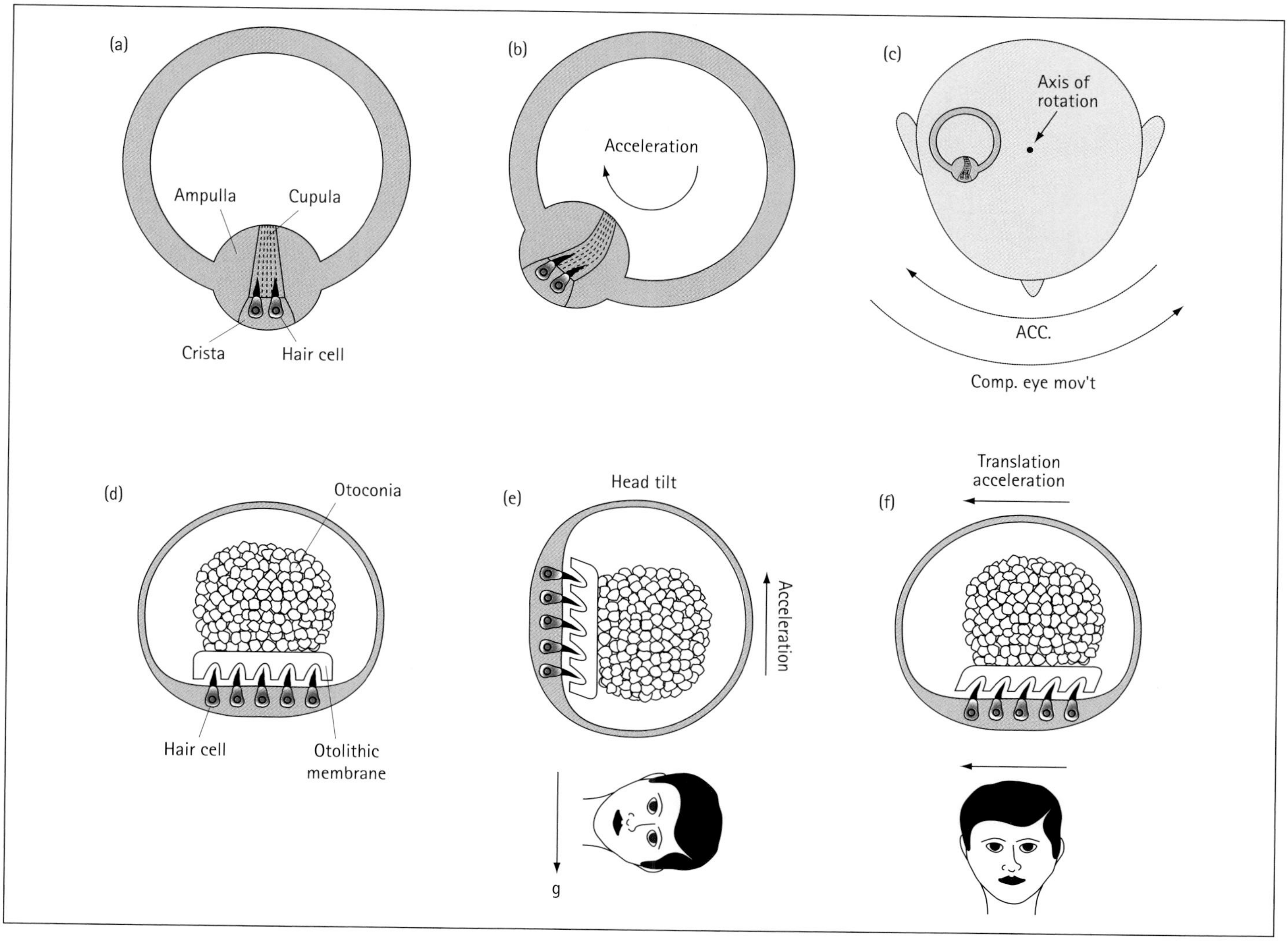

Figure 41.2 (a–c) Representation of the semicircular canal with stereocilia and kinocilia of hair cells on crista embedded in the cupula. (a) Position of the hair cells and cupula with the head stationary. (b) During head acceleration in the clockwise direction, the inertia of the endolymph causes the cupula and hair cell cilia to deflect in the counterclockwise direction. (c) Head rotation to the right about the yaw or long body axis produces a compensatory eye movement to the left over the angular vestibulo-ocular reflex (aVOR). (d) Representation of the utricular macula with the head upright, showing hair cells, otolithic membrane and otoconia. (e) Head tilt to the left causes movement of the otoconia in the direction of gravitational force (g), deflecting the sterocilia and kinocilia of the hair cells. The eyes counter-roll against the head tilt, which tends to maintain the relative position of the retina in space. (f) Linear translation of the head to the right (arrow over head) causes similar deflection of the otoconia and hair cells to the left. For sudden, high-frequency head movements, the linear vestibulo-ocular reflex (lVOR) produces a compensatory eye movement to the left. (Adapted from Hudspeth. *Sci Am* 1983; **248**: 54–64.[89])

based on the resting frequency.[13,14] It has been postulated that the irregularly firing type 1 hair cells, which lie along central portions of the crista (Figure 41.6a, CENT), are largely responsible for producing bursts or pulses of activity that help initiate compensatory head movement when the canals are stimulated.[15] The regularly firing type 2 hair cells, which are located more peripherally on the crista (Figure 41.6a, PER), appear to be more important for generating eye movements through the VOR.[16] Type 1 hair cells are more seriously damaged by ototoxic drugs than are type 2 cells. This may explain why it is relatively rare for vestibulo-ocular function to be completely lost after administration of ototoxic drugs.

Both type 1 and 2 hair cells receive efferent feedback from the brain. The efferent fibers synapse on the chalice-type nerve endings that innervate type 1 hair cells, whereas they make direct synaptic contact with type 2 hair cells (Figure 41.5). Although the functional significance of this difference in efferent endings is unknown, both excitatory and inhibitory effects on afferent input from the semicircular canals have been produced by stimulation of the efferent system. There is broad divergence in the efferent system, with 150 000 fibers originating from just 15 000 cells. This would appear to preclude specificity and to favor a general effect when the system is excited.

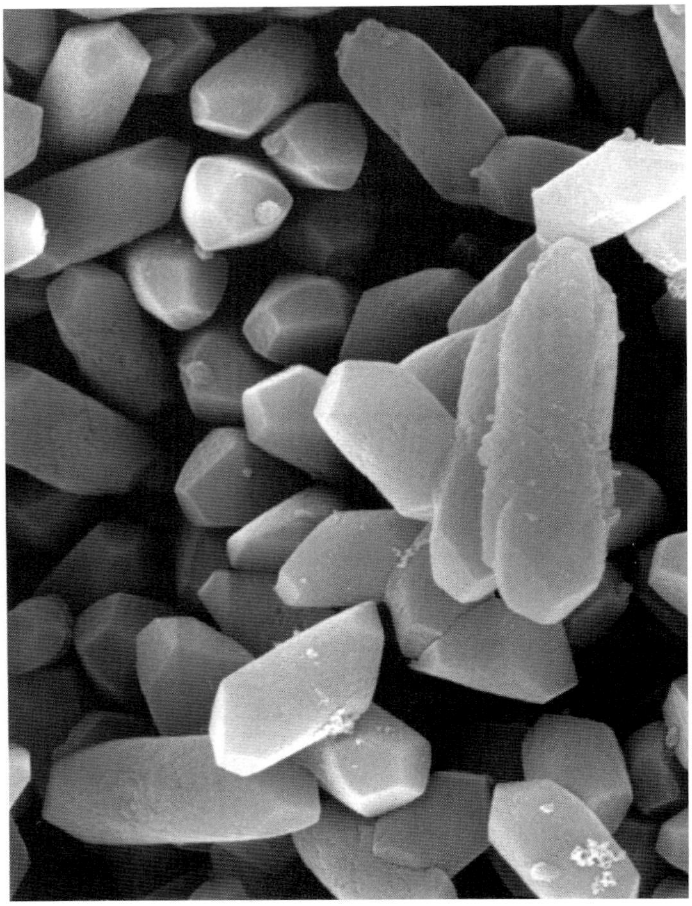

Figure 41.3 Scanning electronmicrograph of otoconia of the ground squirrel, showing polymorphic aragonite crystals of calcium carbonate ($Ca(CO_3)_2$). (Courtesy of Anna Lysakowski.)

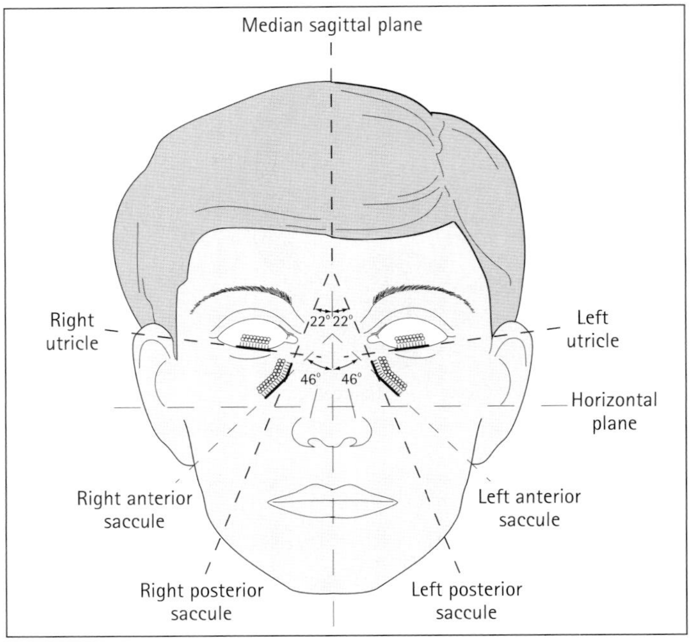

Figure 41.4 Orientation of the utricles and saccules in the head. (From Miller. *Acta otolaryngol* 1962; **54**: 479–501.[2])

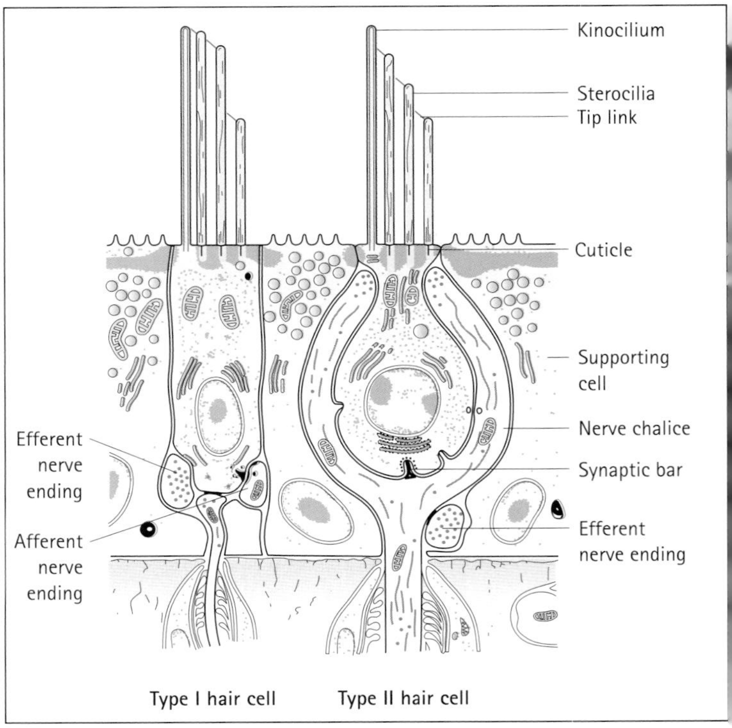

Figure 41.5 Type 1 and type 2 hair cells. (Adapted from Wersall and Bagger-Sjoback. In: Kornhubar, ed. *Handbook of Sensory Physiology*. Berlin: Springer Verlag, 1974; 123–70.[90])

Angular vestibulo-ocular reflex (a VOR)

Ocular compensation for angular head movement originates in the semicircular canals. When the head turns, angular acceleration induces movement of the endolymph relative to the walls of the membranous canals. The fluid presses against the cupula, causing it to bend and deflect the stereocilia and kinocilia of the hair cells embedded in the cupula. In turn, this opens or closes ion channels at the tips of the stereocilia through tiplinks (Figure 41.5).[17] K^+, Ca^{2+} and Cl^- currents are generated in the hair cells and raise or lower the resting potential of the hair cells, activating synapses between the hair cells and fibers in the vestibular portion of the eighth nerve. This activation causes an increase or decrease in the resting discharge of the afferent fibers, signaling to the brain that the head is moving. Compensatory eye movements are then generated over the angular VOR (aVOR) to counter angular head movements and hold gaze stable in space. Vestibulocollic (neck) reflexes produce compensatory head movements and vestibulospinal reflexes readjust the position of the limbs to counter these accelerations and maintain postural stability.

The canal–ocular reflex is uniquely suited to respond rapidly and with precision over a wide range of angular acceler-

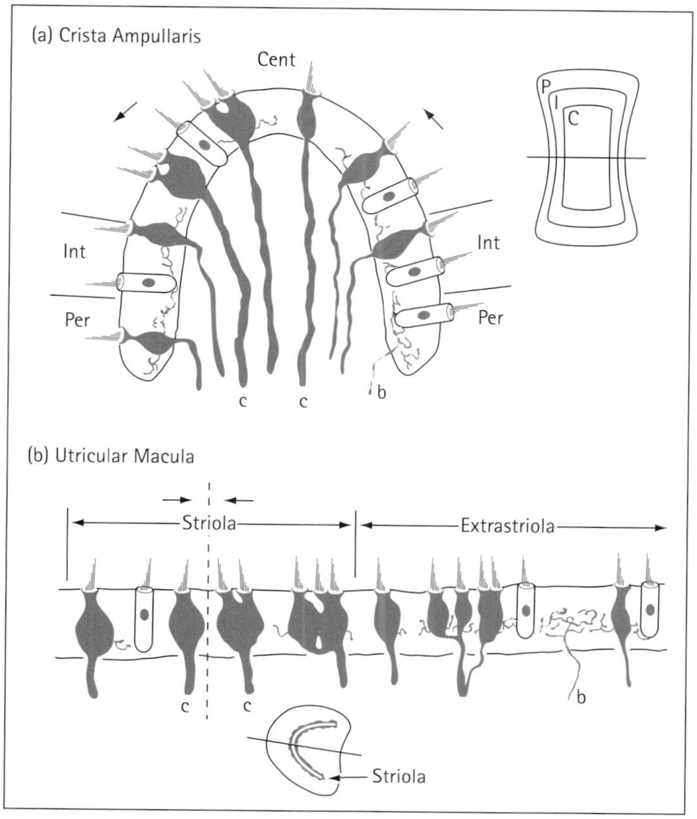

Figure 41.6 Diagram of innervation of semicircular canal crista (a) and utricular macula (b). (a) The crista is divided into central (CENT), intermediate (INT) and peripheral (PER) zones, as shown in the diagram on the right. The horizontal line in the diagram shows the plane of section. (b) The macula of the utricle is divided into striolar and juxtastriolar zones and an extrastriolar zone. The plane of section is shown by the line in the diagram below. The striola is the region where the hair cells reverse their orientation on the macula (dashed vertical line). The arrows on each side of the dashed line show the direction of deflection of the sterocilia and kinocilia that causes excitation. As with the semicircular canals, afferent fibers are excited when the stereocilia are bent toward the kinocilium. In both the crista (a) and macula (b), fibers terminate in boutons (b) or calyces (c). Type 1 hair cells and calyces (black) are more commonly located over the crest of the ampulla and near the striola. Type 2 (cylindrical) hair cells (white) and boutons are present in higher density eccentrically on both structures. (Adapted from Goldberg et al. *Ann NY Acad Sci* 1992; **656**: 92–107.[91])

ations, from about $1°/s^2$ to $10\,000°/s^2$. Low accelerations are normally present while swaying when standing erect, and higher accelerations are present during lateral gaze shifts when the head moves rapidly to the side. Normal head movements generally fall in a frequency range from 0.1 to 8–10 Hz (0.1 Hz indicates a movement repetition rate of once in 10 s, while 8 Hz is a repetition rate of 8/s). Compensatory eye movements can either be smooth or interspersed with oppositely directed rapid eye movements. When there are slow and rapid eye movements, they form a pattern that is known as nystagmus. The slow phases represent the sensory portion of the movement, because vestibular input related to head motion is processed during the slow phases, and the induced slow-phase eye velocity is a function of the velocity of the stimulus. The quick phases are largely restorative, resetting the eyes for the next slow phase. They also function to direct gaze in the direction of turning. Thus, during vestibular nystagmus, the average position of the eyes during the slow and quick phases is usually toward the direction in which the subject is moving. The same principle holds for nystagmus induced by visual motion, known as optokinetic nystagmus (OKN). Slow phases are produced in response to motion of the visual surround, and quick phases are restorative. The velocity of the eyes during the quick phases is determined solely by the size of the movement, and the brain is insensitive to visual input while they are in progress. Typical horizontal OKN in response to a horizontally moving, visual stimulus is shown in Figure 41.7b. This is similar to the 'parade' nystagmus originally described by Purkinje.[18,19] Vestibular nystagmus induced by rotation about a vertical axis in light has similar characteristics.

When the head is rotated, each canal that has a vector of angular acceleration along its canal axis responds. Because of the mechanical characteristics of the endolymph and cupula of the canals, an integration is performed on the head acceleration in the canals and the frequency of firing in the vestibular nerve is related to head velocity, not to head acceleration.[13,20] The mean resting discharge of semicircular canal nerves in many species, including the monkey, is about 90 impulses/s.[21] It is likely to be about the same in humans. When the head is stationary, both nerves should have approximately the same discharge rate. When the discharge rates between the two nerves are balanced, their inputs cancel, and the sum represents zero velocity, signaling to the brain that the head is motionless. As the head moves in the excitatory direction of one of the canals, impulse rates in that canal rise, reaching saturation frequencies of approximately 400–450 impulses/s. This covers rates of angular head velocities up to 800°/s. For movement in the inhibitory direction, impulse rates fall from 90 impulses/s toward zero. Since the resting discharge is not midway between 0 and 450 impulses/s, there is potentially a much larger representation of velocities in the excitatory direction. This asymmetry is not apparent when the reciprocal pairs of canals are functioning in a normal individual, because of their push–pull interaction. That is, when the head moves to one side, excitation from the canal on that side is supplemented by inhibition in the canal in the same plane on the other side. After a unilateral lesion has inactivated the labyrinth on one side, however, head movements to the side ipsilateral to the lesion will be sensed only by inhibition of the resting discharge rate on the contralateral side. Consequently, the range of frequencies sensing such stimulation will be more limited than for movements in the contralateral direction. This asymmetry was first noted by Ewald in his classic monograph on effects of canal stimulation and canal plugging in pigeons.[22] It forms the basis for a useful bedside test for detecting unilateral lesions that has been proposed by Halmagyi and colleagues[23–25] and is described below.

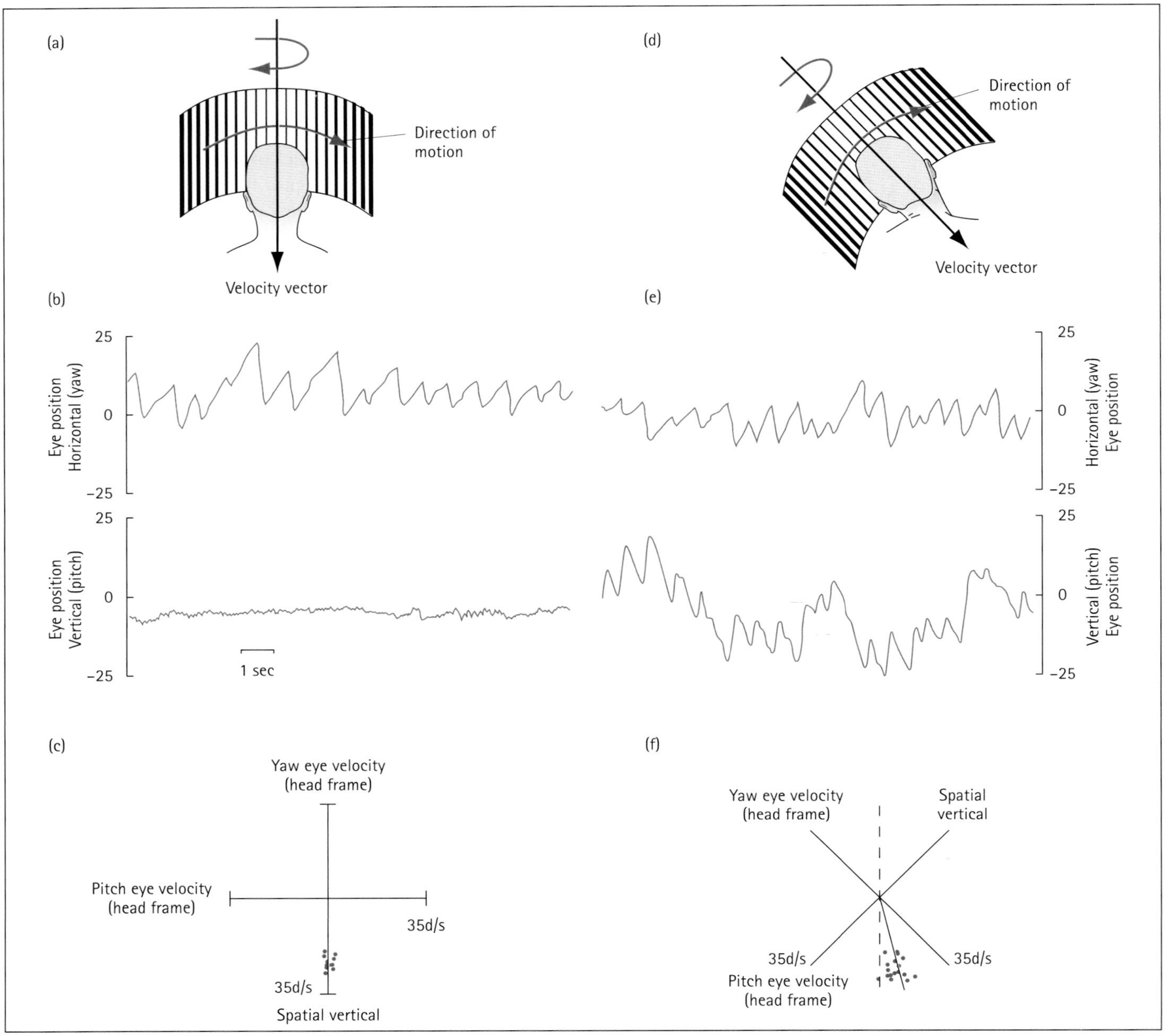

Figure 41.7 Movement of the visual surround at 35°/s about the head yaw axis when this axis is aligned with gravity (a) produced the optokinetic nystagmus shown in (b). The slow phases of nystagmus had no vertical component, and the eyes rotated about a spatially vertical axis. Thus, the slow-phase velocity vectors (dots) aligned with the spatial vertical (c). When the same stimulus was given with regard to the yaw axis of the head, but the head was tilted 45° with regard to gravity (d), a vertical component appeared in the nystagmus (e, bottom trace). This caused the axis of eye rotation and the vector of eye velocity to shift toward the gravitational vertical. In (f), the tilt of the head is shown by the directions of yaw and pitch eye velocity axes in a head coordinate frame (solid lines) with regard to the spatial vertical (dashed vertical line). The dots represent the slow-phase velocity vectors of the nystagmus in (d) with regard to both the head tilt and spatial vertical. The solid oblique line shows the mean vector. Note that the slow-phase eye velocity vector tended to alignment with the gravito-inertial acceleration (spatial vertical) (From Gizzi et al. *Exp Brain Res* 1994; **99**: 347–60.[47])

Planar organization of the canal system

Although there are six semicircular canals, both lateral canals and each anterior and the contralateral posterior canal lie in planes that are approximately parallel (Figure 41.8). Thus, the canals form three reciprocal pairs that sense head angular movement in planes, which are approximately orthogonal to each other. These have been called the lateral, RALP (right anterior–left posterior) and LARP (left anterior–right posterior) planes.[26] When the head rotates in a direction that causes excitation in the fibers of the nerve from one lateral canal, for

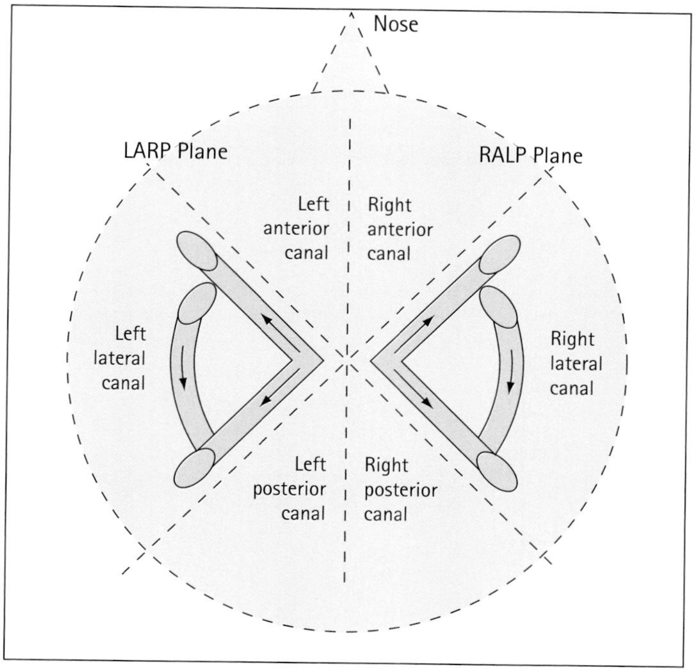

Figure 41.8 Approximate planes of the semicircular canals in the head. The lateral canals lie approximately parallel to each other, as do the left anterior and right posterior canal (LARP) and the right anterior and left posterior canals (RALP). The arrows show the direction of head movement that causes excitation in each canal. (From Yakushin. *Labyrinthine Control of the Vestibular-Ocular Reflex in Three Dimensions*. Brooklyn, New York: CUNY, 1996: p 241.[92])

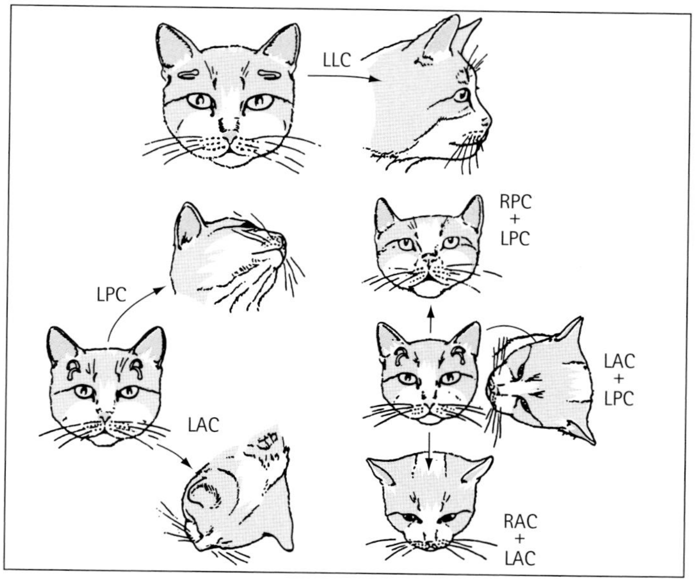

Figure 41.9 Directions of head movement that cause excitation of individual canals. When the head moves to the left, the left lateral canal (LLC) is excited, along with the vertical canals. When the head moves up and to the left, the left posterior canal (LPC) is excited, and when it moves down, the left anterior canal is excited (LAC). The reciprocal canal on the other side is inhibited. Other combinations are shown for upward head movement (RPC + LPC), downward head movement (RAC + LAC) and tilt of the head to the left in roll (LAC + LPC). (From Suzuki et al. *Exp Neurol* 1964; **9**: 137–60.[28])

instance, the reciprocal lateral canal nerve in the same plane in the contralateral labyrinth has a decrease in activity. The same is true for each anterior and contralateral posterior canal. All angular head movements are coded in the vestibular nuclei and vestibulocerebellum in these three semicircular canal planes. The planar organization was obviously highly successful in an evolutionary sense, and the six-canal system is highly conserved and present over a wide range of phylogeny. The same canal structure is present is cartilaginous fish (sharks and rays) and primates, a span of development covering several hundred million years. Even dinosaur skulls have a similar three-canal structure (Clarke, personal communication).

The excitatory directions for eye movements induced from the individual canals were derived by electrically stimulating the canals and recording the induced eye and head movements.[27,28] Data from the cat are shown in Figure 41.9. For the lateral canals, activity increases in the canal nerve when the head is turned toward the same side, causing a movement to the contralateral side. Thus, moving the head to the left causes an increase in activity in the nerve from the left lateral canal (LLC) and a decrease in activity in the nerve from the right lateral canal (RLC), and vice versa. The anterior and posterior canals, which also receive a component of angular acceleration during a lateral head movement, have reciprocal increases and decreases in the activity of their canal nerves. Together, all six canals drive the eyes to the right for leftward head movement, so that gaze is constant in space. The anterior canals are primarily activated when the forehead moves down during a head movement in the sagittal plane, and activity from the posterior canals is inhibited (RAC & LAC). The reverse occurs when the forehead moves up (RPC & LPC).

The three reciprocal canal planes are only approximately orthogonal. In humans, the lateral canals are tilted up anteriorly about 30° from the horizontal stereotaxic plane (the plane made by the line between the inferior orbital ridge of the eye and the external auditory canal) and from Reid's line. (Reid's line is the plane defined by the lateral canthus of the eye and the external auditory meatus.) The vertical canals are tilted posteriorly about 40° from the horizontal stereotaxic plane. Therefore, they are about 10° from being perpendicular to the lateral canals. As a result of the upward tilt of the lateral and vertical canals relative to the head horizontal, the vertical canals receive a component of force during all horizontal head movements and actively participate in producing the horizontal aVOR.[13,20,22] There is very little participation of the lateral canals, however, during pitch head movements.

In practice, it is possible to move the head in specific directions to test for the function of specific pairs of semicircular canals. Halmagyi and Curthoys[23] developed a bedside maneuver utilizing such movements. The basis for the test lies in Ewald's 'Second Law', i.e. in the asymmetry between firing rates in the excitatory and inhibitory directions, described above. Rotating the head back and forth around the long axis of the body, as if to say 'No' (yaw rotation), activates primarily the lateral canals

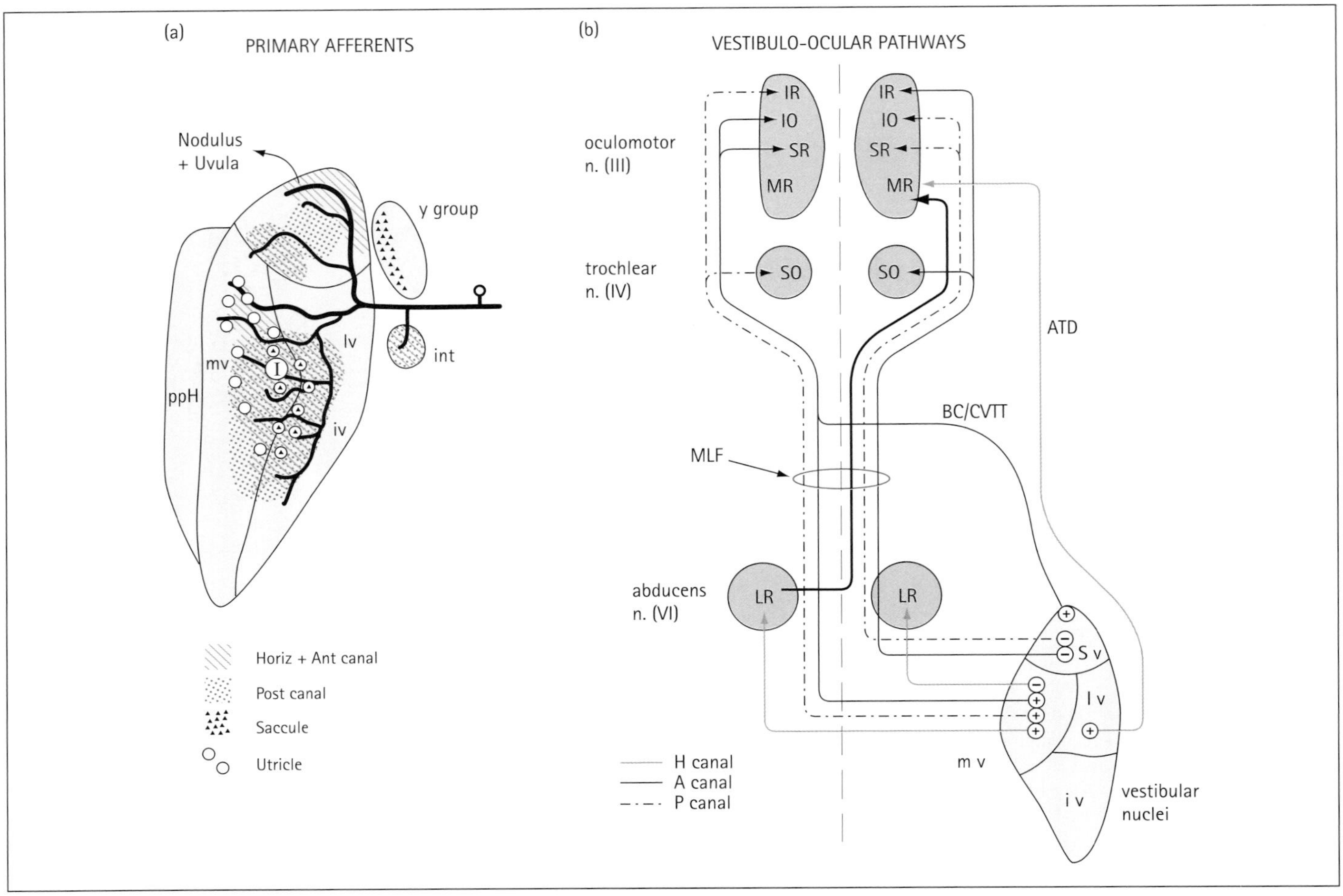

Figure 41.10 (a) Pattern of termination of the left vestibular nerve in the left vestibular nuclei. Canal projections are represented by stripes (LC and AC) and dots (PC). Utricular input is shown by open circles, and saccular input by triangles. Zone I is the only area receiving input from all canals and otoliths. In the superior vestibular nucleus (sv), canal afferents have individual sites of termination and project to the interstitial nucleus of the vestibular nerve (int). Fibers supplying peripheral sv continue on to the nodulus and uvula. The utricle terminates mainly in the medial vestibular nuclei (mv) and the sacculus in the ventral y-group. Additional abbreviations: ppH, prepositus hypoglossi nucleus; iv, inferior vestibular nucleus; lv, lateral vestibular nucleus. (b) Direct pathways from the vestibular nuclei with dominant canal inputs, and their projections to individual eye muscle motoneurons. In monkey and cat, there are also collaterals to other motoneurons. The crossing pathways are excitatory and, with the exception of the ascending tract of Deiters (ATD), the ipsilateral projections are inhibitory. Additional abbreviations: n, nerve; IR, inferior rectus; IO, inferior oblique; SR, superior rectus; MR, medial rectus; SO, superior oblique; MLF, medial longitudinal fasciculus; H, horizontal or lateral; P, posterior; A, anterior; BC, brachium conjunctivum; CVTT, crossing ventral tegmental tract. (From Buettner-Ennever. *Ann NY Acad Sci* 1992; **656**: 363–78.[30])

(Figure 41.9, LLC). Nodding the head forward, around an interaural axis, as if to say 'Yes' (pitch rotation), activates all four vertical canals plus the otolith organs, which also respond to changes in head position with regard to gravity. Nodding the head around an axis shifted 45° from the interaural axis, so that one temple moves down and the contralateral mastoid moves up, moves the head in the plane of one anterior and contralateral posterior canal. The opposite movement activates the reverse anterior and posterior canal pair. If the horizontal, vertical and torsional components of the movement of each eye are recorded during brief head movements of high angular acceleration (5000–10 000°/s^2), it is possible to identify malfunction of single canals, based on an absence of compensatory movement in the plane of a single canal or of a canal pair.[24,25] The same is not true for the otolith organs, where the directions of polarization of the hair cells vary widely over each receptor. This gives each otolith organ the potential for sensing gravitoinertial acceleration in many directions, but it complicates the understanding of central vestibular processing of otolith information as well as detection of lesions of the otolith organs.

The central vestibular system

A detailed description of the central vestibular system is beyond the scope of this chapter (see Brodal,[29] Buettner-Ennever,[30] and

Highstein and McCrea[31] for reviews). Some salient features of central vestibular organization and connectivity will be mentioned, however. The vestibular nuclei are generally separated into four main divisions, the superior, medial, lateral and inferior (or descending) vestibular nuclei—SVN, MVN, LVN and IVN, respectively. Afferent axons from the semicircular canals and otolith organs are widely distributed in the vestibular nuclei (Figure 41.10a). When the axons enter the vestibular nuclei, they bifurcate and send one axon rostrally and another caudally. The anterior canal projects heavily into the SVN, and all six canals send afferents into the MVN, ventral LVN and IVN. The otolith organs also send axons into the SVN, MVN, and IVN. There is some spatial separation between the parts of the vestibular nuclei that control various functions. The VOR is processed through rostral portions of the MVN and SVN. Vestibulospinal pathways arise from more caudal portions of the MVN, from dorsal portions of the LVN, and from the IVN. Vestibular–autonomic pathways are clustered in caudal parts of the MVN and IVN. There are also extensive connections between the vestibular nuclei and the flocculus, paraflocculus, nodulus and uvula. In fact, the vestibular nuclei have frequently been thought of as the deep cerebellar nuclei for these portions of the cerebellar cortex.

The classic vestibulo-ocular arc is composed of three neurons,[32] one from the semicircular canals, a secondary neuron in the vestibular nuclei, which transmits the information to the eye muscle motor nuclei, and the motor neuron itself. The location of second-order neurons in the vestibular nuclei, which are responsible for producing the aVOR, and the projections of their axons to the various oculomotor nuclei are shown in Figure 41.10b. One of these pathways will be illustrated here. Yaw or horizontal head movement causes the eyes to move conjugately to the opposite side to oppose the angular deviation of the head. Activity primarily from the lateral canals, but also from the anterior and posterior canals, excites 'tonic-vestibular-pause neurons' which lie in the rostral portions of the MVN. These TVP neurons project directly to the contralateral abducens nucleus onto lateral rectus motoneurons,[31] which cause the contralateral eye to abduct. The TVP neurons also send activity to abducens internuclear neurons in the contralateral abducens nucleus. Abducens internuclear neurons send their axons back across the mid-line in the medial longitudinal fasciculus (MLF) to the medial rectus motor neurons in the ipsilateral oculomotor (IIIrd) nucleus. This causes the ipsilateral eye to adduct to complete the contralateral compensatory movement. Abducens internuclear neurons also receive activity from burst neurons in the pontine reticular formation that produce adduction during saccadic eye movements. Lesions of the MLF cause paresis or paralysis of adduction or inter-nuclear ophthalmoplegia (INO). The medial longitudinal fasciculus also carries activity from secondary vestibular neurons to the vertical and oblique eye muscles, and lesions in this region also cause deficits in the vertical aVOR.

LVN also receives canal input in its ventral portion, but only the otoliths project into the dorsal portions of the LVN, which is known as Deiter's nucleus. Deiter's cells are very large, and their axons form the lateral vestibulospinal tract that produces extension of the ipsilateral limbs. The Deiter's cells receive heavy inhibitory input from the anterior lobe of the cerebellum that modulates and relaxes limb extension.[33] After anterior lobe lesions, the inhibitory input is reduced, and there is characteristic extension of the limbs, causing 'decerebrate rigidity'.

Velocity-to-position integration

It has been postulated that signals related to angular velocity from the semicircular canals, coding head velocity in space, are mathematically integrated in the vestibular nuclei or the adjacent brainstem to produce a signal for the eye muscle motor neurons that is related to eye position in the orbit.[34] This process has been called 'velocity-to-position integration'. The velocity-to-position integrator is critical for holding the eyes in eccentric positions in the orbit after saccades and is probably utilized by the linear VOR to convert signals related to linear head velocity in the central vestibular system to signals related to eye position in the orbit.[35] Deficits in velocity-to-position integration are manifest by a characteristic deficit in holding eccentric gaze, known as gaze-evoked nystagmus. When patients with this deficit look eccentrically (laterally, up, or down), instead of the eyes being maintained in the eccentric position, they drift slowly back toward the mid-line due to the unopposed mechanical stiffness of the eye muscles. These drifts are the slow phases of gaze-evoked nystagmus, which are interspersed with quick phases that restore the eccentric position. Such nystagmus is a function of the position of the eyes in the orbit, and the nystagmus is more vigorous, i.e. of greater amplitude and frequency, the further the eyes are from the mid-line. Gaze-evoked nystagmus is in contrast to spontaneous nystagmus, which is usually due to an underlying vestibular imbalance that causes the eyes to drift to one side, regardless of their orbital position. Eye velocity is quite different during these different types of nystagmus. The slow phases of spontaneous nystagmus are linear, and eye velocity is generally constant, whereas during gaze-evoked nystagmus, the slow phases are curved, and eye velocity decreases in an exponential fashion as the eyes move toward the mid-position.

Velocity storage

During constant-velocity rotation, the hair cells are initially deflected but soon return to their resting position. This has been modeled by a second-order system with a time constant of 3.5–5 s.[36] When activity of axons in the semicircular canal nerves was recorded, it became clear that the firing rates of the afferent axons, which provide the input to the VOR from the semicircular canals, decayed more rapidly during constant-velocity rotation than did the nystagmus that was induced by the same stimulus.[13,37,38] Comparative time constants of decline in the monkey are 4–5 s for activity from the canals and 15–20 s for the decline in nystagmus slow-phase velocity in response to the same stimulus. Recent evidence indicates that the human canal time constant is also ≈4 s,[39] while the nystagmus time constant is usually 12–20 s. This has led to the recognition that there is a central neural network that holds or stores activity coming from the labyrinth, prolonging the response to low-frequency rotation.

From modeling, it has been shown that the aVOR can be considered to be composed of two components. The first is the short-latency response that stabilizes gaze for high-frequency head movements, which has been considered in some detail above. A second, slower component has been modeled as a leaky integrator that stores eighth nerve activity and outputs a velocity command to produce slow-phase velocity, called 'velocity storage'.[37,38,40] This integrator is separate from that which produces velocity-to-position integration.[41] The dominant time constant of the aVOR largely reflects the velocity storage time constant, not the time constant of afferent activity coming from the semicircular canals, which is shorter. Velocity storage aids ocular compensation during low-frequency head or head-and-body movements, either in light or in the absence of vision.[35,38,40] When subjects rotate in light at a constant velocity, for example, vestibular input at the onset of rotation moves the eyes rapidly to an appropriate compensatory velocity. As rotation continues, however, the input from the canals ceases, and visual input, related to slip of the surround on the retina, generates OKN. This stabilizes images on the retina while the head is moving, and produces optokinetic after-nystagmus (OKAN) that counteracts the after-response of the semicircular canals when rotation ceases. Velocity storage is also activated by the somatosensory system[42] and by otolithic input during rotation about tilted axes[43] to provide a signal related to head and body velocity in space. Such activity is used to generate compensatory gaze velocity during locomotion when there is an angular component.

An interesting aspect of velocity storage is that it is spatially oriented.[35,44–46] If subjects are upright so that their yaw or body axis is aligned with gravity (Figure 41.7a), visual or vestibular stimuli around the long axis of the body produce purely horizontal eye movements (Figure 41.7b). Since eye movements are rotations of a globe in the orbit, these are rotations of the eyeballs around axes that are close to the spatial vertical (Figure 41.7c). If subjects are tilted when the stimuli around the yaw axis are given (Figure 41.7d), however, a vertical component appears (Figure 41.7e). This shifts the axis of rotation of the eyes so that it tends to align with the spatial vertical rather than with the yaw axis of the head and body (Figure 41.7f). Alignment toward the vector sum of the linear accelerations acting on the head, labeled gravito-inertial acceleration (GIA) occurs during both vestibular-induced nystagmus[46] and OKN.[47] In both cases, it depends on the spatial orientation of velocity storage in the vestibular nuclei (see Raphan and Cohen[35,93] for review). Alignment of eye velocity or of the axis of eye rotation to the GIA is important for stabilization of gaze during locomotion along a curved path. During walking or running around an angular track, the GIA swings away from the subject's yaw or long body axis as a result of the addition of centripetal and gravitational linear accelerations. In response, the body is tilted inward as one leans into the turn, so that the long body axis coincides with the GIA. The head and eyes rotate to match this shift of the GIA.[48] The spatial orientation of velocity storage is under control of the nodulus and uvula of the vestibulocerebellum, and the eyes no longer reorient to the GIA vector when these structures are damaged.[49–53]

Linear vestibulo-ocular reflex (lVOR)

The vector sum of linear accelerations acting on the head (GIA) is the stimulus that induces the lVOR. The GIA encompasses the linear acceleration of gravity as well as that generated during forward–backward, side-to-side, or up-and-down translational head movements. The presence of a near target is also essential for producing a compensatory lVOR, since there is no need for ocular compensation against translation if the point of regard is at infinity.[54–56] The lVOR has both compensatory and orienting functions. At high frequencies of head translation (1–8 Hz), the lVOR produces compensatory conjugate eye movements for side-to-side and up–down translation of the head.[57–60] When subjects are moving toward or away from a target (naso-occipital translation), the lVOR also causes the eyes to converge or diverge to help maintain ocular fixation.

Orienting otolith–ocular reflexes, such as ocular counter-rolling (OCR), stabilize the position of the retina in space with respect to gravity during lateral head tilt. OCR also helps to orient gaze toward the GIA during locomotion when turning. This reflex has a low gain, so that there is usually not more than 5–7° of ocular counter-torsion for tilts of the head as large as 60–90°. The tendency of the axis of eye rotation to align with the GIA during vestibular nystagmus and OKN (Figure 41.7d-f) is another example of an orienting function of the lVOR.

Since all linear acceleration is equivalent, theoretically the brain cannot distinguish between tilts due to the linear acceleration of gravity and those due to translational movements. Aside from using other linear acceleration-sensing somatic inputs to make the decision, it has been postulated that this decision is made on the basis of the frequency of the head movement.[61] Tilts of the head with regard to gravity are generally of much lower frequency than translational movements during locomotion. More recently, it has been postulated that canal input, if present, helps also to make this decision.[62]

Gain and phase

An important and useful concept for describing the goodness of function of the VOR is its gain. Gain is defined as the ratio between stimulus input and oculomotor output about a specific axis. Since central processing in the vestibular nuclei, vestibulocerebellum and brainstem is largely in terms of head and eye velocity, VOR gain (G_{VOR}) is generally expressed as a ratio of induced slow-phase eye velocity (V_E) divided by the stimulus (head) velocity (V_H):

$$G_{VOR} = V_E/V_H$$

Gain can also be expressed in terms of head position or head acceleration, as long as the terms of the numerator and denominator are consistent. Note that gain does not specify the velocity at which the subject was rotated. For the angular VOR, the vestibular system is linear within broad limits; that is the gains calculated from eye position, eye velocity and eye acceleration are all the same, and the responses induced by the various frequencies of rotation superpose. The gain of the aVOR of normal humans during rotation in the dark generally lies between 0.4 and 0.7. This is low, considering that compensation must be within several °/s when viewing targets moving with relation to the head if objects are to be fixated on the retina.[63] However, the gain of the aVOR is generally close to unity during active head rotation in darkness. The same is true for rotation in light, where visual input adds eye velocity that accurately compensates for head velocity.

If one attempts to fixate an imaginary target while in darkness, the G_{VOR} becomes close to unity. This demonstrates the powerful effect of cognitive 'set' in determining vestibular reflexes. A unity aVOR gain may not always be desirable, however. If subjects are moving toward or away from objects, the aVOR gains will be lower or higher, to take the combined linear and angular accelerations into account. In addition, viewing distance is of great importance in determining gain of both the aVOR and the lVOR. If the head is rotated with a target at optical infinity, an aVOR gain of 1 is ideal. However, as targets come closer and the eyes converge, higher aVOR gains are necessary to compensate for head movements. Consequently, the aVOR gain rises. In contrast, compensatory lVOR gains are zero when viewing targets at infinity, since there is little or no movement of targets on the retina due to translation of the head. As nearer targets are viewed, however, demands on gain to stabilize vision during translational head and body movements become much higher, and the gain of the compensatory lVOR rises to meet these demands.[54–56]

During testing, head angular velocity is usually induced by rotating the head or the head and body sinusoidally at frequencies from 0.05 to 0.5 Hz. These stimuli cause compensatory changes in eye position and/or nystagmus. As head velocity increases in one direction, slow-phase eye velocity increases in the opposite direction. During sinusoids, the gain is determined from the amplitude of the sinusoidal response, and the phase of the response is expressed relative to the stimulus. Since compensatory eye velocity is oppositely directed, eye and head velocity are generally out of phase by about one half-cycle (180°). There may be shifts in the relationship between the head and eye velocity due to peripheral response time, central neural processing and biases introduced by vestibular lesions. Alternatively, subjects can be rotated at a constant velocity using sudden acceleration at onset and sudden deceleration at the end of rotation (step changes in angular velocity). Because the semicircular canals sense angular acceleration, they only respond to *changes* in angular velocity, not to angular velocity itself. Thus, during constant-velocity rotation, the cupula and hair cells return to their resting positions. If subjects are in the dark, per-rotatory nystagmus elicited by this rotation declines to zero, and individuals no longer feel that they are rotating. At the end of rotation, the hair cells are deflected in the opposite direction, causing oppositely directed, post-rotatory nystagmus, which declines over the same time-course as the per-rotatory nystagmus. The gain (initial slow-phase eye velocity at the onset or end of rotation divided by head velocity (V_E/V_H)) and the rate of decline in eye velocity, expressed as a time constant, are usually the parameters of interest for constant-velocity rotation.

The gain of the lVOR is generally expressed as a function of angular movement of the eyes (in °/s) in response to translational movement of the head (in m/s). In contrast to the gain of the aVOR, which tends to be constant over a wide range of frequencies, the gain of the compensatory lVOR is low for frequencies of head oscillation below 1 Hz and rises dramatically for higher frequencies of oscillation. Orienting movements, induced by alignment to the GIA, have the reverse frequency characteristics. During constant-velocity centrifugation, for example, there are vertical, horizontal and/or torsional changes in eye position that tend to move the eyes in the direction of linear acceleration. Ocular counter-rolling is an example of such a response to lateral head tilt with regard to gravity. The gain of the reflex falls for oscillations above 0.2 Hz, and is approximately constant for oscillations at lower frequencies and for static tilts of the head.

Vision and the VOR

The importance of compensatory eye movements produced by the VOR is perhaps best appreciated when the VOR is acutely lost after hair cell damage due to ototoxic effects of antibiotics such as gentamicin or streptomycin. Vision is normal when the head is held stationary or if the patient is moved smoothly forward with the head held stable in a wheelchair. As soon as the patient begins to walk, however, vision becomes 'jumbled', and the patient is unable to see clearly or to recognize faces. The implication is that natural motion involving the body and head must ultimately be used to test the vestibular system, and that visual tasks that measure the goodness of compensation also form an important part of assessing vestibular function.

Visual information is taken in solely during compensatory movements or the slow phases of nystagmus, and there is no perception during the quick phases. This appears to be largely due to a backward masking effect of a large visual evoked response that accompanies each saccade. The absence of perception during saccades or quick phases is obvious when one looks in a mirror and moves the head back and forth sinusoidally or looks at different points on the image of the eyes in the mirror. It is possible to see the eyes move smoothly with regard to the head, but one never observes the eyes jumping from one position to another in the orbit. As a result of this, patients with peripheral or central vestibular lesions who have spontaneous nystagmus frequently have the illusion of the room moving, and it always moves in the same direction. Patients almost never sense that the visual surround is jumping back during the quick phases. By comparing the perception of movement with the associated nystagmus, it will be noted that the visual surround appears to be moving in a direction opposite to the direction of the slow phases. The reason for this is that the movement of the eyes causes a drift of the visual surround on the retina during the slow phases.

Processing in the VOR is essentially a concatenation of three subsystems. Motion is first sensed in the peripheral vestibular system, which includes the semicircular canals and otolith organs. This activity then reaches central neural circuitry in the vestibular nuclei, which also receives input from the cerebellum, the visual system, and other sensory systems that sense the motion of the body in space. A compensatory movement is generated in the vestibular nuclei, and the activity is passed to the third subsystem, the ocular motor system, for execution. There is no direct feedback from the eye muscles to the semicircular canals to inform them how well the eyes have compensated for head movement. In engineering terms, the job operates in an 'open-loop' fashion. This is an inadequate mode of operation for a system finely tuned to move the eyes to maintain the eyes on target. It is critical that the brain have a constant source of information about the goodness of ocular compensation.

This feedback is provided by vision through pathways involving the flocculus and paraflocculus of the vestibulocerebellum.[64–69] If a target is not stabilized on the retina, there will be an error in eye position (retinal error) and targets will drift across the retina at some velocity (retinal slip). Retinal error induces saccadic eye movements which bring the fovea to the target. Retinal slip induces a pursuit or optokinetic eye movement, causing the eyes to change speed. By changing the amplitude or speed of the eye movement, the target is brought back to the fovea and stabilized on the retina.

There are times when it is advantageous to turn off the aVOR, particularly when one is watching a target moving with the head. In this circumstance, signals generated in the flocculus and paraflocculus counteract the aVOR. The ability to suppress the aVOR during head movement is dependent on the integrity of the systems for ocular pursuit and/or OKN. These have virtually the same characteristics and limitations, namely a latency of about 200 ms, a maximum velocity of about 60°/s and the ability to cancel frequencies only up to about 1 Hz. When the system that produces ocular pursuit or OKN is defective, subjects cannot suppress the aVOR. Thus, patients with cerebellar cortical degeneration may have vigorous nystagmus when they attempt to watch a target moving with the head.

Adaptation of the VOR

Since suppressive drugs are frequently of only limited value in reducing nystagmus and vertigo after lesions, adaptation and VOR plasticity are of great importance in recovery after vestibular lesions. VOR adaptation is produced by the presence of a mismatch between vestibular output and visual input. For example, if the gain of the VOR is low, there is persistent retinal slip when the head moves. Visual input related to this retinal slip activates pursuit and optokinetic pathways to the flocculus and paraflocculus of the vestibulocerebellum. This alters firing patterns of cerebellar Purkinje cells and their target neurons in the vestibular nuclei which project to the eye muscle motor neurons, raising the gain of the VOR.[65–69] As a result, the eyes move faster in response to the same input to hold gaze stable. Adaptive changes can be rapid, but frequently take hours or days to develop and persist for long periods. The amount of adaptation can be striking, and it is even possible to reverse the direction of aVOR at certain frequencies of head movement by wearing reversing prisms.[70] This is remarkable, because the hard-wired aVOR is present from birth, and can even be elicited with caloric stimulation in deep coma. In fact, the absence of ocular deviation in response to head movement or caloric stimulation of the labyrinths over the aVOR is one of the signs used to determine brain death.

There is considerable redundancy across the systems used for ocular compensation for head movement. Vision, vestibular sensation and somatosensory input from the neck and limbs are all utilized. This process also depends on the integrity of the cerebellum and its inputs, the inferior olive and the sources of climbing fiber input to the cerebellum. Exercise and active motion can enhance adaptation of the aVOR and lVOR after central or peripheral lesions.[71–73] VOR gain adaptation does not take place when the flocculus and paraflocculus of the vestibulocerebellum are damaged. The way in which plasticity is realized at the cellular level is still unknown, but possibilities include a change in receptor density or in the amount of transmitter release among others. *N*-methyl-D-aspartate (NMDA) glutaminergic receptors[74,75] and nitric oxide (NO) acting on second messenger systems[76,77] have also been implicated in this process.

Afterword

This chapter is only meant to serve as an introduction to the physiology of the vestibular system, which sits at the heart of the motion-sensing apparatus of the brain. A large body of work was done in the late 19th and early 20th centuries, nicely summarized by Camis and Creed.[78] There has been an explosion of new information in this area since the mid-20th century.[20,79,80] As we have begun to explore vestibular function in freely moving individuals, new physiology and understanding of the vestibular system is beginning to emerge. The reader is referred to a large body of work on vestibular anatomy, physiology and function in recent years, at both peripheral and central levels, for further information on this subject. This includes both general treatments of the subjects[81–83] and symposium volumes.[84–88]

References

1. Okuda M, Bautz A, Membre H et al. Appearance and evolution of calcitic and aragonitic otoconia during plurodeles waltl development. *Hear Res* 1999; **137**: 114–26.
2. Miller EFI. Counterrolling of the human eyes produced by head tilt with respect to gravity. *Acta Otolaryngol* 1962; **54**: 479–501.
3. Curthoys IS, Betts GA, Burgess AM et al. The planes of the utricular and saccular maculae of the guinea pig. *Ann NY Acad Med.* 1999; **871**: 27–34.
4. Goldberg J. Transmission between the type 1 hair cell and its calyx ending. *Ann NY Acad Sci* 1996; **781**: 474–88.
5. Hudspeth AJ, Corey DP. Sensitivity, polarity and conduction change in the response of vertebrate hair cells to controlled mechanical stimuli. *Proc Natl Acad Sci USA* 1977; **746**: 2407–11.
6. Hudspeth AJ, Jacobs R. Stereocillia mediate transduction in vertebrate hair cells. *Proc Natl Acad Sci USA* 1979; **76**: 1506–9.
7. Hudspeth AJ. Extracellular current flow and the site of transduction by vertebrate hair cells. *J Neurosci* 1982; **2**: 1–10.
8. Uchino Y, Sato H, Kushiro K et al. Cross-striolar and commissural inhibition in the otolith system. *Ann NY Acad Sci* 1999; **871**: 162–72.
9. Brichta AM, Goldberg JM. Afferent and efferent responses from morphological fiber classes in the turtle posterior crista. *Ann NY Acad Sci* 1996; **781**: 183–95.
10. Ross MD, Chimento T, Doshay D, Rei C. Computer-assisted three-dimensional reconstruction and simulations of vestibular macular neural connectivities. *Ann NY Acad Sci* 1992; **656**: 75–91.
11. Goldberg JM, Lysakowski A, Fernandez C. Structure and function of vestibular nerve fibers in the chinchilla and squirrel monkey. *Ann NY Acad Sci* 1992; **656**: 92–107.
12. Chimento TC, Ross MD. Evidence of a sensory processing unit in the mammalian macula. *Ann NY Acad Sci* 1996; **781**: 196–212.
13. Goldberg JM, Fernandez C. Physiology of peripheral neurons innervating semicircular canals of the squirrel monkey. I. Resting discharge and response to angular accelerations. *J Neurophysiol* 1971; **34**: 635–60.
14. Goldberg JM, Fernandez C. Physiology of peripheral neurons innervating semicircular canals of the squirrel monkey. III. Variations among units in their discharge properties. *J Neurophysiol* 1971; **34**: 676–84.
15. Goldberg JM, Highstein SM, Moschovakis AK, Fernandez C. Inputs from regularly and irregularly discharging vestibular nerve afferents to secondary neurons in the vestibular nuclei of the squirrel monkey. I. An electrophysiological analysis. *J Neurophysiol* 1987; **58**: 700–18.
16. Minor LB, Goldberg JM. Vestibular nerve inputs to the vestibulo-ocular reflex: a functional ablation study in the squirrel monkey. *J Neuroscience* 1991; **11**: 1636–48.
17. Hudspeth AJ. The cellular basis of hearing: the biophysics of hair cells. *Science* 1985; **230**: 745–52.
18. Purkinje JE. *Beitrage zur naheren Kenntnis des Sehens in subjectiver Hinsicht*, Vol. 6. Prague: Calve, 1819; 79–125.
19. Gruesser O-J. J. E. Purkyne's contributions to the physiology of the visual, the vestibular and the oculomotor systems. *Human Neurobiol* 1984; **3**: 129–44.
20. Wilson VJ, Melvill-Jones G. *Mammalian Vestibular Physiology*. New York: Plenum Press, 1979.
21. Henn V, Cohen B, Young LR. Visual–vestibular interaction in motion perception and the generation of nystagmus. *Neurosci Res Prog Bull* 1980; **18**: 651.
22. Ewald JR. *Physiologische Untersuchungen über das Endorgan des Nervus Octavus*.Wiesbaden: Bergmann, 1892.
23. Halmagyi G, Curthoys I. A clinical sign of canal paresis. *Arch Neurol* 1988; **45**: 737–9.
24. Aw S, Haslwanter Th, Halmagyi GM et al. Three-dimensional vector analysis of the human vestibuloocular reflex in response to high-acceleration head rotations. 1. Responses in normal subjects. *J Neurophysiol* 1996; **76**: 4009–20.
25. Cremer P, Halmagyi GM, Aw ST et al. Semicircular canal plane head impulses detect absent function of individual semicircular canals. *Brain* 1998; **121**: 699–716.
26. Henn V, Straumann D, Hess BJM et al. Three-dimensional transformation from vestibular and visual input to oculomotor output. *Ann NY Acad Sci* 1992; **656**: 166–80.
27. Cohen B, Suzuki J, Bender MB. Eye movements from semicircular canal nerve stimulation in the cat. *Ann Otol Rhinol Laryngol* 1964; **73**: 153–69.
28. Suzuki J, Cohen B, Bender MB. Compensatory eye movements induced by vertical semicircular canal stimulation. *Exp Neurol* 1964; **9**: 137–60.
29. Brodal A. Anatomy of the vestibular nuclei and their connections, In: Kornhuber HH, ed. *Handbook of Sensory Physiology. Vestibular System. Basic Mechanisms*. Berlin: Springer-Verlag, 1974: 239–352.
30. Buettner-Ennever JA. Patterns of connectivity in the vestibular nuclei. *Ann NY Acad Sci* 1992; **656**: 363–78.
31. Highstein SM, McCrea RA. The anatomy of the vestibular nuclei. In: Buttner-Ennever JA, ed. *Neuroanatomy of the Oculomotor System (Reviews of Oculomotor Research)*. Amsterdam: Elsevier 1988: 177–202.
32. Lorente de No R. Vestibular ocular reflex arc. *Arch Neurol Psychiatry* 1933; **30**: 245–91.
33. Ito M. The control mechanisms of cerebellar motor systems. In: Schmitt FO, Worden FG, eds. *The Neurosciences: Third Study Program*. Cambridge Mass: MIT Press, 1974: 293–303.
34. Robinson DA. Oculomotor control signals. In: Lennerstrand G, Bach-y-Rita P. eds. *Basic Mechanisms of Ocular Motility and Their Clinical Implications*. Oxford: Pergamon Press, 1975: 337–74.
35. Raphan T, Cohen B. How does the vestibulo-ocular reflex work? In: Baloh RW, Halmagyi GM eds. *Disorders of the Vestibular System*. New York: Oxford University Press, 1996: 20–47.
36. Steinhausen W. Über die Beobachtung der Cupula in den Bogengansampullen des Labyrinths des lebenden Hechts. *Arch Ges Physiol* 1933; **232**: 500–12.

37. Robinson D. Vestibular and optokinetic symbiosis: an example of explaining by modeling. In: Baker R, Berthoz A, eds. *Control of Gaze by Brain Stem Neurons*. Amsterdam: Elsevier/North Holland, 1977: 49–58.
38. Raphan T, Matsuo V, Cohen B. Velocity storage in the vestibulo-ocular reflex arc (VOR). *Exp Brain Res* 1979; **35**: 229–48.
39. Dai M, Klein A, Cohen B, Raphan T. Model-based study of the human cupular time constant. *J Vestib Res* 1999; **9**: 293–301.
40. Raphan T, Cohen B. Velocity storage and the ocular response to multidimensional vestibular stimuli. In: Berthoz A, Melvill Jones G, eds. *Adaptive Mechanisms in Gaze Control; Facts and Theories*, Amsterdam: Elsevier, 1985: 123–43.
41. Yokota JI, Reisine H, Cohen B. Nystagmus induced by electrical microstimulation of the vestibular and prepositus hypoglossi nuclei in the monkey. *Exp Brain Res* 1992; **92**: 123–38.
42. Solomon D, Cohen B. Stabilization of gaze during circular locomotion in darkness; II. Contribution of velocity storage to compensatory eye and head nystagmus in the running monkey. *J Neurophysiol* 1992; **67**: 1158–70.
43. Cohen B, Suzuki JI, Raphan T. Role of the otolith organs in generation of horizontal nystagmus: effects of selective labyrinthine lesions. *Brain Res* 1983; **276**: 159–64.
44. Raphan T, Cohen B. Organizational principles of velocity storage in three dimensions: the effect of gravity on cross-coupling of optokinetic after-nystagmus. *Ann NY Acad Sci* 1988; **545**: 74–92.
45. Dai M, Raphan T, Cohen B. Spatial orientation of the vestibular system: dependence of optokinetic after nystagmus on gravity. *J Neurophysiol* 1991; **66**: 1422–38.
46. Raphan T, Dai M, Cohen B. Spatial orientation of the vestibular system. *Ann NY Acad Sci* 1992; **656**: 140–57.
47. Gizzi M, Raphan T, Rudolph S, Cohen B. Orientation of human optokinetic nystagmus to gravity: a model based approach. *Exp Brain Res* 1994; **99**: 347–60.
48. Imai T, Moore ST, Raphan T, Cohen B. Stabilization of gaze when turning corners during overground walking. *Soc Neurosci Abstr* 1998; **24**: 415.
49. Waespe W, Cohen B, Raphan T. Dynamic modification of the vestibulo-ocular reflex by the nodulus and uvula. *Science* 1985; **228**: 199–201.
50. Angelaki DE, Hess BJM. The cerebellar nodulus and ventral uvula control the torsional vestibulo-ocular reflex. *J Neurophysiol* 1994; **72**: 1443–7.
51. Angelaki DE, Hess BJM. Organizational principles of otolith and semicircular canal–ocular reflexes in rhesus monkeys. *Ann NY Acad Sci* 1996; **781**: 332–47.
52. Wearne S, Raphan T, Cohen B. Contribution of vestibular commissural pathways to velocity storage and spatial orientation of the angular vestibulo-ocular reflex. *J Neurophysiol* 1997; **78**: 1193–7.
53. Wearne S, Raphan T, Cohen B. Control of spatial orientation of the angular vestibulo-ocular reflex by the nodulus and uvula. *J Neurophysiol* 1998; **79**: 2690–715.
54. Miles FA, Busettini C, Schwarz U. Ocular responses to linear motion. In: Shimazu H, Shinoda Y, eds. *Vestibular and Brain Stem Control of Eye, Head, and Body Movements*. Tokyo: Japan Scientific Societies Press, 1992: 379–95.
55. Schwarz C, Busettini C, Miles FA. Ocular responses to linear motion are inversely proportional to viewing distance. *Science*, 1989; **245**: 1394–6.
56. Schwarz C, Miles FA. Ocular responses to translation and their dependence on viewing distance. I. Motion of the observer. *J Neurophysiol* 1991; **66**: 851–64.
57. Paige GD, Tomko DL. Eye movement responses to linear head motion in the squirrel monkey. I. Basic characteristics. *J Neurophysiol* 1991; **65**: 1170–82.
58. Paige GD, Tomko DL. Eye movement responses to linear head motion in the squirrel monkey. II. Visual–vestibular interactions and kinematic considerations. *J Neurophysiol* 1991; **65**: 1183–96.
59. Telford L, Seidman SH, Paige GD. Dynamics of squirrel monkey linear vestibuloocular reflex and interactions with fixation distance. *J Neurophysiol* 1997; **78**: 1769–90.
60. Telford L, Seidman SH, Paige GD. Canal–otolith interactions driving vertical and horizontal eye movements in the squirrel monkey. *Exp Brain Res* 1996; **109**: 407–18.
61. Mayne R. A systems concept of the vestibular organs. In: Kornhuber HH, ed. *Handbook of Vestibular Physiology. Vestibular System*. New York: Springer-Verlag, 1974: 493–580.
62. Hess BJM, Angelaki DE. Inertial processing of vestibulo-ocular signals. *Ann NY Acad Sci* 1999; **871**: 148–61.
63. Collewijn H, Martins A, Steinman R. Natural retinal image motion: origin and change. *Ann NY Acad Sci* 1981; **374**: 312–29.
64. Ito M. Neural design of the cerebellar motor control system. *Brain Res* 1972; **40**: 81–4.
65. Lisberger SG, Pavelko TA, Broussard DM. Neural basis for motor learning in the vestibuloocular reflex of primates. I. Changes in the responses of brain stem neurons. *J Neurophysiol* 1994; **72**: 928–53.
66. Lisberger SG, Pavelko TA, Bronte-Steward HM, Stone LS. Neural basis for motor learning in the vestibuloocular reflex of primates. II. Changes in the responses of horizontal gaze velocity Purkinje cells in the cerebellar flocculus and ventral paraflocculus. *J Neurophysiol* 1994; **72**: 954–73.
67. Lisberger SG, Pavelko TA, Broussard DM. Responses during eye movements of brain stem neurons that receive monosynaptic inhibition from the flocculus and ventral paraflocculus in monkeys. *J Neurophysiol* 1994; **72**: 909–27.
68. Zhang Y, Partisalis AM, Highstein SM. Properties of superior vestibular nucleus flocculus target neurons in the squirrel monkey. I. General properties in comparison with flocculus projecting neurons. *J Neurophysiol* 1995; **73**: 2261–78.
69. Zhang Y, Partisalis A, Highstein SM. Properties of superior vestibular nucleus flocculus target neurons in the squirrel monkey. II. Signal components revealed by reversible flocculus inactivation. *J Neurophysiol* 1995; **73**: 2279–92.
70. Melvill Jones G. Adaptive modulation of VOR parameters by vision. In: Berthoz A, Melvill Jones G, eds. *Adaptive Mechanisms in Gaze Control*. Amsterdam: Elsevier, 1985: 21–50.
71. Igarashi M, Levy JK, Takahashi M et al. Effect of exercise upon locomotor balance modification after peripheral vestibular lesions

(unilateral utriacular neurotomy) in squirrel monkeys. *Adv Otorhinolaryngol* 1979; **25**: 82.
72. Igarashi M, Levy JK, O-Uchi T, Reschke MF. Further study of physical exercise and locomotor balance compensation after unilateral labyrinthectomy in squirrel monkey. *Acta Otolaryngol* 1981; **92**: 101–5.
73. Igarashi M, Ishiwaka K, Ishii M, Yamane H. Physical exercise and balance compensation after total ablation of vestibular organs. *Prog Brain Res* 1988; **76**: 395–401.
74. Broussard DM, Bronte-Stewart HM, Lisberger SG. Expression of motor learning in the response of the primate vestibulo-ocular reflex pathway to electrical stimulation. *J Neurophysiol* 1992; **67**: 1493–508.
75. Kinney GA, Peterson BW, Slater NT. The synaptic activation of N-methyl-D-aspartate receptors in the rat medial vestibular nucleus. *J Neurophysiol* 1994; **72**: 1588–95.
76. Nagao S, Ito M. Subdural application of hemoglobin to the cerebellum blocks vestibuloocular reflex adaptation. *NeuroReport* 1991; **2**: 193–6.
77. Li J, Smith S, McElligott JG. Cerebellar nitric oxide is necessary for vestibulo-ocular reflex adaptation, a sensorimotor model of learning. *J Neurophysiol* 1995; **74**: 489–94.
78. Camis M, Creed RS. *The Physiology of the Vestibular Apparatus*. Oxford: Clarendon Press, 1930.
79. Kornhuber HH, ed. *Vestibular System, Basic Mechanisms*. *Handbook of Sensory Physiology*, Vol. VI/1. Berlin: Springer-Verlag, 1974.
80. Kornhuber HH, ed. *Vestibular System; Psychophysics, Applied Aspects and General Interpretations*. *Handbook of Sensory Physiology*, Vol. VI/2. Berlin: Springer-Verlag, 1974.
81. Buettner-Ennever JA, ed. *Neuroanatomy of the Oculomotor System*. *Reviews of Oculomotor Research*, Vol. 2. Amsterdam: Elsevier, 1988.
82. Leigh RJ, Zee DS. *The Neurology of Eye Movements*. Contemporary Neurology Series. Philadelphia: FA Davis, 1983.
83. Baloh R, Halmagyi G, eds. *Disorders of the Vestibular System*. New York: Oxford University Press, 1996: 687.
84. Cohen B, ed. Vestibular and Oculomotor Physiology. *Ann NY Acad Sci*. 1981; **374**.
85. Cohen B, Henn V (eds). Representation of three-dimensional space in the vestibular, oculomotor, and visual systems. *Ann NY Acad Sci* 1988; **545**: 239–47.
86. Cohen B, Tomko D, Guedry F eds. Sensing and controlling motion—vestibular and sensorimotor function. *Ann NY Acad Sci*. 1992; **656**.
87. Highstein SM, Cohen B, Buettner-Ennever JA eds. New directions in vestibular research. *Ann NY Acad Sci* 1996; **781**.
88. Cohen B, Hess BJM, eds. Otolith function in spatial orientation and movement. *Ann NY Acad Sci*. 1999; **871**.
89. Hudspeth AJ. The hair cells of the inner ear. *Sci Am* 1983; **248**: 54–64.
90. Wersall J, Bagger-Sjoback D. Morphology of the vestibular sense organ. In: Kornhuber HH, ed. *Handbook of Sensory Physiology*, Vol. VI/1. *Vestibular System. Part 1. Basic Mechanisms*, Berlin: Springer-Verlag, 1974: 123–70.
91. Goldberg JM, Lysakowski A, Fernandez C. Structure and function of vestibular nerve fibers in the chinchilla and squirrel monkey. *Ann NY Acad Sci* 1992; **656**: 92–107.
92. Yakushin S. *Labyrinthine Control of the Vestibulo-Ocular Reflex in Three Dimensions*. Brooklyn, New York: CUNY, 1996: p 241.
93. Raphan T, Cohen B. The vestibulo-ocular reflex in three dimensions. *Exp Brain Res* 2002; **145**: 1–27.

42 Instrumentation and principles of vestibular testing

Floris L Wuyts, Joseph M Furman, Paul Van de Heyning

Introduction

The purpose of vestibular testing is to assess with objective laboratory measures the peripheral and central vestibular functioning of patients suffering from vertigo or disequilibrium. Together with a history and additional investigations such as audiometric data and possibly also imaging, the clinician can better establish a medical diagnosis and hence propose a medical or surgical therapy or a rehabilitative management program.

Since a large number of physiopathological processes underlie symptoms of vertigo and imbalance, the vestibular investigation should primarily enable the differentiation between vestibular system pathologies (central or peripheral) and non-vestibular pathologies, such as cardiovascular or psychogenic disorders. The second most important goal of vestibular testing is the site-of-lesion localization, i.e. which sensory elements, motor output elements or neural pathways are responsible for the reported symptoms. Is the lesion peripheral vestibular, central vestibular, or a mixed type? Is the lesion on the left or right side? Is it recently acquired or has it been present for a long time? What is the degree of function alteration? What is the state of central nervous system compensation, i.e. the alterations made by the central nervous system to account for the flawed information provided by faulty peripheral sensors or neural pathways? It should be noted that this compensatory process may cause the patient's perception of the disease not to correlate closely with the objective measures obtained in the laboratory.

Until recently, most of the vestibular testing has been based on the assessment of the horizontal vestibulo-ocular reflex (VOR). The clinician should be conscious, however, that the vestibular test results only apply to a part of the VOR. Nevertheless, new emerging technologies such as video-oculography enable a more detailed investigation of the VOR.

In addition to the vestibular testing, the authors strongly advocate the assessment of the patient's perspective of his lost quality of life and his psychogenic condition. This is often achieved with validated questionnaires, such as the SF36[1] or the Dizziness Handicap Inventory (DHI).[2]

This chapter focuses on the registration of the VOR with laboratory techniques. Additionally, the chapter provides suggestions to improve the clarity of a quantitative vestibular laboratory examination, by reducing the artefacts that lead to false-positive or false-negative conclusions. Finally, a normative table and meta-analysis is offered for the quantitative outcomes of different vestibular tests.

Recording techniques

Electronystagmography

Electronystagmography (ENG), also called electro-oculography (EOG) has been for many decades the primary technique for eye-movement recording in a clinical setting. It is based on the dipole property of the eyeball, the front of which is positive with reference to the back (Figure 42.1). This corneo–retinal potential is generated by the metabolic processes in the retina. When the eye moves in its orbit, the surrounding electric field is proportionally altered. Thus electrodes (eg. Ag/AgCl) that are placed near the eyeball can record eye position. Either both eyes can be recorded with one pair of electrodes, or each eye can be recorded separately (Figure 42.2). In the latter case, the signals of both eyes are either added together after amplification, which results in a higher signal/noise ratio, or plotted separately. A common ground electrode is usually placed on the forehead. The electrodes should not be placed too close to the lateral canthi, since they can irritate the patient, which leads to more frequent eye blinking.

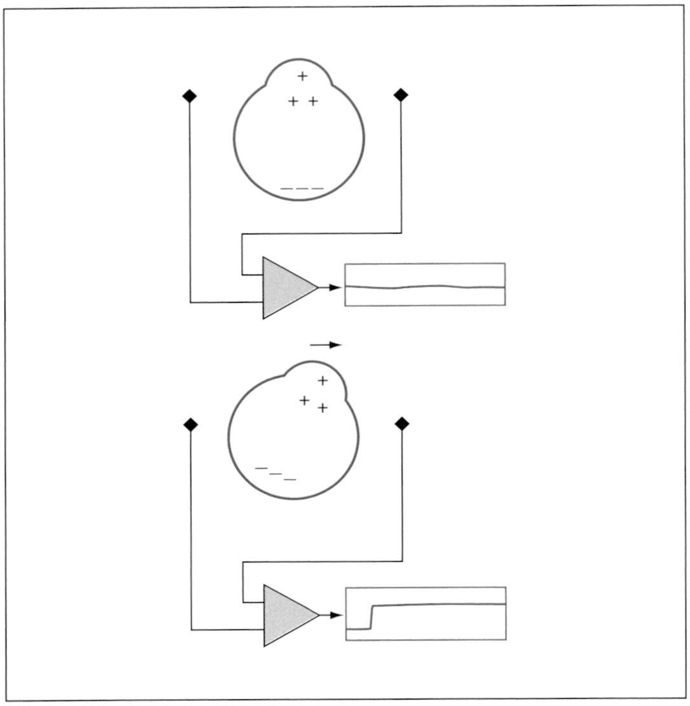

Figure 42.1 The corneo–retinal dipole potential has a magnitude of approximately 1 μV, with the cornea being positive with respect to the retina. The diamonds represent the electrodes. A rightward deviation makes the right electrode more positive, resulting in a positive deflection on the recording.

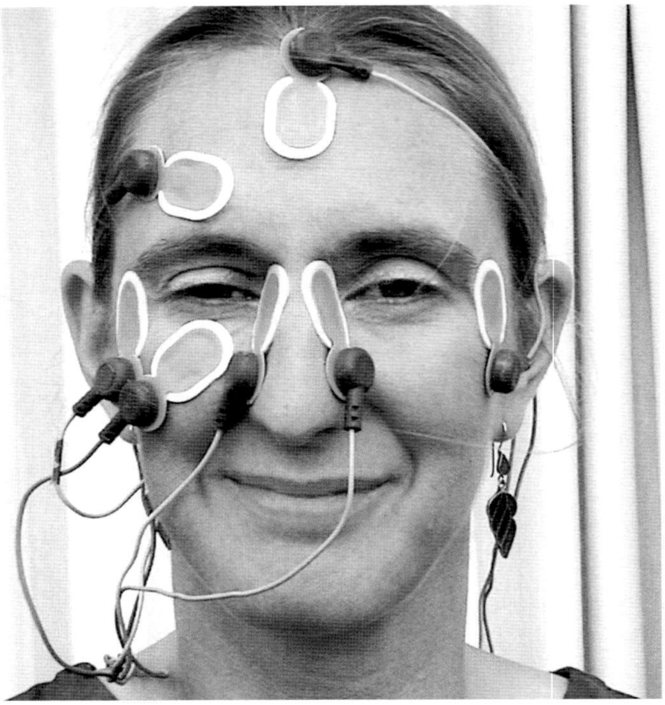

Figure 42.2 Placement of electrodes for horizontal and vertical electro-oculographic eye-movement recording. For horizontal recordings, each eye is recorded separately. The two horizontal signals can be summed by the recording equipment to enhance the signal/noise ratio. The forehead electrode serves as a common ground electrode. The vertical electrodes are typically used for artefact identification only.

Prior to the application of the electrodes, the skin should be thoroughly cleansed by the technician to remove skin oil and cosmetics, by using a fat solvent. Next, the most superficial layer of the squamous epithelium of the epidermis has to be removed, e.g. with a roughened swab. Without these precautions, the electrode–skin impedance will be too high. This decreases the signal/noise ratio, and leads to a direct current (DC) drift. Impedances below 25 kΩ are usually acceptable. Additionally, the impedance difference between the different electrodes should not exceed 10 kΩ.

Proper amplification of the eye signals is preferentially amplified using DC-coupling, since this gives a reliable measurement of eye position, especially during fixation.

Often, an electrode is placed above and below one eye for vertical eye-movement registrations. The information obtained from these vertically placed electrodes is largely qualitative, since eyelid movement, muscular activity near the eyebrow, and eye-blink artefacts cause interference with the dipole potential and render quantitative analysis of vertical EOG questionable (Figure 42.3). Vertical recording can identify artefacts. Frequent blinks can also make the EOG difficult to interpret, as the blinks can be misjudged as quick components of nystagmus. This effect is much enhanced if the horizontal electrodes are misaligned, i.e. not perfectly placed on the inter-pupil line.

The corneo–retinal potential may vary greatly during the examination, especially if the ambient luminance varies during the examination. Additionally, perspiration may alter the skin impedance near the electrodes. Therefore, it is of major importance to perform calibrations repeatedly throughout the entire test, and preferably prior to each sub-test. Calibration is achieved by asking the patient to perform saccades by alternatively fixating dots on a screen. The dots can be placed at 10° left and right of the center, in which case these dots should be placed at $l \tan 10°$ (expressed in meters) from the center dot, where l represents the distance in meters between patient and screen. The output of the recorder can now be adjusted so that the deflection indicates 10° left and right. This yields the calibration factor.

- Changing light conditions dramatically alters the calibration factors.
- It is crucial to perform calibrations repeatedly throughout the entire ENG.

Before the test begins, the patient should be kept in a semi-darkened room for at least 5 min so that the electrode paste or gel can react properly with the skin and the eyes can adapt to the near-darkness. Figure 42.4 shows the corneo–retinal potential during a 105-min-long experiment in one subject where only the light conditions were changed. The results in other subjects were very similar to the presented data. It is striking

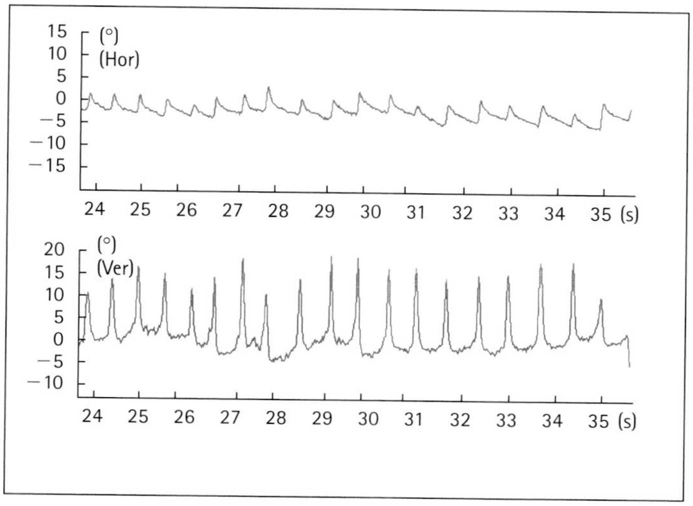

Figure 42.3 The effect of eye blinks on the horizontal electro-oculographic recording (upper trace). The synchrony between the horizontal and vertical peaks as well as the sharpness of the peaks suggest that the apparent horizontal nystagmus is actually artefactual.

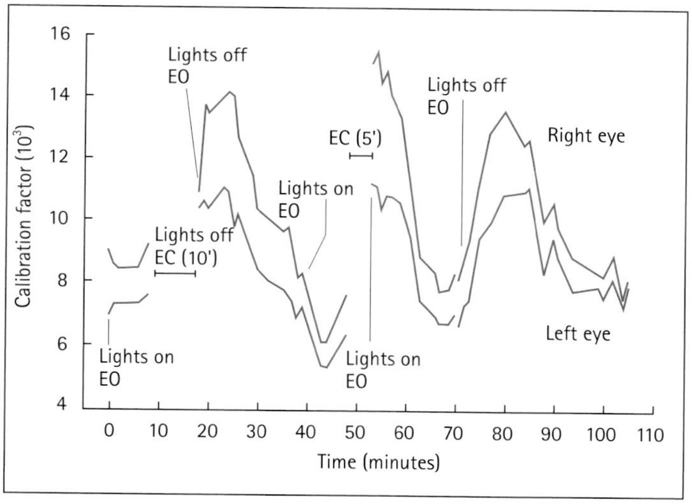

Figure 42.4 Corneo-retinal potential variation during 105 min of recording in one subject. EO, eyes open, EC, eyes closed. A change in ambient luminance produces a change in the corneo-retinal dipole potential of up to 100 %. Note that the eyes did not change equally.

that the calibration alters by 100% throughout the 20 min that follow a lights-out condition or lights-on condition. Metabolic changes in the retina are not controllable, and even under stable light conditions, maintained for 30 min, the potential changed by up to 100%. It is therefore of major importance to calibrate repeatedly throughout the vestibular examination.

Moreover, if a test outcome is based on the analysis of several sub-tests, such as the caloric test that is based on four consecutive sub-tests, it is of great importance to calibrate prior to each individual sub-test. Otherwise, false results may emerge.

Whereas for many years ENG recording systems consisted of amplifiers and chart recorders, most manufacturers now offer PC-based systems with DC-coupled amplifiers. Using a computer, ENG signals can be digitally filtered for noise reduction. Also, a quantitative analysis becomes possible for the calculation of clinically relevant parameters such as rotational gain (response/stimulus), phase (time delay between response and stimulus) or the time constant of the response decay. Moreover, patient traces from the entire test can be stored on digital storage devices for post hoc analysis or archival purposes.

Unfortunately, commercial systems do not adhere to a standardized method of stimulus delivery, response measurement or analysis. It is highly recommended that laboratories use the standards proposed by the ASEM protocol.[3] Additionally, the clinician should never rely blindly on the computer output without inspecting the traces and the calculation results. With very weak responses, in particular, the computer results can be quite misleading.

> The clinician should never blindly rely on the computer output, without inspecting the traces and the calculation results.

Video-oculography

The main component of a video-oculography (VOG) system, also sometimes called video-ENG or VNG, is a small video camera that is placed on a specific mount so that a frontal view of the eye is obtained. The movement of the eye is deduced by means of image processing. Two-dimensional systems (2D) extract horizontal and vertical movements from the video images; three-dimensional systems (3D) additionally extract the torsional component of the eye movements. Most VOG systems function in total darkness by the use of infrared light. VOG systems may be monocular or binocular. Some VOG systems use goggles like ski glasses, where the camera is placed in front of the eye. Others allow unobstructed vision, where the camera can image the eye via a specialized mirror (Figure 42.5).

Most commercial VOG systems have a standard frame rate of 50 or 60 Hz, which may limit the use of VOG for some ocular motor tests such as saccades. Some manufacturers offer high-frame-rate (>200 Hz) cameras, but these are considerably more expensive.

2D VOG, with its reliable vertical movement detection, has the advantage over conventional ENG of enabling an accurate measurement of the vertical eye movements. 3D VOG adds the ability to record torsional eye movements.

2D VOG extracts the horizontal and vertical movements of the eye by exaggeration of the image contrast so that the pupil becomes totally black in an otherwise white field. Extraction of the horizontal and vertical coordinates of the pupil center is then straightforward. To assure accuracy, VOG systems must account for the shape of the pupil when the eyelids are partially closed or when the eye looks eccentrically. With mirror systems that are characterized by a long eye–camera distance, the image

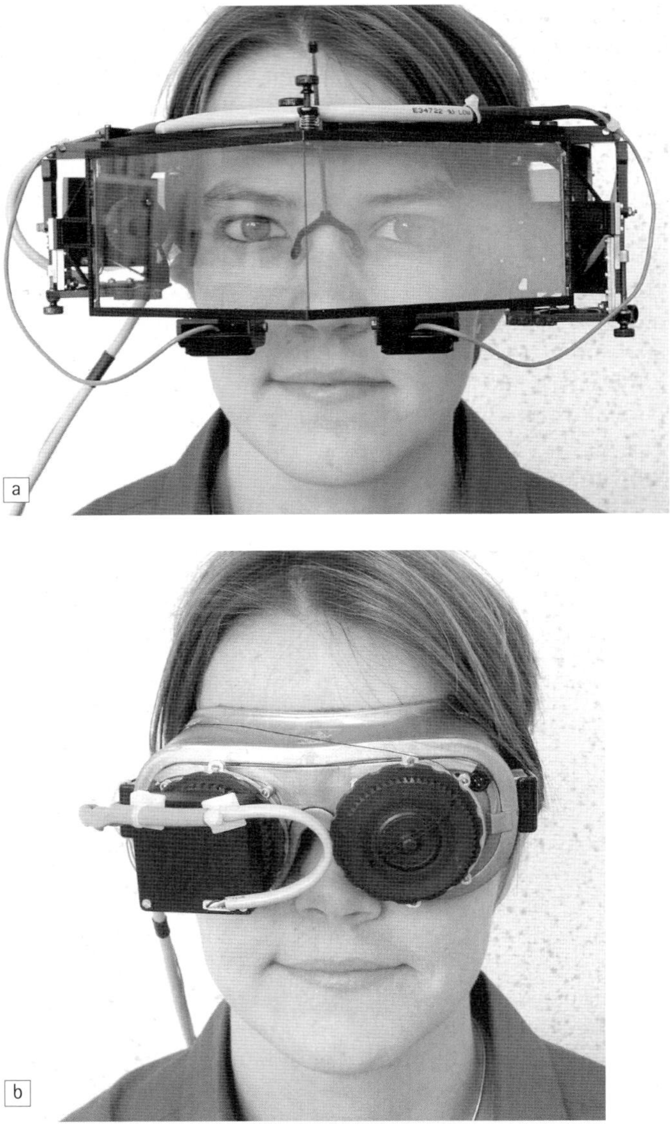

Figure 42.5 A video-oculographic device for eye-movement recording. (a) See-through system. (b) Monocular ski-goggles-type system.

become less deformed[4] with eccentric gaze, as compared to devices that place the camera directly in front of the eye.

3D VOG systems estimate torsional eye movements using either cross-correlation or neural network techniques. Both systems depend upon adequate contrast in the patient's iris. Thus, in some individuals, the estimate of the torsional eye movement is unreliable. Also, in 3D VOG systems, artefacts due to partial eyelid closure and eccentric deflection must be considered.[4,5] With VOG, it is of great importance that the goggles be attached firmly to the patient's head, since any relative movement of the camera with respect to the head will result in a false impression of eye translation or rotation. Thus, some systems are attached to the patient's skull by means of a bite board, but this reduces clinical applicability.[6]

VOG is a new technique that has been developed in the last two decades. 2D VOG is currently evolving from a research tool into a clinical tool, since the evolution in PC technology has reduced the calculation time tremendously. Several manufacturers of standard ENG equipment offer 2D VOG systems at prices that are comparable to those of ENG. Also, the image-processing algorithms are considerably improved to take into account different sources of error, mainly due to geometrical and alignment issues.[7] Most likely, 2D VOG will coexist with ENG for several years, since each technique has its strengths and weaknesses. 3D VOG systems, however, are currently still limited to research facilities, due to the much greater complexity of this technique. Because VOG is new, the need for standardization is again an important issue.

Table 42.1 summarizes the specific properties of ENG, 2D and 3D VOG systems.

Scleral coil

The scleral search coil (SSC) method developed by Robinson[8] is based on the measurement of electric current induced in a small coil of wire placed on the eye by a magnetic field that surrounds the patient. The SSC method has emerged as the gold standard for the accurate recording of eye movements. However, it is an invasive technique that requires that a wired contact lens be placed on the patient's eye. It causes discomfort for the patient, and recording time is limited to approximately 30 min. Consequently, the SSC technique for vestibular testing in general is confined to research rather than clinical settings.

Nystagmus definition

By convention, when eye position is displayed on a computer screen or a chart recorder, a rightward eye movement is reported as an upward deflection and a leftward eye movement as a downward deflection. For the vertical channel, the convention is straightforward, i.e. an upward deflection means an upward eye movement. For torsional eye movements, there is no convention. Therefore, we suggest the following rules: (1) torsional movements are described from the patient's viewpoint; (2) a rightward movement of the upper pole of the eye corresponds with a positive, i.e. upward, deflection on the recording (similar to the corkscrew rule in physics being positive).

A slow eye movement followed by a fast opposite movement is called jerk nystagmus, which is, by convention, named after its fast component. The slow component velocity (SCV) is the parameter of interest, as it reflects the portion of the nystagmus that is generated by the VOR. The fast component is merely a saccadic reset.

Table 42.1 Comparison between ENG, 2D VOG and 3D VOG.

Characteristics	ENG	2D VOG	3D VOG
Recording device	Paste-on electrodes (AgCl/Ag)	Video camera	Video camera
Principle	Corneo–retinal dipole potential	Image processing Contrast enhancement of pupil	Image processing Pupil and iris structure analysis Cross-correlation or neural network
Horizontal eye movement	Reliable	Very reliable	Very reliable
Vertical eye movement	Unreliable	Very reliable	Very reliable
Torsional eye movement	Not possible	Not possible	Reliable
Approximate accuracy	1–2°	1°	1°
Head movement resistant	High	If properly secured	If properly secured
Sampling rate	>150 Hz	25–60 Hz	25–60 Hz
Iris structure dependence	No	No	Yes
Amplifier drift	Yes	No	No
Calibration	Repeatedly	Once	Once
Sensitive to			
Blink artefacts	Yes	Yes	Yes
Changes in room lighting	Yes	No	No
Myogenic activity	Yes	No	No
Vestibular stimuli possible	Yes	Yes	Yes
Functions in total darkness	Yes	Yes	Yes
Patient tolerance	About 1 h	About 30 min	About 30 min

Vestibular function assessment

Effect of medication on the vestibular function assessment

Most patients undergoing testing in the vestibular laboratory use medications either to treat an unrelated medical condition or to treat their dizziness. Unfortunately, many commonly used medications can interfere with vestibular function testing. Some medications, even in therapeutic doses, can produce abnormal eye movements that could be misinterpreted as a sign of vestibular or central nervous system pathology. Moreover, many medications impair alertness, reduce normal nystagmic responses, or suppress abnormal nystagmus, thereby producing misleading laboratory findings. The three most common patterns of medication-related vestibular function test alterations are: (1) the brainstem–cerebellar dysfunction pattern; (2) the central nervous system sedation pattern; and (3) the vestibular system dysfunction pattern.

The vestibular system dysfunction pattern includes eye-movement abnormalities such as reduced caloric and rotational responses associated with bilateral labyrinthine hypofunction and positional nystagmus. Medication-induced bilateral labyrinthine hypofunction may occur as an acute and reversible effect (e.g. aspirin (acetylsalicylic acid) ototoxicity) or as a chronic and irreversible effect (e.g. as a result of gentamicin ototoxicity). Drugs that cause vestibular system toxicity can also produce a pattern of eye-movement abnormalities similar to those caused by central sedation, and it can be difficult to distinguish central nervous system sedation from bilateral labyrinthine hypofunction. Thus, it is critical to maintain alertness in patients who are using or who have used medications capable of producing labyrinthine hypofunction.

Because of the widespread and diverse effects that drugs can have on vestibular function testing, patients referred for ENG examination should be instructed not to take any tranquilizers, sedatives, vestibular suppressants or alcohol for 48 h before testing. Patients should continue to take medications for heart problems, high blood pressure, diabetes, seizure prevention, or other medical conditions. In hospitalized patients for whom it may be impractical to discontinue medications, and patients using medications for serious medical conditions, it is usually best to perform the ENG examination and note the patient's medications. The records should then be reviewed carefully for evidence of any drug effect. Any doubts about the interpretation can then be noted on the report and, if possible, the examination can be repeated again after withdrawal of the presumptive offending medication.

> Patients referred for ENG should not take tranquilizers, sedatives or alcohol for 48 h before testing.

Test battery

Depending on the clinical setting and availability of equipment, vestibular testing consists of several different sub-tests. In most clinical settings throughout the world, the larger part of the following test battery is performed: (1) ocular motor test battery; (2) positional testing; and (3) vestibular test battery, which includes caloric and rotational testing. Each of these tests has its own purpose (Chapter 43). Table 42.2 lists the different tests as well as the relevant outcome parameters to report. The order of tests is designed to reduce possible interference of one test with another. Testing is started with the ocular motor screening battery. First, there is a search for spontaneous (i.e. vestibular) nystagmus, since its presence may greatly influence all the other tests. Next, the ocular motor test battery investigates the integrity of the eye movements in the absence of any vestibular stimulus. Because later tests such as positional and vestibular tests rely upon eye movements, abnormalities of the ocular motor system itself may interfere with other test results. Thus, without an ocular motor screening battery, some vestibular tests can be misinterpreted. The positioning tests should precede the positional test, and both should precede the vestibular tests. The main purpose of performing the positioning test is the detection of paroxysmal positional nystagmus, which might disappear upon repeated positioning. Thus, any maneuver that can reduce paroxysmal positioning nystagmus should be avoided.

Table 42.2 Main parameters of interest of the standard vestibular test protocol

Protocol item	Parameters of interest
Ocular motor screening battery	
Spontaneous nystagmus detection	Nystagmus direction, SCV
Gaze-evoked test (center, 30° left/right, 15° up/down)	Nystagmus at different positions
Saccades	Velocity, latency, accuracy, binocular asymmetry
Optokinetic nystagmus	Gain, left-right asymmetry
Smooth pursuit	Gain, left-right asymmetry, morphology
Position tests	
Positioning testing	Nystagmus direction, latency, fatigability
Positional testing	Nystagmus SCV, fixation suppression
Vestibular tests	
Rotatory chair test	Gain, phase, time constant, asymmetry
Caloric test	Maximum SCV, labyrinth asymmetry, nystagmus asymmetry, total responsiveness

> - Continuous visualization of the patient and monitoring of the eye recordings are essential for test accuracy as well as for patient comfort and safety.
> - Patients alertness greatly influences the VOR. Ensure optimal alertness of the patient throughout the ENG exam.
> - A clinically significant spontaneous nystagmus should appear consistently throughout the ENG test.

It is of great importance that close contact between the investigator and the patient exists in the vestibular function laboratory.

Eyes open in the dark versus eyes closed

When a test requires the absence of visual input, two conditions can be used: (1) eyes open in the dark (EOD); or (2) eyes closed (EC) in a semi-darkened room. The former condition is recommended by the ASEM,[3] since it produces more reliable and reproducible results. Also, closing the eyes induces Bell's phenomenon (transient upward movement of the eyes), which may slightly reduce the nystagmus. However, testing with EOD may lead to excessive eye blinking, which may produce artefacts that should not be confused with ocular movements (see Figure 42.3). Moreover, clinical circumstances do not always allow for a totally darkened room, and it imposes additional problems for the tester. Thus, in some facilities for EOD testing, patients wear darkened goggles that completely occlude the eyes.

In either condition, it is the state of alertness that is most important, since there is a large influence of drowsiness on the vestibulo-ocular reflex.[9] Because drowsiness reduces the magnitude and consistency of the VOR, the patient's alertness should be maintained throughout the tests. This is often accomplished by asking patients to perform simple mental tasks during the non-visual tests.

Ocular motor screening battery

Search for vestibular nystagmus

Spontaneous nystagmus refers to unprovoked nystagmus of vestibular origin, but, for reasons of simplicity, the search for it is incorporated in the ocular motor test battery. To detect a spontaneous nystagmus, the patient is observed while seated in the dark. It is essential that the patient cannot fixate any visual target, since fixation largely reduces nystagmus of vestibular origin. Additionally, the patient should not 'fixate' an imaginary object nearby, since this also suppresses nystagmus. Therefore, instructions to 'look' into the distance are preferable. The patient should be asked to perform some appropriate mental task (e.g. non-trivial multiplications). In our experience, in many cases, especially a few days after the onset of a vestibular neuritis, arousal has elicited a clear nystagmus that was not observed prior to the arousal (Figure 42.6).

Additionally, the patient can be asked to look in the dark at imaginary points left and right. This enables the investigator to see whether the nystagmus changes its amplitude according to Alexander's law. Spontaneous nystagmus can be observed in normal individuals, but the SCV should not exceed 4–7°/s, in which case it is considered as abnormal. Table 42.3 lists normal limits as adopted by several authors. Proctor et al[10] state that a nystagmus frequency of 6 beats per 10 s is the limit for normality. A clinically significant spontaneous nystagmus would be expected to be observed consistently throughout the entire ENG test. A few isolated nystagmus beats should therefore not be considered as abnormal.

Fixation

To investigate the integrity of the ocular motor system and the ability to hold specific eye positions, it is common practice to assess the normal eye movements that are continuously used for our vision, i.e. fixation, saccades, smooth pursuit, and optokinetic movement. Fixation serves to hold the eye on a given point of interest; saccades are used to rapidly jump to a new target; smooth pursuit is needed to follow slowly moving targets; and optokinetic eye movements are induced by full-field movement of the surrounding world, such as occurs when the head moves in space.

In addition to a search for spontaneous nystagmus, the ability to hold the eye fixed on a stationary target that is eccentrically positioned is tested. Traditionally, this property is tested at the beginning of the ocular motor screening battery by the gaze-evoked nystagmus test. The patient is asked to fixate several points at a given distance (at least as far as 1 m away to eliminate convergence, since this reduces nystagmus, if present). These visual targets are in the primary position, i.e. in front of the patient, and 30° left and right, and 15° up and down. If the visual targets are farther away, such as 45° horizontally, a physiological end-point nystagmus may be found. Abnormal findings in the gaze-evoked nystagmus test that occur in the absence of a spontaneous nystagmus strongly suggest central nervous system pathology. See Chapter 47 for a further description of lesions that result in gaze-evoked nystagmus.

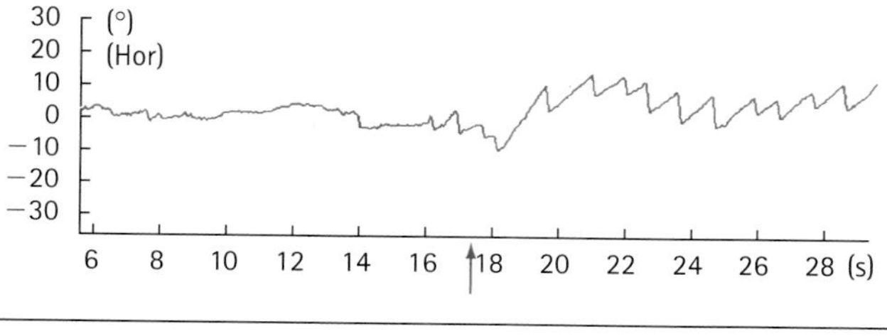

Figure 42.6 The effect of alerting the patient is clearly illustrated by the sudden appearance of a spontaneous nystagmus. At the time indicated by the arrow, the patient was asked 'How much is 12 times 13?'.

Saccades

Saccades are tested by asking the patient to look at small visual targets that move abruptly left and right. To avoid anticipation, the amplitude of the moving target is random, or when a fixed distance is used (e.g. 10° left of the center to 10° right) the pauses between the jumps are random in duration. Attention from the patient is vital for optimum performance. Parameters of interest are latency (time in milliseconds between the stimulus onset and the response), accuracy (if the patient looks systematically too far or too short, followed by a small reset saccade) and velocity. If an inaccuracy is systematically present without the proper correction saccade, the observer should consider a faulty calibration. Table 42.3 lists normal values for peak velocity and latency. Abnormal findings suggest central nervous system pathology, but proper interpretation requires that the patient's age be considered as an important influence, especially for an increase in latency.

> If saccades are consistently overshooting or undershooting the target, without subsequent correction saccades, a faulty calibration is very likely.

Smooth pursuit

During the smooth pursuit test, the patient is asked to follow a gradually moving target, e.g. a small horizontally moving object on a projection screen. The target can move sinusoidally or may follow a triangle wave with speeds that do not exceed 10–30°/s. The total excursion of the target should be restricted to 30°.[11] Attention has a great influence, and often the patient needs encouragement, such as 'please follow carefully the moving dot on the screen, and if you look carefully you can see a small red dot within the yellow one'. The effect of such an instruction is shown in Figure 42.7. Without proper instruction, the traces may suggest central nervous system lesions, especially when the errors are somewhat systematic. Next to the overall shape, the gain (eye velocity/target velocity) is often used as a quantitative measure for abnormality. Table 42.3 represents normal values for the gain of smooth pursuit testing.

Optokinetic test

The optokinetic test is performed by presenting a large visual moving stimulus, such as random dots or stripes, that nearly fills the patient's entire visual field, so that the peripheral retina is stimulated. The stimulus, which typically consists of movement

Table 42.3 Normative data of different papers and reports

Test items	Normative limits (μ ± 2s)	Reference, number of cases
Spontaneous nystagmus	≤4°/s	14,21
	≤5°/s	10,12
	≤6°/s	11,25
	≤7°/s	3,26,27
	≤6 beats/10 s	10
Ocular motor testing		
Saccades		
Peak velocity for 20° saccade: lower limit	210°/s	12,28
	252°/s	29, $N = 20$
	283°/s	24, $N = 38$
Latency for 20° saccade	104–365 ms	30, $N = 34$ (IR method)
	128–255 ms	24, $N = 38$
Smooth pursuit gain at 0.3 Hz	>0.80	14,22,31
Optokinetic nystagmus asymmetry	<13%	24, $N = 38$
	<16%	14, $N = 43$
Positional testing	<6°/s	11
Rotary chair testing		
Sinusoidal harmonic acceleration test		
Gain		
0.05 Hz, 60°/s	0.20–0.80	32, $N = 20$
0.05 Hz, 60°/s	0.13–0.77	33, $N = 10$
0.05 Hz, 50°/s	0.24–0.85	24, $N = 38$
0.05 Hz, 60°/s	0.38–0.98	34, $N = 167$
Phase		
0.05 Hz, 60°/s	6–14°	32, $N = 20$
0.05 Hz, 60°/s	2–20°	33, $N = 10$
0.05 Hz, 50°/s	-1–18°	24, $N = 38$
0.05 Hz, 50°/s	-1.9–24°	35, $N = 50$
0.05 Hz, 60°/s	0.8–20.2	34, $N = 167$
Directional preponderance		
0.05 Hz, 60°/s	≤15%	34, $N = 208$
0.05 Hz, 50°/s	≤24%	24, $N = 38$
Velocity step 90°/s		
Gain	0.33–0.72	36, $N = 20$
Time constant	11–26 s	36, $N = 20$
Directional preponderance	≤22%	36, $N = 20$
Velocity step 100°/s		
Gain	0.27–0.99	14, $N = 43$
Time constant	5–19.4 s	14, $N = 43$
Caloric testing		
Labyrinth asymmetry (%)	≤25%	11, $N = 114$
	≤19.8%	10, $N = 30$
	≤19%	24, $N = 38$
	≤15%	37, $N = 47$

Table 42.3 continued

Test items	Normative limits (μ ± 2s)	Reference, number of cases
Caloric testing		
	≤22%	14,21, *N* = 43
	≤20%	26, *N* = 58
	≤20%	38, *N* = 49
	≤25%	34, *N* = 167
General labyrinth asymmetry limit	≤22%	Meta-analysis
Directional preponderance (%)	≤23%	11, *N* = 114
	≤22.7%	10, *N* = 30
	≤16%	24, *N* = 38
	≤18%	37, *N* = 47
	≤28%	14,21, *N* = 43
	≤26%	26, *N* = 58
	≤27%	38, *N* = 49
	≤31.8%	34, *N* = 167
General directional preponderance limit	≤26%	Meta-analysis

at a constant velocity, should induce circular vection, i.e. the illusion that the patient is moving, not the surrounding world. Both clockwise (CW) and counterclockwise (CCW) stimuli are used. Testing of optokinetic nystagmus by use of a light bar or hand-held rotating drum does not provide true optokinetic stimulation and is really a smooth pursuit task. Asymmetry (see normal values in Table 42.3) and gain of the response to CW and CCW movements are best achieved with stimuli between 20° and 60° per second.[12] Ideally, the patient is gazing straight ahead, so that the passing stripes will produce a small-amplitude 'stare' nystagmus. Both the foveal and retinal pathways are involved in this test. If the patient, however, follows the stripes,

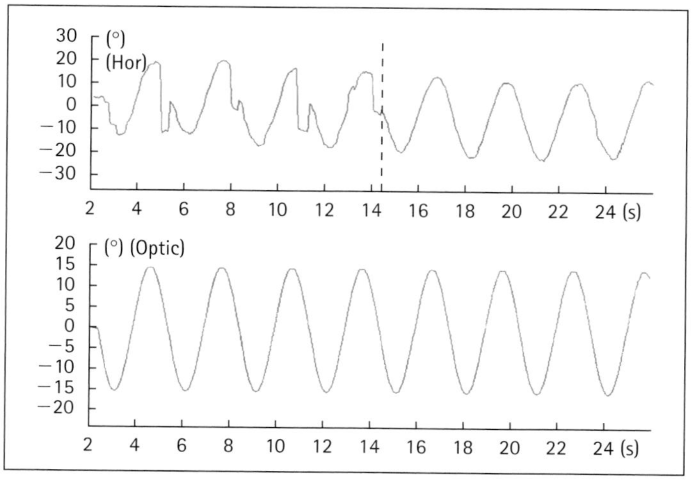

Figure 42.7 Effect of encouragement (after the vertical line) of a patient during smooth pursuit tracking. Apparently consistent saccadic movements to one side can be particularly misleading, as in the first half of the figure. The bottom trace represents the visual target.

then a 'look' nystagmus is induced, which predominantly tests the foveal pathways. According to Honrubia,[13] there is, so far, little evidence in species with a well-developed retinal macula that smooth pursuit and optokinetic nystagmus depend upon very different pathways. Therefore, abnormalities in smooth pursuit should be partially found also in the optokinetic test and vice versa. If this is not the case, either the stimulus was not properly delivered or the cooperation of the patient might be questioned. If both tests are abnormal, there is strong evidence for central nervous system pathology.

A general principle in the administration of the ocular motor test battery is to repeat trials for a given test until maximum performance is achieved from the patient. The rationale is that these tests are looking for signs of failure in the ocular motor pathways. If such a faulty pathway is present, it should be consistent. When a patient is less cooperative, however, an abnormal response could be a false-positive one.

> Failure in the ocular motor pathways lead usually to consistent abnormal patterns. Therefore, either the patient can do it properly, or not at all. Decreased alertness hampers the repeatability.

Positioning and positional tests

The positioning test refers to movement of the patient, while the positional test refers to the sustained position of the patient with respect to gravity. Both tests look for slightly different phenomena. Positioning tests aim to investigate paroxysmal positional nystagmus by means of the Dix–Hallpike maneuver (Chapter 48), whereas positional testing focuses on recording persistent positional nystagmus.

The procedure for positioning tests is as follows. The head of the patient is turned 45° to the right or left while the patient is seated and with eyes opened behind Frenzel's glasses or preferably VOG goggles. Next, the patient is placed supine, rather abruptly, with the head on the bench or head hanging slightly (supported by the examiner). The eye movements also recorded with ENG or VOG are inspected for nystagmus, especially nystagmus that is paroxysmal, i.e. that appears and then decreases, or nystagmus that persists throughout the entire time that the patient is lying in that position. Next, the patient is returned to the seated position. During the test, the patient is asked whether he or she feels dizzy, and if so, when the dizziness occurred, for how long, and whether this dizziness corresponds with the complaint that prompted the visit to the specialist. The same procedure is then repeated for the other side. When the patient's history suggests benign paroxysmal positional vertigo (BPPV), testing should begin with the involved side. Otherwise, the response might be reduced through fatigue and the effect missed.

Additionally, supine, left lateral and right lateral positions can be investigated. For these positional tests the patient is placed in several positions and investigated for persistent response, lasting for as long as the position is maintained. The most frequently used positions are supine, decubitus left and decubitus right, where each position is maintained for at least 30 s. When otoconical debris is adherent to the cupula, the cupula is transformed from a rotational detector into a translation and gravitation detector. This altered physiological state of the cupula may result in persistent positional nystagmus. This nystagmus can be either ageotropic (beating away from the earth), or geotropic (beating towards the earth). VOG is of great use for positional and positioning tests, since vertical and torsional nystagmus may be evident in different positions.

Vestibular tests

Rotary chair test

The major aim of rotary chair tests is the study of the VOR by application of measurable, repeatable and physiological stimuli to the vestibular system. From a systems engineering standpoint, the input is acceleration while the output is slow component eye velocity. The relationship between stimulus and response can be described by gain (response eye velocity/stimulus velocity), phase (time-lag between response and stimulus), and symmetry. These parameters reveal how the entire vestibular system, i.e. end organs, eighth cranial nerve and central pathways, react to the rotational stimulation. More specifically, the rotary chair test demonstrates how clockwise and counterclockwise stimuli are similarly processed by the entire vestibular system. For proper gain and phase calculation, it is strongly recommended to record also the stimulus by means of an accelerometer placed on the patient's head.

During rotary chair testing, which is performed in darkness, mental alertness plays a great role. For this purpose, patients should be systematically asked to perform mental tasks, e.g. to count aloud backwards from 200 to 0 in steps of 3. Speaking to the patient, except through headphones, should be avoided, since this will provide auditory clues regarding orientation, which may jeopardize the validity of the test. Figure 42.8 illustrates the effect of alerting the patient on the response.

- During rotational testing, let the patient perform mental tasks, such as counting backwards in steps of 3.
- Do not talk continuously to the patient because that provides orientation clues that influence the VOR.

Rotary chair tests can be categorized according to the vestibular subsystem that they test, which in general is achieved by changing the axis of rotation with respect to gravity and changing the orientation of the head with respect to the axis of rotation.

Earth vertical axis rotation stimulates both horizontal semicircular canal systems. Some experts[14,15] underline the need for the head to be tilted forward 30° during rotation to bring the horizontal semicircular canals into the plane of rotation. Others remain vague about which head position is preferred for the rotation test. We performed an experiment where 24 normal subjects were rotated (0.05 Hz, 50°/s) in both the upright position and the pitched-down position, in a random order.[16] When analyzed pairwise, the gain was significantly higher in the upright position than in the pitched position. The variances of both conditions were not significantly different. Therefore, since the upright position is also a more natural condition, we recommend rotating the patient in the head-upright position.

Off-vertical axis rotation and eccentric rotation (off-axis vertical rotation) investigate both otoliths and the semicircular canal systems. See Chapter 45 for a further description of this. A mixed type of paradigm exists in a few centers (e.g. Berlin and Antwerp), where during earth vertical axis rotation the axis is displaced gradually 4 cm to each side so that the rotation axis coincides alternately with one of the peripheral vestibular systems of the patient. This stimulus enables the excitation of the otolith organs of one labyrinth at a time.[6,39]

Rotary chair tests differ by their stimulus frequency. Based on the viscoelastic properties of the endolymph and the semicircular canal geometry, the VOR works optimally between 0.1 and 5 Hz,[17] wherein the gain is nearly unity and the phase near zero degrees. That is, between 0.1 and 5 Hz, vestibular-induced eye movement is compensatory, i.e. instantaneous and fully matching the head movement. The predominant frequencies of rotational head perturbations during walking and running are indeed between 0.5 and 5 Hz.[18] At lower frequencies, i.e. below 0.1 Hz, the gain decreases and the phase lead increases. During natural head movements outside the laboratory, visual input works synergistically with vestibular input, resulting again in optimal gaze stabilization.

The optimal stimulus for VOR testing includes stimuli at high frequencies, i.e. above 0.1 Hz, and preferentially above 1 Hz, but the construction of such rotary chair units is mechani-

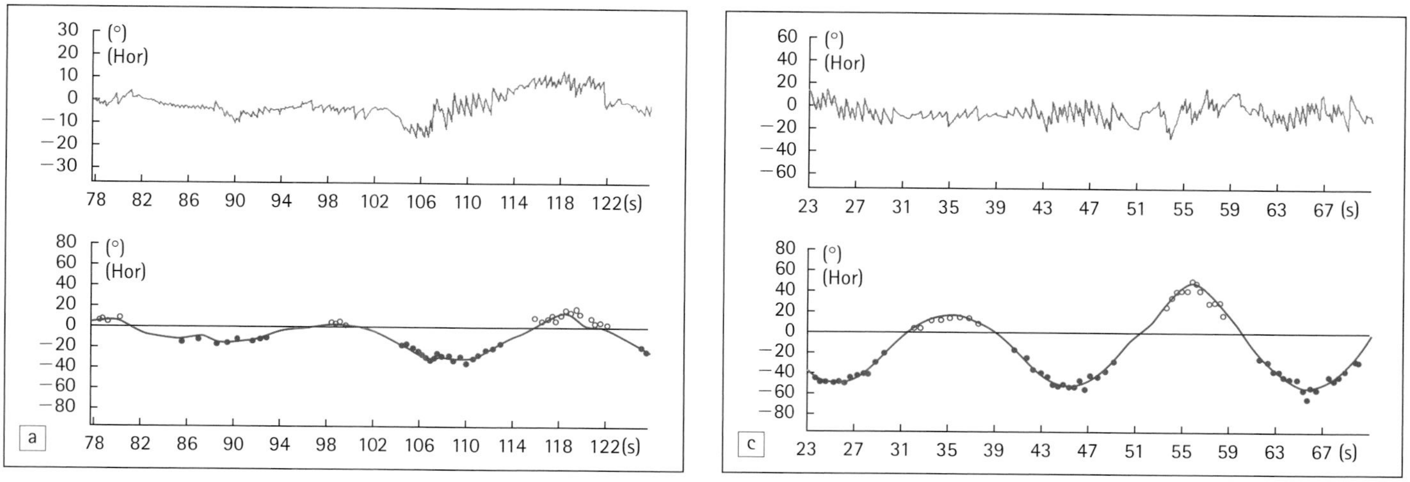

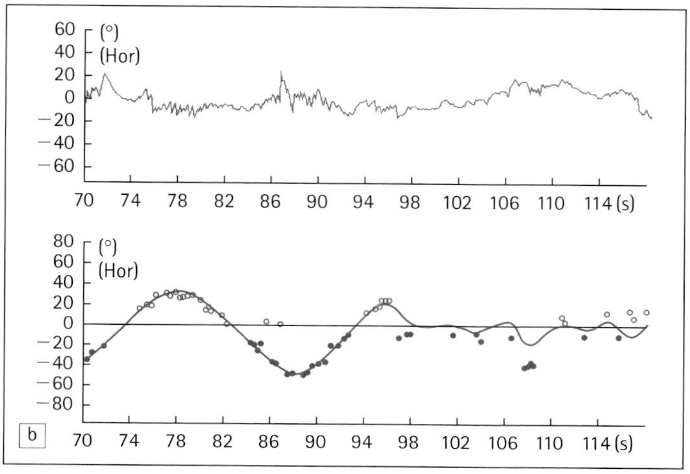

Figure 42.8 The effect of alertness on the rotary chair test is illustrated by the change in gain and asymmetry. The top trace shows the nystagmus, and the bottom trace the slow component velocity. The solid line through the dots is obtained after median filtering. This line should be a simple sinusoid since the stimulus is a simple sinusoid. All tests were at 0.05 Hz with a maximum velocity of 50°/s. (a) During the first part of the test, the patient counted to herself, whereas after second 102 she started counting aloud. Note the effect on the amplitude (i.e. gain). (b) The rotary chair test response where a patient stopped counting after 95 s. The second half of the recording shows that there was no coherent nystagmus response and the gain decreased significantly. The chair, however, did continue rotating. (c) The effect of alertness on response asymmetry. During the first part (until 50 s), the patient did not count, while she did count aloud backward after second 50. The asymmetry during the first part is about 50% whereas in the second part it is about 10%. Caloric testing revealed that the left labyrinth was 38% less active than the right labyrinth. The alertness facilitated the central compensation mechanism so as to make the response more symmetric.

cally cumbersome and expensive, which is the reason why only a few centers have this kind of equipment.[19,20]

Different paradigms have been developed for use with the standard earth vertical axis rotation chairs. The most commonly used stimulus is sinusoidal harmonic acceleration, wherein the patient is rotated alternately to the left and right following a sinusoidal pattern. Usually, the frequency ranges from 0.01 to 1.0 Hz, with a maximum velocity of 50–60°/s. Such a stimulus is usually very well tolerated even by dizzy patients. It should be noted that when the response is too low, characterized by a gain below 0.1, the phase and asymmetry should be interpreted cautiously, since in that case the noise level is too high for proper calculation of phase and asymmetry.

> If the gain is too low, measures of asymmetry or phase are inaccurate, and should be interpreted with caution.

A sinusoidal harmonic acceleration test battery often consists of a combination of successive rotations at different frequencies, depending on the performance of the rotary chair unit. This test only approaches the frequency at which the VOR really functions optimally. Another disadvantage is that the test is lengthy and the patient's level of alertness may decline towards the end of the test, resulting in less reliable responses. To mitigate this problem, a pseudorandom test can be used, where the chair is rotated according to a sum of 3–4 sinusoids with different frequencies. The result is a pseudorandom stimulus in which, for every epoch, all frequencies are present. Fourier analysis allows gain and phase at different frequencies to be computed. However, a frequency-dependent measure of asymmetry cannot be extracted from the results. Also, the reliability of the data at each frequency may be less than that achieved with single-frequency sinusoids.

The velocity step test consists of rotation of the patient at a constant velocity, typically 60–120°/s, until no nystagmus is observed, and then an abrupt stop. The initial acceleration is sometimes chosen to be subliminal (<1 to 2°/s^2) but the brake yields decelerations of 120°/s^2 up to 500°/s^2. This procedure is performed in both CW and CCW directions. When turning CW at suprathreshold acceleration, the nystagmus will beat to the right, since the right labyrinth is excited and the left inhibited. When the rotational velocity remains constant, the nystagmus fades away, due to the relaxing cupula of both horizontal SCCs, although the eye-movement response is prolonged by the velocity storage mechanism (see Chapter 41). When nystagmus is no longer present, the chair is briskly stopped, after which, if the chair was spinning clockwise, the left vestibular system is highly stimulated at high acceleration. The velocity step stimulus has a broad frequency content, which helps render it a relevant VOR stimulus. Following deceleration, nystagmus is observed in which the slow component velocity decreases exponentially over time. When plotted on a log–linear diagram, the SCV follows a linear relationship in time. The intercept with the vertical axis denotes the initial SCV, from which the gain can be calculated. The time at which the response level declines to 37% of its initial response is defined as the time constant. This value is reflected in the slope of the log–linear diagram of the SCV over time. The time constant is analogous to the phase of the sinusoidal response.

Table 42.4 summarizes the advantages and disadvantages of the different rotary chair tests.

Since part of the methodology to obtain the most reliable test results pertains to the instructions given to the patient, examples of instructions for the spontaneous nystagmus detection and the ocular motor test battery are listed in Table 42.5.

Visual–vestibular interaction test

Visual–vestibular interaction testing is performed by asking patients to look at a small target that rotates with them during earth vertical axis rotation or by having them view earth-fixed full-field stripes or dots while undergoing earth vertical axis rotation. In this way, vision is used to either reduce or augment the vestibular response, respectively. Visual–vestibular interaction testing is particularly useful when assessing central vestibular abnormalities, as appropriately combining visual and vestibular information depends on the normal functioning of brainstem and cerebellar structures. Typically, patients are rotated at a single sinusoidal frequency (e.g. 0.05 Hz): (1) in the dark; (2) with a fixation target; and (3) with earth-fixed stripes. A sinusoidal optokinetic stimulus while the patient is stationary may be used as a pure visual stimulus. The responses to these visual, vestibular stimuli are recorded and analyzed in a manner similar to that for measuring the response to sinusoidal rotation tests in darkness, yielding gain and phase.

Caloric test

The caloric test is the preferred test to lateralize a peripheral vestibular lesion. In general, it is used to assess the function of the horizontal semicircular canal. For this test, the patient is placed supine with the head inclined at approximately 30°, such that the horizontal semicircular canal is positioned vertically. After careful inspection of the external auditory canals to exclude perforation or other adverse conditions such as impacted cerumen, both ear canals are consecutively irrigated with warm (44°C) and cool (30°C) water for 30–40 s. This induces a thermal gradient in the vestibular system, and mainly affects the horizontal semicircular canal, which lies closest to the external ear. When the patient is placed properly, this thermal gradient produces a convection current of the endolymph in the horizontal semicircular canal (Figure 42.9). The warm (44°C) irrigation induces a utriculopetal endolymph flow, which corresponds to an excitation of hair cells of the crista in the ipsilateral horizontal canal, resulting

Table 42.4 VOR investigation by rotatory chair tests

Stimulus type	Frequency	Advantage	Disadvantage
Torsion swing	Typically 0.05 Hz	Short examination (2 min) Easy to perform (chair)	Only one frequency, which may be too low
Sinusoidal harmonic acceleration (SHA) test	e.g. 0.01, 0.05, 0.1, 0.5 Hz	Broadband test of the VOR	Time-consuming Alertness may not be equal for all frequencies
Pseudorandom test	Combination of for example, 0.01, 0.05, 0.1, 0.5 Hz in pseudorandom waveform	Broadband test of the VOR Alertness is equal for all frequencies	Time-consuming Technically difficult
Velocity step	High frequency	High frequency stimulus, i.e. close to physiological Less time-consuming than SHA or pseudorandom Time constant is comparable to phase	Two tests must be performed (CW and CCW)
Whole body high-frequency test	1.0–3.0 Hz	Test VOR at its appropriate frequency No neck input No anticipation input	Expensive equipment Patient has to be fastened thoroughly

Table 42.5 Instructions given to the patient during vestibular testing

Protocol item	Comments and instructions to the patients
1. Ocular motor screening battery	
Spontaneous nystagmus detection	In semi-darkened room: 'Please close your eyes, and look in the distance' If eyes open in a total darkened room: 'Please look in the distance' After ±20 s, 'To maintain your alertness: how much is 12 times 13?'
Gaze-evoked nystagmus	'Please fixate carefully on the dot straight ahead' (10 s), 'Look at the left dot' (10 s), and so on for all targets.
Saccades	'The dot will jump back and forth now for a while. Please follow it carefully. Do not jump too soon or too late'
Optokinetic nystagmus	'Look at the stripes and count them as they move past your eyes. Please, do not stare'
Smooth pursuit	'Follow carefully the moving dot. Do not run ahead and do not stay behind'
2. Positioning and positional test battery	
Positioning-positional	'Keep your eyes wide open throughout the maneuver' (if using Frenzel's or VOG goggles). 'Tell us if you are dizzy during the different stages of the maneuver, and for how long'
3. Vestibular tests	
Rotation test	'The chair will turn back and forth. It might make you a bit dizzy. Keep your eyes closed (or open as appropriate). Look to an imaginary horizon and count aloud backward from 200 to 0 in steps of 3 during the entire test'
Caloric test	'We'll put consecutively for 30 to 40 seconds warm and cool water in your ears. This might generate some dizziness, which is perfectly normal. Do not be alarmed. It lasts for nearly half a minute after the irrigation has stopped. This test serves to compare the health of your inner ears with one another. Keep your eyes closed (or open if appropriate) and count aloud from 100 to 0 by 2'

in a nystagmus that beats towards the irrigated ear. The cool (30°C) irrigation induces a utriculofugal movement of the endolymph, resulting in a hyperpolarization of the hair cells in the horizontal semicircular canal crista. Therefore, cool irrigation corresponds to rotational movement to the opposite side, provoking a nystagmus that beats away from the irrigated ear. The mnemonic COWS (Cold Opposite, Warm Same) summarizes the nystagmus direction with caloric stimulation. Although thermal convection accounts for the larger portion of the caloric response, two additional causes for the nystagmus response are to be noted; direct thermal stimulation of the vestibular end organ and neural elements, as shown by microgravity experiments as well as volume expansion of the endolymph.

The caloric stimulation is equivalent to a very low-frequency rotation (0.002–0.004 Hz),[12] in the upright position. During caloric stimulation, the contralateral labyrinth is not simultaneously stimulated. Thus, the patient's central vestibular system is confronted with contradictory information and a false sensation of movement. Therefore, during caloric testing, vertigo may arise. It is very important that the patient is informed about this physiologically normal effect so that he or she does not react with panic or anxiety. Most patients undergo caloric testing with little discomfort. Both open-loop and closed-loop systems are used; the former is inappropriate in the

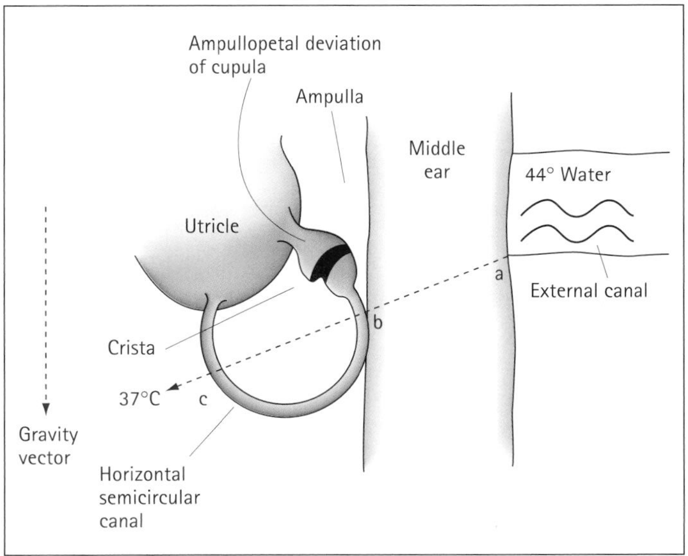

Figure 42.9 Biophysical basis for the caloric test. The thermal gradient (along the line abc) across the semicircular canal produces a convection current, deflecting the ampula. The cupular deflection is exaggerated, since it only deflects 1.5–2.6 µm for cold (10°C) water irrigation. (Adapted from Baloh and Honrubia. *Clinical Neurophysiology of the Vestibular System*, 2nd edn. Philadelphia. FA Davis Company, 1990.[14]).

case of a perforated eardrum. Alternatively, warm and cool air can be used, although this can result in paradoxical results, since air flow across a moist surface such as the ear mucosa creates a cooling effect, even with warm air. Water is a better medium for heat exchange and is preferable.[3] Since warm water induces vasodilatation of the blood vessels in the irrigated region, the thermal conductivity will increase. More heat is delivered to the horizontal semicircular canal as long as the irrigation lasts, but when the irrigation is ceased, the heat will be dissipated faster to the surrounding tissue. Cold water will induce vasoconstriction of the surrounding blood vessels, so that the stimulus is less efficiently transferred to the horizontal semicircular canal but the response will last longer. This biophysical approach explains why the response to the warm stimulus is often higher than that to the cold stimulus. The cold stimulus, however, provokes nystagmus reponses for a longer period.[21]

As an order of irrigation, we suggest warm right, warm left, cold right and finally cold left. A few organizations propose this order (The Dutch Vestibular Society[3]). If a warm irrigation does not induce any nystagmus, that peripheral system is suspected to be hypo- or areflexic. In such a case, cool irrigation with water of 30°C may produce little or no response. In order to ascertain the difference between total absence of excitability and reduced excitability, irrigation with iced water can be chosen as a very strong stimulus. When no nystagmus response is still measured, the probability that the horizontal semicircular canal is entirely areflexic increases considerably. Since an appropriately directed nystagmus may in fact represent an unmasked spontaneous nystagmus, it is critical, if possible, to immediately place the patient in the prone position to search for a reversal in the direction of the nystagmus. In this case, the horizontal canal is likely to be hypoactive but still active.

The amount of water used as well as the duration of irrigation varies in the literature, but in general it consists of 30–40-s irrigation with water of 30° and 44°C, with a flow rate of 350 ± 35 ml/min.[3]

The instructions to the patient are again of great importance, especially those that alter the level of alertness. Different mental tasks are asked, such as naming surnames, cities, flowers etc. starting with the letter ‘A’, then with ‘B’ etc. We prefer to ask the patient to count aloud backwards, such as 100, 98, 96 etc., since this is a very constant mental task that most people can perform. Mental tasks also help the patient not to think excessively about his or her possible vertigo, which may be induced by the irrigation. After each irrigation, at least 5 min are needed to allow temperature stabilization in the labyrinth.

- Warm irrigation corresponds with upright rotation to the right side, for that semi circular canal. Cold irrigation to rotation in the opposite direction.

- Preferred order of irrigation: warm right, warm left, cold right, cold left.
- Maintain alertness throughout the caloric test.
- Calibrate prior to irrigation.
- Caloric responses should be consistent. If one out of four irrigations is not in agreement, it should be repeated.

Most studies agree upon the fact that the most informative variable consists of the maximum SCV. It is determined as the average SCV during a time window of, for example, 5–10 s around the peak response. Other methods of determination consist of a fit of the SCV curve over time to a predicted response. Labyrinth and nystagmus asymmetry are calculated using Jongkees' formula, which has the form: $(A - B)/(A + B) \times 100$. The ‘normalization’ (i.e. dividing by $(A + B)$) reduces the typical biological variability among different individuals. Labyrinth asymmetry is then calculated as $[(RW + RC) - (LW + LC)]/(RW + RC + LW + LC) \times 100$ with RW = right warm, LW = left warm, RC = right cold, and LC = left cold. Table 42.3 provides a list of different limits for asymmetry, according to different authors. In order to provide the reader with a value that takes into account the different studies, we offer a weighted mean, where the weight is determined by the number of cases in each normative group. This approach is used because we did not have access to all the individual measurements. With this method, we obtain a general limit for labyrinth asymmetry of 22%. Nystagmus asymmetry (directional preponderance) is calculated as $[(RW + LC) - (LW + RC)]/(RW + RC + LW + LC) \times 100$. Here the general limit for abnormality, based on the weighted mean of the different studies (see Table 42.3), is calculated as 26%. See Chapter 43 for clinical interpretation of labyrinth and nystagmus asymmetries.

Anatomical temporal bone differences, bloodflow and middle ear fluid differences between the left and right ear are uncontrollable factors that cause variations in the caloric test outcome. Other issues are more controllable, such as calibration (to be performed prior to each irrigation), arousal state of the patient, ensured by the assertive attitude of the technician, identical application of the stimuli, and temperature control of the applied stimulus. If one out of four responses is not in agreement with the other three, it is highly recommended to repeat the ‘faulty’ irrigation. Otherwise, false conclusions may be drawn from this investigation. Figure 42.10a illustrates four responses, of which one was not in accordance with the other three. The butterfly representation of these reponses is depicted in Figure 42.10b. The resulting labyrinth asymmetry was in this case 19%, which is considered as borderline abnormal. Repeating the irrigation resulted in the traces on Figures 42.10c and 42.10d. These responses revealed no labyrinth asymmetry at all (2%).

A caloric fixation–suppression index is obtained by having the patient fixate a visual target, more than 1 m away to avoid suppression due to eye convergence, shortly after the peak response. The fixation–suppression index is defined as the average SCV during fixation divided by the average SCV without fixation. For a further detailed description of caloric testing, see Jacobson et al.

Since the caloric test remains the only tool to evaluate the function of each labyrinth separately, it is very strongly recommended that each laboratory establishes its own set of normative data, to obtain proper normative limits.

Normative data

Although it is repeatedly stated that each vestibular department should establish its own normative limits based on a normative study, it is not common practice, since it is a time-consuming and costly enterprise. However, several studies have reported on normative data. The results of the larger part of these studies are reported in Table 42.3. It is obvious that a considerable variation exists among the different studies. Therefore we performed a meta-analysis on the data for caloric testing, for which there is the most variability. Using this meta-analysis, we determined that a general upper normal limit for labyrinth asymmetry (reduced vestibular response) of 22% is obtained, and a general upper normal limit for directional preponderance of 26% is obtained.

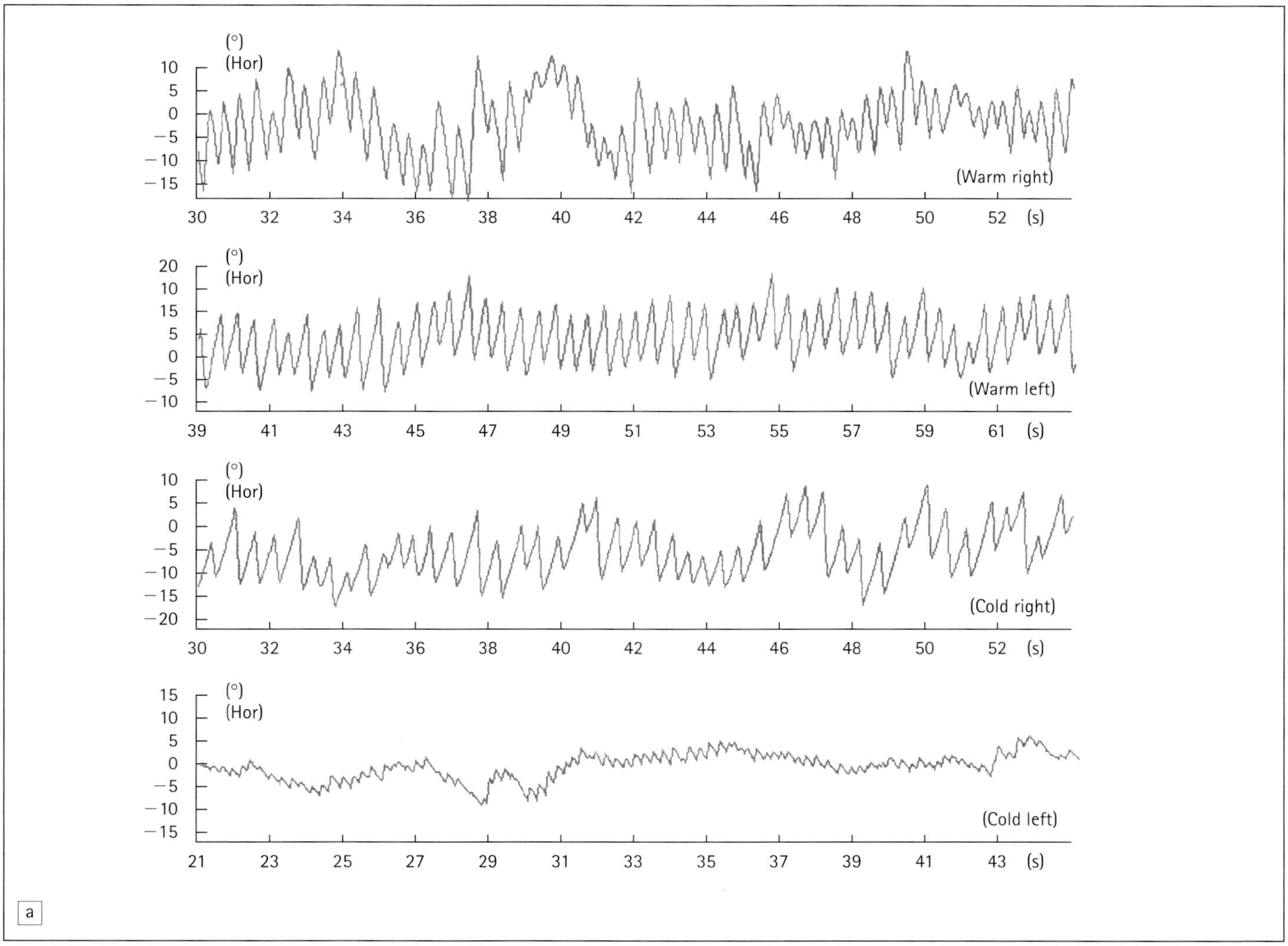

Figure 42.10 (a,b) Caloric responses for which the left cold irrigation is not in accordance with the others. Both raw data traces and butterfly diagrams are shown. The labyrinth asymmetry indicated a left labyrinthine hypofunction of 19%, which in our setting is considered as abnormal. The directional preponderance yielded 2%. The vertical lines indicate the time during which the patient was asked to fixate a point in darkness. The fixation indexes for right and left warm were 10% and 22%, respectively (below 50% is normal). (c,d) The left cold irrigation was repeated, resulting in a normal bilateral response. The labyrinth preponderance yielded 2% and the directional preponderance 12% nystagmus to the right.

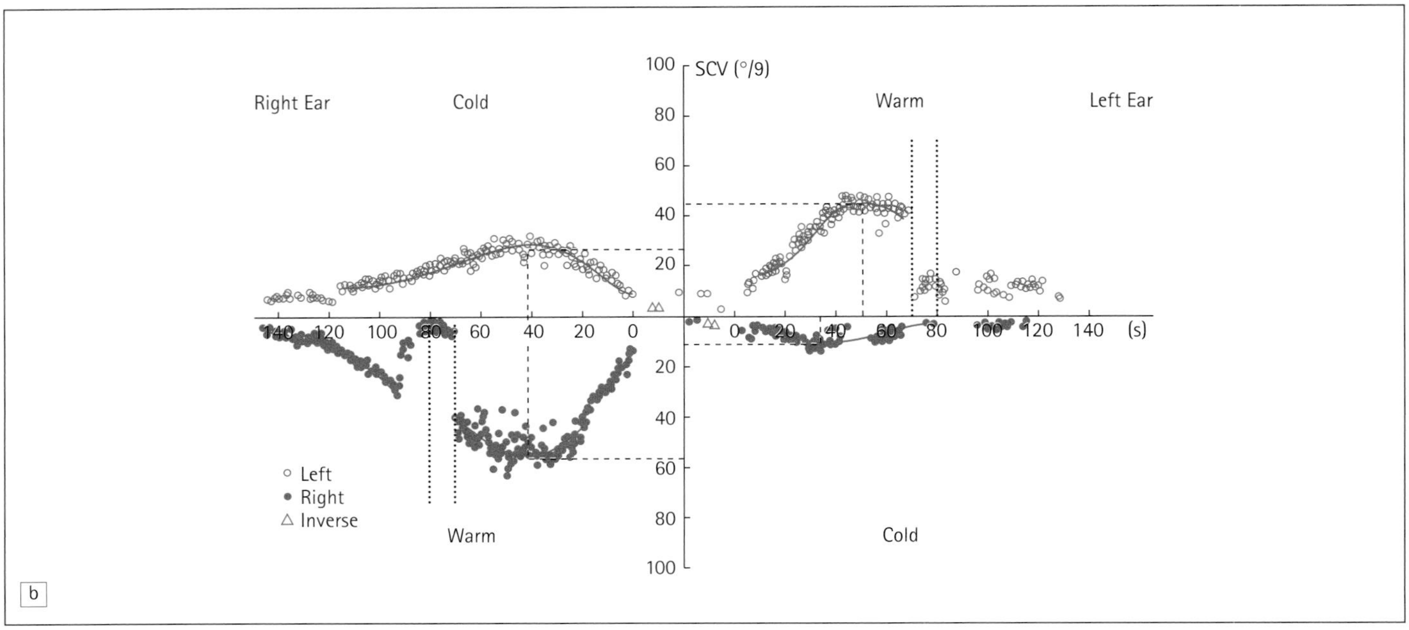
SCV (°/9)
Right Ear
Cold
Warm
Left Ear
Left
Right
Inverse
Warm
Cold
(s)
b

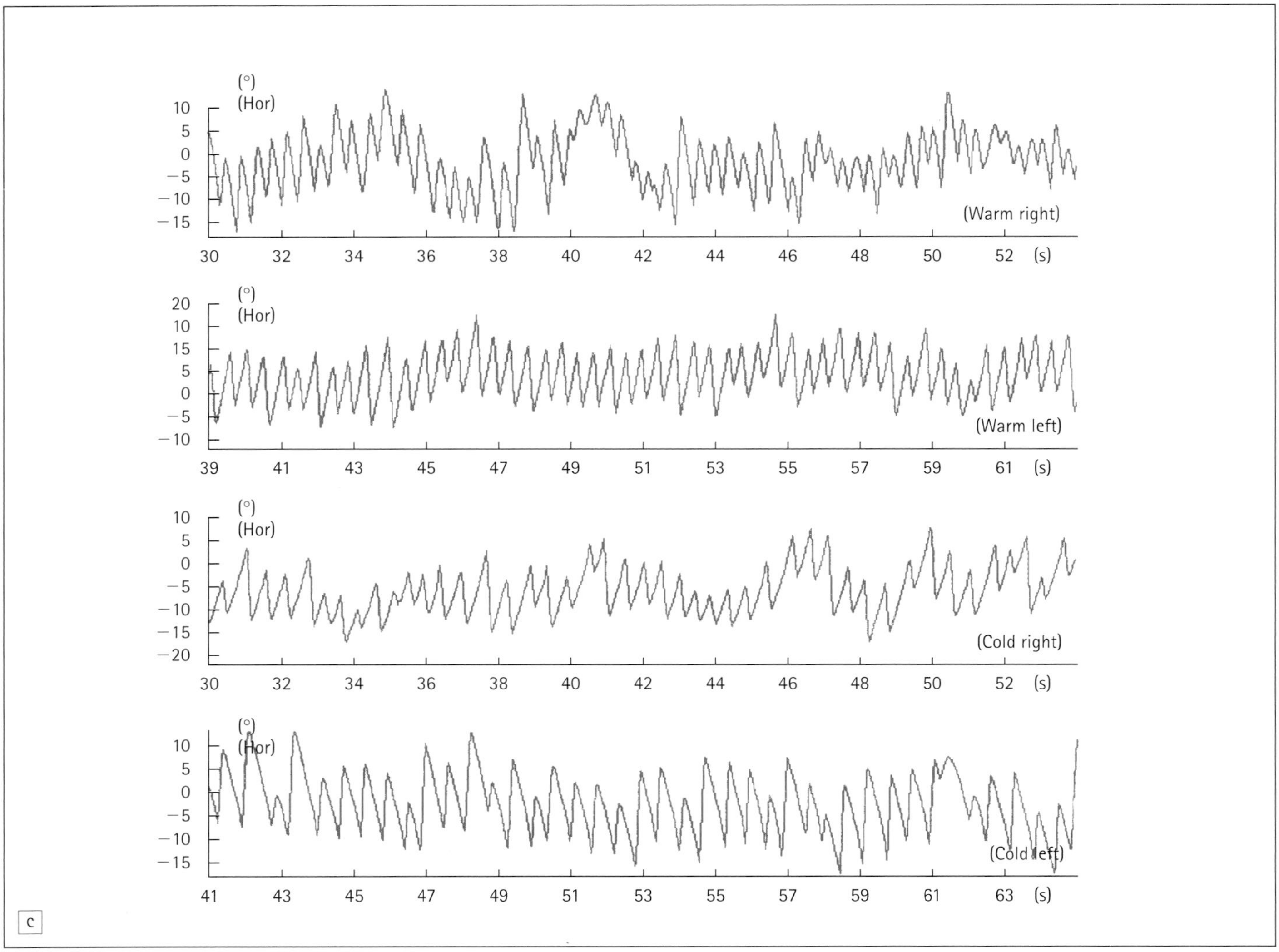
(°)
(Hor)
(Warm right)
(Warm left)
(Cold right)
(Cold left)
(s)
c

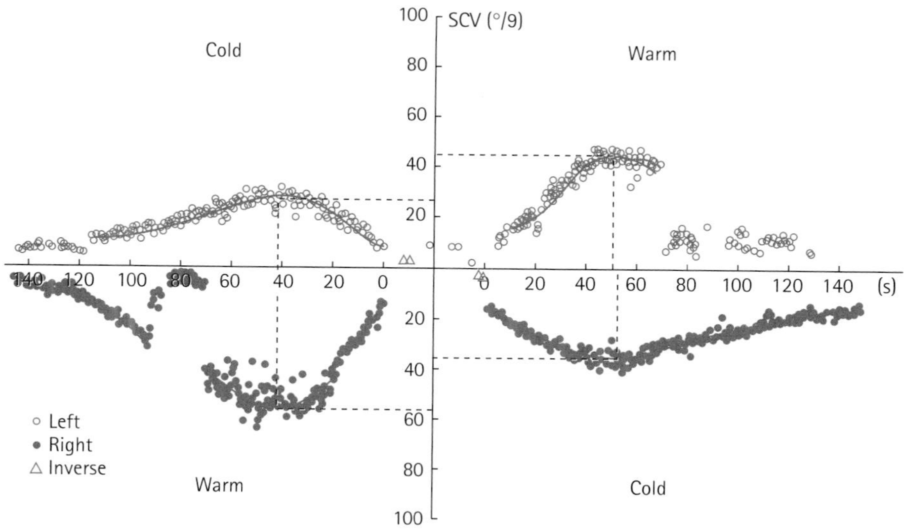

d

- It is strongly recommended that each laboratory establishes its own normative data.
- Meta-analysis indicates an upper normal limit for labyrinth asymmetry of 22% and for directional labyrinth preponderance of 26%.
- A dedicated and well trained technician is crucial for the reliability of vestibular tests.

Conclusion

Both methodological and biological issues, such as calibration or the anatomical differences between the left and right ears, can influence the outcome of vestibular function assessment. These factors should be taken into account so that each laboratory has a standard measurement protocol and a consistent methodology. Apart from the above-discussed methodological issues, it is of major importance that the tests are executed by a well-informed, attentive and dedicated technician. Without the certainty that the vestibular tests are performed by such a well-trained technician, many vestibular test results will be unreliable. Additionally, each vestibular function laboratory should, if possible, establish its own normative data, and follow a strict protocol. Under these constraints, vestibular function testing can reveal crucial information for the clinician to aid in the development of a management strategy for the patient with a suspected vestibular disorder.

Acknowledgement

We wish to thank Mrs Anja Van der Stappen, MD, for her contribution to the normative study. Part of the normative research was funded by FWO grant 3.0305.96.

References

1. Stewart AL, Ware JE. *Measuring Functioning and Well-being: The Medical Outcomes Study Approach*. Durham, NC: Duke University Press, 1992.
2. Jacobson GP, Newman CW. The development of the Dizziness Handicap Inventory. *Arch Otolaryngol Head Neck Surg* 1990; **116**(4): 424–7.
3. Committee on Hearing, Bioacoustics, and Biomechanics. Commission on Behavioral and Social Sciences and Education. National Research Council. Evaluation of tests for vestibular function. *Aviat Space Environ Med* 1992; **63**(2 suppl): A1–34.
4. Moore ST, Haslwanter T, Curthoys IS, Smith ST. A geometric basis for measurement of three-dimensional eye position using image processing. *Vision Res* 1996; **36**(3): 445–59.
5. Haslwanter T, Moore ST. A theoretical analysis of three-dimensional eye position measurement using polar cross-correlation. *IEEE Trans Biomed Eng* 1995; **42**(11): 1053–61.
6. Clarke AH, Engelhorn A. Unilateral testing of utricular function. *Exp Brain Res* 1998; **121**(4): 457–64.
7. Haslwanter T. Measurement and analysis techniques for three-dimensional eye movements. In: Fetter M, Haslwanter T, Misslisch H, Tweed D, eds. *Three-dimensional Kinematics of Eye, Head and Limb Movements*. Amsterdam: Harwood Academic Publishers, 1997: 401–12.
8. Robinson DA. A method of measuring eye movement using a scleral search coil in a magnetic field. *IEEE Trans Biomed Eng* 1963; **10**: 137–45.
9. Moller C, Odkvist L, White V, Cyr D. The plasticity of compensatory eye movements in rotatory tests. I. The effect of alertness and eye closure. *Acta Otolaryngol Stockh* 1990; **109**(1–2): 15–24.
10. Proctor L, Glackin R, Shimizu H, Smith C, Lietman P. Reference values for serial vestibular testing. *Ann Otol Rhinol Laryngol* 1986; **95**(1 Pt 1): 83–90.

11. Barber HO, Stockwell CW. *Manual of Electronystagmography*, 2nd edn. St Louis: Mosby, 1980.
12. Shepard NT, Telian SA. *Practical Management of the Balance Disorder Patient*, 1st edn. San Diego, London: Singular Publishing Group, 1996.
13. Honrubia V. Contemporary vestibular function testing: accomplishments and future perspectives. *Otolaryngol Head Neck Surg* 1995; **112**(1): 64–77.
14. Baloh RW, Honrubia V. *Clinical Neurophysiology of the Vestibular System*, 2nd edn. Philadelphia: FA Davis Company, 1990.
15. Savundra P, Luxon LM. The physiology of equilibrium and its application to the dizzy patient. In: Kerr A, ed. *Scott-Brown's Otolaryngology: Basic Sciences*. Oxford: Butterworth-Heinemann, 1997: 1–65.
16. Van der Stappen A, Wuyts FL, Van de Heyning P. Head position influence on the vestibulo-ocular reflex during rotational testing. *Acta Otolaryngol Stockh* 1999; **119**: 892–4.
17. Wilson BJ, Melville Jones G. *Mammalian Vestibular Physiology*. New York: Plenum Press, 1979.
18. Grossman GE, Leigh RJ, Abel LA, Lanska DJ, Thurston SE. Frequency and velocity of rotational head perturbations during locomotion. *Exp Brain Res* 1988; **70**(3): 470–6.
19. Hyden D, Larsby B, Odkvist LM. Broad-frequency rotatory testing. *Acta Otolaryngol Suppl Stockh* 1988; **455**: 48–52.
20. Dayal VS, Mai M, Tomlinson RD. High frequency rotation test: clinical and research application. *Adv Otorhinolaryngol* 1988; **41**: 40–43.
21. Sills AW, Baloh RW, Honrubia V. Caloric testing 2. Results in normal subjects. *Ann Otol Rhinol Laryngol Suppl* 1977; **86**(5 Pt 3 Suppl 43): 7–23.
22. Jacobson GP, Newman CW, Kartush JM. *Handbook of Balance Function Testing*. 1st edn. San Diego: Singular, 1997.
23. Harada Y, Ariki T. A new theory for thermal influences on endolymphatic flow. *Arch Otorhinolaryngol* 1985; **242**(1): 13–17.
24. Van der Stappen A, Wuyts FL, Van de Heyning P. Computerised electronystagmography: normative data revisited. *Acta Otolaryngol* 2000; **120**: 724–30.
25. Mulch G, Lewitzki W. Spontaneous and positional nystagmus in healthy persons demonstrated only by electronystagmography: physiological spontaneous nystagmus or 'functional scar'? *Arch Otorhinolaryngol* 1977; **215**(2): 135–45.
26. Coats AC. Directional preponderance and spontaneous nystagmus. *Ann Otol Rhinol Laryngol* 1966; **75**: 1135–59.
27. Fischer AJ, Huygen PL, Folgering HT, Verhagen WI, Theunissen EJ. Vestibular hyperreactivity and hyperventilation after whiplash injury. *J Neurol Sci* 1995; **132**(1): 35–43.
28. Baloh RW, Konrad HR, Sills AW, Honrubia V. The saccade velocity test. *Neurology* 1975; **25**(11): 1071–6.
29. Henriksson NG, Pyykko I, Schalen L, Wennmo C. Velocity patterns of rapid eye movements. *Acta Otolaryngol Stockh* 1980; **89**(5–6): 504–12.
30. Abel LA, Troost BT, Dell'Osso LF. The effects of age on normal saccadic characteristics and their variability. *Vision Res* 1983; **23**(1): 33–7.
31. Leigh RJ, Zee DS. *The Neurology of Eye Movements*, 2nd edn. Philadelphia: Davis, 1991.
32. Baloh RW, Sakala SM, Yee RD, Langhofer L, Honrubia V. Quantitative vestibular testing. *Otolaryngol Head Neck Surg* 1984; **92**(2): 145–50.
33. Hess K, Baloh RW, Honrubia V, Yee RD. Rotational testing in patients with bilateral peripheral vestibular disease. *Laryngoscope* 1985; **95**(1): 85–8.
34. Peterka RJ, Black FO, Schoenhoff MB. Age-related changes in human vestibulo-ocular reflexes: sinusoidal rotation and caloric tests. *J Vestib Res* 1990; **1**(1): 49–59.
35. Wall C, Black FO, Hunt AE. Effects of age, sex and stimulus parameters upon vestibulo-ocular responses to sinusoidal rotation. *Acta Otolaryngol Stockh* 1984; **98**(3–4): 270–8.
36. Theunissen EJ, Huygen PL, Folgering HT. Vestibular hyperreactivity and hyperventilation. *Clin Otolaryngol* 1986; **11**(3): 161–9.
37. Jongkees LBW, Philipszoon AJ. Electronystagmography. *Acta Otolaryngol Stockh Suppl* 1964; 189.
38. Boniver-R, Demanez JP. Epreuves rotatoires et caloriques chez le sujet normal. *Med Pharm*, 1975.
39. Wuyts FL, Hoppenbrouwers M, Van de Heyning PH. Unilateral Otolith function testing. In Lacour M, ed. *Posture et Equilibre. Dysfunctionnements da Systeme vestibulaire, compensation et rééducation*. Marseille: Solal, 2001: 257–65.

43 Clinical application of vestibular laboratory testing

Joseph M Furman, Floris L Wuyts

Introduction

This chapter discusses the clinical application of vestibular laboratory testing and focuses on the test techniques discussed in Chapter 42. To make the material more accessible to the reader, the organization of this chapter will follow the organization of Chapter 42. Posturography, discussed in Chapter 44 and emerging technologies, discussed in Chapter 45 will not be addressed in this chapter. First, there will be a discussion of the eye-movement recording techniques that are useful in the clinical setting. Then, there will be discussion of the indications for vestibular laboratory testing. Subsequently, there will be a discussion of the clinical significance of individual vestibular laboratory test abnormalities that may be uncovered during ocular-motor screening, positional and positioning tests, caloric testing, and rotational testing. Various patterns of vestibular laboratory test abnormalities will be discussed. The chapter will conclude with a discussion of laboratory testing abnormalities likely to be encountered in several common balance disorders.

Choice of eye-movement recording technique

As discussed in Chapter 19, vestibular laboratory testing relies almost entirely upon recording eye position. Posturography and some of the emerging technologies (see Chapters 44 and 45) are notable exceptions. Electro-oculography (EOG) has for many decades been the standard eye-movement measurement technique. EOG is a safe, convenient and efficient means of recording eye position in persons of all ages. The primary limitation of EOG relates to its inability to provide consistently reliable vertical eye-movement recording and problematic artefacts caused by eye blinks. Also, fluctuations in the relationship between EOG voltage and eye position can reduce the accuracy and reliability of vestibular laboratory testing. Another drawback of EOG recordings is that a certain level of experience and expertise is required in order to obtain reliable recordings. In particular, electrode impedance can be problematic.

Video-oculography (VOG) will eventually replace EOG as the method of choice for recording eye movements during vestibular laboratory testing. VOG has the advantage of allowing both horizontal and vertical eye-movement recordings with currently available technology. As with EOG, eye-blink artefacts can be problematic. Moreover, relative movement between the VOG goggles and the head can produce artefacts. As with EOG, some expertise is required to obtain reliable recordings, but overall, the ability to record eye position without actually affixing electrodes to the face is a definite advantage. Neither EOG nor currently routinely available two-dimensional VOG provides the ability to record torsional eye movements. However, with advanced image processing, VOG is almost certainly going to be able to provide three-dimensional eye-movement recordings. This ability may allow some of the emerging technologies discussed in Chapter 46 to become clinically useful.

At present, EOG and VOG are alternative techniques that are very comparable. However, as image-processing capabilities improve and camera speeds increase, it is likely that VOG will eventually replace EOG as the preferred eye-movement recording technique during vestibular laboratory testing. Indeed, aside from the ability to record with eyes closed with EOG and not with VOG, and a limited frame rate of VOG, there is no relative advantage of EOG over VOG.

Indications for vestibular laboratory testing

Table 43.1 lists the uses of vestibular laboratory testing. Vestibular laboratory testing is typically ordered by a specialist who has a high level of suspicion that a vestibular disorder may underlie a patient's symptoms. Because of the type of information that can be obtained from such testing, diagnostic accuracy can be improved. In particular, vestibular laboratory testing can aid the clinician in determining whether or not a vestibular system abnormality is present and, if so, whether the problem can be localized to the central or peripheral vestibular system. For patients with peripheral vestibular ailments, laboratory testing can aid in lateralizing the lesion.

Certainly, not all patients with symptoms of dizziness and dysequilibrium should undergo vestibular laboratory testing. However, following a review of appropriate historical and physical examination data, the clinician may determine that vestibular laboratory testing is necessary. Vestibular laboratory testing can provide quantitative information allowing documentation of an abnormality only suspected by bedside evaluation. Moreover, eye movements can be recorded in the laboratory during loss of visual fixation and during stimulation of the labyrinth that is not possible during routine physical examination. Some types of vestibular laboratory testing provide information that may be useful in designing treatment plans, particularly treatment with balance rehabilitation therapy (see Chapter 53). Moreover, some vestibular laboratory tests such as positional testing, rotational testing and posturography can be helpful in the long-term management of patients, because these tests can be repeated intermittently with minimal discomfort to the patient. As noted in Chapter 19 and further described below, vestibular laboratory testing consists of several component parts that may be performed in various combinations. Table 43.2 lists the vestibular test batteries that may be considered, depending upon the suspicions of the clinician regarding the localization of the vestibular system abnormality. If the clinician has a high suspicion of a vestibular system abnormality but does not have a particular idea regarding localization, a more complete vestibular laboratory test battery can be obtained. Overall, as discussed in Chapter 19, vestibular laboratory testing has a somewhat poor sensitivity and specificity.

Table 43.1 Uses of vestibular laboratory testing

Aids in diagnosis
- Localization: central versus peripheral localization
- Lateralization

Documentation of an abnormality suspected by bedside evaluation
Aids in devising a treatment plan
Aids in long-term management

From, Baloh RW, Halmagyi GM, eds. *Disorders of the Vestibular System*. New York: Oxford University Press, 1996, by permission.

Table 43.2 Vestibular test batteries

Suspected peripheral vestibular abnormality
- Ocular motor screening battery
- Search for vestibular nystagmus
- Positional testing
- Caloric testing
- Rotational testing

Suspected central vestibular abnormality
- Ocular motor screening battery
- Search for vestibular nystagmus
- Positional testing
- Rotational testing: visual–vestibular interaction

From, Baloh RW, Halmagyi GM, eds. *Disorders of the Vestibular System*. New York: Oxford University Press, 1996, by permission.

Despite this limitation, vestibular laboratory testing may significantly augment the clinical assessment of the dizzy patient.

Significance of individual vestibular laboratory test abnormalities

Ocular-motor screening battery

Primarily, the ocular-motor screening battery is a means for uncovering ocular-motor system abnormalities that may interfere with the reliability of the vestibulo-ocular reflex (VOR) as a means of assessing peripheral and central vestibular function. Additionally, the ocular-motor screening battery can provide information directly concerning vestibular system abnormalities and, moreover, can provide ancillary information regarding central nervous system structures important for balance function.

Spontaneous nystagmus

The term 'spontaneous nystagmus' is sometimes used to denote a nystagmus that occurs during visual fixation and sometimes used to denote nystagmus that occurs only with loss of visual fixation through eye closure or darkness. However, the term 'spontaneous vestibular nystagmus' is preferred for nystagmus seen only with loss of visual fixation or for nystagmus that is significantly greater in magnitude than that seen with visual fixation (Figure 43.1). The term 'spontaneous nystagmus' is preferred for nystagmus seen with (and without) visual fixation. Spontaneous nystagmus may be either pendular, in which case there are no clearly defined fast and slow components, or jerk, in which there are clearly defined fast and slow components. Pendular nystagmus may be congenital or acquired, and is seen infrequently. Spontaneous nystagmus with clearly defined fast and slow components, i.e. spontaneous jerk nystagmus, is most commonly a

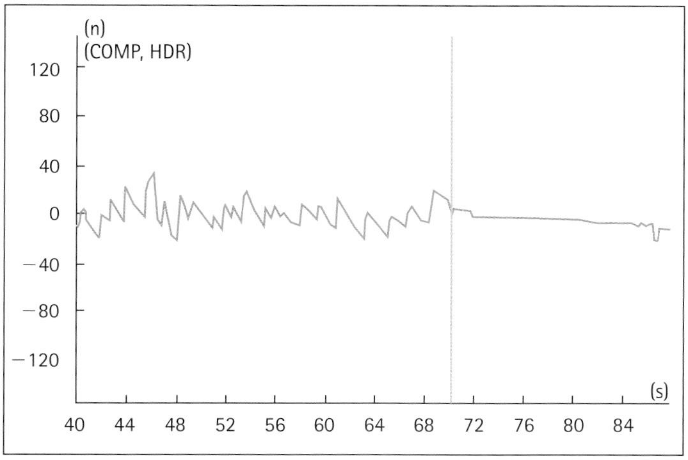

Figure 43.1 Example of spontaneous vestibular nystagmus seen only with loss of fixation. Note that the left side of the figure illustrates right-beating nystagmus recorded with the patient's eyes open in the dark. At timing marker 70 s, the patient was asked to look at a fixation target. Note that the nystagmus is extinguished.

result of an acute vestibular imbalance. In this case, it will have a larger magnitude when visual fixation is absent, and thus should be considered as a spontaneous vestibular nystagmus. A caveat is as follows: patients may manifest spontaneous jerk nystagmus of vestibular origin during visual fixation in the setting of low vision or poor visual fixation abilities or in a very acute phase of neuritis. In these cases, a vestibular nystagmus will be seen with fixation in a manner similar to that seen when a patient with normal visual fixation is placed in darkness.

Spontaneous vestibular nystagmus is typically horizontal or horizontal–torsional. Both EOG and two-dimensional VOG will only record the horizontal component of this nystagmus. The presence of a horizontal–torsional spontaneous vestibular nystagmus does not provide reliable information regarding localization of the abnormality to the peripheral or central vestibular system, and nor does the presence of spontaneous vestibular nystagmus provide reliable information regarding laterality. However, in acute peripheral vestibular lesions, spontaneous vestibular nystagmus typically beats away the impaired labyrinth. For example, an acute right-sided peripheral vestibular lesion will usually be associated with a left-beating spontaneous vestibular nystagmus, because the brain receives a tonic input from the intact (left) labyrinth (about 90 spikes/s) that is not balanced by a tonic input from the impaired (right) labyrinth. The difference is interpreted by the brain as a rotation to the left, so a left-beating nystagmus emerges.

Vertical nystagmus may also be seen both with and without visual fixation. The presence of vertical nystagmus during ocular-motor screening strongly suggests the presence of a central nervous system abnormality. Note that artefacts in the eye-movement recording may simulate vertical nystagmus, especially with EOG.

Gaze-evoked nystagmus

Another component of the ocular-motor screening battery is a search for nystagmus with gaze deviation away from the primary position. That is, it is essential to search for 'gaze-evoked nystagmus'. Gaze-evoked nystagmus may be a result of poor gaze holding on the basis of an abnormal 'ocular-motor integrator'. In this case, gaze-evoked nystagmus will typically be seen with both leftward and rightward gaze and may be seen with upward gaze. The fast component of the nystagmus will be in the direction of gaze. Another type of nystagmus that may be seen with gaze deviation is actually a type of vestibular nystagmus. In particular, because of Alexander's law, a spontaneous vestibular nystagmus may only be evident with gaze deviation. For example, a patient with a recent, but not an acute, right-sided peripheral vestibular lesion may manifest left-beating nystagmus only with gaze to the left, which would accentuate an otherwise unobservable left-beating nystagmus (Figure 43.2). For this reason, it is helpful to search for nystagmus during gaze deviation, both with fixation and in darkness.

Saccadic eye movements

Saccadic eye movements are typically recorded monocularly to uncover abnormalities in voluntary gaze, limitations of gaze and dysconjugacies. Any of the saccadic abnormalities in ocular-motor function may influence vestibular laboratory tests that rely on the VOR. Additionally, an assessment of saccadic eye movements may provide information that is useful in diagnosing specific central nervous system disorders. For further discussion of such saccadic abnormalities, see Chapter 41. Any limitation in eye movements must be noted, since this will obviously influence all subsequent eye-movement recordings during the vestibular laboratory test battery. Moreover, such testing may uncover a previously undiscovered cranial neuropathy or internuclear ophthalmoplegia. A finding of dysconjugate eye movements influences how subsequent data are analyzed. When using EOG recordings, significant ocular-motor dysconjugacies preclude the use of bitemporal EOG, which averages movements of the two eyes. For VOG, the presence of either a limitation of gaze or a dysconjugacy will influence the selection of which eye should be used for subsequent vestibular testing.

Typically, vestibular system abnormalities do not alter saccades. However, in the setting of an acute unilateral peripheral vestibular lesion, there may be a superimposed spontaneous nystagmus seen during attempted gaze holding after completion of each saccade.

Ocular pursuit

Ocular pursuit testing, like saccadic testing, can provide information that supports a diagnosis of a vestibular system abnormality or information that may suggest a central nervous system abnormality. Abnormalities of ocular pursuit are discussed thoroughly in Chapter 47. In the setting of an acute

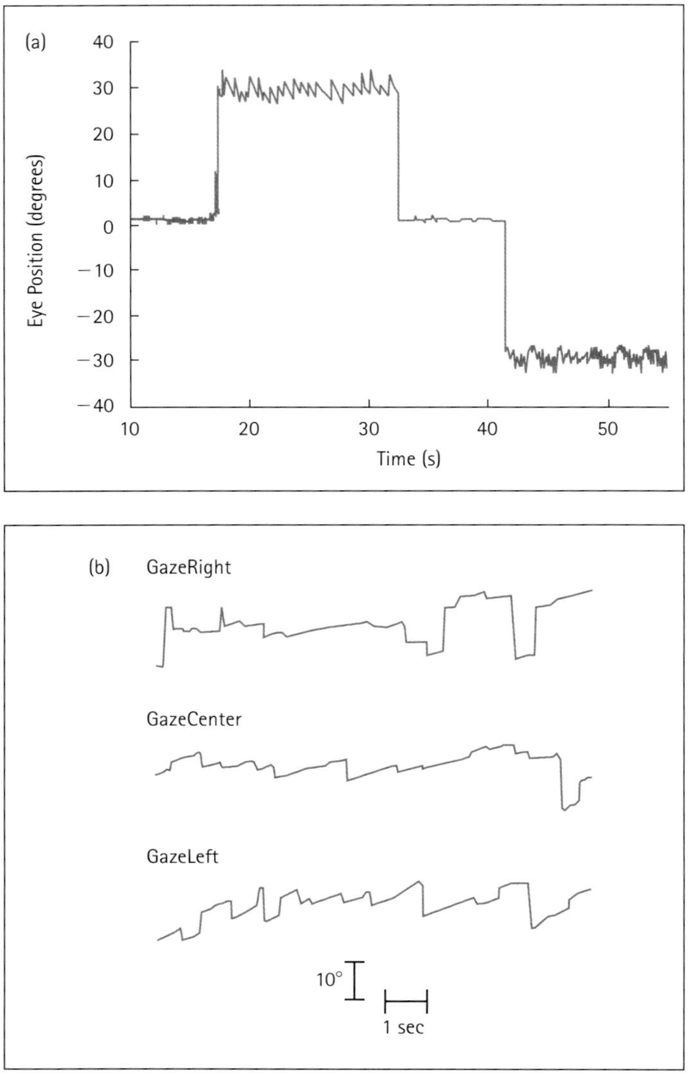

Figure 43.2 Comparison of gaze-evoked nystagmus and third-degree vestibular nystagmus. (a) Gaze-evoked nystagmus. Note right-beating nystagmus on rightward gaze and left-beating nystagmus on leftward gaze, with an absence of nystagmus when looking straight ahead. (b) Third-degree vestibular nystagmus. Note the presence of left-beating nystagmus in leftward gaze, center gaze, and rightward gaze. Note that gaze-evoked nystagmus (a) is bidirectional, whereas third-degree vestibular nystagmus (b) is unidirectional.

peripheral vestibular ailment, patients may show asymmetric pursuit such that the patient has difficulty pursuing away from the side of the lesion (Figure 43.3). This is particularly the case when patients manifest a spontaneous vestibular nystagmus. In this circumstance, the asymmetric pursuit is such that the patient has difficulty pursuing in the direction of the quick component of the spontaneous nystagmus. Without a concomitant spontaneous nystagmus or a history of a recent vestibular insult, asymmetric pursuit, like symmetrically impaired pursuit, indicates a central nervous system abnormality.

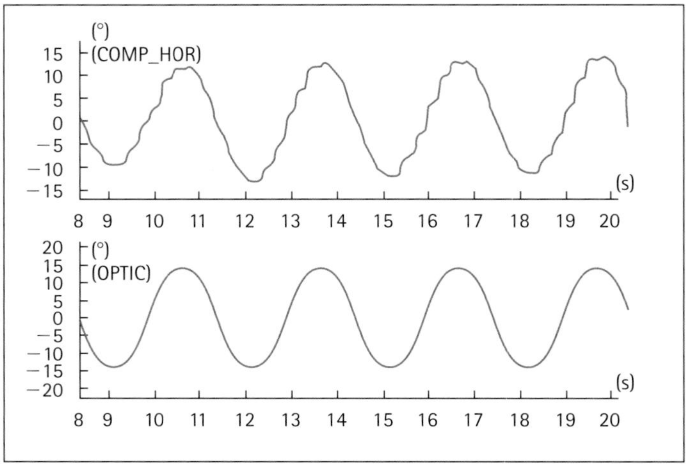

Figure 43.3 Example of asymmetric smooth pursuit eye movements. The lower trace illustrates the position of a small LED target. The upper trace illustrates horizontal eye position and indicates difficulty with pursuit of the target when it is moving to the right.

Optokinetic nystagmus

Optokinetic nystagmus, even when performed using full-field visual stimuli, provides information that largely overlaps that provided by the assessment of ocular pursuit. The clinical significance of abnormal optokinetic nystagmus is comparable to the significance of abnormal ocular pursuit. However, because optokinetic nystagmus induces a large number of quick components, specific information regarding quick component generation can be obtained from optokinetic nystagmus testing

Positional and positioning testing

During positional testing, i.e. searching for a persistent nystagmus with the patient in various fixed positions with respect to gravity, there are several patterns of nystagmus that can be observed. These patterns include direction-fixed positional nystagmus and direction-changing positional nystagmus. With direction-fixed positional nystagmus, the nystagmus beats in the same direction in all positions and often is seen in patients who also manifest a spontaneous nystagmus. Direction-changing positional nystagmus is either geotropic, i.e. the nystagmus beats towards the down ear, or ageotropic, i.e. nystagmus beats away from the down ear. Thus, with geotropic direction-changing positional nystagmus, there is left-beating nystagmus in the head-left and left-lateral positions and right-beating nystagmus in the head-right and right-lateral positions. In some patients, nystagmus may only be seen in a subset of positions, e.g. only in the head-right and right-lateral positions or only in the head-left and left-lateral positions. In such cases, the distinction between direction-fixed and direction-changing becomes less meaningful, unless the patient also manifests a spontaneous nystagmus. In this case, if the spontaneous nystagmus and the positional nystagmus beat in the same direction, the nystagmus can be considered direction-fixed.

The clinical significance of a persistent positional nystagmus is often uncertain.[1] The mechanism of persistent positional nystagmus is uncertain. The change in orientation of the head with respect to gravity necessarily stimulates the otolith organs and may cause nystagmus. Generally, persistent positional nystagmus provides non-specific, non-localizing information, equally suggesting a central or peripheral vestibular abnormality. The ability to suppress positional nystagmus with visual fixation is a useful indicator of central nervous system function. Thus, it is important to assess a patient's ability to suppress positional nystagmus with visual fixation.

It is important to remember that positional nystagmus of low magnitude is seen in normal subjects, especially older individuals.[2] The upper limits of normal for the magnitude of positional nystagmus is 6°/s.[2] Persistent ageotropic horizontal nystagmus, especially when of high magnitude and clearly seen in all ear-down positions, may suggest horizontal semicircular canal cupulolithiasis[3] (Figure 43.4). Paroxysmal, rather than persistent, geotropic horizontal nystagmus seen in the ear-down positions (i.e. left-beating on head-left and left-lateral and right-beating on head-right and right-lateral positions) suggests horizontal semicircular canal canalithiasis[4,5] (Figure 43.5).

Paroxysmal positional nystagmus may be observed during positioning tests, i.e. using the Dix–Hallpike maneuver. The most common type of paroxysmal positional nystagmus is known as benign paroxysmal positional nystagmus, which is considered to be a result of movement of free-floating debris in the posterior semicircular canal, i.e. canalithiasis.[6,7] This nystagmus is largely torsional but also has a vertical upbeating component; that is, the nystagmus beats torsionally, with the upper pole towards the down ear and vertically towards the patient's forehead. Benign paroxysmal positional nystagmus may have a small horizontal component. Because the presence

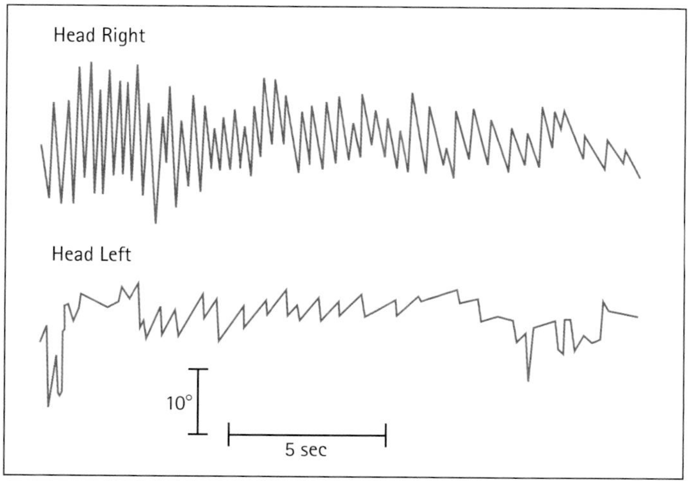

Figure 43.4 Example of persistent positional nystagmus, possibly caused by horizontal semicircular canal cupulolithiasis. The upper trace illustrates left-beating nystagmus in the right-lateral position. The lower trace illustrates right-beating nystagmus in the left-lateral position. Note the persistence of the nystagmus with minimal fluctuation in slow component velocity.

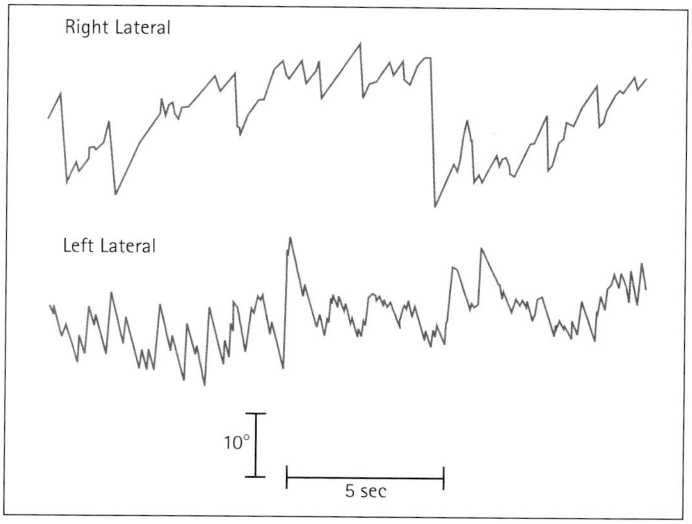

Figure 43.5 An example of paroxysmal horizontal nystagmus in a patient with horizontal semicircular canal benign paroxysmal positional vertigo caused by horizontal semicircular canal canalithiasis. The upper trace illustrates a paroxysmal horizontal right-beating nystagmus seen immediately after the patient's head was rotated from the supine position to the right-ear-down position. The lower trace illustrates a paroxysmal horizontal left-beating nystagmus seen immediately following rotation of the patient's head from the supine position to the left-ear-down position. Note that the right-beating nystagmus seen with the right ear down is of higher magnitude than the left-beating nystagmus seen with the left ear down, suggesting involvement of the right lateral semicircular canal.

of a torsional component is critical for diagnosis, the nystagmus most commonly seen with the Dix–Hallpike positioning test cannot be adequately recorded with EOG or with two-dimensional VOG. Only with three-dimensional VOG can the nystagmus associated with benign paroxysmal positional vertigo be recorded adequately. However, using EOG, recording a paroxysmal upbeating nystagmus can be highly suggestive of benign paroxysmal positional nystagmus, especially if the nystagmus begins shortly (1–2 s) after completion of the Dix–Hallpike maneuver. With some two-dimensional VOG devices, a video tape recording can be reviewed for evidence of torsional nystagmus.

As noted briefly above, a paroxysmal geotropic horizontal nystagmus suggests horizontal semicircular canalithiasis, i.e. free-floating debris in the horizontal semicircular canal. This condition can be diagnosed with a specialized maneuver that has characteristics of both persistent positional testing and the Dix–Hallpike maneuver. Specifically, in patients who are suspected of having paroxysmal positional vertigo, but who have negative Dix–Hallpike tests, a search for horizontal semicircular canal canalithiasis should be undertaken. To do this, the patient should be placed in the supine position and, once any nystagmus or vertigo has subsided, the patient's head should be rapidly turned into the left-ear-down or right-ear-down position. The patient's eye movements are observed for horizontal nystagmus that lasts longer than the maneuver. Then, the patient is returned to the supine position, again waiting for any nystagmus or vertigo to subside. Then, the patient is rapidly moved from the supine position to the opposite-ear-down position, again looking for a horizontal nystagmus.[5] If the induced nystagmus is horizontal, geotropic, and paroxysmal, a diagnosis of horizontal semicircular canal canalithiasis is confirmed.

Rotational testing

As discussed in Chapter 42, the most common type of rotational testing performed clinically is earth-vertical axis rotation using both sinusoidal motion and abrupt decelerations (so-called velocity trapezoids or impulses). Also, rotational stimuli can be combined with visual stimuli to assess visual–vestibular interaction. Both sinusoidal and trapezoidal rotational stimuli can be used to assess the overall sensitivity of the horizontal VOR (gain and magnitude), the dynamics of the VOR (phase lead and time constant), and the left–right asymmetry of the VOR (i.e. directional preponderance). The magnitude of the response to earth-vertical axis rotation, expressed either as gain for sinusoidal stimuli or magnitude for trapezoidal stimuli, reflects the overall sensitivity of the VOR. A modest decrease of gain or magnitude suggests either a significant unilateral peripheral vestibular loss or a mild bilateral loss. When the sensitivity of the VOR is severely reduced, this suggests a bilateral peripheral vestibular loss. These inferences regarding unilateral versus bilateral peripheral vestibular loss can be substantiated by responses during caloric testing (see Chapter 42 and below), except that caloric responses are more variable than rotational testing. It is essential when interpreting responses of low magnitude that the examiner be certain that the patient has a high level of alertness during testing and is not under the influence of vestibular suppressant medication. The gain of the response to rotational sinusoids changes as a function of rotational frequency, typically increasing with increased frequency. This is particularly the case for patients with markedly reduced sensitivity, wherein low-frequency responses (0.02 Hz) may be nearly absent, and high-frequency responses (1 Hz) may be virtually normal.[8] This frequency-dependent behavior reflects the dynamic characteristics of the VOR, which normally works best at about 1 Hz.

Infrequently, the sensitivity of the VOR is found to be increased, as evidenced by high gain and large magnitudes. In such cases, it likely that the normal inhibition of the VOR by the cerebellum is impaired.[9,10]

The dynamics of the VOR, as measured by phase lead for sinusoidal stimuli and time constant for trapezoidal stimuli, provide a non-specific and non-localizing measure reflecting the overall integrity of the vestibulo-ocular system. Increased phase lead and shortened time constant can be seen with unilateral peripheral vestibular loss, bilateral peripheral vestibular loss, (Figure 43.6) and some central vestibular disorders.[8,11]

The symmetry of the VOR can be measured using sinusoidal rotations or trapezoidal rotations. Asymmetry, typically reported as directional preponderance, can reflect the state of central

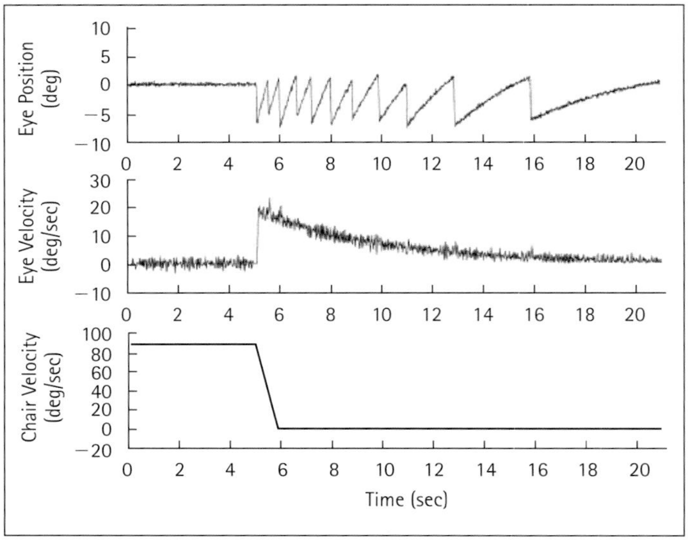

Figure 43.6 Example of a response to an abrupt cessation of constant-velocity rotation, a so-called trapezoidal rotational stimulus. In this example, the time constant of the response is short as compared to normal. The upper trace shows the nystagmoid response. The middle trace shows the slow component velocity of the nystagmus. The bottom trace illustrates the rotational chair velocity.

nervous system compensation for a unilateral peripheral vestibular ailment (Figure 43.7). In patients with a spontaneous vestibular nystagmus (and possibly a direction-fixed persistent positional nystagmus), an asymmetric rotational response is quite common. However, some patients with a peripheral vestibular disorder have an asymmetry on rotational testing but do not manifest a spontaneous or a positional nystagmus.[12] Such patients, therefore, manifest a dynamic VOR asymmetry without a static VOR asymmetry. This suggests incomplete central nervous system compensation. An asymmetry on rotational testing in patients with no evidence of a peripheral vestibular disorder should alert the clinician to a possible central vestibular imbalance. This can be seen in patients with migraine,[13–15] patients with anxiety disorders,[16] and patients without a recognized disorder.

Visual–vestibular interaction testing provides somewhat redundant information with that obtained during ocular-motor screening. In particular, the ability of a patient to inhibit vestibular nystagmus while fixating a head-stationary visual target correlates closely with the ability to pursue a small moving target. Similarly, a patient's ability to augment the VOR with vision correlates with their ability to generate optokinetic nystagmus in response to movement of a visual scene that nearly fills the visual field. An inability to suppress rotational-induced nystagmus suggests a central nervous system abnormality.[17] Such a finding is comparable to an inability to suppress a persistent positional nystagmus with visual fixation (see above) and an inability to suppress caloric-induced nystagmus (see below). When interpreting visual–vestibular interaction, it is essential to be certain that the patient has adequate vision to fixate the target and was alert and cooperative at the time of testing.

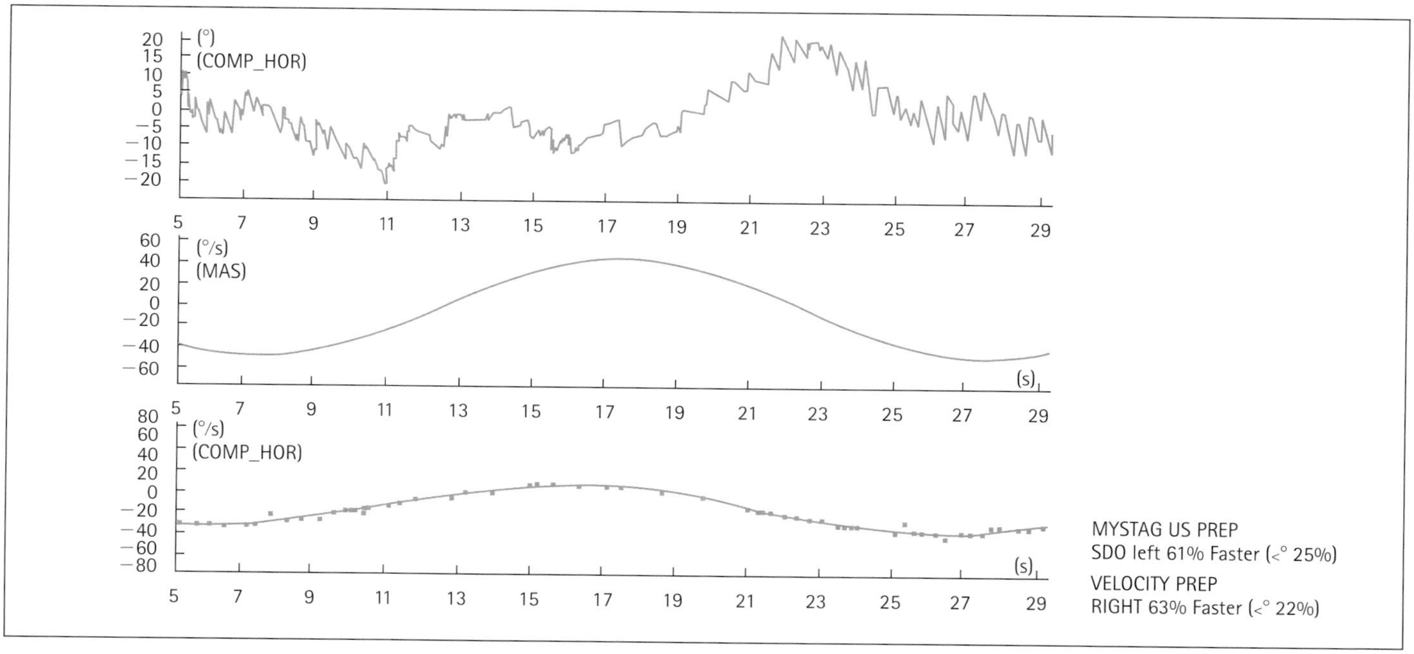

Figure 43.7 Example of directional preponderance seen with rotational testing. The middle trace illustrates the rotational velocity of the patient in a rotational test chair with a frequency of 0.05 Hz and a peak amplitude of 50°/s. The upper trace illustrates the horizontal nystagmus induced by the rotational stimulus. The lower trace illustrates the slow component velocity of the nystagmus. Note the preponderance of right-beating nystagmus in the upper trace and the concomitant asymmetric slow component velocity shown in the lower trace with a preponderance of leftward slow component velocity.

Caloric testing

Caloric testing remains the backbone of vestibular laboratory testing. As discussed in Chapter 42, caloric testing provides information regarding the function of each labyrinth separately. This distinguishes caloric testing from rotational vestibular testing and accounts for its continued popularity. The most physiologically relevant and commonly measured parameter of a patient's response to caloric stimulation is the peak magnitude of the slow component velocity obtained following each irrigation.[18] By comparing the responsiveness of the left and right labyrinths and by comparing the magnitudes of left-beating and right-beating nystagmus, caloric test results can be reduced to a measure of labyrinthine preponderance and a measure of directional preponderance. Additionally, the sum total of responses to each of the four standard caloric stimuli, i.e. left warm, right warm, left cool, and right cool, provides a measure of overall VOR sensitivity. It must be remembered that caloric testing is plagued by high variability, which necessarily reduces its ability to clearly distinguish between normal and abnormal function. By selecting the appropriate threshold for the limits of normality, each laboratory can adjust their false-positive and false-negative rates appropriately.[19,20]

A unilateral caloric reduction outside of normal limits (Figure 43.8) is typically thought to correspond to a unilateral reduction in function. A unilaterally reduced vestibular response is considered, by definition, to represent a peripheral vestibular ailment. In fact, a caloric reduction can be the result of an abnormality in the end organ, the vestibular nerve, or even the vestibular nucleus. However, it must be remembered that caloric testing merely compares the left with the right labyrinth in terms of responsiveness and thus, in patients who have well-defined responses bilaterally, an apparent reduction in responsiveness on one side may, in fact, represent an abnormally increased response contralaterally. In those patients in whom there is no consistent response from an ear, iced-water irrigations should be considered. This matter is discussed in Chapter 19.

A bilaterally reduced response to caloric testing suggests bilateral vestibular loss. However, it must be noted that, because the caloric stimulus is non-physiological and has an equivalent frequency of the order of 0.003 Hz,[21] some individuals who have absent caloric responses, even absent responses to iced-water irrigations, can have preserved rotational responses, especially at higher frequencies.[22] Thus, a diagnosis of bilateral vestibular loss based on caloric testing alone should be made with caution and should be confirmed with rotational testing.

A directional preponderance on caloric testing was at one time considered to represent a central nervous system abnormality.[23] Current thinking, however, has relegated a finding of an isolated directional preponderance on caloric testing to a non-specific, non-localizing abnormality. However, the presence of a directional preponderance on caloric testing (Figure 43.9) may provide additional confirmatory evidence for an ongoing vestibulo-ocular system imbalance. For example, in a

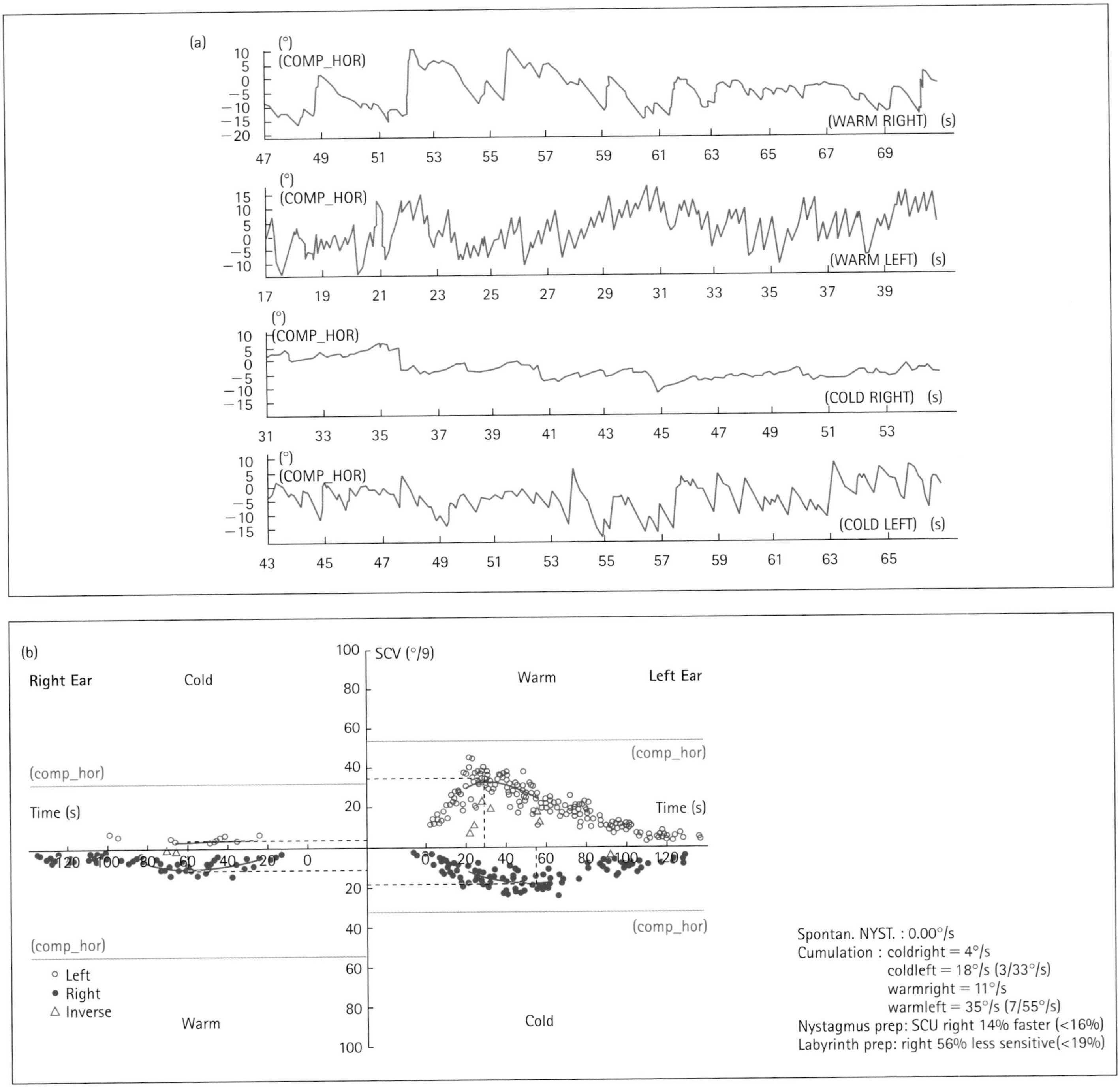

Figure 43.8 Example of caloric responses in a patient with a unilateral reduced vestibular response. (a) Horizontal nystagmus recorded with warm and cold stimulation of the right and left ears. Note the obvious reduction in the magnitude of the response to stimulation of the right ear. (b) 'Butterfly' plots of the slow component velocity response. Again, note the marked reduction of responsiveness of the right ear.

patient who has a spontaneous nystagmus, a direction-fixed positional nystagmus, and/or a directional preponderance on rotational testing, a directional preponderance on caloric testing corroborates the presence of an ongoing vestibular system imbalance. Some electro-nystagmography (ENG) analysis programs allow for a correction of the spontaneous nystagmus by subtracting the slow component velocity (SCV) of the spontaneous nystagmus from the SCV of the four caloric responses. With use of this technique, the directional preponderance may not entirely obscure left–right ear differences.

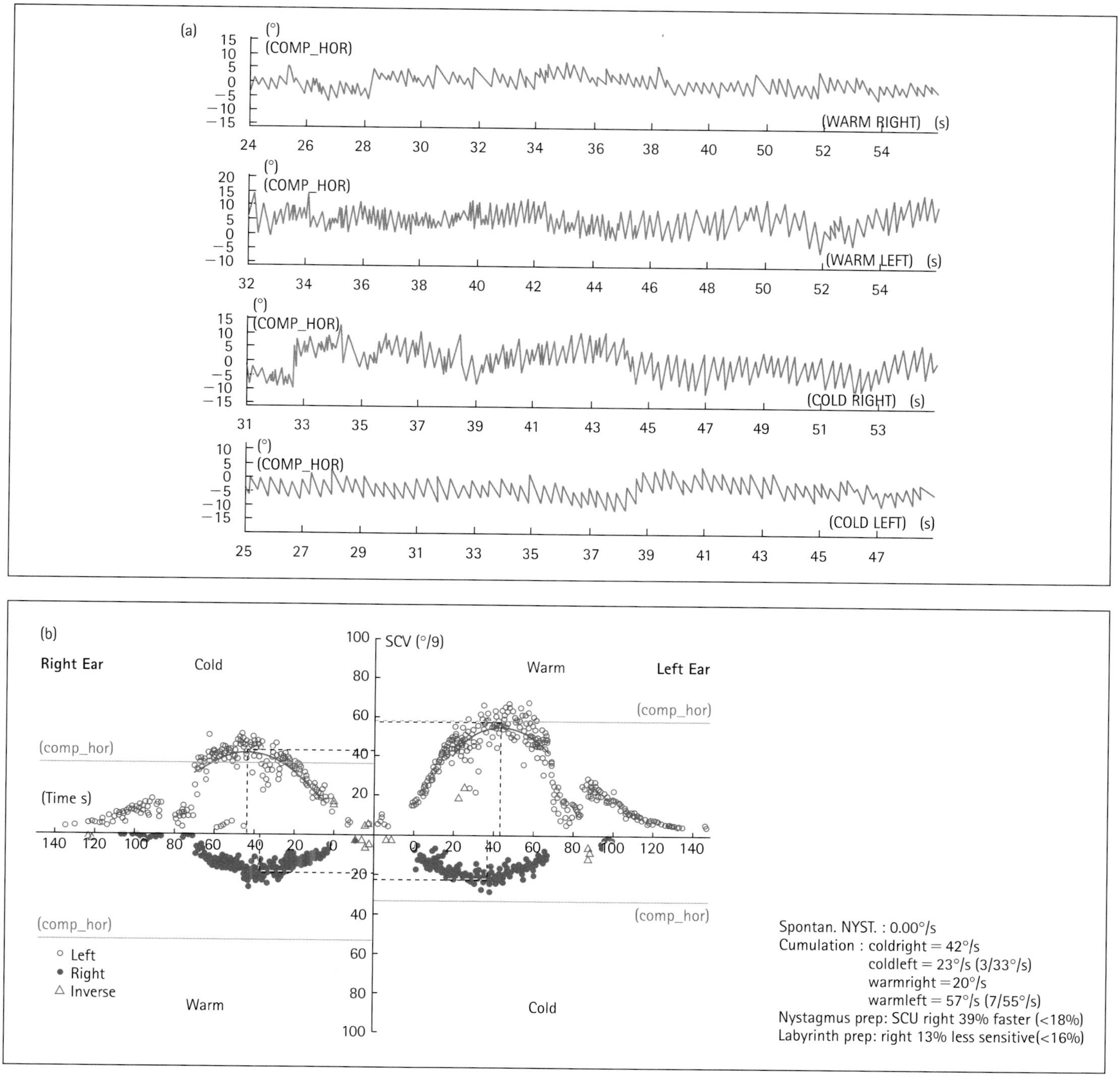

Figure 43.9 Example of a directional preponderance in the response to caloric stimulation. (a) Horizontal nystagmus recorded with warm and cold irrigation of the right and left ears. Note the preponderance of left-beating nystagmus as compared to right-beating nystagmus. (b) 'Butterfly' plots of the responses shown in (a). Again, note the preponderance of the right-cold and left-warm responses as compared to the right-warm and left-cold responses, indicating a left directional preponderance.

Patterns of testing abnormalities

Because vestibular laboratory testing is often performed as a battery of tests, several patterns of test abnormalities have been identified. Combining the results from several test modalities provides more information than any single test result alone. As indicated in Table 43.2, these patterns can help distinguish between central and peripheral vestibular disorders and, in cases of unilateral peripheral vestibular lesions, can help determine the state of central nervous system compensation for the unilateral peripheral vestibular loss. There follows a discussion on the test abnormalities that would be expected with several specific balance disorders.

Laboratory test abnormalities seen with specific balance disorders

This brief discussion of the laboratory test abnormalities often seen with selected balance disorders will attempt to place vestibular laboratory testing in some perspective with regard to its relative usefulness in establishing a diagnosis and in judging the severity of the disorder. Typically, a patient's diagnosis is not known when vestibular laboratory testing is requested. Indeed, as noted earlier in this chapter, vestibular laboratory testing is typically requested when there is a high level of suspicion of a vestibular abnormality but the diagnosis is uncertain. It should be noted that, although in some of the disorders to be discussed below vestibular laboratory testing may be normal, a normal result may still be considered useful in helping to establish a diagnosis, by ruling out other conditions.

Benign paroxysmal positional vertigo

Benign paroxysmal positional vertigo (BPPV) can be diagnosed definitively by observing the characteristic torsional–vertical nystagmus provoked by the Dix–Hallpike maneuver. Unfortunately, unless a laboratory is equipped with three-dimensional VOG, such nystagmus cannot be quantitated in the vestibular laboratory. With use of a two-dimensional VOG system that includes video recording, the patient's eye movements can be evaluated by reviewing the video tape. Although not quantitative, this can aid with diagnosis. With EOG, only the vertical (upbeating) and inconstant horizontal components of the nystagmus associated with BPPV can be recorded. Even if it does not help in obtaining a definitive diagnosis, vestibular laboratory testing can be useful in the assessment of patients with BPPV. That is, a significant percentage of patients with BPPV manifest laboratory abnormalities other than the characteristic paroxysmal positional nystagmus.[24,25] These laboratory abnormalities may include a unilateral reduction of responsiveness to caloric irrigation, a spontaneous nystagmus, and/or a directional preponderance on rotational testing. BPPV is considered to be a disorder localized to the posterior semicircular canal,[26] whereas caloric and earth-vertical axis rotation assess the horizontal semicircular canal. Thus, vestibular laboratory abnormalities other than paroxysmal positional nystagmus in patients with BPPV may suggest a more widespread vestibular disorder beyond simply a posterior semicircular canal abnormality.

Menière's disease

Typically, patients with unilateral Menière's disease will show a unilateral reduction in caloric sensitivity.[27] However, depending upon the clinical progression of the patient's disorder and the time at which laboratory testing is obtained, patients may have normal vestibular testing, much as they may have normal audiometric testing between episodes, especially early in the course of the disorder. Over time, a caloric reduction may or may not be seen.[28] Also, vestibular laboratory testing can provide some inferences regarding either how recently a patient has suffered from a Menière's attack or how well they have compensated for a recent vestibular insult. Specifically, a spontaneous nystagmus and/or a directional preponderance on caloric or rotational testing suggests an incomplete state of central nervous system compensation for peripheral vestibular loss, which is often the case in the early stages of the disease, due to the changing functional status of the peripheral vestibular system. In patients with bilateral Menière's disease, there may be evidence of bilateral vestibular loss. This includes a reduction in the total slow component velocity obtained with binaural bithermal caloric testing and a reduced gain on rotational testing.

In general, vestibular laboratory testing is not particularly helpful for establishing a diagnosis of Menière's disease, because the diagnosis is based primarily on the history and the presence of a characteristic low-frequency hearing loss.

However, vestibular laboratory testing does indicate the functional status of the impaired vestibular system and can be particularly helpful in the management of patients with Menière's disease who are being treated with chemical ablation. For example, following treatment with transtympanic gentamicin, caloric testing of the involved ear may provide information regarding the presence of remaining vestibular function in that ear. It must be remembered, of course, that caloric testing only assesses the horizontal semicircular canal at a very low equivalent frequency.[21] Thus, even in the absence of a response to iced-water irrigation, vestibular function in the involved, treated ear still may be present.

Migraine

There have been several studies that have assessed vestibular function in patients with migraine.[13–15] These studies have suggested a high prevalence of vestibular laboratory abnormalities. The rate of vestibular laboratory abnormalities is high in migraine sufferers who do not have dizziness as well as in those who do have dizziness. A study of patients with migraine-associated dizziness[15] reported a variety of laboratory abnormalities. The authors note that there is no pathognomonic pattern of vestibular laboratory abnormalities in patients with migraine-associated dizziness. Moreover, patients with migraine-associated dizziness may have normal vestibular laboratory testing, evidence of peripheral vestibular abnormality, or evidence of a VOR asymmetry without evidence of a peripheral vestibular abnormality. Despite this wide variability in test results, vestibular laboratory testing can be helpful both diagnostically and with treatment. For example, the presence of a directional preponderance on rotational testing may suggest that a low dose of a vestibular suppressant medication or a course of balance rehabilitation therapy may be beneficial.

Anxiety disorders

Vestibular laboratory abnormalities have been demonstrated in patients with anxiety disorders.[16] Certainly, not all patients with anxiety disorders have a vestibular system abnormality, but there does appear to be an association between anxiety disorders and balance disorders, as evidenced by a particularly high prevalence of vestibular laboratory abnormalities in patients with panic disorder or panic disorder with agoraphobia. Specifically, unilateral caloric reductions have been reported in patients with agoraphobia, as has directional preponderance on rotational testing.[16] The basis for the vestibular laboratory abnormalities in anxiety disorders is unknown.

Cerebellopontine angle tumors

Patients with cerebellopontine angle tumors, including individuals suffering from vestibular schwannomas (acoustical neuroma), may manifest a unilateral caloric reduction on the side of the lesion.[29,30] Often, such patients have minimal, if any, vestibular-related symptoms, because of the gradual nature of the peripheral vestibular loss, which allows central compensation mechanisms to perform optimally. Thus, patients may be found to have a unilateral caloric reduction even if they have no vestibular symptoms. With large cerebellopontine angle tumors, particularly those associated with compression of the cerebellum, patients may exhibit abnormalities on ocular-motor testing, including abnormal smooth pursuit, gaze-evoked nystagmus, and, in some patients, Brun's nystagmus, which consists of a combination of gaze-evoked nystagmus when looking towards the side of the lesion and vestibular nystagmus when looking towards the uninvolved ear.[31] Additionally, torsional eye movements may be present. Thus, although vestibular laboratory testing cannot be considered particularly useful in establishing a diagnosis of an VIIIth nerve tumor, information regarding the amount of remaining peripheral vestibular function may be useful in planning management. Specifically, with surgical treatment, postoperative vertigo would be expected to be more severe in patients with relatively preserved vestibular function preoperatively. However, unilateral caloric areflexia does not necessarily guarantee that postoperatively there will be little to no vertigo. Also, the evolution of VOR gain after surgery is particularly useful for monitoring the rehabilitation process. The role of vestibular laboratory testing in the management of acoustical neuroma patients treated with radiosurgery (gamma knife) is unknown.

Lateral medullary infarction

Patients who have suffered from a lateral medullary infarction, i.e. Wallenberg's syndrome, usually manifest a characteristic pattern of eye-movement abnormalities, including a spontaneous nystagmus, saccadic lateropulsion, and asymmetric ocular pursuit.[32] Vestibular laboratory testing is not particularly useful diagnostically in cases of Wallenberg's syndrome, as the history, neurological examination and brain imaging provide the necessary information. However, vestibular laboratory testing can provide quantitative information regarding how extensively a patient's central vestibular system has been damaged by the infarction.

Ototoxic drug exposure

Patients who have been treated systemically with ototoxic drugs such as aminoglycoside antibiotics or certain chemotherapeutic agents such as cisplatinum may complain of dysequilibrium if they have lost significant peripheral vestibular function bilaterally. During the course of treatment, however, patients may be asymptomatic, since most vestibular symptoms, including vertigo, result from asymmetric vestibular function. Moreover, patients typically adapt quickly to even moderate bilateral peripheral vestibular loss and thus remain essentially asymptomatic. Occasionally, patients exposed to ototoxic drugs systemically may experience vertigo, suggesting asymmetric vestibular involvement. The most common vestibular laboratory abnormalities with ototoxic drug exposure include bilateral caloric reduction and reduced gain on rotational testing.[33] When these are severe, patients with bilateral vestibular loss may have entirely absent responses. Frequently, patients have preservation of high-frequency rotational responses despite absent caloric responses, including absent response to iced-water irrigations. If the magnitude of rotational responses is large enough to obtain a reliable estimate of VOR dynamics, the phase lead of the VOR during sinusoidal stimulation will be increased. Comparably, patients with bilateral vestibular loss, when tested with trapezoidal rotation, will have a reduced magnitude of response and a shortened VOR time constant. Occasionally, patients suffering from ototoxic drug exposure demonstrate an asymmetric vestibular response, i.e. a difference in responsiveness on caloric testing or a directional preponderance on rotational testing. This may relate to asymmetric involvement of the labyrinth and/or reflect some aspect of the compensation process.

Overall, vestibular laboratory testing in patients exposed to ototoxic medications provides highly useful information regarding the severity of the damage and the status of the patient's compensation, including the presence or absence of a VOR asymmetry. Recently, it has been reported that some patients with bilateral vestibular loss may have relatively preserved otolith-ocular responses. The information from vestibular laboratory testing in patients with ototoxic drug exposure may be useful to physical therapists who are designing rehabilitation regimens.[34]

References

1. Brandt T. Background, technique, interpretation, and usefulness of positional and positioning testing. In: Jacobson GP, Newman CW, Kartush JM, eds. *Handbook of Balance Function Testing*. St Louis, MO: Mosby Year Book, 1993: 123–55.

2. Barber HO, Stockwell CW. *Manual of Electronystagmography*, 2nd edn. St. Louis: C.V. Mosby, 1980.
3. Baloh RW, Yue Q, Jacobson K, Honrubia V. Persistent direction-changing positional nystagmus: another variant of benign positional nystagmus? *Neurology* 1995; **45**: 1297–301.
4. McClure JA. Horizontal canal BPV. *J Otolaryngol* 1985; **14**: 30–5.
5. Fife T. Recognition and management of horizontal canal benign positional vertigo. *Am J Otol* 1998; **19**: 345–51.
6. Hall S, Ruby R, McClure J. The mechanics of benign paroxysmal vertigo. *J Otolaryngol* 1979; **8**: 151–8.
7. Epley J. Positional vertigo related to semicircular canalithiasis. *Otolaryngol Head Neck Surg* 1995; **112**: 154–61.
8. Baloh RW, Honrubia V, Yee RD, Hess K. Changes in the human vestibulo-ocular reflex after loss of peripheral sensitivity. *Ann Neurol* 1984; **16**: 222.
9. Baloh RW, Demer JL. Optokinetic–vestibular interaction in patients with increased gain of the vestibulo-ocular reflex. *Exp Brain Res* 1993; **97**: 334–42.
10. Thurston SE, Leigh RJ, Abel LA, Dell'Osso LF. Hyperactive vestibulo-ocular reflex in cerebellar degeneration: pathogenesis and treatment. *Neurology* 1987; **37**: 53–7.
11. Furman JM, Becker JT. Vestibular responses in Wernicke's encephalopathy. *Ann Neurol* 1989; **26**: 669–74.
12. Jenkins HA. Long-term adaptive changes of the vestibulo-ocular reflex in patients following acoustic neuroma surgery. *Laryngoscope* 1985; **95**(10): 1224–34.
13. Toglia JU, Thomas D, Kuritzky A. Common migraine and vestibular function electronystagmographic study and pathogenesis. *Ann Otol* 1981; **90**: 267–71.
14. Kayan A, Hood JD. Neuro-otological manifestations of migraine. *Brain* 1984; **107**: 1123–42.
15. Cass SP, Furman JM, Ankerstjerne J, Balaban C, Yetiser S, Aydogan B. Migraine-related vestibulopathy. *Ann Otol Rhinol Laryngol* 1997; **106**: 181–9.
16. Jacob RG, Furman JM, Durrant JD, Turner SM. Panic, agoraphobia and vestibular dysfunction: clinical test results. *Am J Psychiatry* 1996; **153**: 503–12.
17. Baloh RW, Jenkins H, Honrubia V, Yee R, Lau C. Visual–vestibular interaction and cerebellar atrophy. *Neurology* 1979; **29**(1): 116–19.
18. Luxon LM. Comparison of assessment of caloric nystagmus by observation of duration and by electronystagmographic measurement of slow-phase velocity. *Br J Audiol* 1995; **29**: 107–16.
19. Furman JM, Wall III C, Kamerer DB: Alternate and simultaneous binaural bithermal caloric test: a comparison. *Ann Otol Rhinol Laryngol* 1988; **97**(4): 359–64.
20. Jacobson GP, Newman CW, Peterson EL. Interpretation and usefulness of caloric testing. In: Jacobson GP, Newman CW, Kartush JM eds. *Handbook of Balance Function Testing*. St Louis, MO: Mosby Year Book, 1993: 101–22.
21. Hamid M, Hughes G, Kinney, S. Criteria for diagnosing bilateral vestibular dysfunction. In: Graham MD, Kemink JL, eds. *The Vestibular System: Neurophysicologic and Clinical Research*. New York: Raven Press, 1987; 115–18.
22. Furman JM, Kamerer DB. Rotational responses in patients with bilateral caloric reduction. *Acta Otolaryngol (Stockh)* 1989; **108**: 355–61.
23. Fitzgerald G, Hallpike CS. Studies in human vestibular function. I. Observations on the directional preponderance ('nystagmus-bereitschaft') of caloric nystagmus resulting from cerebral lesions. *Brain*, 1942; 62(part 2): 115–17.
24. Baloh R, Honrubia V, Jacobson K. Benign positional vertigo: clinical and oculographic features in 240 cases. *Neurology*, 1987; **37**: 371–8.
25. McClure J, Lycett P, Rounthwaite J. Vestibular dysfunction associated with benign paroxysmal vertigo. *Laryngoscope* 1977; **137**: 1–9.
26. Furman JM, Cass SP. Benign paroxysmal positional vertigo. *N Engl J Med* 1999; **341**(21): 1590–6.
27. Hulshof JH, Baarsma EA. Vestibular investigations in Meniere's disease. *Acta Otolaryngol* 1981; **92**: 75–81.
28. Hulshof JH, Baarsma EA. Vestibular investigations in Meniere's disease. *Acta Otolaryngol (Stockh)* 1981; **92**: 379–401.
29. Tos M, Thomsen J. Epidemiology of acoustic neuromas. *J Laryngol Otol* 1984; **98**: 685–92.
30. Baloh RW, Konrad HR, Dirks D, Honrubia V. Cerebellopontine angle tumors. *Arch Neurol* 1976; **33**: 507–12.
31. Nedzelski JM. Cerebellopontine angle tumors: bilateral flocculus compression as a cause of associated oculomotor abnormalities. *Laryngoscope* 1983; **93**: 1251–60.
32. Leigh RJ, Zee DS. *The Neurology of Eye Movements*, 3rd edn. New York: Oxford University Press, 1999.
33. Hess K. Vestibulotoxic drugs and other causes of acquired bilateral peripheral vestibulopathy. In: Baloh RW, Halmagyi GM, eds. *Disorders of the Vestibular System*. New York: Oxford University Press, 1996: 360–73.
34. Peterka RJ, Shupert CL, Horak FB. Ocular counterrolling and OVAR tests identify preserved otolith function in some subjects with bilateral vestibular deficits. Abstract. ARO Midwinter Meeting, St Petersburg Beach, FL, 1998.

44 Posturography

Adolfo M Bronstein

Vertigo, dizziness and unsteadiness are common complaints and almost all medical practitioners are likely to encounter patients with these symptoms in their practice. Clinicians with a special interest in these patients, oto-neurologists or neuro-otologists, have different training backgrounds, usually neurology, otolaryngology or audiology. In practice, this introduces a bias in the type of patients seen and in the emphasis placed on different aspects of the clinical examination. It is thus expected that the laboratory investigation of these patients, including posturography, will also be influenced by the clinician's own background.

A 'Medline' literature survey conducted in 1999 with the key words 'posturography' and 'value' (for clinical value), identified 20 papers published between 1984 and 1998. According to the address identifier, 11 of these papers originated from otolaryngology (ORL) departments, three from physical/occupational therapy departments, three from various institutions (psychiatry, basic sciences, orthopaedics) but only two from neurological departments. This limited survey certainly agrees with my impression that ORL/audiology departments are more keen on the use of posturography for clinical purposes than are neurology departments. This could indicate that ORL specialists are either more interested in dizziness or see more dizzy patients than other specialists, but I believe that it indicates that neurologists tend to rely on their own clinical assessment of posture and gait.

Undergraduate and postgraduate neurological teaching places strong emphasis on clinical inspection of postural balance and gait as an important part of the routine neurological examination. Almost all neurological diseases impair gait and posture—common ones such as stroke, spasticity, multiple sclerosis, Parkinson's disease and polyneuropathies, and not so common ones such as the dystonias, and degenerative and inherited disorders. The assessment of posture and gait has been traditionally valued in neurology and is a source of anecdotes. Pierre Marie, one of the masters of early French neurology, was said to be able to diagnose gait disorders by the sound of the patients' gait before they entered the consulting room. This prompted his students to find more and more difficult cases to test Pierre Marie's unusual skill to the limit. Eventually, a French nun with a wooden leg proved too much for the old master (J.E. Burucua, personal communication).

This anecdote, by way of introduction, is just to emphasize the value of the clinical investigation of gait and posture in patients with unsteadiness. I will first summarize the clinical examination of posture and gait, and then address the contribution of posturography.

Clinical examination of balance, posture and gait

Gait unsteadiness is associated with a wide range of disorders.[1] If it has never been associated with vertigo, dizziness, oscillopsia or a hearing disorder it is unlikely to be due to vestibular disease.[2] It is usually possible to establish a topographical diagnosis (site of lesion) in a gait disorder on the basis of clinical observation of gait and a formal neurological examination (Table 44.1).[3–5]

It is beyond the scope of this chapter to describe the many individual diseases with gait disorder. However, the mental 'checklist' required when examining a patient with gait unsteadiness will be reviewed (Table 44.2).

Posture

Observation of head and trunk posture can give immediate useful information. There are abnormal tilts or rotations in dystonia, flexed posture in Parkinson's disease, hyperextension in progressive supranuclear palsy (PSP), and titubation in cerebellar disease. Observation of stance will reveal a broadening of the base of support in diffuse vascular disease, frontal lesions, cerebellar lesions, sensory ataxia, acute vestibular lesions and patients with a cautious gait. Minor degrees of unsteadiness can be brought about by asking the patient to put the feet together or in the heel-to-toe position. A 'bouncy' stance, with head–trunk oscillations c. 2–3 Hz, may be observed in ataxic or ataxic–spastic disorders, typically in multiple sclerosis. A shaky

Table 44.1 Topographical classification of lesions causing stance and gait abnormalities.[3–5]

Lower levels
- Peripheral lesions: mono/polyneuropathies, root lesions and myopathies
- Vestibular and visual lesions

Medium levels
- Spinal and brainstem lesions

Higher levels
- Cerebellar syndromes
- Subcortical disorders (basal ganglia and internal capsule): Parkinson's disease, orthostatic tremor, choreas and corticospinal tract lesions

Highest levels
- Frontal lesions of the cerebral cortex, white matter in the semioval centre and periventricular area (vascular, degenerative diseases, demyelinating diseases, tumours and hydrocephalus)

Cautious gait and psychogenic gait disorders

Table 44.2 Examination of posture and gait.[3–5]

1. Posture
   - Head and neck
   - Trunk
   - Stance and Romberg test
   - Postural reflexes
2. Walking
   - Step initiation
   - Stepping pattern
   - Associated trunk and arm movements
   - Eyes closed walking
3. Neurological and relevant skeletal examination

'tremulous' stance with higher-frequency oscillations, can be seen in some patients with Parkinson's disease and orthostatic tremor (Figure 44.1). The Romberg test, originally described for patients with tabes dorsalis, is positive in patients with dorsal column or severe afferent polyneuropathy. A positive Romberg test means that the patient shows a tendency to actually fall, unlike normal subjects and almost all patients with balance problems, who show a small-to-moderate increase in body sway on eye closure. In a patient with either cerebellar degeneration or polyneuropathy, a high level of unsteadiness on eye closure may indicate the presence of additional bilateral vestibular failure.[6] Patients with anterior lobe cerebellar degeneration may show the characteristic trunk oscillation or titubation only on eye closure; when mild, this may just be visible as a tremor of the ankle extensors ('dancing tendons'). Of practical note, anyone who can stand on either foot unaided, with eyes closed, is unlikely to have any objective postural balance problem. Postural reflexes are examined by gently pushing the upper trunk. This can be done standing behind the patient so that

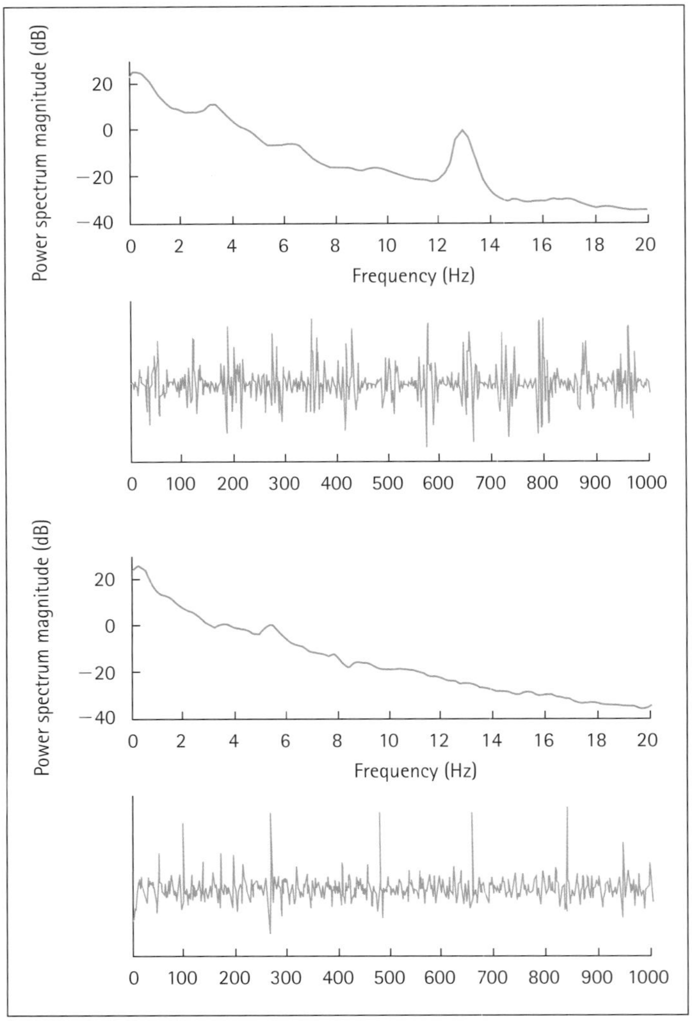

Figure 44.1 Tremulous stance in extrapyramidal disorders. The upper box depicts a patient with orthostatic tremor, showing high-frequency body tremor at 13 Hz and samples of lower-limb EMG. The lower box shows a patient with Parkinson's disease with slight tremor at c. 5.5 Hz. (Modified from Yarrow et al. *Gait Posture* 2001; **13**: 27–34.[88])

they cannot anticipate the precise timing and direction of the push (forwards or backwards) to the shoulders. In akinetic syndromes, these responses may be completely absent, e.g. advanced Parkinson's disease or early PSP, then patients fall rigidly like a log. A few shuffling steps backwards (retropulsion) or forwards can be seen in the early stages. In cerebellar syndromes, particularly anterior lobe disease, the trunk pushes may unmask a trunk titubation, observable as a 'trunk rebound' in response to the push. In the elderly with fear of falling or a cautious gait, trunk pushes trigger a startle, panic-like response.

Walking

Step initiation can be impaired in frontal lesions, including the gait ignition failure syndrome[3,4] and as part of the akinesia in the Parkinsonian syndromes. Initiation of gait is hesitant, the feet appearing to be stuck to the ground (magnetic feet; slipping clutch phenomenon). The steady-state stepping pattern may be less disturbed in patients with difficulty in step initiation, once they are off. In akinetic–rigid Parkinsonian syndromes, steps are often shallow, short and slow but with preserved rhythm. In contrast, cerebellar patients show irregular rhythm, variable length, oscillations and a wide base, giving a lurching, 'drunken' appearance to their walking. Patients with severe loss of sensory information from the lower limbs (sensory ataxia) lift the feet high and place them on the ground under intense visual control; in dorsal column lesions, the heel strikes the ground first (tabetic gait); in cases with ankle extensor weakness (foot drop), the toes make contact first (steppage). In spasticity, the knee extensor and ankle flexor hypertonus leads to the characteristic slow gait with circumduction movements of the leg during the swing phase. The normal associated movements of the arms while walking are lost in Parkinson's disease. Unilateral loss of arm swing can be a useful early sign in Parkinson's disease and hemiparesis. In arteriosclerotic Parkinsonism due to frontal vascular lesions, associated movements and facial expression tend to remain unaffected. Since these patients have a shuffling gait, the condition is sometimes called 'lower-half' Parkinsonism. Patients with cautious gait reach out with their arms as if expecting to fall, and step with apparently unnecessary care, giving the appearance of 'walking on ice'; this gait pattern can be triggered by a vestibular or vascular episode or by a fall, but sometimes is the only finding in elderly patients. Walking with eyes closed in a straight line can reveal a previously unsuspected degree of unsteadiness or a cautious gait in patients with bilateral loss of vestibular function. In unilateral vestibular lesions, at least in the acute stage, patients veer in the same direction as the lesion. In somatosensory ataxia, this task is often impossible.

Summary of the relevant neurological examination

We present a summary of the neurological examination relevant to balance and gait disorders, in the hope that it may guide the non-neurologist who suspects a neurological cause for unsteadiness or gait disorder. Weakness of the legs can be documented by asking the patient to push against the examiner's hands with different muscle groups or by asking the patient to stand/walk on tiptoes and heels, and crouch and rise. Identification of weakness of the ankle extensors is paramount, as these muscles are responsible for toe clearance during the swing phase of the gait cycle. Even if a foot drop is not clinically observed, weakness can cause the toes to get caught when the patient walks fast or under pressure, on uneven ground or with inappropriate footware. Lower-limb weakness is a major contributor to the gait disorder in muscle, root and peripheral nerve disease, and motoneurone and pyramidal tract disease. The osteotendinous reflexes will be exaggerated in pyramidal tract disease and depressed or absent in all the others; extensor cutaneous plantar responses (Babinski sign) can be found in pyramidal lesions. Normal somatosensory function is needed for voluntary placing of the feet while walking, as well as for the proprioceptive reflexes controlling upright posture. At least pin-prick, tuning fork and joint position sense must be examined in the lower limbs. If large fibres carrying proprioceptive input are involved, the ankle and sometimes patella jerks will be absent and the Romberg test will be positive. In peripheral polyneuropathies, the degree of unsteadiness correlates with the decrease in vibration perception rather than with weakness, which testifies to the significance of the somatosensory input in postural control.[7]

NEUROLOGICAL CHECKLIST FOR BALANCE AND GAIT DISORDERS.

- Weakness of legs
- Somatosensory function
  - principle
  - vibration
  - joint position sensation
- Sphincter disturbance
- Cranial nerve dysfunction
- Cellebellar signs
  - nystagmus
  - trunk titubation
  - intention tremor
  - past pointing
- Basal ganglia signs
  - bradykinisia
  - rigidity
  - dytonia

Gait disorders due to neurological involvement at medium or high levels (Table 44.1) will have associated clinical neurological features. In spinal cord compression or lesions, there are often sphincter dysfunction and sensory disturbances in the limbs. At the brainstem level, there is cranial nerve involvement, including central vestibular and ocular–motor disorders; at the cerebellar level, there is trunk titubation, intentional tremor, and abnormal eye movements, including nystagmus; at the basal ganglia level, there are Parkinsonian features (including tremor, cogwheel rigidity, hypomimia, bradykinesia, loss of postural reflexes), dystonic limb or neck posturing and choreoathetosis. It is important to keep in mind the current, unabated weight of the clinical neurological examination in the assessment of balance and gait disorders. Normal CT and MRI scans do not exclude neurological disease (e.g. Parkinson's disease), and posturography findings usually lack topographical and aetiological specificity. In addition, skeletal and cardiovascular examination are mandatory in the elderly. There is an emerging body of evidence that cardiovascular syncope is a major cause for unexplained dizzy spells and falls in the elderly, regardless of whether the patient reports loss of consciousness.[8,9]

Posturography

Strictly speaking, posturography is any means of recording postural activity, not only sway or force platforms, which are indeed the most convenient way. The need for other recording devices arises because 'sway' platforms do not actually measure body sway but only measure foot torque (N_m), conveniently expressed as movement of the centre of foot pressure (c_m). The dissociation between sway and centre of pressure is customarily illustrated with examples of the type shown in Figure 44.2. Imagine a subject standing still on a platform; he suddenly increases activity in his ankle flexor muscles, i.e. he pushes down hard with the ball of his feet and toes. His centre of pressure will move forwards, and this is the signal that a 'sway' platform will initially record. It is clear, however, that, as a result of pushing down on his toes, the subject's centre of mass, its vertical projection (centre of gravity) and the subject as a whole will move backwards. In order to capture the real sway, additional recordings of head or trunk motion would be needed. Simultaneous EMG recordings from the lower limbs would improve the picture, as they would identify the burst of activity preceding the movement of the centre of foot pressure. Goniometric (angle) measurements of the ankle joint would confirm that the ankle moved in flexion rather than extension, thus completing the full postural motion picture.

Although for some standard clinical purposes platform signals alone are acceptable, e.g. comparing a group of patients before and after a treatment, specific questions on the mechanisms involved in postural control require some or all of the recordings mentioned above. Some of the more commonly used in practice are: photo-electrical or electromagnetic recordings of head sway, accelerometric measurements of head or trunk motion, and EMG signals from the lower limbs, alone or in combination with trunk, abdominal and cervical muscle recordings.

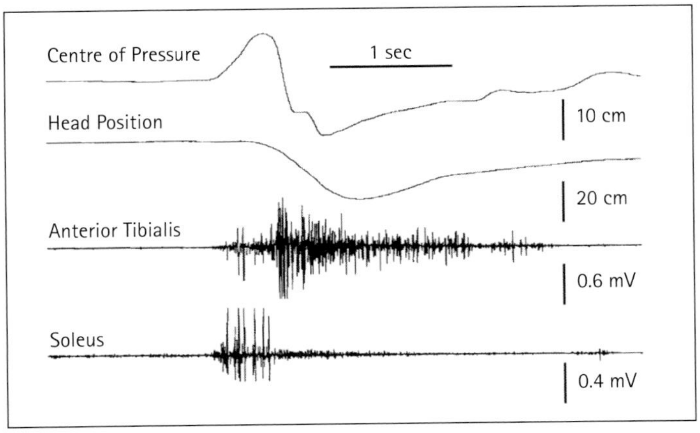

Figure 44.2 Dissociation between centre of pressure and actual body sway. Recordings of a subject's anteroposterior displacement of the centre of foot pressure when standing on a posturography platform during a sudden push-down of toes and ball of the feet. The earliest activity is registered in soleus EMG. Note that although the subject swayed backwards, as shown by head position and late centre of foot pressure traces, the initial movement of the centre of foot pressure was forwards. Upward deflections in the centre of foot pressure and head position displacement indicate displacement forwards; downward deflections indicate displacement backwards.

> If the patient just stands quietly on the platform, with eyes open or closed, the procedure is called *static posturography*. When additional balance perturbations or stimuli (e.g. moving platform, visual stimuli, muscle vibration) are added, it is called *dynamic posturography*.

Three general questions can be asked in the area of posturography: has posturography advanced the knowledge of how postural mechanisms work, has posturography taught us how posture is impaired in patient groups, and does posturography help in the management of an individual patient complaining of a balance problem? The answer to the first two questions is certainly yes, but opinions are divided as to the third.

A detailed discussion on posture and balance mechanisms can be found in Chapters 38 and 46. Posturographic techniques have been useful in defining the contribution of the different sensori-motor components to postural control. The first attempts to generate a comprehensive system approach to postural control were led by Nashner and co-workers.[10–13] They suggested that postural balance is maintained on the basis of a limited repertoire of centrally generated muscle synergies. During slight perturbations to balance, the body behaves essentially as an inverted pendulum, pivoting around the ankle joints. Muscular responses are organized in a distal-to-proximal manner, with activation of distal muscles such as tibialis anterior and soleus occurring earlier than that of proximal ones; this is the 'ankle strategy'. Larger perturbations to balance or lesser possibility of response (e.g. standing on a narrow beam) led to movements around the hip joints and earlier activation of proximal muscles, such as abdominal, paraspinalis, quadriceps and hamstrings; this was called the 'hip strategy'.

These studies were also of value in quantifying adaptability and sensory 'redundancy' in the postural system. The posturography system designed by Nashner consists of a support platform and a visual surround which can be moved angularly about an approximate inter-ankle axis. This setting allows for the ankle and visual information available to the subject to be, at least partly, neutralized by means of coupling the visual surround or the support surface to the anteroposterior sway movements of the subject. This set-up formed the basis of the commercial product 'Equitest', a computerized dynamic posturography (CDP) system, particularly the testing protocol known as the sensory organization test. If patients with vestibular deficits are allowed to stand freely on this system, they show little or no difficulty if the platform is stationary, with normal visual information (e.g. stable surrounds) or with eyes closed. When either or both the platform and visual surround are sway coupled, patients have poor balance performance.[14,15] This led to the hypothesis that the vestibular signal is normally used in postural control as an inertial-gravitational reference system against which conflicts in the other sensory inputs are resolved, i.e. a kind of plumb line. Adaptability of the postural system to stimuli evoking unhelpful postural reactions (toe-up platform rotations which trigger unwanted EMG responses in gastrocnemius) was thought to depend on cerebellar function.[16] A summary of the testing conditions available in the sensory-organization test part of the CDP system is given in Figure 44.3.

Many findings and concepts emanating from the work of Nashner have since been challenged or disproved. Experiments have shown that an important role played by the vestibular system is not 'referential' but in generating fast, short-latency descending vestibulospinal postural responses.[17,18] The role of ankle afferents, as a main afferent source, has also been questioned; trunk and hip movements and proximal EMG responses are critical components in postural stability and seem to be independent of ankle input.[19,20]

In addition, the assumption that torque signals from the ankles can be used to couple the visual surround to head sway, based on the debated concept that the body sways as an 'inverted pendulum', does not seem realistic.[21] Further, cerebellar patients show a number of postural deficiencies but they do not have adaptive difficulties with suppressing 'unwanted' postural responses to visual[22] or support-surface motion[23,24] stimuli. Finally, when presented in a historical context, the findings in vestibular patients seem trivial. Clinicians have known for decades that vestibular patients are usually normal in static conditions and that the way to unveil their unsteadiness is to examine them with eyes closed under conditions of reduced proprioceptive accuracy, e.g. on a mattress.[25] In spite of these criticisms, the systematic approach of the work by Nashner and co-workers was the initial driving force which triggered enormous physiological, clinical and also commercial interest in the field of posturography.

Sensory organization:	1	2	3	4	5	6
Patterns of postural disorientation						
Visually dependent		?	*		?	*
Surface dependent				*	*	*
Vestibular loss					*	*
Sensory selection			*	*	*	*

* = Body sway excessive or falls
? = May or may not show abnormal sway

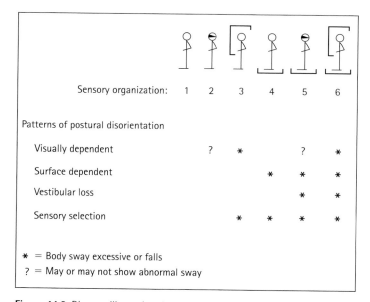

Figure 44.3 Diagram illustrating the testing conditions encountered in the sensory organization test of the CDP. In (1), all sensory inputs are normally available; in (2), subjects close their eyes; in (3), the visual surround is 'sway referenced' (i.e. driven by the movements of the centre of foot pressure and thus providing inaccurate feedback about sway to the subject); in (4), the platform is 'sway referenced'; in (5), the platform is 'sway referenced' and the eyes are closed; and in (6), both the supporting platform and the visual surround are 'sway referenced'. Several of the assumptions underlying this approach have been questioned (see text for details). Underneath, the various patterns of postural disorientation which may be encountered are listed. Identification of these patterns may be useful for rehabilitation but this has not been firmly proven. (From Shumway-Cook et al. In: Bronstein, Brandt and Wollacolt, eds. *Clinical Disorders of Balance Posture and Gait*. London: Arnold 1996: 211–35.[71])

Posturography in peripheral vestibular disorders

Clinical observation of patients with severe acute, unilateral vestibular disorders, e.g. vestibular neuritis, shows that they tend to fall towards the side of the lesion on eye closure—i.e. in the direction of the slow phase of nystagmus.[26] This can be documented by posturography but with little practical clinical benefit for the individual patient. In the compensated state, static posturography with eyes open or closed is usually normal. CDP shows increased sway in conditions in which the support surface, the visual surroundings or both simultaneously are unstable (sway referenced). In some early series, 100% of patients were reported to be abnormal when both visual surround and support surface were sway referenced;[15] in others, this figure dropped to around 50%.[27] In a small but carefully controlled series, 10 patients with severe unilateral caloric reduction were abnormal when tested in the acute stage only under unstable support/visual surroundings.[28] Within 2 weeks, all patients regained total normality in all test conditions. The reasons for these discrepancies are not clear, but the inability to confirm the earlier reports is one of the reasons underlying the current disaffection with the technique.

A problem that is relevant to clinicians is what is the added value of posturography in comparison with traditional testing of the vestibular system. A comparison between posturography and the caloric test showed that the caloric test correlates better with a history of vertigo and that CDP can show abnormalities in patients with normal caloric function.[29] This finding can be interpreted essentially in two ways: either posturography is capable of detecting abnormalities that caloric tests cannot, or posturography can give false-positive results. There is no simple solution to this problem, and, as outlined above, the clinician's beliefs, training background and interests will influence his decision.

A similar problem arises when comparing CDP with inexpensive alternatives. To a large extent, the sophistication of the commercially available CDP systems arises from the fact that the support surface and the visual surround can be moved. Clinical examination of a subject's balance while standing on rubber foam (which makes lower-limb proprioceptive input inaccurate) and with either optically reversing goggles or a Chinese lamp (dome) on their head (which makes visual input unreliable) makes a reasonable, inexpensive approximation to CDP. This is sometimes called the 'clinical test of sensory integration and balance' or simply the 'foam and dome' test (Figure 44.4). A recent study compared CDP with its clinical counterpart and found an excellent correlation between the two sets of results.[30] This is good news for clinicians, particularly in rehabilitation, who may want to assess postural control thoroughly but are not prepared to make a large investment. There was, however, a lower rate of detection of abnormalities in the clinical version of the test. As with the discrepancies observed between caloric tests and posturography, this can be interpreted in two opposite ways. Another comparison between results in moving-platform posturography and clinical analysis of posture with subjects standing on foam also reported significant correlation, with sensitivity and specificity of 90% and over.[31] Surprisingly, static posturography has been reported to have good predictive value in identifying elderly subjects at risk of falls.[32]

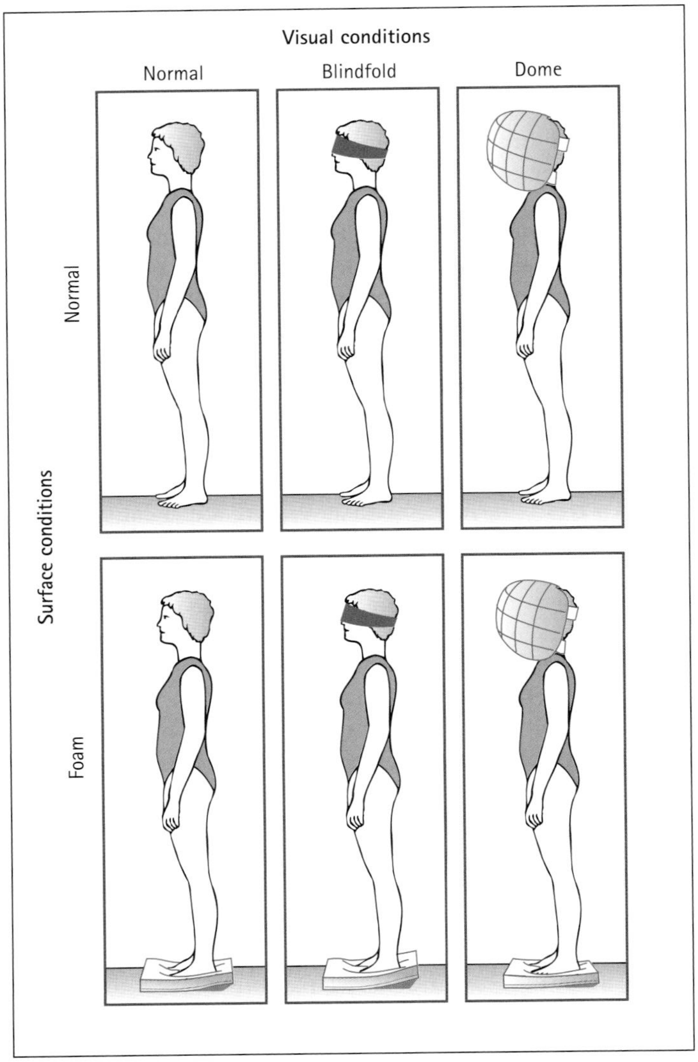

Figure 44.4 The 'clinical test for sensory interaction in balance' or 'foam and dome' test. The conditions increase in complexity from top left (all sensory input available) to bottom right (foam and dome), and are comparable to those shown for CDP in Figure 44.3. (From Shumway-Cook et al. In: Bronstein, Brandt and Wollacolt, eds. *Clinical Disorders of Balance Posture and Gait*. London: Arnold 1996: 211–35.[71])

Bilateral vestibular lesions are easily diagnosed with conventional caloric or rotational tests. Posturography in these patients has limited value in diagnosis, but studies have been of interest in defining the contribution of the vestibular system to postural control. Static posturography is normal in most patients with bilateral vestibular failure.[33,34] It has been known for more than 70 years[25] that a sudden tilt, particularly if the patient is on a mattress and blindfolded, throws these patients off balance. This observation has been confirmed with dynamic posturography, including the fact that rotation of the base of support is more effective than translation in unmasking the postural deficit.[35,36] Although patients tend to use more hip strategy,[36] latencies and muscle synergies are not essentially different from normal. The specific deficit in these patients, which explains why they actually fall during platform tilts, was identified by Allum et al:[17,19,20] EMG amplitudes in lower-limb musculature are reduced by more than 50% during platform tilts. This lack of muscle power is in turn responsible for the reduced ankle torque observed. If the postural responses to movements of the support surface are indeed centrally patterned, these findings indicate that vestibular input is essential for adequate gain setting of early muscular components operating at 80–120 ms.[20] The alternative explanation that independent vestibulospinal or vestibuloreticulospinal pathways mediate the observed effects is equally possible and compatible with known latencies following direct vestibular activation.[18,37] Answering this question may prove difficult when dealing with whole-body postural responses as investigated by posturography. Isolated motion stimuli to the head, which elicit a vestibulocollic response at 20–25 ms before proprioceptive responses take place,[38] may be useful to address this question, and studies in bilateral vestibular patients have shown that short-latency vestibulocollic responses do play a specific role in righting the head during sudden perturbations.[18]

Posturography in neurological disorders

As already emphasized, it would be naive, impractical and expensive to think that a posturography assessment could screen for a neurological deficit. Even if results were abnormal, the topographical and aetiological specificity of the finding would be very low.

Peripheral polyneuropathy

Since the days of Romberg, who reported that patients with tabes dorsallis fall over when closing the eyes, we have known that proprioceptive input is crucial for postural balance in humans. The same cannot be said of the other relevant inputs, visual and vestibular. Patients with peripheral neuropathy have increased sway, and this cannot be compensated for by vestibular and visual input.[7,39,40] The amount of sway correlates with the loss of vibration sense in the lower limbs as measured with calibrated vibration devices (including the bone probe of an audiometer[41]) or with a tuning fork and increases with disease progression.[42] The findings may be clinically relevant, as diabetic patients with neuropathy are at a higher risk of falling than those without.[39] It must be borne in mind that patients with peripheral neuropathy can have involvement of the vestibular nerve and this can contribute to their unsteadiness.[6]

Cerebellum

Early in the twentieth century, views of the postural problem in cerebellar disease were influenced by Gordon Holmes, who saw that 'the main function of the cerebellum was the control of muscular contractions'.[43] The balance disorder was considered solely a consequence of a lack of coordination in the muscles responsible for bringing the centre of gravity of the body within the base of support. We now know that the cerebellum is also a station and a modulatory structure involved in reflex gain control,[44] including vestibular and somatosensory mechanisms involved in postural control, plastic neural adaptation to vestibular loss,[45] recalibration and learning processes.[46]

A comprehensive study with static posturography in large numbers of cerebellar patients was conducted by Diener, Dichgans and co-workers.[47,48] On the basis of comparisons between lateral versus anteroposterior sway, eyes closed versus eyes open (EC/EO, sometimes called Romberg quotient, in order to see the degree of visual stabilization of body sway) and the frequencies of sway involved, these authors defined four sway patterns (Figure 44.5; Table 44.3): lower vermis (vestibulocerebellum), anterior lobe, cerebellar hemisphere and spinalcerebellar (e.g. Friedreich's ataxia) syndromes. Perhaps the single most useful finding is the presence of a body tremor at about 3 Hz in patients with anterior lobe degeneration, either alcohol-induced or degenerative. The origin of this tremor may lie in disinhibited long-latency stretch reflexes, as elicited by toe-up rotation of a tilting platform.[49] In neurological practice, however, this tremor can be detected clinically, and the value of posturography in its diagnosis has been questioned.[50]

Tilting and translating platforms have been used to examine adaptability in the postural control system of cerebellar patients. If someone standing on a platform is pushed forwards from his back, his gastrocnemius experiences a stretch, in turn leading to a stretch response which contributes to restoration of the postural upright. The same effect will be seen if the platform upon which the subject is standing is suddenly translated backwards. If the platform is rotated toes-up, there also is stretch of the gastrocnemius, but, in this case, the resulting stretch

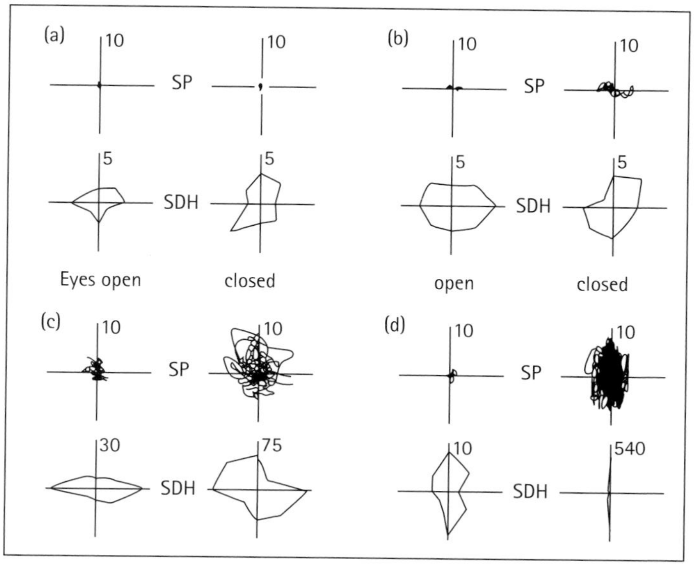

Figure 44.5 Posturography in cerebellar lesions. Recording of sway path (SP) in anterior–posterior and lateral directions and the calculated sway direction histogram (SDH). (a) Normal subject. (b) Increased omnidirectional sway in a patient with haemorrhage of the vestibulocerebellar vermis. (c) Predominantly lateral sway in a patient with Freidreich's ataxia. (d) Predominantly anterior–posterior sway in a chronic alcoholic with atrophy of the anterior lobe. Note the different scalings (a versus b–d) of the axes of the sway direction histogram summing the instantaneous sway directions within each of eight directional bins. (From Diener and Dichgans. In: Bronstein, Brandt and Wollacolt, eds. *Clinical Disorders of Balance Posture and Gait*. London: Arnold 1996: 211–35.[48])

Table 44.3 Results from static posturography in cerebellar diseases.[48]

Lesion	Amount of body sway	Visual stabilization of body sway	Directional preference of sway
Lower vermis	+++	Absent	None
Anterior lobe	++++	Present	Anterior–posterior
Cerebellar hemisphere	+	Absent	None
Spinal lesion	+++	Present	Lateral

response contributes further to the subject's instability: toes-up tilt pushes the subject backwards, and contraction of the gastrocnemius has the same effect. Thus, the response in gastrocnemius is quickly tuned down by central mechanisms to adjust to the new situation. Nashner and Grimm[16] initially reported that this adaptability was impaired in cerebellar patients, but this was not confirmed by Mummel et al,[24] who concluded that the cerebellum is not essential for adaptability to type of surface movement. Adaptability to dynamic conditions is required during full-field visual stimuli. Bronstein et al[22] observed that normal subjects subjected to discrete, full-field, low-velocity visual stimuli sway in the direction of the visual stimulus. This postural response, which is unstabilizing with respect to the real (gravito-inertial) world, is immediately suppressed by normal subjects and cerebellar patients alike but not by patients with Parkinson's disease. It was concluded that the basal ganglia rather than the cerebellum is involved in the suppression of this response. The cerebellum does not appear to be essential for fast adaptability of postural responses.

Parkinson's disease and other basal ganglia disorders

Parkinson's disease is the most common basal ganglia disorder, and approximately one-third of patients report falls.[51] Falls, however, are not common in the early phases of conventional, idiopathic Parkinson's disease, in contrast to other 'parkinsonisms' such as PSP (Steel–Richardson–Olszewski syndrome).[4] There are many contributing factors to the postural instability in Parkinson's disease, and these cannot be reviewed here. Abnormalities during tilting reactions led Purdon Martin to postulate a disorder of central vestibulopostural responses,[25] but direct vestibular (galvanic) stimulation produced normal or even enhanced postural responses.[52] Visual motion stimuli also induced larger than normal responses which patients found difficult to suppress,[22] in agreement with platform motion studies indicating lack of flexibility in switching strategies and scaling responses.[53–55] This fundamental problem in Parkinson's disease suggests that the basal ganglia are implicated in re-weighting the different sensorimotor loops involved in postural control and, more generally, in adaptability in the postural system during changing conditions.[22]

In spite of the significant contribution made by posturography in understanding the nature of the postural disorder in Parkinson's disease, there is very little room for the technique in the practical management of patients. Of possible interest is the fact that the posture and gait problem is not very responsive to L-dopa therapy, and, therefore, in the future, there may be room for objective posturography measurements of the response to new treatments aimed at these specific components of the disease. Another practical point is that in some patients the tremor is recorded by the platform,[22] in which case frequency analysis will show a peak of tremor activity at frequencies between 4 and 6 Hz, well beyond those of body sway (<1–2 Hz).

Other conditions with unsteadiness and high-frequency peaks in posturography recordings include some cerebellar ataxias, with a 3-Hz tremor discussed before,[47,48] and orthostatic tremor.[56] Orthostatic tremor is a relatively newly described condition, so that only the neurologist specializing in movement disorders is very familiar with it.[57] For this reason, these patients do turn up in neuro-otology clinics. This is not surprising, because the chief symptoms in these patients are discomfort while standing up, unsteadiness and 'shakiness' during upright stance due to the leg–trunk tremor. Patients have great difficulty in waiting, e.g. bus stops, and, remarkably, walking often alleviates this discomfort. There are minor or no conventional neurological signs. The standing tremor may just be visible and there are no 'central' vestibulo-oculomotor signs. For these reasons, most of the patients I have seen were initially diagnosed as 'psychogenic'. Keeping the diagnosis of orthostatic tremor in mind is rewarding, since conventional surface EMG recordings—or sway platforms—easily identify the pathognomonic high-frequency tremor (12–20 Hz, typically 16 Hz).[56] It has been suggested[58] that orthostatic tremor deserves to be investigated in all patients with unexplained instability or postural phobia. In that case, Fourier analysis of the sway signals must incorporate frequencies of up to 20 Hz in order to detect the specific tremor peak. This is of practical importance for diagnosis, since an increase in sway frequencies of up to 8 Hz has been reported in some patients with psychogenic unsteadiness.[59] No definitive aetiology for orthostatic tremor has been identified, but some overlap with essential tremor has been suggested.[57] Alcohol and beta-blockers, however, are usually ineffective, whereas primidone and clonazepam can be helpful treatments.

Non-specific abnormalities in dynamic posturography have also been reported in Huntington's disease[60] and in spasmodic torticollis.[61] A possible confounding effect introduced by the excessive abnormal movement in these patients is difficult to exclude, but more specific findings have been described. In Huntington's patients, responses to surface displacements are either delayed or absent.[62,63] In torticollis patients, the normal forwards sway response to dorsal neck vibration is abolished, suggesting that neck-afferent input from the dystonic muscles does not participate in postural control.[64]

Psychological unsteadiness

The relationship between psychological disorders and balance is extremely complex.

> Anxiety can create dizziness and vice-versa, and no clinician can claim to have an easy solution to this common clinical dilemma.

Only a few topics in which posturography has helped to further our knowledge in this area will be mentioned here. As with other patient groups, however, posturography is of less value in the management of the individual patient. Andersson et al[65] examined 16 patients with defined vestibular disorders with posturography during specific and non-specific balance perturbations (calf and arm muscle vibration respectively). Subjective unsteadiness (self-rating), and levels of worry, discomfort, anxiety and arousal (blood pressure and heart rate) were also measured. There was good agreement between subjective and objective unsteadiness and, as expected, the patients had increased levels of coping difficulty, less positive thoughts and increased sensitivity to somatic symptoms. In this group of patients, no evidence of undifferentiated postural responses or disproportionate levels of subjective reporting of unsteadiness was found, in spite of the increased psychological difficulties. This suggests that the psychological findings were genuinely secondary to the vestibular disorder. Both vestibular[66] and anxiety patients[67] show increased sway in response to visual motion. Another study using CDP in patients with symptoms of panic and agoraphobia also showed excessive sensitivity to platform or visual surround motion.[68]

Interestingly, these findings were not correlated with anxiety-related measures, suggesting that they relate more to specific difficulties in postural control than to the anxiety disorder.[68] Some patients report dizziness in surroundings with intense visual motion or repetitive visual patterns, such as driving, supermarkets, crowds, disco lights or ironing striped shirts. We use the term visual vertigo to describe these patients, when there is clinical and/or laboratory evidence of a vestibular lesion without clinically obvious psychiatric disorder.[69] Some of these patients are significantly more unsteady than unilateral vestibular neurectomized patients during visual motion stimuli, particularly if the vestibular disorder is due to a central nervous system lesion or if there is additional strabismus. It was postulated that visual vertigo patients may have pre-morbid high visual dependence for orientation and posture which would interfere with the normal process of vestibular compensation.[69] A recent study by Guerraz et al confirmed that an essential problem in patients with visual vertigo symptoms is one of increased visual dependence.[70] This was documented both at a perceptual and postural level, e.g. by measuring the tilt of the subjective visual vertical and postural responses, respectively induced by a visual stimulus rotating in the frontal plane. In certain conditions, e.g. viewing the rotating disk, the level of unsteadiness induced in these patients was larger than in control patients with complete absence of vestibular function. In contrast, conventional questionnaire assessment of trait anxiety and somatic anxiety showed no difference between these two patient groups, suggesting that primary psychological factors are not the primary problem in the visual vertigo patients.[70]

Visual dependence can also be identified with CDP, or its clinical version the foam and dome test, during testing conditions with sway-referenced visual surroundings.[71] Whether visual dependence identified with CPD correlates with perceptual measures and, in turn, whether they correlate with particular clinical features or outcome in patients has not been established.

It has been reported that posturography can also identify inconsistent and incoherent responses in patients with non-organic dizziness.[35,72–74] In practice, most clinicians rely on a constellation of negative findings (e.g. normal neurological, vestibular and imaging examination), positive malingering or hysteric (conversion) features as well as an appropriate psychological profile of the patient. The tradition of differentiating 'functional' (psychogenic) from organic disease is strongly emphasized in neurological teaching, and, recently, video-taping of patients has helped in establishing clinical criteria for the diagnosis of psychogenic gait disorder.[75] In a difficult patient where the question of organicity arises, it would be unwise to try to find an answer by means of posturography.

Clinical applications of posturography: unfortunately, a personal view

There is intense debate as to the clinical usefulness of posturography for the day-to-day management of patients.[76–79] This is partly due to different medical backgrounds, different interests (e.g. purely clinical or research) and, possibly, financial considerations. Clinicians or researchers linked to the manufacturing companies, clinical departments which have invested relatively large sums from their budget in posturography equipment, and private practitioners, might be biased in their judgement. Admittedly, this is difficult to prove, so the reader will have to reach their own conclusions. In any case, some care with views too enthusiastic about any new technique in medicine—particularly when the claims may come directly or indirectly from the manufacturers—must be exercised.

Probably the first article to appear in a neurological journal with potential to attract the general readership was the 'Special Article' in *Neurology* with the Report on the Therapeutics and Technology Assessment Subcommittee of the American Academy of Neurology.[80] This article remains a good and objective introduction to the topic for non-subspecialized clinicians. The specialist panel concluded in 1993 that dynamic posturography had a promising role in the assessment of balance disorder patients, but the ensuing discussion 8 years later testifies that such potential has not been fully developed. It is my personal experience, shared by many practitioners in academic medicine, that the technique is of no or very limited immediate value for the patient. I am only able to make one diagnosis with posturography which I cannot make by other means, that of orthostatic tremor (and this because I feel it is easier to stand a patient on a platform for

2 min than to obtain surface EMG recordings). However, this is a rare condition. Similarly, good specificity is also seen with the 3-Hz body postural tremor in certain cerebellar lesions but, in agreement with Baloh et al,[50] the tremor is also observed clinically. Unfortunately, all too often papers conclude that a technique is a useful clinical tool when all that it is doing is finding statistically significant differences between normal subjects and a particular patient group or a correlation with disease severity. The rationale behind clinical posturography is that it tests postural control as a whole, with the various sensory inputs interacting in physiological ways or mimicking potential real-life challenges to upright balance. This is its strength and its weakness at the same time, because of its lack of specificity: the findings of a meta-analysis of platform posturography indicated that its overall sensitivity and specificity is of the order of 50%.[81] As expected, the diagnostic aid provided was enhanced if patients with central nervous system lesions were included in the studies. Further debate on this meta-analysis, which was positively reviewed by the NHS CRD database in 1999, can be found in Dobie,[82] Black and Homer[83] and Di Fabio.[84]

It can be argued that posturography can be useful for rehabilitation, and this avenue deserves to be fully explored. Indeed, posturography has been instrumental in proving the value of vestibular rehabilitation.[85,86] However, the daily problem in neuro-otology is the patient who is not particularly unsteady in an objective way but still reports off-balance sensations and dizziness. This is often reflected in the lack of correlation between questionnaire data, such as the Dizziness Handicap Inventory, and posturography data.[87] It can then be argued that what should guide the physiotherapist is not so much how much a vestibular patient sways but how he actually feels. If there was a need for a measure of a clinical outcome, then presumably a questionnaire could be at least as effective and almost certainly cheaper than a posturography system.

References

1. Bronstein AM, Brandt T, Woollacott M (eds). *Clinical Disorders of Balance Posture and Gait.* London: Arnold, 1996.
2. Bronstein AM, Gresty MA, Rudge P. Neuro-otological assessment in the patient with balance and gait disorders. In: Bronstein AM, Brandt T, Woollacott M, eds. *Clinical Disorders of Balance Posture and Gait.* London: Arnold, 1996: 85–113.
3. Nutt JG, Marsden CD, Thompson PD. Human walking and higher-level gait disorders, particularly in the elderly. *Neurology* 1993; **43**: 268–79.
4. Marsden CD, Thompson PD. Frontal gait disorders. In: Bronstein AM, Brandt T, Woollacott M, eds. *Clinical Disorders of Balance Posture and Gait.* London: Arnold, 1996: 188–93.
5. Dominguez RO, Bronstein AM. Assessment of unexplained falls and gait unsteadiness. The impact of age. In: Shepard N, Solomon D, eds. *Practical Issues in Management of Dizzy and Balance Disorder Patient. ORL Clin North Am* **33**: 637–57.
6. Rinne T, Bronstein AM, Rudge P, Gresty MA, Luxon LM. Bilateral loss of vestibular function: clinical findings in 53 patients. *J Neurol* 1998; **245**(6–7): 314–21.
7. Bergin PS, Bronstein AM, Murray NMF et al. Body sway and vibration perception thresholds in normal aging and in patients with polyneuropathy. *J Neurol Neurosurg Psychiatry* 1995; **58**: 335–40.
8. Dey AB, Kenny RA. Orthostatic hypotension in the elderly: aetiology, manifestations and management. *J Ir Coll Phys Surg* 1998; **14**: 182–7.
9. Lawson J, Fitzgerald J, Birchall J et al. Diagnosis of geriatric patients with severe dizziness. *J Am Geriatr Soc* 1999; **47**: 12–17.
10. Nashner LM. A model describing vestibular detection of body sway motion. *Acta Otolaryngol* 1971; **72**: 429–36.
11. Nashner LM. Analysis of movement control in man using the movable platform. In: Desmedt JE, ed. *Motor Control Mechanisms in Health and Disease*. New York: Raven Press, 1983.
12. Nashner LM, McCollum G. The organization of human postural movements: a formal basis and experimental synthesis. *Behav Brain Sci* 1985; **8**: 135–72.
13. Horak FB, Nashner LM. Central programming of postural movements: adaptation to altered support-surface configurations. *J Neurophysiol* 1986; **55**: 1369–81.
14. Black FO, Wall III C, Nashner LM. Effects of visual and support surface orientation references upon postural control in vestibular deficient subjects. *Acta Otolaringol* 1983; **95**: 199–210.
15. Black FO, Nashner LM. Postural control in four classes of vestibular abnormalities. In: Igarashi M, Black FO ed. *Vestibular and Visual Control on Posture and Locomotor Equilibrium*. Basel: Karger, 1985: 271–81.
16. Nashner LM, Grimm RJ. Analysis of multiloop dyscontrols in standing cerebellar patients. In: Desmedt JE, ed. *Cerebral Motor Control in Man: Long Loop Mechanisms*. Basel: Karger, 1996: 300–19.
17. Allum JHJ, Pfaltz CR. Visual and vestibular contribution to pitch sway stabilization in the ankle muscles of normal subjects and patients with bilateral peripheral vestibular deficit. *Exp Brain Res* 1985; **58**: 82–94.
18. Ito Y, Corna S, Von Breven M et al. The functional effectiveness of neck muscle reflexes for the head-righting in response to sudden fall. *Exp Brain Res* 1997; **117**: 266–72.
19. Allum JHJ, Bloem BR, Carpenter MG et al. Proprioceptive control of posture: a review of new concepts. *Gait Posture* 1998; **8**: 214–42.
20. Allum JHJ, Honegger F. Interactions between vestibular and proprioceptive inputs triggering and modulating human balance-correcting responses differ across muscles. *Exp Brain Res* 1998; **121**: 478–94.
21. Di Fabio RP, Emasithi A, Paul S. Validity of visual stabilization conditions used with computerized dynamic platform posturography. *Acta Otolaringol* 1998; **118**: 449–54.
22. Bronstein AM, Hood JD, Gresty MA et al. Visual control of balance in cerebellar and parkinsonian patients. *Brain* 1990; **113**: 767–9.
23. Timmann D, Horak FB. Prediction and set-dependent scaling of early postural responses in cerebellar patients. *Brain* 1997; **120**: 327–37.

24. Mummel P, Timmann D, Krause UWH et al. Postural responses to changing task conditions in patients with cerebellar lesions. *J Neurol Neurosurg Psychiatry* 1998; **65**: 734–42.
25. Martin JP. Tilting reactions and disorders of the basal ganglia. *Brain* 1965; **88**: 855–74.
26. Brandt T, Dieterich M, Woollacott M, eds. *Clinical Disorders of Balance Posture and Gait*. London: Arnold, 1996, 131–46.
27. Burgneay J, Munro KJ. Computerised dynamic posturography: a retrospective analysis of the first 2000 patients tested at the ISVR Hearing and Balance Centre. *J Audiol Med* 1997; **6**: 79–87.
28. Fetter M, Diener HC, Dichgans J. Recovery of postural control after an acute unilateral vestibular lesion in humans. *J Vestib Res* 1991; **1**: 373–83.
29. Goebel JA, Paige GD. Dynamic posturography and caloric test results in patients with and without vertigo. *Otolaryngol Head Neck Surg* 1989; **100**: 553–8.
30. El-Kashlan HK, Shepard NT, Asher AM et al. Evaluation of clinical measures of equilibrium. *Laryngoscope* 1998; **108**: 311–19.
31. Weber PC, Cass SP. Clinical assessment of postural stability. *Am J Otol* 1993; **14**: 566–9.
32. Topper AK, Maki BE, Holliday PJ. Are activity-based assessments of balance and gait in the elderly predictive of risk of falling and/or type of fall? *J Am Geriatr Soc* 1993; **41**: 479–87.
33. Lekhel H, Popov K, Bronstein AM et al. Postural responses to vibration of neck muscles in patients with uni- and bilateral vestibular loss. *Gait Posture* 1998; **7**: 228–36.
34. Sakellari V, Bronstein AM. Hyperventilation effect on postural sway. *Arch Phys Med Rehabil* 1997; **78**: 730–6.
35. Allum JHJ, Shepard NT. An overview of the clinical use of dynamic posturography in the differential diagnosis of balance disorders. *J Vestib Res* 1999; **1**: 11–40.
36. Herdman SJ, Sandusky AL, Hain TC et al. Characteristics of postural stability in patients with aminoglycoside toxicity. *J Vestib Equilibrium Orientation* 1994; **4**: 71–80.
37. Colebatch JG, Day BL, Bronstein AM et al. Vestibular hypersensitivity to clicks is characteristic of the Tullio phenomenon. *J Neurol Neurosurg Psychiatry* 1998; **65**: 670–8.
38. Ito Y, Corna S, Von Brevern M, Bronstein A, Rothwell J, Gresty M. Neck muscle responses to abrupt free fall of the head: comparison of normal with labyrinthine-defective human subjects. *J Physiol* 1995; **489**: 911–16.
39. Cavanagh PR, Simoneau GG, Ulbrecht JS. Ulceration, unsteadiness, and uncertainty: the biomechanical consequences of diabetes mellitus. *J Biomechanics* 1993; **26**: 23–40.
40. Vrethem M, Ledin T, Ernerudh J et al. Correlation between dynamic posturography, clinical investigation, and neurography in patients with polyneuropathy. *Otorhinolaryngol* 1991; **53**: 294–8.
41. Bronstein AM. Audiometry of the ankles. A quick check on the single most important sensory input for balance control. *Br J Audiol* 1996; **30**: 63.
42. Jauregui-Renaud K, Kovacsovics B, Vrethem M et al. Dynamic and randomized perturbed posturography in the follow-up of patients with polyneuropathy. *Arch Med Res* 1998; **29**: 39–44.
43. Holmes G. The Croonian lectures on the clinical symptoms of cerebellar disease and their interpretation. In: Phillips CG, ed. *Selected Papers of Gordon Holmes*. New York: Oxford University Press, 1979: 186–247.
44. MacKay WA, Murphy JT. Cerebellar modulation of reflex gain. *Prog Neurobiol* 1979; **13**: 361–417.
45. Bronstein AM, Mossman SS, Luxon LM. The neck–eye reflex in patients with reduced vestibular and optokinetic function. *Brain* 1991; **114**: 1–11.
46. Ito M. *The Cerebellum and Neural Control*. New York: Raven Press, 1984.
47. Diener HC, Dichgans J, Bacher M et al. Quantification of postural sway in normals and patients with cerebellar diseases. *Electronencephalogr Clin Neurophysiol* 1984; **57**: 134–42.
48. Diener HC, Dichgans J. Cerebellar and spinocerebellar disorders. In: Bronstein AM, Brandt T, Woollacott M, eds. *Clinical Disorders of Balance Posture and Gait*. London: Arnold, 1996: 147–55.
49. Mauritz KA, Scmitt C, Dichgans J. Delayed and enhanced long latency reflexes as the possible cause of postural tremor in late cerebellar atrophy. *Brain* 1981; **104**: 97–116.
50. Baloh RW, Jacobson KM, Beykirch K et al. Static and dynamic posturography in patients with vestibular and cerebellar lesions. *Arch Neurol* 1998; **55**: 646–54.
51. Koller WC, Glatt S, Vetere-Overfield B et al. Falls and Parkinson's disease. *Clin Neuropharmacol* 1989; **12**: 98–105.
52. Pastor MA, Day BL, Marsden CD. Vestibular induced postural responses in Parkinson's disease. *Brain* 1993; **116**: 1177–90.
53. Schieppati M, Nardone A. Free and support stance in Parkinson's disease. *Brain* 1991; **114**: 1227–44.
54. Beckley DJ, Bloem BR, Remler MP. Impaired scaling of long latency postural reflexes in patients with Parkinson's disease. *Electroencephalogr Clin Neurophysiol* 1993; **89**: 22–8.
55. Bloem BR, Beckley DJ, Remler MP et al. Postural reflexes in Parkinson's disease during 'resist' and 'yield' tasks. *J Neurol Sci* 1994;
56. Bronstein AM, Guerraz M. Visual–vestibular control of posture and gait: physiological mechanisms and disorders. *Current Opin Neurol* 1999; **12**: 5–11.
57. Thompson PD. Primary orthostatic tremor. In: Findley LJ, Koller WC, eds. *Handbook of Tremor Disorders*. New York: Marcel Dekker, 1995; 387–99.
58. Mastain B, Cassim F, Guieu JD et al. Primary orthostatic tremor. *Rev Neurol* 1998; **154**: 322–9.
59. Krafczyk S, Schlamp V, Dieterich M et al. Increased body sway at 3.5–8 Hz in patients with phobic postural vertigo. *Neurosci Lett* 1999; **259**: 149–52.
60. Tian JR, Herdman SJ, Zee DS et al. Postural control in Huntington's disease. *Acta Otolaryngol* 1991; **481**: 333–6.
61. Moreau MS, Cauquil AS, Salon MCC. Static and dynamic balance function in spasmodic torticollis. *Move Disord* 1999; **14**: 87–94.
62. Dichgans J, Diener HC. The use of short- and long-latency reflex testing in leg muscles of neurological patients. In: Struppler A, Weindl A, eds. *Clinical Aspects of Sensory Motor Integration*. Berlin: Springer-Verlag, 1987; 165–75.

63. Fetter M, Dichgans J. Vestibular tests in evolution. II. Posturography. In: Baloh RW, Halmagyi GM, eds. *Disorders of the Vestibular System*. New York: Oxford University Press, 1996; 256–73.
64. Lekhel H, Popov K, Anastasopoulos D et al. Postural responses to vibration of neck muscles in patients with idiopathic torticollis. *Brain* 1997; **120**: 583–91.
65. Andersson G, Persson K, Melin L et al. Actual and perceived postural sway during balance specific and non-specific proprioceptive stimulation. *Acta Otolaryngol* 1998; **118**: 461–5.
66. Redfern MS, Furman JM. Postural sway of patients with vestibular disorders during optic flow. *J Vestib Res* 1994; **4**: 221–30.
67. Jacob RG, Redfern MS, Furman JM. Optic flow-induced sway in anxiety disorders associated with space and motion discomfort. *J Anxiety Disord* 1995; **9**: 411–25.
68. Yardley L, Luxon L, Bird J et al. Vestibular and posturographic test results in people with symptoms of panic and agoraphobia. *J Audiol Med* 1994; **3**: 48–65.
69. Bronstein AM. The visual vertigo syndrome. Clinical and posturography findings. *J Neurol Neurosurg Psychiatry* 1995; **59**: 472–6.
70. Guerraz M, Yardley L, Bertholon P et al. Visual vertigo: symptom assessment, spatial orientation and postural control. *Brain* 2001; **124**: 1646–56.
71. Shumway-Cook A, Horak FB, Yardley L, Bronstein AM. Rehabilitation of balance disorders in the patient with vestibular pathology. In: Bronstein AM, Brandt T, Woollacott M, eds. *Clinical Disorders of Balance Posture and Gait*. London: Arnold, 1996: 211–35.
72. Allum JHJ, Huwiler M, Honegger F. Identifying cases of non-organic vertigo using dynamic posturography. *Gait Posture* 1996; **4**: 52–61.
73. Fitzgerald JE, Birchall JP, Murray A. Identification of non-organic instability by sway magnetometry. *Br J Audiol* 1997; **31**: 275–82.
74. Uimonen S, Laitakari K, Kiukaanniemi H et al. Does posturography differentiate malingerers from vertiginous patients? *J Vestib Res Equilibrium Orientation* 1995; **5**: 117–24.
75. Lempert T, Brandt T, Dieterich M et al. How to identify psychogenic disorders of stance and gait, a video study in 37 patients. *J Neurol* 1991; **238**: 140–6.
76. Dobie RA. Does computerized dynamic posturography help us care for your patients? *Am Otol* 1997; **18**: 108–12.
77. Hart CW. Does computerized dynamic posturography help us care for our patients? *Am J Otol* 1997; **18**: 535–7.
78. Stockwell CW. Vestibular testing: past, present, future. *Br J Audiol* 1997; **31**: 387–98.
79. Black FO. Response to Stockwell CW. Vestibular testing: past, present, future. *Br J Audiol* 1998; **32**: 255.
80. American Academy of Neurology. Assessment-posturography. Report of the therapeutics and technology assessment subcommittee of the American Academy of Neurology. *Neurology* 1993; **43**: 1261–4.
81. Di Fabio RP. Meta-analysis of the sensitivity and specificity of platform posturography. *Arch Otolaryngol Head Neck Surg* 1996; **122**: 150–6.
82. Dobie RA. Platform posturography. *Arch Otolaryngol Head Neck Surg* 1996; **122**: 1273.
83. Black FO, Homer LH. Platform posturography. *Arch Otolaryngol Head Neck Surg* 1996; **122**: 1273–4.
84. Di Fabio RP. Platform posturography. *Arch Otolaryngol Head Neck Surg* 1996; **122**: 1274–6.
85. Cass S, Borello-France D, Furman JM. Functional outcome of vestibular rehabilitation in patients with abnormal sensory-organization testing. *Am J Otol* 1996; **17**: 581–894.
86. Brandt T. Vestibular exercises improve central vestibulospinal compensation after vestibular neuritis. *Neurology* 1998; **51**: 838–44.
87. Robertson DD, Ireland DJ. Dizziness handicap inventory correlates of computerized dynamic posturography. *J Otolaryngol* 1995; **24**: 118–24.
88. Yarrow K, Brown P, Gresty MA, Bronstein AM. Force platform recordings in the diagnosis of primary orthostatic tremor. *Gait Posture* 2001; **13**: 27–34.

45 Emerging technologies

Joseph M Furman, Izumi Koizuka

Introduction

This chapter aims to bring the reader up to date regarding several currently promising emerging technologies. The first section concerns assessment of the otolith organs. There are no clinically validated tests for the otolith organs. Discussed in this section are linear acceleration using sleds, eccentric rotation, off-vertical axis rotation, vestibular evoked myogenic potentials, and perception of the subjective visual vertical and horizontal. The second section concerns head-only rotation. The third section concerns galvanic stimulation. The fourth section concerns effects of moving visual scenes on postural sway, and the fifth section concerns high-resolution magnetic resonance imaging of the inner ear. Thus, these technologies span various methodologies looking at the vestibulo-ocular reflex, the vestibulospinal reflex, perception, and new clinical anatomic studies. References are provided so that the reader can delve into these topics more thoroughly, if desired. An attempt was made to approach each of the emerging technologies uniformly. Following a brief description of what the technology entails, each section or sub-section discusses what the technology aims to test, what are its positive attributes, why it might be useful in the future, and what aspect of balance function the technology assesses that is not currently assessed adequately by other techniques. As far as is feasible, the chapter includes a brief description of how the technology is applied, including the current state of development of the technique. Examples of how the technology has been used and what new findings have arisen from the technology are discussed. Additionally, the limitations of the technology are described to account for why the technology is emerging and has not yet 'emerged'. Where possible, some mention is given to whether or not these limitations are surmountable, what improvements are possible, and what other technologies currently available or emerging might be better. Last, the chapter gives an overall opinion as to the likelihood that the technology might become generally available.

Assessment of the otolith organs

Linear translation

Linear translation refers to the use of linear sleds to stimulate the otolith organs. Typically, eye movements and sometimes perceptual responses are measured. Most sleds are horizontal and thus stimulate primarily the utricles if the subject is seated upright. With the subject oriented such that the motion is along the interaural axis, eye movements will be predominantly horizontal. This is the most typically used orientation. With the subject supine, with the motion of the subject along their rostral caudal body axis, the motion will stimulate predominantly the sacculus, with the eye-movement response being predominantly vertical. The advantages of linear translation include the fact that it stimulates the otolith organs directly and naturally, with no concomitant semicircular canal stimulation. In this regard, linear translation has the potential to provide additional information clinically, in that there is no commonly used otolithic stimulus available. Figure 45.1 illustrates a linear sled that has been used primarily for research purposes. Alternative technologies to deliver linear acceleration include the parallel swing[1] and a rotating linear sled that effectively lengthens the sled.[2] Sled length is typically the limiting factor in terms of the lowest frequency of motion that can be applied. Sled length also limits the duration of a step change in linear velocity.

To date, linear translation has been used for research purposes to deduce how otolith stimulation is processed to yield eye movements[2] and perception[1,3–8] of motion using pure otolithic stimuli. Linear translation has been combined with visual stimuli,[7] with vergence eye movements,[5,6] and with the use of imaginary visual targets.[9] These studies have suggested that the point of visual regard greatly influences the eye-movement response to linear translation and that both real and imagined visual targets influence the eye movement response to linear translation. Additionally, linear translation has been used to assess the impact of both peripheral and central vestibular disorders on the otolith–ocular reflex.[10–16] These studies

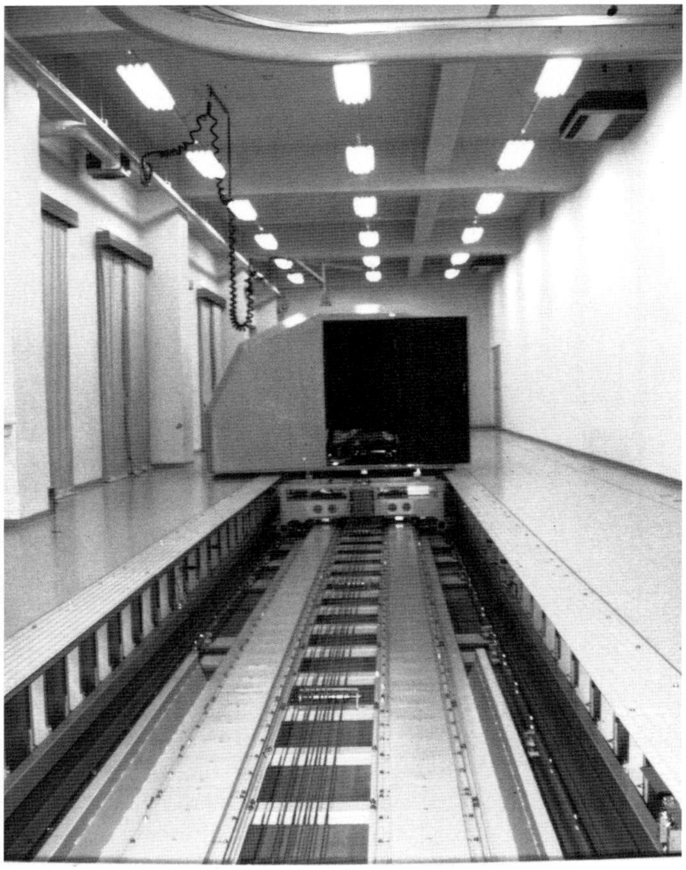

Figure 45.1 Photograph of a linear sled device in Nagoya, Japan. The sled is powered by a magnetic rail. The sled length is 21 m. Translational frequencies of this device range from 0.05 Hz to 0.16 Hz.

have indicated that unilateral peripheral vestibular disease does not significantly influence the otolith–ocular reflex. That is, it appears that a single labyrinth is sufficient to produce the eye movements that result from linear translation. However, with acute unilateral peripheral vestibular loss, asymmetric responses to linear translation have been recorded.[16] Patients with bilateral vestibular loss have been shown to have reduced responses to linear translation. Patients with cerebellar disease have been found to have abnormal visual–vestibular interaction using linear translation.[14]

The limitations of linear translation are many. They include the size and expense of the equipment required to deliver a linear translation stimulus, and the difficulty of coupling the head to the motion device and accurately recording eye movements during the stimulus. Because of the complex nature of the induced eye movements, which may include horizontal, vertical and torsional positions, recording eye movements is difficult. Also, the eye movements induced by linear translation are of small magnitude, further reducing the reliability of the measures. A further limitation of linear translation is that studies to date have indicated that patients with unilateral peripheral vestibular abnormalities exhibit normal responses. Some of these limitations might be overcome with improvements in eye-movement recording methods and development of novel stimuli. However, the likelihood that linear acceleration will be used in routine clinical basis is low. Furthermore, other means of stimulating the otolith organs may be more practical, including eccentric rotation or off-vertical axis rotation. For now, linear translation is a useful stimulus in the research setting to uncover basic information regarding the influence of otolithic stimulation on eye movements and perception of spatial orientation and possibly the influence of vestibular disease on otolithic-dependent responses.

LINEAR ACCELERATION

Major strength

Stimulates the otolith organs directly without stimulating the semicircular canals.

Major weakness

It is technically difficult to deliver a linear acceleration and simultaneously record eye movements.

Eccentric rotation

Eccentric rotation refers to off-axis rotation (not to be confused with off-vertical axis rotation). Eccentric rotation is performed with the subject displaced from the axis of rotation in a manner comparable to a centrifuge. In fact, even with conventional vertical axis rotation, the vestibular labyrinth is typically 'off-axis' because of the location of the labyrinths within the skull. That is, with earth-vertical axis rotation with the subject sitting upright, the axis of rotation cannot physically intersect both labyrinths. Typically, with the patient seated such that the axis of rotation passes through the center of the head, both vestibular labyrinths are eccentric. In a technique popularized by Clarke and Engelhorn[17], the subject is positioned such that the axis of rotation intersects with one or the other labyrinth. In this way, one labyrinth can be subjected to eccentric rotation while the other is subjected only to rotational motion. The physics underlying eccentric rotation is as follows: centripetal accelerations caused by the off-axis location of the labyrinth result in a linear acceleration directed toward the axis. Also, if the rotational velocity is not constant, a tangential linear acceleration is delivered. As a result, eccentric rotation combines a rotational motion with a linear acceleration. Depending upon the orientation of the subject with respect to the axis of rotation and the trajectory of the rotational velocity versus time, various combinations of rotational acceleration and linear acceleration can be delivered. Also, depending upon the particular rotational and linear acceleration delivered to the subject, various types of eye movements are produced. That is, semicircular canal-based responses resulting from the rotational acceleration and otolith organ-based responses based upon the linear acceleration will combine.[18,19] Several studies have suggested that the eye movements induced by this combination of semicircular canal and otolith organ stimulation represent a linear summation of the two effects. For example, the semicircular canal- and otolith organ-induced eye movements can be synergistic or in conflict.[20–22] Alternatively, the two types of eye movements can be in different planes and thus combine, somewhat independently. Eccentric rotational responses can also consist of a perceptual change in the perceived vertical or perceived horizontal.

An advantage of eccentric rotation is that it constitutes an otolith stimulus that can be combined with a semicircular canal stimulus. Also, a visual stimulus can be combined with these various signals. A further positive attribute of eccentric rotation is that the precise nature of the stimulus can be changed by orienting the subject in different ways. Figure 45.2 illustrates an eccentric rotation device with the subject about to undergo a yaw rotational motion. In Figure 45.2a, the subject is either facing the motion or facing away from the motion, whereas in Figure 45.2b, the subject is facing away from the axis of rotation. Thus, the centripetal forces in Figure 45.2a will be oriented through the ears, i.e. they will be interaural. The tangential linear acceleration force, however, will be naso-occipital. Conversely, in Figure 45.2b, the centripetal forces will be naso-occipital, whereas the tangential linear acceleration forces will be interaural.

Eccentric rotation is typically performed using one of two different rotational modalities, either constant-velocity rotation[17] or sinusoidal rotation.[18] With sinusoidal rotation, not only the otolith organs, but also the horizontal semicircular canals, are stimulated simultaneously, and thus the otolith– ocular reflex cannot be evaluated in isolation. The responses obtained during sinusoidal eccentric rotation can be compared with responses obtained during sinusoidal earth-vertical axis rotation. With constant-velocity rotation, it is possible to evaluate the otolith–ocular reflex in isolation, but once constant velocity has been reached, the eye movement induced is essentially the equivalent of just having the patient tilted with respect to gravity.

Studies to date have suggested that eccentric rotation is a complex stimulus producing complex responses that has obvious clinical utility. Responses in patients with unilateral peripheral vestibular disease are not clearly different from responses in normal subjects.[23,24] A study of patients with Menière's disease suggests that there is an abnormal enhancement of eccentric rotational responses in this disorder.[25] Other studies have evaluated conflict between otolith and semicircular canal stimuli and the effects of imagined visual targets. Studies by Clarke and Engelhom[17] have suggested the possibility of using eccentric rotation to assess otolith organs individually. This aspect of eccentric rotation is promising but requires highly specialized equipment.

The limitations of eccentric rotation include the expensive technology required to deliver such a stimulus and the difficulty in recording the complex eye movements elicited by the stimulus. Moreover, clinical studies performed to date have not suggested clear abnormalities, but eccentric rotation has not been evaluated thoroughly. Eccentric rotation, at this time, is one of the candidate methods that might become useful in the clinical setting to evaluate otolith function. The potential technical challenges in delivering eccentric rotation in a clinical setting would appear to preclude this type of stimulus for routine clinical assessment. However, technological advances in eye-movement recording and further research, particularly using very small eccentric distances,[17] may help overcome some of these limitations.

ECCENTRIC ROTATION

Major strength

Both the otolith organs and semicircular canals can be stimulated simultaneously.

Major weakness

Eccentric rotation is technically challenging.

Off-vertical axis rotation

Off-vertical axis rotation (OVAR) is a stimulus wherein persons are rotated while the axis about which they are rotating is tilted with respect to gravity.[26–28] OVAR should not be confused with off-axis rotation, which is another name for eccentric rotation (discussed above). The term OVAR can correctly be used to

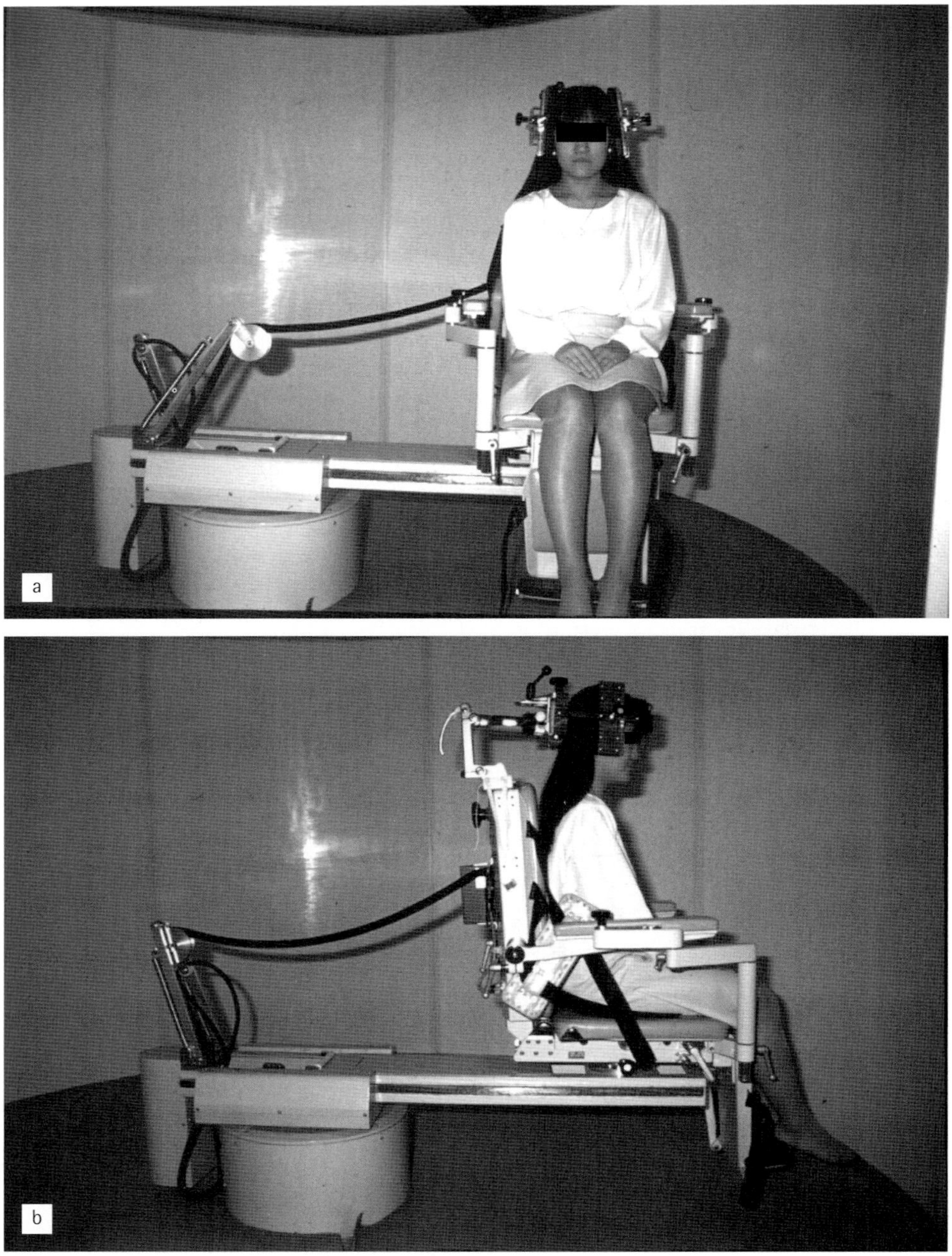

Figure 45.2 Photograph of an eccentric rotation device. (a) Subject is positioned such that the centripetal forces are interaural. Note that the subject may be either facing the motion or have their back to the motion. (b) Subject is positioned on the eccentric rotator with the centripetal acceleration naso-occipital.

describe tilts of the axis of rotation of up to 90°, i.e. so-called 'barbeque' rotation.[29] However, OVAR employs tilts of the axis of rotation of 30° or less.

OVAR has the capability of assessing the otolith–ocular reflex, semicircular canal–otolith interaction, and visual–otolith interaction. In particular, by rotating an individual at constant velocity for a long enough period of time for the semicircular canal responses to decay, OVAR can be used to deliver a pure otolithic stimulus. The most popular OVAR stimulus uses yaw rotation, that is, the subject is rotated in their own horizontal plane, i.e. about a rostral–caudal body axis. In this case, it is probably the utricular organs that are stimulated maximally.

Figure 45.3 shows a diagram of a typical OVAR test device. Note that the orientation of the subject with respect to the axis of rotation produces a yaw stimulus even though the orientation of the axis of rotation is tilted with respect to gravity. Figure 45.4 illustrates a rotate-then-tilt protocol for constant-velocity rotation. The slow-component eye velocity induced by such a stimulus includes the so-called bias and modulation components, each of which reflects the otolith–ocular response.

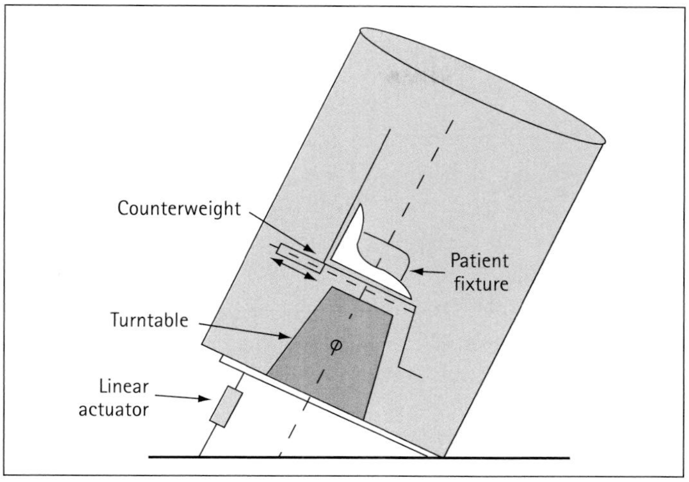

Figure 45.3 Diagram of an off-vertical axis rotation (OVAR) device. Note that the axis of rotation is tilted with respect to gravity.

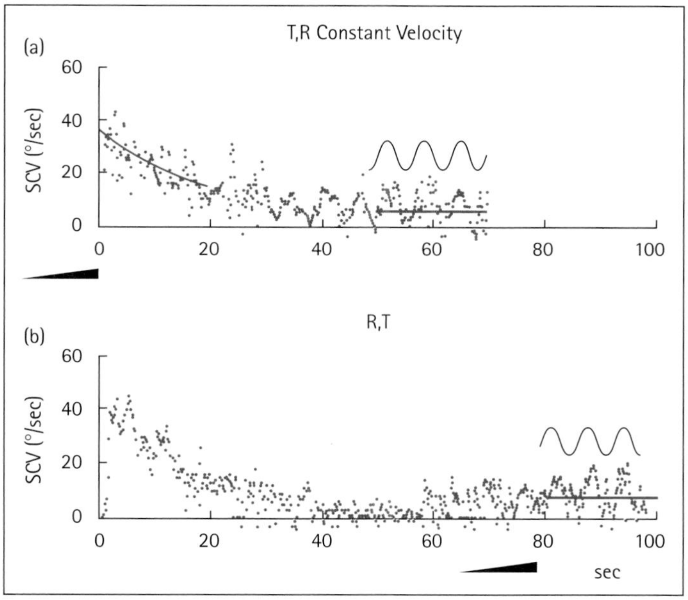

Figure 45.4 Slow-component eye velocity in response to off-vertical axis rotation. A rotate-then-tilt protocol was used to generate purely otolithic-induced eye movements following the tilt. Note the presence of both a bias and a modulation component.

OVAR has been used to assess otolith–ocular function in patients with disorders of the peripheral[30] and central vestibular systems.[31] These studies have suggested that OVAR has the potential to provide clinically useful data. Studies using OVAR have shown that patients with a single functioning labyrinth, e.g. patients with unilateral peripheral vestibular disease, have asymmetric otolith–ocular responses.[30] Patients with central vestibular disease, particularly disease of the vestibulo-cerebellum, have been found to have a reduction in the bias component and an abnormally large modulation component.[31] These studies have provided insights regarding central otolith–ocular processing. Also, patients with bilaterally reduced vestibular responses, even patients with absent responses to ice water caloric stimulation, may have preserved responses to OVAR, suggesting preserved otolith function in patients with severely impaired semicircular canal responses.[32]

Despite the encouraging findings from clinical applications of OVAR, there are several shortcomings of the technique that may limit its widespread applicability. The equipment requirements are somewhat complex. OVAR testing requires a rotational device and a tilt stand with appropriate electronics and safety features. An additional complexity of OVAR is that the induced eye movements are a combination of horizontal, vertical and torsional movements.[33] Further, OVAR is nausea-provoking. Also, since OVAR responses have been shown to be essentially normal in patients with complete unilateral peripheral vestibular loss except for an asymmetry that may be seen with conventional rotation, i.e. earth-vertical axis, the applicability of the technique to patients with partial vestibular disorders is uncertain. This limitation arises from the fact that OVAR stimulates the otolith organs bilaterally. Several areas of research may help to determine the ultimate clinical usefulness of OVAR. In particular, by combining OVAR with certain visual stimuli, important insights may be gained regarding otolith–visual interaction.[34] The clinical usefulness of such information is unknown at the present time. Also, by recording the eye movements induced by OVAR using video-oculography, other aspects of the response to OVAR, i.e. the non-horizontal components, may be uncovered that are clinically useful. Other technologies, some of which are discussed in this chapter, are also designed to assess otolith function. OVAR is relatively easy to perform, certainly as compared to the use of linear sleds, and can be combined easily with visual stimuli.

Overall, OVAR appears to be a promising technology because of its relative ease of use and the ability to combine an otolithic stimulus with vision. Limitations include the somewhat cumbersome equipment required and the nausea produced by the stimulus.

OFF-VERTICAL AXIS ROTATION

Major strength

Both pure otolith organ stimulation and combined semicircular canal and otolith organ stimulation can be delivered.

Major weakness

Off-vertical axis rotation requires a complex device and produces complex eye movements that may be difficult to record.

Vestibular evoked myogenic potentials

Vestibular evoked myogenic potentials VEMPs refer to electrical activity recorded from neck muscles in response to intense auditory clicks.[35–40] VEMPs have been hypothesized to reflect stimulation of the sacculus unilaterally.[39] As a result of this presumed ability of VEMPs to assess the sacculus unilaterally, it has possible clinical applicability. There are no other tests available that are known to assess the sacculus in isolation. As with the other tests of otolith function described in this chapter, the clinical usefulness of VEMP is limited, since otolithic disease in the absence of disease elsewhere in the labyrinth is probably infrequent.

Figure 45.5 provides an example of a VEMP. Studies to date have indicated definite abnormalities in the VEMP in individuals with known peripheral vestibular loss.[35–37,39,40] Moreover, VEMP magnitudes have been found to be elevated in certain unusual inner ear disorders.[38] However, a pure vestibular origin for the VEMP remains controversial. Data are not yet available regarding alterations in VEMPs as a result of partial saccular lesions and it is uncertain how such data can be obtained.

One of the limitations of VEMPs is the technical challenge of obtaining an electromyographic recording from a muscle that has the appropriate amount of background activity. That is, the muscle from which the VEMP is being recorded must be preactivated. Other technical issues that are not resolved include the type of auditory stimulus, the position of the patient, and the exact site of recording. Also, the test may produce unacceptable discomfort in many patients with otologic disorders.

Overall, VEMPs, because they presumably assess function of the sacculus unilaterally, may become more widespread clinically. However, it is likely that even once some of the technical issues surrounding VEMPs, including its test–retest reliability, sensitivity, and specificity, are determined, its usefulness will be limited to special circumstances in which it is clinically necessary to assess saccular function specifically.

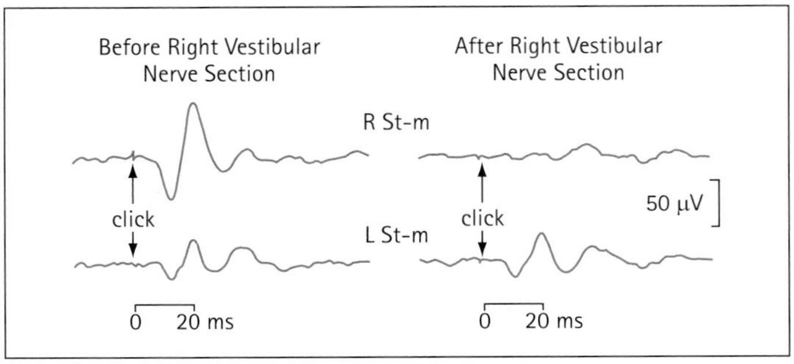

Figure 45.5 The vestibular evoked myogenic potential before and after right vestibular nerve section. (From Colebatch and Halmagyi. *Neurology* 1992; **42**: 1635–6,[35] with permission.)

VESTIBULAR EVOKED MYOGENIC POTENTIALS

Major strength

Vestibular-evoked myogenic potentials appear to allow an assessment of the sacculus, unlike other techniques.

Major weakness

It is technically difficult to adjust the background muscle activity to obtain a useful electromyographic recording; the test may produce unacceptable auditory discomfort.

Perception of the subjective visual vertical/ subjective visual horizontal

Perceptual tests to determine whether or not a patient can accurately judge their orientation with respect to gravity have been available for many years.[41,42] Using very simple instruments, the ability of an individual to judge vertical or horizontal can be assessed. Several perceptual tasks related to vestibular function have been studied, including the subjective visual vertical and horizontal, subjective haptic vertical and horizontal, subjective body vertical, and perceptions of motion and gravito-inertial force during rotation and translation. As with many perceptual tests, precisely which aspects of the balance system are being measured is uncertain. In the case of subjective visual vertical (SVV) and subjective visual horizontal (SVH), there are influences from both the labyrinth and the visual system. Presumably, the labyrinthine sensors most important for accurately setting a test object vertical or horizontal include the otolith organs, i.e. the utricle and saccule. Since the issues pertaining to the SVV and the SVH are identical, further discussion will refer to the SVV.

The technique of assessing SVV in some sense is fully developed, in that no technological advances are required to improve the test technique. However, the use of the SVV has not become widespread, for several reasons. Despite the fact that the SVV is abnormal in acute peripheral vestibular lesions,[43–46] the SVV is normal in chronic lesions.[43,45,47] Central vestibular disorders can also be assessed using SVV.[41,48] The influence of partial vestibular lesions on the SVV is unknown. Also, because of the multifactorial nature of the test technique, the SVV may not provide additional information useful in the clinical setting beyond the information that can be obtained from other methods. A definite advantage, however, of the SVV is its simplicity. Possibly, with future research, SVV will be shown to be a useful adjunct to other clinical techniques. For example, by combining SVV with eccentric rotation, a more sensitive measure of unilateral otolith function may be available.

PERCEPTION OF THE SUBJECTIVE VISUAL VERTICAL AND HORIZONTAL

Major strength

Using simple techniques, a patient's ability to judge spatial orientation can be assessed.

Major weakness

Studies have indicated that the subjective visual vertical is normal in chronic lesions and it relies upon a high level of patient cooperation.

Overall, the measurement of SVV and SVH is a low-technology technique that can be applied easily in the clinical setting. However, because it relies upon the perceptions of the patient and is thus by definition subjective, it is likely to be of limited usefulness clinically.

Head-only rotational testing

Head-only rotational testing is a technique that assesses the vestibulo-ocular reflex using rotation only of the head rather than rotation of the entire body.[49–53] Since the vestibular system is anatomically found in the head, the vestibular stimulus in head-only rotation and in whole-body rotation is identical. As in whole-body rotation, during head-only rotation, eye movements are recorded either with electro-oculography or video-oculography in order to assess the vestibulo-ocular reflex (VOR). Both horizontal and vertical head and eye movements can be recorded, although technical challenges limit the reliability of the test, especially for vertical eye movements. Figure 45.6 illustrates some data obtained using head-only rotational testing. An apparent advantage of head-only rotational testing is that the VOR can be assessed in a frequency range that coincides with natural head movements. This capability is difficult to achieve using whole-body rotation, because of the large moment of inertia of the body and thus the high torque required to rotate an individual at greater than one cycle per second. Also, with whole-body rotation at higher frequencies, it is difficult to assure adequate coupling of the rotational stimulus to the head. Despite these relative advantages, head-only rotational testing, like whole-body rotation, stimulates both labyrinths simultaneously and thus cannot consistently provide information regarding the laterality of a vestibular abnormality. Also, head-only rotational testing may be of limited value in patients with partial vestibular lesions unilaterally.

Some of the limitations of applying head-only rotational testing clinically can be found in the literature.[54] Advantages of head-only rotational testing include the relatively simple equipment that can be used to perform the test, the ability to perform the test at the bedside because the equipment is transportable, and the ability to assess the VOR in its natural frequency range. Limitations include technical problems that can be encountered in rotating the head at high frequency, either actively or passively, the analysis of eye-movement data that contain many small saccadic eye movements, and the possible influence of signals from the neck. Despite these limitations, head-only rotational testing may develop into a clinically useful technique. In particular, head-only rotation may be useful for the assessment of bilateral peripheral vestibular loss, e.g. in patients receiving ototoxic medications such as aminoglycoside antibiotics or certain chemotherapeutic agents.[55] Further research will be required to determine the ultimate clinical applicability of head-only rotational testing.

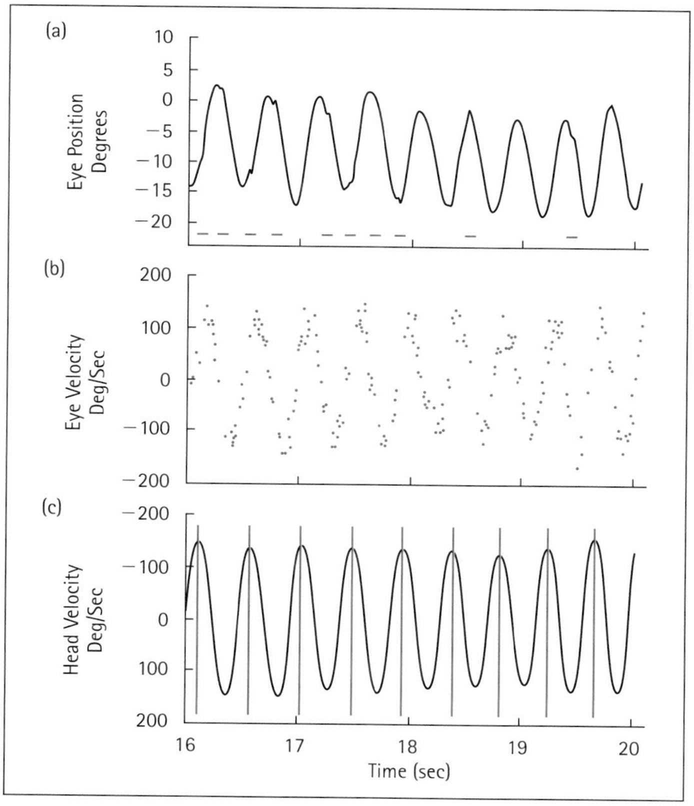

Figure 45.6 Eye movements induced by head-only rotation. Illustrated are eye position, eye velocity and head velocity during head-only rotation. (From Furman and Durrant with permission. *J Vestib Res* 1995; 5: 323–9.[34])

> **HEAD-ONLY ROTATIONAL TESTING**
>
> Major strength
>
> The vestibulo-ocular reflex can be assessed at the bedside using a stimulus that mimics natural head movements.
>
> Major weakness
>
> There are technical problems in rotating the head at high frequency while measuring the small eye movements produced.

Galvanic vestibular stimulation

Galvanic vestibular stimulation is a technique that has been used since the time of Barany, but it has not become a routine clinical measure. Galvanic vestibular stimulation is performed by passing small currents through the vestibular labyrinth using surface electrodes while recording either eye movements[56–60] or postural movements.[61–68] Typical stimulus configurations include placing an electrode on each mastoid, one positive and one negative, to produce medial–lateral sway or horizontal/torsional eye movements. Previous research and clinical application have been limited by the requirement for relatively high, sometimes painful, electric currents to produce recordable horizontal eye movements.[56] More recent studies using lower-intensity currents while recording non-horizontal (i.e. torsional) eye movements[60] or postural movements[66] have led to renewed interest in this technique. A significant advantage of galvanic stimulation is that each labyrinth can be tested separately. However, it is not yet certain which vestibular end organs are responsible for either the eye movements or postural movements induced by such a stimulus. Offsetting this limitation, however, is the fact that galvanic stimulation is believed to excite the synapse between the hair cell and the eighth cranial nerve afferent. As a result, galvanic stimulation can provide information regarding 'neural' versus 'sensory' function. That is, individuals with hair cell damage with preserved eighth nerve function may have normal or increased responses to galvanic stimulation. Thus, galvanic stimulation has promise as an assessment tool for unilateral eighth nerve function. However, it is technically challenging to deliver a well-controlled galvanic stimulus while recording eye movements or postural sway.

A limitation of galvanic stimulation when recording eye movements is similar to the limitation of all previously discussed techniques that rely on eye movements, namely that the technique provides a derived measure of vestibular function that relies upon the ocular motor system. When recording postural responses during galvanic stimulation, there is an additional difficulty based on the complexity of the postural control system, which is neither linear nor time invariant. As for VOR tests, recording postural sway during galvanic stimulation provides only a derived measure of peripheral vestibular function. Further, the stimulus may produce a skin sensation that cues the patient. Additional unresolved issues concerning the effect of galvanic stimulation on postural sway include the influence of head-on-torso position, the waveform of the electrical stimulus, i.e. constant versus sinusoidal, and the timing of the galvanic stimulus with respect to the patient's own sway. Despite these limitations and unresolved issues, however, with the advent of three-dimensional video-oculography and lower-cost motion analysis systems galvanic stimulation may emerge as a clinically useful tool. That is, low-intensity galvanic currents may produce small but recordable non-horizontal eye movements and/or small but recordable postural movements that can be measured reliably using sensitive recording instruments.

GALVANIC VESTIBULAR STIMULATION
Major strength
Galvanic stimulation can assess eighth nerve function unilaterally.
Major weakness
It is uncertain which vestibular end organs are responsive to galvanic stimulation.

Effects of moving visual scenes on postural sway

In response to optic flow stimuli, upright human subjects have been found to alter their postural sway.[69,70] In particular, sinusoidally moving visual scenes have been found to induce periodic postural sway that is of abnormally large magnitude in patients with vestibular disease.[71–73] A limitation of optic flow stimuli is that responses depend upon the postural control system. Additionally, visual influences on postural sway do not directly involve labyrinthine stimulation. Thus, this technique does not assess peripheral vestibular function. Rather, visual effects on postural sway may be influenced indirectly by vestibular function centrally or peripherally. Figure 45.7 shows how visual effects on posture can be assessed in the laboratory. Studies to date have suggested that certain patient groups have abnormal responses to visual stimuli, including patients with vestibular dysfunction,[71–73] children suffering from otitis media,[74] and patients with anxiety disorders.[75] Much research remains to be performed, however. Research issues include the specifics of the visual stimuli that may be most useful in eliciting postural responses and the analysis techniques that may be most useful.

Visual influences on posture may also be important in the nascent field of vestibular rehabilitation using virtual reality.[76–78] Studies of the effects of moving visual stimuli on postural sway may direct the choice of virtual reality scene that is most useful for rehabilitation purposes. Numerous technical and scientific issues remain to be addressed, including the importance of peripheral versus central vision, the direction, speed and complexity of the flow fields, and which aspects of postural sway are most useful to record.

Overall, because of the potential to contribute to both diagnosis and treatment, the use of moving visual stimuli while

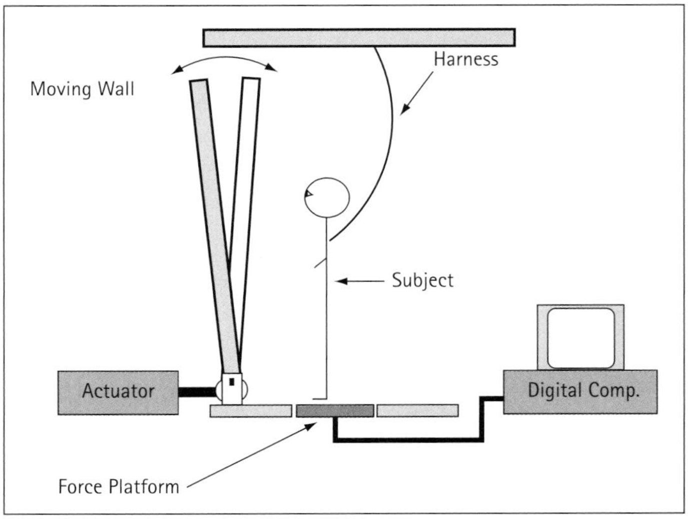

Figure 45.7 Apparatus that can be used for assessing the postural sway response during optic flow stimulation.

recording postural sway is likely to emerge in one form or another as a clinically useful technology.

EFFECTS OF MOVING VISUAL SCENES ON POSTURAL SWAY
Major strength
Postural sway during exposure to moving visual scenes appears to be particularly sensitive to disorders such as anxiety and otitis media.
Major weakness
Multiple neural pathways are involved in the postural response to visual scenes and there are many potential confounding factors that are difficult to control.

High-resolution imaging of the inner ear

High-resolution MRI to assess endolymphatic hydrops

Although the main pathological finding in patients with Menière's disease is distention of the entire endolymphatic system, i.e. endolymphatic hydrops, its diagnosis depends primarily upon a history of fluctuating hearing loss and tinnitus, and episodic vertigo. Therefore, development of a practical tool to obtain objective evidence of the existence of endolymphatic hydrops is important.

Obtaining clear images of the auditory portion of the inner ear is challenging, because the cochlea consists of very small compartments, i.e. the scala vestibuli, scala tympani, and cochlear duct. Moreover, these compartments are separated by thin walls. The scala tympani and cochlear duct are separated by the basilar membrane, which is about 100 µm thick, and the scala vestibuli and cochlear duct are separated by Reissner's membrane, which is only two cells thick (about 10 µm).

The different protein compositions of the cochlear duct versus the scala vestibuli/scala tympani accentuate of the differences in signal intensities from the endolymph and perilymph. This allows the basilar membrane and Reissner's membrane to be located.[79–81] Using such technology, it is possible that Menière's disease can be diagnosed using high-resolution MRI.[82]

The fine structure of the inner ear of a fixed, decalcified, celloidin-embedded human temporal bone determined using high-resolution MRI, including the basilar membrane of each turn of the cochlea, is shown in Figure 45.8. Note that the locations of both the basilar membrane and Reissner's membrane were based on the different protein concentrations of the endolymph versus the perilymph, the scala vestibuli, scala tympani, and cochlear ducts.

A major limitation of high-resolution MRI of the inner ear in the living human is that movement of the head caused by respiration creates movement artefact. Also, to obtain a high-resolution image, the strength of the magnetic field must be high and the frequency of the field must be in the GHz range. Such fields may be dangerous for living humans.

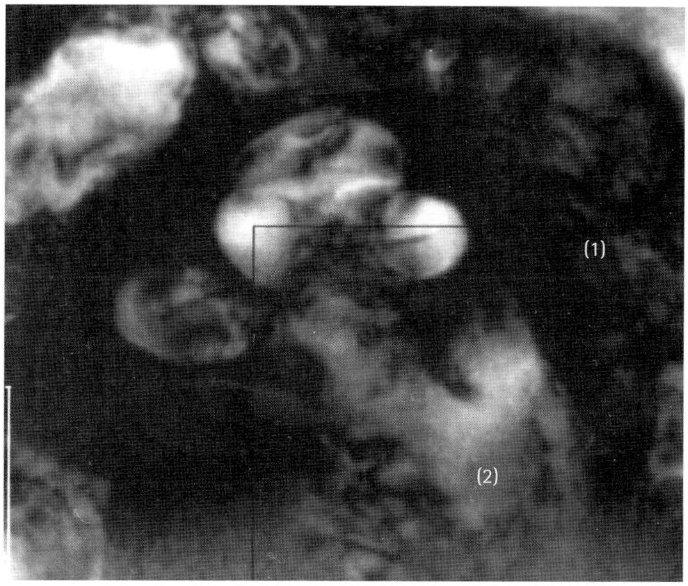

Figure 45.8 High-resolution MR image of the human temporal bone obtained with spin echo (spin echo, time of echo (TE) = 80 ms, time of repetition (TR) = 2500 ms, field of view, (FOV) = 50 mm). (1) The basilar membrane of the basal turn of the cochlea. (2) The internal auditory meatus.

If movement of the subject during MRI scanning could be overcome, it is possible that Reissner's membrane could be imaged and high-resolution MRI could become clinically feasible.

High-resolution CT to assess dehiscence of the superior semicircular canal

Dehiscence of the superior semicircular canal[83] is best identified on parasagittal projections (in the plane of the superior canal) from temporal bone CT scans performed with 0.5-mm collimation. CT scans performed with lower resolution (1.0- or 1.5-mm collimation) are sensitive for identification of a possible dehiscence but are of lower specificity, due to partial volume averaging. Recently, helical CT scans of the temporal bone using a Marconi Medical MxTwin CT scanner (Cleveland, OH, USA) have been used to identify dehiscence of the superior semicircular canal (L Minor, personal communication).

HIGH RESOLUTION IMAGING OF THE INNER EAR
Major strength
Assessment of endolymphatic hydrops and dehiscence of the superior semicircular canal.
Major weakness
Technical issues currently limit the use of high-resolution MRI in vivo.

References

1. Baloh RW, Beykirch K, Honrubia V, Yee RD. Eye movements induced by linear acceleration on a parallel swing. *J Neurophysiol* 1988; **60**: 2000–13.
2. Seidman SH, Telford L, Paige GD. Tilt perception during dynamic linear acceleration. *Exp Brain Res* 1998; **119**: 307–14.
3. Bronstein AM, Gresty MA. Short latency compensatory eye movement responses to transient linear head acceleration: a specific function of the otolith–ocular reflex. *Exp Brain Res* 1988; **71**: 406–10.
4. Watanabe Y, Mizukoshi K, Wasuda K, Ishii M, Sekiguchi C. Eye movement elicited by linear acceleration. *Acta Otolaryngol (Stockh)* 1991; Suppl 481: 34–6.
5. Busettini C, Miles FA, Schwarz U, Carl JR. Human ocular responses to translation of the observer and of the scene: dependence on viewing distance. *Exp Brain Res* 1994; **60**: 2000–13.
6. Gianna CC, Gresty MA, Bronstein AM. Influence of target distance and acceleration level and eye movements evoked by lateral acceleration steps. *Acta Otolaryngol (Stockh)* 1995; Suppl 520, Part I: 65–7.
7. Lathan CE, Wall C, Harris LR. Human eye movement response to z-axis linear acceleration: the effect of varying the phase relationships between visual and vestibular inputs. *Exp Brain Res* 1995; **103**: 256–66.
8. Merfeld DM, Teiwes W, Clarke AH, Scherer H, Young LR. The dynamic contributions of the otolith organs to human ocular torsion. *Exp Brain Res* 1996; **110**: 315–21.
9. Skipper JJ, Barnes GR. Eye movements induced by linear acceleration are modified by visualization of imaginary targets. *Acta Otolaryngol (Stockh)* 1989; Suppl 468: 289–93.
10. Brookes GB, Bronstein AM, Gresty MA. Otolith–ocular reflexes in patients with unilateral and bilateral loss of labyrinthine function. In: Sacristan T, Alvarex-Vicent JJ, Bartual J et al., eds. *Otorhinolaryngology, Head and Neck Surgery*, Amsterdam: Kugler & Ghedini Publications, 1990: 805–8.
11. Fujino A, Tokumasu K, Yosio S, Naganuma H. Sinusoidal linear accelerations test on peripheral vestibular disturbances. *Acta Otolaryngol (Stockh)* 1991; Suppl 481: 67–8.
12. Gresty MA, Bronstein AM. Testing otolith function. *Br J Audiol* 1992; **26**: 125–36.
13. Zee DS, Hain TC. Clinical implications of otolith–ocular reflexes. *Am J Otol* 1992; **13**: 152–7.
14. Baloh RW, Yue Q, Demer JL. The linear vestibulo-ocular reflex in normal subjects and patients with vestibular and cerebellar lesions. *J Vestib Res* 1995; **5**: 349–61.
15. Anastasopoulos D, Lempert T, Gianna C, Gresty MA, Bronstein AM. Horizontal otolith–ocular responses to lateral translation in benign paroxysmal positional vertigo. *Acta Otolaryngol (Stockh)* 1997; **117**: 468–71.
16. Lempert T, Gianna C, Brookes G, Bronstein A, Gresty M. Horizontal otolith-ocular responses in humans after unilateral vestibular deafferentation. *Exp Brain Res* 1998; **118**: 533–40.
17. Clarke AH, Engelhorn A. Unilateral testing of utricular function. *Exp Brain Res* 1998; **121**: 457–64.
18. Koizuka I, Takeda N, Sato S, Kubo T, Matsunaga T. Nystagmus responses in normal subjects during eccentric sinusoidal rotation. *Acta Otolaryngol (Stockh)* 1993; Suppl 501: 34–7.
19. Seidman SH, Paige GD. Perception and eye movement during low-frequency centripetal acceleration. *Ann NY Acad Sci* 1996; **781**: 693–5.
20. Bronstein AM, Gresty MA. Compensatory eye movements in the presence of conflicting canal and otolith signals. *Exp Brain Res* 1991: **85**: 697–700.
21. Bronstein AM, Gresty MA. Eye movements in response to canal and otolith signals in opposing directions. *Ann NY Acad Sci* 1992; **656**: 814–16.
22. Viirre ES, Demer JL. The vestibulo-ocular reflex during horizontal axis eccentric rotation and near target fixation. *Ann NY Acad Sci* 1996; **781**: 706–8.
23. Barratt H, Bronstein AM, Gresty MA. Testing the vestibular–ocular reflexes: abnormalities of the otolith contribution in patients with neuro-otological disease. *J Neurol Neurosurg Psychiatry* 1987; **50**: 1029–35.
24. Odkvist LM, Gripmark MA, Larsby B, Ledin T. The subjective horizontal in eccentric rotation influenced by peripheral vestibular lesion. *Acta Otolaryngol (Stockh)* 1996; **116**: 181–4.
25. Koizuka I, Takeda N, Sato S. Sakagami M, Matsunaga T. Centric and eccentric VOR tests in the patients with Menière's disease and vestibular Menière's disease. *Acta Otolaryngol (Stockh)* 1991; suppl: 55–8.
26. Guedry F. Orientation of the rotation-axis relative to gravity: its influence on nystagmus and the sensation of rotation. *Acta Otolaryngol* 1964; **60**: 30–48.
27. Darlot C, Denise P, Droulez J, Berthoz A. Eye movements induced by off-vertical axis rotation (OVAR) at small angles of tilt. *Exp Brain Res* 1988; **73**: 91–105.
28. Furman JM, Schor R, Schumann T. Off-vertical axis rotation: a test of the otolith–ocular–reflex. *Ann Otol Rhinol Laryngol* 1992; **101**(8): 643–50.
29. Wall III C, Furman JM. Nystagmus responses in a group of normal humans during earth horizontal axis rotation. *Acta Otolaryngol (Stockh)* 1989; **108**: 327–35.
30. Furman JM, Schor RH, Kamerer DB. Off-vertical axis rotational responses in patients with unilateral peripheral vestibular lesions. *Ann Otol Rhinol Laryngol* 1993; **102**: 137–43.
31. Furman JM, Balaban CD, Pollack IF. Vestibular compensation following cerebellar infarction. *Neurology* 1997; **48**(4): 916–20.
32. Peterka RJ, Shupert CL, Horak FB. Ocular counterrolling and OVAR tests identify preserved otolith function in some subjects with bilateral vestibular deficits. Abstract, Association for Research in Otolaryngology Mid-Winter meeting, St Petersburg Beach, FL, 1998.
33. Angelaki DE, Hess BJM. Three-dimensional organization of otolith-ocular reflexes in rhesus monkeys. I. Linear acceleration responses during off-vertical axis rotation. *J Neurophysiol* 1996; **75**: 2405–24.
34. Furman JM, Mendoza J. Visual–vestibular interaction during off-vertical axis rotation. *J Vestib Res* 1996; **6**(2): 93–103.
35. Colebatch JG, Halmagyi GM. Vestibular evoked potentials in

human neck muscles before and after unilateral vestibular deafferentation. *Neurology* 1992; **42**: 1635–6.
36. Robertson DD, Ireland DJ. Vestibular evoked myogenic potentials. *J Otolaryngol* 1995; **24**: 3–8.
37. Murofushi T, Matsuzaki M, Mizuno M. Vestibular evoked myogenic potentials in patients with acoustic neuromas. *Arch Otolaryngol Head Neck Surg* 1998; **124**: 509–12.
38. Ferber-Viart C, Dubreuil C, Duclaux R. Vestibular evoked myogenic potentials in humans: a review. *Acta Otolaryngol (Stockh)* 1999; **119**: 6–15.
39. Heide G, Freitag S, Wollenberg I, Iro H, Schimrigk K, Dillmann U. Click evoked myogenic potentials in the differential diagnosis of acute vertigo. *J Neurol Neurosurg Psychiatry* 1999; **66**: 787–90.
40. Murofusko T, Matsuzaki M, Wu CH. Short tone burst-evoked myogenic potentials on the sternocleidomastoid muscle. *Arch Otolaryngol Head Neck Surg* 1999; **125**: 660–4.
41. Friedmann G. The judgment of the visual vertical and horizontal with peripheral and central vestibular lesions. *Brain* 1970; **93**: 313–28.
42. Friedmann G. The influence of unilateral labyrinthectomy on orientation in space. *Acta Otolaryngol* 1971; **71**: 289–98.
43. Day MJ, Curthoys IS, Halmagyi GM. Linear acceleration perception in the roll plane before and after unilateral vestibular neurectomy. *Exp Brain Res* 1989; **77**: 315–28.
44. Bergenius J, Tribukait A, Brantberg K. The subjective horizontal at different angles of roll-tilt in patients with unilateral vestibular impairment. *Brain Res Bull* 1996; **40**: 385–91.
45. Bohmer A. The subjective visual vertical as a clinical parameter for acute and chronic vestibular (otolith) disorders. *Acta Otolaryngol (Stockh)* 1999; **119**: 126–7.
46. Bohmer A, Mast F. Assessing otolith function by the subjective visual vertical. *Ann NY Acad Sci* 1999; **871**(5): 221–31.
47. Bohmer A, Rickenmann J. The subjective visual vertical as a clinical parameter of vestibular function in peripheral vestibular diseases. *J Vestib Res* 1995; **5**: 35–45.
48. Dieterich M, Brandt T. Ocular torsion and tilt of subjective visual vertical are sensitive brainstem signs. *Ann Neurol* 1993; **33**: 292–9.
49. Jell RM, Guedry FE, Hixson WC. The vestibulo-ocular reflex in man during voluntary head oscillation under three visual conditions. *Aviation Space Environ Med* 1982; **53**: 541–8.
50. Fineberg R, O'Leary DB, Davis LL. Use of active head movements for computerized vestibular testing. *Arch Otolaryngol Head Neck Surg* 1987; **113**: 1063–5.
51. Geobel JA, Fortin M, Paige GD. Headshake versus whole-body rotation testing of the vestibulo-ocular reflex. *Laryngoscope* 1991; **101**: 695–8.
52. Demer JL, Oas JG, Baloh RW. Visual–vestibular interaction during high-frequency, active head movements in pitch and yaw. *Ann NY Acad Sci* 1992; **656**: 832–5.
53. Hoshowsky B, Tomlinson D, Nedzelski J. The horizontal vestibulo-ocular reflex gain during active and passive high-frequency head movements. *Laryngoscope* 1994; **104**: 140–5.
54. Chueng B, Money K, Sarkar P. Visual influence on head shaking using the vestibular autorotation test. *J Vestib Res* 1996; **6**: 411–22.
55. Kitsigianis G, O'Leary DB, Davis LL. Active head-movement analysis of cisplatin-induced vestibulotoxicity. *Otolaryngol Head Neck Surg* 1988; **98**: 82–7.
56. Moore DM, Hoffman LF, Beykirch K, Honrubia V, Baloh RW. The electrically evoked vestibulo-ocular reflex: I. Normal subjects. *Otolaryngol Head Neck Surg* 1991; **104**: 219–24.
57. Straub RH, Thoden U. A modified method of electronystagmography for recording eye movement during the galvanic vestibular test. *ORK* 1992; **54**: 21–4.
58. Zink R, Steddin S, Weiss A, Brandt T, Dieterich M. Galvanic vestibular stimulation in humans: effects on otolith function in roll. *Neurosci Lett* 1997; **232**: 171–4.
59. Zink R, Bucher SF, Weiss A, Brandt T, Dieterich M. Effects of galvanic vestibular stimulation on otolithic and semicircular canal eye movements and perceived vertical. *Electroencephalogr Clin Neurophysiol* 1998; **107**: 200–5.
60. Kleine JF, Guldin WO, Clarke AH. Variable otolith contribution to the galvanically induced vestibulo-ocular reflex. *Neuroreport* 1999; **10**: 1143–8.
61. Coats AC. Limit of normal of the galvanic body-sway test. *Ann Otol* 1972; **81**: 410–16.
62. Benson AJ, Jobson PH. Body sway induced by a low frequency alternating current. *Equilibrium Res* 1973; **3**: 55–61.
63. Nashner LM, Wolfson P. Influence of head position and proprioceptive cures on short latency postural reflexes evoked by galvanic stimulation of he human labyrinth. *Brain Res* 1974; **76**: 255–68.
64. Hlavacka F, Njiokiktjien CH. Postural responses evoked by sinusoidal galvanic stimulation of the labyrinth. *Acta Otolaryngol (Stockh)* 1985; **99**: 107–12.
65. Tokita T, Ito Y, Takagi K. Modulation by head and trunk positions of the vestibulo–spinal reflexes evoked by galvanic stimulation of the labyrinth. *Acta Otolaryngol (Stockh)* 1989; **107**: 327–32.
66. Cass SP, Redfern MS, Furman JM, DiPasquale JJ. Galvanic-induced postural movements as a test of vestibular function in humans. *Laryngoscope* 1996; 106: 423–30.
67. Johansson R, Magnusson M, Fransson PA. Galvanic vestibular stimulation for analysis of postural adaptation and stability. *IEEE Trans Biomed Engng* 1995; **42**: 282–91.
68. Cauquil AS, Gervet MFT, Ouaknine M. Body response to binaural monopolar galvanic vestibular stimulation in humans. *Neurosci Lett* 1998; **245**: 37–40.
69. Lee DN, Lishman JR. Visual proprioceptive control of stance. *J Human Movement Sci* 1975; **1**: 87–95.
70. Bertenthal BI, Dai DL. Infant's postural compensations induced by central versus peripheral optic flow. Paper presented at the 28th meeting of Psychonomic Society, 1987.
71. Bles JMB, de Jong V, de Wil G. Compensation for labyrinthine defects examined by use of a tilting room. *Acta Otolaryngol* 1983; **95**: 576–9.
72. Peterka RJ, Benolken, MS. Role of somatosensory and vestibular cures in attenuating visually-induced human postural sway. In: Woolacot M, Horak F, eds. *Posture and Gait: Control Mechanisms*. Oregon: University of Oregon, 1992: 272–5.

73. Redfern MS, Furman JM. Postural sway of patients with vestibular disorders during optic flow. *J Vestib Res* 1994; **4**(3): 221–30.
74. Casselbrant ML, Furman JM, Rubenstein E, Mandel EM. The effect of otitis media on the vestibular system in children. *Ann Otol Rhinol Laryngol* 1995; **104**(8): 620–4.
75. Jacob RG, Redfern MS, Furman JM. Optic flow-induced sway in anxiety disorders associated with space and motion discomfort. *J Anxiety Disorders* 1995; **9**: 411–25.
76. Viirre ES. Virtual environments: a new technology for vestibular research. *J Vestib Res* 1996; **6**: S74.
77. Kramer PD, Roberts DC, Shelhamer M, Zee DS. A versatile stereoscopic visual display system for vestibular and oculomotor research. *J Vestib Res* 1998; **8**: 363–79.
78. Kim NG, Yoo CK, Im JJ. A new rehabilitation training system for postural balance control using virtual reality technology. *IEEE Trans Rehab Engng* 1999; **7**: 482–5.
79. Koizuka I, Sano M, Kubo et al. Magnetic resonance image of the human temporal bone. *Plact Otolaryngol (Kyoto)* 1990; **83**: 549–55.
80. Koizuka I, Seo R, Sano M et al. High-resolution magnetic resonance imaging of the human temporal bone. *ORL* 1991; **53**: 357–61.
81. Henson MM, Henson OW Jr. Gewalt SL, Wilson JL, Johnson GA. Imaging the cochlea by magnetic resonance microscopy. *Hear Res* 1994; **75**: 75–80.
82. Salt AN, Henson MM, Gewalt SL, Keating AW, DeMott JE, Henson OW Jr. Detection and quantification of endolymphatic hydrops in the guinea pig cochlea by magnetic resonance microscopy. *Hear Res* 1995; **88**: 79–86.
83. Minor LB. Superior canal dehiscence syndrome. *Am J Otol* 2000; **21**: 9–19.
84. Furman JM, Durrant JD. Head-only rotational testing: influence of volition and vision. *J Vestib Res* 1995; **5**: 323–9.

Section V

Vestibular disorders and their management

46 Normal and abnormal balance

Robert W Baloh

Overview

The control of body equilibrium and posture in everyday life is a complex function involving multiple receptor organs and neuronal centers. In particular, vestibular, visual and proprioceptive reflexes must be integrated to ensure postural stability. The prominent role of sensory interaction in orientation can already be appreciated in the behavior of gastropods. The invertebrate *Hermissenda* has only rudimentary vestibular and visual receptors, yet the two systems fully interact to control behavior.[1] Afferent signals from photoreceptors in the eye and from hair cells in the statocyst converge on interneurons in the cerebral plural ganglia, which control a putative motor neuron in each pedal ganglion. Excitation of the motor neuron produces turning of the animal's foot in the ipsilateral direction, consistent with the animal's turning behavior toward light.

The block diagram in Figure 46.1 illustrates the organization of sensorimotor integration within the human brain.[2] Each of the primary sensory systems provides information to a first line of individual central processors which, in turn, pass this information on to a common central processor which provides command signals for eye movements and postural reflexes. The functioning of the overall system is under adaptive control in a manner similar to that involved in other aspects of brain function and behavior. The adaptive processor uses information from cross-sensory modalities in executing automated tasks, such as the repetitive execution of an athletic skill or the adjustment of eye movements to the use of magnifying or minifying lenses.[3] Adaptive mechanisms are also important in selecting orienting strategies, such as maintaining equilibrium after a shift in one's center of gravity by moving knees, hips, arms, or all together. The clinical importance of these adaptive mechanisms is becoming more and more clear, particularly with regard to developing rehabilitative strategies for patients with lesions involving the different sensory systems.[4]

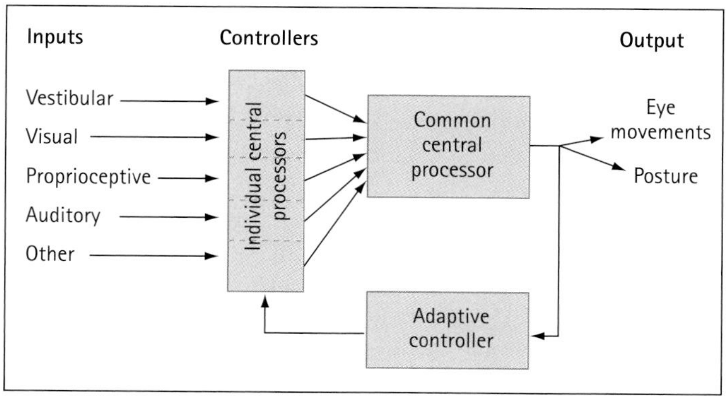

Figure 46.1 Block diagram illustrating the organization of sensorimotor integration within the brain. (From Baloh RW, Honrubia V. *Clinical Neurophysiology of the Vestibular System*, 3rd edn. New York: Oxford, 2001: 19, with permission.)

> Vestibular, visual and proprioceptive reflexes must be integrated in neuronal centers to ensure normal posture.

Organization of postural reflexes

The basic element for the control of tone in the trunk and extremity skeletal muscles is the myotatic reflex or deep tendon reflex. The myotatic reflexes of the antigravity muscles are under the combined excitatory and inhibitory influence of multiple supraspinal neuronal centers (Figure 46.2). In the cat, there are two main facilitatory centers (the lateral vestibular nucleus and rostral reticular formation) and four main inhibitory centers (frontal cortex, basal ganglia, cerebellum, and caudal reticular formation). The balance of input from these different brain areas determines the degree of tone in the antigravity muscles. If one removes the inhibitory influence of the frontal cortex and basal ganglia by sectioning the animal's midbrain, one produces a characteristic state of contraction in the antigravity muscles known as decerebrate rigidity. The extensor muscles increase their resistance to lengthening, and the deep tendon reflexes become hyperactive. The vestibular system is the main contributor to this increase in extensor tone, since bilateral destruction of the inner ears markedly decreases

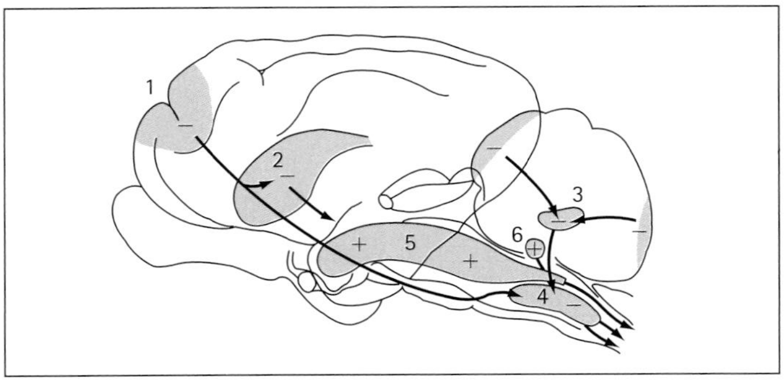

Figure 46.2 Facilitory (+) and inhibitory (−) pathways influencing the myotatic spinal reflex in the cat. Inhibitory pathways are: (1) corticobulboreticular, (2) caudospinal, (3) cerebelloreticular, and (4) reticulospinal. Facilitory pathways are: (5) reticulospinal; and (6) vestibulospinal. (From Lindsley DB, Scheiner LH, Magoun HW. An electromyographic study of spasticity. *J Neurophysiol* 1949; **12**: 197, with permission.)

the tone.[5] Destruction of one inner ear or the lateral vestibular nucleus on that side results in an ipsilateral decrease in tone, indicating that the main excitatory input to the anterior horn cells arises from the ipsilateral vestibular nucleus.[6]

Our earliest understanding of the role of the vestibular system on postural tone was derived from the study of decerebrate animals.[7] The extensor tone in a decerebrate cat can be modulated in a specific way by changing the position of the head in space. The tone is maximal when the animal is in the supine position with the angle of the mouth 45° above horizontal, and minimal when the animal is prone with the angle of the mouth 45° below the horizontal. Intermediate positions of rotation of the animal's body about the transverse or longitudinal axis result in intermediate degrees of extensor tone. If the head of the upright animal is tilted upward (without neck extension), extensor tone in the forelegs increases; downward tilting of the head causes decreased extensor tone and flexion of the forelegs. Lateral tilt produces extension of the extremities on the opposite side.

These tonic inner ear reflexes, mediated by way of the otolith organs, seldom occur in intact animals or human subjects, because of the inhibitory influence of the higher cortical and subcortical centers (as shown in Figure 46.2). They can be seen in premature infants, however, and in adults with lesions releasing the brainstem from the higher neural centers.

The history in a patient with imbalance

Patients often use the term dizziness to describe a sensation of imbalance or disequilibrium that occurs only when they are standing or walking and is unrelated to an abnormal head sensation. Both dizziness and imbalance are commonly associated with lesions involving peripheral and central vestibular structures. The severity of symptoms following a vestibular lesion depends on: (1) the extent of the lesion; (2) whether the lesion is unilateral or bilateral; and (3) the rapidity with which the functional loss occurs. Patients who slowly lose vestibular function bilaterally (e.g. secondary to ototoxic drugs) often do not complain of dizziness but will report oscillopsia with head movements and instability when walking (due to loss of vestibulo-ocular and vestibulospinal reflexes, respectively). If the patient slowly loses vestibular function on one side over a period of months to years (e.g. with an acoustic neuroma), symptoms and signs may be minimal. Such patients often describe a vague feeling of imbalance and unsteadiness on their feet and rarely complain of dizziness. On the other hand, a sudden unilateral loss of vestibular function is usually a dramatic event.[8] The patient complains of severe dizziness and nausea, is pale and perspiring, and usually vomits repeatedly. A brisk spontaneous nystagmus interferes with vision. These symptoms and signs are transient, however, and the process of compensation begins almost immediately. Over time, the patient adapts to the imbalance through a process of compensation that requires intact vision and depth perception, normal proprioception in the neck and limbs, and intact sensation in the lower extremities.[9] Central vestibular pathways are integral to compensation, and damage to these areas results in less effective recovery.

> Both unilateral and bilateral vestibular lesions can present with imbalance without dizziness.

The patient's general state of health prior to the onset of imbalance should be carefully investigated. Most systemic disorders can be associated with dizziness and imbalance, due to either partial involvement of all the body orienting systems or a decreased capacity of the central nervous system to deal with information from these systems. A careful drug history is crucial for evaluating any patient complaining of imbalance. Ototoxic drugs such as the aminoglycosides and salicylates produce abnormalities in gait and balance and oscillopsia from bilateral symmetrical vestibular end-organ damage. Antihypertensive medications can produce dizziness and imbalance after standing, due to postural hypotension. Alcohol and phenytoin produce acute reversible imbalance and chronic irreversible imbalance from cerebellar dysfunction. Sedative drugs (e.g. barbiturates, benzodiazepines and phenothiazines) cause a nonspecific dizziness and imbalance, typically described as a fogginess, cloudiness, or giddiness, that is presumably due to a diffuse depression of the central sensory integrating centers.

Psychiatric illnesses are commonly associated with sensations of dizziness and imbalance. Feelings of dissociation, as though one has left one's own body, are common. Patients use terms such as 'floating', 'swimming', and 'giddiness' to describe the sensation. They may report a feeling of imbalance (commonly a rocking or falling sensation) or even a spinning inside the head—a sensation that can be differentiated from vertigo because it is not associated with an illusion of movement of the environment or with nystagmus. Episodes of dizziness and imbalance can be provoked by certain sensory stimuli (e.g. driving over the brow of a hill, walking on a brightly polished floor, watching a train go by) or by social situations (e.g. eating in a restaurant, shopping in a department store, attending a reception). Symptoms may begin after a period of stress, especially after the death of a loved one or after a patient has been through a severe illness, and may continue for months or years.

Clinical assessment of gait and balance

Maintenance of balance and equilibrium is a complex process requiring integration of diverse sensory signals and multiple brain centers. Considering the many possible loci of dysfunction, the examination of a patient complaining of disequilibrium must include a careful assessment of gait, strength, coordination, reflexes, and sensory function.

> Examination of a patient complaining of imbalance should include a careful assessment of gait, strength, coordination, reflexes and sensory function.

Examination of gait and balance should begin by having the patient walk normally in an open area where there is room for normal stride without fear of bumping into objects. The patient should be asked to walk normally from one end to the other with normal quick turns. One should observe for stride length, base width, overall posture, associated movements, and balance on turning. Having the patient walk heel-to-toe narrows the base and can accentuate imbalance associated with central nervous system disorders, particularly cerebellar lesions (Figure 46.3). However, it is important to keep in mind that normal older people have trouble walking in tandem with eyes open. Romberg[10] first noted that patients with proprioceptive loss from tabes dorsalis were unable to stand with the feet together and eyes closed. Bárány[11] later emphasized the importance of vestibular influences in maintaining the Romberg position with eyes closed. Patients with cerebellar lesions are often unable to stand in the Romberg position even with eyes open.

> Damage to the vestibular, somatosensory or visual systems typically produces subtle gait abnormalities such as slight widening of the base, shortening of the stride, and slow, careful turns.

A variety of semiquantitative bedside measurements of gait and balance have been developed, such as counting the number of steps made in tandem without a side step, timing the subject's ability to stand in the Romberg position or on one foot with

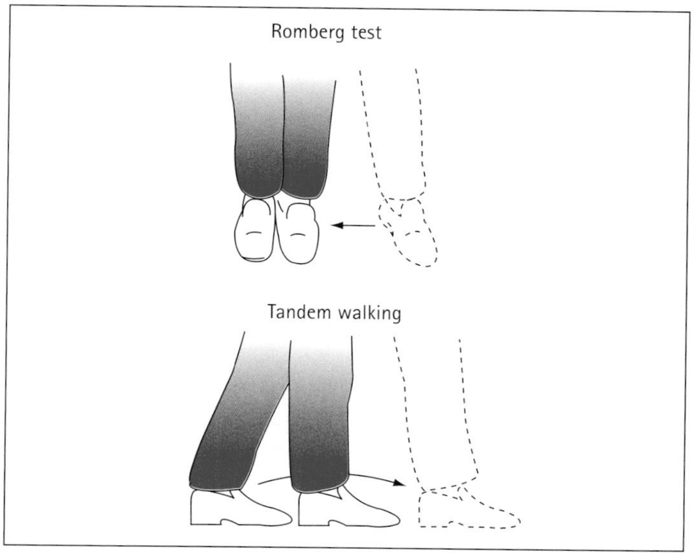

Figure 46.3 Bedside tests of vestibulospinal function.

eyes open and with eyes closed, and timing the subject's ability to walk through a designed obstacle course. Performance on these measurements tends to deteriorate with age, although there is large individual variability, and the sensitivity for identifying balance disorders in a specific patient population has yet to be established. Probably the most widely used semiquantitative bedside test for evaluating gait and balance disorders in older people is the Tinetti gait and balance scale.[12] This scale grades such features as gait speed, stride length and symmetry, and balance on standing, turning, following a nudge and with eye closure. Performance on the Tinetti scale has been correlated with the incidence of falls and other measurements of disequilibrium and imbalance in older people.

Gait and balance features associated with lesions at different sites

Sensory disorders

Since the somatosensory, vestibular and visual systems provide the main source of information about the position of the head and body in space, damage to any of these afferent systems can lead to disequilibrium and gait imbalance. As a general rule, the gait disorders associated with loss of sensory input are milder than other gait disorders and are therefore more difficult to identify on examination. Common features include slight widening of the base, shortening of the stride, and slow careful turns (Table 46.1). Nutt et al[13] called this a 'cautious gait', which they felt was a non-specific response to any cause of disequilibrium. Patients with proprioceptive or vestibular loss become 'visual dependent', so that symptoms and signs are much worse in the dark or with eyes closed (basis of the Romberg test).

Table 46.1 Features of gait disorders in older people

Category	Characteristic features of gait
Sensory loss	'Cautious gait', slightly widened base, shortened stride, slow turns
Musculoskeletal	Difficulty arising, general slowness, limp, decreased elevation of feet, locking of knees
Cerebellar lesions	'Atactic gait', markedly widened base, truncal instability, overactive postural reflexes
Basal ganglia lesions	Difficulty starting, freezing, rigidity, lack of associated movements, turns en bloc
Frontal cortex and subcortical white matter lesions	'Apractic gait', small shuffling steps, feet adhere to the floor, poor reflex control

Somatosensory and visual function are routinely measured as part of the neurological examination. The characteristic stocking/glove distribution sensory loss of a peripheral neuropathy is easily identified. Visual acuity is best measured with the standard Snellen visual acuity chart. Bedside measurement of vestibular function is more difficult, because of overlap of the vestibular system with other sensorimotor systems. Vestibular function testing is extensively reviewed in other chapters but, in my experience, the two most useful bedside tests are the head-thrust test and the dynamic visual acuity test. With the head-thrust test, the patient fixates on the examiner's nose while the head is quickly turned to one side and then the other.[14] Normally, the eyes move smoothly in the orbits, maintaining fixation on the target. Patients with vestibular loss require several quick catch-up saccades to maintain fixation (to one side with unilateral lesions and to both sides with bilateral lesions). For the dynamic visual acuity test, the patient rapidly oscillates the head back and forth (greater than one cycle per second) while reading a standard visual acuity chart.[15] A drop in visual acuity with head-shaking of greater than two lines on the acuity chart suggests bilateral vestibular loss.

> Two useful bedside tests of vestibular function are the head-thrust test and the dynamic visual acuity test.

Musculoskeletal disorders

Examination of any patient complaining of imbalance should include a careful assessment of strength and joint mobility of the lower extremities. In addition to testing the strength of individual muscles, have the patient arise from a chair without using the arms, walk up and down steps, and walk on the toes and heels. Proximal muscle weakness and stiffness are associated with numerous neurological disorders and general systemic illnesses. Musculoskeletal disorders are ubiquitous in older people. The musculoskeletal system is less pliable and there is a general decrease in strength. Deconditioning due to lack of physical exercise can lead to a classic vicious cycle, whereby joint stiffness and decreased strength lead to less activity, which in turn leads to more weakness and stiffness. Patients with musculoskeletal disorders have difficulty arising from a sitting position, and walk in a slow, deliberate fashion. They may show a characteristic limp or lock their knees to overcome proximal weakness (Table 46.1).

Cerebellar disorders

The cerebellum is commonly considered the balance center of the brain, yet how it achieves this function is only partially understood. Cerebellectomized animals retain postural reflexes, although their ability to control these reflexes is impaired. Functionally, the cerebellum can be divided into two major components: the midline structures—the vermis and flocculonodular lobes—which are critical for maintaining equilibrium, and the hemispheres, which control coordination of the limbs. Lesions which produce truncal imbalance invariably involve the midline structures, particularly the anterior vermis or the flocculonodular regions.

> Gait disorders associated with cerebellar lesions are usually much more pronounced than those associated with peripheral sensory loss.

The characteristic wide-based ataxic gait of cerebellar lesions is usually easily differentiated from other gait disorders (Table 46.1). Unlike patients with peripheral neuropathy and bilateral vestibular loss, patients with cerebellar lesions are unable to use vision to stabilize their balance, so that walking is severely impaired, even with vision. Some patients with lesions involving the anterior lobe of the cerebellum show a characteristic three cycle per second postural tremor.[16]

Basal ganglia lesions

The dopaminergic system of the basal ganglia is critical for initiation of gait and for maintaining postural responses. Monkeys who have had this system damaged by the toxin MPTP exhibit a flexed posture, deficient postural reflexes, and freezing.[17] Not infrequently, patients with basal ganglia disorders, particularly patients with Parkinson's disease, will present with frequent falls

> The characteristic gait in patients with basal ganglia lesions is dominated by akinesia and rigidity.

due to disturbed postural responses. The characteristic gait is dominated by akinesia and rigidity (Table 46.1). There is difficulty in starting, freezing, lack of associated movement, and turning en bloc. Festination, retropulsion or propulsion can also occur.

The diagnosis of Parkinson's disease is apparent if one observes the typical gait features along with a pill-rolling tremor, generalized rigidity, and a mask-like facies. On the other hand, early in the disease process, subtle abnormalities of gait may be the only abnormality. Progressive supranuclear palsy is a multisystem disorder that may initially resemble Parkinson's disease, but eventually patients develop other features, including impaired vertical gaze, pseudobulbar signs, and cerebellar signs. An important early differential feature between Parkinson's disease and progressive supranuclear palsy is the posture when walking. Patients with Parkinson's disease have a stooped-forward posture, while patients with progressive supranuclear palsy have increased tone in the extensors of the neck, so that the head and neck are extended backward. The combination of neck extension and impaired down gaze leads to frequent severe falls in patients with progressive supranuclear palsy.

Frontal cortex and subcortical white matter lesions

The characteristic gait associated with frontal cortex and subcortical white matter lesions is the apraxic gait, characterized by small shuffling steps with the feet adhering to the floor almost as though they were stuck to it (Table 46.1). Such patients typically have poor postural reflex control, so that, once they start to fall, they are unable to compensate and often suffer severe injuries. On neurological examination, such patients often exhibit cortical release signs and are unable to relax their limbs voluntarily, a phenomenon called paratonic rigidity. In late stages, such patients cannot walk unassisted and may have difficulty in sitting down from a standing position. They land on the edge of the chair and fall off. Ultimately, they are confined to bed. Although many of these features are similar to those seen with basal ganglia disorders, the apraxia along with paratonia and cortical release signs suggest more generalized involvement, particularly frontal lobe involvement.

> Patients with an apraxic gait shuffle their feet almost as though they are stuck to the floor.

Aging and balance control

The effect of aging on the peripheral and central pathways controlling gait and balance is usually a very subtle process that parallels similar slight changes in memory and other cognitive functions and is generally considered part of the normal aging process. The gait of normal elderly men is characterized by slight anterior flexion of the upper torso with flexion of the arms and knees, diminished arm swing, and shorter step length;[18] the gait of older women tends to be narrow-based, with a waddling quality.[19] The majority of older people recognize that they must walk more slowly, turn more carefully and expect their balance to be less steady than it was in young adulthood. These normal older individuals do not generally present to physicians complaining of imbalance. Only when one or more disease processes occur do overt symptoms develop. It is inappropriate to dismiss symptoms of dizziness and imbalance as due to normal aging or to such non-specific entities as presbyastasis or multisensory dizziness.

> As a rule, dizziness and imbalance in older people should not be attributed to normal aging.

Age-related changes have been identified in each of the special senses and in the cortical centers that integrate these signals. Changes in vestibular function have been documented by numerous investigators.[20] Degeneration of peripheral vestibular structures is known to occur with aging, and neuronal loss has been found in the vestibular nuclei and their cortical projections with aging.[21] Impairment of peripheral sensation of the lower limbs correlates with postural instability, and age-dependent proprioceptive loss has been identified.[22] Visual perception is altered with age, and poor near visual acuity also correlates with postural instability.[23] Slowing of central processing of sensory information may also lead to imbalance in older people,[24] and there is a loss of cerebellar Purkinje cells with age that can reduce coordination and adaptability of visual-vestibular interactions.[25] Cerebral and cerebellar atrophy, ventriculomegaly and subcortical white matter lesions have all been associated with imbalance in older people.[26–28] Cognitive impairment, muscle weakness and the use of certain sedating drugs increase the risk of falls and may play a role in gait disorders in some older people.[29]

Rehabilitation strategies in patients with gait disorders

The treatment of patients with imbalance due to sensory loss is aimed at improving overall sensory function when possible and at training the brain to adjust to the sensory loss. Prevention is the best strategy in managing ototoxic vestibular loss. Potentially ototoxic drugs should be used with great caution, particularly in those with renal impairment. When such drugs are used, patients should be carefully monitored, with daily examinations of gait and balance. Some ototoxic drugs, such as streptomycin and gentamicin, are remarkably selective for the vestibular system, so that monitoring hearing is of little use. Physical therapy programs are aimed at gait and balance training.[30] The goal of these programs is to retrain the brain to use remaining sensory signals to compensate for the areas lost. Patients are taught to understand the nature of their deficits and simple tricks to help overcome them. For example, patients with bilateral vestibular loss cannot see clearly while they are walking, so they are taught to stop and hold their head still whenever they want to read a sign or see the face of a passerby. They are taught which circumstances to avoid and the proper use of aids such as a cane.

> Although treatments for specific balance disorders are limited, most patients will benefit from physical therapy aimed at improving joint mobility and strength and at gait and balance training.

Physical therapy can be very beneficial in patients with musculoskeletal disorders. Joint range of movement and strength can be improved, and the vicious cycle associated with deconditioning can be reversed.

Management of cerebellar gait disorders is usually restricted to helping patients learn to protect themselves from dangerous falls. Gait and balance training often have little effect, since the cerebellum is the key center for adapting postural reflexes. Patients with alcoholic cerebellar degeneration can stop the progression and may even show some improvement after stopping alcohol.

Treatment of Parkinson's disease is aimed at replenishing the damaged dopaminergic system of the basal ganglia. The combination of L-dopa plus a peripheral decarboxylase inhibitor is usually the treatment of choice. The gait disorder is often dramatically responsive to L-dopa therapy. Patients with progressive supranuclear palsy may respond to L-dopa, although the benefit is often minimal. Physical therapy aimed at maintaining strength and joint mobility may slow the rate of progression. With the exception of hydrocephalus, which can be dramatically reversed with the placement of a shunt, most frontal gait disorders are not reversible. They can be helped by improving support with canes or a walker. Tranquilizing medications should be scrupulously avoided, since they can further impair the central integration of sensory information.

References

1. Goh Y, Alkon DL. Sensory, interneuronal, and motor interactions within Hermissenda visual pathway. *J Neurophysiol* 1984; **52**: 156–69.
2. Baloh RW, Honrubia V. *Clinical Neurophysiology of the Vestibular System*. 3rd edn. New York: Oxford, 2001: 17–20.
3. Melvill Jones G. How and why does the vestibulo-ocular reflex adapt? In: Baloh RW, Halmagyi GM, eds. *Disorders of the Vestibular System*. New York: Oxford University Press, 1996; 85–92.
4. Herdman SJ. Role of vestibular adaptation in vestibular rehabilitation. *Otolaryngol Head Neck Surg* 1998; **119**: 49–54.
5. Bach LMN, Magoun HW. The vestibular nuclei as an excitatory mechanism for the cord. *J Neurophysiol* 1947; **10**: 331–47.
6. Fulton JF, Liddell EGT, Rioch DM. The influence of unilateral destruction of the vestibular nuclei upon posture and the knee jerk. *Brain* 1930; **53**: 327–48.
7. Fetter M, Dichgans J. How do the vestibulospinal reflexes work? In: Baloh RW, Halmagyi GM, eds. *Disorders of the Vestibular System*. New York: Oxford University Press, 1996: 105–12.
8. Hotson JR, Baloh RW. Acute vestibular syndrome. *N Engl J Med* 1998; **339**: 680–5.
9. Vidal P-P, De Waele C, Vibert N, Mühlethaler M. Vestibular compensation revisited. *Otolaryngol Head Neck Surg* 1998; **19**: 34–42.
10. Romberg MH. *Lehrbuch der Nervenkrankheit des Menschen*. Berlin: A. Dunker, 1846.
11. Bárány R. Neue Untersuchungsmethoden, die Beziehungen zwichen Vestibularapparat, Kleinhirn, Grosshirn und Rüchenmark betreffend. *Wien Med Wochenschrift* 1910; **60**: 2033.
12. Tinetti ME, Williams TF, Mayewski R. Fall risk index for elderly patients based on number of chronic disabilities, *Am J Med* 1986; **80**: 429–34.
13. Nutt JG, Marsden CD, Thompson PD. Human walking and higher-level gait disorders, particularly in the elderly. *Neurology* 1993; **43**: 268–79.
14. Halmagyi GM, Curthoys IS. A clinical sign of canal paresis. *Arch Neurol* 1988; **45**: 737–9.
15. Demer JL, Honrubia V, Baloh RW. Dynamic visual acuity: a test for oscillopsia and vestibulo-ocular reflex function. *Am J Otol* 1994; **15**: 340–7.
16. Baloh RW, Jacobson KM, Beykirch K, Honrubia V. Static and dynamic posturography in patients with vestibular and cerebellar lesions. *Arch Neurol* 1998; **55**: 649–54.
17. Burns RS, Phillips JM, Chuang CC, et al. The MPTP-treated monkey model of Parkinson's disease. In: Markey SP, Castagnoli N, Trevor AJ, Kopin IJ, eds. *MPTP: A Neurotoxin Producing a Parkinsonian Syndrome*. New York: Academic Press, 1986: 23–46.
18. Murray MP, Kory RC, Clarkson BH. Walking patterns in healthy old men. *J Gerontol* 1969; **24**: 169–78.
19. Finley FR, Cody KA, Finizie RV. Locomotion patterns in elderly women. *Arch Phys Med Rehab* 1969; **50**: 140–6.
20. Baloh RW, Jacobson KM, Socotch TM. The effect of aging on visual-vestibulo-ocular responses. *Exp Brain Res* 1993; **95**: 509–16.
21. Lopez I, Honrubia V, Baloh RW. Aging and the human vestibular nucleus. *J Vestib Res* 1997; **7**: 77–85.
22. Lord SR, Clark RD, Webster IW. Postural stability and associated physiological factors in a population of aged persons. *J Gerontol* 1991; **46**: M69–76.
23. Teasdale N, Stelmach GE, Breunig A et al. Age differences in visual sensory integration. *Exp Brain Res* 1991; **85**: 691–6.
24. Wolfson L, Whipple R, Derby CA et al. A dynamic posturography study of balance in healthy elderly. *Neurology* 1992; **42**: 2069–75.
25. Hall TC, Miller AKH, Corsellis JAN. Variations in the human Purkinje cell population according to age and sex. *Neuropathol Appl Neurobiol* 1975; **1**: 267–92.
26. Thompson PD, Marsden CD. Gait disorder of subcortical arteriosclerotic encephalopathy in Binswanger's disease. *Movement Disord* 1987; **2**: 1–8.
27. Kerber KA, Enrietto JA, Jacobson KM, Baloh RW. Disequilib-

rium in older people. A prospective study. *Neurology* 1998; **51**: 574–80.
28. Whitman GT, Tang Y, Lin A, Baloh RW. A prospective study of cerebral white matter abnormalities in older people with gait dysfunction. *Neurology* 2001; **57**: 990–4.
29. Wild D, Nayak USL, Isaacs B. Prognosis of falls in old people at home. *J Epidemiol Commun Health* 1981; **35**: 200–4.
30. Shumway-Cook A, Horak FB. Rehabilitation strategies for patients with vestibular deficits. *Neurol Clin North Am* 1990; **8**: 441–57.

47 Normal and abnormal eye movements

Christopher Kennard

Introduction

A wide variety of disease processes affecting the central nervous system, from the brainstem to the cortex, can lead to disorders of eye movements. Examination of eye movements at the bedside can often contribute to determining a neurological diagnosis, or provide information regarding anatomical, physiological and neurochemical lesions. This is best achieved with a basic knowledge of the neuroanatomy and neurophysiological concepts of the neural control of the different types of eye movements.

Functional classes of eye movements

The various types of functional classes of eye movements all subserve the same goal, the projection of an image of the object of interest onto the most sensitive part of the retina, the fovea (Table 47.1). Rapid conjugate eye movements, saccades, enable the line of gaze to be redirected to bring the image of a new object of interest onto the fovea, and the dysjunctive or vergence eye movements ensure that these images are simultaneously placed on both foveae regardless of their distance from the observer. There is also a need to stabilize the image of the object of interest on the fovea when the object itself moves, achieved by the smooth pursuit system, or when the subject's head or body moves, as occurs during locomotion, when the vestibular and optokinetic ocular motor reflexes are activated. These different functional types of eye movements can each be rapidly tested at the bedside.[1]

Table 47.1 Goals of various types of eye movements.

To bring the image of a target to the fovea
Saccades
Vergence
To keep the image on the fovea
Pursuit
Vestibular/optokinetic

Saccades

Voluntary saccade initiation should be assessed by instructing the patient to look to the left and then to the right and up and down. The patient is then asked to fixate two targets alternately—e.g. a pen in one hand and a raised finger of the other—so that between each refixation they are briefly moved and their distance from each other varied. This generates reflexive saccades, which are tested in the horizontal and vertical planes, and the examiner should observe saccadic variables such as speed of initiation (latency), velocity and accuracy. Any slowing of saccades can be accentuated by using an optokinetic striped drum or tape, when the repositioning saccades will appear slowed. This is of particular help when showing slowed adducting saccades in a partial internuclear ophthalmoplegia. Another method to accentuate this abnormality is to use oblique targets. Because the velocity is slowed in the horizontal and not the vertical plane, the resulting saccade is L-shaped. Predictive saccades can be tested by alternately raising a finger of one hand and then the other in a predictable regular pattern, and asking the patient to make saccades to the target. Finally, the patient should be observed for any head movements or blinks before making a saccade, as occurs in Huntington's disease and ocular motor apraxia.

Smooth pursuit

Both horizontal and vertical smooth pursuit can be tested by asking the patient to track a small target at a distance of about 1 m while keeping their head still. The target should be moved initially at a slow uniform speed and the pursuit eye movements observed to determine whether they are smooth, or broken up by catch-up saccades. This is a non-specific sign if present in both directions—e.g. due to ageing, drugs or cerebellar disease—or it may indicate a focal posterior cortical lesion if only present in one direction, in which case the abnormal pursuit is in the direction of the lesion. The speed should be gradually increased, but at high velocities all smooth pursuit eye movements will be broken up by saccades even in normal subjects. The OKN drum and tape is a useful method to elicit a series of pursuit movements, and does not elicit true optokinetic eye movements.

Optokinetic nystagmus

The optokinetic system cannot be tested as part of the clinical examination, because the OKN drum and tape commonly used tests smooth pursuit and not the optokinetic system. A full-field revolving striped drum is required to elicit OKN.

Vestibular system

If the vestibulo-ocular system is functioning normally, passive rotation of the patient's head should result in a slow eye movement, so that the eyes deviate in the opposite direction to that of the head movement. This is known as the doll's head (oculocephalic) manoeuvre and should be performed both horizontally and vertically. This technique is valuable not only for assessing vestibular function, but also for differentiating between infranuclear and nuclear from supranuclear gaze palsies, and in the evaluation of brainstem function in comatose patients. It should be noted that the eye movements elicited in unconscious patients by this procedure largely reflect the integrity of the semicircular canals and their central connections, although in conscious patients the effects of visual input on eye movements may influence the response to head rotation.

A rough estimate of any deterioration of vestibular gain (head velocity divided by eye velocity) can be obtained by asking the patient to read a Snellen chart while their head is being passively rotated. If there is an abnormality, the visual acuity will show a deterioration compared with the acuity obtained when the head is stationary. Another bedside test of the horizontal vestibulo-ocular reflex (VOR) is for the examiner to observe the patient's optic disc with an ophthalmoscope while the patient tries to fixate a distant object and shake their head from side to side at the same time. If the gain of the VOR is normal (unity), the examiner will not obscure any movement of the optic disc, and if abnormal the disc will repeatedly slip from view. A further method to test the integrity of the VOR is the head thrust test described by Halmagyi and Curthoys.[2] The patient sits directly in front of the examiner and is instructed to maintain fixation of the examiner's nose, while he or she briefly and rapidly rotates the patient's head first to the left and then to the right. If the VOR is intact, the patient's eyes move smoothly to maintain fixation. However, if there is a unilateral defect, a smooth eye movement interrupted by a refixation saccade is observed.

The VOR can be suppressed by activating the smooth pursuit system. This is tested by asking the patient to hold their arms outstretched and fixate their thumbnail while rotating their head and trunk in harmony. Impaired cancellation of the VOR and hence abnormal smooth pursuit are shown by observing the eye repeatedly moving off fixation due to the VOR, followed by refixation saccades. This is a particularly useful technique for testing pursuit in patients with gaze-evoked nystagmus.

Abnormalities of horizontal and vertical gaze due to brainstem and cerebellar disorders

Anatomy and physiology of horizontal and vertical gaze

There are two main features of the brainstem neural control of horizontal and vertical gaze: an anatomical separation, so that the neural substrate for horizontal gaze is located in the pons and that for vertical gaze in the midbrain, and the requirement to overcome viscous drag and resist elastic restoring forces in the orbit when making dynamic eye movements (Figure 47.1). An understanding of the neural mechanisms which generate a horizontal saccade will serve as an illustration of the principles involved. A rapid phasic contraction of the extraocular muscle e.g. lateral rectus muscle, is required to overcome the orbital viscosity, and a rapid, high-frequency burst of nerve impulses, the pulse, is transmitted to the muscle via the ocular motor nerve (Figure 47.2). The premotor inputs to the motor neurones in the abducens nucleus arise from neurones in a region of the reticular formation that lies ventral and anterior to the nucleus, the paramedian pontine reticular formation (PPRF). The equivalent premotor region for vertical gaze is the rostral interstitial nucleus of the medial longitudinal fasciculus (riMLF) in the midbrain, rostral to the oculomotor nucleus at the level of the red nucleus. The pulse, a velocity signal, is generated by cells called burst neurones, and must be of an appropriate size to ensure that the eye is brought to the target. Once the saccade has been completed, it is necessary to maintain the new position of the globe against orbital elastic restoring forces, which will pull the globe back towards the mid-position. The muscle must, therefore, maintain a sustained

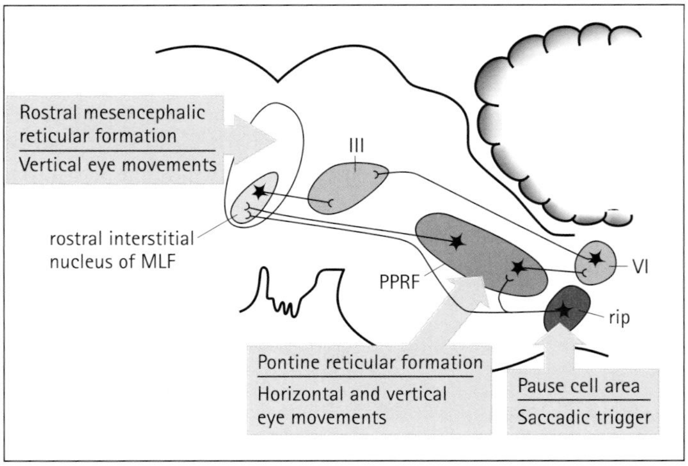

Figure 47.1 Diagrammatic sagittal section of the human brainstem showing a summary of major pathways involved in horizontal and vertical saccade generation. (From Büttner-Ennever and Büttner. In: Büttner-Ennever, ed. *Neuroanatomy of the Oculomotor System*. New York: Elsevier 1988: 119–76.[45])

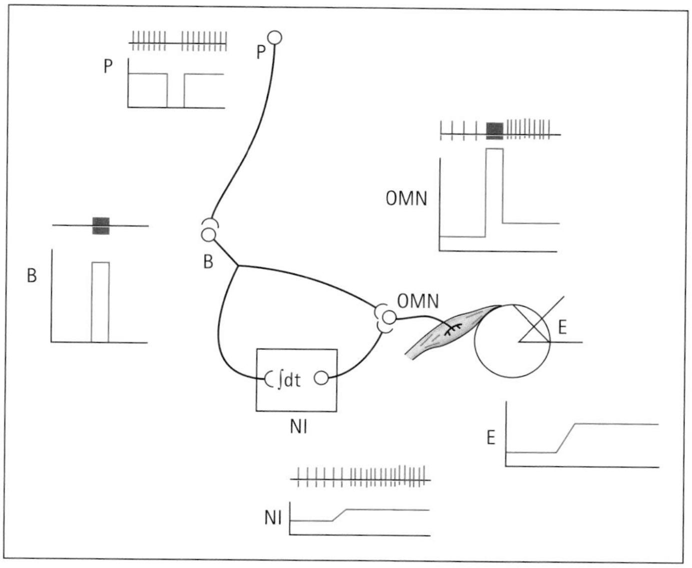

Figure 47.2 The relationship between pause cells (P), burst cells (B), and the cells of the neural integrator (NI), in the generation of the saccade pulse and step. Pause cells cease discharging just before each saccade, allowing the burst cells to generate the pulse. The pulse is integrated by the neural integrator (NI) to produce the step. The pulse and step combine to produce the innervational change on the ocular motor neurones (OMN) that produces the saccadic eye movement (E). Vertical lines represent individual discharges of neurones. Underneath the schematized neural (spike) discharge is a plot of discharge rate versus time. (Redrawn from Leigh and Zee. *The Neurology of Eye Movements.* New York: Oxford University Press © 1999.[43] Used by permission of Oxford University Press, Inc.)

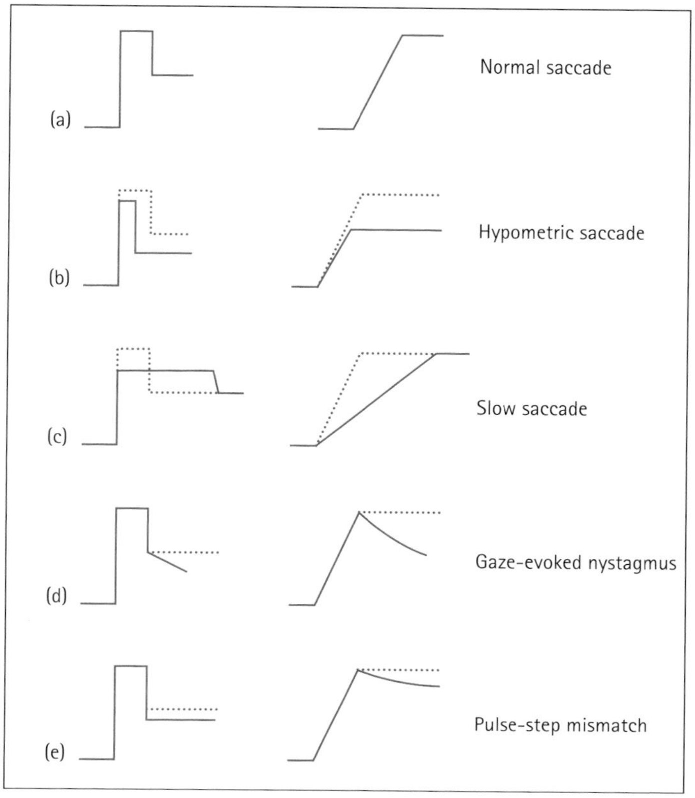

Figure 47.3 Disorders of the saccadic pulse and step. Innervation patterns are shown on the left, eye movements on the right. Dashed lines indicate the normal response. (a) Normal saccade. (b) Hypometric saccade: pulse amplitude (width × height) is too small, but pulse and step are matched appropriately. (c) Slow saccade: decreased pulse height with normal pulse amplitude and normal pulse–step match. (d) Gaze-evoked nystagmus: normal pulse, poorly sustained step. (e) Pulse–step mismatch (glissade): step is relatively smaller than pulse. (Redrawn from Leigh and Zee. *The Neurology of Eye Movements.* New York: Oxford University Press © 1999.[43] used by permission of Oxford University Press, Inc.)

tonic contraction, and this is achieved by the tonic innervation, the step, which is a position signal the motor neurone receives from so-called integrator neurones lying in the nucleus prepositus hypoglossi and the medial vestibular nucleus. The pulse and step must be perfectly matched to prevent drift of the eye back to the primary position at the end of the saccade. Abnormalities of either lead to easily defined eye movement disorders (Figure 47.3). Faulty neural integration leads to an inadequately maintained step, so that after a saccade the eye drifts back in an exponential manner, due to the unopposed orbital elastic restoring forces, followed by a saccade to refixate the target. This pattern leads to gaze-evoked nystagmus and is observed in cerebellar disease and anticonvulsant or sedative intoxication. An abnormal pulse may either be of reduced duration or of reduced firing frequency. If the step is appropriately matched, the former will result in a reduced amplitude (hypometric) saccade and the latter a saccade of reduced velocity which nonetheless has a normal amplitude.

Abnormalities of horizontal eye movements

The abducens nucleus contains two populations of neurones, motor neurones innervating the ipsilateral lateral rectus muscle and interneurones. The axons from the interneurones cross the midline and ascend in the medial longitudinal fasciculus (MLF) to the contralateral medial rectus subdivision of the oculomotor nerve nucleus (Figure 47.4a). The final instructions for horizontal conjugate eye movements, therefore, lie within the abducens nucleus itself, so that its activation results in an ipsilaterally directed horizontal conjugate gaze movement.

Unilateral horizontal gaze palsy

A lesion of the abducens nucleus will, therefore, result in an ipsilateral horizontal gaze palsy for all types of conjugate movements (saccades, pursuit and vestibular). Vergence movements of the eyes are spared, however, so that adduction is possible with a near stimulus.[3] The palsy is usually associated with an ipsilateral lower motor neurone facial nerve palsy due to involvement of the genu of the facial nerve, which passes around the abducens nerve (Figure 47.5). A selective horizontal gaze palsy involving only saccades, including the quick phases of vestibular and optokinetic nystagmus, occurs when the lesion involves the PRRF in isolation, since the vestibular and pursuit inputs pass directly to the abducens nucleus. The

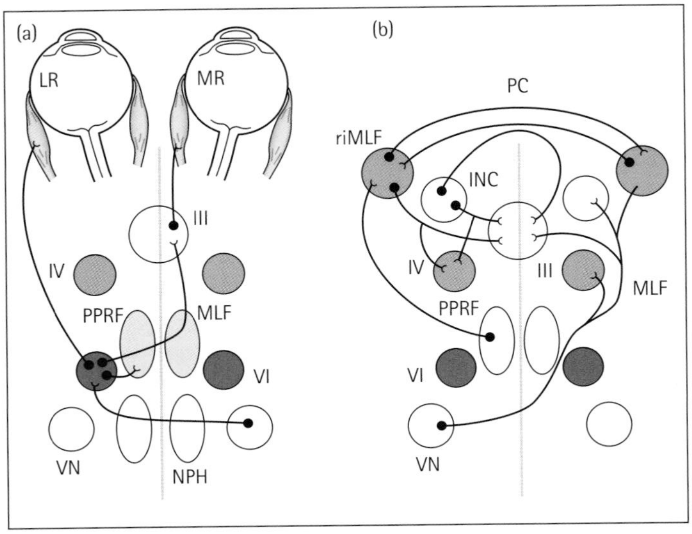

Figure 47.4 Summary of eye movement control. (a) The brainstem pathways for horizontal gaze. Axons from the cell bodies located in the abducens nucleus (VI) travel to the ipsilateral lateral rectus muscle (LR), and the axons of abducens internuclear neurones cross the midline and travel in the medial longitudinal fasciculus (MLF) to the portion(s) of the oculomotor nucleus (III) concerned with the medial rectus (MR) function (in the contralateral eye). (b) The brainstem pathways for vertical gaze. Important structures include the rostral interstitial nucleus of the medial longitudinal fasciculus (riMLF), the paramedial pontine reticular formation (PPRF), the interstitial nucleus of Cajal (INC), and the posterior commissure (PC). Note that axons from cell bodies located in the vestibular nuclei (VN) travel directly to the abducens nuclei and, mostly via the MLF, to the oculomotor nuclei. IV, trochlear nucleus; NPH, nucleus prepositus hypoglossi.

commonest causes of horizontal gaze palsies are either vascular infarction and haemorrhage or demyelination.

Bilateral horizontal gaze palsy

A bilateral pontine lesion involving the PPRF can cause a bilateral selective saccadic palsy with preservation of vestibular and optokinetic eye movements.[4] Such a lesion may impair vertical eye movements, since signals for vertical vestibular and smooth pursuit eye movements ascend in the MLF and other pathways through the pons. The commonest causes for a bilateral horizontal gaze palsy, with sparing of vertical gaze, are neurodegenerative diseases such as Huntington's disease or Gaucher's disease.

Internuclear ophthalmoplegia

A lesion of the MLF produces an internuclear ophthalmoplegia (INO), in which there is a disturbance of adduction ipsilateral to the side of the lesion[5] (Figure 47.6). In a partial INO, adduction will be slowed, but it will be completely absent in a complete lesion (Table 47.2). Since the fibres of the MLF carry the horizontal gaze commands subserving all types of conjugate eye movements, this adduction paresis involves not only saccades but also pursuit and vestibular eye movements. The presence of intact convergence in the absence of voluntary adduction implies that the medial rectus subdivision of the oculomotor nerve is intact, and that the INO is likely to be due to a caudal lesion. Cogan[6] called this a posterior INO, in contrast to an INO and absent convergence, which he called 'anterior'. However, such patients do not necessarily have a lesion involving the medial rectus subdivision of the oculomotor nucleus.

The second major feature of an INO is the nystagmus on abduction in the contralateral eye. This consists of a centripetal (inward) drift, followed by a corrective saccade. Several differ-

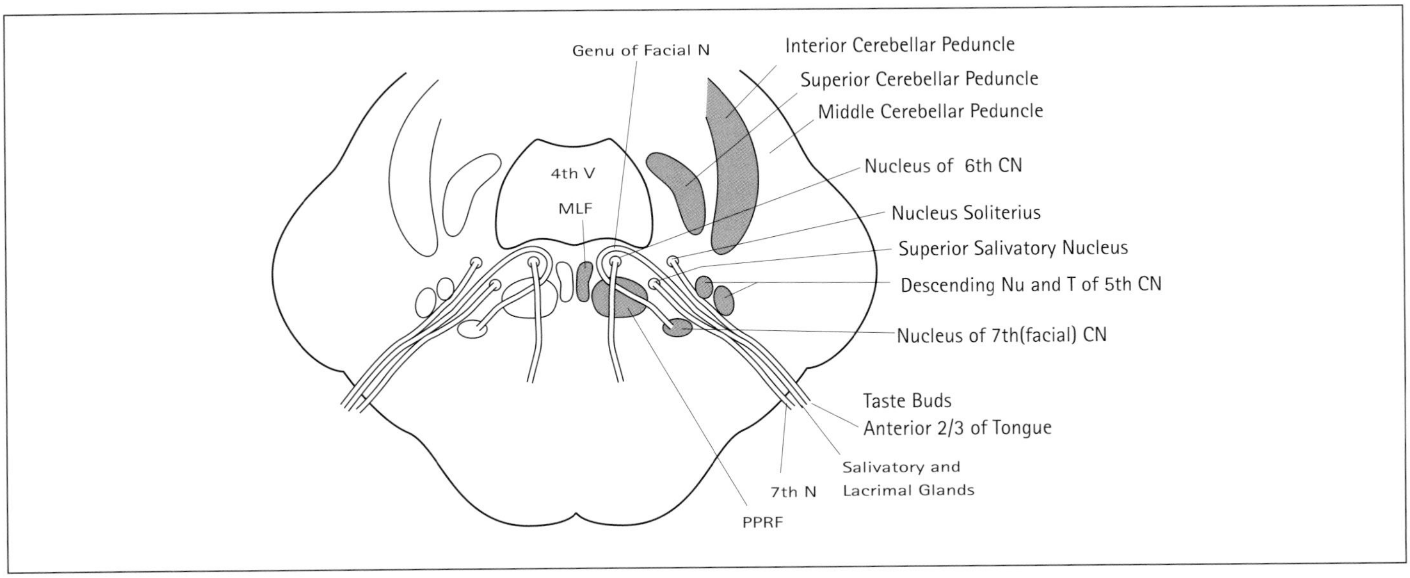

Figure 47.5 Transverse section through the pons at the level of the abducens nucleus to show the relationship of the abducens nucleus to the fascicle of the facial nerve which encircles it.

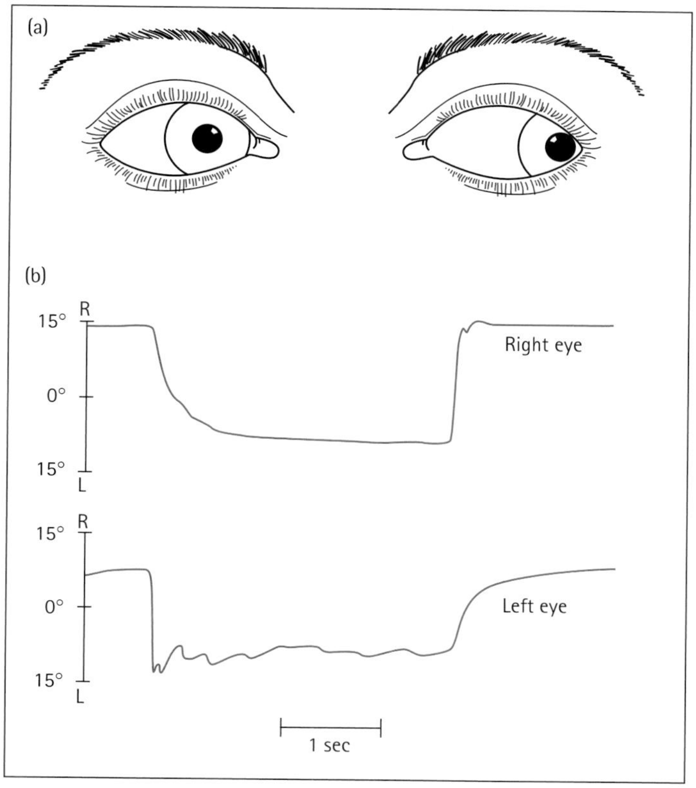

Figure 47.6 (a) A right internuclear ophthalmolplegia showing impaired adduction of the right eye with abducting nystagmus. (b) The eye movement recording of the same patient shows the abducting nystagmus in the left eye and the slowed adducting saccade in the right eye.

ent mechanisms have been proposed to explain the abducting nystagmus.[5] These include: (1) a gaze-evoked nystagmus; (2) impaired inhibition of the medial rectus contralateral to the lesion; (3) an increase in convergence tone; and (4) adaptation to the contralateral medial rectus weakness. The latter is generally considered the most appropriate explanation.

A skew deviation (a vertical misalignment of the visual axes due to a disturbance of supranuclear inputs) is often observed in patients with a unilateral INO, with the higher eye usually on the side of the lesion. However, the eyes are usually orthotropic, even in a complete INO, and if there is any esotropia in the primary position this supports an infranuclear ophthalmoplegia. Patients with bilateral INOs have bilateral adduction weakness and abducting nystagmus. In addition, they also have impaired vertical pursuit and vestibular eye movements, and impaired vertical gaze holding with gaze-evoked nystagmus on looking up or down.[7]

Patients with an INO are usually asymptomatic, although if there is a complete adduction failure they may complain of diplopia, especially during shifts of horizontal gaze. Occasionally, they may complain of oscillopsia. A number of different aetiologies lead to an INO (Table 47.3), but if unilateral the commonest is ischaemia, and if bilateral the commonest is demyelination associated with multiple sclerosis.

A rarer so-called posterior internuclear ophthalmoplegia of Lutz has been described in which there is an impairment of abduction (not adduction) of saccades and pursuit, but not vestibular eye movements. This is different to the posterior INO described by Cogan, in which convergence is intact. The pathogenesis of the posterior INO of Lutz is unclear.[8]

One-and-a-half syndrome

A combined lesion of the abducens nucleus or PPRF and the adjacent MLF on one side of the brainstem results in both an ipsilateral horizontal gaze palsy and INO.[9] The only preserved horizontal eye movement is abduction of the contralateral eye, and the condition is therefore termed the 'one-and-a-half' syndrome. Although the majority of patients have no ocular deviation or an esotropia (convergent deviation) in the primary position of gaze, some patients may habitually fixate with the horizontally immobile ipsilesional eye, which results in exotropia (divergent deviation) of the contralesional eye, which still has an intact lateral rectus innervation. This condition is called paralytic pontine exotropia[10] (Figure 47.7). Some MLF lesions cause an adduction palsy due to INO that is bilateral and isotropic in the primary position, termed a 'wall-eyed' bilateral INO (WEBINO).[11]

The main causes of a one-and-a-half syndrome are brainstem ischaemia, haemorrhage and tumour. The syndrome can be mimicked by a bilateral INO with an ipsilateral abducens nerve palsy.

Table 47.2 Pathogenesis of different signs in internuclear ophthalmoplegia.

Eye	Ocular motor defect	Possible pathophysiology
Ipsilateral eye	Adduction weakness	Interruption of axons of abducens internuclear neurones
Contralateral eye	Abduction nystagmus	Adaptation to impaired (slowed or absent) contralateral medial rectus action
Bilateral eyes	Vertical gaze-evoked nystagmus	Vertical eye position signal inadequate
	Vertical pursuit and vestibular movements impaired	Interruptions of MLF axons carrying these signals

Table 47.3 Aetiology of internuclear ophthalmoplegia.

Multiple sclerosis (commonly bilateral)
Brainstem infarction (commonly unilateral)
Brainstem and fourth ventricular tumours
Arnold–Chiari malformations
Infection
Syphilis
Nutritional disorders, e.g. Wernicke's encephalopathy and pernicious anaemia
Metabolic disorders, e.g. abetalipoproteinaemia, maple syrup urine disease, hepatic encephalopathy
Head trauma
Hydrocephalus
Progressive supranuclear palsy
Drug intoxications: phenothiazines, narcotics, tricyclic antidepressants, lithium, barbiturates
Cancer: carcinomatosis infiltration or paraneoplastic
Pseudointernuclear ophthalmoplegia due to myasthaenia gravis and Fisher's syndrome

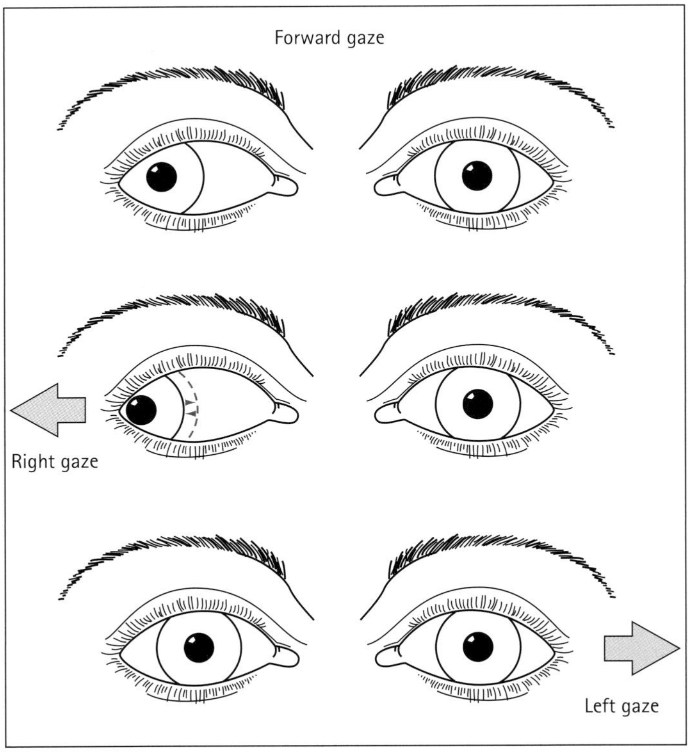

Figure 47.7 Paralytic pontine exotropia. In the primary position, the patient fixates with the horizontally immobile left eye; the right eye is moderately exotropic. On attempted rightward gaze, the right eye abducts normally, but the left eye fails to move. On attempted leftward gaze, the right eye moves to the midline, but the left eye again fails to move. Vertical saccadic movements and vergence movements can be normal. The lesion in this case involves the left pontine paramedian reticular formation and the adjacent left medial longitudinal fasciculus. (From Sharpe et al. *Neurology* 1974; **24**: 1076–81.[10])

Lateropulsion

This is a feature of lateral medullary infarction (Wallenberg's syndrome), in which there is a compelling sensation of being pulled toward the side of the lesion, accompanied by appropriate eye movement signs. During voluntary eye closure and sometimes even during blinks, the eyes deviate toward the side of the lesion, and have to make corrective saccades to refixate the target on eye opening (Figure 47.8). All ipsiversive saccadic eye movements overshoot the target (hypermetric), and saccades directed away from the side of the lesion undershoot the target (hypometric).[12] Vertical saccades have a parabolic ipsiversive trajectory. This ipsipulsion is in contrast to the overshooting of contralateral saccades (saccadic contrapulsion) observed in patients with infarction in the territory of the superior cerebellar artery. The eye signs of lateropulsion are considered to be due to damage to olivocerebellar projections.[13]

Abnormalities of vertical eye movements

Disturbances of vertical gaze are usually associated with damage to one or more of three structures in the mesencephalon, the posterior commisure, the riMLF and the interstitial nucleus of Cajal (INC) (Figure 47.4b). The only exceptions are: an apparent vertical gaze palsy due to mechanical restriction of extraocular muscles in orbital disorders such as thyroid eye disease; large acute pontine lesions involving the PPRF bilaterally producing a temporary vertical saccadic palsy, in addition to the permanent horizontal saccadic palsy; and certain degenerative disorders of the nervous system such as progressive supranuclear palsy or adult Niemann–Pick disease.

Dorsal midbrain syndrome (Parinaud's syndrome)

This syndrome is due to a lesion which involves the posterior commisure and is associated with a variety of aetiologies (Table 47.4) and clinical features (Table 47.5), some of which may not be present in an individual patient.[14] The essential sign is a loss of upward gaze involving all types of eye movement, although the VOR and Bell's phenomenon may sometimes be spared.

Table 47.4 Aetiology of vertical gaze palsy.

Tumour: pineal germinoma or teratoma
Hydrocephalus
Vascular: midbrain and thalamic haemorrhage or infarction
Drug-induced: barbiturates, neuroleptics, carbamazepine
Degenerative: progressive supranuclear palsy, Huntington's disease, corticobasal degeneration, Lytico–Bodig syndrome, diffuse Lewy body disease
Metabolic: Niemann–Pick variants, Tay-Sach's disease, Gaucher's disease, Wilson's disease
Miscellaneous: multiple sclerosis, Whipple's disease, hypoxia, syphilis, encephalitis

Table 47.5 Clinical features of the dorsal midbrain syndrome.
Impairment of upward eye movements (Parinaud's syndrome)
Lid retraction (Collier's sign)
Disturbance of downward eye movements
Disturbance of vergence eye movements
Convergence–retraction nystagmus
Paralysis of convergence
Skew deviation
Pupillary abnormalities (light-near dissociation)

When the syndrome is acute, the eyes may be deviated downwards (the setting-sun sign), and may be observed in premature infants following intraventricular haemorrhage, and when a ventricular shunt becomes acutely blocked. Downward saccades may be of reduced velocity.

The dorsal midbrain syndrome may also be associated with an impairment of convergence, which is usually paralysed but may rarely be excessive and cause convergence spasm, convergence–retraction nystagmus, eyelid retraction (Collier's sign), and a pupillary light-near dissociation.

Selective vertical gaze palsy due to riMLF lesion

A unilateral or bilateral lesion of the riMLF produces a downgaze palsy, mainly affecting saccades, or, more rarely, a complete vertical gaze palsy.[15] Patients with unilateral midbrain lesions can develop combined upgaze and downgaze palsies, isolated upgaze palsies, a uniocular upward ophthalmoplegia with no primary position hypotropia (monocular double elevator palsy), and a vertical one-and-a-half syndrome which describes the combination of a vertical gaze palsy in one direction and a monocular vertical ophthalmoplegia in the other direction, with no primary position heterotropia (ocular misalignments).[16]

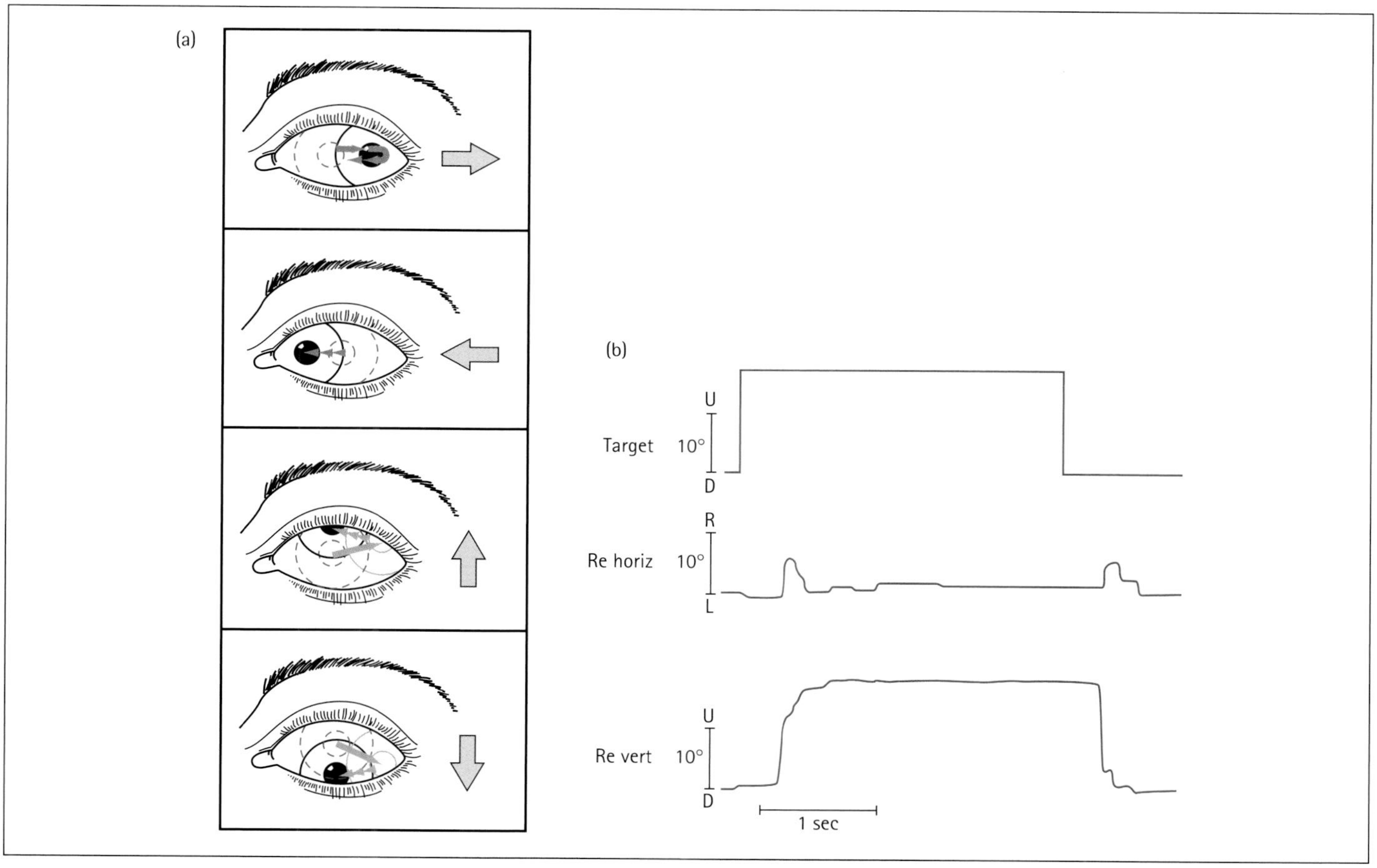

Figure 47.8 Lateropulsion. (a) Leftward lateropulsion in a patient with a left lateral medullary infarct. (Only the left eye is shown, with the direction of gaze indicated by the black arrow.) The single leftward saccade in response to a 20° leftward target overshot the target, so that a single rightward corrective saccade was required in order to fixate the target. Saccades to a 20° rightward target undershot the target, so that three small rightward saccades (each white arrow indicating a saccade) were required in order to fixate the target. Vertical saccades to 20° upward and 20° downward targets also had an unintended leftward component, so that several small rightward saccadic components were required in order to fixate the target. (Adapted from Kommerell G, Hoyt WF.[46]) (b) Rightward lateropulsion in a patient with a left cerebellar infarct: the upward saccade in response to the 20° upward target had an unintended 5° rightward component, which was then corrected by two leftward saccades. U, up: D, down; R, right; L, left; RE HORIZ, right eye horizontal position; RE VERT, right eye vertical position. (From Ranalli and Sharpe. *Ann Neurol* 1986; **20**: 311.[44] Reprinted by permission of John Wiley & Sons, Inc.)

The ocular tilt reaction and lesions of the INC

A lesion of the INC, which lies immediately caudal to the riMLF and rostral to the oculomotor nucleus, produces two distinct deficits: an ocular tilt reaction (OTR), and a deficit in vertical pursuit and vertical gaze holding.[17] The OTR is a head–eye postural synkinesis that consists of a skew deviation with a head tilt (towards the side of the hypometric eye), and torsion of the eyes (incyclotropia of the hypermetric eye and excyclotropia of the hypometric eye) (Figure 47.9). Such patients also show a deviation of their subjective vertical. Although the OTR is produced by a lesion of the INC, it can be found whenever peripheral or central lesions cause an imbalance of otolithic inputs.[18]

Abnormalities of horizontal and vertical eye movements due to thalamic lesions

Lesions of the thalamus can give rise to disorders of both horizontal and vertical eye movements.[19] Conjugate deviation of the eyes contralateral to the lesion (so-called wrong-way deviation) is associated with haemorrhage in the medial thalamus. Thalamic haemorrhage may also lead to forced downward deviation of the eyes, associated with convergence and miosis. Caudal lesions in the thalamus have been associated with unilateral esotropia, which, although usually associated with a downward gaze deviation, may be present as an isolated finding. A paralysis of downgaze is associated with a caudal thalamic infarction, due to occlusion of the proximal portion of the posterior cerebral artery or its perforator branch, the thalamosubthalamic paramedian artery. However, the ocular motor deficit may well be due to damage to the riMLF or its immediate premotor inputs.

The effect of cerebellar lesions upon eye movements

Although it is generally accepted that the cerebellum plays an important role in the control of eye movements in humans, pure lesions of the cerebellum without some brainstem involvement are unusual.[20] This creates some difficulty in determining eye movement abnormalities specific for cerebellar dysfunction. It is appropriate to segregate lesions into

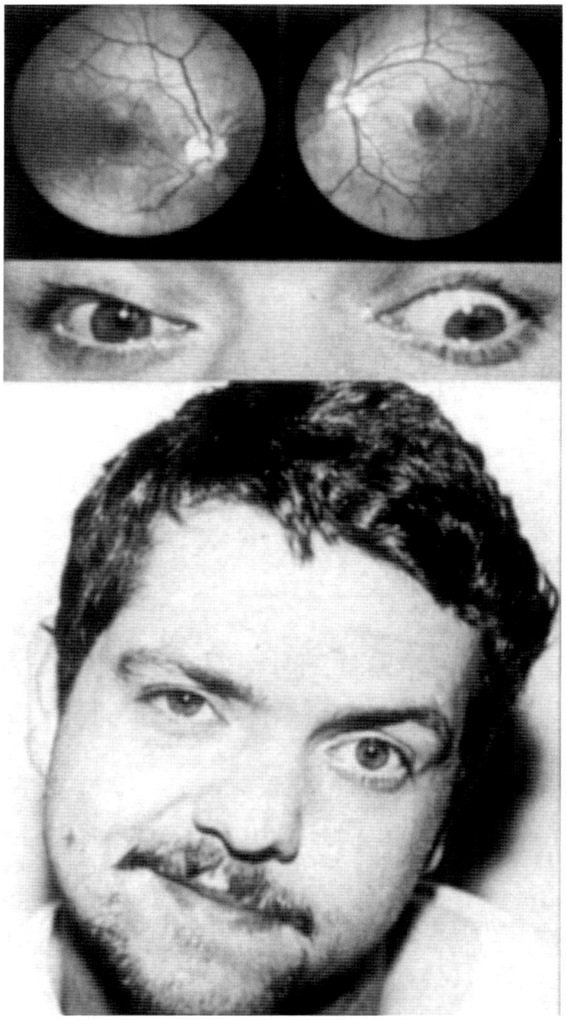
(a)

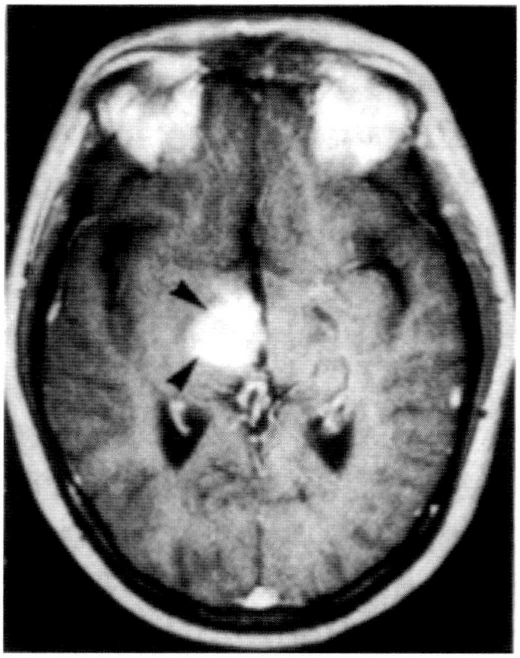
(b)

Figure 47.9 Tonic contraversive ocular tilt reaction caused by a unilateral midbrain–thalamic lesion. (a) The patient had a leftward ocular tilt reaction consisting of a leftward head tilt, left hypotropia, and leftward torsion of each eye, as shown in the fundus photographs. (b) The lesion, a haemorrhage caused by a right (R) midbrain–thalamic arteriovenous malformation, is shown on T_1-weighted parasagittal MRI. (From Halmagyi et al. *Neurol* 1990; **40**: 1503–9.[17])

three main regions of the cerebellum, each of which has a particular ocular motor syndrome: the dorsal vermis and underlying fastigial nucleus, the nodulus and ventral uvula, and the flocculus and paraflocculus. The dorsal vermis and underlying fastigial nucleus are involved in controlling saccadic accuracy and smooth pursuit. Lesions in this region lead to saccadic dysmetria and mild deficits of smooth pursuit. The nodulus and ventral uvula are involved in the control of the low-frequency response of the VOR, and disorders in this region give rise to periodic alternating nystagmus, positional nystagmus and impaired habituation of the VOR, with increased duration of the vestibular responses. The flocculus and paraflocculus are concerned with retinal-image stabilization, e.g. smooth tracking with the head still, gaze holding, control of the VOR and its suppression, and pulse–step matching. Lesions of this region, therefore, lead to impaired pursuit and VOR cancellation with gaze-evoked, rebound, centripetal and downbeat nystagmus, and inappropriate amplitude of the VOR. Other signs which have been associated with cerebellar lesions, although precise localization is not available, include torsional nystagmus during vertical pursuit (lesion in the middle cerebellar peduncle), square wave jerks, esotropia with alternating skew deviation, divergent nystagmus, primary position upbeating nystagmus, and centripetal nystagmus.

The cerebellum is also important in generating long-term adaptive responses that enable eye movements to be kept appropriate to the visual stimulus. For example, when wearing lens corrections there is a magnifying or minifying effect which requires adaptive changes in the gain of the VOR. These take a few hours to days to occur and explain why some individuals experience difficulties when prescribed new lens prescriptions.

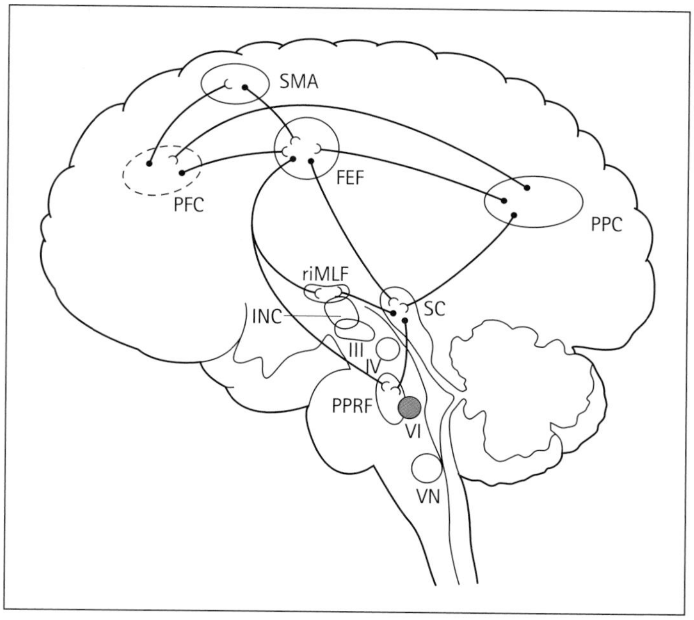

Figure 47.10 Cortical and brainstem saccade centres. The supranuclear connections from the frontal eye fields (FEF) and the posterior parietal cortex (PPC) to the superior colliculus (SC), riMLF and the PPRF are shown. The PPC to SC projection is mainly involved with reflexive saccades, whereas the FEF to SC projection is involved in the production of voluntary saccades.

Disorders of the voluntary control of gaze

Anatomy and physiology of voluntary gaze

The cerebral hemispheres are extremely important for the programming and coordination of both saccadic and pursuit conjugate eye movements. Since different areas are involved in these two types of eye movements, they will be dealt with separately, always realizing that for fully effective ocular motor control, coordination between these subtypes of eye movement is essential.

Saccadic system

There appear to be four main cortical areas in the cerebral hemispheres involved in the generation of saccades (Figure 47.10). In the frontal lobe in humans there is the frontal eye field (FEF), which lies laterally at the caudal end of the second frontal gyrus in the premotor cortex (Brodmann area 8), and the supplementary eye field (SEF), which lies mesially at the anterior region of the supplementary motor area in the first frontal gyrus (Brodmann area 6). The third area is in the dorsolateral prefrontal cortex (DLPFC), which lies anterior to the FEF in the second frontal gyrus (Brodmann area 46). Finally, a posterior eye field (PEF) lies in the parietal lobe, possibly in the superior part of the angular gyrus (Brodmann area 39) and the adjacent lateral intraparietal sulcus. Studies in monkeys reveal that these areas are all interconnected with each other, and they all send projections to the superior colliculus (SC) and the premotor areas in the brainstem controlling saccades.

It appears that there are two parallel pathways involved in the cortical generation of saccades. The first is an anterior system originating in the FEF projecting both directly, and via the SC, to the brainstem saccadic generators. This pathway also passes indirectly via the basal ganglia to the SC. The second or posterior pathway originates in the PEF, passing to the brainstem saccadic generators via the SC. Only after bilateral lesions to both the FEF and SC in monkeys is there a failure to trigger saccades.

Although the precise functions of these various cortical areas in saccade generation have not been determined, a number of general statements can be made. The FEF is involved in triggering volitional saccades, which, for example, may be predictive (in anticipation of the appearance of a target), memory-guided (to a previously seen target), or scanning (searching for a particular target of interest). The PEF is involved in triggering reflexive saccades to the sudden appearance of novel visual or auditory stimuli, and appears to be involved in visuospatial integration. The DLPFC may be responsible for maintaining a spatial map of the environment in short-term memory, providing spatial information for memory-guided saccades and other volitional saccades. There is also evidence that it contains circuits responsible for inhibiting unwanted reflexive saccades made in response to unattended novel visual stimuli. The SEF appears to be involved in the generation of sequences of saccades.

A subsidiary neural circuit related to saccade generation is from the frontal lobe to the SC via the basal ganglia. Projections from the frontal cortex pass to the substantia nigra, pars reticulata (SNpr), via a relay in the caudate nucleus. An inhibitory pathway from the SNpr projects directly to the SC. This appears to be a gating circuit related to volitional saccades, especially of the memory-guided type.

Smooth pursuit system

To maintain foveation of a moving target, the smooth pursuit system has developed relatively independently of the saccadic oculomotor system, although it is essential that there are interconnections between the two. It is first necessary to identify and code the velocity and direction of a moving target. This is carried out in the extrastriate visual area known as the middle temporal visual area (MT) (also called visual area V5), which contains neurones sensitive to visual target motion. In humans, this lies immediately posterior to the ascending limb of the inferior temporal sulcus at the occipitotemporal border (Brodmann area 19/37 junction). Area MT sends this motion signal to the medial superior temporal visual area (MST), which in monkeys is located on the anterior bank of the superior temporal sulcus, but in humans is considered to lie superior and a little anterior to area MT within the inferior parietal lobe. Damage to this area results in an impairment of smooth pursuit of targets moving towards the damaged hemisphere. Evidence of a possible contribution of the FEF to the generation of smooth pursuit has recently been obtained.

Both area MST and the FEF send direct projections to a group of nuclei which lie in the basis pontis of the pons. In the monkey, the dorsolateral and lateral groups of pontine nuclei receive direct cortical inputs related to smooth pursuit. Lesions of similarly located nuclei in humans result in abnormal pursuit. These nuclei transfer the pursuit signal bilaterally to the posterior vermis, contralateral flocculus and fastigial nuclei of the cerebellum. Finally, the pursuit signal passes from the cerebellum to the brainstem, specifically the medial vestibular nucleus and nucleus prepositus hypoglossi, and thence to the PPRF and possibly directly to the ocular motor nuclei. This circuitry, therefore, involves a double decussation, first at the level of the mid-pons (ponto-cerebellar neurone) and second in the lower pons (vestibulo-abducens neurone).

The diagnosis of specific disorders of eye movements

Disorders of saccadic eye movements

Disorders of saccades can be considered in terms of abnormalities of the saccadic pulse–step innervation pattern described previously. A change in the amplitude (width × height) of the pulse, either too big or too small, leads to saccadic hypermetria (overshoot) or hypometria (undershoot), respectively. Such a saccadic pulse dysmetria is associated with a lesion of the dorsal vermis in the cerebellum. A decrease in the height of the pulse, which implies disturbed function of the burst neurones in the PPRF or riMLF, leads to slow saccades. Many causes of slow saccades, several of which involve these areas, have been described (Table 47.6). A mismatch between the size of the pulse and the step (pulse–step mismatch) results in postsaccadic drifts and glissades. They are observed in diseases involving the vestibulocerebellum. If the pulse is not followed by a step (a saccadic pulse), the eye drifts back to its previous position in a decreasing velocity exponential smooth eye movement. Both conjugate and monocular saccadic pulses occur in patients with multiple sclerosis.

Disturbances in the initiation of saccades may lead to a prolonged latency, or the addition of a head movement or blink to initiate the saccade. This may be seen in congenital or acquired oculomotor apraxia, and various degenerative conditions including Parkinson's disease,[21] Huntington's disease[22] and Alzheimer's disease.[23]

Saccades may also occur inappropriately, particularly during attempted fixation. Square wave jerks (SWJ) are small-amplitude (up to 5°) saccades that take the eyes off fixation, followed some 200 ms later by a corrective saccade (Figure 47.11). Many normal subjects have low-frequency SWJ (< 15/min), but elderly subjects often have a higher frequency. They are most prominent in cerebellar disease, progressive supranuclear palsy and multiple system atrophy. Macrosquare wave jerks (5–40°) are encountered in multiple sclerosis and olivopontocerebellar degeneration. Patients with diffuse cerebral

Table 47.6 Causes of slow saccades.

Olivopontocerebellar atrophy
Huntington's chorea
Wilson's disease
Parkinson's disease
Ataxia telangiectasia
Lipid storage disease
Progressive supranuclear palsy
Lesions of the paramedian pontine reticular formation
Internuclear ophthalmoplegia
Peripheral nerve palsy or muscle weakness
Drug intoxications

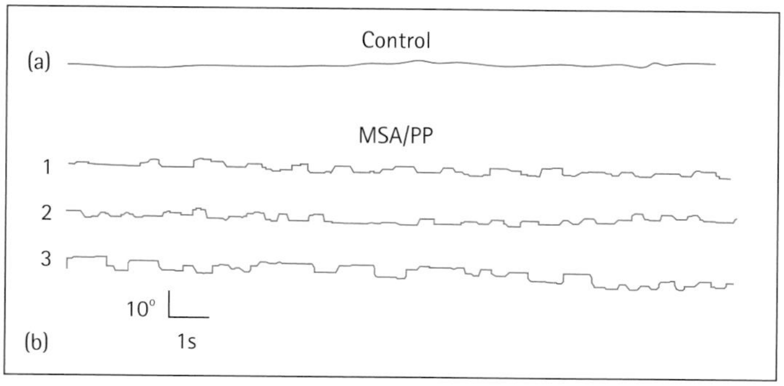

Figure 47.11 (a) A normal eye movement recording of a subject fixating a stationary target. (b) An eye movement recording from a patient with progressive supranuclear palsy fixating a target showing multiple square wave jerks. (Reproduced from Rascol et al. *J Neurol Neurosurg Psychiatry* 1991; **54**: 602 with permission from the BMJ Publishing Group.[47])

cortex damage often exhibit large-amplitude with permission from the BMJ Publishing Group saccades away from the object of regard. After an interval of several hundred milliseconds, the patient makes a saccade back to the target. These anticipatory saccades are particularly observed in Alzheimer's disease.

Ocular motor apraxia is a term used for failure to generate saccades to commands, and may be of a congenital (COMA)[24] or acquired type.[25] COMA may be recognized shortly after birth, when the child does not appear to be fixating upon objects normally. At around 4–6 months, the child develops the characteristic thrusting horizontal head movements, sometimes with blinking, when the child wants to change fixation. This manoeuvre serves to use the intact VOR to drive the eyes into an extreme eccentric position in the orbit. As the head moves past the target, the eyes are dragged along in space until they align with the target. The head then rotates back, and the VOR ensures that fixation is maintained until the eye is in the primary position.[26] The cause of COMA is unknown. It is sometimes associated with developmental abnormalities such as delayed psychomotor development and infantile hypotonia, and with associated anomalies such as agenesis of the corpus callosum, and cerebellar dysplasia and hypoplasia (e.g. as part of Joubert's syndrome). Patients with COMA usually improve with age. In certain diseases affecting the brainstem, a similar clinical syndrome to COMA may occur. These include ataxia–telangectasia, cerebral Whipple's disease, Gaucher's disease, Niemann–Pick disease, vitamin E deficiency and many other storage diseases and aminoacidureas.

Disorders of smooth pursuit

A number of different disturbances of smooth pursuit are found.[27] The commonest abnormality is a low gain (gain = eye velocity/target velocity), which appears as deficient pursuit in which pursuit is broken by small catch-up saccades. Low-gain pursuit can occur as a result of tiredness and inattention, as a side-effect of medications such as sedatives and anticonvulsants, or due to lesions in the vestibulocerebellum. Generally, bilateral low-gain pursuit has no localizing value. This is not the case with asymmetrical low-gain pursuit, which usually occurs as a result of a lesion in the ipsilateral parietal lobe, thalamus, midbrain tegmentum, dorsolateral nucleus of the pons and vestibulocerebellum.[28] Occasionally, a disturbance of pursuit 'tone' (balance) occurs due to cerebral hemisphere lesions, when the eyes drift towards the side of the lesion. Disturbances of direction can occur, for example, in congenital nystagmus, in which there is an apparent 'inversion' of pursuit when the eyes move in an opposite direction to the motion of the target.

Disorders of vergence eye movements

The commonest causes of disturbed vergence are congenital abnormalities. Various forms of convergence or divergence excess or insufficiency are usually accompanied by a concomitant strabismus. Although this may not give rise to diplopia in childhood, it can present as intermittent diplopia later in life. Acquired forms of vergence disorders commonly occur in association with disturbances of vertical gaze, as in the dorsal midbrain syndrome, and in Parkinson's disease and progressive supranuclear palsy. Spasm of the near triad (convergence spasm) is only rarely due to organic disease and is usually a voluntary convergence in patients with a conversion syndrome.[29] The patients often complain of discomfort, and the convergence, which only lasts for a brief period on each occasion, may be associated with visual blurring, diplopia and 'eye strain'. An important clue to this diagnosis is the strong pupillary miosis which accompanies the convergence.

The diagnosis of saccadic oscillations and nystagmus

There is an important distinction between saccadic oscillations, which are sustained oscillations that are initiated by fast saccadic eye movements, and nystagmus, where the oscillations are initiated by smooth eye movements; that is, the fast phase in jerk nystagmus is corrective and not primary (Figure 47.12).

Saccadic oscillations

Saccadic oscillations are bursts of saccades, which may be intermittent or continuous, causing a disruption of fixation. Two main types can be identified, those with normal intersaccadic intervals and those composed of back-to-back saccades with abnormally brief or no intersaccadic intervals.

The oscillations with intersaccadic intervals include square wave oscillations consisting of sequences of SWJ which can occur in Parkinson's disease and progressive supranuclear palsy (Figure 47.13). Macrosaccadic oscillations straddle the intended fixation position. The amplitudes (up to 40°) of

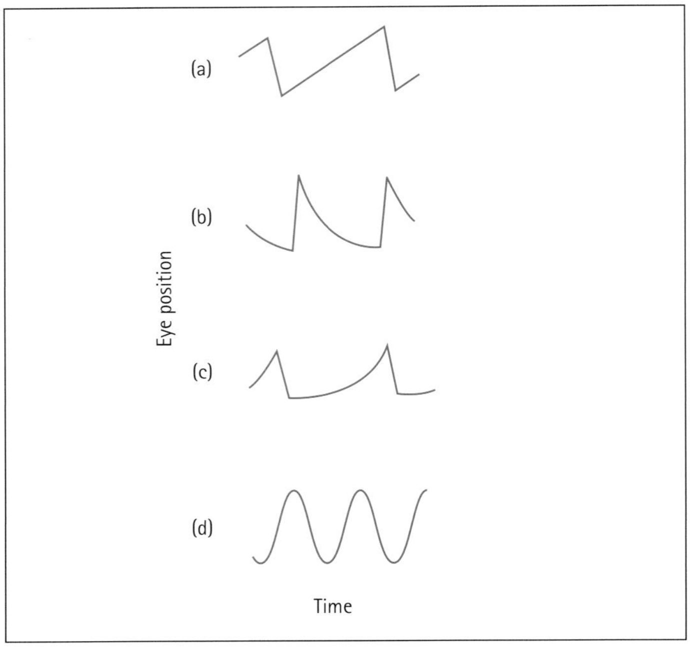

Figure 47.12 Four common slow-phase waveforms of nystagmus. (a) Constant velocity drift of the eyes. This occurs in nystagmus caused by peripheral or central vestibular disease and also with lesions of the cerebral hemispheres. The added quick phases give a sawtooth appearance. (b) Drift of the eyes back from an eccentric orbital position toward the midline (gaze-evoked nystagmus). The drift shows a negative exponential time-course, with decreasing velocity. This waveform reflects an unsustained eye position signal caused by an impaired neural integrator. (c) Drift of the eyes away from the primary position with a positive exponential time-course (increasing velocity). This waveform suggests an unstable neural integrator and is encountered horizontally in congenital nystagmus and vertically in cerebellar disease. (d) Pendular nystagmus, which is encountered as a type of congenital nystagmus and with acquired disease. (Redrawn from Leigh and Zee. *The Neurology of Eye Movements*. New York: Oxford University Press, 1999.[43])

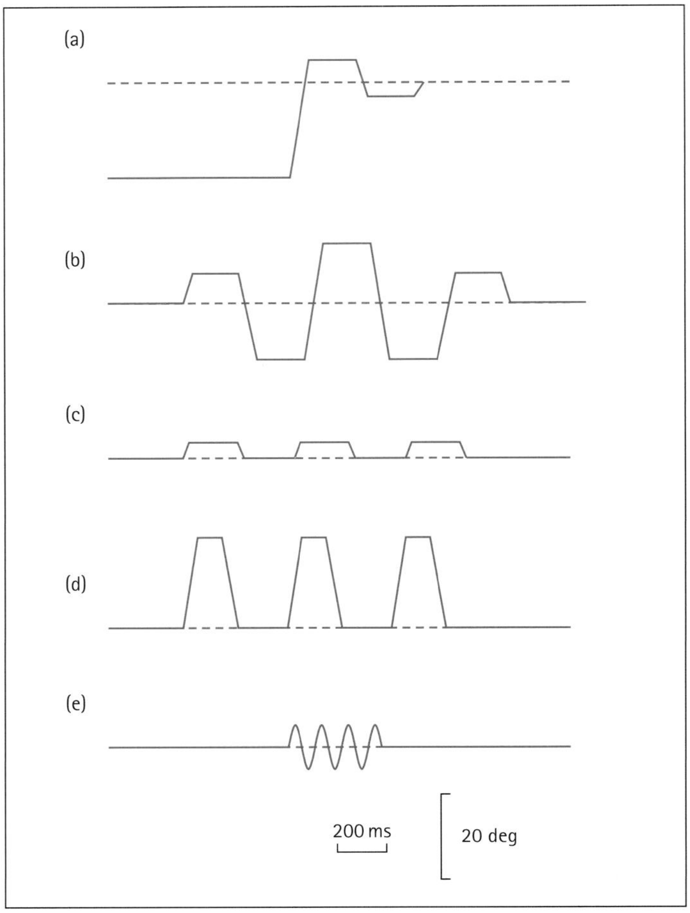

Figure 47.13 Saccadic oscillations. (a) Dysmetria: inaccurate saccades. (b) Macrosaccadic oscillations: hypermetric saccades about the position of the target. (c) Square wave jerks: small, uncalled-for saccades away from and back to the position of the target. (d) Macrosquare wave jerks: large, uncalled-for saccades away from and back to the position of the target. (e) Ocular flutter: to-and-fro, back-to-back saccades without an intersaccadic interval. (Redrawn from Leigh and Zee. *The Neurology of Eye Movements*. New York: Oxford University Press, 1999.[43])

sequential saccades increase in amplitude and then decrease in a crescendo–decrescendo pattern.[30] This type of oscillation is usually observed in acute damage to the dorsal cerebellum involving the deep cerebellar nuclei, as in demyelination, tumour or haematoma.

Oscillations without any intersaccadic interval (back-to-back) include opsoclonus, ocular flutter and convergence–retraction saccadic pulses. Opsoclonus consists of multidirectional (including oblique and torsional) back-to-back saccades of varying amplitude.[31] It has been suggested that the disorder arises due to disordered pause cell function in the PPRF. A variety of posterior fossa disorders can give rise to the condition, including infective agents such as Coxsackie B virus and *Haemophilus influenza* meningitis (Table 47.7). It can also occur in neonates, associated with myoclonus—'dancing eye and dancing feet'. This appears to be a maturational deficit which resolves over approximately 6 weeks. Opsoclonus also occurs as a paraneoplastic (non-metastatic) disorder, which in children is associated with occult neuroblastoma and in adults with small cell carcinoma of the lung and carcinoma of the breast and uterus. Various autoantibodies can be detected in the sera of some patients with opsoclonus, most commonly the anti-Ri antibody. Ocular flutter consists of bursts of back-to-back saccades in the horizontal plane only. It can therefore be observed in patients recovering from opsoclonus. Isolated ocular flutter is most often observed in patients with multiple sclerosis and signs of cerebellar disease. A voluntary form of flutter (voluntary flutter) can be induced by about 8% of the population, usually by convergence. It consists of salvoes of horizontal back-to-back saccades. Lesions of the dorsal midbrain are often associated with upward gaze palsies and convergence-retraction nystagmus.[32] This is incorrectly termed a nystagmus, since it actually consists of adducting saccades and should be redesignated convergence–retraction saccadic pulses. Finally, a further type of saccadic oscillation is ocular bobbing.[33] This consists of rhythmic, sudden, downward jerks of the eyes followed by a slow return to the midposition, either immediately or after a short delay. The typical type, associated with pontine haemorrhage or infarction, is associated with paralysis of horizontal eye movements. Atypical bobbing is similar, except that horizontal eye movements are intact, and occurs in metabolic encephalopathy, obstructive hydrocephalus or cerebellar haematoma. When the fast movement is upward followed by a delayed slow return, the condition is known as reverse bobbing. Several of these types of ocular bobbing and others are observed in unconscious patients, and these are summarized in Table 47.8.

Table 47.7 Aetiology of opsoclonus and ocular flutter.

- Viral encephalitis
- Paraneoplastic
  - Neuroblastoma
  - Other tumours, e.g. small cell lung carcinoma, ovarian carcinoma
- Trauma (in association with hypoxia and sepsis)
- Meningitis
- Intracranial tumours
- Hydrocephalus
- Thalamic haemorrhage
- Multiple sclerosis
- Hyperosmolar coma
- Associated with systemic disease, e.g. viral hepatitis, sarcoid, AIDS. Side-effects of drugs: lithium, amitriptyline, phenytoin, and diazepam. Toxins: chlordecone, thallium, strychnine, toluene, and organophosphates
- Transient phenomenon of healthy neonates ('dancing eyes and dancing feet')

Nystagmus

Nystagmus is an oscillation which is initiated by a slow eye movement. When this slow movement is accompanied by a fast (saccadic) eye movement, it is called jerk nystagmus. Although the direction of the nystagmus is conventionally determined by the direction of the quick phases, it is important to remember that it is the smooth eye movement imbalance which is responsible for the nystagmus. If both phases are smooth eye movements, pendular nystagmus is observed.

The commonest form of jerk nystagmus is vestibular nystagmus, which most frequently results from labyrinth or vestibular nerve dysfunction, but also occurs with central brainstem lesions.

Peripheral vestibular nystagmus

Vestibular nystagmus due to a disturbance of the peripheral vestibular apparatus has a number of typical characteristics, as follows: the form of the nystagmus is usually mixed, i.e. various combinations of horizontal, vertical and torsional components; pure vertical or torsional nystagmus almost never occurs with peripheral vestibular disease; it is always unidirectional, the quick phases beating away from the underactive labyrinth; its intensity increases when the eyes are turned in the direction of the quick phase—Alexander's law; it is markedly suppressed by

Table 47.8 Spontaneous eye movements in unconscious patients.

Term	Description	Causes
Ocular bobbing	Rapid, conjugate, downward movement: slow return to primary position	Pontine strokes; other structural, metabolic or toxic disorders
Ocular dipping or inverse ocular bobbing	Slow downward movement; rapid return to primary position	Unreliable for localization; follows hypoxic–ischemic insult or metabolic disorder
Reverse ocular bobbing	Rapid upward movement; slow return to primary position	Unreliable for localization; may occur with metabolic disorders
Reverse ocular dipping or converse bobbing	Slow upward movement; rapid return to primary position	Unreliable for localization; pontine infarction and with AIDS
Ping-pong gaze	Horizontal conjugate deviation of the eyes, alternating every few seconds	Bilateral cerebral hemispheric dysfunction
Periodic alternating gaze deviation	Horizontal conjugate deviation of the eyes, alternating every 2 min	Hepatic encephalopathy; disorders causing periodic alternating nystagmus and unconsciousness
Vertical myoclonus	Vertical pendular oscillations	Pontine strokes
Monocular movements	Small, intermittent, rapid monocular horizontal, vertical, or torsional movements	Pontine or midbrain destructive lesions, perhaps with coexistent seizures

visual fixation and therefore is accentuated by Frenzel glasses; and it always indicates unilateral or asymmetric bilateral vestibular lesions and is usually associated with vertigo.

Central vestibular nystagmus

Several different types of central vestibular nystagmus are described, all of which show no change in intensity with the removal of fixation (by using Frenzel glasses), in contrast to peripheral vestibular nystagmus. These forms of vestibular nystagmus are often unidirectional, i.e. up- or downbeat, torsional.

Downbeat nystagmus may or may not be present in the primary position. The nystagmus shows a fast phase beating downward which may accentuate in upgaze or downgaze, but particularly in lateral gaze.[34] When it is present in the primary position (even if only apparent on ophthalmoscopy), a bilateral disturbance of the cerebellar flocculus is often found, commonly due to a disturbance at the craniocervical junction, such as a type 1 Chiari malformation (Table 47.9). Other causes include cerebellar degenerations, anticonvulsant drugs, lithium intoxication and intra-axial brainstem lesions. In about half of the patients with downbeat nystagmus, no cause can be found. Many patients with this form of nystagmus experience oscillopsia and postural instability.

Upbeat nystagmus, when present in the primary position, is usually associated with focal brainstem lesions in the tegmental grey matter, either at the pontomesencephalic junction or at the pontomedullary junction, involving the nucleus prepositus hypoglossi or the ventral tegmental pathway of the upward vestibulo-ocular reflex.[35] The commonest causes are multiple sclerosis, tumour, infarction and cerebellar degeneration (Table 47.10).

Torsional nystagmus is a jerk nystagmus around the antero-posterior axis. It is commonly associated with other types of nystagmus. However, when it is pure it indicates a lesion of the lateral medulla involving the vestibular nuclei. Occasionally it may be due to a midbrain–thalamic lesion, involving the INC (Table 47.11).

Periodic alternating nystagmus (PAN) is a primary position horizontal nystagmus that changes direction in a crescendo–decrescendo manner, characteristically approximately every 90 s.[36] Between each directional change there is a null period of 0–10 s. There is a congenital form, and acquired forms are due to Chiari malformations, multiple sclerosis, fourth ventricle tumours, spinocerebellar degenerations and anticonvulsant intoxication. Baclofen has been shown to be an effective treatment.[37]

Gaze-evoked nystagmus is a common clinical observation with limited localizing value. It is a jerk nystagmus which is absent in the primary position and is only present on eccentric gaze. It usually signifies cerebellar parenchymal disease, particularly involving the flocculus or its projections to the brain-

Table 47.9 Aetiology of downbeat nystagmus.

Cerebellar degeneration, including familial periodic ataxia, and paraneoplastic degeneration
Craniocervical anomalies, including Arnold–Chiari malformation, Paget's disease, basilar invagination
Infarction of brainstem or cerebellum
Dolichoectasia of the vertebrobasilar artery
Multiple sclerosis
Cerebellar tumour, including haemangioblastoma
Syringobulbia
Encephalitis
Head trauma
Toxic–metabolic
Anticonvulsant medication
Lithium intoxication
Alcohol
Wernicke's encephalopathy
Magnesium depletion
Vitamin B_{12} deficiency
Toluene abuse
Congenital
Transient finding in otherwise normal infants

Table 47.10 Aetiology of upbeat nystagmus.

Cerebellar degenerations
Multiple sclerosis
Infarction of medulla, midbrain, or cerebellum
Tumours of the medulla, midbrain, or cerebellum
Wernicke's encephalopathy
Brainstem encephalitis
Behçet's syndrome
Meningitis
Leber's congenital amaurosis or other congenital disorder of the anterior visual pathways
Thalamic arteriovenous malformation
Organophosphate poisoning
Tobacco
Associated with middle ear disease
Congenital
Transient finding in otherwise normal infants

Table 47.11 Aetiology of torsional nystagmus.

Syringobulbia, with or without syringomyelia and Chiari malformation
Brainstem stroke (Wallenberg's syndrome) or arteriovenous malformation
Brainstem tumour
Multiple sclerosis
Oculopalatal myoclonus
Head trauma
Congenital
Associated with the ocular tilt reaction

stem. Bilateral horizontal, together with vertical, gaze-evoked nystagmus commonly occurs with structural brainstem and cerebellar lesions, diffuse metabolic disorders and drug intoxication. A variant of gaze-evoked nystagmus is rebound nystagmus, in which gaze-evoked jerk nystagmus changes direction when gaze is returned to the primary position, persisting for 3–25 s. It is also associated with parenchymal cerebellar disease.

Table 47.12 Aetiology of pendular nystagmus.

Visual loss (including unilateral disease of the optic nerve)
Disorders of central myelin
Multiple sclerosis
Pelizaeus–Merzbacher disease
Cockayne's syndrome
Toluene abuse
Oculopalatal myoclonus
Acute brainstem stroke
Whipple's disease
Spinocerebellar degenerations
Congenital nystagmus

Pendular nystagmus is either congenital or acquired due to cerebellar and brainstem disease, usually multiple sclerosis[36] (Table 47.12). Acquired pendular nystagmus may have both horizontal and vertical components, and the amplitude and phase relationships of the two sinewaves determine the trajectory of the eyes, e.g. oblique, circular or elliptical. It can affect one eye or both, equally or unequally, and is often symptomatic, resulting in oscillopsia. It may be associated with oscillations of other structures, such as the palate, head or limbs. When it is present in association with palatal myoclonus, oculopalatal myoclonus, the lesion is usually in Mollaret's triangle, which consists of the red nucleus, dentate nucleus and inferior olivary nucleus.[38] The latter nucleus usually shows pseudohypertrophic degeneration. A combination of a convergence-induced pendular nystagmus and synchronous jaw contractions, called oculomasticatory myorhythmia, is characteristic of Whipple's disease.[39] In see-saw nystagmus, one eye intorts and rises while the other eye extorts and falls in a rapidly alternating sequence. In this pendular form, there is often a bitemporal hemianopia, and the condition is associated with large parasellar masses which have expanded up into the third ventricle and are distorting structures in the mesencephalic–diencephalic region.[40]

Congenital nystagmus is almost invariably a horizontal conjugate nystagmus which is unaltered by vertical position. It is generally of jerk type with accelerating slow phases, and has an eccentric null position. Fixation effort enhances congenital nystagmus, and the patient rarely complains of oscillopsia. Less commonly, the nystagmus is of a pendular type or has a torsional component. Reversed optokinetic nystagmus, beating in the direction of the target motion, is a feature of congenital nystagmus, as is induction of the nystagmus by smooth pursuit or by atttempted VOR suppression. Patients may show a head turn or occasionally a head oscillation.[41]

Latent nystagmus is a type of congenital nystagmus that is only present on monocular viewing and which then beats toward the viewing eye.[42] It is absent on binocular viewing. If the patient has amblyopia in one eye, latent nystagmus is present with both eyes viewing, when it is called manifest latent nystagmus.

References

1. Shaunak S, O'Sullivan E, Kennard C. Eye movements. In: Hughes JAC, ed. *Neurological Investigations*. London: British Medical Journal, 1997: 253–82.
2. Halmagyi GM, Curthoys IS. A clinical sign of canal paresis. *Arch Neurol* 1988; **45**: 737–9.
3. Müri RM, Chermann JF, Kohen L et al. Ocular motor consequences of damage to the abducens nucleus area in humans. *J Neurol Ophthalmol* 1996; **16**: 191–5.
4. Hanson MR, Hamid MA, Thomsak RL et al. Selective saccadic palsy caused by pontine lesions: clinical, physiological and pathological correlations. *Ann Neurol* 1986; **20**: 209–17.
5. Zee DS. Internuclear ophthalmoplegia: clinical and pathophysiological consideration. In: Büttner U, Brandt T, eds. *Ocular Motor Disorders in the Brainstem*. London: WB Saunders, 1992: 455–70.
6. Cogan TG. Internuclear ophthalmoplegia: typical and atypical. *Arch Ophthalmol* 1970; **84**: 583–9.
7. Ranalli PJ, Sharpe JA. Vertical vestibulo-ocular reflex smooth pursuit and eye head tracking dysfunction in internuclear ophthalmoplegia. *Brain* 1988; **111**: 1299–317.
8. Thömke F, Hopf HC, Krämer G. Internuclear ophthalmoplegia of abduction: clinical and electrophysiological data on the existence of abduction paresis of prenuclear origin. *J Neurol Neurosurg Psychiatry* 1992; **55**: 105–11.
9. Wall M, Wray SH. The one-and-a-half syndrome—a unilateral disorder of the pontine tegmentum: a study of 20 cases and review of the literature. *Neurology* 1983; **33**: 971–80.
10. Sharpe JA, Rosenberg MA, Hoyt WF et al. Paralytic pontine exotropia. A sign of acute unilateral gaze palsy and internuclear ophthalmoplegia. *Neurology* 1974; **24**: 1076–81.
11. Komiyama A, Takamatsu K, Johkura K et al. Internuclear ophthalmoplegia and controlled exotropia. Non paralytic pontine exotropia and WEBINO syndrome. *Neuroophthalmology* 1998; **19**: 33–44.
12. Baloh RW, Yee RD, Honrubia V. Eye movements with Wallenberg's syndrome. *Ann NY Acad Sci* 1981; **374**: 600–13.
13. Solomon D, Galetta SL, Liu GT. Possible mechanisms for horizontal gaze deviation and lateropulsion in the lateral medullary syndrome. *J Neuroophthalmol* 1995; **15**: 26–30.
14. Baloh RW, Furman JN, Yee RD. Dorsal midbrain syndrome: clinical and oculographic finding. *Neurology* 1985; **35**: 54–60.
15. Büttner-Ennever JA, Büttner U, Cohen B et al. Vertical gaze paralysis and the rostral interstitial nucleus of the medial longitudinal faxiculus. *Brain* 1982; **105**: 25–49.
16. Hommel B, Bogousslavsky J. The spectrum of vertical gaze palsy following unilateral brainstem stroke. *Neurology* 1991; **41**: 1229–34.

17. Halmagyi GM, Brandt T, Dieterich M et al. Tonic controversive ocular tilt reaction due to unilateral mesodiencephalic lesions. *Neurol* 1990; **40**: 1503–9.
18. Brandt T, Dieterich M. Skew deviation with ocular torsion: a vestibular brainstem sign of topographic diagnostic value. *Ann Neurol* 1993; **33**: 528–34.
19. Clark JM, Albert GW. Vertical gaze palsies from medial thalamic infarctions without mid-brain involvement. *Stroke* 1995; **26**: 1467–70.
20. Lewis RF, Zee DS. Ocular motor disorders associated with cerebellar lesions: pathophysiology and topical diagnosis. *Rev Neurol* 1993; **149**: 665–77.
21. O'Sullivan EP, Kennard C. Neuro-ophthalmology of movement disorders. In: Jankovic J, Tolosa E, eds. *Parkinson's Disease and Movement Disorders*. Williams and Wilkins, 1998: 869–86.
22. Lasker AG, Zee DS. Ocular motor abnormalities in Huntington's disease. *Vis Res* 1997; **37**: 3639–45.
23. Fletcher WA, Sharpe JA. Saccadic eye movement dysfunction in Alzheimer's disease. *Ann Neurol* 1986; **20**: 464–71.
24. Cogan CG. A type of congenital ocular motor apraxia presenting with jerky head movements. *Trans Am Acad Ophthalmol* 1952; **56**: 853–62.
25. Pierrot-Deseilligny C, Gautier JC, Loron P. Acquired ocular motor apraxia due to bilateral fronto-parietal infarcts. *Ann Neurol* 1988; **23**: 199–202.
26. Harris C, Shawkat F, Russell-Eggitt I et al. Intermittent horizontal saccade failure, 'ocular motor apraxia', in children. *Br J Ophthalmol* 1996; **80**: 151–8.
27. Morrow MJ, Sharpe JA. Smooth pursuit eye movements. In: Sharpe JA, Barber HO, eds. *The Vestibular-Ocular Reflex and Vertigo*. New York: Raven Press, 1993: 141–62.
28. Heide W, Kurzidin K, Kõmpf D. Deficits in smooth pursuit eye movements after frontal and parietal lesions. *Brain* 1996; **119**: 1951–69.
29. Sarkies NJC, Sanders MD. Convergence spasm. *Trans Ophthalmol Soc* 1985; **104**: 782–6.
30. Selhorst JB, Hoyt WF, Feinsord M et al. Midbrain correctopia. *Arch Neurol* 1976; **33**: 193–5.
31. Averbuch-Heller L, Remler B. Opsoclonus. *Semin Neurol* 1996; **16**: 21–6.
32. Ochs AL, Stark L, Hoyt WF et al. Opposed adducting saccades in convergence–retraction nystagmus. A patient with Sylvian aqueduct syndrome. *Brain* 1979; **102**: 497–508.
33. Susac JO, Hoyt WF, Daroff RD et al. Clinical spectrum of ocular bobbing. *J Neurol Neurosurg Psychiatry* 1970; **33**: 771–5.
34. Halmagyi GM, Rudge P, Gresty MA et al. Down-beating nystagmus: a review of 62 cases. *Arch Neurol* 1983; **40**: 777–84.
35. Fisher A, Gresty M, Chambers B et al. Primary position up-beating nystagmus. A variety of central positional nystagmus. *Brain* 1983; **106**: 949–64.
36. Fletcher WA. Nystagmus: an overview. In: Sharpe JA, Barber HO. *The Vestibular-Ocular-Reflex and Vertigo*. New York: Raven Press, 1983; 195–215.
37. Halmagyi GM, Rudge P, Gresty M et al. Treatment of periodic alternating nystragmus. *Ann Neurol* 1980; **8**: 609–11.
38. Nakada T, Kwee IL. Oculo-palato-myoclonus. *Brain* 1986; **109**: 431–41.
39. Schwartz MA, Selhorst JB, Ochs AL et al. Oculomasticatory myorhythmia: a unique movement disorder occurring in Whipple's disease. *Ann Neurol* 1986; **20**: 677–83.
40. Daroff RB. See-saw nystagmus. *Neurology* 1965; **15**: 874–7.
41. Dell'Osso LF, Daroff RB. Congenital nystagmus waveforms and foveation strategy. *Doc Ophthalmol* 1975 **39**: 155–82.
42. Gresty MA, Metcalfe T, Timms C et al. Neurology of latent nystagmus. *Brain* 1992; **115**: 1303–21.
43. Leigh RJ, Zee DS. *The Neurology of Eye Movements*, 3rd edn. New York: Oxford University Press, 1999.
44. Ranalli PJ, Sharpe JA. Contrapulsion of saccades and ipsilateral ataxia; a unilateral disorder of the rostral cerebellum. *Ann Neurol* 1986; **20**: 311.
45. Büttner-Ennever JA, Büttner U. The reticular formation. In: Büttner-Ennever JA, ed. *Neuroanatomy of the Oculomotor System*. New York: Elsevier, 1988: 119–76.
46. Kommerell G, Hoyt WF. Lateropulsion of saccadic eye movements. Electro-oculographic studies in a patient with Wallenberg's syndrome. *Arch Neurol* 1973; **28**: 313–20.
47. Rascol O, Sabatini U, Simouetta-Moreau M et al. Square wave jerks in parkinsonian syndromes. *J Neurol Neurosurg Psychiatry* 1991; **54**: 599–602.

48 Peripheral vestibular disorders and diseases in adults

G Michael Halmagyi, Phillip D Cremer, Ian S Curthoys

The symptoms and signs of any lesion involving the nervous system, which includes the vestibular system, are determined by where the lesion is and not by what the lesion is.

> It is the site and not the nature of the lesion that determines the pattern of the functional deficit.

While this is the truth, it is not the whole truth. Two other factors also determine the exact pattern of the functional deficit: the age of the lesion—adaptive processes are particularly vigorous in the vestibular system—and the activity of the lesion—whether the lesion produces underactivity or overactivity of neurones. To illustrate these principles, consider the effects of acute total permanent destruction of one labyrinth. The symptoms and signs at any particular time will depend on whether the lesion has come on suddenly or slowly, and, if it came on suddenly, then the time elapsed since it did. On the other hand, the symptoms and signs will not depend on the nature of the lesion—how the labyrinth was destroyed or damaged will be immaterial to the deficit that is produced.

What happens if one labyrinth is destroyed

Acute destruction or deafferentation of one entire intact labyrinth, in an animal or in a human, by disease or by design, invariably produces an acute, temporary, stereotyped, clinical syndrome of profound motor and sensory abnormalities—for reviews see Curthoys and Halmagyi[1] and Vidal et al.[2] There is, due to otolith deafferentation, a complete, or more often a partial, ocular tilt reaction that is always ipsiversive, i.e. always towards the side of the lesion.

CLINICAL FEATURES OF THE OCULAR TILT REACTION

A leftward complete ocular tilt reaction due to a left peripheral vestibular lesion comprises:

1. A skew deviation with the left eye hypotropic (deviated downwards) producing vertical diplopia.
2. A leftwards head tilt producing no symptoms.
3. Conjugate counterclockwise (from the patient's point of view) torsion of the eyes, evident on fundus photography, producing no symptoms but a leftwards deviation of the visual horizontal or vertical.

The complete ocular tilt reaction (OTR) consists of head torsion, conjugate binocular eye torsion and a hypotropia due to skew deviation—all towards the one side. Owing to semicircular canal (SCC) deafferentation, there is also a spontaneous horizontal–torsional nystagmus with the slow phases toward the side of the lesion, as well as vomiting. Humans, and perhaps animals, experience an illusion of rotation (i.e. vertigo) as well as nausea.

CLINICAL FEATURES OF AN ACUTE UNILATERAL PERIPHERAL VESTIBULOPATHY

1. An illusion of rotation, i.e. vertigo.
2. Nausea.
3. Vomiting.

In a patient with a left vestibulopathy there is:

4. A leftward partial or complete ocular tilt reaction.
5. Horizontal–torsional spontaneous nystagmus with the quick phases to the right, more vigorous with reduced vision (e.g. Frenzel glasses).
6. Leftwards rotation when marching on the spot with the eyes closed (Unterberger test).
7. A positive leftwards horizontal head impulse test.
8. Nos. 1–6 are temporary and recover within 1 week; no. 7 is permanent.

These symptoms and signs make up the syndrome of acute unilateral vestibular deafferentation, which is the same irrespective of the cause. Although normally both humans and animals recover, more or less completely, from the acute unilateral vestibular deafferentation (uVD) syndrome by the process of vestibular compensation, the vestibulo-ocular reflex (VOR) is permanently damaged. From studies of the acute uVD syndrome and of the processes of vestibular compensation in experimental animals, one could infer that peripheral vestibular disorders produce vertigo when they cause asymmetric neural activity between corresponding parts of the left and right vestibular nuclei, and that recovery from the acute uVD syndrome is due to rebalancing of the neural activity in the vestibular nuclei on the two sides. One could also infer that a person not experiencing vertigo, should, at that time, have symmetrical vestibular nucleus activity.

Once vestibular compensation is complete, i.e. there is a chronic, stable uVD, the patient will no longer experience vertigo and most patients will experience no symptoms at all.

In other words, most patients cannot tell whether they have one or two functioning labyrinths. A minority of patients, about 20%, with a chronic stable total uVD will experience ataxia and oscillopsia, symptoms experienced by all patients with bilateral vestibular deafferentation and described in more detail later.

In contrast, chronic progressive unilateral vestibular deafferentation—as would occur with a slowly growing tumour such as a vestibular schwannoma—does not produce the acute uVD syndrome of vertigo, vomiting, OTR and nystagmus. This is presumably because there is never a period of significantly asymmetric neural activity in the vestibular nucleus on each side. In fact, if a patient presents with signs of uVD and categorically denies ever having experienced an attack of acute spontaneous vertigo, one can be almost sure that the uVD has not been acute, and one should therefore look for a potential progressive cause of uVD.

The neural events behind acute unilateral vestibular deafferentation and vestibular compensation

In order to appreciate the mechanisms of vestibular compensation, one needs to consider the changes in vestibular nucleus neural activity that occur after uVD.[1,2]

Normal medial vestibular nucleus activity

Two types of lateral SCC-driven neurones have been found in the medial vestibular nuclei of monkeys, cats and guinea pigs. Both types of vestibular nucleus neurones, just like primary vestibular neurones, discharge spontaneously, i.e. at rest, at rates sometimes in excess of 80 impulses/s. The discharge rate of type 1 neurones increases when the head accelerates ipsilaterally, and decreases when the head accelerates contralaterally. The reverse applies to type 2 neurones; they increase their discharge rate in response to contralateral head accelerations and decrease their discharge rate in response to ipsilateral head accelerations (Figure 48.1). The reason why type 1 and type 2 neurones respond oppositely is that, whereas type 1 neurones are excited by ipsilateral lateral SCC primary afferent neurones and are inhibited by ipsilateral type 2 neurones, type 2 neurones themselves are excited by contralateral type 1 neurones via commissural pathways. Motor and sensory equilibrium requires equal resting activity of type 1 neurones in the two medial vestibular nuclei. Type 1 neurones drive the horizontal VOR by excitatory projections to abducens motorneurones and internuclear neurones in the contralateral abducens nucleus.

Ipsilesional medial vestibular nucleus activity

Immediately after uVD there are changes in the activity of both type 1 and type 2 neurones in the medial vestibular nucleus on the damaged side.[3–10] The resting activity of type 1 neurones decreases, whereas the resting activity of type 2 neurones increases. The decrease in resting activity of type 1 neurones reflects the loss of excitatory drive by lateral SCC primary afferent neurones. The increase in resting activity of type 2 neurones reflects increased excitatory drive by contralesional type 1 neurones which have become disinhibited by the decrease in the activity of contralesional type 2 neurones, which are themselves normally excited by ipsilesional type 1 neurones. As well as showing a reduced resting discharge rate, immediately after uVD, ipsilesional type 1 neurones show a decrease in sensitivity to angular acceleration. The sensitivity of type 2 neurones to angular acceleration remains unchanged.

In the days and weeks that follow, a remarkable series of changes occur in the resting activity of ipsilesional medial vestibular nucleus neurones. The resting discharge rates of both type 1 and 2 neurones are restored to normal even though the medial vestibular nucleus no longer receives any afferent drive

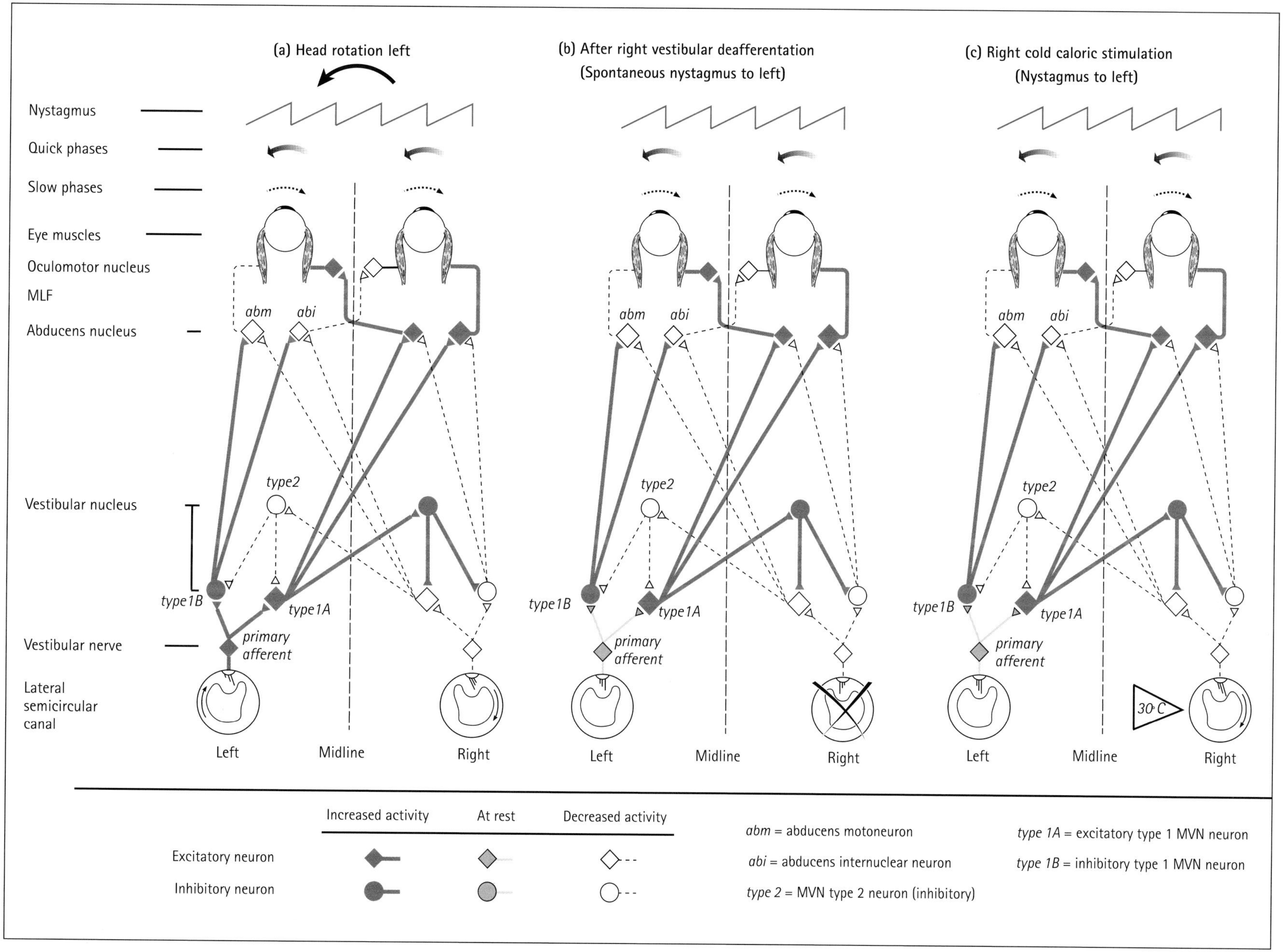

Figure 48.1 Schematic representation of brainstem neurones responsible for the direct, disynaptic vestibulo-ocular reflex (VOR). The activity of these neurones is shown during (a) head rotation to the left, (b) after a right vestibular deafferentation , and (c) during right-ear cold caloric stimulation. In all three situations, there is left-beating nystagmus which is generated by the same pattern of activation and inactivation in two medial vestibular nucleus neurones, type 1 and type 2 neurones. (Courtesy of Dr A. Cartwright, Sydney.)

from its labyrinth. Data so far, mainly from the guinea pig and the gerbil, have shown a limited restoration of sensitivity of type 1 neurones to angular accelerations. This restoration of resting activity in type 1 neurones could also underlie the recovery of humans from the disabling consequences of uVD and the restoration of static equilibrium.

The abrupt loss of peripheral afferent input after uVD results in a large imbalance in average neural resting activity between the two vestibular nuclei. Many neurones in the ipsilesional nucleus become silent, whereas many neurones in the contralesional nucleus fire vigorously, and in so doing indirectly exert greater inhibition than usual of the neurones in the ipsilesional nucleus, via the commissural fibres interconnecting the nuclei. There are widespread changes throughout the brain accompanying this neural imbalance between the vestibular nuclei. In the rat and the guinea pig, the restoration of balanced activity is fast (about 24–48 h) and a host of possible mechanisms have been suggested by which activity returns. That long list is narrowed because balanced activity returns so quickly. Since the initial process is so fast, it suggests that intracellular changes such as adaptation of the high firing rate of the contralesional neurones or changes in the membrane characteristics of neurones in the ipsilesional vestibular nuclei,[11] possibly combined with changes (e.g. downregulation of GABA sensitivity),[12] probably contribute most to the initial recovery process of the recovery of neural activity in the ipsilesional vestibular nucleus.

Contralesional medial vestibular nucleus activity

Immediately after uVD, there is an increase in the resting activity of contralesional type 1 neurones without much change in their sensitivity.[5–10] There is also a decrease in the sensitivity of contralesional type 2 neurones without much change in resting activity. This increase in resting activity of type 1 neurones is due to decreased inhibition by type 2 neurones, which are themselves normally excited by ipsilesional type 1 neurones, now silenced. In the following days and weeks, the resting activity of contralesional type 1 neurones is restored to normal, and the resting activity of contralesional type 2 neurones increases to above normal. These changes in the resting activity of contralesional medial vestibular nucleus neurones occur despite the fact that the ipsilesional vestibular nucleus remains isolated from its labyrinth. However, the remarkable restoration of resting activity in ipsilesional type 1 neurones described above can account for the changes in activity of contralesional medial vestibular nucleus neurones. The restoration of contralesional type 1 resting activity to normal is presumably the result of the increased inhibition by contralesional type 2 neurones, now excited by the restored resting activity of ipsilesional type 1 neurones. Together with the decrease of contralesional type I resting activity to normal, there is a late decrease in contralesional type 1 sensitivity, whereas contralesional type 2 sensitivity remains low.

Normal lateral vestibular nucleus activity

Primary otolithic neurones project to secondary vestibular neurones, mainly in the lateral and the descending vestibular nuclei. The predominant response of lateral vestibular nucleus neurones is an increase in firing rate in response to ipsilateral tilts, i.e. laterally directed linear accelerations, the alpha response. The commissural connections between secondary otolithic neurones are poorly understood. Unlike the commissural connections of the lateral SCC secondary neurones in the medial vestibular nucleus, which are direct and functionally inhibitory, it appears that the commissural connections between the secondary otolithic neurones in the lateral vestibular nucleus are indirect and functionally excitatory. There are also interconnections between the lateral and the medial vestibular nuclei, and some medial vestibular nucleus neurones respond to both semicircular canal and to otolithic stimulation. The changes that occur in the lateral vestibular nucleus after uVD vary between the rostroventral and dorsocaudal areas of the nucleus, which project to the cervicothoracic and lumbosacral segments of the spinal cord respectively.

Ipsilesional lateral vestibular nucleus activity

There is a decrease in the proportion of roll-tilt responsive neurones in the rostroventral area but not in the dorsocaudal area, as well as an overall decrease in the average resting activity of neurones.[13] In contrast, there are increases in the number of position-sensitive neurones, in the tilt sensitivity of dorsocaudal neurones and in the number of beta responses (increases in firing with medially directed linear acceleration). With compensation, there is little recovery in the resting activity of either alpha or beta neurones. The proportion of neurones in the rostroventral areas responsive to roll-tilt increases to normal, while the sensitivity remains normal. The sensitivity of dorsocaudal neurones decreases to normal. The proportions of position-sensitive neurones and beta responses do not change.

Contralesional lateral vestibular nucleus activity

The proportion of roll-tilt sensitive neurones is normal. The overall resting activity is slightly reduced. As in the ipsilesional lateral vestibular nucleus, there is an increase in position-sensitive neurones and in beta responses and a decrease in the roll-tilt sensitivity of neurones in the rostroventral areas. There are scanty data on the changes with compensation, but there appear to be few differences in the contralesional neuronal activity in normal and in uncompensated cats.[14]

What happens if both labyrinths are destroyed

So long as there has been adequate time—about 3 days to have occurred, in a guinea pig and about 1 week in a human—for compensation to have occurred for the first uVD, acute deafferentation of both labyrinths, one after the other, produces two attacks of the acute uVD syndrome. If, however, the second uVD is carried out soon after the first, before there has been a chance for compensation to have occurred, a second uVD syndrome will not develop. In fact, if the second uVD is carried out while the symptoms of the first are at their peak, the uVD symptoms will abruptly terminate. This is called the Bechterew effect.[2,15] It is also important to note that if the two labyrinths are deafferented simultaneously, either suddenly or slowly, the patient will not experience vertigo, since there is never any left-right asymmetry in vestibular nucleus activity.

The long-term effects of bilateral vestibular deafferentation are the same irrespective of whether it has been simultaneous or sequential.[16]

CLINICAL FEATURES OF CHRONIC VESTIBULAR INSUFFICIENCY

1. Sense of imbalance only when standing or walking, especially on uneven surfaces and especially in the dark.
2. A positive modified Romberg test: the patient cannot stand with the feet together and eyes closed on a thick foam mat.
3. Vertical bouncing or simply blurring of vision while the patient is in motion, i.e. oscillopsia.
4. More than three lines' decrement in visual acuity while the patient's head is being vigorously shaken up and down.

The patient will experience the syndrome of chronic vestibular insufficiency (CVI), which has also been called Dandy syndrome,[17] after the American neurosurgeon who pioneered therapeutic vestibular neurectomy, in some cases bilateral, for the treatment of intractable Menière's disease. The three cardinal symptoms and signs of the CVI syndrome derive from the lack of input to vestibulo-ocular, vestibulospinal and vestibulocortical pathways rather than from any asymmetry in input to these pathways, as in patients with vertigo. First, the patient with CVI cannot walk securely in the dark, particularly if the ground is uneven, because there is no input to his vestibulospinal pathways. Second, the patient cannot see clearly while her head is moving quickly, because there is no input to vestibulo-ocular pathways, and she will experience retinal image movement, i.e. oscillopsia on head movement (Figure 48.2). Third, she will be disoriented when visual and proprioceptive sensory input is ambiguous. For example, she will have trouble walking in the dark, particularly if the ground is uneven, and in coming to the surface after she dives underwater, because in these situations there is lack of visual input, ambiguous proprioceptive input and no input to vestibulocortical pathways. It might be some consolation that she will, however, be a fine ship's cook, because she will never be motion sick again, no matter how rough the weather. The difficulty in seeing clearly when the head is rotating quickly is due to retinal image movement, which, fortunately, not every patient with absent vestibular function is aware of in daily life. While some patients will volunteer that their vision bounces up and down when they walk and this is a source of considerable misery, many will deny oscillopsia and will only report blurred vision and only when their head is shaken rapidly by an examiner and not in daily life. How some subjects without vestibular function adapt so quickly and so completely to a degree of image motion that other subjects with the same deficit find intolerable is still an enigma.[18] Some patients with severe unilateral loss of vestibular function will also develop symptoms of CVI.[19,20]

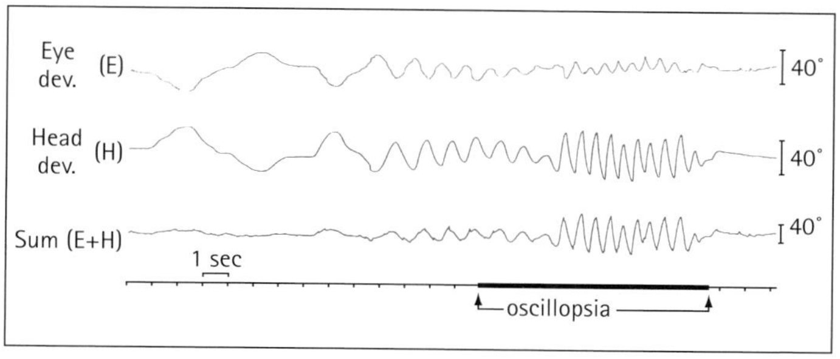

Figure 48.2 Horizontal eye rotations in response to voluntary horizontal head rotations in a patient with bilateral loss of vestibular function. While the patient oscillates the head (H) only slowly, there are adequate compensatory eye rotations (E) generated by the visual system, so that gaze (E+H), called here *SUM*, remains reasonably stable. When the head oscillates faster, compensatory eye rotations become inadequate since the gain of the visual pursuit reflex declines above 1 Hz and the patient has no vestibulo-ocular reflex. Consequently, gaze moves with head and the patient experiences retinal image movement, i.e. 'oscillopsia'. (From Atkin A, Bender MB. Ocular stabilization during oscillatory head movements. *Arch Neurol* 1968; **19**: 559–66.)

What happens if one labyrinth is stimulated

Just as acute deafferentation of one labyrinth invariably produces a stereotyped temporary syndrome of profound ocular-motor abnormalities, mechanical stimulation of one SCC or electrical stimulation of its afferent nerve in an alert animal invariably produces a stereotyped reflex rotation of the head and eyes, in the plane of the stimulated SCC—for a review see Cohen.[21]

For example, stimulation of the left lateral SCC or its nerve produces predominantly horizontal left-beating (i.e. rightward slow-phase) nystagmus, corresponding to the orientation of the lateral SCC within the temporal bone.[22] Similarly, stimulation of the left posterior SCC or its nerve produces upbeating, and, from the patient's point of view, counterclockwise torsional nystagmus, corresponding to the diagonal orientation of the posterior SCCs within the temporal bone.[23] When the entire labyrinth is stimulated, the resulting nystagmus is predominantly horizontal–torsional, since any vertical component is cancelled by the opposing actions of the anterior and posterior SCCs on the same side.

Consequently, each SCC has its signature nystagmus, so that it is possible in some patients, particularly those with irritative peripheral vestibular disorders such as benign paroxysmal positioning vertigo (BPPV) or the Tullio phenomenon, to deduce from an analysis of the nystagmus plane the exact SCC which gives rise to the nystagmus.

For example, in patients with BPPV paroxysmal nystagmus develops in the Dix–Hallpike position, because the ampullary hair cells in one SCC are mechanically stimulated by stray otoconia. If the nystagmus is predominantly horizontal, then the otoconia are in the lateral SCC. If the trajectory of that nystagmus is upbeat and torsional, then the otoconia are in the posterior SCC. Three-dimensional eye-movement recordings confirm that the rotation axis of the nystagmus is orthogonal to the plane of the posterior SCC of the lowermost ear.[24]

In patients with sound-induced vestibular symptoms (the Tullio phenomenon), the axis of the induced nystagmus corresponds to the axis of the anterior SCC on one side; in other words, it has downbeat–torsional quick phases[25–27]—see Figure 48.3A. The problem in these patients appears to be a bony defect or 'dehiscence' in the roof of the superior (i.e. anterior) SCC,[27–29] creating a third window for the membranous labyrinth, so that sound energy is able to deflect the cupula and stimulate ampullary hair cells—see Figure 48.3B.

The standard caloric test is also based on labyrinthine stimulation. Warm or cool water (at 30°C or 44°C) infused into the patient's external auditory canal creates a thermal gradient across the labyrinth and generates a convective movement of endolymph which then deflects the cupula and either increases or decreases the firing rate of SCC primary afferent neurones. The caloric test is mainly a test of lateral SCC function, because the lateral SCC is the closest to the thermal stimulus, and with the patient supine and the head elevated 30° from horizontal, the convective effect is the largest in the lateral SCC canal, since it is earth-vertical.[30] If however, the patient is positioned so that the anterior SCC is earth-vertical, then the axis of the nystagmus becomes more vertical and torsional. The posterior canal is less able to be stimulated by caloric stimuli, perhaps due to its orientation and distance from the heat source. The caloric test can be used to test all three semicircular canals, by positioning the patient so that the canal of interest is earth-vertical, and measuring nystagmus components in each canal plane.[31]

It is also possible to stimulate the otoliths on one side, particularly the utricle. In the cat, electrical stimulation of the utricular nerve produces a contraversive ocular tilt reaction comprising head tilt, conjugate eye torsion and skew deviation with contralateral hypotropia.[32] In humans, galvanic (i.e. DC)

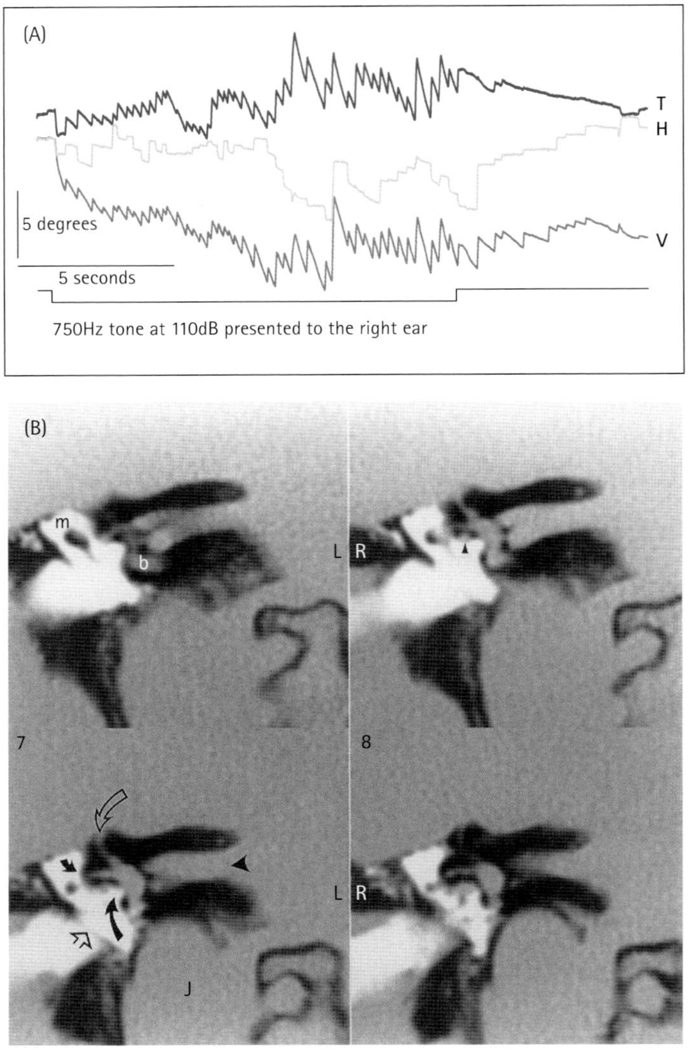

Figure 48.3 (A) Tullio phenomenon from the right ear. A 750-Hz tone at 110 dB produces nystagmus with downward and clockwise (from the patient's point of view) quick phases in darkness, indicating excitation of the right anterior (i.e. superior) semicircular canal by the sound. A three-dimensional search coil recording; H, horizontal, V, vertical, T, torsional. In accordance with the right-hand rule for rotations, the positive direction is leftward, downward and clockwise. The patient had a dehiscence of the right superior (i.e. anterior) semicircular canal. (Courtesy of Dr L. Minor, Baltimore.) (B) Coronal high-resolution CT images of the temporal bone of a patient with Tullio phenomenon of the right ear. There is a deficient bony roof over the superior (i.e. anterior) semicircular canal (curved open arrow). The top left image is most anterior and the bottom right image is most posterior. Other, normal, structures identified are: the head of the malleus (m); the basal turn of the cochlea (b); the jugular bulb (j); the oval window (large solid curved arrow); the tympanic membrane (small straight open arrow); the tympanic segment of the facial nerve (small arrowhead); and the internal auditory canal (large arrowhead). There is normal bony covering over the lateral semicircular canal (small solid curved arrow). The letters 'R' and 'L' refer to the right and left of each image. Compare with Figure 48.12a, which shows the normal bony covering of the superior semicircular canal. (From Watson SRD, Halmagyi GM, Colebatch JG. Vestibular hypersensitivity to sound (Tullio phenomenon). Structural and functional assessment. *Neurology* 2000; **54**: 722–8.)

mastoid stimulation produces a similar, but only partial, OTR comprising conjugate eye torsion and head tilt but no skew deviation.[33,34] Some patients with the Tullio phenomenon have predominantly a contraversive paroxysmal OTR, presumably due to utricular rather than superior (i.e. anterior) SCC activation by sound.[35]

Summary

1. Vertigo is due to asymmetrical vestibular nucleus activity, either an increase in vestibular activity on one side or a decrease on the other.
2. Vertigo is temporary; if it is present all the time and is always the same, then it is not vertigo.
3. Acute total unilateral vestibular deafferentation produces a temporary asymmetry in vestibular nucleus activity and therefore a temporary vertigo.
4. A slowly progressive total unilateral vestibular deafferentation does not produce vertigo, presumably because it does not at any time produce asymmetrical vestibular nucleus activity.
5. A chronic stable total unilateral vestibular deafferentation does not produce vertigo. If the unilateral vestibular deafferentation was acute, then it no longer produces vertigo; if the unilateral vestibular deafferentation was slowly progressive, it never produced vertigo.
6. Bilateral symmetrical vestibular deafferentation does not produce vertigo, but the syndrome of chronic vestibular insufficiency—ataxia and oscillopsia.
7. In some patients, chronic unilateral vestibular deafferentation also produces chronic vestibular insufficiency.

Some common peripheral vestibular diseases

Disorders of the vestibular system produce three main syndromes: the syndrome of acute spontaneous vertigo, the syndrome of provoked vertigo, and the syndrome of imbalance. Each syndrome can be caused by many different diseases. Here we review the diseases most frequently encountered in clinical practice. For the diagnosis of vertigo, the history is critically important, as the patient rarely presents during vertigo attack. The clinical examination of the vestibular system is a specialized skill that requires regular practice. Details of how to take a history and how to examine a patient with a suspected vestibular disorder can be found elsewhere.[36,37]

Acute vestibular neuritis

Definition

Sudden spontaneous, isolated, total or subtotal loss of peripheral vestibular function of one labyrinth is a frequent and usually dramatic clinical event. It is usually ascribed to a viral infection or to a parainfectious event and has been called 'acute vestibular neuritis' as well as 'vestibular neuronitis', 'labyrinthitis' or 'neuro-labyrinthitis'. Some prefer to call it simply 'acute unilateral peripheral vestibulopathy'—for reviews see Strupp and Arbusow[38] or Strupp and Brandt.[39] From the point of view of pathophysiology, vestibular neuritis is a spontaneous acute uVD, and as long as no recovery of peripheral vestibular function occurs, its functional short- and long-term effects are indistinguishable from those of a vestibular neurectomy or labyrinthectomy.

Clinical features

The patient with acute vestibular neuritis experiences spontaneous vertigo as well as nausea and vomiting that can be so intense that she or he cannot get to a doctor and requires either a home visit or admission to an emergency room. The audiological physician is unlikely to see the patient at this stage. The objective vestibular signs are exactly the same as those that occur after a labyrinthectomy or a vestibular neurectomy.

There is a horizontal–torsional spontaneous nystagmus with the slow phases towards the side of the affected ear. The nystagmus is always strictly unidirectional; bidirectional gaze-evoked nystagmus excludes the diagnosis. The nystagmus is to some extent always suppressed by visual fixation, and for that reason it might not be detected on the standard clinical examination but only when some means are used to view the eyes in the absence of visual fixation. This can be done either by ophthalmoscopy with the other eye covered,[40] or with Frenzel's glasses, optical or infrared video. The head impulse test is invariably positive towards the affected side and indicates absent lateral SCC function.[41] Interpretation of the head-impulse test is not confounded by the presence of spontaneous nystagmus. This is because the compensatory saccade, which occurs with a head impulse towards the affected side, will be almost the same size as the head impulse, 20–30°, and therefore much larger than the quick phases of the spontaneous nystagmus, which are usually 3–5° in the presence of visual fixation.

The patient, although unsteady, can, with the eyes open, stand without support, but rotates towards the side of the lesion when trying to march on the spot with the eyes closed—called a positive Fukuda or Unterberger test.

There is also a partial or complete ocular tilt reaction towards the affected side but it is rarely obvious clinically. This is because the head tilt towards the affected side and the skew deviation with the higher image coming from the eye on the side of the affected ear are often absent,[42–46] and the cardinal sign of the ocular tilt reaction, a conjugate ocular torsion towards the affected side, cannot be seen without indirect ophthalmoscopy or fundus photography (Figure 48.4). However, the conjugate ocular torsion can be inferred by testing the subjective visual horizontal.

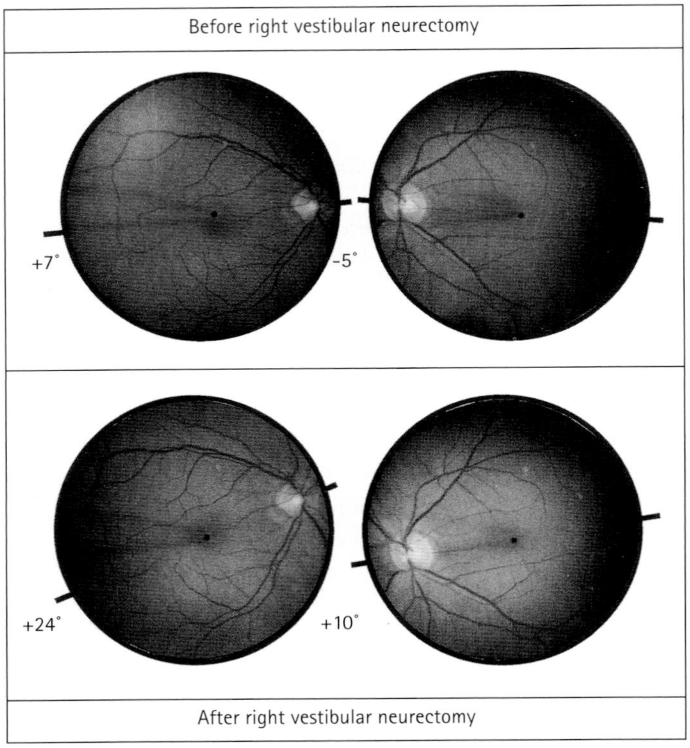

Figure 48.4 The change in torsional eye position before and after unilateral vestibular deafferentation. Fundus photographs of the left and right eye of a patient before (top row) and after (bottom row) right vestibular neurectomy. The right fundus is on the left of the figure, and the left fundus is on the right of the figure. After the operation, there is conjugate tonic rightwards torsion (i.e. clockwise from the patient's point of view) of the 12 o'clock point of each eye. The change in torsional eye position measures 17° in the right eye (from 7° rightwards torsion to 24° rightwards torsion) and 15° on the left (from 5° leftwards torsion to 10° rightwards torsion). The conjugate torsion is part of the ocular tilt reaction.

Investigations

The subjective visual horizontal (SVH) test is the single most useful investigation in the acute phase of suspected vestibular neuritis. Often, perhaps even always, there is a deviation of the SVH, sometimes by more than 20°, and this is always towards the side of the lesion.[47–55] In our laboratory, this test is performed in a dark room, and the seated patient is asked to set, using a push-button controller, a dim-illuminated light-bar until it looks to be aligned with her or his perceived gravitational horizontal. In some laboratories, patients are asked to set a bar to the gravitational vertical, but we find that most patients have a better intuitive understanding of the horizontal than of the vertical and that the settings of the vertical are not the same as those of the horizontal.[56] In any case, in order for the test to be valid, either the room must be totally dark, apart from the light-bar, or there must be some other way that all visual clues are excluded, such as a ganzfeld or a rotating dome.[57]

A normal subject can set such a light-bar within 2–3° of the true gravitational horizontal, every time, and with either eye. Immediately after acute uVD, patients set the bar towards the side of the lesion. They offset the bar by the same amount as the torsional position at which the eye is offset towards the side of the lesion (Figure 48.5). In other words, the SVH is simply an indirect but accurate means of measuring the conjugate ocular torsion, which is the hallmark of the ocular tilt reaction, and which invariably occurs after acute uVD. The conjugate ocular torsion after acute uVD can be thought of as equivalent in the otolithic system to the spontaneous nystagmus in the SCC system. Since the setting of the SVH depends on relative resting activity in the left and right vestibular nuclei, as the patient's brainstem compensates for the uVD, the SVH returns towards normal, although a small offset of the SVH appears to be a permanent stigma of uVD.[51] Therefore, by analogy with spontaneous nystagmus, a return of the SVH towards normal is inevitable, whether or not the labyrinth recovers. It is of interest that after acute uVD in frogs there is head torsion, which follows exactly the same time course as conjugate eye torsion in humans, and has been used to monitor drug effects on vestibular compensation.[58]

Electronystagmography at this stage adds little to clinical observation with Frenzel glasses, but it does create a permanent record in case questions are asked later about whether the nystagmus was really unidirectional and whether it was really suppressed by visual fixation. Caloric testing contributes nothing

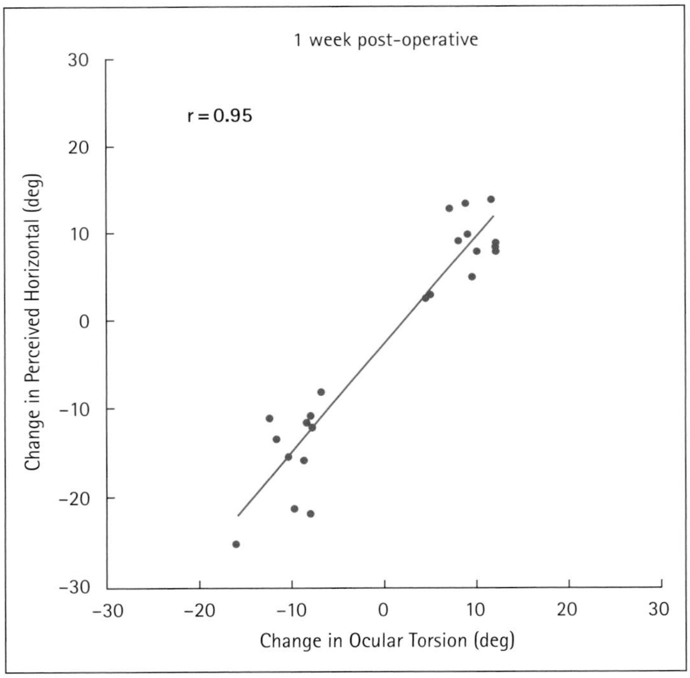

Figure 48.5 Ocular torsion and the subjective visual horizontal. The relationship between the change of ocular torsion and the corresponding change in the subjective visual horizontal (SVH) 1 week after unilateral vestibular neurectomy in 22 patients. The average value of the change in ocular torsion was calculated for each patient and correlated with that patient's average change in the SVH. The correlation (r = 0.95) is significant. (From Curthoys et al. *Exp Brain Res* 1991; **85**: 218–25.[49])

in the acute stage, and it might even produce misleading results. The spontaneous nystagmus might be so vigorous and the adaptive VOR suppression so effective that there might be no response even to 0°C irrigation of either ear. The caloric test will become useful after about 3–4 days.

Natural history

The acute uVD syndrome that occurs with acute vestibular neuritis, i.e. the vertigo, the vomiting, the nystagmus and the ocular tilt reaction, largely resolves within a few days by the process of vestibular compensation. In fact, one can be confident that if the uVD syndrome does not resolve, then the patient has not had acute vestibular neuritis. The uVD syndrome resolves, i.e. the patient gets better, even if the labyrinth does not. That is, a caloric test done at any time after the patient has recovered from the uVD syndrome could show absent or severely depressed warm and cool responses from the affected ear. Superficially, it is as if the patient had a vestibular nerve section. In this regard, sudden unilateral vestibular loss is fundamentally different from sudden unilateral hearing loss. The patient with sudden unilateral hearing loss can tell if his bad ear has not recovered because his hearing would be no better. In contrast, the patient with sudden unilateral vestibular loss cannot tell that his ear has recovered, since his balance will get better, i.e. the acute uVD syndrome will resolve, whether or not the ear itself recovers.

After acute vestibular neuritis, as after surgical uVD, about 20% of patients experience continuing vestibular symptoms, not vertigo but oscillopsia and a persistent subjective imbalance, particularly in the dark and particularly on uneven surfaces. That is, they develop CVI, which is qualitatively the same as that which patients with bilateral loss of vestibular function experience.[19] It seems that, for some patients, one labyrinth is not enough to avoid retinal image slip during head movement and to provide perfect balance in the dark or on uneven ground. Vestibular rehabilitation can be helpful.[59]

As shown by caloric testing, lateral SCC function will progressively recover in only about 50% of patients[60–63] (Figure 48.6). In a few there will be more attacks of acute peripheral vestibulopathy, either on the same side or on the opposite side, a condition called bilateral sequential vestibular neuritis.[64] If the repeated attacks are all on the same side, it will be difficult to be sure that the patient is not developing Menière's disease, especially if there is recovery of vestibular function on caloric tests between the attacks.

After acute vestibular neuritis, about 20% of patients will develop typical posterior SCC-type BPPV. This is of some interest, since it implies that in these patients there must be surviving, functioning receptors and neurones innervating the ampulla of the posterior SCC.[65,66] It is important to distinguish this positional vertigo from the spontaneous vertigo of recurrent vestibular neuritis and from the ataxia that those patients who develop CVI after acute vestibular neuritis experience.

The observation that some patients develop posterior SCC BPPV after acute vestibular neuritis has recently led to work showing that in some, perhaps even in most, patients with acute vestibular neuritis, anterior and lateral SCC function is lost while posterior SCC function is preserved. The most parsimonious explanation of this finding is that in most cases of acute vestibular neuritis only the superior vestibular nerve, innervating the anterior and lateral SCCs and the utricle, is affected, while the inferior vestibular nerve, innervating the posterior SCC and the saccule, is spared.[67,68]

Treatment

There is no effective treatment for acute vestibular neuritis. Despite the fact that peripheral vestibular function will recover in only about half of the patients, they will all recover from the acute uVD syndrome without any treatment. In particular, there is no convincing evidence that corticosteroids shorten or ameliorate the uVD syndrome, help peripheral vestibular function to recover or reduce the chance of the patient developing CVI. Nonetheless, it appears that early mobilization and early vestibular rehabilitation might reduce the incidence of disability from the CVI, which will develop in about 20% of those patients with acute vestibular neuritis whose peripheral vestibular function fails to recover.[59] Like acute facial palsy and some cases of sudden hearing loss, acute vestibular neuritis might be due to viral infection, perhaps with herpes simplex.[69–71]

Differential diagnosis

Cerebellar infarction

The main differential diagnosis of acute vestibular neuritis is acute cerebellar infarction.[72,73] There are several ways to tell the difference clinically. First and foremost is the head-impulse test. In a patient with acute spontaneous vertigo, if the head-impulse test is positive, then the patient has acute vestibular neuritis, and if the head-impulse test is negative, the patient definitely does not have acute vestibular neuritis but might well have had a cerebellar infarct (Figure 48.7).

Second, with a cerebellar infarct the nystagmus might be bidirectional and might not be well suppressed by visual fixation—that is, it will be obvious even without Frenzel glasses. Third, a patient with a cerebellar infarct usually cannot stand without support even with eyes open, whereas the patient with acute vestibular neuritis usually can. If it is not possible to be sure clinically that the patient has acute vestibular neuritis, then it is usually because the examining clinician is insufficiently familiar with the technique of the head-impulse test to show that it is convincingly positive. In that case, imaging will be required, and since many acute cerebellar infarcts are missed by CT, this means MRI (Figure 48.8). Nonetheless, cerebellar infarction is worth diagnosing, for two reasons: first, because about one-third of cases will develop swelling causing potentially lethal, posterior fossa intracranial hypertension requiring urgent neurosurgical decompression, and second, because many cases are due to vertebral artery dissection[74] or cardiogenic embolism and they might require long-term oral anticoagulation or even cardiac surgery in order to prevent recurrences—for a review see Amarenco.[75]

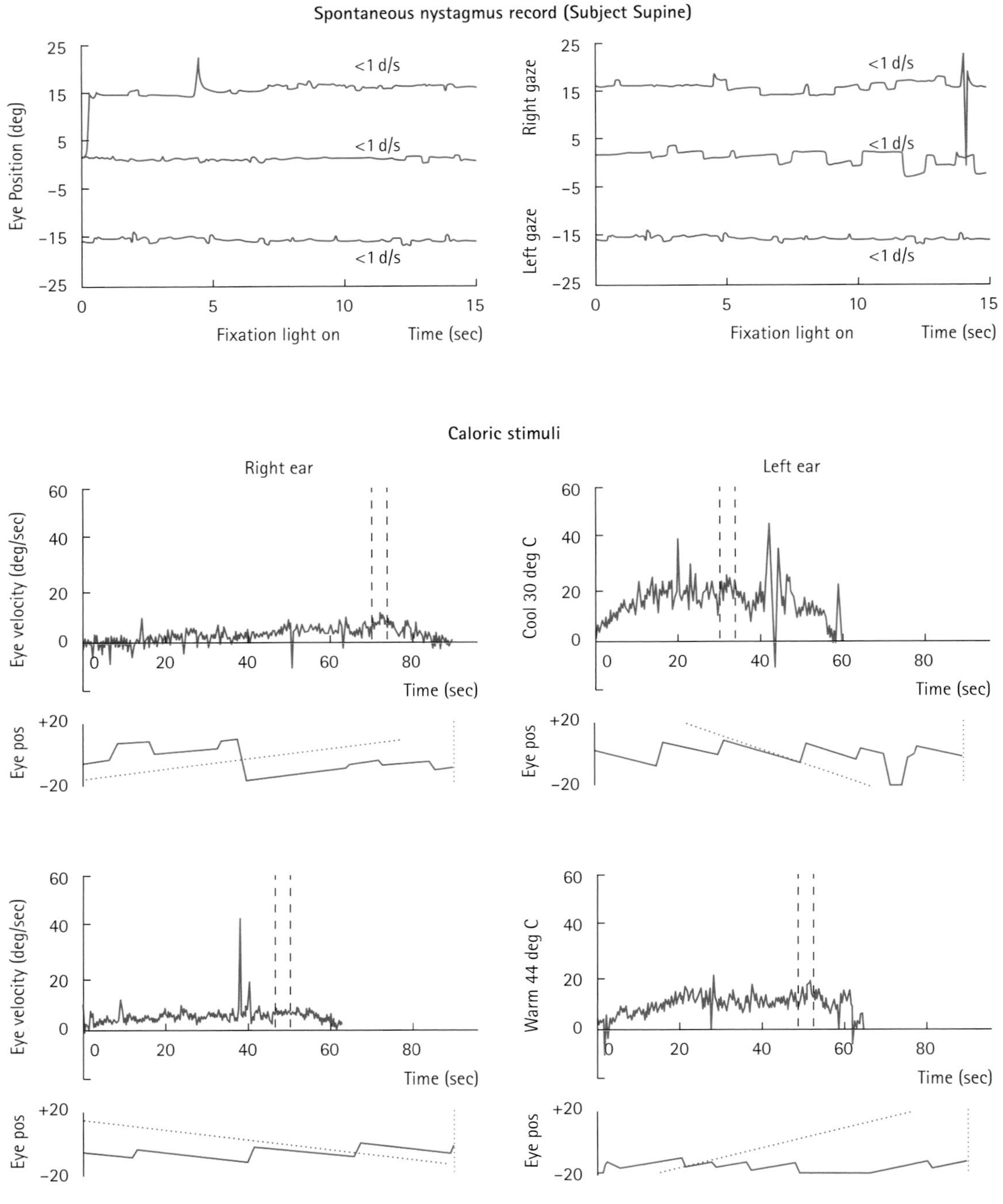

SPON	R30	R44	L30	L44	CP%	DP%	STIMULATOR
<1	8	7	20	14	39	10	Open 25 secs

Figure 48.6 Caloric test in recovered vestibular neuritis. There is a 39% impairment of right lateral semicircular canal function ('canal paresis' or 'CP'), but no spontaneous nystagmus even in the dark and no directional preponderance. The patient had presented to an emergency room 3 months previously with an attack of acute spontaneous vertigo with nausea and vomiting. There had been no loss of hearing, no headache and no other symptoms suggesting brainstem dysfunction. At the time, there was third-degree left-beating nystagmus, and the head impulse test (see Figure 48.7) had been positive to the right. The patient was admitted to hospital but was well enough to go home 3 days later. A caloric test a week later showed a total right canal paresis, but the patient was well enough to return to work. When this caloric test was done 3 months later, there were no clinical abnormalities and the patient was feeling '100%'.

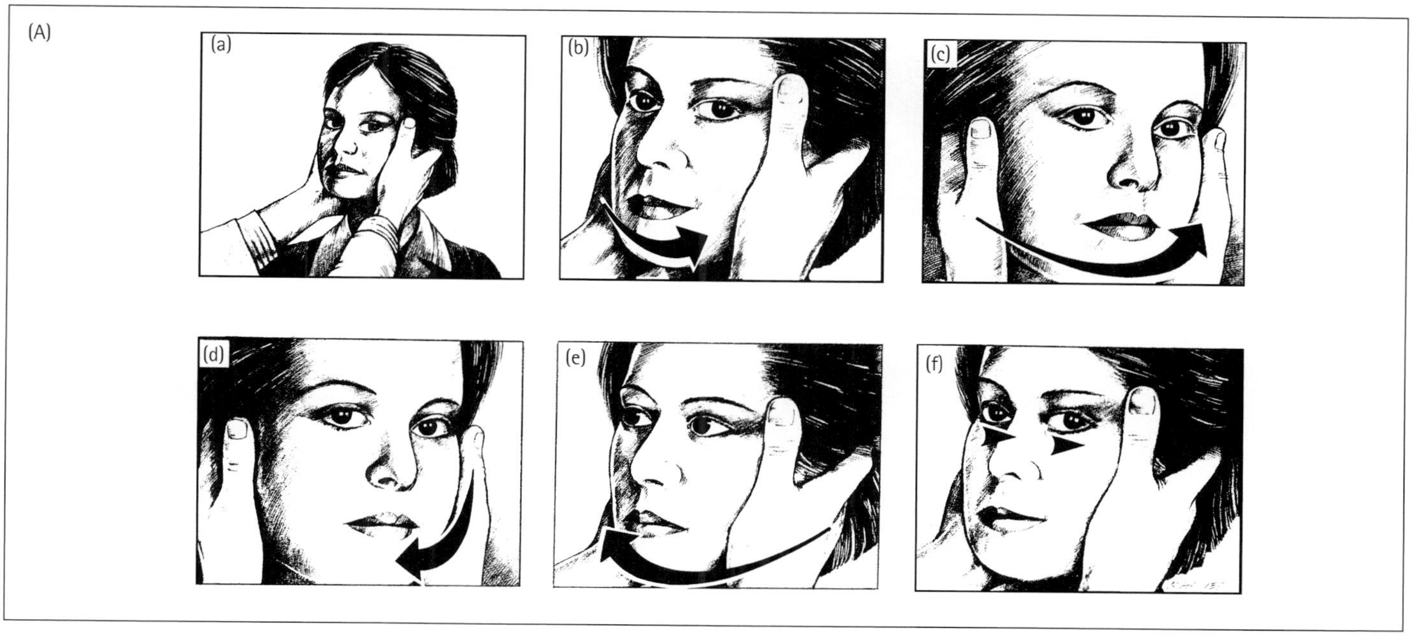

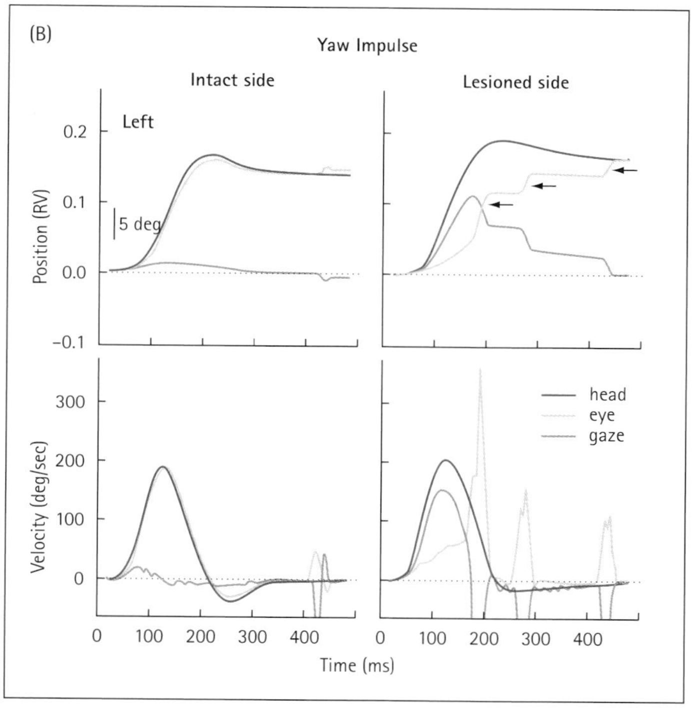

Figure 48.7 (A) Clinical method of the horizontal head-impulse test in a patient who has had a right vestibular nerve section. The examiner turns the patient's head, as rapidly as possible, only about 15° to one side and observes the ability of the patient to keep fixating on a distant target. While the examiner turns the patient's head towards the normal left side (top row), the patient is able to keep fixating on the target. In contrast, when the examiner turns the patient's head to the right, the horizontal vestibuo-ocular reflex fails: the patient cannot keep fixating on the target (e), so that she needs to make a voluntary rapid eye movement, i.e. a saccade, back to target (f) after the head impulse has finished; this can be easily observed by the examiner. This indicates severe loss of right lateral semicircular functions. In doing the test, it is essential that the head be turned as rapidly as possible, as otherwise smooth pursuit eye movements will compensate for the head turn. (From Halmagyi GM, Cremer PD. Assessment and treatment of dizziness. *J Neurol Neurosurg Psychiatry* 2000; **68**: 129–36.) (B) Scleral search coil recordings of a positive-head impulse test in a patient who has had a right vestibular nerve section. Horizontal position (top row) and velocity (bottom row) of the left eye and of the head during a leftwards head impulse (left column) and during a rightwards head impulse (right column). During the leftwards head rotation, the eye rotates by exactly the same amount and at the same velocity as the head, so that the line of sight (gaze) remains almost perfectly stable. In contrast, during the rightwards head rotation, the eye rotates much more slowly, so that gaze shifts with the head, away from the target. The patient needs to make three saccades (arrows) in order to refixate the target. Note that the eye traces have been inverted for ease of comparison with the head traces. (Courtesy of Dr ST Aw, Sydney.)

Labyrinthine infarction

This should not be confused with acute vestibular neuritis, because the internal auditory artery, a branch of the anterior inferior cerebellar artery, also supplies the cochlea, so there should always be a severe or total acute unilateral hearing loss due to cochlear infarction in cases of labyrinthine infarction. That notwithstanding, there are rare cases of acute unilateral vestibulopathy, attributed by some to a branch occlusion of the internal auditory artery, producing infarction of only the labyrinth but sparing the cochlea.[76]

Autoimmune inner ear disease

This is an increasingly popular explanation for obscure cases of bilateral, asynchronous, asymmetrical cochlear hearing loss usually without but sometimes with vestibular involvement.[77] While entities such as Cogan's syndrome have been clearly defined and present with a clinical picture resembling acute vestibular neuritis,[78] autoimmune inner ear disease is not a diagnosis that should be entertained in a patient with acute unilateral loss of vestibular function and normal hearing.

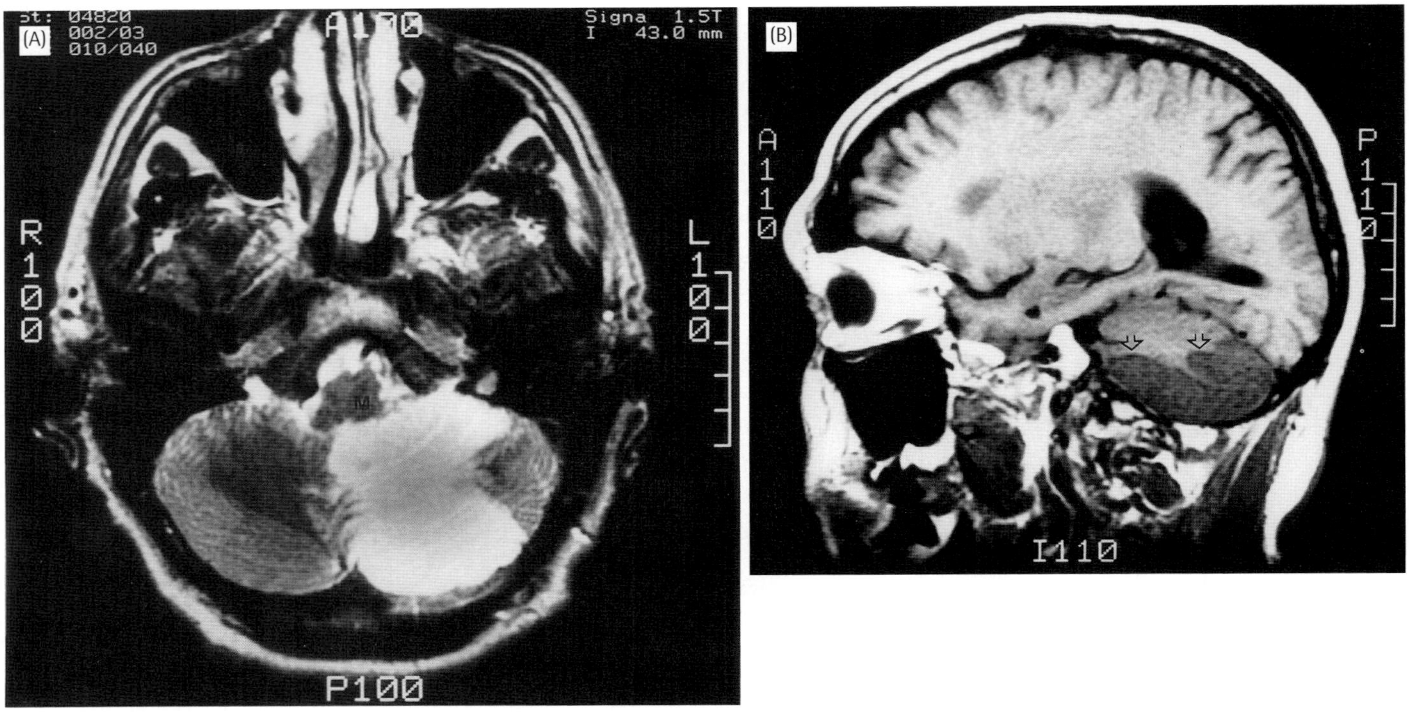

Figure 48.8 Cerebellar infarction. T2-weighted axial (A) and T1-weighted parasagittal (B) MRI scans showing extensive infarction in the territory of the left posterior inferior cerebellar artery. The patient had presented to an emergency room with an attack of acute spontaneous vertigo with nausea and vomiting a week after a 24-h aeroplane flight. At the time, the patient was unable to stand and had third-degree left-beating nystagmus but a negative head-impulse test. A CT scan was normal. The patient was admitted to hospital, and MRI the next day showed not only this cerebellar infarct but also a small right parietal infarct which appeared to be older than the cerebellar infarct. The patient did recall a 4-day episode of numbness in the left hand some three years previously. Note that there is no brainstem infarction but there is compresson of the medulla. The patient made a full functional recovery in a month. Transoesophageal echocardiocardiography showed a small atrial septal defect which was successfully patched non-invasively. This case illustrates the importance of recognizing paradoxical embolism, which can present as a cerebellar infarct, with acute spontaneous vertigo.

Menière's disease

In some patients with Menière's disease, the tinnitus and deafness only begin after many years of repeated vertigo attacks. In our clinic, one patient had recurrent attacks of spontaneous vertigo, with fluctuating lateral SCC function in one ear on caloric testing for 16 years before she developed tinnitus and a fluctuating hearing loss with a positive transtympanic electrocochleogram in the same ear. In general terms, if peripheral vestibular function does not recover after acute unilateral vestibular loss, it is not likely to have been due to Menière's disease.

Menière's disease

Clinical features

Repeated attacks of spontaneous vertigo with nausea and vomiting represent the characteristic early clinical feature of Menière's disease, together with a low-frequency hearing loss (Figure 48.9) a low-frequency tinnitus and fullness, all in the one ear. The vertigo attacks usually last a few hours, but the tinnitus and hearing loss might continue for days. The attacks might occur days, months or even years apart. At first, after each attack of vertigo is over, both vestibular function and cochlear function recover, so that the caloric test and the

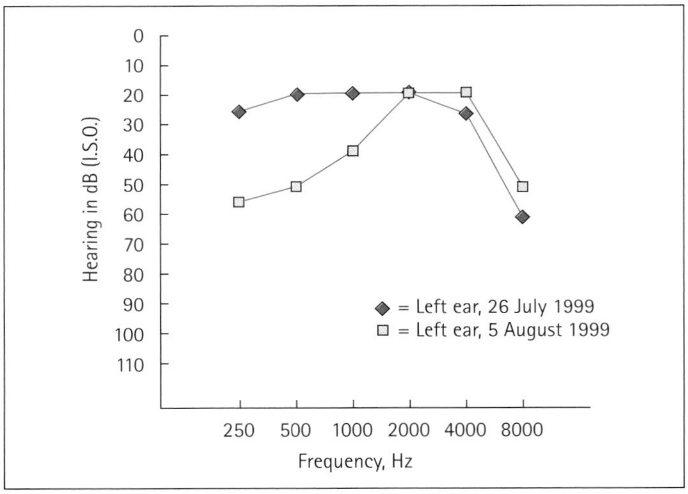

Figure 48.9 Audiogram in Menière's disease. Patient SW, a female aged 44, began to have attacks of acute spontaneous vertigo and left aural fullness and then tinnitus in May 1999. When she was first seen, in between two attacks, in July 1999, the pure-tone audiogram showed only a high-frequency loss, probably due to noise exposure. Two weeks later, she had developed a low-frequency loss on the left. A low-sodium diet was recommended, and the low-frequency loss resolved within 6 weeks and the attacks of vertigo stopped. (Courtesy of Dr M Karlberg, Sydney and Lund.)

pure-tone audiogram will be normal in between attacks. Later, after more attacks of vertigo, a permanent loss of auditory and of vestibular function in the affected ear becomes apparent, even in between attacks. While Menière's disease can remit permanently at any stage, if it does progress, then in the late stages the patient still has vertigo attacks as well as continual tinnitus in a deaf ear that distorts and recruits.

A Menière's attack can have three phases, each defined by the direction of the spontaneous nystagmus.[79] The first is the so-called 'irritative' phase, in which the nystagmus, usually just horizontal, sometimes horizontal–torsional, beats towards the affected ear. This phase lasts less than 1 h, and few physicians ever get to see it. The second is the 'ablative' phase, in which the nystagmus beats away from the affected ear. This phase lasts several hours, sometimes even a day or two. The third is the 'recovery' phase, in which the nystagmus again beats towards the affected side and which lasts about as long as the second phase.

An interesting explanation, based on the nature of vestibular compensation, has been proposed for the recovery phase. Consider a patient with right-sided Menière's disease. During the second phase, the stage of peripheral hypofunction, spontaneous neural activity in the right vestibular nucleus is reduced relative to the left, so that the nystagmus will beat towards the left. After some hours, brainstem compensation will have partly restored the level of spontaneous activity in the right vestibular nucleus, so that the left-beating nystagmus will have abated even though right peripheral vestibular function has not yet begun to recover. As the attack remits and right peripheral vestibular function does recover, the resting activity in the right vestibular nucleus will now be higher than on the unaffected left side so that the nystagmus will now beat towards the right, i.e. there will be a recovery-phase nystagmus.[80]

Some patients, particularly those with advanced Menière's disease, develop drop attacks, also called Tumarkin or otolithic crises. In these, the patient simply drops to the ground without warning, 'like a sack of potatoes', and can sustain a fracture or other injury.[81,82] Lermoyez described patients with Menière's disease whose hearing improved temporarily following a vertigo attack.[83,84]

Natural history

The natural history of Menière's disease is variable. Some patients have a single bout lasting only a few months, with multiple attacks, and never develop any permanent loss of cochlear or vestibular function. Others have a relentlessly progressive course and end up with no useful hearing in one ear. If they are fortunate, they will have no more vertigo attacks and will not have much tinnitus—the so-called burnt-out Menière's disease. Unfortunately, the second ear eventually becomes involved in about half of the patients.[85–87]

Diagnosis

A common clinical problem is the patient presenting with repeated attacks of spontaneous vertigo who is unaware of any temporary hearing loss, or of any temporary tinnitus or any fullness in one ear at the time of the vertigo attacks, and who has no clinical abnormalities, a normal audiogram and a normal caloric test. Could this patient have Menière's disease? The answer is yes. The patient might in fact have had a temporary low-frequency hearing loss during the vertigo attack but would not have noticed it. Patients often do not notice a slight hearing loss in one ear, particularly if the loss is mainly below 1 kHz, the centre of the speech spectrum, and particularly during an incapacitating attack of vertigo and vomiting. On the other hand, there are patients who have repeated spontaneous vertigo attacks for many years before they develop unilateral tinnitus and hearing loss, and the diagnosis finally becomes obvious. The American Academy of Otolaryngology Head and Neck Surgery has published diagnostic criteria for Menière's disease, criteria which are more useful for clinical trials of proposed treatments for Menière's disease than for management of individual patients.[88]

In a patient with repeated attacks of acute spontaneous vertigo, the diagnosis of definite Menière's disease can be made by showing an improvement, either spontaneous or in response to a dehydrating agent such as glycerol—the Klockhoff test—in the unilateral low-frequency hearing loss. It can also be made by showing an improvement in the unilateral vestibular loss on at least two occasions, or by obtaining a positive electrocochleogram. Electrocochleography is most sensitive and most specific for Menière's disease when tone-burst as well as click stimuli are used and when the responses are recorded transtympanically at the promontory (Figure 48.10).[89,90] Giving patients 4 g of oral sodium chloride for 3 days before the ECOG might increase the sensitivity of the test.[91] In the authors' view, the diagnosis of probable Menière's disease can be made if the patient reports two or more attacks of fluctuating unilateral tinnitus, fullness and hearing loss with vertigo all at the same time; the diagnosis of possible Menière's disease is valid even with normal hearing if the patient has had two or more attacks of acute spontaneous vertigo and has a canal paresis on caloric testing, especially if the canal paresis recovers.[92] The patient with many attacks of acute spontaneous vertigo and normal caloric tests is more likely to have vestibular migraine.

Treatment

Strict sodium restriction (urinary sodium less than 50 mmol/day) can be effective in some patients. In our experience, diuretics are not as useful and can produce unwanted side-effects, such as postural hypotension and hypokalaemia.[93] Local pressure treatment might work.[94] Endolymphatic sac surgery (shunting, removal, etc.) is popular but not always effective in stopping either the vertigo attacks or the tinnitus, or in saving the hearing.[95,96] A labyrinthectomy, surgical or preferably pharmacotoxic with intratympanic gentamicin,[97–99] can stop the vertigo attacks and sometimes even the tinnitus.[100] A vestibular nerve section stops the vertigo attacks and also preserves the hearing. Systemic aminoglycosides such as streptomycin or gentamicin have been used in patients with advanced bilateral Menière's

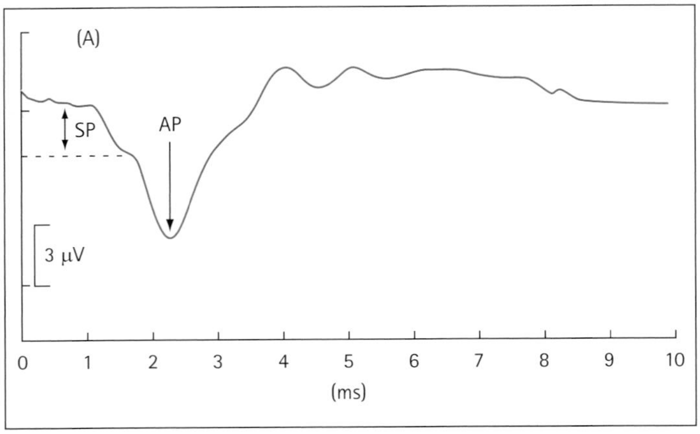

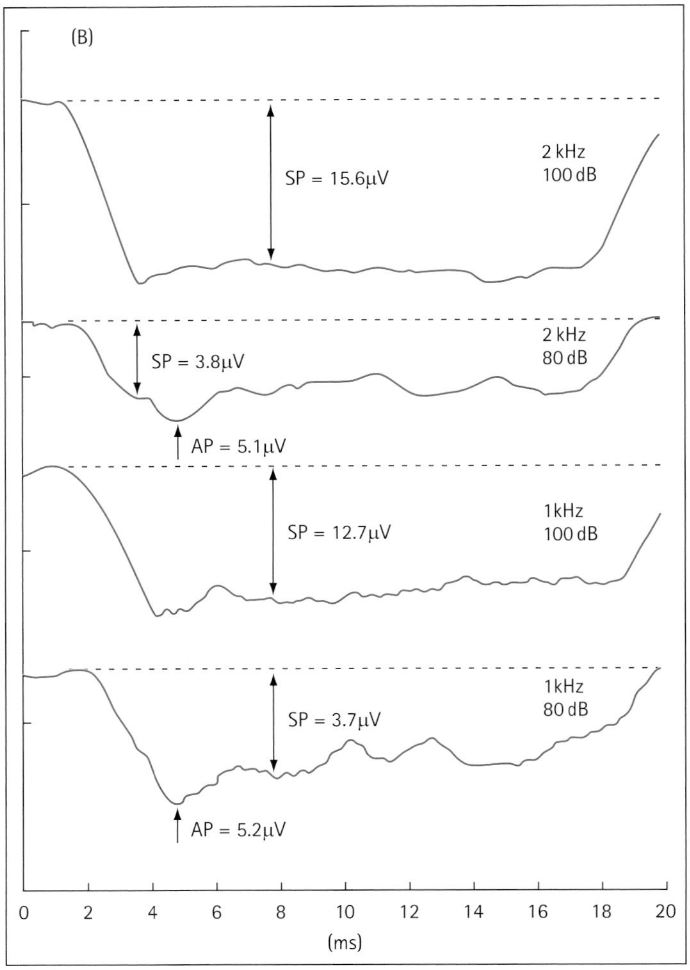

Figure 48.10 (A) Transtympanic electrocochleogram showing averaged responses to 90-dB clicks in August 1999 from the patient whose audiogram is shown in Figure 48.9. The amplitude of the action potential (AP) is 7.5 μV, and the latency is 2.3 ms; the amplitude of the summating potential (SP) is 3.0 μV, giving an SP/AP ratio of 40%. The patient whose audiogram is shown in Figure 48.9 had a subjective threshold of 25 dB nHL for the click stimulus. The mean SP/AP ratio of patients with definite Menière's disease who have subjective click thresholds below 40 dB nHL is 37% (Adapted from Gibson WPR, Arenberg IK. Electrocochleography in the electrophysiologic diagnosis of endolymphatic hydrops. In: Kaufman I, Arenberg IK, eds. *Dizziness and Balance Disorders.* Amsterdam: Kugler, 1993: 477–85).
(B) Transtympanic electrocochleogram showing large negative summating potentials (SP), in response to 16 ms, 1 kHz and 2 kHz tone-bursts at 80 and 100 dB nHL in the same patient as in (A). The mean absolute negative SP levels in patients with definitive Menière's disease, who have subjective thresholds below 40 dB nHL are as follows: 2 kHz, 100 dB > 6 μV; 2 kHz, 80 dB > 4 μV; 1 kHz, 100 dB > 4 μV. These results show that tone burst ECOG responses are more likely to be abnormal in patients with Menière's disease than click-evoked responses.[90] (Courtesy of Prof W Gibson, Sydney.)

disease in order to ablate vestibular function.[101] All ablative procedures on the labyrinth, even if unilateral, carry the risk of producing a mild but permanent chronic vestibular insufficiency, and it is advisable to begin vestibular prehabilitation before any ablative procedures are performed. Those whose hearing is below the reach of standard hearing aids can be helped by cochlear implantation.

Mechanism and aetiology

Endolymphatic hypertension causing enlargement of the cochlear and vestibular ducts, 'endolymphatic hydrops', is generally accepted as the common mechanism of Menière's disease. The endolymph has a total volume of about 100 ml, and is, like intracellular fluid, rich in potassium, while the surrounding perilymph is rich in sodium.[102] The endolymphatic sac, situated under the endosteum of the temporal bone, connects with the cochlea and labyrinth via the endolymphatic duct, which traverses the bony vestibular aqueduct. One theory of the attacks is that the longitudinal flow of endolymph along the cochlear duct[103] becomes obstructed by some 'metabolic debris'. In response, the endolymphatic sac increases its secretion of a hormone called saccin, which in turn increases endolymphatic fluid secretion in the cochlear duct. Endolymphatic pressure builds up, and finally the obstruction is overcome, leading to the vertigo attack.[104] Endolymphatic hydrops supposedly pushes on the basilar membrane and produces an offset of the cochlear summating potential which can be detected by electrocochleography (Figure 48.10).

Many different inner ear or temporal bone diseases such as syphilis, mumps, Cogan's syndrome, trauma, and even chronic suppurative otitis media, can, after many years, produce the clinical picture of Menière's disease. The clinical picture is that of attacks of spontaneous vertigo developing in a patient with a known, often long-standing, unilateral hearing loss. This has been ascribed to delayed endolymphatic hydrops in the deaf ear.[105,106] Sometimes the vertigo develops at the same time as a fluctuating hearing loss in the other previously normal ear, and then this is called contralateral delayed endolymphatic hydrops, and the mechanism is thought to be the development of autoimmunity to inner ear antigens.[107,108] There might also be some evidence that autoimmunity has some role in ordinary Menière's disease, as either cause or effect.[109]

Differential diagnosis

A number of other diseases can produce a clinical picture resembling Menière's disease. Perilymph fistula is a difficult and contentious diagnosis, even at tympanotomy.[110] Some would not make the diagnosis in the absence of obvious trauma or a history of stapes surgery and in the absence of an objective hearing loss, which is usually at the high frequencies. Autoimmune inner ear disease can produce a picture indistinguishable from advanced bilateral Menière's disease, but the vertigo attacks are generally not as violent and the vestibular symptoms are not as obvious.[77] However, the major differential diagnosis of early Menière's disease, before any permanent auditory or vestibular loss has developed, is vestibular migraine.

Vestibular migraine (also called migrainous vertigo)

Those who have migraine headaches have more vertigo than those who do not. Some migraineurs will sometimes have vertigo as their migrainous aura, and will then go on to develop a typical hemicranial headache with nausea and vomiting.[111,112] A few will have a more florid form, with brainstem symptoms and signs including coma and this has been called basilar migraine.[113] Most will have, apart from the attacks of headache, repeated attacks of spontaneous vertigo, typically lasting less than 1 h, with nausea and even vomiting, but without any hearing disturbance or headache at the time.[114,115] The potential mechanism by which migraine might produce vertigo attacks is as contentious as the mechanism of migraine itself. Nevertheless, vertigo attacks in migraineurs can respond to medications used to treat migraine headaches, such as an ergot or a triptan, or even to aspirin. Some patients respond to regular preventative therapy with a beta-blocker, a tricyclic, a calcium channel blocker, sodium valproate or methysergide.[116–118] Since transient neurological events of obscure origin, in the absence of migraine headaches, are common enough in young people,[119] it is likely that migraine can cause vertigo attacks in patients who have never had migraine headaches. Migraine can cause a stroke and a permanent neurological deficit, and there are reports of migraine producing a permanent unilateral loss of vestibular function[120] and of auditory function.[121] There is also a rare dominantly inherited disorder in which patients have migraine headaches as well as repeated attacks of acute spontaneous vertigo which eventually lead to severe or total bilateral loss of vestibular function.[122] Those with migraine appear more likely to develop BPPV than those without.[123]

Benign paroxysmal positioning vertigo

BPPV is the single most frequent cause of vertigo, and in many patients the diagnosis can be made on the history alone.

To understand the mechanism of BPPV and its treatment, it is important to consider what happens if there are otoconia in the duct or on the cupula of an SCC. The otolithic membrane, structurally similar to the tectorial membrane which overlies the organ of Corti, is a gelatinous sheet containing calcium carbonate crystals (relative density 2.7), i.e. otoconia (Figure 48.11). The cilia of the macular hair cells are embedded

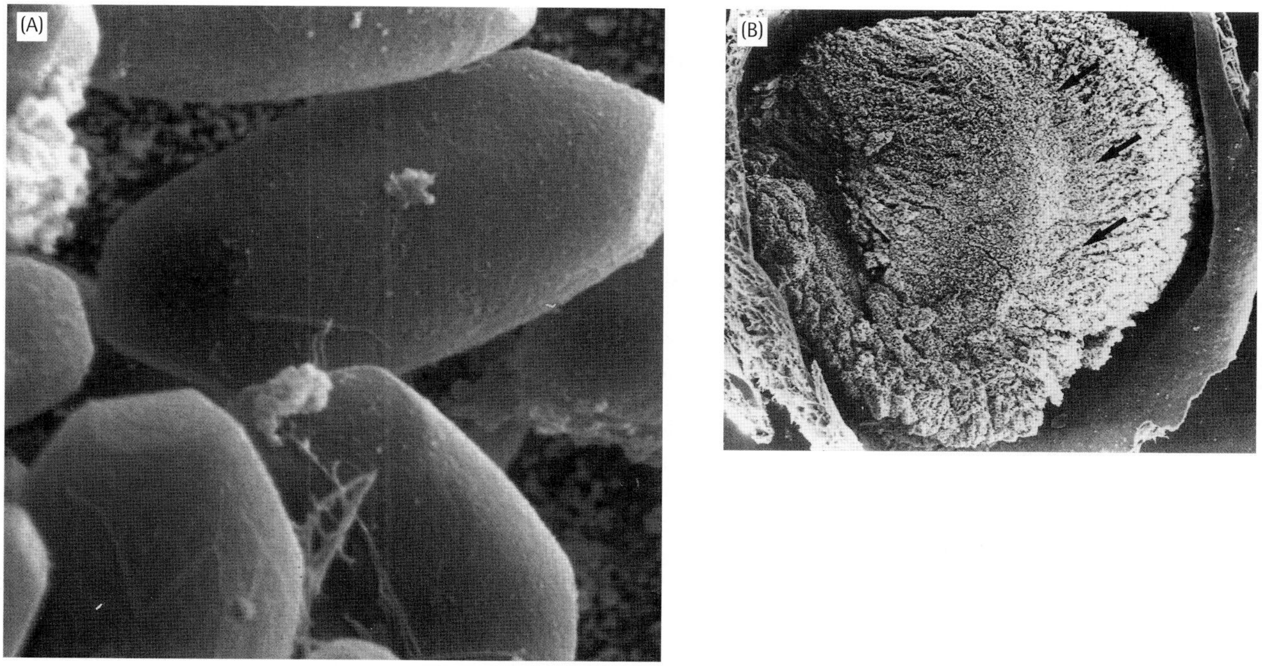

Figure 48.11 (A) Scanning electronmicrograph of human otoconia. Otoconia are 3–5 µm in length; their bodies are rounded and each end is pyramidal. The angle between the faces is about 110–120°. Otoconia in the semicircular canal duct produce benign paroxysmal positioning vertigo. (Courtesy of Professor Y. Harada, Hiroshima.) (B) Scanning electronmicrograph showing otolothic layer of the utricular macula from guinea pig. The thickness of the layer is not even—it is particularly thin at the striola (arrows). Small otoconia predominate on the surface. (From Harada Y. *Atlas of the Ear by Scanning Electron Microscopy*. Lancaster: MTP Press, 1983.)

in this membrane and are displaced by shearing forces applied to the membrane. The shearing forces are produced by linear acceleration, in particular by gravity. If some of these otoconia find their way into a SCC, either the duct (canalolithiasis) or the cupula (cupulolithiasis), changes in head position will shift the otoconia and displace the cupula, either directly in the case of cupulolithiasis, or indirectly by fluid movement in the case of canalolithiasis—for review see Lanska and Remler[124] or Furman and Cass.[125] The cupular displacement produces a sense of rotation, i.e. paroxysmal positioning vertigo, and the paroxysmal positioning nystagmus. The nystagmus will be in the plane of the stimulated SCC.[24] Since the otoconia are almost always in the posterior SCC duct, the nystagmus is almost always vertical–torsional, with the quick phases upwards and towards the affected ear; in gaze towards the affected ear, the nystagmus is mainly torsional, while in gaze away it is mainly vertical. Since the nystagmus produced by otoconia in the posterior SCC is not only torsional but often very vigorous, it is not much suppressed by vision and so is obvious even without Frenzel glasses. If the otoconia are in the lateral SCC, the nystagmus is horizontal.

CLINICAL FEATURES OF BENIGN PAROXYSMAL POSITIONING VERTIGO

A. Left **posterior** semicircular canal

1. Brief vertigo on turning in bed or on looking up.
2. Paroxysmal vertigo with left Dix–Hallpike test.
3. Paroxysmal nystagmus with left Dix–Hallpike test: torsional–vertical quick phases are counterclockwise (from the patient's point of view) and upwards.
4. No vertigo or nystagmus in the right Dix–Hallpike test.

B. Left **lateral** semicircular canal

1. More prolonged vertigo aggravated as well as triggered by lying down.
2. Severe paroxysmal vertigo on turning from right Dix–Hallpike to left Dix–Hallpike position.
3. Prolonged horizontal nystagmus on turning from right to left Dix–Hallpike position—can be left-beating (geotropic—canalolithiasis) or right-beating (ageotropic—cupulolithiasis).
4. Briefer less severe vertigo and horizontal nystagmus on rolling from left to right Dix–Hallpike position; the nystagmus can be right-beating or left-beating.

The history is often unmistakable: 'Doctor, I feel dizzy whenever I turn in bed at night, or I hang out washing on the clothes-line, or look under my car.' Some patients say that they are dizzy all the time, but what they usually mean is that the attacks of BPPV are so frequent and so unpleasant that they still feel unwell in between the attacks. In most patients, the BPPV will occur in bouts lasting several weeks and then it spontaneously remits, only to return weeks, months or even years later.[126] The patient with repeated bouts of vertigo over several decades with no abnormalities on examination most likely has BPPV.

In most patients with BPPV, there are no other symptoms and there is no relevant abnormality of vestibular or auditory function. In a few, BPPV occurs during the course of a progressive inner ear disease such as Menière's disease or Cogan's syndrome.[127] Only rarely is a clinical picture similar to BPPV produced by a posterior fossa tumour, malformation or degeneration.[128]

The positional test, as described by Bárány, developed by Dix, and popularized by Hallpike,[103] is the cornerstone of diagnosis. The principle of the test is to make any otoconia in the posterior SCC move, and so provoke vertigo and nystagmus. Consider a patient with right posterior SCC BPPV, seated on a bed (Figure 48.13). In this position, the posterior SCC is gravitationally vertical, and its ampulla is its lowermost part (Figure 48.12); any otoconia in the duct will have come to rest next to the cupula. The patient's head is now turned to the right and the patient is suddenly pitched backwards (in the plane of the posterior SCC) until the head is hanging over the end of the bed; now the midpoint of the posterior SCC duct, rather than the ampulla, is the lowermost point. The otoconia will now fall down from the cupula and come to rest at the midpoint of the duct. As they fall away from the cupula, they create a negative fluid pressure and so pull on the cupula, producing an ampullofugal deflection, which is excitatory for posterior SCC primary afferent neurones. As a result, there is not only a brief—20 s or so—paroxysm of vertigo but also of nystagmus with upbeating and clockwise quick phases (from the patient's point of view). If the patient is now slowly rotated by 180° about the body long axis towards his left until the left side of his face is on the bed, the posterior SCC will have been inverted, so that the crus communis is now the lowermost point. At this stage, the otoconia should move further along the SCC duct and produce another, less severe, paroxysm of vertigo and clockwise upbeating nystagmus. The patient, still face down, now stands up, and the otoconia will continue along the crus communis back into the vestibule. This is in essence the particle repositioning manoeuvre as described by Epley.[129] Both Epley's[130] and Semont's[131] manoeuvre will stop the BPPV attacks in most patients.[132,133] Patients can even learn to treat themselves.[134] Those who are resistant to repeated repositioning manoeuvres can be cured by surgical occlusion of the posterior SCC.[135,136] Post-traumatic cases in particular can be bilateral and difficult to cure. It is possible, but can be difficult in some patients, to distinguish unilateral from bilateral BPPV.[137]

Lateral canal BPPV is a variant in which the nystagmus is horizontal and usually geotropic—that is, it beats towards the lowermost ear, indicating that the otoconia in the duct are falling towards the cupula.[138] They also fall away from the cupula when the patient rolls onto the normal side, and this produces a less severe vertigo and a less marked, again geotropic, nystagmus. Occasionally, the nystagmus is so brisk in each side as to make it difficult to be certain of the side of the problem.

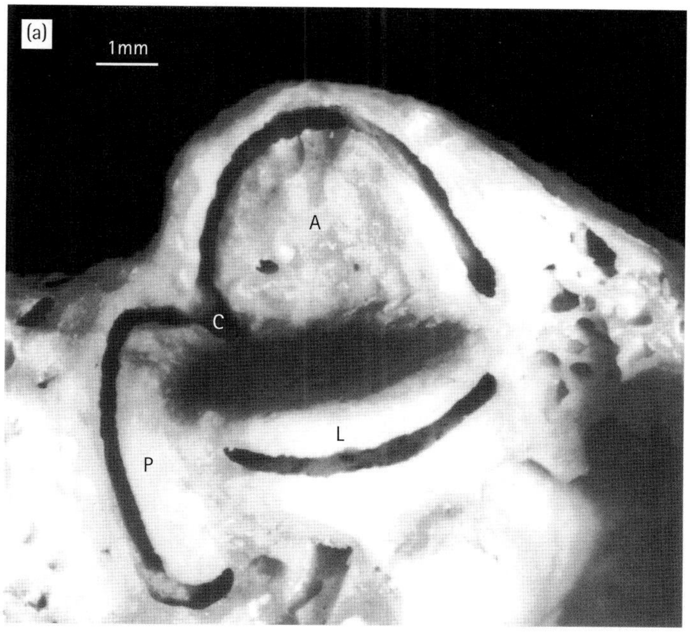

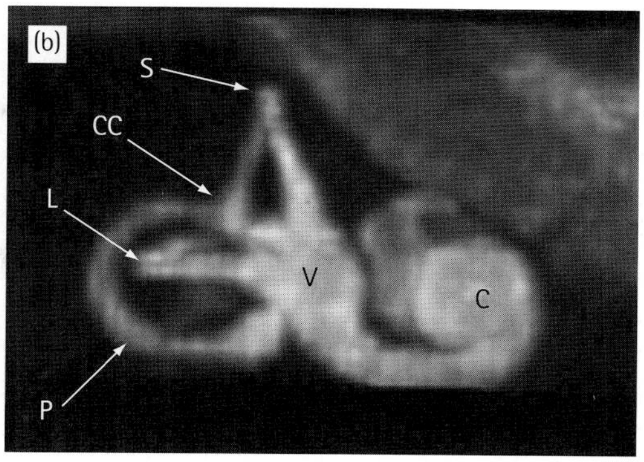

Figure 48.12 (a) Normal human bony labyrinth. Dissection of the right labyrinth in a dry skull showing the relationships of the lateral (L), posterior (P) and anterior (i.e. superior) (A) semicircular canal ducts and the common crus (C) of the anterior and posterior semicircular canals. (b) Normal human membranous labyrinth. Shown in a three-dimensional CISS (Constructive Interference in the Steady State) MR image of the right inner ear, showing the relationships of the lateral (L), posterior (P) and anterior (i.e. superior) (S) semicircular canals, the common crus (CC), the vestibule (V), and the basal, middle and apical turns of the cochlea (C). (Courtesy of M. Todd, Sydney.)

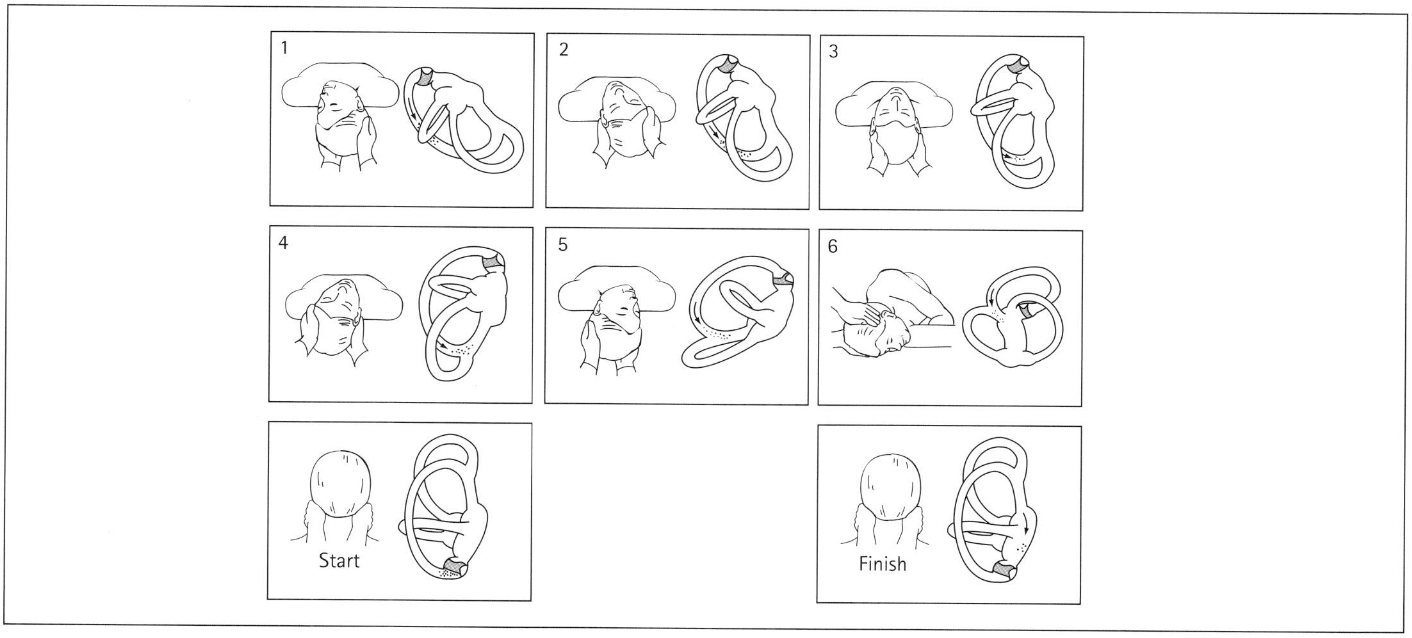

Figure 48.13 The Epley particle repositioning manoeuvre for left posterior SCC BPPV. The patient is rapidly reclined into the left Dix–Hallpike position (1) and remains in that position until both the vertigo and nystagmus have well and truly disappeared and the otoconial particles have settled into the lowest portion of the posterior SCC duct. The patient's head is slowly turned by 90° into the right Dix–Hallpike position (2–5) so that the particles are guided into the common crus. Then the patient slowly rolls onto the right shoulder and the head is turned another 90° so that the particles fall via the common crus back into the vestibule. (From Halmagyi GM, Cremer PD. Assessment and treatment of dizziness. *J Neurol Neurosurg Psychiatry* 2000; **68**: 129–36 with permission from the BMJ Publishing Group.)

Identifying a null head position helps.[139] Treatment of lateral SCC BPPV is less successful than that of posterior SCC BPPV and largely consists of having the patient sleep only on the unaffected side so that the otoconia can find their way out of the lateral SCC back into the vestibule.[140] Sometimes there is a mixed picture, with a conversion of lateral to posterior SCC BPPV or vice versa. Sometimes the otoconia adhere to the lateral SCC cupula, so that the nystagmus and vertigo are persistent and the quick phases are ageotropic—a clinical picture that can suggest a central rather than peripheral vestibulopathy.[141]

Bilateral vestibulopathy

Bilateral loss of vestibular function causes not vertigo but ataxia and oscillopsia, i.e. chronic vestibular insufficiency.[16,142] In the absence of any significant and relevant hearing loss, it can cause some diagnostic difficulties, since an aural cause might not be considered in the differential diagnosis of ataxia.[143] In fact, the patient does not have a cerebellar ataxia, and will be able to walk well heel-to-toe. Thus although the patient will complain of imbalance while walking, the only abnormality will be an inability to keep standing on a soft yielding surface such as a mattress, with the eyes closed, without falling. A bidirectionally positive horizontal and vertical head-impulse test will make the diagnosis on the spot; otherwise, caloric and rotational tests will show bilaterally absent or severely impaired responses. The most common known cause of bilateral vestibular loss without hearing loss is gentamicin toxicity. While systemic gentamicin is not very cochleotoxic in humans, as far as the vestibular system is concerned there is no safe dose, and any patient who notices imbalance after a hospital admission has gentamicin vestibulotoxicity until proven otherwise.[144] In a few patients bilateral vestibular loss is inherited, sometimes in combination with a spinocerebellar ataxia. Their hearing is usually normal. While it will be difficult to recognize a bilateral vestibulopathy in a patient who already has imbalance due to cerebellar ataxia, from examining stance and gait, the compensatory eye movements in response to slow head turning are pathognomonic.[145] Since smooth pursuit is absent due to the cerebellar ataxia, and the vestibulo-ocular reflex is absent due to the peripheral vestibulopathy, even in response to slow head rotations the patient will be unable to make smooth compensatory eye movements and can only produce a series of saccades. The differential diagnosis of the ataxia caused by bilateral vestibulopathy also includes a severe unilateral vestibulopathy, a sensory peripheral neuropathy, hydrocephalus and an early extrapyramidal disorder such as Progressive Supranuclear Palsy or Parkinson's disease.

Diagnoses unlikely to be correct in a patient presenting with vertigo

The purpose of this section is to draw attention to diagnoses that should be made with caution in any patient who has vertigo, and with great caution in a patient who has only vertigo and no fixed loss of auditory or vestibular function and no neurological symptoms or signs.

Middle ear disease

Acute otitis media does not cause vertigo unless there is a suppurative labyrinthitis. Chronic otitis media can, rarely, produce a Menière-like picture due to secondary endolymphatic hydrops or Valsalva-induced vertigo due to perilymph fistula from a cholesteotoma. An oval or round window, post-traumatic or postoperative perilymph fistula can, now and then, produce vertigo, always with a hearing loss, and the cause is always obvious.

Acoustic neuroma

Only rarely does a vestibular schwannoma produce attacks of spontaneous vertigo, and even more rarely without some unilateral loss of auditory or vestibular function.[146]

Vascular compression

Vascular loop compression is a validated cause of paroxysmal symptoms related to the trigeminal and to the facial nerve. While opinions are divided,[147] the evidence that microvascular compression of the vestibular nerve causes paroxysmal vestibular symptoms or any symptoms at all is scanty.[148] The anterior inferior cerebellar artery can normally loop into the internal auditory canal and is not a cause of symptoms. While patients with paroxysmal vertigo and simultaneous paroxysmal tinnitus might respond to treatment with carbamazepine,[149] this does not prove that the cause of the vertigo is compression of the vestibulocochlear nerve.

Perilymph fistula

In almost all patients with perilymph fistula, there will have been an obvious surgical accidental cause or barotrauma and they will all have a unilateral or asymmetrical hearing loss in the affected ear. Spontaneous perilymph fistula is a dubious entity.[110]

Autoimmune ear disease

Autoimmune ear disease is a recognized although difficult-to-prove cause of bilateral, asymmetrical, progressive hearing loss.[66] Patients with immune inner ear disease might also develop vestibular problems but not without hearing problems.

Transient vertebrobasilar ischaemia

Vertebrobasilar ischaemia is a difficult clinical diagnosis to make at any time but unlikely to be correct in a patient whose attacks consist only of vertigo without any other neurological symptoms either at the time of the vertigo or at any other time.[150]

Psychological aspects of vertigo and other vestibular disorders

In all this, it is important to remember that patients with chronic vestibular disorders, especially if the problem remains undiagnosed, untreated and unexplained, and especially if it is all attributed by the doctors to anxiety, tend to oblige and develop major problems with anxiety, panic and even agoraphobia. While the psychological aspects of vestibular disorders are fully discussed in Chapter 53, it is worth emphasizing here that in the anxious dizzy patient one should ask why the patient is anxious, and if one can answer that and treat the cause of the dizziness, one will often relieve the anxiety as well.

Acknowledgements

The long-standing, on-going support of the National Health and Medical Research Council, The Garnett Passe and Rodney Williams Memorial Foundation and the Royal Prince Alfred Hospital Neurology Department trustees is gratefully acknowledged.

References

1. Curthoys IS, Halmagyi GM. Vestibular compensation: a review of the oculomotor, neural, and clinical consequences of unilateral vestibular loss. *J Vestib Res* 1995; **5**: 67–107.
2. Vidal PP, de Waele C, Vibert N, Muhlethaler M. Vestibular compensation revisited. *Otolaryngol Head Neck Surg* 1998; **119**: 34–42.
3. Precht W, Shimazu H, Markham CH. A mechanism of central compensation of vestibular function following hemilabyrinthectomy. *J Neurophysiol* 1966; **29**: 996–1010.
4. Graham BP, Dutia MB. Cellular basis of vestibular compensation: analysis and modelling of the role of the commissural inhibitory system. *Exp Brain Res* 2001; **137**: 387–96.
5. Smith PF, Curthoys IS. Neuronal activity in the contralateral medial vestibular nucleus of the guinea pig following unilateral labyrinthectomy. *Brain Res* 1988; **444**: 295–307.
6. Smith PF, Curthoys IS. Neuronal activity in the ipsilateral medial vestibular nucleus of the guinea pig following unilateral labyrinthectomy. *Brain Res* 1988; **444**: 308–19.
7. Ris L, deWaele C, Serafin M, Vidal PP, Godaux E. Neuronal activity in the ipsilateral vestibular nucleus following unilateral labyrinthectomy in the alert guinea pig. *J Neurophysiol* 1995; **74**: 2087–99.
8. Ris L, Capron B, de Waele C, Vidal PP, Godaux E. Dissociations between behavioural recovery and restoration of vestibular activity in the unilabyrinthectomized guinea pig. *J Physiol* 1997; **500**: 509–22.
9. Newlands SD, Perachio AA. Compensation of horizontal canal related activity in the medial vestibular nucleus following unilateral labyrinth ablation in the decerebrate gerbil. I. Type I neurons. *Exp Brain Res* 1990; **82**: 359–72.
10. Newlands SD, Perachio AA. Compensation of horizontal canal related activity in the medial vestibular nucleus following unilateral labyrinth ablation in the decerebrate gerbil. II. Type II neurons. *Exp Brain Res* 1990; **82**: 373–83.
11. Peusner KD, Gamkrelidze G, Giaume C. Potassium currents and excitability in second-order auditory and vestibular neurons. *J Neurosci Res* 1998; **53**: 511–20.
12. Yamanaka T, Him A, Cameron SA, Dutia MB. Rapid compensatory changes in GABA receptor efficacy in rat vestibular neurones after unilateral labyrinthectomy. *J Physiol (Lond)* 2000; **523**: 413–24.
13. Xerri C, Gianni S, Manzoni D, Pompeiano O. Central compensation of vestibular deficits. I. Response characteristics of lateral vestibular neurons to roll tilt after ipsilateral labyrinth deafferentation. *J Neurophysiol* 1983; **50**: 428–48.
14. Lacour M, Manzoni D, Pompeiano O, Xerri C. Central compensation of vestibular deficits. III. Response characteristics of lateral vestibular neurons to roll tilt after contralateral labyrinth deafferentation. *J Neurophysiol* 1985; **54**: 988–1005.
15. Zee DS, Preziosi TJ, Proctor LR. Bechterew's phenomenon in a human patient. *Ann Neurol* 1982; **12**: 495–6.
16. Hess K. Vestibulotoxic drugs and other causes of bilateral vestibulopathy. In: Baloh RW, Halmagyi GM, eds. *Disorders of the Vestibular System*. New York: Oxford University Press, 1996: 360–73.
17. Syms CA, House JW. Idiopathic Dandy's syndrome. *Otolaryngol Head Neck Surg* 1997; **116**: 75–8.
18. Morland AB, Bronstein AM, Ruddock KH, Wooding DS. Oscillopsia: visual function during motion in the absence of vestibulo-ocular reflex. *J Neurol Neurosurg Psychiat* 1998; **65**: 828–35.
19. Reid CB, Eisenberg R, Halmagyi GM, Fagan PA. The outcome of vestibular nerve section for intractable vertigo: the patients' point of view. *Laryngoscope* 1996; **106**: 1553–6.
20. Waterston JA, Halmagyi GM. Unilateral vestibulotoxicity due to systemic gentamicin therapy. *Acta Otolaryngol (Stockh)* 1998; **118**: 474–8.
21. Cohen B. The vestibulo-ocular reflex arc. In: Kornhuber HH, ed. *Handbook of Sensory Physiology*, vol. 11/2. Berlin: Springer-Verlag, 1974: 477–540.
22. Suzuki J-I, Cohen B. Head, eye, body and limb movements from semicircular canal nerves. *Exp Neurol* 1964; **10**: 393–405.
23. Suzuki J-I, Cohen B, Bender MB. Compensatory eye movements induced by vertical semicircular canal stimulation. *Exp Neurol* 1964; **10**: 137–60.
24. Fetter M, Sievering F. Three-dimensional eye movement analysis in benign paroxysmal positioning vertigo and nystagmus. *Acta Otolaryngol* 1995; **115**: 353–7.
25. Rottach KG, von Maydell RD, DiScenna AO, Zivotofsky AZ, Averbuch-Heller L, Leigh RJ. Quantitative measurements of eye movements in a patient with Tullio phenomenon. *J Vestib Res* 1996; **6**: 255–9.
26. Cremer PD, Minor LB, Carey JP, Della Santina CC. Eye movements in patients with superior canal dehiscence syndrome align with the abnormal canal. *Neurology* 2000; **55**: 1833–41.
27. Minor LB, Solomon D, Zinreich JS, Zee DS. Sound- and/or pressure-induced vertigo due to bone dehiscence of the superior semicircular canal. *Arch Otolaryngol Head Neck Surg* 1998; **124**: 249–58.
28. Minor LB. Superior canal dehiscence syndrome. *Am J Otol* 2000; **21**: 9–19.
29. Brantberg K, Bergenius J, Mendel L, Witt H, Tribukait A, Ygge J. Symptoms, findings and treatment in patients with dehiscence of the superior semicircular canal. *Acta Otolaryngol* 2001; **121**: 68–75.
30. Gentine A, Eichorn J-L, Kopp C, Conraux C. Modelling the action of caloric stimulation of the vestibule. *Acta Otolaryngol (Stockh)* 1990; **110**: 328–33.
31. Aw ST, Haslwanter T, Fetter M, Heimberger J, Todd MJ. Contribution of the vertical semicircular canals to the caloric nystagmus. *Acta Otolaryngol* 1998; **118**: 618–27.

32. Suzuki J-I, Tokumasu K, Goto K. Eye movements from single utricular nerve stimulation in the cat. *Acta Otolaryngol* 1969; **68**: 350–62.
33. MacDougall HG, Brizuela AE, Burgess AM, Curthoys IS. Between-subject variability and within-subject reliability of the human eye-movement response to bilateral galvanic (DC) vestibular stimulation. *Exp Brain Res* 2002; **144**: 69–78.
34. Schneider E, Glasauer S, Dieterich M. Comparison of human ocular torsion patterns during natural and galvanic vestibular stimulation. *J Neurophysiol* 2002; **87**: 2064–73.
35. Dieterich M, Brandt T, Fries W. Otolith function in man. Results from a case of otolith Tullio phenomenon. *Brain* 1989; **112**: 1377–92.
36. Halmagyi GM. The history in the patient with vertigo. In: Baloh RW, Halmagyi GM, eds. *Disorders of the Vestibular System*. New York: Oxford University Press, 1996: 171–7.
37. Zee DS, Fletcher W. Examination of the patient with vertigo. In: Baloh RW, Halmagyi GM, eds. *Disorders of the Vestibular System*. New York: Oxford University Press, 1996: 178–90.
38. Strupp M, Arbusow V. Acute vestibulopathy. *Curr Opin Neurol* 2001; **14**: 11–20.
39. Strupp M, Brandt T. Vestibular neuritis. *Adv Otorhinolaryngol* 1999; **55**: 111–36.
40. Zee DS. Ophthalmoscopy in examination of patients with vestibular disorders. *Ann Neurol* 1978; **3**: 373–4.
41. Halmagyi GM, Curthoys IS. A clinical sign of canal paresis. *Arch Neurol* 1988; **45**: 737–9.
42. Halmagyi GM, Gresty MA, Gibson WPR. Ocular tilt reaction due to peripheral vestibular lesion. *Ann Neurol* 1979; **5**: 80–3.
43. Riordan-Eva P, Harcourt JP, Faldon M, Brookes GB, Gresty MA. Skew deviation following vestibular nerve surgery. *Ann Neurol* 1997; **41**: 94–9.
44. Safran AB, Vibert D, Issoua D, Häusler R. Skew deviation following vestibular neuritis. *Am J Opthal* 1994; **118**: 238–45.
45. Vibert D, Häusler R, Safran AB, Koerner F. Ocular tilt reaction associated in sudden idiopathic unilateral peripheral cochleo-vestibular loss. *ORL* 1995; **57**: 310–15.
46. Vibert D, Häusler R, Safran AB, Koerner F. Diplopia from skew deviation in unilateral peripheral vestibular lesions. *Acta Otolaryngol* 1996; **116**: 170–6.
47. Friedmann G. The judgement of the visual vertical and horizontal with peripheral and central vestibular lesions. *Brain* 1970; **93**: 313–28.
48. Friedmann G. The influence of unilateral labyrinthectomy on orientation in space. *Acta Otolaryngol* 1971; **71**: 289–98.
49. Curthoys IS, Dai MJ, Halmagyi GM. Human torsional ocular position before and after unilateral vestibular neurectomy. *Exp Brain Res* 1991; **85**: 218–25.
50. Böhmer A, Richenmann J. The subjective visual vertical as a clinical parameter of vestibular function in peripheral vestibular disease. *J Vestib Res* 1995; **5**: 35–45.
51. Tabak S, Collewijn H, Boumans LJJM. Deviation of the subjective vertical in long-standing unilateral vestibular loss. *Acta Otolaryngol (Stockh)* 1997; **117**: 1–6.
52. Tribukait A, Bergenius J, Brantberg K. Subjective visual horizontal during follow-up after unilateral vestibular deafferentation with gentamicin. *Acta Otolaryngol (Stockh)* 1998; **118**: 479–87.
53. Vibert D, Häusler R, Safran AB. Subjective visual vertical in unilateral peripheral vestibular diseases. *J Vestib Res* 1999; **9**: 145–52.
54. Vibert D, Hausler R. Long-term evolution of subjective visual vertical after vestibular neurectomy and labyrinthectomy. *Acta Otolaryngol* 2000; **120**: 620–2.
55. Borel L, Harlay F, Magnan J, Lacour M. How changes in vestibular and visual reference frames combine to modify body orientation in space. *NeuroReport* 2001; **12**: 3137–41.
56. Betts GA, Curthoys IS. Visually perceived vertical and visually perceived horizontal are not orthogonal. *Vision Res* 1998; **38**: 1989–99.
57. Dieterich M, Brandt T. Ocular torsion and tilt of the subjective visual vertical are sensitive brainstem signs. *Ann Neurol* 1993; **33**: 292–9.
58. Flohr H, Bienhold H, Abeln W, Macskovics I. Concepts of vestibular compensation. In: Flohr H, Precht W, eds. *Lesion-induced Neuronal Plasticity in Sensorimotor Systems*. Berlin: Springer-Verlag, 1981: 153–72.
59. Strupp M, Arbusow V, Maag KP, Gall C, Brandt T. Vestibular exercises improve central vestibulospinal compensation after vestibular neuritis. *Neurology* 1998; **51**: 838–44.
60. Bergenius J, Perols O. Vestibular neuritis: a follow-up study. *Acta Otolaryngol* 1999; **119**: 895–9.
61. Okinaka Y, Sekitani T, Okazaki H, Miura M, Tahara T. Progress of caloric response of vestibular neuritis. *Acta Otolaryngol Suppl (Stockh)* 1993; **503**: 18–22.
62. Herzog N, Allum JH, Probst R. Follow-up of caloric test response after acute peripheral vestibular dysfunction. *HNO* 1997; **45**: 123–7 [in German].
63. Schmid-Priscoveanu A, Bohmer A, Obzina H, Straumann D. Caloric and search-coil head-impulse testing in patients after vestibular neuritis. *J Assoc Res Otolaryngol* 2001; **2**: 72–8.
64. Schuknecht HF, Witt RL. Acute bilateral sequential vestibular neuritis. *Am J Otolaryngol* 1985; **6**: 255–7.
65. Buchele W, Brandt T. Vestibular neuritis—horizontal semicircular canal paresis? *Adv Otorhinolaryngol* 1988; **42**: 157–61.
66. Murofushi T, Halmagyi GM, Yavor RA, Colebatch JG. Vestibular evoked myogenic potentials in vestibular neuritis: an indicator of inferior vestibular nerve involvement. *Arch Otolaryngol Head Neck Surg* 1996; **122**: 845–8.
67. Fetter M, Dichgans J. Vestibular neuritis spares the inferior division of the vestibular nerve. *Brain* 1996; **119**: 755–63.
68. Aw ST, Fetter M, Cremer PD, Karlberg M, Halmagyi GM. Individual semicircular canal function in superior and inferior vestibular neuritis. *Neurology* 2001; **57**: 768–74.
69. Arbusow V, Schulz P, Strupp M et al. Distribution of herpes simplex virus type 1 in human geniculate and vestibular ganglia: implications for vestibular neuritis. *Ann Neurol* 1999; **46**: 416–19.
70. Arbusow V, Theil D, Strupp M, Mascolo A, Brandt T. HSV-1 not only in human vestibular ganglia but also in the vestibular labyrinth. *Audiol Neurootol* 2001; **6**: 259–62.

71. Gacek RR, Gacek MR. The three faces of vestibular ganglionitis. *Ann Otol Rhinol Laryngol* 2002; **111**: 103–14.
72. Huang CY, Yu YL. Small cerebellar strokes may mimic labyrinthine lesions. *J Neurol Neurosurg Psychiatry* 1985; **48**: 263–5.
73. Norvving B, Magnusson M, Holtas S. Isolated vertigo in the elderly; vestibular or vascular disease? *Acta Neurol Scand* 1995; **91**: 43–8.
74. Iwase H, Kobayashi M, Kurata A, Inoue S. Clinically unidentified dissection of vertebral artery as a cause of cerebellar infarction. *Stroke* 2001; **32**: 1422–4.
75. Amarenco P. The spectrum of cerebellar infarctions. *Neurology* 1991; **41**: 973–9.
76. Kim JS, Lopez I, DiPatre PL, Liu F, Ishiyama A, Baloh RW. Internal auditory artery infarction. Clinicopathologic correlation. *Neurology* 1999; **52**: 40–4.
77. Ryan AF, Keithley EM, Harris JP. Autoimmune inner ear disorders. *Curr Opin Neurol* 2001; **14**: 35–40.
78. Helmchen C, Arbusow V, Jager L, Strupp M, Stocker W, Schulz P. Cogan's syndrome: clinical significance of antibodies against the inner ear and cornea. *Acta Otolaryngol* 1999; **119**: 528–36.
79. Bance M, Nai M, Tomlinson D, Rutka J. The changing direction of nystagmus in acute Menière's disease: pathophysiological implications, *Laryngoscope* 1991; **101**: 197–201.
80. Jacobson GP, Pearlstein R, Henderson J, Calder JH, Rock J. Recovery nystagmus revisited. *J Am Acad Audiol* 1998; **9**: 263–71.
81. Ishiyama G, Ishiyama A, Jacobson K, Baloh RW. Drop attacks in older patients secondary to an otologic cause. *Neurology* 2001; **57**: 1103–6.
82. Kentala E, Havia M, Pyykko I. Short-lasting drop attacks in Menière's disease. Otolaryngol Head Neck Surg. 2001; **124**: 526–30.
83. Schoonhoven R, Schmidt PH, Eggermont JJ. A longitudinal electrocochleographic study of a case of long-standing Lermoyez's syndrome. *Eur Arch Otorhinolaryngol* 1990; **247**: 333–9.
84. Young YJ, Wu CH. Electronystagmographic findings in a case of Lermoyez's syndrome. *Auris Nasus Larynx* 1994; **21**: 118–21.
85. Stahle J, Friberg U, Svedberg A. Long-term progression of Menière's disease. *Am J Otol* 1989; **10**: 170–3.
86. Green JD, Blum DJ, Harner SG. Longitudinal follow-up of patients with Menière's disease. *Otolaryngol Head Neck Surg* 1991; **104**: 783–8.
87. Conlon BJ, Gibson WP. Menière's disease: incidence in the contralateral asymptomatic ear. *Laryngoscope* 1999; **109**: 1800–2.
88. Committee on Hearing and Equilibrium. Guidelines for the diagnosis and evaluation of therapy in Menière's disease. *Otolaryngol Head Neck Surg* 1995; **113**: 181–5.
89. Sass K. Sensitivity and specificity of transtympanic electrocochleography in Menière's disease. *Acta Otolaryngol (Stockh)* 1998; **118**: 150–6.
90. Conlon BJ, Gibson WP. The electrocochleographic diagnosis of Menière's disease. *Acta Otolaryngol* 2000; **120**: 480–3.
91. Gamble BA, Meyerhoff WL, Shoup AG, Schwade ND. Salt-load electrocochleography. *Am J Otol* 1999; **20**: 325–30.
92. Proctor LR. Results of serial vestibular testing in unilateral Menière's disease. *Am J Otol* 2000; **21**: 552–8.
93. Santos PM, Hall RA, Snyder JM, Hughes LF, Dobie RA. Diuretic and diet effects on Menière's disease evaluated by the 1985 Committee on Hearing and Equilibrium guidelines. *Otolaryngol Head Neck Surg* 1993; **109**: 680–9.
94. Barbara M, Consagra C, Monini S, Nostro G, Harguindey A, Vestri A, Filipo R. Local pressure protocol, including meniett, in the treatment of Menière's disease: short-term results during the active stage. *Acta Otolaryngol* 2001; **121**: 939–44.
95. Pensak ML, Friedman RA. The role of endolymphatic shunt surgery in the managed care ear. *Am J Otol* 1998; **19**: 337–40.
96. Thomsen J, Bonding P, Becker B, Stage J, Tos M. The non-specific effect of endolymphatic sac surgery in treatment of Menière's disease: a prospective, randomized controlled study comparing the 'classic' endolymphatic sac surgery with the insertion of a ventilating tube in the tympanic membrane. *Acta Otolaryngol* 1998; **118**: 769–73.
97. Murofushi T, Halmagyi GM, Yavor RA. Intratympanic gentamicin in Menière's disease: results of therapy. *Am J Otol* 1997; **18**: 52–7.
98. Minor LB. Intratympanic gentamicin for control of vertigo in Menière's disease: vestibular signs that specify completion of therapy. *Am J Otol* 1999; **20**: 209–19.
99. Kaplan DM, Nedzelski JM, Al-Abidi A, Chen JM, Shipp DB. Hearing loss following intratypanic instillation of gentamicin for the treatment fo unilateral Menière's disease. *J Otolaryngol* 2002; **31**: 106–11.
100. Eklund S, Pyykko I, Aalto H, Ishikazi H, Vasama JP. Effect of intratympanic gentamicin on hearing and tinnitus in Menière's disease. *Am J Otol* 1999; **20**: 350–6.
101. Balyan FR, Taibah A, De Donato G et al. Titration streptomycin therapy in Menière's disease: long-term results. *Otolaryngol Head Neck Surg* 1998; **118**: 261–6.
102. Sauer G, Richter CP, Klinke R. Sodium, potassium, chloride and calcium concentrations measured in pigeon perilymph and endolymph. *Hear Res* 1999; **129**: 1–6.
103. Salt AN, Thalmann R. Interpretation of endolymph flow results. *Hear Res* 1988; **33**: 279–81.
104. Gibson WPR, Arenberg IK. Pathophysiologic theories in the etiology of Menière's disease. *Otolaryngol Clin North Am* 1997; **30**: 961–8.
105. Schuknecht H, Suzuka Y, Zimmermann C. Delayed endolymphatic hydrops and its relationship to Menière's disease. *Ann Otol Rhinol Laryngol* 1990; **99**: 843–53.
106. Harcourt JP, Brookes GB. Delayed endolymphatic hydrops: clinical manifestations and treatment outcome. *Clin Otolaryngol* 1995; **20**: 318–22.
107. Harris JP, Aframian D. Role of autoimmunity in contralateral delayed endolymphatic hydrops. *Am J Otol* 1994; **15**: 710–16.
108. Schulz P, Arbusow V, Strupp M, Dieterich M, Sautier W, Brandt T. Sympathetic contralateral vestibulopathy after unilateral zoster oticus. *J Neurol Neurosurg Psychiatry* 1999; **66**: 672–6.
109. Atlas MD, Chai F, Boscato L. Menière's disease: evidence of an immune process. *Am J Otol* 1998; **19**: 628–31.
110. Friedland DR, Wackym P. A critical appraisal of spontaneous perilymphatic fistulas of the inner ear. *Am J Otol* 1999; **20**: 261–76.

111. Baloh RW, Neurotology of migraine. *Headache* 1997; **37**: 615–21.
112. Savundra PA, Carroll JD, Davies, Luxon LM. Migraine-associated vertigo. *Cephalalgia* 1997; **17**: 505–10.
113. Bickerstaff E. Basilar artery migraine. *Lancet* 1961; **1**: 15–17.
114. Thakar A, Anjaneyulu C, Deka RC. Vertigo syndromes and mechanisms in migraine. *J Laryngol Otol* 2001; **115**: 782–87.
115. Neuhauser H, Leopold M, von Brevern M, Arnold G, Lempert T. The interrelations of migraine, vertigo, and migrainous vertigo. *Neurology*. 2001; **56**: 436–41.
116. Bikhazi P, Jackson C, Ruckenstein MJ. Efficacy of antimigrainous therapy in the treatment of migraine-associated dizziness. *Am J Otol* 1997; **18**: 350–4.
117. Johnson GD. Medical management of migraine-related dizziness and vertigo. *Laryngoscope* 1998; **108**: 1–28.
118. Reploeg MD, Goebel JA. Migraine-associated Dizziness: Patient Characteristics and Management Options. *Otol Neurotol* 2002; **23**: 364–71.
119. Levy D. Transient CNS deficits: a common benign syndrome in young adults. *Neurology* 1988; **38**: 831–6.
120. Kayan A, Hood JD. Neuro-otological manifestations of migraine. *Brain* 1984; **107**: 1123–42.
121. Viiree ES, Baloh RW. Migraine as a cause of sudden hearing loss. *Headache* 1996; **36**: 24–8.
122. Kim JS, Yue Q, Jen JC, Nelson SF, Baloh RW. Familial migraine with vertigo: no mutations found in CACNAA1A. *Am J Med Genet* 1998; **79**: 148–51.
123. Ishiyama A, Jacobson KM, Baloh RW. Migraine and benign positional vertigo. *Ann Otol Rhinol Laryngol* 2000; **109**: 377–80.
124. Lanska DJ, Remler B. Benign paroxysmal positioning vertigo: classic descriptions, origins of the provocative technique and conceptual developments. *Neurology* 1997; **48**: 1167–77.
125. Furman JM, Cass SP. Benign paroxysmal positional vertigo. *N Engl J Med* 1999; **341**: 1590–6.
126. Zucca G, Valli S, Valli P, Perin P, Mira E. Why do benign paroxysmal vertigo episodes recover spontaneously? *J Vestib Res* 1998; **8**: 325–9.
127. Karlberg M, Hall K, Quickert N, Hinson J, Halmagyi GM. What inner ear diseases cause benign paroxysmal positioninal vertigo? *Acta Otolaryngol* 2000; **120**: 380–5.
128. Büttner U, Helmchen C, Brandt T. Diagnostic criteria for central versus peripheral positioning nystagmus and vertigo: a review. *Acta Otolaryngol (Stockh)* 1999; **119**: 1–5.
129. Epley J. The canalith respositioning procedure for treatment of BPPV. *Otolaryngol Head Neck Surg* 1992; **107**: 399–404.
130. Epley JM. Human experience with canalith repositioning maneuvers. *Ann N Y Acad Sci* 2001; **942**: 179–91.
131. Semont A, Freyss G, Vitte E. Curing BPPV with a liberatory maneuver. *Adv Otorhinolaryngol* 1988; **42**: 290–3.
132. Ruckenstein MJ. Therapeutic efficacy of the Epley canalith repositioning maneuver. *Laryngoscope* 2001; **111**: 940–5.
133. Wolf JS, Boyev KP, Manokey BJ, Mattox DE. Success of the modified Epley maneuver in treating benign paroxysmal positional vertigo. *Laryngoscope* 1999; **109**: 900–3.
134. Radtke A, Neuhauser H, von Brevern M, Lempert T. A modified Epley's procedure for self-treatment of benign paroxysmal positional vertigo. *Neurology* 1999; **53**: 1358–60.
135. Pohl DV. Surgical treatment of benign positional vertigo. In: Baloh RW, Halmagyi GM, eds. *Disorders of the Vestibular System*. New York: Oxford University Press, 1996: 563–74.
136. Walsh RM, Bath AP, Cullen JR, Rutka JA. Long-term results of posterior semicircular canal occlusion for intractable benign paroxysmal positioning vertigo. *Clin Otolaryngol* 1999; **24**: 316–23.
137. Steddin S, Brandt T. Unilateral mimicking bilateral benign paroxysmal positioning vertigo. *Arch Otolaryngol Head Neck Surg* 1994; **120**: 1339–41.
138. Baloh RW, Jacobson K, Honrubia V. Horizontal semicircular canal variant of benign positional vertigo. *Neurology* 1993; **43**: 2542–9.
139. Bisdorff AR, Debatisse D. Localizing signs in positional vertigo due to lateral canal cupulolithiasis. *Neurology* 2001; **57**: 1085–8.
140. Nuti D, Agus G, Barbieri M-T, Passali D. The management of horizontal canal paroxysmal positional vertigo. *Acta Otolaryngol (Stockh)* 1998; **118**: 455–60.
141. Fife T. Recognition and management of horizontal canal benign positional vertigo. *Am J Otol* 1998; **19**: 345–51.
142. Brandt T. Bilateral vestibulopathy revisited. *Eur J Med Res* 1996; **24**: 361–8.
143. Rinne T, Bronstein AM, Rudge P, Gresty MA, Luxon LM. Bilateral loss of vestibular function: clinical findings in 53 patients. *J Neurol* 1998; **245**: 314–21.
144. Halmagyi GM, Fattore CM, Curthoys IS, Wade S. Gentamicin vestibulotoxicity. *Otolaryngol Head Neck Surg* 1994; **111**: 571–4.
145. Migliaccio A, Halmagyi GM, Cremer PD, McGarvie LA, Minor LB. Clinical signs of visual-vestibulo-ocular reflex impairment (submitted).
146. Morrison GA, Sterkers JM. Unusual presentations of acoustic tumor. *Clin Otolaryngol* 1996; **21**: 80–3.
147. Ryu H, Yamamoto S, Sugiyama K, Nishizawa S, Nozue M. Neurovascular compression syndromes of the eighth cranial nerve. Can the site of compression explain the symptoms? *Acta Neurochir (Wien)* 1999; **141**: 495–501.
148. Bergsneider M, Becker DP. Vascular compression syndrome of the vestibular nerve: a critical analysis. *Otolaryngol Head Neck Surg* 1995; **112**: 118–24.
149. Brandt TH, Dieterich M. Vestibular paroxysmia: vascular compression of the eighth nerve? *Lancet* 1994; **343**: 798–9.
150. Oas JG, Baloh RW. Vertigo and the anterior inferior cerebellar artery syndrome. *Neurology* 1992; **42**: 2274–9.

49 Neurological causes of balance disorders

Thomas Brandt

Clinical studies of the differential effects of lesions of the central vestibular pathways have increasingly shown that vestibular syndromes are accurate indicators for a topographic diagnosis.[1,2] These pathways run from the eighth nerve and the vestibular nuclei through ascending fibres, such as the ipsilateral or contralateral medial longitudinal fasciculus (MLF), the brachium conjunctivum, or the ventral tegmental tract to the oculomotor nuclei, the supranuclear integration centres in the rostral midbrain, and the vestibular thalamic subnuclei. From there they reach several cortex areas through the thalamic projection. Another relevant ascending projection reaches the cortex from the vestibular nuclei via vestibular cerebellum structures, in particular the fastigial nucleus.

In the majority of cases, central vestibular syndromes are caused by dysfunction or a deficit of sensory input induced by a lesion. In a small proportion of cases, they are due to pathological excitation of various structures, extending from the peripheral vestibular organ to the vestibular cortex. Since peripheral vestibular disorders are always characterized by a combination of perceptual, ocular motor and postural signs and symptoms, central vestibular disorders may manifest as 'a complete syndrome' or with only single components. The ocular motor aspect, for example, predominates in the syndromes of upbeat or downbeat nystagmus. Lateral falls may occur without vertigo in vestibular thalamic lesions (thalamic astasia) or as lateropulsion in Wallenberg's syndrome.

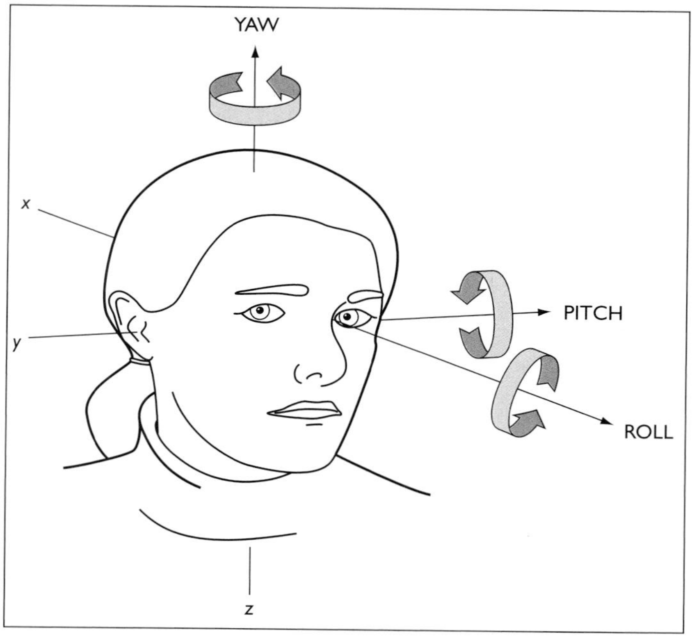

Figure 49.1 Schematic representation of the three major planes of action of the vestibulo-ocular reflex. Horizontal rotation about the vertical *z* axis = yaw; vertical rotation about the binaural *y* axis = pitch; vertical rotation about the *x* axis ('line of sight') = roll.

Clinical classification of central vestibular disorders

The 'elementary' neuronal network of the vestibular system is the di- or trisynaptic vestibulo-ocular reflex (VOR). VOR properties are routinely tested in all patients who complain of dizziness[3] and form part of the examination of the unconscious patient. There is evidence for a useful clinical classification of central vestibular syndromes according to the three major planes of action of the VOR (Figure 49. 1): yaw, roll, and pitch.[4,5]

> The plane-specific vestibular syndromes are determined by ocular motor, postural, and perceptual signs (Figure 49.2):
>
> - Roll plane signs are torsional nystagmus, skew deviation, ocular torsion, tilts of head, body, and perceived vertical, and the ocular tilt reaction.
> - Pitch plane signs are upbeat/downbeat nystagmus, forward/ backward tilts and falls, and vertical deviation of perceived straight-ahead.
> - Yaw plane signs are horizontal nystagmus, past pointing, rotational and lateral body falls, deviation of perceived straight-ahead.

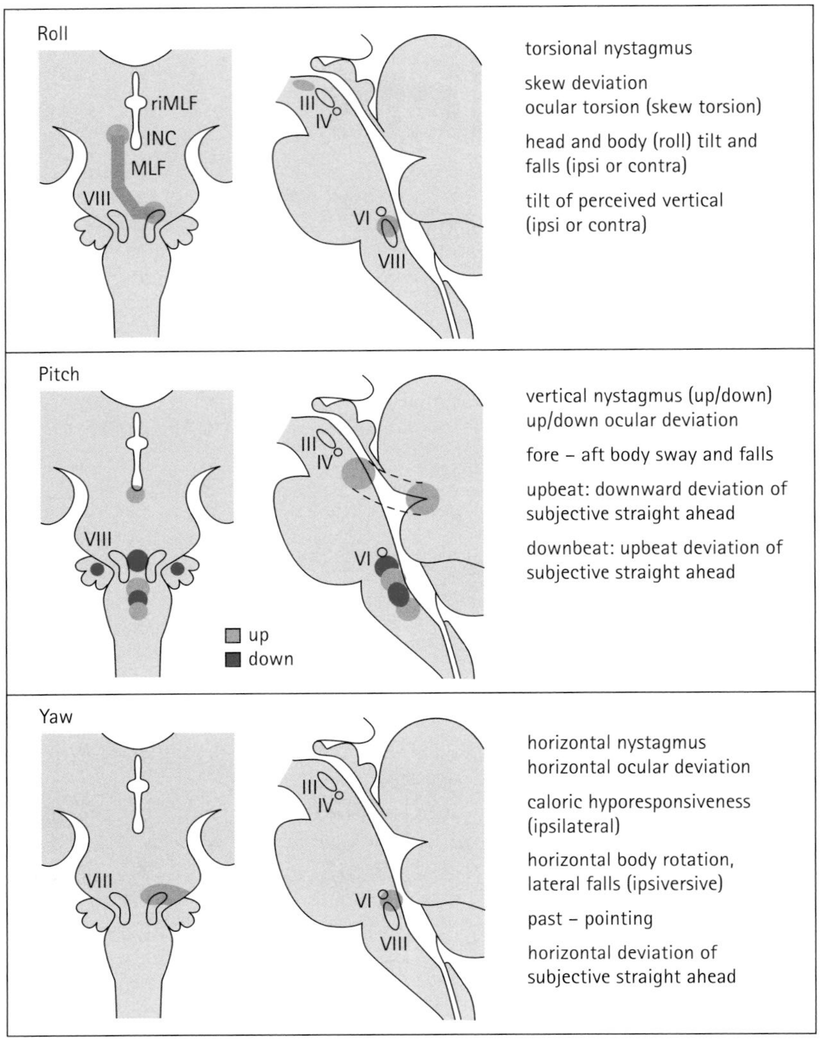

Figure 49.2 Topographic diagnosis of vestibular syndromes in roll, pitch and yaw planes: schematic presentation of the distinct areas within the brainstem and vestibulocerebellum (frontal and sagittal views) in which a lesion induces a vestibulo-ocular tone imbalance in the roll, pitch or yaw plane. Typical ocular motor, postural and perceptual signs are torsional, vertical (up/downbeat) or horizontal nystagmus. A tone imbalance in roll indicates unilateral 'graviceptive' pathway lesions from the medial or superior vestibular nuclei (inducing ipsiversive signs), crossing midline to the contralateral MLF and the rostral integration centres for vertical and torsional eye movements, the INC and riMLF (inducing contraversive signs). A tone imbalance in pitch indicates paramedian bilateral brainstem lesions at the pontomesencephalic or pontomedullary level, the brachium conjunctivum, or the flocculi. It is striking that pontomedullary lesions may induce either upbeat or downbeat nystagmus or transitions between the two, whereas binocular flocculus lesions result only in downbeat nystagmus and a pontomesencephalic lesion only in upbeat nystagmus. A tone imbalance in yaw indicates a unilateral pontomedullary lesion involving the medial and superior vestibular nucleus. This area overlaps with the roll and pitch function of the VOR, which explains the frequency of mixed vestibular syndromes in more than one plane. riMLF, rostral interstitial nucleus of the medial longitudinal fasciculus; INC, interstitial nucleus of Cajal; III, oculomotor nucleus; IV, trochlear nucleus; VI, abducens nucleus; VIII, vestibular nucleus. (Adapted from Brandt. *Neuroopthamology* 1995; **15**: 291–303.[5])

The thus defined VOR syndromes allow for a precise topographic diagnosis of brainstem lesions with regard to their level and side (Figure 49.3).

- A tone imbalance in roll indicates unilateral lesions (ipsiversive at pontomedullary level, contraversive at pontomesencephalic level).
- A tone imbalance in pitch indicates bilateral (paramedian) lesions or bilateral dysfunction of the flocculus.
- A tone imbalance in yaw indicates lesions of the lateral medulla, including the root entry zone of the eighth nerve and/or the vestibular nuclei.

It is hypothesized that signal processing of the VOR in roll and pitch is conveyed by the same rather than separate ascending pathways in the medial longitudinal fasciculus and the brachium conjunctivum. A unilateral lesion (or stimulation) of these 'graviceptive' pathways (which transduce input from vertical semicircular canals and otoliths) affects function in roll, whereas bilateral lesions (or stimulation) affect function in pitch (Figure 49.3). Thus, the vestibular system is able to change its functional plane of action from roll to pitch by switching from a unilateral to a bilateral mode of operation.[5] Pure syndromes in yaw are rare, since the small causative area covering the medial and superior vestibular nucleus is not only adjacent to but overlapped by the structures also subserving roll and pitch function (Figure 49.3). A lesion frequently results in mixed (e.g. torsional and horizontal) nystagmus. The lesional sites of yaw syndromes are restricted to the pontomedullary level because of the short distance between the vestibular nuclei and the integration centre for horizontal eye movements in the paramedian pontine reticular formation. Syndromes in roll and pitch, however, may arise from brainstem lesions located in an area extending from the medulla to the mesencephalon, an area corresponding to the large distance between the vestibular nuclei and the integration centres for vertical and torsional eye movements in the rostral midbrain. Whereas vestibular tone imbalances in pitch — which involve bilateral pathways — may occur with various intoxications or metabolic disorders, this is an unusual aetiology for tone imbalances in yaw or roll which involve vestibular pathways unilaterally.

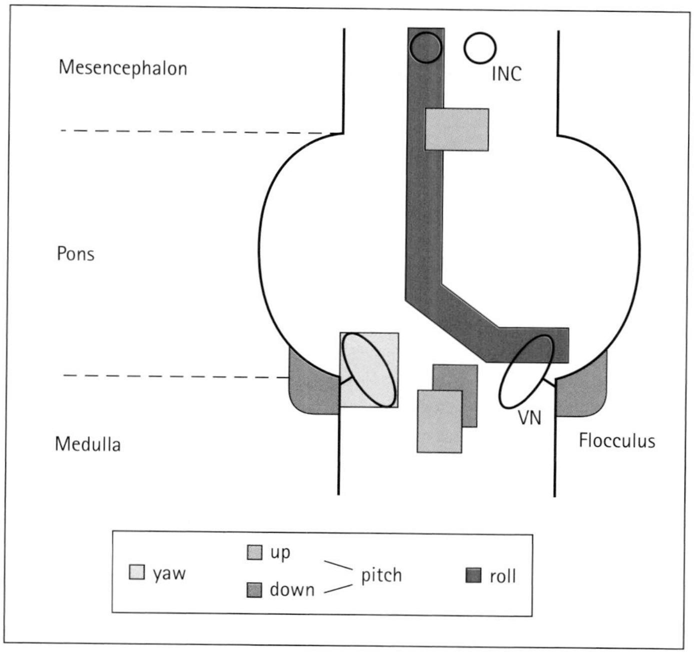

Figure 49.3 Vestibular syndromes in roll, pitch and yaw planes: critical areas are schematically represented based on our current knowledge of vestibular and ocular motor structures and pathways, a lesion of which causes a vestibular tone imbalance in one of the three major planes of action. The mere clinical sign of a vertical, torsional or horizontal nystagmus—if central-vestibular—allows a topographic diagnosis of the lesion, although the particular vestibular structures involved are still under discussion. Whereas a vestibular tone imbalance in the roll plane indicates unilateral brainstem lesions (a crossing in the pons), vertical nystagmus indicates bilateral lesions. Two separate causative loci are known for upbeat nystagmus: medullary or pontomesencephalic. Downbeat nystagmus indicates a bilateral paramedian lesion of the commissural fibres between the vestibular nuclei or a bilateral flocculus lesion. Horizontal nystagmus indicates unilateral pontomedullary lesions involving the vestibular nuclei. The differentiation of vestibular ocular motor signs according to the three major planes of action of the VOR and their mapping to distinct and separate areas in the brainstem are helpful for topographic diagnosis and for avoiding incorrect assignment of clinical signs to brainstem lesions identified with imaging techniques. INC, interstitial nucleus of Cajal; MLF, medial longitudinal fasciculus; VN, vestibular nucleus. (Adapted from Brandt. *Ann Neurol* 1994; **36**: 337–47.[4])

Some vestibular disorders are characterized by a simultaneously peripheral and central vestibular involvement. Examples are large acoustical neurinomas, infarctions of the anterior inferior cerebellar artery, head trauma, and syndromes induced by alcohol intoxication. Others may affect the vestibular nerve root in the brainstem, where the transition between the peripheral and central nervous system has been defined as the Redlich–Oberstein zone (lacunar infarction, focal demyelination in MS).

Cortical vestibular syndromes include vestibular excitation (vestibular epilepsy) and dysfunction due to a lesion, which may manifest with tilt of the perceived vertical, contraversive lateropulsion, and, rarely, rotational vertigo. There is no primary vestibular cortex, but cortical vestibular function is imbedded in a network of multisensory visual–vestibular–somatosensory functions and distributed over several separate and distinct areas in the temporoparietal region. The parieto-insular vestibular cortex[6] seems to act as a kind of main integration centre. Dysfunction of this multisensory and sensorimotor cortex for spatial orientation and self-motion perception may be involved in spatial hemineglect and rare paroxysmal room-tilt illusions.

Most central vertigo syndromes have a specific locus (Table 49.1) but not a specific aetiology. The aetiology may, for example, be vascular, inflammatory, neoplastic, toxic, or traumatic.

Vestibular falls

The following conditions may give rise to *symptomatic falls*: cardiovascular cerebral hypoxia, epilepsy, intoxication, ataxia, movement disorders, paresis, or severe sensory loss. Vestibular dysfunction is, however, a significant differential diagnosis for patients presenting with *unpreventable or unexpected falls*.

Both peripheral and central vestibular disorders cause postural instability with preferred directions of falling. The particular pathological mechanisms that provoke postural instability and cause vestibular falls differ considerably, because they may result from changes in otolith or in horizontal or vertical semicircular canal function.

Vestibular falls may be attributed to either the particular plane of the affected semicircular canal or a central pathway that mediates the three-dimensional VOR in yaw, pitch, and roll. Ipsiversive falls occur in vestibular neuritis or in Wallenberg's syndrome — where they are known as lateropulsion. Contraversive falls are typical for the otolith Tullio phenomenon, vestibular epilepsy, and thalamic astasia. Fore–aft instability is predominantly observed in bilateral vestibulopathy, benign paroxysmal positioning vertigo, and downbeat or upbeat nystagmus syndrome. Falls can be diagonally forward (or backward) and toward or away from the side of the lesion, depending on the site of the lesion (the ocular tilt reaction is ipsiversive in peripheral vestibular and medullary lesions, but contraversive in mesencephalic lesions) and on whether vestibular structures are excited or inhibited.

Peripheral vestibular falls (Table 49.2)

Vestibular neuritis: contraversive rotational vertigo with ipsiversive falls

In vestibular neuritis — due to a vestibular tone imbalance — the fast phase of the spontaneous rotational nystagmus and the initial perception of apparent body motion are

Table 49.1 Central vestibular syndromes.

Site	Syndrome	Mechanism/Aetiology
Vestibular cortex (multisensory)	Vestibular epilepsy	Vestibular seizures are auras (simple or complex partial multisensory seizures)
	Volvular epilepsy	Sensorimotor 'vestibular' rotatory seizures with walking in small circles
	Non-epileptic cortical vertigo	Rare rotatory vertigo in acute lesions of the parieto-insular vestibular cortex
	Spatial hemineglect (contraversive)	Multisensory horizontal deviation of spatial attention with (non-dominant) parietal or frontal cortex lesions
	Transient room-tilt illusions	Paroxysmal or transient mismatch of visual- and vestibular three-dimensional spatial coordinate maps in vestibular brainstem, parietal, or frontal cortex lesions
	Tilt of perceived vertical with body lateropulsion (mostly contraversive)	Vestibular tone imbalance in roll with acute lesions of the parieto-insular vestibular cortex
Thalamus	Thalamic astasia	Dorsolateral vestibular thalamic lesions
	Tilt of perceived vertical (ipsiversive or contraversive) with body lateropulsion	Vestibular tone imbalance in roll
Mesodiencephalic brainstem	Ocular tilt reaction (OTR) (contraversive; ipsiversive if paroxysmal)	Vestibular tone imbalance in roll (integrator-OTR with lesions of the interstitial nucleus of Cajal (INC))
	Torsional nystagmus (ipsiversive or contraversive)	Ipsiversive in INC lesions Contraversive in riMLF lesions
Mesencephalic brainstem	Skew deviation with ocular torsion, i.e. skew torsion (contraversive)	Vestibular tone imbalance in roll with MLF lesions
	Upbeat nystagmus	Vestibular tone imbalance in pitch in bilateral brachium conjunctivum lesions
Pontomedullary brainstem	Tilt of perceived vertical lateropulsion, ocular tilt reaction	Vestibular tone imbalance in roll with medial and/or superior vestibular nuclei lesions
	Pseudo 'vestibular neuritis'	Lacunar infarction or MS plaque at the root entry zone of the eighth nerve
	Downbeat nystagmus	Vestibular tone imbalance in pitch
	Transient room-tilt illusion	Acute severe vestibular tone imbalance in roll or pitch
	Paroxysmal room-tilt illusion in MS*	Transversally spreading ephaptic axonal activity
	Paroxysmal dysarthria/ataxia in MS	Transversally spreading ephaptic axonal activation
	Paroxysmal vertigo evoked by lateral gaze	Vestibular nuclei lesion
Medulla	Upbeat nystagmus	Vestibular tone imbalance in pitch (nucleus prepositus hypoglossi)
Vestibular cerebellum	Downbeat nystagmus	Vestibular tone imbalance in pitch caused by bilateral flocculus lesions (disinhibition)
	Positional downbeat nystagmus	Disinhibited otolith-canal interaction in nodulus lesions
	Familial episodic ataxia (EA1 with Myokymia and EA2 with vertigo)	EA1 = autosomally dominant inherited potassium channelopathy EA2 = autosomally dominant inherited calcium channelopathy
	Encephalitis with predominant vertigo	Viral infection of cerebellum
	Epidemic vertigo	Viral infection of cerebellum

*MS, multiple sclerosis.

directed away from the side of the lesion, and the postural reactions initiated by vestibulospinal reflexes are usually in a direction opposite to the direction of apparent body motion. These result both in the Romberg fall and in pastpointing toward the side of the lesion. There are two sensations, opposite in direction, and the patient may be describing either one (Figure 49.4). The first is the purely subjective sense of self-motion in the direction of the nystagmus fast phases, which is not associated with any measurable body sway. The second is the compensatory vestibulospinal reaction resulting in objective, measurable destabilization in the direction opposite to the fast phases.[7]

Benign paroxysmal positioning vertigo (BPPV): forward falls produced by canalolithiasis of the posterior semicircular canal

Posturographic measurements in patients with BPPV, in whom attacks were elicited by head tilt while standing on a force-measuring platform, reveal a characteristic pattern of postural instability. After a short latency, patients exhibit large sway amplitudes, predominantly in the fore–aft direction, with a mean sway frequency range <3 Hz. Instability decreases over 10–30 s parallel to the reduction of nystagmus and the sensation of vertigo.[8] When subjects close their eyes, the acute destabilization may lead to an almost irresistible tendency to fall. Posturographic data show a shift of the mean position of the centre of gravity forward and toward the direction of the head tilt. The measurable shift of the centre of gravity in the forward direction and ipsiversive to the tilted head can be interpreted as the motor compensation for the initial subjective vertigo in the opposite direction, the diagonal plane corresponding to the spatial plane and working range of the ipsilateral posterior canal.

Menière's drop attacks (Tumarkin's otolithic crisis)

In Menière's disease, periodic endolymphatic membrane ruptures with subsequent transient potassium excitation and palsy of vestibular nerve fibres cause vertigo attacks and postural

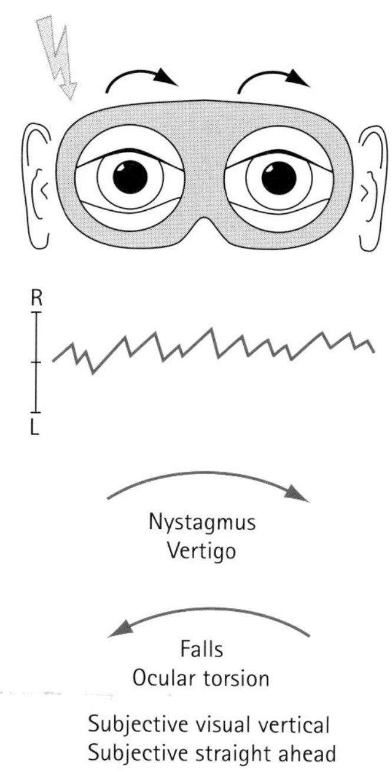

Figure 49.4 Ocular signs, perception and posture in the acute stage of right-sided vestibular neuritis. Spontaneous vestibular nystagmus is always horizontal-rotatory away from the side of the lesion (best observed with Frenzel's glasses). The initial perception of apparent body motion (vertigo) is also directed away from the side of the lesion, whereas measurable ocular torsion and body destabilization (Romberg fall) are always toward the side of the lesion. The latter are the compensatory vestibulo-ocular and vestibulospinal reactions to the apparent tilt. The same is true for adjustments of perceived vertical and subjective straight-ahead.

Table 49.2 Peripheral vestibular falls.

Disorder	Direction	Mechanism
Vestibular neuritis	Lateral ipsiversive	Vestibular tone imbalance (yaw, roll) due to horizontal and anterior semicircular canal paresis and paresis of utricle
Benign paroxysmal positioning vertigo (BPPV)	Forward ipsiversive	Ampullofugal stimulation of posterior canal by canalolithiasis and a heavy clot-induced endolymph flow
Menière's drop attacks (Tumarkin's otolithic crisis)	Vertical	Loss of postural tone due to abnormal otolith stimulation in sudden endolymphatic fluid pressure changes
Otolith Tullio phenomenon	Backward contraversive	Sound-induced mechanical stimulation of utricle by luxated stapes footplate (diagonal)
Vestibular paroxysmia	Forward contraversive	Neurovascular cross compression causing ephaptic stimulation of vestibular nerve (multidirectional)
Bilateral vestibulopathy	Multidirectional fore–aft	Impaired postural reflexes, particularly in darkness

instability with characteristics similar to those in vestibular neuritis. The direction of nystagmus and vertigo changes during the attack and also depends on the location of the membranous leakage in relation to either the posterior or horizontal ampullary nerve.

Rarely, vestibular drop attacks (Tumarkin's otolithic crisis,[9]) occur in early and late stages of endolymphatic hydrops,[10] when sudden changes in endolymphatic fluid pressure cause non-physiological end-organ stimulation (deformation of utricle or saccule membrane?) with a reflex-like vestibulospinal loss of postural tone.

Patients fall without warning; they remain conscious but lose voluntary control of balance. Sometimes during a vestibular drop attack patients have the feeling that they are being pushed or thrown to the ground. However, slower sensations involving apparent tilts of the surroundings also occur, possibly resulting in forward, backward or lateral body tilt.

Otolith Tullio phenomenon: contraversive ocular tilt reaction (OTR) and fall

Sound-induced vestibular symptoms such as vertigo, nystagmus, oscillopsia and postural imbalance in patients with perilymph fistulas are commonly known as the Tullio phenomenon.[11]

An otolith Tullio phenomenon due to a hypermobile stapes footplate typically manifests with the pattern of sound-induced paroxysms of OTR.[12] The patients complain of distressing attacks of vertical oblique and rotatory oscillopsia (apparent tilt of the visual scene) and of falls toward the unaffected ear and backward which are elicited by loud sounds (Figure 49.5).[13] The cause is a non-physiological mechanical stimulation of the otolith. Surgical exploration of the middle ear may reveal a subluxated stapes footplate with a hypertrophic stapedius muscle causing pathologically large-amplitude movements during the stapedius reflex. The otolith lies adjacent to the stapes footplate.

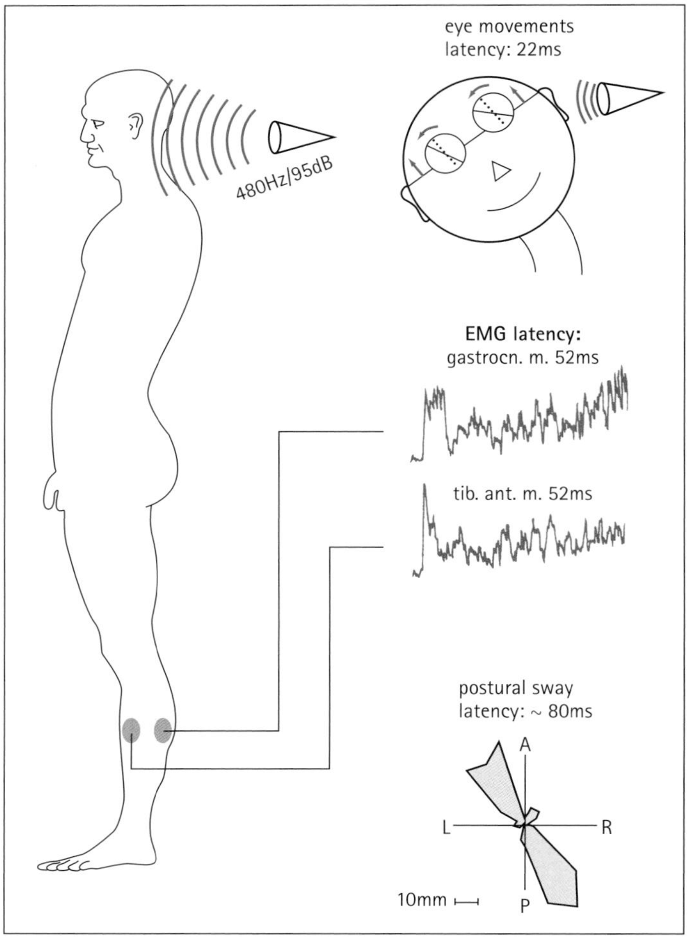

Figure 49.5 An otolith Tullio phenomenon (left) is characterized by a sound-induced ocular tilt reaction (skew deviation with ipsilateral over contralateral hypertropia), ocular torsion counterclockwise, head tilt with ipsilateral ear up (top), and increased body sway predominantly from right–backward to left–forward (bottom). Latencies of dysconjugated eye movements were 22 ms for the left eye; latencies for the vestibulospinal reflex at upright stance were 47 ms in the left tibialis anterior muscle and 52 ms in the left gastrocnemius muscle (centre). Measurable postural sway had a minimal latency of about 80 ms (bottom). (Adapted from Brandt et al. *Adv Otorhinolaryngol* 1988; **42**: 153–6.[13])

Bilateral vestibulopathy with predominant forward and backward falls

Bilateral loss of vestibular function causes unsteadiness of gait, particularly in the dark, and — because of the insufficiency of the VOR at higher frequencies — oscillopsia, associated with head movements or when walking.

These patients complain of oscillopsia and imbalance, and the condition can be identified by the decreased ocular motor responses to caloric irrigation and angular acceleration.[14] Measurements of postural instability show the largest amplitude in the fore–aft direction, corresponding to the predominant direction of fall. In cases of body perturbations, falls may also occur sideways, particularly in darkness when vision cannot compensate sufficiently for the vestibular deficit. The lack of one channel of sensory input — important as it is for demanding balancing tasks in sport — rarely manifests as clinically significant instability. In the absence of sensory information from two of the stabilizing systems, postural control may be severely impaired, as, for example, in a patient with sensory polyneuropathy and/or with bilateral vestibulopathy (Figure 49.6)[15] under restricted visual conditions (darkness).

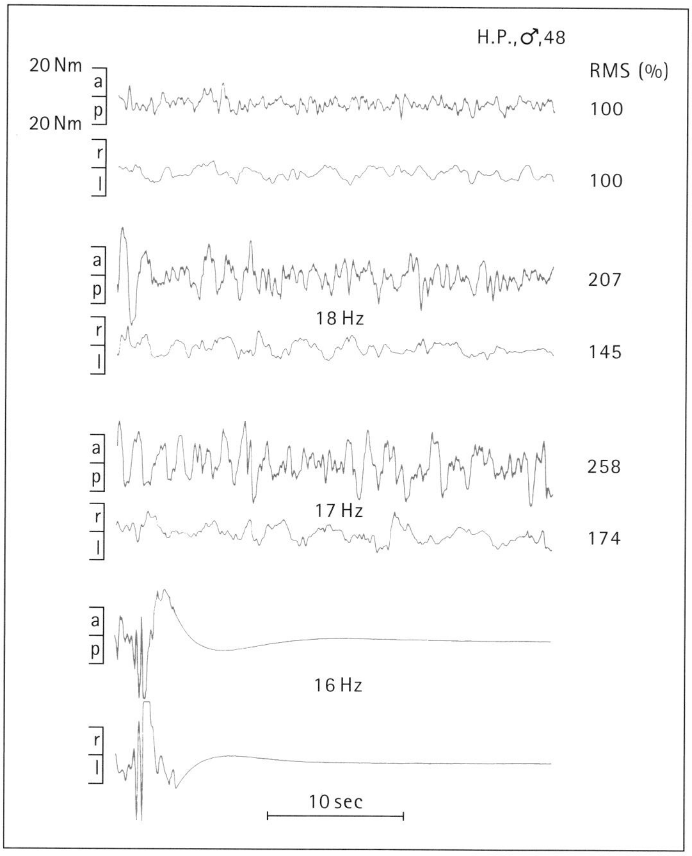

Figure 49.6 Postural imbalance in combined bilateral vestibular failure and sensory polyneuropathy. Original recordings of fore–aft and lateral body sway in a patient (48-year-old male) with almost complete loss of labyrinth function (due to gentamicin treatment) and lower-limb joint position sense (due to sensory polyneuropathy). In contrast to steady room illumination (top), body sway increases with decreasing flicker frequency under stroboscopic illumination. At 16 Hz, balance cannot be maintained even for seconds, as was the case with eyes closed (bottom). (Adapted from Paulus et al. *J Neurol Neurosurg Psychiatry* 1987; 50: 1542–5.[15])

Central vestibular falls

Vestibular epilepsy with contraversive vertigo and falls

From the few detailed reports on the direction of apparent self-motion and surround motion in patients with vestibular epilepsy, it is most likely that the direction of perceived self-motion, measurable body motion and eye deviation is contraversive to the epileptic focus, whereas simultaneously perceived surround motion may be ipsiversive.[16] Actual body movements do not represent vestibulospinal compensations of perceived vertigo but an epileptic response. Rotatory seizures in rare 'volvular epilepsy' are characterized by paroxysmal, repetitive walking in small circles. Vestibular seizures can manifest without any objective eye and body movements, as Foerster[16] described in his stimulation experiments.

Thalamic astasia with contraversive or ipsiversive falls?

There are a few instances of presumed central vestibular dysfunction in which patients without paresis or sensory or cerebellar deficits are unable to maintain an unsupported, upright posture. The conditions are thalamic astasia, lateropulsion in Wallenberg's syndrome, and OTR. Postural imbalance with a transient tendency to fall has been noted following therapeutic thalamotomy and thalamic haemorrhages.[17] Thalamic astasia, as described by Masdeu and Gorelick,[18] occurred as a result of lesions with different causes, all primarily involving superoposterolateral portions of the thalamus but sparing the rubral region. It is our own experience in some 30 patients with thalamic infarctions that the posterolateral type may cause both contraversive and ipsiversive postural instability.[19]

Ocular tilt reaction (OTR): ipsiversive in caudal, contraversive in upper brainstem lesions

OTR is a vestibular tone imbalance involving the vertical VOR in the roll plane (Figure 49.7). It represents a fundamental pattern of coordinated eye–head roll motion and body tilt, is based on both otolith and vertical canal input, and is mediated by the graviceptive pathways from the labyrinths via the rostral medial and superior vestibular nuclei and the contralateral medial longitudinal fascicle to the rostral midbrain tegmentum.

> The OTR consists of lateral head tilt, skew deviation of the eyes (hypotropia of the undermost eye), ocular torsion (clockwise with head tilt left; counterclockwise with head tilt right), and tilt of perceived vertical.

It was first clearly delineated during electrical stimulation of the interstitial nucleus of Cajal.[20]

OTR is not a rare condition. In acute unilateral brainstem infarctions, it can be detected in about 20% of cases if a careful examination for ocular torsion of the eyes (fundus photographs), subtle skew deviation and subjective visual vertical[21] is carried out. OTR and concurrent body tilt are always ipsiversive in patients with pontomedullary lesions,[22] whereas OTR and concurrent body tilt are always contraversive in patients with pontomesencephalic lesions.[23]

Lateropulsion in Wallenberg's syndrome: ipsiversive falls and adjustments of perceived vertical

> Lateropulsion of the body is a well-known transient feature of lateral medullary infarction in which patients cannot prevent ipsiversive lateral falls.

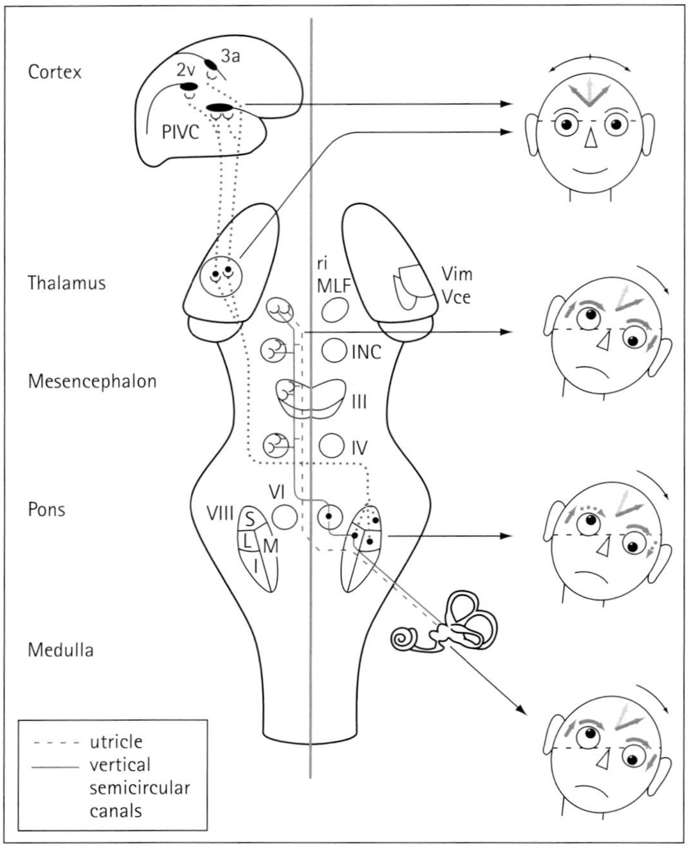

Figure 49.7 Vestibular syndromes in roll plane: graviceptive pathways from otoliths and vertical semicircular canals mediating vestibular function in roll plane. The projections from the otoliths and the vertical semicircular canals to the ocular motor nuclei (trochlear nucleus IV, oculomotor nucleus III, abducens nucleus VI), the supranuclear centres of the INC and the rostral interstitial nucleus of the MLF (riMLF) are shown. They subserve VOR in three planes. The VOR is part of a more complex vestibular reaction which also involves vestibulospinal connections via the medial and lateral vestibulospinal tracts for head and body posture control. Furthermore, connections to the assumed vestibular cortex (areas 2v and 3a and the parietoinsular vestibular cortex, PIVC) via the vestibular nuclei of the thalamus (Vim, nucleus ventro-oralis intermedius; Vce, nucleus ventrocaudalis externus) are depicted. 'Graviceptive' vestibular pathways for the roll plane cross at the pontine level. Ocular tilt reaction (OTR: skew torsion, head tilt, and tilt of perceived vertical, i.e. the subjective visual vertical (SVV)) is depicted schematically on the right in relation to the level of the lesion: ipsiversive OTR with peripheral and pontomedullary lesions; contraversive OTR with pontomesencephalic lesions. In vestibular thalamic lesions, the tilts of SVV may be contraversive or ipsiversive; in vestibular cortex lesions, they are preferably contraversive. OTR is not induced by supratentorial lesions above the level of INC.[5]

We believe that subjective vertigo is usually absent in these patients, because there is no sensory mismatch. The lesion causes a deviation of the perceived vertical. Individual multisensory regulation of posture is then adjusted not to the true vertical but to the pathologically deviated internal representation of verticality produced by the lesion. The more pronounced the lateropulsion, the greater the deviations of subjective visual vertical adjustments. Thus, these patients fall without realizing that it is their active shift of the centre of gravity (lateropulsion) which causes the imbalance. Here also it is the incorrect central computation of verticality (despite correct peripheral sensory signals from the otoliths) that is responsible for postural imbalance.[24]

Downbeat nystagmus syndrome with backward falls

Downbeat nystagmus in the primary gaze position,[25] or in particular on lateral gaze, is often accompanied by oscillopsia and postural instability. Posturographic measurements show a typical postural imbalance with a striking fore–aft body sway[26,27] and a tendency to fall backwards (Figure 49.8). This fore–aft

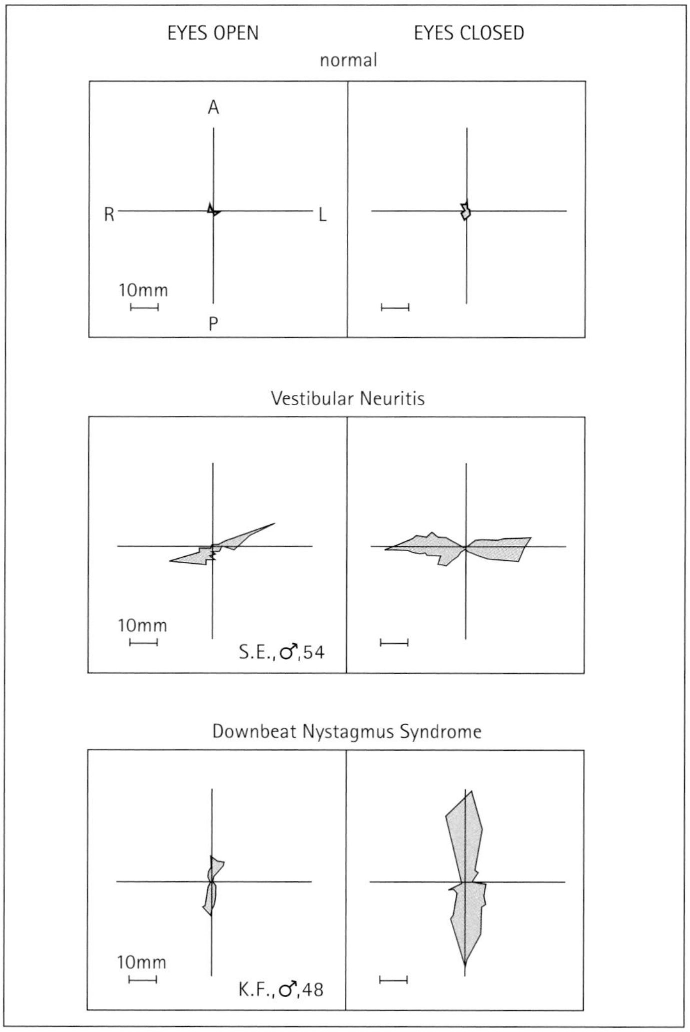

Figure 49.8 Postural instability in vestibular neuritis and in downbeat nystagmus. Histograms for fore–aft (A–P) and lateral (R,L) postural sway during upright stance with eyes open (left) and eyes closed (right) obtained with a force-measuring platform. For comparison, see registrations of body sway in a normal subject (top). The preferred direction of postural instability and body sway is in the lateral direction in patients with vestibular neuritis and in the fore–aft direction in patients with downbeat nystagmus. (Adapted from Brandt and Dieterich. *J Vestib Res* 1993; **3**: 3–14.[27])

postural instability can be interpreted as a direction-specific tone imbalance of the VOR in pitch, due either to a lesion in the floor of the fourth ventricle or to a bilateral lesion of the flocculus. Thus, downbeat nystagmus is not simply an ocular motor syndrome but a central vestibular syndrome comprising ocular motor, postural and perceptual effects.

Cautious senile gait and 'highest-level gait disorders'

Walking is one of the most common of all human movements; it is learned during the first year of life and perfected by around age 7. After age 60, this ability starts to decline, and the elderly gradually slow down.[28]

> A population-based study showed that 15% of the subjects over age 60 had some abnormality of gait,[29] and postural imbalance and gait disorders significantly contributed to the risk of falling.[30]

The so-called senile gait is more appropriately called cautious gait. Many older people adopt it to a greater or lesser degree to

Table 49.3 Classification of gait syndromes.[35]

I Lowest-level gait disorders
A. Peripheral skeletomuscle problems
- Arthritic gait
- Myopathic gait
- Peripheral neuropathic gait

B. Peripheral sensory problems
- Sensory ataxic gait
- Vestibular ataxic gait
- Visual ataxic gait

II Middle-level gait disorders
Hemiplegic gait
Paraplegic gait
Cerebellar ataxic gait
Parkinsonian gait
Choreic gait
Dystonic gait

III Highest-level gait disorders
Cautious gait
Subcortical disequilibrium
Frontal disequilibrium
Isolated gait ignition failure
Frontal gait disorder
Psychogenic gait disorder

Table 49.4 Terminology used to descibe the clinical patterns of gait in this chapter compared with those in previous publications.[35]

Proposed terminology	Previous terms	Lesions
Cautious	Elderly gait Senile gait	Musculoskeletal Peripheral nervous lesions Central nervous lesions
Subcortical disequilibrium	Tottering Astasia–abasia Thalamic astasia	Midbrain Basal ganglia Thalamus
Frontal disequilibrium	Gait apraxia Frontal ataxia Astasia-abasia	Frontal lobe and white matter connections
Isolated gait ignition failure	Gait apraxia Magnetic gait Slipping clutch gait Lower-half parkinsonism Arteriosclerotic parkinsonism Trepidant abasia (Petren's gait)	Frontal lobe, white matter connections, and basal ganglia
Frontal gait disorder	Marche à petits pas Magnetic gait apraxia Arteriosclerotic parkinsonism Parkinsonian ataxia Lower-half parkinsonism Lower body parkinsonism	Frontal lobe and white matter lesions

compensate for arthritis, pain, sensory or vestibular impairment, or simply from fear of falling.[31] When walking, elderly persons responded to a probe auditory reaction time task with greater delays than young adults. This suggests that the elderly have to allocate a greater proportion of attentional resources to the demands of balance.[32]

'Anyone whose balance is insecure, for whatever reason, will attempt to compensate. Normal compensation is best illustrated by our natural reaction to walking on ice. The feet are placed apart to widen the base; the body, hips, and knees are bent to place the centre of gravity firmly over the widened base; the arms are held somewhat abducted and flexed in anticipation of unexpected threats to balance. Locomotion proceeds with small steps on this wide base with a flexed posture. We walk the same way on a rolling deck of a ship.'[31]

Using analysis of covariants, Elble et al[33] found that these changes in gait were distinctly attributable to the reduced stride of older people and not to age per se; they suggest that many gait disturbances in elderly people are similar, regardless of aetiology, because the characteristics of these gait disturbances are heavily veiled by non-specific stride-dependent changes that comprise the syndrome of senile gait. It was also speculated that changes in gait pattern with increasing age are associated with decreasing muscle strength.[34]

Nevertheless, as clinicians we feel that we are able to differentiate the cautious gait of the elderly from other 'highest-level gait disorders'[35] such as frontal disequilibrium, isolated gait ignition failure,[36] or frontal gait disorder (see Table 49.3 for classification and Table 49.4 for terminology). Subcortical disequilibrium has been reported to be an acute consequence of thalamic basal ganglia or midbrain stroke (see thalamic astasia). In frontal disequilibrium there appears to be a breakdown of the organization of leg movements required for locomotion, so that the gait is often bizarre and the feet frequently cross or move in the wrong direction.[31] Frontal disequilibrium is also described as gait apraxia (e.g. in normal-pressure hydrocephalus), frontal ataxia, or astasia–abasia, which indicates dysfunction of the frontal lobe and white matter connections. Isolated gait initiation failure describes an inability to initiate and sustain locomotion with start-and-turn hesitation, shuffling, and freezing, but relatively normal gait once locomotion is initiated; the posture is upright, and there is good arm swing, a normal stride length, and no festination.[36] This makes it different from posture and gait in Parkinson's syndrome.[35,37,38] The so-called frontal gait disorder shares some features of frontal disequilibrium and gait ignition failure; it is characterized by a variable base (narrow-to-wide), difficulty in starting to walk, short steps, shuffling, and hesitation on turns with freezing and moderate disequilibrium.

The crucial questions about these syndromes of highest-level gait disorders are to what extent they are separate entities and how much overlap there is among them.[31,33]

References

1. Baloh RW, Halmagyi GM. *Disorders of the Vestibular System*. Oxford: Oxford University Press, 1996.
2. Brandt Th. *Vertigo: Its Multisensory Syndromes*, 2nd edn. London: Springer-Verlag, 1999.
3. Leigh J, Brandt T. A reevaluation of the vestibulo-ocular reflex: new ideas of its purpose, properties, neural substrate, and disorders. *Neurology* 1993; **43**: 1288–95.
4. Brandt T, Dieterich M. Vestibular syndromes in the roll plane: topographic diagnosis from brainstem to cortex. *Ann Neurol* 1994; **36**: 337–47.
5. Brandt T, Dieterich M. Central vestibular syndromes in the roll, pitch, and yaw planes: topographic diagnosis of brainstem disorders. *Neuroophthalmology* 1995; **15**: 291–303.
6. Guldin W, Grüsser O-I. The anatomy of the vestibular cortices of primates. In: Collard M, Jeannerod M, Christen Y, eds. *Le Cortex Vestibulaire*. Boulogne: Ipsen, 1996: 17–26.
7. Brandt Th, Daroff RB. The multisensory physiological and pathological vertigo syndromes. *Ann Neurol* 1980; **7**: 195–203.
8. Büchele W, Brandt Th. Vestibulo-spinal ataxia in benign paroxysmal positional vertigo. *Agressologie* 1979; **20**: 221–2.
9. Tumarkin A. The otolithic catastrophe: a new syndrome. *Br Med J* 1936; **1**: 175–7.
10. Baloh RW, Jacobson K, Winder T. Drop attacks with Menière's syndrome. *Ann Neurol* 1990; **28**: 384–7.
11. Tullio P. *Das Ohr und die Entstehung der Sprache und Schrift*. München: Urban und Schwarzenberg, 1929.
12. Dieterich M, Brandt Th, Fries W. Otolith function in man: results from a case of otolith Tullio phenomenon. *Brain* 1989; **112**: 1377–92.
13. Brandt Th, Dieterich M, Fries W. Otolithic Tullio phenomenon typically presents as paroxysmal ocular tilt reaction. *Adv Otorhinolaryngol* 1988; **42**: 153–6.
14. Baloh RW, Jacobson K, Honrubia V. Idiopathic bilateral vestibulopathy. *Neurology* 1989; **39**: 272–5.
15. Paulus W, Straube A, Brandt Th. Visual postural performance after loss of somatosensory and vestibular function. *J Neurol Neurosurg Psychiatry* 1987; **50**: 1542–5.
16. Foerster O. Sensible corticale Felder. In: Bumke O, Foerster O, eds. *Handbuch der Neurologie*, Vol. VI. Berlin: Springer, 1936: 358–448.
17. Verma AK, Maheshwari MC. Hyperesthetic-ataxic-hemiparesis in thalamic haemorrhage. *Stroke* 1986; **17**: 49–51.
18. Masdeu JC, Gorelick PB. Thalamic astasia: inability to stand after unilateral thalamic lesions. *Ann Neurol* 1988; **23**: 586–603.
19. Dieterich M, Brandt T. Vestibulo-ocular reflex. *Current Opin Neurol* 1995; **8**: 83–8.
20. Westerheimer G, Blair SM. The ocular tilt reaction: a brainstem oculomotor routine. *Invest Ophthalmol* 1975; **14**: 833–9.
21. Brandt T, Dieterich M. Cyclorotation of the eyes and subjective visual vertical in acute vascular (vestibular) brainstem lesions. *Ann NY Acad Sci* 1992; **658**: 537–49.

22. Brandt T, Dieterich M. Pathological eye–head coordination in roll: tonic ocular tilt reaction in mesencephalic and medullary lesions. *Brain* 1987; **110**: 649–66.
23. Halmagyi GM, Curthoys IS, Cremer PD et al. The human horizontal vestibulo-ocular reflex in response to high-acceleration stimulation before and after unilateral vestibular neurectomy. *Exp Brain Res* 1990; **81**: 479–90.
24. Dieterich M, Brandt T. Wallenberg's syndrome: lateropulsion, cyclorotation and subjective visual vertical in thirty-six patients. *Ann Neurol* 1992; **31**: 399–408.
25. Cogan DG. Downbeat nystagmus. *Arch Ophthalmol* 1968; **80**: 757–68.
26. Büchele W, Brandt Th, Degner D. Ataxia and oscillopsia in downbeat nystagmus/vertigo syndrome. *Adv Otorhinolaryngology* 1983; **30**: 291–7.
27. Brandt T, Dieterich M. Vestibular falls. *J Vestib Res* 1993; **3**: 3–14.
28. Prince F, Corriveau H, Hébert R et al. Gait in the elderly. *Gait Posture* 1997; **5**: 128–35.
29. Newman G, Dovenmuehle RH, Busse EW. Alterations in neurological status with age. *J Am Geriatr Soc* 1960; **8**: 915–17.
30. Tinetti ME, Speechley M, Ginter SF. Risk factors for falls among elderly persons living in the community. *N Engl J Med* 1988; **319**: 1701–7.
31. Marsden CD, Thompson PD. Frontal gait disorders. In: Bronstein AM, Brandt Th, Woollacott M, eds. *Clinical Disorders of Balance, Posture and Gait*. London: Arnold, 1996: 188–93.
32. Lajoie Y, Teasdale N, Bard C et al. Upright standing and gait: are there changes in attentional requirements related to normal aging? *Exp Aging Res* 1996; **22**: 185–98.
33. Elble RJ, Hughes L, Higgins C. The syndrome of senile gait. *J Neurol* 1992; **239**: 71–5.
34. Nigg BM, Fisher V, Ronsky JL. Gait characteristics as a function of age and gender. *Gait Posture* 1994; **2**: 213–20.
35. Nutt JG, Marsden CD, Thompson PD. Human walking and higher-level gait disorders, particularly in the elderly. *Neurology* 1993; **43**: 268–79.
36. Atchison PR, Thompson PD, Frackowiak RSJ et al. The syndrome of gait ignition failure: a report of six cases. *Movement Disord* 1993; **8**: 285–92.
37. Dietz V, Berger W, Horstmann GA. Posture in Parkinson's disease: impairment of reflexes and programming. *Ann Neurol* 1988; **24**: 660–9.
38. Sudarsky L. Geriatrics: gait disorders in the elderly. *N Engl J Med* 1990; **322**: 1441–6.

50 Falls

Joanna Downton

Introduction

Humans are prone to falling because of their upright stance, which results in a relatively high centre of gravity and small base of support. In addition, any movement tends to take that centre of gravity outside the support base. The human nervous system has therefore developed an enormously complex system to maintain balance in static and dynamic situations. Despite this, falls are a universal human experience, though there are particular groups of people who are especially prone to falling. Falls are much commoner at the extremes of life. In children, the maturing nervous system cannot always cope with the demands put upon it by the energetic activities of play, and falls occur frequently, though usually without serious consequences. In the elderly, the depredations of age and disease mean that the neuromuscular balance maintenance system sometimes fails and falls occur. Falls are also much commoner in younger people with diseases which impair the efficiency of the various systems which preserve balance.

Because falls and their complications are so much commoner in the elderly, and because the majority of research on falls has been done in this group, this chapter considers falls in the elderly rather than falls in all age groups, unless stated specifically.

Epidemiology of falls

Much work has been done on the epidemiology of falls over the last 30 years. Despite this, there remains some uncertainty about the prevalence of falling, partly because of the intrinsic difficulties of studying a phenomenon which is frequently unwitnessed, and which tends to occur most commonly in people who may have difficulty describing their experience. As a result, there are widely varying estimates in the research literature of the frequency of falls. It is possible that there are genuine large differences in frequency of falling between and within populations, but studies have been performed inconsistently.[1] Study populations have been selected in ways that make comparisons difficult or impossible; definitions of falls have varied; and not all studies have taken account of the possibility that fallers may forget or not report their falls. Most studies have concentrated on the elderly.

Several large, well-designed population studies of elderly people have now been carried out, and these report fairly consistent estimates of the prevalence of falls in community-dwelling older people (Table 50.1). These methodologically sound epidemiological studies of falls indicate an incidence of falling of 28–35% in those aged 65+,[2–5] 35% in the over-70s,[5,6] and 32–42% in the over 75s.[7,8] Those who have already had a fall have a higher rate of falling (60–70%) in the subsequent year.[9] Some studies have looked specifically at 'healthy elderly' (though there are difficulties defining who these are), who appear to fall less frequently—only about 15% of a group of 'fit elderly' fell over the course of a year.[10] Elderly people in institutional care, who are by definition a frailer group than community-living elderly, fall more frequently, though it is difficult to be certain about the prevalence of falls in this group. It is estimated that at least 50% of elderly people in institutional care are subject to falls.[11]

Complications of falling (Table 50.2)

Death

Most deaths due to falls occur in those aged over 65,[12] and deaths from injury in the over-65s are mainly a result of complications of falls[13] (Figure 50.1). Approximately 2 per 1000 of

Table 50.1 Rates of falling in the elderly (% falling each year).

Community-living elderly	
65+	28–35%
70+	35%
75+	32–42%
Previous fallers	60–70%
'Healthy elderly'	15%
Institutionalized elderly	50%+

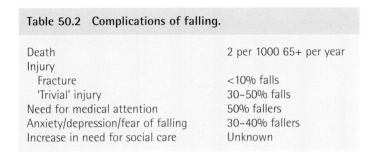

Table 50.2 Complications of falling.

Death	2 per 1000 65+ per year
Injury	
Fracture	<10% falls
'Trivial' injury	30–50% falls
Need for medical attention	50% fallers
Anxiety/depression/fear of falling	30–40% fallers
Increase in need for social care	Unknown

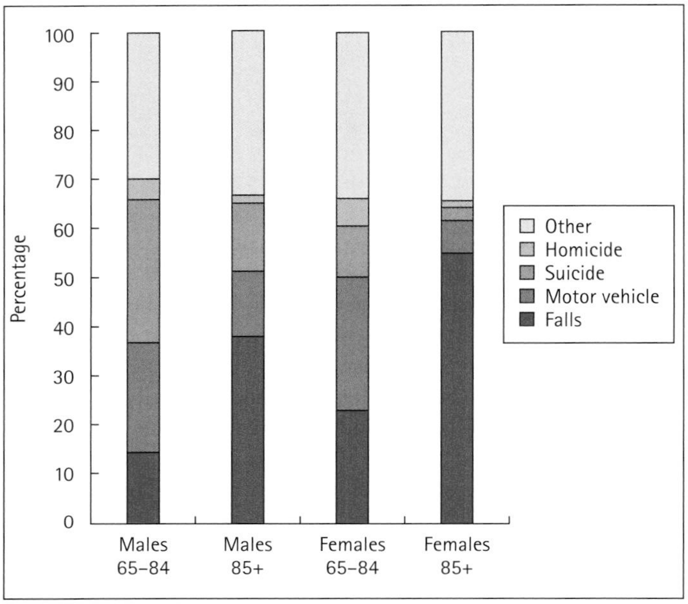

Figure 50.1 Deaths from injury in those aged over 65.[13]

the population over 65 per year die directly as a result of a fall (though these estimates are affected by the inaccuracy of death certification), with men having a higher risk than women. The risk of dying as a result of a fall increases with age[14] (Figure 50.2), and almost half of deaths follow a hip fracture. Falls are also a marker of increased risk of dying from causes other than the direct result of the fall.[15] One study found that fallers had more than double the death rate over 2 years of a matched group of non-fallers.[16]

Although a faller may be uninjured, he or she may be unable to get up without assistance, and may suffer a 'long lie'. The proportion of elderly fallers unable to get up alone has been reported to be as high as 50%.[17] Those who are unable to get up tend to be older and frailer than those who can get up unaided, and are at risk of a number of serious problems such as dehydration, pneumonia, pressure sores and rhabdomyolysis.[18] They have a higher risk of death, of decline in independence and of requirement for institutional care.[17]

Injury

Injuries caused by falling make enormous demands on health and social care systems. Most injuries following falls are relatively trivial, though even 'trivial' injuries in the elderly can have significant functional effects. An injury of some sort occurs in a third to three-quarters of falls.[19] However, more than half of fallers do not present to medical attention.[8] Most serious injuries and the majority of fractures in the elderly are caused by falling,[20] and there is an exponential increase in fractures with increasing age (Figure 50.3). Nonetheless, fractures occur in less than 10% of falls.[8] Although being fit and active reduces

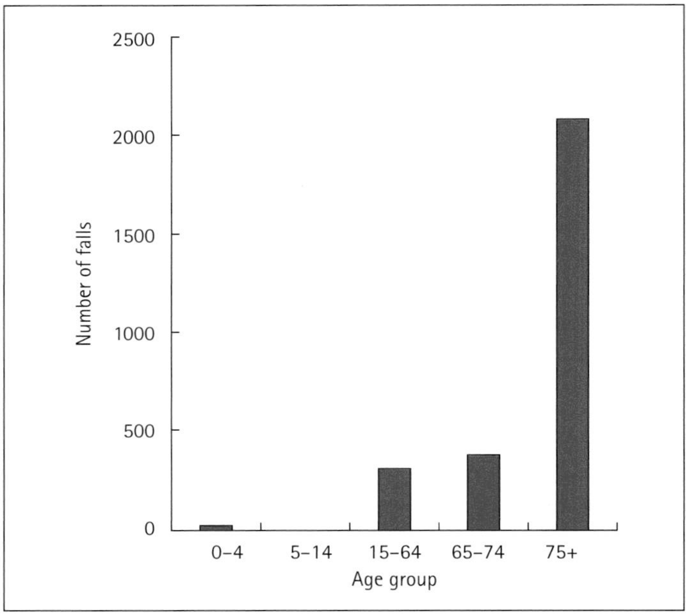

Figure 50.2 Fatal falls in England and Wales 1985 by age group.[100]

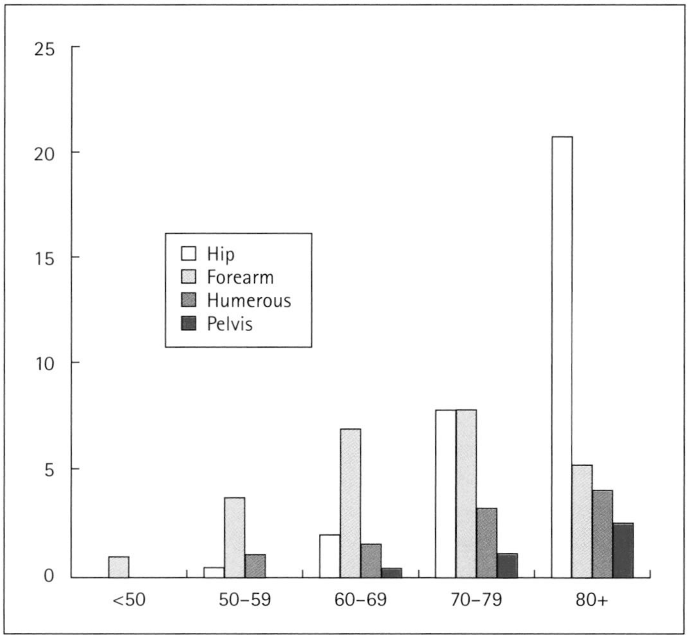

Figure 50.3 Rates (per 1000 women per year) of fall-associated fractures by age group.

the risk of falling, 'healthy elderly' are more likely to suffer a fracture if they do fall.[21]

The commonest fall-related fracture is that of the neck of the femur. Overall, the incidence of fractured femoral neck is reported to be approximately 5 per 1000 population over 65 per year.[22] There are interesting variations in fracture incidence in different parts of the world which are not fully explained[23] (Figure 50.4), though it is thought that they may reflect different patterns of activity at different stages of life. The frequency of osteoporosis also affects the likelihood of a fall-related fracture, though the presence of osteoporosis is a necessary but not a sufficient cause of age-related fracture, and much of the increase in fractures with age reflects the prevalence of falling rather than the prevalence of osteoporosis. The rate of injury following falls is substantially higher in institutionalized elderly than in those living independently.[24]

Fall-related fractures result in substantial costs to health services, though quantification of this is not easy. It is even more difficult to calculate the overall costs of such fractures, given that consequent disability and dependence is frequent, with a substantial demand on social care systems, both formal and informal (Figures 50.5 and Figure 50.6). It is easiest to calculate health service costs for fractured neck of femur, and North American work suggests that the worldwide cost to health systems of treating hip fracture will exceed 130 billion dollars by 2050.[25]

Social and psychological effects of falls

Falls and fear of falling have a huge effect on the quality of life of elderly people. Fear of falling is reported to be at least as common as falling itself.[26] In some cases, such fear can have catastrophic effects on mobility and independence.[27] There is a strong association between falls and fear of falling, but a third of those who had not had a fall in the previous year reported that they limited their activity because of fear of falling.[28] Depressive symptoms are common in patients following hip fracture,[29] and there is some support for the contention that falls themselves produce symptoms of anxiety and depression.[28] Falls and fear of falling may mean that the elderly person makes significant demands on relatives and carers and on formal care

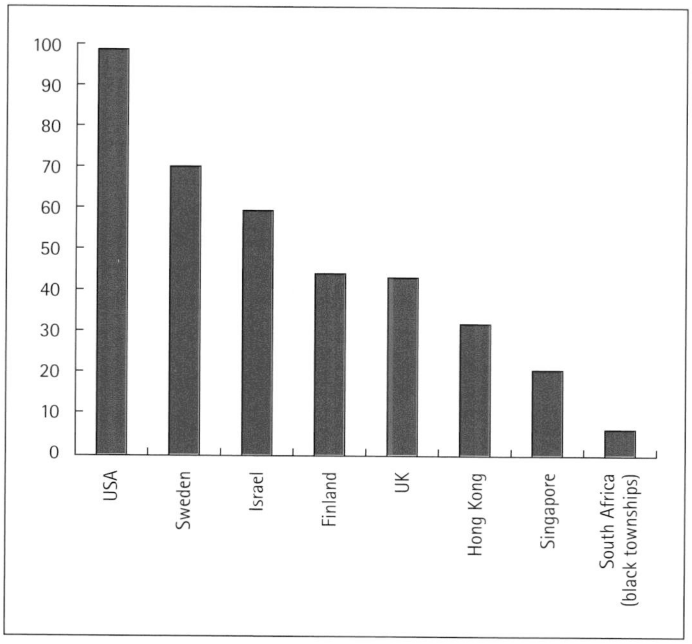

Figure 50.4 Age- and sex-adjusted annual incidence rates of hip fracture.[23]

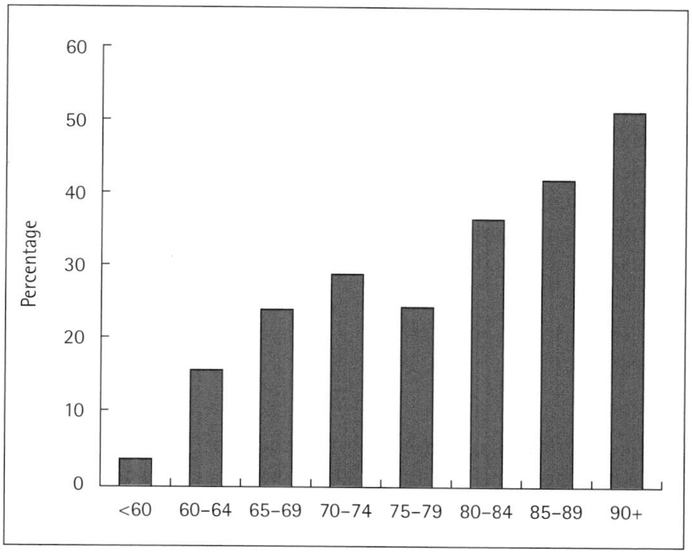

Figure 50.5 Mortality 1 year after fractured neck of femur by age group.[101]

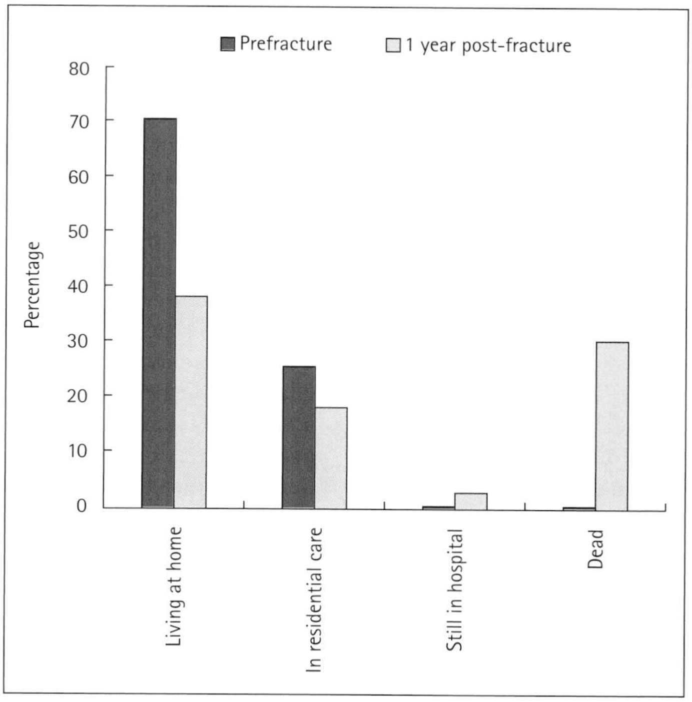

Figure 50.6 Place of residence before and one year after fractured neck of femur in 1000 UK patients.[101]

systems, since falls have been shown to lead to old people restricting their activity.[30]

Fractured neck of femur tends to cause a decline in functional abilities compared with the pre-fracture state,[31] and other fractures can also have a significant effect on independence.[32] Those who are already frail prior to their injury tend to do worse, though thorough assessment and rehabilitation following injury can improve outcome.[33] Fallers, particularly recurrent fallers, are more likely to end up in institutional care than non-fallers.[34]

Causes of falls

It is very difficult to determine the cause of an individual fall, let alone the 'causes of falls'. There will be intrinsic, environmental and temporal factors underlying a fall ('why did this individual fall in this place at this time?'), but even the faller herself, or someone witnessing the fall, may not be able to be certain why it occurred. It is considerably more difficult to ascribe causation at a distance. Despite this, an enormous amount of effort has gone into investigation of 'the causes of falls', partly because of the enormous socio-economic impact of falls and their consequences. Much of the work has identified 'factors associated with falls' rather than causes of falls, though these factors are often then described as causes of falls.

Many factors are implicated in the causation of falls. For reasons related to the complexity of fall aetiology (and sometimes the inadequate quality of some falls research), it is possible to find studies which show an association between practically any medical, psychological, social or environmental factor and falls, and almost as many showing that those factors are not associated. It seems likely that combinations of factors are more important than single problems. A further confounder is that the presence of a factor or factors known to increase the risk of falling does not invariably mean that a fall will occur, so that the predictive value of the presence of an individual factor is far from 100%.

Many factors associated with falls are not independent of each other, e.g. age and cognitive function, confusion and dependency, and neurological disease and abnormal gait, and therefore multivariate analysis is required to determine independent associations. Since this sort of complex statistical analysis has not been done very frequently, particularly in earlier work on falls, the relative risk of any particular factor cannot be estimated. In addition, studies using multivariate analysis have shown limited ability to predict who would be classified as a 'faller' or a 'non-faller', even when used retrospectively on the population from which the factors were derived.[2,4]

There are several factors that have consistently been shown to be associated with a higher risk of falls (Table 50.3), such as increasing age (although in some studies the very elderly have a lower prevalence of falling, possibly because those who reach extreme age may intrinsically be particularly fit and healthy,[3,35]

Table 50.3 Factors associated with increased risk of falling.

Increasing age
Female gender
Having multiple illnesses
Taking multiple medications
High level of functional dependency

female gender (apart from hospitalized subjects, where men have a higher risk than women[36]), and having multiple illnesses. Living alone or spending the greater part of the day alone,[2,3,9] and living in specialized housing for the elderly,[11] have been identified as risk factors for falls, though it is more likely that these merely identify those who have physical or other problems increasing fall risk.

Any fall is the result of an interaction of a number of factors. In order for a fall to occur, there must be an 'opportunity' as well as a 'liability' to fall, and the relative contributions of 'liability' and 'opportunity' vary at different ages, contributing to the different rates of falling with age. They also vary in an individual from moment to moment, depending on tiredness, concentration, health factors, etc. Clinical presentations include the single fall (either a simple trip or a non-trip fall), falls with significant injury, falls associated with loss of consciousness, recurrent falls in those who appear to be otherwise well, and recurrent falls in the frail elderly. Because it can be so difficult to determine the cause of an individual fall, because there are so may different presentations, and because there are so many potential causes of falls, it is perhaps more useful to look at groups of problems that may present with falls.

Clinical problems causing falls (Table 50.4)

Acute medical illness—a 'geriatric giant'

One of the characteristics of illness in the elderly is the tendency of elderly people with acute illness to present with non-specific symptoms and signs. This means that assessment of elderly people can be a considerable diagnostic challenge. There are five so-called 'geriatric giants' which are the commonest non-specific presentations of illness in the elderly—falls, confusion, immobility, incontinence and failure to cope or failure to thrive. Any of these presentations may indicate acute illness of any type. Thus, a fall may be the non-specific presentation of any acute illness.

Specific diseases

Some specific health problems are particularly likely to present with or be associated with falls.

Neuromuscular disease

Impairment of postural control is one of the cardinal features of Parkinson's disease, and so people with this disease are, in general, frequent fallers. Having had a stroke in the past is a risk factor for falling, even where there is little overt residual

Table 50.4 Clinical problems causing falls.

Acute medical illness
Specific diseases
Neuromuscular disease
Loss of consciousness
Autonomic dysfunction
Visual impairment
Age-related gait and balance abnormalities
'Falling syndromes'
Multiple sensory deficits
Cerebrovascular disease
'Frontal lobe gait and balance disorders'
'Drop attacks'
Drugs
Cognitive and affective disorders
Environmental factors

neurological deficit.[37] Lower-limb weakness has been shown to be a risk factor for falls,[38] so myopathies and motor neuropathies, especially those affecting the lower limbs, may result in falls. Sensory neuropathies can contribute to falls because of corruption of postural sensory information. Cervical spondylosis may predispose to falls; impairment of proprioceptive input from the cervical spine mechanoreceptors is a source of symptoms of vague dizziness and imbalance in elderly sufferers,[39] and cervical myelopathy causing lower limb spasticity and weakness is likely to affect gait detrimentally, particularly producing a tendency to trip.

Loss of consciousness
Any disease which results in episodes of loss of consciousness (e.g. epilepsy, cardiac arrhythmia) is liable to be associated with falls, but it should be noted that elderly people may have episodes of loss of consciousness following which they will be aware that they have fallen but may have no recollection that they have lost consciousness.[40] Recent work suggests that a significant number of fallers may have cardiac arrhythmias precipitated by carotid sinus hypersensitivity (Table 50.5).[40,41]

Table 50.5 Types of carotid hypersensitivity.

Cardioinhibitory	Carotid sinus massage produces asystole exceeding 3 s
Vasodepressor	Carotid sinus massage produces fall in systolic blood pressure exceeding 50 mmHg
Mixed	Carotid sinus massage produces both asystole and drop in blood pressure (independent vasodepressor response demonstrated by repeating massage once cardioinhibition has been abolished)

Autonomic dysfunction
This is not very common in healthy community elderly, but when present can be a potent cause of falls because of postural hypotension.[42] Postural hypotension without autonomic failure seems to be commoner, and can be precipitated by drugs, fluid depletion or immobilization.[43]

Visual impairment
This is strongly associated with an increase in risk of falling.[44] In addition to poor visual acuity, other factors such as reduced visual field, impaired contrast sensitivity and the presence of cataract may underlie this association.

Age-related gait and balance changes

Simple observation indicates that many old people do not move about in the same way as their younger peers, and that their balance appears less reliable. Objective measurement has shown some associations between impaired gait and balance and risk of falling,[45] though this is not useful for prediction of falling.[46] Changes in gait and postural stability may be due to age alone, or may be caused by pathology, and it is difficult to determine in individuals or in populations which is responsible. However, some very elderly subjects do seem to retain 'normal' balance and gait.[47] An important age-related change which may predispose older people to falling is that central integrative mechanisms which are important for postural reflexes tend to become slower.[48] Older brains seem to have less processing capacity and reduced ability to divide attention. Thus the appropriate allocation of central processing resources between concurrent tasks is disturbed.[48] If concentration is distracted, e.g. by another cognitive task, there is slower recovery from postural perturbation,[49] and those who struggle to combine walking with another cognitive task are more likely to fall.[50] Where maintaining posture competes with other cognitive demands, impaired postural control is more likely than difficulty with the other cognitive tasks.[51]

'Falling syndromes'

Multiple sensory deficits
Many elderly people have accumulated multiple, often fairly minor, deficits in sensory systems. There is evidence that some of the symptoms of dizziness, imbalance and falls in the frailer elderly are related to these deficits.[52] Individual deficits are associated with an increase in likelihood of falling, but combinations of deficits seem particularly hazardous.

Cerebrovascular disease
A variety of disorders associated with a high risk of falling can be produced by discrete or diffuse vascular disease affecting the brain. Stroke itself significantly increases risk of falling.[37] Multi-infarct dementia almost always produces gait disorder as well as cognitive impairment, and both predispose to falls. Fallers are much more likely to show white matter hypodensity (which is usually due to vascular ischaemic damage) on CT scan than non-fallers.[53]

'Frontal lobe gait and balance disorders'

These are commonly a result of vascular disease and can take a variety of forms.[54] They are often associated with falls, and produce difficulties in gait ignition, unsteadiness on turning, irregularity of gait cadence and/or shuffling gait.

Drop attacks

Although not well understood, these have been recognized for many years.[55] Unfortunately, the term tends to be used as a description for any sudden falling attack, including symptomatic drop attacks due to such things as epileptic fits, cataplexy and focal structural central nervous system lesions.[56] 'Idiopathic' drop attacks have been defined as 'a falling without warning, not associated with loss of consciousness, not apparently due to any malfunction of legs, not induced by changes of posture or movement of the head, and not accompanied by vertigo or other cephalic sensation, not associated with myoclonic jerks'.[57] Aetiology is uncertain, since studies of the phenomenon have rarely been rigorous in excluding symptomatic drop attacks. It is postulated that they are due to transient dysfunction of the brainstem centres in the reticular formation controlling tone in the antigravity muscles.[58] True idiopathic drop attacks appear to have a good prognosis,[59] although there is a substantial risk of injury as a result of the fall.

Drugs

There are good theoretical reasons why some specific drugs might be associated with an increased risk of falling. Any drug which has a tendency to produce postural hypotension (antihypertensives, tricyclic antidepressants, anti-parkinsonian medication, major tranquillizers, diuretics) could be expected to lead to falls in some elderly; drugs with sedative effects (benzodiazepines, anticonvulsants, antidepressants) may impair a range of neurological reflexes and thus threaten postural control. Evidence from a large number of studies (with variable methodological rigour) has been conflicting, however.[2,4,7,60,61] More recent consensus seems to be that it is polypharmacy that is the risk rather than specific drugs,[62,63] though obviously in an individual faller a particular drug may be implicated.

Cognitive and affective problems

There is good evidence that cognitive impairment increases risk of falling,[2,3,64] and dementia sufferers are at significantly higher risk of hip fracture than those with normal cognitive function.[65] Impaired balance mechanisms may occur as part of the neurological deterioration associated with dementia,[66] and being cognitively impaired may make risk-taking behaviour more likely, due to lack of insight into the effects of actions. Although anxiety and depression may result from falls, there is also some evidence that those with affective disorders are more likely to fall.[2,11,67] Again, the explanation for this is uncertain, though those with severe depression do have changes in gait,[68] and their concentration is likely to be impaired, potentially reducing awareness of risks. Rarely, attention-seeking behaviour may result in 'deliberate' falls.[69] Fear of falling may lead elderly people to restrict activity, which can in turn increase risk of falling because of the deconditioning effect of immobility.[43]

Environmental factors

Environmental factors are obviously important in the genesis of falls,[70] though fallers tend to blame external causes excessively, and there is not necessarily a difference between the exposure to environmental hazard of those who fall and those who do not.[71] It seems that environmental factors are a major element in about a third of falls,[72] though the proportion is less in the very elderly.[73] More commonly, the environment combines with intrinsic factors to increase risk of falls. For example, elderly people may have difficulty negotiating stairs if their vision is impaired or if lighting levels are low.[74]

In hospitals and institutions very low staffing levels may be associated with fewer falls because activity is discouraged,[75] while higher staffing levels may reduce fall frequency, presumably because there can be greater supervision of potentially risky activities.[76] Environmental temperature may affect the risk of falling,[77] particularly in thin or undernourished women, perhaps because of a relationship between nutritional state and thermoregulation.[78]

Clinical management of fallers

Table 50.6 Clinical management of fallers.

Assessment
History
Examination
Investigations
Clinical assessment of gait and balance
Treatment of identified diseases/problems
Rehabilitation
Prevention of further falls

Management of fallers involves a range of tasks, including assessment of the faller and the circumstances of the fall, identifying treatable problems, rehabilitation, and prevention of further falls and injury. The first question to be considered is why did this particular person fall at this particular time in this particular place? There will be intrinsic and environmental factors which may be fixed or variable with time. There is always a reason (or more commonly a number of reasons) why someone falls, and with careful assessment it is usually possible to ascertain at least some of the factors that have caused the fall. Contrary to popular opinion it is commonly possible to affect some or all of these to reduce the risk of further falls.[79] However, because of the multiplicity of potential causes of falls, effective assessment requires a systematic approach (considering the factors described above) to make sure that all relevant risk factors are considered.

Assessment of fallers

History

Table 50.7 What to ask an elderly faller.

What were you doing at the time of the fall?
e.g. walking, standing still, getting up from chair
Were you feeling well before you fell?
Did you experience any symptoms before or after the fall?
Did you black out or lose consciousness?

When an elderly faller is questioned about a fall, general questions such as 'why did you fall?' or 'what caused your fall?' are only of relatively limited value. People who have had a straightforward trip or slip are often able to describe the circumstances of their fall in response to such questions, but those who have had a 'non-trip' fall often struggle to describe their experience, or rationalize what happened ('I must have tripped'). A more useful approach is to ask what the person was doing at the time of the fall (e.g. walking, standing still, getting up from a chair), whether they were feeling quite well before they fell, whether they noticed any symptoms (e.g. dizziness, palpitation, chest pain, visual disturbance) prior to, or following, the fall, and whether they blacked out or lost consciousness when they fell, bearing in mind the possibility that they may not remember an episode of loss of consciousness.

Symptoms such as 'dizziness' or 'palpitations' must not be taken at face value, as they may describe a number of different sensations. Although the majority of falls are unwitnessed, if someone else did observe the fall, information should be obtained from the witness, as it is often difficult for the faller to remember or describe the circumstances of the fall. The normal functional status of the faller should be determined, partly because the likely causes of falls in the fit, healthy elderly may be different from those in the frail elderly. A thorough medical history, including drug history, is usually appropriate, given the wide range of potential factors underlying a tendency to fall.

Examination

A full medical examination is usually appropriate, particularly if the fall seems to be due to acute illness or if there are recurrent falls, when the problem or problems may be in any body system. Special attention should be paid to the cardiovascular, neurological and musculoskeletal systems. Specific factors which may be useful in the examination of someone who has fallen are shown in Table 50.8.

Table 50.8 Examination of a faller – specific factors.

Pulse rate and rhythm
Supine and standing blood pressure
Mental status
Visual acuity and visual fields
Muscle power, especially in lower limbs
Neck movements–do these precipitate dizziness, etc.
Knee joint stability
Foot deformities
Romberg test
'Get up and go' test or 'timed up and go' test
Functional reach
Timed walk

Clinical assessment of balance and gait

Simple measures of balance, gait and mobility should be part of the assessment of all elderly fallers. However, many of the assessments of balance, gait and mobility that have been devised are complex and time-consuming and unsuitable for day-to-day use.[80] Nevertheless, a number of simple balance and gait assessments could be carried out routinely in the assessment of elderly fallers. The Romberg test demonstrates stability on standing with the feet together, with eyes open and closed. Severe loss of balance when the eyes are closed suggests vestibular and/or proprioceptive impairment, with reliance on vision to maintain static posture. The addition of a gentle push on the sternum stresses stability further[81] and can indicate the state of the postural and protective responses. 'Functional reach', where the subject stands still and reaches forward as far as possible along a fixed ruler, tests dynamic postural control.[82] Performance in this test has been shown to correlate with other measures of mobility and balance and with risk of falling.[83] The timed walk, either the time taken to complete a given distance or the distance walked in a given time, is a simple assessment of gait and mobility.[84] This can also be used to monitor response to treatment. An overall measure of static and dynamic stability can be made using the 'get up and go test'[85] or the slightly more refined 'timed up and go' test,[86] which again can monitor response to treatment.

Treatment and rehabilitation

Treatment of a faller must be dictated by the assessment of the cause of the fall, as intervention requires identification of possible causes and/or risk factors for falling. Where the cause seems predominantly external, assessment by an occupational therapist to identify potential risks in the immediate environment of the faller can be helpful, though people may be reluctant to make adaptations to their surroundings. It is impossible to remove all risks, and attempts to do so may lead to unacceptable restrictions of the autonomy of elderly people.

Rehabilitation of fallers needs to be matched to individuals and their specific problems. Therefore, the assessments discussed above need to be carried out to determine the particular medical and functional difficulties of the individual. A particular difficulty is that fallers may have a degree of cognitive impairment, and thus may not fully appreciate their limitations, or the changes that may need to be made to improve their function or reduce their risk of falling again. Many fallers demonstrate abnormalities of balance or gait, and input from a physiotherapist, with graded balance and mobility exercises, may be helpful.[87] Teaching someone how to get up after a fall may avoid the potentially dangerous 'long lie' if further falls occur, and can also be of psychological benefit to the faller. Providing a body-worn alarm device may also be of psychological as well as practical benefit, reassuring the faller and relatives or carers that help can be summoned if a fall occurs. It may be useful to visit the home of the faller to look for alterable risk factors in their environment, though recent work suggests that attempts to decrease home hazards have not been particularly effective in reducing falls.[88,89]

Prevention of (further) falls

This is important because of the frequency of falls and their complications in older people. Although primary prevention may be the ideal, secondary prevention (i.e. prevention of further falls in those who have already fallen) is more realistic. For the elderly population as a whole, general strategies in primary prevention should, however, be encouraged. Maintaining physical fitness as far as possible by regular exercise sessions is likely to reduce the risk of falling and injury by improving muscular function,[90] limiting osteoporosis, and possibly maintaining cognitive function.[91]

There is now evidence-based advice available about how to prevent falls in the elderly population. Those at higher risk of falling can be identified by simple assessment of risk factors.[92–95] Multifactorial assessment and intervention seems to benefit the frailer elderly,[16] and the fitter elderly benefit from exercise including a balance component.[96,97] It may be possible to prevent or reduce injury due to falls, for example by using simple hip protectors to reduce the incidence of hip fractures.[98]

Although much can be done to reduce the risk of falling in populations and in individuals, it is not possible to prevent all falls, and attempts to do so may have a deleterious effect on the quality of life of frailer elderly. It is important to remain realistic, and accept that some risk is unavoidable if autonomy is to be retained and life is to remain worth living.[99]

References

1. Downton J. The problems of epidemiological studies of falls. *Clin Rehab* 1987; **1**(3): 243–6.
2. Campbell AJ, Reinken J, Allan BC, Martinez GS. Falls in old age: a study of frequency and related clinical factors. *Age Ageing* 1981; **10**: 264–70.
3. Prudham D, Evans JG. Factors associated with falls in the elderly: a community study. *Age Ageing* 1981; **10**: 141–6.
4. Blake AJ, Morgan K, Bendall MJ et al. Falls by elderly people at home: prevalence and associated factors. *Age Ageing* 1988; **17**: 365–72.
5. Campbell AJ, Borrie MJ, Spears GF, Jackson SL, Brown JS, Fitzgerald JL. Circumstances and consequences of falls experienced by a community population 70 years and over during a prospective study. *Age Ageing* 1990; **19**: 136–41.
6. Campbell AJ, Borrie MJ, Spears GF. Risk factors for falls in a community-based prospective study of people 70 years and older. *J Gerontol* 1989; **44**: M112–17.
7. Tinetti ME, Speechley M, Ginter SF. Risk factors for falls among elderly persons living in the community. *N Engl J Med* 1988; **319**: 1701–7.
8. Downton JH, Andrews K. Prevalence, characteristics and factors associated with falls among the elderly living at home. *Aging* 1991; **3**(3): 219–28.
9. Nevitt MC, Cummings SR, Kidd S, Black D. Risk factors for recurrent non-syncopal falls. A prospective study. *JAMA* 1989; **261**: 2663–8.
10. Gabell A, Simons MA, Nayak USL. Falls in the healthy elderly: predisposing causes. *Ergonomics* 1985; **28**: 965–75.
11. Tinetti ME, Speechley M. Prevention of falls amongst the elderly. *N Engl J Med* 1989; **320**: 1055–9.
12. Waller JA. Injury in aged. Clinical and epidemiological implications. *N York State J Med* 1974; **74**: 2200–8.
13. Sattin RW. Falls among older persons: a public health perspective. *Annu Rev Public Health* 1992; **13**: 489–508.
14. Sattin RW, Lambert Huber DA, DeVito CA et al. The incidence of fall injury events among the elderly in a defined population. *Am J Epidemiol* 1990; **131**(6): 1028–37.
15. Campbell AJ, Diep C, Reinken J, McCosh L. Factors predicting mortality in a total population sample of the elderly. *J Epidemiol Comm Health* 1985; **39**: 337–42.
16. Rubenstein LZ, Robbins AS, Josephson KR, Schulman BL, Osterweil D. The value of assessing falls in an elderly population. A randomized clinical trial. *Ann Intern Med* 1990; **113**(4): 308–16.
17. Tinetti ME, Liu W-L, Claus EB. Predictors and prognosis of inability to get up after falls among elderly persons. *JAMA* 1993; **269**(1): 65–70.
18. Mallinson WJW, Green MF. Covert muscle injury in aged patients admitted to hospital following falls. *Age Ageing* 1985; **14**(3): 174–8.
19. O'Loughlin JL, Robitaille Y, Boivin J-F, Suissa S. Incidence of and risk factors for falls and injurious falls among the community-dwelling elderly. *Am J Epidemiol* 1993; **137**(3): 342–54.
20. Melton LJ III, Riggs BL. Epidemiology of age-related fractures. In: Alvioli LV, ed. *The Osteoporotic Syndrome*. New York: Grune & Stratton, 1987.
21. Speechley M, Tinetti M. Falls and injuries in frail and vigorous community elderly persons. *J Am Geriatr Soc* 1991; **39**: 46–52.
22. Evans JG, Prudham D, Wandless I. A prospective study of fractured proximal femur: incidence and outcome. *Public Health* 1979; **93**: 235–41.
23. Lewinnek GE, Kelsey J, White AA, Kreiger NJ. The significance and a comparative analysis of the epidemiology of hip fractures. *Clin Orthop* 1980; **152**: 35–43.
24. Luukinen H, Koski K, Honkanen R, Kivela S-L. Incidence of injury-causing falls among older adults by place of residence: a population-based study. *J Am Geriatr Soc* 1995; **43**(8): 871–6.
25. Johnell O. The socioeconomic burden of fractures: today and in the 21st century. *Am J Med* 1997; **103**(2A): 20S–25S.

26. Grisso JA, Schwarz DF, Wolfson V, Polansky M, LaPann K. The impact of falls in an inner-city elderly African-American population. *J Am Geriatr Soc* 1992; **40**: 673–8.
27. Murphy J, Isaacs B. The post-fall syndrome. A study of 36 elderly patients. *Gerontology* 1982; **28**: 265–70.
28. Downton JH, Andrews K. Postural disturbance and psychological symptoms amongst elderly people living at home. *Int J Geriatr Psychiatry* 1990; **5**: 93–8.
29. Billig N, Ahmed SW, Kenmore P, Amaral D, Shakhashiri MZ. Assessment of depression and cognitive impairment after hip fracture. *J Am Geriatr Soc* 1986; **34**: 499–503.
30. Kosorok MR, Omenn GS, Diehr P et al. Restricted activity days among older adults. *Am J Public Health* 1992; **82**: 1263–7.
31. Marotolli RA, Berkman LF, Cooney LM. Decline in physical function following hip fracture. *J Am Geriatr Soc* 1992; **40**: 861–6.
32. Greendale GA, Barrett-Connor E, Ingles S, Haile R. Late physical and functional effects of osteoporotic fracture in women: the Rancho Bernardo study. *J Am Geriatr Soc* 1995; **43**(9): 955–61.
33. Bernardini B, Meinecke C, Pagani M et al. Comorbidity and adverse clinical events in the rehabilitation of older adults after hip fracture. *J Am Geriatr Soc* 1995; **43**(8): 894–8.
34. Dunn JE, Furner SE, Miles TP. Do falls predict institutionalization in older persons? *J Aging Health* 1993; **5**: 194–207.
35. Woodhouse PR, Briggs RS, Ward D. Falls and disability in old peoples homes. *J Clin Exp Gerontol* 1983; **5**: 309–21.
36. Berry G, Fisher RH, Lang S. Detrimental incidents, including falls, in an elderly institutional population. *J Am Geriatr Soc* 1981; **29**: 322–4.
37. Forster A, Young J. Incidence and consequences of falls due to stroke: a systematic inquiry. *Br Med J* 1995; **311**: 83–6.
38. Whipple RH, Wolfson LI, Amerman PM. The relationship of knee and ankle weakness to falls in nursing home residents: an isokinetic study. *J Am Geriatr Soc* 1987; **35**: 13–20.
39. de Jong JMBV, Bles W. Cervical dizziness and ataxia. In: Bles W, Brandt T, eds. *Disorders of Posture and Gait*. Amsterdam: Elsevier Science Publishers BV, 1986: 185–206.
40. McIntosh SJ, Lawson J, Kenny RA. Clinical characteristics of vasodepressor, cardioinhibitory, and mixed carotid sinus syndrome in the elderly. *Am J Med* 1993; **95**: 203–8.
41. Kenny RA, Traynor G. Carotid sinus syndrome—clinical characteristics in elderly patients. *Age Ageing* 1991; **20**: 449–54.
42. Mader SL, Josephson KR, Rubenstein LZ. Low prevalence of postural hypotension among community dwelling elderly. *JAMA* 1993; **258**: 1511–14.
43. Creditor MC. Hazards of hospitalization of the elderly. *Ann Intern Med* 1993; **118**: 219–23.
44. Ivers RQ, Cumming RG, Mitchell P, Attebo K. Visual impairment and falls in older adults: the Blue Mountains eye study. *J Am Geriatr Soc*. 1998; **46**(1): 58–64, 1998.
45. Maki BE, Holliday PJ, Topper AK. A prospective study of postural balance and risk of falling in an ambulatory and independent elderly population. *J Gerontol* 1994; **49**(2): M72–84.
46. Baloh RW, Corona S, Jacobson KM, Enrietto JA, Bell T. A prospective study of posturography in normal older people. *J Am Geriatr Soc* 1998; **46**(4): 438–43.
47. Bloem BR, Haan J, Lagaay AM, van Beek W, Wintzen AR, Roos RAC. Investigation of gait in elderly subjects over 88 years of age. *J Geriatr Psychiatry Neurol* 1992; **5**: 78–84.
48. Teasdale N, Stelmach GE, Bard C, Fleury M. Posture and elderly persons: deficits in the central integrative mechanisms. In: Woollacott M, Horak F, eds. *Posture and Gait: Control Mechanisms*. Portland, Oregon: University of Oregon, 1992: 203–7.
49. Stelmach GE, Zelaznik HN, Lowe D. The influence of aging and attentional demands on recovery from postural instability. *Aging* 1990; **2**(2): 155–61.
50. Lundin-Olsson L, Nyberg L, Gustafson Y. Attention, frailty, and falls: the effect of a manual task on basic mobility. *J Am Geriatr Soc* 1998; **46**(6): 758–61.
51. Shumway-Cook A, Woollacott M, Kerns KA, Baldwin M. The effects of two types of cognitive tasks on postural stability in older adults with and without a history of falls. *J Gerontol* 1997; **52A**(4): M232–40.
52. Manchester D, Woollacott M, Zederbauer-Hylton N, Marin O. Visual, vestibular and somatosensory contributions to balance control in the older adult. *J Gerontol* 1989; **44**(4): M118–27.
53. Masdeu JC, Wolfson L, Lantos G et al. Brain white matter changes in the elderly prone to falling. *Arch Neurol* 1989; **46**: 1292–6.
54. Nutt JG, Marsden CD, Thompson PD. Human walking and higher-level gait disorders, particularly in the elderly. *Neurology* 1993; **43**: 268–79.
55. Sheldon JH. *The Social Medicine of Old Age. Report of an Inquiry in Wolverhampton*. London: Oxford University Press, 1948.
56. Lee MS, Marsden D. Drop attacks. In: Bronstein AM, Brandt T, Woollacott M, eds. *Clinical Disorders of Balance, Posture and Gait*. London: Arnold, 1996: 177–87.
57. Stevens DL, Matthews WB. Cryptogenic drop attacks: an affliction of women. *BMJ* 1973; **1**: 439–42.
58. Overstall P. Drop attacks. In: Kenny RA, ed. *Syncope in the Older Patient*. London: Chapman & Hall Medical, 1996: 299–308.
59. Meissner I, Wiebers DO, Swanson JW, O'Fallon WM. The natural history of drop attacks. *Neurology* 1986; **36**: 1029–34.
60. Myers AH, Baker SP, Van Natta ML, Abbey H, Robinson EG. Risk factors associated with falls and injuries among elderly institutionalized persons. *Am J Epidemiol* 1991; **133**(11): 1179–90.
61. Ray WA, Griffin MR, Malcolm E. Cyclic antidepressants and the risk of hip fracture. *Arch Med* 1991; **151**: 754–6.
62. Weiner DK, Hanlon JT, Studenski SA. Effects of central nervous system polypharmacy on falls liability in community-dwelling elderly. *Gerontology* 1998; **44**: 217–21.
63. Close J, Ellis M, Hooper R, Glucksman E, Jackson S, Swift C. Prevention of falls in the elderly trial (PROFET): a randomised controlled trial. *Lancet* 1999; **353**: 93–7.
64. Morris JC, Rubin EH, Morris EJ, Mandel SA. Senile dementia of the Alzheimer's type: an important risk factor for serious falls. *J Gerontol* 1987; **42**: 412–17.
65. Melton LJ, Beard CM, Kokmen E, Atkinson EJ, O'Fallon WM. Fracture risk in patients with Alzheimer's disease. *J Am Geriatr Soc* 1994; **42**(6): 614–19.

66. Visser H. Gait and balance in senile dementia of Alzheimer's type. *Age Ageing* 1983; **12**: 296–301.
67. Granek E, Baker SP, Abbey H et al. Medications and diagnoses in relation to falls in a long-term care facility. *J Am Geriatr Soc* 1987; **35**: 503–11.
68. Sloman L, Berridge M, Homatidis S, Hunter D, Duck T. Gait patterns of depressed patients and normal subjects. *Am J Psychiatry* 1982; **139**: 94–7.
69. Belfield PW, Young JB, Bagnall WE, Mulley GP. Deliberate falls in the elderly. *Age Ageing* 1987; **16**: 123–4.
70. Gibson MJ. The prevention of falls in later life. A report of the Kellogg International Workgroup on the Prevention of Falls by the Elderly. *Dan Med Bull* 1987; **34**: 4–7.
71. Sattin RW, Rodriguez JG, DeVito CA, Wingo PA. Home environmental hazards and the risk of fall injury events among community-dwelling older persons. *J Am Geriatr Soc* 1998; **46**(6): 669–76.
72. Citron N. Femoral neck fractures: are some preventable? *Ergonomics* 1985; **28**: 993–7.
73. Morfitt JM. Falls in old people at home: intrinsic versus environmental factors in causation. *Public Health* 1983; **97**: 115–20.
74. Archea JC. Environmental factors associated with stair accidents by the elderly. *Clin Geriatr Med* 1985; **1**: 555–68.
75. Morris EV, Isaacs B. The prevention of falls in a geriatric hospital. *Age Ageing* 1980; **9**: 181–5.
76. Blake C, Morfitt JM. Falls and staffing in a residential home for elderly people. *Public Health* 1986; 100: 385–91.
77. Campbell AJ, Spears GFS, Borrie MJ, Fitzgerald JL. Falls, elderly women and the cold. *Gerontology* 1988; **34**: 205–8.
78. Bastow MD, Rawlings J, Allison SP. Undernutrition, hypothermia, and injury in elderly women with fractured femur: an injury response to altered metabolism? *Lancet* 1983; **1**: 143–6.
79. Rubenstein LZ, Robbins AS, Schulman BL, Rosado J, Osterweil D, Josephson KR. Falls and instability in the elderly. *J Am Geriatr Soc* 1988; **36**: 266–78.
80. MacKnight C, Rockwood K. Assessing mobility in elderly people. A review of performance-based measures of balance, gait and mobility for bedside use. *Rev Clin Gerontology* 1995; **5**(4): 464–86.
81. Weiner WJ, Nora LM, Glantz RH. Elderly in-patients: postural reflex impairment. *Neurology* 1984; **34**: 945–7.
82. Weiner DK, Duncan PW, Chandler J, Studenski SA. Functional reach: a marker of physical frailty. *J Am Geriatr Soc* 1992; **40**: 203–7.
83. Studenski S, Duncan PW, Chandler J et al. Predicting falls: the role of mobility and nonphysical factors. *J Am Geriatr Soc* 1994; **42**: 297–302.
84. Thapa PB, Gideon P, Fought RL, Kormicki M, Ray WA. Comparison of clinical and biomechanical measures of balance and mobility in elderly nursing home residents. *J Am Geriatr Soc* 1994; **42**(5): 493–500.
85. Mathias S, Nayak USL, Isaacs B. Balance in elderly patients: the 'get up and go' test. *Arch Phys Med Rehabil* 1986; **67**: 387–9.
86. Podsiadlo D, Richardson S. The timed 'up & go': a test of basic functional mobility for frail elderly persons. *J Am Geriatr Soc* 1991; **39**: 142–8.
87. Hogan DB, Berman P, Fox RA, Hubley-Kozey CL, Turnbull G, Wall J. Idiopathic gait disorders in the elderly. *Clin Rehabil* 1987; **1**(1): 17–22.
88. Northridge ME, Nevitt MC, Kelsey JL, Link B. Home hazards and falls in the elderly: the role of health and functional status. *Am J Public Health* 1995; **85**(4): 509–15.
89. Clemson L, Cumming RG, Roland M. Case-control study of hazards in the home and risk of falls and hip fractures. *Age Ageing* 1996; **25**(2): 97–101.
90. Rickli R, Busch S. Motor performance of women as a function of age and physical activity level. *J Gerontol* 1986; **41**: 645–9.
91. Molloy DW, Richardson LD, Grilly RG. The effects of a three-month exercise programme on neuropsychological function in elderly institutionalized women: a randomized controlled trial. *Age Ageing* 1988; **17**: 303–10.
92. Tinetti ME, Williams TF, Mayewski R. Fall risk index for elderly patients based on number of chronic disabilities. *Am J Med* 1986; **80**: 429–34.
93. Nevitt MC, Cummings SR, Hudes ES. Risk factors for injurious falls: a prospective study. *J Gerontol* 1991; **46**(5): M164–70.
94. Tinetti ME, Doucette JT and Claus EB. The contribution of predisposing and situational risk factors to serious fall injuries. *J Am Geriatr Soc* 1995; **43**: 1207–13.
95. Tinetti ME, Inouye SK, Gill TM, Doucette JT. Shared risk factors for falls, incontinence, and functional dependence. Unifying the approach to geriatric syndromes. *JAMA* 1995; **273**(17): 1348–53.
96. Province MA, Hadley EC, Hornbrook MC et al. The effects of exercise on falls in elderly patients. A preplanned meta-analysis of the FICSIT trials. *JAMA* 1995; **273**(17): 1341–7.
97. Lord SR, Ward JA, Williams P, Strudwick M. The effect of a 12-month exercise trial on balance, strength, and falls in older women: a randomized controlled trial. *J Am Geriatr Soc* 1995; **43**: 1198–206.
98. Lauritzen JB, Petersen MM, Lund B. Effect of external hip protectors on hip fractures. *Lancet* 1993; **341**: 11–13.
99. Wynne-Harley D. Living dangerously: risk-taking, safety and older people. Centre for Policy on Ageing, 1991.
100. Consumer Safety Unit. Home and Leisure Accident Research. Department of Trade and Industry, 1988.
101. Keene GS, Parker MJ, Pryor GA. Mortality and morbidity after hip fractures. *BMJ* 1993; **307**: 1248–50.

51 General medical causes of dizziness

Tim Petterson, Rose Anne Kenny

Introduction

Dizziness: What do we mean?

Patients describe their experience of 'sensory dysfunction' using a variety of synonyms, jargon or colloquialisms.[1] Physicians are faced with a colourful array of words and phrases often tainted with medical meaning. Examples include 'funny do's', 'collapse', 'coming over queer', 'about to fall', 'about to faint', 'muzziness', 'unsteadiness', 'vertigo' or 'blackouts'. These descriptions have different meanings for doctor and patient. Dizziness is perhaps the commonest of these presentations and the dizzy patient represents a major diagnostic challenge. A logical approach will help to define an appropriate management strategy (Figure 51.1). The key first step is to encourage the patient to describe their exact experience, by giving the patient time and presenting a series of detailed 'best guess' descriptions. Drachman and Hart[2] reported four types of dizziness: vertigo, lightheadedness, dysequilibrium and others (Table 51.1). The first two descriptions are useful predictors of final diagnostic category and so help to define initial assessment strategies. Vertigo indicates probable vestibular pathology (Chapters 48 and 54) whilst lightheadedness suggests a cardiovascular disorder.[3] Dysequilibrium describes imbalance or unsteadiness and may indicate a central neurological disorder. In practice it is a less useful predictor and its clinical application is therefore limited (Chapter 49). The fourth category of 'others' is a repository for poorly defined dizziness. Significant overlap between these four descriptions may occur. This reflects both the limitations of categorizing subjective data and the multifactorial nature of dizziness in many patients.

There is marked overlap of descriptions and causation.

Epidemiology of dizziness

Dizziness is a common problem, particularly in the elderly. Incidence and prevalence increase with age, more so in females.[4–6] Dizziness affects at least 30% of the UK community aged over 65 years[6–8] and almost half of those aged over 75 years.[9] Twenty per cent of community living elderly people report dizziness severe enough to seek medical advice.[10] In the USA dizziness is the commonest complaint of older people presenting to primary care physicians and emergency rooms.[5]

Vestibular[11] and psychogenic[12,13] causes are prominent in younger people. Medical conditions, particularly cardiovascular disorders, cerebrovascular disease, neuromuscular disorders and drugs are more often implicated in the elderly.

Table 51.1 Classification of dizziness.

Symptom	Possible attributable cause
Vertigo	Vestibular cause
Lightheaded	Cardiovascular cause
Dysequilibrium	Central neurological cause
Others	Miscellaneous causes
	Multifactorial
	Poorly defined

Cardiovascular causes of dizziness

Introduction

Dizziness is difficult to define. Existing studies are in small patient numbers, often retrospective and suffer selection bias. Most use patients attending ENT or neurology clinics rather than population studies. They tend to group patients into vague diagnostic categories or define a single diagnosis which may be contributory rather than causative. There is little emphasis on the assessment of specific interventions to resolve symptoms and reduce disability.[14] Against this background, peripheral vestibular disorders are reported as the commonest cause of dizziness (Chapter 50).

Cardiovascular disorders are increasingly recognized as significant medical causes of dizziness, particularly in older people.[15–17] Specialist centres using detailed cardiovascular

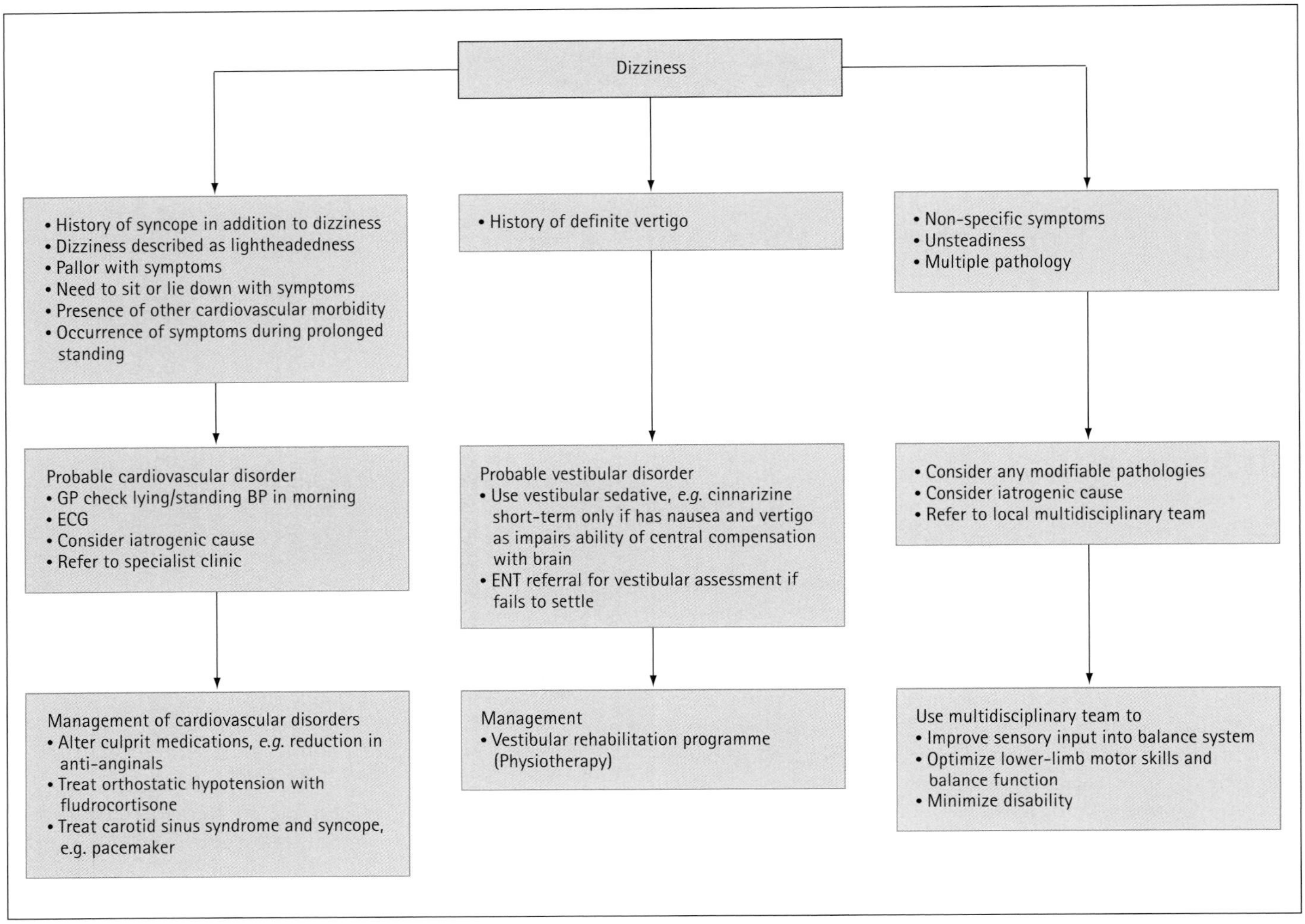

Figure 51.1 Dizziness in older patients: a scheme for basic management.

assessment as part of their evaluation protocol report an overlap between the symptoms of dizziness, syncope and falls.[15,16] Use of phasic blood pressure monitoring (digital photoplethysmography: Portapres), standardized carotid sinus massage (CSM) and head-up tilt testing has implicated three related hypotensive disorders: carotid sinus syndrome (CSS), postural hypotension and vasovagal syncope. Of 169 patients who attended a dedicated facility, over 80% presented with dizziness, usually associated with syncope and/or unexplained falls[15,16,18] (Figure 51.2). Two-thirds of these had an attributable diagnosis, usually CSS and/or orthostatic hypotension (Figure 51.3). These findings from specialist units are supported by a recent prospective study of the causes of severe dizziness in patients over 60 years of age,[3] with marked overlap between carotid sinus hypersensitivity (CSH), orthostatic hypotension and vasovagal syncope (Table 51.2). Predictors of a cardiovascular cause were dizziness described as 'lightheadedness', associated pallor, syncope, prolonged standing, the need to sit or lie down, or co-morbid cardiovascular disease.

CLINICAL PREDICTORS OF CARDIOVASCULAR DIZZINESS

Dizziness described as lightheadedness.
Associated with syncope, pallor, need to sit/lie down.
Symptoms with prolonged standing.
Comorbid cardiovascular disease.

Carotid sinus syndrome

Definition

CSS is diagnosed when CSH is demonstrated in a patient with unexplained dizziness, presyncope or syncope.[19,20] CSH describes 3 s or more of asystole (cardioinhibitory response) or a 50 mmHg fall in systolic blood pressure (vasodepressor response) following 5 s of unilateral CSM. Mixed responses

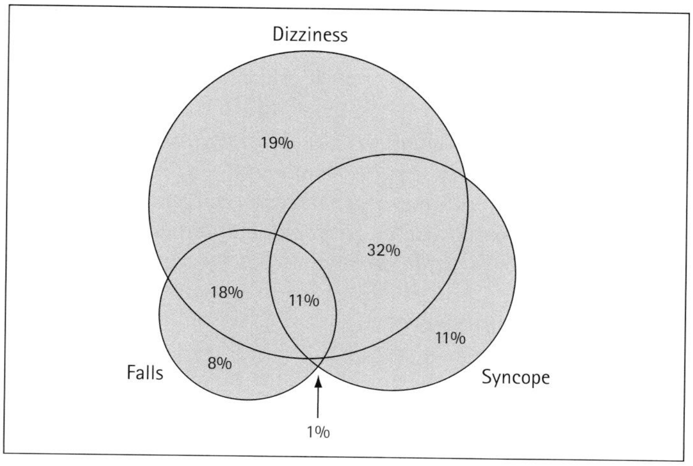

Figure 51.2 Overlap between dizziness, syncope and falls—presenting symptoms in 169 older patients who attended a dedicated facility.

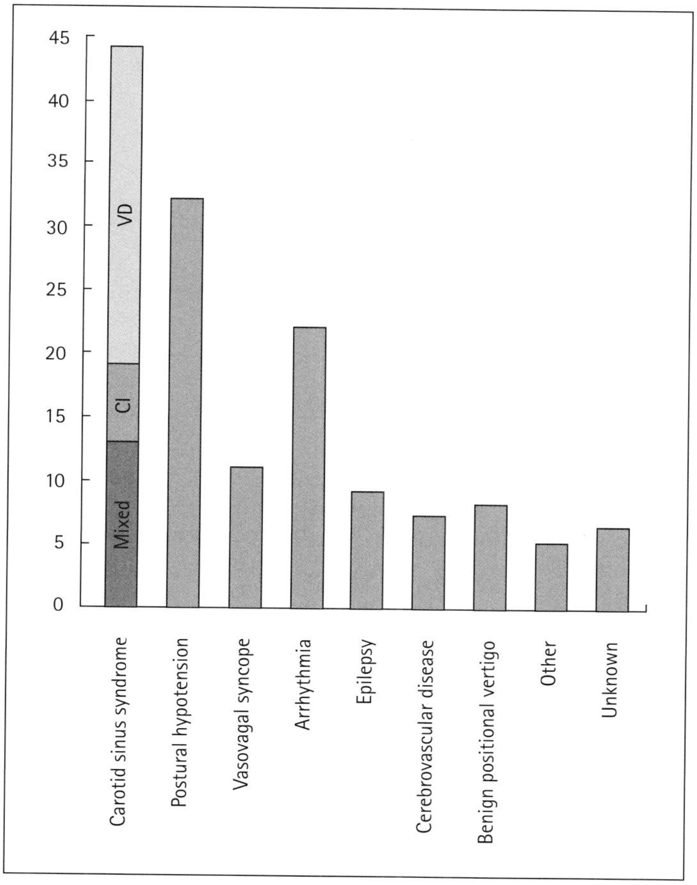

Figure 51.3 Attributable diagnoses in 169 older patients presenting to a dedicated facility with dizziness, syncope and falls.

occur if significant hypotension persists once bradycardia is abolished, either by atrioventricular sequential pacing or intravenous atropine.[21,22] A history of unexplained dizziness and/or syncope is essential, since a hypersensitive response can

Table 51.2 Cardiovascular diagnoses, peripheral vestibular disorders and central neurological disorders in 50 consecutive patients over 60 years presenting with dizziness to the general practitioner.[3]

Diagnosis	*n*
Cardiovascular diagnoses (*n* = 23)	
Total CSH alone or in combination	17
VDCSH	5
CICSH	5
Mixed carotid sinus hypersensitivity	2
Vasovagal	3
VV + VDCSH	2
VV + OH + VDCSH	2
Arrhythmia	2
Orthostatic hypotension	1
Mixed CSH + VV	1
Peripheral vestibular disorders (*n* = 17)	
Vestibular neuronitis	12
Benign paroxysmal positional vertigo	4
Menière's disease	1
Central neurological disorders (*n* = 8)	
Severe cervical spondylosis	2
Drop attacks	2
Stroke disease	2
Migraine	1
Bilateral carotid stenosis (>90%)	1
Associated diagnoses in patients in whom diagnosis remains unknown (*n* = 11)	
Abnormal Romberg	4
Abnormal gait	2
Osteoarthritis lower limbs	2

CSH, carotid sinus hypersensitivity; VDCSH, vasodepressor carotid sinus hypersensitivity; CICSH, cardioinhibitory carotid sinus hypersensitivity; VV, vasovagal syncope; OH, orthostatic hypotension.

be present in asymptomatic individuals, particularly those with coexisting cerebrovascular disease.

Epidemiology

CSS is a disease of older people,[23] especially males with comorbid ischaemic heart disease, cerebrovascular disease, peripheral vascular disease or hypertension.[24] The average age at presentation is 70 years, and it is rare below the age of 50. CSS is a frequent yet overlooked cause of dizziness, syncope and unexplained falls. It is an attributable diagnosis in 20–45% of patients presenting with these symptoms to secondary and tertiary referral centres.[15]

Clinical features

Over two-thirds of patients present with dizziness often associated with syncope and/or unexplained falls.[16] Dizziness, presyncope or syncope can be provoked by manoeuvres which mechanically stimulate the carotid sinus, such as head turning in the presence of tight neckwear or neck pathology. However, this 'Vicar's collar' phenomenon accounts for less than half of presentations. Symptoms are more commonly provoked by stimuli associated with vasovagal syncope or 'fainting'.[16] These include stress, prolonged standing, meals, or raised intra-thoracic pressure (e.g. micturition, defaecation or coughing). Symptoms show marked 'clustering', with variation in frequency both within and between individuals over time.

Pathophysiology

Pathophysiology (Figure 51.4) involves abnormal gain of the baro-reflex, probably at the brainstem level. The afferent pathway runs from the carotid sinus (at the bifurcation of the internal and external carotid arteries) via the glossopharyngeal nerve to the vagal nucleus at the brainstem. The efferent connection is via the vagus nerve to the sinus node and sympathetic nerves to peripheral vasculature. Vagal afferents from other organs are modulated by the brainstem, independent of the sinus. This may explain a hypersensitivity to stimuli unrelated to carotid sinus pressure. Asystole follows sinus arrest due to sinoatrial block and depressed sinoatrial automaticity. Complete heart block may also occur and coexists with sinus arrest in up to 70% of cases.[23] The asystolic response is abolished by atropine.

Diagnosis

Diagnosis is confirmed when symptom reproduction is associated with CSH during CSM. The procedure should be standardized and performed initially in the supine position with the neck slightly extended (Figure 51.5). Longitudinal massage is applied for 5 s over the point of maximal carotid pulsation (usually medial to the sternomastoid muscle at the level of the upper border of the thyroid cartilage) on the right and then left sides, allowing a 30 s interval between stimuli.[24] The heart rate response occurs immediately (Figure 51.6) (mean: 2 s), returns to baseline within 30 s and can be recorded using continuous surface electrocardiography. The blood pressure response lags behind, reaching a nadir at a mean of 18 s and returning to baseline by 30 s.[16] Continuous phasic blood pressure monitoring (Portapres: digital photoplethysmography) (Figure 51.7) is required to detect and monitor the vasodepressor response to CSM. Previous work using conventional mercury or digital sphygmanometry has underestimated the prevalence of vasodepressor and mixed forms of CSH, which are more common than the cardioinhibitory form (Figure 51.2).

In a third of patients, a response is only present during massage at 70° of head-up tilt[25] (Figure 51.8). Upright posture may allow easier location of the carotid sinus and/or alter baro-reflex gain. If the supine response is not diagnostic, CSM should be

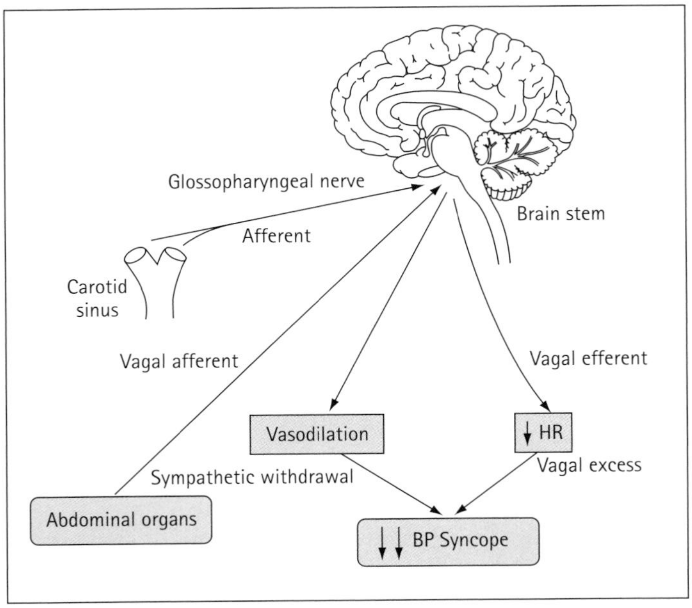

Figure 51.4 Carotid sinus massage: schematic representation of baro-receptor reflex pathways.

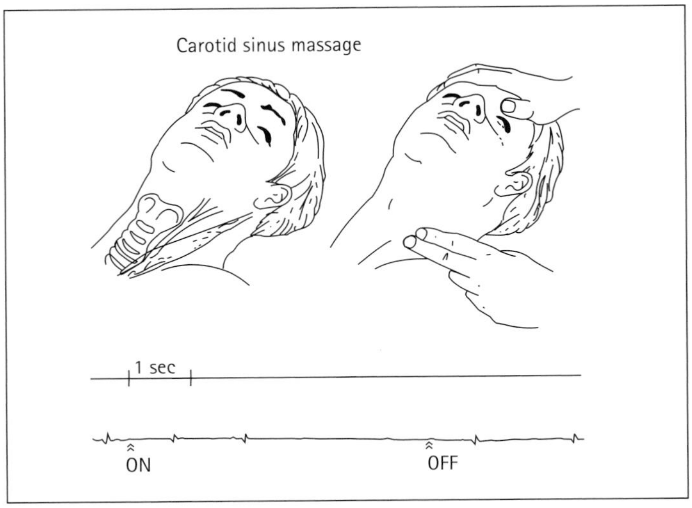

Figure 51.5 Technique of carotid sinus massage: a 5 s longitudinal massage is applied over the point of maximal carotid pulsation (usually 2 cm below the angle of the jaw at the level of the upper border of the thyroid cartilage). The procedure is repeated on the other side after a 30 s interval. Continuous observation of pulse rate (ECG recorder) and blood pressure (digital flowmetry: Portapres) is required.

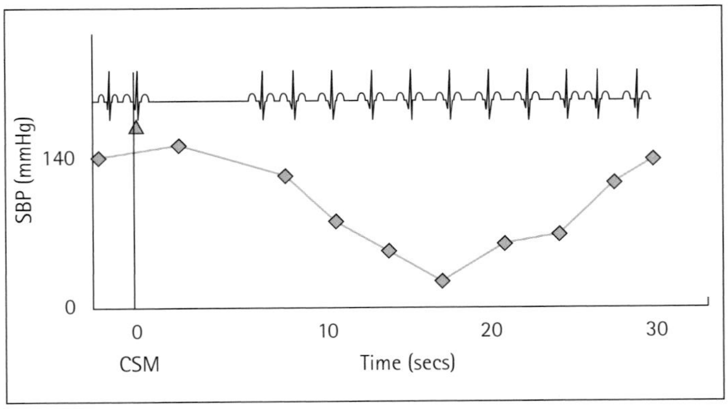

Figure 51.6 Carotid sinus massage: schematic representation of mixed carotid sinus hypersensitivity. Asystole occurs immediately while the blood pressure nadir occurs approximately 18 s later.

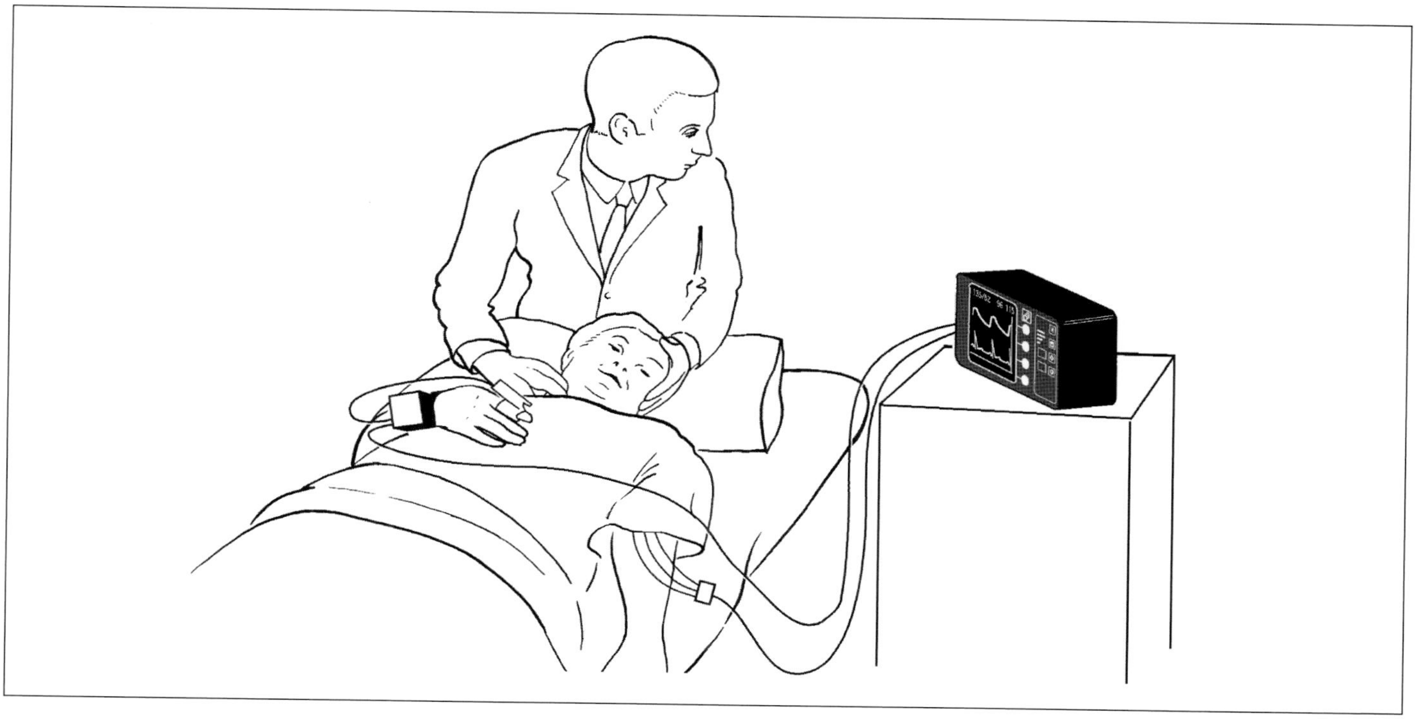

Figure 51.7 Phasic blood pressure monitoring through digital photoplethysmography. Note the ditigal cuff on the first finger of the right hand; the results of pulse, blood pressure and other parameters are visualized on the display screen.

repeated when upright. An abnormal response to CSM may not always be reproduced in those with the syndrome.[22] The procedure should be repeated if massage is negative but clinical suspicion high.

Contraindications to CSM include recent cerebral ischaemia or myocardial infarction, or previous ventricular tachyarrhythmias. Those with carotid bruits or established cerebrovascular disease may undergo CSM if clinically indicated, provided that carotid doppler ultrasonography excludes significant stenosis. Neurological complications following CSM, from arterial occlusion or embolization, are rare, provided that a standardized technique is used and exclusion criteria are respected.[26]

Management

Patients in whom the cardioinhibitory response predominates should have a review of medication. Withdrawal of rate-limiting drugs (digoxin, beta-blockers, diltiazem and others) may render them asymptomatic and CSM negative. Those with syncope in whom drugs are not implicated or cannot be stopped for medical reasons require dual chamber pacing. This abolishes syncope in over 80%, though dizziness may remain unchanged or even exacerbated.[27] Syncopal symptoms are probably converted to less severe dizzy symptoms because an intrinsic vasodepressor response persists despite treatment of the asystolic component. Symptomatic patients with a dominant vasodepressor response are more difficult to treat.[28] They may respond to conservative measures (Table 51.3) and/or drugs aimed at attenuating vasodepressor responses (Table 51.4).

Table 51.3 Conservative measures in vasodepressor syndromes.

Review of all medications
Night-time head-up tilt to 20°
Graded compression hosiery, lower limb or abdominal
Education
Avoid precipitating events/situations
Avoid sudden changes in posture/position
Avoid prolonged standing or sitting
Use evasive actions
Lying down
Limb exercises
Squatting
Know times of lowest blood pressures
Nocturnal
Early morning
Postprandial
Limb exercises before major changes in position/posture
Diet
Caffeine–3-5 cups of strong tea or coffee per day
Salt–high sodium diet
Fluids–drink around 2 l per day
Alcohol–avoid or reduce
Avoid heavy meals (small and frequent)

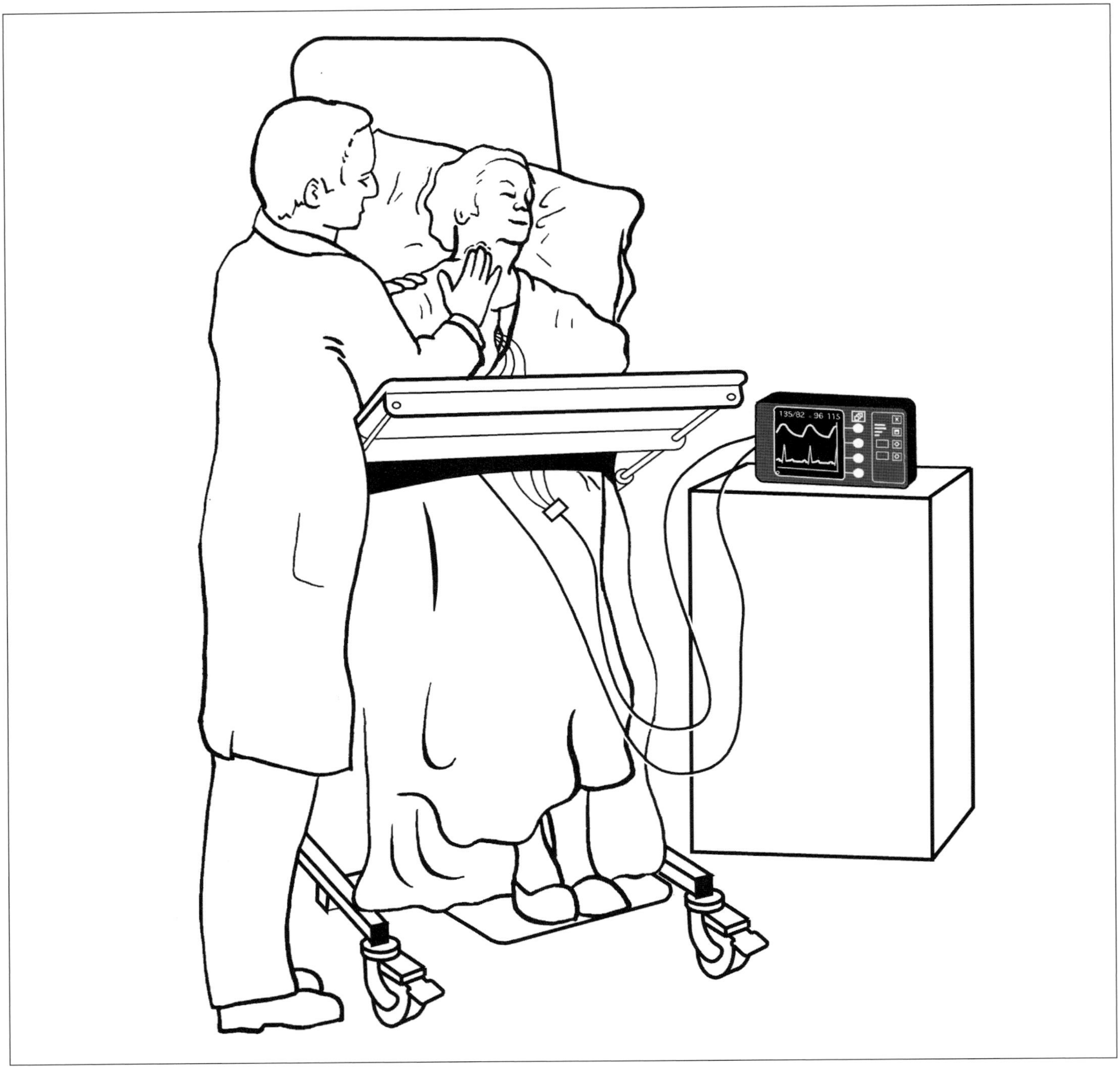

Figure 51.8 Carotid sinus massage at 70° of head-up tilt. One-third of patients are positive only when tilted, probably due to improved anatomical access to the carotid sinus.

Vasovagal syndrome

Definition

Vasovagal syndrome (VVS) describes episodic hypotension and bradycardia resulting in dizziness, pre-syncope or syncope,[29] usually following a classical precipitating event or situation. Both symptoms and haemodynamic changes should be reproducible on head-up tilt testing.[30] As with CSS, the condition may be defined in terms of vasodepressor, cardioinhibitory or mixed responses (Table 51.5).

Prevalence

VVS classically affects younger people between the ages of 20 and 50 years[31] but is now increasingly reported in the elderly.[32] Primary VVS is the commonest cause of vasovagal syncope in

Table 51.4 Drugs most commonly prescribed for the treatment of vasodepressor syndromes.

Drug	Doses	Mechanism(s)	Adverse effects
Fludrocortisone	0.1–1.0 mg (single dose)	Plasma and intracellular volume expander, direct vasoconstrictor, sensitizes α-adrenergic receptors to noradrenaline	Supine hypertension, oedema, heart failure, hypokalaemia
Beta-blockers	Drug dependent—e.g. metoprolol 50 mg tds, atenolol 25–100 mg od	Modulates catecholeamine surge, inhibits Bezold Jarisch reflex, prevents vasodilatation (β-adrenergic blockade)	Lethargy, bronchoconstriction, bradycardia, conduction deficits
Midodrine	2.5–15mg tds	α-Adrenergic agonist (resistance vessels)	Pilomotor reaction, GIT effects, cardiovascular toxicity
SSRIs	Drug dependent—e.g. paroxetine 10–20 mg od	Downregulation of postsynaptic serotoninergic receptors	Peptic ulcer, GIT bleeding, renal impairment
NSAIDs	Drug dependent—e.g. ibuprofen 600mg tds	Prevent vasodilatation (prostaglandin synthetase inhibitors)	Peptic ulcer, gastrointestinal bleeding, renal impairment

SSRI, selective serotonin receptor inhibitor; NSAIDs, non-steroidal anti-inflammatory drug; GIT, gastrointestinal tract.

Table 51.5 Classification of vasovagal syncope.

Type 1 Mixed	Heart rate falls during syncope but the ventricular rate is never less than 40 beats/min, or falls to less than 40 beats/min for less than 10 s with or without asystole of less than 3. Blood pressure falls prior to the fall in heart rate
Type 2A Cardioinhibitory	Heart rate falls at syncope to a ventricular rate less than 40 beats/min for more than 10 s or asystole occurs for more than 30 s. Blood pressure again falls prior to the heart rate fall
Type 2B Cardioinhibitory	Heart rate falls at syncope to a ventricular rate less than 40 beats/min for more than 10 s or asystole occurs for more than 3 s. Blood pressure falls to hypotensive levels (<80 mmHg systolic) only at or after the onset of rapid and severe heart rate fall as previously defined
Type 3 Pure vasodepressor	Heart rate does not fall more than 10% from its peak at the time of syncope. Blood pressure falls to precipitate syncope
Exceptions	The main exceptions to this classification include chronotropic incompetence, an excessive heart rate rise (>130 beats/min) during tilt, and where carotid sinus hypersensitivity is present

Source: Sutton R, Petersen M, Brignole M et al. Proposed classification for tilt induced vasovagal syncope. *Eur J Card Pacing Electrophysiol* 1992; **3**: 180–3.

all age groups, but hypotensive medications, particularly cardiovascular and psychotropic drugs, are implicated in up to 40% of older patients.[2–4]

Pathophysiology

On upright posture, gravity pools around 700 ml of blood in lower limb and splanchnic venous capacitance vessels. This relative central hypovolaemia causes a slight reduction in systolic blood pressure which initiates arterial baro-reflexes. The result is an increase in sympathetic efferent activity and a suppression of vagal outflow to the heart and peripheral vessels. Blood pressure is maintained by the subsequent increase in peripheral vascular resistance through alpha-mediated arteriolar vasoconstriction. Beta-mediated increases in heart rate and myocardial contractility also contribute. The release of several rapidly acting humoral factors such as renin, angiotensin and noradrenaline enhances these effects. Disruption or distortion of this arterial baro-reflex arc results in vasovagal syncope.[33] The precise mechanism remains uncertain but is thought to involve the Bezold–Jarisch reflex (Figure 51.9). Orthostasis (or head-up tilt) reduces venous return and systolic blood pressure. This results in an intense sympathetic response, catecholamine surge (mainly adrenaline) and a small, relatively empty, left ventricular cavity.[34] Vigorous contraction of a small left ventricle initiates the reflex via intracardiac vagal mechanoreceptors. Brain-stem synapsis with vagal efferents produces bradycardia, sympathetic withdrawal and peripheral vasodilatation, leading to profound hypotension and syncope. Other neurohumoral responses may play a part.[35] Serotonin and β-endorphin levels rise before syncope and may initiate central sympatho-inhibitory responses. The adrenaline surge may itself evoke β-adrenergic dilatation of resistance vessels. Central provocation of vasovagal syncope in response to intense emotion, pain and other noxious stimuli may be modulated directly through a limbic sympathoinhibitory pathway or indirectly through the amygdala and its connection with brainstem autonomic nuclei.[36]

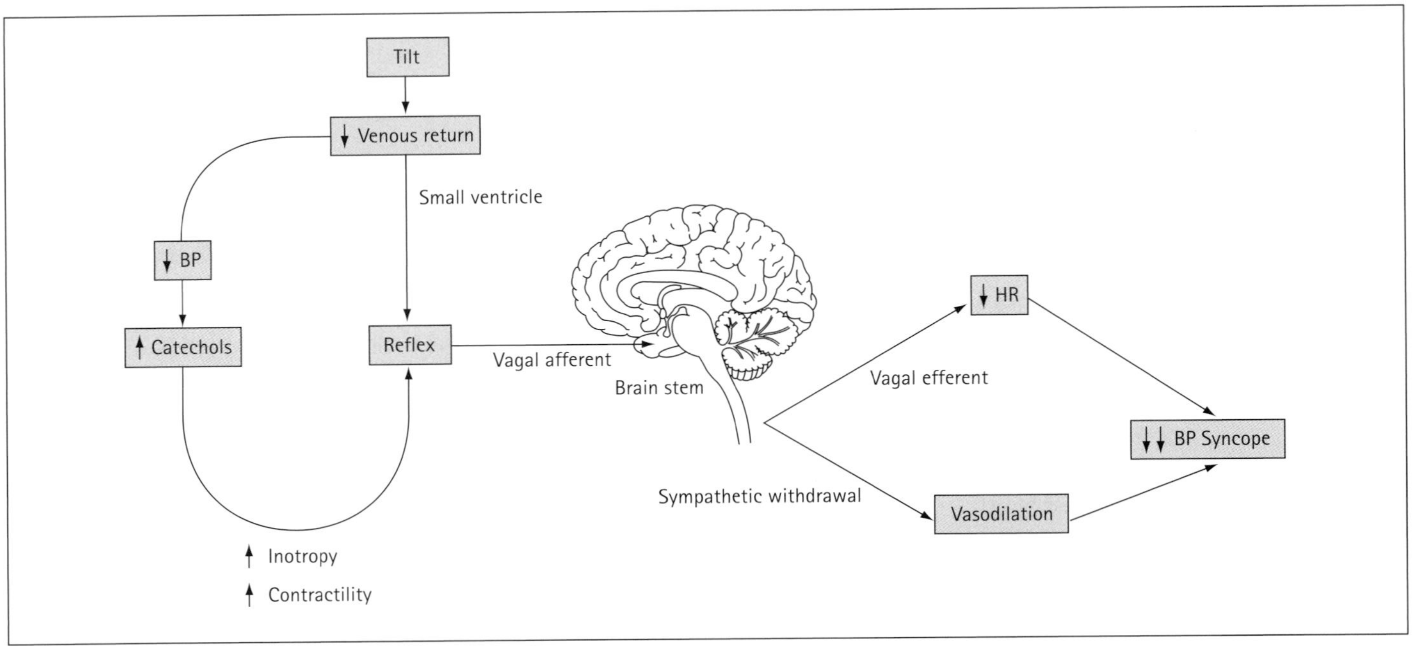

Figure 51.9 Bezold–Jarisch reflex: schematic representation (see text).

Clinical presentation

Symptoms usually (but not exclusively) occur when upright.[35] Classical precipitants include emotional stress, anxiety, exercise, heavy meals, trauma, prolonged standing, a hot stuffy environment, pain or its anticipation. Specific situations may precede an event. These include valsalva manoeuvres implicit in defaecation, straining, coughing or micturition. Prodromal symptoms are common. They include severe dizziness, unsteadiness, vertigo, visual deficits, extreme fatigue, weakness, diaphoresis, nausea, headache, visual or auditory hallucinations and focal neurological deficits. A significant prodrome may warn of impending syncope and allow implementation of successful evasive strategies.

Syncope is associated with extreme pallor, diaphoresis and dilated pupils. Myoclonus, opisthotonos or tonic clonic limb movements (the 'anoxic' or 'convulsive' syncope) may occur. Events are usually brief and recovery rapid. Sequelae include nausea, vomiting, headache, malaise, lethargy, hypersomnolence, confusion and disorientation. Events may be 'clustered', with several occurring together followed by a symptom-free period of days, weeks or months.

Older people with VVS may present atypically.[15] Non-prodromal symptoms and retrograde amnesia associated with cognitive deficits, arthritis and sensory impairment may result in acute presentation with significant injury following a 'fall' or 'drop attack'. If syncope occurs, tonic clonic activity, urinary and/or faecal incontinence and a prolonged post-syncopal state are common, since major organs are usually closer to a failure threshold.

Diagnosis

The diagnosis of VVS should not be one of exclusion. The head-up tilt is the gold standard test for vasovagal syndrome.[37] Symptoms evoked are compatible with those of spontaneous vasovagal events. Prodromal symptoms, haemodynamic responses and changes in plasma catecholamines are almost identical. Estimates of sensitivity (80–90%) and specificity (35–85%) compare favourably with standard cardiological tests, although there is no 'gold standard' tool for comparison, and differences in tilt protocol and haemodynamic monitoring techniques may critically affect results. Reproducibility (62–85%) is better in patients who are severely symptomatic or tilted within 30 days of their last syncopal event. False-positive tests occur in less than 10% of normal patients and may represent enhanced susceptibility to vasovagal events. Exact symptom reproduction must therefore accompany haemodynamic changes if a diagnosis of VVS is to be made with confidence. The test should be mandatory in the investigation of patients with unexplained dizziness, collapse, syncope or seizures. It is also useful in the investigation of elderly patients with unexplained falls, recurrent vague 'neurological' symptoms (often labelled as a 'transient ischaemic attack'), and possible psychogenic or hyperventilation syncope or presyncope. The test is generally safe, but relative contraindications include severe left ventricular outflow obstruction, and mitral valve or proximal coronary artery stenosis.[38]

The test generally uses the physiotherapist's standard tilt table with an electronic foot plate to elevate and lower the bed. The optimal protocol is still a subject of debate. The Newcastle protocol favoured by the authors is described in detail elsewhere.[35] Briefly, blood pressure and heart rate are monitored continuously, initially with the patient supine for 15 min and thereafter during head-up tilt to 70° for 40 min (Figure 51.10). Continuous phasic blood pressure measurements (digital flowmetry; Portapres) are used in preference to standard or automated sphygmomanometry to detect rapid blood pressure changes (Figure 51.7). The test is considered positive only if the patient's original symptoms are reproduced and accompanied by hypotension, bradycardia or both. If initial testing is non-diagnostic but clinical suspicion remains, then further tilting with intravenous cannulation, pharmacological (sublingual glyceryl trinitrate or intravenous isoprenaline) provocation or lower-body negative pressure should be considered.

Treatment

Vasodepressor symptoms may respond to conservative therapy (Table 51.3). Awareness of periods of relative hypotension (at night, early morning, postprandially), avoiding precipitants, and reviewing culprit hypotensive medications may relieve symptoms. Compression hosiery may be useful initially but often proves cumbersome, impracticable or aesthetically unacceptable. Prodromal symptoms should prompt evasive strategies, e.g. lying down, limb exercises, squatting. The patient has usually learned these through experience prior to presentation.

If symptoms persist or are non-prodromal, then additional measures are required.[39] Dual-chamber cardiac pacing is usually reserved for those few patients with malignant VVS.[39] This comprises non-prodromal, frequent, severe or disabling symptoms associated with profound bradycardia (less than 40 beats/min for greater than 10 s) or asystole (greater than 3 s).

Beta-blockers such as metoprolol or atenolol are useful first-line drugs (Table 51.4). Their therapeutic effects are at least partly explained by modulation of the catecholamine surge which occurs prior to syncope. Fludrocortisone is limited by poor tolerability and adverse effects, particularly in older patients, and although prescribed, has not been evaluated in appropriately sized randomized control studies. Midodrine, an alpha-agonist, is currently being evaluated but is contraindicated in those with significant cardiovascular disease and women of child-bearing age.[40] Serotonin reuptake inhibitors such as fluoxetine, paroxetine or sertraline minimize sympatho-inhibitory serotoninergic activity prior to syncope by down-regulating postsynaptic serotonin receptors. Non-steroidal anti-inflammatory drugs may be useful in some patients.

Orthostatic hypotension

Definition

Orthostatic (postural) hypotension (OH) has been arbitrarily defined as a 20 mmHg fall in systolic blood pressure or 10 mmHg fall in diastolic pressure on assuming upright posture.[41,42] However, smaller, often transient changes in blood pressure

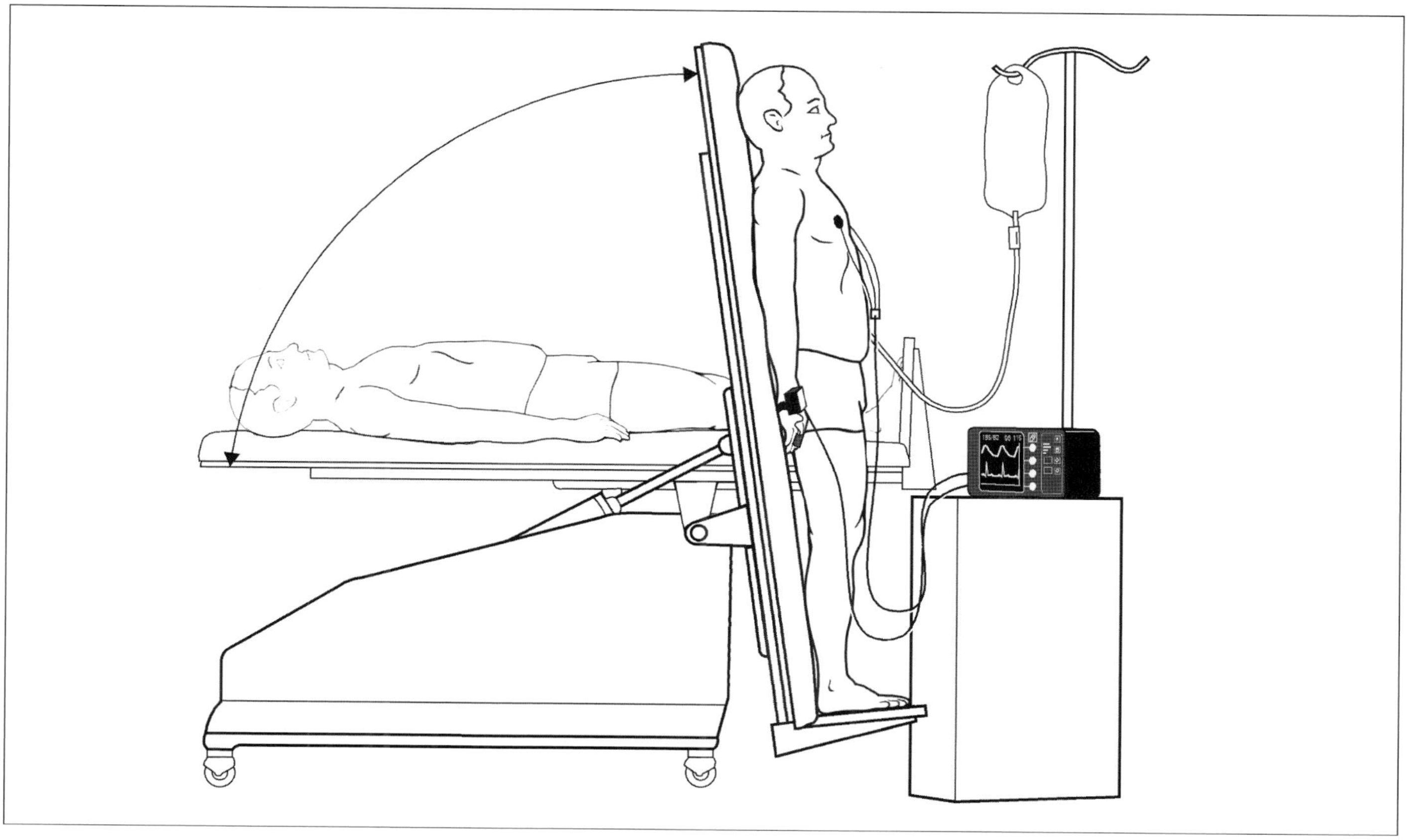

Figure 51.10 The 70° head-up tilt test. Note the digital cuff (right hand) for phasic blood pressure monitoring and the limb leads for ECG recording.

may be significant, particularly in older people with comorbid hypertension and cerebrovascular disease.[43] Conversely, large falls in postural blood pressure may remain asymptomatic in young patients. In practical terms, therefore, diagnosis depends upon the ability to demonstrate a postural fall in blood pressure on active (unassisted) standing associated with symptom reproduction.

Prevalence and the effects of ageing

Older people are much more susceptible to OH.[44] Prevalence in healthy, normotensive, elderly subjects is around 7% but rises in the general elderly population to 24%.[44–46] This is because comorbidity exacerbates age-related physiological changes and blunts compensatory baro-reflex responses.[43] A blunting of the initial heart rate response to OH is compensated for by increased peripheral vascular resistance. Cardiac output is maintained unless the disease process is advanced or compensatory mechanisms are complicated by medication or comorbidity such as neurological disorders, cardiovascular disease (including hypertension)and cerebrovascular disease. Hypertension impairs baro-reflex sensitivity and reduces ventricular compliance. In patients with OH, the normal pattern of 24 h blood pressure behaviour can be reversed. Elderly people with OH are consequently susceptible to symptoms during orthostatic change in the early hours of the morning, on rising from bed, or after meals (Figure 51.11). Hypertension also alters cerebral autoregulation. Symptoms such as dizziness and syncope can occur with even small, transient drops in blood pressure. In older patients with OH and supine hypertension, coexisting cerebrovascular disease further lowers the threshold for cerebral ischaemia and exaggerates symptoms.

In contrast, younger patients retain the ability to maintain cerebral blood flow for systemic blood pressure changes ranging from 90–160 mmHg.[47,48] Severe orthostatic blood pressure changes are asymptomatic or produce only minor symptoms such as dizziness, transient visual disturbance or neck and back discomfort, often in a 'coathanger' distribution. A high index of clinical suspicion is needed to diagnose OH in younger patients.

Pathophysiology

OH results from a transient or persistent failure of the arterial baro-reflex to adapt to postural change.[46] On standing, gravity pools around 500–700 ml of blood in the lower limbs, splanchnic and pulmonary circulations. Venous return falls rapidly and reduces cardiac output and blood pressure. Prolonged standing exacerbates this through interstitial fluid shift and haemoconcentration. The resultant relative hypotension stimulates baro-receptors in the carotid sinus and aortic arch, which activate sympathetic and inhibit parasympathetic activity. Catecholamine release has a net positive inotropic and chronotropic effect, minimizing the fall in cardiac output. Reduced blood volume, cardiac dysfunction, abnormal baro-reflex gain, excessive peripheral blood pooling and impaired sympathetic or parasympathetic activity may precipitate OH.

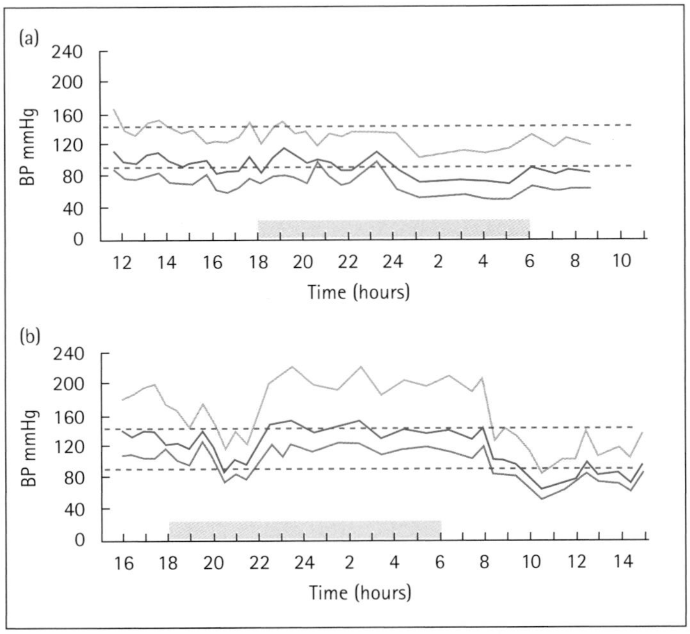

Figure 51.11 Examples of 24-h ambulatory blood pressure profiles: (a) normotensive with nocturnal dip; (b) reversal of diurnal rhythm (nocturnal hypertension) with profound early-morning postural hypotension.

These stresses may result from age-related physiological changes, age-associated diseases or hypotensive drugs.

Causes

Autonomic failure is the commonest pathological mechanism for OH.[49] Underlying causes are listed in Table 51.6. Three primary autonomic failure syndromes are recognized: pure autonomic failure (PAF) (previously idiopathic orthostatic hypotension), multiple system atrophy (MSA) and autonomic failure associated with idiopathic Parkinson's disease (IPD).

Pure autonomic failure presents exclusively with dysautonomia, while the other conditions are distinguished by the presence of additional neurological signs.

Patients with IPD may display autonomic failure, though this is mild and occurs relatively late in the condition. Contributory factors include drugs (for both IPD and comorbid conditions), age-related dysautonomia and autonomic neuropathy complicating other comorbid conditions (e.g. diabetes). MSA is an adult-onset sporadic neurodegenerative condition of unknown cause which is phenotypically diverse and around one-tenth as common as IPD. The median age of onset is around 60 years. It may present with autonomic involvement (Shy–Drager syndrome), with primarily parkinsonian features (striatonigral degeneration type) or with mainly cerebellar and/or pyramidal problems (olivopontocerebellar type). Eventually, features of all three types may coexist, but in the early stages, if parkinsonism predominates, there may be considerable difficulty discriminating MSA from IPD. This is important, since treatment, complications and prognosis are different.

Table 51.6 Causes of autonomic failure.

Primary autonomic failure
- Chronic
  - Pure autonomic failure
  - MSA
    - with Parkinsonian features
    - with cerebellar and pyramidal features
    - with multiple features (combination of above)
- Acute or subacute dysautonomias

Secondary autonomic failure or dysfunction
- Central
  - Brain tumours, especially of the third ventricle or posterior fossa
  - Multiple sclerosis
  - Syringobulbia
  - Elderly
- Spinal
  - Spinal transverse myelitis
  - Transverse myelitis
  - Syringomyelia
  - Spinal tumours
- Peripheral
  - Afferent
    - Tabes dorsalis
    - Holmes–Adie syndrome
    - Guillain–Barré syndrome
  - Efferent
    - Diabetes mellitus
    - Amyloidosis
    - Surgery (such as splanchnicectomy)
    - Dopamine-β-hydroxylase deficiency
    - Nerve growth factor deficiency
  - Afferent/efferent
    - Familial dysautonomia (Riley–Day syndrome)
- Miscellaneous
  - Autoimmune and collagen disorders
  - Renal failure
  - Neoplasia
  - Human immunodeficiency virus infection

Drugs

Neurally mediated syncope
- Vasovagal syncope
  - Carotid sinus hypersensitivity

Source: Adapted from Mathias CJ. Primary autonomic failure in association with other neurological features–the syndromes of Shy–Drager and multiple system atrophy. In: Kenny RA, ed. *Syncope in the Older Patients: Causes and Investigations of Syncope and Falls*. London: Chapman and Hall Medical, 1996: 137–54.

Helpful features differentiating MSA from IPD are given in Table 51.7.

Drugs are a major cause of OH in the elderly.[50] The list of drugs with hypotensive actions is long, and a simple review of medication may be curative.

Table 51.7 Differentiation of multiple system atrophy (MSA) and idiopathic Parkinson's disease: features favouring MSA.

MSA
- Marked OH ± abnormal AFTs
- Levodopa unresponsiveness
- Erectile impotence
- Urinary symptoms
- Mild pyramidal/cerebellar signs
- Nocturnal stridor

OH, orthostatic hypotension; AFTs, autonomic function tests.

Clinical features

In a consecutive series of 40 older patients with OH, over half presented with dizziness, often associated with syncope and/or unexplained falls[17] or 'drop attacks'. In general, symptoms are related to the consequences of low blood flow rates following orthostasis. Other presentations therefore include presyncope, visual disturbance, malaise, lethargy, weakness, neck and back pain in a 'coathanger' distribution, claudication and angina. Precipitating factors include rapid changes in position or posture, prolonged recumbency, vasoactive drugs and 'vagal' stimuli such as a warm environment, raised intrathoracic pressure (coughing, defaecation, micturition) and physical exertion. Patients may report associated dysautonomic symptoms or display focal neurological signs suggestive of MSA.

Guidelines from the American College of Neurology have recommended changes in excess of 20 mmHg in systolic blood pressure during 3 min of standing as diagnostic of OH.[42]

Diagnosis

Diagnosis often depends on symptom reproduction when blood pressure falls during orthostasis. Sphygmomanometer measurement may be as sensitive as more sophisticated phasic blood pressure measurement, and active standing as diagnostic as head-up tilting.[17] Patients should be supine for at least 10 min and erect recordings taken at minute intervals for 3 min during standing using conventional sphygmanometry. In practice, this method is cumbersome. The author's preference is to use continuous phasic blood pressure measurements (digital photoplethysmography: Finapres or Portapres) for 3 min. In this way, rapid or transient changes in blood pressure can be recorded more conveniently. Reproducibility of OH is poor and depends upon time of measurement and autonomic integrity. Repeated measurements may be required in the early morning, 30–60 min after a meal and after exercise.

Baseline tests such as cortisol level, synacthen test, and glucose will exclude secondary causes of OH. Twenty-four-hour ambulatory blood pressure monitoring is useful in defining disturbances in diurnal rhythm and the effects of supine posture, meals and medication. Twenty-four-hour readings can guide therapeutic interventions. Autonomic function tests should also be performed.

Management

Management aims to improve both cerebral and peripheral perfusion.[43] A simple review of medication with rationalization of vasoactive drugs may be sufficient. Conservative measures may help if the cause of OH remains elusive (Table 51.3). Elevation of the head of the bed to 20° during sleep lowers renal artery perfusion pressure, thus activating the renin–angiotensin system. This conserves salt and water, thus increasing intravascular volume. These changes reduce natriuresis and diuresis and elevate morning blood pressures. Patients should be educated about 'vulnerable times' when blood pressure is lowest and take note of possible precipitating factors. Leg exercises before standing can minimize the effects of prolonged recumbency. Graduated pressure hosiery such as stockings or abdominal binders reduce venous pooling but may be poorly tolerated or of only temporary benefit. Increased fluid and salt intake protect against relative volume depletion. Small, frequent meals will reduce the likelihood of postprandial hypotension due to vasodilating effects of insulin and splanchnic pooling. Caffeine is a potent vasoconstrictor of capacitance vessels. An intake of 3–5 cups of strong tea or coffee per day, particularly in the early morning or after meals, may ameliorate symptoms, although haemodynamic tolerance can develop. If conservative treatment fails or there is autonomic failure, then drug treatment is necessary. More than one drug may be required. Therapeutic options are detailed in Table 51.4.

Postural tachycardia syndrome (POTS)

Some patients with orthostatic intolerance do not have significant OH on active standing or head-up tilt testing. Postural tachycardia syndrome (POTS) describes the reproduction of orthostatic symptoms associated with a heart rate increase of >30 beats min (or a maximum heart rate of 120 beats min or greater) in the absence of profound hypotension or generalized autonomic neuropathy.[51,52] The condition usually affects young females and may follow a viral illness or significant weight loss. Patients often describe significant autonomic (profound tremulousness, anxiety, restlessness, palpitations) and somatic (headache, chest wall pain, flushes, chills, fatigue, lethargy) symptoms in addition to those of orthostatic intolerance. Symptoms may be clustered or cyclical and are often mistaken for anxiety, panic attacks, chronic fatigue syndrome, effort syndrome or Da Costa's syndrome. The condition may represent an incomplete or mild autonomic neuropathy. Cardiovascular responses to head-up tilt testing are abnormal.[53] Heart rate usually rises quickly, often with marked variability, to values of between 120 and 170/min within 2–5 min of tilting. Blood pressure response may be normotensive, hypertensive or mildly hypotensive if there is significant venous pooling or relative volume depletion. Autonomic function tests usually define partial peripheral deficits affecting mainly sympathetic innervation. Cardiac innervation remains intact in most patients although β-receptor supersensitivity is described. Patients with peripheral α-receptor hyposensitivity and cardiac β-receptor supersensitivity seem particularly prone to syncope. Defective α-mediated peripheral vasoconstriction limits the increase in total peripheral resistance on assuming upright posture, while β-receptor supersensitivity increases cardiac contractility and may initiate the Bezold–Jarisch reflex. Treatment remains largely empirical, although it may be guided by cardiovascular responses and the type of autonomic dysfunction.[54] Patients with profound tachycardia (>130 beats min) are usually β-receptor supersensitive, and beta blockers are therefore useful. Starting doses should be small, since supersensitivity can exacerbate adverse effects. Excessive lethargy and postural hypotension may occur with conventional doses. Patients with peripheral adrenergic failure may respond to an alpha-blocker (e.g. midodrine). Patients with unstable hypertensive responses to head up tilt may respond to drugs such as phenobarbitone or clonidine at doses which diminish central sympathetic outflow. Those few patients with autonomic deconditioning due to relative volume depletion, prolonged immobility or bedrest often respond to conservative measures (Table 51.3) and fludrocortisone. The natural history of the syndrome remains undefined. In some patients, particularly those with autonomic deconditioning, the disorder may be temporary or show improvement. In others, autonomic dysfunction may show insidious progression over many years.

Dizziness may be a presenting feature of the chronic fatigue syndrome (CFS). Recent work suggests that a partial autonomic neuropathy causes intermittent reductions in cardiac output at rest and/or diminished blood pressure responses to psychosocial stress. The resulting low flow states may be insufficient to support metabolic functions. This may partly explain the heterogeneous nature of CFS and its overlap with postural orthostatic tachycardia.[54,55]

Conduction defects, arrhythmias and outflow obstruction

Bradyarrhythmias and conduction deficits account for most dizzy, presyncopal or syncopal arrhythmic events in older people. These events commonly manifest as sinus node disease or 'sick sinus syndrome', said to be present when sinus rate is inappropriately slow for the physiological conditions prevailing at the time.[56]

Most patients with the sinus node disease or second- or third-degree atrioventricular block are asymptomatic. Incidence is therefore difficult to assess, but is estimated at around 0.2%.[57] The condition usually follows a long erratic course, with an asymptomatic phase detectable on Holter monitoring for many years before clinical presentation.[58] Symptoms are due to the haemodynamic consequences of sinus bradycardia, sinus arrest, sinoatrial block and escape tachyarrhythmias (the so-called 'tachy-brady syndrome').[59] Episodic dizziness, lightheadedness and syncope are the commonest presentations, although subtle features such as fatigue, mild heart failure and intellectual impairment are common in elderly patients with comorbid ischaemic heart and cerebrovascular disease. Palpitations may be prominent if escape tachyarrhythmias such as atrial fibrillation, atrial flutter or atrial tachycardia dominate the clinical picture.

The pathogenesis of the condition is thought to be a combination of age-related sclerosis of the sinus node and comorbid heart disease.[60] The artery to the sinus node is too small to be affected by atherosclerosis. Other conditions such as myocarditis, vasculitis and infiltrations such as haemachromatosis and cardiac amyloid may be implicated.

A high index of suspicion is often needed to make the diagnosis. A 12-lead ECG may provide some clues (in the form of sinus bradycardia, sinoatrial block or underlying ischaemic heart disease) but is often completely normal. Once suspected, the diagnosis is confirmed by ambulatory heart rate monitoring and/or intracardiac electrophysiological studies.

Treatment includes pacemaker implant for the bradycardic component and in some cases antiarrhythmic drugs to control intermittent tachycardia.

One of the commonest causes of syncope in the elderly is failure of atrioventricular (AV) conduction. This can occur as an isolated lesion of the conduction system or as part of a more global abnormality of electrical impulse formation. Electrical block can occur at any point in the specialized conduction system. AV block is classified into two categories—supra-HIS (AV node and proximal HIS bundle) and infra HIS (distal HIS bundle and bundle branches or fascicles).[61] During AV conduction failure, the more proximal the level of block, the more reliable, rapid and therefore better tolerated the ventricular escape rhythm. Although both locations of block may cause symptoms of dizziness and syncope, supra-HIS block is generally more benign than infra-HIS block. In general, if block is established on ECG or by intracardiac electrophysiology, pacemakers are required, whether patients only have symptoms of dizziness or also of syncope.[62] First-degree block is present when there is intact AV conduction but the PR interval is prolonged to more than 200 ms on ECG limb leads. Second-degree block is present when ventricular complexes do not always follow atrial depolarization and beats are 'dropped'. Third-degree block is known as complete heart block and occurs when no atrial depolarization conducts to the ventricles.

Most tachyarrhythmias, except supraventricular tachycardia (both AV reciprocating tachycardia and AV nodal reentrant tachycardia) occur more frequently in the elderly and, if sustained, are less well tolerated.[63] If underlying tachyarrhythmia is suspected as a cause of symptoms, referral for detailed cardiological assessment is necessary.[64,65]

Treatment options for symptomatic tachyarrhythmias include antiarrhythmic drugs and radiofrequency ablation of accessory pathways. Most antiarrhythmic agents can be proarrhythmic and should be used with care. Patients with combined tachy and brady arrhythmias or conduction defects require pacing before starting antiarrhythmic drug therapy. Pacing modes should be selected with care, the most physiological system for the individual patient being preferred.[66]

Cardiovascular conditions causing ventricular outflow obstruction or severely reduced cardiac output may present with dizziness, presyncope or syncope.[67] Symptoms are usually related to exertion but other stresses, such as postural change, OH, vasodilatation or arrhythmia may precipitate events at rest. Aortic stenosis is the commonest structural heart condition. It mainly affects older people through age-related calcification of the valve. Hypertrophic obstructive cardiomyopathy (HOCM) is also being increasingly recognized in older populations. The two conditions have important clinical similarities: a systolic murmur may be the only clinical feature; classical peripheral signs may be completely absent (due to underlying atherosclerosis of the peripheral vessels) and there is a significant risk of sudden death if undetected or untreated. Two-dimensional echocardiography and doppler are needed to confirm diagnosis and will usually assess severity in experienced hands. Obstruction of a prosthetic valve, left-sided atrial tumours (usually a myxoma) and intracardiac thrombus are rare causes of dizziness due to mechanical obstruction. A high degree of clinical suspicion is required for diagnosis, and an unexplained diastolic murmur should alert the physician. Two-dimensional echocardiography may not be sufficiently sensitive, and transoesophageal echocardiography may be required to visualize these conditions. Echocardiography should be performed in any patient presenting with dizziness and/or a murmur to exclude these conditions before proceeding to further provocative tests.

INVESTIGATION OF CARDIOVASCULAR DIZZINESS

Electrocardiography.
Blood pressure and heart rate measurements during standing, head-up tilt, autonomic function tests.
Ambulatory heart rate monitoring.
External or internal loop recorder.
Echocardiography.
Exercise stress testing.
Intracardiac electrophysiological studies.

Non-cardiovascular causes of dizziness

Dizziness in acute medical illness

Dizziness may be a non-specific presentation of acute or subacute medical conditions causing hypotension, cerebral hypoperfusion, hyperventilation or vestibular disturbance. Older people are especially vulnerable, since some organs may operate on the threshold of failure. Major infection, anaemia or acute blood loss, pulmonary embolism, aortic dissection, cerebrovascular disease, metabolic disturbance and adverse drug reactions may all present with dizziness. There are usually other associated symptoms and signs suggesting diagnosis; management is that of the underlying condition.

Non-cardiovascular medical causes of chronic or recurrent dizziness

Peripheral vestibular and psychogenic causes of dizziness dominate in younger people.[11,13] Peripheral vestibular disorders are discussed elsewhere (Chapter 48). Anxiety, depression and panic disorders cause dizziness by hyperventilation, adverse effects of antidepressant drugs or comorbidity. Psychogenic dizziness may be difficult to prove and is often a diagnosis of exclusion. Reproduction of symptoms on head-up tilt testing with overbreathing, stable haemodynamics and an alkalotic, hypocapnoeic, arterial blood gas profile suggests psychogenic (hyperventilation) dizziness or presyncope.[37] Other miscellaneous conditions causing dizziness in younger patients include anorexia nervosa or chronic fatigue syndrome. The latter is particularly heterogeneous and may overlap with the postural tachycardia syndrome.[51,52]

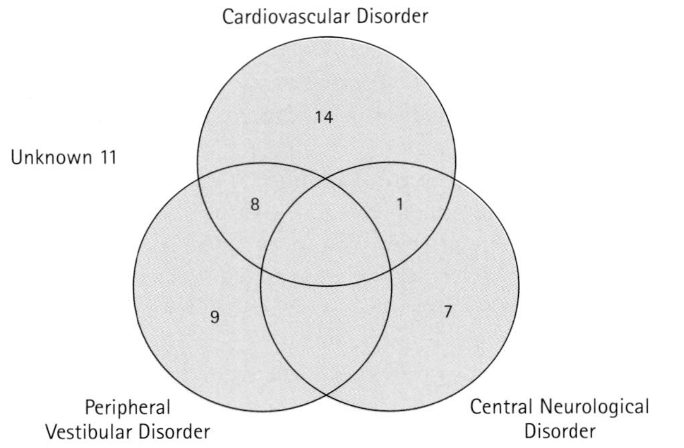

Figure 51.12 Causes of dizziness in 50 consecutive patients presenting to primary care physicians. (Reproduced with permission from Lawson et al. Diagnosis of geriatric patients with severe dizziness. *J Am Geriatr Soc* 1999; **47**: 12–17.[3])

DIZZINESS IN YOUNGER PATIENTS

Is commonly psychogenic and/or vestibular.
Diagnosis of OH requires a high index of suspicion.
A non-medical cause is suggested by:
- Absence of presyncopal or syncopal symptoms.
- Dizzy supine as well as standing.
- No OH or POTS on repeated active stand or head-up tilt.
- An associated psychiatric disorder.
- Head-up tilt with symptom reproduction, hyperventilation and an alkalotic hypocarbic blood gas profile during symptoms.

DIZZINESS IN OLDER PEOPLE

Non-specific presentation of acute medical illness.
Overlaps with syncope and falls.
Retrograde amnesia for events.
Lightheadedness predicts a cardiovascular cause.
True vertigo predicts a vestibular cause.
Cardiovascular causes are the commonest attributable medical cause.
Common non-cardiovascular causes: drugs, peripheral vestibular and central neurological disorders.
Psychogenic causes are rare.
Multifactorial and poorly defined.
Requires multidisciplinary management.

Non-cardiovascular causes of dizziness in older people are heterogeneous and often difficult to define. In contrast to young patients, psychogenic causes of dizziness are uncommon and the significance of peripheral vestibular disorders often overstated[68] (Chapter 48). A major problem is differentiating a causative condition from one which is merely contributory. Many so-called 'provocative tests' are non-specific. For example, symptom reproduction on head and neck movements may be attributable to cervical spondylosis but may equally implicate carotid sinus hypersensitivity or cerebrovascular disease. Many authors have categorized the non-cardiovascular causes of dizziness[3,68] (Figure 51.12) (Chapters 49 and 54).

A prospective case-controlled study by Lawson et al[3] used detailed cardiovascular, vestibular and neuromuscular assessments to define attributable and contributory causes of dizziness in patients over 60 years presenting to their general practitioner. Sixteen per cent of patients had attributable 'central neurological disorders', comprising mainly cerebrovascular disease and cervical spondylosis. A prospective study by Colledge et al[68] recruited older patients with dizziness through local press advertisements and also reported cerebrovascular disease and cervical spondylosis as prominent attributable causes.

Diffuse cerebrovascular disease increases the risk of cerebral hypoperfusion in response to small transient blood pressure reductions difficult or impossible to measure by conventional means. Hypertension, a common comorbid condition, compounds this problem by altering cerebral autoregulation. Dizziness (or vertigo) occurring in isolation cannot be attributed to brainstem ischaemia without a description of additional focal neurological deficits.[69] A combination of dizziness with one or more of dysarthria, diplopia, demianaesthesia or demiparesis (the 'five D's') is required. Absence of these features should prompt investigation for alternative causes of dizziness. In the subclavian steal syndrome, stenosis of the subclavian artery proximal to the origin of the vertebral artery results in transient brainstem ischaemia on physical activity of the affected arm.

POSTERIOR CIRCULATORY DISTURBANCES AS A CAUSE OF DIZZINESS—THE 'FIVE D'S'

Dizziness or vertigo.
Dysarthria.
Diplopia.
Demiparesis.
Demianaesthesia.

Degenerative changes in the cervical spine and paraspinal tissues may disrupt proprioceptive input to central centres, resulting in dizziness and dysequilibrium. This mechanism seems to be more significant than that of intermittent sympathetic interruption or osteophytic vertebral artery occlusion.[70]

Similarly, peripheral disturbances to the sensorium may be caused by a variety of sensory, neurological or locomotor deficits (Figure 51.13). Peripheral neuropathy, degenerative changes in the major weight-bearing joints or muscles[71] and poor visual acuity[72] may contribute to the evolution of dizziness. Twenty-two per cent of patients in Lawson's study had no definitive diagnosis after full evaluation, but a number of peripheral 'somatosensory deficits' were found which may have been contributory.

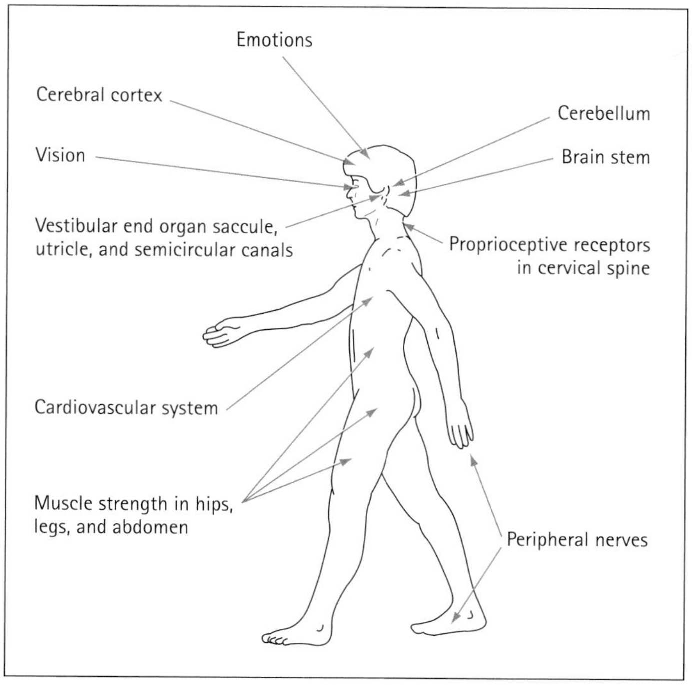

Figure 51.13 The 'sensorium': schematic representation of possible disturbances resulting in dizziness and dysequilibrium.

Ultimately, many if not most elderly patients will have a mixed or multifactorial dizziness, and in a significant proportion no cause will be found, even after comprehensive assessment.

Medical assessment of the dizzy patient

Introduction

A careful clinical history (Table 51.8) and detailed examination (Table 51.9) may direct the physician towards a particular diagnosis or diagnostic category. A logical investigation strategy may then be devised for the individual patient. In many cases, it is difficult to think algorithmically, but a general approach to the dizzy patient is summarized in Figure 51.1.

History

Predictors of a cardiovascular diagnosis[3] include: dizziness described as 'lightheadedness', associated syncope, pallor or unexplained falls, a need to sit or lie down, and symptoms precipitated by prolonged standing or co-morbid cardiovascular disease. A peripheral vestibular disorder is implied by description of vertigo, particularly if associated with other vestibular symptoms such as tinnitus or deafness[1,3] (Chapter 48).

An eyewitness account of a dizzy episode can be invaluable, particularly in older people who may have retrograde amnesia or poor cognitive function.

A detailed past medical history will help to define comorbidity and may identify those likely to have specific, multifactorial or poorly defined causes for their dizziness.

A comprehensive drug review is vital. All drugs (including those obtained 'over the counter') should be regarded as potential causes of dizziness until proved otherwise.

In older people, multifactorial or poorly defined dizziness is common and definitive medical intervention may not be possible. A detailed social and functional review then becomes central to the development of a holistic multidisciplinary strategy designed primarily to maintain function and independence rather than 'cure' dizziness.[14]

Examination

Physical examination should focus on assessment of the cardiovascular, neurological and locomotor systems.[3,17,68] Bradycardia may be drug related or suggest underlying sick sinus syndrome or conduction defects. Systolic murmurs may indicate outflow tract obstruction. Carotid bruits may imply carotid stenosis and

Table 51.8 The dizzy patient: history (key features).

Description of dizziness	
	Vertigo
	Lightheaded
	Others
	Frequency
	Severity
	Duration
	Effect on quality of life
Associated features	
	Cardiological
	Neurological
	Vestibular
Precipitating events	
	Position
	Posture
	Head and neck movements
	Situations
	Valsalva
	Exertion
	Anxiety
Eyewitness account	
	Syncope (pallor, flushing)
	Altered awareness
	Tonic clonic or myoclonic movements
	Post-event states
	Frequency
	Duration and severity of episodes
Past medical history	
	Cardiological
	Neurological
	Vestibular
	Locomotor
	Psychiatric
Drug history	
	Review all drugs (including alcohol and recreational drugs) for potential effects on heart rate, rhythm, blood pressure, mental state, neuromuscular function
Social history	
	Smoking
	Alcohol
	Occupation
	Driver status
	Social and family networks
Functional history	
	Independence in basic and extended activities of daily living

significant cerebrovascular disease. Baseline and orthostatic blood pressure measurements may detect large postural blood pressure deficits. A history of dizziness or presyncope while using an arm, in conjunction with a low-volume radial pulse and a lower blood pressure, would indicate a subclavian steal syndrome.

Table 51.9 The dizzy patient: examination (key features).

General	
	Well or ill
	External stigmata of disease
	Cognitive impairment
	Anxiety state
Cardiovascular	
	Bradycardia or tachycardia
	Systolic or diastolic murmur
	Carotid bruits
	Hypertension
	Postural blood pressure drop
Neurological	
	Cervical radiculomyelopathy
	Peripheral neuropathy
	Stroke disease
	Parkinsonism
	Cerebellar signs
	Gait and balance abnormalities
Locomotor	
	Myopathy
	Arthropathy of cervical spine or weight-bearing joints
Vestibular	
	Hallpike's manoeuvre

Assessment of cognitive function is useful in older patients. Cognitive impairment, due to cerebrovascular disease or Alzheimer's disease, may be a marker of comorbid cardiovascular pathology. Significant cognitive deficits may complicate clinical assessment, make definitive diagnosis difficult and influence management once diagnosis is established. An Abbreviated Mental Test (AMT)[73] is a quick and convenient screen and may be followed by a formal Mini Mental State Examination (MMSE)[74] if indicated.

A full neurological examination should be performed (Chapter 49) and central or peripheral disturbances to the sensorium noted. Pyramidal signs, and an abnormal gait pattern together with vascular risk factors, may suggest a central vascular origin for dizziness. This impression is supported by symptom reproduction during stable haemodynamics on head-up tilt testing. A history of arthritis, neck restriction, mixed motor signs in the upper limbs, pyramidal signs in the lower limbs and an unsteady gait may imply significant cervical radiculomyelopathy as a cause of dizziness and dysequilibrium. Loss of sensory modalities (particularly proprioceptive) in the lower limbs, a positive Romberg's test and gait anomalies suggest a peripheral neuropathy. Patients with OH should be carefully assessed for associated extrapyramidal, pyramidal and cerebellar signs suggestive of MSA. Hallpike's manoeuvre[75] may help to define those in whom benign paroxysmal positional vertigo (BPPV) forms part of their dizziness or balance disorder (Chapter 48).

Examination of the locomotor system may yield evidence of significant arthritis or muscle wasting and weakness. The cervical spine, weight-bearing joints and postural muscles are particularly important in terms of proprioceptive input.

Other physical assessments routinely performed may have little predictive value in terms of diagnosis but may identify minor contributory factors which can direct rehabilitative strategies in those with multifactorial or poorly defined dizziness.[68] Visual acuity should be measured with a Snellen chart. Deficits assume greater significance when associated with vestibular or proprioceptive deficits and may be easily correctible. A positive Romberg's test in the absence of other proprioceptive deficits loosely suggests a primary vestibular problem. A wide range of gait and balance assessments are described.[76] They are non-specific but provide useful information regarding stability, function, judgement and coordination. For example, the 'get up and go test' measures the ability of a patient to rise from a chair, walk a prescribed distance, turn around, stand with eyes shut, walk back to the chair and return to the sitting position. Again, poor performance in various aspects of this and similar manoeuvres may influence rehabilitative intervention.

Investigation

Routine tests, including full blood count, biochemical profile, thyroid function, chest X-ray and 12-lead ECG, are useful in helping to exclude acute general medical causes of dizziness. In older patients with chronic or recurrent dizziness, they help to define significant comorbidity and provide an essential baseline for therapeutic interventions.

Detailed vestibular assessment is usually unhelpful unless a description of true vertigo predominates or there are associated vestibular features.[68] Posturography and formal gait analysis are not generally helpful in diagnosis but may be used as a measure of response to interventions in some patients (Chapter 44). Vestibular review should be directed by an audiology physician with an interest in dizziness and vestibular disorders (Chapter 54).

It is the authors' opinion that all patients presenting with chronic or recurrent dizziness, which does not have vestibular characteristics, should be considered for cardiovascular assessment. This includes provocative testing for common hypotensive disorders, i.e. carotid sinus massage (supine and upright), a 70° head-up tilt test (with provocation if necessary) and orthostatic blood pressure measurements. Non-invasive beat-to-beat blood pressure monitoring (digital plethysmography: Portapres) will detect rapid or transient changes in blood pressure during symptoms. Conventional sphygmomanometry may fail to recognize vasodepressor responses.

Further investigation is individualized by presentation, clinical findings and the results of baseline cardiovascular tests. Most of these have been described in the relevant sections but are summarized here. Ambulatory heart rate (Holter) monitoring is most useful in dizzy patients with associated palpitations, syncope, abnormal 12-lead ECG or other evidence of structural heart disease. If the recording is unremarkable or asymptomatic but clinical suspicion of arrhythmia remains high, then an external (Cardiomemo) or implantable (Reveal: Medtronic Inc) loop recorder may be useful in selected patients. Electrophysiological studies may be useful in a small selected group of patients in whom the suspicion of arrhythmia is high. A 24-h ambulatory blood pressure profile is helpful in further defining vasodepressor syndromes and monitoring response to treatment. Echocardiography should be performed if systolic (aortic stenosis, hypertrophic cardiomyopathy, pulmonary stenosis) or diastolic (left atrial ball thrombus, left atrial myxoma) murmurs are present to exclude mechanical outflow tract obstruction. Other evidence of structural heart disease, particularly left ventricular hypertrophy or dilatation, may provide supportive evidence for dizziness of cardiovascular origin.

Neuroradiography may detail the extent of underlying cerebrovascular disease and exclude other significant intracerebral pathology. Carotid doppler ultrasonography defines the severity of carotid stenosis prior to carotid sinus massage in those with a bruit or recent cerebrovascular events. Retrograde flow in the vertebral artery during upper-limb exercise, if associated with typical clinical features, confirms subclavian steal syndrome. MRI scanning will define the severity of cervical spinal pathology (Chapter 49).

General management of the dizzy patient

Interventions for cardiovascular and specific medical causes of dizziness have been discussed elsewhere. Unfortunately, at least half of all patients remain without a definitive diagnosis even after full evaluation. Many others have dizziness of multifactorial origin.[77] Further detailed investigations are usually unrewarding and often counterproductive. These patients require a holistic multidisciplinary approach. The emphasis should be on defining practical strategies for relieving symptoms and reducing disability rather than finding a panacea for dizziness.[14]

Useful interventions include vestibular rehabilitation exercises and balance re-training (Chapter 54). Provocative exercise programmes encourage habituation to postures and positions associated with dizziness. Such approaches may improve symptoms, proprioceptive input, stability, gait, balance and confidence. Psychological assessment, with anxiety management programmes, may improve hyperventilation or psychogenic symptoms. A detailed home assessment with a physiotherapist and occupational therapist may build confidence and reduce risk of falls through the implementation of various safety strategies.[78–80]

'Traditional' methods of treating the dizzy patient are controversial. In the authors' opinion, soft collars given to prevent osteophytic nipping of the vertebral arteries reduce proprioceptive input and may provoke symptoms of carotid sinus hypersensitivity. Vestibular sedatives should be used with extreme caution. They may exacerbate symptoms if dizziness is not vestibular in origin. Adverse effects may compound comorbidity in older patients. They should be used only after careful thought and stopped after a short trial period if ineffective (Chapter 54). Other regular medications should always be viewed as potential causes of dizziness and reviewed at regular intervals.

Summary

Medical management of the dizzy patient presents a considerable challenge. Physicians should be aware that dizziness may be a non-specific presentation of acute medical illness, particularly in older people. Those with chronic or recurrent dizziness need further careful evaluation. Patients with vertigo and/or other significant vestibular features should be referred to an audiology physician following medical review. Psychogenic dizziness requires specialist intervention by a clinical psychologist once physical causes have been excluded.

Cardiovascular disease is a common but frequently overlooked cause of dizziness in older people. It is suggested by a description of lightheadedness, particularly on prolonged standing, and when associated with syncope, pallor or comorbid cardiovascular disease. Assessment should include carotid sinus massage, a prolonged head-up tilt test and orthostatic blood pressure measurements with continuous phasic blood pressure monitoring.

Non-cardiovascular medical causes of dizziness are heterogeneous and include central neurological disease and peripheral somatosensory deficits. Dizziness is often multifactorial and remains poorly defined in a significant proportion of patients. Those without remediable cause(s) may benefit from rehabilitative strategies to reduce morbidity and maintain independence.

Data to support an evidence-based approach to the dizzy patient remain in short supply. The protean nature of dizziness fosters bias and clouds the assessment of specific interventions. Many views and reviews on the subject must therefore remain personalized rather than evidence-based. The problem is summarized effectively by Sloane and Dallara,[14] who compare the assessment of dizziness to the attempts of three blind men to describe an elephant. Each man feels a different part and so gives a different, accurate, yet biased description of what the elephant is like.

No account of dizziness can therefore be definitive but it is hoped that this text will provide a stimulus to further research and debate. The problem of dizziness impinges on many different medical and paramedical specialities. Collaboration between these groups is essential if we are to develop more effective management strategies for the dizzy patient.

References

1. Orma EJ, Koskenoja M. Dizziness attacks and continuous dizziness in the aged. *Geriatrics* 1957; **12**: 91–100.
2. Drachman DA, Hart CW. An approach to the dizzy patient. *Neurology* 1972; **22**(4): 323–34.
3. Lawson J, Fitzgerald J, Birchall J, Aldren CP, Kenny RA. Diagnosis of geriatric patients with severe dizziness. *J Am Geriatr Soc* 1999; **47**(1): 12–17.
4. Royal College of General Practitioners, Office of Population Censuses and Surveys. *Morbidity Statistics from General Practice.* Table 13. Third National Study, 1981–82.
5. Sloane PD. Dizziness in primary care. Results from the National Ambulatory Medical Care Survey. *J Family Practice* 1989; **29**(1): 33–8.
6. Colledge NR, Wilson JA, Macintyre CC, MacLennan WJ. The prevalence and characteristics of dizziness in an elderly community. *Age Ageing* 1994; **23**(2): 117–20.
7. Sixt E, Landahl S. Postural disturbances in a 75-year-old population: I. Prevalence and functional consequences. *Age Ageing* 1987; **16**(6): 393–8.
8. Evans JG. Transient neurological dysfunction and risk of stroke in an elderly English population: the different significance of vertigo and non-rotatory dizziness. *Age Ageing* 1990: **19**(1): 43–9.
9. Downton J, Andrews K. Postural disturbance and psychological symptoms amongst elderly people living at home. *Int J Geriatr Psychiatry* 1990; **5**: 93–98.
10. Sloane P, Blazer D, George LK. Dizziness in a community elderly population. *J Am Geriatr Soc* 1989; **37**(2): 101–8.
11. Kroenke K, Lucas CA, Rosenberg ML, et al. Causes of persistent dizziness. A prospective study of 100 patients in ambulatory care. *Ann Intern Med* 1992; **117**(11): 898–904.
12. Smith MS. Evaluation and management of psychosomatic symptoms in adolescence. *Clin Pediatrics* 1986; **25**(3): 131–5.
13. Nozawa I, Hisamatsu K, Imamura S, Fujimori I, Nakayama H, Murakami Y. Psychosomatic aspects of healthy young women with orthostatic dysregulation. *Clin Otolaryngol Allied Sci* 1996; **21**(3): 222–5.
14. Sloane PD, Dallara J. Clinical research and geriatric dizziness: the blind men and the elephant. *J Am Geriatr Soc* 1999; **47**(1): 113–14.
15. McIntosh S, Da Costa D, Kenny RA. Outcome of an integrated approach to the investigation of dizziness, falls and syncope in elderly patients referred to a 'syncope'. *Age Ageing* 1993; **22**(1): 53–8.
16. McIntosh SJ, Lawson J, Kenny RA. Clinical characteristics of vasodepressor, cardioinhibitory, and mixed carotid sinus syndrome in the elderly. *Am J Med* 1993; **95**(2): 203–8.
17. Ward C, Kenny RA. Reproducibility of orthostatic hypotension in symptomatic elderly. *Am J Med* 1996; **100**(4): 418–22.
18. Shaw FE, Kenny RA. The overlap between syncope and falls in the elderly. *Postgrad Med J* 1997; **73**(864): 635–9.
19. Thomas JE. Diseases of the carotid sinus—syncope. In: Vinken PJ, Bruyn GW, eds. *Handbook of Clinical Neurology*, Vol II. Amsterdam: North Holland Publishing, 1972: 532–51.

20. Lown B, Levine SA. The carotid sinus: clinical evaluation of its stimulation. *Circulation* 1961; **23**: 766–89.
21. Morley CA, Perrins EJ, Grant P, Chan SL, McBrien DJ, Sutton R. Carotid sinus syncope treated by pacing. Analysis of persistent symptoms and role of atrioventricular sequential pacing. *Br Heart J* 1982; **47**(5): 411–18.
22. Walter PF, Crawley IS, Dorney ER. Carotid sinus hypersensitivity and syncope. *Am J Cardiol* 1978; **42**(3): 396–403.
23. Strasberg B, Sagie A, Erdman S, Kusniec J, Sclarovsky S, Agmon J. Carotid sinus hypersensitivity and the carotid sinus syndrome. *Prog Cardiovasc Dis* 1989; **31**(5): 379–9.
24. Draper AJ. The cardioinhibitory carotid sinus syndrome. *Ann Intern Med* 1950; **32**: 700–16.
25. Parry S, Richardson DA, O'Shea D, Kenny RA. Upright carotid sinus massage is essential. *Heart* 2000; **83**(1): 22–3.
26. Davies AJ, Kenny RA. Frequency of neurologic complications following carotid sinus massage. *Am J Cardiol* 1998; **81**(10): 1256–7.
27. Morley CA, Sutton R. Carotid sinus syncope. *Int J Cardiol* 1984; **6**(3): 287–93.
28. Bexton RS, Davies A, Kenny RA. The rate-drop response in carotid sinus syndrome: the Newcastle experience. *Pacing Clin Electrophysiol* 1997; **20**(3 Pt 2): 840.
29. Lewis T. Vasovagal syncope and the carotid sinus mechanism. *Br Med J* 1932; **1**: 873–6.
30. Kenny RA, Ingram A, Bayliss J, Sutton R. Head-up tilt: a useful test for investigating unexplained syncope. *Lancet* 1986; **8494**: 1352–5.
31. Weissler AM, Warren JV. Vasodepressor syncope. *Am Heart J* 1959; **57**: 786–94.
32. Fitzpatrick A, Sutton R. Tilting towards a diagnosis in recurrent unexplained syncope. *Lancet* 1989; **1**(8639): 658–60.
33. Mark AL. The Bezold–Jarisch reflex revisited: clinical implications of inhibitory reflexes originating in the heart. *J Am Coll Cardiol* 1983; **1**(1): 90–102.
34. Fitzpatrick A, Williams T, Ahmed R, Lightman S, Bloom SR, Sutton R. Electrocardiographic and endocrine changes during vasovagal syncope induced by prolonged head up tilt. *Eur J Cardiac Pacing Electrophysiol* 1992; **2**: 121–8.
35. Sutton R. Vasovagal syncope: clinical features, epidemiology and natural history. In: Blanc JJ, Benditt T, Sutton R, eds. *Neurally Mediated Syncope: Pathophysiology, Investigations, Treatment*. Armonk: Futura, 1996: 71–6.
36. Le Doux JE. Emotion and the amygdala. In: Aggleton JP, ed. *The Amygdala Neurobiological Aspects of Emotion, Memory and Mental Dysfunction*. New York: Wiley Liss, 1992; 339–51.
37. Parry SW, Kenny RA. Tilt table testing. In: Malik M, ed. *Clinical Guide to Cardiac Autonomic Tests*. London: Klewer Academic Publishers, 1998; 67–99.
38. Grubb B, Samoil D. Neurocardiogenic syncope. In: Kenny RA, ed. *Syncope in the Older Patient: Causes and Investigation of Syncope and Falls*. London: Chapman and Hall Medical, 1996; 137–54.
39. Connolly SJ, Sheldon R, Roberts RS, Gent M. The North American Vasovagal Pacemaker Study (VPS). A randomized trial of permanent cardiac pacing for the prevention of vasovagal syncope. *J Am Coll Cardiol* 1999; **33**(1): 16–20.
40. Ward CR, Gray JC, Gilroy JJ, Kenny RA. Midodrine: a role in the management of neurocardiogenic syncope. *Heart* 1998; **79**(1): 45–9.
41. Mathias CJ, Bannister R. Investigation of autonomic disorders. In: Bannister R, Mathias CJ, eds. *Autonomic Failure: A Textbook of Clinical Disorders of the Autonomic Nervous System*. Oxford: Oxford Medical Publications, 1992; 225–90.
42. Anonymous. Consensus statement on the definition of orthostatic hypotension, pure autonomic failure, and multiple system atrophy. The Consensus Committee of the American Autonomic Society and the American Academy of Neurology. *Neurology* 1996; **46**(5): 1470.
43. Dey AB, Kenny RA. Orthostatic hypotension in the elderly: aetiology, manifestations and management. *J Irish Coll Physicians Surgeons*. 1998; **27**: 182–7.
44. Lipsitz LA, Storch HA, Minaker KL, Rowe JW. Intra-individual variability in postural blood pressure in the elderly. *Clin Sci* 1985; **69**(3): 337–41.
45. Caird FI, Andrews GR, Kennedy RD. Effect of posture on blood pressure in the elderly. *Br Heart J* 1973; **35**(5): 527–30.
46. Schatz IJ, Masaki KH, Burchfiel CM, Curb JD, Chiu D. Orthostatic hypotension (OH) as a predictor of two year mortality in elderly men; the Honolulu heart program. *Clin Autonomic Res* 1995; **5**: 321.
47. Sjostrand T. Regulation of blood pressure distribution in man. *Acta Physiol Scand* 1952; **26**: 312.
48. Lassen NA, Christensen MS. Physiology of cerebral blood flow. *B J Anaesthesia* 1976; **48**(8): 719–34.
49. Mathias CJ. Primary autonomic failure in association with other neurological features—the syndromes of Shy–Drager and multiple system atrophy. In: Kenny RA, ed. *Syncope in the Older Patient: Causes and Investigations of Syncope and Falls*. London: Chapman and Hall Medical, 1996: 137–54.
50. Wynne HA, Schofield S. Drug induced orthostatic hypotension. In: Kenny RA, ed. *Syncope in the Older Patient: Causes and Investigations of Syncope and Falls*. London: Chapman and Hall Medical, 1996: 137–54.
51. Schondorf R, Low PA. Idiopathic postural orthostatic tachycardia syndrome: an attenuated form of acute pandysautonomia? *Neurology* 1993; **43**(1): 132–7.
52. Low PA, Opfer-Gehrking TL, Textor SC, Schondorf R, Suarez GA, Fealey RD, Camilleri M. Comparison of the postural tachycardia syndrome (POTS) with orthostatic hypotension due to autonomic failure. *J Autonomic Nervous System* 1994; **50**(2): 181–8.
53. Sandroni P, Opfer-Gehrking TL, Benarroch EE, Shen WK, Low PA. Certain cardiovascular indices predict syncope in the postural tachycardia syndrome. *Clin Autonomic Res* 1996; **6**(4): 225–31.
54. De Lorenzo F, Hargreaves J, Kakkar VV. Possible relationship between chronic fatigue and postural tachycardia syndromes. *Clin Autonomic Res* 1996; **6**(5): 263–4.
55. LaManca JJ, Peckerman A, Walker J et al. Cardiovascular response during head-up tilt in chronic fatigue syndrome. *Clin Physiol* 1999; **19**(2): 111–20.
56. Mazuz M, Friedman HS. Significance of prolonged electrocardiographic pauses in sinoatrial disease: sick sinus syndrome. *Am J Cardiol* 1983; **52**(5): 485–9.

57. Wu DL, Yeh SJ, Lin FC, Wang CC, Cherng WJ. Sinus automaticity and sinoatrial conduction in severe symptomatic sick sinus syndrome. *J Am Coll Cardiol* 1992; **19**(2): 355–64.
58. Hilgard J, Ezri MD, Denes P. Significance of ventricular pauses of three seconds or more detected on twenty-four-hour Holter recordings. *Am J Cardiol* 1985; **55**(8): 1005–8.
59. Short DS. The syndrome of alternating bradycardia and tachycardia. *Br Heart J* 1954; **16**: 208.
60. Kuga K, Yamaguchi I, Sugishita Y, Ito I. Assessment by autonomic blockade of age-related changes of the sinus node function and autonomic regulation in sick sinus syndrome. *Am J Cardiol* 1988; **61**(4): 361–6.
61. Steinhaus D. Atrioventricular conduction disturbance. In: Kenny RA, ed. *Syncope in the Older Patient: Causes and Investigations of Syncope and Falls*. London: Chapman and Hall Medical, 1996: 185–200.
62. Rosen KM, Dhingra RC, Loeb HS, Rahimtoola SH. Chronic heart block in adults. Clinical and electrophysiological observations. *Arch Intern Med* 1973; **131**(5): 663–72.
63. McComb JM. Electrophysiological studies. In: Kenny RA, ed. *Syncope in the Older Patient: Causes and Investigations of Syncope and Falls*. London: Chapman and Hall Medical, 1996: 73–86.
64. ACC/AHA Task Force Report. Guidelines for Implantation of Cardiac Pacemakers and Antiarrhythmia Devices. A Report of the American College of Cardiology/American Heart Association Task Force on the Assessment of Diagnostic and Therapeutic Cardiovascular Procedures (Committee on Pacemaker Implantation). *J Am Coll Cardiol* 1998; **31**(5): 1175–209.
65. Bennett DH. *Cardiac Arrhythmias. Practical Notes on Interpretation and Treatment*, 5th edn. Oxford: Butterworth Heinemann, 1997.
66. Anonymous. Recommendations for pacemaker prescription for symptomatic bradycardia. Report of a working party of the British Pacing and Electrophysiology Group. *Br Heart J* 1991; **66**(2): 185–91.
67. Banning PA, Hall RJC. Structural and mechanical causes of syncope. In: Kenny RA, ed. *Syncope in the Older Patient: Causes and Investigations of Syncope and Falls*. London: Chapman and Hall Medical, 1996: 201–18.
68. Colledge NR, Barr-Hamilton RM, Lewis SJ, Sellar RJ, Wilson JA. Evaluation of investigations to diagnose the cause of dizziness in elderly people: a community based controlled study. *Br Med J* 1996; **313**(7060): 788–92.
69. Sandercock P. Recent developments in the diagnosis and management of patients with transient ischaemic attacks and minor ischaemic strokes. *Q J Med* 1991; **78**(286): 101–12.
70. de Jong PT, de Jong JM, Cohen B, Jongkees LB. Ataxia and nystagmus induced by injection of local anesthetics in the neck. *Ann Neurol* 1977; **1**(3): 240–6.
71. Richmond FJR, Bakker DA, Stacey MJ. The sensorium: receptors of neck muscles and joints. In: Peterson BW, Richmond FJR, eds. *Control of Head Movements*. New York: Oxford University Press, 1988: 49–62.
72. Paulus WM, Straube A, Brandt T. Visual stabilization of posture. Physiological stimulus characteristics and clinical aspects. *Brain* 1984; **107**(Pt 4): 1143–63.
73. Hodkinson HM. Evaluation of a mental test score for assessment of mental impairment in the elderly. *Age Ageing* 1972; **1**(4): 233–8.
74. Folstein MF, Folstein SE, McHugh PR. 'Mini-mental state'. A practical method for grading the cognitive state of patients for the clinician. *J Psychiatr Res* 1975; **12**(3): 189–98.
75. Dix MR, Hallpike CS. The pathology, symptomatology and diagnosis of certain common disorders of the vestibular system. *Ann Otol Rhinol Laryngol* 1981; Suppl 90(1 pt 2): 1–19.
76. Wolfson L, Whipple R, Amerman P, Tobin JN. Gait assessment in the elderly: a gait abnormality rating scale and its relation to falls. *J Gerontol* 1990; **45**(1): M12–19.
77. Tinetti ME, Williams CS, Gill TM. Dizziness among older adults: a possible geriatric syndrome. *Ann Intern Med* 2000; **132**(5): 337–44.
78. Tinetti ME. Where is the vision for fall prevention? *J Am Geriatr Soc* 2001; **49**(5): 676–7.
79. Fabacher D, Pietruszka F, Josephson K. An in-home assessment programme for older adults: preliminary findings. *Gerontologist* 1990; **30**: 46.
80. Tinetti ME, Baker DI, McAvay G et al. A multifactorial intervention to reduce the risk of falling among elderly people living in the community. *N Engl J Med* 1994; **331**(13): 821–7.

52 Balance disorders in children

Claes Möller

At birth, the newborn infant experiences a new world, in which he is exposed suddenly to new kinds of movements and positions. The sensory systems are fully developed at birth; the acquisition of balance is a matter of adaptation and learning, and is achieved using three different systems:

- the proprioceptive system
- the visual system
- the vestibular system.

Afferent signals from all three systems pass into the brainstem, pons and cerebellum, where they are processed, and then modulated neural information is transmitted through efferent nerve fibres to maintain coordinated movements. Assessment of these three sensory systems and the central nervous system is essential when evaluating children with balance disorders.

History

The anamnesis is, as in adults with balance disorders, of the utmost importance. It is, however, difficult to get good case histories from small children or the parents, as a young child, when subjected to attacks of dizziness, can often only respond with crying, pallor and sleepiness. However, the child with a chronic bilateral vestibular dysfunction displays other symptoms, such as delayed motor milestones, which should be established for children with 'dizziness', 'clumsiness', 'funny turns', ataxia or hearing impairment (Table 52.1).

Table 52.1 Early motor milestones.

6 weeks	Hold the head in the plane of the body
12 weeks	Hold the head above the plane of the body
16 weeks	Good head control
6 months	Unsupported sitting
10 months	Standing up with support
12 months	Walking

Questions concerning bilateral vestibular hypofunction or areflexia are simple and straightforward, such as those given in Table 52.2.

If attacks of vertigo or dizziness are suspected in a child, a valuable suggestion is to have the parents keep a diary, in which they should note:

- symptoms (pallor, vomiting, unsteadiness, headache, abnormal movements, falling, loss of consciousness)
- frequency of attacks (increasing, decreasing?)
- duration of attacks and the time of day
- other ear symptoms
- other general medical symptoms
- trauma, drugs, chemicals.

From the general perspective, it is important to obtain a detailed past history regarding the mother's pregnancy, the child's delivery, any perinatal medical history, any history of childhood trauma and/or infections, any previous drug therapy, and a detailed family history of migraine, or neurological or otological disorders.

Balance assessment

Balance assessment is, of course, dependent upon the age of the child, but most balance tests can be performed from a very early age (Table 52.3).

Table 52.2 Questions relevant to vestibular function.

- At what age did the child sit unsupported?
- What was the walking age?
- Did the child experience difficulties in learning to cycle?
- Does the child have problems when walking in darkness or on uneven surfaces?
- Does the child experience motion sickness?
- Does the child have problems in gymnastics and sports activities?
- Is the child considered to be clumsy?

Table 52.3 Balance assessment.

Play
ENT examination
Eye-movement examination
Neurological examination
Romberg test
Video-oculography/electro-oculography
Caloric testing
Standard irrigations
Ice water irrigations
Rotary chair testing

Observation of a child playing can give extremely valuable information regarding vision, position of the head, movement of the arms and legs, and stability (Figure 52.1) although it is time-consuming for the busy clinician. Balls are excellent tools to use in assessment, as they allow evaluation of a number of different skills required for balance.

A detailed ear, nose and throat examination is essential in order to detect dysmorphology of the face, outer ear, ear canal, tympanic membrane and middle ear. A neurological examination, including cranial nerve tests, deep tendon reflexes and assessment of developmental reflexes, allows an overall assessment of central nervous system (CNS) function and may identify specific opthalmological/neurological defects associated with balance dysfunction. Moreover, a detailed clinical examination of eye movements using an 'interesting'—e.g. toy—target should be conducted to assess smooth pursuit, saccades, optokinetic nystagmus and spontaneous and positional nystagmus. The effect of optic fixation can be crudely assessed clinically by using Frenzel glasses or an infrared viewer. Children older than 4 years of age can often perform a sensitized Romberg test, standing on one leg. The performance in younger children displays large standard deviations and depends to a large degree on cooperation between the examiner, the child and the parent.

Objective methods of evaluating vestibular function are important to document the severity of derangements, provide evidence of site(s) of lesion and monitor change. Electronystagmography (ENG) or videonystagmography (VNG) can be performed in small children, but there are difficulties with calibration and interference of eye-movement records by blinks. Eye movements are best recorded in darkness with the direct current (DC) electro-oculography (EOG) technique. Video-oculography is a relatively new method that provides the clinician with good information concerning abnormalities of the vestibulo-ocular reflex, including the presence of spontaneous and induced positional and rotatory nystagmus. This technique is gradually replacing the EOG technique. The easiest way to measure the eye movements is by using Frenzel glasses with infrared TV cameras.

Bithermal binaural caloric testing (250 ml, 30°C, 44°C) should be performed with eyes open in darkness. The velocity of the slow phase is the most physiological parameter to assess. An interaural difference of >20% is considered pathological, and a total sum of four irrigations of <40°/s is considered to indicate bilateral hypoactivity, but each laboratory should define its own

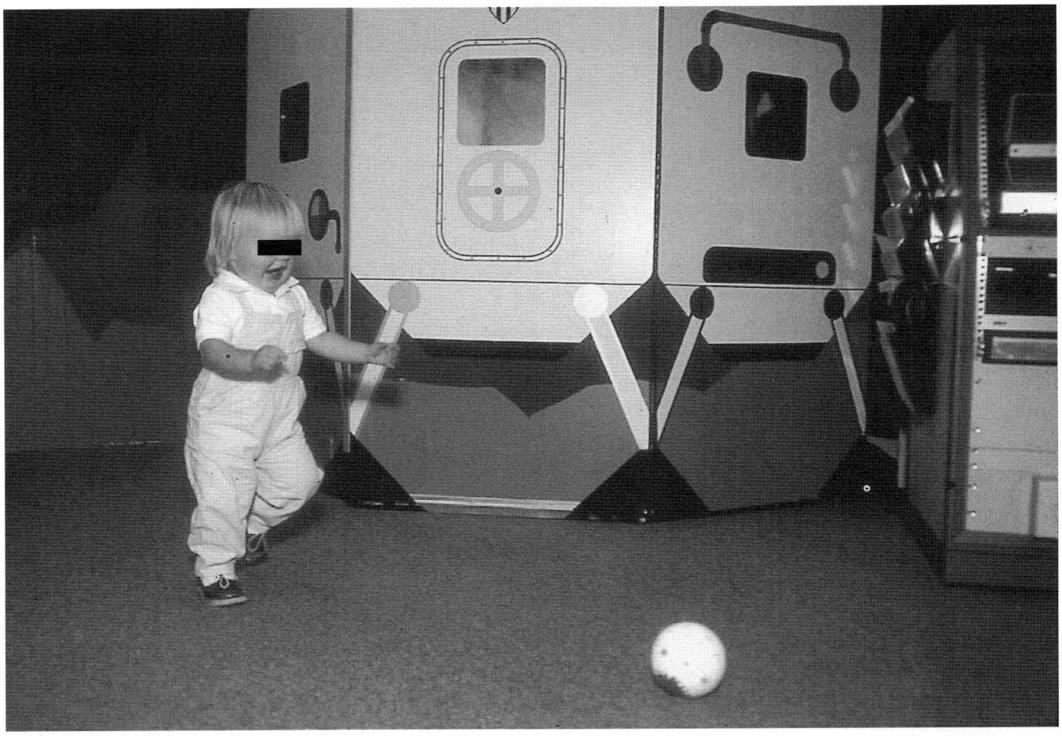

Figure 52.1 Observation of a child playing can give extremely valuable information regarding vision, position of the head, movement of the arms and legs, and stability.

precise normative ranges. Experience dictates that calorics can be performed in children as young as 4–5 years of age. 'Ice-water' calorics performed binaurally (50 ml, 8°C) can be performed in older children who do not show responses during standard caloric tests. This test cannot, however, be quantified but merely indicates the presence or total absence of vestibular function.

Sinusoidal rotatory chair tests are the best tests to evaluate possible bilateral vestibular loss in small children (Figure 52.2). They can be performed using the EOG technique and/or infrared TV monitoring. The tests should be performed in darkness, and if vestibular function is present, a resulting nystagmus will immediately appear. In some cases, a good EOG recording is not possible, and then infrared TV monitoring focused on the eyes of both child and parent will immediately show the difference in response, if bilateral vestibular loss is present. This test may be difficult to quantify, and it is not possible with certainty to differentiate between a unilateral vestibular loss and bilateral normal function.

Depending on the history, examination and balance assessment, other medical and neurological tests such as ECG, EEG, renal ultrasound or genetic typing may be required. Evaluating a child with a balance disorder is often a team effort, in which other specialists such as paediatricians, neurologists and physical therapists are required.

Balance disorders and dizziness, in general and in children in particular, are difficult to diagnose. One of the first approaches is to find out whether the pathology is due to a lesion within the vestibular end organ or the CNS. This differentiation has disadvantages, since the vestibular system is a continuum, which makes it difficult to assess if the lesion is within the labyrinth, the nerve or the vestibular nuclei (Table 52.4).

Table 52.4 Balance disorders–differential diagnosis.

Central nervous system
Epilepsy
Tumour
Migraine
Demyelinating disease
Psychosomatic
Vestibular end organ
Middle ear disease with/without labyrinthitis
Trauma
Sudden vestibular loss (vestibular neuronitis)
Menière's syndrome
Benign paroxysmal vertigo in childhood (BPV)
Meningitis
Ototoxicity
Genetic–with/without auditory impairment

Central nervous system disease

Epilepsy

Children with epilepsy sometimes display symptoms of nausea, vomiting, loss of postural control and loss of consciousness. Most children with dizziness associated with epilepsy do not, however, suffer from grand mal seizures. The epileptic foci are most often located in the temporal lobes. This condition may resemble benign paroxysmal vertigo in childhood (see below), and thus an EEG should be performed in these cases.[1]

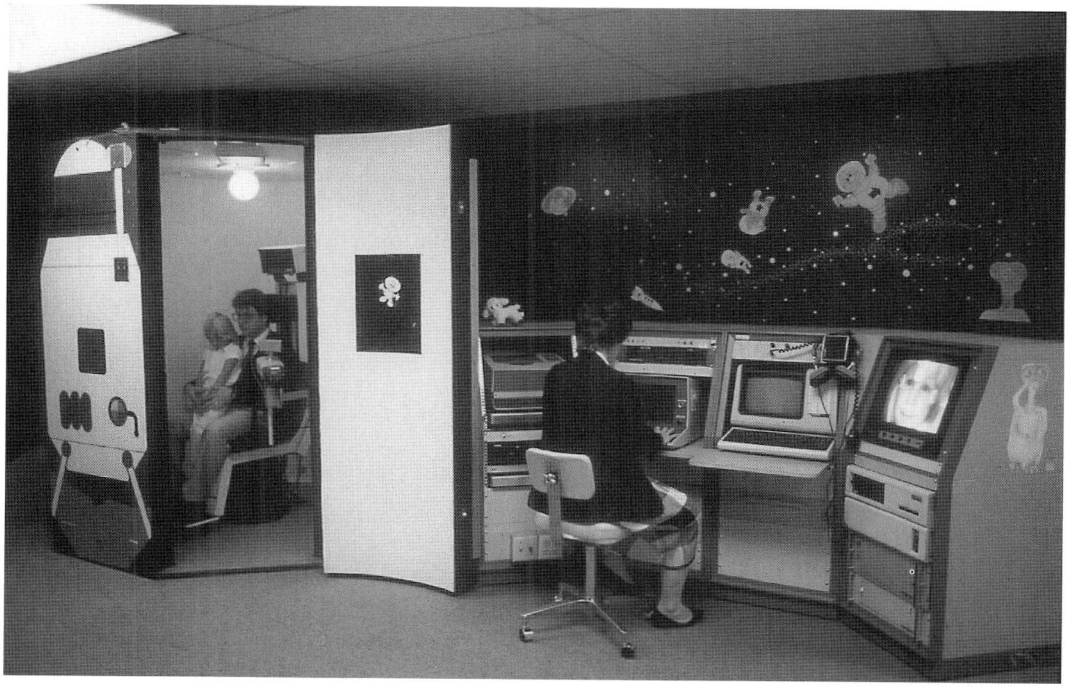

Figure 52.2 Sinusoidal rotatory chair tests are the best tests to evaluate possible bilateral vestibular loss in small children.

Tumour

Any space-occupying tumour along the vestibular system can cause vertigo and dizziness. Brainstem gliomas and cerebellopontine angle tumours occur in childhood but the symptoms often include other neurological abnormalities. If a tumour is located within this region, children, as well as adults, often show pathological smooth pursuit and/or saccadic eye movements. If suspicion is raised, magnetic resonance imaging (MRI) should be performed.

Migraine

Migraine headache is not very common in childhood. It is estimated that 4% of all migraine patients are between the ages of 7 and 15 years. Around 20% of children with migraine complain of dizziness.[2] A general opinion is that these types of migraine may originate within the basilary artery system. The attacks usually start with dizziness or vertigo, followed by headache and insomnia. One associated finding in children with migraine is a high incidence of motion sickness.

It is sometimes difficult to differentiate migraine from benign paroxysmal vertigo (BPV) in childhood. The occurrence of headache and a strong family history of migraine might help to make the diagnosis. A very rare but similar condition is paroxysmal torticollis of infancy. The symptoms are head tilting to one side with pallor and sometimes vomiting. The attacks can last minutes to days. The onset is usually around the age of 1 year, and the symptoms disappear within 1 or 2 years. The pathology is still unclear but, due to the symptoms found, one might expect dysfunction within the vestibular apparatus.[3]

Demyelinating disease

Demyelinating disease (i.e. multiple sclerosis) is rare in childhood. Vertigo may be a symptom if a sclerotic plaque involves the vestibular pathways. The other symptoms do not differ from those in adulthood.

Psychosomatic dizziness

The symptom of dizziness rarely occurs as an isolated entity in children with psychosomatic illness. This diagnosis should be made with caution and only when other diagnoses have been ruled out. This is one of the most difficult diagnoses to make, and requires time, paediatric psychological–psychiatric assessment and therapies.

Vestibular end-organ diseases

Middle ear disease

Serous otitis media is a common cause of vestibular disturbance in children. The reported symptoms include 'falling all over the place' or 'walking clumsily', and the problem is often described as 'unsteadiness' rather than true vertigo. The causes of the symptoms are usually attributed to pressure changes in the middle ear affecting the inner ear through the round and oval windows. The symptoms often disappear following treatment with ventilation tubes or spontaneously.

It is therefore important to examine otoscopically every child with balance disorders and to perform tympanometry. Acute or chronic otitis media rarely produces cases of secondary labyrinthitis with vertigo in the industrialized world, but in debilitated and immigrant populations and the Third World, greater vigilance with regard to this life-threatening condition is required. If vestibular symptoms appear with or without nystagmus, rapid treatment with intravenous antibiotics, myringotomy and mastoidectomy may need to be performed.

Trauma

A head injury in a child may result in different forms of fracture involving the petrous temporal bone. If the fracture involves the labyrinth or the vestibular nerve, severe vertigo will result, together with vomiting and unsteadiness. However, a concussion without a fracture may also result in dizziness. An acute unilateral vestibular destruction will result in a spontaneous nystagmus with the fast phase directed towards the healthy side. The nystagmus and the vertigo will often disappear rapidly due to central compensation and CNS plasticity. Failure of recovery requires rehabilitative treatment, including vestibular rehabilitation by a skilled physiotherapist.

Sudden vestibular loss (vestibular neuronitis)

In the literature, the incidence of vestibular neuronitis in children is very low. The symptoms and course of the disease are the same as in adults, but usually much milder. Thus, the real incidence might be higher. The origin of this disease is still obscure, with viral, vascular, autoimmune and genetic factors having been proposed. The child suffers from acute rotatory vertigo and nystagmus (suggestive of impairment of vestibular function) with the fast phase beating towards the healthy ear. Caloric tests show an asymmetric response. The recovery is usually rapid (2–3 days), with disappearance of spontaneous nystagmus and vertigo, and improved balance. If compensated, the child will not have any sequelae and, in adults, vestibular function may be subsequently totally normal.

Menière's syndrome

Classical Menière's syndrome in children is rare. The symptoms of low-frequency fluctuating hearing loss, rotatory vertigo attacks, tinnitus and fullness are the same as in adults. Auditory and vestibular findings in children with Menière's syndrome indicate the same pathology of endolymphatic hydrops as in adults.[4] The cause of Menière's syndrome remains obscure, although some families have been found to have an inherited tendency, suggesting a genetic factor. Findings in inner ear disorders of genetic origin have demonstrated symptoms resembling Menière's syndrome, showing an autosomal-dominant progressive auditory and vestibular loss. The treatment of Menière's syndrome in children has so far been the same as for adults, including a low-salt diet and diuretics.[5]

Benign paroxysmal vertigo in childhood

This disorder is a distinct clinical entity first described by Basser in 1964.[6] The disorder is characterized by the features listed in Table 52.5.

The diagnosis is made by case history and clinical examination. It is advisable to instruct the parents to make a diary and to teach them to look for nystagmus during the attacks. When examining the child, this condition is associated with *no* hearing loss, normal otoneurological examination and normal EEG. Video/electronystagmography with calorics should be performed, since some authors have reported decreased caloric responses. If the case history is not clear, the differential diagnosis of tumour and epilepsy must be ruled out. Among causes of dizziness in childhood, BPV seems to be one of the most common.[7]

The aetiology of BPV remains unclear. In many cases, the presence of spontaneous nystagmus suggests a vestibular disorder. The possibility of BPV being a migraine equivalent has been raised but not confirmed. In a follow-up study of children with BPV, at least 10 years after diagnosis, migraine was found to be slightly more common than in a normal population. Compared to migraine patients, a positive family history of migraine was much more uncommon in patients who had suffered from BPV. All subjects were free of vertigo and showed normal auditory and vestibular test results at follow-up.[8]

Meningitis

Viral and bacterial meningitis are diseases of early childhood (6–24 months). The main bacterial agents are the *Pneumococcus*, *Meningococcus* and *Haemophilus influenzae*. Viral meningitis, unlike bacterial meningitis, does not cause damage to the inner ear.

Permanent sequelae due to meningitis result from damage to the CNS, including the cranial nerves and the labyrinth. The clinical picture after CNS damage is of mental retardation, motor pareses, seizure syndromes and ataxia. CNS lesions have a prevalence of 1–10%.[9] Sensorineural hearing loss is a manifestation of meningitis in approximately 20% of cases, but involvement of the vestibular end organ is much more common. Not surprisingly, vestibular lesions and vertigo are frequently observed in association with hearing loss due to meningitis. Different studies have shown the prevalence of bilateral vestibular failure to be 40–80%.[10,11] Bilateral vestibular loss can be clinically observed in many cases, while the prevalence of unilateral vestibular loss may pass undetected upon clinical examination.

A child who has suffered from meningitis may have a long period of recovery during which there may be regression of motor milestones. A child who has started to walk may revert to crawling again. The symptoms attributable to vestibular involvement differ, depending upon whether the lesion is unilateral or bilateral. A child with a unilateral vestibular lesion presents symptomatically like a child with vestibular neuronitis, i.e. with spontaneous nystagmus, which disappears quickly, with a rapid recovery provided that there are no major CNS lesions.

A child with bilateral vestibular loss does not suffer from vertigo but rather displays severe unsteadiness and impaired motor milestones. This latter sign is often misinterpreted as the result of CNS involvement rather than reflecting primary vestibular dysfunction. Assessment of vestibular function after meningitis should be undertaken in all cases and, if bilateral lesions are found, appropriate balance retraining should be started as soon as possible.

A summary of the features of meningitis is given in Table 52.6.

Table 52.5 Benign paroxysmal vertigo.[16]

Sex:	No gender difference
Age of onset:	Usually <4 years
Symptoms:	Sudden onset of vertigo, seconds–minutes, pallor, vomiting, nystagmus can occur in any position
	Falling, unable to move, stand or sit
	Complete recovery to normal activities
	Consciousness *not* impaired.
Frequency:	Several times a week to once a year
Prognosis:	Disappears after months to years

Table 52.6 Meningitis.

Sex:	No gender difference
Age of onset:	Usually <2 years
Symptoms:	Vertigo
	Falling
	Increased clumsiness
Unilateral lesion:	Spontaneous nystagmus
	Vertigo
	Rapid recovery
Bilateral lesion:	Retarded motor milestones
	Difficulties in learning to walk
Diagnosis:	Observation of motor milestones
	Caloric testing
	Rotatory tests with video-oculography/ENG
	Bilateral lesion shows no rotatory nystagmus
	Unilateral lesion shows rotatory nystagmus

Ototoxicity

Several groups of drugs are known to be ototoxic, particularly the aminoglycoside antibiotics, chemotherapeutics and some diuretics.

In children, gentamicin and cisplatinum are the most commonly used drugs giving rise to vestibular failure. Both drugs are administered intravenously.

Vestibular damage due to gentamicin arises for two main reasons: the correct dose is difficult to control in small children, and the vestibular part of the inner ear is much more susceptible to gentamicin compared to the cochlea.[12] For these reasons, it is imperative to monitor, very regularly, both serum drug levels and renal function. The mechanism of gentamicin ototoxicity is slow destruction of vestibular supporting cells, and damage may therefore become apparent after treatment has ended. An inherited predisposition to gentamicin-induced susceptibility has been identified. The prevalence of such genes is not yet defined. The symptoms of ototoxicity include dizziness and unsteadiness. If the loss is asymmetric, spontaneous nystagmus may be found, but if bilateral vestibular damage occurs, the picture is that of vestibular failure with retarded motor milestones.

In small, very sick children, such symptoms are very difficult, if not impossible, to observe and interpret. Thus, if ototoxicity is suspected, spontaneous nystagmus, using video-oculography, should be sought. This procedure can be performed at the bedside, although optimal results are achieved in the laboratory with the child seated on the mother's lap in a rotating chair.

Every child who has undergone treatment with ototoxic medication should have a hearing and vestibular assessment performed.

Genetic

Genetic causes of vestibular loss remain obscure. This in part reflects difficulties in diagnosing vestibular dysfunction, both with respect to each of the five receptors in each vestibular labyrinth and with respect to the insensitivity of currently available routine vestibular tests. The vestibular system works closely with vision and the somatosensory system, enabling the CNS to compensate for dysfunction. It is, however, reasonable to believe that there are genetic defects within the vestibular system causing imbalance and dizziness.

The frequency of deafness and severe hearing impairment due to genetic conditions is approximately 50–75% of all hearing losses in children. It is common to identify 'clumsy' deaf children, but rarely, to date, has it been deemed necessary to consider the 'clumsy' element of the child's complaints. Indeed, it is often forgotten, even among physicians, that the inner ear consists of two parts: the cochlea and the vestibular labyrinth. Nonetheless, there is some evidence that deaf children with intact vestibular function are more clumsy than normal children. If this is true, it might be a result of the deafness in itself, with lack of orientation being secondary to auditory responses when crawling, walking and turning.

Provided that vision is adequate and it is light, a deaf person with bilateral vestibular loss can perform nearly normally with respect to balance. On the other hand, in the dark or when walking on an uneven or unstable surface, such as a ploughed field or sand, the loss of the vestibular system can make the same person very clumsy and insecure.

The recent discoveries of different genetic hearing deficiencies have made it necessary to differentiate between similar auditory phenotypes, and vestibular testing has provided valuable, although still limited, information. This is true for both syndromal and non-syndromal hearing loss.

Shambaugh[13] collected information in 1930 from approximately 5000 deaf students and concluded that 70% had normal balance function with no differences between congenital and childhood-onset deafness. He did not, however, perform any vestibular tests. In 1955, Arnvig[14] presented a study of nearly 500 children who were deaf or severely hard of hearing. He found approximately 40% with abnormal caloric reactions. No distinction was made between congenital and

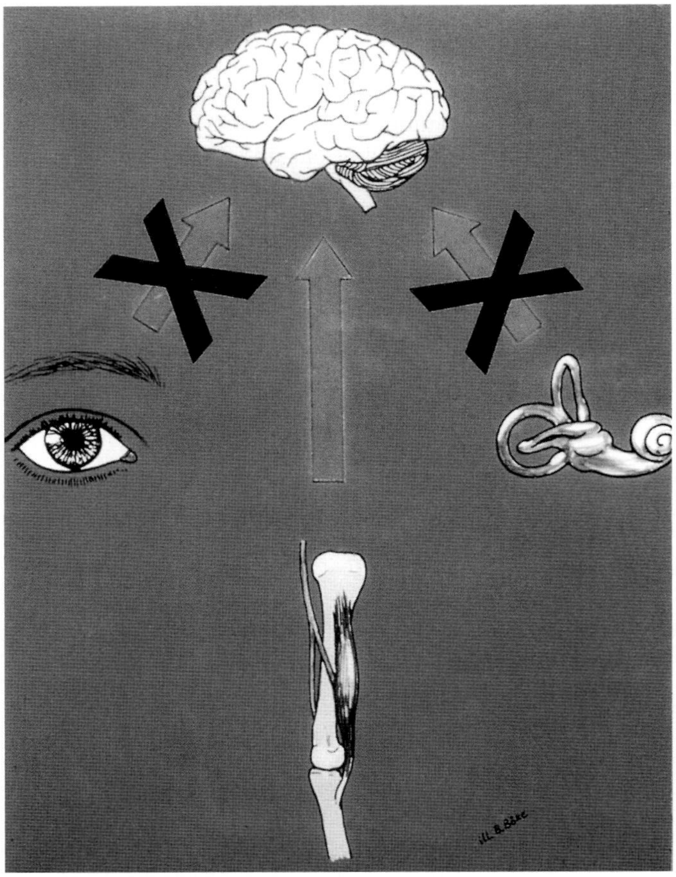

Figure 52.3 Balance relies on information from vision and the somatosensory and the vestibular sysems. Visual problems and vestibular areflexia result in unsteadiness when walking on uneven surfaces or in darkness. (from Möller and Kimberling. *Laryngoscope* 1989; **99**: 73–9.[17])

childhood-onset deafness, and the calorics did not meet present standards.

In 1965, Sandberg and Terkildsen[15] presented results from 57 children who underwent caloric testing according to present standards. They found a positive relationship between the degree of hearing loss and the severity of loss of vestibular function, with vestibular dysfunction being present in 80% of the deaf population.

The author[16] performed a further study of balance in 74 subjects suffering from severe or profound hearing loss. More than 50% of all subjects reported a walking age later than 18 months and significant problems getting around in darkness, especially in winter. Very few had experienced any motion sickness, and none reported motion sickness during car rides. A large majority (75%) remembered problems in sports and gymnastics, and many of these spontaneously reported 'I never cared because I was so clumsy'. All the subjects who had absent vestibular responses on the caloric and rotatory tests reported a walking age later than 18 months. Thus, there are reasons to believe that around 30–40% of all deaf persons suffer from bilateral vestibular areflexia.

Syndromal hearing loss

Vestibular function has been investigated in many different syndromes. One of the first to be characterized was Usher syndrome, in which vestibular function has been found to be the best discriminator between different forms. Table 52.7 summarizes current knowledge of vestibular function in syndromal hearing loss. It is apparent that, in many syndromes, the vestibular end organ shows dysfunction expressed by the same genes which are causing the cochlear deficiency.

Table 52.7 Syndromal hearing losses.

	Vestibular	Other organs	Heredity
Usher type I	+	Eyes	AR
Usher type II	–	Eyes	AR
Usher type III	+/–	Eyes	AR
Alström	+	Eyes	
		Diabetes	AR
		Obesity	
Refsum	+	Eyes	
		Nerves	AR
Waardenburg	?	Skin	
		Eyes	AD
Alports	+	Kidney	AD, AR, X
		Eyes	
BOR	+	Kidney	AD
		Branchial fistulas	
Pendred	+/–	Thyroid gland	AR
Jervell-Lange	?	Heart	AR

+ vestibular hypofunction; – normal; +/–, variable; ?, not known; AD, autosomal dominant; AR, autosomal recessive; X; X-linked.

Usher syndrome

In a study of vestibular function in Usher syndrome (hearing loss/deafness and retinitis pigmentosa),[15] vestibular dysfunction was found to be extremely important in explaining some behavioural patterns, and in helping to classify different types of this condition. In all genetically linked cases of Usher type 1 (deafness + retinitis pigmentosa), bilaterally absent vestibular function has been demonstrated. However, in Usher type II (hard of hearing + retinitis pigmentosa), normal vestibular function bilaterally has been found. Usher type III displays progressive hearing loss and retinitis pigmentosa, and vestibular function seems to follow the hearing loss with a gradual decrease of the vestibular function.

Alström syndrome

Alström syndrome includes early onset of retinitis pigmentosa, which results in blindness in the early teenage years with bilateral symmetrical progressive hearing loss, hyperlipidaemia, elevated triglycerides and early-onset diabetes. Vestibular function shows a progressive decrease, which, together with blindness, results in severe unsteadiness, especially on uneven surfaces.

Conclusion

From a genetic perspective, vestibular tests can discriminate otherwise similar cases of non-syndromal hearing loss into two types: with and without vestibular dysfunction. It is likely that a phenotype reflects an underlying defect which is gene specific. If so, hereditary hearing loss should always be categorized according to whether the vestibular labyrinth is involved or not. If vestibular involvement is consistent within families, then hearing loss with or without vestibular symptoms represents two major clinical categories of hearing impairment. In syndromal hearing loss, it allows the differentiation of subtypes of a syndrome, enabling more accurate prognosis and rehabilitation.

Thus, in order to study hearing disorders and to provide a better mode of classification, vestibular function should be evaluated in all cases of sensorineural and unexplained conductive childhood hearing loss and deafness. This is particularly relevant for children being considered for cochlear implantation, as the presence of good vestibular function may result in vestibular symptoms postoperatively, while the absence of vestibular function emphasizes the need to determine whether the VIIIth nerve is intact.

Moreover, clumsiness and delayed motor milestones in children warrant full balance investigations to establish the presence of isolated vestibular dysfunction, on either an inherited or acquired (ototoxic, traumatic or infective) basis. Thus, appropriate rehabilitation and prognostic advice may be given.

References

1. Eviatar L, Eviatar A. Neurovestibular examination of infants and children. *Adv Otorhinolaryngol* 1978; **23**: 169–91.
2. Prensky A, Sommer D. Diagnosis and treatment of migraine in children. *Neurology* 1979; **29**: 506–9.
3. Parker W. Migraine and the vestibular system in childhood and adolescence. *Am J Otol* 1989; **10**: 364–71.
4. Hausler R et al. Menière disease in children. *Am J Otol* 1987; **8**: 187–93.
5. Akagi H, Yuen K, Maeda Y, Fukushima K et al. Menière's disease in childhood. *Int J Pediatr Otorhinolaryngol* 2001; **61**: 259–64.
6. Basser L. Benign paroxysmal vertigo of childhood. *Brain* 1964; **87**: 141–6.
7. Russel G, Abu-Arafeh S. Paroxysmal vertigo in children—an epidemiological study. *Int J Pediatr Otorhinolaryngol* 1999; Suppl 1: 105–7.
8. Lindskog U, Ödkvist L, Noaksson L, Wallquist J. Benign paroxysmal vertigo in childhood: a long-term follow up. *Headache* 1999; **39**: 33–7.
9. Salvén KM, Vikerfors T, Olecén P. Increased incidence of childhood bacterial meningitis. A 25-year study in a defined population in Sweden. *Scand J Infect Dis* 1987; **19**: 1–11.
10. Van Rijn PM. Causes of early childhood deafness. Theses Nijmegen, The Netherlands, 1990, ISBN 90-9002125-6.
11. Kimberling W, Moller C. Clinical and molecular genetics of Usher syndrome. *J Am Acad Audiol* 1995; **6**: 63–72.
12. Moller C, Ödqvist L, Tell J et al. Vestibular and audiological functions in gentamycin-treated Menière's disease. *Am J Otol* 1988; **9**: 383–91.
13. Shambaugh G. Statistical studies of children in public schools for deaf. *Arch Otolaryngol* 1930; **12**: 190–245.
14. Arnvig J. Vestibular function in deafness and severe hard of hearing. *Acta Otolaryngol* 1955; **45**: 283–8.
15. Sandberg L, Terkildsen K. Caloric tests in deaf children. *Arch Otolaryngol* 1965; **81**: 352–4.
16. Möller C. Balance function and hearing loss. In: Martini A, Read A, Stephen D, eds. *Genetics and Hearing Impairment*. London: Whurr, 1996: 109–17.
17. Möller C, Kimberling W, Davenport S et al. Usher syndrome: an otoneurologic study. *Laryngoscope* 1989; **99**: 73–9.

53 Psychiatric consequences of vestibular dysfunction

Rolf G Jacob, Joseph M Furman, Stephen P Cass

Introduction

Patients with psychiatric symptoms constitute a challenge to the otoneurological clinician. At a minimum, such patients signal extra expenditures of time. Traditionally, therefore, the main reason for otoneurological clinicians to summon psychiatric expertise was to find alternative, 'psychogenic' causes for the dizziness. As we will see, because of its implication that their dizziness is imagined, the patients often resent the resulting psychiatric referral. Furthermore, the receiving psychiatric clinician, ill-informed of the ways of the vestibular system, is not well equipped to care for these patients.

The possibility that psychological or psychiatric symptoms might constitute consequences of vestibular dysfunction is of relatively recent origin. The title of this chapter, therefore, can be seen as recognition of new grounds being broken. Most of the few previous contributions in this area, however, have been more theoretical than practical in nature. The present chapter will therefore focus on qualitative data, i.e. clinical case material. We hope that clinicians – both psychiatric and otoneurological – will be able to recognize, among their own patients, psychiatric symptoms that might be consequences of vestibular dysfunction. Armed with this knowledge, they might be able to cultivate an attitude of recognition and interest. They might be surprised to find that such an attitude by itself has a power of 'healing.'

Sources of qualitative data

Yardley et al performed the only published analysis of qualitative data concerning the psychological or psychiatric function of patients with vestibular disorders.[1] Their report inspired the approach taken in this chapter. Most of the clinical material for the present chapter came from 28 patients with vestibular dysfunction who were referred or sought consultation for psychiatric complications. These patients underwent semistructured psychiatric interview and questionnaire assessments. In the case illustrations, the patients are referred to by a coded name. For easy recognition of patients described on several occasions, first names were chosen to alphabetically code a patient's order of first appearance in the chapter. A few patients provided written material on their experiences. Naturally, excerpts from such autobiographical statements will be in first person format. Another rich source of information about patients with persistent vestibular symptoms is a website designed as a resource for patients with symptoms of Mal de Debarquement (MDD).[2] Many of the autobiographical case descriptions on this website reported reactions similar to those of other patients with unremitting vestibular symptoms. In this chapter we will include some quotes from the website. Such quotes will be designated as 'MDD patient.'

Like the observations by Yardley et al, our observations were in part guided by preconceptions. These included the conclusions by Yardley et al,[1] and our own research on the role of space and motion sensitivity or discomfort.[3–5] An impression that emerged de novo, however, was that certain personality attributes, i.e. perfectionistic tendencies, appeared to increase vulnerability to psychiatric complications and chronicity. Brandt, in his assessments of patients with 'phobic postural vertigo' has already reported this impression.[6] Another insight that emerged was that the spectrum of psychiatric complications in part depends on whether the patient has chronic unremitting or disabling symptoms versus subclinical or intermittent symptoms.[5] Depression and disability appear to be more common in the group with disabling symptoms.

Overview: range of vestibular-psychiatric interactions

The interactions between vestibular symptoms and psychiatric symptoms are complex.[5] This chapter will not cover all of them in detail. Nevertheless, in order to establish an overall context for subsequent discussions, we present an overview of possible interactions in Table 53.1.

> Vestibular and psychiatric symptoms are interrelated at several functional levels

Listed at the top of Table 53.1 is the circumstance where a patient may have a vestibular disorder and a psychiatric disorder simply as a chance co-occurrence. Being afflicted by depression or a psychotic disorder does not immunize patients against vestibular disorders. For example, one of our patients recovered from a vestibular disorder and later developed a depressive episode that appeared to be related to changed work circumstances after his company was sold. Although not a focus of the present chapter, it is important to remember the possibility of such chance co-occurrences, because the presence of psychiatric symptoms may lead to the error of diagnosing the dizziness of such patients as 'psychogenic.'

Dizziness does not always have a vestibular origin. Table 53.1 provides examples of such non-vestibular etiologies to dizziness, including other medical disorders (such as orthostatic hypotension) and psychiatric disorders (such as panic disorder). The latter type of dizziness is referred to as psychiatric dizziness.

In neither of the two scenarios above do psychiatric and vestibular factors influence one another. However, in the next set of circumstances, such interactions do occur. Next in Table 53.1 appears the case where psychiatric symptoms are components of an integrated response to certain types of vestibular dysfunction. We refer to this type of interaction, where psychiatric and vestibular symptoms are based on a common underlying mechanism, as 'linkage.' Psychiatric complications can also occur as psychologically mediated reactions to the perception of vestibular symptoms, or to the distress induced by them. We refer to this interaction as 'somatopsychic' effects. Conversely, certain psychological or behavioral factors can influence vestibular function. We will refer to this interaction as 'psychosomatic' effects.

In our experience, those patients who develop psychiatric complications of vestibular dysfunction also show more intense vestibular symptoms and prolonged recovery. However, not all patients develop psychiatric complications to vestibular dysfunction. We refer to factors that might predispose a patient toward these complications as 'vulnerability factors.' These include anxiety proneness, tendency towards 'somatization,' and obsessive–compulsive personality traits ('perfectionism').

The phenomena discussed thus far have concerned phenomena within a particular patient. However, some psychiatric phenomena are understandable only if we consider the patient in the context of his or her psychosocial environment.

Table 53.1 Overview of vestibular-psychiatric interactions.

Type of interaction	Explication	Example
Chance co-occurrence	Patient with a psychiatric disorder and an unrelated vestibular disorder	Patient with schizophrenia develops BPPV Patient recovered from a vestibular disorder develops depression
Non-vestibular dizziness	Dizziness due to non-psychiatric medical conditions Dizziness that is a symptom of psychiatric disorder: psychiatric dizziness	Orthostatic hypotension Hypoglycemia Dizziness during a panic attack due to hyperventilation
CNS linkage	'Hard wired' neural connections	Primary anxiety, space and motion sensitivity or discomfort
Somatopsychic effects	Psychological reactions to vestibular symptoms	Secondary anxiety, depression
Psychosomatic effects	Vestibular function affected by psychological factors	Reactivating compensated vestibular lesions
Increased vulnerability	Psychiatric conditions predispose to (a) psychiatric complications; (b) delayed recovery from vestibular disorder	Anxiety proneness. Somatoform disorders Perfectionism
'Systems' issues	Interaction between patient's 'illness behavior' and significant other's or provider's 'treatment behavior'	Social withdrawal; anger at provider

These include the behaviors of significant others and treatment providers. The 'systems issues' involved provide a basis for understanding social withdrawal and anger in the patients.

We mentioned earlier that the spectrum of psychiatric complications depends on whether or not the patient has chronic unremitting or disabling symptoms, versus subclinical or intermittent symptoms.[5] This chapter is organized based on this insight. Thus, we will begin with linkage and somatopsychic effects that occur even in patients whose dizziness has diminished or remitted because of central compensation of their vestibular balance. We will then proceed to the additional complications occurring in patients with persistent vestibular symptoms, including 'systems' issues. We will then discuss the role of psychosomatic effects on vestibular function, vulnerability factors, and psychiatric dizziness. The chapter will end with a brief discussion of treatment.

Psychiatric phenomena in with subtle vestibular symptoms

In this section, we will discuss the phenomena of anxiety, panic and a situational specificity of symptoms that we have called 'space and motion discomfort.' These consequences occur not only in patients with active vestibular symptoms, but also in those patients for whom vestibular symptoms are no longer prominent because of the effects of central compensation. In the latter type of patient, psychiatric symptoms may completely mask the remaining subtle vestibular symptoms.

> Panic attacks and phobic avoidance occur frequently in patients with vestibular disorders, including patients with compensated vestibular lesions.

Anxiety and panic

In humans, the experience of anxiety has two components, somatic symptoms and anxious thoughts. These two components are often referred to as 'somatic' and 'cognitive' anxiety symptoms. Somatic anxiety includes autonomic symptoms and symptoms associated with hyperventilation. The autonomic symptoms include heart palpitations, sweating, trembling, nausea or abdominal distress, and chills or hot flashes. Symptoms that resemble the effect of hyperventilation include sensations of shortness of breath or air hunger, chest pain or discomfort, dizziness or feeling faint, depersonalization (feelings of unreality or of being detached from oneself) and paresthesias (numbness or tingling sensations).

Anxious thoughts – also referred to as cognitive anxiety – find their expression as verbal (symbolic) content. This verbal content tells us what the individual is anxious 'about.' The prototypical anxious thought has the form of a 'what if' statement – e.g. 'what if I have a brain tumor?' Because anxious thoughts require verbal competence, they do not occur in preverbal or non-verbal organisms such as infants or animals. Finding out what the patient is anxious 'about' is important if we want to understand the patient. Furthermore, anxious cognitions can be modified by corrective information – 'you don't have a brain tumor.' Cognitive anxiety symptoms represent a hallmark of an anxiety disorder called generalized anxiety disorder. The proverbial 'worry wart' – the individual who worries about the minor daily issues in life – represents the prototype for patients with generalized anxiety disorder.

Most anxiety states have both somatic and cognitive components. Furthermore, the two components are interrelated; an anxious cognition can lead to somatic symptoms and vice versa. Among different forms of anxiety, psychiatrists have singled out one form, the panic attack, as separate from other anxiety responses. The main difference between panic attacks and other forms of anxiety is that somatic symptoms are particularly prominent. Because of their fundamentally somatic or wordless nature, patients experiencing panic attacks often are not able to report what they feel panicky 'about.' This leads to a description of the panic attacks as being unpredictable, uncued, or coming 'out of the blue.' Cognitive anxiety symptoms do occur during panic attacks but can be considered as secondary reactions, reactions in which a significance or 'meaning' is assigned to primary somatic sensations. They include fear of losing control (e.g. 'going crazy') and fear of a catastrophic bodily event (e.g. 'heart attack' or 'death'). The cognitive symptoms can be understood as representing a 'fear of fear' component of the panic attack.

Many patients with panic disorder avoid certain situations because of the panic attacks. They avoid situations in which panic attacks are likely to occur, or situations from which it might be difficult to escape, should a panic attack have occurred. Such patients are said to have panic disorder with agoraphobia.

Anxiety disorder diagnosis

Certain psychiatric disorders will be repeatedly discussed in this chapter. Therefore, we will briefly discuss how psychiatrists diagnose them. In the USA, psychiatric diagnosis follows the criteria codified in the fourth edition of the Diagnostic Manual of the American Psychiatric Association (DSM-IV).[7] Specifically, the DSM-IV lists specific criteria for the diagnosis of each disorder. These criteria were established to maximize reliability of diagnosis, but, unlike traditional medical diagnosis, do not necessarily imply anything about the hypothesized etiology of a disorder. Even so, the DSM-IV is the most authoritive source for descriptive psychiatry.

In the DSM-IV, pathological conditions are organized around three main categories, labeled Axis I, Axis II and Axis III. In addition, Axis IV and Axis V are included to reflect psychosocial stressors and overall functioning, respectively. The five axes were created to ensure that multiple types of information are considered simultaneously in the planning of psychiatric treatment. Axis III involves 'general medical conditions.' Here, diagnostic labels such as 'labyrinthine dysfunction' would be recorded. Axis II was created for conditions that imply enduring predispositions of a person, i.e. characteristics similar to 'temperament' and other traits. This axis includes personality disorders and mental retardation. Axis I is defined as 'clinical disorders' and 'other conditions that may be the focus of clinical attention.' Essentially, the conditions listed on Axis I represent the psychiatric analog to the general medical conditions of Axis III. Having to consider all of the axes in the diagnostic system counteracts our natural tendency of trying to arrive at a single 'correct' diagnosis.

DSM-IV recognizes the existence of 11 different anxiety disorders. Among these, the most important ones for this chapter are panic disorder, generalized anxiety disorder, and 'anxiety disorder due to …' (a specific medical condition). Panic disorder comes in two variants: panic disorder without agoraphobia, and panic disorder with agoraphobia. Panic disorder without agoraphobia is diagnosed if patients report recurrent panic attacks (already described) that lead to either fear of future attacks, worry about the implications of an attack, or other changes in behavior.[7] Panic disorder with agoraphobia also requires the presence of agoraphobia, which we defined in the preceding section.

Generalized anxiety disorder is diagnosed if the patient has been excessively worried – more days than not – for a period of at least 6 months. Furthermore, even though they try, patients cannot stop worrying. In addition, the worries are associated with at least three of six specific symptoms, including restlessness, muscle tenseness, trouble in concentrating, irritability, fatigability and trouble in sleeping. The diagnosis also requires that the worries interfere with the patient's overall functioning or cause significant distress. Finally, generalized anxiety is not diagnosed, if the worries only concern future panic attacks or a medical symptom such as dizziness.

Anxiety disorder due to a medical condition is diagnosed if the clinician judges the anxiety symptoms to be caused by the direct physiological effects of a medical condition. Medical causes of anxiety unrelated to the vestibular system include hyperthyroidism, hypoglycemia, pheochromocytoma and cardiac arrhythmias. The implication of this diagnosis is that if the underlying medical disorder were cured, the anxiety symptoms would completely remit.

Anxiety and panic in patients with vestibular dysfunction

Anxiety symptoms – both somatic and cognitive – are perhaps the most pervasive psychiatric complication of vestibular dysfunction. Several systematic studies conducted in otoneurological settings have documented the high prevalence of anxiety symptoms in vestibular patients.[8–11] For example, in our setting, one-third of consecutive (i.e. unselected) patients with vestibular dysfunction had anxiety symptoms qualifying as panic attacks on a questionnaire assessment.[9] The neurophysiological correlates of the vestibular dysfunction–anxiety link have only recently been explicated.[12] These include convergence between vestibular and visceral afferent inputs in the parabrachial nucleus of the brainstem. The parabrachial nucleus has reciprocal connections with the amygdala, a major way station in the processing of both internal and external fear-inducing stimuli. These basic brainstem circuits are subject to descending cortical inputs. The responsivity of the anxiety-supporting circuitry is further moderated via connections with the locus coeruleus that support responses to novelty.

Especially in patients with compensated vestibular abnormalities, anxiety symptoms can be the principal clinical manifestation; such patients tend to seek psychiatric rather than otoneurological help. In patients with anxiety disorders, vestibular abnormalities have been correlated with the presence of symptoms of agoraphobia, space and motion discomfort (to be discussed further below), and dizziness between panic attacks.[13–15]

The following case illustrates how vestibular symptoms may be missed in patients with panic attacks. The description below came from a research evaluation, conducted by a psychiatric clinician unfamiliar with the ways of the vestibular system. The patient received a diagnosis of uncomplicated panic disorder and mild height phobia.

> Patient: *Arnold S. (as described by psychiatric clinician)*. The patient is complaining of a 3-year history of panic attacks, dating back to the summer of 1991. His initial attacks occurred while at work and were associated with symptoms of lightheadedness, heart palpitations, dry mouth, fear of heart attack and fear of dying. The patient states that attacks are increasing in severity and causing him increasing concern. The patient's current panic symptoms are feelings of breathlessness, nausea, sweating, numb hands, tight chest, heart palpitations, feelings of blacking out and feelings that he is going to die. The attacks are rapid in onset and sometimes occur immediately. Their duration is under 15 min. The patient is unable to identify triggers. He identifies severe distress during current attacks. He worried moderately during the month about having more attacks.

This patient participated in a research study examining the vestibular system in panic disorder. His vestibular laboratory examination revealed a right reduced response of 55%. After the evaluation, he remained asymptomatic for 1 year. When his symptoms recurred, he was examined by one of the co-authors, S.P.C. (otolaryngologist), who reported the following:

> *Arnold S. (as described by S.P.C. (otolaryngologist) 1 year later)*: The patient reports the onset of vertigo beginning approximately 4 years ago. He has had periods of time lasting months when he would have dizziness sensations and then these sensations would disappear for months at a time only to return subsequently. Currently, his symptoms consist of a lightheaded feeling and short bouts of vertigo associated with nausea and lasting from seconds to minutes. Once he begins to feel dizzy, he feels increased anxiety,

which is correlated with increased symptoms. Recently, his spells have been lasting up to hours and have occurred 2–3 times per week. There has been no fluctuation of hearing or aural fullness. There is a bilateral high-pitched tinnitus present.

It is difficult to see that these two descriptions concern the same patient, albeit 1 year apart. There is nothing in the first description that would implicate the vestibular system. In fact, we have found that the symptom profile of a patient's panic attacks do not predict whether or not a patient has vestibular dysfunction. The symptoms occurring between attacks, on the other hand, do predict vestibular dysfunction.[16] These symptoms include feeling like falling, nausea, perceiving the room as spinning, spinning sensations inside the head, and veering.

Even when between-panic vestibular symptoms are more prominent, recognition of vestibular disorder may be delayed.

The patient, *Beatrice S.*, is a 48-year-old physician. One Thursday in October, while attending an art exhibition, she felt a sense of imbalance, started swaying, and had to sit down. Thinking 'Oh my God there is really something wrong with me' she reported 'freaking out,' fearing that she might have a nervous breakdown. The next morning, another episode of excessive swaying occurred. In the afternoon the same day, she had a panic attack. Thereafter, she began to have panic attacks frequently. When not panicky, she would worry about future panic attacks. She also began to dread driving. Because she knew that avoidance leads to agoraphobia, she resisted tendencies to avoid and pushed herself. She began yoga exercises and psychological treatment for panic. However, 3 months later she still felt off balance and went to her internist, who arranged for a CT scan that was negative. Six months after the episode began she went on vacation. She did well until the last day, when she had a migraine followed by a 'huge' panic attack. At the airport coming home, she was so dizzy and off-balance that she needed a wheelchair. The subsequent course was characterized by recovery and further setbacks. In July – 9 months after symptom onset – she was finally referred for vestibular testing. Caloric testing showed reduced left vestibular response. She was sent for vestibular rehabilitation therapy. Examination by the physical therapist revealed impaired performance on dynamic posturography.

Sources for anxiety or panic

The considerations above of brain circuitry linking functions of vestibular processing and anxiety suggest that somatic anxiety is a 'hard-wired' component of responses to vestibular dysfunction. Stated differently, anxiety is a component of the symptomatic response to vestibular dysfunction, just as heart palpitations are part of an integrated response to physical exercise (Table 53.1). However, compared to the heart rate response to exercise, the anxiety response to vestibular dysfunction may be more amenable to the moderating effects from descending, 'cognitive', influences. These latter influences can both increase and decrease the anxiety symptoms or create anxiety symptoms that are only indirectly related to vestibular dysfunction. The various sources for anxiety in vestibular patients are listed in Table 53.2.

We divide the anxiety responses associated with vestibular dysfunction into primary (early, somatic) anxiety and secondary (late, cognitive) anxiety.

Primary anxiety is a correlate of disorientation and loss of physical support associated with vestibular dysfunction. Metaphorically, primary anxiety is equivalent to the startle response that occurs when someone 'has the rug pulled out from under his or her feet.' This type of anxiety has been described as 'almost instinctive'.[1] As stated already by Cawthorne,[17] the symptoms of vestibular injury are

> Often so terrifying ... that observers unused to the ways of the labyrinth may find it difficult to believe that such a profound disturbance can be caused by injury to such a modest organ.

Primary anxiety is not verbally mediated. By this, we mean that the anxiety response would also occur in non-verbal or preverbal organisms. Primary anxiety is different from motion sickness. Whereas motion sickness takes time to build, primary anxiety occurs immediately. Balaban and Thayer report the following situation that illustrates primary anxiety:

Table 53.2 Elicitors of anxiety or panic in patients with vestibular dysfunction.

Type	Characteristics	Source
Primary anxiety	Somatic symptoms, autonomic symptoms	Direct linkage: 'hard-wired' concomitant of vestibular dysfunction Immediate somatopsychic response to disorientation
Secondary anxieties	Cognitions (thoughts) 'What if ...'	Future attacks or dizziness or panic Social consequences (embarrassment) Medical illness (brain tumor) Mental illness ('going crazy') Disability

> Suppose you are stopped at a traffic light on a hillside facing up. In anticipation of the traffic signal changing, a large bus that is alongside your car moves forward slowly, giving you a wide-field optic flow stimulus that you interpret as a backward drift of your car on the hill. You feel an urgent sense of panic as you vigorously depress the brake pedal. This is followed by a sense of relief as you realize that the perceived movement was merely illusory.[12]

This quote illustrates the immediate and reflexive nature of an initial anxiety response, and a secondary response (realizing it was the bus moving, not you) modifying it. This pattern – a primary anxiety 'wave' followed by a second moderating phase – can be described as a 'double take.' That is, the pattern is analogous to the situation where we see a face in a crowd and suddenly realize that it looks familiar and look again for verification.

Returning to the example of waiting at a traffic light next to a bus just quoted, the information gained from the 'second take' of the double take represented good news – it was the bus that was moving, not you. However, good news is not always assured – as the first author once realized after having backed into the car behind him. In patients with vestibular dysfunction, the second take often involves the possibility of bad news. Secondary anxiety begins when patients begin to worry about the meaning or significance about their symptoms. For example, a patient described above (Beatrice S.) expressed a fear of mental disorder. A similar sentiment is expressed in the following autobiographical statement:

> *Cecilia R.*: During my adult life I have had two grand mal seizures. Even though the last one was 17 years ago, I was now afraid that I would become so dizzy that I would faint and have another seizure and possibly die. The fear of seizures has plagued me for 25 years. Was this episode related to seizures? I was very scared . . .

A major source of secondary anxiety is the fear that the dizziness or panic sensations might happen again. This fear can be seen in the patient Beatrice S. just described – when not panicky, she would worry about future attacks. The fear of future panic attacks heralds the onset of panic disorder (see section on diagnosis above). Patients with severe dizziness also fear the return of dizziness per se:

> *Cecilia*: I was afraid to fall asleep, afraid I would wake up and the ceiling would be spinning. The fear was almost as terrifying as the dizziness.

The various sources of panic and anxiety in a patient with dizziness and agoraphobia are apparent in Table 53.3, which reflects a patient's recollection of sensations and thoughts during a panic attack in a shopping mall.

> *Donna P.*: The sequence of events in Table 53.3 can be assumed to extend over a period of 10–30 minutes. They were reported by a 50-year-old female whose problem started with an ear infection at age 48 followed by episodes of dizziness and tinnitus in her left ear ('like a hurricane'). She often staggers and has a tendency to fall to the left. A few times she went into a store and almost passed out. The patient reports panic-like feelings that include the following sensations: severe dizziness or faintness, and nausea; moderate shortness of breath, feeling of choking, feelings of unreality and fear of going crazy. Even when not feeling

Table 53.3 Sequence of subjective events during a panic attack in a patient with agoraphobia and vestibular dysfunction.

Type	Stage	Verbal descriptors or content
1. Primary	A. Prodromal phase	Oh, not again, here it comes! Oh (expletive), here it comes
	B. Somatic symptoms	I'm sick to my stomach My ear is hurting There is buzzing in my head My eyes don't focus My heart is beating fast
2. Secondary	C. Social/appeal for help	Oh God what I'm going to do I'll just have to call somebody to come and get me and take me home
	D. 'Fear of fear'	What if I pass out Oh that is so scary a feeling Oh God, I just want to go home and lie down It is so terrifying
	E. Social/embarrassed	This is embarrassing I feel like an idiot
	F. Social/lonely	Nobody knows how scary it is They look at you like you are crazy

panic-like, she reports the following symptoms as happening often or more: ringing in the ears, veering, lightheadedness, dry mouth, heavy feeling in her chest, nausea, blurred vision, and lump in her throat.

For heuristic purposes, the panic sensations can be divided into the phases of foreboding, somatic symptoms, social/help seeking, fear of fear, social/embarrassed, and social/lonely. The first two phases, foreboding and somatic symptoms, appear to be non-verbal in nature, representing primary anxiety symptoms. Secondary anxiety symptoms occur in the later phases. These include the initial appeal for help ('what if nobody can help me'), followed by further distress from the anxiety symptoms or their possible consequences. As the primary symptoms wane, the patient becomes aware of the possibility of social disapproval (shame and embarrassment).

Space and motion discomfort, fear of heights, and agoraphobia

We mentioned earlier that the symptom profile of panic attacks is unrelated to the presence or absence of vestibular dysfunction but that one indicator of vestibular dysfunction comprised vestibular symptoms occurring between panic attacks. In fact, patients with uncomplicated panic disorder (panic disorder without agoraphobic avoidance or without height phobia or without dizziness between panic attacks) are not any more likely to have vestibular dysfunction than are normal control subjects. Another major theme, however, is that symptoms are situation-dependent; that is, certain situations result in increased symptoms. We refer to this situational pattern as space and motion discomfort (SMD). This discomfort pattern appears to have a physiological basis; we have found that contrived situations with similar characteristics result in increased body sway in patients with balance disorders.[18] We refer to this physiological basis as Space and Motion Sensitivity.[5] Thus, 'discomfort' refers to the tendency to report symptoms, whereas 'sensitivity' refers to increases in objectively measured sway. To facilitate the reader developing a prototypical understanding of the situational patterns involved in SMD, we present the following vignettes obtained from our patients:

> In patients with anxiety disorders, agoraphobia, space and motion discomfort, and dizziness between panic attacks are predictors of abnormalities on clinical laboratory tests of vestibular function.

Donna: The patient whose panic experiences were described in Table 53.3 reported that she avoided the following agoraphobic situations: malls, public transportation, grocery stores, crowds, waiting in line, and going to the hairdresser, and taking elevators. The following symptoms of space and motion discomfort began or worsened after her ear problem began: riding as a passenger in a car (but uphill–downhill), riding on narrow roads, riding in the back seat, supermarkets, tunnels, going down on escalators, rolling over in bed, closing eyes in shower, leaning far back in chair, dancing. She had pre-existing fears of heights but now experiences more dizziness and fear of falling in high places (from three rungs on a ladder and up).

Elisabeth W.: After her symptoms of imbalance started, the patient developed height phobia, including fear of small stepladders. The patient cannot go into a grocery store. In malls she is particularly bothered on the second floor because of the vibrations in the floor on that level.

Fred L.: He does not like bridges, downtown Pittsburgh or New York City (too much motion), the open spaces in Washington DC, the outlook on Mount Washington in Pittsburgh, glass elevators, hotels with large atriums or walkways high up, environmental 'Escher-like' patterns, balconies in restaurants, and theaters with certain spatial characteristics (large balconies and small intimate theatres are OK).

Beatrice: After the dizziness began, she developed new discomfort or anxiety with heights such as standing on a ladder. In addition, she is bothered by department stores, auditoriums, or while walking along a large outdoor open water reservoir. She endorsed the supermarket syndrome (discomfort looking at the shelves while walking down the aisle). She experienced dizziness when closing her eyes in the shower. She reported discomfort while riding in a car, especially on limited access roads, in buses if crowded, in open fields especially if she is in the middle of a field, and in tunnels, especially if curved.

George T.: After the onset of vertigo, the patient began to avoid theaters, restaurants, elevators, and boats. In elevators, he was particularly bothered after the elevator has stopped because the ground still would be moving under him. The patient also developed mild discomfort when looking up at tall buildings.

Hillary G.: She has taken to avoiding going into public places and shopping because her symptoms are brought on there. If her symptoms are brought on while being exposed to a rich visual environment in a store, the symptoms can persist after she leaves. Watching ice-skating and other moving objects can increase her symptoms.

Ivan B.: He was particularly bothered by large drop-offs along the side of the road, particularly on the right side. He is also bothered on bridges, particularly if he is driving in the right lane, and especially on truss or suspension bridges (where the beams on the side provide optokinetic stimulation when driving by).

Additional troublesome situations reported by some of our patients include looking down spiral staircases, looking at Navaho rugs with zigzag patterns, and looking at shiny or backlit surfaces. In addition, watching TV can be problematic, especially when the background is moving (such as when the camera follows a football player running across the field). Some patients are also bothered when working on computers, especially when the screen is scrolling. Other patients report problems driving through an alley of trees when the sun shines from a direction that causes the tree trunks and branches to cast shadows in the form of black stripes across the street. More than one patient complained about the senior author's attire when he was wearing a vertically striped shirt during a session. One of these patients had a hobby of ballroom dancing. She was not able to dance when her husband was wearing shirts with striped patterns.

The phenomena observed by Brandt and coworkers in their studies on a condition they call phobic postural vertigo appear to be consistent with socially disabling SMD. The features of phobic postural vertigo include anxiety and dizziness upon exposure to bridges, staircases, empty rooms, streets, department stores, restaurants, concerts and crowds.[6] The condition was typically preceded by acute vestibular disturbances, such as benign paroxysmal positional vertigo, or traumatic conditions, such as whiplash injury, that could be expected to result in otolith dysfunction.[6] Phobic postural vertigo has been considered to be a form of 'psychogenic' vertigo. However, although the case vignettes above all came from patients referred for psychiatric evaluation, this situational sensitivity is not limited to such patients. In a study in which we assessed anxiety symptoms in consecutive patients with vestibular dysfunction already mentioned,[9] patients with vestibular dysfunction, compared to those evaluated for mild hearing loss, tended to particularly avoid heights and boats.

To assess further the pattern of situations that are problematic for patients with vestibular dysfunction we constructed a questionnaire, the Situational Characteristics Questionnaire.[3] This questionnaire consists of three subscales (the SMD-I, SMD-II and Ag-I). ('SMD' stands for 'space and motion discomfort'; 'Ag' stands for 'Agoraphobia,' reflecting items that would be avoided by patients with agoraphobia even in the absence of vestibular dysfunction.) In patients with anxiety disorders, the SMD-I has been shown to predict the presence or absence of vestibular dysfunction over and above the diagnosis of agoraphobia.[16] Table 53.4 lists the items reflecting situations that bothered the vestibular patients more than patients evaluated for hearing loss.[19] Again, these patients were not specifically selected for psychiatric dysfunction.

Situational fears following the SMD pattern have also been described by others, including fear of heights,[8,20] 'street neurosis',[21] the 'supermarket syndrome',[22,23] the 'motorist vestibular disorientation syndrome',[24] 'visual vertigo'[25] and 'space phobia'.[26,27] Agoraphobia as a syndrome was identified 130 years ago.[28–30] Interestingly, a major theme in the early literature on agoraphobia was whether or not agoraphobia was a form of vertigo.[31] In view of this background, it is of interest that in our study assessing the prevalence of vestibular

Table 53.4 Situations eliciting space and motion discomfort in consecutive otolaryngological patients with dizziness and vestibular dysfunction.

Situation	Aspect of situation inducing more discomfort (SMD-I or Ag-I)	Effect size[b]
Looking up at tall buildings	–	1.1
Closing eyes in the shower	–	1.0
Rolling over in bed	–	0.9
Leaning far back in chair	–	0.8
Riding in a car	Reading versus looking out of the window	0.7
Dancing	–	0.7
Aerobic exercise	–	0.7
Riding in a car	Back seat versus front seat	0.6
Tunnels	Looking at end versus looking at lights on side	0.6
Elevators	Moving versus stationary	0.5
Elevators	Glass versus standard	0.5
Reading newspaper close to face	–	0.4
Riding in a car	Straight roads versus winding roads	0.4
Buses	Moving versus standing still	0.4
Movies	Middle of the row versus aisle[a]	0.4
Supermarkets	Crowded versus empty[a]	0.4
Elevators	Crowded versus empty[a]	0.4
Riding on roller coasters		0.3
Elevators	Stopping versus moving at steady speed	0.3

[a] Item from Ag-I subscale, all other items in this column from the SMD-I. If no item in this column the situation is from the SMD-II
[b] Effect size: Difference between groups divided by the standard deviation of the difference

dysfunction among anxiety patients, the highest-prevalence laboratory vestibular abnormalities were found in patients with agoraphobia.[16]

> Situations triggering space and motion discomfort include long visual distances and busy, 'Escher-like,' wallpaper patterns.

Generally, SMD situations involve one or more of the following: (1) intense vestibular stimulation, such as during abrupt head movements when exercising; (2) neck extension; (3) unfamiliar body accelerations; (4) discordance or incongruence among the information in the vestibular, visual and somatosensory systems,[32] (5) inadequate or confusing visual spatial information, such as those involving long visual distances,[33,34] 'particularly rich or repetitive visual patterns'[25] that provide competing stimuli for visual fixation; or (6) unstable or soft support surfaces.

The mechanism underlying space and motion discomfort can be deduced from the fact that spatial orientation involves an integration of information from three main sensory channels, the visual, somatosensory (proprioceptive), and vestibular. Individuals with vestibular dysfunction may develop a sensory integration strategy in which visual and somatosensory information is used to replace the defective information in the vestibular channel. These individuals would be expected to be unusually sensitive to inadequate or misleading visual information (visual dependence) or unusually sensitive to instability of the support surface (surface dependence). Clinical experience with computerized dynamic posturography, as well as the result of a study examining the response to optic flow stimuli,[18] indicate that many patients with vestibular dysfunction are visually or proprioceptively dependent. In a study of anxiety patients with space and motion discomfort, we found them similarly responsive to optic flow stimuli.[35] Furthermore, agoraphobic patients are characterized by poor performance on dynamic (moving platform) posturography.[36] In our laboratory, we have found that patients with agoraphobia, many of whom had vestibular dysfunction, had a proprioceptively dependent pattern, with poor performance limited to conditions IV–VI on moving platform posturography.[15] Seen in this light, SMD cannot be viewed as an abnormal response to vestibular dysfunction any more than other situational medical symptoms. For example, individuals allergic to cats prudently avoid visiting households with cats.

Patients with unremitting, disabling balance symptoms

Riding a roller coaster is an experience that many individuals choose to have. The situation for the patient with unremitting symptoms, however, can be compared to a roller coaster ride infinite in duration. Besides anxiety and space and motion discomfort, these patients develop psychiatric problems that are related to the unremitting, intrusive nature of the symptoms, or from the disability resulting from the dizziness or imbalance. Although its symptoms are better compared with rides on a boat rather than a roller coaster, the syndrome of MDD[37] can be viewed as a prototype for patients with continuous intrusive symptoms. The intrusiveness of the symptoms can be appreciated in the following quote:

> *MDD patient.*[2] Two hours on the boat. That's all. I now use that cruise as a point of reference in the time line of my life. Pre-boat or post-boat. I remember dates and things I have done in relation to that because I have not been myself since that night.

Among individuals responding to a survey on the Internet focused on MDD, the most common psychiatric symptoms were fatigue, problems in concentrating, anxiety, memory problems, and depression.[2]

> Intrusive or disabling vestibular symptoms often lead to anxiety, decreased ability to concentrate, depression, social withdrawal and anger.

As mentioned already, besides the distress from the symptoms of dizziness or imbalance themselves, restrictions in daily activities provide another source of psychiatric distress. Thus, the patients examined by Yardley et al reported being unable to conduct normal daily activities, including cooking, washing, and shopping.[1] They also restricted their use of transportation (driving or traveling). In addition, the patients reported difficulties in meeting work demands, including the handling of dangerous machinery; there were significant periods of absence, and some patients had to stop working altogether. Even leisure time was affected; the patients reported restrictions in active physical activities such as gardening, dancing, bike riding and other sports restriction, as well as in sedentary pursuits such as reading, knitting, and sewing. Both the distress from symptoms and the disability from behavioral restrictions are illustrated by our patient below:

> *Cecilia*: I could not look up, down, or to the side or bend over without getting uncontrollably dizzy. I could not walk in a dark room with my eyes open or closed. I could not walk without holding on to someone or something. I could not work in my garden, clean, iron, and certainly could not cook. I have always been an avid reader and now I could not read. I could not look at someone or something that was within 2 feet of my vision. I was afraid to fall asleep, afraid I would wake up and the ceiling would be spinning. The fear was almost as terrifying as the dizziness. It was literally impossible to lie on my right side or turn from left

to right while lying down. I have slept only on my left side since last June because I could not lie flat on my back. I could not be in any stores or close places. This meant I could not shop. I could not go inside a mall or movie or even a small room. If I did, the sensations would be a very physical one. A combination of what I would imagine a panic attack would be, along with head pressure, dizziness and motion sickness.

Impaired attention, poor concentration, distractibility, and fatigue

It is impossible for humans to remain standing after falling asleep; control of upright balance requires attention. Maintaining balance under difficult conditions requires more attention than maintaining balance under easy conditions; the former diminish the attentional resources available for other tasks. In a study with normal subjects, reaction time was used as a measure for available attention (with long reaction time implying that less attention was available for the reaction time task).[38] It was found that reaction times were the shortest for sitting, followed by standing with broad support, standing with feet together, and walking, in that order. In another study, evidence for decreased attentional capacity was found when tasks were executed while the subject was standing on a sway-referenced support compared to a stable support surface.[39]

Given these findings on normal subjects, it is not surprising that impaired concentration is a common complaint among patients with balance disorders. The patients have to deploy attention to maintain balance similar to what is required from normal subjects under demanding balance conditions. Complaints by patients therefore include difficulty in maintaining attention on tasks that require planning, difficulty in remembering things, and a subjective sense of one's mind seeming foggy, and 'spacey.'

MDD patient: Probably the worse feeling to me is the fuzzy head, spaciness, or 'Brain Fog' feeling in my head. I feel as if I am not operating on all cylinders ... or that I have a short circuit in the wiring up there. Half of my brain feels like I am here and the other half feels like it is out in 'Ozone Land' somewhere! So hard to concentrate, hard to remember things I just did and just walking in a haze some days.

In addition, persistent attentional demands can lead to fatigue, a common complaint among vestibular patients. Increased attentional demand may be just one pathway to symptoms of fatigue, however. Sleep deprivation is another. Poor sleep may be a consequence of intrusive symptoms of vertigo. Some patients with intense symptoms fear closing their eyes because the vertigo increases.

Jennifer B. is a 32-year-old woman disabled from bilateral vestibular hypofunction and severe oscillopsia. She was unable to sleep because closing her eyes increased her symptoms. One method of coping was to keep her eyes open as long as possible while looking at a small red light on her VCR in darkness. Later she was able to visualize the spot with her eyes closed and this enabled her to fall asleep. A helpful modification of this visualization was to imagine a stick or pole sticking out of the water in a river. The flow of the water would 'model' the environment moving due to vertigo, while the tip of the pole provided a spatially invariant target for visual fixation. Even so, and probably as a result of concomitant depression, she would wake up early. Her total sleep duration was 3 h per night (despite treatment with fluvoxamine, a sedating type of serotonergic reuptake inhibiting antidepressant).

Conversely, fatigue may further decrease attentional capacity and increase symptoms: patients with balance disorders typically report that their discomfort increases as the day progresses (i.e. later during the day[19]).

Depression

Trouble in concentrating, poor sleep and fatigue can also be indicators of another psychiatric consequence of persistent symptoms, depression. Diagnostic criteria for depression appear in Table 53.5. In addition to the three symptoms just mentioned, depression is also characterized by: dysphoric mood; loss of interest in things previously enjoyed; poor appetite (or increased appetite due to 'nervous eating'); agitation or the converse, decreased activity; feelings of worthlessness; and death wishes that can escalate to suicidal ideation.

Jennifer (the patient with bilateral vestibular dysfunction just described), reported depressed mood, difficulty in falling asleep, restlessness, decreased concentration, fatigue, irritability, and guilt over her reduced function in her role as a mother. She had lost 12 pounds in 2 weeks. She did not

Table 53.5 Symptoms and signs of depression.[a]

Symptoms/signs
1. Depressed mood (complains or looks depressed)
2. Loss of interest
3. Weight loss or weight gain
4. Insomnia or hypersomnia
5. Psychomotor retardation or agitation
6. Loss of energy
7. Feeling worthless, guilt feelings
8. Trouble in concentrating
9. Recurrent thought of death or suicidal ideation

[a] Paraphrased and simplified from DSM-IV. To count as a criterion, the symptoms have to be pervasive and occur most of the day and nearly every day.

complain of nausea; nevertheless, she reported that nothing tastes good and that her mouth feels dry. Her concentration is decreased. The patient frequently expresses wishes not to live because she feels like a burden; however, she strongly denies current intent because of the consequences of such an act for her children.

In general, although depression as a psychiatric condition can come on without any apparent external trigger, in many patients depression occurs as a reaction to a psychosocial stressor. One source of depression in vestibular patients comprises the very realistic practical restrictions on lifestyle experienced by the patients, restrictions that deprive them of the rewards of everyday life. Depression represents a state of 'learned helplessness' that has been studied in animal models.[40] Alternatively, the depressed state can be conceptualized as grief over the loss of previous function. Patients with depression often welter in ruminative thoughts. Depressive ruminations can be identified by their characteristic 'if only' verbal structure, e.g. 'If only the doctor could find out why I have these symptoms'. Pervading the state of mind of a depressed person is a sense of hopelessness and demoralization.

Cecilia: Exactly 1 year, 3 weeks and 6 hours ago, on 17 June, 1998, I was diagnosed with benign positional vertigo. In simpler terms ... I was dizzy ... room spinning dizzy .... Too dizzy to sit up, walk or move. This condition would continue in varying degrees throughout this past year and still exists today, in some form .... Imagine turning yourself around 25 times as fast as you can. Now stop. How long would you like to feel that dizzy sensation? Imagine now that it never goes away ... Six months ago, to abate the dizziness, I had begun to use self-inflicted pain as a deterrent. I would pound my head with my fists, scratch my scalp to the bleeding point and bang my head into walls, door frames and windows. One month ago, I lamented that I had just lost a complete year of 'my precious time' ... One whole year. It was over and gone, 365 days stripped from my allotted life span. What a wasted year! This loss was not due to a life threatening illness, or a drug or alcohol addiction, nor was I in prison or in a coma ... That might have been easier to understand.

Once a person is in a depressed state of mind, it tends to be self-perpetuating. Depressed patients tend to attend selectively to things to be depressed about. They view the world from a consistently pessimistic perspective – the proverbial glass is half empty rather than half full. For example, if a patient's symptoms of dizziness have partially improved, the depressed person may selectively focus on the symptoms that remain rather than on the reduction in symptoms. Perhaps this is the reason why many clinicians suspect that the patient's symptoms are caused (entirely) by depression, i.e. are 'psychogenic.' However, the bias for seeing the negative does not mean that their symptoms are self-produced.

Social withdrawal

Studies on patients with balance disorders sometimes reveal social anxiety to be among the most prevalent complications.[1,11] Social fears provide reasons for avoiding public places, in addition to space and motion discomfort already discussed. Specifically, patients may become concerned about appearing intoxicated.

MDD patient: I drive people nuts behind me with my swaying ... It helps to hold on to the cart, it keeps the motion down, but I am sure a few of them think I am drunk!

Jennifer (the patient with bilateral hypofunction) reported that a stranger had once approached her in a shopping mall, confronting her with 'it is a shame that a young women like you should walk around in public, intoxicated'. With persuasion by the therapist (RGJ), the patient was induced to continue going to malls but walk with the assistance of a cane, thereby preventing similar encounters by the use of therapeutic 'impression management'.

Besides social fears, social withdrawal can be the end result of other influences. In the case that the patient is unable to maintain employment, the resulting change in social network naturally results in restrictions in social activities. In addition, patients with persisting vestibular symptoms tend to avoid social activities such as interacting with friends because they are too distracted by their symptoms. Furthermore, depression is often associated with diminished interest in social activities.

Social withdrawal may also occur as an expression of normative influences on illness behavior stemming from the patient adopting the 'sick role.' For individuals succumbing to an acute illness, the sick role social 'contract' permits them to assume the role of a patient, a role that includes license to express distress over symptoms and to be exempted from normal activities.[41] Concurrently, this sick role contract obligates the patient to comply with treatment – e.g. submitting to medical tests and taking medication. The sick role contract also prescribes behaviors for members of the patient's social environment. For example, family members are expected to act supportively in various ways, ranging from showing sympathy to performing the patient's chores.

The sick role contract works well for acute illnesses; if the patient gets better, all participants benefit. Not getting better, however, can be interpreted as a violation of the sick role contract. This transition from acute to chronic disease represents a phase of disappointment for all parties involved. The patient, no longer entitled to the degree of exemption from normal activities bestowed on the acutely ill, is put in a situation of feeling as if he or she is a 'burden.'

Jennifer (the patient with bilateral hypofunction): The patient reports 1 year of feeling anxious, more days than not, with worries about her not being able to respond to family members' needs (e.g. aging parents and children) and finances.

Conversely, family members or friends may indicate their doubt as to whether or not the patient is indeed entitled to the sick role by showing less sympathy:

> *Kathryn H.*: Friends have shown signs of impatience if the patient is weepy. Similarly, her children are not good listeners. Normally, she would have had her husband but he died 10 years ago. The patient has felt a need to talk through her problems with friends of family but they have tended to cut her off with premature advice-giving. Now she puts up a 'good front.'

Patients may attempt to cope with such influences by reducing their demands on the family by withdrawing or by attempting to behave in ways that minimize their illness behaviors.

> *Cecilia*: This pressure to 'keep a stiff upper lip' appears to be particularly pronounced in front of young children or grandchildren.[1] During a session, Cecilia complained that her adult children did not enquire enough about her symptoms. At the same time, however, she would try extra hard to appear free from distress or 'normal' when interacting with her grandchildren.

Anger

The sick role contract just described prescribes behaviors not only for patients and members of their immediate social environments, but also for the health professionals that the patients consult for their problem. In the case of acute illness, the patient's illness behavior is complemented by the clinician's treatment behavior, such that the latter leads to a reduction in the former. Treatment behaviors include the clinician showing interest in the problem, performing appropriate assessments, in due course providing physical explanation for the patient's symptoms, and proceeding and following through with appropriate treatment. If the patient's evaluation is completed and no treatable causes are identified, or if treatment is unsuccessful, clinicians tend to show signs of decreased treatment behavior, in the form of diminished expression of interest, reduction of time spent with the patient, and perhaps suggesting a 'psychogenic' origin of the problem or at least conveying the implication that the patient's vestibular problem is minor. Collectively, we will refer to such behaviors as 'clinician's dismissive behaviors' (CDBs).

CDBs have the untoward effect of further increasing the patient's sick role behaviors. These increases are often accompanied by expressions of anger over the clinician's perceived violation of his or her end of the sick role contract. In fact, outrage over CDBs can be discerned in close to 50% (9/19) of the autobiographical reports published on the website for MDD.[2] CDBs noted by the MDD patients include:

> A clinician's dismissive behavior may cause anger in patients with chronic vestibular symptoms.

1. Failure to recognize that there is a problem:

   MDD patient: There I saw the head of Neurology, who had never heard of MDD and dismissed it immediately .... I found the doctor there to be very indifferent and quite condescending. I get no advice (that I am willing to follow) from my doctors here and not much empathy – perhaps due to my age.

   MDD patient: He looked at it for about 1 minute and handed it back to me saying, 'you don't have this. This happens after an extended boat trip. You were on that boat for 2 hours.' And I said, 'I know that, but the symptoms fit me. It's not BPV.' ... He looked at me and said 'Do you want me to help you or not?' (on the wall behind him was a sign that says 'if you remember who is the doctor and who is the patient, your care will be a success')

2. Minimizing the impact of the problem:

   MDD patient: The doctor in charge of my testing ... said 'if it only happens when I fly, he suggests that I don't fly and even when I do at least I know it will eventually go away.' I have very few kind words to say about ... (the doctor)

3. The degree of CDB is inversely proportional to the amount of time spent with the patient:

   MDD patient: I went armed with all my recent info to the doctor, and I don't know whether his ego was on the line, he just didn't know anything about MDD or just wasn't interested but I couldn't even get him to talk to me for 5 minutes on the phone about this ... not unless I was willing to set up another appointment. I had already paid him $350.00 cash for the tests (no medical insurance), and he would not give me 5 minutes more of his time! .... I was not only insulted that the doctor was not listening to me, but I was mad that he wasn't even interested in an illness or syndrome that he might not have ever heard of before! I gave up on that doctor.

4. 'Insult' is added to 'injury' when suggestions are made that the problem might be 'mental.'

   MDD patient: In six months time I then saw an ear specialist and three neurologists, had CAT scans and an MRI and other neurological tests. All had negative results. There were always hints by the doctors that I was imagining the symptoms or that the condition was stress-related. Finally, I was advised to see a psychiatrist. I related my cruise ship story to the psychiatrist and was sent home with an antidepressant. For 2 years, various antidepressants and other medications were prescribed, none helping to relieve me of this rocking motion.

The opposite of 'dismissive' behaviors is 'validating' behaviors (Table 53.6). Thus, clinician's validating behaviors include: (1) accepting the patient's symptoms even if they do not fit a predetermined pattern and remaining open to the possibility of unknown non-psychiatric conditions or vestibular conditions

Table 53.6 Clinician's dismissive behaviors and validating behaviors.

Clinician's dismissive behaviors	Clinician's validating behaviors
Not acknowledging that there is a problem	Recognize limitations of medical workup, including vestibular laboratory test battery
Minimizing the impact of the problem	Recognize the impact from the perspective of the context provided by the patient
Reducing amount of time spent with patient	Increase the time spent; repetition, patient education.
Suggesting that dizziness is 'psychogenic'	Physical explanations of dizziness etiology as initial 'nidus' of symptom complex

not detected by conventional vestibular laboratory tests;[42] (2) recognizing and showing empathy for the severity of the problem within the context presented by the patient; (3) spending more time with the patient – such time can profitably be spent educating and elaborating on the nature of vestibular symptoms and their consequences (of the kind used by vestibular rehabilitation therapists); and (4) recognizing that unknown etiology does not imply psychiatric etiology. Evidence for the value of clinician validating behaviors can be found in some of the reports from MDD patients:

> *MDD patient*: During our first meeting she evaluated me, listened to my account of my symptoms, and had me do all sorts of balance tests .... Then she told me about this thing called Mal De Debarquement. She pulled a big book off the shelf and read a description of it and I was thinking 'Oh my God. That sounds just like me.'

> *MDD patient*: I once overheard my physical therapist talking to a colleague of hers .... She had called him specifically to ask if he could tell how I would react to flying (I was getting ready to take a trip and was worried about the effects of flying). She said to him, 'this is that patient of mine with MDD I was telling you about.' I know she thinks that is what I have and to hear her actually say it to someone else was like music to my ears. But why can't I get a doctor to tell me that?

Psychosomatic effects on vestibular function

Up to this point, we have discussed psychiatric responses or correlates to vestibular dysfunction. However, psychological factors may also affect vestibular function. Psychosomatic effects on vestibular function can be a result of increased physiological 'arousal,' an effect of hyperventilation, or, possibly, a consequence of sleep deprivation. The latter possibility is speculative and will not be discussed further – see the up-to-date review by Yardley and Redfern.[43]

> Increased arousal and hyperventilation may unmask a previously compensated vestibular lesion.

It is well known that the gain of vestibular responses is dependent on the degree of an individual's arousal or alertness. Low alertness decreases gain; in recognition of this fact, many vestibular tests require alerting tasks such as naming cities or performing calculations. Conversely, high arousal increases gain. High arousal (e.g. elevated heart rate) is a characteristic of anxiety states. These considerations suggest that anxiety or 'stress' might trigger symptoms of vestibular dysfunction. However, the evidence for this possibility is only suggestive. For example, Anderson et al reported a study in which patients with Menière's disease performed daily ratings of 'stress' and 'dizziness'.[44] Using sophisticated time series analysis techniques on each patient's data, the investigators found that the patients reported more dizziness on those days that they also reported more 'stress.' However, they did not find that dizziness was preceded by increases in stress – a finding that stress preceded dizziness would have made a stronger case for a psychosomatic causal relationship. Moreover, the general levels of stress reported by the patients were low.

Hyperventilation is a characteristic of panic attacks. Hyperventilation is also known to affect vestibular function.[45] Sakellari et al found that hyperventilation in normal subjects increased body sway by moderating somatosensory input.[46] Furthermore, in patients with unilateral vestibular hypofunction, hyperventilation led to the re-emergence of nystagmus and to increases in lateral body sway.[46] The latter findings suggest that hyperventilation can reverse the central compensatory processes that had mediated recovery.

> Psychiatric complications resulting from dizziness and dysequilibrium may prolong recovery from a vestibular disorder.

Psychiatric factors such as anxiety states thus may worsen a vestibular disorder in various ways, through increased arousal or hyperventilation. We have already seen, however, that vestibular dysfunction can bring about anxiety through linkage or somatopsychic mechanisms. Thus, vestibular symptoms and psychiatric distress may mutually enhance each other in a vicious circle. This may be why it has been found that the presence of anxiety symptoms predicts poor recovery from vestibular disorders.[47,48] In general, the phenomenon of psychiatric conditions worsening or interfering with the natural course of recovery from a medical disorder is sometimes referred to as 'psychiatric overlay.'

Vulnerability factors

Only some of the patients with vestibular disorders develop psychiatric complications. Little systematic knowledge is available as to whether or not certain patients are more vulnerable than others in these regards. Many of the patients referred to R.G.J. for psychiatric evaluation have commonalities in their pre-vestibular histories. These include pre-existing anxiety symptoms, and obsessive-compulsive personality traits. More rarely, patients showed evidence for somatization, meaning that they had histories of prior non-vestibular medical disorders associated with hypochondriacal preoccupation. It appears that these features provide fertile ground for, or act like a catalyst for, developing psychiatric complications. Alternatively stated, these attributes constitute predisposing or vulnerability factors for psychiatric complications.

Psychiatric complications may in turn be conducive to delayed recovery from the underlying vestibular disorder, as suggested in the previous section. Therefore, psychiatric vulnerability also predisposes for intensified vestibular symptoms or for delayed recovery from the vestibular disorder. For example, symptoms of SMD may escalate from 'discomfort' into phobic reactions, leading us to propose the diagnostic label of 'space and motion phobia'[5] for SMD that is highly intense and socially disabling.

What is not known is the extent to which this impression is a reflection of selection bias. However, our impression of the importance of obsessive-compulsive personality traits parallels that of data by Brandt already published in the reports on phobic postural vertigo.[6] Furthermore, the concept of vulnerability factors (diathesis) is well known in psychiatry. For example, individuals with family histories of anxiety disorders are more likely to react with anxiety disorders to a wide variety of psychosocial stressors, a phenomenon referred to as 'anxiety proneness.'

> Patients with pre-existing anxiety disorders or tendencies toward somatization or perfectionistic personality traits may be particularly vulnerable to developing psychiatric complications.

Pre-existing anxiety

As already discussed, patients with autonomic anxiety symptoms tend to have greater disability and poorer prognosis than vestibular patients without such symptoms.[43,48] In many of the patients referred to R.G.J. for psychiatric evaluation, some of the anxiety symptoms preceded the onset of the vestibular disorder, with new anxiety symptoms being added after onset of the vestibular disorder.

Lena N.: She reports that she always has been afraid of the dark. She also has severe fear of insects, enlisting the aid of neighbors to deal with them at home. She has always worried about the health of relatives. Her two cousins on her father's side recognize that 'we are the same way, it is in our blood; we worry too much.'

Donna (patient in Table 53.3): Most of her anxiety symptoms started after she had the ear symptoms, but some began after an episode of breathing problems that led to an admission for double pneumonia and asthma in 1988. On the other hand, she never liked buses, reading while riding in a car, sitting in the front at the movies, flying, elevators, and roller coasters. She has pre-existing fears of heights but now experiences more dizziness and fear of falling in high places (from three rungs on a ladder and up). She has also always been afraid of thunderstorms and water.

The pre-existing anxiety suggests that the patients are prone to respond with anxiety to a greater number of stimuli than is the case for the average person (anxiety proneness). Therefore, it is not surprising that they respond with anxiety in the presence of vestibular symptoms. Anxiety proneness is genetically determined, as evidenced by the fact that patients with anxiety disorders tend to have positive family histories of anxiety disorders. In other cases, the vestibular symptoms remind the patients of past fearful events and thus elicit conditioned anxiety responses.

Beatrice (the patient whose dysequilibrium had started during an art exhibition) recalled that she had undergone treatment for scoliosis at age 11. After surgical fusion of the mid-thoracic vertebrae, she was put in a body cast for 6 months and then in a smaller cast for 2 months. After this, she was unable to walk and had to learn to walk again. Her vestibular symptoms (described earlier) primed the reoccurrence of emotional states from this time period.

Fred (the patient whose SMD profile included bridges and 'Escher-like' patterns) developed an increased understanding of SMD symptoms and his avoidance was much reduced after a few treatment sessions. However, he remained wary of bridges. During a detailed review of thoughts and symptoms concerning bridges (similar to what was done for the patient in Table 53.3), he described a sequence of cognitions – 'I will be blown away,' 'I feel weightless,' 'It's almost like a drug trip, you are not there, you blend in.' He then realized that these experiences were similar to those from an episode in 1970 in which the patient had a drink that turned out to be laced with LSD – an episode in which he (and other partygoers) experienced extreme panic.

Anxiety and avoidance may also interfere with the functional recovery from vestibular disorders. For example, patients engaging in avoidance behaviors may deprive themselves of input needed for the development of central compensation. They may continue to avoid even though their underlying vestibular disorder has healed, thus maintaining their anxiety disorder. The latter phenomenon is illustrated in the case of a patient with space and motion phobia related to probable benign paroxysmal positional vertigo:

Lena (the patient who had pre-existing fears of insects): About 6 years ago, the patient woke up perceiving the whole room as spinning. This experience was frightening, terrifying. Since then she has had problems with dizziness and SMD. Much of her SMD was height and travel related. In addition, severe dizziness would invariably occur when she was lying on her left side. Consequently, she had not slept on her left side for 3 years. She would avoid rolling over in bed to the left at all cost. For example, she would not roll over on her left side to turn off her alarm clock located on her night table located on the right side of her bed. Instead she had to sit up in bed first.

Because these symptoms were consistent with benign paroxysmal positional vertigo, a session was scheduled with a vestibular rehabilitation therapist for particle repositioning. Because of the patient's high anticipatory anxiety, R.G.J. participated in the session. The patient was equipped with video goggles that documented the occurrence of nystagmus. She was highly anxious with flushed facies prior to the intervention and needed to hold R.G.J.'s hand firmly. Lying down to the right did not elicit nystagmus or dizziness. The patient was then persuaded to lie down with her head turned to the left. No nystagmus was elicited, and the patient did not feel dizzy, much to her surprise. She then lay down on her left side, again without nystagmus or dizziness.

Thus, by consistently avoiding lying on the affected side, the patient had deprived herself of the opportunity to learn that this maneuver now is 'safe.'

Somatization

Somatization refers to the tendency to report and be preoccupied with medical symptoms from varied organ systems. Thus, individuals with tendencies towards somatization report histories of other medical complaints preceding the vestibular disorder.

Maurice R.: Prior to the onset of the patient's vestibular disorder, the patient had an episode of leg pain possibly related to varicose veins. During follow-up sessions, he showed himself preoccupied with his leg pain, a preoccupation that interfered with the discussion of his vestibular symptoms. He reported not wanting his veins stripped 'because I might need the vein in the future' but requested a referral to a surgeon. He also had been concerned about his blood pressure but avoids having it checked, fearing the results.

Ned A.: The patient had a past episode of a painful shoulder with which he was preoccupied for an entire year, until his physician told him that he was healthier than most. He then realized that he had been 'adopting a stance (with respect to somatic symptoms) that turned into fear.'

In a recent study, patients with vestibular disorders were asked to provoke symptoms by engaging in vigorous head movements. Those patients who reported more somatic symptoms during the 2-month period prior to the study responded to the head movements with increased respiration rate.[49] A recent study showed that patients with somatization syndrome had elevated indices of physiological arousal, including salivary cortisol and increased heart rates.[50] Patients with somatization tendencies are prone to form the type of relationship with their medical care providers described under 'anger' above.[41]

Perfectionistic traits and obsessive-compulsive personality disorder

A personality disorder is defined as 'an enduring pattern of inner experience and behavior that deviates markedly from the expectations of the individual's culture.'[7] The pattern is so enduring that it can be identified during adolescence or early adulthood. The requirement that the deviation from cultural expectations should be 'marked' sets a high standard for diagnosis. However, rather than forming distinct pathological categories, personality disorders can also be viewed as maladaptive extremes of fundamental personality dimensions. Many individuals show personality traits similar to these extremes but do not meet the criteria; even so, they still adapt poorly to illness. Thus, whereas these traits may not have caused problems earlier in the person's life, they often interfere with adaptation to illness.

Our clinical experience, as well as that of others, is that of the nine personality disorders in DSM-IV, obsessive-compulsive personality disorder (OCPD) is of particular interest. The behaviors of patients with OCPD are characterized by 'a pervasive pattern of preoccupation with orderliness, perfectionism and mental and interpersonal control' that occurs 'at the expense of flexibility, openness, and efficiency.'[7] Specific criteria include: perfectionism, preoccupation with details, devotion to work, inability to delegate, general inflexibility or stubbornness, a miserly approach to spending money compared to others in similar circumstances, and unwillingness to discard old things even when they have no sentimental value. Again, even if the degree of OCPD traits does not meet strict personality disorder diagnostic criteria, they still seem to affect the person's response to illness. The criteria and descriptions above, however, do not do justice to the fact that the patient with OCPD traits is often highly capable and functional, at least before the onset of their vestibular disorder.

OCPD appears to be so common among patients coping poorly with dizziness that Brandt has included such traits as a definitional criterion of phobic postural vertigo.[6] Many of these patients were reported to have personality disorders, and the majority of those who did had OCPD.[6] On the other hand, the fact that compulsive personality traits were included as a criterion may be part of the reason why it was so commonly reported. However, we share Brandt's impression; a majority of the vestibular patients referred to R.G.J. had obsessive-compulsive traits.

It is not known why OCPD traits seem to put such patients at more risk for continued vestibular symptoms or greater disability from symptoms. One possibility is that these patients tend to be anxiety prone (see above). Many patients with generalized anxiety disorder, for example, have underlying OCPD or traits. A commonality among OCPD patients beyond anxiety is that their thinking style is characterized by a high degree of persistence. Consequently, they have trouble changing their focus of attention – including directing their attention away from their symptoms. The patients try hard to not perceive the symptoms, but in doing so paradoxically increase their awareness of the symptoms. This effect is similar to the consequences of deliberate thought suppression that occur when we are instructed to, for example, 'try not to think about a pink elephant.'

Some patients with OCPD are highly organized ('compulsive') and adhere to high standards of cleanliness and order. They will react with distress when their function is impaired in ways that makes them unable to meet these standards. Some also tend to react negatively when the behavior of others does not meet standards, including those of their clinician. Therefore they may be particularly sensitive to clinician's dismissive behaviors, such as keeping the patient waiting or not returning phone calls (see section on 'anger' above). Finally, patients with OCPD traits tend to have a long time horizon in planning their future; therefore, they respond with distress when vestibular symptoms might necessitate a change in their plans or 'life stories'.[51]

A potential risk with patients with OCPD traits is that they might overcomply with treatment. Our patient, Cecilia, describes the following response to vestibular therapy homework instructions:

> *Cecilia*: I pushed hard and convinced my therapist to give me more and more exercises to do. I would spend up to 2 hours a day, twice a day flipping my head, trying to look down, trying to bend over, trying to roll from side to side. I would march in place while moving my head in all directions. Then, I would stand on a dense foam rubber cushion, march in place, and shake my head until I literally could not shake it one more time. There were countless exercises. And I was to do each one with eyes closed and then open. Each time the dizziness would overwhelm me to the point of tears. I began to chant in my head 'I can do this, I can do this, I can do this', over and over and over. Rest 30 seconds ... begin again. Chant again. This went on for 2 months. It was almost unbearable to exercise but more unbearable to just sit and have the dizziness consume me.

Psychogenic versus psychiatric dizziness

'Psychogenic dizziness,' is a term that until recently pervaded the literature to describe some of the phenomena discussed in this chapter. The reason for our avoiding this term and similar terms, such as psychic dizziness, functional dizziness, and psychophysiological dizziness, is that these imply that the patient does not have a vestibular disorder. The psychogenic dizziness can be traced back to psychoanalytic thinking in which dizziness was seen as an expression of anxiety neurosis that could manifest even without concomitant cognitive anxiety symptoms.[52] Indeed, a clinical practice developed in which the presence of anxiety symptoms constituted a reason to 'rule out' vestibular disorders as a cause for dizziness complaints. As we have seen, however, certain psychiatric symptoms (e.g. space and motion discomfort) actually implicate the vestibular system. This is why the term 'psychogenic' vertigo is inappropriate in most cases. Furthermore, excessive reliance on this concept is counterproductive in the clinical setting. As we have seen, the practice of communicating to a patient that his or her dizziness is psychogenic constitutes a clinician's dismissive behavior that is particularly prone to elicit angry responses from patients.

This chapter would be incomplete, however, without recognizing that the presence of a symptom of dizziness does not always imply vestibular dysfunction. For example, dizziness can be an expression of non-vestibular medical conditions such as orthostatic hypotension or diabetic neuropathy. Similarly, dizziness can be a symptom of certain psychiatric disorders. We have proposed the term psychiatric dizziness for such occasions.[53] The criteria for psychiatric dizziness include:

1. The dizziness occurs exclusively in combination with other symptoms as part of a recognized psychiatric symptom cluster.
2. This symptom cluster is not itself related to vestibular dysfunction.[52]

For example, dizziness is a defining symptom of panic attacks, which represent the defining symptom of panic disorder. Dizziness during panic attacks is a consequence of hyperventilation; the presence of dizziness during a panic attack was not correlated with the presence or absence of vestibular dysfunction.[16] The dizziness that occurs during panic attacks thus fits the definition of 'psychiatric dizziness.' However, vestibular symptoms between panic attacks did predict vestibular dysfunction in our studies. Thus, this form of dizziness does not warrant the label 'psychiatric' – these particular patients have both 'psychiatric' and 'non-psychiatric' dizziness.

The number of psychiatric conditions that can cause complaints of dizziness in the absence of vestibular and other medical conditions associated with dizziness is small (Table 53.7). We have already mentioned panic disorder. Another cause for psychiatric dizziness is conversion disorder, a rare condition in psychiatric settings. Conversion disorder manifests with symptoms or deficits in motor or sensory control; such disturbances in gait can mimic a balance disorder. Still other cases of psychiatric dizziness may be related to verbal labeling phenomena. The experience of dizziness is private in nature and not subject to direct social validation. It is therefore possible that some individuals use the word 'dizziness' idiosyncratically to denote

Table 53.7 Psychiatric dizziness: psychiatric disorders with dizziness or imbalance as a defining or associated symptom.

Phenomenon	Possible mechanism	Associated phenomena	Psychiatric disorder
Dizziness, lightheadedness, faintness	Acute hyperventilation during panic attacks	Pricking sensations, heart palpitations (panic attacks)	Panic disorder
Feeling 'unreal'	Chronic hyperventilation	Anxiety	Panic disorder, generalized anxiety disorder
	'Dissociation'	No panic, no imbalance	Depersonalization disorder
		Extreme 'stress,' numbness	Acute stress disorder
		History of trauma, flashbacks, reports of feeling 'numb'	Post-traumatic stress disorder
Vague complaints, e.g. swimming sensations; no imbalance	Language used for difficulty in concentrating or being fatigued	Poor appetite, trouble in sleeping	Depression
Gait disturbance,	Pharmacological effect	Ataxia	Alcohol/drug intoxication
imbalance	Unknown (dissociation?)	Gait disturbance, no pronounced dizziness	Conversion disorder

vague sensations such as difficulty in concentrating or being fatigued. Still other patients complain of 'feelings of unreality', which might be another manifestation of hyperventilation in panic disorder. This term may also occasionally be used to describe symptoms of dissociation that occur in psychiatric disorders such as post-traumatic stress disorder.

Treatment of patients with vestibular dysfunction and psychiatric complications

Little systematic knowledge is available that is relevant for the treatment of psychiatric complications of vestibular disorders. Clinically, our approach to these patients includes patient evaluation, patient education, vestibular rehabilitation, and medication. Patient evaluation involves a review of both the patient's vestibular and psychiatric symptoms. Because of the complexity of the interrelationships, this often requires a prolonged session of combined questionnaire and interview assessments (e.g. 2 h). This evaluation provides the basic material necessary for the next phase, patient education. This involves providing an internally consistent conceptual structure from which the patient's symptoms can be predicted. In our setting, such education includes handing out literature on vestibular symptoms and space and motion discomfort (such as Jacob et al[3,54]; the present chapter was also written for potential use for our patients). Patient education can extend over several sessions. One focus for continued sessions is to combat and reverse tendencies of avoidance. Furthermore, sources of secondary anxiety are identified and corrective information is given, if indicated. To combat the negative effects of symptom suppression (see section on OCPD), an attitude of acceptance may need to be cultivated in the context of an overall therapeutic approach.[55] Another focus for the patients with intrusive chronic symptoms is the problem of anger (see section on 'anger'), which is validated and placed in perspective.[56]

> Education of the patient using appropriate physiological explanations, exposure to feared situations, vestibular rehabilitation physical therapy, and psychiatric medication are elements of a comprehensive treatment approach to patients who suffer from psychiatric complications of vestibular disorders.

Some patients are also referred for vestibular rehabilitation. The use of vestibular rehabilitation has several advantages. First, symptomatic improvement can be expected from the vestibular rehabilitation exercises. In a recent study, we found that vestibular rehabilitation was helpful for patients with agoraphobia and vestibular dysfunction.[57] Second, the assessment by the rehabilitation therapist provides further details about the patient's functional limitations in a clinically validating context, thus augmenting previous efforts of education.

The third component of treatment is medication. The benzodiazepine clonazepam, in typical doses of 1.0–1.5 mg per day (q.d.) (range 0.25 mg q.d. to 3 mg q.d.), has become the treatment of choice and is often associated with dramatic improvement. At times, 'if needed' dosing of clonazepam is sufficient. However, patients sometimes develop excessive sedation and ataxia, and this is a particularly high risk with elderly patients. Furthermore, although many patients are able to ultimately discontinue the medication, a few develop prolonged rebound anxiety symptoms. An advantage of clonazepam over other benzodiazepines is its longer duration of action, which may minimize withdrawal and rebound symptoms. Clonazepam may have other advantages. For example, the patient below improved significantly after he was switched to clonazepam from diazepam, another long-acting benzodiazepine.

> *George*: The patient had been on diazepam prior to his psychiatric evaluation. This medication was replaced with a combination of clonazepam, 0.5 mg twice per day (bid) and fluoxetine 20 mg q.d. (Eight months later, the fluoxetine was stopped, with no recurrence of dizziness.) After 1 month of treatment, he reported the following:
>
> 'After my appointment with you today, I decided to go biking for the first time this year. I am an avid road bicyclist but have not ridden all year due to my condition .... I found the articles that you wrote quite fascinating, though a lot of it is 'over my head'. I'm also thankful to be able to walk normally, ride elevators, walk across bridges and look over the railing, ride crowded subways facing backwards, eat in crowded restaurants and go to the mall, take trips away from home, etc. My next big step is getting back onto an airplane. Though this was never a fear before the onset of my condition, there is a slight hesitation at this moment .... I do not want to get too optimistic, as I understand that I may have a couple of 'bad days' but I firmly believe the worst is behind me and I am on the road to recovery.'

A second class of drugs that can be considered comprises the serotonin reuptake inhibiting (SSRI) antidepressants. Recent findings of vestibular symptoms in response to withdrawal from SSRIs (Balaban and Thayer[12]) should motivate further study of the effects of such drugs on the vestibular system. However, the SSRIs do not provide benefit for all patients and can be associated with side-effects, such as sexual dysfunction. In our clinical experience, the SSRIs such as fluoxetine (typically 20 mg q.d., but up to 80 mg q.d. may be required) may be particularly useful for underlying obsessive-compulsive personality traits, where they contribute to diminished preoccupation with and disability from dizziness. In addition, the SSRIs, as well as other antidepressants such as imipramine, may be useful in those patients in whom the dizziness is related to migraines.[58] Finally, antidepressants, including the SSRIs, are indicated for symptoms of depression, particularly if the patient shows symptoms of insomnia, loss of appetite, significant difficulty in concentrating, and suicidal ideation.

References

1. Yardley L, Todd AM, Lacoudraye-Harter MM, Ingham R. Psychosocial consequences of recurrent vertigo. *Psychol Health* 1992; **6**: 85–96.
2. Torrie E. Mal de Debarquement: a support page for people with MDD. http://www.etete.com/mdd/).
3. Jacob RG, Lilienfeld SO, Furman JMR, Durrant JD, Turner SM. Panic disorder with vestibular dysfunction: further clinical observations and description of space and motion phobic stimuli. *J Anxiety Disord* 1989; **3**: 117–30.
4. Lilienfeld SO, Jacob RG, Furman JMR. Vestibular dysfunction followed by panic disorder with agoraphobia: a case report. *J Nervous Mental Dis* 1989; **177**: 700–2.
5. Furman JM, Jacob RG. A clinical taxonomy of dizziness and anxiety in the otoneurological setting. *J Anxiety Disord* 2001; **15**: 9–26.
6. Brandt T. Phobic postural vertigo. *Neurology* 1996; **46**: 1515–19.
7. American Psychiatric Association. *Diagnostic and Statistical Manual of Mental Disorders*, 4th edn. Washington, DC: American Psychiatric Association, 1994.
8. Eagger S, Luxon LM, Davies RA, Coelho A, Ron MA. Psychiatric morbidity in patients with peripheral vestibular disorder: a clinical and neuro-otological study. *J Neurol Neurosurg Psychiatry* 1992; **55**: 383–7.
9. Clark DB, Hirsch BE, Smith MG, Furman JMR, Jacob RG. Panic in otolaryngology patients presenting with dizziness or hearing loss. *Am J Psychiatry* 1994; **151**: 1223–5.
10. Stein MB, Gordon J, Asmundson GJG, Ireland D, Walker JR. Panic disorder in patients attending a clinic for vestibular disorders. *Am J Psychiatry* 1994; **151**: 1697–700.
11. Sullivan M, Clark MR, Katon WJ et al. Psychiatric and otologic diagnoses in patients complaining of dizziness. *Arch Intern Med* 1993; 153: 1479–84.
12. Balaban CD, Thayer JF. Neurological bases for balance–anxiety links. *J Anxiety Disord* 2001; **15**: 53–79.
13. Yardley L, Britton J, Lear S, Bird J, Luxon LM. Relationship between balance system function and agoraphobic avoidance. *Behav Res Ther* 1995; **33**(4): 435–9.
14. Jacob RG, Furman JM, Durrant JD, Turner SM. Panic, agoraphobia and vestibular dysfunction: clinical test results. *Am J Psychiatry* 1996; **153**: 503–12.
15. Jacob RG, Furman JM, Durrant JD, Turner SM. Surface dependence: a balance control strategy in panic disorder with agoraphobia. *Psychosom Med* 1997; **59**: 323–30.
16. Jacob RG, Furman JM, Perel JM. Panic, phobia and vestibular dysfunction. In: Yates BJ, Miller AD, eds. *Vestibular Autonomic Regulation*. New York: CRC Press, 1996: 197–227.
17. Cawthorne T. Vestibular injuries. *Proc R Soc Med* 1945; **39**: 270–3.
18. Redfern MS, Furman JM. Postural sway of patients with vestibular disorders during optic flow. *J Vestil Res* 1994; **4**(3): 221–30.
19. Jacob RG, Woody SR, Clark DB et al. Discomfort with space and motion: a possible marker of vestibular dysfunction assessed by the Situational Characteristics Questionnaire. *J Psychopathol Behav Assessment* 1993; **15**: 299–324.
20. Hallam RS, Hinchcliffe R. Emotional stability; its relationship to confidence in maintaining balance. *J Psychosom Res* 1991; **35**(4/5): 421–30.
21. Levy I, O'Leary JL. Incidence of vertigo in neurologic conditions. *Ann Otorhinolaryngol* 1947; **56**: 329–47.
22. McCabe BF. Diseases of the end organ and vestibular nerve. In: Naunton RF, Ed. *The Vestibular System*. New York: Academic Press, 1975: 299–302.

23. Rudge R, Chambers BR. Physiological basis for enduring vestibular symptoms. *J Neurol Neurosurg Psychiatry* 1982; **45**: 126–30.
24. Page NGR, Gresty MA. Motorist's vestibular disorientation syndrome. *J Neurol Neurosurg Psychiatry* 1985; **48**: 729–35.
25. Bronstein AM. Visual vertigo syndrome: clinical and posturography findings. *J Neurol Neurosurg Psychiatry* 1995; **59**: 472–6.
26. Marks I, Bebbington P. Space phobia: syndrome or agoraphobic variant? *BMJ* 1976; **2**: 345–7.
27. Marks I. Space 'phobia': a pseudo-agoraphobic syndrome. *J Neurol Neurosurg Psychiatry* 1981; **44**: 387–91.
28. Benedikt. Ueber 'Platzschwindel'. *Algemeine Wiener Medizinische Zeitung* 1870; **15**: 488–9.
29. Westphal C. Die agoraphobia, eine neuropathische Erscheinung. *Arch Psychiatrie Nervenkrankheiten* 1871; **3**: 138–61.
30. Cordes E. Die Platzangst (Agoraphobie). *Arch Psychiatrie Nervenkrankheiten* 1871; **3**: 521–74.
31. Balaban CD, Jacob RG. Background and history of the interface between anxiety and vertigo. *J Anxiety Disord* 2001; **15**: 27–51.
32. Brandt T, Daroff RB. The multisensory physiological and pathological vertigo syndromes. *Ann Neurol* 1980; **7**: 195–203.
33. Brandt T, Arnold F, Bles W, Kapteyn TS. The mechanism of physiological height vertigo. I. Theoretical approach and psychophysics. *Acta Otolaryngol* 1980; **89**: 513–23.
34. Bles W, Kapteyn TS, Brandt T, Arnold F. The mechanism of physiological height vertigo. *Acta Otolaryngol* 1980; **89**: 534–40.
35. Jacob RG, Redfern MS, Furman JM. Optic flow-induced sway in anxiety disorders associated with space and motion discomfort. *J Anxiety Disord* 1995; **9**: 411–25.
36. Yardley L, Britton J, Lear S, Bird J, Luxon LM. Relationship between balance system function and agoraphobic avoidance. *Behav Res Ther* 1995; **33**(4): 435–9.
37. Murphy Terrence P. Mal de Debarquement syndrome: a forgotten entity? *Otolaryngol Head Neck Surg* 1993; **109**(1): 10–13.
38. Lajoie Y, Teasdale NBC, Fleury M. Attentional demands for static and dynamic equilibrium. *Exp Brain Res* 1993; **97**: 300–10.
39. Andersson G, Yardley L, Luxon L. A dual task study of interference between mental activity and control of balance. *Am J Otol* 1998; **19**: 632–7.
40. Peterson C, Maier SF, Seligman MEP. *Learned Helplessness. A Theory for the Age of Control*. New York: Oxford University Press, 1993.
41. Jacob RG, Turner SM. Somatoform disorders. in: Turner SM, Hersen M, eds. *Adult Psychopathology and Diagnosis*. 1st edn. New York: John Wiley & Sons, 1984: 304–28.
42. Gresty MA, Bronstein AM. Testing otolith function. *Br J Audiol* 1992; **26**: 125–36.
43. Yardley L, Redfern MS. Psychological factors influencing recovery from balance disorders. *J Anxiety Disord* 2001; **15**: 107–19.
44. Anderson G, Hägnebo C, Yardley L. Stress and symptoms of Meniere's disease: a time series analysis. *J Psychosomat Res* 1997; **43**(6): 585–603.
45. Theunissen EJ, Huygen PL, Golgering HT. Vestibular hyperactivity and hyperventilation. *Clin Otolaryngol* 1986; **11**: 161–9.
46. Sakellari V, Bronstein AM, Corna S, Hammon CA, Jones S, Wolsley CJ. The effects of hyperventilation on postural control mechanisms. *Brain* 1997; **120**: 1659–73.
47. Yardley L. Contribution of symptoms and beliefs to handicap in people with vertigo: a longitudinal study. *Br J Clin Psychol* 1994; **33**: 101–13.
48. Clark MR, Sullivan MD, Katon WJ et al. Psychiatric and medical factors associated with disability in patients with dizziness. *Psychosomatics* 1993; **34**(5): 409–15.
49. Yardley L, Gresty M, Bronstein A, Beyts J. Changes in heart rate and respiration rate in patients with vestibular dysfunction following head movements which provoke dizziness. *Biol Psychol* 1998; **49**: 95–108.
50. Rief W, Shaw R, Fichter MM. Elevated levels of psychophysiological arousal and cortisol in patients with somatization syndrome. *Psychosomat Med* 1998; **60**: 198–203.
51. Clark MR, Swartz KL. A conceptual structure and methodology for the systematic approach to the evaluation and treatment of patients with chronic dizziness. *J Anxiety Disord* 2001; **15**: 95–106.
52. Jacob RG, Furman JM, Balaban CD. Psychiatric aspects of vestibular disorders. In: Baloh RW, Halmagyi GM, eds. *Disorders of the Vestibular System*. New York: Oxford University Press, 1996: 509–28.
53. Furman JM, Jacob RG. Psychiatric dizziness. *Neurology* 1997; **48**: 1161–6.
54. Jacob RG, Furman JMR, Clark DB, Durrant JD. Vestibular symptoms, panic and phobia: overlap and possible relationships. *Ann Clin Psychiatry* 1992; **4**: 163–74.
55. Hayes SC, Strosahl KD, Wilson KG. *Acceptance and Commitment Therapy: An Experiential Approach to Behavior Change*. New York: Guilford Press, 1999.
56. Jacob RG, Pelham WH. Behavior Therapy. In: Sadock BJ, Sadock VA, eds. *Kaplan and Sadock's Comprehensive Textbook of Psychiatry*. 7th edn. Vol. 2. Philadelphia: Lippincott Williams & Wilkins, 1999: 2080–123.
57. Jacob RG, Whitney SL, Detweiler-Shostak G, Furman JM. Vestibular rehabilitation for patients with agoraphobia and vestibular dysfunction: a pilot study. *J Anxiety Disord* 2001; **15**: 131–46.
58. Cass SP, Furman JM, Ankestjerne JKP, Balaban CD, Yetiser S, Aydogan B. Migraine-related vestibulopathy. *Ann Otol Rhinol Laryngol* 1997; **106**: 182–9.

54 Medical management of balance disorders and vestibular rehabilitation

Doris-Eva Bamiou, Linda M Luxon

Introduction: vestibular compensation

The balance system in humans has a remarkable capacity to adapt to new situations and to learn new behaviours, which are prerequisites for survival. This capability is characterized by the rapid symptomatic recovery following vestibular damage, referred to as 'vestibular compensation'. Vestibular compensation is not a homogeneous process that affects synchronously all aspects of disordered vestibular function, but consists of a number of subprocesses progressing at different rates and to differing final extents.[1]

Physiology of vestibular compensation

Damage to the labyrinth results in a characteristic syndrome of oculomotor, postural and sensory disturbances that start to recover soon after the damage:

1. Static symptoms include high-frequency spontaneous nystagmus towards the intact side, tonic eye deviation towards the side of the lesion, roll head tilt,[2] and postural imbalance and ataxia,[3] which are present when the only vestibular stimulus applied is gravity.[1] These symptoms are related to the differences in the levels of tonic activity in the vestibular nuclei, as type I excitatory neurones have reduced activity ipsilaterally and increased activity contralaterally to the lesion.[4,5] Static oculomotor recovery is a robust process that starts 3–4 h after onset of the lesion and is complete in a few days,[2] in parallel with the reappearance of active type I neurones ipsilaterally, leading to a return of resting activity and neural rebalancing of the vestibular nuclei. Postural recovery, on the other hand, appears to rely more on propriospinal mechanisms.[6]
2. Dynamic symptoms include abnormalities of the gain, symmetry and phase of the vestibulo-ocular reflex (VOR), as well as deficits of the vestibulospinal responses in response to head movement.[2] These are thought to be related to the loss of one half of the afferent input to the vestibular nuclei, resulting in absent excitation from the lesioned side but persistent disinhibition from the intact side in response to rotation. Horizontal VOR gain is decreased by 50% toward and by 25% away from the side of lesion, while vertical VOR gain is decreased by 66%.[7] Dynamic recovery continues over months or years[8] and seems to be faster for postural than for oculomotor symptoms.[2] Dynamic oculomotor symptoms show incomplete recovery,[9] with deficits becoming more apparent for high velocities of movement.[10]

Current models explain vestibular compensation in terms of central nervous system (CNS) plasticity (flexibility to function under and deal with a variety of conditions), a theory that can accommodate all the proposed subprocesses and that is compatible with the versatility of vestibular function.[11] Following the event of a vestibular lesion, compensatory mechanisms consist of:

1. Adaptation/habituation/plasticity leading to recalibration of the gain of vestibular reflexes. The vestibular nuclei on the side of the lesion are almost devoid of type I neurones immediately after the lesion, and the VOR gain is lower than normal. The VOR gain will partially recover in the following days and months, but it will not reach normal

> **VESTIBULAR COMPENSATORY MECHANISMS**
> **Adaptation/habituation/plasticity**
> → recalibration of gain of vestibular reflexes
> Context-specific process—driven by error signal
> Error signal: retinal image slip and smooth pursuit
>
> **Substitution**
> **of sensory inputs:** visual, proprioceptive, somatosensory and intact labyrinthine input
> **of motor responses:** increased smooth pursuit gain, generation of saccades or blinks
> **of strategies:** based on prediction

pre-lesion levels, as the response to rapid acceleration demonstrates.[3] The restoration of balance in the vestibular nuclei and the resulting recalibration of the gain of the vestibular reflexes are due to adaptation of type I neurones of vestibular nuclei on the intact side, which demonstrate an increased discharge immediately after the lesion, commissural efficacy in effecting inhibition, and cerebellar shutdown of activity on the intact side.[1] Commissural and cerebellar activity seem to affect dynamic rather than static compensation,[2] while the cerebellar flocculus seems to be required for initiating but not for maintaining the compensatory process.[12] The error signal that induces VOR adaptation is a combination of image motion or slip on the retina during head movements[4] and the smooth pursuit which suppresses this retinal slip.[13] Adaptation is context specific;[4] that is the greatest VOR gain change will occur at the adapting frequency.

2. Substitution
   - of sensory inputs, including visual, proprioceptive, somatosensory and labyrinthine input from the intact side.[14] Vision,[15] cervical input[16] and input from the intact labyrinth[14] do not affect static recovery, but are crucial for dynamic recovery. On the contrary, proprioceptive and somatosensory inputs are important for both static and dynamic recovery.[17] There is a critical or sensitive period for substitution mechanisms in vestibular compensation,[18] and sensory deprivation during that time, either by deprivation of light, resulting in reduction in visual stimuli, or by restriction in movement,[19] may have a negative effect on compensation. Patients may rely more on visual or on proprioceptive substitution, depending on the stage, i.e. acute versus chronic, and extent of the lesion, i.e. unilateral versus bilateral failure.[13]
   - of motor responses. The gaze change that is generated by a unilateral vestibular lesion may itself act to restore the neural imbalance between the two vestibular nuclei.[1] In later stages, patients may learn to increase smooth pursuit gain[13] or to generate saccades or blinks during a head movement to the affected side, in order to eliminate the visual blur that occurs due to a deficient VOR gain[20] by suppressing vision during the saccades or the blinks.
   - of strategies. Strategies are highly idiosyncratic and initially conscious actions that are employed to attempt to rectify the dynamic symptoms, after compensation for the static symptoms.[2] They are based on prediction, much as athletes prepare for a race by mentally rehearsing their movements and visualizing the space.[4] Central preprogramming of eye movements results in more significant gain increase for predictable than for unpredictable tasks,[21] and the same may happen for postural reflexes.[13] Some strategies may be inappropriate in the long run, e.g. restriction of head movements to the affected side in order not to challenge an inadequate VOR,[1] which impedes exposure to the error signal that is necessary for adaptation, or use of visual cues to maintain postural stability in the case of bilateral vestibular failure, as eyes are not stable and vision degrades during head movements.[13]

Several theories have been proposed to explain the static and consequently the dynamic compensation by structural and functional neurochemical processes that are distributed throughout the CNS[22] on the basis of behavioural, neurophysiological or neuropharmacological studies.[23] Evidence has recently emerged for a potential spontaneous regenerative capacity in the mature mammalian vestibular system,[24] but no satisfactory evidence of vestibular regeneration contributing towards compensation as yet exists. Darlington and Smith[25] have postulated that intrinsic membrane properties of the neurones in the vestibular nuclei contribute in the (static) compensatory process, with the vestibular nerve being partly responsible for the resting activity in the vestibular nuclei. Furthermore, they explain the initial disappearance of resting activity in terms of a diaschisis phenomenon, i.e. neural shock after the injury due to overstimulation by leakage of neurotransmitters. Curthoys and Halmagyi[3] propose that short-term mechanisms that initiate compensation may include neural adaptation of increased firing in the intact vestibular nuclei, cerebellar shutdown and changes of gaze or spinal input. Reactive synaptogenesis consisting of sprouting of healthy axons,[26] denervation supersensitivity, i.e. neurones becoming more sensitive to the transmitters normally released,[1] increased neurotransmitter release[27] and increased commissural excitability and efficacy[28] are slower-acting processes that may account for later stages of compensation.

Vestibular compensation: clinical perspectives

The majority of patients will learn to function almost normally within a few weeks or months following a peripheral vestibular disorder, although this symptomatic recovery does not parallel recovery of vestibular function, as asymmetry in dynamic gain

FACTORS THAT MAY DELAY COMPENSATION

Central vestibular disorders	Psychological disorders
Cerebellar disorders	Hyperventilation
Progressive vestibular pathology	Somatization
Intermittent vestibular pathology	Autonomic symptoms
Visual impairment	CNS or vestibular suppressant drugs
Impaired proprioception	Restriction of activity
Head injury	Late introduction of vestibular exercises
Other medical comorbidity	

of vestibular reflexes persists.[3] Some patients, however, may have incomplete resolution of symptoms, due to failure of recovery from the initial event, or recurrent episodes of vertigo with no intermittent symptoms or persistent fluctuation of symptoms with improvement and relapses.[11] The reasons for incomplete symptomatic recovery may be single or multiple and need to be addressed prior to or concurrently with rehabilitation. For example, progressive pathology, such as Menière's disease, or intermittent pathologies, such as migraine, may be responsible for recurrence of symptoms and non-recovery.[29] Management in these and similar cases should initially focus on controlling the primary disease before the initiation of vestibular rehabilitation.

Compensation may depend on whether the lesion affects predominantly the vestibular nerve or the labyrinth, and Glasscock et al[30] report a 28% incidence of persistent unsteadiness after labyrinthectomy as opposed to only 14% after vestibular neurectomy. Animal studies suggest that preservation of Scarpa's ganglion in vestibular neurectomy is necessary for vestibular compensation; however, Black et al[31] found similar recovery patterns between those patients who, in the process of unilateral vestibular deafferentation, had Scarpa's ganglion excised and those who had it preserved during the same procedure. Other factors that may delay or impede compensation and symptom recovery include cerebellar damage, impaired proprioception, visual impairment and psychological disorders,[32–35] head injury,[36] hyperventilation,[37] CNS or vestibular suppressant drugs,[33,38] other medical comorbidity,[29] the presence of somatization (i.e. the tendency to complain about unrelated health problems) and autonomic symptoms.[34] Decompensation may occur even in well-compensated patients, due to fatigue, alcohol or drug intake[39] or benign paroxysmal positional vertigo (BPPV).[11] Exercise, on the other hand,[40] vestibular rehabilitation (see Table 54.7 for references and details) and its early introduction[41] have beneficial effects on symptomatic recovery.

A well-compensated patient is able to control and coordinate eye, head and body movements in order to maintain gaze stability and posture, and to achieve vestibular perception, without any adverse symptoms,[42] despite the persisting dynamic asymmetry in the gain of vestibular reflexes.[3] Clinical evaluation of compensation, therefore, is not an easy task, due to the desynchrony between vestibular symptoms, signs and test results.[43–45] Most vestibular tests do not provide an accurate picture of either the extent of impaired function, termed 'disability'[46]/'activity limitation',[47] or the impact of the vestibular disorder on the patient's life, termed 'handicap'[46]/'participation restriction'.[47] Various measures have been employed to quantify compensation from a clinical perspective in order to assess the rehabilitation outcome. These measures include scores calculated by intensity and duration parameters of vertigo induced by positional manoeuvres,[48,49] dynamic posturography,[39] the Clinical Test of Sensory Integration and Balance (CTSIB), which correlates well with posturography results,[50] and standardized, self-report questionnaires.[51–53] Clearly, more than one measure should be employed in order to assess the efficacy of treatment of the vestibular patient.

Treatment of the vestibular patient

Successful management of the vestibular disorder patient depends upon accurate diagnosis, an understanding of vestibular physiology, timing aspects of the intervention, and the physician's awareness of the overlap between the vestibular system and the autonomic and limbic system and of the resulting psychological aspects of the vestibular disorders. Treatment falls into the following main categories:

1. Pharmacological treatment.
2. Vestibular rehabilitation. Theories on vestibular compensation were put into a practical context in the 1940s, when Sir Terence Cawthorne and Dr Harold Cooksey devised the vestibular exercises known as the Cooksey–Cawthorne exercises,[54,55] which still form the basis of vestibular rehabilitation. The development of these exercises was mostly empirical, based on observations of what seemed to benefit patients with unilateral vestibular disorders and head injury patients. However, the Cooksey–Cawthorne exercises became widespread only about 30 years later, when animal studies established the beneficial effect of mobilization and vision on vestibular compensation.[19,56,57] The current rationale for vestibular rehabilitation is based on the concept of the capacity of the vestibular system for adaptation and recalibration of vestibular reflexes by substitution of sensory input, motor responses and strategies in order to achieve symptomatic recovery following a vestibular lesion.[13]
3. Adjunctive treatment: behavioural therapy, relaxation and breathing exercises, treatment aimed to correct vision/proprioception/mobility, environmental modifications and safety measures.
4. Surgery.

Pharmacological treatment of vestibular disorders

Despite our current understanding of vestibular neurochemistry, very few, if any, of the recent discoveries in this field have led to the development of a new anti-vertigo treatment,[58] and most of the drugs that are used today as treatment for vestibular disorders had already become established clinical practice before the era of modern neurochemistry provided information on the vestibular system's neurotransmitters.[59] To date, the treatment of vestibular disorders remains mostly empirical. Causes that hinder major progress in vestibular pharmacology are as follows:

- The potential CNS side-effects of antagonists of vestibular neurotransmitters such as glutamate.[58]
- Difficulties in determining which specific property of a drug is responsible for the drug's anti-vertiginous action.[60]
- The lack of an absolute indicator for compensation and the resulting problems in designing experimental models to judge the anti-vertiginous effect of a drug on animals.[60,61]
- Action of a drug may be species-dependent and animal experiment results do not necessarily indicate a similar action in humans.[61]
- The lack of clinical trials assessing treatment of acute vestibular crisis, due to either the distressing nature of symptoms that necessitate immediate treatment, in which case it is impossible to obtain consent from the patient to take part in a clinical trial, or to the brevity of symptoms, which makes treatment redundant, as it will not be possible to establish effective blood levels of the drug before the symptoms have spontaneously abated.[62]

The ideal anti-vertiginous drug should suppress dizziness, prevent vomiting and help restore normal balance with minimal side-effects and no adverse effects on compensation. However, to date no such drug is available.[62] As a general rule, the aim of pharmaceutical treatment of vestibular disorders is to minimize the patient's symptoms by administering the smallest dose of the drug with the least side-effects for the shortest time possible, and, in the case of an acute vestibular crisis, never for a period longer than a week, as there is strong evidence that vestibular suppressants impede central compensation.[38,63] The drug treatment of a vestibular disorder falls into three main categories:[64]

- Symptomatic treatment of acute vestibular symptomatology.
- Treatment of a specific condition that causes the vestibular symptoms. This may be well documented, e.g. in Menière's disease, migraine, or epilepsy, or emerging but not yet standardized treatment, as in the case of central vestibular disorders.[65]
- Treatment of an underlying or coexisting medical or neurological disorder or of symptoms that developed after the onset and partly as a result of the vestibular disorder (e.g. depression) is mandatory, but beyond the scope of this chapter.
- Experimental drugs e.g. drugs that accelerate compensation.

Symptomatic treatment of acute vestibular crisis

Acute vestibular crisis may be single or recurrent, with symptoms such as vertigo, nausea, vomiting, sweating, pallor or diarrhoea, which can be extremely alarming and debilitating to the patient. Studies that assess the efficacy of the acute vestibular treatment are scarce, and treatment is mostly empirical. The patient has to be reassured and rehydrated, while investigations may be needed in order to exclude a life-threatening condition (e.g. cerebellar haemorrhage) and to plan long-term management. During the acute stage, the patient may need suppression of the vestibular symptoms of vertigo/dizziness, nausea and vomiting. Vestibular suppression should only be initiated if vestibular symptoms last more than 30 min to 2 h,[62] and last no longer than 1 week, as vestibular suppressants hinder compensation and may have severe side-effects, while vestibular rehabilitation should be initiated as soon as the acute symptoms subside.

Drugs that control vertigo seem to target neurotransmitter action, including acetylcholine, histamine, and GABA action, at the level of primary to secondary vestibular neurones and vestibular nuclei,[62] thus suppressing integration of sensory stimuli in the vestibular nuclei.[61] Anti-emetics block input to the medullary vomiting centre from three major afferent pathway that relay the signals of emetic stimuli to the CNS:[60,66]

- the chemoreceptor zone in the area postrema (action blocked by dopamine agonists)
- the gastrointestinal tract (blocked by serotonin ($5HT_3$))
- from the labyrinth, leading to stimulation of the vestibular nuclei (blocked by antihistamine and glutamate antagonists).

Motion sickness is a form of vertigo triggered by travel in which autonomic symptoms such as nausea, vomiting, malaise and increased salivation predominate. It is caused by unusual movements or conflict of sensory stimuli (e.g. visual and vestibular). The neural substrate of nausea is unknown, but may include neurones in the hypothalamus and inferior frontal gyrus of the cerebral cortex.[67]

Treatment should be prophylactic, although it can also be given after the onset of symptoms. Effective drugs for combating motion sickness include antihistamines, antimuscarinics, 5–HT1A (serotonergic) receptor agonists and neurokinin type 1 receptor antagonists,[67] and treatment may include hyoscine, cinnarazine, dimenhydrinate (also appropriate for children) or promethazine.[68]

The properties of the most commonly used vestibular suppressants are given in Table 54.1, while dosage, side-effects and contraindications are given in Table 54.2. Vestibular suppressant drugs include the following.

Anticholinergics

The main drug in this category, hyoscine, was one of the first to be used for treatment of vertigo. Hyoscine is the most effective drug for the treatment of motion sickness.[68] Anticholinergics are thought to act on the CNS, as acetylcholine is the

Table 54.1 Recommended drugs for acute vestibular crises: properties.

Drug	Antagonist of					Sedative action	Anti-emetic action	Anti-vertigo action
	Histamine	Ach	Dopa	$5HT_3$	GABA			
Hyoscine		✓				+ +	+ + +	+ + +
Prochlorperazine		✓	✓			+ +	+ + +	? –
Promethazine	✓	✓	✓			+ + +	+ +	+
Cyclizine	✓	✓				+	+ +	–
Dimenhydrinate	✓	✓				+ + +	+ + +	+
Metoclopramide		✓	✓	✓		+	? + +	–
Cinnarazine[a]	✓					+	+	? + +
Diazepam					✓	+ + +	–	–

[a] Cinnarazine is a calcium antagonist.

Table 54.2 Recommended drugs for acute vestibular crises: dosage, side effects and contraindications.

Drug	Dose	Side-effects	Contraindications/precautions
Hyoscine	*Motion sickness* PO: 300 μg before journey, then by 300 μg/6 h Patch: 500 μg 5–6 h before journey, repeat 72 h after	Dry mouth, drowsiness, constipation, urinary retention	Glaucoma, prostate hypertrophy Caution in elderly: memory disturbance, confusion
Prochlorperazine	PO 5mg TDS up to 30 mg/day IM: 12.5 mg OD followed by oral dose 6 h later if necessary. Per rectum: 25 mg, followed by oral dose 6 h after, if necessary	Sedation, dystonia (0.3%), postural hypotension, extrapyramidal symptoms, dry mouth, blurred vision, constipation, urinary retention, endocrine disturbances	Pregnancy Caution in elderly: more susceptible to postural hypotension, extrapyramidal symptoms
Promethazine	*Motion sickness* PO: 25 mg before journey, then after 5–8 hours as required. *Sedation* PO: 25–50 mg at bed time as a single dose	Sedation, postural hypotension, extrapyramidal symptoms, dry mouth, blurred vision, constipation, urinary retention, endocrine disturbances	Caution in elderly: more susceptible to anticholinergic action, extrapyramidal symptoms
Cyclizine	PO/IV/IM: 50 mg TDS	Drowsiness, dryness, blurred vision, urinary retention, constipation, auditory and visual hallucinations	Heart failure, glaucoma, prostate hypertrophy
Dimenhydrinate	PO: 50–100 mg TDS. *Motion sickness* First dose 30 min before journey, 50–100 mg TDS.	Drowsiness	Caution in glaucoma, hyperthyroidism (anticholinergic action)
Metoclopramide	PO: 5–10 mg TDS	Extrapyramidal symptoms, neuroleptic syndrome, tardive dyskinesia	Renal insufficiency, phaeochromocytoma
Cinnarazine	PO: 30 mg TDS *Motion sickness* First dose 2 h before journey, then 15 mg TDS	Drowsiness, gastrointestinal upset, unsteadiness, headache, extrapyramidal symptoms, depression	Pregnancy Caution in elderly: more susceptible to extrapyramidal symptoms
Diazepam	IV:1–2 mg, continued orally as needed until the acute symptoms subside (smaller dose than for sedation)	Muscle relaxation, sedation, hypnosis, addiction, risk of falls	Caution in acute pulmonary insufficiency, respiratory depression, acute psychosis

predominant neurotransmitter in the efferent feedback from the brainstem to the vestibular labyrinth, to parts of the vestibular cochlear nucleus[69] and at the muscarinic receptors of autonomic effector sites innervated by parasympathetic nerves, both centrally and peripherally.[68] The most common mode of administration is transdermal and it achieves continuous release of the drug into the bloodstream for up to 72 h.[70]

Antihistamines

The phenothiazines are dopamine antagonists with significant antimuscarinic effects that act centrally in the dopamine receptors in the area postrema of the brainstem[69] and are effective in controlling nausea and vomiting.

They include the following:

- Promethazine is a long-acting anti-histamine with anti-emetic, central sedative and anticholinergic properties.
- Prochlorperazine is a dopamine and histamine antagonist, with weak anticholinergic action. It is a very potent anti-emetic and has been reported to be effective in treating vertigo or dizziness in small, uncontrolled studies,[71] but there is no definite evidence that it is more effective than placebo.[72] Buccal prochlorperazine causes less drowsiness and sedation and is slightly more effective than oral prochlorperazine.[73] Prochlorperazine impairs driving, with little subjective appreciation of this impairment.[74] It must be used with caution in the elderly, as it is more likely than other phenothiazines to produce extrapyramidal symptoms.[75] In addition, it slows down compensation in guinea pigs.[38]

Piperazines include cyclizine, a histamine H1 receptor antagonist characterized by a low incidence of drowsiness. Dimenhydrinate (dramamine) is another H1 receptor blocker. Sedation is the most common reported side-effect, and patients who take this drug are advised not to drive. Cyclizine and dramamine have been reported to be similarly effective in preventing the overall subjective symptoms of motion sickness in a double-blind study.[76] The authors postulated that while dramamine's effectiveness may be related to its sedative properties, cyclizine may work more directly on the stomach, leading it to be more effective in preventing or controlling gastrointestinal symptoms.

Metoclopramide is a benzamide closely associated with the parasympathetic nervous control of the upper gastrointestinal system. Combination with phenothiazines should be avoided, due to severe extrapyramidal reactions.[70]

Calcium channel antagonists

Cinnarizine and flunarazine inhibit the influx of calcium intracellularly. Flunarazine has long-lasting vestibulo-suppressant effects in both animals and humans,[77] and residual concentrations in the blood may be detected up to 4 months after administration.[59] In the UK, it is only available on specific specialist request, as it is not included in the British National Formulary; the side-effects of this drug include prolonged extrapyramidal effects and depression.[78] Doweck et al[79] reported significantly reduced seasickness susceptibility and severity in normal subjects who received cinnarizine 50 mg, as opposed to placebo, before travel, with no notable side-effects. However, cinnarizine is less effective than hyoscine in the prevention of motion sickness, but it has fewer side-effects in small doses.[80] Both drugs may have extrapyramidal side-effects,[81] and these adverse reactions preclude their use in older people for more than a few weeks at a time.[59]

Benzodiazepines

Diazepam has no specific action on the vestibular system and acts by reducing neural activity and causing inhibition throughout the CNS, including the vestibular nerve and nuclei.[69] It is an anxiolytic, anticonvulsant, muscle relaxant drug with little autonomic activity. There are anecdotal reports that diazepam during the acute phase of vertigo appears to assist in the early phase of compensation in humans,[64] possibly by allowing for earlier ambulation and head movements. However, the role of diazepam as a vestibular drug is controversial,[63] as its effects on compensation are not entirely clear,[82,83] and its use should be restricted to the initial stage of the acute vestibular crisis.[62]

Other drugs

Ondasetron is a potent, highly selective $5HT_3$ receptor antagonist with highly effective anti-emetic and anti-nausea action, but there are no data to support specific anti-vertigo action.[69] However, it has been reported to help some patients with vertigo due to brainstem stroke.[84] As the precise mode of action in the control of nausea and vomiting is not known, the drug should be reserved for treatment of chemo- or radiotherapy-induced and postoperative nausea and vomiting, and possibly vertigo due to brainstem pathology.

Specific treatment of vestibular disorders

Migraine-associated dizziness

Headache is a common problem that occurs in 91–96% of adults and 51.5% of children, while migraine occurs in 6–18% of adults and 5.7% of children.[85,86] Vertigo, dizziness or imbalance may be migraine-related phenomena that do not necessarily occur at the same time as the headache.[87] Cutrer and Baloh[87] postulate that the short-duration vertiginous attacks, which last for minutes to 2 h and are temporally associated with headache, are due to the same mechanism as other aura phenomena, while longer-lasting attacks of vertigo and motion sickness, with or without headache, result from the release of neuroactive peptides into peripheral and central vestibular structures. Brandt,[88] however, argues that motion sickness symptoms in migraine are due to neuronal hyperactivity and increased bloodflow in the brainstem. Vestibular test results may be normal.[87,89] Benign recurrent vertigo of childhood may also be a migraine precursor, with vertigo replaced by migraine years after the onset of the symptoms, or a migraine equivalent, with simultaneous onset of vertigo and migraine attacks.[90]

DIAGNOSTIC CRITERIA OF MIGRAINOUS VERTIGO[92]

Definite migrainous vertigo

1. Episodic vestibular symptoms
2. Migraine according to HIS criteria
3. At least one of the following during at least two vertigo attacks:
   (a) headache
   (b) photophobia
   (c) phonophobia
   (d) visual/other aura
4. Other causes ruled out by appropriate investigations.

Probable migrainous vertigo

1. Episodic vestibular symptoms
2. Migraine according to HIS criteria
3. Other causes ruled out by appropriate investigations.

Correct diagnosis is essential for treatment. The International Headache Society (IHS) classification of migraine[91] recognizes vertigo as a migrainous symptom only within the framework of basilar migraine; however, more recently there was an attempt to define migrainous vertigo according to a combination of the IHS criteria for migraine and the presence of other specific symptoms.[92] Differential diagnosis from Menière's disease can be difficult to make, while the two conditions may coexist, and diagnosis may only be made following response to treatment.[93] Pharmacological treatment of migraine-related dizziness has a high success rate of up to 92% resolution or improvement of episodic vertigo,[94] while a patient survey study found that the efficacy of pharmaceutical treatment in treating migraine-related dizziness is directly correlated with the ability to alleviate the headache.[95] Treatment of migraine-related vestibular symptoms may include vestibular exercises and pharmacological treatment, as well as dietary measures (avoidance of foods that may trigger the headache), lifestyle adaptation (e.g. regular sleeping patterns) and stress reduction techniques.[89,93,94] Pharmacological treatment of migraine, and, similarly, treatment of migraine-associated dizziness, is primarily symptomatic-abortive or prophylactic when patients have frequent unsatisfactorily treated attacks.[96,97] It may take several weeks in order to choose the single or combination drug and the optimal dose that are most effective for control of the dizziness/vertigo and the headache.[94] Acute abortive treatment may include analgesics such as acetylsalicylic acid, paracetamol or ibuprofen, anti-emetics, ergotamine or serotonin 1D agonists.[88] Prophylactic treatment may include β-blockers, non-steroidal anti-inflammatory drugs, calcium channel blockers, serotonin reuptake inhibitors and amitryptiline.[97] The dosage, side-effects and contraindications of the main anti-migraine drugs are given in Table 54.3.

Symptomatic/abortive treatment This treatment may include anti-vertigo or anti-emetic drugs as well as specific treatment for headache.[98]

Anti-emetics Motion sickness can be a prominent feature of migraine-related dizziness.[87,89] Baloh[98] recommends treating patients with promethazine, because of combined anti-vertigo and anti-emetic properties, dimenhydrinate and meclizine for milder episodes of vertigo, or metoclopramide if vomiting is a prominent symptom. All of these drugs are indicated if symptoms last for more than half an hour, as this is the minimum time needed for the drug to enter the blood.

Over-the-counter medications The vast majority of migraine sufferers may be self-medicating, basing their treatment on information from advertisements and a 'trial and error' method, using drugs such as aspirin, paracetamol, ibuprofen, and other non-steroidal anti-inflammatory analgesics as single or combination drugs that may also include caffeine.[99] The efficacy of this treatment for headache has been established,[100] although its mechanism of action is not fully understood.[99] Sheftell[99] recommends a step-care therapy, starting with a single-ingredient over-the-counter medication and increasing the dose, or replacing with a combination drug if ineffective. He limits use of these agents to three times a week, in order to avoid overuse and rebound phenomena, and avoids using these agents in patients with daily headaches.

Ergot drugs Dihydroergotamine (DHE) has a high clinical efficacy in migraine treatment and has fewer side-effects of arterial constriction and nausea than ergotamine.[101] The DHE abortive treatment dose is 1 mg IM or 2 mg nasal spray, while the ergotamine dose is 2 mg suppository or 2 mg tablets. It is contraindicated in patients with coronary and peripheral

TREATMENT OF MIGRAINE-ASSOCIATED DIZZINESS

General measures	Abortive treatment	Prophylactic treatment
Dietary measures	Anti-vertigo/anti-emetic drugs	β-Blockers
Lifestyle adaptation	Over-the-counter analgesics	Calcium channel blockers
Stress reduction techniques inhibitors	Ergot drugs	Serotonin reuptake
Vestibular rehabilitation	Sumatriptan	Amitryptiline
	Acetazolamide	

Table 54.3 Recommended drugs for migraine: dose, side-effects and contraindications.

Drug	Dose	Side-effects	Contraindications/precautions
Dihydroergotamine[a]	IM:1 mg Spray: 2 mg nasal spray		
Ergotamine	PR: 2 mg supp PO: 2 mg up to 6 mg/day Aerosol: 1–2 up to 6 inhalations per day	Nausea and vomiting, vertigo, diarrhoea, abdominal pain, leg cramps, myocardial ischaemia; pleural or peritoneal fibrosis in prolonged use	Pregnancy, breastfeeding, arteriosclerosis, coronary artery disease, thrombophlebitis, Raynaud, liver or kidney dysfunction, hypertension, porphyria, hyperthyroidism
Sumatriptan	SC: 6 mg—repeat after 1 h if effective and if needed (up to 12 mg/day) 20 mg nasal spray—repeat after 1 h if effective and if needed	Chest pain—throat tightness, arrhythmias, ischaemic ECG changes, myocardial infarction, drowsiness, hypotension, bradycardia, tachycardia, palpitations, pain, tingling, heat sensations	Ischaemic heart disease, coronary vasospasm, peripheral vascular disease, CVA/TIA, hepatic impairment, uncontrolled hypertension, epilepsy, brain lesions
Acetazolamide	PO: 250–1000 mg daily in divided doses	Paraesthesias, loss of appetite, taste disturbance, polyuria, flushing, thirst, fatigue, dizziness, depression, ataxia, gastrointestinal disturbances	Kidney or liver disease, depressed K or Na blood levels, suprarenal gland failure, glaucoma, hyperchloraemic acidosis
Propranolol	PO: 10 mg bd up to 160–180 mg/day	Bradycardia, heart failure, postural hypotension, heart block, cold extremities, dizziness, confusion, psychoses, hallucinations, bronchospasm, fatigue	Bronchial asthma, bronchospasm, bradycardia, cardiogenic shock, hypotension, metabolic acidosis, sick sinus syndrome, untreated phaechromocytoma
Flunarizine[a]	PO: 5–10 mg OD		
Pizotifen	PO: 1.5 mg OD (start with 0.5 mg and increase by 0.5 mg every 3 days)	Drowsiness, increased appetite and weight, dizziness, dry mouth, nausea	Closed angle glaucoma, urinary retention
Methysergide	PO: 1–2 mg TDS	Nausea, heart burn, abdominal discomfort, vomiting, dizziness, drowsiness, fibrosis and vascular reactions	Pregnancy, lactation, peripheral vascular disorders, progressive arteriosclerosis, hypertension, coronary heart disease, pulmonary/ kidney/ liver disease
Amitriptyline	10 mg nocte increased by 10 mg every 2 weeks up to 150–175 mg Usual dose 50 mg nocte	Cardiovascular, CNS and neuromuscular, anticholinergic, gastrointestinal and endocrine reactions, dizziness, weakness, fatigue, weight loss or gain, headache	Arrhythmias, mania, severe liver disease, lactation

[a] Not in ABPI formulary.

vascular disease and in pregnant women. Nausea is a major side-effect. Empirical evidence suggests that it is an appropriate drug for patients with migraine-associated vertigo.[102]

Sumatriptan Sumatriptan is a selective 5-HT receptor agonist that should be used when there is a clear diagnosis of migraine or cluster headache for the acute relief of migraine attack and not for prophylaxis. The drug also relieves symptoms such as nausea, vomiting, and phonophobia, and decreases the need for anti-emetics.[101] The dosage is 6 mg subcutaneously or 20 mg nasal spray into one nostril. The dose can be repeated once in the next 24 h if migraine initially responds but returns at least 1 h after the initial dose. The dose should not be repeated if non-effective but can be taken again for subsequent attacks. Tablets can also be given (50–300 mg per 24 h). Sumatriptan should not be administered with any other acute migraine treatment. Side-effects include chest or throat tightness or pressure as well as dizziness. Bikhazi et al[95] reported that sumatriptan was the single drug that was highly effective in ameliorating both dizziness and headache in a clinical uncontrolled trial of efficacy of a wide range of anti-migrainous drugs used by patients with migraine-related dizziness.

Acetazolamide Acetazolamide stabilizes the transient dysfunction of mutant calcium channels by acidification[103] and has been reported to be effective in controlling vertigo and motion sickness in patients with migraine and vertigo.[87,104]

Prophylactic treatment Prophylactic treatment is appropriate when there are frequent episodes of vertigo or when the severity is not adequately controlled by symptomatic treatment.[98]

β-blockers are the drugs of first choice for migraine prophylaxis,[105] while failure to respond to one drug of this category does not predict failure to respond to another.[97] Propanolol is a β-adrenoreceptor antagonist. A starting dose of 40 mg bd or TDS may be increased by the same amount at weekly intervals according to patient response. An adequate response is usually seen in the range 80–160 mg/day. It must not be used in asthma, atrioventricular conduction defects or brittle diabetes, and it must be withdrawn gradually. Concomitant administration with chlorpromazine increases the plasma levels of both drugs. Side-effects include nightmares and nocturnal hallucinations, fatigue, cold extremities and dizziness. Harker and Rassekh[106] reported that propanolol was effective in abolishing or reducing the frequency of vertigo and migraine attacks and reducing the associated motion sickness in seven of eight treated cases with a diagnosis of basilar migraine, while there is anecdotal evidence suggesting that this drug prevents vertigo as a symptom of migraine aura.[93]

Calcium channel blockers The use of these in migraine prophylaxis has been based on their effect on cerebral blood vessels, protecting from vasospasm, as well as on their protective action against cerebral hypoxia.[97] Flunarazine is of proven efficacy in migraine prophylaxis,[105] while it also has long-lasting vestibulo-suppressant effects in both animals and humans.[77] The standard dose is 10 mg OD, or 5 mg OD if side-effects occur, for at least 2 months.[97] Its main side-effects include weight gain and fatigue, and it is contra-indicated in pregnancy, hypertension and glaucoma.

Serotonin reuptake inhibitors Pizotifen has antiserotonin, antitryptamine and antihistaminic effects as well as some antagonistic activity against quinine. It inhibits the permeability of the migraine-affected cranial vessels, checking the transudation of plasmakinin, so that the pain thresholds of the receptors are maintained at 'normal' levels. Side-effects include drowsiness, increased appetite and weight gain. Pizotifen has been reported to be effective in prophylaxis against migraine that developed after remission of benign recurrent vertigo of childhood.[90] The daily suggested dose is 1.5 mg, starting with 0.5 mg OD, and increasing the dose by 0.5 mg every 3 days until the desired dosage has been established, in order to avoid drowsiness.[97]

DIAGNOSTIC CRITERIA FOR MENIÈRE'S DISEASE (AMERICAN ACADEMY OF OPHTHALMOLOGY AND OTOLARYNGOLOGY, 1995)

Certain Menière's disease:
Definite Menière's disease + histopathological confirmation.

Definite Menière's disease:
≥2 episodes of vertigo of 20 minutes or longer
Documented hearing loss on at least one occasion
Tinnitus or aural fullness in the affected ear
Other cases excluded.

Probable Menière's disease:
One definitive episode of vertigo
Documented hearing loss on at least one occasion
Tinnitus or aural fullness in the affected ear
Other causes excluded.

Possible Menière's disease:
Episodic vertigo characteristic of Menière's disease without documented hearing loss or
Sensorineural hearing loss, fluctuating or fixed with dysequilibrium but without definitive episodes of vertigo
Other cases excluded.

Methysergide (3–6 mg in three divided doses) is a highly effective prophylactic drug, but, due to serious side-effects that include fibrotic disorders with chronic usage, and dizziness, vomiting, sedation and depression with acute use, it should only be used when other prophylactic drugs have not been of benefit.[97]

Amitryptiline Cass et al[89] suggest amitriptyline, a tricyclic antidepressant, as the first drug of choice for migraine-related vestibulopathy, with the second and third choices being β-blockers and calcium channel blockers respectively, and they observe that 30–50% of their patients respond favourably to this treatment. Amitryptyline (10 mg at night, increasing by 10 mg every 2 weeks up to 50 mg, or even 150–175 mg) is the only antidepressant drug with established efficacy in migraine prophylaxis, and its anti-migraine effect seems to be unrelated to its antidepressant effect.[97] Side effects include drowsiness, weight gain and orthostatic hypotension, and contra-indications include glaucoma, urinary retention, pregnancy, breastfeeding and concomitant use of monoamine oxidase inhibitors.

Menière's Disease

The diagnosis of Menière's disease should be based on strict criteria as defined by the American Academy of Ophthalmology and Otolaryngology (AAOO) Committee on Hearing and Equilibrium guidelines.[107] Causes such as migraine,[98] Cogan's syndrome[108] or Menière's disease of syphilitic aetiology[109] have to be differentially diagnosed, as they require specific treatment, which, in the case of Cogan's syndrome and syphilis, needs to be promptly initiated for best hearing results. To date, treatment of Menière's disease remains mostly empirical, as the existence of different theories of pathogenesis, the lack of a universally accepted method of evaluating treatment results despite the AAOO guidelines,[110] and the course of the disease, which has frequent spontaneous remissions, have hindered the development of a widely accepted evidence-based treatment protocol. Furthermore, there is no consensus with regard to prophylactic versus symptomatic treatment.[59] There are a few double-blind randomized studies assessing treatment efficacy,[110,111] which is reported to range between 60% and 80%, but these studies may not be satisfactory after rigorous inspection,[110,112,113] and a placebo effect of treatment cannot be excluded.[111,112] Management of Menière's disease can be medical or surgical. However, destructive surgical treatment must be the last resource after all other options of rigorous medical treatment have failed, as it has non-reversible effects, while it may not prove beneficial in all cases, and the possibility of bilateral Menière's disease as well as the potential of the older patient for postoperative recovery need to be carefully considered.[114] Medical treatment falls into four main categories:

1. Short term—acute vestibular symptom suppression, as described above.
2. Long term—measures that aim to influence endolymphatic hydrops, such as low- or no-salt diet, diuretics, betahistine.
3. Suppression of immunological reactions in the endolymphatic sac.
4. Destruction of the diseased inner ear by intratympanic injection of aminoglycosides.

MANAGEMENT OF MENIÈRE'S DISEASE

Acute phase, short term:
Anti-emetics, anti-vertigo drugs

Chronic phase, long term:
Diet
Diuretics
Betahistine
Vestibular exercises

If evidence for autoimmune aetiology:
Steroid treatment

If medical therapy has failed:
Intratympanic injection of aminoglycosides
Destructive surgery

Measures that aim to influence endolymphatic hydrops

Diet There are no double-blind trials that report on the efficacy of a low-salt diet in treating Menière's disease. Santos et al[115] reported vertigo control in 79% and hearing improvement in 35% of patients with Menière's disease who were evaluated retrospectively with the 1985 AAOO criteria, on a 2-year follow-up after treatment with diuretics and a low-salt diet. However, the study did not attempt to separate benefits derived from diet from benefits due to diuretics, there were no controls, and the number of subjects was small. As a general rule, patients are advised to restrict salt intake to 1 mg[111] or 1.5–2 mg per day.[64] In our experience, strict adherence to a low-salt diet can be sufficient to control a Menière's crisis in many cases. However, the success of this regimen depends on patient compliance as well as on educating the patient about unappreciated sources of salt (e.g. tinned food). Although a low-salt diet is a baseline treatment of Menière's disease in ours as well as in other clinical settings,[64] a study has yet to emerge that convincingly demonstrates the benefits of this regimen.

Diuretics Diuretics (Table 54.4) have been reported to be effective in the long-term control of vertigo but not of hearing loss. However, their beneficial effects are not unanimously accepted, as most efficacy studies have been flawed methodologically, while thiazide diuretics may affect electrolyte levels.[111,116] Significantly, there was only one double-blind placebo-controlled trial between 1978 and 1995, by van Deelen and Huizing,[111,117] and there have been none since.

Bendroflurozide is a thiazide diuretic which reduces the absorption of electrolytes from the renal tubules, thereby increasing the excretion of sodium and chloride ions, and consequently of water. Its main side-effect is hypokalaemia, and a potassium-rich diet or potassium supplements must be administered in conjunction with the drug, which has to be administered with caution to diabetics. There are no data on its efficacy in treatment of Menière's disease.

Dyazide (combination of 50 mg triamterene and 25 mg hydrochlorthiazide) is a potassium-conserving diuretic that has been reported to be effective in controlling vertigo, but not hearing problems.[117]

Chlorthalidone is a sulphonamide derivative that has been reported to be beneficial in uncontrolled studies.[118] Acetazolamide is best avoided, due to ambiguous results and unpleasant side-effects.[119] Loop diuretics such as furosemide should be avoided due to potential ototoxicity.[59]

Betahistine Betahistine (see Table 54.4) is a histamine analogue with weak agonistic action at both H1 and H2 and moderate antagonistic action at H3 histamine receptors. The drug may owe its anti-vertigo properties in Menière's disease to improved microvascular circulation in the stria vascularis of the cochlea which reduces the endolymphatic pressure or inhibits the activity in the vestibular nuclei.[60] In a review paper, Claes and Van de Heyning[111] identified five double-blind trials between 1978 and 1995, three crossover studies and two double-blind comparisons with flunarazine or dihydrochlorthiazide. In a more recent meta-analysis (oral paper) prepared for a systematic review of *betahistine* for the Cochrane library,[110] the authors identified six double-blind subject control trials, excluding crossover if there were no data available before to

Table 54.4 Recommended drugs for Menière's disease: dose, side-effects and contraindications.

Drug	Dose	Side-effects	Contraindications/precautions
Bendroflurozide	PO: 5–10 mg OD or on alternate days early in the morning. Maintenance dose 5–10 mg once or twice per week	May exacerbate/activate lupus erythematosus Hypokalaemia	Renal failure, pregnancy, hypersensitivity to thiazides Caution in Addison disease, hypercalcaemia, diabetes, hepatic impairment.
Dyazide	PO: 1 tablet containing 50 mg triamterene and 25 mg hydrochlorthiazide after the	Dizziness, nausea, vomiting, weakness, headache, dry mouth, hypotension, electrolyte changes	Hyperkalaemia, renal failure, hepatic dysfunction, hypercalcaemia, diabetic ketoacidosis, Addison's disease,
pregnancy	morning meal, thereafter adjusted to patient's needs	with occasional metabolic acidosis, rarely blood dyscrasias	Caution in diabetes
Chlorthalidone	PO: 25–50 mg OD per day at breakfast time	May induce gout, electrolyte changes *Side effects with higher dosage may include:* electrolyte imbalance, dizziness, hypotension and arrhythmias, skin rash, gastrointestinal problems, worsening of glucose intolerance, thrombocytopenia	Anuria, renal/hepatic insufficiency, hypersensitivity, refractory hypokalaemia and hyponatraemia, hypercalcaemia, hyperuricaemia, untreated Addison's disease, lithium therapy Caution in elderly, hyperlipidaemia, coronary disease
Betahistine	PO: 16 mg TDS Maintenance dose: 24–48 mg	Gastrointestinal upset, headache, skin rash, pruritus	Phaeochromocytoma, hypersensitivity Caution in peptic ulcer, pregnancy, bronchial asthma

crossover, as cited on Medline and Embase. None of the trials reported in these review/meta-analysis studies adhered to the AAOO criteria. Claes and Van de Heyning[111] reported unequivocal results, while in a systematic review James and Thorp[112] found conflicting evidence on the effect of betahistine on the symptoms of Menière's disease. However, experimental evidence from animals suggests that betahistine facilitates compensation in cats.[120]

Other drugs include calcium agonists (flunarazine, cinnarazine), but there is no evidence to suggest that these are effective or more effective than betahistine.[111,121]

Suppression of immunological reactions Steroid treatment is based on the assumption of an autoimmune pathogenesis of Menière's disease, as indicated by elevated serum levels of autoantibodies,[122] but there are no double-blind control studies demonstrating the clinical effects of this concept. Steroids can be administered topically or systemically, but topical application achieves a much higher drug penetration and produces fewer side-effects than systemic administration.[123] Shea[124] reported hearing improvement in 35.4% and complete vertigo control in 63.4% of cases treated with 16 mg intratympanic and 16 mg intravenous dexamethasone for 3 consecutive days, followed by oral dexamethasone, in an uncontrolled study that followed the AAOO guidelines. Silverstein et al,[125] however, report no benefit of intratympanic administration of dexamethasone versus placebo in terms of hearing and tinnitus in 22 treated patients with Menière's disease. A recent uncontrolled open trial reported good results for bilateral Menière's disease with methotrexate.[126]

Intratympanic injection of aminoglycosides Streptomycin and gentamicin are selectively vestibulotoxic and act by destroying the dark cells of the secretory epithelium, thus decreasing endolymph production. Gentamicin is currently preferred to streptomycin.[127,128] Although this treatment seems to have a high efficacy in controlling the vertigo in up to 90% of cases,[119,129] there is no consensus as to the best protocol regarding dose, technique of administration and end point of therapy, while deafness may develop in up to 30% of treated cases.[130] This treatment should be reserved for patients who have failed medical therapy,[128] and seems to be of value in patients with incapacitating symptoms of Menière's disease who have not responded to long-term aggressive medical treatment. There are anecdotal reports that if one ear is successfully treated, Menière's disease only rarely develops in the contralateral ear.[127] Although the presence of the A1555G mitochondrial mutation, which increases susceptibility to aminoglycoside ototoxicity,[131] has not been reported so far in patients with aminoglycoside-induced hearing loss following vestibular ablative therapy,[132] patients who are considered for this treatment, and particularly those of Asian origin, should be screened for the mutation, and, if the results are positive, alternative means of treatment (e.g. vestibular neurectomy) should be preferred.

Chronic vertigo

Central vestibular disorders will result in chronic or progressive disability that cannot always be improved by medication, and both the patient and the doctor must have realistic expectations of the treatment. However, alternative gait and posture control strategies in the case of central vestibular patients, and vestibular exercises, in the case of bilateral vestibular failure, as well as implementation of safety measures and assistive devices, may improve the patient's mobility and sense of confidence and should form an integral part of the treatment of the chronic vestibular patient.[35,133,134] Any treatable underlying neurological disease should be treated.

There is some evidence, although inconclusive, that some centrally induced involuntary eye movements can be controlled by medication acting at neurotransmitter sites in the CNS, but drugs have to be titrated against side-effects.[135] One has to bear in mind that the long-term effects of these drugs are unknown, and it is recommended that this treatment be initiated by a neurologist with experience in eye movement disorders. The main drugs available are summarized in Table 54.5.

Psychiatric morbidity is high in patients with vestibular dysfunction,[136] particularly in chronic disorders, and these patients must be identified so that they can be given appropriate treatment. Vestibular sedatives should be particularly avoided as they delay compensation, except in some cases of central neurological conditions that cause intractable vertigo and do not respond to treatment.[137] The drug treatment of the patient with chronic vertigo and falls should be reviewed, in case the falls of the patient are partly caused by medication that can be withdrawn, as, for example, antipsychotic treatment in the older patient is known to predispose to falls and can be prescribed without a solid indication.[138] Table 54.6 summarizes medication that may increase the risk of falls in the elderly. Surgery should only be considered in cases where all other treatment has failed, there is good indication for surgery, and evidence that this may prove beneficial.

Experimental drugs

A novel category of drugs emerging from animal experiments that may potentially be used in the future but has not been fully clinically assessed includes drugs thought to accelerate compensation, such as gingko biloba extract EGb 761, melanotropic peptides[57] and opiates.[139] Schlatter et al,[140] however, found no evidence that EGb 761 accelerates or enhances static compensation, and the authors attributed part of the drug's action to the drug's vehicle. Some homeopathic remedies have also been reported to be effective in reducing the frequency, duration and intensity of vertigo attacks in a double-blind randomized control study that used betahistine as controls.[141] However, the action of homeopathic drugs is poorly understood and their long-term effects are unknown. None of these substances should be used until clinical trials have established their efficacy in treating vestibular disorders and their long-term effects, bearing in mind the UK government's recent directive on the effects of St John's wort.

Table 54.5 Drug therapy of central eye movement disorders.

Condition	Drug	Action	Side-effect
Downbeat nystagmus	Baclofen Clonazepam Scopolamine	GABAergic GABAergic Anticholinergic	Muscle weakness Sedation Drowsiness
Upbeat nystagmus	Baclofen	GABAergic	Muscle weakness
Episodic ataxia	Acetazolamide Sulthiame	Carbonic anhydrase inhibitor Carbonic anhydrase inhibitor	Paresthesia, fatiguability
Periodic alternating nystagmus	Baclofen	GABAergic	Muscle weakness
See-saw nystagmus	Clonazepam Gabapentin	GABAergic Anticonvulsant	Sedation Somnolence, dizziness, ataxia
Congenital nystagmus	Barbiturates Baclofen	 GABAergic	 Muscle weakness
Acquired pendular nystagmus	Baclofen Clonazepam Barbiturate	GABAergic GABAergic	Muscle weakness Sedation

Table 54.6 Drugs that may increase risk of falls in the elderly or adversely affect compensation in the general population.[138]

Drug	Psychomotor impairment	Increased risk of falls	Adverse vestibular effects
Benzodiazepines	+ + + +	+ + +	Delays compensation
Cyclic antidepressants	+ + +	+ +	Induces central vestibular syndrome
Antipsychotics	+ + +	+ +	Delays compensation
Diuretics	?	+?	None reported
Antihypertensives			
Recreational drugs	+ +	+ +	Induces central vestibular syndrome
Alcohol	+ + +	+ + +	Induces central vestibular syndrome
Antihistamines	Drowsiness		Delays compensation
Dimenhydrinate			

Vestibular rehabilitation: key factors

Vestibular rehabilitation should follow a detailed evaluation of the patient. Evaluation should establish:

1. The cause of vestibular lesion, in order to identify and initiate the appropriate medical management, e.g. pharmacological treatment in Menière's disease and migraine or surgery in the case of a vestibular schwannoma.
2. The extent and type of the vestibular lesion. This is essential information in order to choose the most appropriate exercise/manoeuvre regimen. For example, an Epley manoeuvre is appropriate treatment, with very good results for isolated BPPV; however, further coexisting peripheral vestibular pathology will require the appropriate rehabilitation for optimal results.[142] In the case of bilateral vestibular failure, vestibular rehabilitation should be based on exercises that foster substitution of visual and somatosensory cues.[143]
3. Concurrent factors that may affect compensation in order to correct remediable problems, e.g. operation of cataracts for improvement of vision, or to initiate adjunctive therapy, such as behavioural therapy for patients with psychological disorders, or relaxation and breathing exercises for hyperventilation.
4. The patient's particular difficulties, preferred strategies and levels of activity. There is considerable variability among subjects with regard to which mechanisms are used for compensation, and therefore the rehabilitation programme must be based on the type and degree of deficit and on the patient's inherent potential for compensation.[4]
5. Estimate of the prognosis; for example, CVD takes longer than PVD for recovery.[33]

KEY FACTORS OF VESTIBULAR REHABILITATION

Detailed evaluation:
Cause, extent and type of lesion
Identify concurrent factors: medical, vision, proprioceptive, neuro-muscular, musculosceletal, psychological, drugs
Identify patient's main difficulties, preferred strategies, levels of activity

Establish patient's active collaboration:
Explanation of symptoms. Motivation
Realistic outcome targets agreed upon

Timing:
Early introduction of vestibular rehabilitation

Choice of appropriate rehabilitation regimen:
Preset versus customized exercises
Individualized or class instruction
VOR recalibration versus substitution
BPPV manoeuvres

The patient's active collaboration needs to be established. For this reason, an accurate explanation of symptoms and of the purposes of the rehabilitation programme should be given, and time and realistic outcome targets should be set and agreed upon. Motivation, attention, effort and interest have long been recognized as key factors in compensation[144] and may play a specific role, in that the VOR can be adaptively modified by imagination and effort of spatial localization.[4,145]

Timing is a key factor in vestibular rehabilitation, as early onset of the exercises is associated with better outcome,[41] in agreement with animal studies.[18]

Vestibular exercises have to be designed keeping in mind that the vestibular adaptation is induced by an 'error signal' and therefore exposure to situations that produce this is necessary, and that adaptation is context specific, while the VOR is required to have an infinite number of gains for different situations (e.g. looking at objects far/near), and therefore exercises must be done in various contexts and speeds.[13]

Current physical exercise regimens and manoeuvres that are employed in the management of the vestibular patient include:

1. systematic preset exercise programmes
2. 'customized' exercise programmes
3. specific therapies for the treatment of benign peripheral positional vertigo of the posterior, horizontal or anterior semicircular canal.

Systematic preset exercise programmes

Cooksey–Cawthorne exercises

These comprise a series of graded head and body exercises that incorporate eye–head coordination tasks as well as balance tasks that have to be performed at various speeds due to the context specificity of vestibular adaptation, depending on the patient's severity of symptoms. The regimen can be individually tailored by asking the patient to score each exercise according to the symptoms it provokes, from 0 (no symptoms) to 3 (severe symptoms), in order to identify the exercises that elicit dizziness and are therefore required for habituation.[146] The patient is advised to progress to the next exercises on the list when he or she is free of symptoms or after having performed the exercises for 2–3 weeks.

Cawthorne and Cooksey held daily exercise class sessions and encouraged patients to expose themselves to challenging noisy or crowded environments. Classes for Cooksey–Cawthorne exercises are time- and cost-effective and make the best use of limited specialized personnel resources, while the patient's experience is positive as a result of meeting other patients with similar symptoms.[147] Nevertheless, an exercise class may not be ideal for all patients; for example, those with back or psychological problems will require individual instruction.[148]

Cohort observation studies report symptomatic improvement in the majority of patients with vestibular disorders that are managed with Cooksey–Cawthorne exercises.[144,148] However, Szturm et al[149] suggest that dynamic balance measures and VOR asymmetry may benefit more from balance and goal directed eye–head exercises under varied visual and somatosensory input than from the Cooksey–Cawthorne exercises, but potential confounders of their study's results are the non-randomized group assignment and differences in the follow-up arrangements for the two groups. Table 54.7 summarizes major recent studies on the efficacy of vestibular exercises.

Norré's exercises: Vestibular habituation exercises

Vestibular habituation training (VHT) was developed as a treatment for vertigo, induced by movement or change of position, in patients with peripheral vestibular disorders.[150] VHT is based on the concept of the 'error-signal' driven adaptation and on the assumption that repetition of the same stimulus (movement) causes a decline in response (vertigo) which is stimulus specific.[150] VHT consists of 19 positional manoeuvres[151] which are initially performed passively; symptoms of vertigo or dizziness, as well as estimates of their intensity and duration, are noted. The manoeuvres that elicit vertigo are then selected as exercises and the patient is advised to perform these in an active and vivid way.[150] Results in subjects with peripheral vestibular disorders are reported to be excellent with only 8% of patients showing no improvement.[151] A comparison of outcome between subjects who received VHT and controls who received 'sham' exercises or no treatment demonstrated significant improvement in all VHT patients and far better results than in controls.[152] Major disadvantages of VHT are that it does not include eye–head coordination exercises, balance tasks or exercises under challenge of visual/somatosensory input. However, VHT recognizes the significant overlap of vestibular pathology and psychological factors and advocates the use of relaxation exercises[151] and motivation of the patient.[150]

'Customised' exercise programmes

University of Michigan's approach

This regimen combines habituation exercises, balance and gait exercises, and general conditioning exercises suited to age, health and interests.[35,49,153] These are selected for each patient after a detailed neuro-otological multisystem evaluation and more specifically on the basis of posturography findings, gait evaluation and the 'motion sensitivity quotient', which is calculated by tabulating the number of vertigo-producing positions with intensity and duration of symptoms.[35] The selected exercises are then practised in the home environment or under therapist supervision for a period of 2–6 weeks, after which the patient will be reassessed and the exercise programme readjusted. Once the improvement begins to plateau, in 8–10 weeks on average, according to the authors, the patient is offered counselling and a maintenance programme that includes postural control and conditioning exercises. The authors also highlight the importance of educating the patient regarding his or her illness. Outcome results reported in various studies that include patients with different types and degrees of vestibular pathology indicate improvement in up to 90% of patients[33,36,132,153] (see Table 54.7 for details of outcome studies).

The John Hopkins/University of Miami programme

The exercises used by this programme are modifications of the Cooksey–Cawthorne exercises. The programme places particular importance on exercising under limited or altered visual and somatosensory input, on making use of 'central preprogramming', and on making the patient work at the limit of his ability.[154] It includes eye–head, movement and positional exercises, balance and gait training, and a walking programme. The acute vestibular patients are encouraged to start performing eye–head exercises sitting or standing, as early as 2–3 days after the onset of vestibular loss, to gradually increase the duration of exercise over the next few days, and to terminate the exercises only if vomiting. The chronic vestibular patient is encouraged to perform head movements and is taken through a series of balance and gait graded exercises. In bilateral vestibular failure, the treatment approach includes exercises that foster substitution of visual and somatosensory information and the development of compensatory strategies.[143]

Special considerations: central vestibular disorders, Menière's disease, bilateral vestibular failure

Vestibular rehabilitation has been traditionally reserved for patients with a stable peripheral vestibular lesion, but there is evidence to suggest that patients with central vestibular disorders may also benefit from vestibular rehabilitation. Patients with cerebellar lesions have been reported to improve their postural stability after vestibular training.[155] Shepard et al[33]

Table 54.7 Vestibular exercises: outcome evaluation studies.

Study	*N*	Type of trial	Patient groups	Type of treatment	Follow-up	Outcome measures	Main results
Norré[151]	40	Prospective case-control	PVD + BPPV	Vestibular habituation training: subjects 'Sham' exercises: controls No treatment: controls	4 weeks	Vertigo induced by vestibular habituation training manoeuvres	Subjects had dramatically better results than controls
Shepard et al[36]	98	Retrospective before/after	PVD + CVD	Individualized vestibular exercise programme	?	Disability score, symptom score, dynamic posturography, Norré's positioning test with patient's rating of symptoms	Reduction of symptoms in 87% Centrally acting drugs delayed recovery Poorer therapy results for head injury patients, high pre-therapy disability scores, visual and vestibular dysfunction on CDP
Telian et al[133]	14	Prospective	BVF	Habituation, balance retraining, conditioning exercises		Subjective improvement, disability scale, data from therapist, dynamic posturography	73% noted some improvement No improvements in the disability scale 21% improvement in ambulation
Horak et al[196]	25	Prospective case-control	PVD, non-progressive	Individualized vestibular exercise programme: subjects Non-specific exercises: control Medication only: control	6 weeks	Dynamic posturography, duration of standing on one foot, 'dizziness index' for 12 head positions and movements, patient's rating	Patients who received vestibular rehabilitation had the best results. Dizziness improved in all three groups but balance only improved in the vestibular rehabilitation group
Cohen[148]	35	Prospective before/after	PVD + CVD	Vestibular exercises following the Cooksey-Cawthorne paradigm	6–8 weeks	Questionnaire on ability to perform tasks—mailed after end of treatment	Significant improvement/greater independence after physical therapy
Shepard et al[33]	152	Prospective before/after	PVD + CVD including BVF	Individualized vestibular exercise programme	2 years	Disability score, symptom score, CDP, motion sensitivity quotient	85% improvement Prolonged therapy for centrally acting drugs, CVD Poorer therapy results for head injury patients, visual and vestibular dysfunction on CDP, men versus women
Krebs et al[160]	8	Double-blind placebo-controlled	BVF	Individualized vestibular exercise Program: subjects Non-specific exercises: controls	16 weeks	Gait and stairs locomotion, DHI, vestibular function tests	Dynamic stability during locomotion improved significantly more in the subject group DHI scores improved in both groups
Szturm et al[149]	33	Randomized case-control cross-over	PVD	Balance retraining, goal-directed eye head exercises under varied visual/somatosensory conditions: subjects Cooksey-Cawthorne: controls	5 months	VOR, OKN, dynamic posturography	Significant improvement in dynamic standing balance performance in subjects only Reduction in left-right VOR differences in subjects only

Continued

Table 54.7 Continued.

Study	N	Type of trial	Patient groups	Type of treatment	Follow-up	Outcome measures	Main results
Cohen et al[197]	38	Prospective non-randomized case-control	PVD + CVD Non-progress No BPPV	Purposeful activity at hospital and at home: subjects Head exercises at home: controls	3 months	Clinical test of sensory interaction on balance, functional measures, frequency and intensity of vertigo	Both groups had significant improvements in most measures post-therapy Subjects had better functional results than controls
Mruzek et al[198]	24	Randomized case-control	Vestibular ablation patients	Habituation exercises ± social reinforcement: subjects Range of motion exercises: controls	2 months	Dynamic posturography, MSQ, DHI, VOR, asymmetry index	Less motion sensitivity in subjects (± social reinforcement) than controls
Cowand et al[199]	38	Retrospective before-after	PVD + CVD	Gaze stabilization, vest stimulation, gait and proprioceptive retraining, general exercises	1 year	Dizziness Handicap Inventory	Significantly better post- than pre-rehabilitation scores PVD patients had greater improvements in the emotional DHI than CVD patients
Gillespie and Minor[29]	35	Retrospective before-after	BVF	Gaze and postural stability exercises		Snellen chart test, Romberg test, gait velocity, patient's report	51% improved—34% no improvement. Progressive pathology, other medical co-morbidity, lower VOR gain/time constant were more frequent findings in the non-improving group

reported that patients with central vestibular disorders which were predominantly due to brainstem pathology required a lengthier rehabilitation programme, but achieved no worse outcome, than patients with PVD. However, a more recent report suggests a mild-to-moderate reduction in symptoms of patients with central, predominantly cerebellar, lesions in response to vestibular rehabilitation.[156] Rehabilitation of central balance disorders will include retraining of sensory and movement strategies, i.e. training the patient to develop effective motor and sensory strategies in order to maintain stability during any functional tasks, while any coexisting peripheral vestibular pathology should be identified and appropriately rehabilitated.[157] Specific neurological rehabilitation may also be needed in order to restore mobility, either by means of restoring physiological gait functions or by fostering substitute movements and using technical aids.[134] The rehabilitation programme needs to take into account the specific impairments of each patient, underlying pathology, age, cognitive ability, severity of functional deficit and several other factors.[134,157] A patient with central vestibular pathology, e.g. following a traumatic brain injury, may require modified vestibular exercises in order to accommodate impaired motility and cognition, and increased supervision and assistance.[158]

Although vestibular rehabilitation is usually reserved for patients with stable vestibular deficits,[35] it will also benefit Menière patients who have developed unilateral or bilateral vestibular hypofunction, and should be initiated when the frequency of the hydropic attacks has started to decrease.[159]

Patients with bilateral vestibular failure can have different levels of functional impairment.[29] Vestibular rehabilitation will lead to subjective symptomatic improvement as well as improvement of stability during locomotion.[160] However, those with fluctuations in vestibular function will fare worse than the rest.[29] It is essential to educate these patients regarding the functional limitations of their condition, and to counsel them regarding safety considerations (such as working at heights, swimming in the dark, diving in the water) and balance assistive devices.[133,155] Patients with bilateral vestibular failure must be able to use both visual and somatosensory clues, or alternate the use of them, in a variety of challenging or conflicting sensory environments, and their rehabilitation programme must include exercises to foster substitution of alternative strategies for gaze stability as well as exercises that improve static and dynamic stability.[158] Patients with oscillopsia will particularly require eye–head coordination exercises, while posturography findings, as well as the therapist's evaluation, will help to decide whether the patient will benefit more from a customized exercise programme.[133]

Vestibular exercises—conclusion

The decision to refer the patient for preset versus customized exercises will depend on resource considerations, among other factors. Any vestibular exercises are better than no exercises, while a number of studies suggest that customized exercise regimens give significantly better results than preset exercise regimens, particularly in addressing dynamic balance problems. However, not all patients who have experienced vestibular symptoms require vestibular rehabilitation, and not every patient with persistent vestibular symptoms will need customized exercises. It is up to the clinician to decide, depending on clinical judgement, resources available and the presence of prognostic indicators for vestibular rehabilitation outcome, the best available regimen for the patient's needs.

Specific therapies for the treatment of benign paroxysmal positional vertigo of the posterior, horizontal or anterior semicircular canal

Positional vertigo is characterized by vertigo attacks that are triggered by changes in the head's position relative to gravity. The benign or peripheral type has until recently been attributed to 'cupulolithiasis',[161] that is, that degenerative debris adhere to the cupula of the posterior semicircular canal (p-SCC), making it gravity sensitive. More recently, the hypothesis of 'canalolithiasis',[162] i.e. that degenerative debris float freely in the endolymph of the p-SCC, has been considered to explain more effectively the features of benign paroxysmal positional vertigo (BPPV). BPPV most commonly arises from the p-SCC, although it may also arise from the horizontal (h-SCC) or, rarely, the anterior (a-SCC) canals.[163–166] Honrubia et al[166] report the prevalences of p-BPPV, h-BPPV and a-BPPV as being respectively, 93%, 5% and 2%. BPPV may also arise from pathology of more than one canal.[167,168] However, BPPV must be differentially diagnosed from positional vertigo arising from central pathology in the caudal brainstem or vestibulocerebellum[169] with lesions often found dorsolateral to the fourth ventricle or in the dorsal vermis.[170] This localization, together with other clinical features (associated cerebellar and oculomotor signs), generally allows one to easily distinguish central PPV from BPPV, but there are exceptions, and it appears that the direction of nystagmus on testing is the most reliable criterion for differentiation between central and peripheral types.[170,171]

Cawthorne[54] and other authors[172] have advocated vestibular habituation therapy for BPPV, involving repeatedly assuming the position of maximal stimulation in order to gradually habituate to the vertigo-inducing position, while it has been recognized that vestibular suppressants are ineffective treatment.[173] In more recent years, mechanical therapies proposed for the treatment of BPPV, in the form of exercises or single manoeuvres, have been based either on the cupulo- or canalolithiasis hypotheses, and are highly effective in achieving symptomatic relief after a single or short-term application.

Regardless of the chosen set of exercises or manoeuvres, there are three major considerations for the effective treatment of BPPV, which highlight the necessity for detailed neuro-otological testing in all BPPV patients:

1. The following manoeuvres and exercises are only indicated in the presence of BPPV, as diagnosed on the basis of strict criteria[174] (Table 54.8), and by definition are not appropriate for central positional vertigo, which needs to be differentially diagnosed, as it may have life-threatening implications.
2. Concurrent vestibular pathology such as peripheral vestibular hypofunction needs to be appropriately treated. Pollak et al[142] reported that the majority of patients with BPPV and peripheral vestibular hypofunction remain symptomatic after successful treatment of BPPV by single-step manoeuvres and require further vestibular rehabilitation. Herdman[175] also reported that BPPV patients have abnormal postural stability when compared with age-matched controls. This finding may not be related to the debris in the posterior canal and needs to be taken into account when designing the appropriate treatment plan.
3. When deciding on the most appropriate treatment for the BPPV patient, the clinician needs to consider efficacy of the treatment, but also special circumstances in each individual case. For example, the Brandt–Daroff exercises require patient compliance and will not be effective otherwise. Conversely, if the patient has back or neck problems, exercises may be more appropriate than single-step manoeuvres. In addition, anxious patients or those with an avoidance disorder who absolutely refuse to undergo the provoking Hallpike test will require the appropriate psychiatric/behavioural treatment before progress can be made. Our anecdotal observations indicate that most of these patients will comply with and be successfully treated by a single-step manoeuvre after a few sessions with the behavioural therapist.

Specific treatment of p-BPPV

Brandt–Daroff positional exercises In 1980, Brandt and Daroff[176] proposed a mechanical therapy, based on Schucknecht's hypothesis of cupulolithiasis, for BPPV. This consists of a rapid sequence of lateral head/body tilts, starting from the sitting position, rapidly moving to the challenging position (nose up), and remaining in this position for at least 30 s or until vertigo subsides, then sitting up for 30 s, and finally assuming the opposite head and nose down position for 30 s before sitting up (Figure 54.1). The authors reported that 66 of 67 patients experienced complete relief from BPPV within 3–14 days, with the exception of one patient who had a perilymphatic fistula.

Semont's liberatory manoeuvre Semont et al[177] devised a manoeuvre based on the theory of cupulolithiasis, which involves laying the patient on the involved side, with the face turned upwards by 45°, bringing the patient quickly to the sitting position and rapidly swinging the patient to the opposite side, face turned downwards by 45°, maintaining the patient in this position for 5 mins, and then bringing him slowly up to the sitting position (Figure 54.2). The authors reported resolution of symptoms in 92% of patients treated with this manoeuvre.

Table 54.8 Diagnostic characteristics of BPPV.

	p-BPPV	h-BPPV[a]	a-BPPV
History	Vertigo on sitting up from supine, lying down, rolling in bed, extending/flexing neck	Vertigo on rolling from side to side in bed	Onset of symptoms may follow a liberatory manoeuvre
Vertigo	Present on testing	Present on testing	Present on testing
Latency	2–20 s after head tilt	< 5 s	Similar to p-BPPV
Duration	< 40 s	> 20–60 s	Similar to p-BPPV
Nystagmus	Linear-rotatory, geotropic (towards affected undermost ear) or upward when gaze is directed to uppermost ear	Geotropic towards undermost ear—beats stronger to affected ear	Torsional towards unaffected undermost ear
Reversal	On return to sitting position	On rolling to other side	Similar to p-BPPV
Adaptation	Yes	Yes	Yes
Fatiguability	Yes	No	

[a] Atypical h-BPPV may beat towards the uppermost ear (Steddin et al., 1996)[207] and last for minutes when the precipitating position is maintained.

Epley's repositioning manoeuvre In 1992, Epley developed the canalith repositioning procedure (CRP), based on the theory of 'canalolithiasis', as a well-tolerated, non-invasive treatment for BPPV.[178] The canalith repositioning procedure combines head movements and bone vibration in order to induce free canaliths to gravitate out of the p-SCC to the utricle. Patients are premedicated the night before or 1 h before the procedure with a patch of scopolamine or diazepam. The affected p-SCC is identified by the Hallpike manoeuvre, and the latency and duration of nystagmus are noted in order to determine the timing of the procedure. After application of the bone vibrator over the ipsilateral mastoid, the patient is sat on the table and brought down with the head extended over the edge of the table, turned by 45° to the affected side. The head is then turned 90° to the opposite side. This is followed by rotating the head and body 90° facing downwards (135° from the supine position), and the patient is next brought to the sitting position with the head turned 45° to the unaffected side. The CRP finishes with the head turned forward 20° (Figure 54.3). Epley suggested proceeding to the next position of the 5-position CRP until nystagmus approaches termination, or, if there is no nystagmus observed, basing the timing on the last nystagmus latency + duration, with the typical time in each position being 6–13 s. He also advocated repeating the manoeuvre until there is no nystagmus or no progress made in the last two cycles. He reported total resolution of symptoms in 90% of patients and resolution of BPPV but persistence of other symptoms in 10% of patients after the initial CRP treatment. He argued that surgery is elected if there are multiple disabling BPPV recurrences, irrespective of the success of the canalith repositioning procedure. Following Epley's manoeuvre, BPPV symptoms may subside within 72 h in 35% and within 1 week in 74% of treated patients.[179] There are several modifications of this manoeuvre involving longer maintenance at each position and gradual position changing with 30 s intervals.[180,181]

The effect of the duration of symptoms before treatment on CRP success rate is controversial, as some authors report it to be a negative prognostic indicator,[180] while others report no correlation.[179,182] Patients with BPPV due to head trauma tend to benefit less from the treatment than idiopathic BPPV patients,[180] while 'vestibular neuronitis' patients have a better prognosis than patients with BPPV due to other aetiologies.[143] CRP plus mastoid oscillation may achieve better results in terms of symptomatic improvement as well as negative Hallpike test than CRP alone,[183] although this is disputed by other authors.[184]

Complications and adverse reactions Several patients report instability following CRP, possibly due to the new position of the canaliths in the utricle.[185] Complications of CRP include conversion of posterior canal BPPV to anterior or horizontal canal BPPV in about 6% of treated patients.[165]

Moreover, Epley's manoeuvre involves significant neck strain, while Semont's manoeuvre may also strain the spinal column. Modified Brandt–Daroff exercises may constitute an alternative in such cases.[186] Recurrence of BPPV may occur in up to 50% of succesfully treated patients,[164] and in 20% BPPV will recur in the first 2 weeks after treatment.[181]

Treatment of p-BPPV—conclusion BPPV resolves spontaneously within weeks or months, however, if untreated, it will

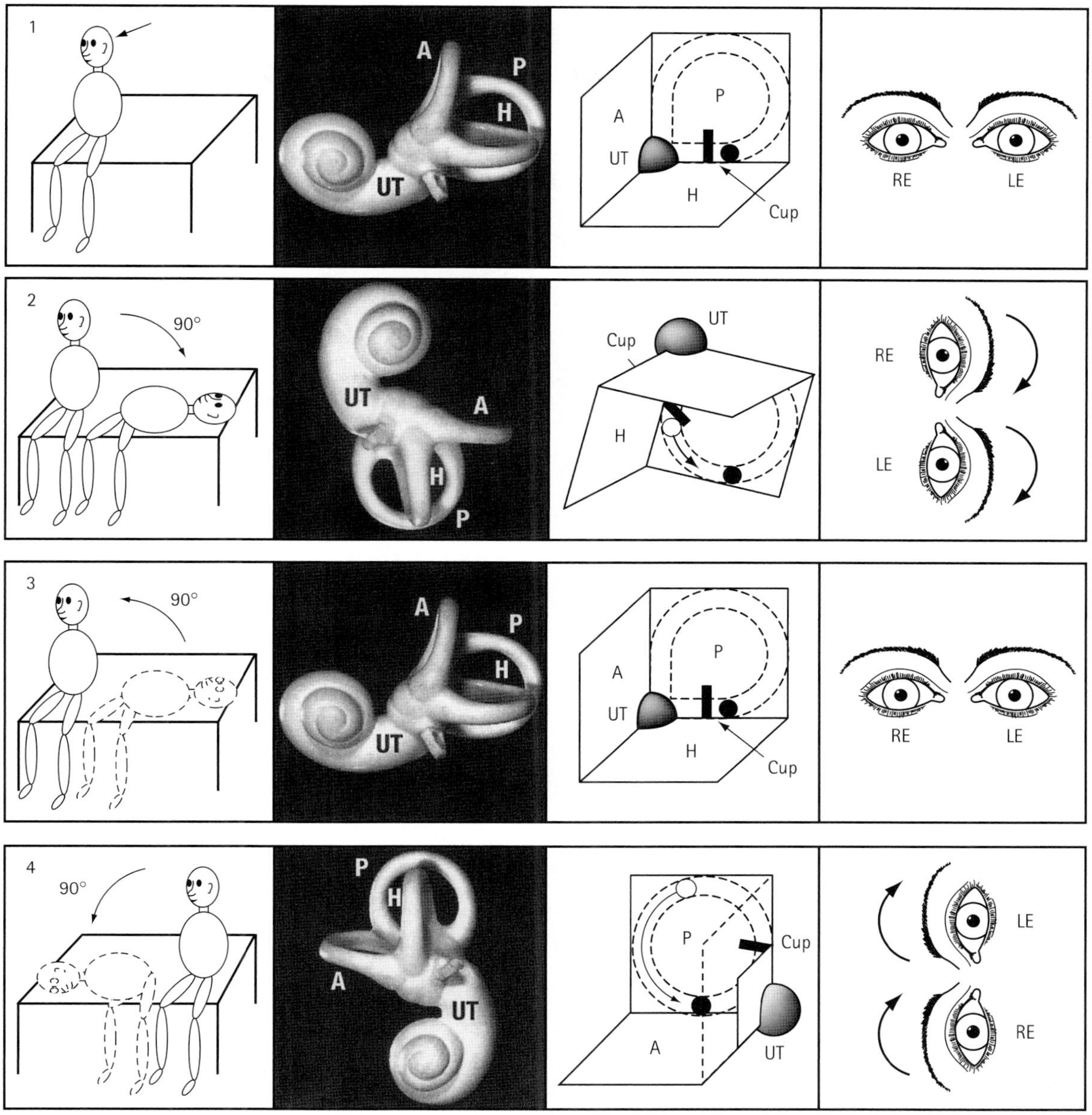

Figure 54.1 Brandt–Daroff positional exercises. For Left BPPV. 1. Sitting position 2. Head and body down to the left (nose up) 3. Sitting position 4. Head and body down to the right (nose down) position. Reproduced from Brandt et al. *Neurology* 1994; **44**: 796–800.[208]

persist in 20–30% of patients.[187] Treatment efficacy by single manoeuvres or exercises is high, as reported by several randomized case–control, non-blinded studies (see Table 54.9 for details), while the complications are few. The patient with p-BPPV should be treated by either of the single-step manoeuvres, except in the case of contraindications such as neck or back problems, vertebrobasilar insufficiency or perilymph fistula. In the case of neck or back problems, modified Brandt–Daroff exercises are indicated. Surgical treatment is only indicated in the few patients who do not respond to appropriate treatment repeated over a long term.

Specific treatment of h-BPPV

Liberatory manoeuvre De la Meilleure et al[167] reported a 100% success rate for this manoeuvre in six patients treated. From the supine position, the head is lifted by 30°, turned to the affected side, and maintained in that position for 5 mins. The head is then turned as fast as possible 180° to the other side and maintained there for 5 mins. The patient is then asked to avoid head shaking and not to lie down for the next 48 h. The authors report that patients may require treatment for bilateral h-SCC or for coexisting p-BPPV. Contraindications for this manoeuvre are cervical spondylosis, vertebrobasilar insufficiency or neck pain during the manoeuvre.

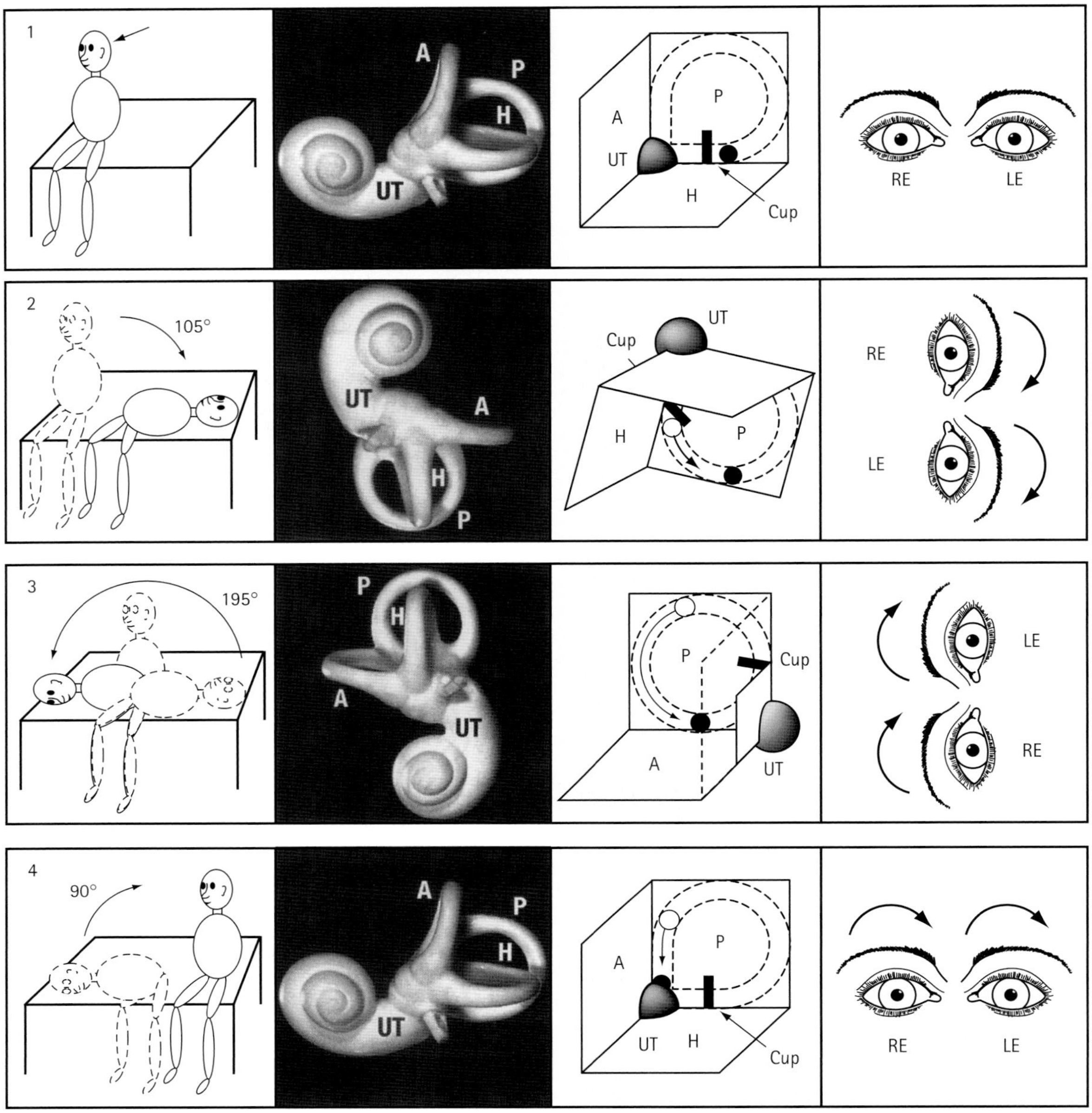

Figure 54.2 Semont's liberatory manoeuvre. For Left BPPV. 1. Sitting position 2. Head and body down to the left (face turned upwards by 45°), neck extended over the couch 3. Rapidly swung to the sitting then head and body down to the right position (face turned downwards by 45°) 4. Slowly up to the sitting position. Reproduced from Brandt et al. *Neurology* 1994; **44**: 796–800.[208]

'Forced prolonged position' on the healthy side Vannuchi et al[188] advise patients with h-BPPV to lie down on the healthy side for 12 h in order to allow the debris in the affected h-SCC to gravitate to the vestibule by maintaining the affected h-SCC uppermost. They report total recovery within 3 days in 74.3% of 35 treated patients and conversion of h-BPPV to homolateral p-BPPV, which they successfully treated with Semont's manoeuvre. By contrast, the rates of recovery within 3 days in the group of patients who received no treatment (15 patients) and in those treated by head shaking (24 patients) were 26% and 16% respectively. Obesity and cervical spondylosis were factors that did not permit maintenance of the position for the time required.

270° 'barbecue' manoeuvre Lempert and Tiel-Wilck[189] report successful treatment of h-BPPV in two patients by an adaptation of Epley's manoeuvre. This consists of turning the patient's head and body from the supine position by three 90° step rotations (total 270°) towards the unaffected ear to assume the lying position on the affected side, and then having the patient sit up. Nuti et al[190] reported that while both the 'barbecue' manoeuvre and the forced prolonged position are effective

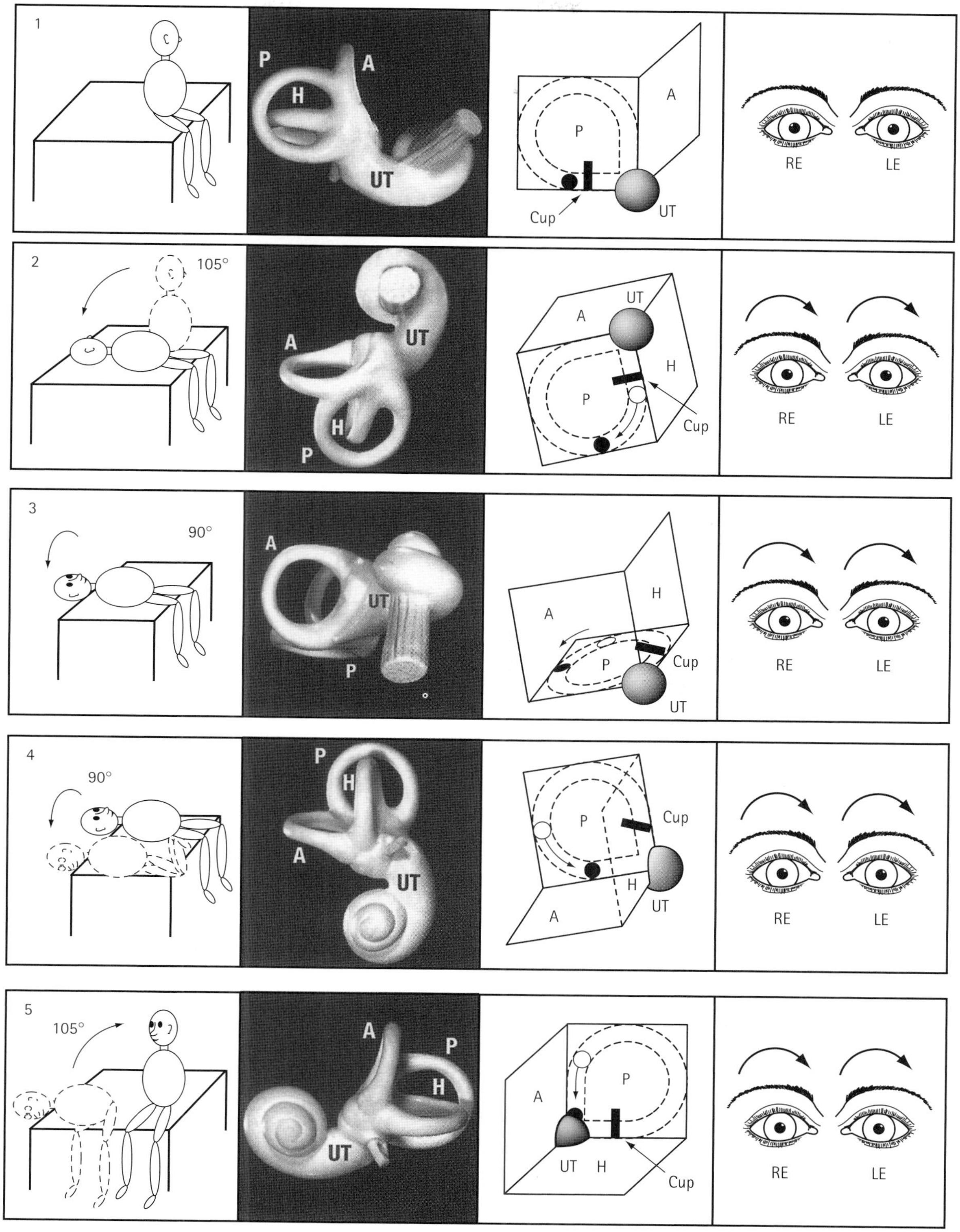

Figure 54.3 Epley's repositioning manoeuvre. For Left BPPV. 1. Sitting position, head turned by 45° to the left. 2. Lying down, neck extended over the couch. 3. Head turned 90° to the right. 4. Head and body rotated 90° facing downwards. 5. Sitting position, head turned 45° to the unaffected side and 20° forward. Reproduced from Brandt et al. *Neurology* 1994; **44**: 796–800.[208]

Table 54.9 BPPV treatment–outcome evaluation studies.

Study	No	Type of trial	Patient groups	Treatment	Other instructions	Results
Norré and Beckers[200]	51	Case-control	BPPV	23–Semont's–if no improvement, habituation exercises 28–habituation exercises		52% free of symptoms after 1 Semont's 32% after 1 week of habituation exercises but 100% after 6 weeks All patients but one who did not improve after Semont's free of symptoms after 6 weeks of habituation exercises
Welling and Barnes[185]	25	Prospective observational	BPPV–no concomittant pathology No controls	Epley's–twice	48 h upright position	84% success rate
Harvey et al[180]	25	Prospective observational	BPPV–various pathologies No controls	Modified Epley's–thrice	48 h upright position Avoid quick head turns Avoid lying on affected ear 1 week	68% significant improvement Duration of symptoms greater in non-responders
Parnes and Price Jones[201]	38	Prospective/ retrospective observational	Uni- and bilateral BPPV	Semont's or modified Epley's	48 h upright position 5 nights' sleep on normal side	88.2% improvement
Massoud and Ireland[202]	96	Randomized case-control	Four groups: two different manoeuvres ± instructions	Semont's ± instructions Epley's manuevre instructions		Similar results for the four groups Success rate of 88%-96%
Herdman et al[181]	60	Randomized case-control	p-BPPV	Semont's versus Epley's	48 h upright position Not to lie on affected side for 5 days Collar	Similar results Semont's: 70% total and 20% partial recovery Epley's: 57% total and 33% partial recovery
Blakley[203]	38	Randomized case-control	p-BPPV	CRP versus no treatment		No differences in subject symptomatic improvement 1 month after treatment in subjects and controls
Li[183]	60	Randomized case-control	p-BPPV	CRP versus CRP + mastoid oscillation versus no treatment	Soft collar	Only patients who received CRP had improved 1 week later–oscillation + CRP achieved the best results
Serafini, et al[204]	160	Prospective observational	p-BPPV	Semont's	Avoid brisk movements	95% cases free of symptoms after maximum five cycles of treatment
Steenerson and Cronin[205]	60	Case control	p-BPPV	CRP versus VHT versus no treatment	Subjects asked to repeat manoeuvre twice weekly	CRP achieved faster relief than VHT–75% untreated subjects unimproved 3 months later
Fung and Hall[182]	65	Observational	p-BPPV–no controls	Epley's	48 h upright position	83.8 % total and14.7% partial improvement
Smouha[206]	27	Observational	p-BPPV–no controls	Epley's		93% improved: 63% due to CRP
Wolf et al[179]	41	Randomised case-control	BPPV for ≥1 month–no previous treatment 30 subjects–11 controls	Epley's: subjects No treatment: controls		Recovery within 72 h in 35%, and within 1 week in 74% of subjects Recovery within 4 weeks in 45% of controls

treatments for h-BPPV, the forced prolonged position may be successful in slightly more cases than the barbecue manoeuvre, which, however, achieves immediate results.

360° yaw rotation Baloh[191] successfully treated two patients with h-BPPV with a 360° yaw rotation performed in 90° steps at 30 s intervals.

Treatment of h-BPPV—conclusion Forced prolonged position is the simplest and possibly the most efficacious treatment for h-BPPV; however, it may be worthwhile to perform a single manoeuvre first, as it may achieve immediate results, and to advise the patient to maintain the forced prolonged position afterwards. If symptoms of h-BPPV persist after 2 days, Brandt[174] advises patients to perform the Brandt–Daroff exercises.

Specific treatment of a-BPPV

BPPV of the anterior canal is a rare variant that may occur as a complication of treatment of p-BPPV by single-step manoeuvres.[165] Owing to the rarity of the syndrome, there are only single-case reports in the literature reporting on treatment. Herdman and Tusa[165] have succesfully treated two patients with a canalith repositioning manoeuvre similar to that for p-BPPV of the contralateral ear (i.e. if there is right a-BPPV, then a left CRP should be performed). Brandt[174] observes that Brandt–Daroff exercises were effective and superior to single-step manoeuvres for patients treated for a-BPPV. In the absence of a clinical trial, either of these approaches can be used, depending on the patient's condition and the physician's personal preference.

Surgical treatment of BPPV

Few patients with BPPV will require surgical treatment, as a last resort. Surgical procedures for treatment of p-BPPV may include singular neurectomy,[192] p-SCC occlusion,[193] and partitioning of the labyrinth.[194]

Adjunctive treatment

Adjunctive treatment, as needed in each case, may include:

1. Behavioural therapy/psychiatric management. Psychiatric disorder is a primary cause in 1:4 to 1:5 of patients presenting with vertigo,[195] while about 50% of patients with peripheral vestibular disorder may experience significant psychiatric symptoms after the onset of the vestibular disorder, which may act as a trigger factor.[136] These patients will require further psychiatric management.
2. Relaxation and breathing exercises. When dizziness is caused or exacerbated by stress, hyperventilation and other similar causes, these exercises may alleviate or remove a cause of the symptoms.[157]
3. Corrective treatment for visual, proprioceptive, neuromuscular and musculoskeletal disorders, as all these disorders may delay vestibular compensation.
4. Safety measures, including environmental modifications and assistive devices.

Surgery

Surgical management of vertigo is indicated if all options of aggressive medical treatment have been employed and failed to alleviate the symptoms, or if the vertigo is due to perilymph fistula or complications of middle ear disease.

References

1. Curthoys IS, Halmagyi GM. Vestibular compensation: a review of the oculomotor, neural and clinical consequences of unilateral vestibular loss. *J Vestib Res* 1995; **5**: 67–107.
2. Smith PF, Curthoys IS. Mechanisms of recovery following unilateral labyrinthectomy: a review. *Brain Res Rev* 1989; **14**: 155–80.
3. Curthoys IS, Halmagyi GM. How does the brain compensate for vestibular lesions? In: Baloh RW, Halmagyi GM, eds. *Disorders of the Vestibular System*. New York: Oxford University Press, 1996.
4. Zee DS. Vestibular adaptation. In: Herdman SJ, ed. *Vestibular Rehabilitation*, Philadelphia: F.A. Davis Company, 1994: 68–79.
5. Halmagyi GM, Curthoys IS. Clinical changes in vestibular function over time after lesions: the consequences of unilateral vestibular deafferentation. In: Herdman SJ, ed. *Vestibular Rehabilitation*, Philadelphia: F.A. Davis Company, 1994: 90–108.
6. Straka H, Dieringer N. Spinal plasticity after hemilabyrinthectomy and its relation to postural recovery in the frog. *J Neurophysiol* 1995; **73**: 1617–31.
7. Allum JHJ, Yamane M, Pfaltz CR. Long-term modifications of vertical and horizontal vestibulo-ocular reflex dynamics in man. *Acta Otolaryngol* 1988; **105**: 328–37.
8. Yagi T, Markham CH. Neural correlates of compensation after hemilabyrinthectomy. *Exp Neurol* 1984; **84**: 98–108.
9. Curthoys IS, Halmagyi GM. Vestibular compensation. *Adv Otorhinolaryngol* 1999; **55**: 195–227.
10. Fetter M, Zee DS. Recovery from unilateral labyrinthectomy in rhesus monkey. *J Neurophysiol* 1988; **59**: 370–93.
11. Luxon LM. Vestibular compensation. In: Davis RA, Luxon LM, eds. *Handbook of Vestibular Rehabilitation*. London: Whurr, 1997.
12. Courjon JH, Flandrin JM, Jeannerod M, Schmid R. The role of the flocculus in vestibular compensation after hemilabyrinthectomy. *Brain Res* 1982; **239**: 251–7.
13. Herdman SJ. Role of vestibular adaptation in vestibular rehabilitation. *Otolaryngol Head Neck Surg* 1998; **119**: 49–54.
14. Precht W, Dieringer N. Neuronal events paralleling functional recovery (compensation) following peripheral vestibular lesions. In: Berthoz A, Mellvill Jones G, eds. *Adaptive Mechanisms in Gaze Control. Facts and Theories* Amsterdam: Elsevier, 1985.
15. Fetter M, Zee DS, Proctor LR. Effect of lack of vision and of occipital lobectomy upon recovery from unilateral labyrinthectomy in rhesus monkey. *J Neurophysiol* 1988; **59**: 399–407.
16. Dichgans J, Bizzi E, Morasso P, Tagliasco V. Mechanisms underlying recovery of eye–head co-ordination following bilateral labyrinthectomy in monkeys. *Exp Brain Res* 1973; 548–62.

17. Lacour M, Xerri C. Vestibular compensation: new perspectives. In: Flohr H, Precht W, eds. *Lesion Induced Neuronal Plasticity in Sensorimotor Systems*. Berlin: Heidelberg, New York: Springer-Verlag, 1981: 240–53.
18. Lacour M. Reapprentissage et periode postoperatoire sensible dans la restauration des fonctions nerveuses. Exemple de la compensation vestibulaire et implications cliniques. *Ann Otolaryngol Chir Cervicofac* 1984; **101**(3): 177–87.
19. Igarashi M, Levy JK, Ouchi T, Reschke MF. Further study of exercise and locomotor balance compensation after unilateral labyrinthectomy in squirrel monkeys. *Acta Otolaryngol* 1981; **92**: 101–5.
20. Berthoz A. The role of gaze in compensation of vestibular dysfunction: The gaze substitution hypothesis. *Prog Brain Res* 1988; **76**: 411–20.
21. Barnes GR. Visual–vestibular interaction in the control of head and eye movement: the role of visual feedback and predictive mechanisms. *Prog Neurobiol* 1993; **41**: 435–72.
22. Igarashi M. Vestibular compensation. An overview. *Acta Otolaryngol* 1984; Suppl 406: 78–82.
23. Smith PF, Darlington CL. Neurochemical mechanisms of recovery from peripheral vestibular lesions. *Brain Res Rev* 1991; **16**: 117–33.
24. Warchol ME, Lambert PR, Goldstein BJ, Forge A, Corwin JT. Regenerative proliferation in inner ear sensory epithelia from adult guinea pigs and humans. *Science* 1993; **259**: 1619–22.
25. Darlington CL, Smith PF. The recovery of static vestibular function following peripheral vestibular lesions in mammals: the intrinsic mechanism hypothesis. *J Vestib Res* 1996; **6**(3): 185–201.
26. Dieringer N, Kunzle H, Precht W. Increased projection of dorsal root fibres to vestibular nuclei after hemilabyrinthectomy in the frog. *Exp Brain Res* 1984; **55**: 574–8.
27. Errington ML, Lynch MA, Bliss TVP. Long term potentiation in the dentate nucleus: induction and increased glutamate release are blocked by D(−) amino phosphorovalerate. *Neuroscience* 1987; **20**: 279–84.
28. Dieringer N, Precht W. Modification of synaptic input following unilateral labyrinthectomy. *Nature* 1977; **269**: 431–3.
29. Gillespie MB, Minor LB. Prognosis in bilateral vestibular hypofunction. *Laryngoscope* 1999; **109**: 35–41.
30. Glasscock ME, Hughes GB, Davis WE, Jackson GC. Labyrinthectomy versus middle fossa vestibular nerve section in Menière's disease. A critical evaluation of relief of vertigo. *Ann Otol Rhinol Laryngol* 1980; **89**: 318–24.
31. Black FO, Wade SW, Nashmer LM. What is the minimal function required for compensation? *Am J Otol* 1996; **17**(3): 401–9.
32. Rudge R, Chambers BR. Physiological basis for enduring vestibular symptoms. *J Neurol Neurosurg Psychiatry* 1982; **45**: 126–30.
33. Shepard NT, Telian SA, Smith-Wheelock M, Raj A. Vestibular and balance rehabilitation therapy. *Ann Otol Rhinol Laryngol* 1993; **102**: 198–205.
34. Yardley L, Luxon LM, Haacke NP. Longitudinal study of symptoms, anxiety and subjective well-being in patients with vertigo. *Clin Otolaryngol* 1994; **19**: 109–16.
35. Shepard NT, Telian SA. Vestibular rehabilitation programmes. In: Shepard NT, Telian SA, eds. *Practical Management of the Balance Disorder Patient*. London: Singular Publishing Group, 1996.
36. Shepard NT, Telian SA, Smith-Wheelock M. Habituation and balance retraining therapy—a retrospective review. *Neurol Clin* 1990; **8**: 459–75.
37. Sakellari V, Bronstein AM, Corna S, Hammon CA, Jones S, Wolsley CJ. The effects of hyperventilation on postural control mechanisms. *Brain* 1997; **120**: 1659–73.
38. Schaefer KP, Meyer DL. Compensation of vestibular lesions. In: Kornhuber HH, ed. *Handbook of Sensory Physiology*, Vol 6/2. Berlin: Springer, 1974: 463–90.
39. Katsarkas A, Segal BN. Unilateral loss of peripheral vestibular function in patients: degree of compensation and factors causing decompensation. *Otolaryngology HNS* 1988; **98**(1): 45–7.
40. Mathog RH, Peppard SB. Exercises and recovery from vestibular injury. *Am J Otolaryngol* 1982; **3**: 397–407.
41. Bamiou DE, Davies RA, McKee M, Luxon LM. Symptoms, disability and handicap in unilateral peripheral vestibular disorders—effects of early presentation and initiation of balance exercises. *Scand Audiol* 2000; **29**: 238–44.
42. Shumway-Cook A, Horak FB. Rehabilitation strategies for patients with vestibular deficits. *Neurol Clin North Am* 1990; **8**: 441–57.
43. Hallam RS, Beyts J, Jakes SC. Symptom reporting and objective test results. *Adv Audiol* 1988; **5**: 129–36.
44. Stephens SDG, Hogan S, Meredith R. The desynchrony between complaints and signs of vestibular disorders. *Acta Otolaryngol* 1991; **111**: 188–92.
45. Spitzer JB. An evaluation of the relationship among electronystagmographic, audiologic, and self report descriptors of dizziness. *Eur Arch Otorhinolaryngol* 1990; **247**: 114–18.
46. World Health Organization. *International Classification of Impairments, Disabilities and Handicaps*. Geneva: WHO, 1980.
47. World Health Organization. *International Classification of Functioning and Disability*. Beta-2 draft. Geneva: WHO, 1999.
48. Norré ME, De Weerdt W. Treatment of vertigo based on habituation. *J Laryngol Otol* 1980; **94**: 971–7.
49. Smith-Wheelock M, Shepard NT, Telian SA. Physical therapy programme for vestibular rehabilitation. *Am J Otol* 1991; **12**: 218–25.
50. El-Kashlan HK, Shepard NT, Asher AM, Smith-Wheelock M, Telian SA. Evaluation of clinical measures of equilibrium. *Laryngoscope* 1998; **108**(3): 311–19.
51. Jacobson GP, Newman WC. The development of the Dizziness Handicap Inventory. *Arch Otolaryngol HNS* 1990; **116**: 424–8.
52. Yardley L, Putnam J. Quantitative analysis of factors contributing to handicap and distress in vertiginous patients: a questionnaire study. *Clin Otolaryngol* 1992; **17**: 231–6.
53. Honrubia V, Bell TS, Harris MR, Baloh RW, Fisher LM. Quantitative evaluation of dizziness characteristics and impact on quality of life. *Am J Otol* 1996; **17**: 595–602.
54. Cawthorne TE. The physiological basis for head exercises. *J Chart Soc Physiother* 1944; **30**: 106–7.
55. Cooksey FS. Rehabilitation of vestibular injuries. *Proc R Soc Med* 1945; **39**: 273–8.

56. Lacour M, Roll JP, Appaix M. Modifications and developments of spinal reflexes in the adult baboon (papio papio) following unilateral vestibular neurotomy. *Brain Res* 1976; **113**: 255–69.
57. Courjon JH, Jeannerod M, Ossuzio I, Schmid R. The role of vision in compensation of vestibulo-ocular reflex after hemilabyrinthectomy in the cat. *Exp Brain Res* 1977; **28**: 235–48.
58. Smith PF, Darlington CL. Can vestibular compensation be enhanced by drug treatment? *J Vestib Res* 1994; **4**(no. 3): 169–79.
59. Rascol O, Hain T, Brefel C, Benazet M, Clanet M, Montastruc JL. Antivertigo medications and drug induced vertigo. A pharmacological review. *Drugs* 1995; **50**(50): 778–91.
60. Timmerman H. Pharmacotherapy of vertigo: any news to be expected? *Acta Otolaryngol* 1994; Suppl 513: 28–32.
61. Lucot JB. Pharmacology of motion sickness. *J Vestib Res* 1998; **8**: 61–6.
62. Foster C, Baloh RW. Drug therapy for vertigo. In: Baloh RW, Halmagyi GM, eds. *Disorders of the Vestibular System*. New York: Oxford University Press, 1996.
63. Zee DS. Perspectives on the pharmacotherapy of vertigo. *Otolaryngol Head Neck Surg* 1985; **111**: 609–12.
64. Shepard NT, Telian SA. Medical therapy for the balance disorder patient. In: Shepard NT, Telian SA, eds. *Practical Management of the Balance Disorder Patient*. London: Singular Publishing Group, 1996.
65. Luxon LM. Modes of treatment of vestibular symptomatology. In: Davis RA, Luxon LM, eds. *Handbook of Vestibular Rehabilitation*. London: Whurr, 1997.
66. Takeda N, Morita M, Hasegawa S, Horii A, Kubo T, Matsunaga T. Neuropharmacology of motion sickness and emesis. *Acta Otolaryngol* 1993; Suppl 501: 10–15.
67. Yates BJ, Miller AD, Lucot JB. Physiological basis and pharmacology of motion sickness: an update. *Brain Res Bull* 1998; **47**(5): 395–406.
68. Nathan A. Products for motion sickness and sleep disturbance. *Pharmaceutical J* 1997; **259**: 929–32.
69. Smith CL, Darlington PF. Drug treatment for vertigo and dizziness. *N Z Med J* 1998; **111**: 332–4.
70. *ABPI Compendium of Data Sheets and Summaries of Product Characteristics 1998–99*. London: Datapharm Publications Limited.
71. Aanta E, Skinhoz A. Controlled clinical trial comparing the effect of betahistine hydrochloride and prochlorperazine maleate for patients with Menière disease. *Ann Clin Res* 1976; **8**: 284–7.
72. Dollery C. Prochlorperazine. In: Dollery C, ed. *Therapeutic Drugs*, London: Churchill-Livingstone, 1999.
73. Bond CM. Comparison of buccal and oral prochlorperazine in the treatment of dizziness associated with nausea and/or vertigo. *Curr Med Res Opin* 1998; **14**(4): 203–12.
74. Betts T, Harris D, Gadd E.The effects of two anti-vertigo drugs (betahistine and prochlorperazine) on driving skills. *Br J Clin Pharmacol* 1991; **32**: 455–8.
75. Rodgers C. Extrapyramidal side effects of antiemetics presenting as psychiatric illness. *Gen Hosp Psychiatry* 1992; **14**(3): 192–5.
76. Weinstein SE, Stern RM. Comparison of marezine and dramamine in preventing symptoms of motion sickness. *Aviation Space Environ Med* 1997; **68**(10): 890–4.
77. Olesen J. Calcium entry blockers in the treatment of vertigo. *Ann NY Acad Sci* 1988; **522**: 690–7.
78. Verspeelt J, De Locht P, Amery WK. Postmarketing study of the use of flunarizine in vestibular vertigo and in migraine. *Eur J Clin Pharmacol* 1996; **51**: 15–22.
79. Doweck I, Gordon CR, Spitzer O, Melamed Y, Shupak A. Effect of cinnarizine in the prevention of seasickness. *Aviation Space Environ Med* 1994; **65**: 606–9.
80. Pingree BJ. INM investigations into drugs for seasickness prophylaxis. *J Royal Naval Med Service* 1994; **80**(2): 76–80.
81. Daniel JR, Mauro VF. Extrapyramidal symptoms associated with calcium-channel blockers. *Ann Pharmacother* 1995; **29**: 73–5.
82. Ishikawa K, Igarashi M. Effect of diazepam on vestibular compensation in squirrel monkeys. *Arch Otolaryngol* 1984; **240**: 49–57.
83. Martin J, Gilchrist DPD, Smith PF, Darlington CL. Early diazepam treatment following unilateral labyrinthectomy does not impair vestibular compensation of spontaneous nystagmus in guinea pigs. *J Vestib Res* 1996; **6**: 135–9.
84. Rice GP, Ebers GC. Ondasetron for intractable vertigo complicating acute brainstem disorders. *Lancet* 1995; **345**: 1182–9.
85. Silberstein SD, Lipton RB. Epidemiology of migraine. *Neuroepidemiology* 1993; **12**(3): 179–94.
86. Sillanpaa M, Anttila P. Increasing prevalence of headache in 7–year-old schoolchildren. *Headache* 1996; **36**(8): 466–70.
87. Cutrer FM, Baloh RW. Migraine-associated dizziness. *Headache* 1992; **32**: 300–4.
88. Brandt T. Migraine and vertigo. In: Brandt T, ed. *Vertigo—its Multisensory Syndromes*, 2nd edn. London: Springer-Verlag, 1999.
89. Cass SP, Furman JM, Ankerstjerne JKP, Balaban C, Yetiser S, Aydogan B. Migraine related vestibulopathy. *Ann Otol Rhinol Laryngol* 1997; **106**: 182–9.
90. Lanzi A, Ballotini U, Fazzi E, Tagliasachi M, Manfrin M, Migra E. Benign paroxysmal vertigo of childhood: a long term follow up. *Cephalalgia* 1994; **14**: 458–60.
91. Headache Classification Committee of the International Headache Society. Classification and diagnostic criteria for headache disorders, cranial neuralgias and facial pain. *Cephalalgia* 1988; **8**: 19–73.
92. Neuhauser H, Leopold M, von Brevern M, Arnold G, Lempert T. The interrelations of migraine, vertigo and migrainous vertigo. *Neurology* 2001; **56**: 436–41.
93. Tusa RJ. Diagnosis and management of neuro-otological disorders due to migraine. In: Herdman SJ, ed. *Vestibular Rehabilitation*. 2nd edn. Philadelphia: FA Davis, 2000.
94. Johnson G. Medical management of migraine-related dizziness and vertigo. *Laryngoscope* 1998; **108**(suppl): 1–28.
95. Bikhazi P, Jackson C, Ruckenstein MJ. Efficacy of antimigrainous therapy in the treatment of migraine associated dizziness. *Am J Otol* 1997; **18**: 350–4.
96. Harker LA. Migraine associated vertigo. In: Baloh RW, Halmagyi GM, eds. *Disorders of the Vestibular System*. New York: Oxford University Press, 1996: 407–17.
97. Tfelt-Hansen P. Prophylactic pharmacotherapy of migraine. *Neurol Clin* 1997; **15**(1): 153–65.

98. Baloh RW. Neuro-otology of migraine. *Headache* 1997; **37**: 615–21.
99. Sheftel FD. Role and impact of over the counter medications in the management of headache. *Neurol Clin* 1997: **15**(1): 187–98.
100. Celentano DD, Stewart WF, Lipton RB, Reed ML. Medication use and disability among migraine sufferers: a national probability sample survey. *Headache* 1992; **18**: 223–8.
101. Mathew NT. Serotonin 1D (5–HT1D) agonists and other agents in acute migraine. *Neurol Clin* 1997; **15**(1): 61–83.
102. Dieterich M, Brandt T. Episodic vertigo related to migraine (90 cases): vestibular migraine? *J Neurol* 1999; **246**: 883–92.
103. Jen JC, Yue Q, Karrim J, Nelson SF, Baloh RW. Spinocerebellar ataxia type 6 with positional vertigo and acetazolamide responsive episodic ataxia. *J Neurol Neurosurg Psychiatry* 1998; **65**: 565–8.
104. Baloh RW, Yue Q, Furman JM, Nelson SF. Familial migraine with vertigo and essential tremor. *Neurology* 1996; **46**: 458–60.
105. Anderson KE, Vinge E. Beta adreno-receptor blockers and calcium antagonists in the prophylactic treatment of migraine. *Drugs* 1990; **39**: 355–73.
106. Harker LA, Rassekh CH. Episodic vertigo in basilar artery migraine. *Otolaryngol Head Neck Surg* 1987; **96**: 239–50.
107. Committee on Hearing and Equilibrium, the American Academy of Opthalmology and Otolaryngology. Committee on Hearing and Equilibrium guidelines for diagnosis and evaluation of therapy in Menière's disease. *Otolaryngol Head Neck Surg* 1995; **113**: 181–5.
108. Bohndorf M, Baykal HE, Plinkert PK, Pleyer U. Cogan I syndrome. Audio-vestibular, ophthalmologic findings and therapy in 6 patients. *HNO* 1996; **44**: 302–6.
109. Pulec JL. Menière's disease of syphilitic etiology. *Ear Nose Throat J* 1997; **76**: 508–27.
110. James AL, Burton MJ. Betahistine for Menière's diseases—a systematic review. *Proceedings of the 4th International Symposium on Menière's Disease*. Hague: Kugler Publications, 2000.
111. Claes J, Van de Heyning PH. Medical Treatment of Menière's disease: a review of literature. *Acta Otolaryngol Suppl* 1997; **526**: 37–42.
112. James A, Thorp M. Menière's disease. *Clinical Evidence* 2001; **5**: 348–55.
113. Ruckenstein MJ, Rutka JA, Hawke M. The treatment of Menière disease: Torok revisited. *Laryngoscope* 1991; **101**: 211–18.
114. Silverstein H, Rosenberg S, Arruda J, Isaakson JE. Surgical ablation of the vestibular system in the treatment of Menière's disease. *Otolaryngol Clin North Am* 1997; **30**(6): 1075–96.
115. Santos PM, Hall RA, Snyder JM, Hughes LF. Diuretic and diet effect on Menière disease evaluated by the 1985 Committee on Hearing and equilibrium guidelines. *Otolaryngol Head Neck Surg* 1993; **109**: 680–9.
116. Arenberg IK, Bayer RF. Therapeutic options in Meniere's disease. *Arch Otolaryngol* 1977; **103**: 589–93.
117. Van Deelen GW, Huizing EH. Use of a diuretic (dyazide) in the treatment of Menière's disease. A double-blind cross-over placebo-controlled study. *ORL J Otolaryngol Relat Spec* 1986; **48**(5): 287–92.
118. Klockhoff I, Lindblom U, Stahle J. Diuretic treatment of Menière's disease. Long term results with chlorthalidone. *Arch Otolaryngol* 1974; **100**(4): 262–5.
119. Brookes GB. The pharmacological treatment of Menière's disease. *Clin Otolaryngol* 1996; **21**: 3–11.
120. Tighilet B, Leonard J, Lacour M. Betahistine dihydrochloride treatment facilitates vestibular compensation in the cat. *J Vestib Res* 1995; **5**: 53–66.
121. Hausler R, Sabani E, Rohr M. The effect of cinnarazine on various types of vertigos: clinical and electronystagmographic results of a double-blind study. *Acta Otorhinolaryngol Belg* 1989; **43**: 177–85.
122. Hamman KF, Arnold WW. Menière's disease. *Adv Otorhinolaryngol* 1999; **55**: 195–227.
123. Parnes LS, Sun Ah, Freeman DJ. Corticosteroid pharmacokinetics in the inner ear fluids: an animal study followed by clinical application. *Laryngoscope* 1999; **109**(suppl 91): 1–17.
124. Shea JJ Jr. The role of dexamethasone or streptomycin perfusion in the treatment of Menière's disease. *Otolaryngol Clin North Am* 1997; **30**(6): 1051–9.
125. Silverstein H, Isaakson JE, Olds MJ, Rowan PT, Rosenberg S. Dexamethasone inner ear perfusion for the treatment of Menière's disease: a prospective, randomized, double-blind, crossover trial. *Am J Otol* 1998; **19**(2): 196–201.
126. Kilpatrick JK, Sismanis A, Spencer RF, Wise CM. Low-dose oral methotrexate management of patients with bilateral of Menière's disease. *Ear Nose Throat J* 2000; **79**: 82–92.
127. Bergenius J, Ödkvist LM. Transtympanic aminoglycoside treatment of Menière's disease. In: Baloh RW, Halmagyi GM, eds. *Disorders of the Vestibular System*. New York: Oxford University Press, 1996: 407–17.
128. Hirsch BE, Kamerer DB. Role of chemical labyrinthectomy in the treatment of Menière's disease. *Otolaryngol Clin North Am* 1997; **30**(6): 1039–49.
129. Blakley BW. Clinical forum: a review of intratympanic therapy. *Am J Otol* 1997; **18**: 520–6.
130. Blakley BW. Update on intratympanic gentamicin for Menière's disease. *Laryngoscope* 2000; **110**: 236–40.
131. Usami S, Abe S, Kasai M, et al. Genetic and clinical features of sensorineural hearing loss associated with the 1555 mitochondrial mutation. *Laryngoscope* 1997; **107**: 483–90.
132. Chen JM, Williamson PA, Hutchin T, Nedzelski JM, Cortopassi GA. Topical gentamycin induced hearing loss: a mitochondrial ribosomal RNA study of genetic susceptibility. *Am J Otol* 1996; **17**: 850–2.
133. Telian SA, Shepard NT, Smith-Wheelock M, Hoberg M. Bilateral vestibular paresis: diagnosis and treatment. *Otolaryngol Head Neck Surg* 1991; **104**: 67–71.
134. Mauritz KH, Hesse S. Neurological rehabilitation of gait and balance disorders. In: Bronstein, Brandt, Woollacott eds. *Clinical Disorders of Balance, Posture and Gait*. New York: Oxford University Press, 1996.
135. Buttner U, Fuhry L. Drug therapy of nystagmus and saccadic intrusions. *Adv Otorhinolaryngol* 1999; **55**: 195–227.
136. Eagger S, Luxon LM, Davies RA, Coelho A, Ron MA. Psychi-

atric morbidity in patients with peripheral vestibular disorders: a clinical and neuro-otological study. *J Neurol Neurosurg Psychiatry* 1992; **55**: 383–7.

137. Lee RJ. Pharmacological and optical methods of treating vestibular disorders and nystagmus. In: Herdman SJ, ed. *Vestibular Rehabilitation*, 2nd edn. Philadelphia: FA Davis, 2000.
138. Thapa BP, Ray W. Medications and falls and fall related injuries in the elderly. In: Bronstein A, Brandt T, Woollacott M, eds. *Clinical Disorders of Balance, Posture and Gait*. New York: Oxford University Press, 1996.
139. Kitahara T, Takeda N, Kiyama H, Kubo T. Molecular mechanisms of vestibular compensation in the central vestibular system. *Acta Otolaryngol* 1998; Suppl 539: 19–27.
140. Schlatter M, Kerr DR, Smith PF, Darlington CL. Evidence that the ginkgo biloba extract, EGb 761, neither accelerates nor enhances the rapid compensation of the static symptoms of unilateral vestibular deafferentation in guinea pig. *J Vestib Res* 1999; **9**: 111–18.
141. Weiser M, Strosser W, Klein P. Homeopathic versus conventional treatment of vertigo: a randomized double-blind controlled clinical study. *Arch Otolaryngol Head Neck Surg* 1998; **124**(8): 879–85.
142. Pollak L, Davies RA, Luxon LM. Effectiveness of the particle repositioning manoeuvre in benign positional vertigo with and without additional vestibular pathology. *Am Otol Rhinol Laryngol* 2002; in press.
143. Herdman SJ. Vestibular rehabilitation. In: Baloh RW, Halmagyi GM, eds. *Disorders of the Vestibular System*. New York: Oxford University Press, 1996: 407–17.
144. Hecker HC, Haug CO, Herndon JW. Treatment of the vestibular patient using Cawthorne's vestibular exercises. *Laryngoscope* 1974; **84**: 2065–72.
145. Jones GM, Berthoz A, Segal B. Adaptive modification of the VOR by mental effort in darkness. *Exp Brain Res* 1984; **56**: 149–53.
146. Foord G, Marsden J. Physical exercise regimes—practical aspects. In: Davis RA, Luxon LM, eds. *Handbook of Vestibular Rehabilitation*. London: Whurr, 1997.
147. Freeman JA, Nairne J. Using a class setting to teach Cawthorne–Cooksey exercises as a means of vestibular rehabilitation. *Physiotherapy* 1995; **81**: 74–9.
148. Cohen H. Vestibular rehabilitation reduces functional disability. *Otolaryngol Head Neck Surg* 1992; **107**: 638–43.
149. Szturm T, Ireland DJ, Lessing-Turner M. Comparison of different exercise programs in the rehabilitation of patients with chronic peripheral vestibular dysfunction. *J Vestib Res* 1994; **4**: 461–79.
150. Norré ME, Beckers A. Vestibular habituation training: exercise treatment for vertigo based upon the habituation effect. *Otolaryngol Head Neck Surg* 1989; **101**: 14–19.
151. Norré ME. Rationale of rehabilitation treatment for vertigo. *Am J Otol* 1987; **8**: 31–5.
152. Norré ME, De Weerdt W. Positional (provoked) vertigo treated by postural training. *Aggressologie* 1981; **22**: 37–44.
153. Shepard NT, Telian SA. Programmatic vestibular rehabilitation. *Otolaryngol Head Neck Surg* 1995; **112**: 173–82.
154. Herdman SJ, Borello-France DF, Whitney SL. Treatment of vestibular hypofunction. In: Herdman SJ, ed. *Vestibular Rehabilitation*. Philadelphia: FA Davis, 1994.
155. Gill-Body KM, Popat RA, Parker SW, Krebs DE. Rehabilitation of balance in two patients with cerebellar dysfunction. *Physical Ther* 1997; **77**: 534–52.
156. Shepard NT, Asher A. Treatment of patients with non-vestibular dizziness and dysequilibrium. In: Herdman SJ, ed. *Vestibular Rehabilitation*, 2nd edn. Philadelphia: FA Davis, 2000.
157. Shumway-Cook A, Horak FB, Yardley L, Bronstein AM. Rehabilitation of balance disorders in the patient with vestibular pathology. In: Bronstein A, Brandt T, Woollacott M, eds. *Clinical Disorders of Balance, Posture and Gait*. New York: Oxford University Press, 1996.
158. Shumway-Cook A. Vestibular rehabilitation in traumatic brain injury. In: Herdman SJ, ed. *Vestibular Rehabilitation*. Philadelphia: FA Davis, 1996.
159. Clendaniel RA, Tucci DL. Vestibular rehabilitation strategies in Menière's disease. *Otolaryngol Clin North Am* 1997; **30**(6): 1145–58.
160. Krebs DE, Gill-Body KM, Riley PO, Parker SW. Double-blind, placebo-controlled trial of rehabilitation for bilateral vestibular hypofunction: preliminary report. *Otolaryngol Head Neck Surg* 1993; **109**: 735–41.
161. Schuknecht HF. Cupulolithiasis. *Arch Otolaryngol* 1969; **90**: 765–8.
162. Epley JM. New dimensions of benign paroxysmal positional vertigo. *Otolaryngol Head Neck Surg* 1980; **88**: 599–605.
163. McLure JA. Horizontal canal BPPV. *J Otolaryngol* 1985; **14**: 30–5.
164. Baloh RW, Jakobson K, Honrubia V. Benign positional vertigo. *Neurology* 1987; **37**: 371–8.
165. Herdman SJ, Tusa R. Complications of the canalith repositioning procedure. *Arch Otolaryngol Head Neck Surg* 1996; **122**: 281–6.
166. Honrubia V, Baloh RW, Harris MR, Jakobson KM. Paroxysmal positional vertigo syndrome. *Am J Otol* 1999; **20**: 465–70.
167. De la Meilleure G, Dehaene I, Depondt M, Damman W, Crevits L, Vanhooren G. Benign paroxysmal positional vertigo of the horizontal canal. *J Neurol Neurosurg Psychiatry* 1996; **60**: 68–71.
168. Suzuki M, Yukawa K, Horiguchi S, et al. Clinical features of paroxysmal positional vertigo presenting combined lesions. *Acta Otolaryngol* 1999; **119**: 117–20.
169. Brandt T. Central positioning vertigo. In: *Vertigo: Its Multisensory Syndromes*, 2nd edn. London: Springer-Verlag, 1999.
170. Buttner U, Helmchen C, Brandt T. Diagnostic criteria for central versus peripheral positioning nystagmus and vertigo: a review. *Acta Otolaryngol* 1999; **119**(1): 1–5.
171. Fife TD. Recognition and management of horizontal canal benign positional vertigo. *Am J Otol* 1998; **19**: 345–51.
172. Norré ME, Forrez G, Beckers A. Vestibular habituation training and posturography in benign paroxysmal positional vertigo. *J Otolaryngol Relat Spec* 1987; **49**: 22–5.
173. McLure JA, Willett JM. Lorazepam and diazepam in the treatment of benign paroxysmal positional vertigo. *J Otolaryngol* 1980; **9**: 472–7.

174. Brandt T. Benign paroxysmal positional vertigo. In: *Vertigo: Its Multisensory Syndromes*, 2nd edn. London: Springer-Verlag, 1999.
175. Herdman SJ. Assessment and management of benign paroxysmal positional vertigo. In: Herdman SJ, ed. *Vestibular Rehabilitation*. Philadelphia: FA Davis, 1994.
176. Brandt T, Daroff RB. Physical therapy for paroxysmal positional vertigo. *Arch Otolaryngol* 1980; **106**: 484–5.
177. Semont A, Freyss G, Vitte E. Curing the BPPV with a liberatory manoeuvre. *Adv Otolaryngol* 1988; **42**: 290–3.
178. Epley JM. The canalith repositioning procedure: for treatment of benign paroxysmal positional vertigo. *Otolaryngol Head Neck Surg* 1992; **107**: 399–404.
179. Wolf M, Hertanu T, Novikov I, Kronenberg J. Epley's manoeuvre for benign paroxysmal positional vertigo: a prospective study. *Clin Otolaryngol* 1999; **24**: 43–6.
180. Harvey SA, Hain TC, Adamiec LC. Modified liberatory maneuver: effective treatment for benign paroxysmal positional vertigo. *Laryngoscope* 1994; **104**: 1206–12.
181. Herdman SJ, Tusa R, Zee DS, Proctor LR, Mattox DE. Single treatment approaches to benign paroxysmal positional vertigo. *Arch Otolaryngol Head Neck Surg* 1993; **119**: 450–4.
182. Fung KF, Hall SF. Particle repositioning maneuver: effective treatment for benign paroxysmal positional vertigo. *J Otolaryngol* 1996; **25**: 243–8.
183. Li JC. Mastoid oscillation: a critical factor for success in the canalith repositioning procedure. *Otolaryngol Head Neck Surg* 1995; **112**: 670–5.
184. Hain TC, Helminski JO, Reis IL, Uddin MK. Vibration does not improve results of the canalith repositioning procedure. *Arch Otolaryngol Head Neck Surg* 2000; **126**: 617–22.
185. Welling DB, Barnes DE. Particle repositioning maneuver for benign paroxysmal positional vertigo. *Laryngoscope* 1994; **104**: 946–9.
186. Beynon GJ. A review of management of benign paroxysmal positional vertigo by exercise therapy and by repositioning manoeuvres. *Br J Audiol* 1997; **31**: 11–26.
187. Brandt T. Benign paroxysmal positional vertigo. *Adv Otorhinolaryngol* 1999; **55**: 195–227.
188. Vannuchi P, Giannoni B, Pagnini P. Treatment of horizontal semicircular canal benign paroxysmal positional vertigo. *J Vestib Res* 1997; **7**: 1–6.
189. Lempert T, Tiel-Wilck K. A positional maneuver for treatment of horizontal canal benign positional vertigo. *Laryngoscope* 1996; 476–8.
190. Nuti D, Agus G, Barbierri MT, Passali D. The management of the horizontal canal paroxysmal positional vertigo. *Acta Otolaryngol* 1998; **118**: 455–60.
191. Baloh RW. Reply to the letter by Lempert: Horizontal benign positional vertigo. *Neurology* 1994; **44**: 2214.
192. Gacec R. Singular neurectomy update. II. Review of 102 cases. *Laryngoscope* 1991; **101**: 855–62.
193. Parnes LS, McLure JA. Posterior semicircular canal occlusion in the normal hearing ear. *Otolaryngol Head Neck Surg* 1991; **104**: 52–7.
194. Anthony PF. Partitioning of the labyrinth: application in benign paroxysmal positional vertigo. *Am J Otol* 1991; **12**: 388–93.
195. Lazko-Schroeder T. Psychological aspects of vestibular rehabilitation. In: Davis RA, Luxon LM, eds. *Handbook of Vestibular Rehabilitation*. London: Whurr, 1997.
196. Horak FB, Jones Rycewicz C, Black O, Shumway-Cook A. Effects of vestibular rehabilitation on dizziness and imbalance. *Otolaryngol Head Neck Surg* 1992; **106**: 175–80.
197. Cohen H, Kane-Wineland M, Miller LV, Hatfield CL. Occupation and visual/vestibular interaction in vestibular rehabilitation. *Otolaryngol Head Neck Surg* 1994; **112**: 526–32.
198. Mruzek M, Barin K, Nichols DS, Burnett CN, Welling DB. Effects of vestibular rehabilitation and social reinforcement on recovery following ablative vestibular surgery. *Laryngoscope* 1995; **105**: 686–92.
199. Cowand JL, Wrisley DM, Walker M, Strasnick B, Jacobson JT. Efficacy of vestibular rehabilitation. *Otolaryngol Head Neck Surg* 1998; **118**: 49–54.
200. Norré ME, Beckers A. Comparative study of two types of exercise treatment for paroxysmal positioning vertigo. *Adv Otorhinolaryngol* 1988; **42**: 287–9.
201. Parnes LS, Price-Jones RG. Particle repositioning maneuver for benign paroxysmal positional vertigo. *Ann Otol Rhinol Laryngol* 1993; **102**: 325–31.
202. Massoud EAS, Ireland DJ. Post-treatment instructions in the non-surgical management of benign paroxysmal positional vertigo. *J Otolaryngol* 1996; **25**: 121–5.
203. Blakley BW. A randomized, controlled assessment of the canalith repositioning maneuver. *Otolaryngol Head Neck Surg* 1994; **110**: 391–6.
204. Serafini G, Palmieri AMR, Simoncelli C. Benign paroxysmal positional vertigo of posterior semicircular canal: results in 160 cases treated with Semont's maneuver. *Ann Otol Rhinol Laryngol* 1996; **105**: 770–5.
205. Steenerson RL, Cronin GW. Comparison of the canalith repositioning procedure and vestibular habituation training in forty patients with benign paroxysmal positional vertigo. *Otolaryngol Head Neck Surg* 1996; **114**: 61–4.
206. Smouha EE. Time course of recovery after Epley's maneuvers for benign paroxysmal positional vertigo. *Laryngoscope* 1997; **107**: 187–91.
207. Steddin S, Ing D, Brandt T. Horizontal canal benign paroxysmal positioning vertigo (h-BPPV): transition of canalolithiasis. *Ann Neurol* 1996; **40**: 918–22.
208. Brandt T, Steddin S, Darroff RB. Therapy for benign paroxysmal positoning vertigo, revisited. *Neurology* 1994; **44**: 796–800.

55 Role of surgery in the management of the dizzy patient

Harold Ludman

This topic can be discussed fully only by consideration of certain separate headings:

1. Diseases of the temporal bone involving the labyrinth, so causing vertigo.
2. The treatment of intrinsic peripheral labyrinthine diseases:
   (a) Menière's disease
   (b) Benign paroxysmal positional vertigo
3. The role of labyrinthine membrane rupture and perilymph fistula.

Temporal bone diseases

Of these, the most urgent and dangerous is cholesteatoma associated with the unsafe variety of chronic suppurative otitis media. Cholesteatoma is stratified squamous keratinizing epithelium like skin,[1,2] which has become involved with, and is invading, the air spaces of the middle ear and, in particular, the attic and antral regions. It may arise in several possible ways. One recognized mechanism is by the retraction of a pocket of tympanic membrane either of the pars flaccida in the attic or of the posterior pars tensa below the posterior malleolar fold (Figure 55.1). There are certainly other possible mechanisms for the development of cholesteatoma.[3,4] It may be congenital; or it might develop from metaplasia of middle ear mucosa, or even by papillary ingrowth through intact tympanic membrane.[5] However it arises, cholesteatoma forms a multiloculated sac of skin wrapping itself around all the complex structures in the attic and middle ear and extending into all the available anatomical air spaces of the middle ear. The importance of cholesteatoma is that it reacts with subjacent bone,[6] and by eroding it can expose the contents of the labyrinth to the effects of pressure wave transmission, and to spreading infection. Many other structures apart from the labyrinth may be exposed and damaged, but vertigo arises if the labyrinth becomes involved. The first way in which this may happen is when the bone over a semicircular canal (usually the lateral) has become thinned until the endosteum within the lumen is exposed to direct contact with the basal layer of the cholesteatoma, which is outermost. At that stage, any pressure changes within the middle ear or the external ear canal are transmitted to vestibular perilymph, causing vertigo and eye movement. This constitutes the basis of the so-called 'fistula sign' (Figure 55.2). Infection within the cholesteatoma may then spread to the interior of the labyrinth causing suppurative labyrinthitis with destruction of labyrinthine function. The effect of this will be severe vertigo with gradual recovery by compensation in the way that happens with any of the other causes of sudden vestibular failure. Apart from the unpleasantness of the vertigo, the danger is that further spread may produce meningitis or other intracranial sepsis.

> The recognition of cholesteatoma, then, is of prime importance, and careful examination of the ears is an essential part of the investigation of any patient complaining of vertigo.

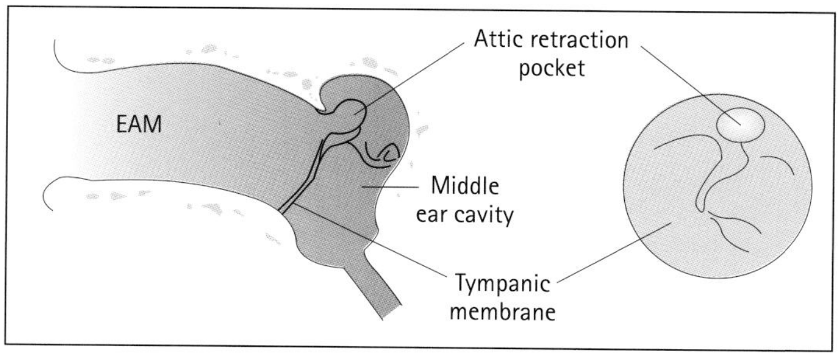

Figure 55.1 Attic retraction pocket.

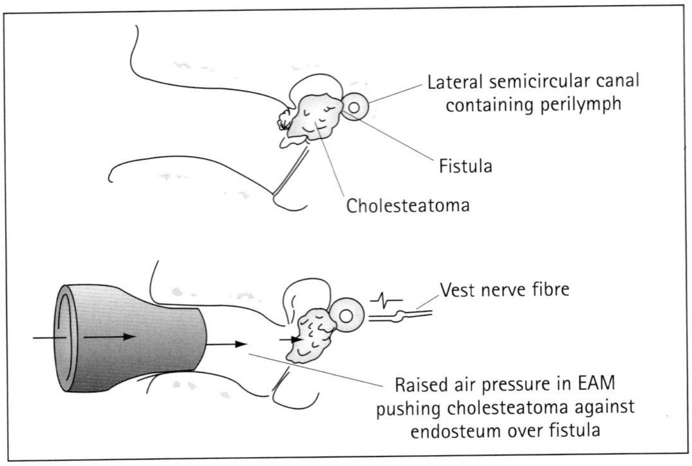

Figure 55.2 Fistula scan.

Examination for a fistula sign is also a cardinal aspect of patient examination. This may be conducted by pressing the tragus into the ear canal to raise the air pressure, but is better conducted by inserting a firmly fitting airtight speculum, and increasing ear canal air pressure with a pneumatic, or Siegle's, speculum. If positive, the patient will complain of vertigo, and jerk away. The eyes must be watched. As pressure increases, the eyes will deviate away from the observer, and if the pressure is maintained, there will then be a rapid jerk back to the mid-line. The actual direction of eye deviations associated with a positive fistula sign depends on the site of the fistula; the commonest site is the lateral semicircular canal.[7] Unfortunately, fistula signs have low predictive power. A false-negative finding arises if a mass of cholesteatoma prevents transmission of sound pressure to the labyrinthine perilymph, while false positives are found as the so-called Hennebert's sign, discussed later in this chapter.

Sometimes an attic cholesteatoma may be hidden from view by a hard crust, acting like a cork, plugging the opening into the cholesteatoma through which the skin has become invaginated (Figure 55.3). Only when such a crust can be removed and the underlying area inspected is it possible to rule out a cholesteatoma, and that inspection should be conducted with a binocular microscope. Occasionally, an ear needs examination under a general anaesthetic. If there is any suspicion of cholesteatoma, even if other causes for vertigo seem probable on historical grounds, the ear must be considered unsafe, and its management will almost always be operative, with the prime purpose of making the ear safe, whereby the patient will be protected from potentially serious disease. There is a role for modern radiological imaging techniques, but the findings can be misleading, and certainty can emerge only from operative inspection.[8,9]

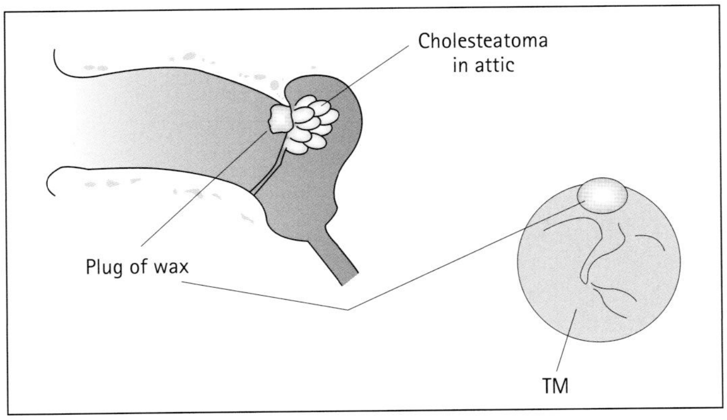

Figure 55.3 Wax plug obscuring cholesteatoma.

The surgical treatment of cholesteatoma

This can follow one of two principles.

> **SURGICAL TREATMENT OF CHOLESTEATOMA**
>
> - Creation of a wide cavity leading into the external ear canal.
> - 'Combined approach tympanoplasty' with the preservation of the posterior meatal bony canal wall and reconstruction of any tympanic membrane defect.

The classical, conventional and most traditional method is creation of a wide cavity opening into the external ear canal. The region occupied by the cholesteatoma is fashioned into as smooth a hemispherical space as possible, within the anatomical constraints. This cavity will become lined with skin that will be histologically identical to that constituting the preceding cholesteatoma. Because of the wide access to the external ear canal, the surface layer of the skin will migrate outwards in the same way as the normal tympanic membrane, and wax within it, together with the surface keratin, will gradually be extruded into the ear canal, and laterally to the exterior. This kind of operation—designated an open cavity operation—includes a number of varieties, such as atticotomy, atticoantrostomy, modified radical mastoidectomy and radical mastoidectomy.

These open cavity procedures differ from each other, and are named according to the extent of anatomical rearrangement necessary to encompass the cholesteatoma and produce a smooth cavity (Figure 55.4). This in turn is determined by the extent of the cholesteatoma, and the damage that it has already done. In an atticotomy (Figure 55.5) the outer attic wall, or scutum, is removed to expose the attic. If the cholesteatoma envelopes the head of the malleus and the body of the incus found therein, it may be necessary to remove the incus and amputate the head of the malleus in order to make a smooth cavity. Hearing efficiency will then rely on displacement of the tympanic membrane medially to adhere to the head of the stapes—an arrangement allowing transmission of sound waves directly from the tympanic membrane to the stapes, called myringostapediopexy. Atticoantrostomy entails more extensive removal of bone backwards, to open both the attic and the mastoid antrum behind it. In the modified radical mastoidectomy

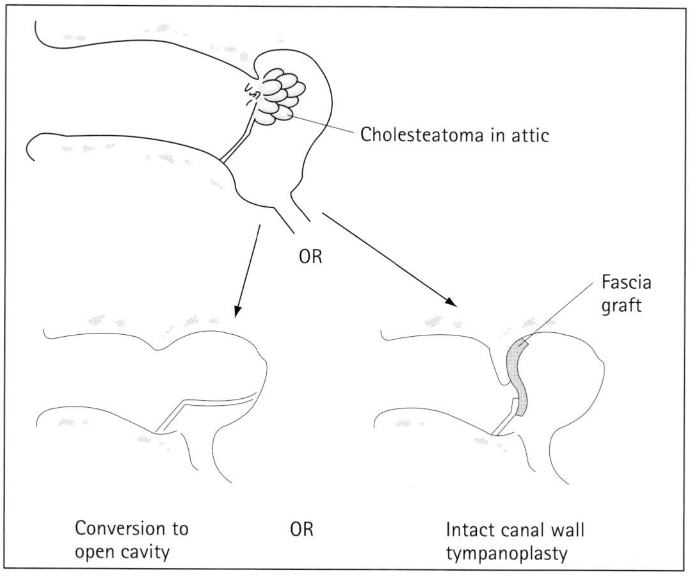

Figure 55.4 Principles of surgical treatment of cholesteatoma.

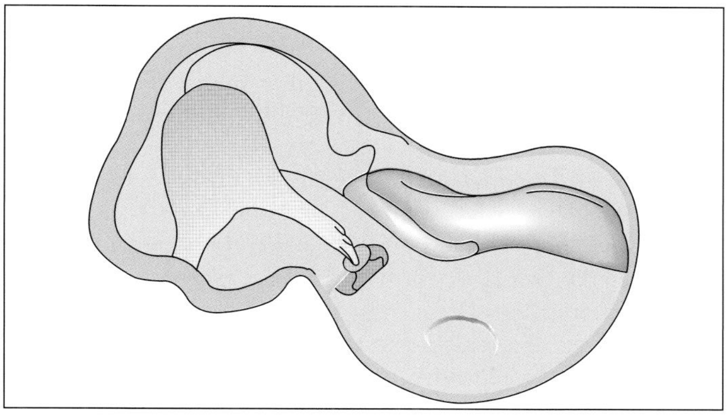

Figure 55.5 Atticotomy, right ear. The tympanic membrane behind the malleus has been lifted forwards. The outer attic wall has been drilled away to expose the body of incus and head of malleus.

the operation extends still further behind and below the mastoid antrum to open any air cells and to follow the cholesteatoma to its limits. In this operation, the remaining incus, which has often lost its long process to erosion, is removed. The head of the malleus must be amputated, and the tympanic membrane displaced medially to lie on the head of the stapes. In this way, the mesotympanum remains as an air-containing cavity, excluded from the attic and the mastoid cavity behind it. A radical mastoidectomy (Figure 55.6) entails removal of much or all of the tympanic membrane as well, to leave the middle ear cavity exposed in continuity with the newly fashioned mastoid cavity. The incus and the malleus are removed, leaving the stapes (or only its footplate if the crura have been destroyed) as the sole remnant of the ossicular chain.

Each of these operations may be performed through an incision behind the ear—postaural—or an incision between the

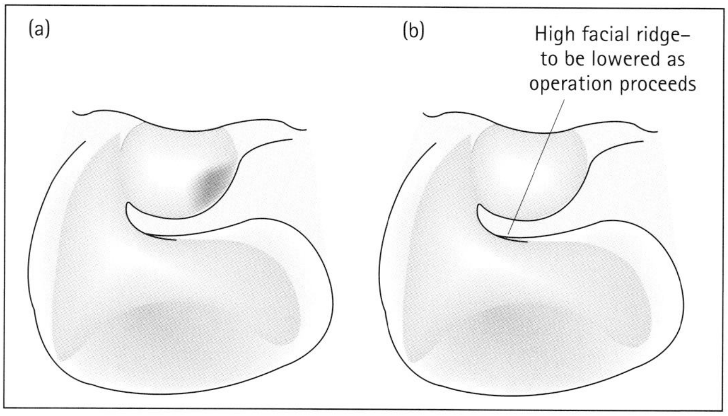

Figure 55.6 (a) Radical mastoidectomy, right ear. Cavity seen behind the facial ridge, over the vertical part of the facial nerve. (b) Modified radical mastoidectomy. The tympanic memebrane and the ossicles have been preserved.

tragus and the crus of the helix—endaural (Figure 55.7). The development of the cavity, by drilling away bone, may (classically) start from behind, by drilling into the mastoid antrum first, and working forwards. Many otologists, including the author, prefer a 'front-to-back' approach, starting by removal of the outer attic wall to expose the attic and its contents, and extending the operation backwards towards the antrum by concentric removals of bone upwards and backwards to reach the limits of the cholesteatoma (Figure 55.8). This technique has the advantages of limiting the size of the cavity to the extent of the disease, and providing assessment of the ossicular chain and the position of the facial nerve early in the procedure. As with all middle ear surgery, there is a risk of damage to other structures, and of these the facial nerve is the most important. It is important to leave the cavity as smooth as possible. The so-called 'bridge', which is the remaining bone of the posterior meatal wall bridging laterally over the aditus ad antrum, is lowered and removed, to leave a smooth vertical bony ridge just covering and protecting the vertical part of the facial nerve. This facial ridge must be carefully reduced, where it abuts against the bony bulge of the lateral semicircular canal. Too high a facial ridge as a result of excessive caution in protecting the facial nerve may leave a pocket of cavity medially not adequately exposed to the meatus, and infected material may accumulate there.

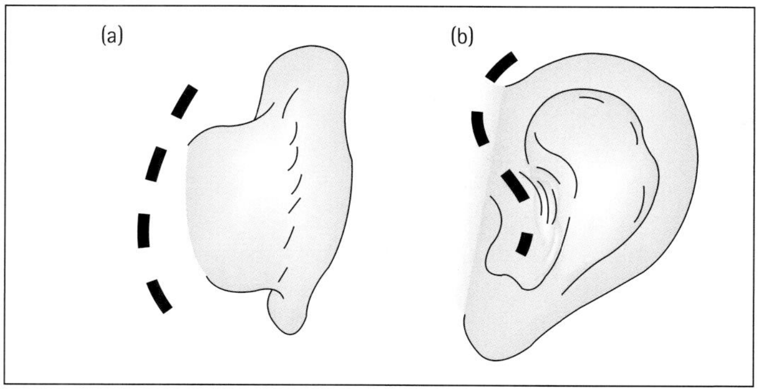

Figure 55.7 (a) Postaural incision. (b) Endaural incision.

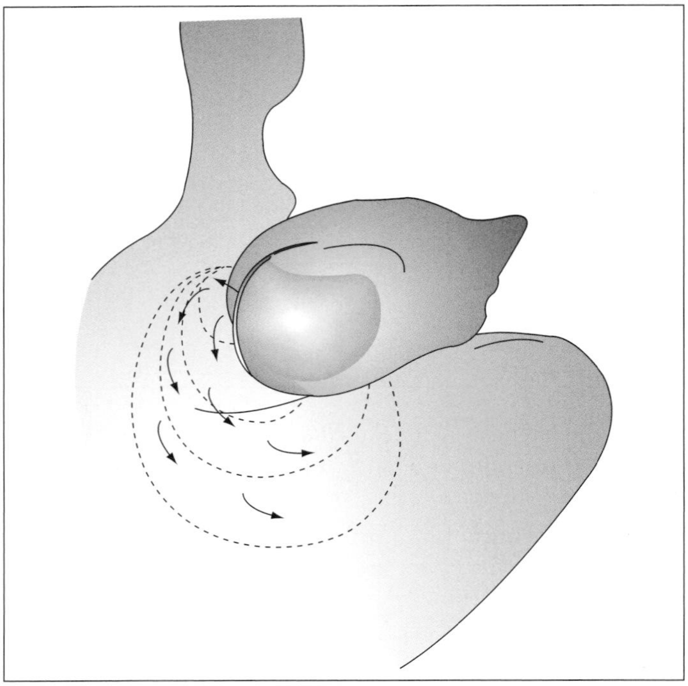

Figure 55.8 Development of mastoid cavity from the attic backwards.

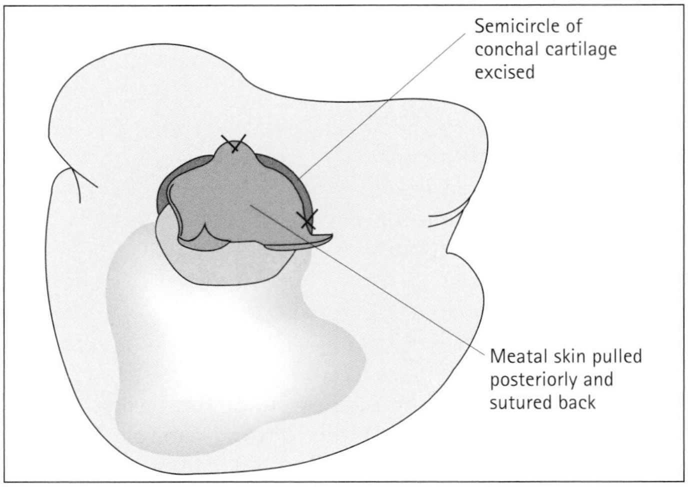

Figure 55.9 Meatoplasty, right ear.

All open cavity operations discharge for some weeks after operation, and many do so continuously, or intermittently if the skin lining becomes infected.[10,11] Indeed, discharge of serum, which easily becomes infected by opportunist commensal organisms, is expected until and unless the whole of the cavity becomes lined with skin. A mastoid cavity is a warm damp chamber uncongenial for the growth and survival of healthy skin, and it is much less likely to develop this healthy skin lining if the volume of the cavity is proportionately large when compared with the diameter of the remaining external meatus. As has already been noted, a healthy mastoid cavity develops a skin lining that is histologically identical to cholesteatoma, but it has no erosive potential, because its surface layer of desquamating keratin can migrate into and through the external ear canal. This desirable behaviour, and easy access to examine and treat by removal of accumulating keratin, is assisted by a wide meatus. Open cavity operations are usually completed by surgically widening the external meatus—meatoplasty (Figure 55.9). Postoperatively, patients need regular outpatient attention, throughout life, for removal of wax and any dead skin that has not cleared itself. Usually, this will become an annual, or less frequent, event. Patients must protect the ear from water, and for this reason should not swim. Open cavity operations require considerable care, skill and experience to produce well-behaved cavities without damaging adjacent structures.

The second approach is called an 'intact canal wall tympanoplasty' or 'combined approach tympanoplasty', and sometimes 'canal wall up surgery'.[12,13] The aim is to remove the cholesteatoma from within the middle ear cleft, while preserving the posterior meatal bony canal wall (Figure 55.10) and reconstructing any defect in the tympanic membrane. It may also be possible to repair the damaged ossicular chain.

Afterwards, there is no residual cavity. The patient is left with a normal external ear canal separated from the middle ear cleft by a reconstructed tympanic membrane. Theoretically, this is a much more satisfactory state than after an open cavity operation, but there are problems.

Intact wall tympanoplasty is carried out through a postaural incision. Extensive removal of bone over the mastoid antrum and the cells behind is needed to provide wide access to the region lateral to the vertical part of the facial nerve. This is a significant disadvantage. If the disease proves to be limited in extent, the bone removal will be much more extensive than would have been needed with an open cavity operation. If, subsequently, because of residual or recurrent disease, it becomes necessary to convert this procedure into a

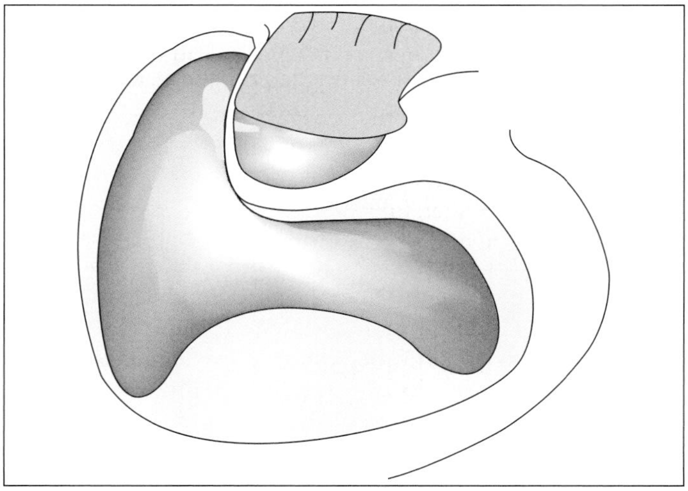

Figure 55.10 Intact canal wall mastoidectomy. The cavity is separated from the meatus by the outer attic wall and the posterior bony meatal wall.

radical mastoidectomy, as sometimes happens, then the resulting cavity will be very much larger than ideal, and more capacious than if a mastoidectomy of the open cavity kind had been formed intentionally to start with. During the intact canal wall procedure, the bridge and posterior bony meatal wall is drilled from its inner surface to paper thickness, but must carefully be left intact. An opening is then made from the mastoid air cell area, which has been uncovered, into the middle ear through a so-called posterior tympanotomy. This is a narrow vertical groove between the air cells behind and the middle ear space in front. Bone is removed from the aditus, just below the region of attachment of the short process of the incus, working downwards, with a fine drill burr, superficial to the vertical part of the facial nerve. Considerable care and skill is needed to avoid damage to the facial nerve, which can be injured thermally by the burr working just fractions of a millimetre away. Laterally, the posterior tympanotomy is limited by the annulus of the tympanic membrane, and this must not be damaged. Through this narrow vertical groove, it is possible to see behind forwards, into the middle ear, medially to the tympanic membrane. When all disease has been removed, and the tympanic membrane defect has been repaired with a temporalis fascia graft, the middle ear and its lateral bony external ear canal should be anatomically virtually normal. It is also possible to reconstruct any parts of the ossicular chain that may have been damaged by disease or by the operative procedure to get access to it. There are differences of opinion about the advisability of conducting reconstruction at the time of the initial operation rather than as a staged procedure later on. Apart from the risk of damage to the facial nerve, which is much greater in intact canal wall procedures, there is also a chance that the cochlea may suffer from vibrations transmitted from the operating drill burr, if it accidentally touches the incus or any other part of an intact ossicular chain. Intact canal wall mastoid surgery carries a higher risk of sensorineural hearing damage than does open cavity operation.

A further risk is that small, even microscopic, particles of cholesteatoma, or skin, may be left behind and later develop into destructive cholesteatoma, hidden from view by the posterior meatal wall and the intact tympanic membrane.[14] For this reason, it is generally accepted that any patient who has had an intact canal wall operation must agree to have the ear opened again some months later, for inspection and the removal of any recurrent or persistent disease. More than one subsequent operation may in fact be needed. These risks, and the disadvantage of further operations, restrict the number of patients suitable for this procedure, since they have to be willing and reliable enough to accept the postoperative plans.

However, intact canal wall surgery does offer the opportunity to leave an anatomically normal middle ear with good hearing. Of even greater importance to many patients is that the ear can be exposed to water while swimming without risk of infection. Open cavity operations should always be protected from water, because the precarious skin lining them is easily infected when it becomes soggy and exposed to external organisms.

Views on the virtues of each of these different types of operation have swung like a pendulum over the past 30 years, and at the present time the mood is more in favour of open cavity operations than it was in the 1970s.[15]

Fistula management

The possibility of discovering a fistula into the labyrinth is particularly high when operating on cholesteatoma in a vertiginous patient. In any mastoid surgery, dissection of cholesteatoma away from otic capsule regions prone to erosion, such as the lateral semicircular canal dome, must be conducted under high magnification, and with care. A fistula will be suspected when the dome is flattened by erosion, and, as the skin of the cholesteatoma—or matrix—is carefully lifted with a fine instrument, the bluish discoloration of the perilymph space within will become visible.

The management of a fistula depends on circumstances. The matrix overlaying the fistula can often be dissected away from the underlying endosteum, but there is a high risk of destroying inner ear function should the endosteum be accidentally transgressed. For this reason, there are many occasions when the surgeon will decide to leave the matrix intact over the fistula. If this decision is made during an intact canal wall operation, then it will need careful management when the ear is explored again. By that stage, the remaining matrix will usually have formed into a so-called 'epithelial pearl'—or skin cyst—which can usually be winkled off the fistula without difficulty.

It is often safer to leave the matrix intact, rather than risking damage to the inner ear, but if it is left in place during an open cavity operation, the patient may afterwards suffer the symptoms of 'perilabyrinthitis' with episodes of vertigo when pressure changes are transmitted to the fistula from outside. This condition was first named by the late Sir Terence Cawthorne, and unfortunately the term is often used incorrectly.[16] Vertigo may be triggered by loud noise (Tullio phenomenon), or even by wind blowing into the fistula from the outside air. The patient may also experience vertigo from time to time, if and when the mastoid cavity lining becomes infected.

If it is thought safe to remove the matrix from the fistula without risk to the endosteum, the fistula can be covered, and protected from subsequent pressure changes, by a graft of mesodermal material such as temporalis fascia.

VERTIGO AFTER MASTOIDECTOMY

- Persistent disease.
- Labyrinthine fistula.
- Poor compensation.
- Residual vestibular epithelium.
- Secondary hydrops.

Vertigo after mastoidectomy

A patient who has undergone open cavity mastoidectomy may experience subsequent vertigo. Of course, this can happen for quite unrelated reasons, but there are a number of different possible mechanisms which may cause vertigo and which can cause diagnostic difficulty.

1. Persisting disease with continuing erosion of the labyrinth. This should be discovered by examination and must be treated by operation
2. Labyrinthine fistula. This should be diagnosed by the fistula test, and by probing the region of a possible fistula (see above).
3. Poor compensation. It is possible that the preoperative condition, or the operation itself, may have destroyed vestibular function, and the patient's recovery from this will have been prolonged and gradual over the course of weeks or months. Recovery by central compensation may later become compromised by other illnesses, old age, or psychological disorders. Under these circumstances, the patient may become dizzy simply because the central mechanism of compensation has broken down. A detailed history of the pattern of any vertigo around the time of the operation may be the only clue to this state of affairs. For instance, the patient may recall a long period of vertigo and imbalance, for days on end, during the initial postoperative recovery period. Cold air caloric testing (since water irrigation would be inadvisable) may demonstrate loss of canal sensitivity.
4. Residual vestibular epithelium. It is theoretically possible for a patient to have lost most vestibular function, but to have retained some vestibular epithelium, which may at random cause episodes of vertigo. Treatment for this relatively rare condition often entailed a labyrinthectomy operation to remove any remaining such epithelium. This kind of labyrinthectomy used to be called a bony labyrinthectomy, in contrast with the membranous labyrinthectomy used in the treatment of Menière's disease to be described later. When it is performed from an open mastoidectomy operation, the medial wall of the vestibule will be left exposed to the cavity. Subsequent vertigo may arise, not because the operation has been inadequate, but because of the development of traumatic neuromas on residual vestibular nerve fibres exposed to the environment.[17] These can sometimes be demonstrated by probing the appropriate part of the cavity and causing vertigo by so doing. Satisfactory relief can be offered by dividing the vestibular nerve. There are particular problems in performing this operation through a potentially infected cavity, and these have been well reviewed.[18]
5. Secondary hydrops. The condition of secondary or delayed hydrops has been recognized for many years.[19] If, for any reason, an inner ear is damaged, with loss of cochlear function and total deafness, but with the survival of some vestibular function, then the patient may develop endolymphatic hydrops in that ear with typical Menière-like attacks of vertigo. The onset, after the initial damage to the inner ear, is on average about 20 years.[20,21] Damage causing secondary hydrops may arise from congenital inner ear abnormalities, viral infections (such as mumps), or indeed trauma—including surgical trauma. The diagnosis after mastoid surgery depends upon a reliable history indicating hearing before the operation and total loss immediately afterwards. The persistence of some vestibular function may be demonstrated by cold air caloric testing. Effective treatment entails radical destruction of the vestibular function of that ear. Total deafness associated with surviving vestibular function will suggest the diagnosis.

It should be clear that the distinction between these different causes rests with a very careful history as well as a detailed examination of the existing state of cochlear and vestibular function.

Surgical treatment of Menière's disease

The general view is that about 20% of patients suffering from Menière's disease cannot be relieved by medication or spontaneous remission, and, for these, operative options are considered.[22]

Radical operations

Relief from vertigo can almost always be achieved by ablating the erratically active labyrinth, (labyrinthectomy), but to do so entails total loss of hearing in the affected ear. For patients who have severe deafness and distortion, this sacrifice may be acceptable, but in some cases the hearing is too valuable to sacrifice, and this is particularly so when there is any doubt about the integrity of the other ear. It might be thought that involvement of the second ear would be easy to establish, but reports in the literature of its frequency are extremely variable because of different criteria used to accept involvement. Some are based on pure tone audiometric tests, others on transtympanic electrocochleography of the normal ear, and yet others on changes in the electrocochleographic findings with glycerol dehydration, or acetazolomide loading. There are many surgeons who take the view that the risk of later involvement of the second ear is too great ever to justify labyrinthectomy, but this seems to be overstating the case. Some patients, particularly those over the age of 60, do not compensate fully for the loss of a labyrinth. Others who have lost a labyrinth earlier in life, for any reason, may experience imbalance from progressive loss of compensation as they grow older. For all these reasons, there are limitations to the role of radical surgery treatment by labyrinthectomy, well reviewed by Pereira and Kerr.[23]

Total destruction of the membranous labyrinth may be achieved by almost any operation that transgresses the membranous labyrinth. Access may be transtympanic through the external auditory meatus, turning forwards a tympanomeatal flap. The incus is removed, and then the stapes is lifted out of its oval window niche, after dividing the fibres of the stapedio-vestibular ligament around the footplate. Fine instruments with hooked ends can then be inserted into the vestibule and used to destroy the utricle and saccule, and to reach into the ampullae of each of the semicircular canals to extirpate the contents (Figure 55.11).

Transmastoid access through a postaural incision allows exposure of the lateral semicircular canal. This can be opened so that the membranous contents may be removed (Figure 55.12). Some surgeons favour an even more radical approach, with destruction of each semicircular canal in turn, possibly followed by extension to the internal auditory meatus in order to divide the vestibular nerve as well.

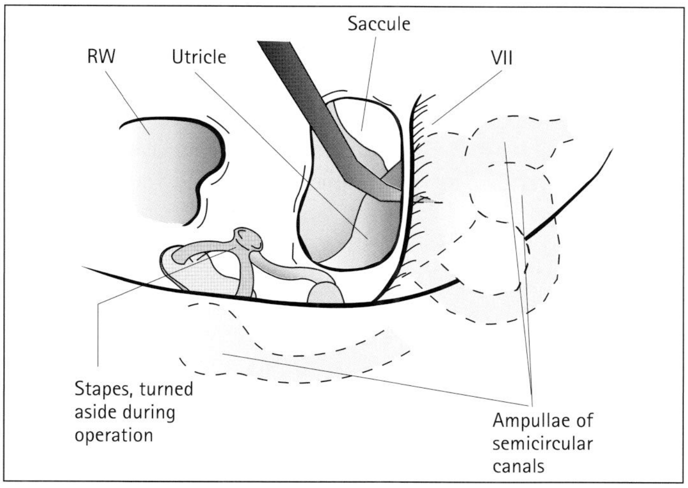

Figure 55.11 Transtympanic labyrinthectomy. A double angled hook has been introduced into the vestibule through the oval window, after displacement of the stapes.

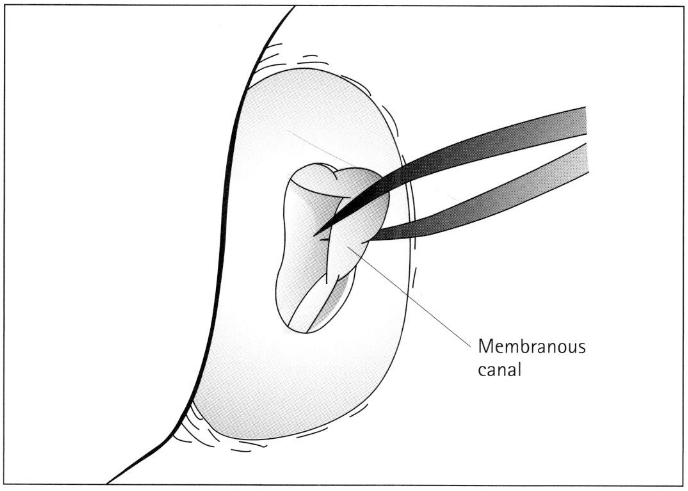

Figure 55.12 Transtympanic labyrinthectomy. The membranous semicircular canal is being removed.

It is also feasible to destroy the labyrinth chemically. In the past, streptomycin injections were used, and today there is a vogue for the use of intratympanic gentamicin.[24,25]

Conservative surgical treatment

The development of so-called conservative operative procedures aimed at relieving vertigo, while attempting to preserve auditory function, is most important. There are two main groups of operation.

1. those addressing a presumed cause of hydrops
2. those eliminating or reducing excitation of the brainstem by the labyrinth, through disconnection of the neural connections between the two, with preservation of the cochlea.

Some procedures that were popular are now obsolete and are of historical interest only. Among these are procedures of dubious rationality. It is axiomatic, in surgical practice, that profusion of surgical solutions is evidence of the efficacy of none. Among the first group of conservative operations, based on a presumed aetiology, one must consider endolymphatic sac decompression as the most important, while noting that in the past there was enthusiasm for cochleostomy or cochleosacculotomy,[26] for cochlear dialysis, for sacculotomy, for the insertion of ventilation tubes into the tympanic membrane, and for cervical sympathectomy. In the second group of conservative procedures vestibular nerve division is the most important. Intratympanic injection of ototoxic drugs deserves mention, and in the past ultrasonic destruction of the vestibular part of the labyrinth was important.

Saccus decompression operation

Operations on the saccus endolymphaticus were first described in the 1920s, but their use relapsed until a renaissance of saccus surgery about 25 years ago. Since then, they have become the most commonly applied techniques of conservative treatment for Menière's disease. A good review of the history of this procedure can be found in the contribution of Lacher.[27]

It is hoped that by dealing fundamentally with the main functional defect of the disorder, the natural history of the disease may be altered, with the preservation of hearing otherwise doomed to inexorable deterioration. It has to be said that it has proved difficult to perform adequate consistently controlled trials of the efficacy of saccus surgery, and the mechanism by which it might work is not understood.

It must even be accepted that there are reasons for doubting whether saccus surgery has any actual effect on the course of Menière's disease, and its benefits to a patient may be those of a placebo.[28–30] Certainly, it is simplistic to believe that endolymph pressure in the pars inferior of the membranous labyrinth is relieved by constant leakage from the opened saccus. The saccus is a flat fan-shaped structure with an alveolar kind of interior, and any incision made in it is likely to become shut off by scarring very soon after operation. It has been suggested that increased vascularity following operative trauma might have some effect on endolymph absorption, but there is as yet no strongly supported explanation. The technique involves exposing the endolymphatic sac, through a cortical mastoidectomy operation, where it is to be found in front of the sigmoid sinus just below the posterior semicircular canal (Figure 55.13). The sac can usually be found without difficulty by following the posterior fossa dura deep to Trautmann's triangle forwards and medially, using a small diamond paste bur to avoid damage to the dura. Sometimes, a bulging sigmoid sinus prevents easy access to the posterior fossa dura and requires compression after the development of a trap door of thin bone on its surface whereby it may safely be pressed medially with a blunt dissector. The saccus can be recognized by its thick texture and whitish colour, contrasting with the thin bluish dura above and below. It can be identified positively by following it medially and identifying the ductus (Figure 55.14). When exposed, the saccus may be left untouched, or opened with a sharp knife into the mastoidectomy cavity. In earlier days, it was usual to place a shunt tube between the lumen of the saccus and the subarachnoid space in the posterior cranial fossa, even

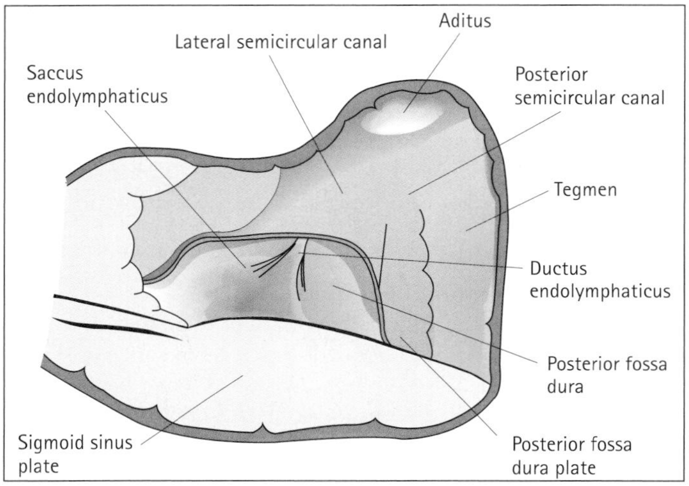

Figure 55.13 Saccus decompression, right ear. The sac has been exposed through a cortical mastoidectomy approach.

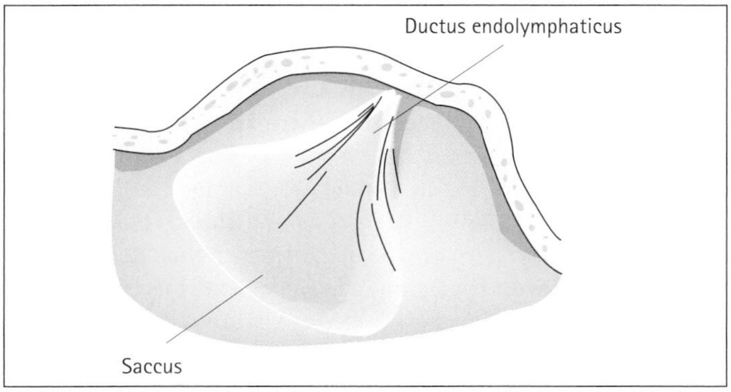

Figure 55.14 Saccus decompression. Demonstration of the endolymphatic duct

though it has been known from earlier structural studies that any lumen in the sac is multiloculated and of minute dimensions. If the saccus is opened, a tube or a sheet of silastic may be placed from the mastoid cavity into whatever lumen it has. It seems that there are no definite differences arising from handling the saccus in different ways. Perhaps this is not surprising, as the effect in helping to cure the disease is not understood, and sham operations seem to be just as good at preventing vertigo.

Recent developments have suggested that the effect of surgery might be due to traumatic destruction of the saccus, and on that basis deliberate saccus ablation has been advocated.[31,32]

Ventilation tube insertion

It seems improbable that the insertion of ventilation tubes into the tympanic membrane could have any effect on Menière's disease, but because of the safety of the procedure it has often been used as a desperate remedy of last resort. The theoretical basis for its possible action has been argued along the following lines. If a patient has intermittent Eustachian tube obstruction, and an abnormally patent aqueductus cochleae, then lowered pressure in the middle ear might displace the round window membrane outwards, drawing cerebrospinal fluid from the subarachnoid space into the labyrinth. Precisely what should happen next is not clear, but this disturbance of intravestibular fluid mechanics might, it is argued, cause changes that disturb the vestibular sense organs. If so, then maintaining pressure equalization with a ventilation tube should protect the patient from this deviant process.

Vestibular nerve section

Division of the vestibular nerve to prevent abnormal sensory labyrinthine stimuli from reaching the vestibular neurones can be performed through a number of different routes—posterior fossa, middle fossa, retrolabyrinthine and retrosigmoid.[33–41] The advantages of different approaches are well documented,[33] and the mechanisms of postoperative recovery have been analysed.[42] Whichever is favoured, the aim is to divide all the vestibular fibres of the cochleovestibular nerve complex without damage to the cochlear nerve or its blood supply (Figure 55.15). It is not always easy to separate the vestibular fibres from those of the cochlear nerve,[35] and one of the main risks of the operation is damage to the cochlear nerve with hearing loss, in about 4–5% of patients.[43] Many of the techniques entail the more serious risks of a neurosurgical operation.[44,45] There are many possible reasons for failure, including inadequate anatomical section.[46]

Benign paroxysmal positional vertigo

It is rare for patients with this disorder to require surgical treatment, but there are two options available for those who are severely incapacitated, and who have not been helped by Epley's particle repositioning manoeuvre.

Posterior ampullary (singular) nerve section

The posterior ampullary nerve carries the sensory fibres of the posterior canal crista to the inferior vestibular nerve. After leaving the internal acoustical meatus, it travels backwards to the posterior semicircular canal ampulla in a channel that takes it just below the lower border of attachment of the round window membrane. It can be reached through a permeatal tympanotomy approach. The bony overhang of the round window niche is drilled away with fine diamond paste burs until the round window membrane is exposed. Drilling further bone below and medially to its inferior edge will expose the singular nerve so that it can be avulsed (Figure 55.16). Accessibility of the nerve depends on its relationship to the round window. If it is too far superomedial, it may not become visible without damage to the cochlea, and although this procedure offers relief for the symptoms of benign paroxysmal positional vertigo, it carries a high risk of severe sensorineural hearing loss.[47,48]

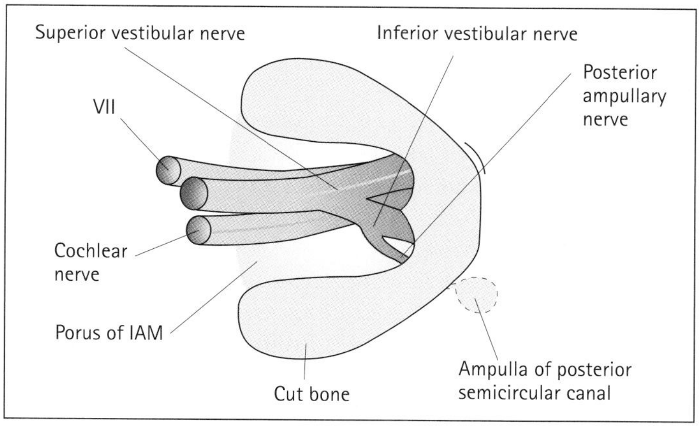

Figure 55.15 Vestibular nerve section. Neural contents of the internal acoustic meatus after removal of its posterior bony wall.

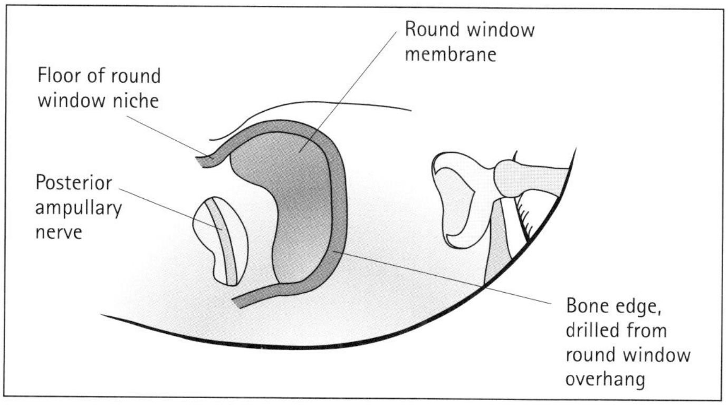

Figure 55.16 Posterior ampullary nerve section, left ear. View through aural speculum after displacing the tympanic membrane forwards.

Posterior canal obliteration

Compression of the membranous posterior semicircular canal can prevent movement of loose material within it.[49–52] The posterior canal is exposed through a cortical mastoidectomy approach (Figure 55.17). Diamond paste burs are used to 'blue line' the canal, which is gently opened. It is important to avoid damage to the membranous labyrinth within. Bone wax or bone paté is then used to fill the perilymph space in order to squash the membranous tube within and prevent movement of its contained endolymph. Recently, lasers have been used to shrink the membranous posterior canal[53] and also to destroy the utricular macula.[54]

Labyrinthine membrane rupture (perilymph fistula)

This condition is controversial, and has exercised otologists for the past 20 years or so. Under certain conditions, the inner ear membranes may be ruptured, and then the oval window or round window may leak perilymph in to the middle ear. The external pressure trauma needed to produce this damage may be severe, as in concussive head injuries and diving barotrauma, or perhaps trivial, as with pressure changes caused by sneezing, straining at stool or light blows to the head briefly raising intracranial cerebrospinal fluid pressure. That perilymph leakages can be caused by the more severe insults is accepted, but there is a great deal of argument about the less violent causes and whether so-called 'spontaneous perilymph fistulae' actually occur.[55,56] The name perilymph fistula is unfortunately misleading, since the damage arising in the inner ear is attributable to tearing of intralabyrinthine membranes, disruption of sensory structures and chemical damage from mixing inner ear fluids. The perilymph leak itself is simply the final evidence, found at operation, of this damage. It cannot rationally be argued that the closure of a fistula which is just the injury at the most peripheral extent of the insult will repair irreversibly disrupted inner ear structures.

The clinical effects of labyrinthine membrane ruptures have never been consistently agreed. This is hardly surprising when the very existence of spontaneous perilymph leaks is uncertain. Suspicion should be directed, it is argued, at all

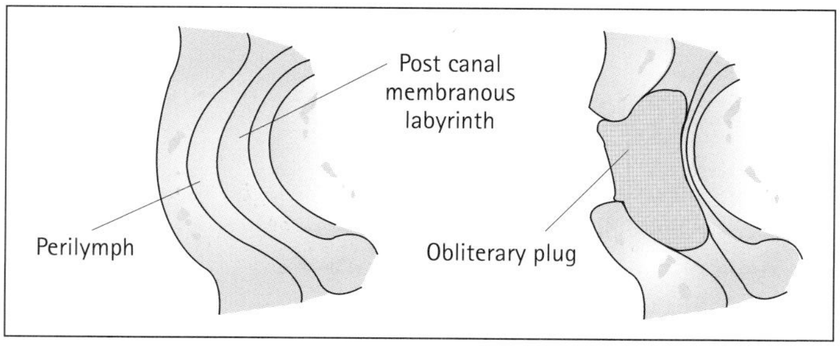

Figure 55.17 Posterior semicircular canal obliteration.

patients who develop sudden sensorineural hearing loss after trauma of the kinds mentioned, and when there are attacks of Menière-like vertigo with atypical features such as persisting imbalance between attacks of proper vertigo. Patients with untypical features and otherwise characteristic benign paroxysmal positional vertigo should also be suspects. There are no useful diagnostic predictable clues beyond the clinician's suspicion.[57] A great deal has been written about the status of a possible fistula sign, but in fact no series of presumed perilymph fistulae has shown the presence of a fistula sign to be more than a useful pointer, and its absence is of no value at all.

Diagnostic proof can be sought only by observation during a tympanotomy operation. Even this is subjective and not as positive a finding as non-surgeons often imagine. False-positive leaks have been described by the observation of fluid accumulating in the round window niche, which actually has come from tissue exudate or preoperative infiltration of the ear canal, while false-negative reports may arise from lowering of perilymph pressure. There have been descriptions of shredding of the round window membrane later shown to be mucosal strands across the round window niche, which normally hides the actual membrane from view. Enthusiasts suggest watching the windows for several minutes with the head lowered on the operating table to raise the cerebrospinal fluid pressure, before the absence of a leak is declared. Absence of leak discovery is sometimes ascribed to spontaneous healing, which is a circular argument in the enthusiasts' armamentarium that is very difficult to gainsay. To see the round window membrane clearly, it is usually necessary to drill away bone overhanging it, but this acutely risks causing a leak.

If a leak is found or suspected, it can easily be patched operatively with a piece of connective tissue or fat from the earlobe. There certainly are reliable anecdotal accounts of immediate relief from ataxia and imbalance after this procedure. There are few reliable accounts of any improvement in the patient's hearing. The rational otologist should keep an open mind about the existence of this syndrome. Any patient developing vertigo or sensorineural hearing loss after diving or definite head injury should be a legitimate suspect for the diagnosis, and ought to be nursed sitting up, since, if healing can occur, it should do so more readily with low cerebrospinal fluid pressure. After a week or so with no improvement, it is reasonable to explore the middle ear surgically, while maintaining scepticism about the findings.

References

1. Youngs R, Rowles P. The spatial organisation of keratinocytes in acquired middle ear cholesteatoma resembles that of external auditory canal skin and pars flaccida. *Acta Otolaryngol (Stockh)* 1990; **110**: 115–19.
2. Lee R, Mackenzie I, Hall B, Gantz B. The nature of the epithelium in acquired cholesteatoma. *Clin Otolaryngol* 1991; **16**: 168–73.
3. Ruah C, Schachern P, Paparella M, Zelterman D. Mechanisms of retraction pocket formation in the pediatric tympanic membrane. *Arch Otolaryngol Head Neck Surg* 1992; **118**: 1298–305.
4. Sadé J, Babiacki A, Pinkus G. The metaplastic and congenital origin of cholesteatoma. *Acta Otolaryngol (Stockh)* 1983; **96**: 119–29.
5. Abramson M, Gantz B, Asarch R, Litton W. *Cholesteatoma Pathogenesis: Evidence for the Migration Theory*. Cholesteatoma. First International Conference. Birmingham: Aesculapius, 1977: 176–86.
6. Kurihara A, Toshima M, Yuasa R, Takasaka T. Bone destruction mechanisms in chronic otitis media with cholesteatoma: specific production by cholesteatoma in culture of bone-resorbing activity attributable to interleukin-I alpha. *Ann Otol Rhinol Laryngol* 1991; **100**: 989–98.
7. McCabe BF. Labyrinthine fistula in chronic mastoiditis. *Ann Otol Rhinol Laryngol Suppl* 1984; **112**: 138–41.
8. Mahmood F, Mafee M. MRI and CT in the evaluation of acquired and congenital cholesteatomas of the temporal bone. *J Otolaryngol* 1993; **22**: 239–48.
9. Leighton S, Robson A, Anslow P, Milford C. The role of CT imaging in the management of chronic suppurative otitis media. *Clin Otolaryngol* 1993; **18**: 23–9.
10. Youngs R. The histopathology of mastoidectomy cavities with particular reference to persistent otorrhoea. *Clin Otolaryngol* 1992; **17**: 505–10.
11. Youngs R. Epithelial migration in open mastoidectomy cavities. *J Laryngol Otol* 1995; **109**: 286–90.
12. Jansen C. The combined approach for tympanoplasty. *J Laryngol Otol* 1968; **82**: 779–93.
13. Glasscock M, Miller G. Intact canal wall tympanoplasty in the management of cholesteatoma. *Laryngoscope* 1976; **86**: 1639–57.
14. Smyth G. Postoperative cholesteatoma in combined approach tympanoplasty. *J Laryngol Otol* 1976; **90**: 597–621.
15. Toner J, Smyth G. Surgical treatment of cholesteatoma: a comparison of three techniques. *Am J Otol* 1990; **11**: 247–9.
16. Cawthorne TE. Perilabyrinthitis. *Laryngoscope* 1957; **67**: 1233–6.
17. Ludman H. Neuronal activity in otology. *J Laryngol Otol* 1986; **100**: 989–1007.
18. Parikh AA, Brookes GB. Vestibular nerve section following previous mastoidectomy. *J Laryngol Otol* 1996; **110**(9): 836–40.
19. Nadol J, Weiss A, Parker S. Vertigo of delayed onset after sudden deafness. *Ann Otol Rhinol Laryngol* 1975; **84**: 841–6.
20. Langman AW, Lindeman RC. Sensorineural hearing loss with delayed onset of vertigo. *Otolaryngol Head Neck Surg* 1995; **112**(4): 540–3.
21. Ludman H. Surgical treatment of vertigo. In: Dix MR, Hood JD, eds. *Vertigo*. Chichester: John Wiley & Sons, 1984: 113–31.
22. Ludman H. Menière's disease. *BMJ* 1990; **301**: 1232–3.
23. Pereira KD, Kerr AG. Disability after labyrinthectomy. *J Laryngol Otol* 1996; **110**: 216–18.
24. Nedzelski JM, Chiong CM, Fradet G, Schessel DA, Bryce GE, Pfleiderer AG. Intratympanic gentamicin instillation as treatment of unilateral Menière's disease: update of an ongoing study. *Am J Otol* 1993; **14**: 278–82.

25. Grant IL, Welling DB. The treatment of hearing loss in Menière's disease. *Otolaryngol Clin North Am* 1997; **30**(6): 1123–44.
26. Giddings NA, Shelton C, O'Leary MJ, Brackmann DE. Cochleosacculotomy revisited. Long-term results poorer than expected. *Arch Otolaryngol Head Neck Surg* 1991; **117**(10): 1150–2.
27. Lacher G. Current and historical perspectives on endolymphatic sac surgery. *Acta Otolaryngol Suppl* 1997; **526**: 50–3.
28. Bretlau P, Thomsen J, Tos M, Johnsen NJ. Placebo effect in surgery for Menière's disease: a three-year follow-up study of patients in a double blind placebo controlled study on endolymphatic sac shunt surgery. *Am J Otol* 1984; **5**(6): 558–61.
29. Kerr AG, Toner JG, McKee GJ, Smyth GD. Role and results of cortical mastoidectomy and endolymphatic sac surgery in Menière's disease. *J Laryngol Otol* 1989; **103**(12): 1161–6.
30. Thomsen J, Kerr A, Bretlau P, Olsson J, Tos M. Endolymphatic sac surgery: why we do not do it. The non-specific effect of sac surgery. *Clin Otolaryngol* 1996; **21**(3): 208–11.
31. Gibson WP. The effect of surgical removal of the extraosseous portion of the endolymphatic sac in patients suffering from Menière's disease. *J Laryngol Otol* 1996; **110**(11): 1008–11.
32. Welling DB, Pasha R, Roth LJ, Barin K. The effect of endolymphatic sac excision in Menière disease. *Am J Otol* 1996; **17**(2): 278–82.
33. Glasscock ME, Thedinger BA, Cueva RA, Jackson CG. An analysis of the retrolabyrinthine vs. the retrosigmoid vestibular nerve section. *Otolaryngol Head Neck Surg* 1991; **104**(1): 88–95.
34. Dufour JJ, Girard L, Mohr G. Selective vestibular neurectomy through the posterior fossa in Menière's disease. *J Otolaryngol* 1988; **17**(6): 311–14.
35. Green JD Jr, Shelton C, Brackmann DE. Middle fossa vestibular neurectomy in retrolabyrinthine neurectomy failures. *Arch Otolaryngol Head Neck Surg* 1992; **118**(10): 1058–60.
36. House JW, Hitselberger WE, McElveen J, Brackmann DE. Retrolabyrinthine section of the vestibular nerve. *Otolaryngol Head Neck Surg* 1984; **92**(2): 212–15.
37. Kemink JL, Telian SA, el-Kashlan H, Langman AW. Retrolabyrinthine vestibular nerve section: efficacy in disorders other than Menière's disease. *Laryngoscope* 1991; **101**(5): 523–8.
38. McDaniel AB, Silverstein H, Norrell H. Retrolabyrinthine vestibular neurectomy with and without monitoring of eighth nerve potentials. *Am J Otol* 1985; **Suppl**: 23–6.
39. Monsell EM, Wiet RJ, Young NM, Kazan RP. Surgical treatment of vertigo with retrolabyrinthine vestibular neurectomy. *Laryngoscope* 1988; **98**(8 Pt 1): 835–9.
40. Ortiz Armenta A. Retrolabyrinthine vestibular neurectomy. 10 years' experience. *Rev Laryngol Otol Rhinol* 1992; **113**(5): 413–17.
41. Pulec JL. Surgical treatment of vertigo. *Acta Otolaryngol Suppl* 1995; **519**: 21–5.
42. Bohmer A, Fisch U. Clinical pathophysiology of vestibular neurectomy. *Otolaryngol Head Neck Surg* 1995; **112**(1): 183–8.
43. Rosenberg SI, Silverstein H, Hoffer ME, Thaler E. Hearing results after posterior fossa vestibular neurectomy. *Otolaryngol Head Neck Surg* 1996; **114**(1): 32–7.
44. Gacek RR, Gacek MR. Comparison of labyrinthectomy and vestibular neurectomy in the control of vertigo. *Laryngoscope* 1996; **106**(2 Pt 1): 225–30.
45. Silverstein H, Wanamaker H, Flanzer J, Rosenberg S. Vestibular neurectomy in the United States—1990. *Am J Otol* 1992; **13**(1): 23–30.
46. Thedinger BS, Thedinger BA. Analysis of patients with persistent dizziness after vestibular nerve section. *Ear Nose Throat J* 1998; **77**(4): 290–2, 295–8.
47. Gacek RR. Singular neurectomy update. *Ann Otol Rhinol Laryngol* 1982; **91**(5 Pt 1): 469–73.
48. Gacek MR, Gacek RR, Martell R. Effect of singular neurectomy on the caloric response. *Am J Otolaryngol* 1995; **16**(6): 362–6.
49. Dingle AF, Hawthorne MR, Kumar BU. Fenestration and occlusion of the posterior semicircular canal for benign positional vertigo. *Clin Otolaryngol* 1992; **17**(4): 300–2.
50. Hawthorne M, el-Naggar M. Fenestration and occlusion of posterior semicircular canal for patients with intractable benign paroxysmal positional vertigo. *J Laryngol Otol* 1994; **108**(11): 935–9.
51. Pace–Balzan A, Rutka JA. Non-ampullary plugging of the posterior semicircular canal for benign paroxysmal positional vertigo. *J Laryngol Otol* 1991; **105**(11): 901–6.
52. Parnes LS. Update on posterior canal occlusion for benign paroxysmal positional vertigo. *Otolaryngol Clin North Am* 1996; **29**(2): 333–42.
53. Kartush JM, Sargent EW. Posterior semicircular canal occlusion for benign paroxysmal positional vertigo—CO_2 laser-assisted technique: preliminary results. *Laryngoscope* 1995; **105**(3 Pt 1): 268–74.
54. Anthony PF. Utricular macular ablation for benign paroxysmal positional vertigo. *Ear Nose Throat J* 1996; **75**(7): 416–21.
55. Shea J. The myth of spontaneous perilymph fistula. *Otolaryngol Head Neck Surg* 1992; **107**: 613–16.
56. Gibson WP. Spontaneous perilymphatic fistula: electrophysiologic findings in animals and man. *Am J Otol* 1993; **14**(3): 273–7.
57. Kohut RI. Perilymph fistulas—clinical criteria. *Arch Otolaryngol Head Neck Surg* 1992; **118**: 687–92.

Index

Page numbers in *italic* denote figures, tables and boxed material where there is no textual reference on the same page. Locators in **bold** denote glossary definitions.

C

D

E

J

K

L

M

N

O

P

Q

R

S

T

U

V

W

X

Y